OXFORD TEXTBOOK OF
CLINICAL
HEPATOLOGY

OXFORD MEDICAL PUBLICATIONS

EDITORS

JOHANNES BIRCHER
Visiting Professor
Department of Clinical Pharmacology
University of Bern
Bern, Switzerland

JEAN-PIERRE BENHAMOU
Professor of Hepatology and Gastroenterology
Hôpital Beaujon
Clichy, France

NEIL McINTYRE
Professor of Medicine
Royal Free Hospital School of Medicine
London, UK

MARIO RIZZETTO
Professor of Gastroenterology
University of Turin
Turin, Italy

JUAN RODÉS
Professor of Medicine
Chief of Liver Unit
University of Barcelona
Barcelona, Spain

OXFORD TEXTBOOK OF
CLINICAL
HEPATOLOGY

SECOND EDITION

VOLUME I
Sections 1–13 and Index

Edited by

Johannes Bircher
Jean-Pierre Benhamou
Neil McIntyre
Mario Rizzetto
Juan Rodés

Oxford   New York   Tokyo
OXFORD UNIVERSITY PRESS
1999

Oxford University Press, Great Clarendon Street, Oxford OX2 6DP

Oxford New York
Athens Auckland Bangkok Bogota Buenos Aires Calcutta
Cape Town Chennai Dar es Salaam Delhi Florence Hong Kong Istanbul
Karachi Kuala Lumpur Madrid Melbourne Mexico City Mumbai
Nairobi Paris São Paolo Singapore Taipei Tokyo Toronto Warsaw

and associated companies in
Berlin Ibadan

Oxford is a trade mark of Oxford University Press

Published in the United States
by Oxford University Press, Inc., New York

© J. Bircher, J.-P. Benhamou, N. McIntyre, M. Rizzetto, J. Rodés, 1999

The moral rights of the author have been asserted

First published 1991
Second edition published 1999

British Library Cataloguing in Publication Data
Data available

Library of Congress Cataloging in Publication Data

1 3 5 7 9 10 8 6 4 2

ISBN 0 19 262515 2 (Two Volume Set)
ISBN 0 19 263039 3 (Vol 1)
ISBN 0 19 263040 7 (Vol 2)
(Available as a two volume set only)

Typeset by Latimer Trend

Printed in Hong Kong

Preface to the second edition

The first edition of the *Oxford Textbook of Clinical Hepatology* enjoyed considerable success and achieved much critical acclaim; we were encouraged, therefore, to produce a new edition, not only to amplify our original aims but also to document the enormous progress made in hepatology and related fields over the last few years. All chapters have been updated, and many have been restructured and expanded. New chapters have been added on topics such as *in vitro* techniques, 'hepatitis G', overlap syndromes, glycogen storage diseases, and intracellular and extracellular lipidosis. To serve the practising hepatologist the focus on clinical medicine has been further strengthened, although the necessary basic science is still included. The initial chapters containing the latter have been directed towards newer techniques and concepts which have developed during the last few years. As before referencing throughout is comprehensive, covering both key sources from the past and the most recent literature.

We thank all our contributors: their patient work and dedication have made the production of the book possible. We also gratefully acknowledge the excellent management of Mrs Christina Wagner in the editorial office and of Dr Irene Butcher and our friends at Oxford University Press.

Johannes Bircher   January 1999
Jean-Pierre Benhamou
Neil McIntyre
Mario Rizzetto
Juan Rodés

Preface to the first edition

We all met several times, in different cities, to plan this book. We wanted to produce a comprehensive account of clinical hepatology, covering not only the common hepatological problems but also the rare conditions which are seen from time to time by hepatologists, gastroenterologists, and general physicians. We thought it important to consider how the liver may be affected in diseases of other systems, and to describe the effects of diseases of the liver on other parts of the body, as these interactions often create a confusing clinical picture; these topics occupy two large sections of the book which should be of particular value to general physicians and specialists in other diseases. We felt a need for a fuller than usual account of the effect of infections on the liver; patients with bacterial, fungal and parasitic infections, and those with viral infections other than the classical viral hepatitides, often have abnormal liver function tests, or symptoms or signs suggesting liver disease.

There are chapters on other topics which have received little attention in other texts, such as symptoms and signs, diagnostic strategy, general management, and prescribing and anaesthesia in liver disease. There are chapters on liver disease in children, in the elderly, and in drug addicts and homosexual men, and one on the history of liver disease.

We also thought it would be helpful to have some appendices: listing non-drug chemicals and toxins causing liver damage, the geographical distribution of infectious diseases, and the rare diseases in which the liver may be involved (particularly in children). Another appendix contains the excellent handouts produced for patients by the American Liver Foundation.

Colleagues often remark that it is irritating, when reading chapters with many references, to have to search at the end of the chapter to find the original sources. We therefore decided to use mainly short 'text references' to enable readers to decide quickly if they are already familiar with the source and, if not, to allow them to jot the reference down with the minimum of effort. We consider this experiment to have been worthwhile, but we hope that readers will tell us if they prefer the conventional approach.

More than 200 authors have contributed to this book; nearly all are acknowledged internationally as experts in their field(s) of interest. We are grateful to all of them. We believe that their expertise is reflected in their contributions, many of which we consider to be quite outstanding.

Our major purpose was to provide a book for practising clinicians. We hope this text will prove useful not only to hepatologists, gastroenterologists, and general physicians, but also to specialists in other fields. It was for this reason that we chose the title 'clinical hepatology'. We believe that this book will provide solutions to many of the hepatological problems which arise in clinical practice, but only our readers can tell whether our belief is justified. If, when using this book, you fail to find the information you are seeking, we would be grateful if you could draw these omissions to our attention (using the cards enclosed), so that they can be corrected in the next edition.

Our book is being brought out in English, French, and Spanish. We would like to thank the staff of the Oxford University Press, Flammarion, and of Salvat, not only for their willingness to publish it but for their help and enthusiasm during the long gestation period. We are particularly grateful to the executive editor for the book, Irene Butcher, who dealt initially with all the manuscripts, and later with the galleys and page proofs of this English edition.

Neil McIntyre
Jean-Pierre Benhamou
Johannes Bircher
Mario Rizetto
Juan Rodés

Contents

Contributors

ALFREDO ALBERTI
Professor of Internal Medicine, University of Padova, Italy
12.1.2.5 Hepatitis C

FRANCIS ANDRÉ
Vice President and Senior Medical Director, SmithKline
Beecham Biologicals, Rixensart, Belgium
12.1.3.1(a) Vaccines against hepatitis A

PETER W. ANGUS
Consultant Hepatologist in Charge, Transplant Unit,
Repatriation General Hospital, Melbourne, Victoria, Australia
*24.2 The effect of gastrointestinal disease on the liver and biliary
tract*
25.5 Effect of liver disease on the gastrointestinal tract

THOMAS ARMBRUST
Junior Scientist in the Department of Gastroenterology and
Endocrinology, Department of Internal Medicine, University
of Göttingen, Germany
2.7.1 Cytokines and the liver

VICENTE ARROYO
Hospital Clinic i Provincial, Barcelona, Spain
8.1 Pathogenesis, diagnosis, and treatment of ascites in cirrhosis
8.2 Renal dysfunction in cirrhosis
24.4 The liver in urogenital diseases
25.7 Effect of liver disease on the urogenital tract

DANIEL AZOULAY
Surgeon, Centre Hepatobiliaire, Villejuif, France
22.2.2 Malignant biliary obstruction
*30.1 General surgical aspects and the risks of liver surgery in
patients with hepatic disease*

CHARLES BALABAUD
Professor of Hepatology, CHU de Bordeaux, Université
Bordeaux II, Bordeaux, France
1.2 Liver and biliary-tract histology

VIJAYAN BALAN
Assistant Professor of Medicine, Divisions of Transplantation
Medicine, Gastroenterology and Hepatology, University of
Pittsburgh Medical Center, Pennsylvania, USA
30.5 Liver transplantation

MICHAEL BARAITSER
Consultant in Clinical Genetics, Hospital for Children,
Great Ormond Street, London, UK
32.3 Rare diseases with hepatic abnormalities

JAMES A. BARROWMAN*
Faculty of Medicine, Memorial University of Newfoundland,
St John's, Canada
2.2 Hepatic lymph and lymphatics

NATHAN M. BASS
Professor of Medicine, University of California, San Francisco
School of Medicine, and Attending Physician, UCSF Hospitals
and Clinics, USA
*2.19 In vitro techniques: isolated organ perfusion, slices, cells, and
subcellular elements*

JEAN-PIERRE BENHAMOU
Professor of Hepatology and Gastroenterology at University of
Paris 7, Service d'Hépatologie, Hôpital Beaujon, Clichy, France
5.4.1 Liver biopsy
6.2 Cirrhosis: clinical aspects
7.3 Intrahepatic portal hypertension
*11.2 Non-parasitic cystic diseases of the liver and intrahepatic
biliary tree*
19 Fulminant and subfulminant liver failure
21.3 Obstruction of the hepatic venous system
21.4 Vascular malformations
22.1.1 Liver haemangioma
22.1.2.2 Benign hepatocellular tumours
*25.1 The effect of liver disease on the cardiovascular system,
lungs, and pulmonary vasculature*

O. BERNARD
Hôpital de Bicêtre, Bicêtre, France
26 Paediatric liver disease

JACQUES BERNUAU
Consultant, Service d'Hépatologie, Hôpital Beaujon, Clichy,
France
19 Fulminant and subfulminant liver failure

H.L.C. BEYNON
Consultant Physician and Rheumatologist, Royal Free
Hospital, London, UK
24.7 Musculoskeletal diseases and the liver
25.9 Musculoskeletal problems in liver disease

PRITHI S. BHATHAL
Professor/Director of Anatomical Pathology, Royal Melbourne
Hospital and University of Melbourne, Victoria, Australia
2.6 Nerve supply and nervous control of liver function

---

* It is with regret that we report the death of Professor J. Barrowman during
the preparation of this edition.

PAULETTE BIOULAC-SAGE
    Professor of Pathology, CHU de Bordeaux, Université de
    Bordeaux II, France
    1.2 Liver and biliary-tract histology

MICHEL BIOUR
    Director, Centre de Pharmacovigilance Paris-Saint Antoine
    and Associate Professor of Pharmacology, Medical School,
    University of Paris VI, France
    17.0 Drug-induced liver injury

JOHANNES BIRCHER
    Visiting Professor, Department of Pharmacology, University
    of Bern, Switzerland
    25.8 The nervous system in liver disease
    29.3 Drug treatment in patients with liver disease

HENRI BISMUTH
    Professor of Surgery, Hôpital Paul-Brousse, Villejuif, France
    1.1 Macroscopic anatomy of the liver
    22.2.2 Malignant biliary tract obstruction
    *30.1 General surgical aspects and the risks of liver surgery in
    patients with hepatic disease*

NORBERT BLANCKAERT
    Professor of Clinical Pathology, University Hospital
    Gasthuisberg, Leuven, Belgium
    2.9 Bilirubin metabolism
    20.6 Hyperbilirubinaemia

ANDRES T. BLEI
    Professor of Medicine, Northwestern University, Chicago,
    Illinois, USA
    9 Hepatic encephalopathy

P. BONNABRY
    Division of Clinical Pharmacology, University Hospital,
    Geneva, Switzerland
    2.5 Hepatic metabolism of drugs

FLAVIA BORTOLOTTI
    Senior Lecturer in Internal Medicine, University of Padova,
    Italy
    12.1.2.5 Hepatitis C

JAIME BOSCH
    Professor of Medicine, University of Barcelona School of
    Medicine and Chief of Hepatic Haemodynamic Laboratory
    and Consultant Physician, Hospital Clinic, Barcelona, Spain
    7.2 Pathophysiology of portal hypertension and its complications
    *7.4 Clinical manifestations and management of bleeding episodes
    in cirrhotics*
    21.2 Obstruction of the portal vein

PIERRE M. BOULOUX
    Department of Medicine, Royal Free Hospital, London, UK
    24.6 The effect of endocrine diseases on liver function
    25.2 The effect of liver disease on the endocrine system

J. BOYER
    Ensign Professor of Medicine and Director, Liver Center,
    Yale University School of Medicine, New Haven,
    Connecticut, USA
    23.3 Intrahepatic cholestasis

F. BRAET
    Faculty of Medicine and Pharmacy, Free University of
    Brussels, Belgium
    1.4 Sinusoidal liver cells

SOLANGE BRESSON-HADNI
    Professor of Hepatology, WHO Collaborating Centre for
    Prevention and Treatment of Human Echinococcoses,
    University Hospital, Besançon, France
    13.4.2 Echinococcosis of the liver

PIERRE BRISSOT
    Professor of Hepatology, University Hôpital Pontchalliou,
    Rennes, France
    2.16.1 Normal iron metabolism
    20.2 Haemochromatosis

MIGUEL BRUGUERA
    Senior Consultant, Hospital Clinic and Professor of Medicine,
    Medical School, University of Barcelona, Spain
    22.1.2.1 Benign biliary tumours
    22.2.3 Malignant mesenchymal tumours of the liver
    *24.5 The effect of haematological and lymphatic diseases on the
    liver*

JORDI BRUIX
    Liver Unit, Hospital Clinic, University of Barcelona, Spain
    22.3.1 Metastatic liver disease

A.D.M. BRYCESON
    Professor of Tropical Medicine, London School of Hygiene
    and Tropical Medicine and Consultant Physican, Hospital for
    Tropical Diseases, London, UK
    13.3.3 Visceral leishmaniasis

A.K. BURROUGHS
    Consultant Physician and Hepatologist, Royal Free Hospital,
    London, UK
    *7.4 Clinical manifestations and management of bleeding episodes
    in cirrhotics*
    28 Liver disease and pregnancy

ALASTAIR D. BURT
    Professor of Hepatopathology, Medical School, University of
    Newcastle upon Tyne, UK
    15.2 Pathology of alcoholic liver disease

J.R. BUSCOMBE
    Consultant in Nuclear Medicine, Royal Free Hospital,
    London, UK
    5.6 Radionuclide investigations of the liver

JOAN CABALLERIA
    Consultant Physician, Liver Unit, Hospital Clinic, University
    of Barcelona, Spain
    15.4 Extrahepatic manifestions of alcoholism

LUIZ CAETANO DA SILVA
Chief, Division of Gastroenterology, Faculty of Medicine, University of São Paulo, Brazil
13.1.2 Leptospirosis
13.4.3 Ascariasis, visceral larva migrans, capillariasis, strongyloidiasis, and pentastomiasis

JOYCE CARLSON
Senior Physician, Department of Clinical Chemistry, Malmö University Hospital, Sweden
20.3 α₁-Antitrypsin deficiency and related disorders

ELLEN CARMICHAEL
Associate Director of Strategic and Corporate Development, Vion Pharmaceuticals, Inc., New Haven, Connecticut, USA
2.14.1 Transcription, RNA processing, liver specific factors, RNA translocation, translation, protein co-translocation, secretion

ANTONI CASTELLS
Gastroenterology Department, Hospital Clinic, University of Barcelona, Spain
22.3.1 Metastatic liver disease

R.W. CHAPMAN
Department of Gastroenterology, John Radcliffe Hospital, Oxford, UK
24.2 The effect of gastrointestinal diseases on the liver and biliary tract
25.5 Effect of liver disease on the gastrointestinal tract

P.P. CHIEFFI
Professor of Preventive Medicine, School of Medicine, University of São Paulo, Brazil
13.4.3 Ascariasis, visceral larva migrans, capillariasis, strongyloidiasis, and pentastomiasis

MARCO CIPOLLI
Consultant Physician, Gastroenterology Service, Cystic Fibrosis Centre, Verona Hospital, Italy
20.4 The liver in cystic fibrosis

PETER COLLINS
Senior Lecturer and Honorary Consultant Cardiologist, National Heart and Lung Institute, Imperial College London, UK
24.1 The liver in cardiovascular and pulmonary disease
25.1 The effect of liver disease on the cardiovascular system, lungs, and pulmonary vasculature

JULIET COMPSTON
Lecturer in Medicine and Honorary Consultant Physician, University of Cambridge School of Clinical Medicine, UK
25.10 The effect of liver disease on bone

L. DA COSTA GAYOTTA
Professor of Pathology, University of São Paulo, Brazil
13.1.2 Leptospirosis
13.4.3 Ascariasis, visceral larva migrans, capillariasis, strongyloidiasis, and pentastomiasis

ROBERT N. DAVIDSON
Consultant Physician, Northwick Park Hospital, Harrow, Middlesex, UK
13.3.3 Visceral leishmaniasis

P. DAYER
Division of Clinical Pharmacology, University Hospital, Geneva, Switzerland
2.5 Hepatic metabolism of drugs

R.B.D. DE ZANGER
Faculty of Medicine and Pharmacy, Free University of Brussels, Belgium
1.4 Sinusoidal liver cells

FRANÇOISE DEGOS
Consultant, Service d'Hépatologie, Hôpital Beaujon, Clichy, France
5.4.1 Liver biopsy

MARIE-HELENE DENNINGER
Head of Haemostasis Laboratory, Hôpital Beaujon, Clichy, France
2.14.3 The liver and coagulation
25.4 Haemostasis in liver disease

VALEER J. DESMET
Emeritus Professor of Pathology, Catholic University of Leuven, Belgium
1.5 Embryology of the liver and intrahepatic biliary tract
3.1 Histological features
3.2 Histological classification of chronic liver disease
11.1 Non-cystic malformations of the biliary tract

JULES DESMEULES
Division of Clinical Pharmacology, University Hospital, Geneva, Switzerland
2.5 Hepatic metabolism of drugs

YVES DEUGNIER
Professor of Hepatology, Université Hôpital Pontchalliou, Rennes, France
2.16.1 Normal iron metabolism
20.2 Haemochromatosis

DANIEL DHUMEAUX
Professor of Hepatology and Gastroenterology, University of Paris XII, France
14.7 The liver in graft-versus-host disease

JULES L. DIENSTAG
Associate Professor of Medicine, Harvard Medical School and Physician, Massachusetts General Hospital, Boston, USA
12.1.2.2 Hepatitis A

TOM DOHERTY
Clinical Scientist, MRC Laboratories, Fajara, Banjul, The Gambia
32.1 Geographic distribution of infections causing liver disease

PETER T. DONALDSON
Head of Immnogenetics, Institute of Liver Studies, King's
College Hospital, London, UK
2.7.2 Immunogenetics of liver disease

JAMES S. DOOLEY
Senior Lecturer in Medicine and Honorary Consultant
Physician, Royal Free Hospital, London, UK
*23.2 Extrahepatic biliary obstruction: systemic effects, diagnosis,
management*
23.5 Cholangitis and biliary tract infections

R. HERMON DOWLING
Professor of Hepatology and Gastroenterology and Consultant
Physician, United Medical and Dental Schools and Guy's
Hospital, London, UK
23.4 Gallstones

GEOFFREY DUSHEIKO
Professor of Medicine, Royal Free Hospital and School of
Medicine, London, UK
12.1.2.3 Hepatitis B

CHRISTOPHE DUVOUX
Physician, Service d'Hépatologie et de Gastroenterologie,
Hôpital Henri Mondor, Paris, France
14.7 The liver in graft-versus-host disease

M. EDDOUKS
Faculty of Medicine and Pharmacy, Free University of
Brussels, Belgium
1.4 Sinusoidal liver cells

C. EMPSEN
Faculty of Medicine and Pharmacy, Free University of
Brussels, Belgium
1.4 Sinusoidal liver cells

MICHAEL J. EPPIHEIMER
Post-Doctoral Fellow, Department of Molecular and Cellular
Physiology, lSU Medical Center, Shreveport, Louisiana, USA
2.2 Hepatic lymph and lymphatics

STEN ERIKSSON
Department of Medicine, University of Lund, Malmö,
Sweden
20.3 α₁-Antitrypsin deficiency and related disorders

SERGE ERLINGER
Professor of Hepatology and Gastroenterology, at University
of Paris 7, Service d'Hépatologie, Hôpital Beaujon, Clichy,
France
6.2 Cirrhosis: clinical aspects

H. FALK
Falk Foundation, Freiburg, Germany
31.0   History of hepatology

NELSON FAUSTO
Professor and Chairman, Department of Pathology,
University of Washington School of Medicine, Seattle, USA
2.8.1 Hepatic regeneration

ALBERTO FERRARI
Assistant Professor of Gastroenterology, Medical School,
University of Modena, Italy
5.4.2 Laparoscopy

V.A. FERREIRA ALVES
University of São Paulo, Brazil
13.1.2 Leptospirosis

JOHAN FEVERY
Chairman, Department of Internal Medicine, University
Hospital Gasthuisberg, Leuven, Belgium
2.9 Bilirubin metabolism
20.6 Hyperbilirubinaemia

JEAN-FRANÇOIS FLÉJOU
Professor of Pathology, University of Paris 7, Service
d'Anatomie Pathologique, Hôpital Beaujon, Clichy, France
22.1.2.2 Benign hepatocellular tumours

NICK FRANCIS
Senior Lecturer in Histopathology, Imperial College School
of Medicine at Charing Cross, London, UK
13.3.2 Malaria

F.H. FRANKEN
Professor, University of Düsseldorf, Germany
31.0 History of hepatology

M. FUCHS
Instructor in Medicine, Department of Internal Medicine,
University of Lübeck, Germany
2.1 Metabolism of bile acids

PETER R. GALLE
Professor of Internal Medicine and Chairman, I. Department
of Internal Medicine, University of Mainz, Germany
2.8.2 Apoptosis in the liver

JUAN CARLOS GARCÍA-PAGÁN
Liver Unit, Hospital Clinic, Barcelona, Spain
7.2 Pathophysiology of portal hypertension and its complications
21.2 Obstruction of the portal vein

JOSÉ M. GATELL
Consultant Physician, Hospital Clinic Barcelona and Associate
Professor of Medicine, University of Barcelona, Spain
13.3.4 Toxoplasmosis

PAUL GENECIN
Director, Yale Health Plan and Clinical Associate Professor of
Medicine (Digestive Diseases), Yale University School of
Medicine, New Haven, Connecticut, USA
2.1 Hepatic blood flow

WOLFRAM H. GERLICH
Professor of Medical Virology ,Institute of Medical Virology,
Justus-Leibig University of Giessen, Germany
*12.1.2.1 Structure, replication, and laboratory diagnosis of
hepatitis viruses*

WOLFGANG GEROK
Emeritus Professor of Internal Medicine, University of
Freiburg, Germany
2.14.2 Protein secretion, degradation, and function

RICHARD GILSON
Senior Lecturer in Sexually Transmitted Diseases, Division
of Pathology and Infectious Diseases, Windeyer Institute of
Medical Sciences, University College London Medical
School, UK
*12.3 Hepatitis and human immunodeficiency virus infection in
homosexual men and injecting drug users*

PERE GINÈS
Staff Member, Liver Unit, University of Barcelona, Spain
8.1 Pathogenesis, diagnosis, and treatment of ascites in cirrhosis
8.2 Renal dysfunction in cirrhosis

PAOLO GIOANNINI
Clinica Malattie Infettive, Ospedale Amedeo di Savoia, Torino,
Italy
12.4 Exotic virus infections of the liver

JONATHAN D. GITLIN
Professor of Pediatrics and Chief, Pediatric Rheumatology,
Washington University School of Medicine, St Louis,
Missouri, USA
2.16.2 Normal copper metabolism
20.1 Wilson's disease

DERMOT GLEESON
Consultant Physician, Gastroenterology and Liver Unit,
Royal Hallamshire Hospital, Sheffield, UK
23.3 Intrahepatic cholestasis

CHRISTIAN GLUUD
Chief Physician, Copenhagen Trial Unit, Copenhagen
University Hospital, Denmark
32.4 The Cochrane Hepato-Biliary Group

D. NEIL GRANGER
Professor and Head, Department of Molecular and Cellular
Physiology, LSU Medical Center, Shreveport, Louisiana,
USA
2.2 Hepatic lymph and lymphatics

A.M. GRESSNER
Professor of Clinical Chemistry, Pathobiochemistry, and
Laboratory Medicine, Institute for Clinical Chemistry and
Pathobiochemistry, RWTH University Clinic, Aachen,
Germany
*2.15 Function and metabolism of collagen and other extracellular
proteins*
*6.1 Cellular and molecular pathobiology, pharmacological
intervention, and biochemical assessment of liver fibrosis*

PAUL GRIFFITHS
Professor of Virology, Royal Free Hospital School of
Medicine, London, UK
12.2 Systemic virosis producing hepatitis

GENY M.M. GROOTHUIS
Assistant Professor of Pharmacokinetics and Drug Delivery,
Groningen Institute for Drug Studies, University Centre for
Pharmacy, University of Groningen, The Netherlands
2.4 Hepatobiliary disposition and targeting of drugs and genes

VOLKER GROSS
Professor of Internal Medicine, University of Freiburg,
Germany
2.14.2 Protein secretion, degradation, and function

HOWARD GROSSMAN
Senior Lecturer in Pathology, University of Melbourne,
Victoria, Australia
2.6 Nerve supply and nervous control of liver function

ROBERTO J. GROSZMANN
Professor of Medicine, Yale University School of Medicine,
New Haven, Connecticut, USA
2.1 Hepatic blood flow

JORGE J. GUMUCIO
Professor of Medicine, Gastroenterology Division, University
of Michigan Medical Center and Veterans Affairs Medical
Center, Ann Arbor, Michigan, USA
2.18 Functional organization of the liver

M. HADCHOUEL
Hôpital de Bicêtre, Bicêtre, France
26.0 Paediatric liver disease

FADI G. HADDAD
Assistant Professor of Pediatric Gastroenterology and
Hepatology, University of Texas Health Science Center,
San Antonio, Texas, USA
2.1 Hepatic blood flow

STEPHANOS J. HADZIYANNIS
Professor of Medicine, Athens University School of Medicine
and Director of the National Reference Centre for
Communicable Liver Disease, Hippokration General
Hospital, Athens, Greece
12.1.2.7 The new 'hepatitis' virus G or GBV-C

A.J. HALL
Reader in Communicable Disease Epidemiology, London
School of Hygiene and Tropical Medicine, UK
32.1 Geographic distribution of infections causing liver disease

D.S. HARRY
Principal Clinical Scientist and Honorary Lecturer, Royal
Free Hospital, London, UK
2.12 Plasma lipids and lipoproteins

D. HÄUSSINGER
Professor of Internal Medicine and Director of Clinic for
Gastroenterology, Hepatology, and Infectiology, Heinrich
Heine University, Düsseldorf, Germany
2.13.2 Ammonia, urea production, and pH regulation

R.J. HAY
Professor of Cutaneous Medicine, United Medical and Dental Schools of St Thomas's and Guy's Hospital, London, UK
13.2 Fungal infections affecting the liver

JENNY HEATHCOTE
Professor of Medicine, University of Toronto and Staff Gastroenterologist, The Toronto Hospital, Ontario, Canada
14.1 Primary biliary cirrhosis
14.6 Overlap syndromes

J. MICHAEL HENDERSON
Department of General Surgery, The Cleveland Clinic Foundation, Ohio, USA
7.1 Anatomy of the portal venous system in portal hypertension

A.J.W. HILSON
Consultant in Nuclear Medicine, Royal Free Hospital, London, UK
5.6 Radionuclide investigations of the liver

K.E.F. HOBBS
Professor of Surgery, Royal Free Hospital School of Medicine, London, UK
23.6 The gallbladder and laparoscopic cholecystectomy

H.J.F HODGSON
Professor of Medicine, Imperial College School of Medicine at The Hammersmith, London, UK
22.3.2 Carcinoid tumours

A.V. HOFFBRAND
Emeritus Professor of Haematology, Royal Free Hospital, London, UK
20.7 The liver in intracellular and extracellular lipidosis

J. HUGHES
Specialist Registrar, Department of Dermatology, Royal Free Hospital, London, UK
24.3 The effect of skin diseases on the liver
25.6 The effect of liver disease on the skin

IRENE HUNG
Pediatric Rheumatology, Washington University School of Medicine, St Louis, Missouri, USA
2.16.2 Normal copper metabolism
20.1 Wilson's disease

D. GERAINT JAMES
Adjunct Professor of Medicine, Royal Free Hospital School of Medicine, London, UK
14.2 Hepatic granulomas

O.F.W. JAMES
Professor of Medicine and Head of School of Clinical Medical Science, University of Newcastle upon Tyne, UK
27 Liver disease in the elderly

P.L.M. JANSEN
Professor of Gastroenterology, University of Groningen, The Netherlands
2.4 Hepatobiliary disposition and targeting of drugs and genes

WLADIMIRO JIMÉNEZ
Hospital Clinic i Provincial, Barcelona, Spain
8.2 Renal dysfunction in cirrhosis

ALBERT L. JONES
Professor of Medicine and Anatomy, University of California, San Francisco, California, USA
1.3 Electron microscopy of the liver

REGINE KAHL
Professor of Toxicology, Institute of Toxicology, University of Düsseldorf, Germany
18.1 Toxic liver injury
32.2 Liver injury in man ascribed to non-drug chemicals and natural toxins

MARK A. KANE
World Health Organization, Geneva, Switzerland
12.1.3.1(b) Hepatitis B vaccines and immunization

EMMET B. KEEFFE
Professor of Medicine, Stanford University School of Medicine; Chief of Clinical Gastroenterology and Medical Director, Liver Transplant Program, Stanford University Medical Center, California, USA
16 Non-alcoholic fatty liver: causes and complications

S. KEIDING
Consultant Physician, Department of Hepatology V and PET Centre, Aarhus University Hospital, Denmark
5.2 Hepatic removal of circulating substances: importance for quantitative measurements of liver function

CHRISTOPHER KIBBLER
Consultant in Medical Microbiology, Royal Free Hospital, London, UK
13.1.1 Bacterial infection and the liver

K. KRAWCZYNSKI
Chief, Experimental Pathology Section, Hepatitis Branch, DVRD/NCID, Centers for Disease Control and Prevention, Atlanta, Georgia, USA
12.1.2.6 Hepatitis E

J.E.J. KRIGE
Associate Professor of Surgery, Department of Surgery and Surgical Gastroenterology, University of Cape Town and Groote Schuur Hospital, South Africa
30.4 Hepatobiliary trauma

YOLANTA T. KRUSZYNSKA
Associate Professor of Medicine, Department of Medicine, University of California at San Diego, La Jolla, USA
2.11 Carbohydrate metabolism
2.13.1 Amino acid metabolism
24.6 The effect of endocrine diseases on liver function
25.2 The effect of liver disease on the endocrine system

F. KUNSTLINGER
Consultant Radiologist, Centre Hépatobiliaire, Hôpital Paul-Brousse, Villejuif, France
1.1 Macroscopic anatomy of the liver

DOMINIQUE LARREY
Professor of Hepatology, Medical School, University of
Montpellier, France
17 Drug-induced liver injury

NICHOLAS F. LaRUSSO
Professor of Medicine and Biochemistry and Molecular
Biology, Mayo Medical School, Clinic, and Foundation,
Rochester, Minnesota, USA
14.4 Sclerosing cholangitis

BERNARD H. LAUTERBURG
Professor of Clinical Pharmacology and Internal Medicine,
University of Bern, Switzerland
*5.2 Hepatic removal of circulating substances: importance for
quantitative measurements of liver function*

BRIGITTE LE BAIL
Maître de Conference des Universités, Praticien Hospitalier
CHU de Bordeaux, Université de Bordeaux II, France
1.2 Liver and biliary-tract histology

DIDIER LEBREC
Director, INSERM, Hôpital Beaujon, Clichy, France
5.7 Splanchic haemodynamic investigations

RANDALL G. LEE
Associate Professor of Pathology, University of Pittsburgh
Medical Center, Pennsylvania, USA
16 Non-alcoholic fatty liver: causes and complications

JOSEP M. LLOVET
Liver Unit, Hospital Clinic, University of Barcelona, Spain
22.3.1 Metastatic liver disease

LAURENCE B. LOVAT
Immunological Medicine Unit (Division of Medicine),
Imperial College School of Medicine, Hammersmith Hospital,
London, UK
14.8 Amyloidosis

ANNA LUCCHINI
Clinica Malattie Infettive, Ospedale Amedeo di Savoia, Turin,
Italy
12.4 Exotic virus infections of the liver

JURGEN LUDWIG
Emeritus Professor of Pathology, Mayo Clinic and Mayo
Medical School, Rochester, Minnesota, USA
14.4 Sclerosing cholangitis
14.5 Vanishing bile duct syndrome

D. LUO
Faculty of Medicine and Pharmacy, Free University of
Brussels, Belgium
1.4 Sinusoidal liver cells

THOMAS T. LUTHER
Medical Student, Medical School, University of
Witten/Herdecke, Germany
*2.19 In vitro techniques: isolated organ perfusion, slices, cells,
and subcellular elements*

R.N.M. MacSWEEN
Professor of Pathology, University of Glasgow; Honorary
Consultant, Department of Pathology, Western Infirmary,
Glasgow, UK
15.2 Pathology of alcoholic liver disease

PIETRO E. MAJNO
Chef de Clinique Associé, Centre Hépatobiliaire,
Hôpital Paul Brousse, Villejuif, Paris, France
1.1 Macroscopic anatomy of the liver
22.2.2 Malignant biliary obstruction
*30.1 General surgical aspects and the risks of liver surgery in
patients with hepatic disease*

S.V. MALLETT
Consultant Anaesthetist, Royal Free Hospital, London, UK
30.2 Anaesthesia and liver disease

FEDERICO MANENTI
Professor of Gastroenterology, Medical School, University of,
Modena, Italy
5.4.2 Laparoscopy

MICHAEL P. MANNS
Medizinsche Hochschule Hannover, Zentrum fur Innere
Medizin und Dermatologie, Hannover, Germany
2.7.2 Immunogenetics of liver disease
5.3 Immunological investigations in liver diseases
14.3 Autoimmune hepatitis

J. WALLIS MARSH
Associate Professor of Surgery, University of Pittsburgh
School of Medicine, Pennsylvania, USA
30.5 Liver transplantation

ADOLFO MARTINEZ PALOMO
Professor of Experimental Pathology, Center for Research and
Advanced Studies, Mexico
13.3.1 Amoebiasis, giardiasis, and cryptosporidiosis

ANTONI MAS
Staff Member, Liver Unit, Hospital Clinic, University of
Barcelona, Spain
18.2 Hepatic injury due to physical agents

GIANNI MASTELLA
Professor of Paediatrics and Scientific Director, Cystic
Fibrosis Centre, Verona Hospital, Italy
20.4 The liver in cystic fibrosis

KEITH P.W.J. McADAM
Wellcome Professor of Tropical Medicine, London School of
Hygiene and Tropical Medicine and Director, MRC
Laboratories, Fajara, Banjul, The Gambia
14.8 Amyloidosis

P. AIDEN McCORMICK
Liver Unit, St Vincent's Hospital, Dublin, Ireland
*10 The spleen, hypersplenism, and other relationships between the
liver and spleen*

NEIL McINTYRE
　Professor of Medicine, Royal Free Hospital School of
　Medicine, London, UK
　2.12 Plasma lipids and lipoproteins
　2.13.1 Amino-acid metabolism
　4.0 Symptoms and signs of liver disease
　5.1 Biochemical investigations in the management of liver disease
　5.8 Diagnostic approach to liver disease
　23.1 Cholestasis
　23.4 Gallstones
　24.1 The liver in cardiovascular and pulmonary disease
　*25.1 The effect of liver disease on the cardiovascular system,
　lungs, and pulmonary vasculature*
　25.3 Haematological abnormalities in liver disease
　29.1 The general management of liver disease

ATUL B. MEHTA
　Consultant Haematologist, Royal Free Hospital, London, UK
　25.3 Haematological abnormalities in liver disease

DIRK K.F. MEIJER
　Professor of Pharmacokinetics and Drug Delivery, Groningen
　Institute for Drug Studies, University Centre for Pharmacy,
　University of Groningen, The Netherlands
　2.4 Hepatobiliary disposition and targeting of drugs and genes

HERMANN MENGER
　Clinic for Neurology and Clinical Neurophysiology,
　University of Witten/Herdecke, Wuppertal, Germany
　25.8 The nervous system in liver disease

YVES MENU
　Professor of Radiology at University of Paris 7, Service de
　Radiologie, Hôpital Beaujon, Clichy, France
　5.5 Imaging of the liver and biliary tract
　*11.2 Non-parasitic cystic diseases of the liver and intrahepatic
　biliary tree*
　22.1.2.2 Benign hepatocellular tumours

KARL-HERMANN MEYER ZUM BUSCHENFELDE
　Professor of Medicine, Johannes-Gutenberg Universität,
　Mainz, Germany
　5.3 Immunological investigations in liver diseases

J.P. MIGUET
　Service d'Hépatologie et de Soins Intensifs Digestifs, CHU
　Jean Minjoz, Besançon, France
　13.4.2 Echinococcosis of the liver

JOSÉ M. MIRO
　Consultant Physician, Hospital Clinic Barcelona and Associate
　Professor of Medicine, University of Barcelona, Spain
　13.3.4 Toxoplasmosis

P.K. MISTRY
　Director of Comprehensive Gaucher Disease Program,
　Department of Human Genetics, Mount Sinai School of
　Medicine, New York, USA
　20.7 The liver in intracellular and extracellular lipidosis
　20.8 Glycogen storage diseases

MARSHA Y. MORGAN
　Senior Lecturer and Honorary Consultant Physician,
　Royal Free Hospital, London, UK
　*15.3 Alcoholic liver disease: natural history, diagnosis, clinical
　features, evaluation, management, prognosis, and prevention*
　29.2 Nutritional aspects of liver and biliary disease

MARTINA MÜLLER
　Department of Internal Medicine IV, Hepatology and
　Gastroenterology, University Hospital, Heidelberg, Germany
　2.8.2 Apoptosis in the liver

MIGUEL NAVASA
　Faculty Member, Liver Unit, Hospital Clinic, University of
　Barcelona, Spain
　25.11 Infections in liver disease

DIETER NEUMANN-HAEFELIN
　Professor of Virology, University Hospital, Freiburg,
　Germany
　12.2 Systemic virosis producing hepatitis

YVES NORDMANN
　Professor of Biochemistry, Faculté Xavier Bichat, University
　of Paris 7, France
　2.17 Haem biosynthesis and excretions of porphyrins
　20.5 Human hereditary porphyrias

ANDREAS OCHS
　Department of Internal Medicine, University of Freiburg,
　Germany
　2.16.3 Trace elements

HIROAKI OKUDA
　Assistant Professor, Institute of Gastroenterology,
　Tokyo Women's Medical College, Tokyo, Japan
　22.2.1 Primary liver cell carcinoma

KUNIO OKUDA
　Emeritus Professor of Medicine, Chiba University School of
　Medicine, Japan
　22.2.1 Primary liver cell carcinoma

ALBERT PARES
　Consultant Physician, Liver Unit, Hospital Clinic, University
　of Barcelona, Spain
　15.4 Extrahepatic manifestions of alcoholism

DOMINIQUE PESSAYRE
　Director of Research, INSERM U481, Hôpital Beaujon,
　Clichy, France
　17 Drug-induced liver injury

RAMÓN PLANAS
　Hospital Clinic i Provincial, Barcelona, Spain
　8.1 Pathogenesis, diagnosis, and treatment of ascites in cirrhosis

JORGE RAKELA
　Professor of Medicine and Chief, Division of
　Gastroenterology and Hepatology, University of Pittsburgh,
　Pennsylvania, USA
　30.5 Liver transplantation

GIULIANO RAMADORI
Professor of Medicine and Chairman of Gastroenterology and
Endocrinology, Department of Internal Medicine,
University of Göttingen, Germany
2.7.1 Cytokines and the liver

JÜRG REICHEN
Professor of Medicine and Chairman, Department of Clinical
Pharmacology, University of Bern, Switzerland
*2.3 Physiology of bile formation and of the motility of the biliary
tree*

ANTONI RIMOLA
Associate Professor, Department of Medicine, Hospital Clinic,
University of Barcelona, Spain
25.11 Infections in liver disease

MARIO RIZZETTO
Professor of Gastroenterology, University of Turin, Italy
12.1.1 Introduction
12.1.2.4 Hepatitis D
12.1.3.2 Therapy of chronic viral hepatitis
12.2 Systemic virosis producing hepatitis

JUAN RODÉS
Professor of Medicine and Chief of Liver Unit, University of
Barcelona, Spain
8.1 Pathogenesis, diagnosis, and treatment of ascites in cirrhosis
8.2 Renal dysfunction in cirrhosis
18.2 Hepatic injury due to physical agents
22.2.3 Malignant mesenchymal tumours of the liver
24.4 The liver in urogenital diseases
25.7 Effect of liver disease on the urogenital tract
30.3 Postoperative jaundice

S.B. ROSALKI
Honorary Consultant in Chemical Pathology, Royal Free
Hospital, London, UK
5.1 Biochemical investigations in the management of liver disease

TANIA ROSKAMS
Professor of Pathology, Catholic University of Leuven,
Belgium
1.5 Embryology of the liver and intrahepatic biliary tract
3.1 Histological features
3.2 Histological classification of chronic liver disease
11.1 Non-cystic malformations of the biliary tract

M. RUSTIN
Consultant Dermatologist, Royal Free Hospital, London, UK
24.3 The effect of skin diseases on the liver
25.6 The effect of liver disease on the skin

MARIE-FRANCE SAINT-MARC-GIRARDIN
Physician, Service d'Hépatologie et de Gastroenterologie,
Hôpital Henri Mondor, Paris, France
14.7 The liver in graft-versus-host disease

MIKKO SALASPURO
Professor of Alcohol Diseases, University of Helsinki, Finland
*15.1 Epidemiological aspects of alcoholic liver disease, ethanol
metabolism, and pathogenesis of alcoholic liver injury*

JUAN M. SALMERON
Staff Member, Liver Unit, Hospital Clinic, Barcelona, Spain
30.3 Postoperative jaundice

JOSE MARIA SÁNCHEZ-TAPIAS
Consultant Physician, Liver Unit, Hospital Clinic and Associate
Professor of Medicine, Medical School, University of Barcelona,
Spain
13.1.1 Bacterial infection and the liver

GIORGIO SARACCO
Associate Professor of Gastroenterology, Azienda Ospedaliera
S. Giovanni Battista, Turin, Italy
12.1.3.2 Therapy of chronic viral hepatitis

PETER J. SCHEUER
Emeritus Professor of Histopathology, Royal Free Hospital
School of Medicine, London, UK
14.2 Hepatic granulomas

DOUGLAS L. SCHMUCKER
Associate Career Research Scientist, Veterans Administration
Medical Center; Professor of Anatomy and Senior
Investigator, Liver Center, University of California,
San Francisco, USA
1.3 Electron microscopy of the liver

J. SCHOLMERICH
Professor and Director, Klinik und Poliklinik für Innere
Medizin I, Universität Regensburg, Germany
2.16.3 Trace elements

DETLEF SCHUPPAN
Medizinische Klinik mit Poliklinik der Friedrich-Alexander
Universität, Erlangen, Germany
*2.15 Function and metabolism of collagen and other extracellular
proteins*
*6.1 Cellular and molecular pathobiology, pharmacological
intervention, and biochemical assessment of liver fibrosis*

SHEILA SHERLOCK
Professor of Medicine, Department of Surgery, Royal Free
Hospital, London, UK
14.1 Primary biliary cirrhosis

ANTONINA SMEDILE
Associate Professor of Gastroenterology, Azienda Ospedaliera
S. Giovanni Battista, Turin, Italy
12.1.2.4 Hepatitis D

WALTRAUD SOMMER
Scientific Assistant, University of Witten/Herdecke, Germany
29.3 Drug treatment in patients with liver disease

HERBERT SPAPEN
Physician, Medical Intensive Care Department, Academic Hospital, Free University of Brussels, Belgium
1.4 Sinusoidal liver cells

EDUARD F. STANGE
Professor of Medicine and Chief, Division of Gastroenterology, Department of Internal Medicine, University of Lübeck, Germany
2.10 Metabolism of bile acids

JOHN TERBLANCHE
Professor and Chairman, Department of Surgery, University of Cape Town; Surgeon-in-Chief, Groote Schuur Hospital Teaching Hospital Group, Cape Town, and Co-Director, Medical Research Council Liver Research Centre, University of Cape Town, South Africa
30.4 Hepatobiliary trauma

JOSEP TERÉS
Professor of Medicine, Hospital Clinic, Barcelona, Spain
21.1 Hepatic arteries

REINER THOMSSEN
Professor of Medical Microbiology and Head of Department of Medical Microbiology, University of Göttingen, Germany
12.1.2.1 Structure, replication, and laboratory diagnosis of hepatitis viruses

JONATHAN M. TIBBALLS
Consultant Radiologist, Royal Free Hospital, London, UK
5.5 Imaging of the liver and biliary tract

DOMINIQUE VALLA
Professor of Hepatology and Gastroenterology at University of Paris 7, Service d'Hépatologie, Hôpital Beaujon, Clichy, France
7.3 Intrahepatic portal hypertension
21.3 Obstruction of the hepatic venous system

J. VAN DEN BOGAERDE
Royal Free Hospital, London, UK
24.7 Musculoskeletal diseases and the liver
25.9 Musculoskeletal problems in liver disease

PETER VAN EYKEN
Consultant Pathologist, Catholic University of Leuven, Belgium
1.5 Embryology of the liver and intrahepatic biliary tract
11.1 Non-cystic malformations of the biliary tract

GIORGIO VERME
Emeritus Professor of Gastroenterology, Azienda Ospedaliera S. Giovanni Battista, Turin, Italy
12.1.2.4 Hepatitis D

D. VERMIJLEN
Faculty of Medicine and Pharmacy, Free University of Brussels, Belgium
1.4 Sinusoidal liver cells

JEAN-PAUL VERNANT
Professor of Haematology, Service d'Hématologie, Hôpital Pitié Salpêtrière, Paris, France
14.7 The liver in graft-versus-host disease

DOMINIQUE VUITTON
Professor of Clinical Immunology, WHO Collaborating Centre for Prevention and Treatment of Human Echinococcoses, University Hospital, Besançon, France
13.4.2 Echinococcosis of the liver

DAVID A. WARRELL
Professor of Tropical Medicine and Infectious Diseases and Director, Centre for Tropical Medicine, University of Oxford, UK
13.3.2 Malaria

K.S. WARREN
The Picower Institute for Medical Research, Manhasset, New York, USA
13.4.1 Blood flukes (schistomes) and liver flukes

ANTHONY F. WATKINSON
Consultant Radiologist, Royal Free Hospital, London, UK
5.5 Imaging of the liver and biliary tract

IAN WELLER
Professor of Sexually Transmitted Diseases, Division of Pathology and Infectious Diseases, Windeyer Institute of Medical Sciences, University College London Medical School, UK
12.3 Hepatitis and human immunodeficiency virus infection in homosexual men and injecting drug users

RUSSELL H. WIESNER
Medical Director, Liver Transplantation, Mayo Clinic and Professor of Medicine, Mayo Medical School, Rochester, Minnesota, USA
14.4 Sclerosing cholangitis

R.M. WINTER
Professor of Dysmorphology and Clinical Genetics, Institute of Child Health, London, UK
32.3 Rare diseases with hepatic abnormalities

EDDIE WISSE
Professor of Cell Biology and Histology, Faculty of Medicine and Pharmacy, Free University of Brussels, Belgium
1.4 Sinusoidal liver cells

GEORGE Y. WU
Professor of Medicine and Chief, Division of Gastroenterology-Hepatology, University of Connecticut Health Center, Farmington, USA
2.14.1 Transcription, RNA processing, liver specific factors, RNA translocation, translation, protein co-translocation, secretion

ELIE-SERGE ZAFRANI
University of Paris XII, France
14.7 The liver in graft-versus-host disease

1

Structure of the liver

1.1 Macroscopic anatomy of the liver

H. Bismuth, Pietro E. Majno, and F. Kunstlinger

The traditional description of the liver in anatomy textbooks, based on its external appearance, is of limited utility in the management of hepatic disease. Modern hepatology, hepatic radiology, and surgery are based upon the functional segmental anatomy of the liver, a sound knowledge of which is essential in the description and localization of hepatic lesions and in the planning of liver resections.

The description of liver anatomy, therefore, can take three forms.

1. Morphological anatomy—this is the classical description of the liver as composed by *lobes* defined by surface markings, of the topographical relations of the organ and of the hepatic vascular and biliary structures.
2. Functional anatomy—this the description of the liver according to the intrahepatic vascular anatomy. It is based on *segments*, which are functional units receiving a portal pedicle. The segments are independent as for their portal and arterial supply, and biliary drainage.
3. Radiological and surgical anatomy—this is the application of the 'ideal' functional anatomy to *each individual liver* by accurate definition of its particular intrahepatic vascular anatomy. This anatomy is visible on radiological investigations such as ultrasound, contrast-enhanced CT, and MRI, and in the operating theatre by the technique of operative ultrasonography.

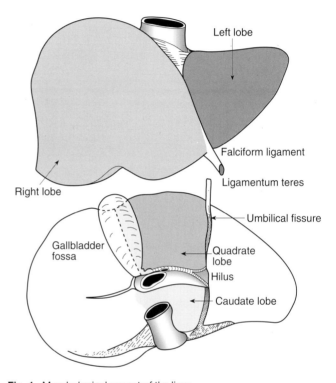

Fig. 1. Morphological aspect of the liver.

Morphological anatomy (Fig. 1)
Peritoneal reflections and ligaments

The liver is situated in the upper part of the abdominal cavity against the diaphragm. It is covered by the visceral peritoneum of Glisson's capsule, which thickens into three folds or ligaments connecting it to the parietal peritoneum: the falciform ligament superiorly, and the right and left triangular ligaments posteriorly. These ligaments circumscribe, on the posterior surface, the bare area of the liver not covered by peritoneum, in which lies the retrohepatic vena cava. On the inferior surface the peritoneum of Glisson's capsule joins into another fold, the lesser omentum, connecting the liver to the lesser curve of the stomach, and reflects around the hepatic pedicle, delimiting Winslow's foramen to the lesser sac. At the hepatic hilum, Glisson's capsule fuses with the connective tissue surrounding the hepatic artery, the portal vein, and the hepatic duct forming the hilar plate, a fibrous structure of surgical importance in the dissection of these structure as they branch into the liver.

Surface marks, hepatic lobes, and their relations

On the inferior surface three markings can be identified: the umbilical fissure medially, into which continues the round ligament, a remnant of the umbilical vein; the gallbladder fossa laterally; and running perpendicularly between them the transverse hilar fissure. This 'H'-shaped configuration defines two main lobes on each side, the right and the left lobes, and two accessory lobes in the middle, the quadrate lobe anteriorly and the caudate lobe posteriorly (Fig. 1).

The left lobe

This is limited on the inferior surface by the umbilical fissure and on the superior surface by the falciform ligament; it is of variable shape, its long axis being sometimes sagittal, sometimes transverse. The superior surface is marked, in the middle, by the inferior

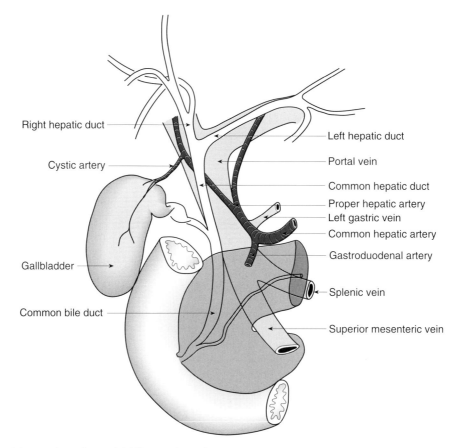

Fig. 2. Representation of the extrahepatic arterial, biliary, and portal anatomy.

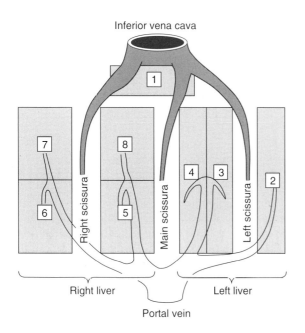

Fig. 3. Schematic representation of the functional anatomy of the liver. There are three main hepatic veins lying within the liver scissurae and dividing the liver into four sectors each receiving a portal pedicle. The hepatic veins and portal pedicles are intertwined as are the finger of two hands.

surface of the heart. The inferior surface lies on the lesser curve of the stomach to which it is connected by the lesser omentum.

The right lobe

This is the bigger of the two main lobes and has three surfaces.

1. The superior surface comprises an upper, convex part, moulded by the diaphragm and forming the dome of the liver, to which surgical access is difficult, and a lower part facing antero-superiorly.
2. The posterior surface is vertical and extends from the right border of the liver to the inferior vena cava.
3. The inferior surface is in relation to the colon anteriorly, and posteriorly to the perirenal fat, from which it is separated by a peritoneal recess, Morisson's pouch (where even a small amount of ascitic fluid collects and can be seen on the ultrasonogram).

The quadrate lobe

This is delimited by the umbilical fissure medially, by the gall-bladder fossa laterally, and by the transverse hilar fissure posteriorly. It lies on the gastric antrum and on the duodenum.

The caudate lobe

This belongs almost completely to the posterior surface of the liver. Laying in a vertical plane, it is limited on the right by the inferior vena cava and on the left by the fissure of Arantius (fissure for the

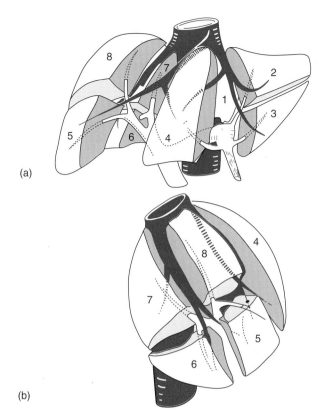

Fig. 4. The functional division of the liver and of the liver segments according to Couinaud's nomenclature: (a) as seen in the patient; (b) the *ex vivo* position.

ligamentum venosum). Its lower border is visible behind the hilum. Two tuberosities can be identified on this border: (i) the caudate tuberosity on the right, which passes towards the right lobe, and (ii) the papillary tubercle on the left, covered by the lesser omentum.

The hepatic artery, the portal vein, and the bile duct

The hepatic artery, the portal vein, and the bile duct run to the liver in the hepatic pedicle. The usual position is the bile duct to the right, at the free edge of the lesser omentum, the artery to the left, and both anterior to the portal vein (Fig. 2).

The hepatic artery

This most frequently originates from the coeliac trunk as the common hepatic artery, then becomes the proper hepatic artery after giving off the gastroduodenal artery behind the duodenum. In the hepatic pedicle it gives off the cystic artery, usually behind the bile duct but sometimes anteriorly. At a variable distance from the hepatic hilum it divides into a left and right branch. Variations of the arterial anatomy are common, and among the most frequent are: the presence a supplementary hepatic artery to the right lobe (together with a right branch of a normal hepatic artery: 10 per cent) or of a replaced hepatic artery (representing the only artery to the right lobe: 8 per cent), or of a main hepatic artery (2.5 per cent), originating from the superior mesenteric artery . In these cases the variant artery may run posteriorly and to the right of the bile duct. A left hepatic artery originating from the left gastric artery may be found in the lesser omentum in 10 per cent of individuals, and very rarely it may be the main hepatic artery (0.2 per cent).

The portal vein runs in the hepatic pedicle after being formed by the confluence of the splenic vein and the superior mesenteric vein behind the neck of the pancreas. On the left it receives the right gastric vein, which is an important route of systemic derivation of portal blood in portal hypertension.

The right hepatic duct, and the left hepatic duct, which has a long and almost horizontal extrahepatic course, form the biliary confluence at the hepatic hilum. The common hepatic duct so formed receives the cystic duct in the hepatic pedicle, and from this point is called the common bile duct. It runs behind the first part of the duodenum, and to the duodenal papilla through the pancreatic head. Anatomical variations in the formation of the hepatic ducts and in the entry of the cystic duct are common, the most important from a surgical point of view being separate entry of an intrahepatic branch into the right hepatic duct or the common hepatic duct, and the insertion of the cystic duct into the right hepatic duct.

The venous drainage of the liver is from the three hepatic veins, the left and the middle hepatic vein joining into a common trunk before exiting into the inferior vena cava (see below). The caudate

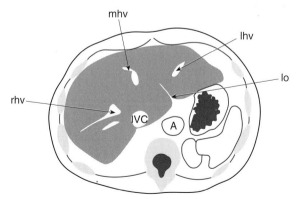

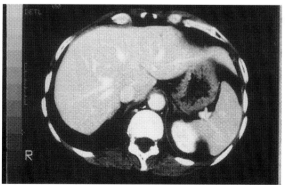

Fig. 5. CT scan: the hepatic veins (intravenous contrast injection). The three hepatic veins (hv) are easily identified following contrast injection and allow the delineation of the right and left livers and the anterior and posterior sectors of the right liver. A fissure can be seen between segments I and II, which represents the attachment of the lesser omentum (lo) and extends to the level of the left branch of the portal vein. A, aorta; IVC, inferior vena cava.

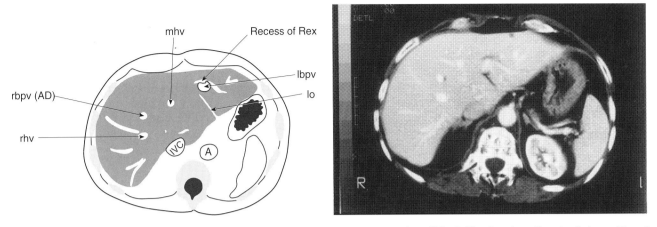

Fig. 6. CT scan: the hepatic veins (intravenous contrast injection). A cut taken 1 cm below that of Fig. 5. The three hepatic veins (hv) are still easily identified and in addition the left branch of the portal vein (lbpv) and the anterior division of the right branch of the portal vein [rbpv (AD)] have come into view. A, aorta; IVC, inferior vena cava; lo, lesser omentum.

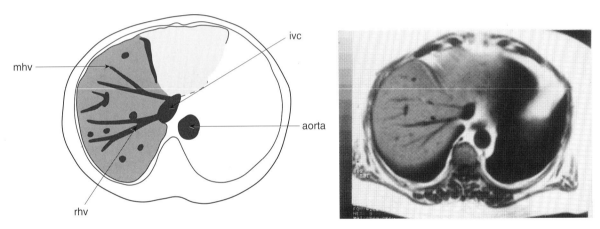

Fig. 7. MRI: the hepatic veins. A very high cut showing the right (rhv) and middle hepatic veins (mhv) and their entry into the inferior vena cava (ivc).

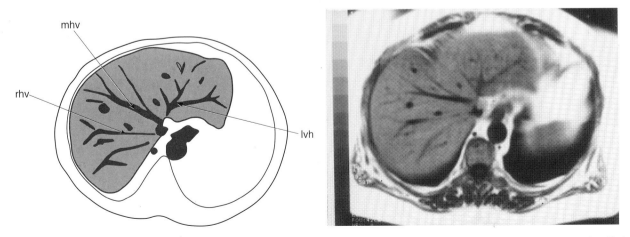

Fig. 8. MRI: the hepatic veins. The three hepatic veins (hv) and the sectors of the liver are clearly seen. Vascular structures are easily identified on MRI without the need for contrast injection. They appear black because the absence of a signal related to the presence of flow.

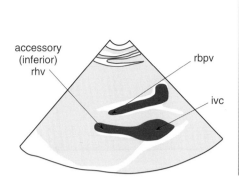
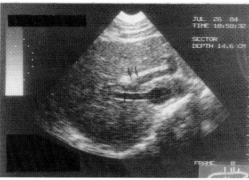

Fig. 9. Ultrasonography: the accessory inferior right hepatic vein. Oblique right subcostal cut showing the portal bifurcation and an accessory (inferior) right hepatic vein (rhv) lying behind the right branch of the portal vein (rbpv). This accessory (inferior) right hepatic vein is present in approx. 10 per cent of the population and is usually associated with another right hepatic vein entering higher than normal into the vena cava at the level of the entry of the middle and left hepatic veins.

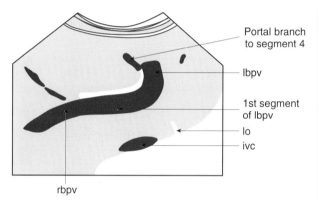
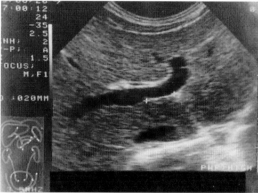

Fig. 10. Ultrasonography: the portal bifurcation. The two white crosses indicate the length of the first segment of the left branch of the portal vein (lbpv). The second segment of the vein continues in the umbilical fissure, which separates the right and left lobes of the liver. The caudate lobe is found between the inferior vena cava (ivc) and the portal bifurcation and is separated from segment II by an echogenic line which corresponds to the lesser omentum (lo) as it comes to merge with the left branch of the portal vein.

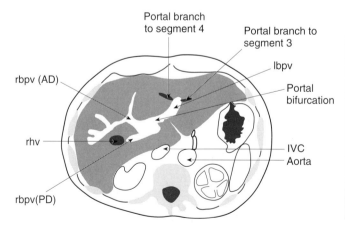
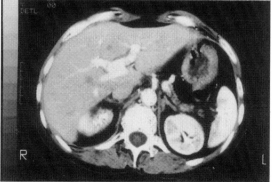

Fig. 11. CT scan (intravenous contrast injection): the portal bifurcation. The portal bifurcation, left and right portal branches (lbpv and rbpv) and the segmental branches are all clearly identified following contrast injection. On this particular cut, the right hepatic vein (rhv) (still to be opacified) can be seen in cross-section between the anterior and posterior divisions of the right branch of the portal vein (rbpv (AD) and rbpv (PD)). IVC, inferior vena cava.

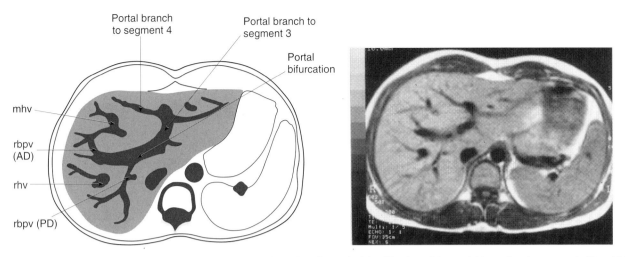

Fig. 12. MRI: the portal bifurcation. This cut through the portal bifurcation allows the identification of the portal branches to segments III and IV to the left and the anterior and posterior divisions of the right branch of the portal vein (rbpv (AD) and rbpv (PD) to the right). The right hepatic vein (rhv) situated between the two divisions of the right branch of the portal vein and the middle hepatic vein (mhv) separating the right and left livers are both easily identified.

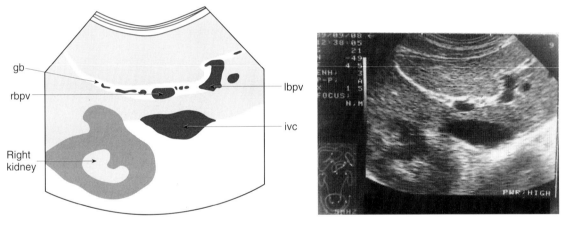

Fig. 13. Ultrasonography: segmental anatomy (segment IV). The flexibility of ultrasonography over both CT and MRI allows cuts to be taken in multiple planes giving a more precise composite picture of liver anatomy. In this cut, segment IV can be precisely delineated by the left branch of the portal vein (lbpv) to the left, the portal bifurcation and the right branch of the portal vein (rbpv) behind, and the gallbladder fossa (gb) to the right. ivc, inferior vena cava.

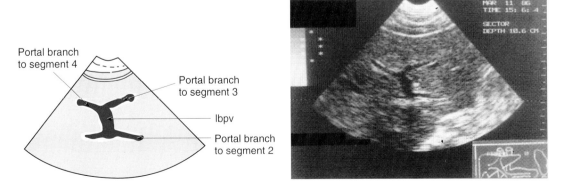

Fig. 14. Ultrasonography: segmental anatomy (segments II, III, and IV and their portal branches). This cut passes through the umbilical segment of the left branch of the portal vein (lbpv) and shows the portal branches to segments II, III, and IV.

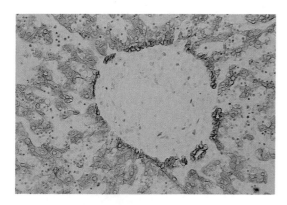

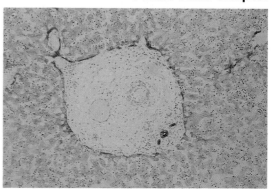

Plate 1. Embryonic ductal plate in liver tissue of a 16-week-old human fetus. The picture shows a branch of the portal vein with its accompanying mesenchyme, surrounded by the 'ductal plate'. The latter corresponds to a partly double layer of epithelial cells, which show smaller size and stronger cytokeratin expression than the surrounding epithelial cells (primitive hepatocyte precursor cells). A more dilated lumen (a tubule) develops in some segments of the ductal plate (between 3 and 4 o'clock, and at 5 o'clock).

Plate 2. Remodelling of ductal plate in liver tissue of a 25-week-old human fetus. A cross-sectioned primitive portal tract is shown, surrounded by the ductal plate which is easily recognized by its stronger cytokeratin expression (brown stain). At 5 o'clock, a tubular duct becomes detached from the ductal plate and is gradually incorporated into the portal mesenchyme, which shows a higher cellularity in that area. (Immunoperoxidase stain with anticytokeratin antibody CAM 5.2, staining cytokeratins 8, 18, and 19. Nuclear counterstain with haematoxylin, × 32.)

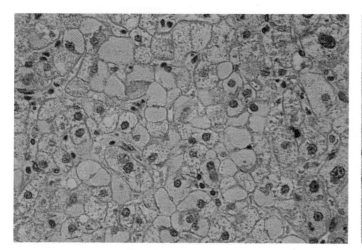

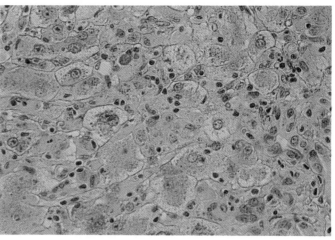

Plate 1. Liver biopsy from a patient with chronic hepatitis B. Numerous ground-glass hepatocytes with homogeneous, pale pink cytoplasm can be seen (haematoxylin and eosin × 65).

Plate 2. Liver biopsy from a patient with acute hepatitis B, characterized by liver cell pleomorphism and parenchymal inflammation. Pleomorphism of hepatocytes is reflected in unequal size and staining quality. Ballooned hepatocytes appear swollen and pale, especially in the peripheral part of their cytoplasm. Two small eosinophilic apoptotic cell fragments lie close to lymphocytes (haematoxylin and eosin × 104).

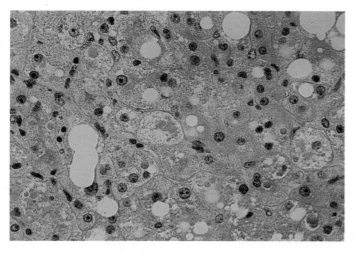

Plate 3. Liver biopsy from a patient with alcoholic liver disease. The picture shows some steatosis vacuoles, two pale, swollen hepatocytes containing an irregularly shaped Mallory body, and several parenchymal cells with one or more round, eosinophilic inclusions: megamitochondria (haematoxylin and eosin × 104).

Plates from Chapter 3.1

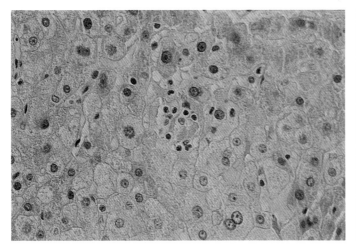

Plate 4. Liver biopsy from a patient with chronic persistent hepatitis B. Small focus of focal (or 'spotty') necrosis, with accumulation of lymphocytes and mononuclear cells around a dying liver cell, of which only two small eosinophilic fragments (apoptotic bodies) are recognizable (haematoxylin and eosin × 104).

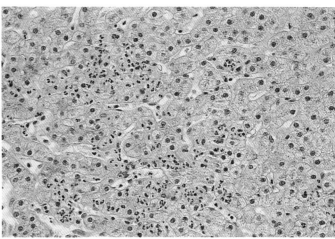

Plate 5. Surgical liver biopsy. 'Surgical necroses' are represented by clusters of accumulating polymorphonuclear neutrophils (haematoxylin and eosin × 65).

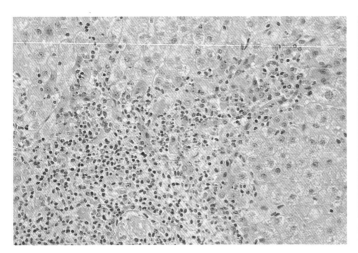

Plate 6. Liver biopsy from a patient with chronic active hepatitis B, characterized by piecemeal necrosis. The portal tract (lower left corner) shows dense mononuclear cell infiltration, which extends into the surrounding parenchyma, creating an irregular connective tissue–parenchymal interphase. A longer extension (up to right upper corner) represents an early stage of active septum formation (haematoxylin and eosin × 65).

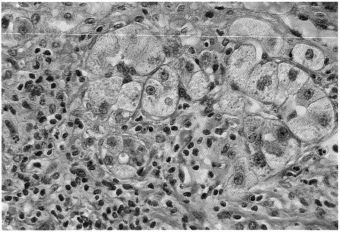

Plate 7. Liver biopsy from a patient with post-hepatitic cirrhosis. Hepatitic liver cell rosettes represent small groups of sequestrated hepatocytes, surrounded by fibrosis and inflammatory infiltration (Masson's trichrome (collagen appears blue) × 104).

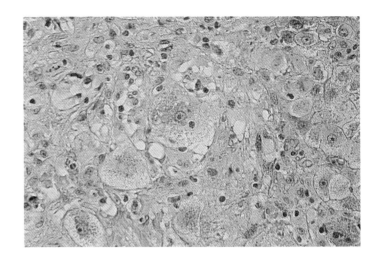

Plate 8. Liver biopsy from a patient with acute hepatitis B. The picture shows liver cell pleomorphism and ballooning, and interrupted continuity of liver cell plates. Note the presence (centre) of a lymphocyte, surrounded by a narrow clear halo, in the cytoplasm of a ballooned hepatocyte: emperipolesis (haematoxylin and eosin × 104).

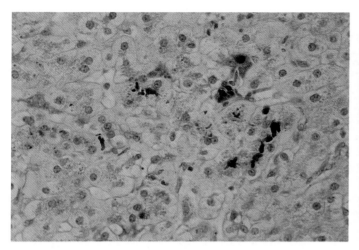

Plate 9. Liver biopsy from an infant with biliary atresia. The picture shows bilirubin granules in a couple of hepatocytes (hepatocellular bilirubinostasis), coarse bilirubin-stained casts in dilated canaliculi (canalicular bilirubinostasis), and coarse bilirubin deposits in hypertrophic, red-stained (PAS-positive) Kupffer (Kupffer cell bilirubinostasis) (PAS-Schiff after diastase digestion (PAS-D), × 104).

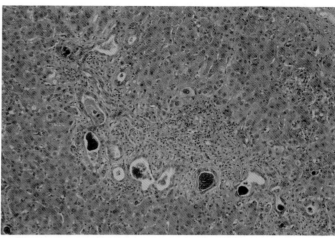

Plate 10. Liver biopsy from a severely jaundiced patient with monilia sepsis. The picture shows an obliquely cut portal tract, extending from the upper left to lower right corner. The upper and lower border is lined by a large number of extremely dilated ductules containing bile concrements in varying degree of inspissation (ductular bilirubinostasis) (haematoxylin and eosin × 26).

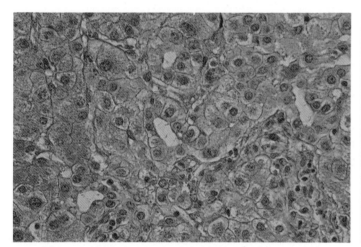

Plate 11. Liver biopsy from a 9-year-old child with incomplete obstruction of the common bile duct by annular pancreas. Chronic cholestasis is reflected in the appearance of cholestatic liver cell rosettes: groups of hepatocytes arranged around a central lumen. In this instance, there are no obvious bile concrements in the lumina (haematoxylin and eosin × 104).

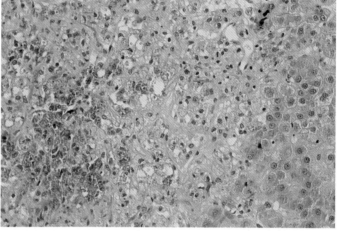

Plate 12. Liver biopsy from a patient with long-standing extrahepatic bile-duct obstruction. The picture shows part of a large paraportal bile infarct (compare with the appearance of relatively normal parenchyma on the right side). The central part of the necrotizing area (left side of picture) is most heavily impregnated with bilirubin pigment (haematoxylin and eosin × 65).

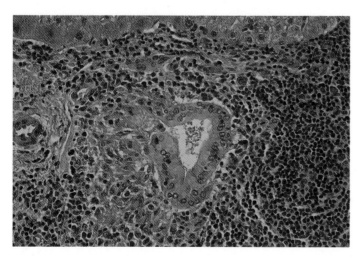

Plate 13. Liver biopsy from a patient with primary biliary cirrhosis. The pictures shows a cross-sectioned interlobular bile duct, lying amidst a densely lymphoplasmocytic infiltrate. Note the focal rupture of the bile-duct lining (near 10'clock) and the development of an epithelioid granuloma on the ruptured side of the duct (haematoxylin and eosin × 65).

Plates from Chapter 3.1

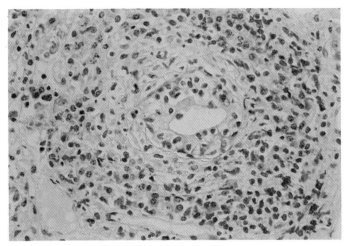

Plate 14. Liver biopsy from a patient with chronic active hepatitis. The picture shows a cross-sectioned interlobular bile duct, in a portal tract with dense infiltration by lymphocytes and plasma cells. The bile-duct lining cells appear swollen and multilayered, and are infiltrated by lymphocytes (haematoxylin and eosin × 104).

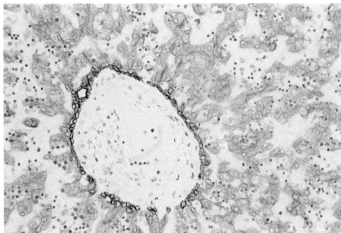

Plate 15. Liver specimen from a 16-week-old human fetus. The picture shows a portal vein branch surrounded with mesenchyme. Adjacent to the latter lies a partly double layer of smaller and darker stainng cells (the ductal plate). A tubular lumen has formed in one of the double layered segments (upper left). The primitive hepatocytes are weakly stained, with stronger positivity near the cell periphery. Interspersed haematopoietic cells are keratin negative (immunoperoxidase stain for cytokeratins (antibody CAM 5.2, which stains cytokeratins nos. 8,18, and 19): counterstain with Harris haematoxylin × 65).

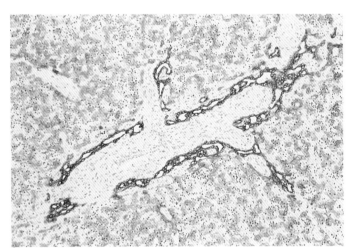

Plate 16. Liver specimen from a 20-week-old human fetus with Meckel syndrome. The picture shows a portal vein with two short side branches surrounded with mesenchyme. Adjacent to the latter lies a double layer of small, darkly-staining cells which form numerous cross-sectioned tubular structures. Persistence of these structures indicates lack of remodelling of the ductal plate, i.e. the ductal plate malformation. The primitive hepatocytes are weakly stained, with stronger positivity near the cell periphery. Interspersed haematopoietic cells are negative for keratin (immunoperoxidase stain for cytokeratins (antibody CAM 5.2, which stains cytokeratins nos. 8,18, and 19): counterstain with Harris haematoxylin, × 65).

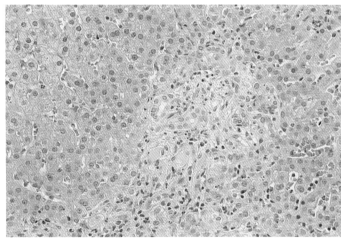

Plate 17. Liver biopsy from a patient with primary sclerosing cholangitis. The portal tract in the centre appears oedematous; an increased number of ductular profiles can be seen extending into the surrounding parenchyma, with a sprinkling of polymorphonuclear and mononuclear inflammatory cells (cholangiolitis) (haematoxylin and eosin × 65).

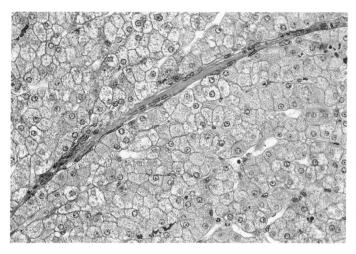

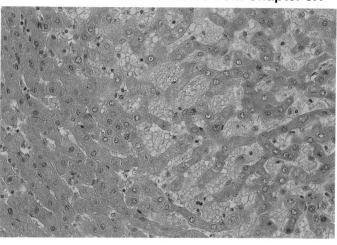

Plate 18. Liver biopsy from a patient with inactive macronodular cirrhosis. A passive septum appears as a sharply delineated blue-stained line. Note the presence of vessels and the absence of inflammatory cells in the septum. The nodular parenchyma appears hyperplastic, with plates of thickness of two or more cells (Masson's trichrome stain × 65).

Plate 19. Liver biopsy from a patient with venous outflow block (heart decompensation). Note the dilatation of the sinusoids, engorged with erythrocytes, and the thinning of the liver cell plates in acinar zone 3 (right side of picture) (haematoxylin and eosin × 65).

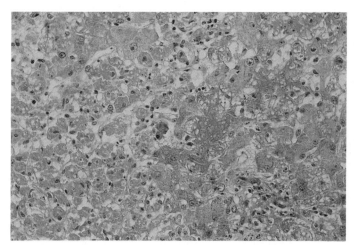

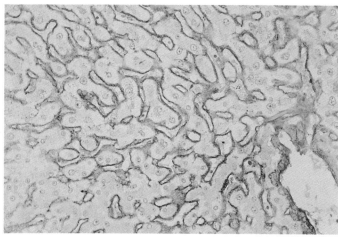

Plate 20. Liver biopsy from a pregnant patient with eclampsia. A small portal tract is located near the lower right corner. Several paraportal sinusoids are blocked with pink fibrin clots (centre and upper right). Note the early stage of ischaemic necrosis of parts of the parenchyma (left side), with increased eosinophilia of the cytoplasm and pyknosis of the nuclei (haematoxylin and eosin × 65).

Plate 21. Liver biopsy from a patient with light chain deposit disease. A terminal hepatic venule (centre vein) is located in the lower right corner. The Disse space between sinusoidal lumina and liver cell plates contains material which is immunoreactive for kappa light chains of immunoglobulin (immunoperoxidase stain for kappa light chains: counterstain of nuclei with haematoxylin and eosin × 65).

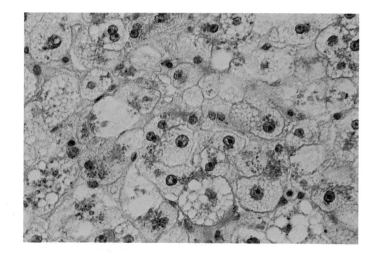

Plate 22. Liver biopsy from a patient with tetracycline intoxication. The picture shows part of the parenchyma, characterized by small droplet steatosis. The hepatocytes contain numerous small fat droplets, and retain their nucleus in central poition. Granular bilirubin pigment also accumulates between the fat vacuoles (hepatocellular bilirubinostasis) (haematoxylin and eosin × 104).

Plates from Chapter 3.1

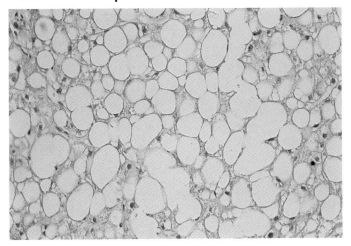

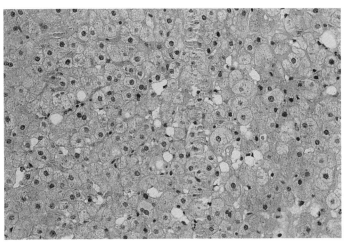

Plate 23. Liver biopsy from a patient with alcohol abuse. Most hepatocytes contain single, large fat vacuoles, pushing the nucleus to the periphery of the cell. Some adjacent vacuoles fuse to larger 'fatty cysts' (haematoxylin and eosin × 65).

Plate 24. Liver biopsy from a patient with vitamin A intoxication. Numerous clear spaces occur between the hepatocytes: they correspond to hyperplastic Ito cells (so-called fat storing cells); they contain fat droplets in their cytoplasm which indent the contour of their nucleus (haematoxylin and eosin × 65).

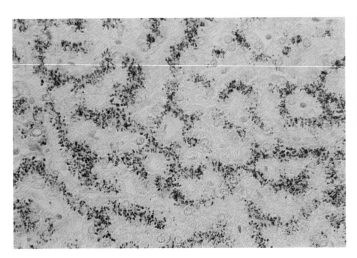

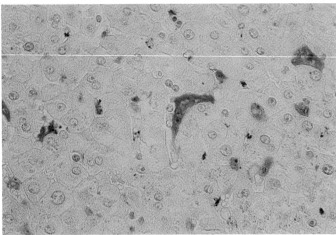

Plate 25. Liver biopsy from a patient with idiopathic (genetic) haemochromatosis. Blue-stained haemosiderin granules accumulate in the pericanalicular region of the hepatocytes (which is a typical localization of lysosomes) (Prussian blue stain for iron; neutral red counterstain, × 104).

Plate 26. Liver biopsy from a patient under chemotherapy for leukaemia. Reticulendothelial siderosis: blue-stained haemosiderin granules accumulate in hyperplastic Kupffer cells; the parenchymal cells are negative (Prussian blue stain for iron; neutral red counterstain, × 104).

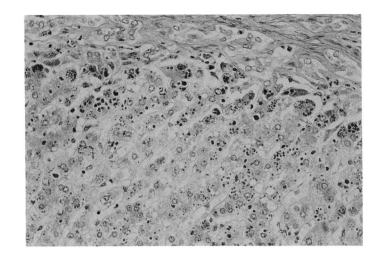

Plate 27. Liver biopsy from a patient with liver cirrhosis and α_1-antitryspsin deficiency. Part of a cirrhotic nodule is shown; red-stained (PAS-positive) inclusions of variable size are present in hepatocytes, especially in the nodular periphery near a connective tissue septum (upper part) (periodic acid-Schiff after diastase digestion (PAS-D), × 65).

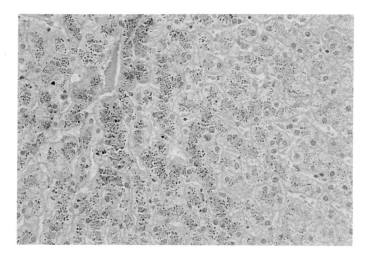

Plate 28. Liver biopsy from a patient with Dubin-Johnson syndrome. A terminal hepatic venule (central vein) is located near the upper left corner. The hepatocytes contain numerous brown pigment granules, especially in acinar zone 3 (haematoxylin and eosin × 65).

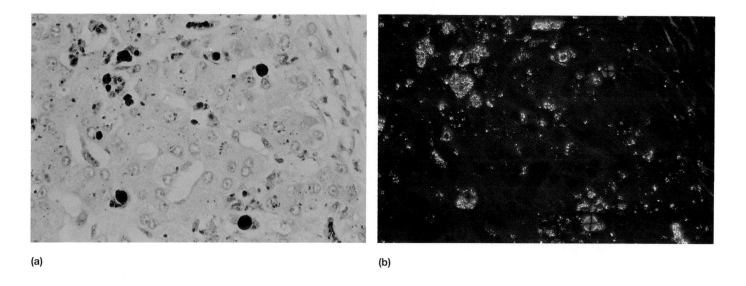

(a) (b)

Plate 29. Liver specimen from a patient with erythropoietic protoporphyria. Brown-black deposits of variable size are seen in hepatocytes, canaliculi, and hyperplastic Kupffer cells. (a) Haematoxylin and eosin, × 104. (b) The same area under polarized light: the deposits show birefringence, in Maltese cross configuration in the larger deposits. (Specimen by courtesy of Dr B. Portmann, London.)

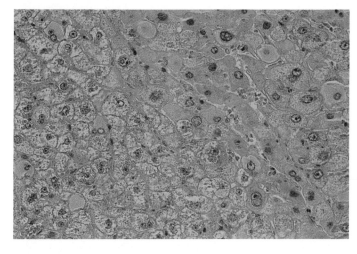

Plate 30. Liver biopsy from a patient with hepatitis B virus positive liver cirrhosis. The upper right half of the picture shows hepatocytes with enlarged cytoplasmic and nuclear size (dysplastic cells). Ground-glass change of the cytoplasm is seen in some of the dysplastic and non-dysplastic cells (haematoxylin and eosin × 104).

Plates from Section 4

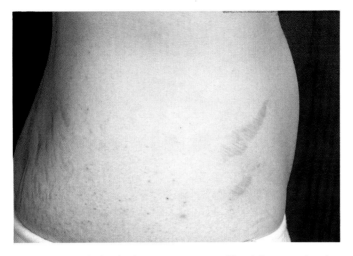

Plate 1. Abdominal striae in a young woman with autoimmune chronic active hepatitis.

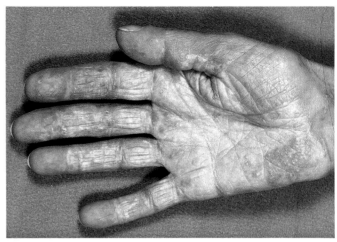

Plate 2. Palmar xanthomas in a patient with long-standing biliary obstruction due to primary biliary cirrhosis.

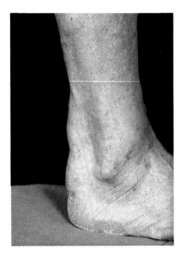

Plate 3. A tendon xanthoma in a patient with primary biliary cirrhosis.

Plate 4. A classical spider naevus in a patient with alcoholic cirrhosis.

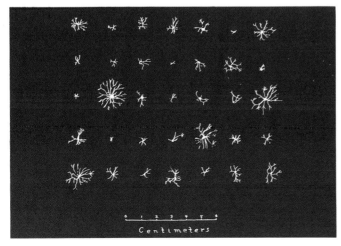

Plate 5. This figure, from Bean's classic paper (Medicine, 1945; 24: 243), illustrates the wide variation that can be seen in the appearance of 'spider naevi'.

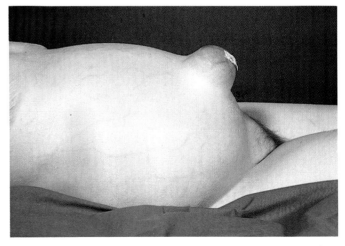

Plate 6. Gross ascites. Note the unusually large distance between the xiphisternum and the umbilicus compared with the distance between the umbilicus and the symphysis pubis.

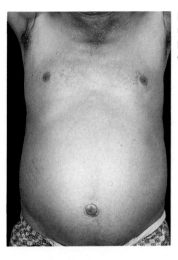

Plate 7. Abdominal collaterals, above and below the umbilicus, which have their origin in the umbilical or para-umbilical veins. They become obvious at some distance from the umbilicus.

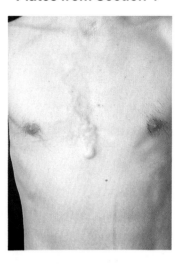

Plate 8. Upper abdominal collaterals, close to the midline, originating in para-umbilical veins, via small veins which penetrate the rectus sheath to reach the surface.

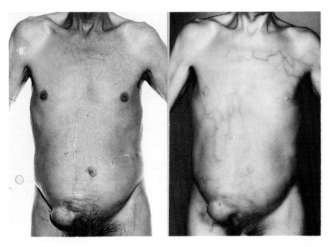

Plate 9. Abdominal collaterals appearing around a scar resulting from previous abdominal surgery, presumably due to adhesions between the viscera and the abdominal wall.

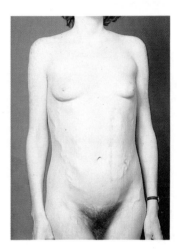

Plate 10. Prominent abdominal wall veins with inferior vena caval obstruction. The blood runs upwards even over the lower abdomen, and the veins are usually most prominent at the sides of the abdomen.

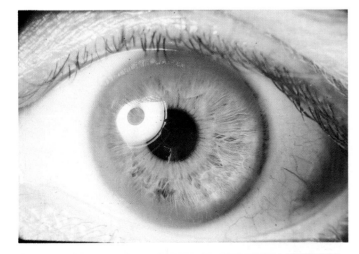

Plate 11. A Kayser–Fleischer ring. It is easy to see in this patient because of the pale iris.

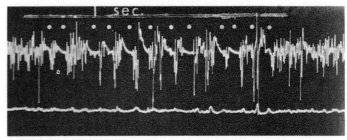

Plate 12. An EMG from a patient with hepatic encephalopathy. Asterixis occurred when longer periods of electrical silence coincided in different muscles (from Leavitt, ArchNeurol, 1964; 10:360).

Plates from Chapter 5.4.2

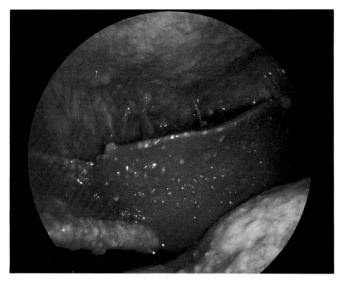

Plate 1. Peritoneal tuberculosis. The whitish nodules are present all over the peritoneal surface (parietal, hepatic, and intestinal). The ascitic fluid is clear and pale yellow.

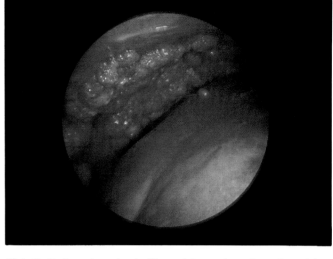

Plate 2. Peritoneal carcinosis. The nodules are irregular, red-greyish, and bigger than tubercula. The picture is strongly suggestive of the diagnosis. Often only an adequate biopsy can distinguish the real nature of the lesion.

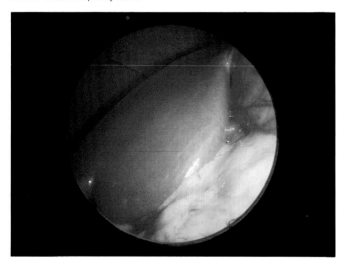

Plate 3. The normal liver (right lobe). The margin is smooth. The surface is regular and lucent with a red-purple colour.

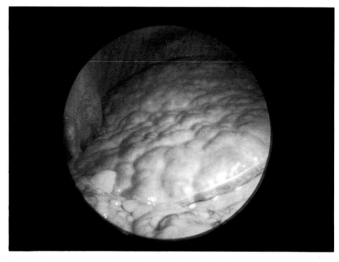

Plate 4. Macronodular cirrhosis (left lobe). The liver is large, with a thick margin, irregular surface, and evident multiple nodules.

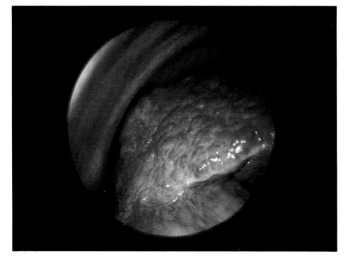

Plate 5. Secondary neoplasm. Typical volcano-like lesion with depressed central zone, surrounded by an hyperaemic halo.

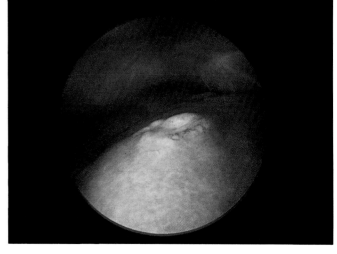

Plate 6. Carcinoma in cirrhosis. The tumour is emerging as a grey-reddish lesion on the convex surface of the right cirrhotic liver lobe.

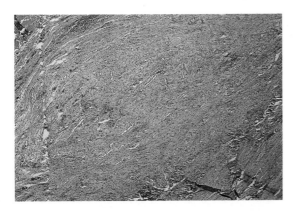

Plate 1. Atresia of extrapatic bile ducts. Fibrous remnant 'Gautier type 1'. Cross-section through fibrous remnant of common hepatic duct which is completely obliterated and reduced to a fibrous cord (haematoxylin and eosin, × 12).

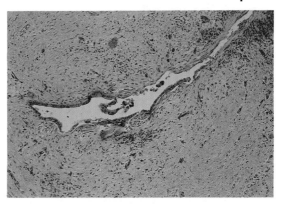

Plate 2. Atresia of extrahepatic bile ducts. Fibrous remnant 'Gautier type 3'. Cross-section through fibrous remnant of hepatic duct. The duct shows partially desquamated and damaged epithelial lining, surrounded by fibrosis and mild inflammatory infiltration (haematoxylin and eosin, × 32).

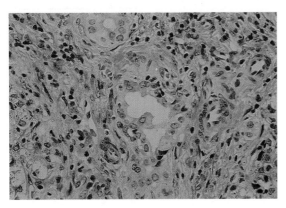

Plate 3. Atresia of extrahepatic bile ducts. Detail from liver biopsy of a baby with EHBDA, showing branches of hepatic artery and interlobular (portal) bile ducts. The duct in the centre shows irregularity and necrobiosis of its lining epithelium. There is mild inflammatory infiltration in the portal connective tissue (haematoxylin and eosin, × 128).

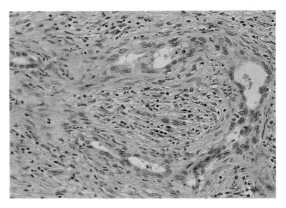

Plate 4. Atresia of extrahepatic bile ducts. Detail from liver biopsy of a 60-day-old baby with EHBDA. The picture shows a portal tract, with obliterating portal vein in the centre, and sprinkling by inflammatory cells. The bile ducts lie in an interrupted circle, corresponding to a partially remodelled ductal plate configuration. The epithelial line of thes ductal plate shows segments of flattening and involution (haematoxylin and eosin, × 80).

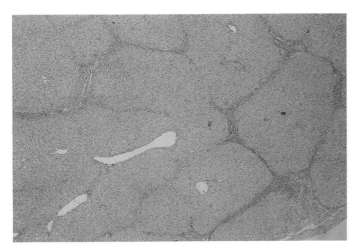

Plate 5. Atresia of extrahepatic bile ducts. Liver biopsy from a patient who is clinically well and jaundice free, 4.5 years after successful hepatic portoenterostomy. The main lesion consists of the development of some periportal fibrosis and portal–portal septa, resembling normal pig's liver (haematoxylin and eosin, × 12).

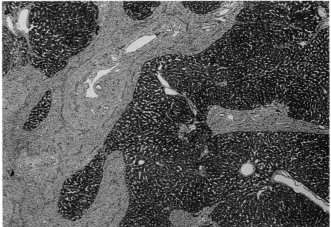

Plate 6. Atresia of extrahepatic bile ducts. Liver biopsy from a patient who is clinically well and jaundice free, 4 years after successful hepatic portoenterostomy. The lesion resembles congenital hepatic fibrosis, with broad porto–portal fibrous connections, but basically preserved lobular architecture. The broad fibrous septa carry excessive numbers of bile-duct structures, many of which appear in circular ductal plate configuration (Masson's trichrome stain (connective tissue in green), × 12).

Plates from Chapter 11.1

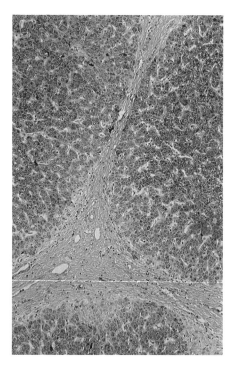

Plate 7. Atresia of extrahepatic bile ducts. Liver biopsy from a patient who is clinically well and jaundice free, 4 years after successful hepatic portoenterostomy. The liver shows advanced biliary fibrosis, with porto-portal fibrous septa. Note absence of portal bile ducts, hypoplastic size of portal veins, and occasional focus of ductular reaction (middle right) (Masson's trichrome stain (connective tissue in green), × 32).

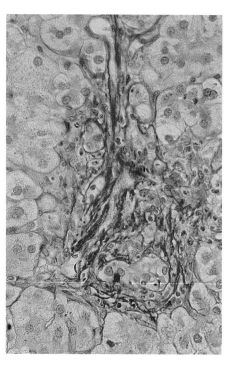

Plate 8. Syndromatic paucity of interlobular bile ducts (Alagille syndrome). Liver biopsy from a 3-month-old baby. Several portal tracts in this biopsy do not contain an interlobular bile duct. The remaining ducts show irregularity and vacuolization of the epithelium and inflammatory infiltration (Sirius red stain (collagen appears in red), × 128).

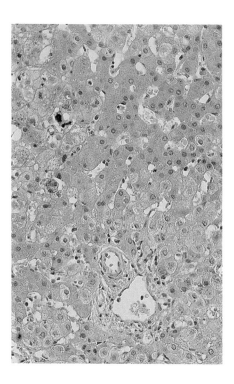

Plate 9. Paucity of interlobular bile ducts. Liver biopsy from a 73-day-old baby. Overview of portal tract (bottom) and parenchyma. The portal tract carries no interlobular bile duct, but is virtually free of inflammatory infiltration and ductular reaction. Bile plugs (bilirubinostasis) appear in the parenchyma (haematoxylin and eosin, × 80).

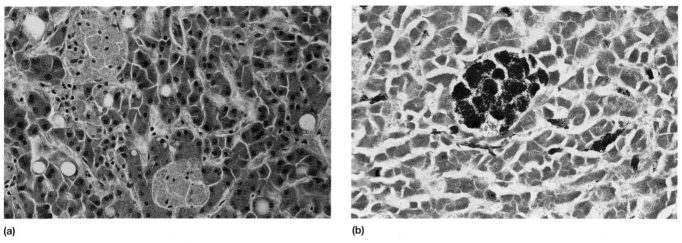

Plate 1. *Mycobacterium avium-intracellulare* complex infection. (a) Discrete, non-necrotic aggregates of unactivated macrophages in the sinusoids. The haematoxyphilic cytoplasm results from the tightly packed mycobacteria (haematoxylin and eosin). (b) The same specimen stained by the Ziehl–Neilsen method showing large numbers of intracellular acid-fast bacilli. (By courtesy of Professor S. Lucas, UMDS Department of Histopathology, London, UK.)

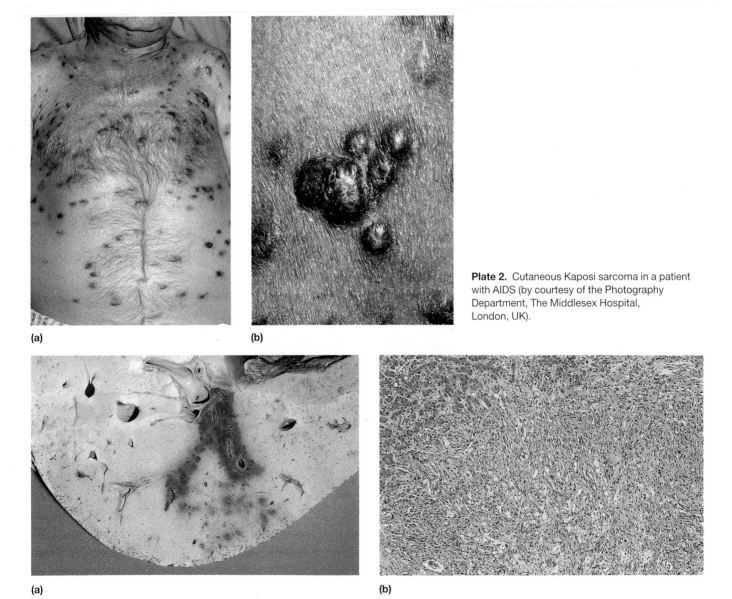

Plate 2. Cutaneous Kaposi sarcoma in a patient with AIDS (by courtesy of the Photography Department, The Middlesex Hospital, London, UK).

Plate 3. Kaposi sarcoma in the liver. (a) Purplish lesion infiltrating the portal tracts and spreading into the parenchyma (fixed liver). (b) Interlacing bands of Kaposi spindle cells infiltrating a portal tract and extending into the parenchyma (haematoxylin and eosin) (by courtesy of Professor S. Lucas, UMDS Department of Histopathology, London, UK).

Plates from Chapter 14.1

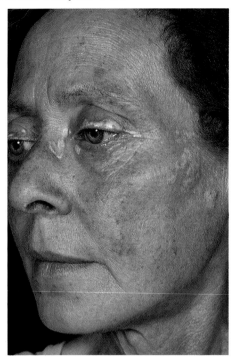

Plate 1. A patient with advanced primary biliary cirrhosis shows pigmentation, jaundice, and xanthelasma.

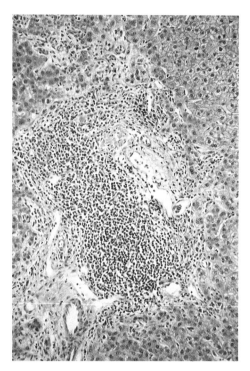

Plate 2. Primary biliary cirrhosis (later stage) shows severe portal inflammation. Portal vein tributaries and hepatic artery branches can be identified but interlobular bile ducts are absent (stained haematoxylin-eosin).

Plates from Chapter 23.6

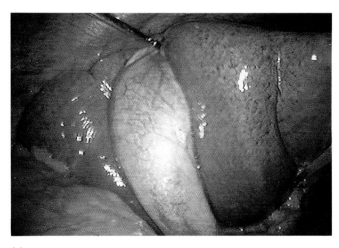

(a)

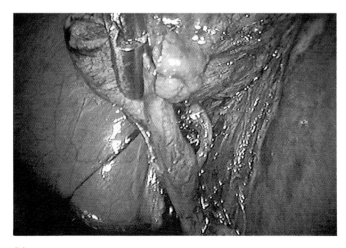

(b)

Plate 1. (a) Appearance of gallbladder and liver at the time of laparoscopy. (b) Cystic duct and artery after dissection during laparoscopic cholecystectomy.

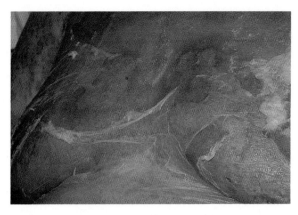

Plate 1. Toxic epidermal necrolysis. There is a background erythema with peeling of the dead epidermis leaving raw denuded dermis.

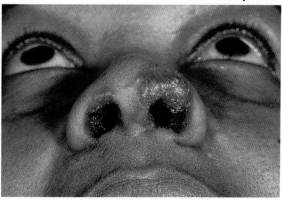

Plate 3. Cutaneous sarcoidosis. Granulomatous papules and nodules on the ala margins and on the columella.

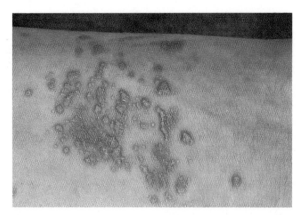

(a)

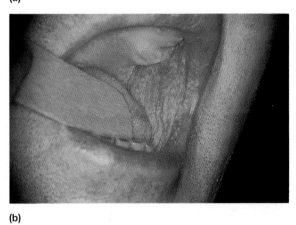

(b)

Plate 2. Lichen planus. Violaceous, polygonal, shiny, flat-topped papules on forearm, some showing evidence of koebnerization (linear lesions occurring at sites of scratching). White lace-like patterning on buccal mucosa, with some areas becoming confluent.

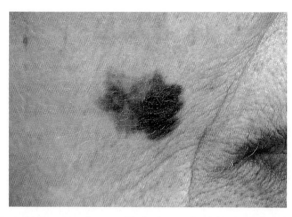

Plate 4. Malignant melanoma. The lesion on the right cheek is variably pigmented and has an irregular outline.

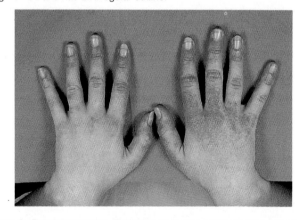

Plate 5. Dermatomyositis. Periungal erythema and papular erythema over the extensor surfaces of the fingers known as Gottron's sign.

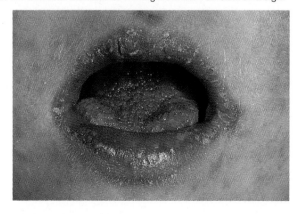

Plate 6. Kawasaki disease. Strawberry red tongue with scaling and fissuring of lips.

Plates from Chapter 25.6

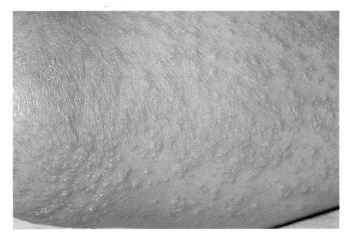

Plate 1. Giannotti–Crosti syndrome. Multiple flesh-coloured monomorphic papules on a thigh.

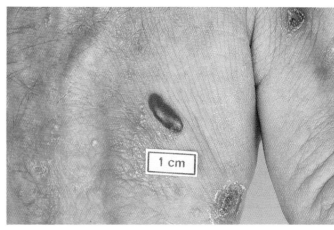

(a)

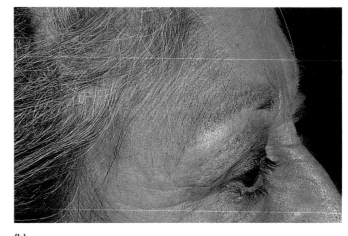

(b)

Plate 4. Porphyria cutanea tarda. Multiple milia (epidermal cysts) and a haemorrhagic blister on the dorsum of the right hand arising after minor trauma. Hypertrichosis of the temple.

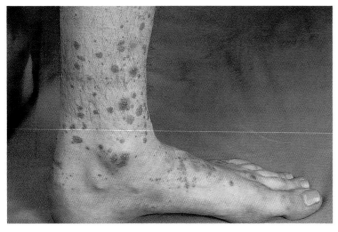

Plate 2. Cryoglobulinaemia. Purpuric areas at peripheral sites corresponding to areas of intravascular thrombosis.

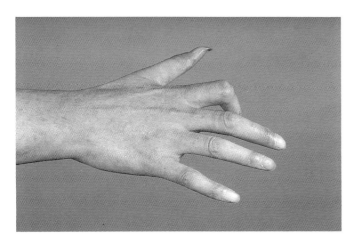

Plate 3. Systemic sclerosis. Sclerodactyly, fixed flexion deformity and loss of finger tip pulp.

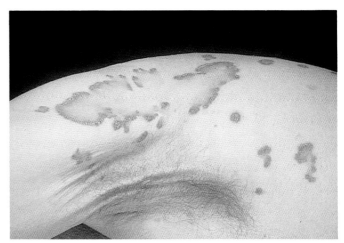

Plate 5. Pseudoxanthoma elasticum-like changes with hanging folds of skin in the axilla and lesions of elastosis perforans serpiginosa on the arm and chest wall characterized by scaly papules arranged in a serpiginous pattern.

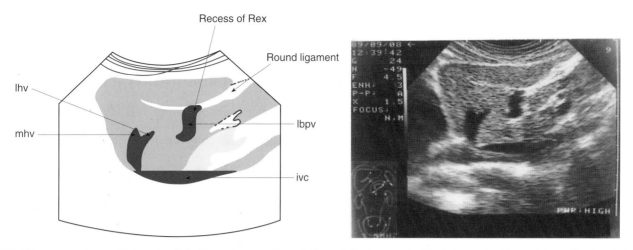

Fig. 15. Ultrasonography: sagittal section (left). This cut passes through the umbilical segment of the left branch of the portal vein (lbpv) and shows the recess of Rex (umbilical recess) and the round ligament (rl). The inferior vena cava (ivc) with the common entry of the middle (mhv) and left hepatic veins (lhv) is seen behind.

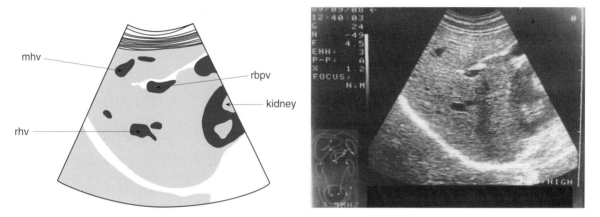

Fig. 16. Ultrasonography: sagittal section (right). This cut shows the right branch of the portal vein (rbpv) and the middle (mhv) and right hepatic veins (rhv) in cross-section.

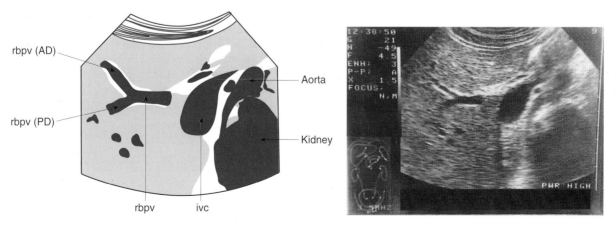

Fig. 17. Ultrasonography: transverse section. This cut passes through the right branch of the portal vein (rbpv) at the level of its bifurcation and clearly shows its anterior and posterior divisions (rbpv (AD) and rbpv (PD)). ivc, inferior vena cava.

lobe is an exception, as it drains directly into the retrohepatic inferior vena cava through several separate veins (spigelian veins).

Functional anatomy

The more recently described functional anatomy of liver can be superimposed upon this classical morphological anatomy. The history of the description of the functional anatomy of the liver starts with the work of Cantlie in 1898 and can be traced through the works of McIndoe and Counseller,[1] Ton That Tung,[2] Hjorstjo,[3] Goldsmith and Woodburne,[4] and Couinaud.[5] Although somewhat complex, the description of Couinaud is the most complete and has formed the basis of modern liver surgery.[6] It is based upon the division of the liver into eight segments following the distribution of the portal pedicles and the location of the hepatic veins (Fig. 3), which interdigitate in an alternation portal pedicle—hepatic vein—portal pedicle. The middle hepatic vein (or better, a plane passing through it, known by anatomists as the main portal scissura, or Cantlie's line) separates the whole liver into a *right liver* (different from the right '*lobe*' of the morphological anatomy) and a *left liver*. The right hepatic vein further separates the right liver into a *right posterior sector* and a *right anterior sector*, and the left hepatic vein separates the left liver into a *left anterior sector* and a *left posterior sector*. In the plane of the middle hepatic vein, the portal vein divides, one branch perfusing the right liver and the other the left liver. The right and left livers separated in this way are totally independent as regards their portal and arterial vascularization and biliary drainage. Each portal branch further divides to perfuse the two sectors of each liver, and in each sector it branches to perfuse two segments. Each segment has an independent supply from a portal pedicle and is therefore a separate functional unit with respect to its portal and arterial perfusion, and biliary drainage.

This gives the complete picture of the segmental anatomy of the liver (Fig. 4), as follows.

The right liver, formed by:

> the *right posterior sector*: segment 6 inferiorly and segment 7 superiorly;
> the *right anterior sector*: segment 5 inferiorly and segment 8 superiorly.

The left liver, formed by:

> the *left anterior sector*: segment 4 medially and segment 3 laterally, separated by
> the umbilical fissure;
> the *left posterior sector*, an exception to the rule 'one sector—two segments'

as it is composed only of segment 2.

The caudate lobe (segment 1) is a case apart, as its venous outflow is independent from the hepatic veins (as mentioned above), and it receives portal blood both from the right and the left branch of the portal vein. For the surgeon, it is defined as the liver tissue that lies between the main bifurcation of the portal vein and the retrohepatic vena cava. The autonomy of this 'third' liver is revealed in the Budd–Chiari syndrome where, as a result of thrombosis of all three main hepatic veins, the entire hepatic venous outflow passes through the caudate lobe, which then undergoes massive hypertrophy.

Radiological and surgical anatomy

Radiological anatomy (preoperative)

The modern radiological investigations, ultrasonography, CT scanning, and MRI are much better at identifying intrahepatic vascular rather than external morphological landmarks and are ideally suited to the study of the functional segmental anatomy of the liver. Lesions can therefore be accurately described in relation to anatomical structures (the hepatic veins and the branches of the portal vein).

Real-time ultrasonography allows a detailed examination of all the liver segments, aided by its ability to generate cuts in all planes. With this instrument, intraparenchymal lesions can be studied rapidly simply by choosing the appropriate plane. In contrast, the CT scan only allows cuts to be taken in a single plane. Each image, however, is a cut through the whole liver, which on occasions simplifies interpretation. Intravenous contrast is used to help identify vascular structures.

In theory, MRI can allow cuts to be taken in different planes. In practice, however, the axes of the vascular structures are unknown and axial cuts are used in sagittal or frontal planes. Unlike in CT scanning, vessels are easily visible with MRI without the need for intravenous contrast.

Figures 5 to 17 illustrate the use of these techniques in studying the liver.

Surgical anatomy (intraoperative ultrasonography)

Intraoperative ultrasonography allows the surgeon to identify accurately the vascular structures, and to adapt the 'ideal' segmental anatomy to the liver he or she is operating upon. This is important in two respects: first, lesions that have been described preoperatively in relation to the main intrahepatic vessels can be accurately localized by using the same landmarks even if they are not palpable or visible on the surface of the liver. Second, resections can be planned and performed respecting the segmental anatomy, allowing the surgeon to work on independent functional units (segments, sectors, and right and left livers). Better vascular control can therefore be achieved, minimizing blood loss, and uninvolved liver tissue can be spared. Although operative ultrasonography is clearly indispensable to accurately define sectors and segments, two landmarks in common between the morphological and the segmental anatomy can help the surgeon in two frequently performed procedures, right hepatectomy and left lobectomy, respectively: (i) the plane that joins the gallbladder fossa to the vena cava, which corresponds to the course of the middle hepatic vein, and to the division between the right and the left liver; (ii) the umbilical ligament, which separates segments 3 and 4—it is in fact embryologically a vessel going to the bifurcation of the portal branch to the left anterior sector; to the left it defines the left lobe according to the segmental anatomy (segments 2 and 3).

Operative ultrasonography resolves the problem of having only few external landmarks corresponding the segmental anatomy. This technique establishes an immediate correlation with preoperative radiological investigations, makes the liver transparent to the surgeon, and renders the segmental anatomy of each individual case immediately accessible.[7]

References

1. McIndoe AH and Counseller VX. A report of the bilaterality of the liver. *Archives of Surgery*, 1927; **15**: 589–96.

2. Thung TT. *Les résections majeures et mineures du foie*. Paris: Masson, 1979.

3. Hjorstojo CH. The topography of the intrahepatic duct systems. *Acta Anatomica*, 1931; **11**: 599–606.

4. Goldsmith NA and Woodburne RT. Surgical anatomy pertaining to liver resection. *Surgery, Gynecology, and Obstetrics*, 1957; **195**: 310–18.

5. Couinaud C. *Le foie. Etudes anatomiques et chirurgicales*. Paris: Masson, 1957.

6. Bismuth H. Surgical anatomy and anatomical surgery of the liver. *World Journal of Surgery*, 1982; **6**: 3–9.

7. Castaing D, Kustlinger F, Habib N, and Bismuth H. Intraoperative ultrasound of the liver: Methodology and anatomical results. *American Journal of Surgery*, 1985; **149**: 676–82.

1.2 Liver and biliary-tract histology

Paulette Bioulac-Sage, Brigitte Le Bail, and Charles Balabaud

General features

Liver and biliary-tract histology, the study of hepatic function, the relation between the structure and function of cells and their organelles and of the extracellular matrix have recently been reviewed in specialized textbooks on pathology,[1] biology and pathobiology,[2] and liver disease.

The liver is a voluminous organ (1200–1500 g) that is highly vascularized. It is surrounded by a thin capsule (Glisson's capsule) composed of collagen fibres, scattered fibroblasts, and small blood vessels. The capsule is thickest around the hilus (or porta hepatis) where blood vessels enter and bile ducts leave the liver. In the parenchyma the capsule merges with the connective tissue surrounding the portal tracts.

Between the incoming vessels of the portal tracts and the central veins lie the hepatic sinusoids, which allow exchange between blood and unicellular sheets of hepatocytes. In histological sections, portal tracts (which contain branches of the hepatic artery and portal vein, one or two bile ducts, lymphatics, nerves, a few lymphocytes, and mast cells in loose connective tissue), centrolobular veins (also called the terminal hepatic venule), and the lobular parenchyma are identified (Figs 1 and 2). The apparent structural unit of the liver is the lobule, a polyhedral prism (0.7 × 2 mm), the boundaries of that are limited by four to five portal triads prolonged by connective tissue septa. The centre of the lobule contains the centrolobular vein (Figs 1, 3). The lobular parenchyma represents approximately 93 per cent of the hepatic parenchyma, portal triads 3 per cent, and hepatic veins 4 per cent (Schroder, JHepatol, 1985; 1: 107).

Human liver biopsy material (needle or surgical) is usually fixed by immersion for a few hours in 10 per cent neutral formalin. For detailed study of the hepatic parenchyma and sinusoidal cells by electron microscopy (transmission and scanning), it is better to use *in situ* perfusion-fixation of the liver through the portal vein or the hepatic artery. For the localization of antigens (immuno-cytochemistry) or the performance of *in situ* hybridization, it is often necessary to use frozen material.

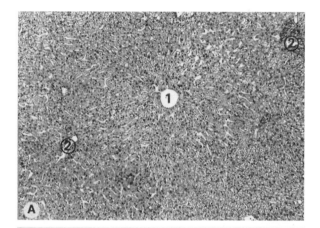

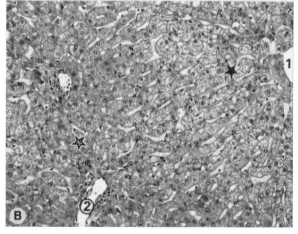

Fig. 1. Hepatic parenchyma: paraffin embedding (5 μm-thick section); haematein eosin saffron; (A) low (×50) and (B) high (×230) magnification. The classic lobule cannot easily be seen. Sinusoids lie, from portal tracts (2) to centrolobular veins (1), in between the unicellular sheets of hepatocytes. In medio- and centrolobular zones (black star), sinusoids are larger and radial; in the periportal zone (white star) they are narrower.

The functional unit of the liver

An adequate description of the liver unit should provide not only structural but also secretory and microcirculatory unity. The acinar organization (zone 1, periportal; 2, mediolobular; 3, centrolobular) based upon a combination of microanatomical, microcirculatory, and metabolic considerations described by Rappaport is now being replaced by the lobular organization proposed by Matsumoto and recently re-evaluated by Ekataksin and Wake.[6]

The architecture of hepatic lobulation is not uniform. A pentagonal lobule is the most typical, rather than the classic hexagonal lobule. In three dimensions the lobule can be schematically represented as a polyhedron with portal tracts in the corners. From the portal vein (in the portal tract) leave perpendicularly, at regular

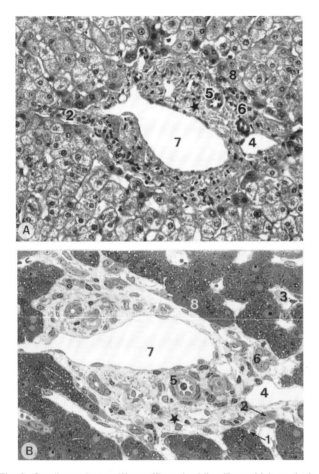

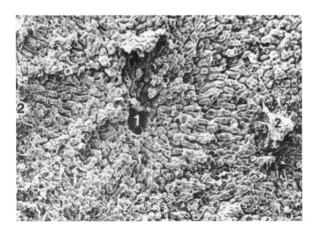

Fig. 2. Small portal tract: (A) paraffin embedding (5 μm-thick section); haematein eosin saffron, ×300; (B) Epon embedding (1 μm-thick section); toluidine blue, ×340. At the periphery of the portal tract several canals of Hering (1), cholangioles (2), and sinusoids (3) with or without Kupffer cells can be seen close to venules (4). In the portal tract, arterioles (5) are close to interlobular bile ducts (6), which are lined by a single layer of cuboidal epithelial cells; some inflammatory cells are present in the stroma (*). (7) portal vein; (8) hepatocytes forming the periportal limiting plate.

Fig. 3. Hepatic lobule: scanning electron microscopy, ×170. A centrolobular vein (1) is visible at the centre of the lobule limited by two portal tracts (2).

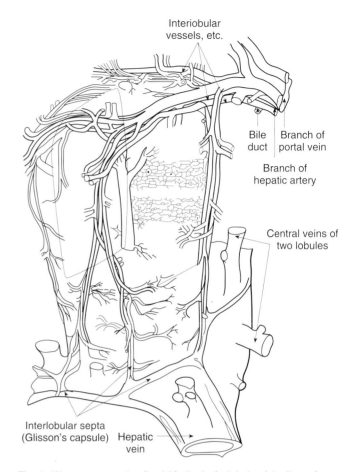

Fig. 4. Wax reconstruction (by A Vierling) of a lobule of the liver of a pig. A portion of the lobule has been cut away to show the centrolobular vein and sinusoids. (After Brauss). (From Bloom and Fawcett. *A textbook of histology*, 1975:689, with permission).

intervals, terminal portal veins that run in the septa (Fig. 4). They are accompanied by arterioles and bile ductules. In man the septa (and the vessels) are not visible by light microscopy. The hepatic lobule is divisible into elementary sectors, called hepatic microcirculatory subunits, of conical shape in three dimensions (Fig. 5). The inlet venules given off at frequent intervals from the portal vein in the portal tracts and the terminal portal venules along the septa penetrate the hepatic microcirculatory subunit and branch out laterally in several sinusoids. This architecture provides the venous system with a resistive site at the inlet venule, followed immediately by an abrupt decrease of vascular resistance, and explains the steep pressure drop between the portal venule and central vein. In the portal zone, sinusoids are interconnected to one another and become radial towards the central vein. Lamers (Hepatol, 1989; 10: 72) proposed a concept of lobular metabolism in which the pericentral zone is circular and discrete whereas the periportal zone is reticular. Seen three-dimensionally the structure of the pericentral zone follows the branching pattern of the terminal hepatic vein, whereas that of the periportal zone envelopes the pericentral compartment, forming an extensive network. In sinusoids, flow is unidirectional, from periportal to centrolobular hepatocytes. The concept of functional heterogeneity has been in part based on this organization.[7]

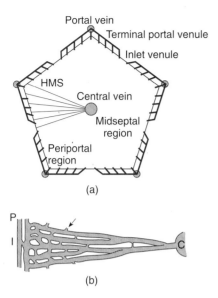

(a)

(b)

Fig. 5. (a) Two-dimensional view of a pentagonal hepatic lobule. In each corner there is a portal tract. On each side of the lobule, in the septum, there are two opposite-running terminal portal venules (accompanied by an arterial branch and a ductule). The hepatic lobule is divisible into elementary sectors, the hepatic microcirculatory subunits fed by the inlet venules derived from the portal vein (in the portal tract) and the terminal portal venules. Compared to the periportal region, the mid-septal region is remote from the portal supply. (From ref. 6, with permission). (b) A typical hepatic microcirculatory subunit shaped like a cone with a portal inlet venule (I) at the base, where one afferent vessel spreads (*) into many sinusoids. The cross-connecting sinusoids (arrows) reduce, or drop-out, while approaching the centrolobular vein (C). (From ref. 6, with permission).

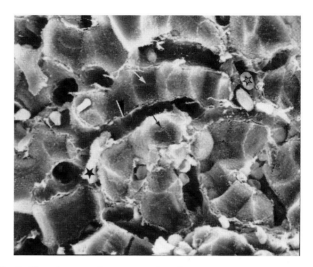

Fig. 6. Hepatic parenchyma: scanning electron microscopy, × 1300. Unicellular sheets of hepatocytes are separated by sinusoids from different planes of sectioning. The block often breaks in between the lateral surface of hepatocytes, allowing visualization of the biliary hemicanaliculi (arrow). In sinusoids, some Kupffer cells (black star), and red blood cells (white star) can be seen. The Disse space can also be identified (arrow head).

The adult human liver contains stem cells located near the junction between hepatocytes and the smallest segments of the biliary tree (ref. 2, p. 1501). It also harbours haemopoietic stem cells but their location has not yet been identified (Taniguchi, NatureMed, 1996; 2: 198).

Hepatocytes

Hepatocytes are arranged in unicellular plates or laminae (Remak's plates). These hepatic laminae branch, and anastomose with one another, to form a complicated walling system, the hepatic muralium, a maze-like arrangement of partitions between which the sinusoids interweave and interconnect in a continuous labyrinth, (Figs 3, 6). Hepatocytes surrounding the portal tract, which constitute an interface between the connective tissue of the tract and the hepatic parenchyma, form the limiting plate (Fig. 2).

The plates are composed of about 20 large, polyhedral epithelial cells, approximately 30 μm long and 20 μm wide. The mean volume density is 5000 μm³. These cells (100 billion) make up approximately 80 per cent of the cell population. The hepatocyte is limited by a membrane in which three domains can be distinguished.

The sinusoidal membrane (70 per cent of the total cell-surface area) is covered with microvilli (0.5 μm long) that increase the surface area sixfold. This membrane burrows in between hepatocytes, delimiting the interhepatocytic space (Figs 7 and 8). Exchange

of materials between the blood and hepatocytes (exo- and endocytosis) through the Disse space is a function solely of the sinusoidal plasma membrane.

The canalicular membrane is the biliary pole of the hepatocyte. It is an intercellular space, formed by the opposition of the edges of gutter-like hemicanals (15 per cent of the total cell-surface area) on the surfaces of neighbouring hepatocytes (Figs 6, 7, 8, and 9). The surface is covered by microvilli. The canalicular surface is isolated from the Disse space by tight junctions.

The lateral membrane (15 per cent of the cell surface area) is more or less straight, separated from the adjacent lateral membranes by an intercellular space of 15 nm. The junctional complexes—desmosomes, gap junctions, intermediate junctions (zonula adherens), and tight junctions—are special membrane differentiations that fix the liver cells together.

The nucleus is spherical and voluminous, occupying 5 to 10 per cent of the cell volume, with one or more prominent nucleoli and scattered chromatin. About 25 per cent of the cells are binucleate. There appears to be a clear correlation between nuclear size and ploidy. As many as 15 per cent can be tetraploid nuclei. The adult liver has a very low mitotic index, with estimates ranging from 2 mitoses per 1000 cells to 1 per 10 000 cells.

Light microscopy of the liver shows a pale-staining, eosinophilic cytoplasm containing granular clumps of basophilic material. This material corresponds to rough endoplasmic reticulum. Near the bile canaliculi, there are fine brown granules of lipofuschin pigment. These are more abundant with age, particularly in the centrolobular zone. A few hepatocytes may contain fat vacuoles. Histochemical procedures are essential to identify such as glycogen, haemosiderin, lipids. Electron microscopy is necessary to visualize organelles: there is an abundant rough and smooth endoplasmic reticulum, a Golgi apparatus close to the biliary pole, numerous mitochondria (1000–1500 per cell) and peroxisomes. The hepatocyte is rich in glycogen, the quantity depending on the time of the last meal. The

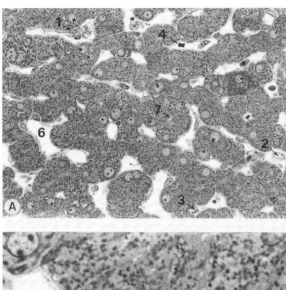

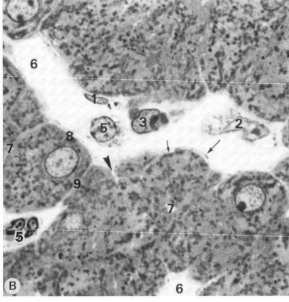

Fig. 7. Sinusoids and sheets of hepatocytes: Epon embedding (1 μm-thick section); toluidine blue (A) × 340; (B) × 1250. It is possible to identify the sinusoidal cells: endothelial cells with the cell body (1) and the barrier (large arrow), Kupffer cells (2) and stellate cells (3); blood cells, red (4) and white (5), in the sinusoidal lumen (6); the Disse space (small arrow) with the interhepatocytic recess (arrow head); bile canaliculi (7); the sinusoidal surface (8) and lateral (9) surface of hepatocytes.

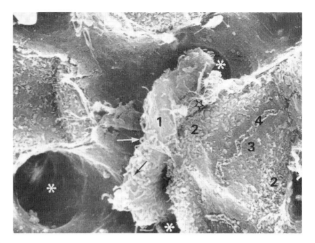

Fig. 8. Kupffer cells: scanning electron microscopy, × 4260. The Kupffer cell (1) with its filipodia (arrow) is located at the branching of several sinusoids (*). The different plasma membranes of the hepatocytes: the sinusoidal with their microvilli (2), the fairly smooth lateral (3) and canalicular (4) membranes are easily recognizable. It is not easy to differentiate collagen bundles from the perisinusoidal cell processes in the Disse space (star).

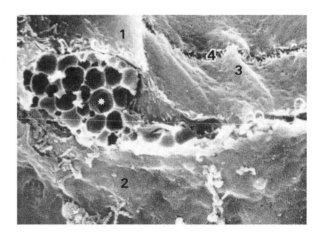

Fig. 9. Stellate cell: scanning electron microscopy, × 7400. The stellate cell in between the hepatocyte (1) and the endothelial barrier (2) contains numerous lipid droplets (star). (3) lateral membrane of hepatocyte; (4) biliary hemicanaliculus.

cytoskeleton of the cell comprises microfilaments, intermediate filaments, and microtubules, which correspond by immuno-cytochemistry to actin, cytokeratin, and tubulin.

The main morphometric data concerning organelles are presented on Fig. 10 (Roessner, ActaHepatoGastroenterol, 1978; 25: 119; Rohr, VirchArch, 1976; 371: 251). The whole cellular machinery performs many functions: uptake, transport, synthesis, biotransformation, degradation (proteins, lipids, carbohydrates, hormones, xenobiotics, bile).

Sinusoids

Sinusoids are special capillaries with (a) a fenestrated endothelial barrier, (b) resident macrophages (Kupffer cells) 'guarding' the entrance of sinusoids, (c) liver-associated lymphocytes, some of which are large, granular lymphocytes, and (d) stellate cells (considered as pericytes) that store vitamin A (Fig. 11(a)). Sinusoids have no genuine basement membrane: this facilitates exchange between incoming blood and hepatocytes through the Disse space, as well as immunological defence mechanisms.

In zone 1, sinusoids are tortuous, narrow, and anastomotic, but tend to become more parallel and larger in zone 3 (Figs 1(b), and 3). The mean diameter (between 7 and 15 μm) is occasionally less than the mean diameter of the red blood cells, which adapt their shape to size differences (Wisse, Hepatol, 1985; 5: 683). The diameter can increase if necessary (up to 180 μm). The mean length is 220 to 480 μm. The sinusoidal lumina occupy approximately 9 to 10 per cent of the lobular parenchyma (Blouin, JCB, 1977; 72: 441).

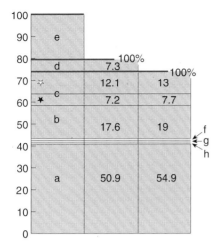

Fig. 10. Morphometric data of hepatocyte organelles. Volumetric composition of the liver expressed as a percentage of the lobular parenchyma (left column), an average hepatocyte (middle column) and hepatocytic cytoplasm (right column). (a) Hyaloplasm; (b) mitochondria; (c) endoplasmic reticulum, rough (white star), smooth (black star); (d) nucleus; (e) extrahepatocytic space (sinusoids and bile canaliculi); (f) lysosomes; (g) lipids; (h) peroxisomes. Lysosomes, lipids, and peroxisome volume density, expressed as percentage of the cytoplasm, are 2, 2.1, and 1.3, respectively.

Sinusoidal cells

These represent about 6 per cent of the lobular parenchyma (2.5, 2, and 1.4 per cent for endothelial, Kupffer, and stellate cells, respectively) and 26.5 per cent of all the plasma membranes of the liver.[8] Observation by light microscopy is difficult. Only transmission and scanning electron microscopy, and immuno-cytochemical methods, allow correct identification.[9]

Endothelial cells (Fig. 12)

These form the barrier of the sinusoid. Their main characteristics are: (a) very thin processes covering a large area (15 per cent of all the plasma membranes of the liver); (b) fenestrations with a mean diameter of 100 nm, grouped in clusters (sieve plates), which allow the passage of molecules of smaller diameters; (d) numerous pinocytotic vesicles, indicating a high endocytic capacity.[10] They show immunoreactivity with monoclonal antibody MS-1, and express the scavenger receptor, Fc IgG receptor, and also the CD4 molecule. In capillarized sinusoids, where sinusoidal endothelial cells have lost their fenestrations, there is a phenotypic shift toward that of vascular-type endothelium: expression of factor VIII-related antigen, *Ulex europaeus* lectin, CD34 molecule.

Kupffer cells

Attached over a (more or less) large area of the endothelial wall, these cells are located within the sinusoidal lumen (Figs 7 and 8). They are more numerous in zone 1 than in zone 3. They contain numerous lysosomes (almost one-quarter of all the lysosomes of the liver). Kupffer cells can be identified with monoclonal antibodies such as KP1 (CD68) (Fig. 13). They phagocytose many substances, such as latex particles, denatured albumin, bacteria, immune complexes. The extent to which Kupffer cells fail to take up colloids in patients with chronic hepatocellular diseases correlates best with indices of the magnitude of portal–systemic blood shunting. Upon stimulation by immunomodulators, Kupffer cells release mediators and cytotoxic agents.[10]

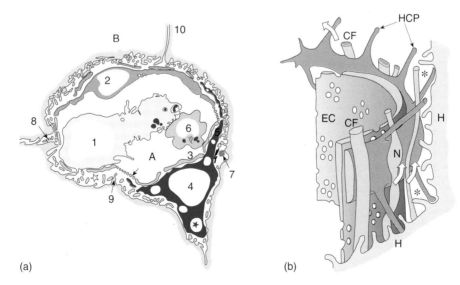

(a)   (b)

Fig. 11. Diagrammatic representation of sinusoids, sinusoidal cells, and Disse space. (a) All four sinusoidal cells are represented in this sinusoid (A) (it is exceptional to see all four, with their nuclei, in the same plane of section)—the Kupffer cell (1), the endothelial cell: cell body (2), processes (3) and fenestrations (arrow); the stellate cell (4) with its lipids (black star) and processes (5); the liver-associated lymphocytes (6). In the Disse space (white star) containing some collagen fibres (7), interhepatocytic recesses (8), sinusoidal membrane microvilli (9), and the lateral membrane (10) of the hepatocyte (B) can be seen. (b) Schema of the sinusoidal wall. Arrows indicate tunnels formed by the processes of the stellate cells and hepatocyte. CF, collagen fibres; H, hepatocyte; HCP, hepatocyte-contacting process of the stellate cell; SP, subendothelial process of the stellate cell; N, nerve fibre; * space of Disse. (From ref.12, with permission).

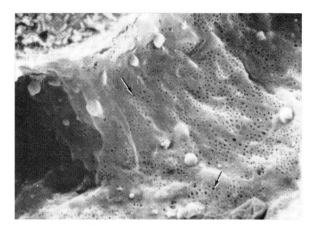

Fig. 12. Endothelial cell: scanning electron microscopy, × 13 440. The endothelial cell processes form the wall of the sinusoid. Fenestrations (arrow) are grouped in clusters, forming so-called sieve plates.

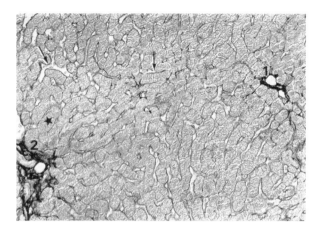

Fig. 14. Identification of the extracellular matrix: paraffin embedding (5 μm-thick section); Sirius red, × 130. This stain allows identification of the thin, perisinusoidal, matricial network (arrow) in between the unicellular, unstained sheets of hepatocytes (star), and of the fibrous tissue around the centrolobular vein (1) and the portal tract (2).

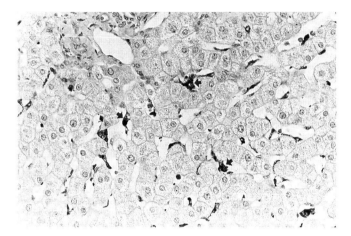

Fig. 13. Kupffer cell identification: paraffin embedding (5 μm-thick section); immunocytochemistry (KP1), × 330. Large Kupffer cells (arrow) are seen in this periportal area.

store vitamin A and participate in synthesis of the extracellular matrix. This latter function increases when they are activated and transformed into α-smooth muscle actin-positive cells.

The Disse space

This lies primarily between the stellate cell sheet and the sinusoidal membrane of the hepatocyte, and represents 2 to 4 per cent of the hepatic parenchyma.[13] The relatively low porosity of the endothelial barrier (9 per cent of the surface) is compensated for by the presence of a great number of hepatocytic microvilli in the Disse space, and particularly since the endothelial cell lacks a genuine basement membrane. In this space, which is not normally discernible in biopsy material by standard light microscopy, one can observe the different components of the extracellular matrix, which can be identified by immunocytochemistry:[14] these are different types of collagens (mainly type III but also type I and IV), proteoglycans, and fibronectin. The presence of laminin is much debated. This whole network can be visualized by silver or Sirius red staining (Fig. 14).The role of the extracellular matrix is complex: it serves to cement the cells, allows intercellular communication, and affects cellular differentiation.

Liver-associated lymphocytes

Far fewer in number (1:10 Kupffer cells), they comprise different types of lymphocytes among which are large, granular lymphocytes (pit cells).[11] They are resident luminal cells, in contact with Kupffer or endothelial cells. Liver-associated lymphocytes differ from peripheral blood lymphocytes (phenotype, cytotoxic activity). They play a role in defence against tumours and viruses.

Hepatic stellate cells

Also called perisinusoidal or Ito cells, they can be identified by: (a) their cell body, which is often located in an interhepatocytic recess and contains lipids (Fig. 9) including vitamin A in most (but 20 per cent of the cells do not contain lipids); (b) their long, thin, cytoplasmic processes, surrounding endothelial cell processes; and (c) their spines, which establish contact with hepatocyte microvilli.[13] This cell, which belongs to the myofibroblast family, can be identified immunocytochemically in rat liver by the presence of desmin, but this protein is not expressed (or only weakly) in man. No basement membrane surrounds the hepatic stellate cell. There are approximately 5 to 20 of these cells per 100 hepatocytes. They

Microcirculation

Blood flows unidirectionally in sinusoids from zone 1 to zone 3. Microcirculation through individual sinusoids is variable in the rat, [15] and might also be so in humans. This irregularity is linked to: (a) the presence of inlet, sinusoidal, and outlet sphincters composed of sinusoidal lining cells bulging into the lumen; (b) transient leucocyte plugging; (c) variations in the morphology of sinusoids in the different zones; (d) the contribution of arterial flow at the beginning of the sinusoid's pathway (Fig. 15) (Yamamoto, Hepatol, 1985; 5: 452).

The average velocity of erythrocyte flow in sinusoids ranges between 270 and 410 μm/s. There are considerable interactions between blood cells and the sinusoidal wall. Soft, fast-moving red blood cells could help fluid- or solid-phase droplets or particles to

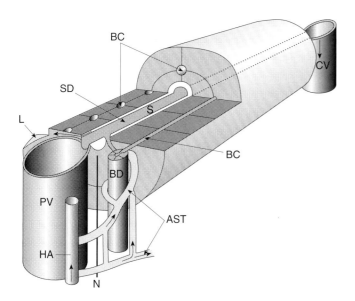

Fig. 15. Diagrammatic representation of the microcirculation and of biliary drainage in the lobule. PV, portal venule; HA, hepatic arteriole; BD, bile ductule; L, lymphatic; N, nerve; AST, arteriosinous twig; S, sinusoid; SD, space of Disse; BC, bile canaliculus; CV, central venule. Arrows indicate direction of flow. Note that the capillaries surrounding the bile duct constitute the peribiliary plexus. (From ref. 14, with permission).

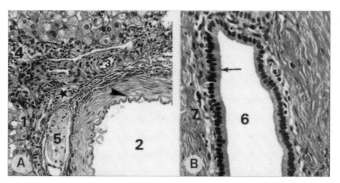

Fig. 16. Large portal tract (partial view): paraffin embedding (5 μm-thick section); haematein eosin saffron; A, ×115; B, ×170. (A) A nerve (5) can be seen inside the connective tissue, not far from the limiting plate of hepatocytes (1), a large artery (2), which is easily identifiable by its internal elastic lamina (arrowhead), an arteriole (3), and biliary ducts (4). (B) This large bile duct (6), which is surrounded by a thick fibrous envelope (7), is limited by a cylindrical epithelium (arrow).

penetrate into the Disse space (forced sieving). Compression of the Disse space by less plastic and larger cells such as white blood cells could displace fluids within this space in a downstream direction, promoting the transport of particles and fluids into and out of the space through the fenestrations (endothelial massage) (Wisse, Hepatol, 1985; 5: 683). Average blood pressure is about 4.8 mmHg in terminal portal branches, 30 to 35 mmHg in arterial blood, and 1.7 mmHg in collecting veins.[4]

Lymphatics (see also Chapter 2.2)

Lymph is collected in lymphatics present in portal triads. Liver lymph is first formed in the perisinusoidal Disse space. The fluid then enters the periportal tissue of the Mall space, which lies between the portal connective tissue and the limiting plate, and then the lymphatic capillaries. Lymph is then conveyed by increasingly large lymphatic vessels to the collecting vessels, which leave the liver at the hilus to reach the thoracic duct. The liver's capsule and stroma contain numerous lymphatic vessels, which form loose plexuses that connect at intervals with underlying lymphatic vessels.

Nerves (see also Chapter 2.6)

Extrinsic innervation of the liver is constituted by:

(a) efferent sympathetic nerve fibres (preganglionic splanchnic fibres and postganglionic fibres after synapse in the coeliac ganglion) and parasympathetic nerve fibres (preganglionic fibres from the vagus); these play a part in the metabolism of hepatocytes (carbohydrate and perhaps lipid metabolism), in haemodynamic regulation, and biliary motility;

(b) afferent fibres, which are thought to be involved in osmo- and chemoreception; at the hilus, amyelinic fibres form the anterior and posterior plexuses, which communicate with each other, and these enter the liver mainly around the hepatic artery.

Intrinsic innervation is composed of fibres mainly associated with vascular and biliary structures in the portal spaces (Fig. 16). Certain fibres enter the liver lobule, where they form a network around hepatocytes and extend into the sinusoidal wall, sometimes reaching the centrolobular vein. Fluorescence histochemistry and immunohistochemistry have revealed different types of nerve fibres: adrenergic (the most numerous in man), cholinergic, and peptidergic. Some neuropeptides have been identified: vasoactive intestinal peptide (in the pathway of cholinergic fibres), neuropeptide Y (in that of adrenergic fibres), substance P, glucagon, calcitonin gene-related peptide (Taniakos, Liver, 1996; in press).

The biliary tract
Intrahepatic biliary tract

The biliary tree contributes to the formation of bile and assures its delivery into the intestine. It consists of the intrahepatic and extrahepatic biliary tract. Biliary epithelial cells present two distinct poles: an apical pole facing the bile-duct lumen, equipped with a variable number of short microvilli, and a basolateral pole in relation to adjacent epithelial cells and the basement membrane.

Bile secreted by hepatocytes flows in the canalicular network (0.4 per cent of the lobular parenchyma), which forms a structurally and functionally coherent system (average diameter, 0.5–1 μm in zone 3 and 1–1.25 μm in zone 1) (Figs 6, 8, 9). Tone is provided by an encircling mesh of contractile microfilaments fixed on the zonula adherens, which follow the outline of the microvilli (Jones, DigDisSci, 1980; 1: 11). Bile flows in the opposite direction to that of plasma flow and enters small ductules or cholangioles. The junction between the last hepatocyte and the first of two spindle-shaped biliary cells is called the canal of Hering.

Cholangioles are lined by three or four cells that become cuboidal; they usually have a diameter less than 15 μm. They are in the vascular axis of the septa. Light microscopy shows that they are at the periphery of the portal triad, and are not accompanied by vessels (Fig. 2). They drain bile into interlobular bile ducts located in portal triads. These ducts (< 100 μm diameter), lined by a cuboidal epithelium, are accompanied by arteries. The confluence of two or more interlobular bile ducts forms the septal ducts (> 100 μm diameter), lined by a cylindrical epithelium.

Segmental ducts (between 400 and 800 μm diameter), as well as left and right bile ducts, are histologically similar. The biliary epithelium, lined by a basement membrane, is surrounded by dense fibrous tissue containing many elastic fibres. A peribiliary plexus (branches of the hepatic artery) supplies all the intrahepatic bile ducts. This plexus drains principally into hepatic sinusoids. In addition to the enterohepatic cycle, a cholehepatic cycle for mono- and dihydroxyl bile acids has been proposed.

Extrahepatic biliary tract

At the exit from the liver, the biliary tract is composed of three portions with many anatomical variations (size, position, orientation), particularly at the different confluences:

(1) the main biliary channel consists of the left and right hepatic ducts located in the hilus, the confluence, the common hepatic duct and the common bile duct;
(2) the accessory biliary apparatus comprises the gallbladder and the cystic duct;
(3) the terminal part of the common bile duct enters the duodenum at the papilla of Vater after traversing the sphincter of Oddi.

Hepatic, cystic, and common ducts

The diameter of these ducts is less than 15 mm and their walls are very thin (0.5–1 mm). The mucosa shows some short folds and is composed of a layer of tall, cylindrical cells resting on loose connective tissue, rich in elastic fibres and containing some small seromucous glands. The muscularis is composed of longitudinal and oblique muscular fibres, reinforced near the duodenum by circular fibres forming the sphincter of Oddi. The muscle layer is most prominent near the cystic duct, in the axis of mucosa folds, where they form the Heister valve (which controls bile flow).

Intra- and extramural peribiliary mucous glands are found in relation to the common hepatic ducts, the hilar ducts, and a portion of the larger septal ducts (Terada, Liver, 1987; 7: 1).

The gallbladder

Located within a fossa (on the undersurface) of the right lobe of the liver, the gallbladder is a pocket firmly attached to the liver. Occasionally the gallbladder is freely suspended from the liver by a mesentery. This spindle-shaped bag, measuring 6 to 12 cm in length and 2.5 to 5 cm in width, may contain 30 to 50 ml of bile and consists of a fundus, a body, an infundibulum, and a neck; the neck forms an 'S' shape that represents the transition from the cystic duct.

The wall is composed of a mucosa (which forms primary and secondary folds when the gallbladder is empty) lying on a plexiform muscularis and an adventitia (Fig. 17). The villosities of the mucosa are separated by depressions and crypts sometimes extending in the entire width of the muscular layer (Rokitansky–Aschoff crypts). The mucosa is lined by a single layer of tall, columnar cells

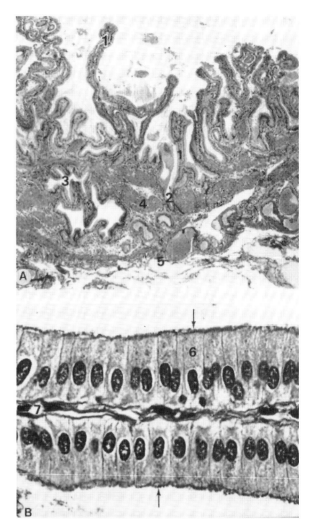

Fig. 17. Gallbladder: paraffin embedding (5 μm-thick section); haematein eosin saffron; A, low magnification (×36) and B, high magnification (×560). (A) The whole gallbladder wall can be seen: the mucosa with its numerous villosities (1) separated by crypts (2) extending into the connective tissue forming Rokitansky sinuses (3), the muscularis (4), and the adventitia (5). (B) The villosities are limited by a single columnar epithelium (6) with an ovoid nucleus near the basal pole of the cell and a striated apical pole (arrow); their axes are of delicate connective tissue (7).

supported by a basement membrane. These cells (Fig. 17) have an ovoid basal nucleus and a pale cytoplasm with microvilli at the apex, only visible by electron microscopy. Some basal cells, rounder and smaller than columnar cells, are located immediately above the basement membrane and should not be confused with intraepithelial lymphocytes, which are more common. Within villosities there is little connective tissue and a few mucous glands can be found in the lamina propria but only near the neck. The muscularis is composed of circular, longitudinal, and oblique smooth-muscle cells in an elastic connective tissue. The adventitia is a connective tissue containing lymphocytes, macrophages, and lipocytes. The gallbladder is richly vascularized by blood and lymphatic plexuses located in the lamina propria and in the adventitia; it is innervated by sympathetic motor fibres and numerous sensory nerve endings. The gallbladder stores and evacuates bile.

The transport properties of biliary epithelial cells and their regulation vary between the various anatomical compartments of the biliary tract. It is usually assumed that intrahepatic ducts are mainly committed to fluid and electrolyte secretion whereas extrahepatic bile ducts and gallbladder are considered to be specialized in absorption and mucin synthesis. The plasticity of the biliary epithelium is important.

References

1. MacSween RNM and Scothorne RJ. Developmental anatomy and normal structure. In MacSween RNM, Anthony PP, Scheuer PJ, Burt AD, and Portmann BC, eds. *Pathology of the liver*. Edinburgh: Churchill Livingstone, 1994; 1–49.
2. Arias IM, Jakoby WB, Boyer JL, Fausto N, Schachter D, and Shafritz DA, eds. *The liver. Biology and pathobiology*. New York: Raven Press, 1994.
3. Millward-Sadler GH and Jezequel AM. Normal histology and ultrastructure. In Wright R and Millward-Sadler GH, eds. *Wright's liver and biliary disease*. London: Saunders, 1992; 12–42.
4. Rappaport AM and Wanless IR. Physioanatomic considerations. In Schiff L and Schiff ER, eds. *Diseases of the liver*. Philadelphia: Lippincott, 1993; 1–41.
5. Jones AL. Anatomy of the liver. In Zakim D and Boyer TD, eds. *Hepatology: a textbook of liver disease*. Philadelphia: Saunders, 1990; 3–30.
6. Gumucio JJ. Bilir BM, Moseley RH, and Berkowitz CM. The biology of the liver cell plate. In Arias IM, Jakoby WB, Boyer JL, Fausto N, Schachter D, and Shafritz DA, eds. *The liver. Biology and pathobiology*. New York: Raven, 1994; 1143–63.
7. Balabaud C., Boulard A, Quinton A, Saric J, Bedin C, Boussarie L, and Bioulac-Sage P. Light and transmission electron microscopy of sinusoids in human liver. In Bioulac-Sage P and Balabaud C, eds. *Sinusoids in human liver: health and disease*. Rijswijk: Kupffer Cell Foundation, 1988; 87–110.
8. Burt AD, Le Bail B, Balabaud C, and Bioulac-Sage P. Morphologic investigation of sinusoidal cells. *Seminars in Liver Disease*, 1993; 13: 21–38.
9. Kuiper J, Brouwer A, Knook DL, and Van Berkel TJC. Kupffer and sinusoidal endothelial cells. In Arias IM, Jakoby WB, Boyer JL, Fausto N, Schachter D, and Shafritz DA, eds. *The liver. Biology and pathobiology*. New York: Raven, 1994; 791–818.
10. Dubuisson L, Fawaz R, Garcia-Barcina M, Neaud V, Winnock M, Balabaud C, and Bioulac-Sage, P. Ultrastructure of human liver-associated lymphocytes *in vivo* and *in vitro*. In Bouwens L, ed. *NK cells in the liver*. Berlin: Springer-Verlag/Landes, 1995; 127–42.
11. Geerts A, De Bleser P, Hautekeete ML, Niki T, and Wisse E. Fat-storing (Ito) cell biology. In Arias IM, Jakoby WB, Boyer JL, Fausto N, Schachter D, and Shafritz DA, eds. *The liver. Biology and pathobiology*. New York: Raven, 1994; 819–38.
12. Wake K. Structure of the sinusoidal wall in the liver. In Wisse E, Knook DL, and Wake K, eds. *Cells of the hepatic sinusoid*. Leiden: Kupffer Cell Foundation, 1995; 241–6.
13. Rojkind M and Greenwel P. The extracellular matrix of the liver. In Arias IM, Jakoby WB, Boyer JL, Fausto N, Schachter D, and Shafritz DA, eds. *The liver. Biology and pathobiology*. New York: Raven, 1994; 843–68.
14. McCuskey RS. The hepatic microvascular system. In Arias IM, Jakoby WB, Boyer JL, Fausto N, Schachter D, and Shafritz DA, eds. *The liver. Biology and pathobiology*. New York: Raven, 1994; 1089–106.

1.3 Electron microscopy of the liver

Albert L. Jones and Douglas L. Schmucker

Preface

Although the scope of this chapter is largely descriptive, brief comments on the functions of the cells and their key components or organelles are provided in order to enhance the understanding of their anatomical relationships. Since the major constituents of the hepatic stroma and vasculature are described elsewhere in this volume, this chapter concentrates on the ultrastructure of liver parenchymal cells (hepatocytes), as well as on that of the biliary and gallbladder epithelium.

Ultrastructure of liver parenchymal cells

Liver parenchymal cells or hepatocytes are large, 10 to 30 μm in diameter, polyhedral cells arranged in plates dispersed between blood vascular channels or sinusoids (Fig. 1). Hepatocytes in mature male rats occupy approximately 87 per cent of the intralobular liver tissue, the remaining volume consists largely of vascular space and sinusoidal cells, for example endothelial, Kupffer, and stellate cells. The volume of the average mononuclear rat hepatocyte is about 6800 μm³, although this varies with sublobular location. Centrally located between adjacent hepatocytes are minute biliary spaces or bile canaliculi which constitute less than 1 to 2 per cent of the extrahepatocyte volume.[1,2] Techniques for the isolation of homogeneous populations of hepatocytes from a variety of species, including rats and humans, and for their maintenance in primary culture have been markedly improved (Arterburn, Hepatol, 1995; 21:175). The role of the basement membrane in regulating hepatocyte development, proliferation, and polarity has been the subject of recent study (Musat, Hepatol, 1993; 18:198; reviewed briefly by Reid, Hepatol, 1992; 15:1198).

Hepatocytes contain almost every organelle found in the animal kingdom due to their wide diversity of functions. Since the distribution of nutrients, biologically active molecules and oxygen is not equitable to all hepatocytes owing to the circulatory pattern, lobular gradients characterized by heterogeneities in cell structure and function are apparent. A description of each of the principal organelles or inclusions in parenchymal cells is given below, including a brief comment on function (see Tables 1 and 2).

Endoplasmic reticulum

Both smooth- and rough-surfaced endoplasmic reticulum (**ER**) are well developed in hepatic parenchymal cells, although their relative

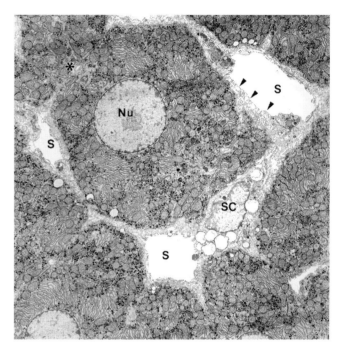

Fig. 1. Low-magnification electron micrograph of rat liver, illustrating the relationships between hepatocytes, sinusoids, and other cell types. Typical liver parenchymal cell architecture and polyhedral shape is demonstrated by the hepatocyte occupying much of the field. Nu, nucleus; S, sinusoid; SC, stellate cell (formerly fat-storing cell); asterisk (*), bile canaliculus; arrowheads, endothelial cell.

Table 1 Volumes of mononuclear rat hepatocyte organelles and inclusions

	Volume (μm³/cell)	Percentage of hepatocyte
Hepatocyte	6791	100
Nucleus	556	8
Cytoplasm	6215	92
ground substance	4720	69
lipid droplets	8	1
mitochondria	1363	20
peroxisomes	101	1–2
dense bodies	32	0.5–1

Table 2 Surface areas of mononuclear rat hepatocyte intracellular membranes		
	Surface (μm^2/cell)	Percentage of total membrane
Total intracellular membrane	78 048	100
Rough endoplasmic reticulum	23 228	30
Smooth endoplasmic reticulum	51 682	66
Golgi	3138	4

quantities, precise positions, and arrangements vary from cell to cell and reflect lobular orientation. In addition to the membrane-bound ribosomes of the rough ER, the hepatocyte contains many free ribosomes and polyribosomes, the number of which fluctuates in response to various conditions.

The rough ER consists of aggregates of parallel, flattened cisternae scattered randomly throughout the cytoplasm, which corresponds to the basophilic bodies or ergastoplasm seen in specially stained histological sections (Figs 2(b), 3). Both rough- and smooth-surfaced ER are prominent in Zones 1 and 2. In the rat, Zone 3 hepatocytes contain between 14 and 42 per cent more surface area of smooth ER than do cells in zone 1 within the same classic liver lobule and depending on animal age.[1,2] This observation is of considerable interest to pathologists since enzymes which convert certain harmless compounds, such as carbon tetrachloride and acetaminophen, into toxic free radicals reside primarily in the smooth ER. Zone 3 hepatocytes, therefore, are much more susceptible to the damaging effects of these metabolites.

The smooth-surfaced ER is composed of an elaborate system of anastomosing tubules (Figs 2(a), b), 4). The rough ER is often found in direct communication with the nuclear envelope and the smooth ER, whereas the smooth ER, itself, frequently communicates with the Golgi complex (Figs 2(b), 4). Contrary to early reports, the endoplasmic reticulum is never in direct contact with any other membrane system, e.g. mitochondria, plasma membranes. However, (1) the rough ER is often found in close association with mitochondria; (2) this rough ER–mitochondrial complex can be isolated intact; and (c) this complex is thought to be involved in the synthesis of haemoproteins, as well as in the biogenesis of mitochondria (Meier, ExpCellRes, 1978; 111:478; Cascarano, Hepatol, 1995; 22: 837; Fig. 5).

Hepatic smooth ER often exhibits local specializations and is almost invariably associated with particulate glycogen (Figs 2(a), b), 4). In spite of the localization of the enzyme glucose 6-phosphatase predominantly to the smooth ER, the functional significance of this relationship remains unclear. The induction of liver microsomal mono-oxygenases, most notably many cytochrome P-450 isoforms, by a variety of drugs and xenobiotics is correlated with the marked proliferation of the smooth endoplasmic reticulum, the primary locus of hepatic phase I drug-metabolizing enzymes (Fouts, Exp-MolPath, 1966; 5:475; Jones, JHistochemCytochem, 1966; 14:215; Orrenius, JCellBiol, 1966; 28:181) (Fig. 6).

Golgi complex

The Golgi complex consists of three to five closely packed, parallel smooth-surfaced cisternae, a variable number of associated vesicles

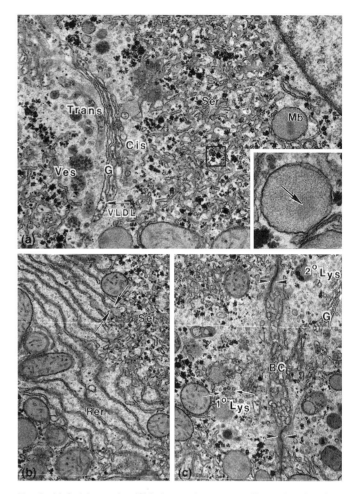

Fig. 2. (a) Golgi complex (G) in human hepatocyte, illustrating the *cis* (convex) and the *trans* (concave) cisternal surfaces and associated vesicles (Ves) containing very low density lipoprotein particles (VLDL). Inset: crystalloid inclusion (arrow) in the matrix of a peroxisome in a human hepatocyte. Square, glycogen rosettes; Mb, peroxisome or microbody; Ser, smooth-surfaced endoplasmic reticulum. (b) Rough (Rer)- and smooth (Ser)-surfaced endoplasmic reticulum in human hepatocytes. Note the anastomosis between these two species of intracellular membranes (arrows). (c) Bile canaliculus (BC) and pericanalicular cytoplasm in human hepatocytes. The blood–bile barrier is maintained by junctional complexes between adjacent hepatocytes (arrowheads). G, Golgi; 2° Lys, secondary lysosomes; 1° Lys, primary lysosomes. (Reproduced from Figs 6–8, Burwen, Hepatol, 1982; 2:426.)

(large and small) and, occasionally, lysosomal elements (Fig. 2(a)). Its *cis*, or convex, surface is considered its forming face, whereas the concave, or *trans*, element is the origin of its secretory vesicles. These structures and the associated cytosol constitute up to 5 per cent of the parenchymal cell volume in the periportal zones and approximately 2 per cent in the centrilobular areas (Claude, JCellBiol, 1970; 47:745). Claude speculated that each hepatocyte may contain as many as 50 such complexes; however, they may be interrelated, representing a single complex with multiple branching.

The associated secretory vesicles usually contain osmiophilic spheres, 500 to 700 Å in diameter, now recognized as triglyceride-rich very low density lipoproteins (**VLDLs**), which play a major

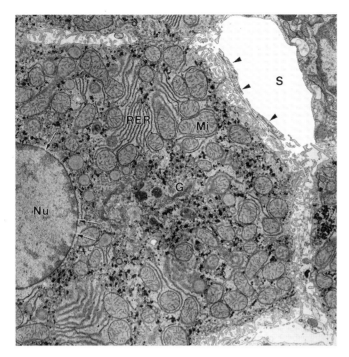

Fig. 3. Mitochondria (Mi), rough (RER)- and smooth-surfaced endoplasmic reticulum occupy much of the hepatocyte cytoplasm. Nu, nucleus; G, Golgi; S, sinusoid; arrowheads, endothelial cell; arrows, nuclear membrane pores.

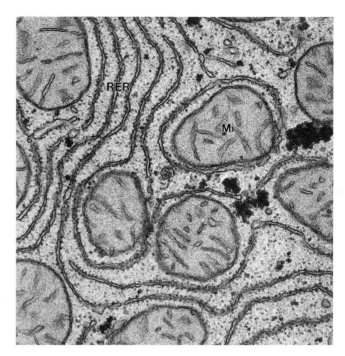

Fig. 5. Close structural and functional relationships can be demonstrated between mitochondria (Mi) and the rough-surfaced endoplasmic reticulum (RER). Intact mitochondrial–RER complexes can be isolated from rat liver using subcellular fractionation techniques.

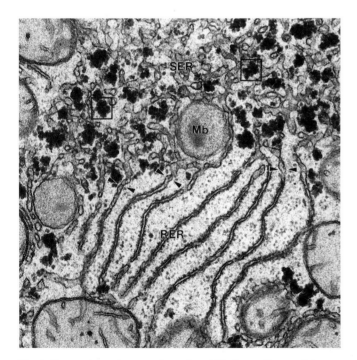

Fig. 4. Frequent anastomoses (arrowheads) between the parallel lamellae of the rough-surfaced (RER) and the tubulovesicular profiles of the smooth-surfaced (SER) endoplasmic reticula illustrate the structural continuity between these two hepatic membrane systems. Mb, peroxisome or microbody; squares, aggregates of glycogen particles in close proximity to SER profiles.

role in systemic lipid transport (Hamilton, LabInvest, 1967; 16:305; Jones, JLipRes, 1967; 8:429). Numerous small, coated vesicles in

the immediate vicinity of the Golgi complex are acid phosphatase-positive primary lysosomes (Figs 2(c), 7). These organelles carry acid hydrolases to secondary lysosomes, such as multivesicular bodies, autophagic vacuoles, etc.

In addition to its role in lipoprotein transport, the Golgi complex plays a major role in the glycosylation of proteins destined for export and in the synthesis of transmembrane glycoprotein receptors. Considerable interest surrounds the recent speculation that bile acid micelles originate as small membrane vesicles from either the Golgi and/or ER, which quickly reach the biliary space. Both physiological and morphological evidence support this concept.[3]

Lysosomes and multivesicular bodies

Lysosomes play an important role in cellular pathology. Hepatic lysosomes increase in viral hepatitis, cholestasis, and cell injury following anoxia. The livers of children with type II glycogenosis (Pompe's disease) lack the enzyme α1, 4-glucosidase and contain large glycogen deposits within their lysosomes (reviewed by Weissman, NEJM, 1969; 273:1084). Hepatic lysosomes also appear to participate in the storage of iron or ferritin. They normally contain ferritin-like substances and accumulate large quantitites in iron-storage diseases, for example haemochromatosis and haemosiderosis.

As discussed above, primary lysosomes are the source of lysosomal enzymes or acid hydrolases which are introduced into other membrane-limited structures (secondary lysosomes) containing effete organelles or unwanted exogenous substances. Liver parenchymal cells contain many secondary lysosomes, predominantly in the cytoplasm immediately surrounding the bile canaliculi and

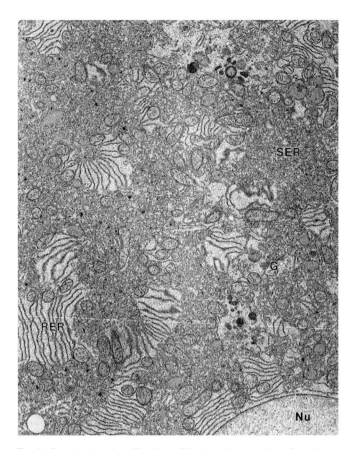

Fig. 6. Drug-induced proliferation of the hepatic smooth-surfaced endoplasmic reticulum (SER) is accompanied by increases in the activities of constituent mono-oxygenases. This hepatocyte is from a rat treated with sodium phenobarbital (50 mg/kg body weight) for 6 days. Much of the cytoplasm is occupied by large lakes of SER causing a condensation of the RER lamellae and other organelles. Nu, nucleus; G, Golgi.

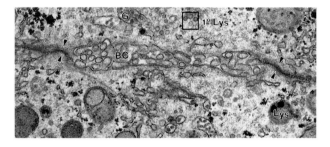

Fig. 7. An electron micrograph of a human liver bile canaliculus (BC). Junctional complexes between the cells, identified by arrowheads, isolate the canalicular system from the blood by excluding the passage of all but very small molecules. G, Golgi; Lys, lysosome; 1° Lys, primary lysosomes.

Golgi complexes (Figs 2(c), 7). Lysosomes at these sites correspond to the peribiliary dense bodies described by early histologists. They are highly pleomorphic organelles, varying in size, number, and position under different conditions (Fig. 8(a), inset). Since no two lysosomes look alike, their positive identification in electron micrographs requires that they (1) be bounded by a single membrane and (2) exhibit a positive staining reaction for acid phosphatase.

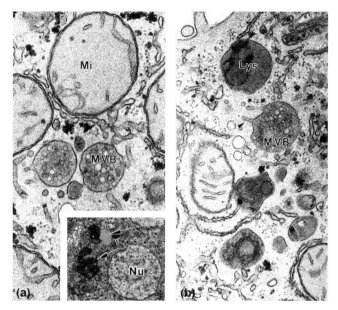

Fig. 8. (a) Multivesicular bodies (MVB) are membrane-bound aggregates of smaller vesicles containing materials endocytosed and destined for degradation. Mi, mitochondria. Inset: secondary lysosomes or residual bodies containing lipofuscin (electron dense) and lipid-like material (electron lucid) in human hepatocytes. Nu, nucleus. (b) Lysosomal degradation involves the fusion of small primary lysosomes with multivesicular bodies (MVB) or other membrane-bound aggregates, as demonstrated by the appearance of a tail-like appendage (arrowhead). Following acidification, hydrolytic activity, and condensation, these inclusions undergo a transition to electron-dense secondary lysosomes (Lys) and, ultimately, residual bodies.

Their contents may be homogeneous, heterogeneous, electron dense, or finely granular and may also include myelin figures, pigment, intact or partially digested organelles, inclusions, or all of the above.

Multivesicular bodies develop as a result of the fusion of endocytic vesicles usually derived via receptor-mediated endocytosis (Cohen, Cancer, 1983; 51:1787). Initially, larger compartments called endosomes are formed, but as the process progresses, the fusing vesicles turn inside-out and enter the larger forming vesicles as multiple inside-out vesicles (Fig. 8). As the intraluminal contents undergo degradation due to lysosomal enzyme activity, these structures become increasingly electron dense until all evidence of the internalized vesicles has disappeared.[4]

Peroxisomes (microbodies)

The peroxisome is a single membrane-bound particle (approximately 0.2–1.0 μm in diameter) with a fine granular matrix (Figs 2(a), 9). Each parenchymal cell has approximately 200 peroxisomes, or one peroxisome for every four mitochondria. They differ from secondary lysosomes in that their matrix consists of a moderate electron-dense homogeneous mass and, in many mammals, a laminated crystalloid core or nucleoid. The structure of the core varies greatly from species to species. In the rat, it consists of tubules of two different sizes; small ones, approximately 45 Å in diameter, and larger ones, 95 to 110 Å in diameter. The core is thought to contain the enzyme urate oxidase, whereas catalase and

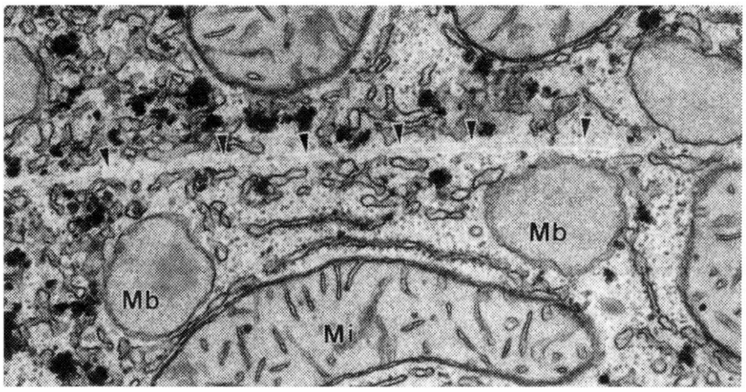

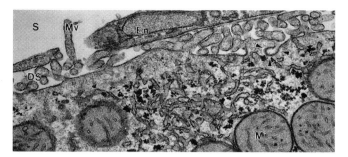

Fig. 9. Rat liver peroxisomes or microbodies (Mb) are characterized by inclusions which, in the appropriate plane of section, yield a uniform crystal lattice appearance attributable to the enzyme urate oxidase. Microtubules (arrowheads) constitute a major component of the hepatocyte cytoskeletal system which is intimately involved in vesicle translocation. Mi, mitochondria.

Fig. 10. Sinusoidal surface of human hepatocyte exhibiting a clathrin-coated endocytic pit (arrowheads), precursor to an endocytic vesicle, and microvilli (Mv) extending into the Disse space (DS) between the parenchymal cell and the adjacent sinusoidal endothelium (En). Note that the endothelial cells are characterized by fenestrae in their thin cytoplasmic extensions which, in this case, permit hepatocyte microvilli to protrude into the sinusoidal lumen. S, sinusoid; Mi, mitochondria.

D-amino acid oxidase activities are present in the matrix. The livers of uricotelic animals, such as humans, have been reported to have peroxisomes deficient in urate oxidase. In support of this, electron micrographs have shown that human liver peroxisomes contain only an occasional nucleoid (Fig. 2(b), inset).

Peroxisomes presumably participate in the disposal of hydrogen peroxide; the metabolism of purines, long-chain fatty acids and alcohols; the oxidation of reduced NAD and gluconeogenesis. Hepatic peroxisomes proliferate during embryological development and early postnatal life, during recovery from partial hepatectomy, during the course of a variety of hepatic diseases, and after the administration of salicylates and certain lipid-lowering agents, such as ethyl-α-p-chlorophenoxyisobutyrate (Clofibrate®).

Plasma membrane

The hepatocyte plasma membrane can be isolated into three distinct domains based on the unique physicochemical features of these different membrane regions (Fig. 1). The plasma membrane limiting the perisinusoidal space or space of Disse contains numerous finger-like projections or microvilli (Figs 3, 10). The microvilli greatly enhance the receptor and transport surface of the liver cell, a fact of considerable importance in view of the multitude of functional responsibilities of the liver. On occasion, microvilli actually protrude through the fenestrae of the sinusoidal endothelium into the sinusoidal lumen. Whether this has functional significance or is merely fortuitous is not known. The lateral plasma membrane has few, if any, microvilli, but does contain regional specializations consisting of desmosomes and gap junctions. Desmosomes apparently add stability to the cell-to-cell interface, whereas the gap junctions are considered the major pathway for intercellular communication via the transfer of chemical and electrical information. Both the basal and lateral membrane domains can be isolated to near homogeneity and identified by electron microscopy and Na^+,K^+- dependent ATPase transport activity.

The bile canaliculus represents the third plasma membrane domain, constitutes approximately 10 per cent of the plasmalemma surface, and marks the beginning of the bile secretory pathway (Arias, Hepatol, 1993; 17:318). The plasma membranes from two or more adjacent hepatocytes limit the defined 1 to 2 μm diameter biliary space (Figs 1, 2(c), 7). The composition and physical characteristics of the bile canalicular membranes are markedly different from those of the basolateral regions. The plasma membranes contribute microvilli and secure the biliary space via tight junctions, the primary permeability barrier between the blood and bile. These junctions are quite strong, since efforts to isolate hepatocytes result in the rupture of cell membranes rather than the tight junction. The cytoplasm within a 1 μm radius of the canaliculus, ie. the pericanalicular cytoplasm, usually contains clear vesicles thought to be involved in the transport of proteins, apoproteins, and various ligands for biliary secretion. Other organelles, such as the Golgi and secondary lysosomes, are also found in the pericanalicular zone. Microfilaments surround the canaliculus and protrude into canalicular microvilli. These contractile filaments maintain the structural integrity of the canaliculus and, based on evidence obtained using isolated hepatocyte 'couplets', may exert force on the biliary space to enhance biliary fluid secretion pressure (Gautam, Hepatol, 1987; 7:216). Thicker intermediate filaments are associated with the microfilaments, but their function and significance remain unresolved.

Microtubules

Microtubules are 250 Å in diameter and vary in length up to approximately 20 μm (Fig. 9). In intact liver parenchymal cells they are scattered randomly throughout the cytoplasm, although they are often seen at the periphery of the cell, as well as near the Golgi and bile canaliculus. These tubules are dynamic organelles capable of depolymerizing at one end and repolymerizing at the other end ('treadmilling'). Recent evidence suggests that they form vectors which direct transport vesicles to their destinations within the cell (Goldman, Gastro, 1983; 85:130; Caron, JCellBiol, 1985; 101:1763). Compounds which either prevent their polymerization (colchicine) or deploymerization (taxol) markedly interfere with vesicle movement. In isolated liver cells, microtubules radiate from the perinuclear Golgi–lysosome region to the cell periphery.

Mitochondria

Liver parenchymal cells contain approximately 800 mitochondria each. Mitochondria are the ATP-producing energy factories of the cell. They are relatively large (up to 1.5 mm in diameter and 4 mm in length); self-replicating, exhibiting a half-life of about 10.5 days; and most contain one or more minute, electron-dense inclusions thought to represent calcium stores (Figs 1, 3, 5). These inclusions disappear rapidly during hypoxia. Other inclusions, including crystalloid structures, have been described in various diseases, but their significance remains obscure. Budding or dividing mitochondria are not usually found in normal hepatocytes, but they are commonplace during recovery from simple riboflavin or dietary iron deficiencies (Tandler, JCellBiol, 1969; 41:477; Dallman, JCellBiol, 1971; 48:79).

Nucleus

Hepatocytes contain one or more spherical nuclei, each containing at least one distinct nucleolus (Figs 1, 3). The nucleus is about 6 to 7 μm in diameter and the karyoplasm is surrounded by a typical nuclear envelope with pores. The tight, coiled chromosomes or heterochromatin can be seen as clumps of electron-dense material scattered throughout the karyoplasm, as well as along the inner border of the nuclear envelope. Mitotic figures are seldom seen in hepatocytes since under normal circumstances only 1 in 20 000 cells is dividing at any time. In fortuitous sections, the outer leaflet of the nuclear envelope can be seen in continuity with elements of the rough ER.

Bile secretory pathway
Intrahepatic ductules and ducts

After entering the bile canaliculus, bile flows toward the periphery of the classic lobule where it enters the proximal end of the biliary duct system, through the canals of Hering (Fig. 11). At first one or two spindle-shaped cells share the periphery of the biliary space with hepatocytes at the terminus of the bile canaliculus. At this point the bile is conveyed through the limiting plate of hepatocytes into the perilobular and interlobular bile ducts in the portal canals. A number of investigators using specific stem cell markers have identified ductal plate cells as precursors to hepatocytes, intrahepatic bile duct epithelial cells (**IBDECs**), and the oval cells characteristic of regenerating liver (Blakolmer, Hepatol, 1995; 21:1510; Golding, Hepatol, 1995; 22:1243; Bisgaard, Hepatol, 1996; 23:62).

The bile ductules and ducts are surrounded by cells which progress rapidly to cuboidal epithelium. A distinct basal lamina surrounds this epithelium except at the point of immediate contact with the bile canaliculus. The nuclei vary from spindle-shaped to round, depending on the configuration of the cells. Each cell has a prominent Golgi complex and numerous cytoplasmic vesicles, but the microvilli are short and sparse in comparison to the relatively long and numerous projections of the canaliculus. These differentiated intrahepatic bile duct epithelial cells have been isolated, partially characterized and maintained in primary culture for *in vitro* studies on bile duct functions (Ishii, Gastro, 1989; 97:1236; Okamoto, Hepatol, 1995; 22:153). Special vascular casting techniques, combined with scanning electron microscopy, have demonstrated that all intrahepatic bile duct epithelium is surrounded by a capillary network derived from tributaries of the hepatic artery and terminating in inlet venules of the portal vein, i.e. peribiliary capillaries. The density of this capillary network varies from animal to animal. Recent studies have shown that development of the

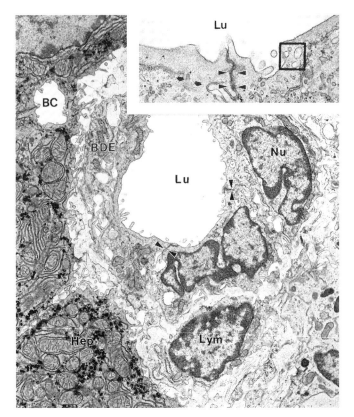

Fig. 11. Electron micrograph of a cross-section of an interlobular bile ductule in rat liver. The intrahepatic bile ductule epithelial cells (IBDECs) undergo a transition from squamous to cuboidal shape between the bile canaliculus (BC) and larger collecting bile ducts. Note the intrahepatic lymphocyte (Lym) in the connective tissue of the portal space. Inset: high magnification of apical cytoplasm of two adjacent biliary epithelial cells. Endocytic vesicles (endosomes) are visible beneath the plasma membrane (square). Nu, IBDEC nucleus; Hep, hepatocyte adjacent to the portal space; Lu, lumen of bile ductule; arrows, microfilaments; arrowheads, junctions between adjacent IBDECs.

human peribiliary capillary plexus occurs in parallel with that of the intrahepatic bile ducts (Haratake, Hepatol, 1991; 14:1196; Terada, Hepatol, 1993; 18:529). Collectively, the observations of prominent Golgi, numerous intracellular vesicles, and elaborate vasculature strongly suggest an important role for this epithelia in the final formation of bile.

Extrahepatic bile ducts

The cells that line the extrahepatic biliary space are similar in morphology to those of the intrahepatic ducts except that they are columnar and the surrounding vasculature is not as well developed. Periodic acid–Schiff-positive cells are found in tubular glands occasionally seen within the epithelium.

Gallbladder

The mucosa of the gallbladder is comprised of a single layer of columnar cells which contain an extensive supranuclear Golgi complex, rough ER, numerous vesicles, and small mitochondria (Fig. 12). Junctional complexes are found in the apical region of the cells. The microvilli are numerous and the lateral plasma membranes are thrown into a series of convoluted folds. During active absorption of fluid from the bile, these intercellular spaces become markedly distended. Human gallbladder epithelial cells have been isolated successfully, maintained in primary culture, and partially characterized (Auth, Hepatol, 1993; 18:546). Autonomic nerve fibres are observed in the serosa, and goblet cell-containing glands, while sparse in the normal gallbladder, are frequently observed in patients with chronic gallbladder inflammation.

Intracellular transport pathways

Plasma-derived proteins bind to specific receptors on the sinusoidal plasma membrane surface of hepatocytes and the protein–receptor complexes are internalized into endocytic vesicles. Proteins that are taken up by the liver are degraded, secreted intact into the bile, or utilized by the liver cell. The receptors determine which proteins are endocytosed, but once uptake has occurred, the intracellular destinations of the proteins dictate which pathway is selected (see ref. 4 and other parts of this textbook for reviews of this process).

The degradative pathway

Some proteins, such as asialoglycoproteins, low density lipoproteins, chylomicron and VLDL remnants, are largely degraded by hepatocytes. They are endocytosed in clathrin-coated pits and vesicles which subsequently fuse to form endosomes (Fig. 10). The endosomes mature into multivesicular bodies which, following fusion with primary lysosomes, form secondary lysosomes. Their contents are degraded by lysosomal enzymes and the degradation products are secreted either back into the blood or into the bile. The specific receptors for these proteins are generally recycled; that is, they uncouple from their ligands in the acidic environment of the endosome compartment and are returned to the sinusoidal plasma membrane. Since they do not travel to the lysosomal compartment, they escape degradation. Microtubules are essential for this process to occur, although their specific role remains unresolved.

The transcellular pathway

Some proteins remain intact and are secreted directly into the bile, such as immunoglobulin A (IgA). The endocytic pits and vesicles may not be clathrin-coated in this transport pathway. The endocytic vesicles do not fuse, but remain a constant size after formation (approximately 1000–1500 Å in diameter) and travel, under the influence of microtubules, directly to the bile canalicular membrane. They do not interact with other organelle compartments *en route* and, consequently, there is no opportunity for lysosomal degradation. These endocytic 'shuttle' vesicles empty their contents into the bile canalicular lumen by exocytosis. IgA is secreted still bound to a portion of its receptor, secretory component. The part of the receptor that remains membrane-associated may be recycled. Shuttle vesicles with membrane-associated secretory component are formed continuously at the sinusoidal surface and translocated to the bile canaliculus even in the absence of internalized IgA.

The intracellular pathway

The uptake of certain endocytosed proteins, such as transferrin, has direct metabolic consequences for hepatocytes. Ferric iron circulates

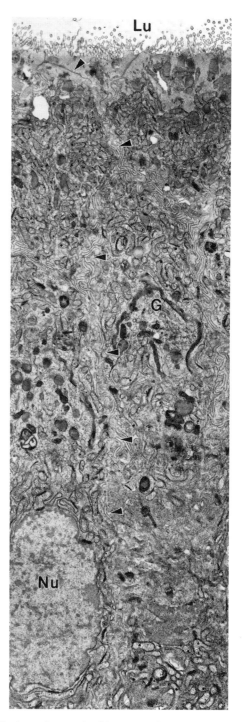

Fig. 12. Electron micrograph of rhesus monkey gallbladder epithelium. These extremely tall columnar epithelial cells are characterized by polarized architecture, with most organelles located in the supranuclear region, and by extensive lateral interdigitations between adjacent cells (arrowheads). Nu, nucleus; G, Golgi; Lu, lumen of gallbladder.

in the blood bound to transferrin. At neutral pH, transferrin-Fe^{2+} binds to its receptor on the sinusoidal plasma membrane and is endocytosed as the transferrin-Fe^{2+}–receptor complex. This complex enters the prelysosomal compartment and, in the acidic environment, Fe^{2+} dissociates from the complex. The transferrin, however, remains bound to its receptor at an acidic pH. The transferrin–receptor complex travels back to the plasma membrane and, upon exposure to the neutral pH at the cell surface, the transferrin dissociates from its receptor and is released back into the blood, whereas the receptor remains associated with the membrane. Meanwhile, inside the cell, following its dissociation from transferrin, iron is released from the transport vesicle by an unknown mechanism and binds to ferritin for storage.

Development

Hepatocytes undergo marked changes during fetal and postnatal development. For example, the bile canaliculi assume the adult appearance during perinatal and early postnatal periods, although bile secretory functions do not fully develop until later (Shaffer, DigDisSci, 1985; 30:558). Hepatocyte plasma membranes characterized by microvilli and endocytic pits, as well as by the uptake of asialo-orosomucoid, appear postnatally in rodents. Qualitatively, rat liver mitochondria resemble the adult organelles by the fifth postnatal day and the volume of this compartment appears to increase during this period (Kanamura, JUltrastructRes, 1985; 93: 195).

The rough-surfaced endoplasmic reticulum is prominent in hepatocytes during gestation and is fully developed by postnatal day 5 in mice. In rodents, the relative concentration of rough ER either (1) remains constant or (2) increases during the late gestational and early postnatal periods (Kanai, AmJAnat, 1986; 175:471). Vesicular smooth ER first appears in mouse hepatocytes between days 18 and 20 of gestation, increases postnatally, and shifts to tubular profiles. The increase in the hepatocellular concentration of smooth ER, which begins immediately after birth, corresponds with a concomitant increase in microsomal drug-metabolizing capacity.

Golgi profiles are readily seen in hepatocytes as early as the tenth day of gestation in rodents and within the first trimester in humans (Franke, CellTissRes, 1985; 242:661). The Golgi initially appears in the perinuclear cytoplasm, migrates closer to the pericanalicular zone by day 20 of gestation, and assumes the adult appearance and position by the fifth postnatal day. In humans, the perinuclear Golgi migrates to the pericanalicular cytoplasm concomitant with the initiation of bile secretion, i.e. during the third gestational month. Peroxisomes first appear in rodent hepatocytes between days 15 and 17 of gestation and the volume of this compartment increases until birth. However, the first appearance of lysosomes in fetal hepatocytes is controversial and ranges between day 15 of gestation and parturition.

Ageing

Ageing is accompanied by changes in cell structure, function, and composition. Unfortunately, much of the information concerning age-related alterations in hepatocyte morphology is qualitative and precludes meaningful correlations with functional changes. The fact that ageing affects the liver is well documented in humans and rodents, and it is generally associated with:

(1) a decline in liver weight or volume;
(2) reduced hepatic blood flow;
(3) an accumulatiopn of 'ageing pigment' or lipofuscin (Fig. 8(a), inset); and
(4) increased fibrogenesis.[5]

Historically, the ageing liver has been characterized by:

(1) fewer and larger hepatocytes;
(2) increased nuclear ploidy; and
(3) a larger binuclear hepatocyte index.

The size of human hepatocytes has either been reported to remain unchanged between 19 and 96 years of age or to increase by 25 per cent beyond 60 years.[6] There have been reports of age-related increases (15–50 per cent) in parenchymal cell volume, as well as a gradual increase during maturation (1–16 months) followed by a decline during senescence (>20 months) in rats.[1,6] The relative volume of the hepatocyte compartment remains stable, i.e. approximately 85 per cent of rat liver volume, but the number of hepatocytes per volume of liver declines during the first 15 months of life, followed by an increase during the remainder of the lifespan. Nuclear volume reflects the changes in cell volume, but increased ploidy levels in human and rodent hepatocytes during ageing are well established. However, Gahan and Middleton reported that no major ploidy shifts occur in the human liver beyond 21 years of age (Gahan, ExpGerontol, 1984; 31:8).

Old mice (30 months) exhibit an increase (60 per cent) in the number of enlarged, vacuolated hepatocyte mitochondria, whereas average mitochondrial volume reportedly declines with age in rats.[6] Other studies have reported:

(1) a decrease in the number of mitochondria per volume of liver;
(2) an increase or a decrease in the number of mitochondria per hepatocyte; and
(3) a decline or no change in the relative volume of this organelle compartment.

The best-documented age-related change in hepatocyte structure is the accumulation of dense bodies, i.e. secondary lysosomes and residual bodies containing lipofuscin. At least five separate studies have reported two- to eightfold increases in the relative volume of this compartment in rodents.[6] Quantitative studies have failed to detect significant age-related changes in the relative volume of the peroxisomal compartment.

Ageing male rats exhibit a 30 per cent reduction in rough ER content between 6 and 20 months, and a subsequent increase such that livers of 1- and 30-month-old animals contain equivalent amounts of membrane.[1] The increase in rough ER in senescent rats correlates with a concomitant increase in the hepatic protein synthesizing capacity of similarly aged animals. Several studies have reported that the hepatocellular concentration of smooth ER in rats gradually increases during development and maturation, but declines thereafter, yielding a significant loss of membrane between maturity and senescence.[1,6] This age-related decline in smooth ER corresponds to lower yields of hepatic microsomes and reduced drug-metabolizing capacity.

References

1. Schmucker DL, Mooney JS, and Jones AL. Stereological analysis of hepatocyte fine structure in the Fischer 344 rat. Influence of sublobular location and animal age. *Journal of Cell Biology*, 1978; **78**: 319.

2. Loud AV. A quantitative stereological description of the ultrastructure of normal rat liver parenchymal cells. *Journal of Cell Biology*, 1968; **37**: 27.

3. Jones AL, Renston R, Schmucker DL, Mooney JL, Ockner RK, and Adler RD. A morphologic evaluation of the pericanalicular cytoplasm in the rat hepatocyte demonstrating possible components of the bile secretory apparatus. In Preiseg R and Bircher J, eds. *The Liver—Quantitative Aspects of Structure and Function*. Aulendorf: Editio Cantor, 1979: 63.

4. Jones AL and Burwen SJ. Pathways and functions of biliary protein secretion. In Forte JG, ed. *Handbook of Physiology, The Gastrointestinal System III*. Bethesda, MD: American Physiological Society, 1989: 663.

5. Popper H. Aging and the liver. In Popper H and Schaffner F, eds. *Progress in Liver Disease*, Vol. VIII. Orlando, FL: Grune and Stratton, 1986: 659.

6. Schmucker DL. Hepatocyte fine structure during maturation and senescence. *Journal of Electron Microscopy Techniques*, 1990; **14**: 106.

1.4 Sinusoidal liver cells

Eddie Wisse, F. Braet, D. Luo, D. Vermijlen, M. Eddouks, C. Empsen, Herbert Spapen, and R. B. De Zanger

Introduction

During recent years, increasing attention has been paid to liver sinusoidal cells. Two waves of fundamental research, starting around 1970, have now passed; the first consisted of morphological studies describing and characterizing the cells and their reactions in normal and experimental conditions[1-7] and the second consisted of biochemical studies using isolation and culture of the cells to provide us with functional data.[8-10] At present, interest is clearly focused on the molecular biology and the medical aspects of this intriguing class of cells (Earnest, p.325 in 11; Tanikawa, p.288 in 11; Ueno, p.293 in 11; Tanikawa, p.131 in 12).

A classical theory, described in textbooks of histology until the mid-1970s, states that sinusoids are bordered by undifferentiated endothelial cells, which are able to develop into Kupffer cells when the proper stimulus is given (see also 1). According to this theory, the two cells mentioned have to be considered as different functional stages of the same cell type. Electron microscopy using perfusion fixation, together with cell-isolation methods, has changed this theory into a more differentiated view. It has become apparent that the normal sinusoid is inhabited by four different types of cell (Wisse, ToxicolPath, 1996; 24:100): endothelial,[4] Kupffer,[5,6] fat-storing (Ito, OkajimasFAnatJap, 1952; 24:243; Wake, IntRevCytol, 1980; 66:303),[1,2] and pit cells.[7,13,14] These cells are located in and around the hepatic sinusoid; each cell type has its own characteristic morphology (Fig. 1), proliferation and population dynamics, and pattern of functions and reactions to disease or experimental situations (Tanikawa, p.131 in 12).[4,6] The cells also differ in enzyme content[10] and the expression of cytoskeletal proteins, adhesion molecules, cytokines, and receptors. No transitional stages between the different cell types are observed in normal, experimental, or diseased livers of different species.

Over the years, methods for the characterization of sinusoidal cells have been developed utilizing morphology, enzyme cytochemistry, reaction to particle injection, and the application of antibodies.[4-6,9,10] Some of these methods can only be applied to cells in intact tissues, or are species dependent and must therefore be applied with some caution. Different antisera have been raised for the immunotyping of sinusoidal cells. Some of these antisera have been raised against a cell type occurring in many tissues of the body (e.g. endotheloial cells) and are therefore not exclusive for the cell types in the sinusoid (Morris, JCellBiol, 1988; 106:649; Daemen, p.400 in reference 11; Hardonk, p.434 in reference 11). A monospecific antiserum (3.2.3) raised against the cytolysis-triggering molecule NKR-P1 on natural killer (**NK**) cells can be used to identify pit cells (Chambers, JExpMed, 1989; 169:1373; Luo, Hepatol, 1995; 21:1690). With this antibody, the number of pit cells in frozen sections of rat liver was counted as $13.7/mm^2$. Kupffer cells are immunostained with Ki-M2R, a rat antimacrophage monoclonal antibody (Yamaguchi, DigDisSci, 1995; 40:548), with ED2 (Daemen, p.400 in reference 11; Van Rooijen, CellTissRes, 1990; 260: 215), and monoclonal anti-KCA-1 (Sugihara, AmJPath, 1990; 136: 345). A monoclonal antibody RECA-1 against rat endothelial cells was developed, which also reacts to hepatic sinusoidal endothelial cells (Duijvestijn, LabInvest, 1992; 66:549). For future research, it would be useful to have more specific antibodies against different types of sinusoidal cells.

New data have become available which demonstrate a co-operation between sinusoidal cells (Van Berkel, p.10 in reference 11). For instance, sinusoidal cells seem to be involved in the synthesis and/or secretion of hepatocyte growth factor or scatter factor (Noji, BBResComm, 1990; 173:42; Schirmacher, Hepatol, 1992; 15:5; Maher, JCI, 1993; 91:2244; Masumoto, CellStructFunc, 1993; 18: 87; Yamane, Oncogene, 1994; 9:2683). Also, sinusoidal cells influence the release of glucose by parenchymal cells (Kuiper, BBActa, 1988; 959:143; Decker, p.171 in reference 11; Van Berkel, p.10 in reference 11). The majority of cytokines produced by sinusoidal cells are cleared by parenchymal cells, which metabolize the compounds and/or partly secrete them in bile (Tran-Thi, JHepatol, 1987; 5:322). The activity of inducible glucuronosyltransferases was higher in Kupffer and endothelial cells than parenchymal cells (Oesch, BiochemPharm, 1992; 43:731). The infusion of insulin into rats enhances the use of glucose by parenchymal cells by about 50 per cent, whereas uptake by endothelial cells increased 100 per cent and by Kupffer cells up to 600 per cent (Spolarics, BBResComm, 1992; 186:455). However, parenchymal cells have more insulin-binding sites than Kupffer and endothelial cells, which only contributed an estimated 10 to 15 per cent of the total hepatic insulin degradation (Kolaczynski, Metabolism, 1993; 42:477). The cytochrome P-450 in Kupffer cells was induced more than 10-fold by acetone treatment. The specific activity of Kupffer cell homogenates from acetone-treated rats was nearly equal to that for

Our work was financially supported by the Belgian Science Foundation NFWO, grants 3.00053.92, 3.00050.95 and G0038.96 and the Research Council of the Free University of Brussels (VUB), grants 195.332.1310, 196.322.0140, 02R230.

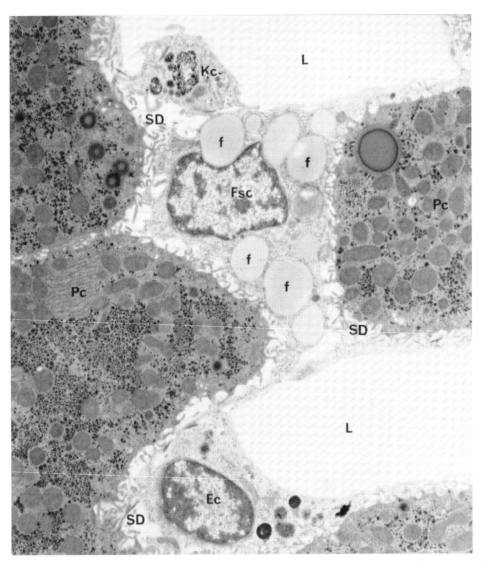

Fig. 1. Low magnification of two sinusoids showing four liver cell types: parenchymal cells, an endothelial cell, a fat-storing cell, and part of a Kupffer cell. The endothelial cell is characterized by its continuity with the fenestrated endothelial lining, which is shown better in Fig. 2. The fat-storing cell has numerous and large fat droplets and is located in the space of Disse. The Kupffer cell (of which only a fraction is shown here) normally has the characteristics of a macrophage, which consist of pseudopodia, lysosomes, and a variable shape. Abbreviations used in Figs 1–5: ci, cilium; co, collagen bundle; Ec, endothelial cell; end or e, endothelial lining; f, fat droplet; Fsc, fat-storing cell; g, Golgi apparatus; Kc, Kupffer cell; L, sinusoidal lumen; m, mitochodrion; N, nucleus; Pc, parenchymal cell; R, rod-cored vesicle in a pit cell; s, lysosomes; SD, space of Disse. All figures are from perfusion-fixed rat liver.

the parenchymal cells (Koop, JPharmExpTher, 1991; 258:1072). These observations lead to the conclusion that sinusoidal cells might share some functions with parenchymal cells, but normally will exert their specific functions in a well-differentiated functional and histological unit together with the parenchymal cells.

Endothelial cells

Endothelial cells constitute a sieve (Fig. 2), filtering the fluids which are exchanged between the sinusoidal lumen and the space of Disse (Horn, Hepatol, 1987; 7:77). Endothelial fenestrae measure 150 to 175 nm in transmission electron microscopy preparations, occur at a frequency of 9 to 13/μm^2, and occupy 6 to 8 per cent of the total endothelial surface in scanning electron microscopy preparations

(Wisse, Hepatol, 1985; 5:683). Endothelial fenestrae have a lobular gradient in diameter and frequency along a portal to central axis (Wisse, Hepatol, 1985; 5:683), resulting in a higher porosity in centrolobular regions. The diameter of fenestrae can be influenced by different agents, such as serotonin, CCl$_4$, alcohol, nicotine, pantethine, and pressure (Horn, 1987; Fraser, BrJExpPath, 1988; 69:345; Braet, LabInvest, 1994; 70:944; Braet, JMicrosc, 1996; 181: 10; Fraser, p.335 in reference 11).[15,16] Recently, endothelial fenestrae were visualized in endothelial cells with atomic force microscopy straight after fixation *in vitro*, before further preparation for scanning electron microscopy. In principle, this type of microscopy has the potential for studying fenestrae in living endothelial cells *in vitro*.

The fenestrated lining blocks the passage of particles larger than

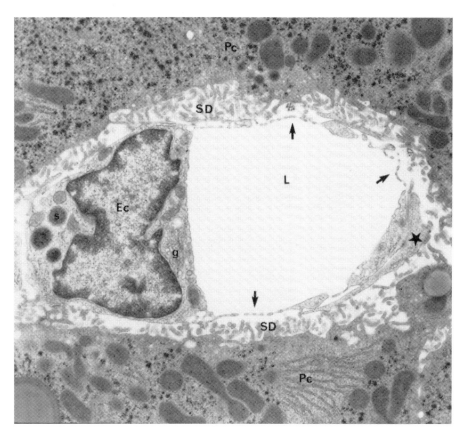

Fig. 2. An endothelial cell surrounding the sinusoidal lumen. The endothelial lining is clearly fenestrated and separates the space of Disse from the lumen. It is thought that all transport between the lumen and the parenchymal cells has to pass through this filter. The endothelial lining seems to be supported by processes of fat-storing cells (asterisk). Endothelial cells of the sinusoids have a high endocytotic and digestive capacity, here reflected by the presence of lysosomes, which are quite abundant in these cells. For abbreviations see Fig. 1.

about 0.2 μm, such as chylomicrons and their remnants (Naito, CellTissRes, 1978; 190:371; Wright, Artscler, 1983; 3:344). Chylomicron remnants that enter the space of Disse have selectively lost their triglycerides and are enriched in cholesterol and cholesterol esters (Wisse, Hepatol, 1985; 5:683; Fraser, Hepatol, 1995; 21:863). Perturbations of the endothelium influence the metabolism of lipoproteins (Fraser, Hepatol, 1995; 21:863). The transport of chylomicron remnants will also mediate the influx of vitamin A to the parenchymal and fat-storing cells (Blomhoff, PNAS, 1982; 79: 7326; Hendriks, Hepatol, 1988; 8:276), which determines the level of activation of fat-storing cells and fibrogenesis in liver tissue. In addition, the uptake of cholesterol by parenchymal cells inhibits the *de novo* synthesis of cholesterol in the liver and contributes to both the production of bile acids and the synthesis of lipoproteins (VLDL). We think that the hepatic uptake of cholesterol is controlled by fenestrae during the access of chylomicron remnants to the space of Disse. The fenestrae are therefore thought to play an important role in the balance and distribution of lipids, cholesterol, and vitamin A.

It is known that rabbits have smaller fenestrae than rats (Wright, Artscler, 1983; 3:344), which might explain why these animals are more sensitive to atherosclerosis, supposing they have equally sized circulating lipoprotein particles. Smaller fenestrae cause cholesterol-rich remnants to circulate longer before they are taken up by the liver. Acute ethanol administration opens the fenestrae,[15]

which supports the admission of fat and the development of fatty liver. Partial hepatectomy (66 per cent) induces a 10-fold increase in porosity of the endothelial lining and a 20-fold increase of fat droplet volume in parenchymal cells (Morsiani, Hepatol, 1995; 21: 539). To the contrary, livers from long-term alcohol-fed animals showed a massive loss of fenestrae. Endotoxin (lipopolysaccharide or endotoxin) administration also decreased fenestration and accentuated the alcohol alterations (Sarphie, AlcoholClinExpRes, 1995; 19:221). Chronic alcohol abuse defenestrates the endothelial lining (Horn, Hepatol, 1987; 7:77) resulting in hyperlipidaemia (Clark, Lancet, 1988; 26:1225) and inhibits transport of cholesterol and vitamin A to parenchymal and fat-storing cells. Smoking of cigarettes or nicotine narrows the fenestrae (Fraser, BrJExpPath, 1988; 69:345), which might contribute to coronary disease. It might be concluded that the present data indicate a role for the fenestrae in the distribution of cholesterol and other components of lipoproteins, such as vitamin A and triglycerides, within tissues and cells. It is, however, difficult to assess the long-term role of the liver sieve in the balance of triglycerides, cholesterol, cholesterol esters, and vitamin A in different body compartments such as the vessel wall, blood, liver, and bile.

The rat liver sinusoid is a quite narrow type of capillary, with a diameter in the range of 5 to 7 μm. White blood cells overlap or exceed this size (Wisse, Hepatol, 1985; 5:683), resulting in regular, mechanical interaction between blood cells and the sinusoidal wall or straightforward plugging, as can be seen by *in vivo* microscopy. This interaction results in two physiologically relevant phenomena— endothelial massage and forced sieving (Wisse, Hepatol, 1985; 5:683). These are considered to be driving forces in the exchange of particles and fluids between the blood and the space of Disse with the parenchymal cells. Forced sieving is promoting the escape of lipoprotein particles into the space of Disse, whereas endothelial massage is supporting the mixing, transport, and refreshing of fluids within the space of Disse (Wisse, Hepatol, 1985; 5:683). Flow resistance decreases from zone 1 to 3. The narrow diameter and the tortuous path of sinusoids and resistance factors appear to contribute to the slow velocity in zone 1 (Komatsu, MicrovascRes, 1990; 40:1). Due to the narrowness and tortuosity of the periportal sinusoids, the interaction with white blood cells is greatest in zone 1, the periportal region (Wisse, SEM, 1983; iii: 1441).

Because of the limited porosity (<10 per cent) of the endothelial cells, they constitute a barrier which protects the parenchymal cells from direct contact with the blood. Endothelial cells might be involved in the protection of parenchymal cells from viral infections (Kirn, Biomedicine, 1978; 29:25), because a viral particle, having a diameter of about 45 nm and more, will be inhibited from reaching the parenchymal cell by the presence of the lining together with defensive cells, such as the Kupffer cells. Keller (p.308 in reference 11) demonstrated an antiviral activity in cocultures of endothelial and parenchymal cells after a stimulus with endotoxin, which induces the release of interleukin 1 (**IL-1**) and interferon from endothelial cells. In contrast, endothelial cells were found to be permissive for mouse hepatitis virus 3 (Steffan, Hepatol, 1995; 22: 395).

Fenestrae are surrounded by a filamentous, fenestrae-associated cytoskeleton ring with a thickness of 16 nm. The diameter of this ring is narrowed during serotonin-induced contraction. When endothelial cells *in vitro* are treated with cytochalasin B or latrunculin A, the number of fenestrae is doubled in about 10 min; at the same time, each of the newly formed fenestrae is provided with a (new) fenestrae-associated cytoskeleton ring (Braet, Hepatol, 1995; 21:180; Braet, Hepatol, 1996; 24:627). Cytochalasin B and latrunculin A interfere strongly with the actin cytoskeleton by different mechanisms, leading to the conclusion that the actin cytoskeleton is important in the numerical dynamics of endothelial fenestrae. Because the fenestrae-associated cytoskeleton ring opens and closes like fenestrae in response to ethanol and serotonin treatment, and at the same time becomes thinner or thicker, it is suggested that this ring is composed of a contractile protein, probably regulating the size changes of the fenestrae. The contraction of fenestrae after serotonin administration is associated with an increase of Ca^{2+}, derived from extracellular sources, by way of a serotonin-activated channel (Brauneis, BBResComm, 1992; 186: 1560).

Sinusoidal endothelial cells possess Fc receptors II (Tomita, Hepatol, 1994; 20:317) and III, but there is no direct evidence for antigen presentation by these cells. The monoclonal antibody 2E1 against the Fc receptor II reacts with endothelial cells, except in the periportal area (Muro, AmJPath, 1993; 143:105). Circulating immune complexes were found to be ingested by Kupffer cells and endothelial cells, according to Fc receptor distribution (Ito,

VirchArchCP, 1990; 58:417; Kosugi, JHepatol, 1992; 16:106). Endothelial cells appear to be a major site of IgM catabolism (Chrones, ArchBiochemBiophys, 1995; 319:63). A monoclonal antibody SE-1 against a surface antigen on rat sinusoidal endothelial cells did not cross-react with other types of endothelial cells or non-endothelial cells (Ohmura, Cytochemistry, 1993; 41:1253). Antisinusoidal endothelial cell antibody occurred in the sera of patients with autoimmune hepatitis type 1 (Han, DigDisSci, 1995; 40:1213). Endothelial cells also express CD14, involved in endotoxin binding, together with CD4 and intercellular adhesion molecule 1 (**ICAM-1**), which may be involved in the adhesion of Kupffer cells (Scoazec, Hepatol, 1991; 14:789).

Endothelial cells possess specialized endocytotic mechanisms in addition to receptors for mannose/N-acetylglucosamine, N-acetylneuraminic acid, and scavenger receptors (for a review see De Leeuw, p.94 in reference 11), together supporting a well-developed endocytotic apparatus. In morphometric studies it was found that endothelial cells possess about 45 per cent of the volume of all pinocytotic vesicles in the liver (Blouin, JCellBiol, 1977; 72:441). Because of the presence of these receptors, a number of substances are taken up specifically by endothelial cells, such as transferrin, caeruloplasmin, transcobalamine II, glucosaminoglucans, modified high-density lipoprotein (**HDL**) and low-density lipoprotein (**LDL**), formaldehyde-treated serum albumin, liver lipase, collagen, remnant ApoE, very low-density lipoprotein (**VLDL**), horseradish peroxidase, hyaluronic acid, chondroitin sulphate, lysosomal hydrolases, invertase, amylase A, asialoorosomucoid, and ovalbumin (Praaning-Van Dalen, FEBSLett, 1982; 141:229; Eskild, JGastro, 1987; 22:1263; Praaning-Van Dalen, Hepatol, 1987; 7:672; De Leeuw, p.94 in 11; Smedsrod, p.69 in reference 11).

Besides specific uptake, endothelial cells have the capacity to endocytose all kinds of molecules and small particles up to the size of 0.1 μm (Wisse, p.33 in reference 17). This capacity, together with the presence of fenestrae without a diaphragm and the absence of a regular basal lamina, makes these endothelial cells different from other types of endothelial cells in the body. Endothelial cells in culture still display their main morphological and functional characteristics, such as fenestrae and pinocytotic vesicles, and respond to agents such as alcohol and serotonin (Steffan, Hepatol, 1987; 7: 1230; Braet, LabInvest, 1994; 70:944; Braet, JMicrosc, 1996; 181: 10). Endothelial cells cultured in collagen gels invaded the gel and formed three-dimensional tubes when laminin was present. Without laminin, the cells stayed on top of the gel. Endothelial cells cultured on Matrigel had many fenestrae and formed tubes (10 μm) (Shakado, Hepatol, 1995; 22:969), indicating that extracellular matrix components also determine the phenotype of endothelial cells.

Smedsrod demonstrated the clearance of procollagen and (denatured) collagen by high-affinity receptors on endothelial cells (Smedsrod, p.69 in reference 11). Also, the C-terminal propeptide of type I procollagen is rapidly cleared, mainly by endothelial cells through their mannose receptors (Smedsrod, BiochemJ, 1990; 271: 345). The NH_2-terminal propeptide of type I procollagen appears to be cleared by the scavenger receptor of endothelial cells (Melkko, JExpMed, 1994; 179:405). It might be assumed that endothelial cells have the task of protecting the circulation from components of the extracellular matrix which have been secreted into the space of Disse by fat-storing cells. Collagen is well known to be an inducer of platelet aggregation and the presence of such products in the sinusoidal lumen might disturb liver blood flow. Uptake *in vitro* by endothelial cells was mainly mannose specific, whereas uptake in parenchymal and Kupffer cells was mainly galactose specific. Apparently there are more mannose receptors on endothelial cells than on Kupffer cells. Whereas endothelial cells have become well known for their endocytotic capacity, they have also been shown to display retroendocytosis. This endocytosis involves a partial processing of ingested molecules, instead of a total digestion within lysosomes. The rate of retroendocytosis was found to be about four times higher in endothelial than in parenchymal cells. Binding to the scavenger receptor causes decreased retroendocytosis. Retro-endocytosis is based on incomplete dissociation of ligands from receptors before receptor recycling to the cell surface (Magnusson, BiochemJ, 1992; 287:241). Tumour necrosis factor-α and IL-1β enhance endocytosis in endothelial cells via the scavenger and mannose receptors (Martinez, BBResComm, 1995; 212:235).

Clearance of hyaluronic acid appears to be a useful test for liver endothelial cell function (Deaciuc, Hepatol, 1993; 17:266; Imamura, Gastro, 1995; 109:189), for instance in the case of ischaemic liver preservation (Sutto, JHepatol, 1994; 20:611). The uptake of hyaluronan by endothelial cells is receptor mediated (Fraser, ExpCellRes, 1991; 197:8), and is inhibited by heparin, which competes for the receptor (Deaciuc, Hepatol, 1993; 17:266). The hyaluronan receptor is composed of a heterodimer (Yannariello, JBC, 1992; 267: 20451). Antiserum against a 100-kDa protein that binds hyaluronan on endothelial cells inhibits the binding of hyaluronan (Forsberg, BBActa, 1991; 1078:12). The elevated plasma hyaluronan in septicaemia cannot be attributed to a change in receptors on endothelial cells (Fraser, ExpCellRes, 1991; 197:8). Three days after liver transplantation in rats, endothelial cells of rejectors showed elevated hyaluronic acid levels and endothelialitis. Impairment of endothelial cell function can be measured by hyaluronan clearance and occurs earlier than traditional indicators (Yokoi, Transpl, 1994; 57:27).

Endothelial cells seem to be vulnerable cells; a fact which becomes obvious during preparation for electron microscopy[3] and during procedures for liver transplantation (Fratte, Hepatol, 1991; 13:1173; Rauen, Transpl, 1993; 55:469). Endothelial cells are apparently sensitive to ischaemia and elevated pressure. Preparation for electron microscopy preferably should be performed by perfusion fixation at physiological pressure and room temperature, starting within seconds after laparotomy and cannulating the portal vein. This seems to be obligatory for the preservation of the fine structure of the endothelial lining, such as intact fenestrae and sieve plates (Wisse, Hepatol, 1985; 5:683).[3,18] With retarded perfusion, or immersion fixation, the endothelial lining will develop large, irregular gaps; probably, the endothelial cytoskeleton is destabilized and fenestrae fuse and turn into gaps. Comparable effects occur during the start of warm oxygenated reperfusion after cold ischaemic storage, which apparently damages endothelial cells (Caldwell, Hepatol, 1991; 13:83; Fratte, Hepatol, 1991; 13:1173; Rauen, Transpl, 1993; 55:469; Carles, Liver, 1994; 14:50). Neutrophils and Kupffer cells contribute to the damage by releasing O_2^- (Jaeschke, JLeukBiol, 1992; 52:377). In severe cases, reperfusion injury leads to complete de-endothelialization and the formation of blebs by parenchymal cells. These changes occur when warm reperfusion starts, which probably indicates that switching from a cold anoxic state to a warm oxygenated state induces the damage. Parenchymal cells seem to be intact and surviving even after 48 to 96 h of cold

storage (Lemasters, p.277 in reference 11). Addition of potassium cyanide (KCN) to the perfusion fluid increased survival of the endothelial cells (Rauen, Transpl, 1993; 55:469).

Endotoxin can reduce the porosity of the endothelium to 40 per cent, with a decrease in diameter and number of fenestrae (Dobbs, Liver, 1994; 14:230). Endothelial cells can probably change into continuous endothelial cells and start the formation of a basal lamina, a process called capillarization, which occurs during fibrosis (Martinez, Hepatol, 1991; 14:864; Arai, Gastro, 1993; 104:1466; Dobbs, Liver, 1994; 14:230). Factor VIII-related antigen and UEA-1 appear in endothelial cells during capillarization in chronic liver diseases (Urashima, Alcohol, 1993; 28:77). Capillarization should lead to decreased parenchymal cell uptake (Martinez, Hepatol, 1991; 14:864).

A variety of lectin–FITC complexes have been used to demonstrate the presence of glucose, mannose, galactose, *N*-acetyl-neuraminic acid, and *N*-acetyl-glucosamine reactive sites on endothelial cells, especially in the periportal zone (Barbera Guillem, Hepatol, 1991; 14:131). Endothelial cells in normal liver possess limited adhesion molecules, but express two integrins, α_1, β_1 and α_5, β_1. No selectin could be detected in normal cells, but endotoxin-induced massive synthesis of E- and P-selectin in endothelial cells and Kupffer cells (Essani, BBResComm, 1995; 211:74). In normal liver, the selectins ELAM-1 and CD62 are present on portal and central vein endothelial cells (Steinhoff, AmJPath, 1993; 142:481). These endothelial cells possess a basal lamina, but lack fenestrae. LFA-1 and VLA-4 seem to be important for lymphocyte–endothelial adhesion in liver sinusoids (Garcia-Barcina, AmJPath, 1995; 146:1406). ICAM-1 may be responsible for the accumulation and proliferation of inflammatory cells in the liver of MRL/lpr mice (Ohteki, ImmunolLett, 1993; 36:145). Without stimulation, ICAM-1 was weakly expressed, but after tumour necrosis factor, IL-1, or endotoxin stimulation, the expression of ICAM-1 in endothelial and Kupffer cells was increased (Mccourt, JBC, 1994; 269: 30081; Ohira, JHepatol, 1994; 20:729; Essani, BBResComm, 1995; 211:74). ICAM-1 was also expressed on sinusoidal endothelial cells of diseased MRL/lpr mice (Ohteki, ImmunolLett, 1993; 36:145), or could be induced by injection of IL-6. Interestingly, ICAM-1 on rat liver endothelial cells was found to be identical to the hyaluronan receptor (Mccourt, JBC, 1994; 269:30081). The adhesion molecules of endothelial cells are modified during capillarization (Couvelard, AmJPath, 1993; 143:738). Cirrhotic, capillarized endothelial cells displayed PECAM-1 and laminin receptors α_6 β_1 and α_2 β_1 (Couvelard, AmJPath, 1993; 143:738). Treatment of endothelial cell monolayers with lymphoma cells or their conditioned medium (4 to 6 h) enhanced the adhesion of lymphoma cells; this was abolished by anti-IL-1β monoclonal antibody (Yoneda, JpnJCancerRes, 1994; 85:723). Sialyl Le(x), a ligand for ELAM-1 and anti-ELAM-1 monoclonal antibody blocked the enhanced adhesion of lymphoma cells to endothelial cells. Anti-VCAM-1 monoclonal antibody did not affect adhesion (Yoneda, JpnJCancerRes, 1994; 85:723). Tumour cell adhesion to (stimulated) endothelial cells is apparently mediated by ELAM-1 on endothelial cells (Yoneda, JpnJCancerRes, 1994; 85:723).

The release of cytokines and other biologically active substances by endothelial cells is not well known, the focus is typically on Kupffer cells. However, production of platelet-activating factor by endothelial cells is affected by IL-1 and arachidonic acid metabolites

(Mizoguchi, JGastHepatol, 1991; 6:283). Endothelial cells also produce IL-1 and IL-6, with an amount and kinetics similar to Kupffer cells (Feder, JLeukBiol, 1993; 53:126).

Kupffer cells

Kupffer cells (Fig. 3) (or 'Sternzellen', stellate cells) are anchored to or are inserted into the endothelial lining and have irregular outlines, but are basically stellate in shape.[5] The cell surface has microvilli or lamellipodia and a hairy, fuzzy coat after direct osmium fixation, in addition to peculiar invaginations, such as worm-like structures that are apparently involved in endocytosis.[5] In the cytoplasm there are a variety of intracytoplasmic vesicles, mitochondria, an extensive Golgi apparatus, vacuoles, fuzzy-coated vacuoles, and dense bodies, with varying shape, diameter, and electron density. The dense bodies and vacuoles together constitute the well-developed lysosomal apparatus of the Kupffer cell.[5] These cells also have microfilaments, microtubules, and vimentin filaments (Marugg, JStructBiol, 1990; 105:146). Kupffer cells *in situ* do not possess fat droplets, glycogen particles, autophagic vacuoles, or multivesicular bodies.[5] In rat liver, Kupffer cells can be stained for peroxidase, which shows a positive reaction product in dispersed cisternae of rough endoplasmic reticulum, the nuclear envelope, and annulate lamellae. This staining differs from monocytes, which show a positive reaction for peroxidase only in granules.[5] In the rat, therefore, Kupffer cells can be characterized by electron microscopy, staining for peroxidase, and the uptake of latex particles,[5] in addition to immunostaining with ED2. These characteristics distinguish Kupffer cells from other sinusoidal cells and monocytes.[19] However, these criteria should be used with caution because endothelial cells also endocytose latex particles *in vitro* (Dan, ExpCellRes, 1985; 158:75; Steffan, Hepatol, 1986; 6:830) and show peroxidase staining in the mouse. Kupffer cells form the largest population of macrophages in the body and are located preferentially in the periportal area of the liver lobule (Sleyster, LabInvest, 1982; 47:484; Bouwens, Hepatol, 1986; 6:718). They form the centre of erythroblastic islands during fetal haemopoiesis (Morris, JCellBiol, 1988; 106:649; Naito, p.497 in reference 17). Kupffer cells can be isolated, purified, and cultured.[8,10]

Kupffer cells function as a waste receptacle for all kinds of old, unnecessary, damaged, altered, or foreign material circulating in the blood, such as old blood cells, cellular debris, parasites, bacteria, viruses, and tumour cells. Kupffer cells bear Fc receptors (Muro, Gastro, 1987; 93:1078; Tomita, Hepatol, 1994; 20:317; Tanikawa, p.288 in reference 11) and complement receptors (Munthe-Kaas, ExpCellRes, 1976; 103:201) on their surface and react vigorously to foreign material by attachment and phagocytosis. It has been demonstrated also that fibrin fibres attach to Kupffer cells during disseminated intravascular coagulation, but no phagocytosis occurs, although the cells take up fibrin degradation products (Emeis, AmJPath, 1981; 103:337).

Different endocytotic mechanisms have been described (Munthe-Kaas, ExpCellRes, 1976; 103:201; Wisse, p.33 in reference 17). Coated pits, macropinocytotic vesicles, worm-like structures, fuzzy-coated vacuoles, and phagosomes are well-known instruments for the uptake of intravenously injected molecules and particles of various sizes. These structures, which so obviously play a role during endocytosis of visible marker particles, are also present in the livers of untreated animals and one might ask what these structures are endocytosing in normal conditions. Which circulating molecules and particles are normally taken up by endocytotic structures in the liver? We do not know.

Apparently, phagocytosis by Kupffer cells is facilitated by opsonization of particles by plasma fibronectin or opsonin. Phagocytosis of gelatinized red blood cells was increased by preopsonization with fibronectin (Cardarelli, JLeukBiol, 1990; 48:426). The binding of serum fibronectin to Kupffer cells was demonstrated to be specific; about 2800 to 3500 binding sites for fibronectin were found on the Kupffer cell membrane (Cardarelli, JLeukBiol, 1990; 48:426). Receptors such as the galactose particle receptor of the Kupffer cell (Schlepper-Schäfer, BloodCells, 1988; 14:259; Hardonk, p.434 in reference 11) and the scavenger receptor of the endothelial cell (Eskild, JGastro, 1987; 22:1263; De Leeuw, p.94 in reference 11) are involved in the uptake of molecules and particles with different properties, such as chemical composition, surface charge, and fluid or solid phase. Observations indicate that D-galactosyl groups of plasma fibronectin react with the lectin-like galactose-specific binding site of membrane-associated C-reactive protein and integrin receptor(s) synthesized by and present on Kupffer cells (Kempka, JImmunol, 1990; 144:1004; Kolb-Bachofen, CarbohydrRes, 1991; 213:201; KolbBachofen, JCI, 1992; 90:1819; Egenhofer, Hepatol, 1993; 18:1216).

It has been demonstrated that sinusoidal cells in cholesterol-fed rabbits took up as much LDL as parenchymal cells did, on a per cell basis. In controls, parenchymal cells took up about six times more LDL per cell than endothelial or Kupffer cells. Thus, 30 per cent of the hepatic uptake of LDL in the cholesterol-fed rabbits was by sinusoidal cells, compared with 6 per cent in controls (Nenseter, JLipRes, 1992; 33:867). LDL was bound to the specific LDL receptor on human parenchymal and Kupffer cells. The lysosomal degradation of LDL by human Kupffer cells was 18-fold higher (on a per milligram of cellular protein basis). Kupffer cells also clear Ox-LDL from the circulation by a specific binding protein (Derijke, JBC, 1994; 269:824).

Alcohol was found to depress the endocytotic capacity of cultured Kupffer cells (Earnest, p.325 in reference 11), as described earlier for the reticuloendothelial system. The reason for such a depression is less clear. Kupffer cells specifically take up endotoxin (Ruiter, LabInvest, 1981; 45:38; Brouwer, JHepatol, 1988; 6:36; Van Bossuyt, JHepatol, 1988; 7:45,325; Fox, p.305 in reference 11; Van Bossuyt, p.297 in reference 11). This uptake cannot be saturated (Fox, p.305 in reference 11), nor can it be influenced by colchicin; it is temperature dependent, inhibited by deoxyglucose, and requires ATP. Kupffer cells are negative for CD14, a receptor for endotoxin and endotoxin-binding protein (Tomita, Hepatol, 1994; 20:317). After the uptake, Kupffer cells partly digest the endotoxin and secrete a product that contains less sugar and more lipid, but which is still toxic and is probably identical with the lipid A component of endotoxin (Fox, p.305 in reference 11). Parenchymal cells might take up this material and finally detoxify the endotoxin, or secrete what remains of it into the bile together with bile salts (Van Bossuyt, JHepatol, 1988; 7:325; Ueno, p.293 in reference 11). It has become an accepted view that endotoxin toxicity is indirect and mainly based on the secretory products of Kupffer cells or other macrophages, rather than a direct toxic effect of endotoxin *per se*. It has

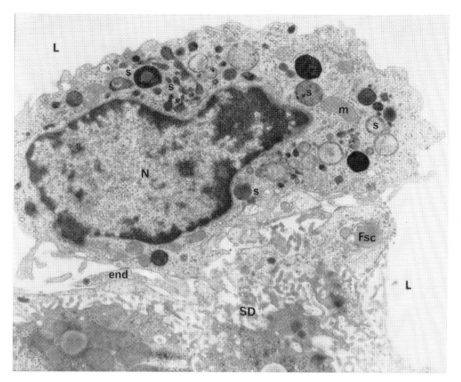

Fig. 3. A Kupffer cell showing its many lysosomes of different density, shape, and diameter, indicating the enormous endocytotic and digestive capacity of these cells. Endothelial cells have lysosomes that are more uniform in shape and diameter. Kupffer cells can penetrate the endothelium and touch the parenchymal or fat-storing cells. For abbreviations see Fig. 1.

been demonstrated that endotoxin does not induce any toxic effects on Kupffer cells in culture (Van Bossuyt, p.388 in reference 11).

Kupffer cell activation has been the subject of many studies over the past decade. Endotoxin of *Escherichia coli* or other bacteria is the most frequently used stimulator to activate Kupffer cells. Besides endotoxin, other activating substances or conditions have been reported, such as sepsis or shock (Ertel, Blood, 1991; 78:1781), zymosan, glucan (Sherwood, JLeukBiol, 1987; 42:69), OK432, interferon-γ, arachidonic acid (Eyhorn, JHepatol, 1988; 6:23), phorbol meristate acetate, colony-stimulating factor, A23187, tumour necrosis factor, and liposomal muramyldipeptide.

Signs of activation are considered to be the release of a list of products, mostly cytokines, mitosis, and increased surface roughness. Activated Kupffer cells secrete products with potent biological effects, such as oxygen radical species or superoxide anions including H_2O_2, nitric oxide, proteases (Decker, p.171 in reference 11), tumour necrosis factor, IL-1, IL-6, IL-10 (Knolle, JHepatol, 1995; 22:226), transforming growth factor-β, interferon-α or -γ (Decker, EurJBioch, 1990; 192:245; Decker, p.171 in reference 11), eicosanoids such as prostaglandin D_2, hydroxyeicosatetraenoic acid (HETE), prostaglandin A_2, prostaglandin E_2, and arachidonic acid (Duyster, JCellBiochem, 1992; 48:288).

It is obvious that some of the products released by Kupffer cells are also activators of the cells themselves and therefore take part in an autocrine loop. On the other hand, the released products can be part of a negative feedback loop and are sometimes also able to depress the release of other products (Decker, p.171 in reference 11). For instance, tumour necrosis factor stimulates the production of prostaglandin E_2, which inhibits the release of tumour necrosis

factor in its turn; interferon-γ stimulates prostaglandin E_2 production and enhances tumour necrosis factor production, but suppresses IL-1 release (Kawada, Liver, 1991; 11:42), whereas IL-6 release is suppressed by prostaglandin E_2 (Callery, JSurgRes, 1990; 48:523). Inhibitors like indomethacin, dexamethasone, chloroquine, staurosporin, K252a, acetylsalicylic acid, and polymyxin are reported mostly to inhibit, but sometimes also to stimulate, the release of a variety of cytokines.

Kupffer cells are thought to be the only source of tumour necrosis factor-α in the sinusoid (Hoffmann, JHepatol, 1994; 20: 122). The pattern and time course of this and other products seem to depend on the stimulus, meaning that different stimuli initiate the secretion of a different spectrum of products with a dissimilar time course (Hoedemakers, JImmunother, 1994; 15:265). Unstimulated Kupffer cells produce negligible IL-6 and prostaglandin E_2 (Callery, JSurgRes, 1990; 48:523). Kupffer cells treated with endotoxin show a rapid but transient release of tumour necrosis factor (Busam, JHepatol, 1990; 11:367; Peters, EurJBioch, 1990; 191:583; Chensue, AmJPathol, 1991; 138:395), followed by a slow, steady synthesis of prostaglandin E_2 (Callery, 1990; Peters, 1990) and IL-1β, IL-1α, and IL-6 (Busam, JHepatol, 1990; 11:367; Callery, 1990; Chensue, 1991; Ayala, JSurgRes, 1992; 52:635; Callery, CircShock, 1992; 37:185).

Nitric oxide is released from Kupffer cells after stimulation with interferon-γ or endotoxin, which also causes the release of tumour necrosis factor-α and prostaglandin E_2. Neither tumour necrosis factor-α nor IL-1β stimulates nitric oxide synthesis. Antitumour necrosis factor-α antibody as well as antiprostaglandin E_2 antibodies reduce the release of nitric oxide after endotoxin stimulation. The effect of endotoxin on nitric oxide production seems to be in part due to the stimulating effect of prostaglandin E_2 and some cytokines produced by Kupffer cells (Gaillard, Pathobio, 1991; 59:280; Gaillard, BiolChemHS, 1992; 373:897). In another study, prostaglandin E_2 was found to inhibit the nitric oxide synthesis of Kupffer cells in a dose-dependent fashion (Harbrecht, JSurgRes, 1995; 58: 625). Nitric oxide derived from Kupffer cells was also triggered by contact with hepatoma cells and probably induced killing of tumour cells (Curley, JLeukBiol, 1993; 53:715; Kurose, CancerRes, 1993; 53:2676).

The activation and cytokine release situation seems to be different when rat and human Kupffer cells are compared. Endotoxin-stimulated human Kupffer cells released IL-1, IL-6, tumour necrosis factor-α, transforming growth factor-β, and prostaglandin E_2. In contrast to rat Kupffer cells, no nitric oxide production could be detected. Indomethacin prevented prostaglandin E_2 release, while upregulating tumour necrosis factor-α, IL-1, and IL-6, but not transforming growth factor-β. In human Kupffer cells, the cytokine response to endotoxin was not downregulated by prostaglandin E_2. Many features are shared by rat and human Kupffer cells, but differences apparently exist (Roland, AnnSurg, 1994; 219:389). Freshly isolated human Kupffer cells also secrete IL-10 in response to endotoxin. IL-10 downregulates IL-6 and tumour necrosis factor-α by Kupffer cells after endotoxin stimulation (Knolle, JHepatol, 1995; 22:226). Kupffer cells are activated in liver diseases as shown by the novel expression of CD14 and Fc γRI (Tomita, Hepatol, 1994; 20:317).

Kupffer cell secretory products can be toxic for the liver parenchyma (Schlayer, JHepatol, 1988; 7:239; Shiratori, p.313 in reference 11), showing cellular ballooning and blebbing necrosis, causing fever, and blocking biochemical processes. The release of tumour necrosis factor (Hoffmann, JHepatol, 1994; 20:122) induces the swelling of endothelial cells and the adherence of white blood cells (Schlayer, JHepatol, 1988; 7:239; Van Bossuyt, CellTissRes, 1988; 251:205; Decker, p.171 in reference 11). Tumour necrosis factor appears to induce the adherence of polymorphonuclear leucocytes to endothelial cells, after which the leucocytes might degranulate and release oxygen radicals, causing further damage to the tissue (Schlayer, JHepatol, 1988; 7:239). Acute-phase reactants seem to protect the tissue against these toxic effects of tumour necrosis factor. Fat-storing cells (Ramadori, p.49 in reference 11) and parenchymal cells (Kurokawa, JClinLabImmunol, 1988; 25: 131) were both found to produce the acute-phase product α_2-macroglobulin.

Long-term activation by particulate glucan leads to the formation of hepatic granulomas. In monocytopenic mice, Kupffer cells formed granulomas and transformed into epithelioid cells and further into multinuclear giant cells (Naito, LabInvest, 1991; 64:664; Yamada, JLeukBiol, 1991; 47:195).

The interaction between bile acids and endotoxin has been reported (Ueno, p.293 in reference 11; Van Bossuyt, p.297 in reference 11). Patients with cholestasis or cirrhosis have a higher incidence of endotoxaemia (Tanikawa, p.288 in reference 11). Endotoxin clearance by Kupffer cells is inhibited by bile acids (Tanikawa, p.288 in reference 11; Thomas, p.302 in reference 11; Ueno, p. 293 in reference 11). Phagocytosis by Kupffer cells *in vitro* is also inhibited by the presence of bile acids (Takiguchi, VirchArchCP, 1988; 54:303; Tanikawa, p.288 in reference 11; Van Bossuyt, p.297 in

reference 11). On the other hand, endotoxin inhibits bile secretion. Endotoxin and bile salts therefore mutually inhibit each other's clearance or secretion. Patients with jaundice have, by definition, low intestinal concentrations of bile acids. Bile acids are known to inhibit bacterial growth, so that in cholestasis, more bacteria and more endotoxin are produced. It has been observed that the uptake of endotoxin from the intestine increases in cholestasis. Apparently, bile acids inhibit the uptake of endotoxin by the intestinal mucosa. Bile acids form complexes with endotoxin, which then loses its toxicity and can no longer be demonstrated by the *Lymulus* lysate test (Van Bossuyt, p.297 in reference 11). In conclusion, the complexing of endotoxin and bile acids renders a non-toxic product in the blood, bile, and intestinal lumen, inhibits the uptake by the mucosa and Kupffer cell, and promotes the removal of endotoxin in the faeces. These observations imply that a vicious circle of increasing amounts of endotoxin and bile acids can start as soon as the concentration of one of these products is raised in the portal blood. These data suggest that oral substitution of certain bile acids or endotoxin-complexing agents might forestall the increase of intestinal endotoxin uptake and endotoxaemia in cholestasis.

Despite the use of immunophenotyping with monoclonal antibodies, the controversy concerning the origin and kinetics of Kupffer cells persists. Different models are used to study either the proliferation of resident macrophages or the influx of macrophages into the liver. Several authors have confirmed the mitotic potential of Kupffer cells *in situ* (Bouwens, Hepatol, 1984; 4:213; Bouwens, JLeukBiol, 1986; 39:687; Yamada, JLeukBiol, 1990; 47:195; Koudstaal, p.281 in reference 11; Naito, p.394 in reference 11; Naito, p.497 in reference 17).[6] Naito (p.394 in reference 11) reported the proliferation of Kupffer cells during severe monocytopenia caused by strontium-89. Freudenberg (VirchArchA, 1986; 410:1) presented evidence for the recruitment of sinusoidal macrophages from the bone marrow after heavy irradiation of the resident Kupffer cell population and reported that, following bone marrow grafting, most liver macrophages were of the donor type, whereas after 35 weeks the donor-type cells had disappeared from the liver. Other tissues, such as the spleen, bone marrow, and yolk sac, might also provide precursors of resident macrophages (Bouwens, JLeukBiol, 1986; 39:687; Bouwens, CellTissKinet, 1986; 19:217; Wacker, VirchArchCP, 1986; 51:71; Daemen, p.400 in reference 11). Kupffer cells also proliferate and migrate to injured areas in the early stages of fibrosis (Geerts, JHepatol, 1986; 6:50). According to Hardonk and Daemen (Daemen, p.400 in reference 11; Hardonk, p.434 in reference 11), local proliferation and extrahepatic recruitment occurs after intravenous injection of liposome-encapsulated muramyldipeptide, which also induces activation.

The reduced production of macrophage colony-stimulating factor in the liver of protein-deprived mice results in numerical reduction, maturation failure, and decreased proliferative capacity of Kupffer cells. The administration of this factor re-establishes the proliferative capacity of Kupffer cells (Honda, LabInvest, 1995; 72: 696), whereas rhIL-2 does not (Hoedemakers, Hepatol, 1994; 19: 666).

The conclusion of Bouwens (Hepatol, 1984; 4:213) still holds: Kupffer cells can proliferate locally and can also be supplemented by the immigration of resident-type macrophages from an extrahepatic origin. The relative importance of these mechanisms seems to depend on experimental or pathological conditions; local proliferation is prominent during liver regeneration, whereas extrahepatic recruitment seems to be important when the Kupffer cell population has been wiped out. The evidence of cell population kinetic studies is compatible with the existence of two types of macrophages in the liver: a resident type (like the Kupffer cell) and a monocyte-derived type of macrophage. To distinguish these two: Kupffer cells have rough endoplasmic reticulum that is positive for peroxidase, they are strongly phagocytic for 0.8-μm latex particles, and have a 'large' and irregular cytoplasm with many lysosomes, whereas monocytes have peroxidase-positive granules, are less phagocytic for latex when in the liver, are smaller, and have a different morphology.[19] Kupffer cells as well as monocytes are able to proliferate in hepatic sinusoids (Bouwens, JLeukBiol, 1985; 37:531; Wacker, VirchArchCP, 1986; 51:71; Daemen, p.400 in reference 11; Koudstaal, p.281 in reference 11) and both can probably migrate into and out of the liver.

Isolated Kupffer cells can be separated into classes of decreasing size by elutriation, reflecting a portal to central vein gradient (Sleyster, LabInvest, 1982; 47:484; Hardonk, p.434 in reference 11). Smaller, centrolobular Kupffer cells express more Ia, release more IL-1, possess a lower phagocytic capacity, and show increased levels of tumour cytotoxicity for longer periods of time (3 to 4 days) after stimulation with liposomal muramyldipeptide. Larger Kupffer cells ingest more latex, can only be activated to tumour cytotoxicity up to day 2 after stimulation, and secrete more tumour necrosis factor and prostaglandin E_2 (Ito, Liver, 1992; 12:26; Hoedemakers, JImmunother, 1994; 15:265). One of the intriguing questions here is whether or not the small Kupffer cells are precursors of the larger ones.

An interesting experimental tool is given by the elimination of the Kupffer cell population using a single intravenous injection with dichloromethylene diphosphonate liposomes. This treatment selectively eliminates the Kupffer cells from the liver, but not the resident macrophages in other tissues. Within 2 days, repopulation occurs (Van Rooijen, CellTissRes, 1990; 260:215; Bogers, ClinExpImmun, 1991; 85:128; Heuff, CancerImmunTher, 1993; 37:125; Imamura, Gastro, 1995; 109:189). Gadolinium chloride also blocks phagocytosis and eliminates the large Kupffer cells of the periportal zone; this leads to a repopulation starting on day 4 (Hardonk, JLeukBiol, 1992; 52:296). Elimination of Kupffer cells also elucidates their role in tissue damage and experimental situations. The absence of Kupffer cells prevents elevated levels of serum aspartate aminotransferase (**AST**) and liver cell death after the application of CCl_4 (Edwards, ToxApplPharmacol, 1993; 119:275), and also prevents alcohol-induced serum AST, liver tissue fatty changes, inflammation, and necrosis (Adachi, Hepatol, 1994; 20:453). Absence of Kupffer cells does not modify the effect of 24-h cold ischaemia/reperfusion on the rat liver (Imamura, Gastro, 1995; 109:189), but it does promote metastatic tumour growth (Heuff, CancerImmunTher, 1993; 37:125).

During recent years it has become apparent that Kupffer cells, with their repertoire of cytokines, are able to influence parenchymal cell metabolism. Kupffer cell-conditioned medium inhibits albumin synthesis in parenchymal cells. IL-1, IL-6, and tumour necrosis factor-α also inhibit albumin synthesis. IL-6 induces the well-known acute-phase reaction in parenchymal cells (Kowalski, Hepatol, 1992; 16:733).

Fat-storing cells

Fat-storing cells (Fig. 4) (synonyms: Ito cells, lipocytes, peri- or parasinusoidal cells, 'Perizyten', stellate cells) have a morphology similar to fibroblasts, except for the presence of fat droplets. Fat-storing cells are located in the space of Disse and are always separated from the lumen by endothelial cells. They can therefore only communicate with the sinusoidal lumen through the endothelial filter. Long branched processes of the cells underly the endothelial lining (Wake, CellTissRes, 1993; 273:227; Takahashi-Iwanaga, p.59 in reference 12; Wake, p.23 in reference 12) and are studded with thorn-like microprojections. Fat-storing cells contain a number of fat droplets, which store considerable amounts of vitamin A (Hendriks, ExpCellRes, 1985; 160:138; Hendriks, Lipids, 1987; 22:266; Tsutsumi, Hepatol, 1987; 7:277; Yumoto, BiomedRes, 1988; 9:147). On the basis of this vitamin, the cells show a characteristic, quickly fading autofluorescence in the fluorescence microscope. The cells are thought to play a major role in the production of connective tissue components in the normal liver and during fibrosis and cirrhosis. The cells stain for desmin in some species (Yokoi, Hepatol, 1984; 4:709; Burt, JPath, 1986; 150:29; Ogawa, AmJPathol, 1986; 125:611; Tsutsumi, 1987; Ballardini, VirchArchCP, 1988; 56:45; Takase, JHepatol, 1988; 6:267; Wake, 1993; Ballardini, p.462 in reference 11) and α-smooth muscle actin when they become activated. Unmyelinated nerve fibres in the human space of Disse are located close to fat-storing cell processes and parenchymal cells (Bioulac-Sage, JHepatol, 1990; 10:105).

The current interest in fat-storing cell biology is their role in liver fibrosis. An aspect of particular interest is the final outcome of a variety of hepatic diseases: cirrhosis. However, the process can occur at different places in the tissue (periportal, pericentral) and involves several cell types, many cytokines, many different extracellular molecules in various forms of organization (fibrils, aggregates, adhesion molecules), and synthesis as well as degradation, which can be both stimulated or inhibited.

Fat-storing cells display heterogeneity in desmin, α-smooth muscle actin, and cytokeratin staining, as well as the length of dendritic processes and vitamin A storage, relative to their zonal location (Greenwel, LabInvest, 1993; 69:210; Wake, CellTissRes, 1993; 273:227). This has been attributed to clonal heterogeneity (Greenwel, 1993) as fat-storing cell lines could be developed *in vitro* with heterogeneity in proliferation, collagen α-chains, IL-6, and transforming growth factor-β mRNAs (Greenwel, 1993). Some authors report the occurrence of desmin-negative fat-storing cells in pericentral areas and conclude that desmin cannot be used as a specific cell marker (Ballardini, Hepatol, 1994; 19:440). Others report that fat-storing cells in normal liver are devoid of desmin and exceptionally stain for α-smooth muscle actin, in contrast to embryonic or adolescent fat-storing cells (Schmittgraff, AmJPathol, 1991; 138:1233). Freshly isolated fat-storing cells are postive for vimentin, some are positive for desmin, but all are negative for α-smooth muscle actin. Staining for α-smooth muscle actin increases at day 7 of culture (Ramadori, VirchArchCP, 1990; 59:349). In fibrotic liver, septal (fibroblastic) cells are positive for vimentin and desmin and negative for α-smooth muscle actin (Bhunchet, Hepatol, 1992; 16:1452). In adult human liver, fat-storing cells are positive for α-smooth muscle actin (Enzan, VichArchA, 1994; 424:249), but

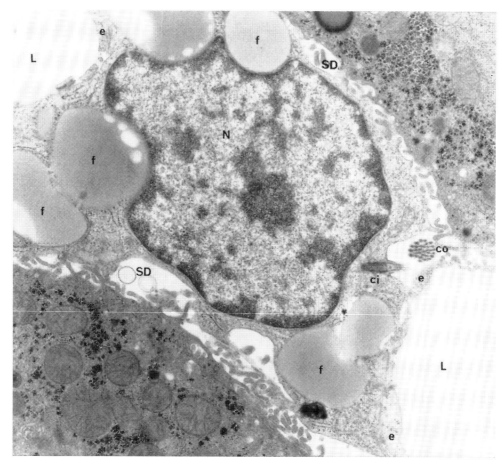

Fig. 4. A fat-storing cell with many and large fat droplets, which are partly dissolved due to the treatment with alcohol in the histological procedure. Fat-storing cells are always located in the space of Disse and are therefore always covered by endothelial cells. In this picture you might notice the presence of a cilium. For abbreviations see Fig. 1.

show no staining for desmin in normal and pathological livers (Enzan, 1994).

Fat-storing cells contain a high percentage of the body's vitamin A. Retinoids are transported from the intestine to the liver within chylomicrons or their remnants, which also carry triglycerides, cholesterol, cholesterol ester, and apoproteins to the parenchymal cells (Blomhoff, PNAS, 1982; 79:7326; Fraser, Hepatol, 1995; 21: 863). Because retinoids are only soluble in lipids, they need special binding proteins to handle them during transport at the cellular level. A number of specific retinoids and their binding proteins have been identified in serum, parenchymal cells, and fat-storing cells (Knook, p.16 in reference 11). It has become obvious that the parenchymal cells represent the first stage of uptake and handling of retinoids (Blomhoff, 1982; Hendriks, Hepatol, 1988; 8:276), whereas the fat-storing cells are the final destination. Endothelial and Kupffer cells do not seem to be directly involved, nor do they possess binding proteins (Senoo, p.29 in reference 11). Rats which were fed a vitamin A-depleted diet did not have fat droplets in their fat-storing cells. Administration of retinoic acid restored the presence of fat droplets (Yumoto, p.33 in reference 11), whereas retinol and/or retinyl ester promoted an increase in the number and diameter of the fat droplets.

The distribution of vitamin A over different cell types might be influenced by disease processes. The importance of this line of

research lies in the fact that vitamin A appears to influence vital cell functions. There is clinical evidence to correlate a high daily intake of vitamin A in any form (food, medication) with the occurrence of fibrosis (Jacques, Gastro, 1979; 76:599). It might be concluded, therefore, that vitamin A in high doses has a toxic influence on parenchymal cells (Seifert, p.43 in reference 11). On the other hand, the level of vitamin A is considerably lower in livers which have been damaged by alcohol abuse and which might proceed to develop fibrosis (Leo, NEJM, 307:597). Since fibrosis and cirrhosis occur as an final stage of a variety of liver pathologies, it might be concluded that fibrosis results from parenchymal cell damage that leads to mesenchymal cell activation. The exact role of vitamin A in these cellular interactions is not yet clear (Koudstaal, p.281 in reference 11).

Fat-storing cells proliferate in conditions such as partial hepatectomy and fibrosis (Burt, JPath, 1986; 150:29; Ogawa, AmJPathol, 1986; 125:611). They can be isolated, but seem to behave differently from endothelial and Kupffer cells in culture because they become activated, proliferate, and produce progressively increasing amounts of extracellular matrix components *in vitro* (De Leeuw, Hepatol, 1984; 4:392; Shiratori, JHepatol, 1986; 3:294; Shiratori, DigDisSci, 1987; 32:1281; Friedman, AnalBioch, 1987; 161:207; Davis, Hepatol, 1988; 8:788; Zerbe, ExpMolPath, 1988; 49:87; Davis, p.39 in reference 11). By doing so, fat-storing cells transform into myofibroblast-like cells (Tsutsumi, Hepatol, 1987; 7:277; Ballardini, VirchArchCP, 1988; 56:45; Takase, JHepatol, 1988; 6:267; Ballardini, p.462 in reference 11; Davis, p.39 in reference 11; Geerts, p.20 in reference 11). This development includes the loss of fat droplets and vitamin A, together with the expression of α-smooth muscle actin (Schmittgraff, AmJPathol, 1991; 138:1233). High doses of vitamin A cause injury to parenchymal cells. Transport of retinoids to parenchymal cells might be rate limited by dynamic changes of endothelial fenestrae. The loss of endothelial fenestrae, causing reduced transport of retinoid-containing remnant chylomicrons, has been described in chronic alcoholic damage of liver tissue (Horn, Hepatol, 1987; 7:77; Fraser, Hepatol, 1995; 21:863).

Fat-storing cells in culture secrete a spectrum of extracellular matrix products (Gressner, JHepatol, 1987; 5:299; Schafer, Hepatol, 1987; 7:680; Gressner, JHepatol, 1988; 7:310; Gressner, Gastro, 1988; 94:797; Gressner, p.64 in reference 11; Yumoto, p.33 in reference 11). Obviously, secreted protein products have to accumulate for 2 or 3 days in these cultures before biochemical analysis can be performed. During this time, the phenotype of the cells starts changing into myofibroblast-like cells and they have an increasing rate of synthesis for protein and other extracellular matrix products. Northern blots of freshly isolated fat-storing cells are sensitive enough to analyse the expression of mRNAs for different matrix products in unaltered cells. Fat-storing cells synthesize collagen types I, III, and IV, fibronectin, laminin, chondroitin sulphate, dermatan sulphate, and hyaluronic acid (Shiratori, DigDisSci, 1987; 32:1281; Tsutsumi, LabInvest, 1988; 58:88; Moshage, Hepatol, 1990; 12:511; Friedman, Hepatol, 1992; 15:234; Maher, Hepatol, 1994; 19:764; Davis, p.39 in reference 11). Interestingly, collagen type I and pro-III were found to be colocalized by immunocytochemistry within collagen fibrils in the space of Disse (Geerts, Hepatol, 1990; 12:233). Several agents induce activation and proliferation in fat-storing cells, for example: acetaldehyde (Moshage, Hepatol, 1990; 12:511; Casini, JHepatol, 1993; 19:385; Gressner, JHepatol, 1995; 22:28), CCl_4 (Shiratori, JHepatol, 1986; 3:294; Shiratori, DigDisSci, 1987; 32:1281), eicosanoids (Gressner, JHepatol, 1995; 22:28), insulin-like growth factor 1 or 2 (Gressner, Liver, 1993; 13:86), in vitro cell culture (Friedman, Hepatol, 1992; 15:234), Kupffer cell secretory factors (Shiratori, 1986; Shiratori, 1987; Shiratori, p.313 in reference 11), Kupffer cell- or polymorphonuclear leucocyte-derived superoxide (Shiratori, p.313 in reference 11), lactate (Gressner, JHepatol, 1995; 22:28), oxygen species (Gressner, 1995), and Spanish toxic oil (Hernandez-Munoz, Gastro, 1994; 106:691).

Differences in the DNA binding proteins that interact with the 1(I) collagen gene were found in activated fat-storing cells (Rippe, Hepatol, 1995; 22:241). The cellular vitamin A content of fat-storing cells determines the level of activation and/or differentiation of the cell. Higher intracellular retinoid levels reduce collagen synthesis and proliferation in myofibroblast-like cells (Pinzani, JHepatol, 1992; 14:211; Sato, ExpCellRes, 1995; 217:72). Vitamin A potentiates tissue damage by CCl_4 or ethanol (Leo, Hepatol, 1983; 3:1; Seifert, p.43 in reference 11) and causes high rates of lethality when given before or in combination with CCl_4 (Seifert, p.43 in reference 11). However, if vitamin A is given after CCl_4 treatment, at the onset of fibrosis, it helps dissolving fibrotic septa and excludes necrosis and lethality (Seifert, p.43 in reference 11). Isolated fat-storing cells from vitamin A-treated rats have depressed rates of

proliferation and collagen synthesis in vitro (Shiratori, JHepatol, 1986; 3:294). The differentiation of fat-storing cells into myofibroblast-like cells is also observed in culture, where it seems to be reversible by the addition of vitamin A (Geerts, p.20 in reference 11). Protein synthesis, including collagen synthesis and cellular proliferation, could be inhibited in vitro by treating the cells with retinol (Davis, Hepatol, 1988; 8:788; Davis, p.39 in 11; Geerts, p.20 in reference 11). These reactions are promising and indicate the possibility of low-dose retinoid administration as a therapeutic agent against fibrosis.

Fat-storing cells transform into activated myofibroblast-like cells by a loss of fat droplets, expression of α-smooth muscle actin, and loss of retinyl palmitate, together with proliferation and enhanced matrix synthesis (Bachem, JHepatol, 1993; 18:40) and increased mRNA for collagen type I, lesser amounts for type III and pro-IV, laminin, and fibronectin (Weiner, Hepatol, 1990; 11:111; Knittel, Gastro, 1992; 102:1724; Ramadori, Gastro, 1992; 103:1313; Weiner, Matrix, 1992; 12:36). As a result of fat-storing cell activation in vivo, matrix deposition is exaggerated and causes bridging of connective tissue between central or portal veins. At this stage, an irreversible cirrhosis has developed, with a disturbance of the hepatic microcirculation. One of the peculiar phenomena in the development of fibrosis is the creation of straight septa which follow strictly linear or planar patterns in the tissue (French, AmJPathol, 1988; 132:73; Seifert, p.43 in reference 11) as is also seen in the histology of the normal pig liver. This phenomenon might be the result of microcirculatory conditions, which might indicate that the extracellular matrix is deposited at regions of minimal flow, where conditions for collagen fibre formation are optimal.

Heparan sulphate, dermatan sulphate, and chondroitin sulphate are synthesized mainly by activated fat-storing cells and are increased about fourfold in fibrotic human and rat liver. Stimulated synthesis rather than reduced breakdown is most probably the main reason for enhanced deposition. Fat-storing cells also produce proteoglycans, such as decorin, biglycan, and syndecan, under the stimulation of tumour necrosis factor-α, transforming growth factor-α, epidermal growth factor, platelet-derived growth factor, and fibroblast growth factor. These effects depend on the presence of receptors for these cytokines on fat-storing cells in transformation (Gressner, PSEBM, 1991; 196:307; Gressner, PatholResPract, 1994; 190:864).

A major cause, common to all conditions leading to liver fibrosis, seems to be damage to the parenchymal cell, resulting in the release of a mitogen for fat-storing cells. During subsequent inflammation, activated Kupffer cells release factors supporting the transformation of fat-storing cells into myofibroblasts. Activated fat-storing cells display paracrine stimulation, which contributes to self-perpetuation of fibrogenesis even after the disappearance of the pathogenetic event (Gressner, JHepatol, 1995; 22:28).

Transforming growth factor-β, which has three isoforms and a number of family members, is at present a heavily investigated key molecule in liver fibrosis. It was found that this factor is mainly expressed in Kupffer cells of normal rat liver.[20] In cells isolated from fibrotic livers, transforming growth factor-β is enhanced in Kupffer cells (Matsuoka, Hepatol, 1990; 11:599), endothelial cells, and fat-storing cells, but fat-storing cells increase their content by 12-fold over normal ones.[20] Transforming growth factor-β was also found in the mesenchymal cells of the fibrotic septa (Krull,

Hepatol, 1993; 18:581). Fat-storing cells possess receptors (type I) for transforming growth factor-β and bind it, whereas my-ofibroblast-like cells display a greater variety of receptors (types I, II, and III) and bind more of it. Binding activity in these cells correlated with responsiveness to transforming growth factor-β₁ (Friedman, JBC, 1994; 269:10551).

Transforming growth factor-β has major effects on fat-storing cells:

1. It stimulates the transformation of fat-storing cells into myo-fibroblasts *in vitro* (Bachem, JCI, 1992; 89:19; Bachem, Virch-ArchCP, 1993; 63:123).
2. It stimulates the production of extracellular matrix products *in vitro* (Weiner, Hepatol, 1990; 11:111; Gressner, PSEBM, 1991; 196:307; Armendariz-Borunda, JBC, 1992; 267:14316; Bachem, 1992; Ramadori, Gastro, 1992; 103:1313; Gressner, Pathol-ResPract, 1994; 190:864). It seems to regulate collagen type I gene expression at the transcriptional level (Armendariz-Borunda, 1992).
3. It inhibits proliferation of fat-storing cells (Bachem, JHepatol, 1993; 18:40; Davis, p.39 in reference 11), but it does not affect the growth of myofibroblast-like cells (Bachem, 1993).
4. It increases the expression of transforming growth factor-β in cultured fat-storing cells (Weiner, 1990; Bachem, 1992; Weiner, Matrix, 1992; 12:36).
5. It downregulates inducible nitric-oxide synthase mRNA, which was enhanced after IL-1, tumour necrosis factor-α, endotoxin, and interferon-γ administration, or bile duct ligation (Rockey, JCI, 1995; 95:1199).

Other important growth factors seem to be involved as well: transforming growth factor-α stimulated the proliferation of fat-storing cells, but not myofibroblast-like cells (Bachem, JHepatol, 1993; 18:40); insulin-like growth factor 1 was mitogenic for fat-storing and myofibroblast-like cells.

The effects of these growth regulators apparently depend on the phenotype (Bachem, JHepatol, 1993; 18:40). The administration of tumour necrosis factor-α to cultured fat-storing cells is reported to increase (Weiner, Hepatol, 1990; 11:111) or decrease (Armendariz-Borunda, JBC, 1992; 267:14316) collagen production and to stimu-late the transformation and proliferation of fat-storing cells into myofibroblast-like cells (Bachem, VirchArchCP, 1993; 63:123). Platelet-derived growth factor is a potent mitogen for fat-storing cells (Mallat, Hepatol, 1995; 21:1003) or myofibroblasts (Bachem, JHepatol, 1993; 18:40). Fat-storing cells secrete bioactive platelet-derived growth factor, suggesting an autocrine effect of this factor on fat-storing cell proliferation (Marra, Gastro, 1994; 107:1110). Apart from this factor, fat-storing cells also secrete platelet activating factor (Pinzani, Gastro, 1994; 106:1301) and insulin-like growth factor 1 (Pinzani, Endocrinol, 1990; 127:2343). Proliferation in-duced by platelet-derived growth factor depends on the expression of the platelet-derived growth factor-β receptor and is inhibited by prostaglandin E and transforming growth factor-β (Davis, Bio-chemJ, 1991; 278:43; Beno, BBActa, 1994; 1222:292).

Most studies on liver fibrosis deal with the synthesis of extra-cellular matrix components. Although the general impression is that fibrosis mainly results from exaggerated synthesis, the aspect of matrix degradation should also be taken into account. In fibrosis there is a decrease in collagenase activity (Iredale, ClinSci, 1995;

89:75). It is known that activated fat-storing and Kupffer cells synthesize matrix metalloproteinases, interstitial collagenase, type IV collagenase/gelatinase, and possibly stromelysin. Fat-storing cells also secrete tissue inhibitor of metalloproteinase 1 and α₂-macroglobulin, an acute-phase protein and a scavenger of pro-teinases and transforming growth factor-β (Ramadori, Hepatol, 1991; 14:875; Iredale, JCI, 1992; 90:282; Arthur, PatholResPract, 1994; 190:825; Arthur, p.57 in reference 11). Kupffer cell-derived gelatinase B rapidly degraded denatured collagens (gelatin) as well as native collagen types III, IV, and V, but not collagen types I and VI (Winwood, Hepatol, 1995; 22:304).

Therapeutic approaches to stop the fibrotic process have had limited success so far. However, interferon-γ seems to have some interesting qualities, because it blocks fat-storing cell activation (Rockey, JCI, 1993; 92:1795) and proliferation in culture and also reduces expression of α-smooth muscle actin. The interferon-γ effect extended to extracellular matrix gene expression and reduced collagen types I and IV and total fibronectin mRNAs to very low levels without affecting total protein synthesis (Rockey, Hepatol, 1992; 16:776; Mallat, Hepatol, 1995; 21:1003). Also, the cytosolic-binding proteins of cyclosporin A and FK506 merit consideration for the therapy of hepatic fibrosis (Ikeda, Hepatol, 1995; 21:1161).

Although most of the attention given to fat-storing cells has been focused on their role in hepatic fibrogenesis and the implications of vitamin A transport and metabolism, we should not forget their potential role in regulating sinusoidal blood flow (Housset, PNAS, 1993; 90:9266). Microscopic studies show that fat-storing cells embrace the sinusoids with a spider-like network of branching cytoplasmic processes, underlying the endothelium (Takahashi-Iwanaga, p.59 in reference 12; Wake, p.23 in reference 12). The well-developed cytoskeleton contains actin (De Leeuw, Hepatol, 1984; 4:392; Ogawa, AmJPathol, 1986; 125:611; Ballardini, Virch-ArchCP, 1988; 56:45; Ballardini, p.462 in reference 11) and desmin, which make the cells candidates for sphincter function. The ques-tion remains as to whether the cells are indeed able to contract and whether they respond to vasoactive substances or nerve stimuli. Contacts between nerves and fat-storing cells have been described for human liver (Lafon, p.230 in reference 11).[1] Endothelin types 1, 2, and 3, as well as serum, were found to induce fat-storing cell contraction *in vitro*. Cytochalasin B and interferon-γ inhibited contraction (Housset, 1993; Rockey, JCI, 1993; 92:1795). Normal fat-storing cells are non-contractile, but activation as indicated by the acquisition of α-smooth muscle actin is associated with contractility. Therefore, fat-storing cells might contribute to va-soregulation in injured, but not normal, liver (Rockey, JCI, 1993; 92:1795). The endothelin-1 induced contraction of fat-storing cells was inhibited by acetaldehyde (Kawahara, Alcohol, 1993; 28:9). Endothelin 1 causes a transient increase of intracellular Ca^{2+}. Iloprost, prostaglandin E₂, and sodium nitroprusside promoted fat-storing cell relaxation. Iloprost and sodium nitroprusside induced the disappearance of actin stress fibres in contracted cells (Kawada, EurJBioch, 1993; 213:815). Localization of radioactively labelled endothelin by autoradiography revealed grains located above the cytoplasm of fat-storing cells (Furuya, AnatEmbryol, 1992; 185:97).

Pit cells

Pit cells (Fig. 5) were described for the first time in 1976 (Wisse, SemLivDis, 1997; 17:265).[7] The cells are situated on or are

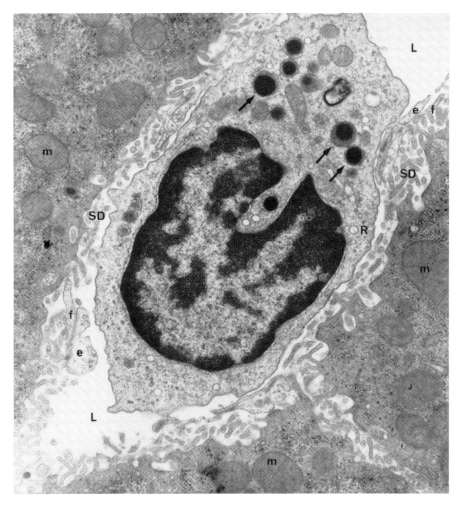

Fig. 5. Pit cell with a typical structure showing specific granules (arrows), polarity of the cell (i.e. all organelles on one side of the nucleus), a dense nucleus, and pseudopodia touching endothelial and parenchymal cells. One rod cored vesicle ® can be seen at the right-hand side of the cell. For abbreviations see Fig. 1.

embedded in the endothelial lining. Their organelles lie on one side of the nucleus, giving polarity to the cells. Pit cells possess characteristic granules[7] and rod-cored vesicles (Kaneda, p.77 in reference 21). After their initial description, no key to their function could be found on the basis of their morphology until Kaneda suggested that there is a resemblance in structure between pit cells and large granular lymphocytes, known to possess natural killer (NK) activity (Kaneda, BiomedRes, 1983; 4:567). A method for the isolation of pit cells from rat liver and proof of their spontaneous cytotoxicity against Yac-1 cells, a natural killer characteristic, was presented by Bouwens (EurJImmun, 1987; 17:37). The spontaneous and MHC class II-unrestricted killer activity of pit cells against tumour cells, and possibly virus infected cells, occurs without activation of any kind and defines the pit cell as the resident natural killer cell of the liver.

The different definitions of pit cells, natural killer and large granular lymphocyte, largely refer to the same class of cells, although the terms come from different disciplines, such as electron microscopy (pit cell), immunology or tumour biology (NK cell), and haematology (large granular lymphocyte). It is obvious that the criteria used to characterize the cells in these different disciplines are not the same, which in most cases will not lead to controversies, but which might in some instances lead to discordancies.

Pit cells can be isolated from rat liver by a simple washout technique: sinusoidal lavage with physiological saline at an elevated pressure of 50 cmH$_2$O (Bouwens, EurJImmun, 1987; 17:37). This physiological saline does not contain enzymes and so preserves cell surface antigens and markers during isolation. A yield of about 1 million pit cells per gram of liver tissue was obtained, providing suspensions of pit cells that were 27 per cent pure (Bouwens, 1987). Other cells in the washouts were lymphocytes and monocytes. Pit cells can be recognized in cytospin preparations by light microscopy, owing to the presence of small azurophylic granules that stain darkly with Giemsa. Pit cells can be enriched in cell suspensions by Ficoll-Paque density-gradient centrifugation, followed by nylon wool filtration and Percoll gradient centrifugation (Bouwens, 1987). With this method, about 60 per cent pure preparations of pit cells were obtained. The highest level of purification could be obtained by magnetic cell sorting.[22] Pit cells have also been isolated from human liver (Bouwens, p.471 in reference 11).

Isolated pit cells possess a very high level of natural killer activity. This level is comparable with that of IL-2 activated blood or spleen NK cells. When pit cells are coincubated with Yac-1 leukaemia cells, we observe the adherence of effector cells to target cells. NK cells penetrate with pseudopodia into the cytoplasm of the tumour cells. After 4 h of interaction at an effector to target cell ratio between 10/1 and 20/1, about 40 per cent of the chromium-51 bound to Yac-1 cells is released, which is considered to be a measure of cytolysis, and which parallels degenerative changes such as mitochondrial swelling and changes in the nucleus (Bouwens, Eur-JImmun, 1987; 17:37). A relationship between the concentration of pit cells in the effector cell population and the rate of lysis of Yac-1 cells has been demonstrated. The cytotoxicity can be suppressed by treating the cells with anti-asialo-GM1 serum, which inhibits NK activity (Bouwens, 1987; Kanai, ClinImmunPath, 1993; 69:23). Isolated rat pit cells can be immunophenotyped as OX8+, OX19-, whereas the typical NK marker, asialo-GM1, seems to be present on about a one-quarter to one-half of the cells (Bouwens, Eur-JImmun, 1987; 17:1423; Kanai, 1993), the remaining cells being CD3+ T cells and a few B cells (Kanai, ClinImmunPath 1993; 69: 23). The pattern of immunotyping distinguishes pit cells from monocytes (OX8–), B lymphocytes (OX8–), and T lymphocytes (OX19+) and confirms the NK nature of liver pit cells. Human liver-associated lymphoid (LAL) cells express CD3+ and CD56+. LAL cells from patients with benign liver disease showed high levels of NK and LAK activity, whereas those from patients with liver metastases did not differ from blood NK cells (Winnock, Gastro, 1993; 105:1152). LAL cells have increased CD11b+, CD54+, CD56+, and CD58+ and decreased CD2+ compared with peripheral blood lymphocytes. The increase in adhesion molecule expression in LAL cells, together with their increased NK and LAK activities, supports the fact that LAL cells are in an activated state compared with blood lymphocytes (Garcia-Barcina, Immunol, 1994; 82:95).

Pit cells not only have NK activity (demonstrated by 4-h co-incubation with YAC-1 cells), but also possess natural cytotoxicity (NC) activity, which is defined as the cytotoxicity expressed at 16 h of incubation against cells isolated from solid tumours (Bouwens, p.215 in reference 11). These cells are resistant to 4 h of co-incubation. The pit-cell mediated spontaneous cytolytic effect differs from the cytotoxicity observed with Kupffer cells, which become cytolytic after activation by a proper stimulus (Stukart, CancerRes, 1987; 47:3880; Bouwens, CancerImmunTher, 1988; 27: 137; Phillips, Hepatol, 1988; 8:1046; Daemen, p.400 in reference 11; Hardonk, p.434 in reference 11). The distinction between NK and NC activity also makes sense, because different tumour cell lines have a different sensitivity to these two forms of cytotoxicity (Bouwens, p.215 in reference 11). NK activity is thought to be based on the release of pre-existing products, located in specific granules, whereas NC activity might be dependent on the *de novo* synthesis of cytolytic molecules. Tumour cell killing is apparently not the result of tumour necrosis factor secretion, because cell lines resistant to tumour necrosis factor are killed by pit cells (Bouwens, p.215 in reference 11). Cyclosporin treatment of rats suppressed the tumour cell killing by pit cells (Bouwens, p.215 in reference 11). The NC activity includes the spontaneous killing of solid tumour-derived cell lines, such as colon carcinomas. It is interesting that colon cancer cells which resisted the cytotoxic potential of activated

Kupffer cells were found to be sensitive to pit cell-mediated lysis (Bouwens, p.215 in reference 11).

Vanderkerken and Bouwens have shown that pit cells form a heterogeneous population, which can be separated into two density fractions with a 45 per cent Percoll gradient, one of high density and the other of low density (Vanderkerken, p.456 in reference 11). It seems that a gradient in NK characteristics exists between large granular lymphocytes from the blood and liver high-density and low-density NK cells. Low-density cells express lower levels of asialo-GM1, and have more, but smaller, granules than large granular lymphocytes in the blood. Low-density pit cells are 5 to 8 times more cytotoxic against Yac-1 cells and colon carcinoma cells than blood NK cells. Low-density cells are able to lyse P-815 cells, a known LAK target cell, normally resistant to blood NK cells (Vanderkerken, Hepatol, 1990; 12:70; Kanai, ClinImmunPath, 1993; 69:23; Tanaka, p.451 in reference 11). These observations suggest that NK cells in different compartments, such as the bone marrow, peripheral blood, and liver, relate to one another (Bouwens, Hepatol, 1988; 8:46; Tanaka, p.451 in reference 11; Vanderkerken, p.456 in reference 11). In the case of pit cells, this would mean that hepatic low-density (pit) cells are derived from hepatic high-density cells, which are in their turn derived from large granular lymphocytes in the blood. Experiments based on irradiation, intravenous injections with asialo-GM1 antiserum, and adoptive transfer of fluorescent cells, followed by cell sorting of washouts after 3 days, strongly support the hypothesis that large granular lymphocytes in the blood localize in hepatic sinusoids to become high-density cells, which further differentiate into low-density cells or pit cells (Vanderkerken, Hepatol, 1993; 18:919). The transfer of large granular lymphocytes from the blood to the liver is supported by CD2 and CD11a/CD18 adhesion molecules on the large granular lymphocytes, as treatment of rats with antibodies against these surface markers strongly inhibits the recruitment of pit cells in the liver. Treatment of endothelial cells *in vitro* with tumour necrosis factor-α induces a marked increase in the adherence of NK cells. Treatment of mice with neutralizing antisera to tumour necrosis factor-α eliminates the hepatic influx of NK cells. Therefore, this factor seems to be a major cytokine involved in the recruitment of NK cells in the liver (Pilaro, JImmunol, 1994; 153:333).

Kupffer cells play an important role in the differentiation of NK cells in the liver sinusoids as becomes evident when Kupffer cells are eliminated with liposomes containing dichloromethylene diphosphonate. These liposomes are specifically taken up by Kupffer cells and digested in the lysosomes, which frees the drug, but kills the macrophages (Van Rooijen, CellTissRes, 1990; 260:215). Such removal of Kupffer cells also induces a gradual disappearance of pit cells within 2 weeks. Also, Kupffer cell-conditioned medium enhances the viability, tumour cytotoxicity, and adherence of pit cells to liver sinusoidal endothelial cells *in vitro* (Vanderkerken, Hepatol, 1995; 22:283). Other observations also support the transfer of large granular lymphocytes from the blood to the liver during liver transplantation (Lukomska, JHepatol, 1991; 12:332) and labelling experiments (Matsunaga, Liver, 1990; 10:325).

Pit cells are able to proliferate locally (Bouwens, Hepatol, 1990; 12:1365).[7] With continuous infusion of rhIL-2 over 7 days, there is an increase of pit cells in the liver of up to 43 times (Bouwens, 1990). Biological response modifiers, such as *C. parvum*, Zymosan, or OK432, activate pit cells and also increase their number

(Bouwens, Hepatol, 1988; 8:46; Tanaka, p.451 in reference 11). Pit cell proliferation occurs mainly in the liver, although extrahepatic recruitment from the bone marrow is indicated (Bouwens, 1988). Anti-asialo-GM1 antiserum decreases the number of pit cells in the liver (Shiratori, Hepatol, 1992; 16:469).

Pit cells also display a remarkable behaviour during regeneration after partial hepatectomy. The number of pit cells is restored 3 days after partial hepatectomy. During the early period of liver regeneration, parenchymal cells appear to be sensitive to lysis by pit cells of normal rats, whereas pit cells of partially hepatectomized rats are unable to mediate cytotoxicity. Depletion of pit cells by treatment with anti-NKR-P1 monoclonal antibody augments liver regeneration after partial hepatectomy, clearly indicating that pit cells play a role in liver regeneration (Vujanovic, JImmunol, 1995; 154:6324).

Large granular lymphocytes seem to play a role in killing virus-infected cells. At present, the mechanism by which parenchymal cells die in virus-infected livers is not known exactly. The antiviral role of pit cells, therefore, needs further investigation. For further details on pit cells see Wisse, SemLivDis, 1997; 17:265.

Sinusoidal cells and liver cancer

The subject of sinusoidal cells and cancer may be split into three parts: (i) the reaction of sinusoidal cells during the development of a primary liver tumour, such as hepatocellular carcinoma, (ii) the tumours which develop from each of the sinusoidal cell types, and (iii) the reactions of sinusoidal cells against immigrating haematogenic tumour cells, metastasizing from an extrahepatic origin, such as the colon, the skin (melanoma), or other sources.

Sinusoids in hepatocellular adenoma and carcinoma were comparable to those in normal liver. In hepatocellular carcinoma, fenestrae disappeared and a continuous basement membrane developed, according to the process of capillarization (Ichida, Cytopath, 1990; 22:221). Fat-storing cells lost their lipid droplets. Kupffer cells and pit cells were not seen inside the sinusoid (Haratake, Cancer, 1990; 65:1985; Ichida, 1990; Haratake, ArchPathLabMed, 1992; 116:67; Shoji, JpnJCancerRes, 1994; 85: 491). Sinusoids in normal liver could not be stained with *Ulex europaeus* lectin, but stained positively in intratumoural vessels, suggesting a change in endothelial cell surface glycoproteins (Haratake, 1990).

Reports on tumour formation in different types of sinusoidal cells are rare, but mostly concern endothelial cells. Different causes are given for the transformation of normal endothelial cells into (benign) haemangioendothelioma and (malignant) angiosarcoma (Bannasch, RecResCancRes, 1986; 100:1). The recognition of sinusoidal cells is difficult using light microscopy only, owing to their small size in comparison with parenchymal cells. Morphological methods for characterizing the cells should therefore use electron microscopy and/or immunocytochemical staining (Abe, ActaPathJpn, 1987; 37:1653). Cases of epithelioid haemangioendothelioma have been described (Ichida, JClinElectronMicrosc, 1981; 14:5; Fukuyawa, VirchArchA, 1984; 404:275; Dean, AmJSurgPath, 1985; 9:695; Bellmunt, JpnJClinOncol, 1989; 19: 153; Scoazec, HumPath, 1989; 20:673; Fedeli, ItalJGastr, 1991; 23: 261; Bancel, AnnPath, 1993; 13:23) and were found to be immunoreactive for factor VIII-related antigen BNH9, and vimentin and

demonstrate so-called Weibel–Palade bodies (dense granules, positive for factor VIII). This disease seems to develop after taking oral contraceptives for 4 to 7 years. Haemangioendotheliomas were induced in rat livers after a 12-week treatment with quinoline (Hasegawa, Carcinogenesis, 1989; 10:711). Angiosarcoma is a malignant endothelial cell tumour that progresses to tumorous vascular masses (Fortwengler, Gastro, 1981; 80:1415; Nguyen, ActaCytol, 1982; 26:527; Goodman, AnnClinLabSci, 1984; 14:169; Noguchi, JpnJClinOncol, 1987; 17:275; Balazs, ActaMorphHung, 1991; 39: 201) having a peculiar vasculature with capillarization of sinusoids and several layers of basement membrane (Balazs, 1991). Angiosarcoma development may possibly be related to the use of arsenic (Roat, AmJMed, 1982; 73:933), long-term androgen therapy (Balazs, ActaMorphHung, 1991; 39:201), vinyl chloride (Fortwengler, Gastro, 1981; 80:1415), or thorotrast and arsenic (Popper, AmJPathol, 1978; 92:2). Hepatic angiosarcomas could be induced by 1,2-dimethylhydrazine dihydrochloride in experimental animals with 100 per cent incidence (Sato, CancerLett, 1984; 24:313). Isolated liver cells of rats given diethylnitrosamine developed angiosarcomas after transplantion into young rats (Luquette, LabInvest, 1985; 53:546). Hepatic angiosarcomas were also found in a relatively large number of patients within 40 years after the intravenous injection with thorotrast, a preparation stored in endothelial cells[4] and used to increase X-ray contrast, but containing α-emitting thorium dioxide (Jennings, JClinPath, 1978; 31: 1125; Manning, ArchPathLabMed, 1983; 107:456; Tateno, GanNoRinsho, 1984; 30:23; Kojiro, ArchPathLabMed, 1985; 109:853; Abe, ActaPathJpn, 1987; 37:1653)

Kupffer cell tumours appear to be rare. Kupffer cell sarcoma has been reported to show diffuse or nodular proliferation of Kupffer cells, with giant cells present (Chopra, p.457 in reference 21). These Kupffer cells contained peroxidase activity in the rough endoplasmic reticulum (Chopra, p.457 in reference 21). Undifferentiated (embryonic) sarcoma was found as a rare, primary liver tumour of children and young adults. It shows undifferentiated stellate and spindle cells (Goodman, AnnClinLabSci, 1984; 14:169).

Benign spongiosis hepatis (spongiotic pericytoma) in livers of rats treated with *N*-nitrosomorpholine originates from fat-storing cells, as indicated by positive desmin and vimentin staining (Bannasch, LabInvest, 1981; 44:252; Bannasch, RecResCancRes, 1986; 100:1; Stroebel, AmJPathol, 1995; 146:903). While the preneoplastic or neoplastic nature of spongiosis hepatis is discussed, further development of spongiosis hepatis into pericytoma has been suggested (Bannasch, RecResCancRes, 1986; 100:1).

With regard to the transformation of pit cells into tumour cells, a recent report describes an Epstein–Barr virus-associated, hepatosinusoidal, NK cell leukaemia/lymphoma. Patients with NK cell leukaemia/lymphoma were found to have liver dysfunction and enhanced lactate dehydrogenase levels. Most patients displayed cells with positive reactions for CD2, CD7, CD16, CD56, and Ia, and negative reactions for CD3, CD4, CD8, CD19, and CD25. Epstein–Barr virus transcripts were detected in these cells (Ohshima, HemOnc, 1995; 13:83).

The reaction of sinusoidal cells against tumour cells has been investigated primarily *in vitro*. It was found that pit cells have spontaneous cytotoxicity against a variety of tumour cell lines. Kupffer cells were found to have a lower level of cytotoxicity, which was increased after activation (Daemen, JImmunther, 1991; 10:200;

Daemen, p.400 in reference 11). Recently, a synergistic effect of pit cells and Kupffer cells against CC531 colon carcinoma cells was demonstrated (Thomas, CellHepSin, 1995; 5:130).

Immigrating tumour cells adhere to the sinusoidal endothelium, whereas mechanical trapping of tumour cells in narrow sinusoids can be assumed, but could not be confirmed (Kan, Hepatol, 1995; 21:487). Antibodies against the IL-1 receptor reduced the IL-1-mediated adhesion of B16 melanoma cells to sinusoidal endothelial cells in mice and reduced the number of hepatic metastases (Vidal, CancerRes, 1994; 54:2667). Endothelial cell-conditioned medium contains migration-stimulating activity for tumours that are highly liver metastatic (Hamada, CancerRes, 1993; 53:4418).

Kupffer cells seem to become activated soon after inoculation of syngeneic rats with CC531 colon carcinoma cells (Thomas, JLeukBiol, 1995; 57:617). Free radicals derived from nitric oxide appear to play a significant role in Kupffer cell cytotoxicity, because NG-monomethyl-arginine reduced the number of injured tumour cells during coincubation (Yonei, Liver, 1994; 14:37). Kupffer cell-mediated cytotoxicity correlated with the amount of nitric oxide produced (Aono, BBResComm, 1994; 201:1175). Superoxide dismutase did not prevent the tumouricidal effect (Yonei, 1994), indicating the absence of oxygen radical toxicity. The cytotoxicity of Kupffer cells could be enhanced by the administration of human granulocyte/monocyte colony-stimulating factor (Schuurman, CancerImmunTher, 1994; 39:179), interferon-γ (Phillips, Cancer-MetRev, 1989; 8:231; Schuurman, CancerImmunTher, 1994; 39:179), muramyl peptide (Phillips, CancerMetRev, 1989; 8:231), and intravenous OK432 (Zhang, JSurgRes, 1993; 55:140) or IL-2, or both (Sasaoki, CancerImmunTher, 1992; 35:75). Antitumour necrosis factor-α blocked Kupffer cell cytotoxicity (Schuurman, CancerImmunTher, 1994; 39:179). In addition, paraformaldehyde-fixed Kupffer cells were also able to lyse certain tumour cells. These observations indicate that cell membrane-bound tumour necrosis factor-α is a cytolytic mechanism of Kupffer cells (Schuurman, CancerImmunTher, 1994; 39:179). Also, the number of developing metastases seems to correlate with a treatment that stimulates Kupffer cells (OK432, reducing the number of tumour foci) or that depresses Kupffer cell function (GdCl$_3$ or carrageenan, increasing the number of tumour nodules) (Zhang, JSurgRes, 1993; 55:140). Although such treatment seems to involve Kupffer cells directly, it is advisable to bear in mind that pit cell activity also correlates with Kupffer cell function (Vanderkerken, Hepatol, 1995; 22:283), in addition to the possible synergism of both cells in killing tumour cells.

Kupffer cells rapidly clear haematogenic tumour cells from the circulation by phagocytosis (Phillips, CancerMetRev, 1989; 8:231; Rushfeldt, CancerRes, 1993; 53:658; Kan, Hepatol, 1995; 21:487). The major binding proteins between Kupffer cells and colorectal cancer cells seem to be galactose-binding lectins (Meterissian, CancerLett, 1994; 81:5). Desialylation of tumour cells inhibits hepatic metastasis (Petrick, ClinExpMet, 1994; 12:108). After 24 h, a great proportion of labelled tumour cells is engulfed by Kupffer cells, transferring the fluorescein label to the Kupffer cell lysosomes (Rushfeldt, CancerRes, 1993; 53:658). In tumour-bearing livers, the number and the phagocytic capacity of Kupffer cells seems to be increased in non-tumorous areas, but is decreased inside the tumours (Kan, Hepatol, 1995; 21:487).

In the future it may be possible to develop an immunostimulating protocol, protecting patients with a resection of a primary tumour in the gastrointestinal tract. These patients are at risk for liver metastasis, but if they were given biological response modifiers perioperatively (such as interferon-γ or muramyl peptides), Kupffer and pit cells might become stimulated to kill haematogenic tumour cells (Oka, Surgery, 1994; 116:877; Vanderkerken, Hepatol, 1995; 22:283). Such a strategy seems to be appropriate because surgical stress depresses the cytotoxic activity of NK cells and enhances the growth of metastatic liver tumours. Such Kupffer cell-directed therapeutic intervention would probably be limited to situations in which tumour cells are still contained within the vasculature of the lumen of the sinusoid, in other words very early stages of metastasis. Well-developed intraparenchymal tumour nodules, surrounded by inflammation and hiding behind a wall of connective tissue, appear to be unreachable by intravenous preparations and do not seem to involve reactions of sinusoidal cells. Therefore, such treatment may only be of benefit to patients with early, minimal tumour load, typically during surgical intervention, rather than patients with established, radiologically detectable liver tumours (Phillips, CancerMetRev, 1989; 8:231).

Sinusoidal cells and HIV

Human immunodeficiency virus (**HIV**) was found to infect endothelial (Steffan, PNAS, 1992; 89:1582) and Kupffer cells (Schmitt, AIDSRes, 1990; 6:987; Gendrault, Pathobio, 1991; 59:223; Lafon, AIDS, 1994; 8:747). Therefore, endothelial and Kupffer cells constitute a target and a reservoir for HIV. Three out of seven patients with HIV were found to have Kupffer cells that were infected with HIV-1 (Hufert, JAIDS, 1993; 6:772). The infection of endothelial and Kupffer cells is probably facilitated by the presence of CD4 surface antigen on both cells as shown by immunogold-electron microscopy (Scoazec, Hepatol, 1990; 12:505; Steffan, ANAS, 1992; 89:1582). Treatment with anti-CD4 antibody abolishes the infection of endothelial cells *in vitro* (Steffan, ANAS, 1992; 89:1582), whereas morphine increases the reproduction of HIV (Schweitzer, ResVirol, 1991; 142:189). Endothelial and Kupffer cells were found to display budding of new viral particles, indicating the production of new viruses (Gendrault, Pathobio, 1991; 59:223; Steffan, ANAS, 1992; 89:1582). Infection of Kupffer cell cultures with HIV-1 induced the formation of syncytia or giant cells (Schmitt, AIDSRes, 1990; 6: 987; Gendrault, Pathobio, 1991; 59:223). Virus released from Kupffer cells could infect lymphocytes, but could also be neutralized by the serum of a patient with HIV seropositivity or with anti-gp120 antibody (Schmitt, AIDSRes, 1990; 6:987). Simian immunodeficiency virus was also found in Kupffer cells of macaques (Persidsky, Hepatol, 1995; 21:1215); it budded from the surface and induced the formation of multinucleated giant cells.

Conclusion

Sinusoidal cells play a crucial role in homeostasis and are involved in the pathogenesis of a number of human liver diseases.

Kupffer cells clear endotoxin and other substances from the blood. These substances activate Kupffer cells, which then secrete a number of cytokines that cause a variety of different, and not completely analysed, effects such as portal hypertension, glucose release, activation of other cells, and cellular necrosis.

Endothelial cells are highly endocytotic, filter the fluids that enter the space of Disse, and are involved in regulating the liver/body fat balance. Forced sieving and endothelial massage help refresh fluids in the space of Disse.

Fat-storing cells contain the major part of the body's depot of vitamin A. They produce extracellular matrix components and contribute to fibrosis and cirrhosis after being activated to become myofibroblast-like cells. The cells are contractile and embrace the sinusoid with long branched processes.

Pit cells possess natural killer activity and cytotoxicity against colon carcinoma and other tumour cells and are involved in the hepatic antineoplastic defence.

References

1. Ito T and Shibasaki S. Electron microscopic study on the hepatic sinusoidal wall and the fat-storing cells in the normal human liver. *Archives of Histology and Cytology*, 1968; **29**: 137–92.

2. Wake K. Sternzellen in the liver: perisinusoidal cells with special reference to storage of vitamin A. *American Journal of Anatomy*, 1971; **132**: 429–61.

3. Wisse E. An electron microscopic study of the fenestrated endothelial lining of rat liver sinusoids. *Journal of Ultrastructural Research*, 1970; **31**: 125–50.

4. Wisse E. An ultrastructural characterization of the endothelial cell in the rat liver sinusoid under normal and various experimental conditions, as a contribution to the distinction between endothelial and Kupffer cells. *Journal of Ultrastructural Research*, 1972; **38**: 528–62.

5. Wisse E. Observations on the fine structure and peroxidase cytochemistry of normal rat liver Kupffer cells. *Journal of Ultrastructural Research*, 1974; **46**: 393–426.

6. Wisse E. Kupffer cell reactions in rat liver under various conditions as observed in the electron microscope. *Journal of Ultrastructural Research*, 1974; **46**: 499–520.

7. Wisse E, Van't Noordende JM, Van Der Meulen J, and Daems WT. The pit cell: description of a new type of cell occurring in rat liver and peripheral blood. *Cell Tissue Research*, 1976; **173**: 423–35.

8. Knook DL and Sleyster EC. Separation of Kupffer and endothelial cells of the rat liver by centrifugal elutriation. *Experimental Cell Research*, 1976; **99**: 444–9.

9. Knook DL, Blansjaar N, and Sleyster EC. Isolation and characterization of Kupffer and endothelial cells from the rat liver. *Experimental Cell Research*, 1977; **109**: 317–29.

10. Knook DL and Sleyster EC. Isolated parenchymal, Kupffer and endothelial rat liver cells characterized by their lysosomal enzyme content. *Biochemical and Biophysical Research Communications*, 1980; **96**: 250–7.

11. Wisse E, Knook DL, and Decker K, eds. *Cells of the hepatic sinusoid*. PO Box 5815, 2280 HV Rijswijk, The Netherlands: Kupffer Cell Foundation, 1989.

12. Motta PM, ed. *Biopathology of the liver, an ultrastructural approach*. Dordrecht: Kluwer, 1988.

13. Wisse E, *et al.* The role of pit cells in the defense of the liver against metastasizing tumor cells. In Wisse E, Knook DL, and Wake K, eds. *Cells of the hepatic sinusoid*. PO Box 2215, 2301 CE Leiden, The Netherlands: The Kupffer Cell Foundation, 1995: 90–5.

14. Wisse E, *et al.* On the tumoricide function of pit cells, the NK cells of the liver. In Vidal Vanaclocha F, ed. *Functional heterogeneity of the liver tissue*. Austin: Medical Intelligence Unit, RG Landes Co., 1996: 207–35.

15. Charels K, De Zanger RB, Van Bossuyt H, Van Der Smissen P, and Wisse E. Influence of acute alcohol administration on endothelial fenestrae of rat livers: an *in vivo* and *in vitro* scanning electron microscopic study. In Kirn A, Knook DL, and Wisse E, eds. *Cells of the hepatic sinusoid*, Vol 1. PO Box 5815, 2280 HV Rijswijk, The Netherlands: The Kupffer Cell Foundation, 1986: 497–502.

16. Wisse E, Van Dierendonck JH, De Zanger RB, Fraser R, and McCuskey RS. On the role of the liver endothelial filter in the transport of particulate fat (chylomicrons and their remnants) to parenchymal cells and the influence of certain hormones on the endothelial fenestrae. In Popper H, Bianchi L, Gudat F, and Reutter W, eds. *Communications of liver cells, Falk Symposium 27*. Lancaster, UK: MTP Press Ltd, 1980: 195–200.

17. Wisse E and Knook DL, eds. *Kupffer cells and other liver sinusoidal cells*. Amsterdam: Elsevier, 1977.

18. Wisse E, De Wilde A, and De Zanger R. Perfusion fixation of human and rat liver tissue for light and electron microscopy. In O'Hare AMF, ed. *Science of biological specimen preparation*. Chicago: SEM Inc., 1984: 31–8.

19. Daems WT, Wisse E, Brederoo P, and Emeis JJ. Peroxidatic activity in monocytes and macrophages. In Van Furth R, ed. *Mononuclear phagocytes in immunity, infection and pathology*. Oxford: Blackwell Scientific, 1975: 57–83.

20. De Bleser P, *et al.* Distribution of TGF-$\beta_{1,2,3}$ gene transcripts in cells of normal and CCl$_4$ treated rat liver. In Knook DL, Wisse E, eds. *Cells of the hepatic sinusoid*, Vol. 4. PO Box 430, 2300 AK Leiden, The Netherlands. The Kupffer Cell Foundation, 1993: 214–17.

21. Knook DL and Wisse E, eds. *Sinusoidal liver cells*. Amsterdam: Elsevier Biomedical Press, 1982.

22. Kanellopoulou C, *et al.* Isolation of pure pit cells with a magnetic cell sorter and effect of contaminating T cells on their cytolytic capability against CC531. In Wisse E, Knook DL, Balabaud C, eds. *Cells of the hepatic sinusoid*, Vol. 6. PL Box 2215, 2301 CE Leiden, The Netherlands. The Kupffer Cell Foundation, 1997: 471–3.

1.5 Embryology of the liver and intrahepatic biliary tract

Valeer J. Desmet, Peter Van Eyken, and Tania Roskams

Introduction

The past decade has witnessed a rekindled interest in the embryonic development of the liver and the biliary tree. Until then, theories on hepatic embryogenesis were based on routine light and electron microscopic observations. The advent of new techniques including immunohistochemistry, *in situ* hybridization, and cell isolation and culturing has opened up new avenues to address issues of cell lineage and differentiation during development. As a result, a wealth of new data on the normal development of the liver has become available. It has become clear that a better insight into liver and bile duct development is relevant to our understanding of the functioning of the postnatal liver and of congenital diseases of the biliary tree (see Chapters 11.1 and 11.2).

This chapter summarizes the currently prevailing and most plausible theories of hepatic development. An overview of the sequence of events during hepatic development is given in Table 1. The reader should realize that chronology, when indicated, is at best approximate. Unlike the case in laboratory animals, there is a wide range of normal variation in actual human embryonic or fetal age for a given Carnegie stage, crown–rump length, or body weight.[1] Furthermore, it is impossible to identify the exact time at which a certain event occurs because descriptions in the literature differ appreciably among investigators. Moreover, often it is not clear whether the ages described in published reports refer to fertilization age or to menstrual age, and most reports do not specify whether the age indicated refers to the nearest or completed week of gestation.[1]

Hepatic primordia and early development

The liver is formed from two distinct primordia: the parenchyma and bile duct system derive from the hepatic diverticulum of endoblastic origin, while the mesenchymal framework of the liver derives from the septum transversum (a transverse sheet of cells which incompletely separates the pericardial and peritoneal cavities), with a contribution from cells of the mesenchymal lining of the associated celomic cavity which actively invade the septum transversum.[2,3] In the human embryo, the first sign of the formation of the hepatic diverticulum or liver bud is a thickening of the endoblastic epithelium in the ventral wall of the foregut (the future duodenum), near the origin of the yolk stalk (this area is termed the anterior intestinal portal). This occurs around the 7-somite stage (2.5 mm) on the 18th day. In the 19-somite embryo (3 mm, 22nd day), the diverticulum is formed (Fig. 1).[4] In the 22-somite embryo, the hepatic diverticulum is a well-defined hollow structure. From the ventral and lateral surfaces of the diverticulum, where the endoderm is in contact with the bulk of the mesoderm, short sprouts of endodermal cells extend into the septum transversum (Severn, AmJAnat, 1972; 133:85). The septum transversum consists of a mass of loosely arranged mesodermal cells in which appear small isolated spaces; the mesodermal cells bordering the larger spaces are flat and evenly aligned, and form an endothelial boundary; these endothelium-lined spaces resemble capillaries or sinusoids. Dorsolateral to the diverticulum, some of the endothelium-lined spaces are continuous with the larger omphalo-mesenteric (vitelline) vessels. The endodermal sprouts from the diverticulum extend between the endothelium-lined spaces, thus establishing the basic composition of liver tissue—epithelial cords between sinusoidal vessels. In the 23-somite embryo, the diverticulum acquires a T-shaped cephalic end, with more pronounced growth of epithelial sprouts from the lateral walls, creating the early outline of right and left lobes of the liver (Severn, AmJAnat, 1972; 133:85). In the 25-somite embryo (3.6 mm, 28th day), the irregular outgrowths of endodermal cells have invaded the ventral portions of the septum transversum and grow laterally into the direction of the vitelline veins; the cells are often loosely connected or even completely detached in the peripheral parts of the proliferating masses.[2] Endodermal cells spreading into the septum transversum are observed as far distally as the junction of the hepatic diverticulum with the foregut.[5]

Once established, the liver grows rapidly. It soon extends beyond the confines of the septum transversum in whichever direction it can. It bulges dorsally on each side of the midline, into the peritoneal cavity. It also grows ventrally and caudally into the mesenchyme of the anterior abdominal wall, extending down to the umbilical ring.[3] Initially, the stomach and duodenum are in broad contact with the septum transversum. While the liver develops, these organs draw away from the septum transversum, producing a midsagittal sheet of mesoderm—the ventral mesogastrium or future lesser omentum. As the duodenum withdraws from the septum transversum, the stalk of the hepatic diverticulum is also drawn out and forms the epithelial components of the extrahepatic bile ducts

Table 1 Human hepatic embryogenesis

Component	First start of development in embryonic stage		
	Length of embryo (mm)	Gestation time	Somite stage
First sign of liver anlage	2.5	18 days	7
Hepatic diverticulum formed	3[2] 4[4]	22 days	19
Outgrowth of parenchyma	3.6[2]	28 days	25
Pars caudalis (cystica) of hepatic diverticulum	5[2,20]		
Canaliculi	10[11]	7–8 weeks[12]	
Haematopoiesis	10[4]		
Bile secretion		3 months[20] 4 months	
Bile acid synthesis		12 weeks[a]	
Intrahepatic bile ducts	22–30[11] 18[4]	5–9 weeks[2]	
Ductus venosus	6[2] 10[b]		
Definitive fetal pattern of liver circulation	17	6 weeks (approximately)	

Modified from ref. 18 with permission. Superscripts refer to ref. no.
[a] Suchy, SemLivDis, 1987; 7:77.
[b] Lassan, AnatClin, 1983; 5:97.

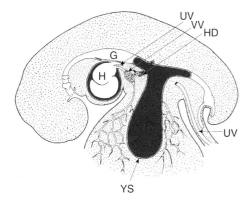

Fig. 1. Human embryo of 4 mm. G, gut (sectioned in the intestinal region); H, heart; HD, hepatic diverticulum growing in the septum transversum (finely stippled zone); UV, umbilical vein; VV, vitelline vein; YS, yolk sac, partially open. (Redrawn from ref. 2, with permission.)

within the lesser omentum (see below). The liver becomes partly detached from its initial broad contact with the septum transversum by extensions of the peritoneal cavity, so that, in the adult, direct contact with the diaphragm persists only as the bare area of the liver. The latter is bounded by the attachments of peritoneal reflections, which form the coronary and falciform ligaments.[3]

Parenchyma and canaliculi

Most authors agree that primitive hepatocyte precursor cells (hepatoblasts) derive exclusively from the endodermal outgrowths of the hepatic diverticulum,[2] without participation of mesodermal cells from the celomic lining which on occasion were claimed to be

'recruited' into parenchymal precursors (Elias, ActaHepatolJpn, 1955; 3:1).[4] Taken together, all data available indicate that the liver primordium is made up of a uniform population of at least bipotential progenitor cells that will give rise to both liver parenchymal cells and biliary epithelial cells (Desmet, Hepatol, 1990; 12:1249; Fausto, CurrOpinCellBiol, 1990; 2:1036; Shiojiri, CancerRes, 1991; 51:2611; Desmet, MedTher, 1995; 1:227).[6-10] In man, the progenitor cells are immunoreactive for cytokeratins 8, 18, and 19 of the catalogue of Moll *et al.* (Shah, ArchPathLabMed, 1989; 113:1135; Desmet, Hepatol, 1990; 12:1249; Stosiek, Liver, 1990; 10:59).[7] From 10 to 14 weeks of gestation, progenitor cells express in addition cytokeratin 14 (Haruna, Hepatol, 1994; 20:210A). There is some discrepancy between different studies as to whether the primitive hepatoblasts are arranged in tubules or in plates.

Muralia

According to some authors the parenchymal precursor cells are arranged in plates (Lipp, ZMikroskAnatForsch, 1952; 59:161).[2,4] The 'tubules' illustrated by Bloom[11] are interpreted by Elias (ActaHepatolJpn, 1955; 3:1) as 'plates'. Initially, the liver cell plates are three to five cells thick (muralium multiplex). Junctional assembly, indicating maturation of lateral domains of hepatocytes, most probably is a major factor inducing cell polarization and organization of hepatocytes into plates as suggested generally for epithelial polarization (Stamatoglou, FASEBJ, 1994; 8:420). At the time of birth, and for a considerable time in postnatal life, the liver cell plates or muralia are two cells thick (muralium duplex). It is not until the child's fifth year that the typical form of the adult human liver, the one-cell thick plate or the muralium simplex is achieved (Morgan, ArchPath, 1961; 71:86). In contrast, several studies (including more recent electron microscopic investigations) describe tubular arrangements of primitive hepatoblasts in the developing liver.[11-14] Tubular arrangements were more frequently described by authors who studied the development of bile canaliculi.

Canaliculi

In 1898, developing bile canaliculi were first described by Hendrickson using Golgi's staining method. The canaliculi were seen to develop first as networks in the vicinity of branches of the portal vein, to appear first at the hilum and then to spread through the rest of the liver (Hendrickson, JohnsHopkHospBull, 1898; 9: 220). Using Eppinger's stain, Bloom obtained comparable results.[11] He described the first canaliculi in a 10-mm embryo, quite some time before the development of intrahepatic bile ducts which occurs at about the 22- to 30-mm stage. The canaliculi were found to be lined by between three and seven cells, in contrast to bile canaliculi in adult liver which are lined by only two or, exceptionally, three hepatocytes. Comparable observations were made on the embryogenesis of the mouse liver.[13] Electron microscopic investigations on human liver development have added some further specification.[12,14] It appears that intercellular canaliculi are rarely observed before 2 months but are readily seen from 9 weeks onwards.[12] Classic bile canaliculi, lined by two hepatocytes and thus occurring in liver cell plates, are found mainly in the vicinity of draining veins.[14] In contrast, 'hepatocellular tubules' (i.e. bile canaliculi lined by several—more than 3 and up to 14—parenchymal cells) occur more frequently in the region surrounding the portal veins. The lumina are lined by microvilli and sealed by junctional complexes.[14] Apparently, the periportal 'hepatocellular tubules' are those that differentiate into 'bile tubules'[15] in the limiting plate or ductal plate in order to give rise to ductules and ducts (see below under development of intrahepatic bile ducts). A reasonable conclusion seems to be that the architecture in the fetal liver corresponds to a muralium multiplex, but with variations between different livers and even inside the same liver.[16] In neonatal rats, dilated canaliculi without microvilli have been described (Jezequel, LabInvest, 1965; 14:1894; De Wolf-Peeters, ExpMolPath, 1974; 21:339) which are quite similar to those observed in adult cholestasis. This was suggested to represent a cholestatic episode in neonatal rats (De Wolf-Peeters, PediatRes, 1971; 5:704). More recent studies have confirmed the bile secretory immaturity or physiological cholestasis of the liver at birth (Suchy, SemLivDis, 1987; 7:77). Chronologically sequential analysis of canalicular changes in fetal and neonatal rats have led to a proposal for the mechanism of canalicular development between adjacent hepatocytes, by a series of membrane foldings appearing between junctional complexes (De Vos, ExpMolPath, 1975; 23:12). This model of canalicular development has largely been confirmed by studies on hepatocyte monolayers in vitro (Gebhardt, EurJCellBiol, 1982; 29:68; Feltkamp, JCellSci, 1983; 63:271).

Hepatocytes

The majority of progenitor cells differentiate into liver parenchymal cells. During this process, they gradually lose cytokeratins 14 and 19 (Stosiek, Liver, 1990; 10:59). Cytokeratin 19 is no longer detectable in human hepatoblasts after 20 weeks of gestation (Shah,

ArchPathLabMed, 1989; 113:1135; Stosiek, 1990). The histochemical and ultrastructural characteristics of embryonic and fetal hepatocytes have been investigated in a number of studies. Hepatic synthesis and secretion of α_1-fetoprotein begins during the very earliest period of morphological differentiation of the fetal liver, as early as 29 days after conception. α_1-Fetoprotein is synthesized and secreted by the primitive liver cell precursors, and by intestinal and yolk sac cells (Gitlin, JCI, 1969; 48:1433). Human α_1-fetoprotein synthesis is repressed immediately after birth. Glycogen granules were observed in fetal parenchymal cells at about 8 weeks by electron microscopy.[12] Most studies have described the onset of glycogenesis in human liver occurring between the end of the 3rd month and the beginning of the 4th month of intrauterine life. An influence of the hypophyseal–adrenal hormonal sequence on fetal hepatic glycogenesis has been demonstrated. The fetal liver reaches its maximal glycogen reserve at birth. In relation to the onset of glucose-6-phosphatase activity, hepatic glycogen decreases rapidly after birth; within 2 to 3 h, only 10 per cent of the maximum store remains.[2]

Fat appears early in the liver of all mammals studied; in man, its appearance coincides with the start of glycogenesis at about the 4th month of intrauterine life. The increase in hepatocellular lipids is at first slow, but accelerates rapidly at the end of gestation, at which time the hepatic lipid reserve becomes enormous.[2] Although haemosiderin granules are seen in hepatocytes quite early, appreciable hepatocellular iron storage coincides with the slowing down and disappearance of hepatic haematopoiesis. Iron storage reaches its peak at the end of gestation. The haemosiderin granules are almost exclusively located in the hepatocytes in the limiting plate (or ductal plate). The same hepatocytes are also the storage sites for copper and zinc.[2] A number of mitochondrial, microsomal, and lysosomal enzymes were demonstrated by enzyme–histochemical techniques in the parenchymal cells of the liver of a 3-month-old human embryo (Wegmann, ArchMalAppDigNutr, 1965; 54:215). Immunohistochemical investigations on carbamoyl phosphate synthetase, arginase, and glutamate dehydrogenase demonstrated a heterogeneity between rat fetal hepatocytes between days 16 and 20 of gestation. This heterogeneity is related to the vascular architecture of the liver, and disappears perinatally as a result of strong stimulation of enzyme synthesis (Gaasbeek, JHistochemCytochem, 1988; 36:1223).

Morphometric studies have demonstrated major changes during development in the volume density of organelles, especially in the perinatal period (Rohr, LabInvest, 1971; 24:128; Daimon, ExpPath, 1982; 21:237). Morphometric studies on parenchymal zonal gradients in newborn mouse liver revealed that ultrastructural heterogeneity between periportal and centrolobular hepatocytes (in terms of volume density of organelles) is not present in newborn mice but gradually develops during the first 10 days of postnatal life (Asada-Kubota, AnatRec, 1982; 202:395). Canalicular motility is disordered and actin investment of fetal hepatocytes is immature, but rapidly develops after birth (Miyari, PediatRes, 1985; 19:1225). The Golgi apparatus of fetal hepatocytes in very young embryos is located near the nucleus; it moves towards the canaliculus at about 3 months, when bile secretion is said to begin.[12] The literature on fetal bile acid metabolism and the development of bile formation has been summarized (Suchy, SemLivDis, 1987; 7:77). In its initial phase, hepatocyte-specific gene expression is subject to a complex regulation at the transcriptional and translational level (Van Roon, DevBiol, 1989; 136:508). Hepatocyte differentiation requires interactions between hepatic endoderm and mesenchyme (Houssaint, CellDiff, 1980; 9:269). Changes in the extracellular matrix are likely to play a key role in the regulation of liver cell phenotype and in the maintenance of hepatocyte polarity during development (Reif, Hepatol, 1990; 12:519).

Sinusoids, sinusoidal lining cells, Kupffer cells, and hepatic stellate cells

Minot coined the term 'intercrescence' for the process involved in establishing the relationship between the early developing parenchyma and the blood vessels in the septum transversum (Minot, ProcBostonSocNatHist, 1900; 29:185).'Intercrescence' implies a reciprocal interaction between pre-established blood vessels and the liver parenchyma, in such a manner that large vessels are broken down by the invasion of the growing parenchymal cords. Most authors, however, reject this interpretation and adhere to the concept that sinusoids develop in situ.[2,4] Small endothelium-lined spaces develop in the septum transversum, near the hepatic diverticulum. The parenchymal cords projecting from the walls of the diverticulum into the mesenchyme of the septum transversum anastomose around these pre-existing endothelium-lined vesicles. The parenchymal sprouts nearest the diverticulum surround the largest of these vesicles, while those cords further away from the diverticulum surround either smaller endothelial-lined spaces or small masses of mesenchyme. The older the embryo and the greater the amount of parenchymal proliferation, the more well-defined become the endothelium-lined spaces. The spaces nearest the diverticulum start to coalesce, resulting in anastomosing vessels. It appears that, once the mesenchyme is isolated by anastomosing parenchymal cords, cellular rearrangement occurs with subsequent formation of small vessels. It has become the classical concept that the liver parenchymal cells invade the mesenchyme of the septum transversum and surround pre-existing sinusoids (Lipp, ZMikroskAnatForsch, 1952; 59:161; Elias, ActaHepatolJpn, 1955; 3:1), a phenomenon termed 'interstitial invasion'.[4] During early developmental stages, the sinusoidal endothelium shows large intercellular gaps allowing passage of haematopoietic cells.[17] By 18 weeks of gestation, small-sized fenestrae often provided with a diaphragm appear.[17]

More specific cell types of the sinusoidal lining become identifiable during the second half of the 3rd month: Kupffer cells with active phagocytosis appear, and hepatic stellate cells (fat-storing cells, Ito cells) located in the Disse spaces contain one or two fat droplets.[18] The origin of Kupffer cells has not been settled: they may originate from primitive macrophages derived from the yolk sac which colonize the liver or, alternatively, may develop in loco from haematopoietic stem cells (Naito, JLeukBiol, 1990; 48:27). The number of Kupffer cells increases during gestation, reaching normal adult values in the neonatal period (Cope, ClinExpImmun, 1990; 81:485).

Haematopoiesis

From the 6th gestational week (10-mm stage) the liver begins to assume haematopoietic activity, when the first haemocytoblasts appear.[2] The first blood-forming islands are found in the 12-mm, or 7th week, embryo. These increase in number and volume and invade all of the hepatic parenchyma, but are more pronounced in the right lobe of the liver.[2] By the 12th week, the liver is the main site of haematopoiesis superseding the yolk sac.[3] Haematopoiesis in the liver attains its maximal activity towards the 6th to 7th month,[2] and then regresses rapidly as the bone marrow becomes haematopoietic. The fetal liver at birth contains only a few disseminated islands, which disappear during the first weeks after birth. Hepatic haematopoiesis in man is essentially erythropoietic, mainly forming definite erythroblasts, although the stem cells also give rise to granulocytes, megakaryocytes, and monocytes. Cells of the erythroid lineage form circumscribed clusters in the hepatic parenchyma (Timens, VirchArchA, 1990; 416:429). Sorenson (AmJAnat, 1960; 106:27) described the close contact between primitive hepatoblasts and haematopoietic cells, with indentations in the cellular membrane of erythroblasts, which were considered to be the morphological expression of the exchanges taking place between the two types of cells—an intercellular pinocytosis or 'rhopheocytosis' (Policard, CRAcadSci, 1958; 246:3194). The transcription factor erythroid Kruppel-like factor (EKLF) appears to be essential for the final steps of definitive erythropoiesis in fetal liver (Nuez, Nature, 1995; 375:316). Cells of the myelomonocytic lineage appear from about 6 weeks of gestation onwards and are mainly present in the mesenchymal tissue surrounding the portal vein branches (Timens, VirchArchA, 1990; 416:429). Lymphoid cells become detectable from 14 weeks of gestation. Hepatocytes may play an active role in T lymphopoiesis in the fetal liver (Nanno, JImmunol, 1995; 155:2918). According to Timens et al., the presence of immature blast cells displaying exclusive reactivity with the monoclonal antibody MT1 appear to be a unique feature of fetal liver haematopoiesis. In the mouse, the stem cells develop de novo in the blood islands of the yolk sac, proliferate, and migrate to colonize the fetal liver and other lymphoid and myeloid organs.[3] During its haematopoietic phase, the liver produces a stimulator that in vitro can switch quiescent mouse marrow stem cells into active mode (Dawood, JAnat, 1990; 168:209).[3] In mouse liver, declining production of this stimulator in late gestation and after birth correlates with a decrease in haematopoietic stem cell numbers in the liver (Dawood, 1990).[3]

Different populations of haematopoietic precursors expressing SR-1 Ad, the c-kit receptor, CD33, CD34, and the 'homing' receptor CD44 have been isolated from fetal liver (Papayannopoulou, Blood, 1991; 78:1403). Interestingly, epithelial cells of ductal plates and immature bile ducts are immunoreactive to c-kit, CD33, and CD34 (Blakolmer, Hepatol, 1995; 21:1510). The expression of the latter three antigens, which are usually regarded as early haematopoietic markers by liver progenitor cells, raises the question of whether the relationship between the liver parenchyma and the haematopoietic system may be closer than previously thought. Likewise, the expression of the rat oval cell antigens OC2 and OC3 by both hepatic and haematopoietic precursor cells (Sigal, Hepatol, 1994; 19:999) suggests a close relationship between liver cells and haematopoietic cells. The complement regulatory proteins decay-accelerating factor (DAF), membrane cofactor protein (MCP), and CD59 are differentially expressed by the haematopoietic and epithelial cell compartments in the developing human liver (Simpson, Immunol, 1993; 80:183).

Hepatic vasculature and circulation

As previously mentioned, the earliest anlage of the liver in the 3- to 4-mm embryo develops in connection with the vitelline (omphalomesenteric) veins. The latter form a capillary plexus which soon becomes invested in a muralium formed by the outgrowing primitive hepatoblasts. Beginning cranially, anastomotic capillaries connect the umbilical veins with the vitelline venous plexus. This is possible because between the anterior intestinal portal and the sinus venosus, the septum transversum unites the body wall (in which the umbilical veins run) with the splanchnopleure which harbours the vitelline veins.[4] The vitelline veins play a role in the development of the portal vein (which drains the blood from the intestine), whereas the umbilical veins (draining the blood from the placenta and becoming the principal source of blood entering the liver) play the major role in organizing the intrahepatic vasculature and determining hepatic segmentation. During the 5-mm stage, three large anastomoses are established between the caudal portions of the vitelline veins. The most cranial one is situated within the liver; the other two are inferior to it. The middle communicant vessel passes dorsally, and the caudal anastomosis passes ventrally to the gut (Fig. 2). In this way two venous rings are formed, one above the other. By the 9-mm stage, the right half of the upper ring and the left half of the lower ring disappear. The end result is an S-shaped vessel, which later becomes the portal

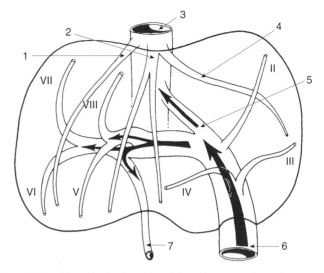

Fig. 3. Portal hepatic circulation in a 17-mm human embryo. 1, vena hepatica dextra; 2, vena hepatica media; 3, vena cava inferior; 4, vena hepatica sinistra; 5, ductus venosus; 6, vena umbilicalis sinistra; 7, vena portae. (Redrawn from Lassau, AnatClin, 1983; 5:97–102, with permission.)

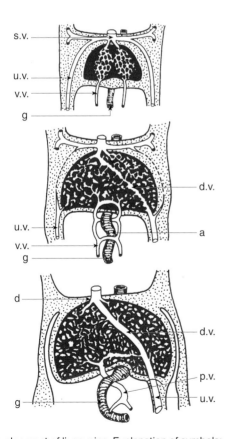

Fig. 2. Development of liver veins. Explanation of symbols: a, caudal anastomosis of distal vitelline veins; d, diaphragm; d.v., ductus venosus; g, gut; p.v., portal vein; s.v., sinus venosus; u.v., umbilical veins; v.v., vitelline veins. Liver parenchyma in black. (Redrawn from ref. 2, with permission.)

vein.[2] Cranially to the liver, the stems of the vitelline veins enter into the primitive sinus venosus as the hepatocardiac channels. The right channel later becomes greatly enlarged to form the right hepatic vein, the main drainage from the liver. The left channel regresses.[2,4,16]

In the 6- to 7-mm embryo, the right umbilical vein and the proximal portion of the left umbilical vein disappear rapidly. The distal portion of the left umbilical vein persists and becomes the main source of blood entering the liver, partly because of the disappearance of its partner on the right side so that it has to carry all the oxygenated blood coming from the placenta, and partly because the volume of blood returning from the gut in the vitelline veins is small. In the 6-mm embryo, a large venous trunk develops in the sinusoidal system and shunts blood directly from the umbilical vein to the inferior vena cava, probably in response to the obliquely directed stream of placental blood.[2-4,16] This ductus venosus Arantii persists until birth; at that time it atrophies and after 10 to 20 days it leaves as a vestige the ligamentum venosum. The definitive vascular pattern of the fetal liver becomes established around the 6th week (embryos 17-mm long) (Fig. 3) (Lassau, AnatClin, 1983; 5:97). At this stage the umbilical vein reaches the anteroinferior margin of the liver and bends backwards at a right angle to penetrate the hepatic mass. The vein bifurcates to anastomose with the inferior vena cava by means of the ductus venosus and to merge with the left branch of the developing portal vein. Blood in the left umbilical vein has a choice of three routes through the liver: (i) through branches which enter the sinusoidal plexus of the left half of the liver; (ii) through the sinusoidal plexus of the right half of the liver, by retrograde flow through its connection with the left branch of the portal vein; and (iii) through the ductus venosus directly into the inferior vena cava. In the fetus, therefore, the umbilical vein is the major component of the portal system, as indeed it must be since the placenta is the sole source of nutrients.[3]

Study of the differences in calibre of the venous structures can give an idea of the direction and form of blood flow through the embryonic liver. From such studies it appears that the portal segmentation[19] appears to be initiated and maintained uniquely by the direction and force of blood flow through the left umbilical vein. This represents a haemodynamic concept rather than the vestigial theory of the development of liver vasculature and hepatic segmentation (Lassau, AnatClin, 1983; 5:97). Data on the development of the hepatic arterial system are more sparse. In the 10-mm embryo, a hepatic branch of the celiac artery can be followed up to the ductus hepaticus. The branch to the cystic duct develops first, so that the hepatic artery first seems to be the artery for the gallbladder.[20] Its further branchings follow those of the portal system. Compared with their appearance in the fully developed liver, the arterial branches are fairly large relative to the portal vein branches.[16] At birth, a sphincteric mechanism closes the ductus venosus at its proximal end, blood flow ceases in the umbilical vein, and the left side of the liver receives blood which now flows from right to left through the left branch of the portal vein. Through the directness of the entrance of the portal vein into the right end of the great umbilical arch, portal blood supply to the right side of the liver is excellent, but flow to the left occurs by circuitous routes. This impairment of blood flow to the left side of the liver has usually been considered to be the main cause for the relative retardation of growth of the left and quadrate lobes.[4] Recent studies, however, indicate an intrinsic hepatic asymmetry throughout the embryonic period with a greater proportion of the liver mass being to the right of the median plane (Hutchins, PediatPath, 1988; 8:17). After birth, the segment of the umbilical vein between the umbilicus and the liver regresses into a fibrous cord—the ligamentum teres hepatis.

Innervation

The development of nerves in the human fetal liver has been studied by Tiniakos et al.[21] using immunohistochemistry. A few neurofilament-containing fibres are present at the liver hilum as early as 8 weeks, but portal tract innervation is not observed before 12 weeks.[21] The density of the fibres (detected using antibodies to PGP 9.5, S-100 protein, neurone-specific enolase, and neurofilament) progressively increases towards term although intra-sinusoidal fibres appear late in gestation.[21] Galaninergic and somatostatinergic fibres are present from 22 weeks of gestation onwards but are no longer detectable at birth and are absent in the adult liver.[21] In contrast, neuropeptide-Y-ergic fibres cannot be detected in fetal livers at any gestational age but are present at term and in adult liver.[21] Developmentally regulated expression of neuropeptides such as galanin and somatostatin may play a role in morphogenesis and control of physiological processes during fetal development.

Cholangiogenesis: development of bile ducts

Development of extrahepatic bile ducts and the gallbladder

The development of the extrahepatic bile ducts in the human has only recently been documented in two meticulous studies by Tan and Moscoso.[5,22] The primitive extrahepatic bile duct originates from the hepatic foregut diverticulum. It is in contact with the hepatic anlage from the start of organogenesis and remains so throughout gestation.[5] In the 34-day embryo, the common bile duct is a tube lined by columnar epithelium. At this stage, the common hepatic duct is a broad funnel-like structure in direct contact with the liver, without a recognizable left or right hepatic duct.[5] During the 5th week, a rapid endodermal proliferation occurs in the funnel-shaped common hepatic duct, giving rise to multiple channels at the level of the porta hepatis.[5] Tan and Moscoso speculate that this remodelling may explain in part the many normal variants of right and left hepatic duct morphology.[5] Up to 8 weeks of gestation, the extrahepatic biliary tree develops by lengthening of the caudal part of the hepatic diverticulum and remains completely patent.[5] The observations by Tan and Moscoso disprove the long-held concept that there is a 'solid stage' of endodermal occlusion of the common bile duct lumen. It follows that extrahepatic bile duct atresia cannot be caused by a failure of recanalization of the common bile duct.[5] The distal portions of the right and left main hepatic ducts develop from the extrahepatic bile ducts and are clearly defined tubular structures by 12 weeks of gestation.[22] The proximal portion of the hilar bile ducts derives from the intrahepatic ductal plate.[22] The extrahepatic bile ducts and the developing intrahepatic biliary tree maintain luminal continuity from the very start of organogenesis throughout further development.[22] Following the rotation of the gut, which occurs at about the 5th week, the attachment of the common bile ducts becomes displaced to the dorsal side of the duodenum.[2]

The gallbladder anlage is already seen at 29 days postfertilization as a right anterolateral dilatation along the distal half of the hepatic diverticulum.[5] No primitive liver cells are seen in continuity with the gallbladder anlage.[5] The cystic duct is already present at 34 days postfertilization.[5] At that stage, a narrow lumen is patent throughout the gallbladder and the cystic duct. From 11 weeks of gestation onwards, the gallbladder epithelium reacts with a monoclonal antibody directed against a 40-kDa autoantigen in ulcerative colitis (Das, JClinGastro, 1992; 15:311). This unique epitope appears simultaneously in the gut and the skin.

Development of intrahepatic bile ducts

During the first 7 weeks or so of embryonic life, there is no intrahepatic bile duct system in the liver.[4,11] Different authors give varying reports of the precise moment of its first appearance. Its formation sets in at about the 18-mm[4,16] to 22-mm stage[11] or between the 5th and 9th gestational week.[2] Several theories have been advanced on the development of the intrahepatic duct system. One theory maintains that the intrahepatic bile ducts are derived exclusively from proliferation and ingrowth of the epithelium from the large hilar duct structures.[23] This concept is now abandoned, and most authors adhere to the hepatocytogenic origin of intrahepatic bile ducts, originally proposed by Kölliker.[24] A combined theory has attempted to reconcile both points of view and suggests that the larger ducts up to and including the interlobular ducts are derived from the primitive hepatic duct whereas the remaining part of the system, the ductules or cholangioles, are derived from parenchymal cells.[16,25] The predominant view nowadays, with increasing supportive evidence,

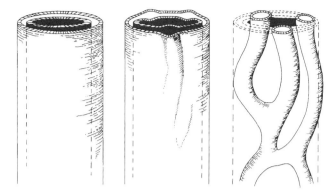

Fig. 4. Schematic representation of intrahepatic bile duct development. Left panel: ductal plate. The central axis (containing a branch of the portal vein with its surrounding mesenchyme) is encircled by a double cylinder of bile duct-type cells (in reality, the double-walled cylinder is perforated). Middle panel: early remodelling of ductal plate. Dilated lumina appear in some segments of the cylindrical perimeter. These dilated parts remain, whereas the intervening parts of the ductal plate disappear (see also Plate 1). Right panel: network of interlobular bile ducts incorporated into the connective tissue of the portal tract, representing the end result of ductal plate remodelling (see also Plate 2).

is that the ductal epithelium is derived from hepatoblasts. This hepatocytogenic interpretation of the development of intrahepatic bile ducts will be adhered to in the following description.

Most workers agree with the following basic observations: the development of the intrahepatic bile duct system starts geographically at the porta hepatis, and afterwards proceeds to the periphery of the liver;[7,8,13,15,22] a formed section of the system always seems to be in continuity with segments more distal to it;[11,13,22] and the bile duct system develops in close relationship with the developing afferent vascular system of the liver (Shiojiri, AnatEmbryol, 1992; 185:17). Although the afferent veins comprise the umbilical vein branches as well as the portal vein ramifications (see above), in the following description all afferent veins will be termed 'portal' (for reasons of simplicity and also because they are located in the future portal tracts). Indeed, in contrast to the efferent veins of the liver, which remain thin-walled, the afferent 'portal' vessels are surrounded by a cuff of mesenchyme (Mollier, GegenbaursMorphJahrb, 1939; 83:569). In the developing liver, the continuous further branching of the portal veins induces the constant creation of new perivenous mesenchymal sheets, which are the forerunners of future portal tract connective tissue strands. The fetal hepatic cells in contact with the mesenchyme surrounding a portal vein branch are smaller and more darkly staining than the remaining primitive hepatoblasts. This is interpreted as a transformation of primitive parenchymal cells into bile duct-type cells (arguments in favour are discussed below) (Fig. 4). This periportal layer of transformed hepatocytes forms a cylindrical sheet, or more appropriately a perforated sheet or sleeve of epithelium, around the portal mesenchyme. This epithelial sleeve corresponds to the 'ductal plate',[23] or the 'limiting plate'.[2] There is general agreement that primarily this plate is one cell thick. This is the layer of cells also rich in haemosiderin and copper granules.[2]

Soon afterwards, a second interrupted or discontinuous layer of cells shows a similar transformation into bile duct-type cells, resulting in a partly double epithelial sleeve delineating a slit-like lumen, and encircling the portal mesenchyme (Plate 1). Here some controversy arises. Apparently, it is too schematic to describe the ductal plate simply as a continuous circular double-layer of epithelium. Hammar himself, using three-dimensional reconstruction models, describes his ductal plate as being single layered in the more peripheral parts of the liver, as consisting of a double layer outlining a slit-like circular lumen in areas more proximal to the liver hilum, and as assuming a string of pearl-like appearance in areas still closer to the hilum.[23] Thus, with progressing development, the plate showed an increasing number of holes of increasing size. These holes were traversed by vessels with associated connective tissue. Horstmann insists that there is no continuous circular double-layer, but a closely meshed network of 'tubules' surrounding the portal mesenchyme.[15] Others share this view.[14] These 'bile tubules' are transitory embryonic structures as precursors of the future bile ducts.[13] It appears that species differences may also determine the detailed appearance of the ductal plate: for instance it appears more as a network of tubules (resembling a string of pearls in cross-section) in the rat[8] than in man.[7] It seems an acceptable summary that the ductal plate can be viewed as a perforated double-layered epithelial sleeve.[26] The number, size, and spacing of the holes or 'perforations' in the sleeve determine the appearance on microscopic sections—either as a closely set series of tubules, or as curved epithelium-lined segments, or as a combination of both. The issue is not of extreme importance; even if there is an early stage in which the ductal plate is continuously cylindrical, it must be very transient.

Very soon, 'remodelling' of the ductal plate sets in: some parts of the slit-like lumen become more dilated, and the dilated parts become separated by ingrowing mesenchyme, resulting in the progressive 'perforation' of the sleeve or, in other words, resulting in a network of tubules as shown in the wax models of Hammar (Fig. 4).[23] The important issue in this process is that the developing network of tubules remains in luminal continuity with the parenchymal network of canaliculi through multiple connections between the mesenchymal interruptions. Further 'remodelling' of the ductal plate into portal bile ducts involves the gradual incorporation of the 'tubule' into the expanding mesenchyme, with separation of the tubule from the parenchyma by interposition of mesenchyme so that the future bile duct comes to lie more centrally in the broadening portal connective tissue (Plate 2). Remodelling further implies a relative decrease in the number of tubules. This seems to be brought about by preferential development of some parts of the network,[15] by stretching of the network due to concomitant liver growth,[13] and also by breakdown and resorption of the excess of early embryonic structures.[16]

This process results in the appearance of an anastomosing network of individualized portal bile ducts (Fig. 4). It first occurs in larger portal spaces, and proceeds from the hilar region to the periphery of the liver. The first generation of ducts (left and right hepatic ducts) are present from 12 weeks onwards.[22] Second and third generation ducts are observed at 15 weeks and between 17 and 25 weeks, respectively.[22] The gradient from hilum to periphery explains why, in a liver of a given gestational age, several stages of development of intrahepatic bile ducts are observed simultaneously, with mature ducts in older (hilar) portal tracts and more or less immature duct structures in more peripheral parts of the liver.[7,8, 15] It is interesting that, even at 40 weeks of gestation, some of the smallest portal vein branches are not yet accompanied by an individualized mature bile duct, but are still in a stage where they are surrounded by a discontinuous ductal plate.[7,8] This indicates that the intrahepatic bile duct system is still immature at the time of birth, and that further development of the finest ramifications of the intrahepatic biliary tree proceeds during the first few weeks of life.[7] This observation has implications for the early histo-pathological diagnosis of diseases characterized by paucity of intrahepatic bile ducts, in which determination of the bile duct-to-portal tract ratio is of diagnostic significance (Kahn, Hepatol, 1989; 10: 21).

In summary, the entire system of intrahepatic bile ducts and ductules develops from hepatoblasts in the limiting plate, and the process proceeds for some time after birth in the peripheral areas of the liver. The divergent theory of Hammar claims that the intrahepatic bile ducts derive from ductal epithelium growing in from the porta hepatis and 'sliding' or 'skating' along the portal mesenchyme. Hammar's conclusions were based on the same findings as those described here. It is important to determine which observations allow us to discard his concept, and to prefer the hepatocytogenic interpretation of intrahepatic bile duct development when faced with identical findings. A histological argument is that the formation of the bile ducts always takes place at the junction between the muralia of the liver sponge and an afferent portal vein with its surrounding cuff of mesenchyme, that is, always in the most intimate contact with primitive hepatoblasts (Shiojiri, AnatEmbryol, 1992; 185:17).[7,16] At the cytological level, an argument in favour of the hepatocytogenic origin of the ducts can be found from the observation of intermediate or transitional types between the parenchymal cells and the smaller, darker, bile duct cells. Such intermediate cell types were observed by some of the early investigators using the light microscope[4,15] but denied by others.[4, 15,20,23,25] Later electron microscopic investigations repeatedly identified intermediate cell types (Enzan, ActaPathJpn, 1974; 24: 427),[14] thus confirming their existence as reported by earlier light microscopic studies.

The presence of glycogen in cells of the ductal plate[12,23] can also be taken as an indicator of their derivation from hepatocytes. Enzyme–histochemical staining revealed transitional forms between hepatocytes and cells of the ductal plate (Wegmann, Arch-MalAppDigNutr, 1965; 54:215). Recent immunohistochemical studies on developing human and rat liver have provided irrefutable evidence that the cells forming the ductal plates are hepatoblasts which gradually acquire (through a stage of 'transitional cells') the full set of phenotypic characteristics of mature intrahepatic bile duct cells (Germain, CancerRes, 1988; 44:4909; Gall, JGastHepatol, 1989; 4:241; Shah, ArchPathLabMed, 1989; 113:1135; Fausto, CurrOpinCellBiol, 1990; 2:1036; Marceau, LabInvest, 1990; 63:4; Ruebner, PediatPath, 1990; 10:55; Shiojiri, CancerRes, 1991; 51: 2611; Mathew, JClinPath, 1992; 45:679).[7,8] Throughout development, cells of the ductal plates and of the interlobular bile ducts show a strong immunoreactivity for cytokeratins 8 and 18 and stain for cytokeratin 19 (Plates 1 and 2). At around 20 weeks of gestation, individual bile ducts in large portal tracts show a weak apical positivity for cytokeratin 7 (thereby acquiring the full set of cytokeratins characteristic of normal biliary epithelial cells, i.e. cytokeratins 7, 8, 18, and 19) (Fig. 5) (Blakolmer, Hepatol, 1995; 21:1510). [7] Over the following weeks of gestation, bile ducts and ductal plate cells display an increasing inmmunoreactivity for cytokeratin 7, but 'adult' staining intensity is reached only at 1 month after birth.[7]

Ductal plate cells are reactive with antibodies directed against α_1-antitrypsin and α-fetoprotein (Blakolmer, 1995). New carbohydrate chain structures gradually emerge as intrahepatic bile ducts develop and mature (Terada, Hepatol, 1994; 20:388). Before birth, biliary epithelial cells express the apomucin (mucin core protein) **MUC1**. By contrast, in the postnatal liver, MUC1 expression is lost and epithelial cells of intrahepatic large bile ducts constantly express MUC3 (Sasaki, AmJPathol, 1995; 147:574). The pancreatic enzymes α-amylase, trypsinogen, and lipase are expressed in developing and mature hilar bile ducts and in immature hepatocytes (9 to 25 weeks of gestation) (Terada, Gastro, 1995; 108:1236). These enzymes are not detectable in peripheral ductal plates or bile ducts. These data lend support to the concept that the cell lineage of the intrahepatic hilar bile ducts and hepatocytes is similar or identical to that of the pancreatic ducts and exocrine pancreatic cells (Terada, 1995). The potential of hepatoblasts to transform into biliary epithelium has also been confirmed in cell culture experiments (Germain, CancerRes, 1988; 48:4909) and by transplanting fragments of fetal liver not yet containing bile ducts (Shiojiri, JEmbrExpMorph, 1984; 79:25, Gall, JExpPath, 1990; 71:41).

It is interesting that in the adult liver, in several pathological conditions associated with chronic cholestasis, a similar phenotypic shift from hepatocytes into bile duct-type cells occurs, suggesting the reappearance of an ontogenic phenomenon in pathological conditions.[27] It is important to determine which factor(s) determine(s) the differentiation of primitive hepatoblasts into bile duct cells. Several authors have emphasized the modulating role of the portal mesenchyme.[2,11,15] This is supported by experiences with tissue cultures of liver cells which on addition of fibroblasts changed in appearance and growth pattern towards structures resembling bile ducts (Doljanski, VirchArchA, 1934; 292:256). For Horstmann this was a strong argument in favour of the hepatocytogenic theory.[15] Ductal plate cells are accompanied by laminin and type IV collagen throughout all stages of formation and remodelling (Shah, ArchPathLabMed, 1990; 114:597; Terada, Histopath, 1994; 25:143). The extracellular matrix glycoprotein tenascin may be involved in the development of the hilar bile ducts (Terada, Histopath, 1994; 25:143). Various growth factors may be involved in bile duct development. Biliary epithelial cells of all developmental stages are immunoreactive for transforming growth factor-α and its receptor, allowing for proliferation and differentiation of bile duct cells via an autocrine mechanism (Terada, VirchArch, 1994; 424: 669). Parathyroid hormone–related peptide (**PTHrP**) may also function as a growth and differentiation factor for growing and maturing bile ducts (Roskams, IntHepatolComm, 1994; 2:121). PTHrP is the product of a growth factor regulated gene. Remodelling ductal plates and bile ducts in neonates are strongly immunoreactive for PTHrP. Immunoreactivity decreases and is no longer present by the age of 4 years

Others (Aron, CRMemSocBiol, 1921; 85:110) have suggested a morphogenetic influence from a factor in the portal blood; this

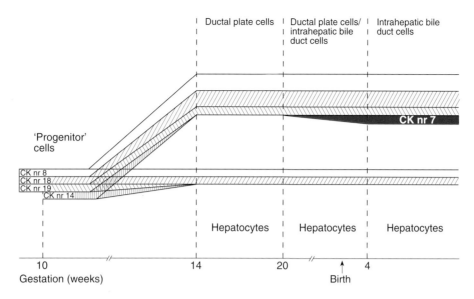

Fig. 5. Schematic representation of the cell lineage relationships in developing human liver and the development of the intrahepatic bile ducts as determined by cytokeratin-immunohistochemistry (Stosiek, Liver, 1990; 10:59; Haruna, Hepatol, 1994; 20:210A).[7] For detailed discussion see text.

remains a valid, but still unproven, hypothesis. Incipient bile formation and secretion in the embryonic liver has been suggested as a factor inducing the development of the ducts. However, at first sight this is difficult to accept, because bile secretion cannot be demonstrated until the 3rd[20] or the beginning of the 4th fetal month,[25] as judged from bile staining (bilirubin) of the gut content. Bile acid synthesis begins near week 12 in the human fetus, and on day 11 of the 22-day gestation in the rat. In the latter, bile acid synthesis thus starts before the first signs of development of intrahepatic bile ducts, which occurs on day 16.[8] Although the start of bile duct formation is observed earlier than week 12 in the human embryo, it is conceivable that a low level of unusual bile acid synthesis plays a role, in view of the complexity of the ontogeny of bile acid synthesis in man (Suchy, SemLivDis, 1987; 7:77).

Recently, the hypothesis has been raised that a small number of bipotential progenitor cells persist in the adult human and rat liver (Sell, CancerRes, 1990; 50:3811; Shiojiri, CancerRes, 1991; 51: 2611).[10,28] This would have tremendous implications for liver carcinogenesis and regeneration (Marceau, LabInvest, 1990; 63:4; Sell, 1990).[27,28] Evidence to support this hypothesis is currently accumulating and excellent reviews have been devoted to this topic (Sell, 1990).[10,28] Studies supporting the concept of a stem cell (Sell, AmJPathol, 1983; 134:1347) locate this still hypothetical element in the smallest ductules or canals of Hering. The canal of Hering is the smallest, terminal ramification connecting the bile draining ducts with the canalicular network.[29] It is partly lined by bile duct cells, and partly by hepatocytes. The early embryonic ductal plate, with its first layer of ductal cells and its interrupted second layer developing from hepatocytes, is the most primitive type of embryonic duct and at the same time the first edition of a structure equivalent to the canal of Hering. It will be interesting to discover whether this parenchymal–ductal junction does indeed encompass stem cells in the adult organ as it does in the embryonic stage.

Terada and Nakanuma (AmJPathol, 1995; 146:67) have recently presented data suggesting that balanced cell proliferation and apoptosis (programmed cell death) are involved in the normal development of intrahepatic bile ducts and hepatocytes. The number of apoptotic cells as detected by *in situ* nick end labelling was high in the remodelling ductal plates. The *fas* antigen, c-myc protein, and Lewis[y] antigen (thought to be stimulators of apoptosis) were detected by immunohistochemistry in hepatocytes, ductal plates, remodelling ductal plates, and bile duct cells throughout development (Terada, AmJPathol, 1995; 146:67). The Bcl-2 protein, an inhibitor of apoptosis, was only very weakly expressed by remodelling ductal plates. Imbalance between apoptosis and cell proliferation during fetal development of the intrahepatic bile ducts may lead to congenital diseases of the intrahepatic bile ducts characterized by the 'ductal plate malformation' (see Section 11). Appropriate secretion and balanced activation and inactivation of matrix proteinases (matrix metalloproteinases, serine proteinases, cysteine proteinases) may also be essential for the normal development (and in particular the 'remodelling') of the biliary tree (Terada, AmJPathol, 1995; 147:1207).

Development of the peribiliary glands and the peribiliary capillary plexus

The large intrahepatic bile ducts contain both intra- and extramural peribiliary glands (Terada, Liver, 1987; 7:1). According to Terada and Nakanuma, both types of peribiliary glands arise from the ductal plates at the liver hilum (Terada, LabInvest, 1993; 68:261). Their formation starts at 10 weeks of gestation with epithelial buds growing from the ductal plates. Tan and Moscoso hold a slightly different view and describe the formation of peribiliary glands from epithelial evaginations of tubular structures (i.e. a more advanced stage of bile duct formation).[22] By 30 weeks the buds are completely transformed into small tubules. At birth, incomplete or immature peribiliary glands are present. Mucus acini containing neutral mucin, sialomucin, and sulphomucin only appear 3 months after birth. An adult state with a normal density of peribiliary glands is only reached by the age of 15 years.

The intrahepatic bile ducts are nourished by the peribiliary capillary plexus (a capillary network derived from the hepatic artery) (Terada, JHepatol, 1989; 8:139). Using immunohistochemistry for von Willebrand factor and lectin histochemistry (*Ulex europaeus* lectin, succinylated wheat germ agglutinin), Terada and Nakanuma (Hepatol, 1993; 18:529) have documented the development of the peribiliary capillary plexus. It appears that the plexus arises from spindle-shaped 'angioblasts' in the mesenchyme surrounding the portal vein branches. Gradually, vessels are formed which—through successive stages termed 'immature' and 'premature' peribiliary plexus—finally develop into mature peribiliary plexus. The development of the plexus thus occurs at the same rate as that of the intrahepatic bile duct system. Again, development first starts at the liver hilum and only later spreads to the peripheral portions of the liver. The 'mature' stage is reached at 15 years.

Hepatic growth and lobular development

The embryonic liver develops very quickly and tends to occupy all the space not used by neighbouring organs. The liver is already bilobed in the 7.5-mm embryo. The caudate lobe develops at 6 weeks, the quadrate lobe somewhat later. The hepatic volume increases consistently, but the ratio of hepatic volume to body volume is not constant (5 per cent in the 10-mm embryo, 10 per cent at the 30-mm stage, 5 per cent in the newborn, and 2 per cent in the adult). The curve of the relative liver weight is comparable with that of the relative volume.[2] Scatter factor/hepatocyte growth factor (**SF/HGF**) appears to be essential for the development of the liver. Mice lacking SF/HGF die *in utero* with livers markedly reduced in size and showing extensive loss of parenchymal cells (Schmidt, Nature, 1995; 373:699). Using Northern blot analysis, fetal human liver contains an 11- to 22-fold increased HGF mRNA (hepatotrophin mRNA) level compared with adult human liver (Selden, FEBSLett, 1990; 270:81). Other factors such as basic fibroblast growth factor and transforming growth factor-α (**TGF-α**) (Fausto, AnnNYAcadSci, 1990; 593P: 231; Hoffman, JCellPhysiol, 1990; 142:149) may also be important in regulating normal growth and development of the liver. The latter two factors are hepatotrophic mitogens. During human liver development, immature hepatocytes display moderate immunoreactivity for both TGF-α and its receptor (Terada, VirchArch, 1994; 424:669). In the postnatal liver, TGF-α immunoreactivity gradually decreases to become negative in adult hepatocytes while immunoreactivity for the TGF-α receptor increases and is strongly positive in adult human liver. These data suggest an important role for TGF-α and its receptor in the control of proliferation of fetal hepatocytes. Transforming growth factor-β$_1$, on the other hand, may act as an inhibitor of hepatocyte DNA replication (Fausto, AnnNYAcadSci, 1990; 593P:231).

Mitotic inhibitory activity also resides in a group of proteins of low molecular weight, called hepatocyte proliferation inhibitor (**HPI**), isolated from the cytosolic fraction of adult human liver

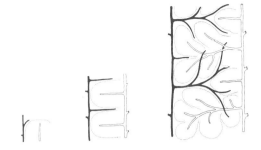

Fig. 6. Scheme representing three successive stages of liver lobule development. Black vessels, portal vein branches; white vessels, hepatic vein branches. Note that this scheme refers to the lobular concept of liver architecture (with draining veins in the centre of the lobule). (Redrawn after ref.[20].)

(Chen, Cytobios, 1989; 59:79). In a study of developing human liver, HPI activity was first noticed in the cytosolic fraction of a 20-week-old fetal liver and thereafter increased with liver maturation (Geetha Devi, BiochemCellBiol, 1993; 71:241). An inverse correlation between the ontogeny of HPI activity and mitotic counts of hepatocytes during human liver development was established. During development, modulation of extracellular matrix proteins takes place as documented by Reif *et al.* (Hepatol, 1990; 12:519). In developing rat liver, the content of type I and type II collagen and laminin decreases in the perinatal period (from 17 days of gestation onwards). The higher laminin and collagen content of the fetal liver may be related to a stimulatory role in cell proliferation. Moreover, the fetal liver shows a diffuse and punctate staining of extracellular matrix proteins in contrast to the more restricted localization (around vascular networks and in the perisinusoidal area) seen in adult liver. The development of the structural and functional units of the liver has been studied from the point of view of the classical hexagonal liver lobule of Kiernan (PhTrRoySoc, 1833; 123:711) (Fig. 6). Although today this concept is replaced by the acinar unit of liver structure (Rappaport, BeitrPath, 1976; 157:215), and the latter itself is subject to further modifications (Lamers, Hepatol, 1989; 10:72), the basic principle remains that development of new parenchymal units is determined by the development of further branches of the afferent veins and their interdigitation with the newly forming branches of the draining veins (Johnson, AmJAnat, 1919; 25:299).[20]

References

1. Nishimura H. Introduction. In Nishimura H, ed. *Atlas of Human Prenatal Histology*. Tokyo: Igaku-Shoin, 1983: 1–4.
2. Dubois AM. The embryonic liver. In Rouiller C, ed. *The Liver*. New York: Academic Press, 1963: 1–39.
3. MacSween RNM and Scothorne RJ. Developmental anatomy and normal structure. In MacSween RNM, Anthony PP, Scheuer PJ, Burt AD, and Portmann BC, eds. *Pathology of the Liver*. Edinburgh: Churchill Livingstone, 1994: 1–49.
4. Elias H and Sherrick JC. *Morphology of the Liver*. New York: Academic Press, 1969.
5. Tan CEL and Moscoso GJ. The developing human biliary system at the porta hepatis level between 29 days and 8 weeks of gestation: a way to understanding biliary atresia. Part 1. *Pathology International*, 1994; **44**: 587–99.

6. Desmet VJ and Van Eyken P. Embryology, malformations and malpositions. In Haubrich W and Schaffner F, eds. *Bockus Gastroenterology*, 5th edn. Philadelphia: WB Saunders Company, 1995: 1849–57.

7. Van Eyken P, Sciot R, Callea F, Van der Steen K, Moerman P, and Desmet VJ. The development of the intrahepatic bile ducts in man: a keratin-immunohistochemical study. *Hepatology*, 1988; **8**: 1586–95.

8. Van Eyken P, Sciot R, and Desmet V. Intrahepatic bile duct development in the rat: a cytokeratin-immunohistochemical study. *Laboratory Investigation*, 1988; **59**: 52–9.

9. Van Eyken P and Desmet VJ. Development of intrahepatic bile ducts, ductular metaplasia of hepatocytes, and cytokeratin patterns in various types of human hepatic neoplasms. In Sirica AE, ed. *The Role of Cell Types in Hepatocarcinogenesis*. Boca Raton: CRC Press, 1992: 227–63.

10. Marceau N, Blouin MJ, Noël M, Török N, and Loranger A. The role of bipotential progenitor cells in liver ontogenesis and neoplasia. In Sirica AE, ed. *The Role of Cell Types in Hepatocarcinogenesis*. Boca Raton: CRC Press, 1992: 121–49.

11. Bloom W. The embryogenesis of human bile capillaries and ducts. *American Journal of Anatomy*, 1926; **36**: 451–62.

12. Koga A. Morphogenesis of intrahepatic bile ducts of the human fetus. Light and electron microscopic study. *Zeitschrift für Anatomie und Entwicklungsgeschichte*, 1971; **135**: 156–84.

13. Wilson JW, Groat CS, and Leduc EH. Histogenesis of the liver. *Annals of the New York Academy of Sciences*, 1963; **111**: 8–24.

14. Picardi R, Gardiol D, and Gautier A. Etude de la cholangiogénèse chez le foetus human. II Aspects histologiques et ultrastructuraux de la génèse des canaux biliaires intrahepatiques. *Zeitschrift für Zellforschung*, 1968; **84**: 319–27.

15. Horstmann E. Entwicklung und Entwicklungsbedingungen des intrahepatischen Gallengangsystems. *Wilhelm Roux' Archiv für Mikroskopisch-Anatomische Forschung*, 1939; **139**: 363–92.

16. Jørgensen MJ. The ductal plate malformation. A study of the intrahepatic bile duct lesion in infantile polycystic disease and congenital hepatic fibrosis. *Acta Pathologica et Microbiologica Scandinavica*, 1977; **257** (Suppl.): 1–88.

17. Macchiarelli G, Makabe S, and Motta PM. Scanning electron microscopy of adult and fetal liver sinusoids. In Bioulac-Sage P and Balabaud C, eds. *Sinusoids in Human Liver: Health and Disease*. Rijswijk: The Kupffer Cell Foundation, 1988: 63–85.

18. Semba R, Tanaka O, and Tanimura T. Digestive system. In Nishimura H, ed. *Atlas of Human Prenatal Histology*. Tokyo: Igaku-Shoin, 1983: 171–234.

19. Couinaud C. *Le Foie. Etudes Anatomiques et Chirurgicales*. Paris: Masson, 1957.

20. Lewis FT. Die Entwicklung der Leber. In Keibel F and Mall FP, eds. *Handbuch der Entwicklungsgeschichte des Menschen*, Vol. Band 2. Leipzig: Engelmann, 1911: 391–418.

21. Tiniakos D, Mathew J, Tiniakos G, and Burt AD. Development of intrahepatic nerves in human fetal liver. In Shimazu T, ed. *Liver Innervation*. London: John Libbey, 1996; in press.

22. Tan CEL and Moscoso GJ. The developing human biliary system at the porta hepatis level between 11 and 25 weeks of gestation: a way to understanding biliary atresia. Part 2. *Pathology International*, 1994; **44**: 600–10.

23. Hammar JA. Über die erste Entstehung der nicht kapillaren intrahepatischen Gallengänge beim Menschen. *Zeitschrift für Mikroskopisch-Anatomische Forschung*, 1926; **5**: 59–89.

24. Kölliker A. Handbuch der Gewebelehre des Menschen für Aerzte und Studierende, 5th edn. Leipzig: Engelmann, 1867.

25. Streeter GL. Developmental horizons in human embryos. *Carnegie Institution of Washington Publication No. 575, Contribution to Embryology*, 1948; **32**: 133–204.

26. Bernstein J. Hereditary renal disease. In Churg J, Spargo BH, Mostofi FK, and Abell MR, eds. *Kidney Disease. Present Status*. Baltimore: Williams & Wilkins, 1979: 295–326.

27. Desmet VJ. Modulation of biliary epithelium. In Reutter W, Popper H, Arias IM, Heinrich PC, Keppler D, and Landmann L, eds. *Modulation of Liver Cell Expression*. Lancaster: MTP Press, 1987: 195–214.

28. Fausto N. Liver stem cells. In Arias IM, Boyer JL, Fausto N, Jakoby WB, Schachter DA, and Shafritz DA, eds. *The Liver: Biology and Pathobiology*. New York: Raven Press, 1994: 1501–18.

29. Hering E. Ueber den Bau der Wirbeltierleber. *Sitzungsberichte der Akademie der Wissenschaften in Wien, Mathematisch-Naturwissenschatige Klasse*, 1866; **54**: 496–515.

2

Functions of the liver

2.1 Hepatic blood flow

Fadi G. Haddad, Paul Genecin, and Roberto J. Groszmann

This chapter describes hepatic blood flow (which consists of contributions from the portal vein and hepatic artery), techniques for its measurement, and factors that affect it. The reader is referred to the chapters covering liver anatomy, aspects of hepatic removal of circulating substances, haemodynamic studies, vascular abnormalities, and the section on portal hypertension and gastrointestinal bleeding for discussions of closely allied subjects.

The methods for measurement of hepatic blood flow can be divided into clinical techniques (some of these techniques are also used in investigational studies in laboratory animals) and those reserved only for investigational use in laboratory animals (Table 1).

Clinical techniques

Indicator dilution technique

This method requires catheterization of the hepatic artery, or of the portal vein, superior mesenteric artery or splenic artery (any one of these vessels is sufficient if the splanchnic circulation is normal), as well as of the hepatic vein. Because of its invasiveness, it has limited clinical application. However, it has an important advantage over clearance methods because it is not dependent on liver function (Reichman, JCI, 1958; 37:1848). A known dose of an indicator that

---

Table 1 Hepatic blood-flow measurement

Clinical techniques

Indicator dilution

Clearance techniques

Constant infusion method

Single injection method

Inert gas wash-out

Echo-Doppler and related techniques

Oral–intravenous pharmacokinetics

Magnetic resonance

Techniques applicable only to animal studies

Distribution of cardiac output (radioactive-labelled microspheres)

Ultrasonic pulsed-Doppler flowmetry and related methods

Outflow collection

---

is not metabolized by the liver is injected into the portal vein or hepatic artery with adequate mixing. Hepatic blood flow is proportional to the amount of hepatic blood that has diluted the indicator (Cohn, AmJMed, 1972; 53:704).

Frequently used indicators include ^{131}I-labelled human serum albumin and ^{51}Cr-labelled erythrocytes. Hepatic blood flow is calculated from the equation $HBF = l \times 60 \div C_m \times t$, where HBF = hepatic blood flow per minute, l is the injected dose of indicator, C_m is the mean amount of indicator measured in the hepatic vein, and t is the total duration of the time curve in seconds. With a normal hepatic circulation, injection into the hepatic, superior mesenteric, or splenic artery leads to recovery of the same amount of indicator in the hepatic vein (Fig. 1). Thus, any one of these injection sites may be used for a correct calculation of an indicator dilution curve for the measurement of hepatic blood flow.

When portal–systemic shunts are present, a certain percentage of the injected indicator will bypass the liver through collaterals and will not be collected in the hepatic venous blood. A modification of the indicator dilution method has been devised for calculating portal–systemic shunting: the indicator concentration is measured in the hepatic vein following selective injection of the splenic, superior mesenteric, and hepatic arterial circulations (Fig. 2) (Groszmann, AmJMed, 1972; 53:715). By using this technique, the amount of blood flow shunted into each regional vascular bed can be measured.

Clearance techniques

These methods rely on the injection of dyes or radioactively labelled particles that are avidly extracted by liver cells (indocyanine green, bromosulphthalein, [^{14}C]taurocholate) or reticuloendothelial cells ([^{32}P]colloidal chromic phosphate, heat-denatured ^{131}I-labelled albumin). If the substance is totally extracted by the liver in one pass, its clearance equals total hepatic blood flow. However, no substance has actually been shown to have this property. Therefore, catheterization of the hepatic vein is mandatory to measure hepatic blood flow accurately. This is particularly obvious in patients with liver disease in whom the extraction of the indicator is diminished (Groszmann, Hepatol, 1983; 3:1039).

Constant infusion method

The clearance technique, which was reported by Bradley in 1945, is based on the Fick principle.[1] Under steady-state conditions, the amount of plasma perfusing the liver (litres/min) can be expressed as the ratio of the amount of indicator taken up by the liver

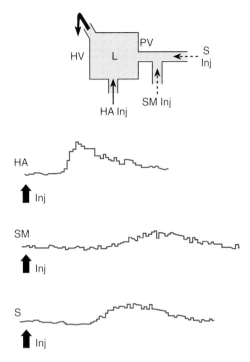

Fig. 1. Indicator dilution technique for measuring liver (L) blood flow with diagrammatic representation of blood-flow patterns in the absence of portal–systemic shunting: [^{131}I]albumin is injected into the hepatic artery (HA), superior mesenteric artery (SM), and splenic artery (S) of a normal human, with the isotope concentration recorded in hepatic vein (HV). Calculation of flow from the area under each curve yields hepatic blood flow. (Reprinted from Groszmann, AmJ Med, 1972; 53:715 by permission.)

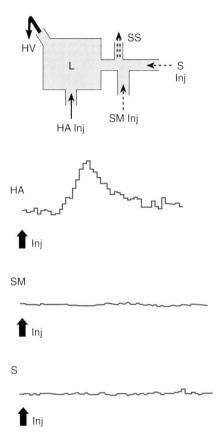

Fig. 2. Indicator dilution technique in presence of nearly total portal–systemic shunting due to alcoholic cirrhosis and portal hypertension in a human: radioactivity is not detected in hepatic vein (HV) following injections into superior mesenteric artery (SM) or splenic artery (S), indicating complete portal–systemic shunting (SS), as depicted diagrammatically. (Reprinted from Groszmann, AmJ Med, 1972; 53:715, by permission.)

per min (R) to the difference in concentration of the indicator in the plasma entering the liver (peripheral arterial or portal blood) and in plasma leaving the liver (hepatic venous blood; C_i–C_0):

$$\text{Hepatic plasma flow} = \frac{R}{C_i - C_0}$$

This method requires a catheter in the hepatic vein for blood sampling, a constant peripheral intravenous infusion of the indicator, and a peripheral arterial catheter for blood sampling. At steady state, that is, when the plasma indicator concentration is constant, the rate of infusion is equal to the rate of hepatic uptake (R) and arterial plasma concentration is taken to equal C_i. This leaves only C_0 to be measured by sampling of hepatic venous blood. Most commonly used substances are distributed exclusively in plasma. Conversion from plasma flow to blood flow (litres/min) is expressed as:

Hepatic blood flow = hepatic plasma flow × 1 ÷ 1 – (packed cell volume).

Indocyanine green has little extrahepatic uptake, negligible extrahepatic metabolism, and relatively (but not completely) preserved hepatic uptake even in liver disease, making it the dye of choice despite its cost and instability (Winkler, ScaJCLI, 1965; 17:423). Bromosulphthalein, in contrast, has the disadvantages of extrahepatic uptake and enterohepatic recirculation (Ohnhaus,

BrJClinPharm, 1979; 7:223) as well as relatively less liver extraction in the presence of hepatic disease.

The disadvantages of these methods include invasiveness and inaccuracy in the case of markedly impaired liver function (Villeneuve, AmJGastr, 1982; 77:233). However, the continuous infusion clearance techniques, especially with indocyanine green, are reliable and technically simple when the liver is normal. Sorbitol clearance may also be a safe, non-invasive, and accurate means of measuring parenchymal liver plasma flow in patients with normal or diseased livers (Zeeh, Gastro, 1988; 95:749).

Single injection method

Based on the same principles as the continuous infusion method, the single injection method can also employ the same indicators (indocyanine green, bromosulphthalein). A single, carefully measured bolus of the indicator is injected. Over 15 min, paired blood samples are withdrawn at frequent intervals (every 3–5 min) from both an hepatic vein and a peripheral artery. Following assay of dye concentrations in plasma from both sources, each set of data is plotted on semilogarithmic paper and hepatic blood flow is calculated as follows (Villeneuve, AmJGastr, 1982; 77:233).

1. Hepatic blood flow = dye clearance from whole blood ÷ hepatic dye extraction ratio
2. Dye clearance = injected bolus dose ÷ area under peripheral artery decay curve × [1-(packed cell volume)]
3. Hepatic dye extraction ratio = area under peripheral artery decay curve − area under hepatic vein decay curve ÷ area under peripheral artery decay curve.

Although less reliable than the constant infusion method, the single injection method has the advantage of speed, which permits repetition. The method also permits better estimation of the extraction ratio in the presence of liver disease because dye saturation is less probable. However, with severe hepatocyte dysfunction, both clearance methods are inaccurate. In general, there is satisfactory agreement between the continuous infusion and single injection methods (Caesar, ClinSci, 1961; 21:43; Villeneuve, AmJGastr, 1982; 77:233).

A variation of the single injection technique is the use of radioactively labelled colloid substances that are cleared by the reticuloendothelial system (Kupffer cells) rather than by the hepatocytes (Dobson, ActaMedScand (Suppl 273), 1952; 144:1). Particles in use include radiolabelled [^{32}P]chromic phosphate, [^{131}I]heat-denatured human serum albumin, and [^{99}Tc^{m}]sulphur colloid. In theory, these methods bypass the limitation of impaired dye extraction by hepatocytes in liver disease because reticuloendothelial function is often relatively preserved despite poor hepatocellular function. However, the extraction of these compounds is usually lower than that of dyes and measurements in patients with liver disease have yielded disappointing results.

Inert gas wash-out

Inert gases such as krypton-85 and xenon-133 are used in this technique. These gases establish immediate equilibrium between tissues and blood according to a specific partition coefficient. The inert gas may be administered by intraparenchymal injection (Hall, ScaJCLI, 1975; 35:635), intrasplenic injection (Lam, ActaChirScand, 1979; 145:95) or portal vein injection (Sheriff, Gut, 1977; 18:1027). Better suited to clinical studies, however, are less invasive methods employing inhalation (Schmitz-Feuerhake, ActaHepatoGastroenterol, 1975; 22:150) and, particularly, intraluminal administration in the gastrointestinal tract (Cassell, Gastro, 1969; 57:533). This technique may be adapted to estimate portal–systemic shunting as well (Shiomi, JNuclMed, 1988; 29:460).

After the establishment of equilibrium between blood and liver, the rate of wash-out of the inert gas is measured with an external counting device. This rate is proportional to hepatic blood flow. Although reproducible and accurate, this method must be employed with great caution in patients with fatty liver and other conditions affecting liver composition. These conditions can introduce an important source of error by changing the coefficient of partition for the inert gas. The coefficient of partition must also be adjusted for the haematocrit. In addition, this method measures only blood perfusing the hepatic sinusoids. Therefore, flow may be underestimated in the presence of hepatic arterial–venous shunts. Finally, care must be taken to avoid inclusion of the right lung in the counting field.

Echo-Doppler and related techniques

The sonographic technique of pulsed-Doppler flowmetry is increasingly used in clinical practice. Scepticism has been expressed about the reliability and the methodology of available studies, which may be subject to bias and subjectivity (Burns, Gastro, 1987; 92: 824). Nevertheless, this method is inexpensive, non-invasive, and capable of efficiently obtaining serial measurements (Sabba, Gastro, 1992; 102:1009).

Based on the Doppler effect, the echo-Doppler test yields information derived from the movement of red blood cells. It measures the direction and velocity of flow. In addition, through the use of B-mode ultrasonography to measure the cross-sectional area of a blood vessel, volume can be derived by the expression (velocity × area). Portal vein measurements alone are not very reliable due to wide variations in blood flow and vessel diameter under physiological conditions such as respiration and the Valsalva manoeuvre. However, the superior mesenteric artery provides 75 per cent of the blood flow entering into the portal system and experimental studies have shown that changes in mesenteric blood flow are a reliable indicator of blood flow changes in the portal vein (Kroeger, Hepatol, 1985; 5:97). Moreover, mathematical elaboration of the velocity waveform in arteries yields the pulsability index (**PI**):

$$PI = \frac{\text{Peak to peak velocity}}{\text{Mean velocity}}$$

This ratio has been related to the resistance in the vascular bed under examination (Qamar, USMedBiol, 1986; 12:773). Recent studies have demonstrated that this principle can be applied to the human superior mesenteric artery (Buonamico, Hepatol, 1995; 21: 134).

The colour-Doppler method simultaneously provides a B-mode image of the blood vessel and two-dimensional flow signals that are converted into colours. It permits rapid determination of the presence of blood flow. It can distinguish flow direction and can differentiate laminar from turbulent flow.[2] (Additional information on ultrasonography and hepatic blood flow (in particular colour-Doppler) is presented in Chapter 5.5.)

Oral–intravenous pharmacokinetics

This method is based on the principle that hepatic drug clearance depends on two important variables. One is blood flow and the other is the intrinsic ability of the liver to metabolize the drug in question (Wilkinson, ClinPharmTher, 1975; 18:377).[3] Drugs such as propranolol, indocyanine green, and lidocaine are avidly extracted by the liver and their clearance is determined by blood flow. In contrast, poorly extracted drugs such as warfarin and antipyrine undergo blood flow-independent hepatic clearance; their clearance depends instead on the metabolic activity of hepatic enzymes (Kornhauser, ClinPharmTher, 1978; 23:165).

A method for measuring hepatic blood flow has been developed that employs simultaneous oral and intravenous doses (one of them radiolabelled) of a highly extracted drug that is completely absorbable by the gastrointestinal tract and metabolized only by liver (Perrier, JPharmExpTher, 1974; 191:17; Kornhauser, ClinPharmTher, 1978; 23:165). dl-Propranolol has been used for this purpose (^{3}H-labelled propranolol intravenously and unlabelled drug orally; Kornhauser, ClinPharmTher, 1978; 23:165), with the equation for total liver blood flow in the presence of normal hepatic blood flow given as:

$$Q = \frac{D_{iv}D_0}{AUC_{iv}D_0 - AUC_0D_{iv}}$$

where Q = liver blood flow, D_{iv} = intravenous dose (^{3}H-labelled propranolol), D_0 = oral dose (unlabelled propranolol), AUC_{iv} = area under the blood concentration/time curve for intravenous (^{3}H-labelled) propranolol, and AUC_0 = area under the blood concentration/time curve for oral (unlabelled) propranolol.

Simultaneously administered doses of indocyanine green (hepatic blood flow-dependent clearance) and antipyrine (low extraction ratio) have also been used to estimate both liver blood flow and the fraction of blood that is shunted in the presence of liver disease (McLean, ClinPharmTher, 1979; 25:161).

Techniques applicable to animal studies

Distribution of cardiac output (radioactive-labelled microspheres)

The injection of radiolabelled microspheres with reference blood sampling is a technique commonly used in animal studies for the measurement of cardiac output as well as regional blood flows (Malik, JApplPhysiol, 1976; 40:4792; Groszmann, AmJPhysiol, 1982; 242:G156). While a known number of microspheres is being injected into the left ventricle, a sample of peripheral arterial blood (the reference blood sample) is simultaneously withdrawn. Organ radioactivity can thus be compared with the activity of the reference sample and regional blood flow can be calculated.

Hepatic blood flow can be estimated by adding the hepatic arterial flow, yielded by the above method, to the portal venous inflow, calculated by adding the separate flows to the splanchnic organs that drain into the portal vein. In normal animals, this sum is a fair estimate of hepatic blood flow. However, in the presence of portal hypertension with portal–systemic shunting, the sum of hepatic arterial and portal venous inflow will overestimate hepatic blood flow by the amount of blood that is shunted through collaterals. To correct for shunting, a technique has been developed for estimating its extent (Groszmann, AmJPhysiol, 1982; 242: G156): the spleen or mesenteric venous system is injected with a second radiolabelled microsphere. Radioactivity is assessed in the organs of the dead animal (radioactive c.p.m.).

Cardiac output (**CO**) (ml/min) and organ blood flow (**OBF**) are calculated from the systemic microsphere injection (Malik, JApplPhysiol, 1976; 40:4792):

CO = injected radioactivity × reference blood flow (ml/min) ÷ reference blood radioactivity
OBF = organ radioactivity × reference blood flow ÷ reference blood radioactivity
Portal–systemic shunting (**PSS**) (per cent) is calculated from the splenic or mesenteric venous injection (Groszmann, AmJPhysiol, 1982; 242:G156):

$$PSS = \frac{lung\ radioactivity}{lung + lung\ radioactivity}$$

As stated above, this method does not directly measure portal blood flow; therefore the 'portal venous flow' or, in this case, the more accurately named portal venous inflow (**PVI**) is calculated by adding the flows to spleen, pancreas, stomach, and intestines. In the presence of portal–systemic shunting, the hepatic fraction of portal venous blood inflow is defined as $PVI - PSS$ (ml/min), where

$$PSS = \frac{PVI \times PSS}{100}.$$

Hepatic blood flow is calculated by adding hepatic arterial flow and the hepatic fraction of portal venous blood inflow. The calculation of portal–systemic shunting will differ according to whether the microspheres are injected into the spleen (which overestimates shunting) or into the mesenteric venous system (which underestimates shunting). For this reason, calculations of hepatic blood flow using the correction for portal–systemic shunting are actually estimates and not true measurements. However, multiple studies have demonstrated this technique to yield a reliable and detailed evaluation of the systemic and splanchnic circulations in animals with and without portal hypertension.

Ultrasonic pulsed-Doppler flowmetry and related methods

The radioactive microsphere method provides only instantaneous haemodynamic information; it is therefore unsuited to the study of changes in blood flow over time. Other techniques have been developed for the longer-term evaluation of blood flow. In the past, electromagnetic flowmeters have been the method of choice, mainly for short-term experiments. Disadvantages of these devices include cumbersome design, baseline or zero instability, and unsuitability for small blood vessels, low-flow states, and long-term preparations.

The continuous-wave Doppler flow probe is an improvement over the electromagnetic flowmeter because it has a stable baseline and is simpler to calibrate. It has been employed in animal studies (Franklin, Science, 1961; 134:564; Vatner, JCI, 1971; 50:1950) and is available in multichannel versions. However, the probe is also large and unwieldy, especially for the study of the hepatic circulation in small animals, in which the portal vein and hepatic artery are in close proximity.

The multichannel, directional, pulsed-Doppler principle has recently been adapted for measuring flow in multiple vessels in small animals (Hartley, JApplPhysiol, 1974; 37:626). The pulsed-Doppler transducer uses a minute piezoelectric crystal that serves alternately as receiver and transmitter. This crystal receives echoes from blood cells after transmitting bursts of sound. The echo produced by moving blood cells returns at a slightly different frequency than that which is transmitted. This difference is expressed by the equation

$$fD = \frac{2fv}{c \times \cos \alpha}$$

where fD is Doppler shift frequency, f is transmitted frequency (constant), v is velocity of the fluid, c is the velocity of sound in the fluid (constant), and cos α is the cosine of the angle between the flow axis and the acoustic axis (constant).

Since all but fD and v are constants, Doppler shift frequency and velocity are linearly related (Hartley, JApplPhysiol, 1974; 37: 626). As with continuous-wave Doppler flowmetry, the zero or baseline of the pulsed-Doppler flowmeter is stable. These flow probes are implanted directly on to blood vessels and several regional flows can be monitored simultaneously for long periods of time (days–months) in conscious, unrestrained rodents (Haywood, AmJPhysiol, 1981; 241:H273).

The echo-Doppler flowmeter measures blood-cell velocity, not actual blood flow, but a linear relation between flow and velocity has been demonstrated (Haywood, AmJPhysiol, 1981; 241:H273; VanOrden, AmJPhysiol, 1984; 247:H1005). Although the curve relating Doppler shift and volume flow may be straight for an individual animal, the slopes for different animals may not be the same (Hartley, JApplPhysiol, 1974; 37:626). Therefore, caution must be exerted in interpreting anything more than percentage changes in velocity when comparing groups of animals. Pulsed-Doppler flowmetry has recently been applied to the chronic study of the hepatic artery, portal vein (Braillon, AmJPhysiol, 1988; 255: G194), and superior mesenteric artery and iliac artery (Colombato, Hepatol, 1991; 15:323) in awake, unrestrained, portal-hypertensive rats.

Outflow collection

Outflow collection applies to the measurement of liver blood flow in the isolated perfused liver (Gores, Hepatol, 1986; 6:511). It has importance for *in vitro* studies of hepatic extraction, excretion, liver metabolism, as well as pharmacological experiments and other applications.[4]

Magnetic resonance

Magnetic resonance has recently been applied to the study of blood flow; so far its application to hepatic blood flow has not been widespread, although studies in the rat (Ackerman, PNAS, 1987; 84:4099) and dog (Pettigrew, AmJRoent, 1987; 148:411) have appeared. At present, the dynamic flow range of available magnetic resonance hardware limits the accuracy of blood-flow measurements under conditions of rapid velocity (Pettigrew, AmJRoent, 1987; 148:411). Although human vascular anatomy can be detailed with magnetic resonance, studies of hepatic blood flow in man have been disappointing. For example, magnetic resonance can accurately detect portal vein thrombosis and the patency of surgical shunts, yet it cannot distinguish anterograde from retrograde portal venous flow (Torres, AmJRadiol, 1987; 148: 1109). A prospective study with axial, breath-held, multiplanar spoiled-gradient echo magnetic resonance to measure hepatic volume and a cine phase-contrast sequence perpendicular to the portal vein to measure flow showed a good correlation between biochemical measures of hepatic dysfunction and the hepatic index (hepatic mass corrected for body surface area) and portal flow index (portal flow corrected for hepatic mass) in liver transplant candidates (Kuo, Surgery, 1995; 117:373).

Physiology of hepatic blood flow
Overview

The liver receives a large volume of blood: roughly 25 per cent of the cardiac output perfuses the liver under resting conditions.[5] Approximately one-third is contributed by the hepatic artery (Tystrup, JCI, 1962; 41:447), with the remaining two-thirds supplied by the portal vein, which receives venous drainage from the stomach, intestines, spleen, omentum, and pancreas. Hepatic arterial and portal venous blood are freely mixed in the hepatic sinusoids. Total hepatic blood flow, as measured by plasma clearance of indocyanine green, is approx. 1860 ml/min in young, healthy males and 1550 ml/min in females.[6]

Hepatic blood flow varies significantly under physiological conditions. Feeding increases splanchnic and portal venous blood flow, whereas sleep decreases flow (Villeneuve, AmJGastr, 1982; 77:233).[7] Respiration results in a pattern of decreased hepatic venous flow with inspiration (Horvath, AmJPhysiol, 1957; 189: 573) and increased flow with expiration (Brauer, JPhysiol, 1960; 3:28), possibly contributing to a constant inflow of blood to the right heart from the inferior vena cava (Moreno, AmJPhysiol, 1967; 213:455). Several studies have indicated that splanchnic, and therefore hepatic, blood flow decreases with upright posture and exercise. However, a recent study using $^{99}Tc^m$-labelled red blood cells suggests that a less marked haemodynamic effect may occur with upright exercise than was previously thought (Froelich, JNuclMed, 1988; 29:1714). Age results in reduced liver volume and blood flow (by indocyanine green clearance) (Wynne, Hepatol, 1989; 9:297).

Physiological regulation of hepatic arterial flow

An important concept in understanding hepatic blood flow is that oxygen demand in the liver does not determine the supply of arterial blood.[8] With normal liver blood flow, the liver extracts less than half of the supplied oxygen (4.6 mg/min; 100 g liver).[9] In most situations where oxygen demand is increased, the liver extracts more oxygen rather than augmenting blood flow. In fact, in chronic ethanol-fed rats, oxygen requirement by the liver increased markedly (45 per cent) without causing hepatic arterial vasodilatation or increased flow, but an increase in portal blood flow was observed (Bredfeldt, AmJPhysiol, 1985; 248:G507).

Hepatic arterial autoregulation

Vascular autoregulation is said to occur when blood flow is regulated in a pressure-dependent manner. Over at least part of the physiological range of pressures, resistance rises with increased pressure, and reductions in pressure result in a lowering of resistance in order that a constant blood flow be maintained. Autoregulation in the hepatic artery has been demonstrated by several investigators, but probably does not have major physiological importance.[10] More recent evidence from using adenosine antagonists in cats suggests that pressure-flow autoregulation in the hepatic artery may be mediated by adenosine (Ezzat, AmJPhysiol, 1987; 252:H836).

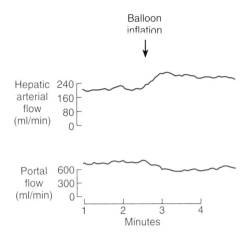

Fig. 3. Simultaneous tracings of mean hepatic arterial flow and mean portal venous flow during reduction of portal flow by balloon catheter inflation in the superior mesenteric artery of an anaesthetized dog. An immediate increase in hepatic arterial flow follows the decrease in portal flow. Blood flow was measured by electromagnetic flowmetry and verified by the blood collection method. (Reprinted from Groszmann, Gastro, 1978; 75:187, by permission.)

Relation between hepatic arterial and portal venous blood flow

It has been known for many years that reduction of portal flow in several species results in hepatic arterial hyperaemia.[10,11] In fact, in humans, the prognosis for recovery following portocaval anastomosis appears to correlate with hepatic arterial hyperaemia after the diversion of the portal flow (Burchnell, AnnSurg, 1978; 184:289). The hepatic artery has the capacity to increase its flow in the range of 22 to 100 per cent in response to decreased portal blood flow (Groszmann, Gastro, 1978; 75:187) (Fig. 3).

Hepatic blood flow in the studies cited was not restored to normal by hepatic arterial hyperaemia. Nevertheless, the drop in hepatic arterial resistance (with ensuing increase in flow) that results from decreased portal venous inflow has clear physiological importance: it tends to increase total hepatic blood flow in compromising situations such as haemorrhage (Greenway, JPhysiol, 1967; 193:375).

The mechanism determining the relation between hepatic arterial and portal venous flow is undefined. One theory postulates that it is a mechanical consequence of the convergence of a fast-flowing and a slow-moving stream (Tennberg, Science, 1965; 150:1030). Accordingly, decreased portal flow is tantamount to removal of the impedance to hepatic arterial flow. Possibly a more plausible view is that any increase in sinusoidal pressure (which may result from increased hepatic arterial, portal venous or hepatic venous pressure) leads to an increase in pressure in the hepatic arteries. This in turn elicits a myogenic constriction and decreased hepatic arterial flow.[10] More recently, the existence of a so-called hepatic arterial 'buffer response' has been postulated, based on experiments in cats.[12] According to this hypothesis, hepatic arterial vasodilation is mediated by an accumulation of adenosine in the space of Mall under conditions of decreased portal flow. Support for this hypothesis is provided by the following factors: (a) adenosine is a potent hepatic arterial vasodilator; (b) infusion of

adenosine into the portal vein causes hepatic arterial vasodilation; (c) the adenosine-uptake blocker, dipyridamole, potentiates vasodilatation; and (d) pharmacological adenosine blockers attenuate the buffer response.[12] A specific site of adenosine secretion has not been identified and it is unknown whether such production might be constant or perhaps subject to regulation by physiological factors such as oxygen deficit, local metabolites, or endogenous vasodilator substances.

Constriction of the hepatic arterial bed with elevated hepatic venous pressure

The increase (up to 43 per cent) in hepatic arterial resistance and decrease in flow in the presence of stepwise elevation of hepatic venous pressure from 1 to 11 mmHg is attributed to a myogenic mechanism.[10] The possibility that adenosine plays a part is so far unexplored. According to the adenosine theory, stasis of blood in the sinusoids might be predicted to increase the concentration of adenosine in the region of presinusoidal resistance vessels and induce vasodilatation rather than vasoconstriction. Constriction of the hepatic artery with elevation of hepatic venous pressure may be modulated by the interplay of decreased mesenteric (and therefore portal) flow with resulting arterial vasodilation (Lautt, CircRes, 1977; 41:787).

Portal vein flow

In contrast to the flow in the hepatic artery, blood flow in the portal vein is not subject to pressure-dependent autoregulation and the portal system is generally thought to be a passive vascular bed. Whereas reduced flow in the hepatic artery results in a drop in resistance, decreased portal venous flow leads to a passive collapse of the portal vasculature and a corresponding increase in portal venous resistance. Likewise, increased pressure results in diminished portal vein resistance, indicating the absence of autoregulation.[10]

Moreover, the relation between hepatic arterial and portal venous flow that mediates a decrease in arterial resistance and increased arterial flow when portal flow decreases (Greenway, JPhysiol, 1967; 193:375) is not reciprocal. Hence, in most experiments, portal flow does not increase with curtailment of hepatic arterial flow.[12] Likewise, the response of the portal vein to increased hepatic venous pressure does not appear to be autoregulated.[10]

Physiological factors governing portal venous blood flow are predominantly those that control the supply of blood to the intestines and spleen. For example, feeding dramatically enhances hepatic blood flow due to increased splanchnic, and therefore portal, hyperaemia (Hopkinson, Surgery, 1968; 63:970).

Resistance to flow in the portal vein in the normal liver is generally agreed to be minimal at the precapillary and sinusoidal level. Resistance sphincters at the level of the hepatic vein have been demonstrated in the dog[4] and suggested in the cat (Lautt, AmJPhysiol, 1986; 14:G375). However, the existence of such sphincters in man is unexplored and speculative.

Hepatic blood volume

The liver contains a disproportionately large amount of blood (10–15 per cent of the total blood volume). Blood comprises 25 to

20 per cent of the total liver volume.[8] The liver subserves an important capacitance function. With elevation of hepatic venous pressure, sinusoidal pressure passively increases. Liver blood volume may also expand up to 4 ml/100 g of liver for each mmHg increase in hepatic venous pressure. Hepatic blood volume may passively expand to as much as 60 ml/100 g of liver in heart failure.[13] Moreover, in blood volume-expanded cats, the liver is capable of engorging to absorb up to 20 per cent of the added volume (Greenway, JPhysiol, 1974; 237:279).

The role of the liver as a blood reservoir has importance during haemorrhage (Lautt, CanJPhysPharm, 1980; 58:1049). Sympathetic nerve stimulation can result in the rapid discharge of as much as 50 per cent of the total hepatic blood volume. In the cat, up to 7 per cent of the total circulating volume can be mobilized from the liver. In the dog, a 60 per cent decrease in liver blood volume can be achieved within seconds of sympathetic nerve stimulation. (Carneiro, CircRes, 1975; 40:150; Carneiro, AmJPhysiol, 1977; 232:H67). The topic of nervous control of hepatic arterial flow has been previously reviewed.[14]

Pathophysiological regulation of hepatic blood flow

This discussion will mainly centre around the circulatory disturbances observed in liver cirrhosis and the development of portal hypertension. Portal hypertension is the main abnormal circulatory manifestation of the alterations observed as a consequence of abnormalities in the liver circulation. With rare exceptions, portal hypertension is almost always due to an increase in intrahepatic vascular resistance caused by a disease process affecting the liver and/or its vascular structures. Increased blood flow in the portal vein is an uncommon cause of portal hypertension, but it is an important contributor to the severity of portal hypertension that develops in cirrhosis. Portal hypertension is the result of increased intrahepatic vascular resistance and increased splanchnic blood flow.

Intrahepatic vascular resistance

Increased resistance to portal venous flow may be localized to prehepatic, intrahepatic, or posthepatic sites. In prehepatic and posthepatic portal hypertension, this increased resistance is secondary to obstruction of the portal venous inflow or hepatic venous outflow, respectively. Intrahepatic portal hypertension is more complex and is usually a consequence of anatomical derangements of the hepatic lobule and the liver microcirculation.

While structural alteration in the hepatic microcirculation due to fibrosis and nodular regeneration is the most important factor, a primary increase in vascular tone similar to that observed in arterial hypertension may also contribute to the increased intrahepatic resistance observed in chronic liver disease. Hepatic stellate cells have been shown to play a part in hepatic fibrogenesis. In addition, there is evidence that they may act as liver-specific pericytes, a type of cell that regulates blood flow in other organs (Pinzani, JCI, 1992; 90:642). In acute and chronic liver injury, stellate cells acquire contractile characteristics similar to those of myofibroblasts and may contribute to the dynamic modulation of intrahepatic resistance.[15] These cells, which also may be the chief source of collagen synthesis in chronic

liver disease, may contribute to the regulation of hepatic blood flow at the microcirculatory level. Stellate cells are strategically located in the sinusoids, with perisinusoidal and interhepatocellular branching processes containing actin-like filaments. They also express the α-actin gene that is characteristic of vascular smooth muscle. Myofibroblast-like cells occur in fibrous septa around sinusoids and terminal hepatic venules in cirrhotic livers where their density may correlate with vascular resistance. These cells are thought to have a role in the regulation of vascular resistance in the isolated perfused liver of the cirrhotic rat (Bhathal, JHepatol, 1985; 1:325).

Normal stellate cells when activated in culture acquire contractile properties with an enhanced response to endothelial-derived vasoconstrictors such as endothelins (Rockey, Hepatol, 1992; 16:316). There are three known endothelins. Their effects are mediated by endothelin-A and -B receptors. One of the most important effects is the modulation of vascular tone. Endothelin 1 and sarafotoxin S6C (an endothelin-B receptor agonist) induced contractility in the stellate cells that was proportionate to the degree of liver injury, thus being the most pronounced in cirrhotic livers. During the process of liver injury, there is an activation of stellate cells that comprises the expression of α-actin and increased collagen production. The physiological translation (effect on portal pressure) of this action on to stellate cells was different for different endothelins. While endothelin 1 caused a pronounced and rapid increase in portal pressure in both normal and cirrhotic rats, sarafotoxin S6C induced a greater increase in portal pressure in cirrhosis than in normal liver. Bosantan, an endothelin-A and -B receptor antagonist, reduced the portal pressure by a small percentage, suggesting that factors in addition to endothelins are involved in the increased vascular tone observed in cirrhotic livers (Rockey, Hepatol, 1996; 24:233).

The vascular endothelium also synthesizes potent vasodilators (prostacyclin and nitric oxide) (Rubanyi, JCellBiochem, 1991; 46:27). Nitric oxide (NO) regulated intrahepatic resistance in normal and cirrhotic rat livers (Gupta, Hepatol, 1994; 20:200A; Mittal, AmJPhysiol, 1994; 267:G416). Nitric oxide, being a vasodilator that exerts its action locally, is considered a major 'fine tuner' of vascular tone. In fact, one of the most important vascular roles of NO is to balance the effect of humoral and local vasoconstrictors. Vascular beds with defective NO synthesis demonstrate an abnormally increased vascular resistance. There are several different processes that impair endothelial cell function and the local synthesis of NO. These include trauma, arteriosclerosis, and arterial hypertension (Mayhan, AmJPhysiol, 1990; 259:H1455; Raij, AmJMed, 1991; 90:13S). We have recently demonstrated that NO contributes to the regulation of intrahepatic resistance in the normal rat liver (Mittal, AmJPhysiol, 1994; 267:G416). Mechanisms that regulate the production of NO in the hepatic microcirculation and the part NO plays in pathological states such as cirrhosis remain to be determined. Preliminary data suggest that NO production is deficient in the hepatic microcirculation of cirrhotic livers (Mittal, Gastro, 1993; 104:A956).

Splanchnic blood flow

A syndrome characterized by generalized vasodilatation and a hyperdynamic splanchnic and systemic circulatory state is

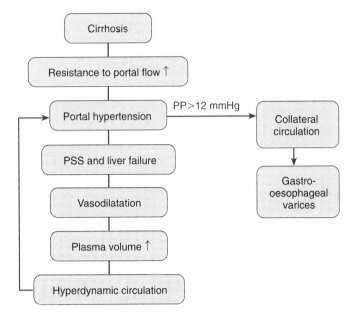

Fig. 4. The hyperdynamic state contributes to the severity of portal hypertension (see text). PP, portal pressure; PSS, portosystemic shunt. (Modified from Groszmann RJ. Vasodilatation and hyperdynamic circulatory state in chronic liver disease. In: Bosch J and Groszmann RJ, eds. *Portal hypertension pathophysiology and treatment*. Oxford: Blackwell Science, 1994.)

observed in chronic liver diseases associated with extensive portosystemic shunting and/or hepatic failure (Vorobioff, AmJPhysiol, 1983; 244:G52).[16,17] In most cases, portal hypertension is a main feature of this syndrome and a hyperdynamic splanchnic circulation that results in an increase portal venous inflow is a major contributor to the severity of portal hypertension.[16,18] The aetiology of the hyperdynamic circulation is still controversial, although it is most probably initiated by vasodilatation induced by an increase in activity of endothelial-dependent and -independent vasodilators. Vasodilatation leads to central hypovolaemia, sodium retention, and increased intravascular volume (Schrier, Hepatol, 1988; 8:1151; Colombato, Hepatol, 1993; 18:100A).[19,20] The combination of vasodilatation and an expanded intravascular volume is necessary for the full expression of the hyperdynamic state (Fig. 4).

References

1. Bradley SJ *et al*. The estimation of hepatic blood flow in man. *Journal of Clinical Investigation*, 1945; **24**: 890–7.

2. Becker CD and Cooperberg PL. Sonography of the hepatic vascular system. *American Journal of Roentgenography*, 1988; **150**: 999–1005.

3. Rowland M, Benet LZ, and Graham GG. Clearance concepts in pharmacokinetics. *Journal of Pharmacokinetics and Biopharmacology*, 1973; **1**: 123–6.

4. Bradley SE. The hepatic circulation. In Hamilton WF, Dow P, eds. *Handbook of physiology*. Washington DC: American Physiological Society, 1963: 1387–428.

5. Bradley SE. Variations in hepatic blood flow in man during health and disease. *New England Journal of Medicine*, 1949; **240**: 456–61.

6. Wynne HA *et al*. The effect of age upon liver volume and apparent liver blood flow in healthy man. *Hepatology*, 1989; **9**: 297–30.

7. Orrego J, Mena I, Baraona E, and Palma R. Modifications in hepatic blood flow and portal pressure produced by different diets. *American Journal of Digestive Disease*, 1965; **10**: 239–48.

8. Lautt WW. Hepatic vasculature: a conceptual review. *Gastroenterology*, 1977; **73**: 1163–9.

9. Myers JD. The hepatic blood flow and splanchnic oxygen consumption in man: their estimation from urea production or bronsulphalein excretion during catheterization of the hepatic veins. *Journal of Clinical Investigation*, 1947; **26**: 1130–7.

10. Hanson KM and Johnson PC. Local control of hepatic arterial and portal venous flow in the dog. *American Journal of Physiology*, 1966; **211**: 712–20.

11. Greenway CV and Oshiro G. Intrahepatic distribution of portal and hepatic arterial blood flows in anesthetized cats and dogs and the effects of portal occlusion, raised venous pressure and histamine. *Journal of Physiology (London)*, 1972; **227**: 473–485.

12. Lautt WW, Legare DJ, and D'Almeida, MS. Adenosine as putative regulator of hepatic arterial flow (the buffer response). *American Journal of Physiology*, 1985; **248** (Heart Circ Physiol 17): H331–8.

13. Hanson KM. Liver. In Johnson PC, ed. *Peripheral circulation*. New York: Wiley, 1978: 285–314.

14. Richardson PDI and Withrington PG. Liver blood flow. 1. Intrinsic and nervous control of liver blood flow. *Gastroenterology*, 1981; **81**: 159–73.

15. Rudolph R, McClure WJ, and Woodward M. Contractile fibroblasts in chronic alcoholic cirrhosis. *Gastroenterology*, 1979; **76**: 704–9.

16. Groszmann RJ. Hyperdynamic circulation of liver diseases forty years later: Pathophysiology and clinical consequences (Editorial). *Hepatology*, 1994; **20**: 1359–63.

17. Murray JF, Dawson AM, and Sherlock S. Circulatory changes in chronic liver disease. *American Journal of Medicine*, 1958; **24**: 358–67.

18. Genecin P and Groszmann RJ. Biology of portal hypertension. In Arias I, Boyer JL, Fausto N, Jakoby W, Schachter D, Shafritz D, eds. *The liver: biology and pathophysiology*. New York: Raven Press, 1994: 1327–42.

19. Henricksen JH *et al*. Reduced central blood volume in cirrhosis. *Gastroenterology*, 1989; **97**: 1506–13.

20. Albillos A, Colombato LA, Lee FY, and Groszmann RJ. Chronic octreotide treatment ameliorates peripheral vasodilatation and prevents sodium retention in portal hypertensive rats. *Gastroenterology*, 1993; **104**: 568–72.

2.2 Hepatic lymph and lymphatics

James A. Barrowman, Michael J. Eppiheimer, and D. Neil Granger

Anatomical considerations

Liver lymphatics and the hepatic interstitium

In humans and all other species examined, initial lymphatics—the smallest lymphatic capillary vessels whose wall consists of only a single endothelial cell layer—arise in the portal tracts but are not found within the hepatic lobule. In the smallest portal tracts, they may be absent or difficult to detect. Of the portal tract structures, the lymphatic capillaries are most closely related spatially to branches of the hepatic artery. In the central venous region of the lobule, some less conspicuous initial lymphatics have been described.[1] A third network of lymphatics has been observed in relation to the liver capsule; this network consists of three layers.[2,3] Some uncertainty exists regarding the presence of communications between the capsular lymphatic network and the vessels of the portal tracts and central veins. Major lymph trunks leave the liver at the hilum and pass in the hepatoduodenal ligament, draining eventually to the cisterna chyli. Other vessels are found in relation to the hepatic veins and drain to the thoracic duct and retrosternal lymph trunks. In dogs, it has been estimated that the hilar lymphatics carry approximately 80 per cent of liver lymph, the remainder passing via those vessels that accompany the hepatic veins (Ritchie, AmJ-Physiol, 1959; 196:105).

The function of lymphatics is to drain excess tissue fluid and protein from the interstitial spaces of an organ. What are the relevant tissue spaces in the liver? Interstitial spaces are recognized in the portal tracts, around the central veins, and below the liver capsule, but the most prominent hepatic interstitial space is the perisinusoidal space of Disse (Fig. 1).

The space of Disse in the perisinusoidal cleft is bordered by the endothelial cells of the sinusoid and the sinusoidal spaces of the hepatocytes. It has long been assumed that the space of Disse is a major source of hepatic lymph.[3] Raising venous pressure in an organ increases capillary pressure and the resulting increase in capillary filtration leads to enhanced lymph flow. The width of the space of Disse (0.2 to 0.5 μm) may change under various pathological conditions, such as hepatic venous obstruction, to increase lymph

It is with regret that we record the death of Dr J. A. Barrowman since the publication of the first edition. Much of his chapter has been retained in this edition.

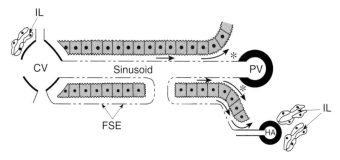

Fig. 1. Schematic diagram of blood–lymph barrier in the normal liver. CV, central vein; PV, portal vein; HA, hepatic artery; IL, initial lymphatics; FSE, fenestrated sinusoidal endothelium. The perisinusoidal space of Disse lies between the fenestrated sinusoidal endothelium and the hepatocytes. The arrows indicate the flow of filtrate towards the portal tract. The asterisks indicate that part of the pathway for the fluid and solute movement towards the lymphatics which is incompletely defined (after Henriksen, Liver, 1984; 4:221).

flow. The high protein content of liver lymph, approximately 80 per cent of plasma protein concentration, suggests a major contribution from a highly porous microcirculation, which clearly points to the sinusoids. The liver sinusoids are approximately 300 μm in length, 5 μm in width, and total 1.85×10^9 in number. The sinusoids are lined with fenestrated endothelium that forms sieve plates. There are approximately 25 sieve plates/mm^2 of sinusoidal endothelium and 30 fenestrations per sieve plate, which corresponds to a total of 200 000 fenestrae/sinusoid and a porosity of 20 per cent. It is possible that the fenestrae of the endothelium permit a free bi-directional exchange of macromolecules, which suggests that the space of Disse is a perivascular space rather than a lymphatic space. In addition, the sieve effect produced by the fenestrae may not be relevant for the passage of most of the plasma proteins, as only molecules with an M_r of less than 1×10^6 and a diameter of less than 20×10^{-9}m may pass through the fenestrae. The notion of the space of Disse as the principal source of liver lymph, however, has been called into question on the morphological grounds that a plate of hepatocytes separates this space from the portal tract lymphatics; thus the ultrastructure of the pathway between the perisinusoidal space of Disse and the portal tract lymphatics has not been fully elucidated. Another assumption is that a contribution to hepatic lymph is provided by a filtrate from the peribiliary capillary plexus found in the portal tracts, but this has been estimated to account for less than 10 per cent of the total lymph flow from the liver. These microvessels have endothelium of the continuous type and are presumably much less permeable to macromolecules than the sinusoids. Thus, peribiliary capillaries probably play a role in regulating arterial flow in addition to water and solute transport across the biliary epithelium.[4,5] A protein-poor filtrate from the peribiliary microcirculation has been considered to dilute the protein of the sinusoidal filtrate whose composition is believed to be similar to that of plasma. The concept of liver lymph being largely derived from sinusoid filtrate with a small contribution from other less permeable microcirculations has generally served as a framework for an understanding of liver lymph physiology. There is a need, however, to re-examine the underlying assumptions in this concept and test these with novel experimental approaches.

Gallbladder lymphatics

Three interconnected lymphatic networks—mucosal, muscular, and subserosal—are found in the gallbladder. The mucosal vessels are located deep in that layer, suggesting that they may play a major role in the transport of fluid absorbed by the gallbladder. There is evidence that anastomotic connections exist between gallbladder and liver lymphatics, and between pancreatic lymphatics and vessels associated with the biliary tract.[1]

Physiological considerations

Liver lymph and interstitial fluid homeostasis

Lymph flow from a tissue serves to maintain the homeostasis of the interstitium of that tissue by quantitatively removing fluid and protein which accumulates by transmicrovascular filtration; in most tissues a small amount of fluid is constantly passing from the plasma to the interstitium. Therefore, lymph flow opposes a tendency for oedema to form.[3] The structure of the lymphatics in the liver is similar to those found in other tissues. In most tissues, lymph flow is mediated by factors such as muscular activity, pulsation of blood vessels, venous pressure, and/or gravity. In addition to these factors, lymph flow along the thoracic duct may be influenced by respiratory movements or pressure on the abdominal wall. Given that lymphatics have valves which permit drainage in one direction, compression of the lymphatics by any of the latter factors acts to propel the lymph along the lymphatic vessels.

The liver is characterized by a very high blood flow and a highly permeable microcirculation, the sinusoids. One important feature distinguishing the liver from other tissues is that its interstitium, in addition to being drained by lymphatic vessels, is in communication with the peritoneal cavity via its capsule. Thus, two routes exist for the disposal of accumulated interstitial fluid in the liver. The driving force for filling of initial lymphatics is generally considered to be simply the hydrostatic pressure of the interstitial fluid, and the lymphatic endothelial wall which lacks a basement membrane is believed to offer no restriction to protein movement. This also means that no transmural oncotic pressure gradient is developed across the lymphatic wall. The other route for lymph disposal, leakage across the liver capsule, is also likely to involve a hydrostatic pressure gradient, the difference between the hepatic interstitial

pressure or the subcapsular lymphatics and the intraperitoneal pressure, which may be aggravated in the diseased state.

Fluid filtration across the microcirculatory vessels of any tissue is enhanced by a disturbance of the hydrostatic or oncotic forces operating across these vessels. Thus an increase of microvascular pressure resulting from an elevation of venous pressure or a fall in transcapillary oncotic pressure by dilution of plasma protein enhances filtration. This is opposed to some extent by a rise in interstitial hydrostatic pressure and a fall in interstitial fluid oncotic pressure. As capillary filtration increases, the flow of lymph rises, driven by increased tissue fluid pressure, and oedema is opposed. When the opposing forces—enhanced lymph flow and readjustments of forces across the capillary wall—are overcome at a certain change in net transmicrovascular pressure, termed the 'total oedema safety factor', oedema results. In the dog liver, a rise of only 1 to 2 mmHg in net transmicrovascular pressure is sufficient to cause gross liver oedema with transcapsular fluid filtration. Every tissue responds to such a disturbance with its own particular readjustment of forces. Because of low tissue compliance in the liver, the interstitial pressure rises rapidly in response to increased fluid filtration. This opposes further filtration and drives up liver lymph flow. No contribution is made by alterations in the transcapillary (trans-sinusoidal) oncotic pressure because the sinusoidal wall is totally permeable to proteins and no effective oncotic pressure gradient is thought to exist.[6,7]

From these considerations one can predict the physiological consequences of acute hepatic venous obstruction occurring in an experimental or a clinical setting: it is evident that the liver is exquisitely sensitive to small rises in venous pressure. Thus, the resulting hepatic vascular congestion and increased intrasinusodial pressure with enhanced fluid filtration would lead to dilatation of the space of Disse and a sharp rise in interstitial pressure, enhancing liver lymph flow.

Flow of liver lymph

It is difficult to obtain a quantitative measure of total liver lymph flow. However, in the various species in which it has been measured, lymph flows from the liver are high and are often estimated to be between 25 and 50 per cent that of total thoracic duct flow. A rough estimate of total hepatic lymph flow obtained from various species is approximately 0.5 ml/kg of liver per min; the ratio of liver lymph–blood flow, therefore, is approximately 1:2000.[8]

Proteins of liver lymph

Of all regional lymphs, that of the liver has the highest protein concentration. All species of plasma protein are present. It is generally agreed that the high protein concentration, approximately 80 per cent of that in plasma, reflects its origin from a highly permeable microcirculation. There is no evidence that hepatic lymph serves as a specific route for the delivery of newly synthesized proteins from the liver to the general circulation (Smallwood, ClinSci, 1968; 35:35).

Although the protein concentration of liver lymph is high, it is not identical to plasma and there is some evidence for sieving of plasma proteins by the hepatic blood–lymph barrier. The concentration in the lymph compared with that in the plasma of the various species of plasma protein falls with increasing molecular size suggesting that there is some permselectivity of the blood–lymph barrier in the liver.[9] Where is this sieving occurring? Morphological evidence suggests that it is not likely to be at the level of the sinusoidal wall, which is perforated by openings of 100 to 200 nm in diameter;[10] furthermore, the sinusoidal wall has no well-defined basement membrane. It is possible that there is an extravascular sieve formed by structures such as collagen fibres in the perisinusoidal space of Disse. Another possibility is that while no permselectivity towards proteins is exerted by the sinusoid, the restrictive properties of the peribiliary microcirculation whose filtrate contributes to total liver lymph are responsible for the apparent permselectivity.

In most organs, as lymph flow rises in response to venous pressure elevation, the concentration of protein in lymph progressively falls to a minimum level. The liver is an exception: here, the concentration of protein rises with increased lymph flow resulting from a rise in hepatic venous pressures, and permselectivity for large protein species is lost (Granger, Gastro, 1979; 77:103). The explanation for this is not clear. It is possible that venous pressure elevation selectively enhances sinusoidal filtration, which can be anticipated in view of the absence of a trans-sinusoidal oncotic pressure gradient. Thus, the sinusoidal filtrate component of total liver lymph would predominate at such high flows. Alternatively, the postulated sieve in the perisinusoidal space of Disse might be opened by increased hydration of this space reducing its sieving properties. Whatever the mechanism, it is difficult to determine which of these two possibilities is responsible.

Pathophysiological considerations
Schistosomal hepatic fibrosis

This condition is usually considered to cause presinusoidal portal hypertension as a result of extensive periportal fibrosis. Theoretically this should not be expected to produce sinusoidal hypertension or enhanced liver lymph flow, though splanchnic bed hypertension and increased splanchnic lymph flow might be anticipated: the latter is the case. However, dilated liver lymphatics in the subcapsular and hilar regions have been observed in patients with schistosomal liver disease suggesting that the pathological process, in addition to causing splanchnic venous congestion, probably also produces a degree of sinusoidal hypertension, presumably due to an element of postsinusoidal obstruction (Aboul-Enein, JCardiovascSurg; 14:529).

Cirrhosis

In contrast to schistosomal hepatic fibrosis where the principal resistance to blood flow is believed to be presinusoidal, the resistance in cirrhosis is considered to be at the sinusoidal and postsinusoidal levels. Fibrotic changes in the perisinusoidal space of Disse and in the region of the central veins are responsible for this flow resistance. Thus in cirrhosis, sinusoidal hypertension is a characteristic feature. Splanchnic hypertension is also found, the result of resistance to flow in the liver and of enhanced arterial inflow into the splanchnic bed.

Lymph flows in the thoracic duct in cirrhosis are greatly elevated.[11] Flows as high as 15 ml/min have been recorded in patients with cirrhosis with pressures rising to 30 mmHg on obstruction (normal flow is about 1 ml/min). These enhanced flows are due to lymph contributions from both the liver and splanchnic organs as a result of raised hydrostatic pressures in the respective microcirculations (see Section 7). In experimental cirrhosis in rats, 30-fold elevations of hepatic lymph flow have been recorded (Barrowman, Gastro, 1984; 87:165). The liver is unique in that in addition to draining its lymph into the interstitium via lymphatics vessels, it may leak its excess lymph from its surface into the peritoneal cavity. In general, the peritoneal cavity is free of lymph suggesting that the rate of formation and the absorption of fluid in the lymphatics is in balance. In patients with cirrhosis, the formation of fluid in the peritoneal cavity is a prominent feature and has also been suggested as a cause for renal dysfunction (Witte, Gastro, 1980; 78:1059). Traditionally, it is believed that lymph imbalance begins with intrahepatic obstruction of blood flow (producing an elevation in microvascular pressure), which leads to a disruption of the equilibrium in the Starling forces within the hepatic circulation and, ultimately, an increased production of hepatic lymph. It has been demonstrated that an elevation in blood pressure by 1 mmHg may increase lymph production by 50 per cent.[7] This elevation in lymph flow is initially compensated by an increased return of fluid to the superior vena cava via the hepatic lymph vessels. With a sustained elevation in hepatic vascular pressure, the lymph flow exceeds the capacity for absorption via the lymphatic vessels and hepatic lymph passes from the liver surface into the peritoneal cavity as ascites. The resulting decrease in vascular volume may activate baroreceptors to initiate the retention of water and sodium by the kidneys. When excessive, this compensatory mechanism may augment portal hypertension and thereby exacerbate the formation of lymph in the peritoneal cavity.

The sinusoidal endothelium undergoes characteristic morphological changes in cirrhosis: the term 'capillarization' has been applied to the finding of a basement membrane, normally not present, and a reduction in porosity, resulting from loss of many fenestrae (Schaffner, Gastro, 1963; 44:239). In addition, considerable amounts of collagen are deposited in the space of Disse. These changes result in a decrease in the hydraulic conductivity of the sinusoidal wall; this should be expected to reduce fluid filtration across the vessel. However, the rise in sinusoidal hydrostatic pressure is considerable and more than offsets the reduced permeability; thus filtration increases and hepatic lymph flows rise. The protein concentration of liver lymph falls and the sieving characteristics of the liver microcirculation come to resemble those of capillary vessels of other organs, such as the intestine. Where an acute rise in hepatic venous pressure causes the protein concentration of liver lymph in the normal condition to rise towards that of plasma, a similar rise in hepatic venous pressure in the cirrhotic liver causes a fall in lymph protein. These changes in the permeability of the hepatic microcirculation can be ascribed to 'capillarization' of the sinusoids.[12]

Biliary obstruction

It has long been recognized that in acute biliary obstruction, reflux of conjugated bilirubin and other bile constituents into blood occurs via lymphatics of the liver and biliary tract.[1] Radiological contrast material injected under pressure into the biliary system in experimental animals promptly appears in liver lymph. Ligation of

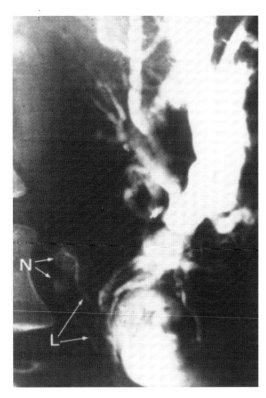

Fig. 2. Percutaneous transhepatic cholangiogram demonstrating partial obstruction of the distal common bile duct and opacification of associated lymphatic vessels (L) and lymph nodes (NL).

the common bile duct causes a large rise in liver lymph flow and the lymph is visibly bile-stained. The anatomical pathway from bile to lymph in the liver has not yet been clarified.

In the case of chronic biliary obstruction, there is also evidence that bile enters the lymph.[1] It is probable that this occurs both within the liver and in relation to the extrahepatic biliary tree. At percutaneous transhepatic cholangiography in patients with extrahepatic biliary obstruction, radiological contrast medium has

frequently been demonstrated to pass from the dilated biliary system to neighbouring lymphatic vessels (Fig. 2), and in one remarkable case of complete, chronic, common bile-duct obstruction, lymphatics running alongside the common bile duct discharged their contents into the duodenum, the flow being sufficient to prevent jaundice (Stair, SouthMedJ, 1984; 77:91). Observations such as this have suggested the possible use of lymphaticoenteric anastomosis as a means of treating biliary atresia. This has been explored but has proved unsuccessful on account of fluid, protein, and electrolyte losses.

References

1. Barrowman JA. *Physiology of the gastro-intestinal lymphatic system.* Cambridge: Cambridge University Press, 1978.
2. Comparini L. Lymph vessels of the liver in man. *Angiology*, 1969; **6**: 262–74.
3. Trutmann M and Sasse D. The lymphatics of the liver. *Anatomy and Embryology*, 1994; **190**: 201–9.
4. Barrowman JA. and Granger DN. Effects of experimental cirrhosis on splanchnic microvascular fluid and solute exchange in the rat. *Gastroenterology*, 1984; **87**: 165–72.
5. Rappaport A. The acinus-microvascular unit of the liver. In Iautt WW, ed. *Hepatic circulation in health and disease.* New York: Raven Press, 1981: 175–92.
6. Granger DN and Barrowman JA. Gastrointestinal and liver edema. In Staub NC and Taylor AE, eds. *Edema.* New York: Raven Press, 1984: 615–56.
7. Laine GA, Hall JT, Laine SH, and Granger HJ. Transsinusoidal fluid dynamics in canine liver during venous hypertension. *Circulation Research*, 1979; **45**: 317–23.
8. Brauer RW. Liver circulation and function. *Physiological Reviews*, 1963; **43**: 115–213.
9. Dive ChC, Nadalini AC, and Heremans JF. Origin and composition of hepatic lymph proteins in the dog. *Lymphology*, 1971; **4**: 133–9.
10. Wisse E. An electron microscopic study of the fenestrated endothelial lining of rat liver sinusoids. *Journal of Ultrastructural Research*, 1970; **31**: 125–50.
11. Dumont AE and Mulholland JH. Flow rate and composition of thoracic duct lymph in patients with cirrhosis. *New England Journal of Medicine*, 1960; **263**: 471–4.
12. Witte MH, Witte CL, and Dumont AE. Estimated net transcapillary water and protein flux in the liver and intestine in patients with portal hypertension from hepatic cirrhosis. *Gastroenterology*, 1981; **80**: 265–72.

2.3 Physiology of bile formation and of the motility of the biliary tree

Jürg Reichen*

The formation of bile represents the exocrine function of the liver; both hepatocytes and bile ductules/ducts participate in its elaboration. In some but not all species bile is temporarily stored in the gallbladder and released into the duodenum upon digestive demands by an intricate interplay of gallbladder contraction and relaxation of the sphincter of Oddi. The formation of bile serves many different functions (Table 1); thus it provides micelles for the activation of lipase and facilitation of lipid absorption in the duodenum. Bile represents the predominant excretory pathway for many endobiotics such as cholesterol, bilirubin, and aged proteins. Together with the kidney, bile is the main excretory pathway for xenobiotics; due to the specialized organization of the liver circulation and the enzymatic make-up of the hepatocytes, lipophilic and highly protein-bound drugs are preferentially excreted into bile. Maintenance of the ionic milieu in the duodenum is achieved by the elaboration of a bicarbonate-rich secretion by the ductules. Finally, the liver is a major part of the mucosal defence system. Depending on the species, the hepatocytes or biliary ductules excrete secretory immunoglobulin A (**IgA**) and thereby contribute to the mucosal integrity. This review will be restricted to consideration of the physiological processes leading to the elaboration of hepatocellular and ductular bile, the absorptive capacity of the gallbladder, and the motility of the gallbladder and sphincter of

Oddi. For immunological and pharmacological aspects of biliary function the reader is referred to other chapters in this textbook.

Primary, hepatocellular, or canalicular bile is elaborated by the hepatocytes by a process of osmotic filtration. This primary secretory product remains inaccessible *in vivo* for direct analysis but hepatocyte couplets have provided an important tool in biliary physiology since they allow direct visualization and electrophysiological studies (Graf, JHepatol, 1990; 10:387). The canalicular bile is then modified by reabsorption and secretion of organic and inorganic ions in the collecting system, the biliary ductules and ducts. The best known function of these structures is the elaboration of a bicarbonate-rich secretion under the influence of secretin (Preisig, JCI, 1962; 41:1152). Here again, technological advances such as the isolation of primary secretory units (Roberts, PNAS, 1993; 90:9080) and of stable cell lines of cholangiocytes (Strazzabosco, Hepatol, 1994; 19:145) have permitted a much better understanding of the molecular physiology of this process. Finally, bile is concentrated up to 20-fold by the gallbladder mucosa and released into the duodenum depending upon the metabolic demands in species with gallbladders.

Normal man produces approximately 600 ml of bile per day; the different fractions are shown in Fig. 1. Bile is usually isotonic with plasma; its cation composition is very similar to that of plasma (Fig. 2). The biliary pH depends on hormonal influences. Secretin leads to an increase in bicarbonate and to an alkaline pH (Fig. 2). The anion composition depends markedly on the feeding state and on bile acids. The presence of bile acids and their capacity to form micelles and mixed micelles together with phospholipids and cholesterol, make the osmotic behaviour of bile rather complex. The role of the cation–anion gap indicated for the basal state in Fig. 2 will be considered later.

Hepatocellular bile formation

The hepatocytes elaborate primary bile by a process of osmotic filtration; hydrostatic pressure does not influence bile formation within the physiological range and the bile secretory pressure is higher than the perfusion pressure, for example in perfused livers (Brauer, AmJPhysiol, 1954; 177:103). Sperber[1] was the first to demonstrate the osmotic origin of bile using different model anions. The principle of osmotic filtration and its anatomical requirements are shown in Fig. 3. Different carriers for organic and inorganic

---

Table 1 Functions of bile formation

Digestion
  Bile salt secretion (activation of lipase and micelles)
  Duodenal ion homeostasis (HCO_3^-)
Enterohepatic circulation
  Bile acids
Excretion of endobiotics
  Cholesterol
  Bilirubin
  Aged proteins
Excretion of xenobiotics
  Drugs
  Environmental toxins
  Heavy metals
Mucosal immunity
  Secretory IgA

* Supported by SNF grant (No. 32–45349.95).

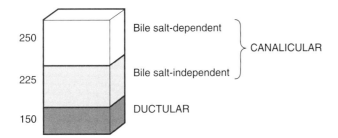

Fig. 1. The three fractions of bile in man. Approximately 75 per cent of bile is of canalicular origin, consisting in equal parts of bile salt-dependent and bile salt-independent bile. Ductular bile accounts for approximately 25 per cent and is secreted mostly under the influence of the gastrointestinal hormone, secretin.

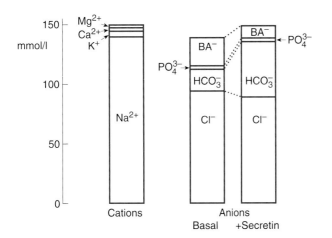

Fig. 2. Ionic composition of bile in secretin-responsive species. Under basal conditions, a cation–anion gap is frequently observed. This has been ascribed to the existence of choleretic anionic compounds in bile (Klos, AmJPhysiol, 1979; 236:E439), part of which are accounted for by glutathione and glutathione disulphide (GSSG) (Ballatori, AmJPhysiol, 1989; 256:G22). Under the influence of secretin, the concentration of bicarbonate markedly increases at the expense of chloride and bile acids.

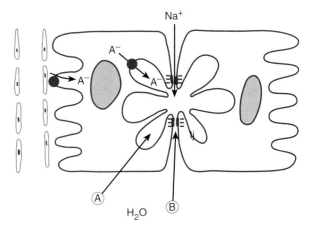

Fig. 3. Osmotic filtration of bile: the active transport of anions (A-) occurs transcellularly. Negative charges on the tight junctions (tj) prevent back-diffusion of the actively secreted anions. Cations such as sodium follow passively across the tight junction. Water will follow passively (A) transcellularly or (B) paracellularly to keep the bile isotonic.

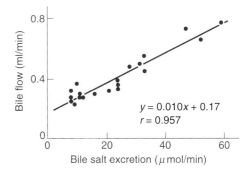

$$y = 0.010x + 0.17$$
$$r = 0.957$$

Fig. 4. Correlation between bile salt secretion and bile flow in a patient with a T-tube. The slope of this linear relationship expresses the osmotic activity of bile acids; the intercept with the ordinate (at zero bile salt secretion) is taken as bile salt-independent bile flow.

anions on the sinusoidal and canalicular membranes are able to transport them against a concentration gradient. As in other epithelia, the tight junction between the hepatocytes has a negative charge and is thus cation-selective (Bradley, AmJPhysiol, 1978; 235:E570; Graf, AmJPhysiol, 1983; 244:G233). Therefore, cations follow the actively secreted anions passively into the canaliculus. The negative charges on the tight junction are thought to prevent back-diffusion of the actively secreted anions. Water follows passively—transcellularly and/or paracellularly. The electrical characteristics of this system have been elucidated using micropuncture techniques (Graf, JMembrBiol, 1987; 95:241). In hepatocyte couplets, the basolateral and canalicular membrane resistance averaged 0.15 and 0.78 GV, respectively, while the paracellular (tight junctional) resistance was only 25 MV. The luminal potential ranged from −4.3 to 5.9 MV.

Different compounds are responsible for the osmotic filtration of bile, foremost among them the bile acids. As shown in Fig. 4, for most species, including man, there is a linear relationship between bile salt excretion and bile formation (Wheeler, JCI, 1960; 39:161).

The slope of this line expresses the choleretic activity of a given bile acid and is in the range of 8 to 15 ml/mmol for most physiological bile acids in the different species. Bile flow in the absence of bile acids exists as can be demonstrated in the perfused rat liver (Boyer, Gastro, 1970; 59:853). It is estimated by the intercept of the regression line with the ordinate at zero bile acid secretion (in Fig. 4) and is often referred to as the bile salt-independent fraction of bile. This concept is somewhat misleading since the slope can change with the rate of bile salt secretion (Balabaud, JLabClinMed, 1977; 89:393). Moreover, bile acids can interfere with the different ion pumps involved in the formation of the bile salt-independent fraction (Strasberg, JLabClinMed, 1983; 101:317).

Bile salt-dependent fraction

The hepatic excretion of bile acids depends on at least three steps, as schematically indicated in Fig. 5. They are uptake (Fig. 5(A and F)), translocation and eventual binding to intracellular binding proteins (C in Fig. 5(C)), and, finally, carrier-mediated excretion into the bile (D in Fig. 5(D)).

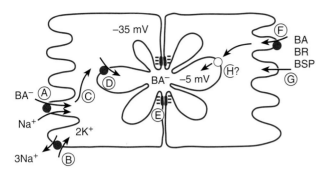

Fig. 5. Elaboration of bile salt-dependent canalicular bile: (A) bile acids are taken up by a sodium-dependent, secondary active transport system mediated by Na⁺-dependent taurocholate transport protein (**ntcp**); (B) this process is energized by the Na,K-ATPase. (F) A second process involving oatp; termed **MOAT** for multispecific organic anion transporter by some authors. (G) Finally, bile acids can enter the hepatocyte by passive diffusion. (C) After uptake bile acids are translocated across the hepatocyte and (C) extruded via an adenosine 5′ triphosphate (**ATP**)-dependent transport protein. The driving force is ATP for the carrier D and perhaps the cell potential of -35 mV. (E) Back-diffusion of bile acids is prevented by the negative charges on the tight junctions.

Hepatic uptake of bile acids

Hepatic uptake is a saturable, carrier-mediated, sodium-dependent process (Reichen, AmJPhysiol, 1976; 231:734; Inoue, Hepatol, 1982; 572; Duffy, JCI, 1983; 72:1470). Simple diffusion (Fig. 5(G)) may play a role in the uptake of unconjugated bile acids. The carrier-mediated sodium-dependent uptake has been cloned in the rat (Hagenbuch, PNAS, 1991; 88:20629) and in man (Hagenbuch, JCI, 1994; 93:1326) their mRNA encoding for peptides of 48 and 38 kDa in the two species, respectively. The proteins exhibit over 75 per cent homology and are thought to act as a sodium–bile acid symport leading to secondary active transport since it is activated by the sodium gradient established by the activity of the Na,K-ATPase (Fig. 5(B)). Thus, the sodium gradient is one of the main determinants of bile salt uptake. Alterations in the membrane lipid composition can alter bile salt transport via a modulation of Na,K-ATPase activity (Rosario, Biochem, 1988; 27:3939). In addition, microfilaments have been shown to be involved in the hepatocellular uptake of taurocholate by mechanisms as yet unknown (Reichen, BBActa, 1981; 643:126). A second protein with a molecular weight of 74 kDa called organic anion transporting protein (**oatp**) has been cloned and sequenced (Jacquemin, PNAS, 1994; 91:133); it is responsible for the sodium-independent uptake of bile acids and organic anions such as sulphobromopthalein and presumably mediates the uptake of these organic anions by facilitated diffusion (Fig. 5(F)).

Intracellular binding and translocation

Different cytosolic bile acid-binding proteins have been identified, some of them exhibiting glutathione-*S*-transferase activity (Sugiyama, JBC, 1983; 258:3602). At high bile salt loads, vesicular traffic and involvement of the Golgi apparatus has been observed (Lamri, JCI, 1988; 82:1173). At physiological doses, an intact microfilament but not microtubule function appears to be required for translocation of bile acids across the hepatocyte (Kacich, Gastro,

1983; 85:385). Unconjugated bile acids, either administered exogeneously or reabsorbed after bacterial deconjugation in the intestine, are usually completely amidated with glycine or taurine prior to excretion; this process is not rate limiting under normal conditions. For certain tertiary and some synthetic bile acids, however, conjugation has been shown to be rate limiting (Zouboulis-Vafiadis, AmJPhysiol, 1982; 243:G208). An important regulatory mechanism for canalicular excretion is the insertion of carrier protein-containing vesicles into the canalicular plasma membrane, a process which has both, microtubule-dependent and -independent facets (Boyer, Gastro, 1995; 109:1600).

Canalicular secretion

Like hepatic uptake, canalicular excretion is a saturable process normally characterized by a transport maximum which is conventionally determined by measuring the bile salt secretion at increasing bile acid concentrations. The maximal canalicular transport rate is lower than the maximal uptake velocity (Reichen, AmJPhysiol, 1976; 231:734); this method does not reveal the true transport maximum but rather is a reflection of both the toxicity and maximal transport capacity (Hardison, AmJPhysiol, 1981; 241: G337). The canalicular secretion of bile acids is driven by two processes, one dependent on the membrane potential and the other independent of sodium (Inoue, JCI; 1984; 73:659; Meier, BiochemJ, 1987; 242:465; Ruetz, PNAS, 1988; 85:6147). More recently, an ATP-dependent mechanism mediated by a 110 kDa protein has been described independently by different groups (Müller, JBC, 1991; 266:18920; Nishida, PNAS, 1991; 88:6590; Stieger, BiochemJ, 1992; 284:67). The affinity of different bile salts to this transporter is influenced by the charge of the bile acid molecule, its hydroxylation and conjugation but not by the side-chain length (Nishida, Hepatol, 1995; 21:1058). It has been suggested that only the ATP-dependent transport resides on the canalicular membrane the potential-dependent carrier being localized in the endoplasmic reticulum (Kast, JBC, 1994; 269:5179) and its role—if any—in canalicular secretion remains unclear.[2]

Bile salt-independent canalicular bile flow

Different mechanisms contribute to the bile salt-independent elaboration of canalicular bile. Bile formation in the perfused rat liver depends in part on the presence of bicarbonate (Hardison, AmJPhysiol, 1978; 235:E158). A potential mechanism for this is depicted in Fig. 6: metabolically-formed CO_2 leads to the formation of bicarbonate and protons mediated by carbonic anhydrase (Fig. 6(A)). The bicarbonate is extruded into the canaliculus by a canalicular chloride–bicarbonate exchanger (Fig. 6(B)) (Meier, JCI, 1985; 75: 1256). To maintain the intracellular pH, the proton formed is excreted across the sinusoidal membrane by a sodium–proton antiport (Fig. 6(C)). This mechanism could contribute to the bicarbonate-rich choleresis induced by bile acids such as ursodeoxycholate (Renner, AmJPhysiol, 1988; 254:G232).

Bile often exhibits a cation–anion gap (Klos, AmJPhysiol, 1979; 236:E434; see also Fig. 2). A small molecular-weight anion has been isolated from bile salt-depleted bile and shown to exhibit choleretic properties. Part of this phenomenon is due to carrier-mediated

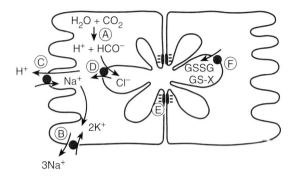

Fig. 6. Elaboration of bile salt-independent canalicular bile: (A) metabolically formed CO_2 is used to generate protons and bicarbonate under the influence of carboanhydrase. (D) The bicarbonate is excreted into the canaliculus via a chloride–bicarbonate exchanger. (C) The proton is extruded by a sodium–proton antiporter activated by the Na, K-ATPase. (F) A second step potentially important in the generation of bile salt-independent bile could be the carrier-mediated excretion of GSSG or glutathione conjugates.

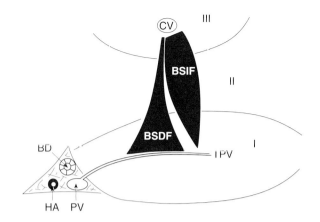

Fig. 7. Acinar organization of canalicular bile flow: the acinus according to Rappaport is shown; it is determined by the terminal portal venule (**TPV**) and the central vein (**CV**). Bile salt-dependent flow (**BSDF**) is mainly a function of zone I and bile-salt-independent flow (**BSIF**) a function of zone II and III hepatocytes, respectively.

biliary glutathione excretion (Ballatori, AmJPhysiol, 1989; 256:G22) (see also Fig. 6(F)). Glutathione conjugates are excreted into bile via an ATP-dependent mechanism (Akerboom, JBC, 1991; 266: 13147). At least part of this activity is due to the multidrug resistance protein (**MRP**) (Mayer, JCellBiol, 1995; 131:137) which is absent in mutant rats with congenital jaundice (Jansen, Hepatol, 1987; 7:71; Büchler, JBC, 1996; 271:15091) and in patients with Dubin–Johnson syndrome (Kartenbeck, Hepatol, 1996; 23:1061). Besides bilirubin the endogeneous substrates for this carrier protein are cysteinyl leukotrienes (Leier, JBC, 1994; 269:27807). Finally, a recently cloned nucleoside transporter could play a role in maintaining bile salt-independent bile formation (Che, JBC, 1995; 270:13596).

Acinar organization and bile formation

Several metabolic processes, including those involved in bile formation, show acinar specialization. While the bile salt uptake seems to be equally distributed from zones I to III, the hepatocytes of zone I excrete bile acids much more efficiently than those from zone III (Groothuis, AmJPhysiol, 1982; 243:G435). This contention is supported by studies where zone I or zone III were selectively destroyed. This zonal difference appears to be changed by alterations in the bile acid load, for example induced by bile acid feeding (Reichen, Experientia, 1989; 45:135) or biliary drainage (Baumgartner, Gastro, 1991; 100:1054) and is abolished after partial hepatectomy (Baumgartner, JHepatol, 1995; 22:454). These studies suggest that the formation of bile salt-dependent bile is mainly a function of zone I (see Fig. 7); in contrast, the bile salt-independent fraction of bile appears to be predominantly a function of zone III; this has been ascribed to a flushing function for this fraction of bile (Gumucio, JLabClinMed 1977; 91:350).

Role of the cytoskeleton in bile formation

Microfilaments are involved in the regulation of hepatic taurocholate uptake (Reichen, BBActa, 1981; 643:126). Bile acid translocation across the hepatocyte also depends on intact microfilament function (Kacich, Gastro, 1983; 85:385). Lipid and protein secretion, in contrast, depend on microtubules (Goldman, Gastro, 1983; 85:130; Barnwell, BiochemJ, 1984; 220:723; Sewell, AmJPhysiol, 1984; 246: G8). As in other epithelia, microfilaments are thought to be involved in the regulation of tight junctional permeability. A close interplay between the microtubules and microfilaments is responsible for receptor-mediated endocytosis (Novikoff, JCellSci, 1996; 109:21). The 'motor' for this movement—kinesin—has been isolated and, interestingly, is inhibited by cholestatic bile acids (Marks, Gastro, 1995; 108:824). Actin is enriched in the pericanalicular area and presumably responsible for the canalicular contractions initially observed in hepatocyte cultures (Oshio, Science, 1981; 212:1041). These contractions are dependent upon an increase in intracellular calcium (Watanabe, LabInvest, 1985; 53:275) and are accelerated by choleretic bile acids such as taurocholate (Miayiri, Gastro, 1984; 87: 788). Finally, transcytosis of inert solutes appears to depend on the microtubules (Jaeschke, BiochemJ, 1987; 241:635).

Biliary permeability

The importance of the negative charge on the tight junctional complexes has been described in the introduction to this chapter (Fig. 3). In contrast to other epithelia, paracellular resistance in the liver cannot be measured directly. The use of inert solute markers as a probe of paracellular permeability has fallen into some disrepute following the realization that part of their movement occurs across the cell (Lake, JCI, 1985; 76:676; Tavoloni, Gastro, 1988; 94:217). This may be mediated by a novel tubuloreticular pathway of transcytosis (Sakisaka, Gastro, 1988; 95:793). Newer techniques such as compartmental analysis, observation of the re-entry of inert solutes from the bile into the perfusate in isolated organ preparations (Jaeschke, BiochemJ, 1987; 241:635), and the use of the biliary indicator dilution technique (Reichen, AmJPhysiol, 1985; 249:G48) will permit the quantitation of paracellular events in the future. A very thorough stereological analysis of junctional depth, strand number and horseradish peroxidase permeation into junctional complexes has shown a very good correlation between cholestasis, junctional alterations and permeability changes (Rahner, Gastro, 1996; 110:1564). The most satisfying method for addressing this important problem in biliary physiology has, however, yet to be found. From recent studies using these novel techniques, as well as from older studies, the following conclusions may be drawn.

1. An increase of biliary permeability—in contrast to the suggestions of earlier investigations—is not necessarily associated with cholestasis. Thus, taurocholate increases the biliary permeability at choleretic doses well below the toxic range (Reichen, JCI, 1988; 81:1462). In other instances, hypercholeresis in the face of increased biliary permeability has been described (Accatino, JLabClinMed, 1981; 97:525).
2. Under the influence of calcium-mobilizing hormones such as vasopressin, the biliary permeability may be altered without a change in bile flow (Lowe, AmJPhysiol, 1988; 255:G454).
3. An increase in the biliary permeability appears to be a universal phenomenon in cholestasis; at present it is unclear whether this represents a final common pathway or whether under certain circumstances an increase in the permeability or a loss of negative surface charge can be pathogenically important in cholestasis (see Chapter 23.1).
4. A close correlation is found between the microstructure of the junctional complexes and alterations in the biliary permeability in intra- and extrahepatic cholestsis (Rahner, Gastro, 1996; 110:1564).

Biliary lipid secretion

A major function of bile is to excrete excess cholesterol (Table 1); to keep this practically water-insoluble molecule in solution, cholesterol is incorporated into mixed micelles and vesicles (Donovan, Biochem, 1987; 26:8125; Somjen, JLipRes, 1985; 26:699; Halpern, JLipRes, 1986; 27:295). Consideration of the physicochemical properties of bile is beyond the scope of this chapter; the reader is referred to work by the pioneers in this fascinating field (Mazer, Biochem, 1980; 19:601; Carey, JCI, 1978; 61:998; Carey, Gastro, 1988; 95:508; Holzbach, Hepatol, 1986; 6:1403).

Biliary lipid secretion is regulated by the bile salt secretion rate (Mazer, JLipRes, 1984; 25:932; Schersten, EurJClinInv, 1971; 1:242) and by the hydrophobicity of the secreted bile salts (Bilhartz, Gastro, 1988; 95:771). The main lipid species are cholesterol and phospholipids, mainly lecithin. Both are derived from specialized presumably intracellular pools (Gregory, JCI, 1975; 55:105). In the case of cholesterol there is a clear dissociation between cholesterol synthesis and secretion (Stone, JCI, 1985; 76:1773; Turley, JLipRes, 1979; 20:923), esterification playing a major regulatory role (Nervi, JCI, 1984; 74:2226). Similarly, phospholipids are derived from an intracellular, specialized pool rather than being eluted by the detergent action of bile acids from the canalicular membrane (Kawamoto, BBActa, 1980; 619:35). It has been suggested that this pool is located close to the Golgi apparatus; its turnover appears to be regulated by bile acid flux across the hepatocytes (Rahman, BiochemJ, 1986, 234:421).

From these findings it appears that biliary lipid secretion is due to some sort of vesicular traffic rather than to simple dissolution of the canalicular membrane by the detergent action of bile acids. This contention is supported by the finding that an intact microtubule function is required for biliary lipid secretion (Gregory, Gastro, 1978; 74:93). The translocation of phospholipids requires a flippase which has recently been identified to be the mdr2 P-glycoprotein (Smit, Cell, 1993; 75:451). Interestingly, mice with the gene for mdr2 knocked out develop a cholestatic picture with nonsuppurative cholangitis (Mauad, AmJPathol, 1994; 145:1237). This points to the protective role of phospholipids against bile acid toxicity and could lead to a better understanding of different inborn errors of metabolism associated with cholestasis. This fascinating model permitted another insight into the physiology of biliary lipid secretion: in the knockout mice there was increased cholesterol secretion suggesting that in the absence of phospholipids cholesterol is removed from the canalicular membrane by the direct detergent activity of bile salts (Oude Elferink, JCI, 1995; 95:31).

An elaborate mathematical model, taking into account a wealth of information from experimental animals and man, has been proposed to explain the coupling of lecithin and cholesterol to bile salt secretion (Mazer, JLipRes, 1984; 25:932). This model predicts that bile salt secretion directly induces lecithin secretion by an unknown mechanism; lecithin secretion in turn activates cholesterol secretion. The model correctly predicts a hyperbolic relationship between the three major components involved in biliary lipid secretion, namely bile acids, lecithin, and cholesterol.

Protein secretion

Protein secretion has long been considered to be negligible, representing just accidental elution of proteins from the canalicular membrane by the detergent action of bile acids and filtration of plasma proteins. Some proteins appearing in bile, for example alkaline phosphatase, are clearly linked to the bile salt secretion rate and are probably derived from the canalicular plasma membrane (Hatoff, Hepatol, 1982; 2:433). In the past 10 years, a quite different picture has emerged ascribing different important functions to biliary secretion in protein and bile homeostasis (see Table 1). The protein composition of bile and the canalicular membrane exhibit marked differences suggesting that most biliary proteins are not derived from the canalicular membrane (Evans, BiochemJ, 1976; 154:589). Up to six different pathways for protein entry into bile have been postulated (Kloppel, Hepatol, 1986; 6:587).

One of these pathways involves lysosomal secretion of proteins and their degradation products via receptor-mediated endocytosis. This receptor, termed the asialoglycoprotein receptor or hepatic binding protein (Stockert, Hepatol, 1983; 3:750), recognizes galactose-terminated proteins. Constitutive lysosomal proteins, in contrast, are excreted in a coordinated fashion suggesting exocytotic bulk discharge corresponding to approximately 3 per cent of the total hepatic protein per day (LaRusso, JCI, 1979; 64:948).

Another important function of biliary proteins relates to mucosal immunity. The secretory component, an integral membrane protein, serves as a receptor for IgA (Fisher, PNAS, 1979; 76:2008). The resulting secretory IgA is extruded into bile via a vesicular process (Renston, Science, 1980; 208:1276). Marked species differences exist in this pathway (Delacroix, Hepatol, 1983; 3:980); while humans and dogs express the secretory component predominantly on ductular cells, in rodents IgA transfer is a function of the hepatocyte.

A very important aspect of biliary protein secretion concerns pro- and antinucleating proteins which play a key role in the pathogenesis of cholesterol and, as recently demonstrated, of pigment gallstones. This aspect will be covered elsewehere in this volume.

The collecting system

The collecting system consists of the bile ductules, bile ducts, common hepatic and common bile ducts, cystic duct, and the gallbladder. Its main functions are as follows.

1. The modification of hepatic bile by reabsorption and secretion, mostly under the influence of gastrointestinal hormones.
2. To store bile and to extrude it into the duodenum upon digestive demands, under the influence of gastrointestinal feedback mechanisms.
3. The damping of pressure within the biliary tree.

Modification of hepatic bile
Bile ducts and ductules[3]

The ductules and ducts represent the collecting system for canalicular bile. Their main function is to modify canalicular bile further by reabsorption and secretion. The latter function is mainly under the influence of secretin, which is released following vagal stimuli and the arrival of acid gastric contents in the duodenum. Elicited by secretin, a bicarbonate-rich secretion is formed (Wheeler, AmJPhysiol, 1966; 210:1153; Chenderovitch, AmJPhysiol, 1972; 223:695). This activation is cAMP dependent and, at least in the rat liver, achieved by activation of luminal chloride channels (Alvaro, JCI, 1993; 92:1314; McGill, AmJPhysiol, 1994; 266:G731). There are different populations of cholangiocytes in rat liver, with only large and medium sized ducts expressing secretin receptors and the cystic fibrosis gene product CFTR (Alpini, Gastro, 1996; 110:1636). In some species, this is associated with a loss of cytoplasmic vacuoles (Buanes, Gastro, 1988; 95:417). The secretin effect is abolished by somatostatin via enhanced reabsorption of bile (Rene, Gastro, 1983; 84:120). In addition to promoting bicarbonate secretion, secretin also induces exocytosis of preformed vesicles (Kato, JBC, 1992; 267: 15523). Besides the secretin receptor and cystic fibrosis transmembrane (CFTR), human cholangiocytes express type II anion exchanger protein on their luminal surface (Martinez-Anso, Hepatol, 1994; 19:1400). In contrast to hepatocytes, cholangiocytes express both type 1 and type 2 isoforms of the sodium–proton exchanger (Marti, JHepatol, 1996; 24:498); the functional significance of this is not clear. Also in contrast to hepatocytes, cholangiocytes express water channels of the channel-forming integral membrane (CHIP) family (Yano, JBC, 1996; 271:6702).

The ductular epithelium is permeable to a variety of inert solutes (Smith, AmJPhysiol, 1982; 242:G52). This permeability is regulated by bile acids (Reichen, JCI, 1988; 81:1462). As in the hepatocytes this could occur via transcytosis since a similar tubulovesicular pathway has recently been functionally and structurally demonstrated (Benedetti, Hepatol, 1993; 18:422). A potentially important role has been ascribed to the ductular system to explain hypercholeresis induced by certain short-chain bile acids invoking a so-called 'cholehepatic shunt pathway' (Palmer, AmJPhysiol,

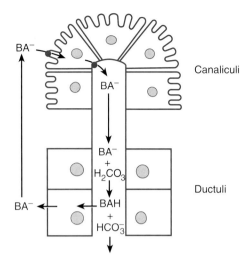

Fig. 8. The cholehepatic shunt pathway: certain bile acids such as ursodeoxycholate and short-chain bile acids are actively excreted into the canaliculi. In the ductules they are protonated, reabsorbed, and the resulting bicarbonate is excreted during each cycle. Bile acids therefore lead to an increased excretion of bicarbonate in excess of their own secretion.

1987; 252:G219). This mechanism is demonstrated in Fig. 8: bile acids are excreted into the canaliculi as anions and in the bile ducts they are protonated and therefore reabsorbed. During each cycle of the bile acid, one molecule of bicarbonate is formed and excreted explaining the bicarbonate-rich bile observed following the administration of such bile acids. Another important role of the ductule may be the reabsorption of glucose and amino acids (Moseley, AmJPhysiol, 1988; 255:G253; Guzelian, JCI, 1974; 53: 526). For sugar reabsorption, functional evidence for the existence of at least two transport systems has been provided (Lira, Gastro, 1992; 102:563).

The surface of the bile ducts is enlarged by a plexus of convoluted glands around the large ducts (Yamamoto, LabInvest, 1985; 52: 103). This plexus may serve as a gallbladder equivalent in species which have no gallbladder. Its functions and the control thereof remain largely unknown but it is important to recognize their anatomy to avoid mistaking them for dilated bile ducts in different imaging procedures (Baron, AJR, 1994; 162:631).

Gallbladder epithelium

The gallbladder epithelium has served as a paradigm to physiologists because of its marked concentrative capacities. Concentration can be achieved in any two-membrane system when the hydraulic water permeability is different between the two membranes and if at least one of the membranes has an active transport system. While earlier studies, in particular by Diamond (Nature, 1966; 210:817), have postulated the existence of a standing osmotic gradient, more attention has been given lately to transcellular ion transport as the basis for the concentrative capacity of the gallbladder.

Based on theoretical calculations, Spring (JExpBiol, 1983; 106: 181) demonstrated that an osmotic gradient of 3 mosmol/l could achieve the concentrative activity of the gallbladder observed *in vitro*. Two pump systems are required for the concentrating capacity, either a sodium–chloride symport or a sodium–proton, chloride–

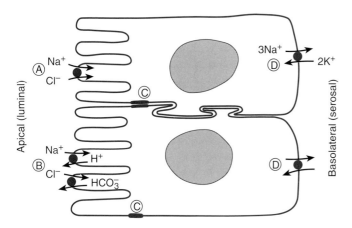

Fig. 9. Absorption in the gallbladder; concentration by an epithelium can occur every time an ion pump is situated on either of two membranes with differing permeabilities. (D) The active transport is basolaterally represented by the Na,K-ATPase. Conductive potassium channels also exist in the basolateral membrane. (A) The apical membrane pumps sodium and chloride either by a sodium–chloride symport or (B) by a system of two antiports. See the text for further details. (C) Back-diffusion of chloride is prevented by the negative charge on the tight junction.

bicarbonate antiport system on the apical membrane and the Na,K-ATPase on the basolateral membrane (Fig. 9).

The symport hypothesis is favoured by the observation that bumetanide, a sodium–chloride symport inhibitor, abolishes the concentrating capacity of the gallbladder (Larson, JMembrBiol, 1983; 74:123). Similarly, the anion transport inhibitor SITS abolishes the concentrating ability of the gallbladder (Ericson, AmJPhysiol, 1982; 243:C140).

On the other hand, there is abundant information supporting the coupled antiport system schematically shown in Fig. 9(B). Thus, in the *Necturus* gallbladder, there is a dissociation of sodium and chloride entry into the cell (Reuss, JGen Physiol, 1984; 84:423). Short-chain fatty acids, which can substitute for bicarbonate, maintain fluid transport in bicarbonate-free media, also suggesting an important role for a chloride–bicarbonate antiporter (Petersen, JMembrBiol, 1981; 62:183). Lowering the luminal pH increases transport; this finding has also been taken as support for the antiport system (Whitlock, AmJPhysiol, 1969; 217:310). However, this observation could also be explained by the secretion of metabolically formed CO_2 and reabsorption of bicarbonate. Finally, the finding that transport in the human gallbladder is rheogenic argues against an electroneutral sodium–chloride pump (Gelarden, JMembrBiol, 1974; 19:37). The development of specific chloride channel blockers has recently permitted the demonstration of the existence of both electroneutral and electrogenic bicarbonate secretion in the guinea-pig gallbladder (Peterson, JPharmExpTher, 1993; 266:65).

As discussed above for liver, it is still unclear whether water follows the transported ions transcellularly or whether it reaches the basolateral side via the tight junction. The gallbladder epithelium is leaky with a transmural resistance of $100\,\Omega/cm^2$ (Suzuki, PfluegersArchPhysiol, 1982; 394:302). As in other epithelia, the paracellular pathway is cation selective and has long been thought to provide free passage to many solutes; the diameter of the junctional

barrier has been estimated at 10 to 20 Å by different probes (Fromter, JMembrBiol, 1972; 8:259). A role for the paracellular pathway is suggested by the following observations.

1. The cation selectivity is different from the diffusion coefficients of cations in free solution and shows the following order: K > Rb > Na > Li > Cs (Moreno, JMembrBiol, 1974; 15:277).
2. The cation selectivity is regulated by cAMP; this mediator decreases the junctional permeability rapidly and reversibly (Zeldin, JMembrBiol, 1985; 84:193). This decrease in permeability is associated with an increase in the number of strands and of tight junctional depth.
3. The relative exclusion of chloride by the tight junction increases the gradient against which chloride can be absorbed by the epithelial cells since there is very little back-diffusion.
4. The interjunctional cleft markedly dilates during fluid absorption (Fig. 9(D)); this has been cited in favour of paracellular fluid movement (Diamond, Nature, 1966; 210:817).

On the other hand, when one considers that the surface area of the apical membrane is 10 000 times larger than that of the tight junction (Blom, JMembrBiol, 1977; 37:45), it appears likely that water entry occurs mostly transcellularly. This consideration is an oversimplification, however. Direct puncture of the intercellular space by micropipettes has shown that the paracellular pathway accounts for 30 per cent of the transepithelial resistance (Ikonomov, PfluegersArchPhysiol, 1985; 403:301).

The gallbladder absorptive capacity is mostly regulated by the second messenger cAMP. This is achieved by a decrease in the junctional permeability, an increase in the apical bicarbonate conductance, and a decrease in the basolateral potassium conductance leading to depolarization (Zeldin, JMembrBiol, 1985; 84:193). Vasoactive intestinal peptide (**VIP**) induces secretion (Jansson, Gastro, 1978; 75:47) while octreotide—a somatostatin analogue—promotes fluid absorption (Moser, Gastro, 1995; 108:1547).

The gallbladder epithelium absorbs sugars and amino acids by sodium-dependent processes (Mirkovitch, PfluegersArchPhysiol, 1975; 355:319). The epithelium is impermeable to taurocholate and bromosulphophthalein but permeable to the less-ionized, unconjugated bilirubin (Ostrow, JCI, 1967; 46:2035). Unconjugated bile acids are injurious and can leave the lumen by simple diffusion (Ostrow, JLabClinMed, 1971; 78:255). Bile supersaturated with cholesterol enhances gallbladder absorption in prairie dogs (Roslyn, AmJMedSci, 1986; 292:75). Recently, it has been recognized that lysophosphatidyl choline decreases absorption and can even lead to net secretion (Neiderhiser, JLabClinMed, 1983; 101:699). Furthermore, different bile components, in particular bile acids, modify mucin secretion by the gallbladder (Klinkspoor, Gastro, 1995; 109: 264). These mechanisms may be important in the pathogenesis of gallstone formation and will be discussed in another chapter.

Motility

The biliary system is a low-pressure, low-flow system. The gallbladder and sphincter of Oddi contract and relax reciprocally under different hormonal influences (Fig. 10). While the common bile duct is not thought to have any intrinsic motility, the situation is less clear for the cystic duct. Observations that the pressure in the cystic duct can change independently of that observed in the

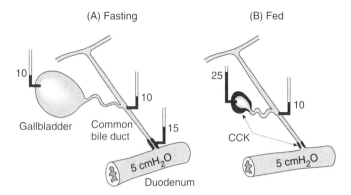

Fig. 10. Coordinated motility of the gallbladder and sphincter of Oddi: the pressures in gallbladder, common bile duct, and sphincter of Oddi are schematically represented (A) during fasting and (B) in the fed state. The duodenal pressure is usually 5 cm of water and always lower than pressure in the sphincter of Oddi. (B) Cholecystokinin (**CCK**) is the main messenger leading to gallbladder contraction and sphincter of Oddi relaxation in the fed state. The system is not entirely passive during fasting. See the text for further details.

gallbladder raise the possibility of the existence of a cystic duct sphincter.

Traditional teaching considers the gallbladder to be mainly under hormonal control; the organ is richly innervated, however and several neurotransmitters are involved in control of the tone and contraction; the effects of different neurotransmitters on gallbladder and sphincter function have been reviewed (McKirdy, PharmTher, 1988; 38:429) (see also Table 2).

The motility of the gallbladder has been studied by oral cholecystography and marker perfusion techniques; the modern techniques of real-time ultrasound (Everson, Gastro, 1980; 79:40) and nuclear scintigraphy (Klingensmith, Radiol, 1981; 141:771) have permitted more accurate analysis of the kinetics of gallbladder

emptying. Using these techniques, gallbladder emptying has been described as an exponential process obeying the equation.

$$V_t = V_0 \exp^{(-kt)}$$

V_0, the fasting volume, ranges from 10 to 50 ml in humans, the normal range being 20 to 30 ml. Physiological stimuli or CCK induce 50 to 75 per cent emptying over 30 to 45 min with a $t/2$ of 10 to 20 min. Combining the two modalities, sonography and biliary scintigraphy, the normal pattern of gallbladder filling and emptying can be studied non-invasively in health and disease (Jazrawi, Gastro, 1995; 109:582).

The sphincter of Oddi can be studied by manometry during ERCP and by cineradiography, electromyography, or nuclear scintigraphy. Geenen (Gastro, 1980; 78:317) defined the sphincter in man by manometry during ERCP as an area 4 to 6 mm long with pronounced phasic contractions superimposed upon a basal tone which is consistently 4 mm higher than either the pressure in the common bile duct or the duodenum (see also Fig. 10). The most popular animal model for the study of the sphincter of Oddi is the opossum sphincter since it is a well-defined muscular layer situated extraduodenally (Toouli, JCI, 1983; 71:208).

Interdigestive motility

Initially, it was assumed that during the interdigestive phase the gallbladder exhibited little motor activity and that bile reaching the duodenum was of purely hepatic origin (Peeters, Gastro, 1980; 79:678). More recent investigations, however, have demonstrated rhythmic activity of both the gallbladder motility and bile flow into the duodenum (Itoh, Gastro, 1982; 83:645; Traynor, AmJPhysiol, 1984; 246:G426). Gallbladder contraction is associated with phase 2 of the migrating motor complex in man. On relaxation there is an increase in hepatic bile formation with a consequent dilution of the gallbladder contents. An increase in gallbladder pressure has been

Table 2 Effects of different neurotransmitters and gastrointestinal hormones on contraction (C) or relaxation (R) of the biliary tree		
	Gallbladder	**Sphincter of Oddi**
CCK	C (Malagelada, Gastro, 1973; 64:950)	R (Geenen, Gastro, 1980; 78:317; Sandbloom, AmJPhysiol, 1935; 93:175; Toouli, Surgery, 1982; 92:497; Wiley, JCI, 1988; 81:1920)
Motilin	C (Svenberg, Gut, 1982; 23:1024)	C (Behar, Gastro, 1988; 95:1099)
Secretin	R (Ryan, AmJPhysiol, 1976; 230:553)	C, R (Geenen, Gastro, 1980; 78:317)
Pancreatic polypeptide	R (Conter, Gastro, 1987; 92:771)	R (Greenberg, DigDisSci, 1979; 24:11)
VIP	R (Sundler, Gastro, 1977; 72:1375)	R (Wiley, JCI, 1988; 81:1920)
Neurotensin	R (Walker, AnnSurg, 1985; 201:675)	
Peptide YY		R (Conter, AmJPhysiol, 1987; 252:9736)
Glucagon	R (Geenen, Gastro, 1980; 78:317; Behar, Gastro, 1988; 95:1099; Ponce, DigDisSci, 1989; 34:61)	
Acetycholine	C (Pallin, ActaPhysiolScand, 1964; 60:358; Marzio, EurJClinPharmac, 1987; 33:151; Fisher, Gastro, 1985; 89:716; Davison, Digestion, 1975; 13:251)	
α-Adrenergics	C (Pallin, ActaPhysiolScand, 1964; 60:358)	C (Persson, BrJPharmacol, 1971; 42:447)
β-Adrenergics	C (Pallin, ActaPhysiolScand, 1964; 60:358)	C (Persson, BrJPharmacol, 1971; 42:447)
Histamine	C(H_1); C, R (H_2) (Wise, JSurgRes, 1982; 33:146)	
Endorphins	C (Saveri, LifeSci, 1988; 42:2373)	

observed to be directly associated with the delivery of bile into the duodenum (Scott, AmJPhysiol, 1985; 249:G622).

In humans, an emptying of the gallbladder of up to 30 per cent is observed during fasting (Svenberg, Gut, 1982; 23:1024); this is associated with an increase in the serum concentration of motilin and associated with phase 2 of the migrating motor complex as in animal models. The goal of these fasting contractions could relate to a housekeeping function of the gallbladder and serve to prevent accumulation of cholesterol microcrystals.

As in the gallbladder, rhythmic contractions associated with the migrating motor complex are observed in the sphincter of Oddi in dogs (Scott, Gastro, 1984; 87:793) and opossums. In man, rhythmic contractions have been observed during the interdigestive phase also, 60 per cent of which occur in antegrade, 14 per cent in retrograde, and 26 per cent in bidirectional fashion (Toouli, Surgery, 1982; 92:497). These rhythmic contractions appear to evolve from some proximal area in the common bile duct with an assumed pacemaker function and then extend into the high pressure zone of the sphincter.

The sphincter is thought by some to act as a peristaltic pump to promote bile flow into the duodenum (Toouli, JCI, 1983; 71:208). By others, it is regarded rather as a resistor to permit gallbladder filling. It probably has both functions.

Digestive motility [4]

During digestion, contraction of the gallbladder occurs in response to a meal reaching the duodenum or to exogenous CCK (see Fig. 10(B)). Ivy and Goldberg (AmJPhysiol, 1928; 86:599) were the first to demonstrate the release of a humoral factor after the instillation of acid into the duodenum. This substance was later identified by Jorpes (Gastro, 1968; 55:157) as CCK, a polypeptide of 28 amino acids; two other physiologically active forms exist, CCK-33 and the carboxy-terminated CCK-8. It is believed that CCK-33 is the biologically active molecule. Earlier investigations reporting that CCK-8 is biologically more active are probably erroneous and due to avid binding of CCK-33 in the absence of protein. The development of sensitive and specific radioimmunoassays has shown CCK to increase within 2 min of administration of a fatty meal and to reach a peak after 16 min. Maximal gallbladder contraction occurs approximately 5 min later.

CCK relaxes the sphincter of Oddi in dogs (Sandbloom, AmJPhysiol, 1935; 93:175) and man (Sarles, DigDisSci, 1986; 31: 208) by decreasing both the tonic and phasic contractile response. When given as a bolus, however, CCK may transiently increase the sphincter of Oddi motility. This relaxing effect appears to be mediated by a release of VIP (Wiley, JCI, 1988; 81:1920), the second messenger being cAMP.

Many gastrointestinal hormones modulate the contractile and relaxing responses of the gallbladder and sphincter of Oddi, respectively (see Table 2). Both the gallbladder and the sphincter are richly innervated by vagal, sympathetic and non-adrenergic, non-cholinergic (**NANC**) nerve fibres.

Stimulation of the vagus increases gallbladder motility (Pallin, ActaPhysiolScand, 1964; 60:358); during the cephalic phase of digestion cholinergic stimuli are responsible for gallbladder contraction in man (Fisher, Gastro, 1986; 90:1854). This can also be elicited by antral distension; this pylorocholecystic reflex is blocked by atropine (Debas, AnnSurg, 1979; 190:170). Vagotomy decreases gallbladder motility and leads to a doubling of the fasting gallbladder volume (Johnson, Surgery, 1952; 32:591). Conversely, the resistance of the sphincter of Oddi increases after vagotomy in prairie dogs (Pitt, Surgery, 1981; 90:418). The cephalic phase decreases the resistance to bile flow across the sphincter of Oddi via NANC inhibitory neuropeptides. After vagotomy, the response to CCK decreases, the dose–response curve being shifted to the left (Malagelada, Gastro, 1973; 64:950). Therefore, it is thought that the full action of CCK depends on an intact cholinergic input (Pallin, ActaPhysiolScand, 1964; 60:358; Davison, Digestion, 1975; 13:251). Nitric oxide is an important mediator of sphincter of Oddi relaxation (Kaufmann, AmJSurg, 1993; 165:74; Wells, AmJPhysiol, 1993; 265:G258).

Adrenergic fibres also appear to modulate gallbladder and sphincter of Oddi tone, β-adrenergic stimuli having a relaxing and α-adrenergic stimuli a contracting effect on both organs (Persson, BrJPharmacol, 1971; 42:447).

Motilin increases pressure in the sphincter of Oddi by an increase in spike burst activity; this is achieved by activation of a local excitatory pathway involving serotonin, acetylcholine, and endorphins (Behar, Gastro, 1988; 95:1099).

Gallbladder and sphincter of Oddi motility have received increasing attention lately because of their pathogenic role in gallstone formation and the recognition that dysfunction of the sphincter of Oddi can lead to biliary-type colic in certain patients. An extensive discussion of the effects of early gallstone formation on the absorptive and motor activity of the gallbladder can be found in a recent review (Carey, Gastro, 1988; 95:508).

References

1. Sperber I. Biliary secretion of organic anions and its influence on bile flow. In Taylor EW, ed. *The biliary system*. Oxford: Blackwell, 1965: 457–67.
2. Meier PJ. Molecular mechanisms of hepatic bile salt transport from sinusoidal blood into bile. *American Journal of Physiology*, 1995; 269: G801–12.
3. Boyer JL. Bile duct epithelium: frontiers in transport physiology. *American Journal of Physiology*, 1996; 270: G1–5.
4. Toouli J and Baker RA. Innervation of the sphincter of Oddi: Physiology and considerations of pharmacological intervention in biliary dyskinesia. *Pharmacology and Therapeutics*, 1991; 49: 269–81.

2.4 Hepatobiliary disposition and targeting of drugs and genes

Dirk K. F. Meijer, P. L. M. Jansen, and Geny M. M. Groothuis

General aspects of drug transport in the liver

Introduction

In evolution the living organisms have been exposed to many toxic xenobiotics, mainly as food components. Examples are plant alkaloids of which many are readily absorbed and can be extremely toxic due to interaction with neural and hormonal receptor systems and/or genetic material. In the evolutionary processes, excretory organs such as the kidney, gut, and liver became adequately equipped with detoxifying mechanisms. These include metabolic conversion processes and secretory systems for potentially toxic compounds to remove such potential life-threatening agents from the body.[1,2]

At the same time, selective transport mechanisms for essential nutrients are necessary to maintain hepatic cell function and the production of vital physiological substrates. Against this background, it is not surprising that multiple carrier-mediated transport systems for endogenous and exogenous compounds evolved at the hepatic uptake and excretion level.

Many of these processes are genetically related to well characterized transport systems in micro-organisms, such as bacteria and fungi, and several superfamilies of transporters are present (Doige, AnnRevMicro, 1993; 47:291; Germann, SemCellBiol, 1993; 4:63). Apart from the many transport processes in the sinusoidal and canalicular domains of the hepatocyte plasma membrane, intracellular transport sites have been identified in organelles such as endosomes, lysosomes, mitochondria, and probably the cell nucleus.[1,3] Therefore, hepatobiliary transport of drugs and diagnostic agents can be envisioned as a number of sequential transport steps (see Fig. 1): uptake, intracellular binding and sequestration, metabolism, sinusoidal secretion, and biliary excretion. Each of these steps may determine the rate of hepatobiliary transport. In addition, blood flow, plasma protein binding, and possibly canalicular reabsorption may influence this rate.

Knowledge of hepatic drug traffic and the transporters involved has increased substantially in the past decade. However, many gaps in this knowledge impair our full understanding of the hepatobiliary transport processes. More attention should be paid to a systematic

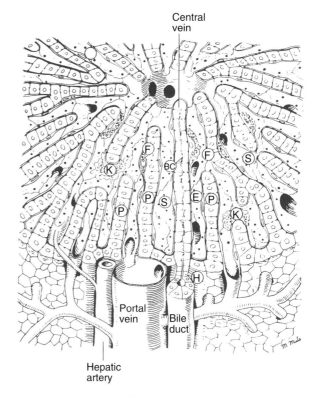

Fig. 1. Schematic representation of the cellular liver structure with fenestrated endothelial lining of the sinusoids (S) that receive blood from the hepatic artery (HA) and terminal portal venules (PV). Bile is primarily excreted in the bile canaliculi draining into the bile ductules (BD). Four cell types are indicated: hepatocytes (H), endothelial cells (EC), Kupffer cells (KC), and fat-storing cells or stellate cells (FSC). Sinusoids finally drain their contents in the central veins (CV).

structure–transport relationship for the various categories of substrates. More detailed knowledge of the cloned carrier-proteins, their DNA, and antibodies will provide more fundamental insight into membrane translocation on the molecular level. Moreover, this information will stimulate research on the regulation of the transport processes, not only in the normal liver but also in the diseased liver. In addition, it may add to the elucidation of the intra-acinar localization and the regulation of this heterogeneity in drug transport.

Future research will have to shed light on the black box of intracellular transport from the sinusoidal to the canalicular membrane. Also, the involvement of non-parenchymal cell types in the regulation of transport activity in the liver is a poorly studied aspect.

Most of the available knowledge on drug transport in the liver is at present obtained from animal studies. The recent development of *in vitro* techniques aimed at measuring drug transport in the human liver (Sandker, BiochemPharm, 1994; 47:2193; Groothuis, JHepatol, 1996; 24:3)[4] will provide the opportunity to gather more information on qualitative and quantitative aspects of drug traffic transport in the hepatobiliary system in man. Adequate *in vitro* to *in vivo* extrapolations and interspecies comparisons will be needed here. This may also stimulate the development of novel diagnostic function tests with an improved predictive value in liver disease and in liver transplantation. Such tests should include 'on-line' measurements of the disposition of several substrates simultaneously and will need an advanced pharmacokinetic analysis.

Finally, in the area of cell-specific drug delivery that is reviewed in the last section of this chapter, knowledge of membrane transport and receptor-mediated endocytosis will have to reach a higher integration level in order to gain more insight into the factors that determine the residence time of targeted drugs in the targeted cell type.

Liver structure

The liver occupies a strategic place in the body: it is interposed between the digestive tract and the general circulation and receives 20 to 25 per cent of the cardiac output (about 1.5 l/min per 70 kg body weight) via the portal vein and hepatic artery. Nutrients, drugs, and other potentially toxic xenobiotics that are absorbed in the gastrointestinal tract have to pass this chemically active organ before they reach the other tissues in the body. Only substrates absorbed in the buccal cavity or the lower part of the rectum, of which the venous outflows directly drain into the general circulation, can bypass the liver and escape first-pass elimination (De Boer, ClinPharmacokin, 1982; 7:285).

A number of factors favour the role of the liver in the exchange of blood components to maintain body homeostasis. The large size of the organ (about 3 per cent of body weight) allows a relatively long residence time of substrates in spite of the impressive blood flow mentioned above. The highly branched capillary systems (Fig. 1) (the hepatic sinusoids) enable efficient exposure to the sinusoidal cell types—Kupffer cells (2.5 per cent of the total liver cell volume), endothelial cells (3.3 per cent), stellate cells (1.6 per cent), and the hepatocytes (92.5 per cent).[5] The fenestrated endothelial lining, in principle, permits direct contact of soluble blood constituents with the villous plasma membranes of the hepatocytes.

About 15 per cent of the total liver volume consists of intravascular space, the space of Disse (between the endothelial lining and the hepatocytes), bile canaliculi, and ductules, as well as lymphatic vessels. The space of Disse, although optically empty, contains the components of the extracellular matrix, such as collagens and glycosaminoglycans (predominantly heparan sulphates and fibronectin). These components may influence the elasticity of the fenestrated blood vessel wall and probably also the rate of exchange of substrates. Development of perisinusoidal fibrosis may create an extra diffusion barrier for compounds to be taken up in hepatocytes.[5]

The hepatocyte (80 per cent of the total liver volume) is a highly polarized cell which possesses distinct regions: one is oriented towards the sinusoids and is involved in exchanges with the plasma; the other forms the biliary canaliculus with an adjacent hepatocyte and is involved in bile secretion. These two cellular domains are separated by tight junctions so that substances excreted in the biliary canaliculus do not flow back into the plasma.

Bile secreted by hepatocytes flows through bile canaliculi, which are small channels, 1 µm in diameter. In the canalicular region, the plasma membrane has short microvilli that account for approximately 13 per cent of the cell surface and contains carrier proteins as well as specific enzymes. Canalicular bile flows in a direction opposite to sinusoidal plasma flow from perivenous to periportal regions. Canaliculi from several hepatocytes end at the periphery of the lobule in the canal of Hering, a channel of two to four cells in length that is made up of both hepatocytes and biliary cells and is prolonged by ductules (or cholangioles) formed by biliary epithelial cells (cholangiocytes).

The lateral domain of adjacent hepatocytes, which accounts for 15 per cent of the cell surface, constitutes an intercellular cleft of 20 nm in width that opens in the space of Disse. This portion of the plasma membrane contains numerous gap junctions that allow communication between cells.

The plasma membrane of the sinusoidal domain bears numerous microvilli and accounts for approximately 70 per cent of the cell surface. This region contains numerous specialized proteins: carrier proteins, and receptors for endocytosis of glyco- and lipoproteins, hormones, and growth factors.

Disposition of drugs and macromolecules in the liver

The various cell types in the organ deal not only with nutrients from the gut and endogenous metabolic products from other parts of the body but also with drugs, toxins, immune complexes, and denatured proteins, as well as low density lipoprotein (**LDL**) and high density lipoprotein (**HDL**) particles. After primary uptake of material by the liver, a versatile metabolic apparatus for degradation and biotransformation is available in intracellular organelles such as lysosomes and the endoplasmic reticulum. Further disposition may be by secretion of the products from the organ via at least three pathways: the systemic circulation, the biliary system, and the lymphatic system. Apart from many carrier systems for inorganic ions (Na^+, K^+, Ca^{2+}, SO_4^{2-}, Cl^-, and HCO_3^-) (Stieger, p.25 in reference 6), hepatocytes possess uptake mechanisms for bile acids, fatty acids,[7] various types of amino acids, sugars (i.e. glucose and galactose) (Stieger, p.25 in reference 6), and oligopeptides,[8] as well as nucleosides (Plagemann, BBActa, 1988; 947:405). Such endogenous compounds are translocated into the cell by carrier-mediated facilitated diffusion. Although these processes are considered to be quite specific for the particular type of agents, they are in theory also suitable for exogenous compounds, provided that sufficient structural similarity with endogenous substrates is present.

In principle, all of the cell types mentioned can take up a large variety of organic compounds. First of all, passive permeation of lipid-soluble (hydrophobic) drugs occurs due to the large membrane surface that is present on the various cell types. For polar drugs and macromolecules that cannot pass through the bilayer lipid membranes by 'dissolving', more or less specific receptors or carrier proteins are available for translocation of the particular molecules into the interior of the cells. Receptor-mediated endocytosis and carrier-mediated (facilitated) diffusion are very different types of membrane transport phenomena, yet both display saturability, competition between structurally related compounds, and require some form of cellular 'activity' to maintain or drive the transport into the cell.[9] Carrier or receptor molecules may have quite specific binding sites for a particular category of substrates and often association of substrates is helped by the presence of inorganic ions such as Na$^+$ and Cl$^-$. Similar types of receptor- or carrier-mediated processes may play a role in intracellular sequestration into organelles and exocytosis or excretion from the cells.

The relative rate at which a certain organic compound is taken up in the liver and is subsequently metabolized or excreted, determines its storage in the particular cell type and, if a drug is involved, this determines the local therapeutic activity or toxicity in the tissue. Distribution of compounds in the liver is inherently inhomogeneous since the cells may differ intrinsically in transport characteristics (Groothuis, AmJPhysiol, 1982; 243:G455; Groothuis, TrendsPharmacolSci, 1985; 6:322). Apart from such cellular differences, their unequal localization in the hepatic acinus (in periportal as opposed to perivenous areas) may imply that the more distant cells are exposed to lower concentrations than those in the first part of the sinusoids[10] since substrates are removed progressively from the blood during passage through the liver.

The fact that each cell type contains specialized uptake mechanisms for drugs or macromolecules can be used to deliver drugs, enzymes (Meijer, SemLivDis, 1995; 15:202), and even genes or antisense oligonucleotides (Poznansky, PharmRev, 1984; 36:277; Ledley, Hepatol, 1993; 18:1263; Chang, Gastro, 1994; 106:1076)[11, 12] specifically to certain cell types in the liver. This is achieved by linking these agents covalently via biodegradable bonds to the particular carrier molecules. The fate of the drug/gene in the body is then dictated by the properties of the chosen carrier as a result of specific cell recognition, internalization, and subsequent intracellular transport and biodegradation (Meijer, SemLivDis, 1995; 15:202).

The enterohepatic circulation and its consequences for drug clearance

The clearance function of the liver consists of metabolic conversion and/or excretion into bile. Although biliary excretion mostly leads to removal of the drug from the body in the faeces (Fig. 2), in the gut the drug (-conjugates) may undergo a reversed type of metabolic conversion through deconjugation to the parent compound, which in principle is followed by reabsorption from the gastrointestinal tract into the general circulation. These processes may lead to multiple, more or less complete, enterohepatic cycles (Watkins, p.357 in reference 13). For example, the antibiotic ceftriaxone owes its long half-life to extensive enterohepatic circulation and, for this reason, can be administered once daily. As a consequence, in spite of a primary abundant biliary excretion, this may finally result in prominent urinary excretion of the drug or its metabolites (Watkins,

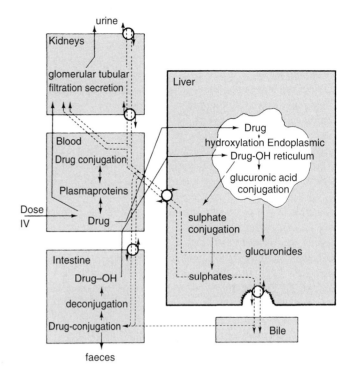

Fig. 2. Schematic representation of sulphate and glucuronide formation, biliary and sinusoidal secretion, enterohepatic circulation, and renal excretion processes. Drugs are taken up in the liver, some are hydroxylated and subsequently conjugated. Sulphate conjugates tend to be excreted into the general circulation, whereas glucuronides are mainly excreted in the biliary system. Excretion of these polar conjugates from the liver into plasma and bile is likely to be carrier mediated. Conjugates entering the circulation can finally be excreted into urine and the gut lumen. Conjugates secreted into the intestine via bile or blood may undergo deconjugation to phenolic drugs, which may be extracted and absorbed by the liver. Inhibition of sinusoidal secretion of anionic drug conjugates by other organic anions may lower urinary excretion and increase biliary excretion.

p.357 in reference 13).[14] If reabsorption of a drug from the gut is relatively small, and thus biliary excretion is a major elimination route, inhibition of biliary clearance of the drug prolongs its elimination half-life (Harrison, JPharmaceutSci, 1976; 65:1346). In contrast, in cases where drugs are rapidly excreted in bile but undergo major intestinal reabsorption in the parent form, inhibition of the biliary excretion process paradoxically may shorten the elimination half-life of the drug, since inhibition of the enterohepatic cycling in that case only reduces the distribution volume of the drug and leaves the real clearance process (via the urine) unchanged (Colburn, DrugMetDisp, 1979; 7:100).

Biliary excretion and the enterohepatic circulation of drugs and their metabolites can have important implications for their local action on the gastrointestinal tract, for example in the case of antibiotics (Ambrose, JDrugDevel, 1989; 1:233), laxatives, and immunoglobulins. Toxic effects related to excretion into the gut have been reported for non-steroidal anti-inflammatory drugs, oestrogens, lithocholate, and methotrexate among others.[14] For instance, the duration of action of cardiac glycosides, the coumarin type of anticoagulants, and progesterone, as well as the systemic toxic effects of cardiac glycosides and chloramphenicol, can be largely influenced by the process of enterohepatic cycling (Watkins, p.357 in reference 13). Both interactions between rifampicin antibiotics and oral contraceptives at the level of biliary excretion and the induction of metabolism of contraceptive drugs by antiepileptics can lead to failure of contraceptive treatment.[14]

Activated charcoal, aluminium hydroxide, and cholestyramine can influence the intestinal (re-) absorption of drugs and thereby enterohepatic cycling (Siegers, p.389 in reference 13). Dietary components and inhibition by antibiotics of microfloral enzymes can greatly influence microbial biotransformation and thereby enterohepatic circulation of various drugs (Siegers, p.389 in reference 13). Although the liver is the principal site for the disposal of macromolecules and metabolism of drugs in the body, excretion from the organism is a concerted action of the liver, kidneys, intestine, and to a lesser extent of the lungs and skin. One consequence of inhibition of hepatobiliary transport is that the excretion rate in the urine and the fraction of renally excreted drug will increase. This is not due to an increased renal clearance function *per se*, but rather to the elevated plasma levels that are produced as a consequence of inhibition of biliary excretion (excretion rate = clearance × plasma concentration). If total body clearance (Cl) is calculated for instance by using the equation $Cl = \text{Dose}/\mathbf{AUC}$ (Area Under the plasma concentration/time Curve), renal clearance can be found easily by multiplying the fraction of the dose finally excreted unchanged in the urine (f_e) multiplied by the total body clearance. It is often assumed that non-renal clearance is performed mainly by the liver and, therefore, is called hepatic clearance (hepatic clearance = total body clearance – renal clearance). This assumes that intestinal secretion (from blood to the intestinal lumen) or excretion via the skin and lungs is relatively small. However, the latter is not negligible with volatile drugs such as general anaesthetics. Intestinal secretion can be a major elimination pathway for some lipophilic drugs such as digoxin and doxycycline, especially in the absence of renal function (Israili, DrugMetabolRev, 1984; 15: 1123). Passive diffusion of lipophilic drugs directly from the blood across the large surface area of the intestinal mucosa can occur and net transport to the gut in such cases is helped either by ion trapping (i.e. basic drugs excreted into the stomach) or binding to the intestinal contents and ingested activated charcoal. Alternatively, secretion into the gut can be mediated by carrier transport across the intestinal mucosal cells (i.e. sulphonic acids and quaternary amines).[15]

Relation between chemical structure of drugs and their excretion routes

The chemical structure of drugs, that is, the number of charged groups and the lipophilicity/hydrophilicity balance of the molecules, enables a rough prediction of renal, intestinal, and biliary excretion patterns.[16,17] Generally, drugs with a high level of plasma protein binding and relatively high lipophilicity are mainly disposed of by the liver (Meijer, JHepatol, 1987; 4:259; Oude Elferink, BBActa, 1995; 1241:251).[16,18] Substrates that are only partially bound to plasma proteins can be easily removed via the kidneys by glomerular filtration and/or tubular secretion (Ullrich, BBActa, 1994; 1197:45). Passive and carrier-mediated tubular reabsorption can counteract this renal elimination process. Tubular reabsorption may be influenced largely by the extent of dissociation of the drug molecules and thus by the pH of the urine and pK_a values of the dissociable groups in the drug molecule (Van Ginneken, ClinPharmacokin, 1989; 16:38).[19] For instance, the urinary excretion rate of weakly basic compounds such as nicotine and amphetamine-like substances is very low due to the extensive tubular reabsorption, especially if the urine is made alkaline by the ingestion of $NaHCO_3$ (Van Ginneken, 1989).[19] This 'shunting' of the glomerular removal process may lead finally to more extensive hepatic metabolism. An efficient type of renal transport is through carrier-mediated tubular secretion via carrier systems for anionic, uncharged, and cationic substrates that partly overlap in their substrate specificity (Rennick, AmJPhysiol, 1981; 240:F83; Somogyi, Trends-PharmacolSci, 1987, 8:354; Ullrich, 1994). These processes resemble intestinal and hepatobiliary carrier systems. In all of these excretory processes at least two steps are involved: uptake into the cells and secretion from the cells (Rennick, 1981; Somogyi, 1987; Van Ginneken, 1989).[19] The affinity of a given drug for the various carriers in these organs may vary greatly and is probably one of the major factors that determines the relative contribution of the excretory organs in its overall removal from the body.[16] The organ clearance is an adequate parameter to express the absolute excretory activity of an organ *per se*, while the relative contribution to drug excretion is properly reflected in the fraction of the dose of the non-metabolized (parent) form that is eliminated by the particular organ.

The presence of large hydrophobic rings in the molecular structure of agents with a relatively high molecular weight, in combination with charged groups in the molecule, probably favours recognition by the hepatic carrier molecules in the sinusoidal and especially canalicular membranes (Neef, Naunyn-Schmiedb-ArchPharm, 1984; 328:111) (Fig. 3). In spite of the fact that plasma protein binding is often high, the liver is well equipped to remove anionic and cationic agents with a 'bulky' molecular structure from the bloodstream. In addition, association of such amphipathic compounds with biliary micelles may help in preventing reabsorption from the biliary tree and/or facilitate net transport to the canalicular lumen (Scharschmidt, JCI, 1978; 62:1122; Kuipers, p.215 in reference 13). It is important to note that it is not the molecular weight itself but rather the balance between hydrophilic (often charged) groups and hydrophobic moieties of the molecule that provides the best prediction of the distribution and elimination patterns in the whole body (Hirom, BiochemSocTrans, 1974; 2: 327).[16,17] This point was clearly demonstrated in studies with series of cationic (Neef, 1984) and anionic (Hirom, 1974) drugs. Like the hepatic transport systems, renal tubular uptake and secretion processes are also 'sensitive' to variations in lipophilicity of the transported drugs, but they tend to differentiate more on the basis of the type of charge and number of charged groups (Rennick, AmJPhysiol, 1981; 240:F83; Somogyi, TrendsPharmacolSci, 1987, 8:354; Ullrich, ClinInvest, 1993; 71:843).[19] The intestinal mucosal secretory systems take an intermediate position in this respect (see Fig. 4). Since hydrophobicity is a general feature of cholephilic drugs irrespective of their charge, the liver transport systems for anionic, cationic, and uncharged organic compounds will exhibit more overlapping substrate specificity than similar processes in other organs.

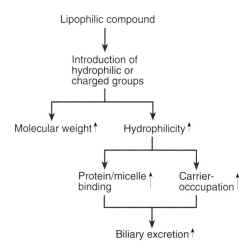

Fig. 3. Factors which explain the empirical finding that drugs with molecular weights of more than 400 are excreted into the bile to a considerable extent (the so-called 'molecular weight threshold hypothesis'). A proper balance of hydrophilic and hydrophobic properties increases the affinity for carrier-mediated transport, promotes net canalicular transport through micelle binding, and increases association with plasma proteins, which in the whole body improves presentation to the liver and limits renal excretion.

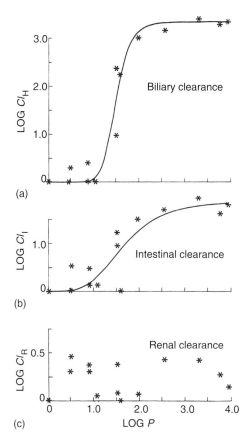

Fig. 4. Relation between lipophilicity (P) (measured by partition between octanol and Krebs' buffer, and expressed relative to the value of tetramethylammonium) and carrier-mediated clearance of 14 monovalent organic cations (drugs with a quaternary ammonium group) via biliary (Cl_H), intestinal (Cl_I), and renal (Cl_R) routes in the rat. The clearance values depicted by an asterisk for each individual compound are corrected for passive fluxes (glomerular filtration, etc.) and indicate carrier-mediated transport in the organs. Between log P = 1 and 2, biliary clearance increases about 1000 and intestinal clearance about 100 times compared with renal clearance, which shows no such correlative pattern.

Studies on structure–excretion relationships have been performed for organic cations such as monovalent (Ryrfeldt, ActaPharmTox, 1971; 30:59; Hughes, BiochemJ, 1973; 136:967; Neef, Naunyn-SchmiedbArchPharm, 1984; 328:111) and bivalent quaternary amines (Wassermann, Naunyn-SchmiedbArchPharm, 1971; 270:R154; Hughes, BiochemJ, 1973; 136:979),[3] organic anions such as sulphonamides (Despopoulos, AmJPhysiol, 1971; 220:1755; Hirom, Xenobiot, 1972; 2:205), penicillin (Hirom, 1972), bile acids (Anwer, Naunyn-SchmiedbArchPharm, 1978; 302:19; Hardison, AmJPhysiol, 1984; 246:G477; Poupon, BiochemPharm, 1988; 37: 209; Aldini, Hepatol, 1989; 10:840),[20] hepatic immino-diacetic acids (**HIDA** radioscanning agents) (Lan, Gastro, 1988; 95:1625; Krishnamurthy, Hepatol, 1989; 9:139), dyes (Hirom, BiochemJ, 1972; 129:1071; Hirom, BiochemSocTrans, 1974; 2:327; Tokumo, Hepatol, 1988; 8:1265), and uncharged cardiac glycosides (Marzo, Naunyn-SchmiedbArchPharm, 1977; 298:51).[17,21] In general, hepatobiliary clearance of organic compounds increases with increasing lipophilicity. Bile acids (Poupon, 1988; Aldini, 1989) and cardiac glycosides (Marzo, 1977) are exceptions to this rule: hepatic uptake strongly benefits from the introduction of hydrophilic groups (Poupon, 1988), while conjugation of bile acids with glycine and especially with taurine promotes canalicular transport (Poupon, 1988). In fact an inverse relation between lipophilicity and overall hepatobiliary transport was found for both groups of agents that basically have a prominent hydrophobic steroid nucleus in common. Glucuronide and sulphate conjugation of steroidal hormones promotes biliary excretion, yet the metabolites of the relatively more hydrophobic steroids are more readily excreted in bile than metabolites of polar steroids (Younes, p.273 in reference 13). Furthermore, also for some amphiphilic cationic drugs that are substrates for the Multi-Drug-Resistance (MDR) system, it was postulated that hydrophobic properties play a crucial role in the accommodation of the agents by P-glycoprotein and/or other potential drug carrier proteins in the canalicular membrane (Smit, BrJPharmacol, 1998, in press). In general, it can be concluded that a proper balance between hydrophobic and hydrophilic properties (charged groups or sugar groups) in the molecular structure of all of the above-mentioned agents is a prerequisite for efficient biliary excretion.

Accumulation of organic compounds in the liver is not only determined by the relative rates of membrane transport into and out of the cells but also by binding to cytosolic proteins and intracellular organelles (Meijer, JPharmacokinBiopharm, 1984; 12: 43).[18] Binding to proteins is often also favoured by hydrophobic properties.[16,22] Drugs that are hydrophilic and of low molecular weight can generally enter hepatocytes easily either by passive diffusion or carrier-mediated transport, but are minimally excreted into bile. This may be due to a relatively low affinity for the canalicular carriers or to secondary loss from the biliary tree. Passage from primary bile into blood can occur across the epithelial cells of the ductules or directly via passage through the 'permselective' channels (Bradley, AmJPhysiol, 1978; 235:E570) in the tight junctions that seal off the canalicular space (see Fig. 1).

Variability in hepatobiliary transport

Hepatobiliary transport can vary greatly depending on a number of experimental, genetic, and environmental factors.[16,17,21] These factors include sex and pregnancy, age differences (especially at the extremes of life), feeding conditions or diet, exercise, circadian variation and/or diurnal rhythms, species variations, adaptive responses on exposure to chemicals, and hepatic regeneration, as well as genetically determined deficiencies in hepatobiliary transport. Relatively scarce information on humans is available with regard to these various factors.

Sex differences

Differences in the hepatobiliary transport rate between male and female animals have been widely described (Persico, JHepatol, 1988; 6:343; Sorrentino, BiochemPharm, 1988; 37:3119; Weisiger, AmJPhysiol, 1988; 255:G822).[17,21] Male rats excrete chlorothiazide and phenol red–glucuronide more rapidly into bile than females, but they excrete indocyanine green, tartrazine, bromosulphthalein (**BSP**), BSP–glutathione, digoxin, and taurocholate less rapidly than females (Sorrentino, 1988).[14,21] Differences in net hepatic uptake rate may often underlie this sex variability and this phenomenon in animals can be manipulated by treatment with sex hormones and castration (Persico, 1988). Sex hormones may influence membrane fluidity and also the membrane potential of hepatocytes, which is on average –25 mV in females and –30 mV in males (Weisiger, 1988). The higher membrane potential in males may retard the net hepatic uptake rate of organic anions like BSP, but probably promotes Na^+-coupled uptake of bile acids that occurs in an electrogenic manner through cotransport with multiple Na^+ ions. In the human, sex variability has been reported for indocyanine green and bilirubin, plasma clearance being higher in females (Tiribelli, ClinSci, 1986; 71:1).

Pregnancy can be associated with a lower biliary output of organic anions, probably due to the influence of oestrogens or toxic oestrogen metabolites, whereas lactation may promote bile flow and biliary excretion.[14,21] Oestrogen-induced cholestasis involves perturbation of transport processes at multiple levels in the hepatocyte: changes in membrane fluidity occurs both at the sinusoidal and canalicular level. Both Na^+-dependent taurocholate uptake and voltage-dependent taurocholate efflux in canalicular membrane vesicles are affected. Fluidity changes and direct (non-) competitive interactions between oestrogen and its metabolites may underly inhibition of the organic anion and bile acid transport steps in addition to changes in Na^+K^+-ATPase. Glucuronide conjugates (in the D-ring) of oestradiol have a prominent effect on canalicular transporters and, recently, a high affinity for P-glycoprotein and the MRP2 (cMOAT) carrier was demonstrated (Vore, ToxApplPharmacol, 1993; 118:2).

Age differences

Many investigations have shown considerable age-related variability in hepatobiliary transport. Most of these studies were performed in rats. When studying the influence of age during the total life-time of rats, it should be emphasized that the first 6 months of life in a rat is a developmental period and studies should be followed for up to 2 years to investigate senescence.

Hepatobiliary transport of substances such as BSP is depressed, although moderately, in old age in rats and humans (Kitani, LifeChemRep, 1988; 6:143). In addition, age-dependent changes in bile acid output in bile as well as bile acid composition have been reported. In rats, the maximal transport rate of organic anions and taurocholate declines with age, independent of sex differences. Hepatic clearance of taurocholate and ouabain decreases linearly with age, probably due to a decline in the uptake rate, as shown in hepatocytes isolated from rats between 4 and 40 months of age, in which a 50 per cent decrease was found after 24 months (Kitani, p.417 in reference 13). Reduction in indocyanine green clearance with age was shown to be due to a decrease in blood flow rather than in hepatic extraction.

During fetal development, hepatic excretion processes develop slowly and, together with a limited intestinal reabsorption and lack of defecation, may result in entrapment of transplacentally acquired xenobiotics that may even cause postnatal toxicity. This has been suggested for valproic acid and diethylstilboestrol and carcinogenic polycyclic aromatic hydrocarbons such as benzpyrene (Gregus, p.401 in ref. 13). At parturition, biliary excretion may be severely challenged due to a sudden lack of placental removal and decrease in hepatic oxygenation.

After birth, bile is formed at a relatively low rate but gradually increases to adult levels by the end of the first month. In the neonate rat, hepatic uptake of bile acids, organic anions, colchicine, and cardiac glycosides is low initially but may develop rapidly within a few days. Likewise, the biliary excretion rate of drugs and drug conjugates is deficient in neonates of various animal species and gradually improves postnatally (Gregus, p.401 in reference 13). There is often a reduced capacity of the liver to accumulate compounds, pointing to deficiencies at the level of uptake and intracellular binding (Gregus, p.401 in reference 13). In the case of taurocholate, an underdeveloped canalicular transport system is the major factor explaining the slower biliary excretion rate in early life, but decreased uptake into the hepatocytes has also been found (Suchy, PediatRes, 1982; 16:282). Since biliary excretion rates of some organic anionic drugs such as BSP and indocyanine green are bile acid dependent, the deficient bile acid transport is one of the factors explaining the above-mentioned low excretion of organic anions. The carrier protein for Na^+-dependent bile acid uptake (ntcp) is not functionally expressed in the rat fetus throughout gestation but, as indicated by mRNA levels, is suddenly expressed just prior to birth on fetal day 20, with a progressive increase in the 4 weeks after birth (Hardikar, p.120 in reference 6). The mRNA expression for the organic anion transporter (oatp) precedes that of ntcp and can be detected on fetal day 16. Thereafter, the oatp-mRNA expression remains stable during the perinatal period and increases after weaning (Debuisson, JHepatol, 1996; 25:932). ATP-dependent bile acid transporter(s) at the canalicular level reach 50 per cent of adult transport V_{max} at 7 days old. The maturing of this process may be partly related to gradual N-glycosylation of the particular carrier proteins in addition to the rate of transcription.

Scarce data are available on age dependency of hepatobiliary transport in the human liver. In a study with isolated human hepatocytes, Olinga *et al.* showed a clear age-dependency of tauro-cholate uptake.[31] Studies on hepatic clearance of indocyanine green and BSP in humans showed an age-dependent decline in hepatic blood flow (Kitani, p.417 in reference 13), while liver weight also decreased with age in humans. Deficiency in biliary elimination has been demonstrated for compounds such as BSP and cefoperazone in human neonates (Rosenfeld, AntimicrobAgents-Chemother, 1983; 23:866; Gregus, p.401 in reference 13). In this situation, relatively higher amounts may be found in the urine (Rosenfeld, 1983).

Food

Food intake may indirectly affect the rate of hepatobiliary transport of drugs through stimulation of the enterohepatic cycling of bile acids, especially in species with gallbladders. As a consequence of this, hepatobiliary transport of anionic dyes is stimulated.[14] Conversely, interruption of bile acid cycling, for instance in patients with T-tubes, depresses anion excretion into bile (Meijer, EurJClin-Pharm, 1983; 24:549). Fasting induces a marked decrease in hepatic clearance of bilirubin, BSP, indocyanine green, and bile acids that may be secondary to decrease in blood flow, intracellular content of binding proteins, and changes in affinity for the carrier systems.[14, 21] Often the influence of fasting and food composition is much more pronounced in drug metabolism than in hepatic drug transport *per se*.

Circadian variations and exercise

Variability in the hepatobiliary transport of organic anions due to night and day time variations have been reported in rat (Vonk, ClinSciMolMed, 1978; 55:399). Since part of the observed effects are secondary to food intake, motility, blood flow, posture, and body temperature, such variations are inherently species dependent. Rodents are night animals and will display different diurnal rhythms to carnivores or mammals. Acute exercise can, in principle, affect a number of rate-limiting steps in hepatobiliary clearance (Martin, p.497 in reference 13). A decrease in hepatic blood flow as measured by initial plasma clearance of indocyanine green was found after 3 h of treadmill walking in humans. Little information is available on the influence of exercise on biliary clearance: while the secretin and cholecystokinin levels in plasma rise in humans during acute exercise, bile flow and bile acid output seem to be unaffected, at least in rodents. With regard to chronic exercise, virtually no data are available.

Species differences

There are extensive species differences in the hepatobiliary clearance of organic compounds. These appear to be largely determined by the molecular weight and thus the hydrophobicity–hydrophilicity balance in the particular drug molecule.[17] For instance, interspecies differences in the clearance of dyes of high molecular weight like (D)BSP or indocyanine green and substances such as cromoglycate are relatively small,[17] whereas very marked species variations have been reported for cardiac glycosides (Marzo, Naunyn-SchmiedbArchPharm, 1977; 298:51)[14,21] and indomethacin (Duggan, DrugMetabolRev, 1979; 9:21), among others. Cumulative biliary excretion of indomethacin, for instance, was reported to be 362 per cent (enterohepatic cycling!), 134 per cent,

26 per cent, 21 per cent, 13 per cent, and 10 per cent of the dose in dogs, rats, monkeys, guinea pigs, rabbits, and humans, respectively (Duggan, 1979). In general, rats, mice, dogs, and hens are considered as relatively efficient biliary excretors, cats and sheep as intermediate, and rabbits, guinea pigs, and humans as poor biliary excretors. Dogs and humans are poor excretors of small (type I) organic cations as well as of ouabain.[21] Such variations are at least partly based on differences in the carrier systems at the membrane level, as was shown in uptake studies using isolated human and rat hepatocytes (Sandker, BiochemPharm, 1994; 47:2193) (4). Considerable species differences were also found in the affinities of various substrates for the organic cation transporter in the sinusoidal membrane (Olinga, DrugMetabDisp, 1998; 26:in press; Gorboulev, DNACellBiol., 1997; 16:871). In addition, differences in the expression of the various Multi-Drug-Resistance proteins are evident in man and rat (Müller, AmJPhysiol, 1997; 272:G1285). Secondary factors such as bile acid output, bile flow, rate of metabolic conversion, or other competing elimination mechanisms may also play a role.[14,17,21]

Genetic factors

In various animal species and also in humans, marked genetic disorders in hepatobiliary transport have been reported, albeit in relatively small populations.[23] Such interindividual transport mutations provide interesting study objects for investigators of transport mechanisms with regard to the cellular synthesis, degradation, and membrane expression of the carrier systems involved (Sorrentino, SemLivDis, 1988; 8:119). Well known are the patients with Dubin–Johnson syndrome (defective canalicular organic anion transport), Gilbert syndrome (in some but not all cases, deficient hepatic uptake of organic anions), and Rotor syndrome (deficient hepatic clearance of coproporphyrine and conjugated bilirubin), and the Corriedale sheep (deficient canalicular transport of non-bile acid organic anions). More recently, a transport mutant rat (TR⁻, GY rat, or EHBR rat) was found with very low biliary excretion of glutathione, glutathione conjugates, and various bivalent organic anions such as bilirubin (Jansen, Hepatol, 1987; 7:71). Such defects can be quite specific: patients with Dubin–Johnson syndrome, Corriedale sheep, and the mutant rats have normal bile acid transport, while transport of hydrophobic dyes such as indocyanine green and BSP, but especially that of the more hydrophilic anions (reduced glutathione, DBSP, and BSP–glutathione), is abnormally low. In these transport mutant rats with deficient anion excretion, hepatobiliary transport of type I cationic drugs is normal but that of ouabain is moderately depressed (Jansen, 1987). The molecular mechanisms explaining this selective dysfunction of the carrier-mediated transporter have been clarified as a defect in the so-called canalicular multispecific organic anion transporter (**cMOAT**). This carrier protein, of which the gene has recently been cloned (Kartenbeck, Hepatol, 1996; 23:1061; Paulusma, Science, 1996; 271:1126; Yamazaki, PharmaceutRes, 1996; 13:495), has a molecular mass of 170 kDa in rats and 190 kDa in humans, and is encoded by the *mrp2/MRP2* gene (Büchler, JBC, 1996; 271:15091; Paulusma, Science, 1996; 271:1126). A point mutation in the 3′-end of the coding region of the gene is responsible for the genetic defect in transport mutant rats. In Dubin-Johnson patients, as in TR⁻ rats, the expression of the gene product is not detectable in the canalicular membrane (Kartenbeck, Hepatol, 1996; 23:1061; Müller, AmJPhysiol, 1997; 272:G1285), due to a mutation in the gene coding for this protein (Paulusma, Hepatol, 1997; 25:1539).

Adaptive changes

Hepatic clearance of drugs can be markedly influenced by long-term changes in physiological conditions or by persistent exposure to agents that induce hypertrophy and/or hyperplasia of liver tissue.[14,16,21] Partial hepatectomy, selective biliary obstruction, liver regeneration, and chronic exposure of the liver to cholephilic substrates may lead to adaptation of the hepatic transport system.[14,16,21,24] Many potential rate-limiting factors in hepatic transport can be affected. Enzyme-inducing agents such as phenobarbital may at the same time affect hepatic blood flow (Wilkinson, ClinPharmTher, 1975; 18:377), body temperature,[21,24] and probably nervous control. They also induce cytosolic-binding proteins (Meijer, JPharmExpTher, 1977; 202:8; Wolkoff, AmJPhysiol, 1979; 236:E638)[18,21] as well as drug-metabolizing enzymes involved in drug oxidation and conjugation.[16] At the same time they can cause extra bile flow (Meijer, 1977)[21] and may also stimulate membrane transport itself by somehow increasing the expression of carrier proteins (Gonzalez, JCI, 1979; 63:684; Simon, JCI, 1982; 70:401).

The time sequence of these changes after exposure to such agents can be very variable.[21] The duration of the pretreatment and the type and dose of the inducing agents, as well as the dosage regimen and the category of the transported drug, can greatly influence the outcome of the particular interaction.[16] For instance, phenobarbital pretreatment exerts much more effect on the hepatobiliary transport of BSP and DBSP than on that of indocyanine green or rose bengal,[14,21] pointing to multiplicity in organic anion transport mechanisms.

A number of possible adaptive mechanisms can be proposed. Exposure to xenobiotic compounds may lead to an increase in liver weight. Many of the effects of 'inducing' agents on the hepatic uptake rate of biliary clearance of drugs are parallel to this change: transport rate expressed per unit of liver weight is not often affected (McDevitt, BiochemPharm, 1977; 26:1247; Meijer, JPharmExpTher, 1977; 202:8).[24] However, the induced extra liver mass is not always functional with regard to drug transport (Meijer, 1977).[24] Most of the inducing compounds increase total hepatic blood flow but not blood flow per unit of liver weight (McDevitt, 1977; Meijer, 1977). This increase in blood flow may explain many of the observed changes in the initial plasma-disappearance rate, [21,24] reflecting a more rapid distribution to the liver of drugs with a high initial extraction ratio (McDevitt, 1977; Meijer, 1977). Besides proliferation of endoplasmic reticulum or other cell organelles, these agents generally increase the concentration of drug-binding cytosolic proteins and thus hepatic storage of many anionic drugs (Meijer, 1977; Wolkoff, AmJPhysiol, 1979; 236:E638).[25] This factor may add to the influence of the elevated liver volume on hepatic drug content.

The increased bile flow may stimulate the net flux of organic anions into bile at high doses.[16,21] 3-Methylcholantrene, an enzyme inducer that does not produce choleresis, has no effect on the biliary excretion of organic anions.[21,24] The inducing agents may further stimulate synthesis or inhibit degradation of functional carrier proteins or alternatively may change the membrane environment of the carrier and improve its translocating function (Gonzalez, JCI, 1979; 63:684; Simon, JCI, 1982; 70:401). This mechanism may be responsible for the increase in bile acid transport by pretreatment with phenobarbital (Simon, JCI, 1982; 70:401) and stimulation of ouabain excretion by pretreatment with pregnenolone-16β-carbonitril (PCN) (Klaassen, JPharmExpTher, 1974; 191:201,212).

Hepatectomy (Klaassen, JPharmExpTher, 1974; 191:25; Uesugi, BiochemPharm, 1976; 25:1361) or selective biliary obstruction (i.e. obstruction of one major liver lobe) (Adler, Gastro, 1977; 73:129) does not lead to a proportional decrease in hepatobiliary clearance of various organic anions.[21,24] This may be partly due to the relatively greater supply of bile acids to the remaining functional cells. If bile salts are depleted prior to the experiment, the transport of organic anions, on a liver weight basis, is much less increased (Uesugi, BiochemPharm, 1976; 25:1361).

Adaptation of hepatobiliary transport after exposure to high concentrations of bile salts has been reported in studies with intraduodenal infusion (Simon, JCI, 1982; 70:401), repeated oral administration (Watkins, JPharmExpTher, 1981; 218:182), and selective biliary obstruction (Adler, Gastro, 1977; 73:129). An increased synthesis of bile acid-transport proteins may play a role. The adaptive response can be blocked by cycloheximide (Gonzalez, JCI, 1979; 63:684). Such adaptive increases in biliary excretion rate, however, have not been demonstrated for non-bile salt organic anions (Fischer, ArchInternatPharmTher, 1983; 264:135).

Adaptive changes also occur in pathological conditions such as blockade of the common bile duct. In this case, the expression of the bile acid uptake and excretion carriers are down regulated, probably to protect the hepatocytes from high, toxic bile acid concentrations (Müller, AmJPhysiol, 1997; 272:G1285).

The hepatic transport rate of drugs and peptides that are accommodated by the bile acid system may therefore adapt in situations of extra demand. These mechanisms require further study, especially with regard to the molecular mechanisms at the level of protein synthesis and membrane transport.

In general, studies on the regulation of transport under physiological and pathological conditions are still in their infancy. Transcription regulation of transport has been demonstrated for steroid hormones, glucagon, cAMP and phorbol esters, thereby regulating the activity of the transporting proteins. However, the picture is far from clear and more research is needed fully to elucidate the regulation of transport in the liver.

Zonal heterogeneity in transport in the hepatic acinus

The microcirculatory and functional unit of the liver is the acinus (Rappaport, IntRevPhysiol, 1980; 21:1), a small parenchymal mass, irregular in size and shape (see Figs 1 and 5). The vascular axis consists of a terminal portal venule and a hepatic arteriole, a bile duct, lymph vessels, and nerves. The periphery of the acinus is formed by two terminal branches of the hepatic vein that drain the acinar blood. The liver receives 70 to 75 per cent of its blood supply through the portal vein and 25 to 30 per cent through the hepatic artery (Campra, p.911 in reference 26). These vessels join somewhere in the acinus: in human liver the arterioles terminate in the

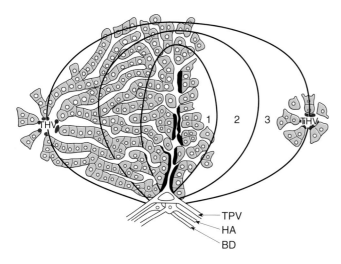

Fig. 5. Schematic representation of the microcirculatory unit of the liver: the hepatic acinus. An arbitrary division into three zones is indicated. BD, bile ductule; HA, hepatic artery; TPV, terminal portal venule; THV, terminal hepatic venule.

first part of the sinusoids adjacent to the portal tracts (Yamamoto, Hepatol, 1985; 5:452; Campra, p.911 in reference 26).

The acinus is commonly divided into three zones: zone 1 or the periportal cells, zone 3 or the perivenous cells, and the intermediary zone 2 (Groothuis, TrendsPharmacolSci, 1985; 6:322; Gumucio, Hepatol, 1989; 9:154). Many structural differences exist between the zones. Bile flows from zone 3 to zone 1, hence cholestasis might be observed sooner upon zone 1 damage than in zone 3 toxicity (Gumucio, AmJPhysiol, 1983; 244:G578; Baumgartner, LabInvest, 1987; 56:576) if this damage leads to canalicular obstruction. On the other hand, substances excreted into bile in zone 3 in principle can be reabsorbed from the canaliculi in zone 1. Along the sinusoids, several structural differences exist. This is partly due to the presence of other cell types such as Kupffer cells and endothelial cells. Kupffer cells are more abundant in the periportal area (Bouwens, Hepatol, 1986; 6:718). The endothelial lining in the hepatic sinusoids displays fenestrae that can be arranged in groups, named sieve plates. The density and the diameter of the fenestrae, and hence porosity, is significantly larger in zone 3 (Wisse, Hepatol, 1985; 5: 683). A higher porosity could favour uptake of relatively large solutes or particles in zone 3. Many factors alter the fenestrae *in vivo*: pore diameter increases after exposure to alcohol (Fraser, Pathology, 1980; 12:371; Mak, Hepatol, 1984; 4:386; Horn, Hepatol, 1987; 7:77), pressure (Fraser, BrJExpPath, 1980; 61:222), hypoxia, irradiation, and endotoxin.[27] Moreover, cytochalasin B influences pore diameter as well as the number of fenestrae (Steffan, Hepatol, 1987; 7:1230), pointing to an involvement of the cytoskeleton in their formation. The number of fenestrae also decreases after alcohol treatment (Mak, 1984), mainly in zone 3 (Horn, 1987).

Periportal sinusoids are narrower and more tortuous than perivenous sinusoids (Miller, Gastro, 1979; 76:965). Furthermore, the vascular space in zone 3 is twice as large as in zone 1 (Miller, 1979). As a result, the higher uptake of many substances in periportal hepatocytes due to a larger supply to these cells might be partly offset by the lower blood flow and more favourable

perivenous sinusoidal structure for uptake and exchange processes (Wisse, Hepatol, 1985; 5:683). On the other hand, a higher surface to volume ratio in zone 1 might favour periportal uptake (Miller, 1979).

Metabolic zonation

Many substances are removed from blood during passage through the liver, while other compounds are released by the cells into the blood. This results in sinusoidal concentration gradients, increasing or decreasing towards the hepatic vein. If hormones or mediators are absorbed or secreted at different rates, concentration ratios will be different in the acinar zones, leading to a different metabolic regulation (Thurman, PharmRev, 1980; 31:229; Jungermann, Hepatol, 1982; 2:385; Gumucio, AmJPhysiol, 1983; 244:G578; Groothuis, TrendsPharmacolSci, 1985; 6:322; Thurman, Hepatol, 1985; 5:144).

In addition to hormones, many other substrates enter the liver. Of those, oxygen is vital. An acinar gradient of O_2 exists due to its consumption by the cells (Matsumura, AmJPhysiol, 1983; 244:656; Gumucio, Hepatol, 1989; 9:154). Oxygen tension decreases from about 250 torr in the periportal area to 70 torr perivenously (Matsumura, 1983). Concomitantly, periportal O_2 uptake is two- to threefold higher than perivenous uptake (Matsumura, 1983). When zone 1 or zone 3 O_2 concentrations (13 and 4 per cent O_2, respectively; Wölfle, EurJBioch, 1983; 135:405) are applied to parenchymal cells in culture, the lower O_2 pressure appears to delay ageing of the hepatocytes by adapting DNA and protein content to the new environment (Holzer, JCellPhysiol, 1987; 144:297). By reversing the flow in perfused liver (Thurmann, DrugMetabolRev, 1988; 19:263), both urea synthesis (Kari, EurJBioch, 1987; 163:1) and gluconeogenesis (Anundi, JBC, 1987; 262:9529) shifted to the upstream zone, the oxygen-rich area. However, this observation can also be explained as a higher availability of substrate in upstream cells due to a concentration gradient.

Cell damage can be expected in hypoxia because oxygen is vital to every cell. Hypoxia is seen in zone 3 predominantly, for instance upon chronic ethanol treatment.[28] The relatively low O_2 concentration renders zone 3 more susceptible to changes in Po_2. On the other hand, mid-zonal cell death was described to occur during low-flow hypoxia (Marotto, Hepatol, 1988; 8: 585), supposedly due to gradients of both O_2 and glutathione resulting in highest concentration of oxygen radicals in zone 2.

Also in amino acid metabolism acinar gradients exist which are regulated among others by blood pH (Lenzen, EurJBioch, 1987; 166:483) and ammonium concentration (Thurman, Hepatol, 1985; 5:144; Thurman, DrugMetabolRev, 1988; 19:263).

An acinar gradient of substrates may thus arise due to their uptake or release by the liver. Zonal tissue concentration gradients of ammonia, amino acids, and glucose may well have direct or indirect effects on intrahepatic drug distribution, excretion, or metabolism. For instance, local differences in pH may influence drug binding and net membrane transport,[29] while the zonal availability of certain amino acids (Lenzen, EurJBioch, 1987; 166:483) and glucose may determine relative rates of drug conjugation (Thurman, Hepatol, 1985; 5:144; Thurman, Drug-MetabolRev, 1988; 19:263).[16] Zonal differences in hepatobiliary transport will be treated in later sections of this chapter.

Techniques to study hepatic transport function

A spectrum of liver preparations seems necessary to study transport processes ranging from the intact liver *in vivo* to the isolated perfused organ, isolated hepatocytes, liver slices, and membrane vesicles, as well as cloned and reconstituted carrier proteins. Transport characteristics measured *in vitro* at the membrane level cannot always be translated to the situation in the integrated whole organism. The recent availability of mutant animals with selective deficiencies in transport functions has been very useful in this respect. The combined use of *in vivo* and *in vitro* systems, especially, enables useful extrapolation and interpolation for a more definite elucidation of hepatobiliary transport in animals and humans (Blom, BiochemPharm, 1982; 31:1553; Meijer, p.165 in reference 30).[10]

In vivo studies

When the hepatobiliary transport of drugs is examined in the intact organism, useful data on the relative rates of uptake and excretion can be obtained and the involvement of the liver in the clearance of the compound under study under optimal conditions of liver function can be assessed quantitatively. For evident ethical and toxicological reasons, the majority of the *in vivo* studies on drug transport are performed in laboratory animals, mostly in the rat and to a lesser extent in the mouse.

A number of factors such as the influence of extrahepatic distribution of the compound under study, the involvement of other organs in the overall elimination, the influence of the toxicity of the drug under study, and the impossibility of studying the influence of changes in blood and bile flow and of protein binding complicate the interpretation of *in vivo* studies, especially in man. Therefore, *in vitro* studies are neccesary to obtain more detailed kinetic data on the mechanisms involved in uptake and excretion of drugs by the liver.

The isolated perfused liver

Studying drug transport in the isolated perfused liver (Meijer, MethodsEnz, 1981; 77:81; Nijssen, Hepatol, 1992; 15:302; Meijer, p.165 in reference 30; Pang, p.259 in reference 30; Reichen, p.149 in reference 30) combines the advantages of elimination of the extrahepatic influences and an intact liver structure with the opportunity to manipulate medium flow, composition, temperature, and perfusion direction. This allows studies on, for instance, the substrate specificity of putative carriers by determining drug–drug interactions, the influence of protein binding (Meijer, JPharmExpTher, 1977; 202:8; Nijssen, 1992; Proost, JPharmacokinBiopharm, 1993; 21:375), the flow dependency of drug clearance (Pang, JPharmacokinBiopharm, 1988; 16:595), the influence of temperature on drug transport (Nijssen, BiochemPharm, 1991; 42:1997), and the acinar heterogeneity of hepatocytes in transport functions (Jones, AmJPhysiol, 1980; 238:G233; Groothuis, AmJPhysiol, 1982; 243:G455; Groothuis, TrendsPharmacolSci, 1985; 6:322).[10] It should be noted that the isolated liver is a denervated organ and that autonomic nervous regulation is no longer present.

Important information was obtained by combining normal (with medium flow from the portal to central vein) and retrograde (from the central to portal vein) perfusions with the determination of the acinar localization of the substrate under study by autoradiography (Groothuis, AmJPhysiol, 1982; 243:G455; Van der Sluijs, Hepatol, 1988; 8:1521),[10] fluorescence microscopy (Braakman, Hepatol, 1987; 7:849; Braakman, Hepatol, 1988; 8:1386; Nijssen, Hepatol, 1992; 15:302), or histochemistry (Groothuis, BiochemPharm, 1983; 32:2721). To ascertain blood supply to the biliary ductules and peribiliary plexus, a double perfusion set up with portal as well as arterial blood supply has been developed (Gardemann, AmJPhysiol, 1987; 253:238; Reichen, JCI, 1988; 81:1462; Than, JSurgRes, 1989; 47:251; Pang, Hepatol, 1994; 20:672).

The limited number of experiments that can be performed with one perfused liver preparation, the constraints of liver viability to about 3 to 4 h, and the limitation imposed by the size of the liver, which does not allow the use of this technique for the human liver and larger animals, initiated the development of other techniques such as isolated cells, plasma membrane vesicles, and more recently, precision-cut liver slices.

Liver slices

The recent development of the Krumdieck tissue slicer, allowing the reproducible production of slices of 200 to 300 μm in thickness (Krumdieck, AnalBioch, 1980; 104:118), initiated a revival in the use of liver slices in research on liver functions. The advantages of this technique are evident: the liver structure with the various parenchymal and sinusoidal liver cells remains intact and the hepatocytes retain their polarity, as in the perfused liver, but now many experiments can be performed in one liver. In addition, the localization of periportal and perivenous cells in the acinus is maintained, but in contrast to the intact liver, where acinar gradients of substrates are inevitable due to the unidirectional flow, all cells in the slices are exposed to the same substrate concentrations.[10] The technique is easily applicable to the livers of various species including that of man, making this technique very useful for studying drug transport in human liver *in vitro* and to assess interspecies differences in drug metabolism and transport (Connors, Toxicology, 1990; 61:171; Dogterom, DrugMetDisp, 1993; 21:705; Olinga, ATLA, 1993; 21:466).[4]

The slices can be used after 24 h of cold storage in University of Wisconsin organ preservation solution (Olinga, p.91 in reference 31 and Olinga, Xenobiot, 1998; in press). Cryopreservation was reported to result in appreciable but variable loss in metabolic function (Fisher, Cryobiology, 1991; 28:131; Wishnies, Cryobiology, 1991; 28:216; Ekins, CryoLett, 1996; 17:7), but very recently a successful methodology for long-term preservation of animal and human liver slices was reported (de Kanter, ATLA, 1995; 23:653; de Kanter, p.107 in reference 31 and de Kanter, Xenobiot, 1998; in press).

Human liver slices can be prepared with success from pieces of livers that are left over after tranplantation of a part of a donor liver and from pieces of liver obtained after partial hepatectomy. The liver tissue may be stored for up to 24 h in an adequate storage solution (Olinga, p.91 in reference 31 and Olinga, Xenobiot, 1998, in press). Human liver slices are comparable with isolated cells in their reflection of drug metabolism rate (Powis, DrugMetabolRev, 1989; 20:379; Olinga, ATLA, 1993; 21:466), but transport studies are still in their infancy (Olinga, p.149 in reference 31, and Thompson, JLipidRes, 1993; 34:553; Worboys, DrugMetabDisp, 1995; 23:393).

Isolated hepatocytes

Isolated hepatocytes are widely used to investigate the mechanisms of drug transport and the results of such studies show that isolated cells exhibit similar transport characteristics to isolated perfused livers and livers *in vivo* (Schwenk, ArchToxicol, 1980; 44:113; Blom, BiochemPharm, 1982; 31:1553; Berry, LifeSci, 1992; 51:1; Miyauchi, PharmaceutRes, 1993; 10:434; Sandker, BiochemPharm, 1994; 47:2193). This technique is very versatile in determining the K_m and V_{max} and the driving forces for uptake of a drug under study, competition by other drugs, and the influence of protein binding (Wolkoff, JCI, 1987; 79:1259; Mol, JPharmExpTher, 1988; 244:268; Berry, LifeSci, 1992; 51:1).[32]

The loss of cell polarity and the redistribution of canalicular membrane proteins over the entire cell surface (Groothuis, EurJCellBiol, 1981; 26:43),[33] and the impossibility of discerning between excretion via the sinusoidal and canalicular membrane, make isolated cells less suitable for studying drug excretion, although biliary excretion processes can certainly be detected (Tarao, AmJPhysiol, 1982; 243:G253; Oude, Elferink, AmJPhysiol, 1990; 258:G699).

Drug transport studies are limited to freshly isolated cells. Cultured cells and hepatocyte-derived cell lines do not seem to be adequate models for studying drug transport. In culture, the cells rapidly dedifferentiate and exhibit decreased or even lack of membrane transport functions, whereas hepatocyte-derived cell lines often lack liver-specific transport functions (Petzinger, BBActa, 1988; 937:135; Kwekkeboom, BBResComm, 1989; 162:619; Föllmann, AmJPhysiol, 1990; 258:C700; Liang, Hepatol, 1993; 18:1163).

Isolated cells can be stored for at least 24 h in organ preservation solution, for example the University of Wisconsin solution or modifications thereof, without loss of transport (Sandker, BiochemPharm, 1992; 43:1479; Sandker, BiochemPharm, 1993; 46:2093) or metabolic functions (Olinga, JHepatol, 1997; 27:738). Cryopreservation in general leads to a considerable loss of metabolically viable cells after thawing (Chesné, ToxicolInVitro, 1991; 5:479).

Separation of isolated hepatocytes into fractions enriched in periportal and perivenous cells can be achieved by a brief, zone-selective perfusion with digitonin (Lindros, BiochemJ, 1985; 228:757; Quistorff, BiochemJ, 1987; 243:87) or by fluorescence-activated cell sorting after selectively labelling one of the zones (Braakman, Hepatol, 1991; 13:73). The obtained cell fractions can be used to study intrinsic differences in drug transport functions between periportal and perivenous hepatocytes (Groothuis, TrendsPharmacolSci, 1985; 6:322).[10,34]

Canalicular bile secretion is successfully studied by applying fluorescence microscopy (Fentem, ToxicolInVitro, 1990; 4:452; Verkade, BiochemJ, 1992; 284:259), confocal microscopy (Graf, JHepatol, 1990; 10:387; Nathanson, CellCalcium, 1992; 13:89), and time-lapse video recording (Watanabe, JCellBiol, 1991; 113:1069) to couplets of hepatocytes: pairs of cells that are not separated from each other during collagenase treatment and that have conserved their bile canaliculus in between them (Bayer, MethodsEnz, 1990; 192:501; Wilton, Hepatol, 1991; 14:180).

Human hepatocytes can be isolated from human donor liver material and from liver material obtained after partial hepatectomy.

However, the reproducibility of the isolation procedure with respect to yield and viability is much less than with rats, which seems to be partly due to the different isolation procedures used[35] and partly to the variability in the human liver tissue. Despite this, after removal of non-viable cells by Percoll density separation (Groothuis, ToxicolInVitro, 1995; 9:951), human hepatocytes have been used successfully for drug metabolism and toxicity studies (Sandker, Xenobiot, 1994; 24:143).[35] Drug transport studies with human hepatocytes are still scarce, but the available data show that the isolated cells are a good model to study interspecies differences and the mechanisms of drug transport in man (Azer, BiochemPharm, 1993; 46:813; Sandker, Xenobiot, 1994; 24:143; Sandker, BiochemPharm, 1994; 47:2193).

Plasma membrane vesicles

The development of techniques to prepare closed membrane vesicles from either the sinusoidal (basolateral) or canalicular membranes allowed the separate study of drug transport at each pole of the cells (Blitzer, JBC, 1984; 259:9295; Meier, JBC, 1984; 259:10614). However, cross-contamination with cytoplasmic proteins, other plasma membranes, or endosomal membranes has to be taken into account (Hardikar, Hepatol, 1993; 18:1278). The orientation of the vesicles and the integrity of the transport proteins and their membrane environment are difficult to assess. Nevertheless, the use of such membrane vesicles has evident advantages enabling the study of electrogenic features, energy dependency, and ion requirements for transport of drugs (Adachi, Hepatol, 1991; 14:655). Interference of intracellular events such as toxic influence on liver cell function, metabolism, and binding to intracellular binding proteins and organelles is excluded. Moreover, plasma membrane vesicles can be successfully prepared from human livers (Novak, Hepatol, 1989; 10:447; Wolters, JCI, 1992; 90:2321; Sandker, BiochemPharm, 1994; 47:2193).

Isolated transport proteins

In order to assess the molecular features of membrane transport, many attempts have been made to isolate and characterize the carrier proteins involved. Various techniques have been used, such as affinity chromatography with immobilized substrates (Reichen, BBResComm, 1979; 91:484; Wolkoff, JCI, 1980; 65:1152; Stremmel, JCI, 1983; 71:1796; Von Dippe, BBActa, 1986; 862:352) and photo-affinity labelling (Mol, ArchPharm, 1989; 322:613; Mol, BiochemPharm, 1992; 43:2217),[36] but the most successful results have been obtained with molecular biological techniques.

Molecular biological techniques

Expression cloning of proteins in, among others, *Xenopus laevis* oocytes has proved a very powerful technique in the study of carriers involved in uptake of drugs for which the oocyte itself has low uptake capacity (Hagenbuch, PNAS, 1991; 88:10629; Jacquemin, JCI, 1991; 88:2146; Xie, Hepatol, 1992; 16:147A; Meier, JHepatol, 1996; 24:29). With this approach, the sodium-dependent taurocholate transporter from rat (ntcp) and man (NTCP) (Hagenbuch, JCI, 1994; 93:1326), the rat and human organic anion transporter (oatp₁, OATP) (Jacquemin, JCI, 1991; 88:2146), the organic cation transporter (oct1) (Zhang, MolecPharm, 1997; 51:913; Gorboulev,

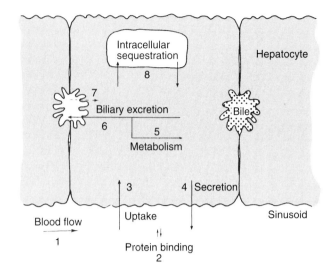

Fig. 6. Potential rate-limiting steps in the rate of hepatobiliary transport. Hepatic uptake rate can be influenced by hepatic blood flow (1), protein binding (2), and net sinusoidal membrane transport: primary uptake (3) and sinusoidal efflux (secretion) (4). Elimination rate from the cells is composed of metabolism (5) and net canalicular excretion: membrane transport to the lumen (6) and vice versa (7). Rate of metabolism as well as efflux at sinusoidal and canalicular levels is at the same time determined by intracellular binding to proteins and sequestration to organelles (8) (hepatic distribution volume).

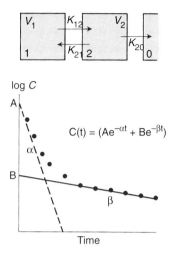

Fig. 7. Schematic presentation of a pharmacokinetic two-compartmental model with a central compartment (V_1) and a runoff compartment (V_0) attached to the peripheral (liver) compartment (V_2). k values indicate transport rates for transport from perfusate to liver (k_{12}), from liver to perfusate (k_{21}), and from liver to bile (k_{20}). The curve is composed of two exponential phases with slopes α and β, while A and B are intercepts. From these four parameters the three rate constants and distribution volumes can be calculated from the equations $k_{12} = (A\alpha + B.\beta) / (A + B)$; $k_{20} = \alpha.\beta / k_{12}$; and $k_{21} = (\alpha + \beta) - (k_{12} + k_{23})$; $V_1 = D/(A + B)$; and $V_2 = V_1 \{1 + [k_{12} / k_{21} + k_{20}]\}$.

DNACellBiol., 1997; 16:871), and the sinusoidal glutathione transporter (Yi, PNAS, 1995; 92:1495) were cloned, sequenced, and functionally characterized. The study of carriers involved in excretion is hampered by the existence of relatively high endogenous export capacity of the oocytes (Shneider, JBL, 1993; 268:6985). Transport characteristics of carrier proteins can also be investigated successfully in transfected cell-lines, including COS-7 (Boyer, AmJPhysiol, 1994; 266:G382), CHO (Stieger, Gastro, 1994; 107: 1781), Hela (Shi, JBL, 1995; 270:25591), V79 and HPCT-1E3 (Platte, EurJCellBiol, 1996; 70:54), and LLC-PK1 (Van Helvoort, Cell, 1996; 87:507) cells. These heterologous expression systems permit comparison of substrate specificities and functional transport properties of cloned proteins. Finally, baculovirus expression systems permit the production of large quantities of proteins and provide high expression levels for direct transport measurements.

Pharmacokinetic analysis of drug transport in the liver

In the hepatobiliary transport of drugs a number of rate-limiting steps are theoretically possible: rate of supply via the blood, uptake into the parenchymal cells by either passive diffusion or carrier-mediated processes, association with cytosolic proteins, metabolism, and secretion across the canalicular membranes (Fig. 6). To be able to characterize the mechanisms involved in the various processes, or to identify possible interactions between substances to be transported, an experimental design should be chosen that enables a quantitative analysis of these different transport steps (Carson, NEJM, 1979; 300:1016).

Compartment analysis

In practice, a limited number of rate-limiting steps can be detected by inspection of the profiles of plasma disappearance and biliary excretion rate of drugs and diagnostic agents (Meijer, JPharmacokinBiopharm, 1984; 12:43) after a single intravenous injection. Since both the concentration profiles in blood and in bile reflect these transport processes, it is preferable to analyse bile and plasma data in a simultaneous fitting procedure. This yields a set of parameters that describe the transport rate at the uptake and secretion level (Meijer, p.344 in reference 37).[3] Classic examples of such parameters are rate constants indicating the fraction of the drug removed per unit of time from one of the defined compartments (Richards, ClinSci, 1959; 18:499; Häcki, JLabClinMed, 1976; 88:1019; Meijer, JPharmExpTher, 1977; 202:8).[25] In many clinical and experimental studies, the plasma disappearance and biliary excretion rates of dyes like BSP and DBSP have been interpreted on the basis of a two-compartment model with elimination from the peripheral compartment (the liver) (Richards, 1959; Carson, NEJM, 1979; 300:1016). A peripheral compartment is postulated as a certain volume of tissue(s) in the body that relatively slowly exchanges significant amounts of drug with the central (plasma) compartment to which the drug was initially administered (see Fig. 7). Consequently, one or more initial distribution phases are seen in the plasma decay curve (Richards, 1959; Häcki, 1976).

A number of rate constants as well as the distribution volumes can be calculated and can then be used to simulate the biliary excretion after a single injection or constant infusion and to compare this with the experimental data (Richards, ClinSci, 1959; 18:499; Häcki, JLabClinMed, 1976; 88:1019). Both fitting the plasma disappearance using the integrated exponential functions and fitting with a number of differential equations, indicating the rate of change in the various compartments, are used (Meijer, p.344 in reference 37).[3] Two-compartment models do not always provide a satisfactory fit with the experimental data. Three-compartment models using a 'deep' compartment in the liver have been proposed for ouabain (Blom, BiochemPharm, 1982; 31:1553), taurocholate (Kroker, NaunynSchmiedbArchPharm, 1978; 303:287), and vecuronium (Meijer, p.344 in reference 37)[3] and provided more optimal fits with the experimental data. Efficient storage in intracellular organelles and slow exchange of material from such pools may underlie this deep storage phenomenon. Another reason for introducing a third compartment in models describing hepatobiliary transport can be an extensive but relatively slow distribution to extrahepatic tissue (Blom, BiochemPharm, 1982; 31:1553). In such cases a third, slow component is observed in the plasma disappearance curves.

In either of the above-mentioned models the liver is pictured as a compartment that relatively slowly equilibrates with the plasma compartment (in other words as a peripheral compartment) from which elimination occurs by metabolism or biliary excretion (see Fig. 7). In the two-compartment analysis, four primary parameters are used: two slopes and two intercepts from a biexponential disappearance curve. The four parameters allow calculation of three rate constants (Richards, ClinSci, 1959; 18:499): k_{12} (fraction transferred from blood to liver per unit of time) as well as k_{21} and k_{20} (fractional rate constants for hepatic reflux to plasma and for biliary excretion respectively). The initial plasma clearance by hepatic uptake Cl_{12} is $V_1 * k_{12}$ in which V_1 is the volume of the central compartment. The rate of membrane transport process itself is dependent on the maximal rate of transport and, consequently, the maximal number of carriers available (V_{max}) and the affinity of the transported substrate for these carriers that is expressed as the so-called Km value. The Km is defined as the concentration at which the transport rate is half maximal. The membrane transport process for a certain substrate at low concentration is determined by the ratio of these parameters (V_{max}/Km), also called the intrinsic clearance value (Cl_i).

Although rate constants may characterize the particular transport steps, it should be stressed that apart from the membrane transport processes, *per se*, hepatic uptake and efflux rate may also be influenced by the rate of supply to the liver through hepatic blood flow (Q_H) and on protein binding in plasma and liver:[18] k_{12} is, therefore, flow dependent if $Cl_i \gg Q_H$ and is influenced by plasma protein binding, especially if $Cl_i \ll Q_H$. If the test substance accumulates in tissues other than the liver, initial clearance Cl_{12} ($k_{12}.V_1$) can no longer be used as a simple parameter for hepatic uptake. Such an extrahepatic event is often unnoticed since the particular compartment may be reflected in a third component in the disappearance curve only at very low plasma levels. The calculated elimination rate constant (k_{20}) can be checked in animal experiments directly by measuring the amount in the liver and the biliary excretion rate at a given time point, since by definition the k_{20} is the fraction of the amount present in the liver that is excreted into bile per unit of time (Richards, ClinSci, 1959; 18:499; Meijer, JPharmacokinBiopharm, 1984; 12:43).

The net uptake of compounds in the liver, as determined by the k_{12} and k_{21} values, also influences the biliary clearance or the hepatic clearance by metabolism. This must be so as the elimination rate is governed by the intrahepatic concentration, being the driving force for elimination. This is expressed in the following equation for steady-state hepatic clearance of drugs ($Cl_H{}^{SS}$): $Cl_H{}^{SS} = [k_{12}.k_{20}/(k_{21} + k_{20})].V_1$ (Richards, ClinSci, 1959; 18:499; Meijer, JPharmacokinBiopharm, 1984; 12:43). Only for drugs of which distribution to the hepatocytes is completely flow limited, $k_{12}.V_1$ is equal to Q_H. Since $Cl_H = Q_H.E$, in this extreme condition the equation mentioned above shows that hepatic extraction (E) in that case is equal to $k_{20}/(k_{21} + k_{20})$. This condition, however, should not be assumed in normal individuals and certainly not in individuals with chronic liver disease, as was done in a study on indocyanine green (Kawasaki, ClinPharmTher, 1988; 44:217; Meijer, EurJClinPharm, 1988; 35:295).

Since the value k_{12} can be influenced by hepatic blood flow and by extent of protein binding, $Cl_H{}^{SS}$ is also influenced by these parameters. However, changes in binding within the liver will influence k_{20} and $(k_{21} + k_{20})$ to the same extent and consequently will not affect the steady-state hepatic clearance: only the amount in the liver at the steady-state plasma concentration (or V_2) will be altered. The hepatic uptake step will also be reflected in the biliary excretion profile. Plotting the biliary excretion rate per unit of time against time affords a biexponential curve with ascending and descending phases (Richards, ClinSci, 1959; 18:499; Meijer, JPharmExpTher, 1977; 202:8). If hepatic uptake is rapid compared with excretion, the ascending phase will reflect the uptake process. However, if uptake in the liver is relatively slow relative to the excretion process, the rate of hepatic uptake will be reflected predominantly in the descending and terminal phase of the excretion curve (Meijer, EurJClinPharm, 1988; 35:295; Shinohara, Hepatol, 1996; 23:137).

Multiple indicator dilution techniques

The compartment approach may give a fair impression on uptake and excretion rate and may even allow a characterization of the particular membrane transport process involved (if correction for influence of blood flow and protein binding can be made) (Blom, BiochemPharm, 1982; 31:1553). It is clear, however, that the compartment (lumped) models have limitations since they do not take into account the fall of concentration of substrates during passage of the liver from the portal to central vein (Forker, AmJPhysiol, 1983; 244:G573).

An alternative is the multiple-indicator dilution procedure that has been applied for calculation of hepatic uptake of galactose (Goresky, Hepatol, 1985; 5:805), bile salts (Reichen, AmJPhysiol, 1976; 231:734), and many other compounds (Reichen, AmJPhysiol, 1976; 231:734; Goresky, Hepatol, 1985; 5:805; Wolkoff, AnalBioch, 1987; 167:1; St Pierre, Hepatol, 1989; 9:285). The method was also employed for detection of changes in microcirculation in patients with cirrhosis (Huet, JCI, 1982; 70:1234). Portal injections of the compound to be tested together with reference compounds that are confined to the vascular lumen and extracellular fluid (labelled erythrocytes and labelled albumin, respectively) are followed by taking sequential venous samples at intervals of a few seconds, providing three outflow curves. Fitting of the curves and proper mathematical treatment of the data affords rate constants for uptake, efflux, and clearance (metabolic and/or biliary) as well as for blood flow and volume of the sinusoids and space of Disse (Reichen, 1976;

Goresky, 1985; Wolkoff, 1987; St.Pierre, 1989). Apart from being very time-consuming and the implicit requirement to collect samples from the venous outflow, errors can also be introduced with this method since, as in the two-compartment model, one assumes uniform sinusoids, while the influence of extralobular vasculature and inhomogeneous behaviour of transporting systems in various parts of the liver acinus is ignored (Forker, AmJPhysiol, 1983; 244: G573). In addition, technical problems may evolve because the slow efflux of solute that entered the hepatocytes may result in a tailing of the outflow curve at concentrations that cannot be reliably detected. When used *in vivo*, recirculation artefacts will decrease the fidelity of the estimates. It should be noticed that the terminal part of the curve, especially, contains most of the information on the clearance processes (Reichen, 1976; Wolkoff, 1987).

Liver perfusion models

The 'well stirred' liver perfusion model has been extensively used to calculate hepatic clearance as influenced by hepatic blood flow and plasma protein binding as well as the liver first-pass elimination of drugs (Rowland, JPharmacokinBiopharm, 1973; 1:123).[24] This model assumes that substrates entering the liver are immediately ideally mixed in the organ and all of the cells are in equilibrium with the venous outflow concentration of the substrate (the 'well stirred' model therefore is also called the 'venous equilibration model') (Rowland, 1973).[24]. Although attractive in its simplicity, this model has limitations because, especially for high clearance substrates, it has been shown that sinusoidal and tissue concentrations in the liver are not homogeneous (Groothuis, AmJPhysiol, 1982; 243:G455).

Alternatives to the single-compartment and 'well stirred' liver models are models that describe the liver as an array of parallel tubes (the sinusoids) (Keiding, JHepatol, 1987; 4:393). In the tubes a gradual decline of substrate concentration occurs, going from portal to venous sites due to the removal of the substrate through metabolism and/or biliary excretion (see Fig. 8). Mathematical equations have been derived for sinusoidal (parallel tube) liver models, taking into account the exponential decrease of concentration along the acinar axis (Forker, AmJPhysiol, 1983; 244: G573; Keiding, 1987). These models have even been refined, including parallel sinusoids of unequal radius and length (Forker, 1983) as well as longitudinal heterogeneity of the sinusoids with regard to rate of flow (Forker, 1983; Bass, BiochemPharm, 1988; 37:1425) and enzyme distribution (Bass, 1988) along the acinar axis (clearance of flow distribution models).

More recently, a liver dispersion model was introduced (Roberts, JPharmacokinBiopharm, 1988; 16:41). The latter model pictures the liver as a flow reactor in which residence time of substrates in the liver depends on the degree of axial mixing and dispersion. By varying the dispersion factor from 0 to 1.0, the extremes of the well stirred model and sinusoidal zero-mixing model, as well as all the cases in between, can be accommodated (see Fig. 8).

Three groups (Sawada, ChemPharmBull, 1985; 33:319; Roberts, JPharmacokinBiopharm, 1988; 16:41; Smallwood, JPharmacokinBiopharm, 1988; 16:377) tested the above-mentioned perfusion models in a systematic way and arrived at the general conclusion that the dispersed and clearance/flow distributed models provide the most satisfying prediction of changes in elimination rate or bioavailability at variations in protein binding or liver blood flow.

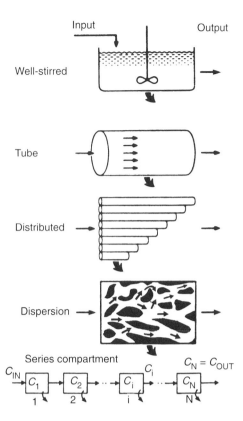

Fig. 8. Pharmacokinetic perfusion models proposed to describe the flow dynamic clearance system of the liver (modified from Morgan, ClinPharmacokin, 1990; 18:61).

An alternative to the dispersed and parallel-tube distributed models is the series compartment model (Groothuis, BiochemPharm, 1983; 32:3069; Gray, DrugMetDisp, 1987; 15:27; Mendel, Endocrinol, 1988; 123:1817; Braakman, JPharmExpTher, 1989; 249:869). The liver is described as a series of pharmacokinetic compartments that if necessary can be individually defined by volume (intracellular binding), uptake, reflux, and secretion/or metabolism rates (Braakman, 1989). Such models provide an empirical interpretation of the decreasing concentrations of substrates along the acinar axis and enable modelling of acinar heterogeneity in binding, deep compartment sequestration, and 'activity' of enzymes or carrier proteins. This model based on a series of compartments satisfactorily fitted the outflow curves of substrates earlier generated by the multiple-indicator dilution technique (Gray, 1987). A similar, somewhat more expanded model also explained the time-dependent intrahepatic distribution and typical plasma disappearance pattern of the lipophilic organic cation rhodamine B (Braakman, 1989).

Recently, several models for the hepatic uptake of protein-bound ligands have been described, in order to explain the changes in clearance as a result of changes in protein concentration. These will be described in the section on the influence of protein binding on hepatic uptake.

Liver models in practice

The question arises of which liver model should be preferred for practical purposes. In general, models should not be trivialized by an excess of adjustable parameters, but should be physiologically reasonable and also clinically relevant (Bass, BiochemPharm, 1988; 37:1425). The more complex the model (increasing number of variables), the more demands should be made on the number of sample points in order to define the exact kinetic profiles and to test the validity of the model with changes in physiological conditions such as blood flow and protein binding (Smallwood, JPharmacokinBiopharm, 1988; 16:377; Morgan, ClinPharmacokin, 1990; 18:61).

Hepatic extraction of propranolol, lidocaine, and meperidine was found to be compatible with the simple venous equilibration model (Wilkinson, ClinPharmTher, 1975; 18:377; Roberts, JPharmacokin-Biopharm, 1988; 16:41; Smallwood, JPharmacokinBiopharm, 1988; 16:377), whereas galactose, diazepam, and ethanol kinetics were more adequately described by the undistributed sinusoidal perfusion model (Keiding, JHepatol, 1987; 4:393). For taurocholate, neither model could satisfactorily explain the effect of protein binding on hepatic uptake rate (Forker, AmJPhysiol, 1983; 244: G573; Bass, BiochemPharm, 1988; 37:1425). This might be explained by the independent observation that for this substrate sharp acinar gradients occur and also intrinsic cellular differences exist with a lower rate of biliary excretion from pericentral cells (Jones, AmJPhysiol, 1980; 238:G233; Groothuis, AmJPhysiol, 1982; 243: G455; Groothuis, TrendsPharmacolSci, 1985; 6:322). Recalculation of the original data concerning taurocholate, taking into account the extent of plasma protein binding and the dispersed and clearance/flow distributed models (Sawada, ChemPharmBull, 1985; 33:319; Smallwood, 1988), provided the best prediction of the kinetic behaviour of this substrate. However, even such sophisticated models do not guarantee a watertight analysis of what happens in the intact body. For instance, flow patterns in the intact animal may be largely influenced by factors such as interlobular flow patterns, ventilation movements, and changes in arterial supply.

At the moment, therefore, it is advisable to employ the equations depicted in Fig. 9 in practical situations. These equations are based on the 'well stirred' and the 'parallel tube' model and relate the measured hepatic clearance to the intrinsic clearance (enzymatic process or carrier transport in the absence of supply limitation of blood flow or protein binding). They represent a very useful set of equations in which the three potential rate-limiting steps (protein binding, blood flow, and intrinsic clearance) in the clearance process are reflected. The choice for either model should be based on knowledge concerning the hepatic extraction and acinar disposition of the substance to be analysed as observed *in vivo*. Within certain limits with regard to the hepatic extraction value, predictions on the basis of both models are not greatly different (Wilkinson, ClinPharmTher, 1975; 18:377; Roberts, JPharmacokinBiopharm, 1988; 16:41; Smallwood, JPharmacokinBiopharm, 1988; 16:377; Morgan, ClinPharmacokin, 1990; 18:61) and the most simple one, the well stirred, would suffice. At a high hepatic extraction (> 0.90) the parallel tube model should in general be preferred on physiological grounds.

Measurement of hepatic blood flow and shunting

In spite of the ongoing dispute on this topic, clearance concepts in hepatology have led to a more quantitative approach and eventually

'Well-stirred model'

$$Cl_H = Q_H \left(\frac{f_u Cl_i}{Q_H + f_u Cl_i} \right) \quad (1)$$

'Parallel-tube model'

$$Cl_H = Q_H \left(1 - e^{-f_u Cl_i / Q_H} \right) \quad (2)$$

Cl_i = intrinsic clearance (V_{max}/K_m) in absence of flow limitation and protein binding, due to metabolism or unidirectional transport (hepatic uptake or biliary excretion)

Cl_H = hepatic plasma clearance measured (l/h)

Q_H = hepatic plasma flow (l/h)

f_u = fraction unbound in the blood plasma

Note: terms in parenthesis represent hepatic extraction fraction (*E*), since $Cl_H = Q_H E$

$$V = V_P + \frac{f_u}{f_{u_T}} (V_T) \quad (3)$$

V = total distribution volume
V_P = total volume of blood plasma
V_T = total tissue volume to which the drug distributes
f_{u_T} = fraction unbound in V_T

Fig. 9. Equation describing hepatic clearance (Cl_H) as influenced by intrinsic cellular function (Cl_i), blood flow (Q_H), and extent of protein binding (indicated by f_u as the unbound fraction).

may lead to the design of model compounds to estimate liver blood flow (Wilkinson, ClinPharmTher, 1975; 18:377) as well as the degree of intrahepatic shunting and functional liver mass by non-invasive means (McLean, ClinPharmTher, 1979; 25:161; Gillette, Pharmacol, 1981; 23:237). In principle, a number of techniques can be employed to quantify hepatic blood flow pharmacokinetically. The classic method is to sample arterial and hepatic venous blood during constant infusion of a model substrate and directly determine hepatic extraction under steady-state conditions (the Fick principle). Since hepatic clearance is equal to hepatic bloodflow times extraction ratio ($Cl_H = Q_H.E$) and clearance is equal to the known infusion rate R_0 divided by the steady-state blood concentration ($Cl_H = R_0/C_{ss}$), Q_H can be calculated from Cl_H and E and represents total hepatic bloodflow, including a possible shunting fraction.

The other approach uses the equation depicted in Fig. 9 that can be transformed into: $Q_H = 1/(1/Cl_H - 1/f_u.Cl_i)$ (Morgan, ClinPharmacokin, 1990; 18:61). If a model compound is employed that is completely absorbed after oral dosing and is only eliminated by the liver, Cl_H can be calculated from $Cl_H = D/AUC_{iv}$ and Cl_i from $Cl_i = D/AUC_{oral}$. In other words Q_H can be estimated by administering a model compound with the aforementioned features both intravenously and orally and subsequent calculation of the area under the blood concentration/time curves (George, ClinPharmacokin, 1979; 4:433; Wilkinson, PharmRev, 1987; 39:1). This assumes that the liver microcirculation is normal and without shunts, because otherwise part of the oral dose would not be exposed to the liver tissue and the produced AUC_{oral} would be incorrectly high. Also, the dose should be low enough to ensure linear (non-saturating) kinetic conditions in the hepatic clearance process. The presence of intrahepatic shunts may depend on the nature and stage of the hepatic disease. In acute liver disease, cellular damage rather than portosystemic shunting would be anticipated. If the hepatocytes were functionally affected but the hepatic microcirculation was normal (the sick cell hypothesis), the above-mentioned calculation would still be valid even in cirrhotic conditions. However, if only a proportion of the hepatocytes were exposed to incoming blood due to portosystemic shunts and the cells were functionally intact (intact cell hypothesis), major errors could be introduced with kinetic calculations. It is preferable to estimate functional hepatic blood flow via galactose or sorbitol clearance because, even in diseased livers, clearance of these compounds is so rapid that it reflects effective hepatic blood flow. The difference between total hepatic flow obtained through the Fick principle and functional hepatic blood flow as indicated by galactose clearance may indicate the degree of intrahepatic portosystemic shunting (McLean, ClinPharmTher, 1979; 25:161; Wilkinson, 1987; Vaubourdolle, ScaJGastr, 1989; 24:467; Morgan, ClinPharmacokin, 1990; 18:61;).

Hepatobiliary clearance can also be studied under steady-state conditions through constant infusion where, by definition, the rate of biliary excretion is equal to the rate of infusion. If organic anions are infused at a rate exceeding the operative biliary transport maximum, a constant biliary output can be found, with a linear increase in both the plasma concentration and liver content over time (Wheeler, JCI, 1960; 39:1131). The latter observation indicates first-order kinetic conditions for net hepatic uptake over a wide range of concentrations at which biliary excretion is already saturated. Since the concentration ratio between liver and plasma (hepatic storage) remains constant, saturable binding of the anionic dye to plasma proteins as well as to macromolecules in the hepatocytes apparently change to the same extent. The methods have been used previously to calculate hepatic storage (S) and the operative biliary excretion maximum (T_m) in patients. However, various complicating factors such as extrahepatic distribution and elimination of the dye corrupt interpretation of the data (Klaassen, CanJPhysPharm, 1975; 53:120; McIntyre, p.417 in reference 38).

During constant infusion, below T_m conditions, ultimately an equilibrium will be reached in which the rate of drug input (infusion rate) will equal biliary excretion rate at constant plasma levels in the plasma and in the liver. Assuming a steady state for a drug A in blood plasma, liver, and bile, the introduction of a competing drug B will lead to a new steady state with an increased plasma level of A. By definition, in the new 'steady state', the rate of output of A should again be equal to the dosing rate. However, hepatobiliary clearance of A (excretion rate/plasma concentration) will be decreased by the competitive action of B. If transport competition occurs solely at the hepatic uptake level, the liver content of A in the steady state should not be changed compared with the situation before the interaction (bile/liver concentration). In contrast, if mainly canalicular transport was competitively inhibited, both liver concentration and plasma concentration should be higher. If B only displaced A from intracellular binding sites, plasma concentration in the new steady state would not change, but liver content would be lower. Since interactions both at the level of plasma proteins and cytosolic proteins may occur simultaneously with interactions at the membrane level, knowledge about the unbound concentrations both in the plasma and liver is necessary to identify the exact mechanism underlying the change in tissue concentration.

Rate-limiting steps in hepatobiliary transport

Hepatobiliary transport of drugs can be envisioned as a number of sequential transport steps (see Fig. 7). In the following section these potential rate-limiting processes will be treated separately and clinical implications in the perturbation of these processes will be discussed.

Hepatic blood flow

For drugs with a very efficient cellular elimination (high V_{max}/K_m ratio) the liver removes all of the substrate that is supplied via the bloodstream. Even in situations where liver clearance is favoured, for instance when the metabolic process is induced or if protein binding of the drug in the blood plasma is decreased, hepatic clearance will not increase because the liver cannot remove more than is supplied via the bloodstream either in bound or unbound form (Wilkinson, ClinPharmTher, 1975; 18:377). Since the blood flow in an adult man is about 1 ml/min per 1 g of liver (1.1 to 1.8 l/min), this represents the upper limit of hepatic clearance for any given substrate. Concentrations of such high clearance substrates in the hepatic sinusoids and the surrounding cells will exponentially decrease from periportal to perivenous tissue. This has been clearly demonstrated for taurocholate and lipophilic drugs by autoradiographic and fluorescence microscopy respectively showing sharp acinar concentration gradients that are reversed on retrograde perfusion (Jones, AmJPhysiol, 1980; 238:G233; Groothuis, AmJPhysiol, 1982; 243:G455; Gumucio, AmJPhysiol, 1983; 244:G578; Groothuis, TrendsPharmacolSci, 1985; 6:322; Braakman, Hepatol, 1987; 7:849) (Fig. 10). For efficiently extracted compounds that are highly bound to plasma proteins, this implies that dissociation of the drug from the protein must have occurred in the sinusoids or space of Disse.[18]

For drugs with an extraction ratio exceeding 0.80, blood flow is therefore the rate-limiting step in the hepatic uptake and clearance process. This implies that hepatic clearance is altered with changes in blood flow, for instance through changes in the cardiac output (Wilkinson, ClinPharmTher, 1975; 18:377). However, if the intrinsic cellular removal of such a drug is largely decreased by a competitive interaction or a process such as enzyme inhibition, blood flow no longer is rate limiting and the plasma disappearance rate of the substrate in the new situation tends to be unaffected by changes in blood flow, but can be modified further through changes in cellular function. Blood flow limitation in hepatic clearance is relevant in the use of high extraction compounds such as galactose (Goresky, Hepatol, 1985; 5:805; Keiding, Gastro, 1988; 94:477) and indocyanine green (Meijer, EurJClinPharm, 1988; 35:295; Shinohara, Hepatol, 1996; 23:137) to measure hepatic blood flow. In normal individuals, extraction of these compounds is between 0.8 and 1.0 and the clearance calculated from the initial plasma disappearance rate is indicative of total hepatic blood flow (Rowland, JPharmacokinBiopharm, 1973; 1:123; McLean, ClinPharmTher, 1979; 25:161; Meijer, EurJClinPharm, 1988; 35:295). However, if as a result of liver disease the cellular clearance function of high clearance drugs is decreased, the calculated clearance no longer solely reflects hepatic blood flow but also the intrinsic cellular function (Wilkinson, 1975). The increase in hepatic clearance of

(a)

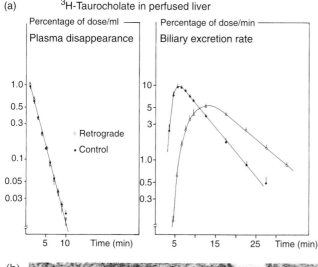

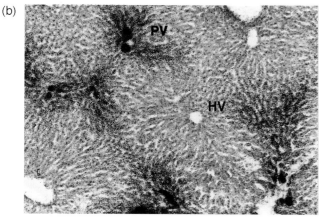

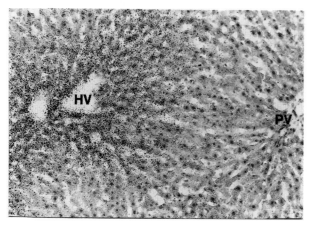

Fig. 10. (a) [³H]Taurocholate kinetics in isolated perfused livers with normal and retrograde direction of perfusate flow after addition of a tracer dose (0.4 nmol) of [³H]taurocholate. Plasma decay (hepatic uptake rate) is identical but biliary excretion rate is markedly lower after retrograde loading of zone 3. (b) Light microscopic autoradiograph of rat liver, 30 s after injection of a tracer dose (7 nmol) of [³H]taurocholate into the portal vein *in vivo*. A steep gradient of grains is apparent from the periportal (zone 1) to the perivenous (zone 3) region. The distribution during antegrade perfusion of isolated rat liver was similar. (c) Autoradiograph of a liver, perfused in the retrograde direction (from hepatic vein to portal vein), 30 s after injection of a tracer dose of [³H]taurocholate. The gradient is now completely reversed: grains are concentrated in zone 3 and are virtually absent in zone 1. PV, terminal portal venule; HV, terminal hepatic venule; Bar = 100 μm.

high extraction substances like indocyanine green and DBSP observed after pretreatment with phenobarbital can be at least partly explained by an increase in hepatic blood supply (McDevitt, BiochemPharm, 1977; 26:1247; St Pierre, Hepatol, 1989; 9:285). Much less of an effect is seen in the isolated perfused organ with standardized blood flow or with compounds with a less efficient hepatic uptake (Meijer, JPharmExpTher, 1977; 202:8). For the same reason, the magnitude of the effect of phenobarbital is dependent on the dose of indocyanine green as hepatic extraction of the dye decreases with increasing dose (Wilkinson, 1975; McDevitt, 1977).

Hepatic blood flow is influenced by posture, exercise, and food intake, mostly through influences on the autonomic nervous system (George, ClinPharmacokin, 1979; 4:433). Drugs that have major vascular or cardiac effects implicitly change hepatic perfusion. This may not only influence the clearance of drugs but also hepatic first-pass effects and systemic bioavailability after oral dosing (Wilkinson, ClinPharmTher, 1975; 18:377; Pond, ClinPharmacokin, 1984; 9:1). It can be intuitively understood that hepatic extraction decreases at an increased hepatic blood flow when it is realized that hepatic residence time of the substrate will decrease and opportunity to escape the eliminating system consequently increases. Therefore, an increase in hepatic blood flow may increase bioavailability, especially if hepatic extraction is relatively high. Since the removal rate from the bloodstream will increase at the same time, it can be predicted that after oral administration the peak concentrations will be higher but the elimination half-life shorter (Wilkinson, 1975). In fact, the venous equilibration perfusion model predicts an unchanged area under the plasma concentration/time curve (AUC) as the effects cancel each other (Wilkinson, 1975; Pond, 1984; Rowland, ClinPharmacokin, 1984; 9(Suppl. 1):10). Therefore, oral clearance (Dose/AUC_0) is independent of blood flow and reflects the intrinsic clearance and thus the cellular elimination process (Wilkinson, 1975; Pond, 1984). Other liver perfusion models deviate from this rule in the sense that at a high extraction ratio (low bioavailability), they predict a much larger variation in bioavailability with changes in blood flow or protein binding (Pond, 1984; Wilkinson, PharmRev, 1987; 39:1; Morgan, ClinPharmacokin, 1990; 18:61). This impact of changes in blood flow and protein binding on the bioavailabitlity of drugs remains to be tested in the human situation, yet it may provide important clues as to the validity of the proposed perfusion models for the liver.

One of the consequences of clearance limited by blood flow is that drugs may alter their own kinetic patterns and those of other drugs via their influence on the general circulation (haemodynamic drug interactions) (George, ClinPharmacokin, 1979; 4:433). The systemic clearance of the active L-isomer of propranolol *in vivo*, but not in isolated perfused liver, is lower than that of the inactive D-isomer because of its negative effect on cardiac output (Wilkinson, ClinPharmTher, 1975; 18:377). A similar phenomenon was reported for verapamil (Wilkinson, 1975). For example, glucagon and iso-proterenol elevated the clearance of lidocaine and propranolol through their stimulating effect on hepatic blood flow (Wilkinson, 1975).

In conclusion it should be stressed that the measurement of hepatic uptake rate and bioavailability of high extraction drugs *in vivo* can be largely determined by haemodynamic influences. Such factors should be taken into account as potential mechanisms when observing pharmacokinetic drug interactions as well as variable

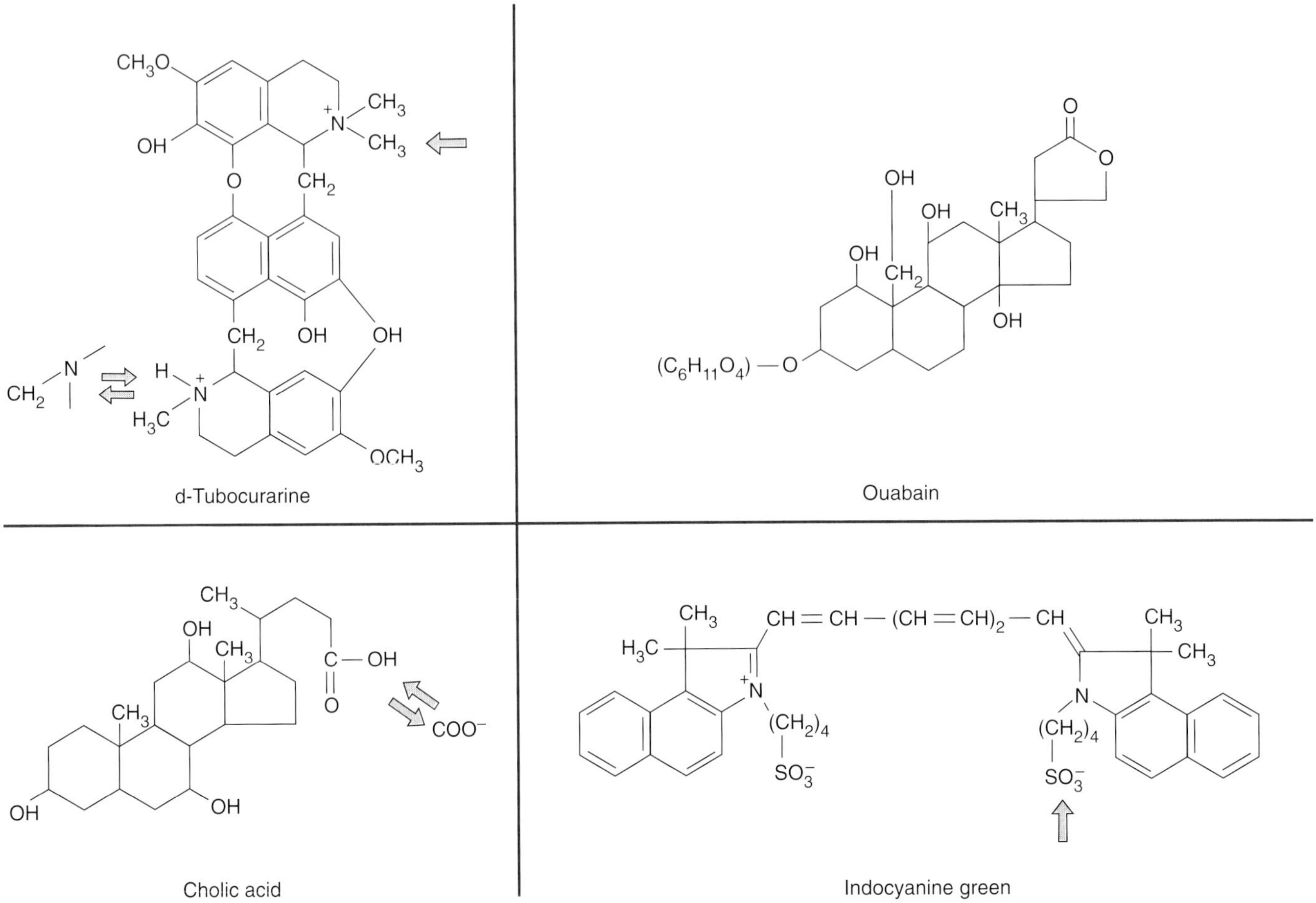

Fig. 11. Chemical structures of bulky cholephilic model compounds. d-Tubocurarine is a bivalent organic cation, ouabain an uncharged steroidal glycoside, cholic acid a steroidal compound with a weakly acidic carboxyl group, and indocyanine green (ICG) has two strong anionic centres and one cationic centre (zwitterion).

clearance patterns of model compounds that dose-dependently affect cardiac function, hepatic vascular resistance or peripheral blood circulation.

Plasma protein binding

Many kinetic studies in animals and man have been performed in the past to investigate the hepatic transport function for endogenous and exogenous compounds. Often conclusions were drawn with regard to liver function or kinetic interactions of such agents without taking into account possible changes in the extent of protein binding of the agents studied (Wilkinson, ClinPharmTher, 1975; 18:377; Blaschke, ClinPharmacokin, 1977; 2:32; Grainger-Rousseau, Int-JPharmaceutics, 1989; 54:1; MacKichan, ClinPharmacokin, 1989; 16:65).[18,22] Nevertheless, many drugs undergoing hepatic metabolism or hepatobiliary transport are to a large extent protein-bound. This is partly related to their amphipathic character which favours hepatobiliary transport and/or metabolism but at the same time also may promote association with plasma proteins[18,22] (Fig. 11).

In plasma at least two different proteins are responsible for most of the binding: albumin and α_1-acid glycoprotein (orosomucoid) (Table 1). Roughly speaking, the first protein, which has a relatively high plasma concentration (4.0 per cent or 600 µmol), binds acidic (anionic) drugs (Gumucio, AmJPhysiol, 1984; 246:G86),[22] and the second protein, which occurs at a much lower plasma concentration (0.1 per cent or 22 µmol), binds predominantly basic (cationic) drugs, including tertiary (Piafsky, ClinPharmacokin, 1980; 5:246)[22] and quaternary amines (Van der Sluijs, JPharmExpTher, 1985; 234:703). Both proteins are synthesized in the liver and especially during chronic liver diseases and/or loss via the urine in renal disease, plasma albumin levels can be abnormally low (Grainger-Rousseau, IntJPharmaceutics, 1989; 54:1). During acute-phase reactions such as inflammation, tumours, and burns, the concentration of α_1-acid glycoprotein in plasma may be greatly elevated through increased hepatic synthesis (Piafsky, 1980).[22]

Drug binding to these proteins is a saturable phenomenon and can be characterized by determining the number of binding sites (n) per protein molecule as well as the affinity for these binding sites.[22] The unbound fraction of a drug (f_u) will therefore be determined by the total plasma concentration of the drug and protein and the binding capacity of the protein as well as the affinity of the drug for the particular binding sites. The unbound fraction (f_u) multiplied by the total drug concentration (C) yields the unbound concentration (C_u). For anionic drugs at least two separate classes of binding sites

Table 1 Plasma protein binding of drugs		
	Albumin	**α₁-Acid glycoprotein (orosomucoid)**
Molecular weight	65 000	44 000
pI	4.8; 5.6	2.7
Sugars (%)	<2	40
Plasma level	600 μmol	15 μmol
Variation (+)	Exercise Benign tumours Hypothyroidism Psychiatric disorders	Stress Inflammatory diseases Burns, trauma, surgery Myocardial infarction Tumours
Variation (−)	Nephrotic syndrome Chronic liver disease Pregnancy Age Gastrointestinal disease Malignant tumours	Liver cirrhosis Nephrotic syndrome Oral contraceptives
Drugs bound Category I	Bilirubin Coumarines Pyrazolinones Thiazide diuretics	Quinidine, disopyramide Local anaesthetics Narcotic analgesics Psychotropic drugs β-Blocking agents Anticholinergic agents Peripheral muscle relaxants
Category II	Tryptophan Benzodiazepines Arylacetic acid analgesics Sulphonic acid dyes Ethacrynic acid Clofibrate-like agents	

are present on the albumin molecule, although the binding sites for acidic drugs often have an overlapping substrate specificity (Blaschke, ClinPharmacokin, 1977; 2:32).[22] Saturation of these binding sites will occur for albumin only after relatively high doses of drugs, whereas α₁-acid glycoprotein can be saturated at low concentrations of drugs.[22]

It is fairly easy to determine the f_u in plasma directly by ultra-filtration, ultracentrifugation, or dialysis of plasma. However, this requires good reproducibility of such methods and often sensitive bioanalytical methods (Blaschke, ClinPharmacokin, 1977; 2:32; Piafsky, ClinPharmacokin, 1980; 5:246; Levy, ClinPharmacokin, 1984; 9(Suppl.1):1; Rowland, ClinPharmacokin, 1984; 9(Suppl. 1): 10; Grainger-Rousseau, IntJPharmaceutics, 1989; 54:1; MacKichan, ClinPharmacokin, 1989; 16:65). For instance, the relatively low-dosed indomethacin is about 99.8 per cent bound to plasma protein and thus the f_u is in the order of 0.002. A slight displacement by another drug leading to a new binding percentage of 99.0 increases the f_u fivefold. Such a change is readily detectable in an ultrafiltrate of plasma. Especially for drugs which are over 90 per cent bound to plasma protein, displacement interactions or changes in protein concentration will produce large relative changes in the f_u (MacKichan, ClinPharmacokin, 1989; 16:65). The influence of such changes in plasma protein binding on hepatic clearance can be predicted by using various perfusion models of the liver (see Fig. 9).

Protein binding and clearance

Variations in the unbound fraction of the drug in plasma may also alter the clearance of drugs by the liver (Wilkinson, ClinPharmTher, 1975; 18:377; Rowland, ClinPharmacokin, 1984; 9(Suppl. 1):10). If clearance is relatively low compared with hepatic blood flow, in principle the clearance may vary linearly with the f_u, as the driving force for the metabolic and excretion processes is the free concentration of the drug. However, if clearance is high compared with blood flow, the latter may become rate limiting, and an increase in the f_u can only moderately affect hepatic clearance (Rowland, 1984). The equations describing the relation of the f_u with clearance for two commonly used perfusion models are depicted in Fig. 9. Both equations refer to steady-state conditions in hepatic clearance: a situation in which equilibrium between the plasma and liver compartments is reached and as much drug is cleared from the body as is entering the body per unit time.

The initial rate of distribution of a drug to the liver after an intravenous bolus injection can also be influenced by protein binding and, in principle, the above-mentioned concepts can also be applied to this process (Meijer, JPharmExpTher, 1977; 202:8). It follows that for drugs with a very rapid distribution to the liver, this uptake process will have the tendency to be more limited by blood flow and less influenced by changes in protein binding than the actual clearance process (either metabolism or biliary excretion or both) (Meijer, 1977).

From these considerations one can conclude that variations in protein binding will be reflected in changes in hepatic disposition of drugs, but the extent of such a change is not only dependent on the magnitude of change in the f_u, but also on the type of clearance of the particular drug. If this aspect is not taken into account, major misinterpretations in the estimation of liver function can be made. For instance, if as a result of liver disease the albumin concentration is abnormally low, the decreased intrinsic clearance function may be partly or even completely masked by an increased f_u (Grausz, NEJM, 1971; 284:1403). This effect may be even more prominent if under these pathological conditions endogenous compounds accumulate in plasma and compete with the drug for binding to plasma proteins (Grainger-Rousseau, IntJPharmaceutics, 1989; 54:1). Also, drug interactions on the cellular level may not be clearly expressed if the drugs mutually compete for binding to plasma proteins and changes in the f_u are more pronounced than interactions on the level of hepatocellular metabolism or excretion.

Differences in protein binding should also be taken into account if one compares transport capabilities in isolated hepatocytes with liver function in the intact animal (Blom, BiochemPharm, 1982; 31:1553). In the absence of albumin, the uptake rate of BSP is considerably higher than its glutathione derivative BSP–glutathione (Schwarz, AmJPhysiol, 1980; 239:C118). In the presence of albumin (Yam, JLabClinMed, 1976; 87:373), however, hepatic uptake of BSP–glutathione occurred more rapidly than for BSP. This apparent discrepancy can be explained by the large difference in protein binding: BSP–glutathione is bound to albumin at a level of 10 to 100 times less than BSP (Baker, JCI, 1966; 45:281).

For these reasons it is preferable to determine the unbound instead of the total concentration of drugs to characterize liver function for diagnostic purposes or for the characterization of kinetic drug interactions at the level of plasma proteins or cellular disposition. For example, hepatobiliary clearance of anionic dyes was shown to be higher at lower plasma albumin concentrations, as observed in man (Grausz, NEJM, 1971; 284:1403), intact animals (Inoue, Hepatol, 1985; 5:892), isolated perfused rat liver (Meijer, JPharmExpTher, 1977; 202:8), and isolated hepatocytes (Blom, BiochemPharm, 1981; 30:1809). Under these various conditions, clearance is inversely related to the albumin concentration. The same can be concluded for metabolic clearance of drugs by the liver (Rowland, ClinPharmacokin, 1984; 9(Suppl. 1):10).

Protein binding and volume of distribution

In the whole body, lower binding to albumin or other plasma proteins also leads to an increase in distribution volume of the drug. The effect of changes in the free fraction f_u on the distribution volume can be described by equation 3 of Fig. 9. If the plasma volume (V_p) is small compared with the total distribution volume (V), V_p in equation 3 can be neglected and V changes linearly with f_u.

A twofold increase in the f_u of a drug with a capacity-limited type of hepatic clearance would lead to a twofold increase both in apparent clearance and distribution volume. This implies that the rate of elimination (for instance expressed as half-life) would be unchanged. However, for a drug with a flow-limited type of clearance, distribution volume would increase twofold but, in contrast, clearance would be unchanged as total hepatic blood flow is limiting

and clearance cannot be increased further. Consequently, an increase in the f_u in such a case would lead to an increased half-life of elimination (Wilkinson, ClinPharmTher, 1975; 18:377; Rowland, ClinPharmacokin, 1984; 9(Suppl. 1):10; Grainger-Rousseau, IntJPharmaceutics, 1989; 54:1). This illustrates not only that one should not use parameters that depend on distribution volume (such as half-life) for characterizing clearance function, but also that diagnosis of abnormal transport function would be improved by measuring the unbound drug concentration (Levy, ClinPharmacokin, 1984; 9(Suppl.1):1).

The influence of plasma protein binding on hepatic transport

Many organic compounds, both anions like bile acids, free fatty acids (e.g. oleate), and cholephilic dyes (e.g. rose bengal, BSP, and DBSP) and cations like methyldeptropine, are avidly bound to serum albumin or α_1-acid glycoprotein in the general circulation (Meijer, JPharmExpTher, 1977; 202:8; Meijer, JPharmacokin-Biopharm, 1984; 12:43; Van der Sluijs, JPharmExpTher, 1985; 234:703; Berk, Hepatol, 1987; 7:165; Van der Sluijs, JPharmExpTher, 1987; 240:668). Despite their very high plasma protein binding, these ligands are effectively removed from the circulation by the liver. Because uptake is not accompanied by a significant removal of albumin (Goresky, p.807 in reference 26),[39] except for a small quantity extracted through fluid-phase endocytosis, ligands have to dissociate from their extracellular carrier before hepatic uptake can occur (Fig. 12). According to the classic theory, only unbound ligand is taken up by the liver and an instantaneous equilibrium between bound and unbound ligand is assumed (Weisiger, PNAS, 1985; 82:1563; Berk, Hepatol, 1987; 7:165; Bass, BiochemPharm, 1988; 37:1425).[18] This theory still holds for most of the substrates presented to the liver. However, it has been shown on various occasions (starting as far back as 1966) that uptake of certain highly bound ligands exceeded the amount of unbound substrate that could dissociate during a single-pass passage through the liver, based on in vitro measurements of the dissociation rate constants (Forker, JCI, 1981; 67:1517; Weisiger, PNAS, 1985; 82:1563; Berk, Hepatol, 1987; 7:165).[18]

Several hypotheses were therefore proposed to explain this phenomenon, the most important ones being the 'albumin–receptor hypothesis' (Forker, JCI, 1981; 67:1517; Weisiger, PNAS, 1985; 82:1563) and the dissociation limitation theory (Weisiger, 1985; Van der Sluijs, Hepatol, 1987; 7:688) that later on was elaborated into the so-called 'extended diffusion limitation theory'or the 'unstirred water layer model' (Bass, BiochemPharm, 1988; 37:1425). In the albumin-receptor hypothesis it is postulated that in spite of the fact that binding to albumin lowers the unbound concentration of the substrate (and thereby should decrease carrier occupation and their uptake rate), the protein at the same time 'helps' the substrate to diffuse into the unstirred layer at the sinusoidal membrane and thereby prevents a major depletion of substrate at the vicinity of the membrane. This allows even very poorly water-soluble compounds to be efficiently exposed to the plasma membrane (Barnhart, AmJPhysiol, 1983; 244:G630; Weisiger, AmJPhysiol, 1989; 257:G904). This situation in the liver is fundamentally different to that in the kidney where the endothelial lining lacks fenestrae and plasma proteins cannot be rapidly presented to the uptake carrier systems.

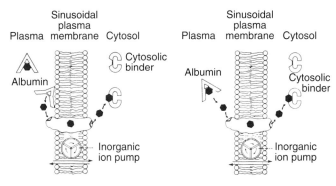

Fig. 12. Schematic representation of organic anion uptake (left) and sinusoidal secretion mechanisms (efflux to the bloodstream, right). The anionic substrate binds to albumin in the plasma and to cytosolic binding proteins in hepatocytes. After dissociation from albumin (dissociation constant K_d), binding to a transmembrane channel-like carrier protein occurs. Translocation is helped by phosphorylation through ATP hydrolysis (active transport). Once translocated, the substrate binds to the cytosolic binding protein, resulting in a lower free concentration in the cytosol. The efflux process exhibits the same binding and debinding processes but in a reversed direction. Carrier-mediated, facilitated, efflux is not ATP dependent but is supposed to be helped by chloride gradients built up by an associated Cl⁻ pump. The rate of efflux can be association rate limited (see k_a for binding to albumin).

That the passage of unstirred layers may become a rate-limiting step in the uptake (instead of membrane transport itself) is exemplified by experiments in hepatocytes, oocytes, and membrane vesicles in which substrate concentration and albumin concentration are varied in a fixed molar ratio. In spite of the fact that this procedure keeps the unbound concentration constant, an apparent 'saturation' pattern is observed. Many studies misinterpreted this as a 'Michaelis–Menten type of kinetics' allowing calculation of K_m and V_{max} values of membrane transport whereas, in fact, rate limitation in diffusion is seen (Sorrentino, JHepatol, 1996; 25:178).

These models were recently tested in anaesthetized pigs *in vivo* using a constant infusion of indocyanine green (ICG). These experiments showed that for ICG the dissociation limitation model and additionally the effects of an unstirred water layer could predict the observed changes in clearance, while they rejected the influence of an albumin-receptor (Ott, Hepatol, 1997; 26:679; Ott, AmJPhysiol, 1997; 273:G227).

Protein binding may have great implications for the contribution of the various zones of the acinus to transport of protein-bound substrates. This was shown for BSP (Gumucio, AmJPhysiol, 1984; 246:G86) and DBSP (Nijssen, Hepatol, 1992; 15:302): in the absence of albumin the extraction is so high that in normal perfusions only zone 1 cells, and in retrograde perfusions only zone 3 cells, are initially involved in uptake and transport. However, in the presence of albumin the extraction is normally much lower and all acinar cells are involved in transport of BSP (Groothuis, BiochemPharm, 1983; 32:3069) and DBSP (Nijssen, 1992). In addition, it has been demonstrated that protein binding strongly influences sinusoidal excretion of drugs and their metabolites back into the blood. Proteins do not only affect the unbound concentration of drugs but may also have a direct influence on the hepatocyte sinusoidal membrane. For instance, albumin somehow improves the unbound clearance of prazosin and antipyrine in the *in vitro* perfused liver

(Oie, JPharmExpTher, 1985; 234:636), compounds that bind poorly to the protein. A facilitating effect was also seen for organic anions in isolated hepatocytes (Barnhart, AmJPhysiol, 1983; 244:G630) and for taurocholate in isolated membrane vesicles (Blitzer, AmJPhysiol, 1985; 249:G34; Zimmerli, JPharmExpTher, 1989; 250:301). Apart from the above-mentioned effect on passage of unstirred layers, this promoting effect may also be explained by albumin-specific protective effects against *in vitro* damage of the membrane,[18] either due to the physical coating of the membrane or through the scavenging of reactive oxygen species by albumin (Di Simplicio, FreeRadicResComm, 1991; 14:253).

Implications of plasma protein binding for clinical pharmacokinetics

Care should be taken in extrapolating data on plasma protein binding from the *in vitro* to the *in vivo* situation. Although, as discussed above, binding to albumin will to some extent decrease clearance, lowering of plasma albumin *in vivo* may at the same time lead to a markedly increased distribution volume (V) of the drug (Wilkinson, ClinPharmTher, 1975; 18:377; George, ClinPharmacokin, 1979; 4:433; Grainger-Rousseau, IntJPharmaceut, 1989; 54:1). In other words, *in vivo* albumin also serves to keep the drug in the plasma compartment and more efficiently exposes the drug to the hepatic elimination systems. In analbuminaemic rats, the biliary excretion rate of anionic substrates is highly stimulated if albumin is administered (Inoue, Hepatol, 1985; 5:892).

Perturbation of plasma protein binding may also corrupt the interpretation of drug interaction data. The lack of an anticipated competition during hepatic uptake between two compounds may be due to simultaneous interactions at the level of uptake and protein binding in plasma or liver. For instance, indocyanine green and DBSP probably compete for carrier-mediated uptake in the liver. In the presence of albumin, however, indocyanine green inhibits uptake of DBSP whereas, in contrast, DBSP enhances uptake of indocyanine green. This was explained by the displacement of indocyanine green from albumin by DBSP. In the case of the highly bound indocyanine green, this relatively large effect on its free fraction in plasma could completely mask the concomitant competition for membrane transport (Meijer, JPharmacokinBiopharm, 1984; 12:84).

In liver cirrhosis, albumin concentration in plasma is often lowered and metabolic functions are decreased (Blaschke, ClinPharmacokin, 1977; 2:32). The latter aspect does not only imply that the rate of drug metabolism can be decreased, but also that many substrates that are no longer efficiently removed by the liver accumulate in the general circulation (Grainger-Rousseau, IntJPharmaceut, 1989; 54:1). This in turn may affect plasma and tissue binding or even the therapeutic and/or side-effects of drugs directly. It follows that not only the nature but also the stage of the pathological condition will determine the final outcome on drug clearance and unbound plasma concentration.

In general it can be stated that a decrease in protein binding will facilitate drug distribution out of the plasma compartment and, at the same time, will lead to increased clearance, that is if clearance is not already close to its maximum value (i.e. about equal to blood flow). In general, therefore, unbound drug levels in the plasma in steady state that determine the therapeutic effect will be only moderately changed, if at all. Nevertheless, the total plasma concentration of drugs that is often determined in routine drug monitoring will be decreased. It obviously would be wrong in this case to increase the dose on the basis of the total plasma concentration data (Levy, ClinPharmacokin, 1984; 9(Suppl.1):1; Grainger-Rousseau, IntJPharmaceutics, 1989; 54:1).

This is true irrespective of the route of administration (oral or intravenous) because, theoretically, the bioavailability of a drug with a low extraction ratio is only slightly affected by changes in protein binding ($F = 1 - Cl_H/Q_H$) even if clearance were to increase due to the decrease in protein binding. However, for drugs with a high hepatic extraction ratio due to displacement interactions (MacKichan, ClinPharmacokin, 1989; 16:65), unbound steady-state concentrations will increase while average total drug concentration is predicted to be unchanged. The therapeutic effect in the latter case may increase or even, at the same time, may give rise to toxic reactions. Therefore, the drug dose should be decreased if the drug is given intravenously. In contrast, after oral administration, the decreased bioavailability (higher first-pass effect) of such a drug will fully compensate for the displacement effect (Wilkinson, ClinPharmTher, 1975; 18:377) and the dosage regimen can, therefore, be left unchanged. These considerations refer to changes in steady-state conditions. It should be stressed that, apart from the above-mentioned effects on clearance and bioavailability, plasma protein displacement interactions always lead to an immediate and often drastic rise in the unbound concentrations of the displaced drug in plasma. This occurs because it takes some time before the suddenly liberated drug can diffuse completely out of the plasma compartment and the increased clearance can take care of the displaced drug (Blaschke, ClinPharmacokin, 1977; 2:32; Piafsky, ClinPharmacokin, 1980; 5:246; Rowland, ClinPharmacokin, 1984; 9(Suppl.1):10; Grainger-Rousseau, IntJPharmaceut, 1989; 54:1; MacKichan, 1989).

Some aspects of drug therapy in liver disease in clinical practice (see also Chapter 29.3)

The pharmacokinetic behaviour of many drugs is altered in liver disease. The volume of distribution, the plasma half-life, and drug clearance may all be changed in these patients and due to changes in plasma protein binding, hepatic drug metabolism, liver blood flow, and/or intestinal absorption are usually altered to some extent (McLean, ClinPharmacokin, 1991; 21:42).[40]

Drugs which are slowly cleared from the circulation are mostly affected by decreased hepatic metabolism, drugs with a fast clearance are affected more by changes in hepatic blood flow. In practice, therefore, one often concludes that it is prudent to reduce the dose or to change the dosing interval of drugs whose metabolism depends on the liver. However, patients with liver disease can be critically ill and their lives may depend on proper and adequate drug therapy. In addition, one has to realize that in patients with severe decompensated liver disease, other organs are also involved, such as the brain, kidney, and intestine. Hepatic encephalopathy, functional renal failure, hepatorenal syndrome, and gastrointestinal haemorrhage frequently accompany severe liver disease. Very often these life-threatening conditions are elicited iatrogenically through the inadvertent use of drugs.

Intestinal absorption is most affected in cholestatic liver disease and in conditions of insufficient bile production. The intestinal absorption of cyclosporin is dependent on the presence of bile salts and therefore it is better to administer the drug intravenously in the early days after liver transplantation or during cholestatic episodes.

Changes in the volume of distribution are mainly due to decreased protein binding. For example, frusemide is firmly bound to albumin, but in the case of hypoalbuminaemia, as occurs in liver cirrhosis, its volume of distribution is increased (Verbeeck, ClinPharmTher, 1982; 31:719). Administration of frusemide together with albumin in these conditions increases its renal delivery and enhances its efficacy.

The functional liver mass is usually decreased in liver disease. Benzodiazepines should be used with caution or not at all in these conditions. During acute hepatitis, monitoring of central nervous system function is clinically important to differentiate between acute and fulminant hepatitis. This parameter can be lost for days after a single dose of benzodiazepines. If sedation is necessary, for example during endoscopic sclerotherapy, a benzodiazepine with a short half-life, such as midazolam, is the best choice (Trouvin, BrJAnaesth, 1988; 60:762).

Portal hypertension causes the shunting of blood from the splanchnic area to the systemic circulation. A considerable fraction of the blood from the splanchnic area can now bypass the liver, and drugs, particularly those which under normal conditions are cleared from the blood during the first passage through the liver, now enter the systemic circulation (Pomier-Layrargues, Gastro, 1986; 91:163). A patient can be particularly sensitive to such a drug. Propranolol and lidocaine belong to this category.

In Table 2 the half-lives and clearances of some frequently used drugs and the alterations caused by liver disease are shown. A significant increase in half-life calls for prolongation of the dosing interval, whereas a reduction of the dose is the appropriate answer to a decrease in clearance. Often both are affected in liver disease.

Whether a dose reduction is necessary also depends on the toxicity of a drug. For example, for adequate antibiotic coverage in a patient with spontaneous bacterial peritonitis, one does not need to reduce the dose of ampicillin because this drug has a wide safety margin. However, for aminoglycosides, the dose needs to be reduced and the interval changed to twice daily instead of three times a day. Also for some cephalosporins such as cefotaxim, ceftriaxone, and cefoperazone, drugs that are predominantly cleared via the bile, a dose reduction of about 30 per cent is recommended (Moore, AmJMed, 1986; 80:1093). Antimycotic drugs that can be given to patients with liver disease without the need for dose reduction include amphotericin and nystatin. Ketoconazole is metabolized by the liver and the monitoring of serum values is recommended. The tuberculostatic drugs ethambutol and para-aminosalicylic acid can be given and appear to be safe. The doses of isoniazid and rifampicin need to be reduced (rifampicin maximally 6 to 8 mg/kg). Pyrazinamide and ethionamide are metabolized by the liver but data about their use in patients with liver disease are lacking (Holdiness, ClinPharmacokin, 1984; 9:511). Penicillins are safe. For metronidazole, dose reduction to 50 per cent is recommended.

Table 2 Drug therapy in liver disease

	Half-life (h)		Clearance (ml/min)		Recommendation
	Liver cirrhosis (controls)	Change (%)	Liver cirrhosis (controls)	Change (%)	
Low clearance drugs					
Ampicillin	1.9±0.6 (1.3±0.2)	+46#	280±140 (324±80)	−13.6	Normal dose
Chlordiazepoxide	63±27 (24±12)	+162#	9±1 (18±5)	−50#	Reduce dose by 50% and prolong interval to every other day or third day
Cimetidine, ranitidine	3±1 (2.3±0.7)	+30	460±150 (510±90)	−9.8	Normal dose,[c] inhibits cytochrome P450 and may interfere with metabolism of other drugs (13) (e.g. theophylline, propranolol, and anticoagulants). CNS effects have been described
Diazepam	106±15 (47±14)	+125#	14±2 (27±4)	−48#	prolonged half-life, not recommended
Frusemide	2±1 (1.2±0.3)	+67#	120±40 (140±40)	−15.5	Efficacy may be decreased because of low albumin, dose should then be increased
Lorazepam	32±10 (22±5)	+45#	57±34 (53±16)	+7.5	Normal dose
Naproxen			9±2 (9±1)	No change	Use not recommended in patients with liver disease
Oxazepam	6±3 (6±2)	No change	156±70 (136±13)	+14	Normal dose
Prednisone[a]	3±1 (3±1)	No change	280±80 (260±60)	+8	Normal dose
Theophylline	29±14 (6±2)	+383#	22±13 (74±34)	−70#	Not recommended; if needed, serum levels should be monitored
Tolbutamide	4±1 (6±1)	−33#	30±6 (21±3)	+44#	Normal dose, enhanced risk for hypoglycaemia
Warfarin[b]	23±5 (25±3)	−8	102±15 (102±12)	No change	Caution because of already existing bleeding tendency, normal dose
High clearance drugs					
Lidocaine	6±4 (1.8±0.1)	+217#	360±150 (640±60)	−43#	Dose reduction
Metoprolol	7±4 (4±3)	+71	600±400 (800±300)	−23	Normal dose
Morphine	2±1 (3±2)	−12	1150±350 (1230±430)	−7	Because of CNS actions, the use of this drug and this group of drugs is not recommended
Pentazocine	7±2 (3.8±0.5)	+72#	680±300 (1250±240)	−46#	Has CNS actions, paracetamol (maximum 4 g/day) is better alternative
Propranolol	11±8 (4.0±0.9)	+175#	600±400 (900±300)	−33	Dose reduction
Verapamil	14±9 (3±1)	+379#	500±200 (1600±400)	−65#	Dose reduction

[a] Chronic active hepatitis.
[b] Acute hepatitis.
[c] In another study, dose reduction is recommended because of impaired renal clearance of cimetidine in patients with liver cirrhosis.
Significantly different from control ($p<0.005$).
Table adapted and modified from Williams, NEJM, 1983; 309:1616).

Apart from altered pharmacokinetics, adverse drug reactions frequently occur in patients with liver disease, more often than, for example, in patients with chronic renal failure. In patients with liver disease there is a delicate balance between normal and abnormal function of various organs. Prostaglandin synthesis inhibitors easily tip this balance. In patients with liver disease, they cause a decrease in renal perfusion, in particular in volume-depleted patients. This can precipitate functional renal failure. Furosemide is another drug that is frequently used in patients with liver disease and ascites. However, this drug frequently causes volume depletion, hyponatraemia, and hypokalaemia in liver disease, with mental disturbances or frank hepatic encephalopathy as a result. In fact, diuretics more often induce hepatic encephalopathy than benzodiazepines. Spironolactone is the diuretic drug of choice in liver disease, despite the fact that its use can be hampered by cumbersome and painful gynaecomastia (Verbeeck, ClinPharmTher, 1982; 31:719).

In conclusion, one has to think twice before giving a particular drug to a patient with liver disease. In particular, patients with decompensated liver cirrhosis are sometimes in a precarious equilibrium. The inadvertent use of drugs like sleeping pills, analgesics, or diuretics, which in normal patients have a considerable safety, can cause severe and even life-threatening complications such as hepatic encephalopathy, hepatorenal syndrome, and gastrointestinal haemorrhage in patients with liver disease.

Uptake at the sinusoidal plasma membrane (transport from blood into the hepatocyte)

In principle, four entirely different mechanisms can accomplish the uptake of organic solutes into hepatocytes:

(1) passive diffusion of uncharged lipophilic drugs through the lipid phase of the membrane;
(2) passive diffusion of relatively small, charged drugs through aqueous pores in the membrane;
(3) carrier-mediated primary transport;
(4) carrier-mediated active or secondary active transport.

Only the last two processes are saturable and, in these cases, the rate of transport is not linearly related to drug concentration over the entire concentration range.

Passive lipoid diffusion is a common transport mechanism not specific to the liver and involves 'dissolution' of a lipophilic drug molecule in the lipid bilayer of the membrane. Penetration into the cells occurs down a chemical gradient and net transport is helped by intracellular binding or maintenance of a concentration gradient by metabolic conversion. Classic studies demonstrated a clear-cut relationship between lipophilicity and penetration rate of drugs in isolated perfused livers (Kurz, NaunynSchmiedbArchPharm, 1966; 254:33).

Passive diffusion through pores in structural membrane proteins, in principle, may occur for relatively small hydrophilic compounds (MW < 150) such as urea, but is not important for the majority of drugs.[9,41]

For relatively small, polar or charged substrates representing many of the common drugs, carrier-mediated membrane transport is necessary for substantial penetration into the cell (Berk, Hepatol, 1987; 7:165; Meijer, JHepatol, 1987; 4:259).[16,17,42,43] Carriers are probably single or grouped structural membrane proteins that form pores or undergo conformational changes so as to shuttle substrates through the lipid bilayer (see Figs 12 and 13). It is not known whether this shuttling process involves passage through gated channels, or positional changes of closely associated pairs of proteins (Berk, Hepatol, 1987; 7:165; Sorrentino, SemLivDis, 1988; 8:119).[9,42,43] Nevertheless, much progress has been made in the identification of potential carrier proteins, in particular by molecular cloning and functional expression techniques (Meijer, JHepatol,

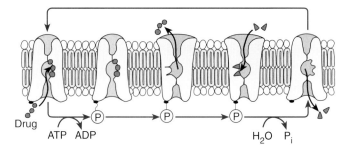

Fig. 13. Schematic diagram depicting one possible mechanism of translocation of a drug through binding to a transmembrane protein (consisting of a single polypeptide or a combination of them). Membrane translocation occurs through conformational changes in the protein by phosphorylation with ATP. The carrier protein can only return to its original conformation through binding of extracellular inorganic ions. Overall, these events result in an antiport of the drug and the particular ions. The number of charged groups in the drug and the number of antiported ions determine whether the transport is electrogenic or not.

1996; 24:29), but also by more conventional procedures like specific photoaffinity labelling and protein isolation (Berk, 1987; Frimmer, BBActa, 1988; 947:75; Sorrentino, 1988; Kurz, p.267 in reference 37; Levy, p.279 in 37).[3,43] Antibodies raised against synthetic sequences of cloned carrier proteins can be employed to study cellular and tissue localization. Some of the isolated carrier proteins have been reconstituted in proteoliposomes (Sottocasa, BBActa, 1982; 685:123; Von Dippe, BBActa, 1986; 862:352; Levy, p.279 in reference 37)[43] and the complete amino acid sequence of some of these proteins, as well as the genetic material involved in their synthesis, has been identified (see Table 3) (Sottocasa, 1982; Von Dippe, 1986).[43]

Passive carrier-mediated transport involves recognition by a specific carrier on the basis of the physicochemical features of the substrate.[9,16] Transport occurs along the (electro-) chemical concentration gradient. This process is saturable, displays competition between structurally related ligands, and transstimulation or accelerated exchange diffusion (Berk, Hepatol, 1987; 7:165).[9,42,43] The latter phenomena can be demonstrated in isolated cells or membrane vesicles by preloading them with a transportable agent and observing an increased initial rate of uptake of a chemically related compound under these conditions. This preloading effect is supposed to be due to reorientation of the carrier binding site to the outer layer of the membrane, a process that is supposed to occur only in the drug-bound form (Berk, 1987; Sorrentino, SemLivDis, 1988; 8:119).[9]

Vectorial transport of charged compounds can lead to an unequal concentration on either side of the membrane simply due to equilibration according to the membrane potential.[16] For instance, organic cations can reach a fourfold higher intracellular concentration[3,16,41] as a result of the inside negative membrane potential of the hepatocyte (30 to 40 mV), while organic anions can be driven out of the cell at the canalicular level for the same reason (Weinman, AmJPhysiol, 1989; 256:G826).[42,43] Real 'uphill transport' against an electrochemical gradient requires energy-rich co-substrates such as ATP (primary active transport) or may operate via existing gradients of organic ions (H^+, OH^-, HCO_3^-, Na^+, or K^+) that drive the translocation process, since such ion gradients can only be built up through the use of energy-rich compounds. Transfer of the organic solute via ion gradients is called 'secondary active transport'. In the latter category, one finds clear examples of Na$^+$-linked transport of bile acids,[43] fatty acids (Stremmel, JHepatol, 1989; 9:374), and certain amino acids (Christensen, Adv-Enz, 1979; 49:41). One or more Na$^+$ ions are supposed to be bound to the carrier together with the substrate. After translocation to the intracellular site where Na$^+$ concentration is much lower, Na$^+$ dissociates from the carrier and the drug is released because affinity of the bile acid for the Na$^+$-free carrier is reduced.[9,43]

For uptake of solutes into hepatocytes, primary active transport using ATP is definitely established for Na$^+$K$^+$ transport (the electrogenetic Na$^+$K$^+$-ATPase pump system). Sugiyama and co-workers have published some data suggesting ATP-dependent uptake of several anionic and cationic compounds such as the Na-independent component of bile acid transport, dibromo-sulphophthalein (DBSP), benzylpenicillin, 1-anilino-8-naphthalene-sulphonate (ANS) (Yamazaki, AmJPhysiol, 1993; 264:G693; Yamazaki, JHepatol, 1992; 14:41), some H$_2$ receptor antagonists (Nakamura, JPharmExpTher, 1994; 269:1220) and more recently the quinolone antibiotic grepafloxacin (Sasabe, JPharmExpTher, 1997; 282:162). However, these findings have not yet been confirmed by others.

Facilitatory role of intracellular proteins in uptake

Binding of the drug molecule to a carrier is necessary for vectorial transport. Yet, dissociation from the carrier at the opposite side of the membrane is also required for net transport. This would, in principle, imply that binding proteins within the cell or outside the cell could be essential for an efficient net transport in either direction (Meijer, JPharmExpTher, 1977; 202:8; Tipping, BiochemJ, 1981; 195:441).[44] Association with such non-membrane proteins might, therefore, help dissociation of the ligand from the (mobile) carrier, enabling reorientation of the membrane carrier in its original state (see Fig. 12). Such a mechanism may operate in the sinusoidal secretion (efflux) of organic anions out of the cell that is accelerated by albumin in the extracellular medium (Nijssen, Hepatol, 1989; 10:593). A facilitatory mechanism has also been proposed for cytosolic proteins in the uptake process (Tipping, 1981).[44] For instance, the glutathione transferase B (ligandin) and fatty acid binding (Z) proteins have been linked to such a role in the translocation of bilirubin and BSP (Levi, JCI, 1969; 48:2156).[45] The recent observations that these cytoplasmatic binding proteins display saturation, mutual competition between similar substrates and counter transport, supports the idea that these proteins can be considered as true intracellular carrier systems (Weisiger, Hepatol, 1996; 24:1288). The fact that intracellular concentrations of these binding proteins poorly correlate with the uptake rate of these agents, at first sight, does not favour this idea.[21,42] Nevertheless, the relation between the concentration of such proteins and transport rate could be essentially non-linear and it is possible that such a role could only be demonstrated in a range of protein concentrations that cannot be manipulated in the intact

cell. Experiments in isolated plasma membrane vesicles should provide more definite clues here.

Multiplicity in hepatic uptake mechanisms

Traditionally, hepatocellular uptake of organic compounds was classified according to the charge of the substrate and was divided into carrier systems for uncharged substrates, organic cations, and organic anions (Mol, JPharmExpTher, 1988; 244:268; Meier, JHepatol, 1996; 24:29).[3] However, at present, the overall picture emerging from the available studies, using a variety of experimental systems, is that multiple mechanisms exist for the hepatic uptake of each of these classes of compounds (see Fig. 11) (Berk, Hepatol, 1987; 7:165; Steen, p.239 in reference 13).[3,43] This classic subdivision, on the basis of net charge of the transported substrates, has also been questioned because many (competitive) interactions during uptake were observed for compounds originating from the different classes defined above (Frimmer, TrendsPharmacolSci, 1982; 3:395; Steen, p.239 in reference 13).[3,34] However, such interactions are often observed at relatively high substrate concentrations and can, apart from overlapping substrate specificity, be explained by the involvement of a multispecific carrier system that, under such conditions, largely contributes to overall uptake rate. This postulated carrier system may accommodate relatively hydrophobic amphipathic compounds irrespective of charge (Frimmer, 1982; Steen, BiochemPharm, 1992; 44:2323; Bossuyt, JPharm-ExpTher, 1996; 276:891).[3,34] The relative contribution of such a multispecific system to total hepatocyte uptake of a certain substrate thus increases with increasing sinusoidal concentration of the particular compound and predicts transport interactions with a broad variety of organic substrates under these conditions.

Apart from interactions of charged groups exposed on the drug and the carrier protein, hydrophobic interactions may also play an important role in the affinity of organic solutes for the particular carrier systems. As discussed previously, structure/kinetic studies with organic anions and cations clearly indicate that the liver parenchymal transport system favours relatively hydrophobic (lipophilic) drugs. These are often compounds with a relatively high molecular mass and their bulky ring structures render them hydrophobic. Since the various carrier proteins in the hepatocyte probably possess hydrophobic binding sites, it is not surprising that many cholephilic ligands interact, at least non-competitively, during hepatic uptake in spite of their different overall charge. A direct influence on the lipid bilayer and consequently on carrier mobility may also play a role in transport interaction. Treatment of rats with ethinyl oestradiol, for example, leads to a cholestatic condition and impaired bile acid transport that may be due to an increased rigidity of the sinusoidal plasma membrane. It has been shown that membrane fluidity and transport of bile acids and BSP can be restored by administration of certain detergents (Simon, JCI, 1980; 65:851; Miccio, BiochemPharm, 1989; 38:3559).

A major complicating factor in the study of hepatic transport is the use of rather 'hybrid' model compounds: molecules that can be present in more than one form in the body, either dissociated and undissociated or in the form of couples with counter ions.

In practice this means that many substrates will be transported by more than one carrier system at the same time, as determined by their relative concentration in relation to the K_m of the particular processes. The presence of counter ions and the extent of protonation of the molecules in the microclimate of the cells[2,3] may influence the fraction of the transportable form present.

Uptake of organic anions

The organic anions readily taken up in hepatocytes represent a widely varying group of molecular structures. Often they are more or less hydrophobic compounds with one or more negative charges. Among this class of compounds are many that are therapeutically or diagnostically relevant. Organic anions taken up by the liver are commonly divided into three subclasses: bile acids, non-esterified (free) fatty acids, and non bile-acid cholephilic anions (including bilirubin, BSP, DBSP, radioscanning HIDA compounds, and iodinated radiocontrast media) (Stremmel, PNAS, 1986; 83:3584; Berk, Hepatol, 1987; 7:165; Meier, JHepatol, 1996; 24:29; Kuipers, p.215 in reference 13).[2] Class-specific, integral membrane, binding proteins have been identified that may represent the putative carriers for uptake into hepatocytes (Frimmer, TrendsPharmacolSci, 1982; 3:395; Berk, 1987; Yamazaki, PharmaceutRes, 1996; 13:495; Zeigler, p.317 in reference 37; Yi, PNAS, 1995; 92:1495; Bossuyt, JHepatol, 1996; 25:733; Müller, AmJPhysiol, 1997; 272:G1285; Meier, Hepatol, 1997; 26:1667) (see Table 3).[7,34,46]

Uptake of organic anions into rat liver can be roughly divided into sodium-dependent and sodium-independent transport mechanisms (Berk, Hepatol, 1987; 7:165; Zimmerli, JPharmExpTher, 1989; 250: 301; Meier, Hepatol, 1997; 26:1667).[43,46] Kinetics corresponding with sodium-coupled carrier-mediated transport have been shown both *in vivo* and *in vitro* for bile acids (Frimmer, TrendsPharmacolSci, 1982; 3:395; Zimmerli, 1989; Buscher, JHepatol, 1991; 13:169),[43] ethacrynic acid, iodipamide (Mol, JPharmExpTher, 1988; 244:268),[2] fatty acids (Stremmel, PNAS, 1986; 83:3584; Berk, Hepatol, 1987; 7:165), and several other compounds.[2] Sodium-independent carrier-mediated uptake of organic anions has been shown for rose bengal (Wang, BiopharmDrugDispos, 1992; 13:647), 1-anilino-8-naphthalenesulphonate (ANS) (Chung, JHepatol, 1990; 11:240), bilirubin (Berk, Hepatol, 1987; 7:165), and indocyanine green, as well as for BSP (Chen, Hepatol, 1984; 4:467; Berk, Hepatol, 1987; 7:165; Wolkoff, JCI, 1987; 79:1259) and DBSP (Blom, BiochemPharm, 1981; 30:1809; Yamazaki, PharmaceutRes, 1996; 13:495). This sodium-independent system may also mediate uptake of taurocholate, although it has a lower affinity for taurocholate than the sodium-dependent systems (Jacquemin, JCI, 1991; 88:2146).[34] However, even within this category of cholephilic dyes, differences were found in regard to the ATP dependency of uptake: indocyanine green, rose bengal, and BSP uptake seem to be independent of cellular ATP content and may reflect carrier-mediated facilitated diffusion. In contrast, uptake of DBSP, ANS, and benzylpenicilline is clearly ATP dependent (Yamazaki, JHepatol, 1992; 14:41; Yamazaki, AmJPhysiol, 1993; 264:G693; Yamazaki, PharmaceutRes, 1996; 13: 495).

Recently, Sandker *et al.* (BiochemPharm, 1994; 47:2193), using hepatocytes and plasma membrane vesicle isolated from human liver, showed that also in man taurocholate uptake is mediated by a sodium-dependent and a sodium-independent mechanism. The overall uptake rate in human cells is about 10-fold lower than in rat cells. This interspecies difference in uptake rate measured *in vitro*

appeared to represent the *in vivo* clearance adequately (Sandker, 1994).

The Na⁺-dependent bile-acid carrier system both for the rat and for human liver was recently cloned and expressed in oocytes (Hagenbuch, JBC, 1990; 265:5357; Hagenbuch, PNAS, 1991; 88: 10629). The rat carrier protein (ntcp) produced in this cell system, which mediates Na⁺ cotransport of predominantly but not exclusively conjugated bile acids. It also mediates transport of oestrogen conjugates, cyclic oligopeptides, and certain drugs (Meier, AmJPhysiol, 1995; 269:G801). It exhibits a molecular mass of 51 kDa and is dissimilar to the 48-kDa proteins that were originally claimed from photoaffinity labelling studies to be responsible for this transport (Zeigler, p.317 in reference 37).[34,43,47] This 48-kDa protein, however, was found to be identical to microsomal epoxide hydrolase and a bifunctional role was suggested (Alves, JBC, 1993; 268:20148).

The human Na⁺-dependent taurocholate carrier (**NTCP**) cloned in oocytes showed a higher affinity for taurocholate than the rat protein ($K_m = 6.3 \, \mu$mol for NTCP and 25 μmol for ntcp) (Hagenbuch, JBC, 1990; 265:5357; Hagenbuch, PNAS, 1991; 88: 10629).

The Na⁺-independent taurocholate carrier is probably identical to the organic anion transporter identified in rat liver (oatp₁) (Jacquemin, JCI, 1991; 88:2146)[34] of which the human variant has also been cloned recently (Kullak-Ublick, Gastro, 1995; 109: 1274; Bossuyt, JHepatol, 1996; 25:733). This 80-kDa carrier not only mediates the transport of anions such as BSP, DBSP, indocyanine green, drugs such as pravastine (Yamazaki, PharmaceutRes, 1996; 13:1495), and unconjugated and conjugated bile acids, but also accommodates uncharged compounds, steroids and large bulky cations (Shi, JBC, 1995; 43:25591; Meier, Hepatol, 1997; 26:1667). The uptake of such compounds appeared to be Na⁺-independent and electrogenic.[2,46] Several attempts to isolate and identify the proteins involved in the uptake of these anions indicate that several polypeptides are probably responsible. Apart from the organic anion transporting polypeptide (oatp₁) cloned by Jacquemin *et al.* (1991), the role of organic anion transport was also ascribed to the 37-kDa bilitranslocase (BTL) isolated from liver plasma membranes by Sottocasa *et al.* (1985; Sottocasa, MethodsEnz, 1989; 174:50). After reconstitution in liposomes, the latter protein showed electrogenic transport of BSP, albeit in a reversed direction, taking into account the inside negative membrane potential in hepatocytes (Sottocasa, BBActa, 1982; 685:123; Sottocasa, 1985). In addition, a 55-kDa BSP/bilirubin binding protein (BBBP) (Reichen, BBResComm, 1979; 91:484; Stremmel, JCI, 1983; 71:1796) and a separate 55-kDa organic anion binding protein (**OABP**) (Wolkoff, JCI, 1980; 65: 1152)[7] were isolated independently. The OABP is identical to the β-subunit of mitochondrial F1-ATPase but may also be present in the plasma membrane (Wolkoff, p.179 in reference 48) as detected by antibody reaction. However, the relative roles of all of these organic anion transporters in animals and humans have not been elucidated yet.

These 'anion' transport systems such as oatp₁ do not only transport anions but have an overlapping substrate specificity and also accommodate uncharged cardiac glycosides, steroids, and amphipathic cations, as well as various oligopeptides (Hunter, Hepatol, 1990; 12:76; Shi, JBC, 1995; 43:2559; Zeigler, p.317 in reference

Table 3 Functional properties of cloned hepatic transport proteins involved in bile formation

Name	Species	Alternative names	Substrates	K_M (μmol)	Driving force	Localization	mRNA	Amino acids	Mr
NTCP	Human	BSBT	Monovalent bile salts	6 (TC)	Na$^+$	BLM	1.7	349	50
Ntcp	Rat		Monovalent bile salts	25 (TC)	Na$^+$	BLM	1.8	362	51
oct1	Rat		Small organic cations	95 (TEA)	?	BLM	1.9/3.4	556	62
OATP	Human		Bulky amphipathic compounds	1.5 (BSP) 50 (TC)	?	BLM	2.7	670	180
oatp1	Rat		Bulky amphipathic compounds	20 (BSP) 60 (TC)	?	BLM	2.7	670	80
MDR1	Human		Bulky hydrophobic compounds		Mg^{2+}/ATP	CM	4.5	1280	170
mdr1a	Mouse	mdr3	Bulky hydrophobic compounds		Mg^{2+}/ATP	CM	4.3	1276	150
mdr1b	Mouse	mdr1	Bulky hydrophobic compounds		Mg^{2+}/ATP	CM	4.3	—	—
mdr1a	Rat	pgp3	Bulky hydrophobic compounds		Mg^{2+}/ATP	CM	?	?	?
mdr1b	Rat	pgp1	Bulky hydrophobic compounds	10 (APDA) 20 (Dau)	Mg^{2+}/ATP	CM	4.3	1282	150
MDR3	Human	MDR2	Phospholipids, PC		Mg^{2+}/ATP	CM	4.5	1279	170
mdr2	Mouse		Phospholipids, PC		Mg^{2+}/ATP	CM	4.5	1276	150
mdr2	Rat	pgp3	Phospholipids, PC		Mg^{2+}/ATP	CM	4.5		
spgp	Rat		Monovalent bile acids		Mg^{2+}/ATP	CM	5.4	?	180
mrp2	Rat	cmoat cmrp	Anionic conjugates	0.25 (LTC$_4$)	Mg^{2+}/ATP	CM	6.5 6.5	1541	200
MRP2	Human		Anionic conjugates		Mg^{2+}/ATP	CM	6.5	1545	200
MRP1	Human	LTEC GS-X pump	Anionic conjugates	0.097 (LTC$_4$) 93 (GSSG)	Mg^{2+}/ATP	LM, BDE	6.5	1531	190
mrp1	Mouse		Anionic conjugates	0.070 (LTC$_4$)	Mg^{2+}/ATP	LM	6.0/6.2	1528	185
cBAT		BSEC	Monovalent bile salts	7–10 (TC)	Mg^{2+}/ATP	CM	?	?	?

Carrier systems for liver uptake (in the basolateral domain of the plasma membrane: BLM) or biliary excretion (in the canalicular membrane domain: CM) are indicated; K_M is the concentration at the half maximal transport rate indicated per substrate; mRNA, messenger RNA; Mr, molecular radius; LM, lateral membrane domain of hepatocytes; BDE, bile duct epithelial localization; TC, taurocholate; TEA, tetraethylammonium; BSP, bromsulphophthalein; APDA, azidopropyldeoxy-ajmalinium; Dau, daunomycin; LTC$_4$, leukotriene C$_4$; GSSG, oxidized glutathione; NTCP, Na$^+$-dependent taurocholate transporting peptide; oct1, organic cation transporter; OATP, organic anions transporting peptide; MDR, multidrug resistance protein; spgp, sister of P-glycoprotein; mrp, multidrug resistance-related protein; cBAT, canalicular bile acid transporter.

37).[8] Interestingly, transport of compounds such as BSP in hepatocytes shows Cl$^-$ dependency (Blom, BiochemPharm, 1981; 30: 1809; Jacquemin, JCI, 1991; 88:2146; Min, JCI, 1991; 87:1496) that is probably due to an improved dissociation of BSP from albumin rather than to an influence of a transmembrane Cl$^-$ gradient, *per se*. A similar effect of Cl$^-$ on organic anion uptake rate was observed in oocytes (Jacquemin, 1991) and HeLa cells (Shi, JBC, 1995; 270: 25591) transfected with mRNA coding for the above-mentioned 80-kDa carrier oatp$_1$, but this was observed only in the presence of albumin. The latter study also indicated that oatp can mediate bi-directional transport. The unglycosylated oatp$_1$ is a 65-kDa polypeptide which has multiple isoforms (Meier, AmJPhysiol-GastroLivPhysiol, 1995; 269:G801). The protein consistes of 670 amino acids with 10 to 12 transmembrane-spanning domains (Meier, JHepatol, 1996; 24:29). The role of the organic anion transporters (oatp/OATP) in the transport of bilirubin and its conjugates is still unclear, but Kanai *et al.* (AmJPhysiol, 1996; 270: F319) found that these compounds were not transported in Hela cells that were transiently infected with oatp$_1$. The involvement in bilirubin transport of the BTL mentioned above was hypothesized, but its contribution can only be definitively established when this protein is cloned.

Recently, another member of the rat oatp-family was cloned (Noe, PNAS, 1997; 94:10346) and was called oatp$_2$. Oatp$_2$ is a polypeptide of 661 amino acids and has 77 per cent homology with oatp$_1$. Oatp$_2$ is expressed in brain, liver, and kidney and exhibits a similar substrate specificity as oatp$_1$, but has a higher affinity for digoxin.

Human OATP shows a 67 per cent amino acid identity with rat liver oatp$_1$. Qualitatively, the human and rat protein show a similar but not identical substrate specificity, but, qualitatively, significant differences exist with respect to K_m and V_{max} values. Human OATP shows a lower transport rate for bile acids and organic anions, but a higher transport rate for cations, compared to rat oatp$_1$ (Kullach-Ublick, Gastro, 1995; 109:1274; Bossuyt, JHepatol, 1996; 25:733).

Uptake of cationic drugs

The category of organic cations is composed of a wide variety of chemicals containing one or more tertiary/quaternary amine or other positively charged groups (Fig. 14). The quaternary ammonium compounds possess a strongly basic nitrogen centre that is permanently positively charged at physiological pH. Tertiary amine groups acquire a cationic charge by protonation and consequently the fraction of total amount present in the body in the cationic form is dependent on the pK_a value of the particular tertiary group as well as on the pH of the biological milieu. Some compounds contain both a quaternary and tertiary aminic group and the extent of protonation of the tertiary amine function in such compounds may largely influence the rate of hepatic uptake and biliary secretion (Mol, BiochemPharm, 1992; 44:1453).[3]

Endogenous organic cations that are transported by the liver include thiamine, choline, and *N*-methylnicotinamide (Moseley, AmJPhysiol, 1990; 259:G973; Moseley, AmJPhysiol, 1992; 263: G775). Certain net positively charged peptides,[8] carnitine,[49] sphingoid bases (Liscovitch, BiochemPharm, 1991; 42:2071), and polyamines (Byers, BiochemJ, 1990; 269:35; Khan, CellBiolIntRep, 1991; 15:9; Toninello, JBC, 1992; 267:18393) can also be considered as endogenous cationic compounds. Exogenous organic cations are also abundant. It has been estimated that at least 50 per cent of the therapeutic agents available at present have a (partly) cationic character. Among others, certain antineoplastic agents, (anti)-histaminergic, (anti)cholinergic, (anti)adrenergic, (anti)dopaminergic, (anti)serotoninergic, and antiarhythmic drugs as well as certain local anaesthetic, antihelmintic, and neuromuscular blocking drugs contain tertiary or quaternary nitrogen groups.

Multiple transport processes have been identified for the above-mentioned endogenous cations. These systems, in general, poorly accommodate the exogenous organic cations, although overlapping substrate specificity may exist. In addition, at least five different uptake mechanisms have been postulated to date for exogenous cationic compounds (mostly drugs) (Steen, p.239 in reference 13)[1, 3] (Fig. 14). The relative contribution of these multiple cation transporters to the overall uptake and secretion rate of a given compound is dependent on the (unbound) concentration of the particular agent in relation to the affinity for the various transporting modalities.

Mechanisms for hepatic uptake of organic cations have been studied in human liver (Fig. 15) (Meijer, EurJPharm, 1971; 14:280; Agoston, ActaAnaesthScand, 1973; 17:267; Meijer, Anesthesiology, 1979; 51:402; Sandker, BiochemPharm, 1994; 47:2193; Steen, p.239 in reference 13), but most investigations have been in rat liver employing a large variety of techniques such as *in vivo* studies,[3] isolated perfused livers,[3] isolated hepatocytes (Aarons, JPharm-Pharmacol, 1979; 31:322; Mol, JPharmExpTher, 1988; 244:268; Sandker, BiochemPharm, 1994; 47:2193; Steen, p.239 in reference 13), basolateral plasma membrane vesicles (Moseley, AmJPhysiol, 1990; 259:G973; McKinney, AmJPhysiol, 1992; 263:G939; Moseley, Gastro, 1992; 103:1056; Moseley, AmJPhysiol, 1992; 263:G775), and photoaffinity labelling studies (Mol, BiochemPharm, 1992; 43: 2217; Steen, p.239 in reference 13).[3,36] Recently, expression cloning of potential organic cation carriers in oocytes has also been successful (Xie, Hepatol, 1992; 16:147A; Gründemann, Nature, 1994; 372:549; Gorboulev, DNACellBiol, 1997;16:871; Zhang,

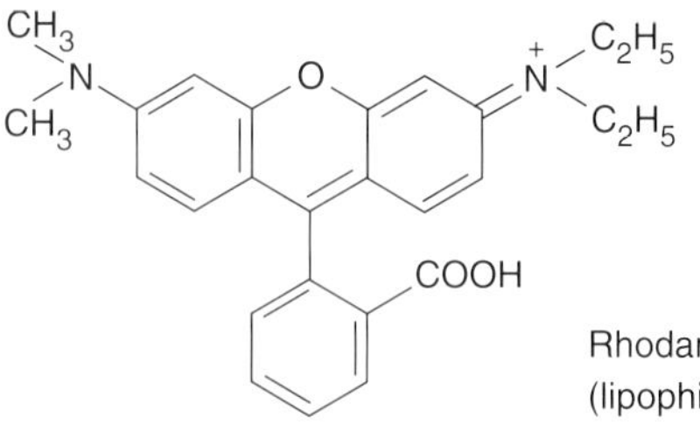

Rhodamine B
(lipophilic)

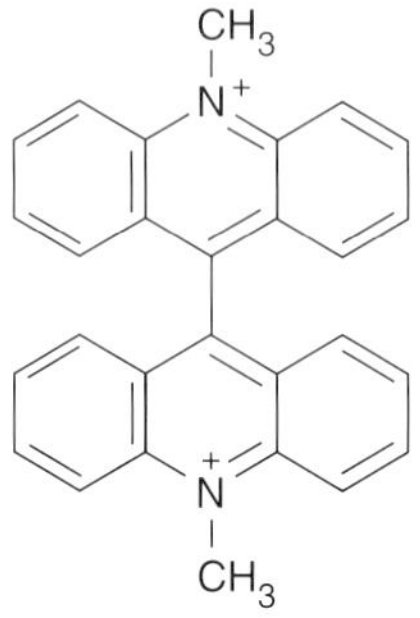

Lucigenin
(hydrophilic)

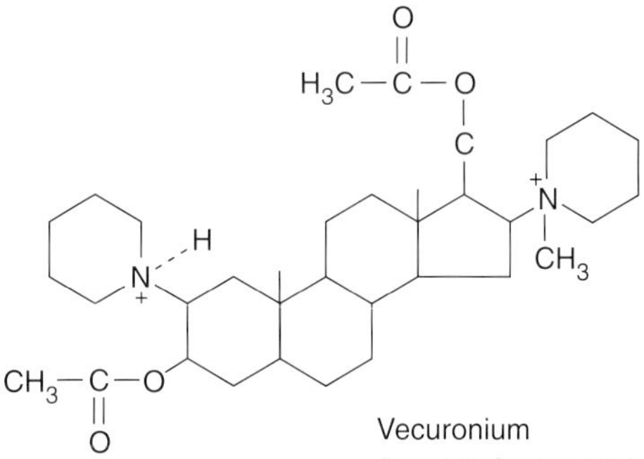

Vecuronium
(lipophilic/hydrophilic)

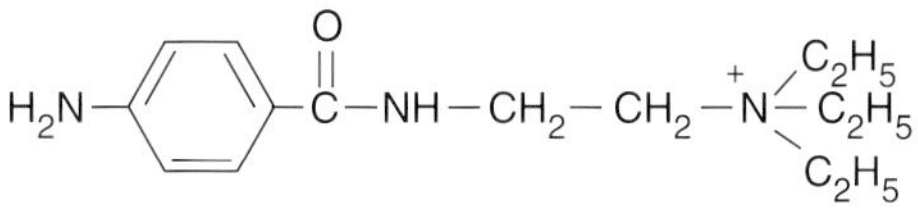

Procainamidoethobromide

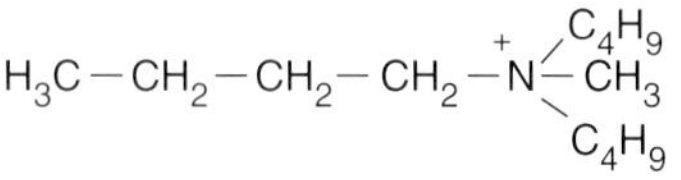

Tributylmethylammonium

Fig. 14. Chemical structures of organic cation model compounds with entirely different physicochemical and transport properties. The fluorescent dye rhodamine B is very lipophilic and enters cells by passive lipoid diffusion. The fluorescent dye lucigenin is very hydrophilic and charged and can only enter cells by adsorptive endocytosis. Vecuronium is an organic cation of intermediate lipophilicity, especially in its deprotonized form. It displays high affinity for uptake and secretion carriers for organic cations. Procainamidoethobromide (PAEB) is a classic type 1 organic cation with a cationic group distant from an aromatic ring. Tributylmethylammonium (TBuMA) is a small aliphatic cation with bulky butyl groups that give the drug an intermediate lipophilicity among this category of agents. PAEB and TBuMA are both substrates for type 1 uptake carriers such as oct1.

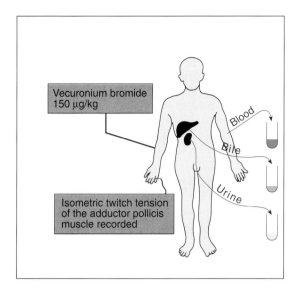

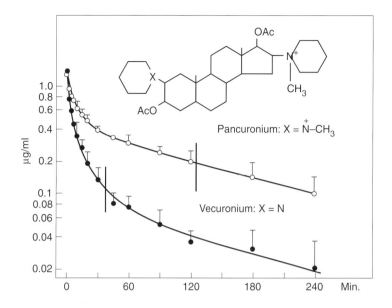

Fig. 15. Relationship between the pharmacokinetics and neuromuscular blocking effects of the organic cations pancuronium and vecuronium which only differ by one methyl group on the nitrogen centre (indicated by × in the chemical structure). Pancuronium is a permanently bivalent cation whereas vecuronium can be partly present as a monovalent cation leaving a large hydrophobic ring structure in the molecule. This unequal structure results in a marked difference in plasma disappearance in the first phase: vecuronium concentration decreases much more rapidly (right). This has been shown in patients to be due to efficient hepatic uptake. In contrast, the hydrophilic pancuronium exhibits much less affinity for the uptake carrier and is poorly extracted by the liver and largely excreted by the kidneys. In patients, these elimination patterns were determined by taking blood, bile, and urine samples while the muscle relaxation was measured by the muscle twitch tension (left). The vertical bars in the curves indicate the concentration range of the agents at which the muscle contraction is restored, indicating that at equipotent doses, vecuronium has a short duration of action (30 min) and pancuronium is a long-acting compound (2 h).

JPharmExpTher, 1997; 51:913). A liver-specific isoform of the renal organic cation uptake carrier ($rOCT_1$) was identified and exhibits a substrate specificity similar to the functionally defined type I carrier system (Gründemann, Nature, 1994; 272:549; Busch, JBC, 1996; 271:32599; Martel, NaunynSchmiedbArchPharm, 1996; 354:320; Zhang, MolPharm, 1997; 51:913) (see Table 3). The overall picture emerging from these studies is that multiple mechanisms exist for the hepatic uptake of these organic cations. Widely overlapping substrate specificity may exist and, depending on the concentration of the organic cation studies, often more than one system will contribute to the overall uptake rate of a given compound. Nevertheless, the individual transport systems exhibit quite different features with regard to maximal transport rate, energization, and ion dependency as well as to the influence of inhibitors.

Non-carrier-mediated mechanisms in cation uptake

Although carrier-mediated transport is the major mechanism for uptake of organic cations, it should be emphasized that passive uptake can occur for very lipophilic organic cations. Examples are the fluorescent probe rhodamine B (Braakman, Hepatol, 1987; 7:849; Braakman, JPharmExpTher, 1989; 249:869) and the anticholinergic drug methyl-deptropine (Van der Sluijs, JPharmExpTher, 1987; 240:668). As a consequence of its passive transfer mechanism, uptake rate of rhodamine B is not inhibited by other cationic compounds.[50]

In contrast, the hydrophilic fluorescent compound lucigenin, which cannot pass the sinusoidal plasma membrane by passive transport or carrier-mediated mechanisms, is probably internalized via a vesicular uptake process (Braakman, MolPharm, 1989; 36: 532,537). This was inferred from fluorescence microscopy studies showing a clustered intracellular distribution of lucigenin with dots of fluorescence close to the plasma membrane. Partial inhibition by microfilament inhibitors such as cytochalasin B and nocodazole, as well as by competitors for membrane adsorption such as poly-L-lysine (Braakman, 1989), indicated a process of adsorptive endocytosis. Such a phenomenon has also been described for basic drugs at the renal tubular level (Tulkens, EurJClinMicrob, 1991; 10:100).

Carrier-mediated uptake mechanisms for exogenous organic cations

Hepatic uptake of cationic drugs seems to occur by at least two facilitated diffusion carrier processes that are Na^+ independent and of which one may be stimulated by proton gradients. The electrogenicity of the uptake systems for exogenous cations currently remains unresolved. ATP dependency could not be demonstrated. The inhibitory effects on uptake of cations by metabolic inhibitors may be explained by direct interaction with the supposed carriers rather than by depletion of ATP (Mol, JPharmExpTher, 1988; 244:268; Steen, JPharmExpTher, 1991; 258:537; King, Gastro, 1993; 104:A927; Steen, BiochemPharm, 1993; 45:809).

Facilitated (carrier-mediated) diffusion mechanisms are the most likely candidates (Mol, 1988; Steen, 1991; McKinney, AmJPhysiol, 1992; 263:G939; Mol, BiochemPharm, 1992; 43:2217; Moseley, AmJPhysiol, 1992; 263:G775; King, 1993). For the endogenous cations thiamine and N-methylnicotinamide, separate H^+-antiport systems appear to be operating at the sinusoidal level. For uptake of choline in the hepatocyte, at least two transport systems are available of which one is Na^+ dependent. Whether choline shares at least one uptake mechanism with thiamine and whether some exogenous cations are also accommodated by the choline carrier systems remains to be established (Meijer, AdvDrugDelRev, 1997; 25:159).

The cationic drugs as a whole show clear heterogeneity in hepatocyte uptake mechanisms. The relatively small cations such as tetraethylamine (McKinney, AmJPhysiol, 1992; 263:G939; Moseley, AmJPhysiol, 1992; 263:G775), tributylmethylamine (Steen, PharmExpTher, 1991; 258:537), and procainamidoethobromide (Steen, p.239 in 13) and its azido analogue azido-procainamide methyliodide (Mol, BiochemPharm, 1992; 43:2217) are transported by a system that is inhibited by choline and lipophilic (amphipathic) cations but not by cardiac glycosides and bile salts (Steen, BiochemPharm, 1992; 44: 2323; Steen, p.239 in 13). They were categorized as type I organic cations and comprise either aliphatic quaternary ammonium compounds or molecules in which the cationic amine group is at some distance from the aromatic ring structure. Larger cationic drugs with the positively charged group included in or situated close to large, aromatic ring structures (called type II compounds) behave differently: hepatic uptake is not affected by a large excess of choline or the type I compounds but can be largely blocked by cardiac glycosides and bile salts. This is explained by competitive inhibition for multispecific systems which recognize bulky amphipathic compounds irrespective of their charge (Steen, 1992). It is at present unknown whether type II transport is performed by one multispecific carrier or by two different carrier proteins. It is of interest that hepatocyte uptake of both type I and type II organic cations is stimulated by inorganic counter anions (Mol, JPharmExpTher, 1988; 244:268; Steen, 1991) such as HCO_3^- and Cl^-. This effect may be due to an improved presentation of the cations to the membrane carriers via ion-pair formation rather than to facilitation through cation/anion symport (Steen, 1991).

Photoaffinity labelling studies with azido-procainamide methyliodide (**APM**) (Mol, ArchPharm, 1989; 322:613; Mol, BiochemPharm, 1992; 43:2217) showed predominant labelling of 50-kDa and 72-kDa proteins in plasma membrane fractions of rat liver, while labelling studies with the bulky type II compound azo-N-pentyl-deoxy-ajmalinium (**APDA**) showed labelling of 48-kDa and 50-kDa proteins.[36] Incorporation of label in the APM studies was inhibited by type II compounds (an interaction also found in isolated hepatocytes), while labelling of potential carrier proteins with APDA was strongly reduced by cardiac glycosides and bile salts. Prior photoaffinity labelling of hepatocytes with APDA reduced the V_{max} without changing the K_m of N-propyl-deoxy ajmalinium uptake into hepatocytes, indicating that part of the carriers was inactivated through covalent labelling.

More definite identification of the putative carrier proteins for organic cations has come from studies using molecular biological techniques. Expression cloning of the carrier protein for organic cation uptake has been performed (Xie, Hepatol, 1992; 16:147A; Gründemann, Nature, 1994; 372:549). A 1.8-kb mRNA fraction

seems to encode for a protein that was called OCT1 and mediates potential-dependent tetraethylamine uptake in *Xenopus laevis* oocytes, which was inhibitable by other cationic drugs like tetramethylammonium and N-methylnicotinamide (Gründemann, 1994). Uptake is inhibited by hydrophilic type 2 organic cations but it is uncertain whether the latter category of compounds is also transported by the carrier (Koepsell, AnnRevPhysiol, 1998, in press).

Therefore, hepatic uptake of organic cations seems to occur by at least three facilitated-diffusion carrier processes in the rat (see Fig. 16). One is an electroneutral proton antiport system for N-methylnicotinamide and thiamine (Moseley, AmJPhysiol, 1990; 259:G973; Moseley, AmJPhysiol, 1992; 263:G775). The recently cloned OCT1 carrier functions as a H^+- independent and electrogenic uptake system for a wide variety of organic cationic drugs and endogenous cations (Gründemann, Nature, 1994; 372:549; Busch, JBC, 1996; 271:32599). The above-mentioned unspecific carrier protein oatp$_1$ may be partly involved in the uptake of especially bulky cationic drugs (Bossuyt, JHepatol, 1996; 25:733; Bossuyt, JPharmExpTher, 1996; 276:891). However, the substrate specificity of the latter protein with regard to cation transport remains to be definitely established. Interference of cardiac glycosides and bile acids with hepatic uptake of bulky organic cations may reflect this carrier modality (Bossuyt, 1996) (see Table 3).

Acinar heterogeneity in uptake of organic anions and cations

For a growing number of substrates, a possible heterogeneous involvement of periportal and perivenous cells in uptake was investigated.[10] For many high clearance compounds, such as conjugated bile salts, DBSP (in the absence of albumin), rhodamine B, parathion, asioloorosomucoid, and cysteine, very steep concentration gradients that declined from zone 1 to zone 3 were observed, indicating a heterogeneity in the involvement of the cells in these zones in uptake of these compounds. For most of these compounds these gradients reverse on retrograde perfusion, suggesting that the *in vivo* heterogeneity is due to the steep concentration gradients in the sinusoids and thus to the localization of the cells in the acinus. From these studies it also became clear that the distribution of drugs within the acinus may be dependent on the dose, on the albumin concentration, and can even be time dependent (Groothuis, AmJPhysiol, 1982; 243:G455; Braakman, Hepatol, 1987; 7:849; Buscher, JHepatol, 1989; 8:181; Buscher, JHepatol, 1991; 13:169; Nijssen, Hepatol, 1992; 15:302; Buscher, Hepatol, 1993; 17:494).[10,34]

For taurocholic acid more detailed studies have been performed in order to investigate possible intrinsic acinar differences in uptake rate. We (Groothuis, AmJPhysiol, 1982; 243:G455; Groothuis, TrendsPharmacolSci, 1985; 6:322) and others (Jones, AmJPhysiol, 1980; 238:G233; Buscher, JHepatol, 1991; 13:169)[34] showed that under normal physiological conditions only zone 1 cells participate in taurocholate uptake because of this high uptake rate (Fig. 10). Zone 3 cells exhibit the same K_m for uptake as zone 1 cells, as was demonstrated by Buscher *et al*.[34] Only when the bile salt load is increased are zone 3 cells recruited for transport of taurocholic acid (Groothuis, 1982; Buscher, JHepatol, 1989; 8:181). Zone 3 cells appeared to have a 50 per cent lower V_{max} for the sodium-dependent

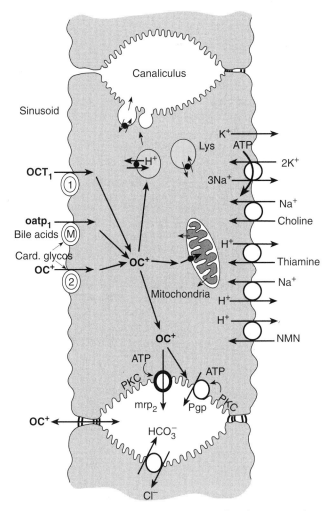

Fig. 16. Tentative scheme depicting carrier-mediated transport of organic cations at the sinusoidal and canalicular level of the hepatocyte. Three uptake systems are indicated for exogenous cations: type I carrier system (1) which was recently identified as oct_1, a multispecific (M) uptake system $oatp_1$, that recognizes amphipatic drugs irrespective of charge, and an as yet unidentified carriersystem (2). Transport processes for choline and thiamine exhibit Na^+ dependency in cells and for N-methylnicotinamide a H^+ dependency in basolateral plasma membrane vesicles. Sinusoidal membranes contain the Na^+/K^+ pump and the Na^+/H^+ antiporter. The canalicular membrane possesses a Cl^-/HCO_3^- antiport system and at least two cation carriers: the multidrug resistance P-glycoprotein carrier protein and the multidrug-resistance related protein (mrp_2).

No major intrinsic differences between periportal and perivenous hepatocytes in uptake rate have been reported for non-bile acid organic anions. Both periportal and perivenous cells avidly take up these compounds and in the absence of albumin very steep acinar gradients have been found (Gumucio, AmJPhysiol, 1984; 246: G86; Nijssen, Hepatol, 1992; 15:302) which disappear at increasing albumin concentrations.

Due to the efficient uptake process of the cation rhodamine B, initially sharp tissue concentration gradients are observed for this agent *in vivo* and perfused livers. This periportal to perivenous concentration gradient reverses over time due to a time-dependent redistribution and a higher binding capacity for dye in the pericentral (zone 3) hepatocytes (Braakman, Hepatol, 1987; 7:849; Braakman, JPharmExpTher, 1989; 249:869). In retrograde perfusions the gradient is the exact mirror image of that in antegrade perfusions, indicating no intrinsic difference in uptake, which is in line with the proposed mechanisms of passive diffusion.

Adsorptive endocytosis of the hydrophilic di-cation lucigenin leads to an initial hepatic extraction of 60 per cent in perfused livers and extensive clustering in cytoplasmic organelles, probably endosomes, lysosomes, and mitochondria (Braakman, Hepatol, 1988; 8:1386; Braakman, MolPharm, 1989; 36:537). The zonal distribution is mainly perivenous due to the influence of taurocholate (see Fig. 10), which inhibits uptake of the cation predominantly in zone 1. This represents one of the few examples of the distribution of a xenobiotic compound in the liver being influenced by an endogenous substrate. At retrograde perfusion the fluorescent compound is mainly present in zone 1, because in that condition taurocholate will mainly enter zone 3 cells. This also indicates that the heterogeneous distribution of lucigenin is not due to primary intrinsic cellular differences in uptake rate.

Similarly, for acridine orange (Gumucio, Gastro, 1981; 80: 639; Braakman, Hepatol, 1991; 13:73),[51] propranol (Anderson, JPharmExpTher, 1978; 206:172), the alkaloid dehydrocorydaline (Fujii, EurJDMPharm, 1984; 9:235), chlorpromazine, and imipramine (Fujii, 1984), steep gradients are observed in antegrade perfusions. Although retrograde perfusions and quantification of the gradients are missing, this heterogeneity is probably, as in the case of rhodamine B, due to the very efficient uptake of these lipophilic cations. Aminotriazole showed a much lower extraction and no clear acinar gradient was seen shortly after injection (Fujii, EurJDMPharm, 1984; 9:257). For the type I and type II model compounds, no studies concerning the acinar heterogeneity in uptake have been published.

Intracellular protein binding and sequestration

Net hepatic uptake is not only influenced by extracellular protein binding but also by intracellular binding. After primary uptake, extensive binding of drugs to proteins and organelles within the cell occurs both for organic anions and cations (Meijer, JPharmacokinBiopharm, 1984; 12:43; Berk, Hepatol, 1987; 7:165).[1–3, 18,52] This intracellular binding may result in high liver/blood concentration gradients.

It is important to note that these liver/blood concentration gradients under steady-state conditions, even when corrected for

uptake carrier.[34] However, because they exhibit a fivefold higher V_{max} of the sodium-independent uptake compared with zone 1 cells, at very high bile salt concentrations the contribution of zone 3 cells may even exceed that of zone 1 cells (Buscher, 1991).

Similar concentration gradients have been found for glycocholic acid as for taurocholic acid. However, for the unconjugated cholic acid, only shallow portal to central gradients were found upon injection of a tracer dose (Groothuis, unpublished observation). As cholic acid represents the major part of the bile salts in the portal vein, the involvement of zone 3 cells in normal bile acid transport is possibly larger than was anticipated from the above-mentioned studies with taurocholate.

extracellular and intracellular protein binding, do not merely reflect the uptake process since they are the result of the relative rates of uptake, biliary and sinusoidal excretion, and sequestration into organelles (Mol, BiochemPharm, 1990; 39:383). The latter processes may provide sink conditions, especially if hepatic uptake rate is relatively low.

Intracellular protein binding and sequestration of organic anions

Three types of cytosolic binding proteins have been identified for organic anions. The Y-protein or 3α-hydroxysteroid dehydrogenases are important binding proteins for bile acids and drugs such as indomethacin (Takikawa, Hepatol, 1996; 23:1642). Glutathione-S-transferase B (also called ligandin) constitutes 4 to 5 per cent of the cytosolic protein and is the major binding protein for non-bile acid anions (Capron, JHistochemCytochem, 1979; 27: 961; Meijer, JPharmacokinBiopharm, 1984; 12:43; Berk, Hepatol, 1987; 7:165). The Z fraction contains the fatty acid binding protein (also called Z-protein) (Meijer, JPharmExpTher, 1977; 202:8; Suzuki, JPath, 1987; 153:385; Bass, Hepatol, 1989; 9:12) and binds not only organic anions such as bilirubin and fatty acids but also uncharged compounds such as sex steroids. Both glutathione-S-transferases and fatty acid binding proteins probably facilitate net hepatic uptake of organic anions. Kinetic studies using two-compartment kinetic analysis (Meijer, 1977) and the multiple indicator dilution technique (Wolkoff, JCI, 1987; 79:1259) in isolated perfused liver indicated that this effect is due to reduction of sinusoidal efflux rather than to stimulation of the actual uptake process.

Binding to the cytosolic proteins is saturable and thus concentration dependent (Meijer, JPharmacokinBiopharm, 1984; 12: 43), and mutual competition for binding is found for similar substrates (Weisiger, Hepatol, 1996; 24:1288). Increasing the dose of organic anions results in higher binding to intracellular membranes and organelles. These structures have such a high binding capacity that the unbound fraction of organic anions in the cytosol remains almost constant with increasing hepatic content (Meijer, 1984). It is important to note that normally the binding of water-soluble substrates to cytosolic proteins keeps the intracellular free concentrations of these agents low and, thereby, prevents excessive binding or accumulation in cellular organelles. Proteins may also bind water-insoluble compounds and help to keep them in aqueous solution, thereby serving as intracellular carriers for such agents (Weisiger, Hepatol, 1996; 24:1288). For instance, it has been suggested that cytosolic proteins are important in the intracellular transport of fatty acids to the endoplasmic reticulum for further metabolism (Bass, Hepatol, 1989; 9:12). The bile-acid binding proteins that have been identified could function in the vectorial transport to conjugative sites (Sugiyama, JBC, 1983; 258:3602; Takikawa, Hepatol, 1996; 23:1642).

Organic anions such as BSP and indocyanine green at high intracellular concentrations interfere with mitochondrial respiration and the production of ATP (Laperche, JPharmExpTher, 1976; 197: 235; Burr, BiochemPharm, 1977; 26:461; Laperche, ToxApplPharmacol, 1977; 41:377). There is evidence that this is due to association with or accumulation in mitochondria, probably because the anionic drugs occupy carrier sites for naturally occurring substrates of an anionic character. Uptake in this organelle against

an evident electrochemical gradient could be explained by anion exchange or antiport systems. For instance, OH⁻ and inorganic phosphate may provide electroneutral transport, while binding to macromolecules within the mitochondrial compartments may lead to further accumulation and toxicity. It is interesting that taurocholate prevents the association of cholephilic anions with mitochondria (Fischer, ArchToxicol, 1980; Suppl. 4:343; Gregus, p.401 in reference 13). The resulting reduction in toxicity may improve cellular function and thereby elevate the apparent transport maximum of the dye.

Intracellular sequestration of organic cations

Following uptake at the sinusoidal domain of the hepatocyte, organic cations can reach high concentrations in the cytoplasmic compartments (Steen, p.239 in reference 13).[1–3,52] Transmembrane (cytoplasm to blood plasma) concentration gradients of 15 and more have been calculated, both for monovalent (Meijer, Naunyn-SchmiedbArchPharm, 1972; 273:179) and bivalent positively charged model compounds (Mol, BiochemPharm, 1990; 39:383). For many compounds this value greatly exceeds the gradient that would occur by passive equilibration of cations according to the membrane potential (−35 mV in hepatocytes). For some organic cations the sinusoidal uptake process is rate limiting in overall hepatobiliary transport (Meijer, 1972; Mol, BiochemPharm, 1990; 39:383). In such cases cytoplasm/blood plasma concentration gradients below unity have indeed been reported (Meijer, 1972; Mol, 1990). However, real 'uphill transport' against an electrochemical gradient of the cationic species is difficult to prove because many of these studies rely on subcellular distribution studies after whole liver homogenization and redistribution from the particulate fractions to the cytosol fractions cannot entirely be prevented.

Cell fractionation studies of livers taken from animals that were injected with organic cations *in vivo* revealed enrichment of the mitochondrial, lysosomal, and nuclear fractions (Meijer, Naunyn-SchmiedbArchPharm, 1972; 273:179; Meijer, JPharmExpTher, 1976; 198:229; Weitering, Naunyn-SchmiedbArchPharm, 1977; 299:277; Mol, BiochemPharm, 1990; 39:383).

Lysosomal/endosomal accumulation was confirmed by electron microscopy of electron-dense precipitates of such agents (Weitering, Naunyn-SchmiedbArchPharm, 1975; 289:251) as well as by more recent uptake studies in acidified multivesicular membrane preparations (Van Dyke, JPharmExpTher, 1992; 261:1). This sequestration process of permanently charged quaternary amines seems to be fundamentally different from the processes proposed for lysosomal uptake of tertiary organic bases such as chloroquine (MacIntyre, JPharmaceutSci, 1988; 77:196; Ward, TrendsPharmacolSci, 1988; 9:241). The latter agents can pass the lysosomal membrane passively in the uncharged form and subsequently become protonated in the acidified intraorganelle space. It was shown that organic cation transport into lysosomes is partly ATP dependent and sensitive to proton-dissipating agents such as monensin as well as to H⁺-ATPase inhibitors. Consequently, an ATP-driven proton antiport or a cation/hydroxyl symporter was proposed (Van Dyke, JPharmExpTher, 1992; 261:1) (Fig. 16).

This endosomal compartment appears to have a relatively small functional size, as displacement of the cations from the endosomes by primaquine did not lead to an increased rate of biliary excretion

(Weitering, Naunyn-SchmiedbArchPharm, 1977; 299:277; Van Dyke, JPharmExpTher, 1992; 261:1).

A number of factors determine mitochondrial sequestration: (i) the considerable intracellular volume of mitochondria; (ii) the presence of mitochondrial DNA, to which the cationic drugs can bind; and (iii) the sizeable negative membrane potential of the organelle (–220 mV) that drives the uptake process (Woolley, FEBSLett, 1987; 224:337; Steen, BiochemPharm, 1993; 45:809). Fluorescent cationic probes are widely used for measurement of the organelle membrane potential (Bunting, BiophysJ, 1989; 56:979). Initial uptake rate of various organic cations into isolated rat liver mitochondria was shown to be highly sensitive to agents that dissipate the mitochondrial membrane potential such as lipophilic cationic dyes and to ionophores such as CCCP and valinomycin (Steen, 1993). Electrogenic transport into the inner mitochondrial space was found to be (at least partly) carrier mediated and mutual competitive inhibition was demonstrated for various model organic cations.[53] Apart from electrogenic uptake, electroneutral proton antiport (or OH$^-$ symport) systems have been identified (Krämer, BBActa, 1986; 855:201).

Uptake rate into the mitochondria depends on the lipophilicity of the cationic model compounds.[53] This is supposed to be due to the relative affinity for putative carriers in the mitochondrial membranes. Carrier-mediated mitochondrial transport processes were described for choline and quinidine (Porter, JBC, 1992; 267: 14637) as well as spermidine (Toninello, JBC, 1992; 267:18393). Saturable and electrophylic choline transport was competitively inhibited by hemicholiniums, quinidine, and quinine, the latter agent being a 10-fold stronger inhibitor compared with quinidine (Porter, 1992). The polyvalent polyamines are also transported via a uniport system or channel that is membrane potential dependent (Toninello, 1992) and indirectly coupled to transport of inorganic phosphate. Interestingly, photoaffinity labelling studies with lipophilic (type 2) organic cations in hepatocytes consistently reveal labelling of the mitochondrial protein carbamoyl synthetase that is inside the mitochondrial matrix, suggesting an intraorganelle localization of the probe.[54,55]

The mitochondrial pool of organic cations can be largely mobilized by addition of inhibitors of mitochondrial function. In isolated perfused livers, addition of the proton ionophore CCCP or the K$^+$-ionophore valinomycin leads to massive efflux of the intracellularly stored organic cations back into the perfusion medium. This confirms that mitochondria constitute a major component of the hepatic storage compartment for organic cations (Steen, BiochemPharm, 1993; 45:809).

In conclusion it can be said that although the outer membrane of mitochondria provides some barriers against the effects of especially hydrophylic cationic agents (Diwan, BiochemPharm, 1988; 37:957), more lipophilic basic drugs may easily reach the mitochondrial matrix, where they may exert toxic effects (Koch, BiochemPharm, 1960; 3:231; Mannella, BBActa, 1989; 981:363). Both passive (membrane potential driven) equilibration (Woolley, FEBSLett, 1987; 224:337; Steen, BiochemPharm, 1993; 45:809) and carrier-mediated transport across both the outer and inner mitochondrial membranes (Woolley, FEBSLett, 1987; 224:337; Porter, JBC, 1992; 267: 14637)[53] may play a role in this process.

Apart from the lysosomal/endosomal and mitochondrial sequestration of organic cations, the cell nuclear material may bind considerable amounts of these agents. Nuclear staining with fluorescent cations such as propidium bromide, ethidium bromide, and acridine dyes is generally used in cytofluorometric analysis (Yeh, JImmunol, 1981; 43:269; Ronot, BiolCell, 1986; 57:1; Zimmermann, AngewChemIntEdEngl, 1986; 25:115). The relative amount of cationic drugs in the cell nucleus is dependent on the liver load (Mol, BiochemPharm, 1990; 39:383). Therefore, the extent of nuclear binding of cationic drugs does not only depend on the inherent affinity of the cationic drugs for the polyanionic DNA but also on 'saturation' of the lysosomal and mitochondrial pools. The strong intercalation of some cytostatic drugs with double-strength DNA is partly explained by their cationic character.

It was earlier assumed that quaternary probes such as ethidium bromide passively pass through pores in the nuclear envelope and bind to the polyanionic polynucleotides through electrostatic forces. Although nuclear membranes are punctured by up to 60 pores/ μm^2, simple equilibration of small anionic or cationic drugs between cytoplasmic and intranuclear compartments, according to pore diffusion, is unlikely. In fact, considerable transnuclear concentration gradients of inorganic ions as well as small organic molecules such as insulin, saccharose, and glutathione were observed (Csermely, BBActa, 1995; 1241:425). Regulated ion channels and nuclear ion pumps associated with the nuclear pore complex are operating while even proteins, bearing a nuclear localization signal (a certain amino acid sequence), can be transported across the nuclear membrane via receptor binding (Csermely, BBActa, 1995; 1241:425).

Acinar heterogeneity in intracellular binding

The acinar distribution of ligandin has been studied by several groups of investigators. The results show either a higher content in the perivenous region or a uniform distribution both in humans and rats (see Traber, Gastro, 1988; 95:1130 and references therein). The fatty acid binding protein (Z-protein) shows a zone 1 to zone 3 concentration gradient of 1.6 in male and of 1.1 in female rats (Bass, Hepatol, 1989; 9:12) indicating that the zonal distribution of net transport of fatty acids, bilirubin, and sex steroids may differ between male and female rats. For the bile acid binding protein no acinar distribution has been published yet. However, Baumgartner et al. (AmJPhysiol, 1986; 251:G431) found indications for a higher binding of the bile acid taurodeoxycholate in zone 3. Cellular organelles involved in binding also show acinar gradients: the smooth endoplasmic reticulum and lysosomes are more abundant in zone 3, mitochondrial volume is higher in zone 1, but total mitochondrial membranes are more abundant in zone 3 (Loud, JCellBiol, 1968; 37:27). The effects of this heterogeneity on hepatobiliary transport are unknown.

Kinetic analysis of the rhodamine B kinetics in livers loaded either in zone 1 or zone 3 (Braakman, Hepatol, 1987; 7:849) showed that binding of rhodamine B to organelles and membranes was higher in zone 3. Although the lower biliary excretion rate of taurocholic acid by zone 1 cells can be explained by a lower transport rate across the canalicular membrane, a possible higher binding in zone 3 might play an additional role in the heterogeneity in biliary excretion rate of taurocholic acid (Groothuis, AmJPhysiol, 1982; 243:G455). Normal and retrograde perfusion with DBSP in the absence of albumin showed steep acinar gradients (Nijssen, Hepatol, 1992; 15:302) and no difference in the kinetic pattern of biliary excretion, suggesting no acinar difference in intracellular binding of DBSP (Groothuis, unpublished results).

Sinusoidal efflux of organic compounds

Subsequent to hepatic uptake, xenobiotics (or their metabolites) can be excreted into the bile or back into the general circulation. The latter transport process is called sinusoidal efflux (Fig. 12). Sinusoidal efflux of the organic anion DBSP was inferred kinetically from data obtained *in vivo* (Meijer, JPharmExpTher, 1977; 202:8) and in isolated perfused rat liver experiments (Meijer, 1977; Meijer, JPharmacokinBiopharm, 1984; 12:43). Increasing the albumin concentration in the perfusion medium of livers preloaded with DBSP strongly increased the DBSP concentration in perfusate, which could only be explained by the bidirectionality of transport across the sinusoidal membrane (Meijer, 1984; Wolkoff, JCI, 1987; 79: 1259).

The net sinusoidal efflux rate, as measured in the perfusate of the isolated perfused rat liver, by definition is the difference between the actual sinusoidal efflux and the reuptake of ligand secreted into the sinusoid by downstream cells. Pharmacokinetic modelling indicated that albumin may have two effects (Nijssen, Hepatol, 1992; 15:302; Proost, JPharmacokinBiopharm, 1993; 21:375). First, it binds the released anion and thereby prevents reuptake. This process is association rate limited and probably occurs under non-equilibrium conditions. Second, albumin may directly stimulate the carrier-mediated transport process by unloading the efflux carrier (Nijssen, Hepatol, 1992; 15:302; Proost, JPharmacokinBiopharm, 1993; 21:375). Several investigations (Weisiger, PNAS, 1985; 82: 1563; Van der Sluijs, Hepatol, 1987; 7:688) have suggested that binding of highly extracted compounds to albumin is not at equilibrium within the sinusoid. A series of compartments model was used to simulate the hepatic handling of DBSP (Proost, 1993) (Fig. 17). These simulations showed that the net sinusoidal efflux process is association rate limited, which means that it is not the ligand–protein binding equilibrium but the rate of binding which determines the net sinusoidal efflux rate.

Interestingly, in order to mimic the experimental results accurately, both the dissociation and association rate constant of the ligand–BSA complex had to be increased compared with the *in vitro* values. This possibly indicates altered binding characteristics of the complex upon passage through the liver. Such an acceleration might be due to conformational changes of the protein following an interaction of albumin with low-affinity binding sites at the plasma membrane. Conformational changes due to interaction with isolated rat hepatocytes have been claimed (Horie, AmJPhysiol, 1988; 254: G465; Reed, JBC, 1989; 264:9867).

The data on the biliary excretion rate in the above-mentioned experiments indicated that the biliary excretion process and inusoidal efflux process occur from pharmacokinetically different ompartments (Proost, JPharmacokinBiopharm, 1993; 21:375). Pharmacokinetic modelling showed that the hepatic handling of the dye could be simulated accurately only if an intracellular 'storage' compartment was incorporated (Proost, 1993). The physiological

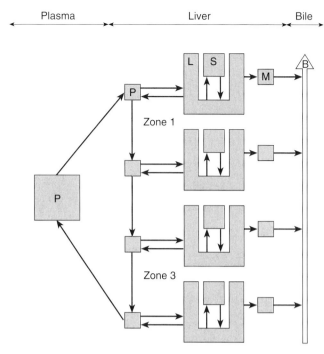

Fig. 17. Multicompartment model picturing the liver as a series of four compartments (L) each containing a slowly exchanging storage compartment (S). Drugs are taken up from sinusoidal plasma compartments (P). In the liver compartments, biotransformation to a metabolite (M) occurs, which is subsequently excreted into a run-off biliary compartment (B). Such models can simulate adequately the decreasing concentration gradients in hepatic sinusoids and liver tissue as well as biliary excretion rate patterns. Through numerical procedures they can be used to fit experimental data and establish the various rate constants for hepatic uptake, storage, and excretion in health and disease.

significance of this intracellular compartmentalization in relation to efflux at the two domains of the cell remains to be clarified.

Binding to albumin, therefore, is essential for the net efflux of anionic drugs and drug conjugates from the organ. This phenomenon may at least partly explain the predominant sinusoidal excretion of sulphate conjugates compared with glucuronide conjugates. Sulphate conjugates bind more avidly to albumin than glucuronide conjugates (Mizuma, JPharmPharmacol, 1991; 43:446).

Sinusoidal efflux of organic anions has also been demonstrated for glutathione and glutathione conjugates (Ookhtens, JCI, 1985; 75:258; Fernandez-Checa, AmJPhysiol, 1988; 255:G403; Wright, AmJPhysiol, 1988; 255:G547; Akerboom, MethodsEnz, 1989; 173: 523; Kobayashi, JBC, 1990; 265:7737) as well as for the glucuronide and sulphate conjugates of benz[*a*]pyrene (Meijer, p.165 in reference 30), morphine,[56] and harmol (De Vries, BiochemPharm, 1985; 34:2129). Harmol is conjugated in the rat by glucuronidation and sulphation only. Harmol sulphate is secreted predominantly into the general circulation and finally into the urine, whereas harmol glucuronide is equally well excreted into the bile and urine (De Vries, 1985). It has been shown that DBSP can inhibit the sinusoidal excretion and thus the urinary excretion of harmol sulphate and vice versa (De Vries, 1985).

Many studies have been focused on the sinusoidal efflux of the anionic tripeptide glutathione, a physiologically important compound in intra- and extrahepatic detoxification reactions (Nicotera,

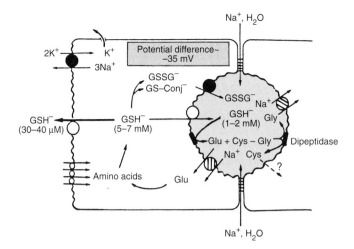

Fig. 18. Transport systems for glutathione (GSH) and glutathione conjugates at the sinusoidal and canalicular level. Glutathione transport at both poles of the cell is down an electrochemical gradient. Oxidized glutathione (GSSG) produced by oxidative stress and other glutathione conjugates may leave the cell via a carrier separate from that for glutathione at the canaliculus, but with a common mechanism at the sinusoidal level. Within the canalicular lumen, glutathione is split by dipeptidase and γ-glutamyl transferase, and glycine and glutamine are reabsorbed by Na^+-dependent mechanisms (after Meier, ref. 43).

JBC, 1985; 260:1999; Ookhtens, JCI, 1985; 75:258; Fernandez-Checa, AmJPhysiol, 1988; 255:G403; Wright, AmJPhysiol, 1988; 255:G547; Akerboom, MethodsEnz, 1989; 173:523; Kobayashi, JBC, 1990; 265:7737; Oude Elferink, AmJPhysiol, 1990; 258:G699). Over 90 per cent of total glutathione in the general circulation originates from efflux from the liver (Ookhtens, 1985; Akerboom, 1989). Sinusoidal efflux of glutathione in the isolated perfused liver can be inhibited reversibly in a dose-dependent manner by several organic anions such as oxidized glutathione, glutathione conjugates, (D) BSP, rose bengal, indocyanine green, and unconjugated bilirubin, but not by taurocholate (Ookhtens, 1985; Ookhtens, JCI, 1988; 82:608; Garcia-Ruiz, Hepatol, 1991; 14:154A). It was concluded that these anions exert their effect from inside the cell (Ookhtens, 1988) (Fig. 18).

The sinusoidal efflux of BSP, DBSP, and bilirubin is sensitive to replacement of Cl^- by gluconate in perfusion media (Wolkoff, JCI, 1987; 79:1259; Min, JCI, 1991; 87:1496; Nijssen, BiochemPharm, 1991; 42:1997) in contrast to that of glutathione (Ookhtens, JCI, 1988; 82:608). This was explained by the direct effect of the Cl^- gradient on the efflux carrier (Nijssen, 1991). In contrast, the chloride effect on BSP uptake appeared to be more of an effect on the albumin binding of BSP than on the uptake process itself. The efflux process of glutathione conjugates (Kobayashi, JBC, 1990; 265:7737; Oude Elferink, AmJPhysiol, 1990; 258:G699) and DBSP (Nijssen, 1991) is relatively insensitive to ATP depletion compared with hepatic uptake and canalicular secretion (Akerboom, MethodsEnz, 1989; 173:523; Oude Elferink, 1990). Glutathione efflux is probably driven by the negative membrane potential in contrast to that of the above-mentioned organic anions (Kobayashi, 1990; Oude Elferink, 1990; Nijssen, 1991). This points to separate efflux processes for glutathione compared with glutathione conjugates (Akerboom, MethodsEnz, 1989; 173:523; Kobayashi, JBC, 1990; 265:7737) and other organic anions. Nevertheless, *cis*-inhibition and

trans-stimulation suggest at least overlapping substrate specificity (Ookhtens, 1988; Garcia-Ruiz, Hepatol, 1991; 14:154A). The sinusoidal transporter is only expressed in liver, is clearly *cis*-inhibited by BSP–glutathione conjugate, and is sensitive to thiol reduction and oxidation. In contrast, the 'canalicular' transporter is found in many organs, is not *cis*-inhibited by glutathione conjugates, and it is resistant to thiol-modifying agents. Cloning of the sinusoidal excretion carrier has not yet been successful. However, the involvement of oatp$_1$ seems likely since expression cloning of this protein demonstrated that it might function as a bi-directional carrier.

Acinar heterogeneity in sinusoidal efflux

Zonal heterogeneity in the sinusoidal efflux process has not been investigated extensively. Braakman *et al.* (Hepatol, 1987; 7:849; JPharmExpTher, 1989; 249:869) measured the sinusoidal efflux of rhodamine B in zone 1 by retrograde perfusion of livers previously loaded in zone 1 by antegrade perfusion, and in zone 3 by antegrade perfusion of livers loaded in zone 3 by retrograde perfusion, in order to prevent reuptake of excreted substrates in the non-loaded zones. They found a 1.4-fold higher excretion rate constant for zone 3 than zone 1.

Nijssen *et al.* (Hepatol, 1992; 15:302), using a somewhat different technique, could not find an acinar heterogeneity in the sinusoidal excretion of DBSP. Sinusoidal efflux of bile acids is very low in normal conditions, but increases for taurodeoxycholic acid after 4 days of bile drainage to a similar degree in zone 1 and zone 3 (Baumgartner, Gastro, 1991; 100:1054).

Canalicular transport of organic compounds

The final, and for most drugs rate-limiting, step in hepatobiliary transport is excretion across the canalicular membrane. This transport step results in large concentration gradients between the canalicular space and the liver, which may amount to bile/liver concentration ratios of about 1000, as was shown for bile acids, DBSP,[2] and organic cations (Mol, BiochemPharm, 1990; 39:383; Mol, BiochemPharm, 1992; 44:1453).

A number of mechanisms may explain this cell to bile 'uphill' transport. Anionic compounds may be driven out of the cell by the negative membrane potential (Meier, BiochemJ, 1987; 242:465; Weinman, AmJPhysiol, 1989; 256:G826),[43] whereas cationic drugs may at least partly be excreted by countertransport with inorganic cations (Ruifrok, BiochemPharm, 1982; 31:1431; Moseley, JPharmExpTher, 1996; 276:561). However, the bile/liver concentration gradients of organic anions are larger than can be explained by the hepatocyte membrane potential. One factor to explain this is that net transport into bile is helped by association of the excreted compounds with biliary micelles and/or vesicles in the primary bile (Scharschmidt, JCI, 1978; 62:1122). However, recently, it became clear that for bile acids and other anionic compounds as well as for cationic agents, ATP-dependent (electroneutral) transport systems operate in the canalicular membrane (Kamimoto, JBC, 1989; 264:11693; Ishikawa, JBC, 1990; 265:19279; Oude Elferink, AmJPhysiol, 1990; 258:G699; Adachi, Hepatol, 1991; 14:655; Kobayashi, BBResComm, 1991; 176:622; Sinicrope, JBC, 1992;

267:24995; Müller, FEBSLett, 1994; 343:168; Müller, AmJPhysiol, 1997; 272:G1285).

An alternative to such active transport mechanisms of biliary components is intracellular vesicular transport. Some have suggested that at least part of the micelles and vesicles composed of cholesterol, phospholipids, and bile acids, are formed within the cells in the vicinity of the Golgi system (Crawford, SemLivDis, 1988; 8:105; Erlinger, BiomedPharmacoth, 1990; 44:409; Nathanson, Hepatol, 1991; 14:551), and that these vesicles would subsequently be transported to the canalicular membrane through an active effort of the microtubular system (Nathanson, 1991). Exocytosis of the vesicles would then result in extrusion into the biliary lumen. In principle this may also form a pathway for any hydrophobic organic compound as the affinity of such agents for biliary micelles is positively correlated with their hydrophobicity (Tokumo, Hepatol, 1988; 8:1265). However, for bile acids, vesicular transport may only be important quantitatively at a relatively high, non-physiological, bile salt flux. Bilirubin conjugates formed within the endoplasmic reticulum may partly join this transport route although the relative contribution to the total biliary secretion may be modest. Autoradiographic pictures of taurocholate in liver tissue and bile ductules shortly after *in vivo* injection of tracer do indicate a transit time of considerably less than 1 min (Fig. 10) (Groothuis, AmJPhysiol, 1982; 243:G455). For several substrates, for which vesicular transport is clearly demonstrated, the transcellular transport takes more than 10 min. Therefore, the transport of bile salts into bile may occur predominantly from the cytoplasm directly across the canalicular membranes through active carrier-mediated transport.[43]

Canalicular transport of organic anions

Distinct carrier systems appear to operate for bile acids and for non-bile acid organic anions. This was inferred from studies with mutant rats with a clearly deficient biliary excretion of most non-bile acid organic anions but with normal bile acid output, the so-called TR⁻ or GY rat (Jansen, Hepatol, 1987; 7:71; Kuipers, JLipRes, 1989; 30:1835; Oude Elferink, Hepatol, 1989; 9:861; Oude Elferink, JCI, 1989; 84:476). The results of these studies were in line with the findings in studies with mutant Corriedale sheep (Barnhart, Hepatol, 1981; 1:441) and in patients with the Dubin–Johnson syndrome (Javitt, Gastro, 1978; 75:931). Transport of non-bile acid organic anions at the canalicular level occurs through exchange with one or more HCO_3^- or SO_4^{2-} ions (Anwer, AmJPhysiol, 1988; 255:G713).[2]

Two bile acid carriers were shown to be present in the bile canalicular membrane. The putative bile acid carrier for monovalent bile acids was proposed to be a 110-kDa glycoprotein and operates as an ATP-dependent transporter with a low K_m (in the micromolar range) for taurocholate (Stieger, BiochemJ, 1992; 284:67). It was supposed to transport taurine- and glycine-conjugated bile salts as well as unconjugated bile salts (Nishida, PNAS, 1991; 88:6590; Stieger, 1992), and was called cBAT. The transport of bivalent anionic bile salts appeared to be mediated by cMOAT (see below). More recently, a so-called sister gene of Pgp (Spgp) was identified by isolating a cDNA clone from a rat library, homologous to the pig Spgp-cDNA. By expressing this cDNA in oocytes, ATP-dependent transport of taurocholate was shown to be mediated by Spgp. Also,

in membranes of baculovirus-infected Sfg cells, similar results were found (Gerloff, Hepatol, 1997; 26:358A). These results strongly suggest that cBAT and Spgp are identical and that Spgp is the bile salt transporter in the canalicular membrane. In man, deficiency in bile salt transport was found in PFIC1 and PFIC2 patients, suggesting a mutation in the human Spgp gene in these patients.

There is growing evidence that multiple anion carriers are operable at the canalicular domain of the cell. On the basis of interaction studies *in vivo* and canalicular membrane vesicles (Sathirakul, JPharmExpTher, 1993; 268:65), a differentiation was made between a 'DBSP system' that also accommodates leukotriene metabolites and cephalosporins, and an indocyanine green system (Sathirakul, 1993). Indocyanine green and (D)BSP excretion into bile are also affected differently in TR⁻ mutant rats (Kuipers, p.215 in reference 13), mutual inhibition studies (Meijer, JPharmacokinBiopharm, 1984; 12:43), and in patients with a genetic defect in organic anion transport (Okuda, Gut, 1976; 17:588).

Many organic anions have been shown to be substrates for the so-called canalicular organic anion transporter (cMOAT). This protein has been cloned recently (Kartenbeck, Hepatol, 1996; 23:1061; Paulusma, Science, 1996; 271:1126; Yamazaki, PharmaceutRes, 1996; 13:495) (Table 3). As concluded from studies with the transport mutant rats (TR⁻ or GY), which lack the activity of cMOAT, many bivalent anionic compounds like BSP, DBSP, glutathione, oxidized glutathione, glutathione conjugates, bilirubin conjugates, and leukotriene C4 are transported into bile by cMOAT in an ATP-dependent way (Yedkitschky, BiochemJ, 1997; 327:305). This transporter is probably regulated through protein kinase C-mediated phosphorylation (Oude Elferink, JHepatol, 1996; 24:94). In addition, divalent anionic bile salts as sulphated taurolithocholic acid appear to be substrates for cMOAT (Kuipers, JCI, 1988; 81:1593). It has been suggested that cMOAT could be identical to the so-called MDR-related proteins (**MRP₁**), an ATP-dependent carrier system that is overexpressed in tumour cells, apart from P-glycoprotein itself (Mayer, JCellBiol, 1995; 131:137). However, recent studies indicate that cMOAT is not identical to MRP₁. In fact, MRP₁ is expressed in many tissues in the body but poorly in the liver. Instead, a closely related and liver-specific isoform was detected, which was called MRP₂ (Fig. 19). Sequence analysis in normal and TR⁻ (GY) rats as well as substrate specificity indicate that MRP₂ is identical to cMOAT. The functional defect in the mutant rat strain was shown to be due to a point mutation in the particular carrier protein (Büchler, JBC, 1996; 271:15091; Paulusma, Science, 1996; 271:1126) (Table 3). Both the rat and human MRP₂ were cloned and appeared to have homology with MRP₁/mrp₁. They both exhibit similar specificity and transport a broad range of amphipatic anionic conjugates with similar kinetic parameters (Ishikawa, JBC, 1990; 265:9279; Jedlitsckky, CancRes, 1996; 56:988; Oude Elferink, BBA RevBiomembranes, 1995; 1241:215). In analogy with the TR- rat, Paulusma *et al.* (Hepatol, 1997; 25:1539) recently demonstrated that the Dubin–Johnson syndrome in man is based on mutations in the cMOAT-gene.

Earlier suggestions for vesicular transport of bile acids combined with other biliary components (Crawford, LabInvest, 1994; 71:42; Crawford, JLipRes, 1995; 36:2147; Erlinger, JHepatol, 1996; 24:88), through presequestrations in the endoplasmic reticulum or Golgi vesicles and vectorial transport to the canaliculus followed by exocytosis, have been dismissed recently (Crawford, 1994;

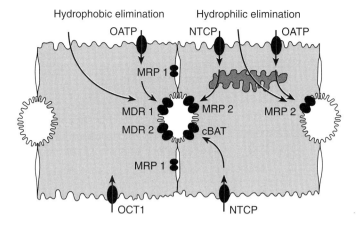

Fig. 19. Current concepts on carrier-mediated transport of organic compounds in the liver. A sinusoidal uptake system that has been cloned recently is the organic anion transporting polypeptide (OATP), which also may accommodate amphiphilic cations and uncharged compounds. OCT_1 represents the organic cation transporter that is responsible for uptake of a wide variety of endogenous and exogenous cations. NTCP stands for the Na^+ taurocholate cotransporting polypeptide that accommodates mostly conjugated bile acids. At the canalicular level, the P-glycoproteins MDR_1 and MDR_2 are involved in the excretion of bulky organic cations and phospholipids, respectively. MRP_2 (multidrug resistance-related protein) is identical to cMOAT (the canalicular multispecific organic anion transporter). MRP_1 is only present in lateral plasma membranes and possibly in intracellular organelles. Finally, cBAT is the canalicular bile acid transporter, which was recently identified as being identical to the sister of P-glycoprotein (Spgp) (Gerloff, Hepatol, 1997; 26:358A).

Crawford, 1995; Erlinger, 1996). Instead, the observed interactions of bile acids with intracellular organelles may have a regulatory role, for instance in the vesicular trafficking of bile acid carrier proteins from the Golgi/endoplasmic reticulum to the canalicular membranes and vice versa (Erlinger, JHepatol, 1996; 24:88; Oude Elferink, JHepatol, 1996; 24:94). There is now abundant evidence that bile acid/phospholipid/cholesterol vesicles present in bile arise from bile salt-induced vesiculation of lipid microdomains in the canalicular membrane (Crawford, JLipRes, 1995; 36:2147; Oude Elferink, JHepatol, 1995; 23:617) (Table 3).

Canalicular transport of organic cations

Many studies have described the inhibition of biliary excretion of organic cations by structurally related compounds *in vivo* and isolated perfused livers (Steen, p.239 in reference 13).[1,3,10] In some cases, mutual inhibition for pairs of cationic drugs was observed. These studies pointed to the involvement of carrier-mediated transport. More recently, interaction studies with compounds that are known substrates or inhibitors of P-glycoprotein (MDR) pump systems (Zamora, MolPharm, 1988; 33:454; Speeg, Hepatol, 1992; 15:899; Watanabe, JHepatol, 1992; 16:77; Gottesman, AnnRevBiochem, 1993; 62:385; Speeg, CancChemoPharm, 1993; 32:434; Thalhammer, EurJPharm, 1994; 270:213)[57] have suggested the involvement of P-glycoprotein and/or a related ATP-dependent translocator(s) in the biliary excretion process of organic cations. The canalicular localization of P-glycoproteins (mdr1a, mdr1b, and mdr2) that was demonstrated by immunochemistry and

photoaffinity labelling in rodent liver (Fojo, PNAS, 1987; 84:265; Thiebaut, PNAS, 1987; 84:7735; Bradley, JCellPhysiol, 1990; 145:398; Buschman, JBC, 1992; 267:18093) may support such a hypothesis.

In addition, a number of other observations, albeit indirectly, support the hypothesis that P-glycoprotein is one of the putative cation carriers responsible for biliary excretion of bulky (amphiphilic) organic cations. In the first place, ATP-dependent transport has been demonstrated in canalicular membrane vesicles and in plasma membrane vesicles of MDR-transfected cells for various amphiphilic basic drugs such as daunomycin (Kamimoto, JBC, 1989; 264:11693; Sinicrope, JBC, 1992; 267:24995), as well as quinidine, deoxyajmalinum, and their quaternary N-pentyl derivatives (Müller, FEBSLett, 1994; 343:168). Second, excretion of cationic antineoplastic agents but also type I cations such as TBuMA and type II cations as rocuronium in bile in the intact organ is greatly inhibited by verapamil and other so-called MDR-reversal agents (Speeg, Hepatol, 1992; 15:899; Watanabe, JHepatol, 1992; 16:77; Thalhammer, EurJPharm, 1994; 270:213; Smit, BrJPharmacol, 1998; in press).[57] In addition, it was found that induction of mdr1a through partial hepatectomy and regeneration leads to induction of an increased biliary clearance of vinblastine (Schrenk, Hepatol, 1993; 17:854). Finally, photoaffinity labelling of canalicular membranes and plasma membranes of mdr1b-transfected cells revealed a protein of 140 kDa, being in the range of deglycosylated P-glycoprotein.

There is evidence that the basal activity of P-glycoprotein is modulated through phosphorylation/dephosphorylation reactions mediated through protein kinase and probably other kinases (Grunicke, PharmTher, 1992; 55:1; Versantvoort, BrJCanc, 1993; 68:939). Therefore, protein kinase may also be involved in the short-term regulation of canalicular drug transport. A recent study demonstrates that protein kinase modulators affect the biliary excretion rate of the monovalent organic cation tributylmethylammonium (Steen, Hepatol, 1993; 18:1208). A dose-dependent stimulation was found for phorbol esters that stimulate the enzyme. Vasopressin, which indirectly increases enzyme activity, also increased biliary output of the quaternary amine, whereas the protein kinase C inhibitor staurosporine blocked these effects and also lowered the basal excretion rate. These effects were observed in the intact (isolated perfused) liver and were unrelated to moderate changes in bile flow and uptake rate of the organic cation (Steen, 1993). The fact that MDR-reversal agents such as verapamil and quinidine almost completely inhibit tributylmethylammonium excretion into bile at an unchanged bile flow[57] indicates that such lipophilic amines not only interact with P-glycoprotein but also with other organic cation carriers. In this respect it is important to note that excretion of both type 1 and type 2 organic cations into bile is 60 to 70 per cent reduced in mice with disrupted *mdr1a* and *mdr1b* genes, directly demonstrating the excretory role of these proteins. Yet, even in the complete absence of both P-glycoproteins in these mice, there is still a residual excretion of the cationic drugs (Smit, Hepatol, 1996; 24:214A; Smit, Hepatol, 1998, in press; Smit, BrJPharmacol, 1998, in press). These observations point to at least one additional organic cation transport system at the canalicular level that is not identical to mdr1a or mdr1b. A non-ATP-dependent H^+-antiport system for tributylmethylammonium was earlier identified in canalicular membrane vesicles (Moseley, JPharmExpTher,

1996; 276:561). This carrier system might be related to a 110-kDA protein that, apart from the P-glycoprotein, is consistently photolabelled in these canalicular membrane preparations.[36] Another candidate for canalicular transport of cationic drugs is the aforementioned MRP$_2$ carrier system that, as well as accommodating organic anions, may also have affinity for more lipophilic organic cations (see Table 3).

The general picture emerging from the above-mentioned studies is that supposed cation transport systems in the canaliculus are multispecific and display overlapping substrate specificity, depending on the hydrophobicity/hydrophilicity balance in the particular molecules. Even hydrophobic bile acids and organic anions such as oestradiol glucuronide (Gosland, CancerRes, 1993; 53:5382; Vore, ToxApplPharmacol, 1993; 118:2) may, therefore, inhibit both the P-glycoprotein and MRP$_2$ transport systems (Arias, Hepatol, 1993; 18:216).

Acinar heterogeneity in canalicular transport of anions and cations

Both for taurocholate and taurodeoxycholate it was shown (Fig. 10) that, after a single dose, excretion is slower in retrograde perfusions, where zone 3 cells are mainly involved in biliary excretion, than in antegrade perfusions, where zone 1 cells are mainly involved (Groothuis, AmJPhysiol, 1982; 243:G455; Baumgartner, AmJPhysiol, 1986; 251:G431; Reichen, Experientia, 1989; 45:135). Two explanations can be given: either zone 3 cells have less canalicular carriers or zone 3 cells have more bile acid-binding protein, resulting in a lower free concentration and thus slower biliary excretion. Probably both effects may contribute to these zonal differences. After increasing the bile salt load over several days by either choledochocaval shunting (Baumgartner, AmJPhysiol, 1987; 252:G114), cholate feeding (Reichen, 1989), or partial hepatectomy (Baumgartner, JHepatol, 1995; 22:474), zone 3 cells appear to excrete moderate doses of bile salts almost as fast as zone 1 cells, indicating increased carrier activity (Simon, JCI, 1982; 70:401). However, in this situation a tracer dose is excreted at an even lower rate than in control rats, indicating an induction of binding protein. Bile drainage on the contrary results in a decreased transport rate in zone 1 and thus in loss of heterogeneity (Baumgartner, Gastro, 1991; 100:1054). Both the lower excretion rate and the higher binding capacity lead to a higher residence time of bile acids in zone 3. For taurodeoxycholic acid this results in a higher percentage of the load excreted as metabolites by zone 3 cells than by zone 1 (Baumgartner, 1986). In contrast, zone 3 cells have a higher excretion rate of more polar and detergent metabolites of tauro-lithocholate. The higher metabolic rate of the cholestatic taurolithocholate in zone 3 cells results in lower concentrations of this toxic compound in zone 3 and this explains why tauro-lithocholate has a high cholestatic potency in antegrade perfusions and hardly any cholestatic potency in retrograde perfusions (Baumgartner, LabInvest, 1987; 56:576). The excretion rate of glycocholic acid appears similar in zone 1 and zone 3 (Sherman, Hepatol, 1986; 6:444; Groothuis, unpublished observations).

Interestingly, preliminary experiments indicated that the biliary excretion rate of a tracer dose of glycocholic acid is similar or even slightly faster in retrograde perfusions than in normal perfusion. This indicates that zone 3 cells have similar or even higher excretion

rate for glycocholate. The biliary excretion rate of the anion DBSP appeared not to be different between the zone 1 and zone 3 cells (Nijssen, Hepatol, 1992; 15:302). The results from studies using selective acinar toxicity were not in line with the above-mentioned results (Groothuis, NaunynSchmiedbArchPharm, 1983; 322:298, 310). However, in these studies, both adaptation of the non-damaged zone and specific inhibition of the carriers by the zone 1 toxin may have influenced the outcome significantly.

The T_{max} for the excretion rate of the glutathione conjugate of BSP is lower in zone 3 than in zone 1 (Chen, Hepatol, 1984; 4:467). Using intravital televisual microscopy, Sherman and Fisher (Sherman, Hepatol, 1986; 6:444) found indications that zone 1 cells excrete fluorescein much faster than zone 3 cells.

The only cationic substrate for which zonal heterogeneity in biliary excretion was studied is rhodamine B (Braakman, Hepatol, 1987; 7:849; Braakman, JPharmExpTher, 1989; 249:869). A higher rate constant for biliary excretion was found in zone 1. Taking into account the higher intracellular binding and sinusoidal excretion in zone 3 for this substrate, the biliary excretion rate might be even more different than expected from the difference in rate constant only.

Biliary reabsorption

Substrates excreted into the primary bile become associated with biliary micelles. Compounds of relatively low molecular weight, especially the hydrophilic ones, will be partly present in bile in the unbound form (Scharschmidt, JCI, 1978; 62:1122; Reuben, Hepatol, 1984; 4:15S).[58] This would provide a driving force for diffusion back into the cells or across the tight junctions in between the cells back into the blood. The tight junction channels (Fig. 18) have a diameter that allows compounds of less than 200 Da in molecular mass to pass (Boyer, YaleJBiolMed, 1979; 52:61). By their inner net negative charge they may only favour the passage of cationic molecules (Bradley, AmJPhysiol, 1978; 235:E570). Such a 'perm-selective' passage may lead to a loss of drug molecules from the primary bile, but in principle also allows a direct passage from blood into the biliary spaces (Boyer, 1979). Such processes may operate for small organic cations that are poorly recovered from bile (Neef, BiochemPharm, 1984; 33:3977). Taurocholate was shown to increase biliary output of certain organic cations without stimulating their uptake into the liver. Transport of the cations may, therefore, occur via direct transfer from plasma into the canaliculi (Neef, 1984).

Data on transport of reduced glutathione, oxidized glutathione, and bile acids in canalicular vesicles point to potential bidirectional fluxes across the canalicular membrane. The net flux of drugs and organic solutes may therefore be largely influenced by the relative intra- and extracellular binding to proteins and (biliary) micelles, apart from being determined by the membrane potential and coupling to gradients of inorganic ions.

The possibility of canalicular reabsorption (also called back-flux) of organic solutes is relevant in relation to the mechanism of stimulation of biliary output of drugs by choleretic agents. Biliary excretion of indocyanine green, BSP, and DBSP, especially after relatively high doses, can be strongly stimulated by infusion of bile salts and some non-bile salt choleretics.[14,16,21,24,42] Dilution of the concentration in primary bile would decrease the bile-to-cell gradient and in principle could explain this phenomenon.[58] However, while for some organic anions the stimulatory effect is highly correlated with bile flow,[58] for others this is not the case. Some potent non-bile salt choleretics (mostly glucuronides) leave biliary output of organic anions virtually unchanged (Erlinger, Gastro, 1974; 66:281; Forker, p.326 in reference 38). This lack of effect cannot be fully explained by concomitant competitive inhibition at the canalicular membrane or to an unequal acinar and/or intracellular compartmentalization of the choleretics and the dyes. The bile salt effects discussed above may also be explained by allosteric membrane effects (Forker, p.326 in reference 38) or alternatively attributed to recruitment of pericentral cells in biliary excretion (Goresky, CanJPhysPharm, 1974; 52:389). However, bile salts fail to increase transport of dyes out of isolated hepatocytes, which would be expected if allosteric effects play a role (Vonk, BiochemPharm, 1978; 27:397). Also, the bile salt stimulatory effect on organic anion secretion is maintained even after selective destruction of zone 3 cells (González, BiochemPharm, 1985; 34:507).

It is important to note that the bile salt effect is most prominent at 'transport maximum conditions' of the dyes, a situation in which the liver is loaded with the model compound and aspecific toxic effects on the plasma membranes or intracellular organelles can be anticipated. There is evidence that taurocholate prevents accumulation of, and toxic effects of, BSP in mitochondria (Gregus, ArchInternatPharmTher, 1979; 238:124) and also prevents precipitation of aggregating dyes at the canaliculi (Vonk, Naunyn-SchmiedbArchPharm, 1974; 282:401). It may thereby increase the 'apparent transport maximum of dyes', a phenomenon that probably represents a labile equilibrium between maximal membrane transport of the dyes and the inherent negative influence on cell metabolism.

Apart from this effect, bile salts induce the formation of drug-binding micelles and thereby promote 'sink conditions' for removal of the compounds (Scharschmidt, JCI, 1978; 62:1122). However, this cannot be a general mechanism, since non-micelle forming bile salts can also have a major stimulatory effect (Delage, AmJPhysiol, 1976; 231:1875). The conclusion is that more than one mechanism may play a role in the stimulation of biliary output, depending on the nature and dose of the bile salts and the type of cholephilic compound studied. Choleresis does not lead uniformly to improved biliary elimination as shown for some organic cations and cardiac glycosides[58] while, as mentioned above, the effect for organic anions is variable, depending on the bile salt or non-bile salt choleretics used.

Reabsorption of organic solutes from the biliary tree has been demonstrated for amino acids *in vivo* (Ballatori, AmJPhysiol, 1988; 254:G1). Reversed transport from bile into the hepatocytes and/or from bile directly into the bloodstream may underlie the observed reabsorption of various organic compounds, as studied by the technique of segmented retrograde biliary injection.[56] The loss from the biliary tree with the latter technique was negatively correlated with the molecular weight of the compounds and suggests some form of pore transport. Both back transport across the canalicular domain of the hepatocytes via the tight junctions in between the cells or alternatively across the ductular epithelia is possible (Strazzabosco, JHepatol, 1996; 24:78) (Fig. 20). The arterial supply to the peribiliary plexus may be essential in the exchange of bile and blood constituents at the ductular level. A cholehepatic shunt

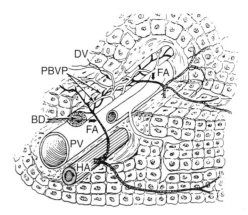

Fig. 20. Schematic representation of the portal tract with the peribiliary vascular plexus (PBVP). HA, hepatic artery; PV, portal vein; FA, feeder artery for PBVP; DV, drainage vein for PBVP.

pathway in which undissociated non-bile acids are reabsorbed at this level has been suggested (Hofmann, p.553 in reference 26). Such a local circulation of these bile salts may explain their potent choleretic effects on a molar basis (Hofmann, p.553 in reference 26).

It has been claimed that epithelial cells of the bile ductules possess a transport system for organic anions that is probably carrier mediated (Sleyster, LabInvest, 1982; 47:484; Stremmel, BBActa, 1989; 1014:108; Elsing, JHepatol, 1996; 24:121). Transport of such agents out of the bile to the general circulation could be mediated by such a process. It may correlate with the carrier-mediated tubular reabsorption system in the kidney. Such 'active' reabsorption processes in the bile ducts deserve further study in relation to the regulation of enterohepatic cycling and biliary elimination of organic compounds.

Hepatic disposition of macromolecules in relation to targeting of drugs and genes to the liver

Drug targeting to the liver can be achieved either by coupling therapeutic agents to macromolecules or by enclosing drugs into particles that have a high affinity for one of the cell types within the organ (Poznansky, PharmRev, 1984; 36:277; Fallon, AdvDrugDelRev, 1989; 4:49; Fiume, AdvDrugDelRev, 1994; 14:51; Meijer, AntiviralRes, 1992; 18:215; Monsigny, AdvDrugDelRev, 1994; 14:1). Distribution of the drug in the whole organism is now dictated by the nature of the chosen macromolecular carrier rather than by the physicochemical features of the parent drug. The more specific distribution in the body and delivery of the particular drug to the intended cell type can improve drug efficacy and at the same time reduce the side-effects that normally occur during single or chronic administration of the parent drug. Obviously, this concept is only useful if the drug is released within the particular cells in an active or preactive form. After intracellular release it should not be rapidly redistributed to other tissues. Neither the carrier nor its degradation products should exhibit overt toxicity to the organ, nor induce immunological reactions or general side-effects.

Many drugs by themselves reach high concentrations in the liver. This is due to a rapid uptake from the bloodstream by the aforementioned passive- or carrier-mediated processes.[1,2] Orally absorbed drugs with a high first-pass distribution in the liver are efficiently taken up in this organ. Generally, however, no cell specificity is obtained and, after a steady state has been reached, redistribution from the liver to other tissues will occur.

Drug targeting to the liver is performed for diagnostic and therapeutic purposes. Liver disorders or liver metabolism can be influenced by various agents. Agents for antiviral, antiparasitic, antineoplastic, or antilipidaemic effects, drugs counteracting liver fibrosis or hepatotoxic reactions, and genetic material (DNA) to correct genetic enzyme deficiencies can be specifically targeted to hepatocytes, Kupffer cells, and endothelial and stellate cells (formerly called Ito cells, fat-storing cells, or lipocytes).

Drug targeting implies the manipulation of drug distribution in the whole body. Therefore, drug delivery and drug targeting are research areas in which *in vivo* studies in animals and patients are crucial for the demonstration of targeting efficacy. Yet, *in vitro* studies with potential target cells can be helpful to study the relative rate of endocytosis, carrier degradation, and intracellular release of the targeted drug. Clearly, investigations in the intact organism (including studies in the diseased state) should provide more definite clues with regard to the cell specificity of the chosen carrier system as well as its toxicity and immunogenicity. In addition, the potential to pass anatomical barriers en route to the target cells can only be controlled *in vivo*.

Currently, carrier systems include particle-type carriers such as liposomes, lipid particles (LDL, HDL), microspheres, and nanoparticles as well as soluble carriers. Soluble carrier systems can be derived from monoclonal antibodies, modified plasma proteins, polyamino acids, polysaccharides, and other biodegradable polymers. In some cases the carrier can be designed such that it contributes to the therapeutic effects (Meijer, AntiviralRes, 1992; 18:215). Examples are modified enzymes that can deal with certain aspects of inflammation and fibrosis (superoxide dismutase, alkaline phosphatase, collagenases), antiviral proteins (interferons, negatively charged albumins), and certain growth factors and monoclonal antibodies.

The mechanisms responsible for the disposition of oligopeptides and proteins in the body include carrier-mediated transport (in the liver, kidneys, gut, and central nervous system), filtration, and reabsorption (in the kidneys) as well as receptor-mediated endocytosis (in the liver and various other tissues), while phagocytosis (in macrophages) occurs for particles (Fig. 21). Important features determining the fate of these macromolecules in the body are chemical composition, spatial conformation, overall size, net charge, presence of sugars, aggregation state, and possible opsonization by blood components.

Small peptide carriers (up to 12 amino acids) can be efficiently cleared by the liver depending on hydrophobicity and charge through different carrier systems, some of which are bile acid transporters. Time- and dose-dependent (saturation) kinetics, extremely short half-lives, and low bioavailability can therefore result.[8]

Larger carrier molecules (up to about 50 kDa) are easily filtrated by the kidney. Peptide carriers of that size are often fully reabsorbed and degraded in lysosomes of the renal tubules. Such proteins of low molecular weight can therefore be used as drug carriers for renal-specific drug delivery. Targeting to the kidney of anti-inflammatory drugs, antimicrobial agents, angiotensin-converting enzyme inhibitors, and dopaminergic compounds has been studied (Franssen, AdvDrugDelRev, 1994; 14:67).

Glycoproteins can be recognized by sugar-specific receptors or scavenger receptors in various cell types in the body. For instance, the extent and type of glycosylation can be crucial for the elimination of monoclonal antibodies. Complex formation of antibodies with circulating antigens can largely determine their fate in the body through removal via Fc receptors on macrophages. Glycoconjugates can be used for cell-specific targeting of antiviral drugs to the liver (viral hepatitis) (Molema, AdvDrugDelRev, 1994; 14:25; Meijer, p.303 in reference 59)[8] and blood cells (HIV infections) (Meijer, AntiviralRes, 1992; 18:215). Such drug targeting devices can also be used for delivery of antisense nucleotides and genes to reprogramme various cell types in the body *in vivo* to produce proteins with therapeutic activity (Wu, JBC, 1989; 264:16985; Meijer, 1992; Keegan-Rogers, p.105 in reference 60).

Endocytosis in various cell types of the liver

The liver contains several cell types of which the arrangement in the hepatic acinus is depicted in Fig. 1, showing hepatocytes, endothelial cells, Kupffer cells, and stellate cells. Their contribution to total liver volume is 78, 2.8, 2.1, and 1.4 per cent (Hendriks, Hepatol, 1987; 7:1368; Brouwer, p.665 in reference 26)[5] and to the total liver cell volume 92.5, 3.3, 2.5, and 1.6 per cent, respectively. Disposition of low molecular weight xenobiotics (including most of the commonly used drugs) mainly occurs by the hepatocytes. However, non-parenchymal cells as well as hepatocytes play a prominent role in handling macromolecules.

Endothelial cells

The sinusoidal endothelial cells form the sinusoidal lining and this endothelium forms a sieved wall with fenestrations of diameter 50 to 150 nm (Brouwer, p.665 in reference 26). The arrangement of endothelial cells enables hepatocytes to exchange substances with plasma via the space of Disse. However, because of the limited size of the pores, there is a distinct selection of substances by size. Molecules with a molecular weight exceeding 250 kDa cannot pass through the pores (Brouwer, p.665 in reference 26),[5] and therefore do not interact significantly with hepatocytes. This can only partly protect the hepatocytes against direct injuries caused by bacteria and viruses. However, the dimensions of this barrier are dynamic (Fraser, Hepatol, 1995; 21:863) and are influenced by pathological conditions as well as properties of the micro-organisms and cells that infiltrate by chemical activation or deformation.[5]

These endothelial cells express most of the functions of Kupffer cells and possess prominent vacuolar structures that are indicative of a well developed endocytic apparatus operating in the removal of plasma-borne substances. Endothelial cells express most of the functions of the Kupffer cells and produce thromboxane and prostaglandins among other mediators but do not form coagulation factor VI in contrast to endothelial cells of other tissues. The hepatic capillaries or sinusoids contract through their endothelial lining and fat-storing cells after nerve stimulation or administration of vasoactive hormones and other mediators (Fraser, Hepatol, 1995; 21:863).[5]

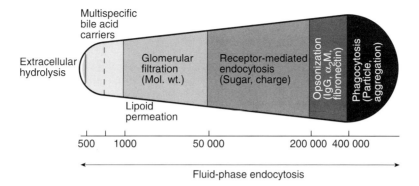

Fig. 21. Clearance mechanisms for small peptides (oligopeptides) and larger peptides (proteins) in the body; these are dependent on size, charge, exposed sugars (in glycoproteins), aggregation, and opsonization of the proteins in the circulation. Relatively small peptides can be filtrated passively in the kidneys, hydrolysed in the blood at cell surfaces, or be recognized by sinusoidal membrane carriers. For larger (glyco-) proteins, binding to receptors leads to cellular uptake. The relative contribution of these processes in distribution and elimination is dependent (among other factors) on the size of the peptide molecule. Functional groups (terminal sugars), charge, and hydrophobicity determine the affinity of monomeric proteins for various receptor-mediated endocytotic processes. Phagocytosis is the removal mechanism for aggregated and opsonized proteins. Fluid-phase endocytosis occurs over the entire range of molecular weight.

Kupffer cells

These are located in the sinusoidal lumen at intersections of sinusoids and are anchored to the endothelial cells by long processes. The prominent location of Kupffer cells in zone 1 of the acinus suggests that blood entering the sinusoid is monitored for material that can be endocytosed. It appears that in analogy to hepatocytes there is also a functional heterogeneity in the Kupffer cell population, for instance with regard to endocytic and tumouricidal capacities (Smit, Hepatol, 1991; 12:1192; Moghimi, CritRevTherDrugCarrSys, 1994; 11:31; Brouwer, p.665 in 26). Kupffer cells are part of the reticuloendothelial system and represent 80 to 90 per cent of all resident macrophages in the body. Kupffer cells also modulate certain hepatocyte functions through the release of peptide and lipid mediators, demonstrating a local and chemical communication between these cell types (Brouwer, p.665 in reference 26; Jones, p.683 in reference 26).[5] The liver macrophages are activated by agents such as β-interferon, endotoxins, platelet-activating factor, phorbol esters, zymosan, and Ca^{2+}-ionophores. Following activation they produce cytokines such as interleukin 1 and 6, tumour necrosis factor-α, and β-interferon as well as lipid mediators (platelet-activating factor, leukotrienes, and prostaglandins).[5] In addition, they liberate oxygen-derived radicals and lysosomal enzymes. The composition of the mixture of agents released from Kupffer cells is largely determined by the nature of the stimulatory agent. The released factors may subsequently affect microcirculation and production of glucose and acute-phase proteins by hepatocytes, among others (Brouwer, p.665 in reference 26; Jones, p.683 in reference 26). The surface of Kupffer cells displays a wealth of receptors that are involved in the endocytosis of macromolecules (Moghimi, 1994).

Hepatic stellate cells (fat-storing cells, lipocytes)

These cells are situated in the space of Disse between endothelial cells and hepatocytes (Hendriks, Hepatol, 1987; 7:1368; Brouwer, p.665 in reference 26), and they have a well defined role in vitamin A metabolism and collagen biosynthesis (Hendriks, 1987; Brouwer, p.665 in reference 26). Recently, more became known about the disposition of macromolecules in this cell type (Friedman, AmJPhysiol, 1993; 264:G947; Ohata, AmJPhysiol, 1997; 35:G258). They store retinyl esters of vitamin A and their cytoskeletal system may have close contacts with nerve endings. This cell type synthesizes and secretes collagen and may play an important role in fibrosis, although not an exclusive one. During the fibrotic process they are transformed to myofibroblasts that express receptors for endothelin, which is a powerful endogenous vasoconstrictor. This leads to an increase in the portal resistance in periportal areas and slows down portal blood flow.[5]

Other cells

Some consider monocytes and T and B lymphocytes as hepatic sinusoidal cells because commonly they are present in the sinusoids both under normal and pathological conditions (Brouwer, p.665 in reference 26). The so-called pit cells have the morphology of natural killer cells, show cytotoxicity, and may therefore represent a defence system against tumour and virus-infected cells in co-operation with the Kupffer cells.[5]

Mechanisms for hepatic clearance of macromolecules and particles

The liver is involved in the disposition of a variety of macromolecules, both in the form of particles and as soluble species. Solid, often opsonized, particles such as bacteria, viruses, parasites, tumour cells, and damaged blood cells are removed from the bloodstream by a process called phagocytosis (Moghimi, CritRevTherDrugCarrSys, 1994; 11:31). Many particulate drug carriers such as liposomes, nanoparticles, and microspheres are also cleared by such phagocytotic processes, which are mainly situated in Kupffer and endothelial cells.

Soluble material, such as lipid particles, immune complexes, bacterial toxins, and certain lysosomal enzymes as well as denatured or otherwise abnormal glycoproteins, can be handled by the liver by a versatile apparatus for receptor-mediated endocytosis and subsequent degradation. Endocytosis is not specific to liver cells but occurs in all eukaryotic cells except mature red blood cells.

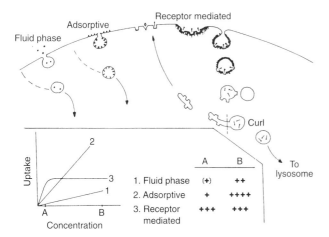

Fig. 22. Three potential mechanisms for cellular endocytosis: (1) aspecific fluid-phase endocytosis (non-saturable, small capacity), (2) adsorptive endocytosis (non-saturable, large capacity), and (3) receptor-mediated endocytosis (saturable, relatively large capacity at low doses). The inset shows the relative contributions of these processes at a relatively low dose (A) and at a much higher dose (B) at which the receptor-mediated process is overwhelmed by the other mechanisms and consequently cell specificity of uptake is decreased (after Ryser and Shen, ref. 61).

At least three different endocytotic mechanisms can be involved in the internalization of such materials (Fig. 22):[61]

1. Fluid-phase endocytosis or pinocytosis is a non-saturable process that does not require membrane binding and involves the engulfment of a small amount of extracellular fluid packed in a piece of the plasma membrane. Up to 20 per cent of the plasma volume in the body is endocytosed within 24 h in this process of 'cell drinking' and substances are taken up at rates proportional to their concentration in the extracellular fluid. Markers that are commonly used to measure fluid-phase uptake are horseradish peroxidase and polyvinylpyrrolidone (Jones, p.683 in reference 26). Binding to the cell's surface is not involved in this uptake process. Apart from fluid-phase uptake, horseradish peroxidase is also taken up by a receptor system in the Kupffer cells (Jones, p.683 in reference 26).

2. Adsorptive endocytosis operates through an aspecific binding of the substrate to the membrane. As a consequence, the substrate becomes concentrated and is endocytosed more efficiently than via a fluid-phase mechanism. As is the case for the fluid-phase process, adsorptive endocytosis cannot be saturated easily because of the intrinsic high capacity of the process.[61] Adsorptive uptake thus operates as a selective and concentrating process whereby cells can internalize large amounts of a solute without ingesting a correspondingly large volume of solution. Consequently, competition through binding of chemically related molecules can in principle occur. Binding of certain ligands to mammalian cells can even stimulate adsorptive endocytotic activity, particularly if the ligand is bivalent or multivalent in its interaction with the cell surface (Silverstein, AnnRevBiochem, 1977; 46:669).

3. Receptor-mediated endocytosis is an important mechanism that involves binding to a more specific receptor (Shepherd, TrendsPharmacolSci, 1989; 10:458; Forgac, p.207 in reference 26; Jones,

p.683 in reference 26). Among the macromolecules that undergo receptor-mediated endocytosis are growth factors, hormones, transport proteins (e.g. transferrin), proteins destined for degradation (α_2–macroglobulin), and proteins to be transported across polarized cells (pIgA) as well as toxins and viruses. Lateral movement leads to clustering of the receptor–substrate complex in a specialized coated part of the membrane (coated pits), inducing formation of coated vesicles within the cell. This process can be partially inhibited by hypotonic media and acidification of the cytosol (Sugiyama, PharmaceutRes, 1989; 6: 192; Burwen, JElectronMicrosc, 1990;14:140). A fundamental difference to carrier-mediated translocation of small organic and inorganic substrates is that following internalization the transported ligand remains segregated from the cytoplasm within vesicular structures. Receptor molecules possess a hydrophilic extracellular (ligand-binding) domain with various glycosylation sites, a hydrophobic membrane-spanning region, and a cytoplasmic tail. The intracellular part may exhibit protein kinase activity (for instance in the case of insulin and epidermal growth factor) (Sugiyama, 1989; Burwen, 1990). For some receptors (LDL, transferrin, asialoglycoproteins), internalization occurs even without ligand binding (constitutive endocytosis), for others such as epidermal growth factor and insulin, ligand–receptor formation is necessary (triggered endocytosis) (Shepherd, 1989; Burwen, 1990).

Endocytosis is an energy-requiring process in which the microfilament system is involved in the invagination process (Sugiyama, PharmaceutRes, 1989; 6:192; Burwen, JEMTech, 1990; 14:140; Forgac, p.207 in reference 26; Jones, p.683 in reference 26). The intracellular vesicles formed in this process are uncoated through an uncoating ATPase and form endosomes or phagosomes that are acidified through an ATP-dependent proton pump (Yamashiro, JCellBiol, 1983; 97:929; Yamashiro, JCellBiochem, 1984; 26: 231) (Fig. 23). This process is essential in the dissociation of the substrate and its receptor (Mellman, AnnRevBiochem, 1986; 55: 663; Schwartz, AnnRevPhysiol, 1986; 48:153). From the endosomal compartment, vesicles containing the receptor molecules often recycle to the membrane, whereas the endocytosed ligand in the smooth endosomes is trafficked to the lysosomes (Geuze, Cell, 1983; 32:1277). This acidic organelle contains a variety of aggressive enzymes to degrade proteins, lipids, and oligosaccharides, among others (De Duve, AnnRevPhysiol, 1966; 28:435). Some vesicles escape this pathway and return to the plasma membrane. They exocytose their contents back to the plasma in a short-circuit process (Russel, Gastro, 1983; 85:225; Regoeczi, ExpCellRes, 1985; 157: 495) or diacytose the material at the other pole of the cell (Ahnen, Gastro, 1985; 89:667; Brown, Hepatol, 1989; 9:763), to the bile canaliculi. The signals for the intracellular sorting and routeing remain to be defined (Geuze, Cell, 1983; 32:1277; Shepherd, TrendsPharmacolSci, 1989; 10:458; Stoorvogel, JCellBiol, 1989; 108:2137). After internalization, asialoglycoproteins, transferrin, and epidermal growth factor are present in primary endosomes. Yet the asialoglycoprotein is trafficked to lysosomes and after uncoupling of the ligand its receptor recycles to the plasma membrane. The transferrin molecules recycle completely, still combined with their receptors, whereas much of the epidermal growth factor receptor ends up in lysosomes associated with its ligand (Marti, Hepatol,

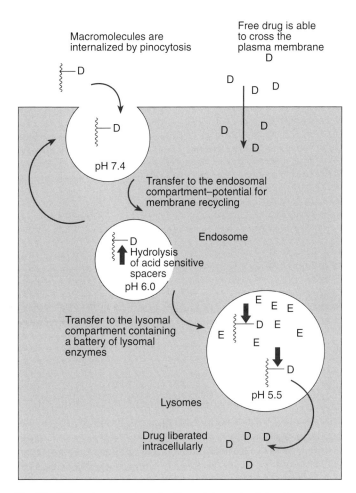

Macromolecules are internalized by pinocytosis

Free drug is able to cross the plasma membrane

pH 7.4

Transfer to the endosomal compartment–potential for membrane recycling

Endosome

Hydrolysis of acid sensitive spacers
pH 6.0

Transfer to the lysomal compartment containing a battery of lysomal enzymes

Lysomes

pH 5.5

Drug liberated intracellularly

Fig. 23. Different mechanisms for the uptake and cellular disposition of free drug (D) and carrier–drug conjugates. Following phagocytosis, pinocytosis, or endocytosis, the targeted drug enters acidified endosomes enabling hydrolysis of acid-sensitive drug–carrier linkages. Alternatively, the endocytosed drug conjugate is routed to lysosomes containing proteolytic or hydrolytic enzymes (E) by which the drug is released and diffuses into the cytoplasmic compartment (after Duncan, AntiCancDrugs, 1992; 3:175).

1989; 9:126). These different patterns of uncoupling and sorting may be related to maturation of the early endosomes (Shepherd, 1989; Stoorvogel, 1989). Since the average pH of the vesicles initially drops rapidly from 7.4 to 6.3, followed by a further gradual acidification to 5.0, differences in the pH dependency of receptor–ligand dissociation may induce unequal sites of escape from the endosomes and thus an unequal probability of recycling and/or modification of the proteins in the trans-Golgi reticulum (Shepherd, 1989; Stoorvogel, 1989). Also, the sequence of changes in Ca^{2+} content, membrane potential, and membrane fluidity of the endosomes may underlie such receptor- and ligand-specific intracellular routeing.

Ligand–receptor dissociation, endosome sorting, and transcellular movements can be affected by temperature, metabolic inhibitors, and weakly basic compounds that interfere with acidification of the endocytotic vesicles (NH_4Cl and tertiary amines such as chloroquine). Agents that dissipate H^+ gradients (nigericin and monensin), inhibitors of microfilament function (cytochalasin

B), and disassemblers of the microtubular tubulin polymers (colchicine and vinblastine) consequently can also influence these processes (Van der Sluijs, BiochemPharm, 1985; 34:1399; Sugiyama, PharmaceutRes, 1989; 6:192; Burwen, JEMTech, 1990; 14:140; Nishida, PharmaceutRes, 1991; 8:1253; Forgac, p.207 in reference 26).

Receptor-mediated endocytosis in various cell types of the liver

A large number of receptor-mediated processes have been identified on hepatocytes, endothelial cells, stellate cells, and Kupffer cells (Table 4). On hepatocytes one finds the asialoglycoprotein receptor, which recognizes galactose- and N-acetyl-galactosamine-terminated glycoproteins (Ashwell, AnnRevBiochem, 1982; 51:531; Schwartz, CritRevBiochem, 1984; 16:207),[62] a receptor for polymeric IgA/IgM (called secretory component) (Ahnen, Gastro, 1985; 89:667; Brown, Hepatol, 1989; 9:763),[63] and receptors for HDL particles (Goldstein, AnnRevBiochem, 1977; 46:879; Havel, Hepatol, 1988; 8:1689), epidermal growth factor (Burwen, JCellBiol, 1984; 99:1259; Marti, Hepatol, 1989; 9:126), transferrin (Stoorvogel, JCellBiol, 1989; 108:2137; Forgac, p.207 in reference 26),[62] haemopexin, chylomicron remnants, haemoglobin, insulin, and peptide hormones (Sugiyama, PharmaceutRes, 1989; 6:192; Burwen, JEMTech, 1990; 14:140), as well as for lysosomal proteases (after complex formation with α_2-macroglobulins) (Barret, MethodsEnz, 1981; 80:737).[64]

On Kupffer cells, receptors for immune and complement complexes (Fc and C_3 receptors) and for fibronectin were detected that were also able to mediate endocytosis of opsonized particulate material (Jones, p.683 in reference 26). In addition, a galactose particle receptor is described, recognizing cells and other particles (Kolb-Bachofen, BiolCell, 1984; 51:219; Biessen, p.157 in reference 63) that expose galactose groups. In contrast to the asialoglycoprotein receptor on hepatocytes, this galactose-specific receptor (that is identical to membrane-associated C-reactive protein; Kolb-Bachofen, p.143 in reference 63) is highly sensitive to size. Affinity for the receptor rises sharply when particle size increases from 1 to 12 nm and plateaus above this value. This 'optimal' size may reflect the absolute size of the pentameric receptor (Biessen, p.157 in reference 63). As in other macrophages, a mannose/N-acetylglucosamine/fucose receptor has been identified (Stahl, TrendsBiochemSci, 1980; 5:194) that not only recognizes terminal mannose and N-acetylglucosamine groups on glycoproteins but may also accommodate (neo-)glycoproteins with terminal glucose and fructose groups (Sano, JHepatol, 1990; 10:211; Smedsrod, BiochemJ, 1990; 266:313; Stahl, AmJRespirCellMolBiol, 1990; 2:317). Apart from this system, specific receptors for fucose-terminated glycoproteins (α_1-3 fucose residues) were identified on parenchymal cells, while on Kupffer cells a receptor that binds Fuc-β albumin was found distinct from the mannose/N-acetyl glucosamine receptor (Jones, p.683 in reference 26). Kupffer cells, along with hepatocytes, can also endocytose lysosomal proteases by complex formation with circulating α_2-macroglobulin (Barrett, MethodsEnz, 1981; 80:737).[64] The latter receptor may also accommodate certain lipid particles (Gliemann, p.273 in reference 63) and tissue-type plasminogen activator (Bu, PNAS, 1992; 89:7427).

Table 4 Receptors for endocytosis of proteins on different liver cell types

On hepatocytes	On Kupffer cells	On endothelial cells	On stellate cells
Asialoglycoprotein (<10 nM, galactose recognition)	Agalactoglycoprotein (mannose recognition)	Agalactoglycoprotein (mannose recognition)	Ferritin
Insulin	Galactose particle (>10 nM, galactose recognition)	Scavenger (negatively charged proteins)	IGF-II/mannose 6-phosphate
Epidermal growth factor	LDL	Sulphated polysaccharide (chondroitin sulphate, hepatin)	α_2-Macroglobulin
IgA (polymeric IgA)	Macrophage enzyme (tissue-derived enzymes)	Fc (immune complexes)	
Transferrin (transferrin/Fe complexes)	α_2-Macroglobulin (α_2-Macroglobulin/protease complex)		
LDL	Fibronectin (opsonized material)		
HDL	Fc (immune complexes, opsonized particles)		
	C_3b (complement factors)		

HDL, high-density lipoprotein; LDL, low-density lipoprotein.

Finally, Kupffer cells exhibit receptors for positively charged (Bergmann, ClinSci, 1984; 67:35; Nishida, IntJPharmaceut, 1992; 80:101; Fujita, JDrugTarget, 1994; 2:157) and for negatively charged proteins (scavenger receptors) (Smedsrod, BiochemJ, 1990; 266: 313; Jansen, PharmaceutRes, 1993; 10:1611; Takakura, IntJ-Pharmaceut, 1994; 105:19). Although the above-mentioned receptors in Kupffer cells had once been supposed to be specific for this cell type, it is now agreed that many of them are also present on endothelial cells (Praaning-Van Dalen, Gastro, 1981; 81:1036; Van der Laan-Klamer, ScaJImmunol, 1986; 23:127; Smedsrod, BiochemJ, 1990; 266:313). The endothelial cells also have receptors for LDL particles (Goldstein, AnnRevBiochem, 1977; 46:879). Scavenger receptors may even be localized predominantly on the endothelial cells (Smedsrod, 1990; Praaning-Van Dalen, 1981; Van Berkel, p.49 in reference 65). Kupffer cells can greatly increase in number upon exposure to, for instance, inflammatory stimuli through recruitment from peripheral blood and bone marrow. The phagocytotic function can be upregulated by various cytokines or endotoxin, but can also be reduced by repeated administration of particulate and polymeric material owing to receptor loss and/or defects in surface attachment. Carbon colloids, dextran sulphate, and opsonized gadolinium chloride are well known examples (Moghimi, CritRevTherDrugCarrSys, 1994; 11:31).

Relatively little information is available on cell-surface receptors and endocytosis in hepatic stellate cells. Various cytokine receptors involved in the activation of this cell type have been defined (i.e. receptors for several growth factors). Cellular internalization and degradation processes for macromolecules have only been described for ferritin (Ramm, JCI, 1994; 94:9), for mannose-6-phosphate containing ligands (Nissley, MolReprodDev, 1993; 35:408), and for α_2-macroglobulin (Kasza, EurJBiochem, 1997; 248:270). However, such receptors are unlikely to be specific for this hepatic cell type; they have also been found on extrahepatic fibroblasts.

In the intact organism, the relative contribution of the various cell types to the clearance of a certain substrate will be determined by the receptor density and exposed surface of the cell types involved, by the acinar localization of the cells, and their activation status, as well as by the presence of competing endogenous substrates and the amount of the substrate administered. The latter factor should be seen in relation to the receptor capacity and affinity (V_{max}/K_m ratio) of the endocytotic processes. These parameters are not necessarily constant because on chronic administration of substrates down-modulation of the receptors can occur (Sugiyama, PharmaceutRes, 1989; 6:192).[66] Since various cell types may 'compete' for the same substrate, dose dependency should be taken into account in measuring the relative clearance of macromolecules by the various cell types.

Receptor-mediated uptake of macromolecules requires a preceding selective binding of these substances to the plasma membrane of either the hepatocytes or the sinusoidal cell types. The binding is determined by a number of structural properties of the molecule such as size, charge, terminal sugar, and the capability of the molecule to form complexes with other circulating proteins such as α_2-macroglobulin, fibronectin, and immunoglobulins (Table 4). Progress has been made in the characterization of various receptor systems for endocytosis of glycoproteins on the functional and molecular level (Forgac, p.207 in reference 26). Most of the receptor proteins have been isolated and purified to homogeneity using affinity chromatography and other protein separation techniques. Molecular mass, degree of glycosylation, and amino acid composition, as well as functional clustering of the receptor complexes determined by radiation inactivation, have been reported (Smedsrod, BiochemJ, 1990; 266:313; Stahl, AmJRespir-CellMolBiol, 1990; 2:317; Forgac, p.207 in reference 26). The number of receptor complexes per cell and the maximal internalization rate of the particulate ligands was estimated from kinetic cell studies. For instance, each rat hepatocyte contains 250 000 dimeric asialoglycoprotein surface receptors (molecular weight of subunits about 48 000) with a K_d for asialo-orosomucoid of 10^{-7} mol. At the maximum rate, each cell can internalize 5 million glycosylated molecules per hour (Ashwell, AnnRevBiochem, 1982; 51:531; Forgac, p.207 in reference 26). Part of the receptor molecules may also be detected in intracellular pools, relating to the processes of synthesis, repair, recycling, and degree of down-modulation.[66] It should be realized, however, that remarkable differences in receptor characteristics can occur between *in vivo* and *in vitro* (cell culture) conditions (Dunn, MethodsEnz, 1983; 98: 225).

Influence of sugar density and sugar clustering on endocytosis of glycoconjugates

The efficiency of endocytosis and degradation of glycoproteins can be influenced by the number, density, and geometric clustering of sugar groups on the protein molecule (Nishikawa, PharmaceutRes, 1995; 12:209). For instance, in the case of the natural mannose-terminated glycoproteins on macrophages, mainly the proteins with tetra-antennary oligosaccharide structures are endocytosed (Maynard, JBC, 1981; 256:8063; Taylor, AmJPhysiol, 1987; 252: E690; Jones, p.683 in reference 26). That sugar clustering is important for uptake into hepatocytes was shown in studies on naturally occurring glycoproteins containing the typical tetra-, tri-, bi-, or monoantennary oligosaccharide structure (Fig. 24). In hepatocytes, triantennary asialoglycoproteins have a much higher affinity for the hepatic lectin than the bi- and monoantennary derivatives (Baenziger, Cell, 1980; 22:611; Connolly, JBC, 1982; 257:939). The latter may partly undergo 'short-circuit' exocytosis or retro-endocytosis and after primary endocytosis are again released from the cells in the intact form (Evans, Hepatol, 1981; 5:452; Townsend, PNAS, 1984; 81:466; Regoeczi, ExpCellRes, 1985; 157:495; Magnusson, p.189 in reference 63). This may lead to repeated cycles of endocytosis and exocytosis and an overall slow clearance of the macromolecule. Efflux from the cells of glycoproteins is also stimulated by high concentrations of bile salts (Russel, Gastro, 1983; 85:225), GalNAc, and EGTA (Townsend, PNAS, 1984; 81:466) without destruction of the cells. It has been suggested that recycling of (asialo-) glycoproteins is related to some kind of repair through resialylation in the Golgi system, a process that may only occur at a low concentration range of such glycoproteins (Evans, 1981; Townsend, 1984). Retroendocytosis of internalized glycoproteins in endothelial cells may be even faster than in hepatocytes (Magnusson, p.189 in reference 63).

Receptor affinity of complex oligosaccharides and efficiency of receptor-mediated endocytosis, therefore, is much higher than for neoglycoproteins with a similar number of randomly distributed monosaccharides. A high density of the sugar molecules and thereby the possibility of binding to several receptor sites clustered in coated pits may explain the more efficient triggering of endocytosis. For instance, this was shown for tracer doses of asialo-orosomucoid and lactosaminated albumin, each with about 25 'terminal' sugars (L_{25}-**HSA**) (human serum albumin) (Van der Sluijs, BiochemPharm, 1985; 34:1399; Van der Sluijs, Hepatol, 1986; 6:723; Van der Sluijs, Hepatol, 1987; 7:688; Van der Sluijs, Hepatol, 1988; 8:1521). The half-time for internalization in perfused rat liver was 3.4 min for

asialo-orosomucoid and 34.9 min for the lactosylated serum albumin. Evidently, neoglycoproteins which are prepared by reductive amination (Schwartz, ArchBiochemBiophys, 1977; 181:542) or amidination (Stowell, AdvCarbChemBiochem, 1980; 37:225) with simple sugars have a lower affinity for the asialoglycoprotein receptor than the natural glycoproteins. On the other hand, neoglycoproteins prepared through thiophosgene activation of *p*-aminophenyl sugars (Kataoka, Blood, 1985; 65:1165) will contain extra negative charge and this may lead to partial capturing by scavenger-like receptors on non-parenchymal cell types (Jansen, JBC, 1991; 266:3343). The extent of endocytosis of such glycoproteins by non-parenchymal cells is probably inversely related to the relative affinity of the particular neoglycoprotein for the asialoglycoprotein receptor in the hepatocytes.[18]

The presence of specific sugar groups on a protein molecule can also inhibit lysosomal proteolysis (Taylor, AmJPhysiol, 1987; 252: E690; Sano, JHepatol, 1990; 10:211; Jones, p.683 in reference 26). Density and clustering of the sugar groups and microheterogeneity of the oligosaccharide chains will therefore largely affect cellular degradation rate. Consequently, the composition as well as the geometry of the glycoprotein structure will influence the overall involvement of certain cells in the disposition of a particular glycoprotein. Interaction of clustered galactosyl residues with the asialoglycoprotein receptor *per se* is insufficient to elicit irreversible endocytosis: monomeric tris-galactosyl conjugates of low molecular weight drugs did not provide an improved hepatic targeting (Eichler, BiochemPharm, 1992; 44:2117). Apparently, a macromolecular structure with appropriate spacing of galactosyl residues as present in natural and neoglycoproteins is a prerequisite for recognition by a number of the dimeric receptors.

Drug targeting to the liver with hepatotrophic carriers

The previous sections underline that macromolecules, depending on their size, charge, and carbohydrate structure, can be recognized by various cell types within the liver. The particular physiological processes can be exploited for cell-specific delivery of drugs (Poznansky, PharmRev, 1984; 36:277; Fallon, Hepatol, 1985; 5:899; Monsigny, AnnNYAcadSci, 1988; 551:399)[18,67] on the basis of receptor-mediated endocytosis and subsequent (proteolytic) degradation of the drug–carrier complex. The endocytotic processes may operate in concert with aspecific fluid-phase endocytosis (pinocytosis) and adsorptive endocytosis.

Fluid-phase endocytosis takes place for any material in the bloodstream but is relatively slow. Adsorptive endocytosis is important for ligands that have a multivalent interaction with the plasma membrane due to charge and is quantitatively important after large doses of macromolecules. Such processes may to some extent corrupt specific receptor-mediated drug delivery. However, due to the high affinity of the drug carriers for the receptor systems actually aimed at, receptor-mediated processes can often compete easily with these more aspecific mechanisms if their maximal uptake capacity is not exceeded.

Potential carrier systems for liver targeting

Both soluble and particle types of carriers have been employed for the purpose of drug targeting to the various cell types in the liver.

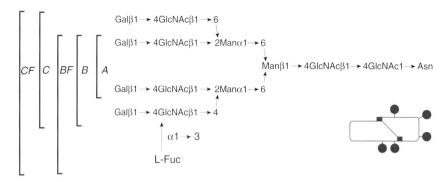

Fig. 24. Characteristic structure of an oligosaccharide side chain of natural occurring glycoproteins, such as α_1-acid glycoprotein (orosomucoid) and fetuin. Normally, the major part of the galactose group is substituted by *N*-acetylneuraminic acid (sialic acid). However, microheterogeneity of the antennary structure and sialic acid substitution exists under pathological conditions and acute-phase reactions. A, B, and C denote bi-, tri- and tetra-antennary structures, respectively. In the CF and BF forms L-fucose is present at the indicated site. The inset shows localization of five of these chains at the protein core of the acute-phase protein α_1-acid glycoprotein.

Relevant in this respect is the endothelial barrier: particles of more than 100 to 150 nm cannot pass through the fenestrae (pores) in the endothelial lining (Brouwer, p.665 in reference 26). This is the case for normal-sized liposomes and nanoparticles, and consequently such carriers can only reach Kupffer, pit, and endothelial cells. Small-sized liposomes and HDL particles can, in principle, be used for delivery of lipophilic (pro-)drugs to hepatocytes and stellate cells (Bijsterbosch, Biochem, 1994; 33:14073; Van Berkel, p.49 in reference 65).[68] These agents can also be enclosed in the lipid core of LDL particles or in liposomes and be delivered to the sinusoidal cell types (Storm, p.333 in reference 59; Van Berkel, p.49 in reference 65). After degradation of the carrier, such drugs could act locally in these cells or be slowly released from the cells to reach the other cell types in the liver. Reuptake of the parent drugs in these cells, however, may not be efficient enough to reach therapeutic concentrations and at the same time prevent toxic levels in extra-hepatic tissues.

The type of carrier is chosen on the basis of a number of considerations (Poznansky, PharmRev, 1984; 36:277):[18]

1. The cost of the chosen carrier is considered, taking into account that clinical application is the final goal.
2. Can the target cell type really be reached in sufficient amounts (endothelial barriers, 'competitive' removal by the reticuloendothelial system)?
3. Does the carrier allow sufficient drug loading, taking into account the drug potency as well as the capacity of the particular endocytic process?
4. Is the carrier really cell specific when administered *in vivo* (does reaction with opsonic factors occur?) and is specificity unaltered after linkage of the drug?
5. Is the carrier biodegradable (proper release rate of the drug and toxicity to the reticuloendothelial system of the carrier itself)?
6. Are degradation products of the carrier material non-toxic?
7. Do immunogenic reactions occur after chronic administration?
8. Is the drug released in its active form and at an adequate rate (proper cellular residence time in relation to therapeutic effects)?
9. Is the receptor pathway that is aimed at also expressed in pathological conditions and is it influenced by concomitantly administered drugs?

Intracellular release of active drug from the protein carrier

The final goal in drug targeting is to make the active form of the drug available in a particular cell type. Drugs such as doxorubicin that are covalently linked via their $-NH_2$ groups to -COOH groups of the carrier protein can only be released slowly because the amide bond is quite resistant to enzymatic attack. Introduction of amino acid spacers between the drug and the protein can improve release rate and such spacers can be used for a programmed release and optimization of the cellular concentration profile (Shen, BBRes-Comm, 1981; 102:1048; Trouet, PNAS, 1982; 79:626; Schneider, p.1 in 69). Drugs with functional -COOH groups or isothiocyanate moieties can be linked to lysine-NH_2 groups of proteins, but the final degradation product will contain at least one amino acid (lysine) because this linkage cannot be split from the drug by the lysosomal enzymes (Van der Sluijs, BiochemPharm, 1985; 34:1399). An example is fluorescein isothiocyanate covalently coupled to asialo-orosomucoid, which is taken up quantitatively by the parenchymal cells of the liver. After degradation the dye is released still bound to lysine and after conjugation with glucuronic acid it is excreted into bile (Fig. 25). The excretion rate of the fluorescent material in bile reflects the rate-limiting lysosomal degradation of the glycoprotein carrier (Van der Sluijs, 1985). Uncoupling of the drug can also happen too fast: trifluorothymidine covalently linked to the hepatotrophic carrier asialofetuin is released so rapidly from lysosomes in the hepatocytes that substantial amounts escape from the liver to the general circulation and reach toxic concentrations in non-target tissues such as bone marrow (Fiume, p.1 in reference 70).

The chemical bond that links the drug to the carrier protein should be stable in the bloodstream but labile in acidic compartments within the target cells (Shen, BBResComm, 1981; 102: 1048; Monsigny, AnnNYAcadSci, 1988; 551:399). The antiviral nucleoside analogues in their mono- or diphosphate forms can be linked to a lysine-NH_2 group and histidine nitrogen via a pH-sensitive phosphoamide group (Fig. 26). Introduction of phosphorylated nucleosides into the cell via covalent binding to carrier proteins may also improve the rate of cellular activation to triphosphate forms that is necessary before any inhibition of DNA

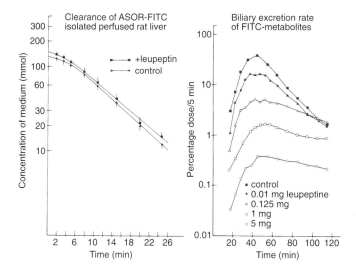

Fig. 25. Perfusate disappearance of asialo-orosomucoid coupled to fluorescein isothiocyanate in isolated perfused rat liver. Either 1 ml of phosphate buffered saline (controls, $n = 6$) or 1 ml of phosphate buffered saline plus 5 mg leupeptin ($n = 6$) was added to the medium followed 20 min later by the administration of 14.4 nmol of asialo-orosomucoid–fluorescein isothiocyanate. Right panel: the influence of various doses of leupeptin on the biliary excretion rate of fluorescent degradation products in the isolated perfused rat liver. Leupeptin appears to leave hepatic uptake unchanged (left panel) but dose dependently inhibits lysosomal degradation of the glycoprotein, a process that produces fluorescein–lysine metabolites that are excreted in bile (right panel) (after Van der Sluijs, BiochemPharm, 1985; 34: 1399).

polymerase can be achieved. Such activation may occur only slowly by the cellular kinases of hepatocytes, and phosphorylation via kinases derived from hepatitis B virus does not take place (Fiume, p.1 in reference 70). Alternatives to acid-sensitive linkages are biodegradable spacer moieties composed of sugars[71] or amino acids (Trouet, PNAS, 1982; 79:626; Trouet, p.19 in reference 70).

Alternatively, drug peptide carriers can be designed with a simpler structure than the naturally occurring plasma proteins. Various types of polylysines with different charge can be tailor-made and even provided with clustered sugar groups (Arnold, MethodsEnz, 1985; 112:270; Fiume, FEBSLett, 1986; 203:203; Monsigny, AnnNYAcadSci, 1988; 551:399; Biessen, JHepatol, 1994; 21:806; Martinez-Fong, Hepatol, 1994; 20:1602; Di Stefano, BiochemPharm, 1995; 49:1769; Fiume, Hepatol, 1995; 22:1072).

An important factor determining the rate of release from lysosomes is probably the extent of protonation of the delivered drug in the lysosomal compartment. Basic drugs such as chloroquine will be largely protonated at the relatively low internal pH of this organelle (pH 5 to 6) and consequently will undergo persistent storage and relatively slow release. In contrast, weakly acidic drugs will be present mainly in the undissociated form and therefore will leave these organelles easily. This was shown for the protease inhibitor pepstatin that was covalently coupled to asialofetuin (Furuno, JBiochem(Tokyo), 1983; 93:249). This carboxylic tripeptide was delivered properly to hepatocyte lysosomes, but after carrier degradation was excreted rapidly into bile. However, in spite of this rapid release, intralysosomal levels remained high enough for the inhibition of cathepsin for 6 h after injection, demonstrating the extreme potency of the pepstatin molecule.

It follows that knowledge about receptor- and carrier-mediated transport should be integrated in drug targeting. From the moment that a targeted drug is released in the target cell, detailed information on membrane transport mechanisms is necessary to understand the relative rates of cellular export and subcellular (organelle) distribution, factors that apart from the delivery process determine the cellular concentration profile in relation to the pattern of the pharmacological response (Fig. 27).

Hepatic targeting of diagnostic agents

Many of the macromolecular carriers that have been discussed above for targeting of drugs can also be employed for diagnostic

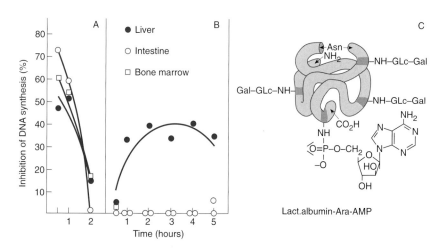

Fig. 26. Targeting of the anti-HBV drug adenine arabinoside monophosphate (ara-AMP) coupled to lactosaminated HSA via an acid-sensitive phosphoamide bond (C). Intravenous administration in ectromelia virus-infected mice of the ara-AMP itself leads to short-lasting inhibition of (viral) DNA synthesis in the liver, but also to depression of endogenous DNA synthesis in intestinal mucosa and bone marrow cells (A). The targeted conjugate, however, yields a sustained inhibition pattern in the liver without major effects on the extrahepatic tissues (B) (adapted from Fiume, AdvDrugDelRev, 1994; 14:51).

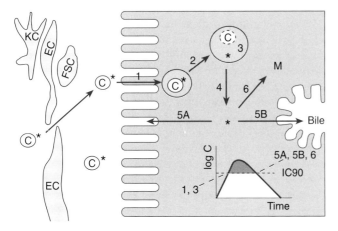

Fig. 27. Rate-limiting processes that determine the intracellular concentration profile of a targeted drug (indicated as *) which is delivered to hepatocytes via a carrier (C). The carrier is taken up by receptor-mediated endocytosis (1) and, after routeing of endosomes (2) to lysosomes, is degraded (3) and releases the targeted drug (4). The released drug will be removed from the cell by sinusoidal (5A) and canalicular secretion mechanisms (5B) or eliminated by metabolism (6). The inset shows the time course of the intracellular drug concentration of which, depending on the carrier and carrier–drug coupling techniques, the ascending phase can be determined either by the rate-limiting step of endocytosis or by the lysosomal degradation process. The descending phase is determined by the three indicated elimination pathways. The amount of drug targeted to the cells should provide intracellular concentrations that, for an adequate period, exceed the IC_{90} value (concentration at which 90 per cent inhibition of the targeted process occurs).

purposes including liver imaging. The traditional tests with hepatotrophic dyes, bile acids, iodinated contrast agents, HIDA compounds, and galactose are based on carrier-mediated membrane transport processes.[1,2] More recent is the interest in receptor-mediated (endocytic) processes as targets to probe liver functions. The asialoglycoprotein receptor (also called hepatic binding protein) is instrumental in this approach. For this purpose $^{99}Tc^m$-galactosyl-neoglycoalbumin (**NGA**) was developed as a substrate for estimation of liver functional mass, and liver blood flow under physiological and pathological conditions. Vera and colleagues developed this receptor radiopharmaceutical agent via elegant *in vitro* (Radiol, 1984; 151:191) and *in vivo* studies (JNuclMed, 1985; 26:1157; JNuclMed, 1989; 30:1519; JNuclMed, 1991; 32:1169), and the probe was chemically applied in several studies (Vera, 1989; Virgolini, BrJCanc, 1990; 61:937; Virgolini, BrJClinPharm, 1990; 29:207; Vera, 1991; Virgolini, NuclMedComm, 1991; 12:507; Virgolini, Hepatol, 1992; 15:593). A Japanese group (Hazama, JpnJNuclMed, 1986; 23:917; Kawa, JpnJNuclMed, 1986; 23:907; Kawa, JNuclMed, 1991; 32:2233) independently developed a similar technetium-labelled ligand, $^{99}Tc^m$-labelled serum galactosyl albumin, with a more stable *in vivo* binding of the technetium via chelation by diethyltriaminepentaacetic acid that was covalently coupled to the carrier.

Development of an adequate non-linear pharmacokinetic model enabled a proper analysis of the γ-radiation liver-time and heart-time activity data that can be collected non-invasively through γ-camera imaging (Kudo, JNuclMed, 1991; 32:1177; Vera, JNuclMed, 1991; 32:1169). Of considerable value is that this analysis allows the

determination of both the hepatic receptor concentration as well as the association constant for the binding of hepatic binding protein (Vera, IEEETrBiomedEng, 1985; BME-32:312; Vera, 1991). This is accomplished by fitting the parameters of the model iteratively to the collected experimental data as applied by Virgolini *et al.* (BrJ-Canc, 1990; 61:937; NuclMedComm, 1991; 12:507; Hepatol, 1992; 15:593). This approach yielded useful data on receptor characteristics in patients with acute viral hepatitis, showing a high liver specificity of the probe (Virgolini, 1992). Tracer accumulation studies indicated that the degradation products of NGA, together with some intact protein, are excreted via the bile rather than via the urine.

In patients with acute viral hepatitis, hepatic binding protein concentrations were about 50 per cent of the normal values in the acute phase. During the recovery phase the hepatic binding protein concentration rose as did the association constant and blood flow and fairly good correlations were found with other laboratory tests in the course of the disease.

Hepatic targeting of antiviral drugs

Using receptor-mediated endocytosis of drug–protein conjugates in the liver, selective drug delivery of antiviral drugs has been accomplished *in vivo*, including in patients, resulting in an increase in drug potency and in therapeutic safety. This is seen as an important alternative therapy along with interferon treatment (Mutchnick, AntiviralRes, 1994; 24:245). Examples are the delivery of the antiviral drugs trifluorothymidine (Fiume, p.1 in reference 70), adenine arabinoside monophosphate (**ara-AMP**) (Fiume, Gut, 1984; 25:1392; Fiume, BiochemPharm, 1986; 35:967; Jansen, Hepatol, 1993; 18:146), acyclovir (Plourde, DrugDel, 1995; 2:136), iodo-deoxyuridine (Bijsterbosch, Biochem, 1994; 33:14073), and dideoxyguanosine (Korba, Hepatol, 1996; 23:958). In the case of ara-AMP, a single administration of a conjugate with lactosylated albumin (L_{30}-HSA) (Fiume, BiochemPharm, 1986; 35:967) yielded a stronger and longer lasting inhibition of ectromelia virus DNA replication in the liver compared with the parent drug (Fig. 26). Virtually no effects of the ara-AMP conjugate on bone marrow and intestinal mucosa cells were found. Recently, Ponzetto *et al.* showed a clear reduction of woodchuck hepatitis virus DNA replication *in vivo* after treatment with ara-AMP and acyclovir monophospate conjugated to lactosaminated albumin. These effects occurred at a significantly lower dose compared with that of the free drugs (Ponzetto, Hepatol, 1991; 14:16), without showing signs of general toxicity. The ara-AMP–albumin conjugate does not seem to evoke major immunogenic reactions after chronic administration if homologous albumin is used (Fiume, CancerDrugDeliv, 1987; 4:145).

As mentioned earlier, antiviral nucleoside analogues in their mono- or diphosphate forms can be linked to lysine-NH_2 and histidine nitrogen via a pH-sensitive phosphoamide group (Fiume, FEBSLett, 1980; 116:185). The initial one-step coupling reaction (Fiume, p.1 in reference 70), in which the nucleoside monophosphate is activated with carbodiimide in the presence of the neoglycoprotein, was replaced by a two-step procedure in which the phosphate group is activated at pH 4.5 and after the albumin is added the pH is raised to 7.5. This prevents simultaneous activation of -COOH groups in the protein leading to formation of dimers and trimers (Jansen, Hepatol, 1993; 18:146). Such multimeric conjugates will tend to be taken up in liver endothelial and Kupffer cells (Fiume, CancerDrugDeliv, 1987; 4:11) and thus may corrupt the specificity of the carrier. Virtually all monomeric ara-AMP-lactosaminated albumin (L_{27}HSA-ara-AMP) is taken up by the hepatocytes (Jansen, 1993) and almost none by the sinusoidal cell types (Jansen, 1993).

Crucial for keeping the drug inside the cells may be the release of the polar, monophosphated form of drugs such as azidothymidine (**AZT**) or araA (Fiume, p.1 in reference 70). Yet, some ara-AMP that is released in the liver is effluxed and reaches other organs, albeit to a much lower extent than after administration of ara-AMP itself (Fiume, JHepatol, 1994; 20:681). Ara-AMP is remarkably stable in lysosomal fractions of liver homogenates. After incubation of ara-AMP–L-HSA conjugates, ara-AMP was released predominantly in the cells after degradation of the carrier rather than araA itself (Jansen, Hepatol, 1993; 18:146).

Acyclovir was linked to asialo-orosomucoid or polylysine-coupled asialo-orosomucoid through a γ-aminobutyryl ester, through a succinyl ester, and via a monophosphoryl linkage using acyclovir monophosphate (Plourde, DrugDel, 1995; 2:136). The latter conjugate inhibited replication of hepatitis B virus (**HBV**) DNA in cultured cells and was 80 times more potent than unconjugated acyclovir. The monophosphate conjugate was more potent than the ester conjugates probably because acyclovir monophosphate is released through a combination of acid hydrolysis and phosphatase activity on the phosphoramidate linkage, whereas acyclovir itself is released from the ester conjugates. The bypass of monophosphorylation may be crucial here (Plourde, 1995). Recently, an alternative coupling method for nucleoside monophosphates was described by Fiume *et al.* in which the imidazolide phosphoric ester of the drug was employed for linking the drug to L-HSA (Fiume, AnalBioch, 1993; 212:407). It was reported that the conjugation via the imidazolide did not cause any cross-linking of L-HSA in contrast to the conjugates prepared by these authors using EDCI. In addition, the new conjugate is more water soluble and biodegradable because it did not produce lysosomal vacuoles as found for the ara-AMP-L-HSA conjugates made with the EDCI method. The latter phenomenon occurs in rat liver at doses 5 to 10 times in excess of the usual therapeutic dose (Fiume, JHepatol, 1992; 15:314) and is due to osmotic swelling of secondary lysosomes as a consequence of the lysosomal incapacity to digest such high amounts of the conjugate. The improved conjugate prepared by the imidazolide method enters both parenchymal and sinusoidal cells in the liver to an equal extent. Apart from the earlier mentioned charge effects (see glycoprotein carriers), the rather high density of the lactose groups in this preparation may play a role as a high degree of lactosylation may increase the affinity for the Kupffer cell galactose-particle receptor (Biessen, JHepatol, 1994; 21:806).

In a clinical study, 13 patients chronically infected with HBV were treated with L_{30}-HSA-ara-AMP (one to three courses of 1.5 mg of coupled ara-AMP/kg per day for 3 to 7 days). In all patients, the plasma levels of HBV DNA dropped significantly. In most patients they returned to pretreatment values when the administration was discontinued. However, in some patients, plasma HBV DNA remained undetectable during the follow-up period of 1 year (Fiume, Lancet, 1988; 332:13; Fiume, AdvDrugDelRev, 1994; 14:51).

By a kinetic analysis of the plasma conjugate concentrations, using the data of Fiume *et al.* (Lancet, 1988; 332:13), we calculated a surprisingly long half-life of 1.5 h for the ara-AMP-L-HSA conjugate. In healthy volunteers, the blood plasma half-life of galactose-terminated albumin was reported to be only 0.2 h (Vera, JNuclMed, 1989; 30:1519).

One of the factors involved could be a down-regulation of the hepatic galactose receptor in the case of HBV infection (Virgolini, Hepatol, 1992; 15:593) and liver inflammation (Sawamura, Gastro, 1981; 81:527). Although non-HBV-infected human hepatoma cells such as HepG2 normally express the galactose receptor, data from various laboratories show that HBV DNA-transfected cells (HepG2 2.2.15) have a lower expression of this receptor. Thus HBV-infected cells may have altered receptor characteristics depending on the state of the disease (Virgolini, 1992). As mentioned above, the hepatic receptor density in patients with an acute HBV infection, as calculated from neoglycoalbumin clearance, is about 50 per cent of normal. In spite of this lower expression of the galactose receptor in these patients, endocytosis and further cellular disposition of the lactosaminated HSA is sufficiently retained for an adequate delivery of the coupled antiviral drug.

An interesting approach in the design of liver-specific drug carriers was recently taken in the production of ara-AMP–arabinogalactan conjugates (Groman, BioconjugChem, 1994; 5: 547; Enriquez, BioconjugChem, 1995; 6:195). Arabinogalactan is a simple uncharged polysaccharide of arabinose and galactose from the tree *Larix occidentales*. The compound is commercially available in a highly purified form at a cost of at least 100 times less than albumin. The sugar polymer, after initial reduction, is coupled with ethylenediamine and to the resulting arabinogalactan-amine molecule about 8 mol of ara-AMP were coupled through the above-mentioned two-step procedure (Jansen, Hepatol, 1993; 18:146). The combination of the monophosphate groups that introduce one negative charge per coupled drug molecule and the positive charges of the remaining single (-NH$_2$) groups produced an electroneutral complex that is unlikely to be recognized by scavenger receptors on non-parenchymal cells. Although the conjugate is stable in blood, part of it will be lost via the urine because the observed molecular radius of this conjugate, of 40 kDa at most, does not prevent glomerular filtration. Yet, the affinity for the asialoglycoprotein receptor is in the same range as lactosaminated HSA and predicts efficient delivery to the liver. Daily injections of the conjugate (3 mg ara-AMP/kg for 14 days) decreased serum levels of woodchuck HBV DNA in the woodchuck *in vivo* while, in contrast to treatment with the parent drug, viral DNA serum levels remained depressed for 42 days after administration ceased (Enriquez, 1995). Clinical studies with this interesting conjugate will probably be performed in the near future. In addition to its application in therapies, arabinoglycan-based conjugates may also be useful for diagnostic purposes. Magnetic resonance imaging (MRI) agents coated with arabinoglycan have been applied to visualize functional asialoglycoprotein receptors in rats after partial hepatectomy and endotoxaemia (Leveille-Webster, Hepatol, 1996; 23:1631) This may be a tool to assess hepatic damage and regeneration in patients with liver diseases.

Other carriers for hepatic delivery of nucleoside analogues that have been recently described are lactosaminated poly-L-lysine, as tested in mice (Di Stefano, BiochemPharm, 1995; 49:1769) and woodchucks (Fiume, Hepatol, 1995; 22:1072; Fiume, JHepatol, 1997; 26:253), as well as reconstituted HDL particles (Bijsterbosch, Biochem, 1994; 33:14073). Intramuscular administration of poly-L-lysine–AMP markedly lowered viraemia and this conjugate generates hepatic concentrations of the antiviral drug that are at least three times higher than in other organs. Advantages compared with glycoprotein carriers are the lower immunogenicity and the high loading capacity of the poly-L-lysine, apart from the more patient-friendly intramuscular route of administration (Di Stefano, 1995; Fiume, 1995). Reconstituted HDL particles were employed to incorporate lipophilic prodrugs of iododeoxyuridine (Bijsterbosch, 1994). After lactosylation, the carrier directed more than 75 per cent of the dose to the liver. Further intrahepatic disposition or antiviral efficacy was not studied. A similar approach was taken by Korba et al. (Hepatol, 1996; 23:958), including lipophilic phosphatidyl prodrugs of nucleoside analogues in liposomes. This preparation showed remarkable activity in a woodchuck model where it reduces serum levels of hepatitis virus DNA more efficiently than the parent compound.

Recent studies have addressed the specific delivery of the anti-HIV drug AZT to macrophages and T lymphocytes using neoglycoproteins as drug carriers. Neoglycoproteins with human serum albumin as the protein backbone and various types of sugar were synthesized. AZT, in its monophosphate form, was covalently attached to the albumin using a water-soluble carbodiimide as a linking agent (Molema, JMedChem, 1991; 34:1137). The number of AZT monophosphate molecules per protein molecule varied between one and six and the charge of the protein did not alter upon conjugation (Molema, BiochemPharm, 1990; 40:2603; Molema, 1991).[72] In an in vitro anti-HIV assay using the HIV-III$_B$ strain of the virus and the MT-4 human T-lymphocyte cell line as the target cells, mannosylated albumin–AZT monophosphate conjugates were shown to have a remarkably high activity against HIV-1-induced cytopathogenicity (Molema, 1990). The galactosylated and fucosylated HSA–AZT monophosphate conjugates exhibited anti-HIV-1 activity in the same concentration range. All of these conjugates were significantly more potent against HIV-1 than the non-glycosylated albumin–AZT monophosphate conjugate and selectivity indices (the ratio of the 50 per cent cytotoxic concentration and the 50 per cent inhibitory concentration) were comparable with or higher than those of AZT and AZT monophosphate administered in a free form.

Some of the particular neoglycoproteins with relatively low sugar density (less than 10 galactose groups per albumin molecule) exhibit a favourable pharmacokinetic profile: they are only slowly eliminated from the bloodstream and will therefore be adequately exposed to the target cells. A relatively low galactose substitution and minimal change in net charge will prevent recognition by the hepatic and splenic endocytic systems, while negatively charged (glyco-) proteins or mannosylated proteins can deliver AZT-like drugs to endothelial cells and Kupffer cells, respectively. Both cell types are CD4+ and become infected by HIV. The conjugates with mannose substitution in the range of 15 sugar groups per albumin molecule are especiallly attractive candidates for targeting to liver macrophages.

The possible mechanisms of action of these neoglycoprotein–AZT monophosphate conjugates that were proposed are: (i) extracellular hydrolysis of the phosphoamide bond between AZT monophosphate and the neoglycoprotein at the surface of the cells, followed by diffusion of the AZT into the cells; (ii) sugar-specific recognition and internalization of the AZT monophosphate conjugates by the target cells, followed by intracellular release of the drug; (iii) coendocytosis of virus and AZT monophosphate conjugates following sugar-specific interaction between virus and neoglycoprotein–AZT monophosphate conjugate; and (iv) a combination of the above-mentioned mechanisms.

Extracellularly, the phosphoamide bond between AZT monophosphate and protein appears to be fairly stable. Experiments with ^{125}I-labelled AZT monophosphate conjugates showed that uptake of some of the conjugates was temperature dependent and could be partially inhibited by excess unlabelled conjugate, indicating a receptor-mediated uptake process.[72] In addition, direct binding of (neo-)glycoproteins to envelope proteins of HIV and possibly coendocytosis with HIV particles may play a role.

Interestingly, the neoglycoprotein carrier containing a high ratio of mannose to protein (40:1) had its own activity against HIV-1-induced cytopathogenicity.[72] It was considered that this intrinsic activity of the carrier might be caused by mannose-mediated inhibition of the interaction between HIV-1 gp120 and the target cells. However, another explanation for the strong anti-HIV-1 effect was found: the increased negative charge of the carrier, introduced by the p-aminophenyl sugars (Jansen, MolPharm, 1991; 39:818). More drastic derivatization by removing the positive charge of –NH$_2$ groups and adding anionic –COOH groups in human serum albumin, using the reaction of albumin with succinic anhydride or aconitic anhydride, turned the protein into highly negatively charged polypeptides (**suc-HSA** and **aco-HSA**, respectively). Aco-HSA exhibited an anti-HIV-1 activity of 10 to 40 times that of AZT on a molar basis (Jansen, 1991; Jansen, MolPharm, 1993; 44: 1003). The mechanism of this charge-based antiviral activity was demonstrated to be on the virus–cell fusion level (Jansen, 1991; Jansen, 1993). It was found that the negatively charged albumins interact with the V3 loop of the gp120 envelope glycoprotein, which has been demonstrated to be essential for virus–cell fusion (Swart, AntiviralNews, 1994; 2:69). This mechanism was also proposed earlier for the polyanionic agent dextran sulphate (Callahan, JVirol, 1991; 65:1543; Batinic, JBC, 1992; 267:6664). However, in contrast to dextran sulphate, suc-HSA inhibits syncytium formation in a 100-fold lower concentration than that at which it affects virus binding, pointing to a selective effect on virus–cell and T4-cell fusion. In concentrations above the antiviral inhibitory concentration range, a prolonged residence time in the circulation was found and rapid penetration of the lymphatic system (Swart, 1994; Jansen, PharmRes, 1993; 10:1611).

The peculiar mechanism of action of negatively charged albumin was also reported in a study on maleylalbumin (Takami, BBActa, 1992; 1180:180). At present, these proteins are investigated as potential carriers for AZT-like compounds, producing conjugates that provide inhibition of HIV replication at the level of virus–cell fusion as well as of RNA transcription. Such 'dual targeting' with intrinsically active carriers could lead to synergistic effects and prevention of drug resistance (Meijer, AntiviralRes, 1992; 18:215; Swart, AntiviralNews, 1994; 2:69). High activity was found against syncytium-inducing variants of HIV-1 that predominate in the terminal phase of HIV infection. Syncytium-inducing HIV-1 clinical isolates have been shown to have an increased positive charge in the V3 loop of the gp120 domain due to changes in amino acid composition and were shown to be largely inhibited by the modified albumins (Swart, 1994), in contrast to monoclonal antibodies raised against this part of the envelope protein (Callahan, JVirol, 1991; 65:1543; Batinic, JBC, 1992; 267:6664).

The negatively charged albumins may also bind toxic gp120 molecules shed during viral entry into the cell. Furthermore, they are readily biodegradable and exhibit very low immunogenicity, while they do not affect blood coagulation as is the case for dextran sulphate (Jansen, MolPharm, 1991; 39:818; Jansen, MolPharm, 1993; 44:1003).

Hepatic targeting of antineoplastic drugs

Cytostatic agents such as daunomycin, vindesine, methotrexate, cyclophosphamide, and treminon and toxins such as ricin, abrin, and gelonin as well as diphtheria toxins have been studied in relation to hepatoma targeting (reviewed in: Fallon, AdvDrugDelRev, 1989; 4:49; Wu, p.1303 in reference 13)[18,73]. (Neo-)glycoproteins (Trouet, PNAS, 1982; 79:626; Bodmer, MethodsEnz, 1988; 112: 298; Monsigny, AnnNYAcadSci, 1988; 551:399; Truet, p.19 in reference 70), tumour-specific antibodies (Adler, Hepatol, 1995; 22:1482),[74] poly-L-lysine (Arnold, MethodsEnz, 1985; 112:270; Ponpipom, p.53 in reference 69),[61,67] and various other synthetic polymers, liposomes, and particles as well as cells or virus coats were used as carriers. These carriers differ in molecular weight, size, and spatial conformation, lipophilicity, possibilities for derivatization with either specific targeting devices or drugs, cell specificity of binding and intracellular handling, and, as a consequence of all these features, whole body distribution and immunogenicity. These categories of targeting systems are not strictly separated, as demonstrated by the use of galactosylated monoclonal antibodies (Kojima, EurJNuclMed, 1990; 16:781; Ong, CancerRes, 1991; 51:1619) or liposomes (Haensler, GlycoconjugJ, 1991; 8:116; Yamazaki, MethodsEnz, 1994; 242:56), immunoliposomes (Storm, p.333 in reference 59) as well as neoglycoprotein liposomes (Kamps, PNAS, 1997; 94:11681).

With regard to hepatoma-specific drug targeting with (neo-)glycoproteins, however, the success of drug delivery with these galactose-terminated polymers *in vivo* depends on the difference in expression of the asialoglycoprotein between healthy hepatocytes and hepatoma cells, as well as on the internalization kinetics and sensitivity towards the drug. In a study of biopsy samples from patients with hepatocellular carcinoma, it was reported that 7 out of 10 biopsies retained at least some of the galactose-recognizing receptor, suggesting that asialoglycoprotein is a feasible route to deliver anticancer agents to hepatoma cells (O'Hare, Hepatol, 1989; 10:207). However, in many of the efficacy studies with galactosylated polymer conjugates, quite disappointing antitumour effects were reported if compared with proper controls. This is partly due to the fact that the polymer delivers the cytostatic drugs to the healthy hepatocytes and to a lesser extent to the tumour cells. Concomitant administration of inhibitors of the various lectins involved in hepatocyte uptake was therefore suggested to improve the tumour/liver tissue ratio (Ong, CancerRes, 1991; 51:1619; Seymour, AdvDrugDelRev, 1994; 14:89).

A crucial factor here is the saturability of the receptor-mediated uptake systems. It was calculated, on the basis of number of

receptors per hepatocyte and the maximal endocytic capacity, that at most 2 µg doxorubicin/g liver per hour can be delivered using an asialoglycoprotein carrier. At higher saturating doses, a more general tissue distribution occurs because aspecific fluid-phase endocytosis overwhelms the receptor-mediated uptake. In such conditions, the copolymers would concentrate passively in the solid tumour (partly due to a lack of lymphatic removal) (Seymour, CritRevTherDrugCarrSys, 1992; 9:135). It was claimed that the more optimal intracellular distribution of the passively endocytosed anticancer agents in the tumour cells could be beneficial (Duncan, AntiCancDrugs, 1992; 3:175; Seymour, AdvDrugDelRev, 1994; 14: 89). In addition, the hepatocytes surrounding the tumour and loaded with the targeted drug could function as a local slow-release compartment for the antitumour drugs. However, anticancer drug delivery to hepatoma cells with HPMA polymers without galactose derivatization showed a higher tumour to blood concentration than the galactosylated equivalent, making the asialoglycoprotein-mediated delivery of anticancer drugs to hepatomas of questionable benefit. Therefore, for specific tumour delivery, the use of antibody fragments, smaller proteins or peptides with specificity for the tumour cells attached to HPMA–drug conjugates, perhaps affords a better opportunity (Duncan, 1992; Adler, Hepatol, 1995; 22: 1482). Recently, adriamycin was coupled to a panel of monoclonal antibodies via a dextran bridge and tested in human hepatocellular carcinoma that was intrahepatically transplanted into mice. This led to detectable drug concentrations in the intrahepatic tumours but not in normal liver and myocardial tissue. The efficacy of the conjugate to lower α-fetoprotein levels was superior to the effect of mixtures of the individual compounds. This therapeutic effect of immunotargeting combined with the reduced systemic toxicity may provide attractive opportunities in the therapy of hepatocellular carcinoma.

Interestingly, the fact that hepatoma cells have a relative lack of asialoglycoprotein receptors can be used to rescue non-cancer cells from the toxic effects of high doses of methotrexate (Wu, p.1303 in reference 13). This was accomplished by coupling folinic acid to asialoglycoproteins and combining the conjugate with methotrexate. Only the receptor-negative cells are killed by the combination. It can be concluded from these data that the rescue factor, after release from the carrier, does not redistribute rapidly to the cancer cells. This targeting concept was expanded afterwards to prevent hepatoxicity of acetaminophen (Wu, Hepatol, 1985; 5:709) and galactosamine (Wu, JBC, 1988; 263:4719) through covalent coupling of *N*-acetylcysteine and uridine monophosphate, respectively, to asialoglycoproteins. In these studies it was assumed that *in vivo* the particular antitoxicant preparations are delivered equally to all the hepatocytes. However, studies on the acinar distribution of injected asialoglycoproteins exhibited zonal heterogeneity with relatively low concentrations in the central (zone 3) cells (Van der Sluijs, Hepatol, 1988; 8:1521; Burwen, JEMTech, 1990; 14:140). This would mean that the drug may only be presented adequately to the central cells, if the portal concentration of the carrier exceeds the K_m for receptor-mediated uptake. Fortunately, the affinity of most galactose-terminated neoglycoproteins for the receptor, as well as the hepatic extraction, is considerably lower than for the naturally occurring asialoglycoproteins. Therefore, a major heterogeneity in intrahepatic distribution of the neoglycoproteins is not anticipated (Van der Sluijs, p.235 in reference 60).

A special case of drug targeting to hepatocellular carcinomas is the use of Lipiodol. This derivative of poppy seed oil is administered intra-arterially into the hepatic artery. It is retained in the vasculature of the tumour for many days. Since Lipiodol is radio-opaque, this agent can be used for diagnostic purposes. Areas in the liver wherein the agent is retained for 2 to 3 weeks after administration are likely to be hepatocellular carcinomas. Tumours with diameters of 2 cm or greater can be visualized in this way. The specificity and the sensitivity of this method, however, is limited. Drugs like doxorubicin and cisplatin can be dissolved in Lipiodol and, for these drugs, Lipiodol serves as a slow-release system from where the cytostatic drugs are slowly delivered to the tumour cells. These methods are used in combination with chemoembolization. Inhibition of tumour growth has been reported using this technique (Izumi, Hepatol, 1994; 20:295).

Hepatic targeting of anti-inflammatory drugs

The sinusoidal cell types such as endothelial cells, stellate cells, and Kupffer cells play a central role in acute inflammatory reactions, septic shock, and liver rejections as well as in chronic fibrotic processes. The release of lipid mediators, cytokines, nitric oxide, and reactive oxygen species is a central aspect in these pathological conditions. Many drugs were developed to influence the production and cellular effects of these agents but often their efficacy is limited due to dose-limiting side-effects and lack of cell specificity. Therefore, cell-specific drug delivery formulations for the liver were developed.

The anti-inflammatory agent naproxen was covalently coupled to human serum albumin and to galactose- and mannose-terminated HSA to deliver this drug selectively to different cell types of the liver (Fig. 28) (Franssen, BiochemPharm, 1993; 45:1215). The liver to kidney ratios of the drug and the protein after injection of the conjugate were increased compared with the uncoupled drug, indicating an improved delivery of both protein and drug to the target site (Franssen, 1993).

Immunohistochemical staining of liver slices and cell separation studies revealed that the endothelial cells, and to a lesser extent Kupffer cells, were the sites for hepatic uptake of the naproxen–HSA conjugate. Further pharmacokinetic studies of naproxen$_{20}$-HSA in isolated perfused rat livers showed a saturable uptake process. The uptake in the liver could be inhibited by various polyanionic probes, indicating the involvement of a scavenger receptor system in the internalization mechanism of naproxen$_{20}$-HSA. This uptake via the scavenger receptor system was shown to be related to the increased negative charge and hydrophobicity of the naproxen–albumin conjugate as revealed by anion exchange chromatography. Studies in the intact organ and in purified liver lysosomal lysates indicate that, after internalization, naproxen$_{20}$-HSA is proteolytically degraded leading to the formation of the lysine conjugate of naproxen. This amino acid conjugate of naproxen was shown to be equipotent to naproxen itself with regard to inhibition of prostaglandin-E_2 synthesis (Franssen, PharmaceutRes, 1991; 8:1223).

A pronounced alteration in the intrahepatic distribution was observed when naproxen was coupled to lactosaminated and mannosylated HSA. Coupling of naproxen to Lac$_{27}$-HSA and Man$_{10}$-HSA resulted in a major shift in intrahepatic distribution from endothelial cells to the hepatocytes and Kupffer cells, respectively (Franssen, BiochemPharm, 1993; 45:1215). We conclude that conjugation of naproxen to HSA in itself results in a selective delivery to sinusoidal cells and that the local proteolysis of the conjugate produces an active catabolite. Selective delivery to endothelial, Kupffer, and parenchymal cell types of the liver can thus be achieved by attaching naproxen to (neoglyco-) proteins with an appropriate charge and sugar group (Fig. 28).

A cell protective effect of naproxen–HSA as a model targeting preparation was recently demonstrated *in vitro* and *in vivo* (Lebbe, Hepatol, 1994; 19:89I; Albrecht, Hepatol, 1996; 24:187A; Albrecht, Hepatol, 1997; 26:1553; Lebbe, JDrugTarget, 1997; 4:303). The effects of naproxen–HSA in isolated perfused liver of rats pretreated with *Corynebacterium parvum* and challenged with endotoxin were tested. A dose-dependent protection of the liver by naproxen–HSA in this model of acute hepatotoxicity could be observed. The highest dose of naproxen–HSA tested was as protective as a conventional dose of naproxen, but the effect was attained at a 30 times lower dosage (Lebbe, 1994). *In vivo*, an effective conventional dose of uncoupled naproxen at chronic administration induces toxic effects on renal function, while this side-effect is absent after administration of the albumin-conjugated drug. *In vivo* studies showed that coupling of naproxen to human serum albumin favourably altered the distribution and the kinetics of the drug. Pharmacokinetic analysis showed that the apparent volume of distribution and plasma half-life of naproxen–HSA in rats were markedly reduced compared with the parent compound (Lebbe, 1994). Naproxen–HSA taken up by the liver was metabolized to naproxen–lysine. This active metabolite was found in the liver 30 min after administration. It is excreted into the bile over a relatively long period of time at a constant elimination rate in contrast to the rapid excretion after injection of naproxen–lysine itself. Degradation of the carrier and release of naproxen–lysine is probably rate-limiting in this elimination process. Only a small amount of naproxen itself reappeared in the plasma. Preferential uptake into endothelial and Kupffer cells compared with hepatocytes could be demonstrated by cell isolation and immunocytochemical studies. It was recently shown that a low dose of the naproxen–albumin conjugate greatly increased survival rate of lipopolysaccharide (LPS)- infused rats with ligated bile ducts. This effect may be due to a decrease of prostaglandin production in the activated liver macrophages in this model. The combined release of prostaglandins and tumour necrosis factor-α is supposed to be lethal to the rats owing to overt lung toxicity (Albrecht, JHepatol, 1996; 25:130).

These investigations may lead to an alternative therapeutic approach in the treatment of acute and chronic liver disease; thus, more effective anti-inflammatory drugs such as corticosteroids or leukotriene synthesis inhibitors could be targeted to different liver cell populations. This may not only provide more effective treatment with less side-effects but could also help to elucidate the role of different cell populations in the pathogenesis of chronic liver disease.

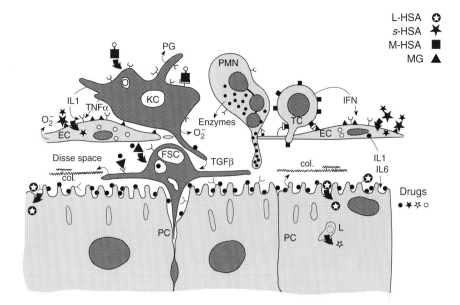

Fig. 28. Potential carriers in drug targeting to various liver cell types: parenchymal cells (PC) are targeted with lactosaminated HSA, endothelial cells (EC) with succinylated HSA, Kupffer cells (KC) with mannosylated HSA, and stellate cells with modified forms of certain globulins (MG).

Targeting of genes and antisense material to the liver

The process of receptor-mediated endocytosis and the above-mentioned drug targeting technology can in principle also be employed for delivery of small fragments of DNA/RNA or antisense oligonucleotides to certain cell types. This concept has been reviewed recently (Ledley, Hepatol, 1993; 18:1263; Chang, Gastro, 1994; 106: 1076).[11] The aim is to correct genetic deficiencies or to induce the production of essential proteins such as peptide hormones, plasma proteins, and membrane carriers/receptors. DNA in the form of suitable plasmids should be delivered to the cytoplasmic compartment or be integrated into the cellular genome. Transcription to mRNA as well as the final translation into polypeptides can be monitored to detect the cellular expression of the targeted gene. Gene targeting was first attempted for a proinsulin gene that was included in small liposomes (Nicolau, CritRevTherDrugCarrSys, 1989; 6:239), but many other studies have been reported to date (Frese, AdvDrugDelRev, 1994; 14:137; Grasso, AdvPharmacol, 1994; 28:169; Monsigny, AdvDrugDelRev, 1994; 14:1; Perales, PNAS, 1994; 91:4086; 14:113; Wagner, AdvDrugDelRev, 1994). In order to test the suitability of the targeted gene product, foreign 'reporter' genes such as the bacterial gene coding for chloramphenicol acetyltransferase (**CAT**) are often used. *In vitro*, genes can be introduced into cultured cells by microinjection or calcium phosphate-mediated permeation of the plasma membrane. Fusion of plasmid-containing liposomes (Nicolau, 1989) with cells and cellular penetration by adeno- or retroviruses (Wilson, p.149 in reference 65) are also employed. Evidently, cellular transfection is much more difficult to perform in the intact organism. However, recent developments in gene targeting to the liver *in vivo* indicate that persistent expression of genes might be achieved (Wu, Hepatol, 1988; 8:1251; Wu, Biochem, 1988; 27:887; Wilson, Hepatol, 1989; 10:631; Wu, Hepatol, 1989; 10:618; Frese, 1994; Wagner, 1994). Receptor-mediated endocytosis is used to introduce the gene, in spite of the fact that most of the endocytosed material is usually trafficked to a degradative compartment: the lysosomes. The crucial question here is how the endocytosed plasmid can be engineered to escape this abortive route. There is evidence for some internalized ligands that a small proportion of the endocytotic vesicles may become associated with the Golgi system, may recycle to the plasma membrane, or can undergo transcytosis (Russel, Gastro, 1983; 85: 225; Townsend, PNAS, 1984; 81:466). For growth factors such as epidermal growth factor, vectorial transport to the cell nucleus is normally a minor route. During liver regeneration following hepatectomy, complete perturbation of cellular routeing is observed in the sense that much less of the ligand is trafficked to lysosomes and much more to the cell nucleus (Marti, Hepatol, 1989; 9:126). Whether this is true for other macromolecules remains to be studied. Nevertheless, integration of targeted DNA and also its expression can be greatly enhanced by prior partial hepatectomy (Wu, Hepatol, 1988; 8:1251; Wu, Hepatol, 1989; 10:618), probably as a consequence of rapid cell replication. Also, agents that induce hyperplasia of the liver can be used to improve integration of the foreign DNA. Pretreatment of rats with the hypolipidaemic agent nafenopin, which induces marked growth of the liver (Meijer, JPharmExpTher, 1977; 202:8), leads to persistent expression of the CAT gene injected *in vivo* (Wu, Hepatol, 1990; 12:871).

Major research efforts are devoted at present to the design of a suitable carrier for targeting DNA to organs *in vivo*. The DNA–carrier complex should be sufficiently stable in the bloodstream, non-covalent binding of DNA should be preferred, and the complex should be water soluble. Various groups have used the basic polypeptide polylysine that strongly binds DNA. In the studies of Wu *et al.* the polylysine matrix was covalently coupled to asialoorosomucoid to obtain hepatocyte specificity (Wu, p.1303 in reference 13). Direct galactosylation of polylysine is an alternative (Biessen, JHepatol, 1994; 21:806; Martinez-Fong, Hepatol, 1994; 20:1602; Monsigny, AdvDrugDelRev, 1994; 14:1), while galactosylated liposomes (Koike, AnnNYAcadSci, 1994; 716:331) and

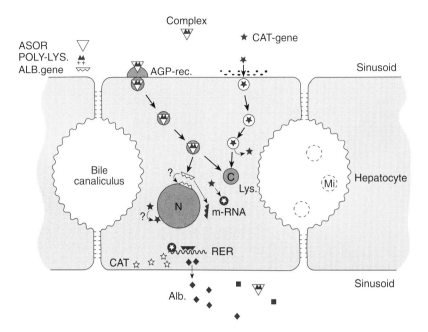

Fig. 29. Targeting of genes to the hepatocyte with macromolecular carriers. In principle, two transfection procedures can be used: cationization of the plasma membrane leading to adsorptive endocytosis of the DNA fragments, for instance by cationic liposomes (indicated for the chloramphenicol acetyltransferase (CAT) gene); or non-covalent binding of the plasmid to poly-L-lysine, covalently coupled to the asialoglycoprotein asialo-orosomucoid (indicated for the albumin gene). After receptor-mediated or adsorptive endocytosis an unknown part of the endocytosed material escapes the abortive lysosomal route. This DNA remains in the cytoplasmic compartment and is translated into mRNA. Integration into the cellular genome presumably does not take place, but persistent expression was detected by mRNAs and synthesis of the coded proteins (see Wu, p.1537 in reference 48).

histones (Chen, HumGeneTher, 1994; 5:429) have also been proposed. Depending on the size of the plasmid, polylysine polymers of different length can be employed. Careful titration is necessary to keep the complex in solution. This concept was applied to target a foreign gene (CAT) combined with various promoters to the liver and clear expression of the gene was demonstrated (Wu, Biochem, 1988; 27:887), especially after partial hepatectomy (Wu, Hepatol, 1988; 8:1251). Excess asialo-orosomucoid prevents DNA targeting to the liver, probably through competition with the asialo-glycoprotein receptors. Both viral promoters and human promoter genes can be used. Wu *et al.* succeeded in using gene targeting to correct genetic analbuminaemia in the so-called Nagase rat model (Wu, Hepatol, 1989; 10:618) (Fig. 29) and cholesterolaemia due to an LDL receptor deficiency in the rabbit (Wilson, Hepatol, 1989; 10:631). A gene coding for human serum albumin was expressed in rats within 48 h after injection, raising the albumin concentration in the plasma from 0 to 18 mg/100 ml. Persistent expression was seen until 4 weeks postinjection. A gene coding for the LDL receptor protein was targeted to the rabbit liver *in vivo* resulting in a 25 to 50 per cent decrease in cholesterol plasma concentration lasting for 2 days after injection of the plasmid–polylysine–asialo-orosomucoid preparation (Wilson, Hepatol, 1989; 10:631).

Another technology that could lead to specific inhibition of HBV and HCV replication is cellular delivery of antisense DNA (Blum, Lancet, 1991; 337:1230; Stein, Science, 1993; 261:1004).[12] This approach has been taken in a number of studies (Goodarzi, JGen-Virol, 1990; 71:3021; Blum, 1991; Wu, JBC, 1992; 267:12436; Offensperger, EMBOJ, 1993; 12:1257; Lu, JNuclMed, 1994; 35: 269) and an effective block of viral replication occurred via multiple translational steps, such as RNA processing and translation as well as arrest of viral gene expression. These 'code blockers' have been shown to be very effective *in vitro* and incidentally also *in vivo* as shown in the Peking duck (Offensperger, 1993). *In vivo* application requires efficient hepatocyte uptake and cytoplasmic/nuclear delivery of the polyanionic antisense material. However, it can be anticipated that the negatively charged polynucleotides will either be largely taken up by scavenger systems in endothelial and Kupffer cells and/or be excreted renally, so that antiviral efficiency will be limited. Consequently, some sort of encapsulation or targeting device is required. Similar to the above-mentioned targeting of DNA, this can be achieved by complexation with lactosaminated poly-L-lysine (Martinez-Fong, Hepatol, 1994; 20:1602; Monsigny, AdvDrugDelRev, 1994; 14:1) or asialoglycoprotein–poly-L-lysine conjugates (Wu, 1992; Lu, JNuclMed, 1994; 35:269).[12] The latter approach, at least *in vitro*, yielded a long-lasting inhibition of HBV replication. Further studies in the intact organism, including improved preparations that at least partially escape the abortive route to lysosomes, need to be undertaken. An alternative to the use of antisense nucleotides is the use of ribozymes. These are enzymes that are provided with specific cRNA sequences that link to DNA. When linked to DNA, the ribozyme cuts it and so prevents transcription. In this way the transcription of unwanted RNA, such as viral RNA, is prevented and this represents a potentially powerful antiviral therapy (Zaia, AnnNYAcadSci, 1992; 660:95; Blum, AdvDrugDelRev, 1995; 17:321). However, delivery of the ribozyme to the cells of choice needs to be established. Cationized liposomes are employed for this purpose (Konopka, AntiviralRes, 1995; 26:A266).

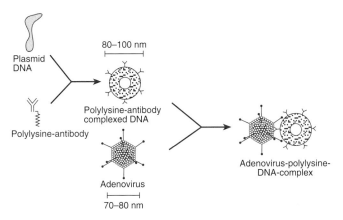

Fig. 30. Schematic representation of the approach to target adenovirus–polylysine–DNA complexes containing heterologous DNA attached to an exterior adenovirus capsid. To accomplish linkage of an adenovirus and a polycationic DNA-binding domain, a chimeric adenovirus containing a heterologous epitope in the exterior domain of its hexon protein was employed in conjunction with the monoclonal antibody specific for this epitope. The monoclonal antibody was rendered competent to carry foreign DNA sequences by attaching a polylysine moiety. Interaction of the polylysine–antibody complexed DNA with adenovirus occurs via the specificity of the conjugated antibody (see Wagner, AdvDrugDelRev, 1994; 14:113).

The particular RNA or DNA-targeting complexes bear a resemblance to enveloped viruses both with regard to size and entry functions. However, viruses have an additional feature: the release of viral DNA from the endosomal compartment into the cytoplasm and subsequent targeting to the cell nucleus. Endosomal acidification activates viral coat proteins that trigger the disruption of the endosomal membrane (adenovirus) or induce fusion of the viral and endosomal membranes (influenza virus) (Fig. 30). Virus-free targeting preparations in which the endosome-disruptive proteins are included are being developed at present (Frese, AdvDrugDelRev, 1994; 14:137; Heard, Hepatol, 1994; 20:253; Monsigny, AdvDrugDelRev, 1994; 14:1; Wagner, AdvDrugDelRev, 1994; 14:113; Zhang, Hepatol, 1994; 20:271A). In addition, engineered (recombinant) DNA and RNA virus particles have been designed for hepatic targeting of genetic material (Huber, PNAS, 1991; 88:8039; Cardoso, HumGeneTher, 1993; 4:411; Morsy, JCI, 1993; 92:1580; Basu, Hepatol, 1994; 20:1640; Bralet, AmJPathol, 1994; 144:896; Branchereau, HumGeneTher, 1994; 5:803; Chang, Gastro, 1994; 106:1076; Drazan, Surgery, 1994; 116:197; Grasso, AdvPharmacol, 1994; 28:169; Kolodka, SomCellMolGen, 1994; 20:251; Prager, Gastro, 1994;104:974A; Shaked, Transpl, 1994; 57:32, 1508). A promising gene transfer vector in this respect is the genome of human adeno-associated virus type 2, while chicken adenovirus I that cannot replicate in human cells can also be used (Ledley, Hepatol, 1993; 18:1263; Bowles, AdvDrugDelRev, 1995; 17:293; Wilson, AdvDrugDelRev, 1995; 17:303).

For the purpose of *in vivo* DNA targeting, recombinant viruses are produced in which all the viral sequences are present except the inverted terminal repeats at both ends of the genome that were replaced by heterologous genes.[11] Random integration in the cellular genome of various cell types has been reported in proliferating cells (i.e. in hepatocytes during regeneration) and also in non-proliferating cells (Ledley, Hepatol, 1993; 18:1263; Bowles,

AdvDrugDelRev, 1995; 17:293; Wilson, AdvDrugDelRev, 1995; 17: 303).[11] The advantage of this methodology is that the transgene expression is transient (up to 6 to 8 months), while the expression level can be sufficient even in quiescent cells (via extrachromosomal persistence). Disadvantages of adenoviral vectors are potential insertional mutagenesis (albeit less likely than in the case of retroviral vectors) and low cell specificity *in vivo* (Ledley, 1993; Bowles, 1995).[11] Also, repeated administration can be severely hampered by major immune responses. Recently, Ilon (JCI, 1997; 99:1098) showed that oral tolerization with adenoviral antigen was successful in permitting long term gene expression. Co-administration of anti-inflammatory drugs may also be an option to solve this problem. Chronic immunosuppression by cyclosporin (Fang, HumGeneTher, 1995; 6:1039) or even temporal down-regulation of B and T cell responses by cyclophosphamide during adenovirus vector administration (Jooss, HumGeneTher, 1996; 7:1555) strongly prolongs transgene expression in mice. It should also be realized that the upper limit in size of the gene to be transfected is 8 kilobase pairs.[11]

An alternative is the use of amphotrophic retroviruses, in which integration of the viral genome in chromosomal DNA results in a stable and lifelong expression, assuming that the promotion sequence that directs the expression remains active.[11] Although *in vivo* cell specificity is low, the use of a cell type-specific promoter may provide satisfactory tissue selectivity. Although the random integration may invite mutagenesis, the practical risk seems to be low. Promoters derived from genes originating from the liver, such as the β-actin promoter, produce more persistent gene expression than viral promoter sequences. Very promising, in this respect, are synthetic promoters including a binding site for hepatocyte nuclear factor 3 (Hafenrichter, JSurgRes, 1994; 56:510).

As mentioned above, non-viral gene transfer systems like polylysines, provided with receptor-directed recognition modalities (glycoproteins, antibodies), combined with endosome-disrupting viral capsid molecules or endosomeolytic peptides can be very elegant carriers for genes and antisense material (Wagner, PNAS, 1990; 87:3410; Midoux, NucAcidRes, 1993; 21:871; Chang, Gastro, 1994; 106:1076; Wu, p.1537 in reference 48).[11] The advantages are that viral recombinant events, theoretically leading to replication-competent viruses, cannot occur and relatively large expression cassettes (up to 40 kilobase pairs) can be transfected. Nevertheless, the expression level is relatively low even if intracellular distribution is favourably influenced by endosomolytic peptides (Ledley, Hepatol, 1993; 18:1263).

A number of measures can be taken to increase the efficiency of transfection *in vivo* including: 30 to 70 per cent hepatectomy (Wilson, JBC, 1992; 267:11483; Wu, p.1537 in reference 48), portal vein injection during hepatic in-flow occlusion (Rettinger, PNAS, 1994; 91:1460), induction of liver regeneration by pretreatment with hypolipidaemic drugs (Wu, Hepatol, 1990; 12:871), or transfection of hepatocytes with a urokinase gene that leads to hepatocyte degeneration and regeneration (Lieber, PNAS, 1995; 92:6210). Other procedures are the concomitant use of inhibitors of endosomal and lysosomal function with chloroquine (Yamamoto, Hepatol, 1995; 22:847) and microtubule/microfilament-disrupting agents (Chowdhury, Gastro, 1993; 104:A981).

In the case of adenoviral and retroviral vectors, major problems arose either through opsonization by complement factors (Squinto,

AdvDrugDelRev, 1995; 17:213)[11] or other immunological re- actions that hamper repeated administration. A combined immuno- suppressive treatment with cyclosporin (Fang, HumGeneTher, 1995; 6:1039) or soluble cytotoxic lymphocyte antigen-4 that inter- feres with the interaction between T cells and antigen-presenting cells has been reported to cope with this problem (Kay, NatureGen, 1995; 11:191).

Alternatives to viral and non-viral targeting systems to be used *in vivo* are *ex vivo* protocols (Chowdhury, Science, 1991; 254:1802) in which a portion of the liver is removed, the hepatocytes isolated and transfected, and subsequently reintroduced into the body via the portal vein or injection into the spleen (Wu, p.1537 in reference 48). From the spleen the cells later translocate to the liver. Although this method is feasible, only up to about 5 per cent of the liver may be derived from a hepatocellular graft of which, at most, 20 per cent can be transfected with a retroviral vector. Consequently, only up to 1 per cent of the hepatocyte volume of the liver can be transduced by a heterologous gene (Grossman, HumGeneTher, 1992; 3:501; Grossman, JLabClinMed, 1993; 120:472). Recently it was shown that, when liver cell damage was induced before cell transplantation, a proper proliferating stimulus may result in extensive repopulation of the liver with the transfected cells.

In addition, direct injection of naked DNA, DNA-coated microprojectiles, and cationized DNA-containing-liposomes that induce adsorptive endocytosis have been reported (Hickman, Adv- DrugDelRev, 1995; 17:265). Intraparenchymal injection *in vivo* and direct intratumoural injection (Chen, PNAS, 1995; 92:2577) can be employed to overcome the low specificity of, for instance, adenoviral vectors for dividing cells. This treatment can be considered for slowly growing hepatocellular carcinoma and liver metastasis (Hick- man, 1995).[11] Other potential types of improved tumour speci- ficity are the use of retroviral vectors (expressed in proliferating cells) and the inclusion of a carcinoma-specific promoter in the gene construct. Either the introduction of a suicide gene such as one that codes for thymidine kinase (Mullen, PharmTher, 1994; 63:199) and leads to rapid conversion of nucleoside analogue prodrugs to their active triphosphate derivatives in proliferating tumour cells, or inclusion of an α-fetoprotein promoter combined with such a suicide gene (Macri, HumGeneTher, 1994; 5:175; Ido, CancerRes, 1995; 55:3105) are promising technologies in hepatic antitumour therapy (Ledley, Hepatol, 1993; 18:1263; Macri, 1994).

Major problems to be solved in the above-mentioned techniques are the generally low expression levels, the transient character of gene expression, and the lack of 'therapeutic' regulation of the expressed genes (negative or positive feedback by gene products or pathology markers). Nevertheless, long-lasting expression of the production of therapeutic proteins has been reported recently. For instance, canine factor IX gene transfer led to a 9-month influence on clotting time (Kay, PNAS, 1994; 91:2353) and therapeutic levels of factor IX persisted for 6 to 8 months in mice transfected with an adenoviral vector (Kaleko, JCellBiochem, 1995; 21A:C6) and for about 5 months in rats treated with a galactosylated poly-(L)- lysine–DNA complex (Perales, PNAS, 1994; 91:4086).

Applications in the correction of genetic disorders such as enzyme deficiencies and receptor/carrier protein deficiencies as well as the *in vivo* production of pharmacologically active polypeptides represent novel options in the study of liver metabolism and therapy.

References

1. Meijer DKF and Groothuis GMM. Hepatic transport of drugs and proteins. In McIntyre N, Benhamou JP, Bircher J, Rizzetto M, and Rodes J, eds. *Oxford textbook of clinical hepatology*, Vol. 1. Oxford: Oxford University Press, 1991: 40–78.
2. Meijer DKF. Transport and metabolism in the hepatobiliary system. In Schultz SG, Forte JG, and Rauner BB, eds. *Handbook of physiology*, Sect. 6, Vol. III. New York: Oxford University Press, 1989: 717–58.
3. Meijer DKF, Mol WEM, Müller M, and Kurz G. Carrier-mediated trans- port in the hepatic distribution and elimination of drugs, with special reference to the category of organic cations. *Journal of Pharmacokinetics and Biopharmaceutics*, 1990; **18**: 35–70.
4. Olinga P, Meijer DKF, Slooff MJH, Groothuis GMM. Liver slices in *in vitro* pharmaco-toxicology with special reference to the use of human liver tissue. *Toxicology In Vitro* 1997;**12**:77–100.
5. Ballet F. Hepatic circulation: potential for therapeutic intervention. *Phar- macology and Therapeutics*, 1990; **47**: 281–328.
6. Wehner F and Petzinger E, eds. *Cell biology and molecular basis of liver transport*. Dortmund: Projekt Verlag, 1995.
7. Sorrentino D, Potter BJ, and Berk PD. From albumin to the cytoplasm: the hepatic uptake of organic anions. In Popper H and Schaffner F, eds. *Progress in liver diseases*. Philidelphia: WB Saunders, 1990: 203–24.
8. Meijer DKF and Ziegler K. Mechanisms for the hepatic clearance of oligopeptides and proteins. Implications for rate of elimination, bio- availability and cell-specific drug delivery to the liver. In Audus KL and Raub TJ, eds. *Biological barriers to protein delivery*. New York: Plenum Press, 1993: 339–408.
9. Stein WD. *Transport and diffusion across cell membranes*. Orlando: Academic Press, 1986.
10. Groothuis GMM and Meijer DKF. Hepatocyte heterogeneity in bile formation and hepatobiliary transport of drugs. *Enzyme*, 1992; **46**: 94–138.
11. Alt M and Caselmann WH. Liver-directed gene therapy: molecular tools and current preclinical and clinical studies. *Journal of Hepatology*, 1995; **23**: 746–58.
12. Lee-Young AW, Wu GY, and Wu CH. Delivery of polynucleotides to hepatocytes. In Lee YC and Lee RT, eds. *Neoglycoconjugates: preparation and applications*. San Diego: Academic Press, 1994: 511–37.
13. Siegers C-P and Watkins JB, III, eds. *Biliary Excretion of Drugs and Other Chemicals*. Stuttgart: Gustav Fischer Verlag, 1991.
14. Gregus Z and Klaassen CD. Enterohepatic circulation of toxicants. In Roxman K and Hänninen O, eds. *Gastrointestinal toxicology*. Amsterdam: Elsevier Science Publishers BV, 1986: 57–118.
15. Lauterbach F. Intestinal permeation of organic bases and quaternary am- monium compounds. In Csaky TZ, ed. *Handbook of experimental phar- macology, Vol. 70/II. Pharmacology of intestinal permeation*. Berlin: Springer Verlag, 1984: 271–84.
16. Groothuis GMM and Meijer DKF. Drug traffic in the hepatobiliary system. *Journal of Hepatology* 1996; **14**: 3–28.
17. Smith RL. Excretion of drugs in bile. In Brodie B and Gilette JG, eds. *Handbook of experimental pharmacology*. Berlin: Springer-Verlag, 1971: 354– 89.
18. Meijer DKF and Van der Sluijs P. Covalent and noncovalent protein binding of drugs: implications for hepatic clearance, storage, and cell-specific drug delivery. *Pharmaceutical Research*, 1989; **6**: 105–18.
19. Weiner IM. Organic acids and bases and uric acid. In Seldin DW and Giebisch G, eds. *The kidney: physiology and pathophysiology*. New York: Raven Press, 1985: 169–84.
20. Hofmann AF. Enterohepatic circulation of bile acids. In Forte JG, ed. *Handbook of physiology. Section 6: the gastrointestinal system. Vol. III. Sa- livary, gastric, pancreatic and hepatobiliary secretion*. New York: American Physiological Society, Oxford University Press, 1989: 567–96.
21. Klaassen CD and Watkins JB, III. Mechanisms of bile formation, hepatic uptake and biliary excretion. *Pharmacological Reviews*, 1984; **36**: 1–67.
22. Tozer TN. Implications of altered plasma protein binding in disease states. In Benet LZ, ed. *Pharmacokinetic basis for drug treatment*. New York: Raven Press, 1984: 173–93.

23. Roy Chowdhury N, Roy Chowdhury J, Bizzaro W, and Arias IM. Bile pigment metabolism. In Arias IM, Frenkel M, and Wilson JHP, eds. *The liver annual 6.* Amsterdam: Elsevier Science Publishers BV, 1987: 478–504.

24. Levine WG. Biliary excretion of drugs and other xenobiotics. *Progress in Drug Research*, 1981; **25**: 361–419.

25. Lauterbach F. Intestinal secretion of organic ions and drugs. In Kramer M, ed. *Intestinal permeation.* Amsterdam: Excerpta Medica, 1977: 173–95.

26. Arias IM, Jakoby WB, Popper H, Schachter D, and Shafritz DA, eds. *The Liver: biology and pathobiology.* 2nd edn. New York: Raven Press, 1988.

27. Frenzel H, Kremer B, and Hucker H. The liver sinusoids under various pathological conditions. A TEM and SEM study of rat liver after respiratory hypoxia, telecobalt-irradiation and endotoxin application. In Wisse E and Knook DL, eds. *Kupffer cells and other liver sinusoidal cells.* Amsterdam: Elsevier, 1977: 213–22.

28. Fukui H, *et al.* Effect of ethanol on hepatic oxygenation: evidence of hepatic hypoxia. In Pijper J, Goldstick TK, and Meyer M, eds. *Oxygen transport to tissue XII.* New York: Plenum Press, 1990: 691–6.

29. Sugiyama Y and Kato Y. *In vitro* models of hepatic uptake: methods to determine kinetic parameters for receptor-mediated hepatic uptake. In Taylor MD and Amidon GL, eds. *Peptide-based drug design: controlling transport and metabolism.* Washington, DC: American Chemical Society, 1994: 525–51.

30. Ballet F and Thurman RG, eds. *Research in perfused liver: clinical and basic applications.* London: INSERM/John Libbey, 1991.

31. Olinga P. Human liver slices and isolated hepatocytes in drug disposition and transplantation research. Thesis, University of Groningen, 1996.

32. Berry MN, Edwards AM, and Berritt GJ. Utilization of hepatocytes for drug studies. In Burdon RH vKH, ed. *Isolated hepatocytes preparation, properties and applications.* 1st edn. Amsterdam: Elsevier, 1991: 182–4.

33. Gebhardt R. Use of isolated and cultured hepatocytes in studies on bile formation. In Guillouzo A and Guguen-Guillouzo C, eds. *Research in isolated and cultured hepatocytes.* London/Paris: John Libbey Eurotext Ltd./INSERM, 1986: 353–76.

34. Buscher HP, *et al.* Hepatic transport systems for bile salts: localization and specificity. In Paumgartner G, Stiehl A, and Gerok W, eds. *Bile acids and the liver.* Lancaster, England: MTP Press, 1987: 95–110.

35. Rogiers V. Cultures of human hepatocytes in *in vitro* pharmaco-toxicology. In Rogiers V, Sonck W, Shephard E, and Vercruysse A, eds. *Human cells in* in vitro *pharmaco-toxicology.* Brussels: VUB Press, 1992: 77–115.

36. Mol WEM. Transport mechanisms for cationic drugs in the hepato-biliary system. A pharmacokinetic and cell biological study. Thesis, University of Groningen, 1988.

37. Petzinger E, Kinne RKH, and Sies H, eds. *Hepatic transport of organic substances.* Berlin: Springer-Verlag, 1989.

38. Paumgartner G and Preisig R, eds. *The liver. Quantitative aspects of structure and function.* Basel: Karger, 1973.

39. Goresky CA. The lobular design of the liver: its effect on uptake processes. In Lundgvist F and Tygstrup N, eds. *Regulation of hepatic metabolism.* Copenhagen: Munksgaard, 1974: 808–22.

40. Bass NM and Williams RL. Hepatic function and pharmacokinetics. In Zakim D and Boyer TD, eds. *Hepatology. A textbook of liver disease.* 2nd edn. Philadelphia: WB Saunders; Harcourt Brace Jovanovich, 1990: 235–54.

41. Schanker LS. Transport of drugs. In Hokin LE, ed. *Metabolic pathways. Vol. VI. Metabolic transport.* 3rd edn. New York: Academic Press, 1972: 543–79.

42. Boyer JL. Mechanisms of bile secretion and hepatic transport. In Andreoli TE, Hoffman JF, Fanestil DD, and Schultz SG, eds. *Physiology of membrane disorders.* 2nd edn. New York: Plenum Medical Book Company, 1986: 609–36.

43. Meier PJ. Transport polarity of hepatocytes. *Seminars in Liver Disease*, 1988; **8**: 293–307.

44. Meuwissen JATP, Ketterer B, and Heirwegh KPM. Role of soluble binding proteins in overall hepatic transport of bilirubin. In Berk PD and Berlin NI, eds. *Chemistry and physiology of bile pigments.* Bethesda: National Institutes of Health, 1977: 323–37.

45. Wolkoff AW. The glutathione *S*-transferases: their role in the transport of organic anions from blood to bile. In Javitt NB, ed. *Liver and biliary tracts physiology I.* Baltimore: University Park Press, 1980: 151–69.

46. Petzinger E. Transport of organic anions in the liver. An update on bile acid, fatty acid, monocarboxylate, anionic amino acid, cholephilic organic anion, and anionic drug transport. *Reviews of Physiology, Biochemistry and Pharmacology*, 1994; **123**: 47–211.

47. Petzinger E, Fischer K, and Fasold H. Role of the bile acid transport system in hepatocellular ouabain uptake. In Erdmann E, Grieff K, and Akou JC, eds. *Cardiac glycosides 1785–1985. Biochemistry, pharmacology, clinical relevance.* Darmstadt: Steinkopf Verlag, 1986: 297–304.

48. Arias IM, Boyer JL, Fausto N, Jakoby WB, Schachter DA, and Shafritz DA, eds. *The liver: biology and pathobiology.* 3rd edn. New York: Raven Press, 1994.

49. Brass EP. Carnitine transport. In Ferrari R, DiMauro S, and Sherwood G, eds. L-*Carnitine and its role in medicine: from function to therapy.* London: Academic Press; Harcourt Brace Jovanovich, 1992: 21–36.

50. Braakman I. Hepatocyte heterogeneity in organic cation transport. Thesis, University of Groningen, 1988.

51. Thalhammer T, Fellinger A, Meijer DKF, Groothuis GMM, and Graf J. Separation of periportal and centrilobular rat liver parenchym cells in a fluorescence activated cell sorter after acridine orange staining. In Davison JS and Shaffer EA, eds. *Gastrointestinal and hepatic secretions: mechanisms and control.* New York: University of Calgary Press, 1988: 82–4.

52. Meijer DKF. The mechanisms for hepatic uptake and biliary excretion of organic cations. In Kramer M and Lauterbach F, eds. *Intestinal permeation.* Amsterdam: Excerpta Medica, 1976: 196–207.

53. Steen H. Mechanisms for the hepatic disposition of cationic drugs. Molecular aspects of membrane transport in the hepatocyte. Thesis, University of Groningen, 1992.

54. Müller M. Membrantransport von organischen kationen in hepatocyten. Ein beitrag zur aufklärung von hepatischen transportvorgängen. Dissertation, Universität von Freiburg, 1988.

55. Buscher H-P, *et al.* Membrane transport of amphiphilic compounds by hepatocytes. In Greten H, Windler E, and Beisiegel U, eds. *Receptor-mediated uptake in the liver.* Berlin: Springer-Verlag, 1986: 189–99.

56. Fujimoto JM. Some *in vivo* methods for studying sites of toxicant action in relation to bile formation. In Plaa G and Hewitt WR, eds. *Toxicology of the liver.* New York: Raven Press, 1982: 121–45.

57. Smit JW, Steen H, and Meijer DKF. Modulators of protein kinase C as well as MDR reversal agents have a major influence on the biliary excretion of the cationic drugs tri-N-butylmethyl-ammonium (TBuMA) and doxo-rubicin. In Keppler D and Jungermann K, eds. *Transport in the liver.* Heidelberg: Falk Symposium No. 74, 1994: Abstract no. 27.

58. Vonk RJ, Van Doorn ABD, and Meijer DKF. The influence of bile salts on hepatocellular transport. In *Falk Symposium No. 26. V. Bile Acid Meeting. Biological effects of bile salts.* Lancaster: MTP, 1978: 121–6.

59. Claassen V and Timmerman H, eds. *Trends in drug research.* Amsterdam: Elsevier Scientific, 1990.

60. Wu GY and Wu CH, eds. *Liver diseases. Targeted diagnosis and therapy using specific receptors and ligands.* New York: Marcel Dekker, 1991.

61. Ryser HJ-P and Shen W-C. Drug–poly(lysine) conjugates: their potential for chemotherapy and for the study of endocytosis. In Gregoriadis G, Senior J, and Poste G, eds. *Targeting of drugs with synthetic systems.* New York: Plenum Publishing, 1986: 103–21.

62. Steer CJ and Ashwell G. Hepatic membrane receptors for glycoproteins. In Popper H and Schaffner F, eds. *Progress in liver diseases*, Vol. VIII. New York: Grune & Stratton, 1986: 99–123.

63. Windler E and Greten H, eds. *Hepatic endocytosis of lipids and proteins.* München: W. Zuckschwerdt Verlag, 1992.

64. Sottrup-Jensen L. α-Macroglobulin and related thiol ester plasma proteins. In Putman FW, ed. *The plasma proteins: structure, function, and genetic control*, Vol. 5. 2nd edn. Orlando: Academic Press, 1987: 192–291.

65. Tomlinson E and Davis SS, eds. *Site-specific drug delivery.* Chichester: John Wiley, 1986.

66. Weiss P and Ashwell G. The asialoglycoprotein receptor, properties and modulation by ligand. In Bauman P, Eap CB, Muller WE, and Tillement JP, eds. *α1–Acid glycoprotein. Genetics, biochemistry, physiological functions and pharmacology*. New York: Alan Liss, 1989: 169–84.

67. Shen TY. Preferential membrane permeation and receptor recognition in drug targeting. In Roche EB, ed. *Bioreversible carriers in drug design. Theory and application*. New York: Pergamon Press, 1989: 214–25.

68. Roerdink FH, Daemen T, Bakker-Woudenberg IAJM, Storm G, Crommelin DJA, and Scherphof GL. Therapeutic utility of liposomes. In Johnson P and Lloyd-Jones JG, eds. *Drug delivery systems. Fundamentals and techniques*. Chichester: VCH, 1987: 66–80.

69. Gregoriadis G, Poste G, Senior J, and Trouet A, eds. *Receptor-mediated targeting of drugs*. New York: Plenum Press, 1984.

70. Gregoriadis G, Senior J, and Trouet A, eds. *Targeting of drugs*. New York: Plenum Press, 1982.

71. Molteni L. Dextrans as drug carriers. In Gregoriadis G, ed. *Drug carriers in biology and medicine*. New York: Academic Press, 1979: 107–25.

72. Molema G and Meijer DKF. Optimization of the synthesis of neo-glycoprotein-AZTMP conjugates. Influence on stability, hepatic clearance and anti-HIV activity. In Delivery of the anti-HIV drug azidothymidine (AZT) to T-lymphocytes with neoglycoprotein carriers. Thesis, University of Groningen, 1992: 91–104.

73. Blakey DC and Thorpe PE. Prevention of carbohydrate-mediated clearance of ricin-containing immunotoxins by the liver. In Frankel AE, ed. *Immunotoxins*. Boston: Kluwer Academic Publishers, 1988: 457–73.

74. Ghose T, Blair AH, Vaughan K, and Kulkarni P. Antibody-directed drug targeting in cancer therapy. In Goldberg EP, ed. *Targeted drugs*. New York: John Wiley, 1982: 1–22.

2.5 Hepatic metabolism of drugs

J. Desmeules, P. Bonnabry, and P. Dayer

Pathways of drug metabolism

In order to cross biological membranes and to have access to their target tissues, most drugs and other biologically active xenobiotics share the common characteristic of lipophilicity and remain un-ionized or only partially ionized at physiological pH. On the other hand, major physiological excretion pathways, such as the renal and biliary routes, because of their hydrophilic nature, have the capacity to eliminate hydrophilic compounds only. Drugs and related xenobiotics would therefore have a prolonged duration of activity in the absence of an efficient biotransformation system capable of altering them to hydrophilic derivatives. Drug metabolism is an alternative process that may lead to the termination of biological activity, but during this process of chemical biotransformation the risk of generating powerful reactive and toxic intermediate products is very high. Hepatic metabolism of drugs and toxins thus represents a critical determinant of xenobiotic-induced tissue toxicity.

Major enzyme systems

The toxication/detoxification process of xenobiotics is achieved by a group of enzymes with broad substrate specificity (Table 1).[1–4]

It is noteworthy that some of these enzymes are implicated predominantly in physiological processes and appear to metabolize xenobiotics as alternatives to their endogenous substrates (e.g. the liver mono-oxygenase responsible for hydroxylation of steroids is also implicated in the metabolism of several drugs).

Although each tissue possesses some ability to metabolize drugs, the liver is the principal organ where this metabolism takes place. Most drug-metabolizing enzymes are located in the lipophilic domain of the membranes of the endoplasmic reticulum (e.g. the oxidative enzymes, the glucuronyltransferases), but metabolism also can take place in the mitochondria, the cytosol (e.g. some phase II enzymes), or in lysosomes. Other tissues where drug biotransformation may occur include the skin, intestine, lungs, blood, central nervous system, kidneys, and placenta.

Biotransformation has been divided into two distinct phases (Tables 2 and 3). Phase I usually converts the parent drug to a more polar metabolite by the addition or unmasking of a specific functional group, resulting in 'functionalization' of the drug molecule. If phase I derivatives are sufficiently polar, they can be readily excreted. In most cases, however, phase I products undergo a subsequent biosynthetic reaction, called a phase II reaction, the product of phase I being in an appropriate chemical state to be acted upon by the phase II enzymes. An endogenous substrate such as glucuronic acid or an amino acid combines with the product of the phase I reaction to form a highly polar conjugate. A common feature of phase II reactions is the requirement for an activated intermediate (cofactor or drug). Phases I and II are often co-ordinated, although some parent drugs may already possess a functional group which may form a conjugate directly (e.g. NSAIDs).

In general, drug metabolism can be considered as a detoxification process in that it converts active compounds into inactive metabolites. However, metabolic bioactivation can sometimes occur and be a pathogenic mechanism of adverse drug reactions. Both phase I and phase II enzymes are responsible for some drug bioactivation where the xenobiotic biotransformation leads to products with enhanced activity or toxicity, including mutagenicity, teratogenicity, and carcinogenicity. An imbalance between bioactivation and bio-inactivation may be acquired as a result of environmental factors or a genetically determined enzyme deficiency and may lead to tissue injuries.

Of the wide variety of enzymes that participate in xenobiotic metabolism listed in Table 1, only the major enzymes will be discussed. It should be noted that many drugs can undergo several of the reactions listed above simultaneously. The relative importance of a particular pathway depends on many factors, including chemical, physiological, pathological, and exogenous factors.

Oxidations

Cytochrome P-450-dependent mono-oxygenase system

The cytochrome P-450-dependent mono-oxygenase system is the product of a multigene family of central importance. The cytochrome P-450 enzymes are determinants in oxidative, peroxidative, and reductive metabolism of exogenous (drugs, environmental chemicals like carcinogens and pollutants) and endogenous compounds such as steroids, bile and fatty acids, prostaglandins, biogenic amines, and retinoids. Each individual organism possesses a number of different cytochromes P-450, many of which are selectively inducible by a variety of foreign compounds.

The key enzymatic components of the system are the flavoprotein NADPH-cytochrome P-450-oxidoreductase and cytochrome P-450.

Table 1 Some examples of enzymes involved in xenobiotic biotransformation
Acetyltransferase
Dehydrogenase
Esterase, amidase
Flavin-containing mono-oxygenase
Glutathione-S-transferase
Methyltransferase
Mixed function oxidase
Reductase
Sulphotransferase
UDP-glucosyltransferase
UDP-glucuronyltransferase

Cytochromes P-450

Cytochrome P-450, the terminal electron acceptor and substrate-binding site of the microsomal mixed-function oxidase system, is probably the most versatile and unique biological catalyst known.

In 1962, Omura and Sato described a pigment with unusual spectral properties when studying rabbit liver microsomes; they called it cytochrome P-450 because this haemoprotein pigment, containing protoporphyrin IX as the prosthetic group, exhibits a spectral absorbance maximum at 450 nm when reduced and complexed with carbon monoxide (Omura, JBC, 1964; 239:2370). Later, Estabrook *et al*.[5] revealed the key role of this haemoprotein in the hydroxylation of steroids, drugs, and carcinogens.

The human cytochromes P-450 are located within the membrane of the endoplasmic reticulum of the liver (also called hepatic microsomes, the vesicles formed from the endoplasmic reticulum membranes upon cellular disruption). Some cytochromes P-450 are also expressed in other tissues such as the intestine, kidney, skin, lung, and central nervous system, and individual forms are heterogeneously distributed within a given tissue: for example, in the liver, some forms are more abundant in the centrilobular than in the periportal regions. Cytochromes P-450 are also present in animals, plants, and bacteria.[6,7]

Multiplicity and nomenclature

The ancestral gene of the P-450 family existed before prokaryote–eukaryote divergence. Cytochrome P-450 was originally thought to be a single haemoprotein with a broad substrate specificity, but subsequently it became apparent that there exists a large family of closely related isozymes, the members of which catalyse the oxygenation of numerous endogenous and exogenous hydrophobic substrates, and which display different but overlapping substrate specificities (Lu, PharmRev, 1980; 31:277). These isozymes are distinguishable by their physical, chemical, and immunological properties; only minor variations of the amino-acid sequence may be associated with major differences in substrate specificity. A great deal of progress has been made in the identification and characterization of human liver cytochromes P-450 with immunological and recombinant DNA technology, revealing the magnitude and complexity of the P-450 superfamily, and confirming that each P-450 enzyme is derived from a different gene.[8] On this basis, the cytochromes P-450 have been classified into families and subfamilies related to their degree of sequence similarity. Foundations of the nomenclature system for the P-450 superfamily were laid with the

Table 2 Subclassification of major phase I reactions
Oxidations
Alcohol oxidation
Alcohol/aldehyde dehydrogenations
Amine oxidation
Aromatic/aliphatic hydroxylations
Dehalogenation
Epoxidation
N-, *S*-, *O*-dealkylations
N-, *S*-Oxidations
Oxidative deamination
Phosphothionate oxidation
Xanthine oxidation
Reductions
Hydrolysis
Amide, ester hydrolysis
Hydrazine and carbamate hydrolysis
Hydration
Isomerization

first report published by Nebert and Gonzales (Nebert, AnnRevBiochem, 1987; 56:945) and frequently updated since then (Nelson, Pharmacogenet, 1996; 6:1). To date the P-450 superfamily contains 74 gene families of which 14 families exist in all mammals examined today. These 14 families comprise 26 mammalian subfamilies of which 20 have been mapped in the human genome. This nomenclature is based on divergent evolution of the P-450 superfamily. P-450 protein sequences from one gene family are defined has having more than 40 per cent amino-acid identity to each other, and more than 55 per cent within the same subfamily (Whitlock, ISIAtlasSci: Pharmacol, 1988:351). These originally arbitrary decisions turned out to be useful because, so far, genes within a defined subfamily have been found lying within the same gene cluster. Cytochromes P-450 were first designated with letters representing the substrates that led to their discovery. Today, an alphanumerical nomenclature is defined. For human genes, an italicized root symbol *CYP* is used (*cy*tochrome *P*-450), followed by an Arabic number denoting the family, a letter designating the subfamily, and an Arabic number representing the individual gene.

In humans, cytochrome P-450 gene families 1 to 3 are the major isozymes implicated in the inactivation of xenobiotics such as drugs and endogenous substrates (see Table 4). On the basis of their expression in the liver, it appears that they represent 70 per cent of total cytochromes and among them CYP3A4 is the most abundant (30 per cent), followed by CYP2C (20 per cent), CYP1A2 (13 per cent), CYP2E1 (7 per cent), CYP2D6 (2 per cent), and CYP2B6

Table 3 Subclassification of major phase II reactions (conjugation reactions)
Acetylation
Amino-acid conjugation
Condensation
Fatty-acid conjugation
Glucuronidation
Glutathione conjugation
Glycosylation
Methylation
Sulphation

Table 4 Human drug-metabolizing cytochrome P-450 genes that have been characterized to date

Family	Subfamily	Isoform	Trivial name	Chromosome	Relative quantity (%)	Remarks
1	A	1A1	P1	15		Extrahepatic isoform, inducible
		1A2	PA, P3	15	13	Inducible
2	A	2A6	IIA3, IIA4	19	<1	
	B	2B6	LM2, IIB1	19	<1	Inducible
		2B7	HIIB2	19		Absent in the liver, present in lungs
	C	2C8	IIC2, MP-12	10		Bimodal distribution
		2C9/10	TB, IIC1, MP-8	10	10	
		2C18	29c, 6b	10		
		2C19	MP, 11a	10	1	Genetic polymorphism
	D	2D6	DB1, BUF1	22	2	Genetic polymorphism
	E	2E1	J	10	7	Inducible
3	A	3A3/4	NF, PCN1	7	30	Inducible
		3A5	hPCN3	7	15–30 if present	Present in 20–30% of the population
		3A7	HFLa, HFL33	7	30–50 of fetal liver P-450	Major fetal isoform, absent in adult liver

(less than 1 per cent) (Shimada, JPharmExpTher, 1994; 270:414). Some of them will be discussed separately.

The CYP1 gene family

A comprehensive review of the animal data on the CYP1 gene family has been published (Ioannides, DrugMetabRev, 1990; 22:1). Those cytochromes P-450 were isolated from B6 mouse liver and their production was induced by 3-methyl cholanthrene. CYP1A1 was specific for the oxidation of benzo[a]pyrene while CYP1A2 was specific for acetanilide oxidation. These enzymes are ubiquitous in mammals and seem to play an important role in carcinogen activation.

The CYP1A subfamily

The CYP1A subfamily has only two members in humans with a great overlap in substrate specificity. The human *CYP1A* genes, located on the chromosome 15, were sequenced (Jaiswal, NucAcidRes, 1985; 13:4503 and 1986; 14:6773).

Unlike CYP1A2, which is constitutively expressed in human liver, CYP1A1 appears to be expressed only in extrahepatic tissues such as lung and placenta (Wong, CancerRes, 1986; 46:999; Shimada, MolPharm, 1992; 41:856; Murray, Carcinogenesis, 1993; 14:585). This enzyme does not contribute significantly to the hepatic metabolism of drugs. The activation of heterocyclic amines benzene to mutagenic products by this isozyme is well documented (Nebert, DNA, 1989; 8:1; Edwards, Carcinogenesis, 1994; 15:829). Polymorphism in CYP1A1 expression has been reported in a number of ethnic populations and it has been associated with a putative increase in susceptibility to lung cancer in Japanese people who smoke cigarettes (Nakachi, CancerRes, 1993; 53:2994), whereas a recent case–control study does not support the hypothesis of CYP1A1 polymorphism as a risk factor for lung cancer development in Europeans (Bouchardy, Biomarkers, 1997; 2:131).

The CYP1A2 isozyme represents approximately 10 per cent of total cytochrome P-450. It has a high level of catalytic activity towards arylamines and is responsible for the N-demethylations of caffeine and theophylline (Table 5) (Nebert, IntJBiochem, 1989; 21:

Table 5 Some xenobiotics whose biotransformation is mediated by CYP1A2

Aflatoxin B1
Caffeine
Clomipramine
Clozapine
Imipramine
NNK (4-(methylnitrosamino)-1-(3-pyridyl)-1-butanone)
Ondansetron
Paracetamol
Phenacetine
Propranolol
Tacrine
Theophylline
Warfarin

243).[8] The levels of expression vary 40-fold in different hepatic samples and reflect the variability observed in caffeine N^3-demethylation (Butler, Pharmacogenet, 1992; 2:116). Although a polymorphism has been claimed, it is still a matter of debate (Kalow, ClinPharmTher, 1991; 49:44). If a polymorphism exists, it could be at the level of the regulatory system and not the structural gene, compatible with the known racial difference in inducibility.[9] The isoenzyme is induced by environmental factors such as smoking, omeprazole, phenobarbital, phenytoin, charbroiled food, cruciferous vegetables, and dioxin. It can also be inhibited by a number of xenobiotics such as amiodarone, ciprofloxacine, norfloxacine, fluvoxamine, and furafylline. In addition to theophylline and caffeine, the clinical contribution of this enzyme to the metabolism of drugs has been underlined for tacrine therapy, which is associated with an unpredictable hepatotoxic reaction in up to 50 per cent of patients (Murray, Carcinogenesis, 1993; 14:585; Spaldin, BrJClinPharm, 1994; 46:13).[8] *In vitro* studies have demonstrated that microsomal enzyme-dependent bioactivation of tacrine to the electrophilic protein-reactive quinone is CYP1A2 dependent (Madden, BiochemPharm, 1993; 46:13). This quinone can be reduced by the addition of cellular thiols such as glutathione or react with macromolecules such as protein or DNA to initiate cell damage.

Clozapine *N*-demethylation correlates with CYP1A2 activity (Pirmohamed, JPharmExpTher, 1995; 272:984), but the putative bio activation of clozapine in liver or leucocytes is mediated by enzymes other than CYP1A2. This isozyme is also responsible for the activation of mutagenic products like aflatoxin B1 or NNK (4-(methylnitrosamino)-1-(3-pyridyl)-1-butanone), a procarcinogen found in cigarette smoke.

The CYP1B subfamily

The catalytic function of the recently discovered subfamily CYP1B has still to be determined.

The CYP2 gene family

The CYP2 gene family contains at least 8 subfamilies and 57 individual isoforms (Gonzales, TrendsPharmacolSci, 1992; 13:346).

CYP2A6 and CYP2B6 isozymes, for which genes are located on chromosome 19, are both expressed in human liver (less than 1 per cent) (Mimura, DrugMetDisp, 1993; 21:1048). A genetic polymorphism has been described for the *2A6* gene, but the incidence of the deficient allele is low (less than 2 per cent) (Fernandez Salguero, AmJHumGen, 1995; 57:651). The clinical contribution in the metabolism of drugs appears to be minimal. The CYP2A6 isozyme is known to catalyse the 7-hydroxylation of coumarine, which could serve as a non-invasive assay for the enzyme (Fernandez Salguero, AmJHumGen, 1995; 57:651). This isozyme also metabolizes a number of carcinogens including aflatoxin B1.

The CYP2C subfamily

The CYP2C subfamily constitutes a major group of expressed cytochrome P-450 in human liver, with four isozymes identified up to now (CYP2C8, CYP2C9/10, CYP2C18, CYP2C19). Their genes are located on chromosome 10 and each of them have more than 80 to 90 per cent sequence homology with the others.

P-450 *2C8* has been cloned (Ged, Biochem, 1988; 27:6929). The 6α-hydroxylation of taxol and the 4-hydroxylation of retinoic acid have been identified as being catalysed by this isozyme (Leo, ArchBiochemBiophys, 1989; 269:305; Harris, CancerRes, 1994; 54:4026) (Table 6). However, since most antibodies or nucleic acid probes cannot discriminate among members of this subfamily, the metabolic reactions catalysed by this isozyme are not yet characterized.

P-450 2C9/10 are the most abundant proteins of the CYP2C subfamily expressed in the liver and represent 10 per cent of total cytochrome liver content. The protein-coding sequence of CYP2C10 differs from that of CYP2C9 in only two codons and may be an allelic variant of CYP2C9 or a library artefact.[9]

A few years ago, *in vitro* findings suggested that tolbutamide and *S*-mephenytoin hydroxylations were catalysed by the same enzyme; however, the *in vivo* disposition of tolbutamide does not differ between extensive and poor metabolizers for the mephenytoin-type polymorphism. The yeast-based expression system using a cDNA clone (MP-8) related to the cytochrome 2C subfamily displayed tolbutamide hydroxylase and hexobarbital 3′-hydroxylase activities in *Saccharomyces cerevisiae*, but no mephenytoin 4′-hydroxylase activity. These results led to the suggestion that the hydroxylations of mephenytoin and tolbutamide are catalysed by similar but distinct cytochromes P-450 (Brian, Biochem, 1989; 28:4993). Other authors

Table 6 Some xenobiotics whose biotransformation is mediated by the CYP2C subfamily		
2C8	2C9/10	2C19
Taxol	Hexobarbital	Antidepressants
Tolbutamide	Losartan	Amitriptyline
Retinoic acid	NSAIDs	Clomipramine
	Diclofenac	Imipramine
	Flurbiprofen	Moclobemide
	Ibuprofen	Diazepam
	Mefenamic acid	Lansoprazole
	Naproxen	S-mephenytoin
	Oxicams	Omeprazole
	Oral anticoagulants	Propranolol
	S-acenocoumarol	
	S-warfarin	
	Phenytoin	
	Sulphamethoxazole	
	Tienilic acid	
	Tolbutamide	
	Torasemide	

confirmed this observation (Relling, JPharmExpTher, 1990; 252:442; Veronese, BBResComm, 1991; 175:112). In addition to tolbutamide, this isozyme also catalyses the hydroxylation of tienilic acid (Lopez Garcia, JBioch, 1993; 213:223), the 4-hydroxylation of phenytoin (Veronese, BBResComm, 1991; 175:112), the 7-hydroxylation of *S*-warfarin and *S*-acenocoumarol (Rettie, ChemResTox, 1992; 5:54), and the oxidation of a number of non-steroidal anti-inflammatory drugs (**NSAIDs**) like diclofenac, tenoxicam, piroxicam, ibuprofen (Leemann, DrugsExpClinRes, 1993; 19:189; LifeSci, 1993, 52:29), and flurbiprofen (Tracy, BiochemPharm, 1995; 49:1269) (Table 6). Sulphaphenazole and fluvastatine appear to be strong and selective inhibitors of P450 2C9 (Miners, BiochemPharm, 1988; 37:1137; Transon, ClinPharmTher, 1995; 58:412; EurJClinPharm, 1996; 50:209).

P450 2C18 appears to be a minor member of the CYP2C subfamily and to date no reaction has been identified to be catalysed preferentially by this isozyme.

P450 2C19 (Romkes, Biochem, 1991; 30:3247) is the polymorphic isozyme responsible for *S*-mephenytoin 4-hydroxylation as demonstrated with a recombinant isozyme (Goldstein, Biochem, 1994; 33:1743). This genetic polymorphism shows the expected pattern of mendelian inheritance which affects about 2 to 5 per cent of Caucasian (Kupfer, EurJClinPharm, 1984; 26:753) and 13 to 23 per cent of Asian populations (e.g. 19 per cent in the Japanese). Two defective CYP2C19 alleles have been described which account for 87 per cent of Caucasian and more than 99 per cent of Oriental PM alleles (De Morais, JBC, 1994; 269:15419; MolPharm, 1994; 46:594). The major defects responsible for this polymorphism were identified as a splice variation of CYP2C19 (called m1), a single base change in exon 4 leading to a premature stop codon (called m2), and recently, a single base change in the initiation codon (called m3), which affects the initiation of translation and contributes to the PM polymorphism in Caucasians (Goldstein JA, personal communication). A number of drugs of clinical importance cosegregate with *S*-mephenytoin hydroxylase activity, such as diazepam *N*-demethylation (Zhang, ClinPharmTher, 1990; 48:496)

Table 7 Some xenobiotics whose biotransformation is mediated by CYP2D6	
Antidepressants	Bufuralol
Amitriptyline	Metoprolol
Citalopram	Propranolol
Clomipramine	Timolol
Desipramine	**Antiarrythmics**
Doxepine	Ajmaline
Fluoxetine	Encainide
Fluvoxamine	Flecainide
Imipramine	Propafenone
Maprotiline	Sparteine
Mianserine	**Opioids**
Nortriptyline	Codeine
Paroxetine	Dextromethorphan
Trimipramine	Dihydrocodeine
Venlafaxine	Ethylmorphine
Neuroleptics	Hydrocodone
Clozapine	Levomethorphan
Haloperidol	Tramadol
Perphenazine	**Others**
Risperidone	Methoxyamphetamine
Thioridazine	Methoxyphenamine
Zuclopenthixol	Ondansetron
β-Blockers	Phenformin
Alprenolol	Ritonavir
Bopindolol	Tropisetron

and omeprazole hydroxylation, the polymorphism of which correlates closely with that of mephenytoin in Caucasian and Chinese populations (Andersson, Pharmacogenet, 1992; 2:25). Omeprazole could also decrease CYP2C19 activity and slow the clearance of diazepam (Caraco, ClinPharmTher, 1995; 58:62). *In vivo*, the metabolism of propranolol to naphtoxylacetic acid cosegregates with *S*-mephenytoin 4-hydroxylase activity (Ward, ClinPharmTher, 1989, 45:72), but *in vitro* data with recombinant isozymes revealed that the *N*-desisopropylation of *S*-(-)-propranolol is partially inhibited by selective inhibitors of CYP1A2 (Yoshimoto, BrJClinPharm, 1995; 39:421) and the mean partial clearance of propranolol to naphtoxylacetic acid was twice as high in those who smoke (inducing CYP1A2) than in non-smokers (Walle, BrJClinPharm, 1984; 18: 741). In conclusion, both CYP1A2 and CYP2C19 seem to catalyse the *N*-deisopropylation of propranolol. Other important reactions appear to be catalysed by the CYP2C19 isozyme (Table 6).

The CYP2D gene subfamily

This subfamily is associated with a common human defect in drug oxidation known as the debrisoquine/sparteine polymorphism, the target enzyme of this polymorphism being cytochrome P-450 debrisoquine 4-hydroxylase. Unlike many other cytochrome P-450 enzymes, debrisoquine 4-hydroxylase is not inducible. About 20 years ago, the defect was simultaneously and independently discovered by two groups for debrisoquine and sparteine respectively, and was followed by population studies (Mahgoub, Lancet, 1977; ii:584; Eichelbaum, EurJClinPharm, 1979; 16:183). It was found that 5 to 10 per cent of Caucasians failed to oxidize these drugs, and developed exaggerated pharmacological responses. Subsequent studies showed that poor metabolizers also exhibit an impaired capacity for the oxidation of the compounds listed in Table 7.

The clinical significance of this polymorphism is well established and there is now convincing evidence that poor metabolizers represent a subgroup in the population with a propensity to develop adverse drug reactions or inability to activate drugs. Moreover, studies have also indicated that a link may exist between the debrisoquine/sparteine-type polymorphism and some neuropsychological traits, 'spontaneous' neurodegenerative disease like Parkinson's, and pulmonary cancer (Ayesh, Nature, 1984; 312:169; Armstrong, Lancet, 1992; 339:1017; Bouchardy, CancerRes, 1996; 56:251).

The deficiency is inherited as an autosomal recessive trait. The identification of this genetic polymorphism of drug oxidation related to mono-oxygenase function permitted a more detailed study of the mechanisms causing interindividual variations in drug metabolism and was followed by extensive investigations at the protein and gene level (Meyer, PharmTher, 1990; 46:297). Initial studies led to the identification of CYP2D6 (P-450 DB1, P-450 BUF1) as the deficient enzyme (Gut, FEBSLett, 1984; 173:287; Gut, JBC, 1986; 261: 11734; Dayer, BiochemPharm, 1987; 36:4145). Immunoquantification of cytochrome P-450 2D6 in human liver then provided evidence for the specific absence of debrisoquine hydroxylase as the cause of debrisoquine polymorphism. A cDNA probe for human cytochrome P-450 2D6 has been cloned and sequenced, and has subsequently led to the discovery of several aberrant splicing patterns of CYP2D6 pre-mRNA in the liver of poor metabolizers (Gonzalez, Nature, 1988; 331:442). The analysis of leucocyte DNA from *in vivo* phenotyped poor and extensive metabolizer individuals, for restriction fragment length polymorphisms (**RFLP**), allowed the identification of mutant alleles of the P-450 *2D6* gene (Skoda, PNAS, 1988; 85:5240). It was further pointed out (Gonzales, ClinPharmTher, 1991; 50:233) that using the polymerase chain reaction (**PCR**) and RFLP (Gonzales, ClinPharmacokin, 1994; 26: 59) allows the detection of some 20 different haplotypes causing CYP2D6-dependent drug metabolism of normal, decreased, increased, or absent catalytic activities (see refs in[10]). Using PCR and RFLP, three genotypes stand out from epidemiological studies on 410 healthy European volunteers, the homozygous D6/D6 (44 per cent) and heterozygous D6/D6B (29 per cent) among the extensive metabolizers, while the homozygous D6(B)/D6(B) accounts for the majority of poor metabolizers (4.84 per cent) (Broly, DNA, 1991; 10:545). Among the poor metabolizers, three major defective alleles were described—CYP2D6(B) (21 per cent; Kagimoto, JBC, 1990, 265:17209), CYP2D6(D) (5 per cent; Gaedigk, AmJHumMet, 1991; 48:943), and CYP2D6(A) (2 per cent; Kagimoto, JBC, 1990; 265:17209), as well as four mutations of minor importance. There is a pronounced interethnic difference in the distribution of the defective alleles, for example CYP2D6B and CYP2D6A are almost exclusively present in Caucasians while CYP2D6D is harmoniously distributed between Oriental, black, and Caucasian populations. Further sequencing of the *CYP2D6* locus on chromosome 22 revealed the existence of two homologous pseudogenes: *CYP2D7* and *CYP2D8* (Kimura, AmJHumGen, 1989; 45:889). Finally, subjects requiring higher doses of CYP2D6 substrates were identified (ultrarapid metabolizers) and were shown to possess duplicated or amplified active *CYP2D6* genes (Johansson, PNAS, 1993; 90:11825; Dahl, JPharmExpTher, 1995; 274:516).

Table 8 Some xenobiotics whose biotransformation is mediated by CYP2E1

Chlorinated hydrocarbons
Chlorzoxazone
Ethanol
Paracetamol
Volatile anaesthetics
    Enflurane
    Halothane
    Isoflurane
    Methoxyflurane
    Sevoflurane

The CYP2E gene subfamily

An ethanol-inducible form of cytochrome P-450, CYP2E1, has been purified in human liver, reconstituted, and expressed from its cDNA (Bouchardy, Biomark, 1997; 2:131).[8] The gene is localized on chromosome 10. This enzyme has a catalytic activity against exogenous, hydrophobic, small compounds such as ethanol, short-chain alcohols, and N-nitrosodimethylamine (Guengerich, TrendsPharmacolSci, 1989; 10:107). Induction of this enzyme is likely to play a role in the development of cancers (nitrosamine-induced cancers, tobacco–alcohol neck, and head cancers). Preliminary evidence indicates that CYP2E1 displays large interindividual variability (Lieber, NEJM, 1988; 319:1639). CYP2E1 expression is also correlated with glucose homeostasis; it seems to be regulated by starvation or insulin treatment and could play a role in gluconeogenesis (Johansson, BBResComm, 1991;173:331).[10] Chlorzoxazone is 6-hydroxylated *in vitro* specifically by human CYP2E1 (Peter, ChemResTox, 1990; 3:566) and was proposed as a probe of the *in vivo* metabolic potential of CYP2E1 (Vesell, Pharmacogenet, 1995; 5:53). Other metabolic reactions appear to be catalysed by CYP2E1 (Table 8.)

The CYP3 gene family
The CYP3A gene subfamily

The human liver CYP3 family is clinically important because it is responsible for the biotransformation of a large number of drugs (Table 9). In man, four genes inducible by anticonvulsants, rifampicin, and barbiturates are known. One member of this gene subfamily, CYP3A4, has been isolated on the basis of its oxidase activity towards nifedipine and related dihydropyridines (Guengerich, JBC, 1986; 261:5051; Gonzalez, PharmTher, 1990; 45:1). This subfamily is of particular interest as it is the most abundant in man and because its substrate specificity is low. At least 20 other dihydropyridines are oxidized to pyridine by this enzyme.[6]

This enzyme or a closely related protein is also implicated in the metabolism of several endogenous substances such as 17β-oestradiol, testosterone (Guengerich, MolPharm, 1988; 33:500), and cortisol, as well as numerous xenobiotics such as quinidine, cyclosporin (Kronbach, ClinPharmTher, 1988; 43:630), lidocaine (Bargetzi, ClinPharmTher, 1989; 46:521), midazolam (Kronbach, MolPharm, 1989; 36:89), and other benzodiazepines and several anticancer drugs (see Table 9).

The extremely variable metabolism (more than 10-fold) of nifedipine suggested the existence of a genetic polymorphism, but characterization of the enzyme at the molecular level and population studies (Porchet, ClinPharmTher, 1990; 48:155) showed no difference in the enzyme between individuals who were deficient in the oxidation of this drug and controls (Gonzalez, DNA, 1988; 7:79). Environmental factors thus seem to contribute to the variability in the catalytic activity of the cytochrome P-450 3A4 enzyme.

Other members of this subfamily are CYP3A3, CYP3A5, and CYP3A7. CYP3A3 differs from CYP3A4 by only 11 amino acids and no differences in activity between these two isoforms have been identified. CYP3A5 is expressed in only 20 to 30 per cent of the population. Its metabolic capacity is less important than CYP3A3/4, but it shares with them a similar substrate profile; for example, it also metabolizes midazolam, nifedipine, and steroids, but does not catalyse the oxidation of quinidine and erythromycin. Finally, CYP3A7 is the major cytochrome P-450 expressed in fetal liver. Its role is not well understood and this isoform is totally absent from adult liver.

Catalytic cycle of cytochrome P-450

Although cytochrome P-450 plays a major role in the activity of mixed-function oxidase, it does not act alone. The overall process of oxidation catalysed by cytochrome P-450 requires cytochrome P-450, NADPH-cytochrome P-450 reductase, molecular oxygen, and lipids for substrate binding and interaction between cytochrome P-450 and NADPH-cytochrome P-450 reductase molecules. This last enzyme consists of 1 mol of flavine mononucleotide and 1 mol of flavine adenine dinucleotide per 1 mol of apoprotein and exists in close association with cytochrome P-450 in the endoplasmic reticulum. The flavoprotein transfers reducing equivalents from $NADPH + H^+$ to the oxygenated form of cytochrome P-450. One flavoprotein molecule is present for 10 to 100 molecules of cytochrome P-450, and thus the cytochrome P-450 haem reduction is the rate-limiting step in many hepatic drug oxidations.[1,3]

In the course of the reaction, one molecule of substrate reacts with one molecule of molecular oxygen and NADPH to yield the oxidized substrate and NADP. One molecule of oxygen is reduced per substrate molecule, one oxygen atom being incorporated into the substrate, and the other reduced to water (White, AnnRevBiochem, 1980; 49:315).[6]

The initial step in the cycle involves the drug binding to the oxidized form of cytochrome P-450, to form a binary complex. In the second step, the substrate–P-450 binary complex is reduced by a single electron provided by NADPH through the action of the flavoprotein, NADPH-cytochrome P-450 reductase. The ferrous haemocytochrome P-450–substrate binary complex then binds oxygen to form an 'activated-oxygen' complex. This complex transfers 'activated oxygen' to the drug substrate to form the oxidized product. The last steps involve electron rearrangement, introduction of a second electron, oxygen insertion, and product release. The overall reaction and its stoichiometry can be illustrated as follows, RH symbolizing the substrate:

$$RH + O_2 + NADPH + H^+ \rightarrow ROH + H_2O + NADP^+$$

The potent oxidizing properties of the activated oxygen complex together with very low specificity allows oxidation of a large number of substrates that share a high lipid solubility.

Table 9 Some xenobiotics and endogenous compounds whose biotransformation is mediated by CYP3A4 or a closely related isozyme

Antidepressants
  Amitryptiline
  Clomipramine
  Imipramine
  Mianserine
  Sertraline
  Venlafaxine
Anti-infectious drugs
  Dapsone
  Erythromycin
  Indinavir
  Josamycin
  Ketoconazole
  Primaquine
  Ritonavir
  Sagrinavir
  Troleandomycin (TAO)
Antihistamines H1
  Astemizole
  Loratadine
  Terfenadine
Benzodiazepines and related drugs
  Alprazolam
  Clonazepam
  Diazepam
  Midazolam
  Triazolam
  Zolpidem
  Zopiclone

Cardiovascular drugs
  Amiodarone
  Diltiazem
  Losartan
  Lovastatin
  Nifedipine and related dihydropyridines
  Quinidine
  Simvastatin
  Verapamil
Cytostatics
  Carmustine
  Cyclophosphamide
  Etoposide
  Fluorouracil
  Fosphamide
  Lomustine
  Tamoxifen
  Taxol
  Teniposide
  Vinblastine
  Vincristine
  Vindesine
  Vinorelbine
Gastrointestinal drugs
  Cisapride
  Granisetron
  Lansoprazole
  Omeprazole
  Ondansetron
  Tropisetron
Local anaesthetics
  Bubivacaine
  Cocaine
  Lidocaine
  Ropivacaine

Opioids
  Alfentanil
  Codeine (N-demethylation)
  Dextromethorphan (N-demethylation)
  Ethylmorphine
  Fentanyl
  Methadone
  Sulphentanil
  Tramadol
Steroids
  Cortisol
  Dexamethasone
  Oestradiol
  Ethinyloestradiol
  Gestodene
  Medroxyprogesterone
  Mifepristone (RU486)
  Prednisolone
  Testosterone
Others
  Aflatoxin B1
  Bromocriptine
  Carbamazepine
  Cyclosporin
  Ergotamine
  Finasteride
  Haloperidol
  Paracetamol
  Tacrolimus (FK506)
  Theophylline
  Warfarin

Structure–activity relationships of substrates

Some recent developments have been used to investigate the active sites of major drug-metabolizing cytochromes P-450. For three major isozymes, for which a great number of substrates are known, the tridimentional structure of the active site was modelled, in order to discover essential elements for the fixation and the oxidation of substrates (Smith, BiochemPharm, 1992; 44:2089; Smith, EurJDM-Pharm, 1994; 3:193). It was shown that substrate binding to CYP2C9 and CYP2D6 is controlled primarily by ionic bonds, whereas hydrophobic bonds are responsible for CYP3A4 substrate fixation.

All CYP2D6 substrates are basic nitrogenated drugs, positively charged at physiological pH, and possessing a hydrogen-bond acceptor site 7 Å away from the nitrogen atom. It now seems very probable that an ionic bond is formed primarily between the basic site of substrates and an anionic site of the enzyme, which is an aspartate amino acid situated in position 301 of the protein sequence. This first bond is indispensable to the catalytic activity, as demonstrated by the loss of the activity when the enzyme is synthesized with a deleted anionic site.

A similar situation exists for CYP2C9, but in this case, an acidic function is needed in the chemical structure of the substrate. An ionic bond with a basic site of the enzyme is postulated, but the precise mechanism remains to be identified. The study of tridimentional structures of CYP2C9 substrates showed the existence of a relatively constant distance (7 to 11 Å) between the acidic function and the oxidation site.

Concerning CYP3A4, actual data are much less accurate, and the major common point between substrates is their lipophilicity. As binding to the active site is mediated by hydrophobic bonds, substrates possess a greater liberty to find an orientation favourable to the oxidation.

The prediction that an isozyme may metabolize a drug on the basis of its chemical structure is today embryonic, but physicochemical characteristics of the substance can guide the investigator toward a specific isoform. This field is quite promising and should lead to very interesting results in the future.

Role in activation and toxification

Although originally this enzyme system was thought to function principally for detoxification, it is now known that it can metabolize many drugs and procarcinogens to active, even toxic, metabolites that initiate toxic and carcinogenic events.[11] An example of such metabolic activation is the biotransformation of the hepatocarcinogen acetylaminofluorene (Johnson, JBC, 1980; 255:304). In fact, numerous chemicals are dependent on metabolism for the expression of their carcinogenicity (including aflatoxins, aromatic amines and nitrosamines, benzene, halothane, isoniazid, and cyclophosphamide). However, it should be noted that factors other than

Table 10 Some powerful inducers of hepatic microsomal drug metabolism in humans

Alcohol
Barbiturates
Carbamazepine, oxcarbamazepine
DDT
Dioxin (TCDD)
Glucocorticoids
Griseofulvin
Phenytoin
Polycyclic hydrocarbons
Rifampicin, rifabutine
Tobacco smoke

metabolism are also likely to play a role in the expression of carcinogenicity.

Variation of activity

Humans are exposed, intentionally or accidentally, to many chemical substances able to alter the activity of drug-metabolizing enzymes, either by enhancing or reducing it. The increase in cytochrome P-450-dependent metabolism has been termed induction, while a diminution of enzyme activity is termed inhibition. As the duration and intensity of effect of many drugs is related primarily to their rate of metabolism, induction or inhibition phenomena would be expected to alter radically the pharmacological effect of many drugs.[12]

Various currently used drugs, carcinogens, and other chemicals have been shown to stimulate the components of the microsomal enzyme system in man and thereby to induce either their own metabolism or the biotransformation of other drugs (Table 10).

For instance, exposure to environmental pollutants such as benz[a]pyrene, present in tobacco smoke and charbroiled meat, is known to induce specific forms of cytochrome P-450 isozymes. Enhanced elimination of antipyrine, diazepam, theophylline, and other drugs has been demonstrated in those who smoke. Other inducers are encountered in nature, such as coumarins, safrole, and steroid hormones.[4]

The process of induction generally requires *de novo* protein synthesis, the precise molecular mechanism of cytochrome P-450 induction being partially understood for some cytochromes. Five mechanisms have been implicated in the regulation of cytochrome expression: gene transcription, processing, mRNA stabilization, translation, and enzyme stabilization (Porter, JBC, 1991; 266: 13469). In the case of phenobarbitone induction, it has been suggested that this phenomenon takes place through binding of the inducer to a specific receptor in the nucleus which initiates formation and translation of new cytochrome P-450-specific mRNA, resulting in protein synthesis (Okey, PharmTher, 1990; 45:241). Induction is dose and time dependent and is present only after chronic exposure.

The common feature of inducers is their lipophilicity, slow elimination, and relatively restricted biotransformation. The process of induction generally takes a few days, some time being required for *de novo* protein synthesis. The phenomenon of induction (extent, time of appearance, and disappearance) is difficult to quantify for each individual.

The clinical consequences of induction can be difficult to appraise. Induction results in an increased rate of metabolism, and usually a decrease in the pharmacological action of the inducer and of some concomitantly administered drugs. This phenomenon has been used with success to treat neonatal hyperbilirubinaemia (Yaffe, NEJM, 1966; 255:1461). Alternatively, this phenomenon may aggravate drug-mediated toxicity due to the excess formation of reactive intermediates (e.g. paracetamol) (Slattery, ClinPharmTher, 1996; 60:241). In some clinical situations it may be extremely dangerous when the inducing agent is withdrawn, since the time to recover a normal microsomal activity is difficult to predict and can take days or weeks.

It should be noted that, although induction has been investigated most intensively for the cytochromes P-450 (in animals, inducers have been used as a tool for defining specificity and differentiation of P-450 isozymes), other enzymes such as the glucuronyl-transferases or the glutathione-S-transferases may be induced simultaneously.

The inhibition of drug metabolism by other drugs or xenobiotics is another well-recognized phenomenon. It is of major concern in drug–drug interactions. The enzymes implicated most here are also the components of the microsomal mixed-function oxidase system.[12] Enzyme inhibition can take place through several mechanisms, including competition for binding sites, destruction of pre-existing enzymes (by olefinic and acetylenic derivatives, e.g. acetylene, vinyl chloride), inhibition of enzyme synthesis (by metal ions, e.g. cobalt), or formation of an inactive complex with the enzyme. In the latter case, the complex-forming inhibitors are metabolized by cytochrome P-450, resulting in an intermediate that binds tightly, but irreversibly, to the haemoprotein. Such an inhibition is seen with some macrolide antibiotics, such as troleandomycin: concomitant administration of this antibiotic with theophylline may produce theophylline intoxication; when given with oral contraceptives, cholestasis may result. Troleandomycin acts by inducing its own demethylation and its subsequent oxidation to a metabolite that forms an inactive complex with cytochrome P450 3A4.[13]

The largest group of inhibitors is represented by substances that act competitively, and reversibly displace other compounds from their substrate-binding site on the cytochrome P-450. Mutual competitive inhibition of two compounds strongly suggests that they are metabolized by the same isozyme, whereas lack of inhibition implies that different enzymes are implicated. An example is the spectacular selective blockade of the polymorphic cytochrome P-450 2D6 in extensive metabolizers by quinidine, a powerful inhibitor both *in vitro* and *in vivo* (Otton, LifeSci, 1984; 34:73; Leemann, EurJClinPharm, 1986; 29:739). It was also shown that neuroleptics and some selective serotonin reuptake inhibitors are potent inhibitors of the hydroxylation of tricyclic antidepressants, a reaction mediated by the polymorphic CYP2D6. Another example is the interaction between cyclosporin and ketoconazole, an azole antifungal agents, which leads to a decreased clearance of cyclosporin (First, Transpl, 1991; 51:365).

The specificity of inhibitors towards cytochrome P-450 isoforms is very variable, ranging from drugs inhibiting one isozyme very selectively to substances blocking the activity of a large number of isoforms (see Table 11). Carbon monoxide binding to the Fe^{2+} in protoporphyrin IX is a typical feature of all cytochrome P-450

Table 11 Non-specific inhibitors of the cytochrome P-450 isozymes

Allopurinol
Antibiotics (chloramphenicol, isoniazide)
Cardiovascular agents (amiodarone, diltiazem, verapamil)
Antacid (cimetidine)
Hormones (oestrogens, progestagens)
Protease inhibitors (ritonavir)
Others
Solvents (e.g. carbon tetrachloride)
Insecticides (e.g. parathione)
Alcohol

enzymes and inhibition of mono-oxygenation reactions by carbon monoxide is often used as a general, non-selective test to identify the catalyst as a cytochrome P-450 enzyme. Recently however, it was demonstrated that carbon monoxide differentially inhibits the activity of three human cytochromes P-450, its affinity for CYP2D6 being greater than for CYP2C9 and much greater than for CYP3A4 (Leemann, LifeSci, 1994; 54:951). Carbon monoxide may be considered now as a useful tool for screening new substrates of specific human cytochrome P-450 isozymes, by means of simple experimental procedures.

It is noteworthy that drug–drug interactions are usually only of importance for drugs with a narrow therapeutic index (i.e. anticoagulants, anticonvulsants, cyclosporin), where a relatively minor alteration in their metabolism may lead to either an ineffective or a harmful response.

Clinical implications of cytochrome P-450 induction and inhibition will depend upon the relative activities of the parent drug and the metabolites produced by the oxidative pathway. Apart from drug–drug interactions, changes in metabolism of endogenous substrates, as well as drug toxicity, may result from induction and inhibition. For instance, it has been demonstrated that cortisol 6β-hydroxylation is induced by phenytoin and rifampicin. Toxicity, arising from enzyme induction by one drug and increased production of toxic metabolites of a second drug, should also be considered.

Other oxidases

Microsomal flavin-containing mono-oxygenase (FMO)

This enzyme is a polymeric protein present in many species and located in several tissues, the highest concentrations being found in the microsomal fraction of the liver. It was originally named 'microsomal mixed-function oxidase' in view of the fact that many amines were N-oxidized by this enzyme. However, the enzyme also catalyses the S-oxidation of a variety of xenobiotics.

Five distinct FMO isozymes have been cloned from human and animal tissues and their DNA sequences have been determined (see refs in Gasser, ExpToxPath, 1996; 48:467). The entire gene family is clustered in chromosome 1q (McCombie, Genomics, 1996; 34:426). The proposed nomenclature is based on comparison of amino acid sequences and evidence for a single gene family composed of five different genes (Lawton, ArchBiochemBiophys, 1994; 308:254). Human FMO1 is subject to developmental regulation since it is more abundant in fetal than in adult human liver (Dolphin, JBC, 1991; 266:12379). FMO2 is expressed predominantly in lungs, whereas FMO3, -4, and -5 were isolated from human liver (Dolphin, BiochemJ, 1992; 287:261; Phillips, ChemBiolInteract, 1995; 96:17). FMO3 accounts for the majority of FMO expressed in the human liver and exhibits stereoselectivity for oxygenation of various compounds (Cashman, ChemBiolInteract, 1995; 96:33).

The FMOs catalyse the direct insertion of oxygen without forming intermediate radicals. However, as for cytochromes P-450, some reactions catalysed by FMO result in the formation of potentially toxic metabolites. These enzymes are distinct from cytochrome P-450 and can oxidize a variety of substances that possess a nucleophilic hetereoatom, including phenothiazines, imipramine, ephedrine, N-methylamphetamine, and cimetidine, as well as thioether and carbamate-containing pesticides.[1,2,4] Many of these substances are potential substrates for both mono-oxygenase systems and there is no clear distinction between the types of oxidations carried out by FMOs and those carried out by cytochromes P-450. The final oxidation products are usually different, and the reaction is rarely mediated by both enzymatic systems (Gasser, ExpToxPath, 1996; 48:467).

These N- and S-oxidations yield amine oxides (which form N-hydroxyammonium ions), hydroxylamines, sulphoxides, and sulphones. The FMO system also plays a major role in the oxidative toxification and detoxification of thiol compounds.

Prostaglandin endoperoxide synthetase

Prostaglandin synthetase is an enzyme system present in nearly all mammalian cell types, and is partially responsible for prostaglandin synthesis as epoxidation of arachidonic acid is also catalysed by CYP2C8 and CYP2C9 (Daikh, JPharmExpTher, 1994; 271:1427). It has been demonstrated that in the course of conversion of arachidonic acid to prostaglandin H_2, mediated by the prostaglandin synthetase (cyclooxygenase), drugs such as aminopyrine, benzphetamine, paracetamol, as well as chemical carcinogens, (i.e. benzidine, benz[a]pyrene) are co-oxidized.[2] The mechanism underlying this co-oxidation is not entirely understood; for paracetamol, which also undergoes substantial metabolism by the cytochrome P-450 system, the postulated reaction mechanism is a one-electron oxidation leading to hydrogen abstraction and yielding the phenoxy radical of paracetamol during the reduction of prostaglandin G_2 to prostaglandin H_2. The phenoxy radical then reacts with cellular glutathione and forms a glutathione conjugate derivative.

The prostaglandin synthetase system seems to be significant for several compounds, particularly in tissues lacking in cytochrome P-450-dependent mixed-function oxidation activity. Prostaglandin synthetase may play a role in the metabolic activation of several bladder and renal carcinogens.

Alcohol dehydrogenase

This is considered to be the major enzyme responsible for alcohol metabolism; it oxidizes alcohol to acetaldehyde with a zero-order kinetic energy, using NAD as a cofactor. Twin studies revealed a genetic contribution to the control of alcohol metabolism. Three classes of alcohol dehydrogenase enzymes were identified: pyrazole sensitive (class I), insensitive (class II), and class III. The class I enzymes are responsible for alcohol metabolism. They are composed by the association of two forms of dimers and three types of polypeptide subunit, α, β, and γ, whose genes are mapped on chromosome 4 (Smith, BiochemSocTrans, 1988; 16:227). There are 21 possible combinations of these subunits (see refs in[14]). One of those corresponds to the variant and more active form of alcohol dehydrogenase in man described by Von Wartburg in 1965 (CanJBiochem, 1965; 43:889). This atypical alcohol dehydrogenase has an important ethnogeographic variation and is represented in 5 to 20 per cent of Caucasian compared with 90 per cent of Oriental people. This could confer a better ability to oxidize alcohol. Different ethnic groups metabolize alcohol at different rates; Orientals have higher rates of metabolization than Caucasians and a much greater propensity to develop vasomotor responses to alcohol consumption.[14]

Hydrolysis
Esterases and amidases

Xenobiotics which contain ester and amide bonds can be hydrolysed readily by various enzymes. The specificity of the esterases and amidases depends on the nature of the radical groups rather than on the adjacent atom (oxygen or nitrogen). The esterases have been classified into three categories based on their interaction (role of substrate, of inhibitor, or no interaction) with organophosphates. Several of these enzymes are inducible by phenobarbital. The hydrolysis of esters can take place in the plasma (non-specific acetylcholinesterase, pseudocholinesterase) or in the liver (specific esterases). Numerous drugs contain an ester likely to be hydrolysed as a functional group, such as acetylsalicylic acid, atropine, heroin, procaine, and pethidine. The selectivity for substrates between species is interesting: for example atropine is rapidly detoxified by hydrolysis in the rabbit but not in man.[1,4]

Amides are hydrolysed preferentially in the liver, but more slowly than the corresponding esters. Among xenobiotics which can undergo this type of reaction are lidocaine, phenacetin, and chloramphenicol.

Epoxide hydrolases

Epoxide hydrolases are a group of catalytic enzyme proteins existing in multiple forms and located in numerous tissues and organs, principally in the liver, but also in the kidneys, lungs, testes, ovaries, and skin, with unique biochemical and structural properties (Krishna, ClinPharmacokin, 1994; 26:144). In the liver, epoxide hydrolase activity occurs predominantly in the endoplasmic reticulum, cytosol, and nuclear membranes (Bentley, FEBSLett, 1975; 59:291; Cresteil, EurJBioch, 1985; 151:345). The enzyme is induced by most classical inducers of the hepatic metabolism.

Epoxides are reactive electrophilic species formed during the cytochrome P-450-mediated oxidative metabolism of xenobiotics (e.g. carbamazepine, cyproheptadine), endogenous compounds (e.g. androstene), and environmental pollutants from the polycyclic aromatic hydrocarbon class. The epoxide hydrolases play a critical role in detoxication/toxification processes of epoxides. These enzymes take part in the metabolism of endogenous compounds such as leukotrienes and the cyclization of squalene epoxide during cholesterol synthesis. Among several metabolic pathways, including

spontaneous decomposition, formation of phenols by rearrangement, irreversible binding to components of the cell, conjugation with glutathione, and further oxidation, enzymatic hydration by epoxide hydrolases is a major route for the biotransformation of epoxides. These enzymes, also called epoxide hydrases or hydratases, catalyse the hydration (a specialized form of hydrolysis where water is added without dissociation of the drug) of epoxides yielding dihydrodiols. The reaction is stereoselective, resulting in the predominant formation of diols with a *trans*-configuration.

The idiosyncratic, severe, systemic, adverse reactions due to phenytoin (pseudolymphoma, eosinophilia, hepatotoxicity, haemolysis, and fever) are putatively the consequence of a highly reactive toxic intermediate metabolite (arene oxide) produced by oxidation via a cytochrome P-450 enzyme. Normally this process is prevented by the immediate destruction of this toxic metabolite by epoxide hydrolase to form arene dihydrodiols.[15] Experimental data suggest that a deficiency in epoxide hydrolase could lead to this clinical syndrome of adverse reactions (Spielberg, NEJM, 1981; 305:722). An association to major birth defects has been suggested, resulting from a suspected partial deficiency in epoxide hydrolase in a mother who was exposed to phenytoin during pregnancy (Strickler, Lancet, 1985; ii:746). Usually, end-products of the hydration are less reactive and are more readily excreted. However, the reaction can also proceed to a metabolic activation, as seen with the biotransformation of benz[a]pyrene to a mutagenic diol-epoxide derivative, which forms covalent bonds with nucleic acids.[1,2]

Conjugations

The conjugation reactions of parent drugs or their phase I metabolites with an endogenous compound generally yield more water-soluble conjugates that are usually inactive and readily excreted. Unlike many products of phase I metabolism, those of phase II reactions have no common link, except that all conjugate formations require some energy-rich intermediates (activated cofactor or drug).

Conjugation occurs if a xenobiotic with an appropriate functional group (usually polar and relatively large) meets a cosubstrate able to combine with it and specific transfer enzymes (transferases). Such enzymes can be found in the endoplasmic reticulum (UDP-glucuronyltransferase, glutathione-S-transferase), in the cytosol (sulphotransferase, acetyltransferase, glutathione-S-transferase), or in the mitochondria (CoA activation for amino-acid conjugation). Depending on the available functional group in the chemical structure of a potential substrate for conjugation, one or more transferases may convert the xenobiotic to a conjugate. The major factors determining the result of the action of several of these transferases on a xenobiotic have been reviewed extensively.[16,17] They include the substrate specificity of the enzyme involved, the pharmacokinetics of the substrate, and the cosubstrate availability (nutritional supply).

It must be emphasized that although conjugation reactions have been associated in the past with terminal drug inactivation or detoxification, it is now apparent that in certain cases, depending on special structural characteristics of the substrate, conjugation reactions may result in the formation of active metabolites (e.g. morphine) or of more reactive and toxic derivatives.

Uridine diphosphoglucuronyltransferases and glycosyltransferases

Human hepatic microsomal uridine diphosphate (**UDP**)-glucuronyltransferases are involved in metabolic reactions in balance either with sulphation or with glutathione conjugation.

In glucuronidation, the cosubstrate UDP 2α-D-glucuronic acid generated in the cytoplasm is coupled with a substrate containing the suitable functional group to form the β-pyranosiduric acid or glucuronide. Numerous xenobiotics are substrates for UDP-glucuronyltransferases, such as morphine, oxazepam, amitriptyline, cyproheptadine, and chlorpromazine. As with many phase II enzymes, the UDP-glucuronyltransferases display low substrate specificity. The most important functional groups forming glucuronides are hydroxyl, carboxyl, amino, and sulphydryl groups.[19]

The *O*-glucuronides are the most commonly encountered conjugates; they are generally stable at physiological conditions. However, the *N*-glucuronides lack this stability. The *S*-glucuronides represent a minor pathway, except for thiol compounds (e.g. antabuse). Exceptionally, very stable *C*-glucuronides are synthesized, as observed for phenylbutazone. Endogenous compounds that are substrates for the transferases include bilirubin, steroid hormones, thyroxine, serotonin, and catechols. The importance of glucuronidation of endogenous compounds is illustrated by the known genetic defect of bilirubin glucuronidation in Gilbert's and Crigler–Najjar syndromes. These conditions are characterized by elevated bilirubin levels and reduction or loss of bilirubin UDP-glucuronyltransferase activity, but most xenobiotics are glucuronidated normally in these patients.

Drugs habitually lose their pharmacological activity during the glucuronidation process, but in some instances, glucuronidation may lead to a more active compound. A well-documented example is morphine-6-glucuronide, which is some 10-fold more potent than morphine itself at the receptor level (Mori, LifeSci, 1972; 11:525; Osborne, ClinPharmTher, 1990; 47:12). Glucuronides sometimes serve to transport biologically active compounds. Bisacodyl is glucuronidated in the liver, then secreted into bile and hydrolysed at its site of action in the colon by β-glucuronidases. This property is used as a therapeutic tool by means of inactive glucuronides (prodrugs), which are further activated by deconjugation, using β-glucuronidases targeted to tumour cells by antibodies (Wang, CancerRes, 1992; 52:4484).

Glucuronyltransferases are found mostly in the liver but they are also present in the kidneys, small intestine, lungs, skin, adrenal glands, and spleen. The pattern of isozymes is variable in different tissues. Like the cytochrome P-450-dependent mono-oxygenases, the UDP-glucuronyltransferases are an integral part of the endoplasmic reticulum. Their catalytic activity is strongly influenced by the presence of phospholipids. The subcellular localization among the UDP-glucuronyltransferases varies in related to their function; the enzymes have been found in rough and smooth endoplasmic reticulum, the nuclear envelope, mitochondria, the Golgi apparatus, and plasma membranes (Burchell, PharmTher, 1989; 43:261).

The heterogeneity of these enzymes has been confirmed by physiological and physicochemical criteria, as well as with studies on the tissue specificity; each isozyme exhibits individual but sometimes overlapping specificities. These studies indicated that distinct

Table 12 Human liver UDP-glucuronyltransferases
pI 7.4 UDP-glucuronyltransferase (oestriol)
pI 6.2 UDP-glucuronyltransferase
Bilirubin UDP-glucuronyltransferase
Morphine UDP-glucuronyltransferase
6-Hydroxy bile acid UDP-glucuronyltransferase
Tertiary amine UDP-glucuronyltransferase
Phenol UDP-glucuronyltransferase

populations of human UDP-glucuronosyltransferases exist which specifically glucuronate bilirubin, bile acids, 5-hydroxytryptamine, and drugs such as morphine, clofibrate, and chloramphenicol. Little information on the characteristics of the human enzymes was available until recently because of the difficulty in purifying the enzymes (instability, sensitivity to detergents). However, distinct forms have been purified to apparent homogeneity (Irshaid, MolPharm, 1987; 31:27). More recently, the cloning and expression of human UDP-glucuronosyltransferase cDNA has been used as an alternative approach to the study of these enzymes. Different cDNA species have been isolated from human livers and two of these clones have been expressed in tissue culture cells, permitting the study of the substrate specificities of the individual enzymes (Harding, PNAS, 1988; 85:8381; Tephly, TrendsPharmacolSci, 1990; 7: 276) (Table 12). Cloning, sequencing, and expression of cDNAs in cultured cells has brought to light the existence of a supergene family of isozymes.[17,18] At the latest count more than 110 distinct cDNAs in yeast, plants, bacteria, and animal species, including human varieties, have been sequenced to date (see references cited in reference 18). In mammals, 47 cDNA genes, belonging to three families have been described.[18] Two families, UGT1 and UGT2 are comprised of four subfamilies of which two have have been mapped in the human and mouse genomes.[18] The proposed classification is similar to that developed for cytochromes P-450. The root symbol **UGT** is proposed, followed by the Arabic number denoting the family, a letter designating the subfamily, and the Arabic number representing the individual gene.[18] Members of family 1 are derived from one gene located on chromosome 2, the bilirubin/phenol UGT gene complex. All family 1 isozymes are characterized by a unique exon 1 and share the mRNAs for exons 2 to 5. Each exon 1 is preceded by its own promoter, and each isozyme appears to be regulated independently (Owens, ProgNucAcidResMolBiol, 1995; 51:305). Four human isozymes have been characterized in this family: UGT1,1 and UGT1,4 conjugating bilirubin, ethinyloestradiol, and oestriol; UGT 1,6 conjugating planar phenols; and UGT 1,7 conjugating planar and bulky phenols (Wooster, BiochemJ, 1991; 278:465). Various mutations of the gene complex have been shown to be responsible for the Crigler–Najjar syndrome types I and II (Robertson, JInherMetDis, 1991; 14:563; Owens, Pharmacogenet, 1992; 2:93). Family 2 UGTs appears to be clustered on chromosome 4.

UGT1,1, UGT 1,6, and UGT 2,4 show some substrate selectivity whereas other forms accept a broad range of substrates (UGT1,7, UGT 2,7, and UGT 2,11).

A number of major UGT have not been cloned to date, for instance those responsible for the glucuronidation of morphine, tertiary amines, and tricyclic antidepressants.

UGT 1,1 and 1,4, i.e. bilirubine glucuronidation are induced by phenobarbital-type inducers. 3-Methylcholantrene-type inducers appear to enhance glucuronidation of drugs like paracetamol by UGT 1,6.[17] However, paracetamol is an overlapping substrate for several UGTs.

In most species, the major route of sugar conjugation is conjugation with glucuronic acid (glucuronidation), although in insects, plants, or vertebrates, conjugation with glucose is more important. Glucosidation of several drugs including barbiturates and sulphonamides has also been observed in man. The reaction is the same as for glucuronide formation but involves UDP-glucose transferase instead of UDP-glucuronyltransferase. Similarly O-, N-, and S-glucosides are formed. Conjugation with UDP-xylose or UDP-ribose is also possible (Tang, PharmTher, 1990; 46:53).

Methyltransferases

N-, O-, or S-methylations are conjugation reactions predominantly seen with endogenous substrates, such as histamine, amino acids, proteins, and carbohydrates. They are relatively minor pathways for xenobiotics and the resulting metabolites are generally less polar.

Many forms of methyltransferases are located in various tissues including the liver, adrenal glands, lungs, kidneys, skin, nervous tissue, and pineal gland. In humans, catechol-O-methyltransferase, thiopurine methyltransferase, and N-methyltransferase are controlled by genetic polymorphisms (Weinshilbloum, PharmTher, 1989; 43:77; refs in[20]). The activity of several methyltransferases is age related: in the newborn, theophylline is highly N-methylated yielding caffeine, a reaction which decreases during neonatal development and becomes low in adults (Aranda, NEJM, 1976; 295:413).

The methyltransferase-catalysed conjugations require the cofactor S-adenosylmethionine. Some of these reactions are stereoselective: the $(R)(+)$-enantiomer of nicotine, for example, is methylated preferentially .

S-Methyltransferase is an important pathway in the biotransformation of sulphydryl drugs. It is performed by two different enzymes, thiopurine methyltransferase which catalyses the S-methylation of azathioprine and 6-mercaptopurine, and thiol methyltransferase which catalyses the biotransformation of 2-mercaptoethanol, captopril, penicillamine, and N-acetylcysteine.[20] Thiopurine methyltransferase is submitted to a balanced polymorphism, with a trimodal frequency distribution of its activity in human erythrocytes (88.6, 11.1, and 0.3 per cent or high, intermediate, and low activity, respectively) (Weinshilbloum, AmJHumGen, 1980; 32:651). A correlation exists between enzyme activity in erythrocytes and the liver.[20] An interethnic variability has been observed in the ratio of intermediate to high activity phenotypes from 0.034 for Chinese people to 0.37 for black people from Florida (Jones, ClinPharmTher, 1993; 53:238; Lee, ClinPharmTher, 1993; 54:28). This could be of clinical interest since the deficiency of thiopurine methyltransferase leads to an increased rate of side-effects with 6-mercaptopurine and azathioprine (Lennard, ClinPharmTher, 1989; 46:149; Schutz, Lancet, 1993; 341:436).

O-Methylation of a phenolic group is implicated in the metabolism of neurotransmitters and any structurally related drugs, involving the cytosolic enzyme catechol-O-methyltransferase. This enzyme is one of the two catecholamine-inactivating enzymes. It is controlled by a genetic polymorphism which follows a mendelian transmission, the gene being located on chromosome 22 (Grossman, Genomics, 1992; 12:822). Catechol-O-methyltransferase contributes to the metabolism of levodopa, methyldopa (Campbell, ClinPharmTher, 1984; 35:55; Da Prada, Experientia, 1984; 40:1165), and isoprenaline (see refs in[20]).

N-Methylation is mediated by several enzymes, such as nicotinamide-N-methyltransferase and histamine-N-methyltransferase. The distribution of the activity of these enzymes in human liver is bimodal.[20]

Sulphotransferases

In parallel with the formation of glucuronides, sulphation is a major conjugation pathway for phenols, alcohols, hydroxylamines, and to a lesser extent, for thiols. It requires the activated donor 3′-phosphoadenosine-5′-phosphosulphate (**PAPS**). The sulphotransferases are a family of enzymes that catalyse the transfer from the activated sulphate donor to a nucleophilic acceptor, either possessing a hydroxyl or amino group (see refs in reference 21).

Sulphotransferases are cytosolic enzymes widely distributed in mammalian tissues such as liver, gut, kidney, and platelets (Pacifici, Pharmacol, 1988; 36:411).

They catalyse the sulphation of a variety of endogenous compounds (e.g. steroids, carbohydrates, and proteins) and the resulting products are important cellular constituents. They also esterify numerous lipophilic xenobiotics to more readily excreted metabolites. β_2-Adrenoceptor agonists like fenoterol, salbutamol, and terbutaline are eliminated in the urine essentially as sulphate conjugates. The estimation of sulphation could be essential in predicting the elimination rate of these drugs that are administered by inhalation.[21] The sulphation of salbutamol is believed to be catalysed by catechol-sulphotransferase (Walle, BrJClinPharm, 1993; 35:413). This sulphoconjugation is stereoselective since in human lung the more active (-)-salbutamol is a better substrate for sulphotransferase than (+)-salbutamol (Pacifici, EurJClinPharm, 1996; 49:299). The rate of sulphation in the lung is similar to that found in the liver (Pacifici, ChemBiolInteract, 1994; 92:219). Other drugs like methyldopa, paracetamol, and diflunisal undergo sulphation in man (see refs in reference 21).

Sulphotransferases exist in many forms and have been divided into five groups according to their substrates (aryl, alcohol, estrone, tyrosine, and bile-salt sulphotransferases). Unlike most of the detoxication enzymes, sulphotransferases are not inducible by the known inducers of drug metabolism, but can be inhibited by several compounds (e.g. pentachlorophenol). Several food constituents such as apple juice or dry residues of red wine are strong inhibitors of phenol sulphation (Gibb, BiochemPharm, 1987; 36:2325). Drug competition can also inhibits sulphation reactions. Tertiary amines like cyclizine, promethazine, and chlorpromazine are inhibitors of endogenous steroid sulphation (Bamforth, EurJPharm, 1992; 228:15). The inhibition can also results from a PAPS depletion.

There are species, sex, and developmental differences in sulphate conjugation. Sulphotransferases develop prenatally and are well expressed in the liver and extrahepatic tissues after the second trimester of fetal life. Catechol-sulphotransferase develops earlier than phenol-sulphotransferase and the activity of the former is higher in the fetal than in the adult human liver (see refs in[21]). The expression of phenol-sulphotransferases are genetically controlled, whereas catechol-sulphotransferases seem more dependent on environmental factors (Reveley, JPsychiatRes, 1983; 17:303). The level of activity of phenol-sulphotransferase seems to be regulated by a major genetic polymorphism in conjunction with polygenic inheritance (Price, Genetics, 1989; 122:905).

It must be remembered that sulphate formation can compete with glucuroconjugation for most endo- and xenobiotics, since similar functional groups are conjugated by enzyme systems. Sulphotransferases exhibiting high affinity and low capacity predominate at low substrate concentration, while glucuronyl-transferases are more important at high substrate concentration (Pacifici, DevPharmacolTher, 1990; 14:108).

In general, the sulphoconjugates are end-products of metabolism and are readily excreted. In some instances, however, the conjugates are more reactive than their parent compounds and can bind to cellular macromolecules after transformation into reactive intermediates. The classic example of a metabolic activation by sulphation is the biotransformation of *N*-hydroxy-2-acetyl-aminofluorene to an unstable sulphate derivative which decomposes to a nitrenium ion capable of covalent binding to macromolecules.

Glutathione-S-transferases (GSTs)

GSTs are a group of multifunctional proteins which play an important role in the biotransformation and detoxication of many endogenous and exogenous compounds. The detoxication processes can be divided into reductions and the much more frequent conjugation reactions. Owing to its high nucleophilicity, the sulphur atom of glutathione will bind almost any lipophilic molecule containing a functional group with strong electrophilicity (epoxides, polycyclic aromatic hydrocarbons, haloalkanes, nitroalkanes, alkenes, aromatic halogen, and nitro compounds).[22,23] The glutathione conjugates may then be excreted directly in urine or bile, but more often undergo further enzymatic biotransformation resulting in the urinary or biliary excretion of mercapturic acids.

GSTs can also act as 'ligandins' (intracellular binding proteins), that is, they can bind xenobiotics on the enzyme surface without metabolizing them, thereby preventing these compounds from interfering with proteins or nucleic acids. In addition, the enzymes possess the capacity to form covalent bonds between reactive compounds and the enzyme's active site, a mechanism called 'suicide inactivation'. Because glutathione and GSTs are so abundant, they have often been referred to as a protective system. The metabolism of paracetamol illustrates this property: the hepatotoxicity of paracetamol is mediated by an enzymatic reaction catalysed by CYP2E1, leading to a reactive electrophilic *N*-acetyl benzoquinone imine intermediate; this reacts with the nucleophilic glutathione, and toxicity is prevented as long as reduced glutathione is available (see Section 17).

Although once thought to provide protection against xenobiotics, it should be noted that glutathione conjugation may increase markedly the toxicity of certain compounds, such as halogenated alkenes whose glutathione conjugates are nephrotoxic.[1] GSTs, in spite of their high basal intracellular concentration in many tissues, may have their synthesis increased by various inducers, including phenobarbitone and several polycyclic aromatic hydrocarbons.

GSTs exist in many isozyme forms in the organism or even in a single tissue. Most of these have broad overlapping substrate specificities. They are grouped into distinct classes on the basis of their primary structures.[22] Four classes of different types of proteins have been identified in mammalian tissues: α, μ, π, and θ. The cytosolic GSTs are dimeric with two subunits, the name of the enzyme depending on the subunits composition. Each subunit is denoted by a letter indicating the class and an Arabic number distinguishing the subunit.

Genes of cluster μ are located on chromosome 1 whereas those of class α are on chromosome 6. GST M1-1 is genetically polymorphic and is present in only 50 per cent of individuals in a large number of racial groups. Except for the null phenotype, the enzyme can occur in three forms corresponding to two alleles of the active gene, with no known differences in their functional properties (Widersten, BiochemJ, 1992; 285:377). Individuals lacking this enzyme are less protected against the toxic effects of epoxides.

Some studies support the idea that GST M1-1 individuals may have an increased susceptibility to DNA adduct formation (Liu, Carcinogenesis, 1991; 12:2269), whereas susceptibility for pulmonary carcinoma is still a matter of debate.[22] Carcinogenic arene oxides are detoxified more efficiently by other GSTs. Propenals (acrolein) are detoxified by GST P1-1, and 4-hydroxyalkenals, generated by lipid peroxidation, could be detoxified by human isoenzymes with similar activities to animal ones. Another perspective of GST is that tumour cells, as a resistance mechanism, may express new forms of this enzyme with an enhanced capacity to inactivate cytostatic drugs. In fact, some alkylating agents are known to be conjugated by GST A1-1 as observed with chlorambucil (Ciacco, BiochemPharm, 1991; 42:1504; Meyer, BrJCanc, 1992; 66:433) or by GST M3-3 as reported for 1,3-bis(2-chloro-ethyl-1-nitrosurea) (Berhane, CancerRes, 1993; 53:4257). One possible therapeutic approach could be the inhibition of GST or the development of cytostatic prodrugs that release a nitrogen mustard after activation by GST present in tumour cells (Lyttle, JMedChem, 1994; 37:1501 see refs in[22]).

Amino-acid conjugation

Many carboxylic acid-containing xenobiotics, including NSAIDs, diuretics, analgesics, and hypolipidaemic agents, are conjugated with endogenous amino acids such as glycine (for refs see[24]). The reaction leading to amide formation requires metabolic activation of the carboxyl group to its acyl coenzyme A derivative. This conjugation reaction occurs principally in the liver. The glycine mechanism is used by the majority of species for the conjugation of aliphatic, aromatic, heteroaromatic, and phenylacetic acid congeners. The conjugation of benzoic acid with glycine resulting in excretion of hippuric acid has been used in chemical tests of liver function. Amino acids other than glycine can be involved in this conjugation reaction (e.g. glutamine, ornithine, arginine, and taurine); 10 of the 20 amino acids are known to be implicated.

N-Acetyltransferases

The *N*-acetyltransferases catalyse the acetylation of a number of commonly used drugs and foreign compounds which are arylamine, hydrazine, or hydrazide derivatives. They are also involved in the amide formation of endogenous primary aliphatic amines. The

Table 13 Some xenobiotics whose biotransformation is primarily or partially mediated by *N*-acetyltransferase

Arylamines and hydrazines	Secondary aromatic amines	Mutagens and carcinogens
Aminoglutethimide	Acebutolol	2-Aminofluorene
Amrinone	Caffeine	2-Aminonaphthalene
Dapsone	Clonazepam	(β-Naphthylamine)
Hydralazine	Nitrazepam	Benzidine
Isoniazid	Salazosulphapyridine	2-Chloroaniline
Phenelzine		3,3-Dichlorobenzidine
Procainamide		
Sulphamethazine		

activities of these enzymes vary widely between individuals. Forty years ago, a large variation in the metabolism of the antituberculous drug isoniazid suggesting a genetic polymorphism was reported (Bonicke, ArchExpPatholPharmakol, 1953; 220:321). Some years later, further studies produced evidence of a clearly bimodal frequency distribution of the isoniazid-acetylating capacity (Biehl, TransConfChemotherTuberc, 1957; 16:108; Evans, BMJ, 1960; ii: 485). The rate of acetylation of several drugs and certain carcinogenic arylamines has been shown to be under the same genetic control as isoniazid (Table 13). Slow acetylators are homozygous for an autosomal recessive gene, whereas rapid acetylators are either homozygous or heterozygous for the dominant allele.[25,26]

The cytosolic polymorphic enzyme is mainly distributed in liver and intestinal mucosa (Jenne, JCI, 1965; 44:1992). The acetylation reaction requires the cofactor acetyl coenzyme A (**CoA**), and involves the transfer of the acetyl group from acetyl CoA to the arylamine substrate. A different enzyme, found in the kidneys, spleen, and blood, is responsible for the acetylation of drugs such as para-aminosalicylic acid, for which the acetylating capacity shows a unimodal distribution.

A first step towards a direct understanding of the molecular basis of the human acetylation polymorphism has been achieved with the partial purification of an *N*-acetyltransferase (**NAT**) from human liver tissue showing that this enzyme is markedly decreased or absent in livers of slow acetylators. Further characterization studies of the defect have been performed at the molecular level. The cloning, nucleotide sequencing, and functional expression of three human arylamine *N*-acetyltransferase genes has recently been achieved; they correspond to the polymorphic human liver *N*-acetyltransferase (Blum, DNA, 1990; 9:193). Human genetic loci encode two distinct and independently expressed NATs: NAT1 and NAT2, which are both polymorphic.[27] They differ by only 55 amino acids, but have different substrates specificities. The *N*-acetylation of sulphamethazine and procainamide appears to be catalysed mainly by NAT2, whereas NAT1 and NAT2 both contribute to the *N*-acetylation of the carcinogen 2-aminofluorene. NAT1 seems implicated principally in the *N*-acetylation of *p*-aminosalicylate and *p*-aminobenzoate. cDNA expression studies using NAT1–NAT2 chimeras combined with site-directed mutagenesis studies have been used to map sites involved in substrate selectivity and stability. The sulphydryl group of Cys68 appears to be involved in the transfer of acetate from acetyl CoA. The functional significance of the allelic variants encoded by *NAT1* and their ethnovariability remain to be investigated. Genetic variability at the *NAT2* locus accounts for the well known individual variability in

the acetylation of isoniazid and sulphamethazine. More than 10 variant alleles for the *NAT2* locus have been identified in various ethnic populations (Lin, AmJHumGen, 1993; 52:827).[27] *In vitro* studies suggest that slow acetylation of those substrates by variant NAT2 enzymes may be linked to impaired efficiency in translation of mutant NAT2 mRNA and to the enhanced degradation of mutant NAT2 protein resulting in a substantial decrease in cytosolic NAT2 content (Blum, PNAS, 1991; 88:5237; Deguchi, JBC, 1992; 267: 18140; Abe, BBResComm, 1993; 191:811). Ethnogeographic studies have been performed for NAT2. A correlation between *NAT2* genotype and acetylator phenotype have been found in three ethnic groups: Japanese (Deguchi, JBC, 1992; 267:18140; Mashimo, HumGenet, 1992; 90:139; Abe, BBResComm, 1993; 191:811;) Caucasians (Hickman, Pharmacogenet, 1992; 2:217), and African-Americans (Bell, Carcinogenesis, 1993; 14:1689). The failure to find a perfect correlation between genotype and phenotype could be linked to experimental or non-genetic factors that can influence the rate of acetylation, such as hepatic and renal diseases, coadministration of certain drugs, and alcohol intake. These factors should be taken into account when phenotyping patients.

Ethnic differences in the drug-acetylating capacity have been recognized; Caucasians have a 50:50 distribution of the phenotypes, whereas Japanese and Eskimo populations show a predominance of the fast acetylator phenotype (more than 90 per cent). The main clinical interest is the putative association of the phenotype with therapeutic response, adverse drug reactions, and disease association. Slow acetylators have higher risks of variation in drug response, susceptibility to adverse drug effects, and occurrence of 'spontaneous' (not drug-induced) disorders. Studies have demonstrated, for instance, that the acetylator phenotype influences isoniazid cerebrospinal fluid concentrations in children with tuberculosis meningitis, but this did not prevent therapeutically effective concentrations to be achieved in rapid acetylators when conventional treatment schedules were applied (Donald, Pediat, 1992; 89:247). The same results have been obtained repeatedly with various forms of tuberculosis and neither the outcome of the disease nor the resistance to drugs is dictated by acetylator phenotype when standard daily schedules dosages are applied (see references cited in reference 26).

Present evidence suggests that a metabolite derived from acetylhydrazine and hydrazide, two metabolites of isoniazid, could be responsible for the hepatotoxicity of isoniazid. Both metabolites could accumulate in slow metabolizers, the fate of acetylhydrazine being dependent on NAT. In Caucasian and Indian subjects the slow metabolizer phenotypes are more prone to severe hepatotoxicity following isoniazid treatment.[26] As for isoniazid, dapsone efficacy does not correlate with the acetylator phenotype except for indirect evidence in dermatitis herpetiformis (Forstrom, AnnClinRes, 1974; 6:308). The acetylator status has been associated with bladder cancer and drug-related lupus erythematosus.

Since the rate of acetylation may be a critical determinant of the toxicity of several xenobiotics, knowledge of the acetylator status may be clinically relevant in a few selected conditions (Clark, Drugs, 1985; 29:342).

Ontogeny of drug-metabolizing enzymes

Early studies on the hepatic drug-metabolizing capacity of fetal and newborn animals (mostly rodents) appeared to show that the fetus lacks such ability or at least had a very markedly lower activity of oxidizing as well as conjugating enzymes. However, with immunological tools and more sensitive analytical methods which could detect low levels of activity, it was found during recent decades that the human fetus possesses the major hepatic drug-metabolizing enzymes.[28,29] In contrast, attempts to demonstrate hepatic glucuronidation in the human fetus have been unsuccessful.

Investigations with different substrates and using various tissues have indeed demonstrated many enzyme activities very early during human development, that is, the 5th or 6th week. Usually these activities increase as gestation advances to reach a plateau by the end of the second trimester. In contrast to CYP3A4, the polymorphic isozyme CYP2D6 is not expressed until late gestational age, and only in about one-third of specimens examined (Ladona, BrJClinPharm, 1991; 32:295; Treluyer, EurJBioch, 1991; 202:583). There is in fact a clear-cut difference in the expression of cytochrome P-450 between adult and fetal human liver (Cazeneuve, BrJClinPharm, 1994; 37: 405; see references cited in reference 30); CYP3A7 is the major cytochrome P-450 in fetal liver, representing 30 to 50 per cent of total content, but this isozyme is absent in adult liver.

To date there is still very little information about the key factors (the rate-limiting steps) in the ontogenesis of fetal drug-metabolizing capacity: hormonal changes during development are thought to have a profound effect on drug metabolism. Thus the fetal adrenal gland, which produces the glucocorticoids, appears to be of considerable importance for fetal drug metabolism as it not only contains a number of drug-metabolizing enzymes with higher specific activities than the fetal liver, but is proportionally much larger than in the adult.

Fetal and neonatal enzyme activities may differ from those in the adult. For example, limited activity of one pathway may result in more extensive use of another. Thus, deficient glucuronidation in the neonate seems to be compensated for by sulphation activity or methylation by methyltransferase. Several reactions are markedly reduced (e.g. hydroxylation of amylobarbitone), but other activities are just as efficient (reduction) or even increased (methylation, sulphation) compared with the adult. Only very few of the well characterized cytochrome P-450 enzymes responsible for the major pathways of drug biotransformation have been detected. Some well-defined drug-metabolizing enzymes or prototype activities which have been identified in the early human conceptus are summarized in Table 14.

Table 14 Some drug-metabolizing enzymes or prototype activities identified in human fetal liver during early gestation

Oxidations
  Aldrin epoxidase
  Aniline hydroxylase
  Benz[a]pyrene hydroxylase
  Benzphetamine N-demethylase
  Dehydroepiandrosterone-16α-hydroxylase
  Dextromethorphan N-demethylase
  7-Ethoxycoumarin-O-deethylase
  Ethylmorphine-N-demethylase
  4-Nitroanisole-O-demethylase
  Testosterone-6β-hydroxylase
  Midazolam-4'-hydroxylase
Hydrolyses
  Epoxide hydrolase
Conjugations
  Glutathione-S-transferase
  Monomorphic N-acetyltransferase (NAT1)
  Polymorphic N-acetyltransferase (NAT2)
  Sulphotransferase
  UDP-glucuronyltransferase[a]

[a] Enzyme responsible for 5-hydroxytryptamine glucuronidation (not for bilirubin).

Model systems for drug-metabolizing enzymes

During drug development as well as clinical practice many situations require studies of drug metabolism. The objectives of the investigations could be of various types, including the determination of pharmacokinetic parameters, the identification of metabolic profile, the characterization of isozyme(s) involved, and the investigation in patients or volunteers of ability to metabolize a drug. The characterization of isozymes involved in a biotransformation pathway is of particular interest in drug development, because it allows the early prediction of interindividual variability due to genetic polymorphism, drug interactions, or social habits (e.g. alcohol, coffee, and cigarettes).

To assess drug-metabolizing enzyme activity in humans, several *in vitro* and *in vivo* approaches are used (Table 15). Additionally, the prediction of *in vivo* biotransformation and pharmacokinetic behaviour on the basis of simple *in vitro* experiments has been investigated for at least 20 years. Early work showed good correlations between metabolic clearance predicted from *in vitro* data

Table 15 Models for human drug metabolism studies

In vivo
  Pharmacokinetics of drug and metabolites—urinary metabolite pattern

In vitro
  Perfused organs
  Tissue slices
  Isolated cells: hepatocytes (cultures and cocultures)
  Subcellular fractions: S9, microsomes, cytosol
  Purified enzymes
  cDNA-expressed enzymes (in bacteria, yeast, or mammal cells)

In vitro to *in vivo* extrapolation

and those measured *in vivo* and gave support to the idea that such predictions were indeed feasible. Recent years have seen a growing interest for the potential of *in vitro* to *in vivo* predictions in the area of drug interactions, with promising results.[31]

The choice of the model of investigation depends first on the type of question asked and second on tool availability. Generally, the more distant a model is from the human situation *in vivo*, the more specific can be the investigation, but this may make extrapolation to the patient more difficult. The different approaches are complementary to each other, and all have advantages and drawbacks.

In vivo probes

In vivo approaches are attractive because they take into account all the determinants of drug disposition—absorption, distribution, metabolism (phases I and II), and elimination. However, the mechanisms involved are numerous and complex, and the use of probes in answering specific questions is generally not adequate. They are very useful for the determination of pharmacokinetics, for the identification of metabolite profiles, and to a lesser extend for the characterization of isozymes involved in the biotransformation of drugs. Today, the development of test compounds (i.e. probe drugs) reflecting the activity of one or several metabolic enzyme(s) are very promising, because they might allow the 'mapping' of patients or volunteers in regard to their ability to metabolize drugs.

In vivo studies imply administration of a compound, which might be the drug under investigation or a probe drug, followed by urine collection or blood sampling. The elimination half-life, the fractional clearance of the drug to its various metabolites, and more frequently the determination of a metabolic ratio (Jackson, JClinPharm, 1989; 28:647) are then calculated.

A probe drug is devised to provide information that exceeds information on the drug itself, that is, it can be extrapolated to other important issues, such as enzyme activity or rate of metabolism of other compounds. There is no consensus on the properties that are required from a probe drug, but nevertheless one can devise a list of properties which might be useful for most or many purposes:[32] metabolite formation determined predominantly by metabolism (not by liver blood flow or protein binding), full characterization of its biotransformation in man (including chemical reactions, *in vivo* and *in vitro* characterization), enzyme specific, not inhibitory to other enzymes of interest, safe (including application in patients and children), analytical methodology not too demanding, worldwide availability, and full validation of the method. A large number of drugs have been proposed as test compounds for specific metabolizing enzymes, but the degree of validation of these methods is variable and sometimes poor. Some of the best-documented *in vivo* probes now available to assess genetic and environmental variations in drug-metabolizing enzyme activity are listed in Table 16.

When *in vivo* models are used to characterize the isozyme(s) responsible for the elimination of a drug, four major approaches might be used: (i) correlations between metabolic activity of the drug and those of specific markers administered separately; (ii) correlations between metabolic activity and the status of poor or extensive metabolizer determined by phenotyping or genotyping (when a genetic polymorphism exist); (iii) inhibition by specific inhibitors (e.g. fluvoxamine for CYP1A2, sulphaphenazole for

CYP2C9, quinidine for CYP2D6, or TAO for CYP3A4); and (iv) induction by specific inducers, like rifampicin or carbamazepine for CYP3A4.

One of the limitations of any marker drug currently used to measure drug-metabolizing enzyme activity *in vivo* is that the results obtained with one drug have predictive values only towards a small number of drugs metabolized by the same enzyme. The multiplicity of the cytochrome P-450 isozymes, for instance, implies that several substrate probes are required to obtain a good estimation of the global enzyme activity in oxidative drug metabolism. This leads to a strategy termed 'cocktail approach', which involves the administration of a combination of substrate probes simultaneously, allowing the determination of the 'metabolic status' of patients or volunteers (Breimer, TrendsPharmacolSci, 1990; 11:223). In some instances, a single drug might be useful to determine the activity of several isozymes, which is very useful to limit the number of components in the cocktail. For example, caffeine could be used to determine the activity of CYP1A2 and NAT2 (Kalow, ClinPharmTher, 1993; 53:503), and dextromethorphan may reflect CYP2D6 (*O*-demethylation) and CYP3A4 (*N*-demethylation) (Gorski, BiochemPharm, 1994; 48:173).

Methods which do not require administration of a probe drug, but where the disposition of an endogenous substance is monitored, are sometimes used. For instance, 6β-hydroxycortisol, a minor metabolite of cortisol formed by hepatic mixed-function oxidases and excreted in urine, provides a sensitive marker of CYP3A4 activity (Watkins, Pharmacogenet, 1994; 4:171).

A major limitation, however, of any *in vivo* system is linked to the difficulty in interpretation of the data obtained, since they are affected also by the influence of several non-hepatic factors. Additionally, the description of new but poorly validated methods increases the complexity of the interpretation, because their reliability is generally unknown. For example, a poor correlation was found between three putative probes (erythromycin, dapsone, and cortisol) of CYP3A4 activity in man (Kinirons, ClinPharmTher, 1993; 54:621), leading to a confusing situation where it becomes very difficult to choose the appropriate tool to determine metabolic capacity. Another example of discrepancy is the dissociation observed in a Chinese population between debrisoquine hydroxylation phenotype determined on the basis of metabolic ratio and genotype determined directly from DNA. In this case, the reason could be the presence of additional enzyme activities in non-Caucasian subjects (Yue, Lancet, 1989; ii:870). To limit these problems, it is always recommended to perform assays with the best-documented and validated probe drugs and to perform corroborating *in vitro* assays where needed.

In vitro models

The *in vitro* approach allows more direct insight and can provide more information on mechanisms of drug biotransformation than *in vivo* studies. Several *in vitro* systems are available today, which vary in complexity from the entire organ to systems expressing a single isozyme (Rodrigues, BiochemPharm, 1994; 48:2147). They can be used to study specific reactions involved in the biotransformation of a drug or the mechanism of a particular reaction. Most commonly the liver is used for drug metabolism studies, because it is quantitatively the most important organ and has a high

Table 16 Some *in vivo* probe drugs for drug-metabolizing enzymes

Enzyme	Probe drug	Selective inhibitor
Phase I		
CYP1A2	Caffeine	Furafylline
		Fluvoxamine
CYP2C9	Diclofenac	Sulphaphenazole
	Tolbutamide	Fluvastatine
CYP2C19	Mephenytoin	
	Omeprazole	
CYP2D6	Dextromethorphan	Quinidine
	Codeine	
	Debrisoquine	
	Sparteine	
CYP2E1	Chlorzoxazone	Diethyldithiocarbamate
CYP3A4	Erythromycin	Troleandomycin (TAO)
	Midazolam	Ketoconazole
	Cortisol (endogeneous)	Grapefruit juice
	Nifedipine	
Phase II		
N-Acetyltransferase	Caffeine	
	Dapsone	
	Isoniazid	
	Sulphamethazine	
Glucuronyltransferases	Lorazepam	
	Paracetamol	
Glutathione transferase	Paracetamol	
Sulphotransferase	Paracetamol	

enzyme activity towards most drugs (Beaune, PharmTher, 1988; 37:193).

At cellular level: perfused organs, organ slices, and intact cells

Compared with purified enzymes and subcellular fractions, perfused organs, organ slices, and intact cells seem to be the more suitable systems for *in vitro* to *in vivo* extrapolations. The normal spatial distribution of enzymes and cofactors is maintained, allowing entire metabolic pathways to be followed, and production rates of metabolites correspond more closely to those observed *in vivo*. In contrast, subcellular fractions often give higher activities because conditions are optimized for a particular enzyme (e.g. saturating levels of substrate and cofactors).

For several reasons, studies with perfused organs are rarely performed in man. They could be used for clearance and extraction experiments, because they maintain the original structure of the organ, but their poor availability and very short lifespan markedly limit their use.

Organ slices were used frequently before isolated cells became available. However, interest in organ slices was boosted at the end of the 1980s as a result of improved cutting techniques which allow the reproducible production of thin and regular slices (200 μm thick) (Smith, LifeSci, 1985; 36:1367) suitable for studying toxicology, transport, and enzyme induction. The functional heterogeneity of the liver is maintained, including its polarity, which allows the study of active transport and biliary excretion. On the other hand, oxygen penetration inside slices is poor, incubation times are long, and viability is short.

Systems involving isolated cells are very attractive because they are more reproducible and more easily characterized than perfused organs or organ slices while conserving the complexity of metabolic pathways. They are very useful for studying metabolism, drug interactions, and toxicology, as well as intracellular transportation systems. They can be used either in freshly isolated suspensions or in cultures. The preparation of isolated hepatocytes from freshly excised livers is now rapid and simple. The drawbacks of such a system are its short lifespan (5 to 7 h), the use of a high oxygen tension in the incubation medium that may alter some drug-metabolizing activities, and the loss of organ structure during isolation and incubation. The primary cultures of hepatocytes have longer lifespans (several days), but they loose drug-metabolizing capacities within the first 2 to 3 days, possibly by dedifferentiation of cells (Skett, Xenobiot, 1996; 26:1). Recent developments partially overcome this problem by using cocultures of hepatocytes with fetal rat liver epithelial cells (Guillouzo, ToxicolInVitro, 1990; 4:415) or within two layers of extracellular matrix components (collagen) to simulate the *in vivo* environment of the liver (Bader, Xenobiot, 1994; 24:623). The authors of these experiments report an unchanged catalytic activity for at least 1 week. Another very attractive alternative is the use of cryopreserved hepatocytes. As a result of major progress in this field, it is now possible to measure high metabolizing activities in such cells (Loretz, Xenobiot, 1989; 19: 489).

For all these systems involving intact cells the cofactors are endogenous, but the cells must have a sufficient energy production to allow their synthesis and regeneration. In some situations endogenous supply is not sufficient and additional exogenous co-substrates are required (e.g. addition of inorganic sulphate for sulphate conjugation; addition of cysteine to the incubation or perfusion medium for glutathione synthesis). Finally, in these models there is a coupling between phase I and phase II reactions and, consequently, identification of products of phase I reactions becomes complicated.

At subcellular level: S9, microsomes, and cytosol

Subcellular fractions can be obtained by differential centrifugation of cellular homogenates. The supernatant (**S9**) of a low-speed centrifugation (9000 g) contains cytosol and reticulum membranes, which are further separated by an ultracentrifugation (100 000 g). The supernatant (cytosol) and the pellet (microsomal fraction) are among the most frequently used *in vitro* systems, whereas experiments with S9 are only occasionally performed. Studies on subcellular fractions include measurements of enzyme activity, kinetic studies, correlation studies, characterization of isozyme(s) responsible for a metabolic pathway, inhibition studies, interspecies comparison of activities, and identification of metabolites formed from specific reactions.

The rapid and easy preparation from liver frozen deeply for several years is a major advantage of these techniques, as well as the opportunity to preserve subcellular fractions for several months at –80°C, without a dramatic fall in their activities.

In vitro assays with subcellular fractions require the addition of cofactors, such as NADPH or NADP for cytochrome P-450-dependent oxidations, acetyl CoA for *N*-acetylation, and UGD-α-D-glucuronic acid for glucuronidations.

A feature of such *in vitro* systems is that they permit the study of specific reactions without interference from others. Microsomes contain cytochromes P-450 and other membrane-bound enzymes (e.g. FMO, glucuronyltransferases), whereas cytosol contains soluble enzymes, that is, the majority of the other transferases. Depending on the fraction used and the cofactor added, it is therefore possible to study a family of enzymes independently of the others. Of particular interest are the studies made in human liver microsomes on the cytochrome P-450 system responsible for the conversion of numerous xenobiotics and endogenous compounds into a variety of possible products, including inactive metabolites, as well as toxic and carcinogenic intermediates.

The use of specific substrates at low concentration (high affinity reactions) allows the distinction between different forms within families of drug-metabolizing enzymes. Since the discovery of genetic defects in drug oxidation, the use of a probe drug in liver microsomes has, for instance, permitted the identification of a large number of compounds whose metabolism is mediated by the polymorphic cytochrome P-450 isozyme responsible for the debrisoquine hydroxylation. Moreover, the use of selective chemical or immunological (antibodies) inhibitors can improve the ability of appropriate substrates to probe for particular types of drug-metabolizing enzymes. Quinidine is an example of such an inhibitor which at low concentration selectively inhibits the activity of CYP2D6. The combined use of isozyme-selective substrates and -specific inhibitors is a powerful means of measuring functionally active individual forms of drug-metabolizing enzymes.

At protein level: purified enzymes

A higher level of specificity is reached when only one catalytic activity is present. Many enzymes have now been purified and characterized in animals and in man using electrophoretic technology. Studies of isolated enzymes have provided the strongest evidence for the existence of multiple forms of cytochrome P-450 and have allowed determination of the individual forms involved in particular reactions. To date, more than 10 human liver cytochrome P-450 isozymes have been purified. Other purified enzymes are the microsomal flavin-containing mono-oxygenases, epoxide hydrolases, prostaglandin synthetases, glucuronyltransferases, glutathione-*S*-transferases, and sulphotransferases.

Important advances in the understanding of structure and function of drug-metabolizing enzymes have resulted from studies of purified enzyme systems which permit the identification and characterization of various isozymes, the study of their sequencing, regulation, induction, and molecular reaction mechanisms.

There are, however, many drawbacks to purification of enzymes. For example, the purification of membrane-bound enzymes leads to a loss of the membrane environment, which may have a profound impact on the catalytic activity of the enzyme. This is the case for the cytochrome P-450-mediated oxidation of drugs, which is dependent on addition of a fraction containing electron donors. The complexity of isolation procedures, associated with the development of biotechnology, has led the investigators to focus on DNA cloning rather than on enzyme purification.

At gene level: DNA cloning

The limitations encountered with the *in vitro* systems previously described have been partially overcome by developments in molecular biology. These permit the study of genetic factors involved in drug metabolism, as well as the regulation and expression of the drug-metabolizing enzymes. In this respect, the application of DNA recombinant technology to problems relevant to drug metabolism has led to a tremendous advance in our understanding in this field. Most of the major drug-metabolizing cytochromes P-450 have been cloned and are today available as expression systems. They have been successively expressed in bacteria (*Escherichia coli*), yeasts (*Saccharomyces cerevisiae*), and mammal cells (COS, CHO, HepG2, V79) (Gonzalez, AnnRevPharmTox, 1995; 35:369). Among these systems, yeasts seem to offer the best profile: the expression level is high, the preparation of microsomes with an environment similar to the natural situation is possible, and the culture is not costly (Renaud, Toxicology, 1993; 82:39).

These expression systems generate very accurate information on the isozymes involved in specific biotransformation pathways, yet the interpretation of results is sometimes difficult. The *in vitro* system only partially mirrors the *in vivo* situation, thus a major metabolic pathway identified *in vitro* might correspond to a minor biotransformation step *in vivo*, such as when the concentration of the implicated enzyme in the liver is low. In conclusion, investigations with systems expressing a single isozyme are very useful, but they should be completed with microsome or hepatocyte studies to obtain a better reflection of *in vivo* metabolism.

Perspectives

Major developments in the future should be concerned with the extrapolation of *in vitro* data to the *in vivo* situation. Once the validation of these techniques is improved, they promise to be very useful for the integration of data obtained in partial systems to the whole organism. The major drawback of *in vitro* technology is that it offers only a partial similarity to the *in vivo* situation. Forecasting from *in vitro* data to *in vivo* situations by means of new computer approaches (e.g. modelling) will be a very powerful tool to improve the understanding of drug metabolism pathways, and to avoid useless investigations in man.

References

1. De Bethizy JD and Hayes JR. Metabolism: a determinant of toxicity. In Hayes AW, ed. *Principles and methods of toxicology*. New York: Raven Press, 1989: 29–66.

2. Gibson GG and Sket P. *Introduction to drug metabolism*. London: Chapman & Hall, 1986.

3. Correia MA. Drug biotransformation. In Katzung BG, ed. *Basic and clinical pharmacology*. 4 edn. Norwalk, Connecticut: Appleton & Lange, 1995: 48–59.

4. Bechtel P and Testa B. Biotransformation des médicaments: voies bio-moléculaires et pharmacologie clinique. In Giroud JP, ed. *Pharmacologie clinique. Bases de la therapeutique*. Paris: Expansion Scientifique Française, 1988: 25–55.

5. Estabrook *et al.* In Hess B and Staudinger H, eds. *Colloquium der Gesellschaft für Biologische Chemie* 19th edn. Berlin: Springer-Verlag, 1968: 142.

6. Guengerich FP. Cytochrome P-450 enzymes and drug metabolism. In Bridges JW, Chasseaud LF, and Gibson GG, eds. *Progress in drug metabolism*. London: Taylor & Francis, 1987: 1–54.

7. Black SD and Coon MJ. Comparative structures of P-450 cytochromes. In Ortiz de Montellano PR, ed. *Cytochrome P-450. Structure, mechanism and biochemistry*. New York: Plenum Publishing, 1986: 161–216.

8. Gonzalez FJ. Molecular genetics of the P-450 superfamily. *Pharmacology and Therapeutics*, 1990; **45**: 1–38.

9. Guengerich FP. Cytochromes P-450 of human liver. Classification and activity profiles of the major enzymes. In Pacifici GM and Fracchia GN, eds. *Advances in drug metabolism in man*. Luxembourg: European Commission, 1995: 179–231.

10. Ingelman Sundberg M, *et al.* Genetic polymorphism of human drug metabolizing enzymes. Recent aspects on polymorphic forms of cytochromes P450. In Alvan G, *et al.*, eds. *COST B1 Conference on Variability and Specificity in Drug Metabolism*. Brussels: European Commission, 1995: 93–110.

11. Guengerich FP. Analysis and characterization of enzymes. In Hayes AW, ed. *Principles and methods of toxicology*. New York: Raven Press, 1989: 780–814.

12. Park BK and Kitteringham NR. Relevance and means of assessing induction and inhibition of drug metabolism in man. In Gibson GG, ed. *Progress in drug metabolism*. London: Taylor & Francis, 1988: 1–60.

13. Babany G, Larrey B, and Pessayre D. Macrolide antibiotics as inducers and inhibitors of cytochrome P-450 in experimental animals and man. In Gibson GG, ed. *Progress in drug metabolism*. London: Taylor & Francis, 1988: 61–97.

14. Evans DAP. Alcohol and alcoholism. In Evans DAP, ed. *Genetic factors in drug therapy. Clinical and molecular pharmacogenetics*. Cambridge University Press, 1993: 780–814.

15. Evans DAP. Phenytoin. In Evans DAP, ed. *Genetic factors in drug therapy. Clinical and molecular pharmacogenetics*. Cambridge University Press, 1993: 119–131.

16. Mulder GM. The interrelationship between different conjugating enzymes *in vivo*. In Benford DJ, Bridges JW, and Gibson GG, eds. *Drug metabolism— from molecules to man*. London: Taylor & Francis, 1987: 121–34.

17. Bock KW. Human UDP-glucuronosyltransferases. Classification and properties of isozymes. In Pacifici GM and Fracchia GN, eds. *Advances in drug metabolism in man*. Luxembourg: European Commission, 1995: 289–309.

18. Mackenzie PI, Owens IS, Burschell B, *et al.* The UDP glycosyltransferase gene superfamily: recommended nomenclature update based on evolutionary divergence. *Pharmacogenetics*, 1997; 7:235–69.

19. Siest. In *Cellular and molecular aspects of glucuronidation*. London: John Libbey Eurotext, 1988: 1.

20. Pacifici GM and Fracchia GN. Human methyltransferases. Classification and metabolic profile of the major forms. The point of view of the clinical pharmacologist. In Pacifici GM and Fracchia GN, eds. *Advances in drug metabolism in man*. Luxembourg: European Commission, 1995: 461–93.

21. Pacifici GM and De Santi C. Human sulphotransferase. Classification and metabolic profile of the major isoforms. The point of view of the clinical pharmacologist. In Pacifici GM and Fracchia GN, eds. *Advances in drug metabolism in man*. Luxembourg: European Commission, 1995: 311–49.

22. Mannervik B and Widersten M. Human glutathione transferases: classification, tissue distribution, structure and functional properties. In Pacifici GM and Fracchia GN, eds. *Advances in drug metabolism in man*. Luxembourg: European Commission, 1995: 407–59.

23. Hayes JD, *et al.* Human glutathione-*S*-transferase. In Benford DJ, Bridges JW, and Gibson GG, eds. *Drug metabolism—from molecules to man*. London: Taylor & Francis, 1987: 82–94.

24. Caldwell J. The conjugation of carboxylic acid drugs and xenobiotics with amino acids. In Pacifici GM and Fracchia GN, eds. *Advances in drug metabolism in man*. Luxembourg: European Commission, 1995: 495–512.

25. Weber WW and Hein DW. *N*-Acetylation pharmacogenetics. *Pharmacological Review*, 1985; **37**: 25–79.

26. Evans DAP. *N*-Acetyltransferase. In Evans DAP, ed. *Genetic factors in drug therapy. Clinical and molecular pharmacogenetics*. Cambridge University Press, 1993: 211–85.

27. Weber WW and Vastis KP. Human *N*-acetyltransferases. Genetic polymorphism and metabolic profiles of the major isoforms. In Pacifici GM and Fracchia GN, eds. *Advances in drug metabolism in man*. Luxembourg: European Commission, 1995: 351–405.

28. Netter KJ. Comparison of fetal and adult drug metabolizing enzymes. In Benford DJ, Bridges JW, and Gibson GG, eds. *Drug metabolism—from molecules to man*. London: Taylor & Francis, 1987: 317–29.

29. Pelkonen O, Pasanen M, and Vahakangas K. Metabolic activation by the fetus and placenta. In Benford DJ, Bridges JW, and Gibson GG, eds. *Drug metabolism—from molecules to man*. London: Taylor & Francis, 1987: 734–46.

30. Rane A. The major physiological factors that modulate drug metabolism in man. Implication for drug effects and toxicity. In Pacifici GM and Fracchia GN, eds. *Advances in drug metabolism in man*. Luxembourg: European Commission, 1995: 149–76.

31. Leemann TD and Dayer P. Quantitative prediction of *in vivo* drug metabolism and interactions from *in vitro* data. In Pacifici GM and Fracchia GN, eds. *Advances in drug metabolism in man*. Luxembourg: European Commission, 1995: 783–830.

32. Pelkonen O, Rautio A, and Raunio H. Specificity and applicability of probes for drug metabolizing enzymes. In Alvan G *et al.*, eds. *COST B1 Conference on Variability and Specificity in Drug Metabolism*. Brussels: European Commission, 1995:

2.6 Nerve supply and nervous control of liver function

Prithi S. Bhathal and Howard Grossman

Introduction

The influence of the autonomic nervous system on liver function was first postulated by Claude Bernard in 1849, who demonstrated that 'wounding' of the floor of the fourth venticle stimulated release of glucose from the liver. In further experiments in 1893, the Cavazzani brothers showed that hyperglycaemia could be provoked by stimulating the coeliac plexus. The presence of vasomotor control of the hepatic circulation via the nervous system was first established by Pal in 1888, and later confirmed by Bayliss and Starling (1894) and in a series of studies by Burton-Opitz (1910–1915). Historically, the major emphasis has been on investigating the efferent nerve supply to the liver. Afferent (sensory) nerves from the liver have long been recognized but their function remains poorly understood.

Anatomy

The autonomic nerves of the liver form two intercommunicating plexuses surrounding the structures of the porta hepatis as they enter the liver. The anterior plexus is formed around the hepatic artery, the posterior plexus surrounds the portal vein and bile duct. Sympathetic nerve fibres are derived from the coeliac ganglion and parasympathetic from the vagus nerve. Some fibres also enter the liver with the hepatic veins and via the lesser omentum.

Within the liver, nerve fibres supply the biliary system and the parenchymal cells as well as the hepatic arterial and portal vascular beds. While the biliary system and parenchymal cells are both sympathetically and parasympathetically innervated, the blood vessels receive mainly sympathetic fibres. The fibre types found in the liver are predominantly monoaminergic and peptidergic. In recent years, somatostatin, neurotensin, vasoactive intestinal peptide, substance P, neuropeptide Y, glucagon- and glucagon-like peptide-, gastrin/cholecystokinin C-terminus-, serotonin-, and galanin-immunoreactive nerve fibres have also been identified in human liver (El-Sahy, ScaJGastr, 1993; 28:809), while calcitonin gene-related peptide-reactive fibres have been reported in rat and cat liver. There is also evidence of a cholinergic innervation in some species.

Unfortunately, histological identification of these fibre types has not yet been matched by a knowledge of their function and physiological significance. Studies to date have involved electrical stimulation of fibres at various levels from the hypothalamic centres to the perivascular plexuses at the porta hepatis. This frequently involves non-selective stimulation of all of the autonomic nerves present in a nerve trunk or plexus. Species differences have also limited progress in this area. Anatomical studies of human livers have demonstrated an extensive parenchymal innervation in contrast to the sparse nerve supply in laboratory animals such as the rat, in which many functional studies have been performed.

In the human liver, adrenergic, dopaminergic, and cholinergic nerve fibres are found within the wall of blood vessels and extend from the portal tracts into the space of Disse. Adrenergic fibres have also been observed within the walls of terminal hepatic venules and larger hepatic veins (Burt, Hepatol, 1989; 9:839). Neuropeptide Y also appears to be localized within the sympathetic nerves. Substance P- and vasoactive intestinal peptide-immunoreactive fibres are concentrated in the portal tracts, but are also found along the sinusoids and around terminal hepatic venules (Ueno, AmJGastr, 1991; 86:1633). Hence, nerve terminals with a variety of putative transmitter substances lie in close proximity to the smooth-muscle cells, fibroblasts, biliary epithelial cells, and sinusoidal lining cells of the liver, as well as the parenchymal cells.

Presumptive sensory nerve endings have also been found within the lobules of human liver. Sensory nerves are present around the central veins and bile ducts, as well as in the liver capsule and ligaments. The majority of afferent fibres from the liver run via the vagus and splanchnic nerves, but some fibres also run to the right phrenic nerve. Fifty per cent of the sympathetic fibres in the splanchnic nerve and up to 90 per cent of all fibres in the abdominal vagus are thought to be afferent. The afferent nerves of the liver may register information from osmoreceptors, ionic receptors, baroreceptors, and metabolic and nociceptive receptors. For example, it has been demonstrated experimentally that intrahepatic glucose sensors exist that influence pancreatic and adrenal function via vagal afferent fibres (Gardemann, EurJBioch, 1992; 207:399).

Nervous control of hepatic circulation

Stimulation of the hepatic nerves causes hepatic arterial constriction and a fall in the total liver blood flow. These responses are largely mediated by α-adrenergic receptors. In addition, vasodilator β_2-adrenergic receptors are present (Poo, Hepatol, 1992; 15:459) and branches of the hepatic artery are innervated by a subpopulation of vasodilator dopaminergic fibres (Mann, ClinAutonomRes, 1991;

1:141). Experimental evidence suggests that vasomotor tone to the hepatic arteries is generally low and that autoregulatory escape from prolonged nerve stimulation occurs, thus assuring the supply of arterial blood to the liver. The situation in the human liver is not known, but extrinsic nervous regulation appears to be of minor physiological importance compared to intrinsic autoregulation of hepatic arterial flow, except under conditions of stress.

Stimulation of the hepatic sympathetic nerves does not alter portal flow, since this is determined by events outside the liver. However, it does induce an increase in hepatic vascular resistance and hence a rise in portal pressure. Studies of the liver *in vivo* have confirmed that stimulation of sympathetic nerves induces a graded constriction of the terminal portal venules and sinusoids (McCuskey, SemLivDis, 1993; 13:1). This response is mediated by α-adrenoreceptors. Since the sinusoids lack smooth-muscle cells, constriction of these vessels may be due to contraction of the perisinusoidal stellate cells or possibly the endothelial cells. The portal vein and its branches are capacitance vessels with an important role in the regulation of splanchnic venous return. Hence, activation of sympathetic nerves also results in a rapid expulsion of blood from the liver into the systemic circulation.

Nervous control of hepatic metabolism and bile formation

It has been shown in patients undergoing surgery that stimulation of hepatic sympathetic nerves results in a release of glucose from the liver [Nobin, ActaPhysiolScand, 1977; 452 (Suppl. 103)]. A similar clear-cut response occurs in a wide variety of species and is thought to provide the organism with a source of energy under conditions of stress. However, studies of the effects of autonomic nerve stimulation on hepatic metabolism in the intact organism are often difficult to interpret because this procedure also induces changes in liver blood flow and alters circulating levels of hormones such as insulin, glucagon, and catecholamines.

The isolated perfused liver preparation has often been used in an effort to simplify the problems of interpretation. The findings in this system have been ably reviewed (Gardemann, EurJBioch, 1992; 207:399) and are summarized in Table 1. Thus, electrical stimulation of perivascular autonomic nerves increases glucose and lactate output, but decreases urea formation, ketone-body formation, and xenobiotic metabolism. Portal flow and oxygen consumption are also reduced and the blood flow within the liver is redistributed. These actions are mediated predominantly by sympathetic adrenergic nerves through α_1-receptors. Most of these metabolic effects (except urea and glutamine synthesis) are preserved even when concomitant vascular changes are prevented pharmacologically. Nerve effects can be modulated by circulating hormones such as insulin, glucagon, and somatostatin, demonstrating the interplay of these two regulatory systems, the autonomic nervous and the endocrine. In the isolated rat liver, parasympathetic stimulation (perivascular stimulation in the presence of α- and β-blocking agents) has little effect on basal hepatic glucose balance, yet it antagonizes the effects of glucagon on glucose output.

The gallbladder, and extra- and intrahepatic bile ducts are all innervated. Stimulation of hepatic nerves reduces bile flow, but it is not clear if this effect is secondary to changes in blood flow. In the

Table 1 Regulation of hepatic metabolism and bile secretion by the autonomic nervous system

	Sympathetic nerve	Parasympathetic nerve
Metabolism		
Glucose release	⇑	⇓
Glycogenolysis	⇑	⇓
Glycogen synthesis	⇓	⇑
Urea output	⇓	?
Glutamine output	⇓	?
Ammonia uptake	⇓	?
Ketogenesis	⇓	?
Oxygen consumption	⇓	?
Bile formation		
Bile flow	⇓	?
Bile-acid secretion	⇓	?

⇑, activation; ⇓, inhibition; ?, uncertain.

isolated rat liver, sympathetic nerve stimulation leads to a decrease in bile flow and bile-acid secretion mediated by α_1-receptors. This appears to be a direct effect but may not be completely independent of changes in blood flow (Beckh, AmJPhysiol, 1991; 261:G775). Prostaglandins synthesized by the non-parenchymal cells have been postulated as mediators of the nervous effects on bile secretion (see also Mechanism of nerve action below). Prostaglandins $F_{2\alpha}$ and D_2 are themselves able to decrease the bile flow and bile-acid secretion. It is possible that circulating factors, such as hormones and endotoxins, also influence bile secretion via this mechanism.

Mechanism of nerve action

As mentioned above, there are species differences in the density of nerve endings in the hepatic parenchyma, with little direct innervation in the rat. However, signal propagation between hepatocytes may be achieved via gap junctions and the release of mediators from non-parenchymal cells. Experimental data suggest that, in spite of these species differences, the mechanism of sympathetic nerve action involves all three cell populations, namely neurones, parenchymal, and non-parenchymal cells. Besides noradrenaline as the neurotransmitter of the sympathetic nervous system, prostanoids synthesized only by the non-parenchymal cells seem to be mediators of intercellular communication. It has been shown that prostaglandins $F_{2\alpha}$ and D_2 are probably involved in the actions of sympathetic hepatic nerves regulating carbohydrate metabolism (Iwai, EurJBioch, 1988; 175:45).

Possible clinical implications of hepatic nerves

In patients suffering from inflammatory or neoplastic liver disease, or following biopsy or acute distension of the liver, a dull pain and tenderness may be experienced in the right upper quadrant, presumably due to stimulation of the nociceptive fibres referred to earlier. The route of these afferent nerves is poorly understood. It is of interest that when the liver is biopsied laparoscopically no pain is reported on puncturing the capsule. Pain referred to the shoulders implies that the pathological process has extended beyond the liver to involve the diaphragm (i.e., the cervical roots of C3–C5).

Parasympathetic nerves may have a role in the pathogenesis of non-obese, type 2 diabetes. It has been postulated that a neuropathy may result in impairment of the glucose-induced activation of parasympathetic nerves, leading to an impairment of insulin secretion from the pancreatic islets and to a reduced direct stimulation of glycogen synthesis as a very early manifestation of diabetes.

An hepatorenal baroreceptor reflex has been postulated in which an increase in sinusoidal pressure results in an increase in afferent hepatic nerve activity and in efferent renal sympathetic nerve activity. Since it has been shown that this reflex persists in cirrhotic rats, a role has been postulated for hepatic afferent nerves in the pathogenesis of the systemic haemodynamic disturbances associated with cirrhosis (DiBona, AmJPhysiol, 1995; 269:G29).

Chronic liver disease is associated with striking changes in the distribution of hepatic nerves. In the cirrhotic human liver, the number of nerve fibres is increased in the portal areas and fibrous septa, but reduced within regenerative nodules (Miyazawa, AmJ-Gastr, 1988; 83:1108). The functional significance of these changes is uncertain but may be considerable. Animal studies suggest that the metabolic response to sympathetic nerve stimulation may be reduced, but the haemodynamic response (increased hepatic vascular resistance) may be enhanced, even in early cirrhosis (Gardemann, Hepatol, 1993; 18:1544). In addition to haemodynamic and metabolic responses, regeneration may be impaired, since the regenerative response of the liver following experimental partial hepatectomy is reduced by vagotomy.

Following transplantation the liver is effectively denervated. Hepatic blood flow is often increased in the early stages of the recovery period. It has been suggested that this is due to a loss of vasomotor tone in the transplanted liver (Henderson, Hepatol, 1988; 10:288; Paitaud, Therapie, 1992; 47:47; Navasa, Hepatol, 1993; 17: 355). However, this suggestion has not been supported by recent evidence. In the rat liver, total hepatic blood flow and the distribution of blood flow within the liver were reportedly normal 4 weeks after transplantation and as soon as 1 week after chemical denervation (Wheatley, JHepatol, 1993; 19:442). A study of 68 transplant recipients identified numerous factors that may disturb hepatic and systemic haemodynamics at this time, including persistence of portosystemic shunting (Gadano, Hepatol, 1995; 22: 458). This work showed that liver blood flow was not enhanced after transplantation for acute liver failure and gradually returned to normal over the first year after transplantation for cirrhosis.

No significant regeneration of nerve fibres takes place in the transplanted liver within the first few years (Boon, JPath, 1992; 167: 217). In spite of this, there are no data showing an obvious deficiency of the regulation of liver metabolism and bile formation. It would appear from these findings that, under normal circumstances, control of the liver is achieved by hormones and substrates reaching the organ via the circulation, and that the role of the hepatic nerves is restricted mainly to situations of physiological stress.

Bibliography

1. Forssmann WG and Ito S. Hepatocyte innervation of primates. *Journal of Cell Biology*, 1977; **74**: 299–313.
2. Lautt WW. Hepatic nerves: a review of their functions and effects. *Canadian Journal of Physiology and Pharmacology*, 1980; **56**: 679–82.
3. Lautt WW. Afferent and efferent neural roles in liver function. *Progress in Neurobiology*, 1983; **21**: 323–48.
4. Gardemann A, Puschell GP, and Jungermann K. Nervous control of liver metabolism and hemodynamics. *European Journal of Biochemistry*, 1992; **207**: 399–411.
5. Niijima A. Neural control of blood glucose level. *Japanese Journal of Physiology*, 1986; **36**: 827–41.
6. Shimazu T. Neuronal regulation of hepatic glucose metabolism in mammals. *Diabetes/Metabolism Reviews*, 1987; **3**: 185–206.
7. Sawchenko PE and Friedman MI. Sensory functions of the liver—a review. *American Journal of Physiology*, 1979; **225**: R5–20.
8. Lautt WW and Greenway CV. Conceptual review of the hepatic vascular bed. *Hepatology*, 1987; **7**: 952–63.
9. Richardson PDI and Withrington PG. Liver blood flow. 1. Intrinsic and nervous control of liver blood flow. *Gastroenterology*, 1981; **81**:159–73.

2.7 Immunology

2.7.1 Cytokines and the liver

Giuliano Ramadori and Thomas Armbrust

Introduction

The term cytokine denotes peptides that are released from certain cells to act upon others. They represent one of the ways cells communicate with each other over long and short distances via specific cytokine receptors. A variety of functions have been attributed to cytokines such as the survival, growth, activation, and differentiation of cells and the induction of certain cellular functions. Several types of cytokines have been proposed according to their target (for example interleukins), function (haematopoietic growth factors), or structure (chemokines).

Cytokines form a complex network connecting organ systems and the cells therein. They may be produced by single cell types or almost every cell of the body and may affect single as well as a variety of cell types. Some cytokines may be constitutively produced in the normal state, in particular those that regulate physiological responses, whereas others are detectable only under certain circumstances. The complexity of the cytokine network is becoming increasingly apparent, constantly raising more and more questions. Nevertheless, an increasing body of knowledge is available about how cells can affect other cells via cytokines. It permits the statement that cytokines are crucial factors in most physiological and pathophysiological responses.

The acute phase reaction represents one of the best known phenomena about how cytokines can affect the function of the liver. In addition to hepatocytes, which are the target in this case, the liver contains the bulk of the fixed tissue macrophages, the Kupffer cells, which are capable of synthesizing cytokines in response to stimulatory agents. From this example alone, it may be concluded that the liver must not only be regarded as an important target for but also an important source of cytokines. This chapter summarizes the effects of cytokines on the liver, in particular in liver diseases, while also taking into account the fact that the liver is an important source of cytokines (Table 1).[1]

Liver cells and cytokines

The liver is composed of parenchymal cells, that is hepatocytes and non-parenchymal or sinusoidal cells. The latter, approximately 30 per cent of all liver cells, comprise a heterogeneous group of sinusoidal lining cells, sinusoidal endothelial cells, Kupffer cells, fat-storing cells, and pit cells, as described in detail elsewhere.

Table 1 Cytokines and their abbreviations

Cytokine	Abbreviation
Interleukin-1	IL-1
Interleukin-6	IL-6
Tumour necrosis factor-α	TNF-α
Tumour necrosis factor-β	TNF-β
Interleukin-11	IL-11
Leukaemia inhibitory factor	LIF
Ciliary neurotropic factor	CNTF
Transforming growth factor-β	TGF-β
Interferon-α	IFN-α
Interferon-γ	IFN-γ
Epidermal growth factor	EGF
Fibroblast growth factor	FGF
Platelet-derived growth factor	PDGF
Hepatocyte growth factor	HGF
Insulin-like growth factor	IGF

Hepatocytes make up most of the liver mass and most of the liver cells. They must be regarded as one of the most important cell types of the liver upon which cytokines can act when considering the observation that they are supplied with various cytokine receptors. Nevertheless, hepatocytes are also capable of synthesizing cytokines, in particular when there is a need for multiplying (growth factors in development and liver regeneration).

The largest group of non-parenchymal liver cells, the sinusoidal endothelial cells, are highly specialized endothelial cells with various morphological and functional characteristics enabling an intensive exchange of molecules between the blood and the hepatocytes. They are the cells which initiate the immigration of inflammatory cells from the bloodstream when hepatocellular damage occurs by displaying adhesion molecules, a process that is controlled by cytokines. They are also capable of endocytosis and may take part in immunological reactions indicating that the sinusoidal endothelial cells are of importance in the effects of cytokines on the liver.

Kupffer cells represent approximately 80 per cent of all fixed tissue macrophages of the body and therefore may hold a key role in the function of the mononuclear phagocyte system (**MPS**). They are exposed to blood arriving from the gut, which may contain more pathogenic substances and micro-organisms than blood from other organs. Therefore, the clearance of particulate material is suggested to be the main function of these macrophages. Phagocytosis by Kupffer cells (and other macrophages) initiates a broad spectrum of defence mechanisms that culminate in the release of a variety of cytokines. Many other events are also capable of inducing cytokine production by macrophages implying that these cells (including the Kupffer cells) belong to the most important cellular sources of cytokines.

Fat-storing cells are well-differentiated, perisinusoidal cells which have attracted great interest since the discovery of their pivotal role in liver fibrogenesis. Not much is known about their function in the 'normal' state, but increasing information is available regarding their activation and transformation into myofibroblast-like cells, presumably caused by certain cytokines which may also be produced by the fat-storing cells themselves.

The pit cells are located in the sinusoids exhibiting natural killer (**NK**) activity against tumour cells and virus-infected cells with no need for activation. Representing a subset of lymphocytes, the close relation between the pit cells and cytokine network is obvious.

Effect of cytokines on the liver
Acute phase reaction

The acute phase response comprises a cascade of systemic responses upon tissue injury or infection (Baumann, ImmunolToday, 1994; 15:74). It is characterized by a variety of changes in organ functions such as fever, leucocytosis, and major laboratory changes. One of the most striking changes is a change in the plasma concentration of a group of proteins denoted as the acute phase proteins (**APPs**) which may increase (positive APPs) or decrease (negative APPs) in the plasma during the acute phase reaction. The pattern of the APPs as well as the degree of change in the plasma levels differ from species to species. In the last decade it has become clear that these changes are mediated by blood-borne effectors (cytokines) that modulate protein synthesis by hepatocytes. The major acute phase cytokines have now been identified as IL-1, IL-6, and tumour necrosis factor-α (**TNF-α**); nevertheless the participation of several other cytokines as well as hormones (for example, corticosteroids) must be considered. The origin of the acute phase mediators has not so far been fully elucidated. Although macrophages and blood monocytes rank as the main cellular source of acute-phase cytokines, it remains to be elucidated whether cytokines in the circulation are produced locally at the site of tissue injury or are derived from distant sources.

The acute phase mediators act via highly specific cytokine receptors present on the surface of hepatocytes. Receptors for IL-1 (**IL-1R**; Sims, Science, 1988; 241:585), IL-6 (**IL-6R**; Yamasaki, Science, 1988; 241:825), and TNF-α (**TNF-αR**; Schall, Cell, 1990; 61:361) have been characterized. While the IL-1R and IL-6R belong to the immunoglobulin superfamily, the TNF-αR exhibits the structural features of the nerve growth factor receptor which is also present in soluble form (Heller, PNAS, 1990; 87:6151).

IL-1 comprises two different proteins, IL-1α and IL-1β, each synthesized by a variety of cells such as mononuclear phagocytes, leucocytes, and endothelial cells as 31 kDa (pro-IL-1α) or 34 kDa (pro-IL-1β) precursor proteins. Both IL-1α and IL-1β share biological effects by binding to the same cell surface receptor. While pro-IL-1α exhibits biological activity, pro-IL-1β needs to be activated by proteolytic cleavage, a process that is not yet understood in detail. Although a specific enzyme has been described that is capable of cleaving pro-IL-1β (IL-1β converting enzyme), the way in which mature IL-1β is released from the synthesizing cells remains to be elucidated. In recent years, evidence has accumulated indicating that the occurrence of mature IL-1β may be associated with apoptosis or cellular necrosis (Armbrust, BBResComm, 1995;

Table 2 Cytokines of the acute phase response

Cytokine	Effect on the liver
IL-6-type cytokines	
IL-6	Stimulation of most of the acute phase
IL-11	proteins
LIF	
CNTF	
IL-1-type cytokines	
IL-1	Synergists with IL-6-type cytokines in
TNF-α	the stimulation of the APPs
TNF-β	inhibition of negative APPs

207:637). IL-1 affects a variety of organ systems inducing fever, leucocytosis, and T-cell and B-cell activation and is involved in the immune response.

TNF-α was first identified by its cytotoxicity to fibrosarcoma *in vivo*. Cytotoxic effects on further tumour cell lines were demonstrated thereafter, but revealed that this monokine affects various functions of normal cells. Mainly secreted by macrophages in response to stimuli such as viruses and bacteria, it is involved in the inflammatory response during host defence (Cerami, RecProgHormRes, 1987; 43:99; Le, LabInvest, 1987; 56:234; Perlmutter, JCI, 1987; 78:1349). TNF-α is strongly associated with mortality during sepsis (Beutler, Science, 1985; 229:869; Tracey, Nature, 1987; 330:662). TNF-α was also shown to induce hepatocyte apoptosis in the presence of transcriptional inhibitors such as D-galactosamine (Decker, GastrJap, 1993; 28(S4):20; Leist, JImmunol, 1994; 153:1778).

IL-6 is a cytokine with a central role in host defence enabling growth-inducing, growth-inhibiting, and differentiation-inducing activity in cells of the immune sytem and in the induction of the hepatic acute phase response (Akira, FASEBJ, 190; 4:2860) (Table 2).

IL-6 was shown to induce most of the changes in the APP plasma levels seen *in vivo*. The hepatocyte synthesis of fibrinogen, C-reactive protein, serum amyloid A, haptoglobin, α_1-antitrypsin, α_1-antichymotrypsin, α_1-acid glycoprotein, and caeruloplasmin is increased by IL-6 (Castell, FEBSLett, 1988; 232:347; Gauldie, PNAS, 1987; 84:7251; Baumann, JBC, 1987; 262:9756; Ramadori, EurJImmun, 1988; 18:1259). Similar effects are induced by leukaemia inhibitory factor (**LIF**) (Baumann, JImmunol, 1989; 143:1163; Waring, JCI, 1992; 90:2031), IL-11 (Baumann, JBC, 1991; 266:20424), oncostatin M, and ciliary neurotrophic factor (**CNTF**) which were denoted as IL-6-type acute phase mediators. It has been suggested that the common action of these structurally distinct cytokines is mediated by the membrane protein gp130 which is capable of modulating the affinity of the receptors for each of the IL-6-type cytokines (Taga, FASEBJ, 1992; 6:3387; Gearing, Science, 1992; 255:1434). By means of IL-6-deficient mice, a major role of IL-6 has been demonstrated in localized inflammation, whereas in systemic tissue damage lipopolysaccharide (**LPS**) knocked out IL-6 might be reparable by the effect of other cytokines such as TNF-α (Fattori, JExpMed, 1994; 180:1243; Libert, EurJImmun, 1994; 24:2237).

In contrast to the IL-6-type cytokines, IL-1, TNF-α, and TNF-β (IL-1-type cytokines) stimulate the synthesis of a different set of positive APPs such as complement factors C3 and B and affect mainly negative APPs such as albumin, transferrin, and α-feto-protein (Ramadori, JExpMed, 1985; 162:930; Perlmutter, JCI, 1986; 78:1349; Darlington, JCB, 1986; 103:787; Andus, EurJImmun, 1988; 18:739).

Glucocorticoids although able to stimulate some APPs directly, mainly act on most APPs through enhancing the effect of acute phase mediators (Prowse, MolCellBiol, 1988; 8:42). Their effects may be facilitated in part by glucocorticoid-mediated induction of the 80 kDa IL-6R (Sayers, PNAS, 1990; 87:2830).

Furthermore, transforming growth factor-β (**TGF-β**) attenuates the effects of IL-1 on APPs, but augments that of IL-6 (Mackiewicz, PNAS, 1990; 87:1491) and insulin-like growth factor (**IGF-I**) (and insulin) decreases the effect of both IL-1 and IL-6 (Campos, MolCellBiol, 1992; 12:1789).

Cytokines in hepatic protein metabolism

During acute phase conditions or in the normal state, cytokines affect the uptake and metabolism of amino acids. *In vivo* studies have revealed a stimulatory effect of IL-1 and TNF-α on amino acid uptake by the liver (Argiles, BiochemJ, 1989; 261:357; Roh, Metabolism, 1986; 35:419). *In vitro* experiments only demonstrated enhanced amino acid uptake by IL-6 (Bereta, IntJBiochem, 1989; 21:361), while TNF-α was capable of increasing amino acid uptake only in the presence of glucagon (Warren, PNAS, 1987; 84:8619). Furthermore, epidermal growth factor (**EGF**), alone or in combination with IL-6, stimulates amino acid uptake in hepatocyte cultures (Moule, BiochemJ, 1987; 247:233), whereas TGF-β (Bereta, FEBSLett, 1990; 266:48) and IGF-I (Jakob, JCI, 1989; 83: 1717) inhibit liver amino acid uptake.[2]

In analogy to the uptake of amino acids, hepatic amino acid degradation may also be affected by cytokines. IL-1 and EGF increase the degradation of amino acids by stimulating histidine decarboxylase and ornithine decarboxylase activity (Endo, BiochemPharm, 1989; 38:1287; Moriarity, BBActa, 1970; 204:578).

Cytokines in hepatic lipid metabolism

Cytokines may modulate hepatic lipid metabolism. The synthesis of fatty acids is increased by interferon-α (**IFN-α**), IL-1, and IL-6 (Feingold, JCI, 1986; 80:184). The application of TNF-α to rats induced a strong, rapid increase of hepatic fatty acid synthesis accompanied by a rise in the triglyceride levels (Feingold, Endocrinol, 1989; 125:267). It was found that increased hepatic fatty acid synthesis induced by TNF-α is mediated by elevated citrate levels which activate acetyl-CoA carboxylase. Otherwise, IFN-α is capable of increasing fatty acid synthesis independently of the citrate levels suggesting that there may be another regulatory pathway of fatty acid synthesis. Furthermore, IL-4 was found to inhibit the increase of fatty acid synthesis induced by IL-1, IL-6, and TNF-α, but not that induced by IFN-α (Grunfeld, CancerRes, 1991; 51: 2803).

Furthermore, the modulation of hepatic cholesterol synthesis has been shown to be mediated by IL-1, TNF-β, and IFN-γ which might be due to an induction of HMG-CoA reductase, the rate-limiting enzyme of cholesterol synthesis (Klasking, JNutr, 1988; 118:1436). A negative regulation of cholesterol synthesis by EGF and platelet-derived growth factor (**PDGF**) may be suggested,

since these cytokines have been shown to upregulate low-density lipoprotein (**LDL**) receptors in human hepatoma cells. Cholesterol synthesis may then be reduced via feedback mechanisms (Grove, 1991, JBC; 266:18194).

Cytokines in hepatic carbohydrate metabolism

The metabolism of carbohydrates is regulated in part by cytokines. IL-6 has been shown to enhance glucose uptake by cultured hepatocytes (Ritchie, AmJPhysiol, 1990; 258:E57), which was also observed *in vivo* after the application of IGF-I (Jakob, JCI, 1989; 83: 1717), whereas IL-1 and TNF-α had no effect on glucose uptake by primary cultures of hepatocytes. Glycolysis is enhanced by the action of EGF through the inhibition of pyruvate kinase (Moule, BiochemJ, 1988; 255:361).

On the other hand, gluconeogenesis may be reduced by IL-1 through a decrease in steroid receptors and the subsequent decreased induction of phosphoenolpyruvate carboxykinase (Hill, JImmunol, 1986; 137:858). TNF-α had no effect on hepatocyte gluconeogenesis *in vitro* (Rofe, BiochemJ, 1987; 247:789).

The synthesis of glycogen may be affected by EGF, which is stimulatory in fetal hepatocytes together with IGF-I and IGF-II (Freemark, Endocrinol, 1986; 119:522; Parkes, BBResComm, 1986; 134:427) and inhibitory in adult hepatocytes (Chowdhury, BiochemJ, 1987; 247:307) by counteracting the effect of insulin.

The liver as a source of cytokines

Under certain circumstances, the liver may be an important source of cytokines. During development, circulating EGF and IGF-II (Laborde, AmJPhysiol, 1988; 255:E28; Brown, JBC, 1986; 261: 13144) have been reported to derive from the liver. Under acute phase conditions, the origin of the acute phase mediators still has to be elucidated. It must be considered that Kupffer cells, the major population of tissue macrophages, may be an important source of cytokines in this situation even when tissue damage or infection occurs at other sites than in the liver. Circulating metabolites may lead to the activation and induction of cytokine production in this important macrophage population. Concordantly, it has been shown *in vitro* that Kupffer cells are capable of synthesizing inflammatory mediators in response to endotoxin which is suggested to be the main inducer of the acute phase response (Magilavy, JExpMed, 1988; 168:789; Busam, JHepatol, 1990; 191:575; Decker, EurJBioch, 1990; 192:245). The relevance of these findings remains unclear, since TNF-α was not found in the liver after endotoxin administration *in vivo* by use of a transgenic mouse model (Giroir, JCI, 1992; 90:693). Furthermore, the peripheral vein injection of endotoxin yielded higher arterial TNF-α concentrations than mesenteric vein application of endotoxin (Badger, Gut, 1992; 33: 694). Similarly, IL-6, although found to be produced by cultured Kupffer cells after the *in vivo* application of endotoxin, was not detected in non-parenchymal cells after the *in vivo* application of turpentine (Billiar, ArchSurg, 1992; 127:31) suggesting that IL-6 production may occur locally at the site of tissue damage.

During liver regeneration due to liver damage or partial hepatectomy, TGF-α, TGF-β, and fibroblast growth factor (**FGF**), each of which is supposed to be crucial in the initiation and regulation of

Table 3 Cytokines of liver fibrosis

Cytokine	Effect on liver cells
PDGF	Transformation of fat-storing cells into
IGF-1	myofibroblasts
TGF-β	Stimulation of extracellular matrix synthesis

Table 4 Cytokines of liver regeneration

Stimulatory effect	Inhibitory effect
HGF	TGF-β
EGF	
TGF-α	
IL-6	

regeneration, have been shown to be produced by the regenerating liver (Kan, PNAS, 1989; 86:7432; Mead, PNAS, 1989; 86:1558) (see Table 4).

Fat-storing cells are capable of producing IGF-I (Murphy, Endocrinol, 1987; 120:1279) and TGF-β1 during liver fibrogenesis (Nakatsukasa, JCI, 1990; 85:1833). Sinusoidal endothelial cells may produce basic FGF (Rosenbaum, BBResComm, 1989; 164:1099). The liver produces erythropoietin in anaemia (Bondurant, MolCellBiol, 1986; 6:2731). IFN-α is produced in hepatocytes in chronic viral and non-viral liver disease (Sutherland, JClinPath, 1989; 42:1065).

Cytokines in liver diseases

Cytokines in alcoholic liver disease

Cytokines have been suggested to be pathogenetic factors in alcoholic liver disease. Elevated production and serum levels by peripheral leucocytes of TNF-α (Bird, AnnIntMed, 1990; 112:917; Khoruts, Hepatol, 1991; 13:267), IL-1 (McClain, SemLivDis, 1993; 13:170), IL-6 (Deviere, ClinExpImmun, 1989; 77:221; Hill, JLabClinMed, 1992; 119:547), and TGF-β (Annoni, JHepatol, 1992; 14:259) have been reported. Presumably, these elevated peripheral cytokine concentrations parallel increased levels of hepatic cytokines (McClain, SemLivDis, 1993; 13:170) which are suggested to result from increased endotoxin levels in the circulation due to an alcohol-induced increase of the gut permeability (Bode, JHepatol, 1987; 4:8; Bjarnason, Lancet, 1984; i:179). Alcohol itself does not directly increase cytokine production.

Cytokines in autoimmune hepatitis

Patients with autoimmune hepatitis have higher levels of activated T cells expressing IL-2R and HLA-DR antigens as compared to patients with other liver diseases, which may explain the increased immune reactivity in this liver disease. In contrast, the expression of the inflammatory cytokines IL-1, IL-6, and TNF-α is markedly reduced in such livers, whereas the IFNs were similar in normal livers and autoimmune hepatitis (Tovey, Experientia, 1987; 67:95).

Cytokines in chronic viral hepatitis

Persisting viral infections have been thought to be due to an impaired cell-mediated immune response which, in chronic viral hepatitis, is still strong enough to provoke hepatocellular necrosis. An impaired production of IFN-α as well as an impaired response to IFN-α may underly this hypothesis which is derived from the observation that patients with chronic hepatitis B virus (**HBV**) infection have a partial deficiency of IFN-α and IFN-β production (Kato, Hepatol, 1982; 2:789; Pointrine, Hepatol, 1985; 5:171; Twu,

JVirol, 1989; 63:3065, Onji, Hepatol, 1989; 9:92). Exogenous IFN-α is able to provoke T-cell activation (Alexander, JHepatol, 1986; 3:S269) which is reduced in chronic HBV infection (Anastassakos, Gastro, 1988; 94:999).

Cytokines in liver fibrogenesis

Chronic liver diseases tend to lead to the development of liver fibrosis and subsequently, to liver cirrhosis. Due to sustained hepatocellular necrosis, inflammatory cells such as mononuclear phagocytes and platelets accumulate in the liver and, by the release of inflammatory mediators, activate fat-storing cells which start to synthesize and secrete increasing amounts of extracellular matrix proteins which are then deposited in developing fibrous septa. The activation of fat-storing cells and transformation into myofibroblast-like cell types has been considered to be the crucial event in liver fibrogenesis. Several cytokines have been identified as supporting this process; among them TGF-β and PDGF are suggested as the most important. TGF-β is synthesized by liver mononuclear phagocytes (Matsuoka, Hepatol, 1990; 11:599) and is stored in the granules of platelets and has been shown to increase extracellular matrix synthesis by fat-storing cells dramatically *in vitro* (Knittel, Gastro, 1992; 102:1724). DNA synthesis in fat-storing cells is increased mainly by PDGF, whereas TGF-β has been reported to inhibit fat-storing cell proliferation (Czaja, JCB, 1989; 108:2477; Matsuoka, Liver, 1989; 9:71). IGF-1 seems to be another cytokine that promotes fat-storing cell transformation and DNA synthesis (Pinzani, Endocrinol, 1990; 127:2349). TGF-β may also act in an autocrine fashion by stimulating its own synthesis in fat-storing cells (Weimer, Hepatol, 1990; 11:111). Furthermore, TGF-β may not only be responsible for increased matrix protein synthesis, but also for reduced matrix degradation by the induction of protease inhibitors (Edwards, EMBOJ, 1987; 6:1899) (Table 3).

Cytokines in liver regeneration

Liver regeneration is the compensatory hyperplasia after chemical, viral, ischaemic, or immunological injury or after partial hepatectomy. Within a short time the original liver mass is fully restored as a result of multiple cell divisions by all the liver cell types. A large number of regulatory processes and complex interactions is involved in the organization of liver regeneration. Many early biochemical events have been identified so far which are detectable within a few min after, for example, partial hepatectomy, resulting in an ultimate stimulation of DNA synthesis at least 10 to 20 h later. Nevertheless, the linkage between these events and the major mechanisms responsible for liver regeneration have still to be clarified (Table 4).

Several growth factors enhancing the DNA synthesis of hepatocytes have been identified in the last decade, but in the later years most attention has been paid to the so-called hepatocyte growth factor (**HGF**) which is suggested to be the most powerful stimulator of liver mitogenesis. HGF (Michalopoulos, Hepatol, 1992; 15:149) is not only a mitogen for hepatocytes and bile duct cells, but also for the bronchial epithelium, endothelial cells, mammary duct epithelial cells, melanocytes, and various neoplastic cells (Michalopoulos, GastrJap, 1993; 2(S4):36). It is synthesized by the mesenchymal cells of various organs and binds to the proto-oncogene c-*met* (Naldini, Oncogene, 1991; 6:501) which is also present in most organs.

The plasma levels of HGF increase dramatically within 1 h after experimental partial hepatectomy (Lindroos, Hepatol, 1991; 3:743) and remain elevated for longer than 24 h. This is also observed in humans after surgical liver resection (Tomiya, Gastro, 1992; 103: 1621). However, HGF was also found to be elevated in the sera of patients with acute hepatitis and chronic liver disease (LaBrecque, Gastro, 1992; 103:1686). Unilateral nephrectomy led to an increased HGF messenger RNA content in the intact kidney (Nagaike, JBC, 1991; 266:22781) and elevated serum levels of HGF are found after various surgical interventions (Tomiya, Gastro, 1992; 103:1621) being well correlated with peripheral leucocyte counts and C-reactive serum levels indicating that this cytokine may be better classified as an acute phase mediator.

This cytokine meanwhile has been shown to possess pleiotropic effects not only stimulating hepatocyte growth, but also being involved in the inflammatory reactions of other organs.

Hitherto, the involvement of several other cytokines in the regulation of liver regeneration has been reported. Although the serum levels of EGF do not increase after partial hepatectomy, its growth-promoting ability has been shown *in vivo* and *in vitro* (Skov-Olsen, Hepatol, 1988; 8:992; Rasmussen, ScaJGastr, 1992; 27:372; Blanc, Gastro, 1992; 102:1340). EGF may not be important in liver regeneration, since neutralizing antibodies did not prevent regeneration *in vivo* (Vesey, Gut, 1992; 33:831). TGF-α is also capable of augmenting liver growth after partial hepatectomy (Mead, PNAS, 1989; 86:1558), and the growth of hepatocytes *in vitro* (Brenner, DNA, 1989; 8:279). It was found to be elevated in models of regenerating liver (Evarts, MolCarcin, 1992; 5:25). Nevertheless, the serum levels of TGF-α first increase when DNA synthesis has already started.

A recent study has shown the importance of IL-6 in liver regeneration by means of IL-6-deficient mice (Cressman, Science, 1996; 274:1373). The IL-6-deficient mice had an impaired regenerative response after partial hepatectomy characterized by massive liver necrosis and subsequent liver failure. Hepatocyte DNA synthesis was reduced compared with wild-type animals, whereas DNA synthesis remained unchanged in sinusoidal cells. The alterations in IL-6-deficient mice were fully prevented by application of IL-6 prior to partial hepatectomy indicating the direct involvement of this cytokine.

FGF is another cytokine exhibiting hepatocyte growth-promoting abilities *in vivo* and *in vitro* (Houck, JCellPhysiol, 1990; 143: 129; Kan, PNAS, 1989; 86:7432). FGF gene expression after partial hepatectomy increases prior to increases of TGF-α suggesting that FGF may initiate hepatocyte growth in the early phase after injury (Presta, BBResComm, 1989; 164:1182).

In addition to promoters of liver growth, inhibitory factors are suggested as regulating the extent of regeneration, for example TGF-β inhibits the proliferation of hepatocytes *in vitro* and *in vivo* (Wollenberg, CancerRes, 1987; 47:6595; Strain, BBResComm, 1987; 145:436). Concordantly, TGF-β gene expression in regenerating livers peaks after DNA synthesis has reached its peak. TGF-β may act in part by terminating the effect of growth-promoting factors (Russell, PNAS, 1988; 85:5126).

Cytokines in the pathogenesis of hepatocellular carcinoma

Hepatocellular carcinoma is closely related to chronic hepatitis, implying that changes in the growth control mechanisms during regeneration which are mediated in part by cytokines may be involved in hepatic carcinogenesis. The involvement of cytokines as mitogens for hepatocytes has therefore been studied in detail in this context. As stated above, HGF is a considerable hepatic mitogen during liver regeneration. Nevertheless, the transformation of the HGF gene in hepatoma cells gene resulted in a strong decrease of proliferation (Shiota, PNAS, 1992; 89:373) weakening the role of this cytokine in hepatocarcinogenesis. IGF-II, another strong mitogen for hepatocytes found in the liver during development, was detected in hepatocellular carcinoma and hepatoma cells (Su, CancerRes, 1989; 49:1773; Cariani, Hepatol, 1991; 13:644). It is expressed in precancerous lesions (Schirrmacher, CancerRes, 1992; 52:2549) and is suggested to be closely related to hepatocarcinogenesis (Cariani, JHepatol, 1991;13:220). Furthermore, TGF-α is expressed in hepatoma cells (Liu, CancerRes, 1988; 48: 850). TGF-α overexpressing mice develop multifocal hepatocellular carcinoma (Lee, CancerRes, 1992; 52:5162).

The treatment of hepatocellular carcinoma with IFN-α has not been established. Although some authors have reported a benefit in the median survival time in inoperable hepatocellular carcinoma (Lai, BrJCanc, 1989; 60:928), others could not confirm this effect (Kardinal, Cancer, 1993; 71:2187).

References

1. Ramadori G and Meyer zum Büschenfelde K-H. Liver cells and cytokines. *Current Opinions in Gastroenterology*, 1993; 9: 359–66.
2. Gerok W, Decker K, Andus T, and Gross T. *Cytokines and the liver.* Dordrecht, Boston, and London: Kluwer Academic Publishers, 1995.

2.7.2 Immunogenetics of liver disease

Peter T. Donaldson and Michael P. Manns

General introduction

The immune system consists of a network of cellular and humoral components that contribute to the basic function of the system—the distinction between 'self' and 'non-self'. Because of this, the organism can identify infectious agents (such as viruses) and attack virus-infected cells, thereby eliminating the virus. Effector T lymphocytes recognize viral antigen only if it is presented on the surface of the infected cell by autologous HLA molecules. Disturbances in this highly specific distinction between 'self'and 'non-self' may lead to an autoimmune response towards 'self', which may end in autoimmune diseases. A key role in the diversified network of the immune system is played by the interaction between an HLA molecule, the antigenic peptide presented in its groove, and the T-cell receptor. All three components may be highly polymorphic, the HLA molecule in particular. HLA class I molecules present antigenic peptides to CD8+ cytotoxic T lymphocytes, and HLA class II molecules present peptides to CD4+ T-helper lymphocytes. While our knowledge is limited concerning the polymorphism of the T-cell receptor and the antigen in particular, the HLA system has been extensively studied. HLA typing has reached everyday clinical practice, for instance in transplant medicine to identify organ donors. As far as immunogenetics in liver diseases are concerned, we are just beginning to understand the genetic background that predisposes to some chronic liver diseases, in particular those of a presumed autoimmune background. Recently, our knowledge has grown concerning the immunogenetic background in viral hepatitis B and C in regard to clinical outcome, severity, prevalence, and vaccine failure. Significant recent advances in our knowledge of HLA molecules are due to the dramatic technological developments in this area, which are based on the introduction of molecular biological techniques. This has changed the nomenclature of the whole system and taught us that the results obtained by the old serological typing method were frequently insufficient. Now that immunogenetics has become everyday clinical practice, not only in transplant medicine, we recognize that immunogenetics will contribute significantly to our understanding of liver diseases.

Immunogenetics is a hybrid science which brings together both immunology and genetics. Though in theory this definition encompasses all polypeptides with an immune function, in practice most of the published data relates to the genes which encode the three immunoglobulin supergene family molecules—the T-cell receptor (**TCR**, chromosomes 7 and 14), the immunoglobulins (**Ig**, chromosome 14), and the human leucocyte antigens (**HLAs**), also referred to as major histocompatibility antigens (**MHC**, chromosome 6p21.3). These three molecules are required for antigen processing and presentation and are therefore essential for both T- and B-cell immunity.

All three of these complex genetic systems exhibit extensive polymorphism, though much of the TCR and immunoglobulin polymorphism is generated by somatic mutation and recombination and there is only limited germ-line polymorphism. In contrast, the genes of the human MHC have very extensive interindividual (i.e. germ-line) polymorphism. Indeed it is the barrier that these major histocompatibility antigens (or HLA antigens) pose for organ/tissue transplantation between individuals of the same species that gave rise to their name and the generic description MHC, which is applied to the gene complex encoding them in different animal species. As a consequence of their importance in clinical transplantation, the human MHC antigens (or HLA antigens) and their genes (the HLA genes) have been more widely studied and have become easier to investigate than either the TCR or Ig genes.

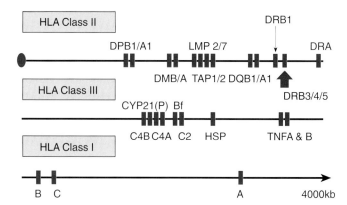

Fig. 1. An abridged version of the human MHC gene map based on Campbell and Trowsdale, Immunol Today, 1997; 18:43. Only expressed HLA genes are illustrated.

In this chapter we will describe the genetic organization of the *HLA* and other immunogenes and their functions, review the various clinical immunogenetic studies of both autoimmune and viral liver disease, and explore a number of hypotheses to explain the disease associations which we describe. This chapter will concentrate on recent developments and new areas of research and only briefly touch on the early studies which have been reviewed elsewhere.[1-3]

Genetic organization of the HLA region

The human MHC is located on the short arm of chromosome 6 spanning approximately 4 million base-pairs in the 6p21.3 band (Fig. 1).[4] By convention the region is divided into three subregions referred to as HLA class I (telomeric), HLA class II (centromeric), and HLA class III (located between class I and class II). The divisions are largely historical and were originally based on structural and functional similarities between the polypeptides encoded by the genes within the three subregions.

HLA class I genetics, structure, and function

There are presently more than 100 genes or gene sequences mapped to the HLA class I region. Of these, six genes encode cell surface HLA glycoproteins including the classical HLA antigens A, B, and Cw and also the non-classical HLA E, F, and G. The other class I genes include numerous short sequences, some without functional products (i.e. pseudogenes) and others whose function is unknown.[4] Included among these are the *HUMORMHC-FAT11* and *-OL42* and *MCHOR2* olfactory MHC genes which may be important in mate selection and also a number of genes encoding metal-dependent DNA-binding proteins.

The classical class I genes HLA A, B, and C are highly polymorphic with at least 84 recognized alleles of *HLA A*, 186 of *HLA B*, and 42 of *HLA C*.[5] Each of these genes encodes a single polypeptide α-chain of 45 kDa which forms a non-covalent bond with a 12-kDa β₂-microglobulin molecule (the β-chain, encoded on chromosome 15).

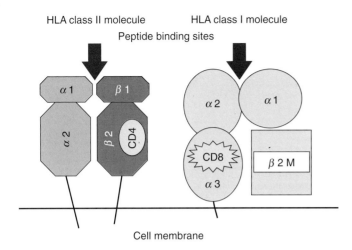

Fig. 2. Simple illustration of the expressed HLA class I and class II molecules. The site of the class I and class II antigen-binding grooves is indicated by the arrows.

Table 1 Organization of the *HLA DRB* genes in different haplotypes split according to the *DRB1* genomic group (genes underlined are pseudogenes)

DRB1 allelic group	Genomic organization				
DRB1*01, DRB1*10	DRB1	DRB6		DRB9	DRA
DRB1*15, DRB1*16	DRB1	DRB6	DRB5	DRB9	DRA
DRB1*03, DRB1*11, DRB1*12, DRB1*13, DRB1*14	DRB1	DRB2	DRB3	DRB9	DRA
DRB1*04, DRB1*07, DRB1*09	DRB1	DRB7 DRB4	DRB8	DRB9	DRA
DRB1*08	DRB1			DRB9	DRA

HLA A, B, and C molecules are constitutively expressed on all nucleated cells, though they are only weakly expressed on hepatocytes. In contrast, HLA E, F, and G have only limited polymorphism and limited tissue expression. HLA E has four alleles and is expressed at low levels on placenta, fetal liver, and resting T cells; HLA G also has four alleles and is expressed on placenta (Carosella, ImmunolToday, 1996; 17:407); and HLA F is non-polymorphic with only one identified allele and is found on fetal liver only.[4,5]

Expressed HLA class I molecules form an α/β-heterodimer spanning the plasma membrane with four extracellular domains, three from the α-chain (α_1, α_2, and α_3) with β_2-microglobulin providing the fourth (β_1) (Fig. 2(a)). The two domains closest to the cell membrane, namely α_3 and β_1, form a supporting platform on which the remaining two domains (α_1 and α_2) form a complex structure composed of criss-crossed β-pleated sheets surmounted by opposing α-helices resulting in an enclosed groove of 25 Å long, 10 Å wide, and 11 Å deep.[6,7] This groove or cleft is now known to be the actual site at which antigen (peptide) is bound for presentation to the TCR.

Class I molecules present antigenic peptides derived from within the cell cytoplasm (endogenous antigens) to CD8+ T cells. This interaction is favoured by the presence of a CD8-binding site on the α_3- domain. The CD8–MHC interaction helps to stabilize the MHC–peptide–TCR complex and it is this which is the basis of so-called HLA restriction which was originally described by Doherty and Zinkernagel.[8]

HLA class II genetics, structure, and function

The HLA class II region encodes more than 30 genes, including those which encode the classical 'transplantation antigens' HLA DR, DQ, and DP, genes encoding the intracellular proteins TAP (*TAP1* and *TAP2*), LMP (*LMP2* and *LMP7*), and DM (*DMA* and *DMB*), a collagen gene (*COLL11A2*), as well as a number of pseudogenes.

HLA DR, DQ, and DP

Though there are less genes mapped to the HLA class II region, the genetic arrangement of HLA class II is more complex than that of the class I region and the DR subregion is the most confusing. In contrast to the HLA class I molecules, both the α- and β-polypeptides of the HLA class II molecules are encoded on chromosome 6. The DR subregion has a single, essentially non-polymorphic, *DRA* gene (encoding a 32-kDa α-chain) and nine *DRB* genes, five of which (*DRB2, DRB6, DRB7, DRB8,* and *DRB9*) are pseudogenes and four of which (*DRB1, DRB3, DRB4,* and *DRB5*) are expressed (each encoding a different 28-kDa β-chain). The number of *DRB* genes that an individual may possess varies according to the *DRB1* allelic group (Table 1) which is inherited as a discrete unit or haplotype from each parent. The *DRB* genes are highly polymorphic with more than 220 alleles listed at present.

In contrast to HLA DR each of the DQ and DP subregions encodes a single pair of functional *A* genes and *B* genes, both of which have extensive polymorphism. Presently there are more than 18 alleles of *DQA*, 31 alleles of *DQB*, 10 alleles of *DPA*, and 77 alleles of *DPB*.[5]

HLA DR, DQ, and DP molecules are constitutively expressed on specialized antigen-presenting cells, B cells, monocytes, tissue macrophages, dendritic cells, and also to some extent on endothelial and bile-duct epithelial cells, but rarely if at all on hepatocytes. Class II molecules may be induced by interferon-γ (Germain, Cell, 1994; 76:287). As with HLA class I, the class II molecule is expressed as an α/β-heterodimer folded to form four extracellular domains (α_1, α_2, β_1, and β_2) (Fig. 2(b)). X-ray crystallography reveals a similar secondary structure to that of the HLA class I molecule with an antigen-binding groove formed from the membrane distal α_1- and β_1-domains.[9] In contrast to HLA class I where the peptide-binding groove has closed ends favouring the binding of peptides of 8 to 9 amino acid residues, the class II groove is an open-ended structure allowing the linear binding of peptides of up to 24 amino acid residues. Peptide binding to both class I and class II HLA molecules may be enhanced by specialized binding pockets at particular positions that provide additional anchors for side chains on the antigenic peptides (Madden, AnnRevImmunol, 1995; 13: 587).[10]

Class II molecules present antigenic peptides derived from the outside of the cell (i.e. exogenous antigens). This interaction is favoured by the presence of a CD4-binding site on the β_2-domain of the HLA class II molecule. Exogenous antigens enter the cell through endocytosis and may undergo proteolytic cleavage in acidic endosomes before binding newly assembled HLA class II molecules. The class II molecule is expressed at the plasma membrane only after peptide binding and neither HLA class I nor class II molecules are expressed with the peptide-binding groove unoccupied.

TAP, LMP, and DM

The *TAP1/2*, *LMP2/7*, and *DMA/B* genes encode proteins which are expressed intracellularly and their expression is required for antigen processing and presentation. Peptide antigens destined to be presented at the cell surface by class I molecules are derived from endogenous antigens and are 'processed' to short peptide units of eight or nine amino acids by proteolytic cleavage by the large multifunctional protease or proteasome. LMP2 and LMP7 are proteasome-β components that modify proteasome activity, though their exact function is unknown. A processed peptide is transported to the endoplasmic reticulum with the help of the transporter heterodimer **TAP** (transporter associated with antigen processing). This heterodimer is the product of the *TAP1* and *TAP2* genes.

Class II molecules are synthesized in the endoplasmic reticulum where they are prevented from binding to intracellular peptides by association with the invariant chain (**Ii**) a 'molecular chaperone'.[11] The stable class II heterodimer/invariant chain complex migrates via the trans-Golgi to an acidic compartment where a second heterodimer, DM, enables the Ii chain to dissociate from the class II molecule, thereby making the binding groove accessible for interaction with antigenic peptides (Sloan, Nature, 1995; 375:802; Roche, Science, 1996; 274:526; Weber, Science, 1996; 274:618). The DM heterodimer is the product of the *DMA* and *DMB* genes.

The *LMP*, *TAP*, and *DM* genes are all located between the HLA DQ and DP subregions. *DM* and *LMP* are of limited interest to the immunogeneticist since they are non-polymorphic, but there are five alleles of *TAP1* and four alleles of *TAP2*.

HLA class III genetics, structure, and function

The HLA class III region encodes more than 70 genes amongst which there is a diverse array encoding immunologically active proteins including: the complement proteins C2, C4 (A and B), and factor B (**Bf**); tumour necrosis factor-α (**TNF-α**) and lymphotoxin-α and -β (**LT-α and -β**) and heat shock proteins (**HSP-70**, HSP-71, HSP-72), as well as a number of enzymes and pseudogenes.

The complement proteins C2 and C4 are classical complement pathway polypeptides required for the conversion of C3 to C3d (C3-convertase) and C5 to C5d (C5 convertase). Factor B (Bf) has a similar catalytic function and combines with C3b to form a C3 convertase in the alternative complement pathway (Fig. 3). There are two isotypes of C4, C4A and C4B, which may have differing affinities for amino and carboxyl groups. The genes for C2, C4A, C4B, and Bf are all polymorphic. Abnormal complement function has been demonstrated in chronic liver disease, though whether this is secondary to liver damage is uncertain. Individuals with null or non-expressed complement genes (either deleted or otherwise) are

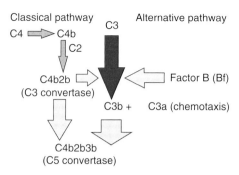

Fig. 3. Illustration of the HLA class III complement C4, C2, and Bf gene function in conversion of C3 to C3b. C3b complexes with the C4b2b forming C4b2b3b (C5 convertase), which converts C5 to C5b, the first subunit in the membrane attack complex. C3a, the other C3 fragment, has weak chemotactic properties.

more likely to develop a lupus-like illness and those who are homozygous for null C2 and C4 may have complement deficiencies which may be lethal.

Tumour necrosis factor is a proinflammatory cytokine and an important mediator of inflammation and tissue damage in a number of diseases including acetaminophen- and alcohol-induced liver injury.[12,13] There is very extensive polymorphism of both the *TNF-α* and *LT-α* gene region and, though not all of the polymorphism which has been described has functional significance, two *TNF* polymorphisms, *TNF308* and the uncommon *Nco*I restriction fragment of *LT-α*, have been associated with serum TNF levels.[12]

Practical considerations

The significance of HLA–disease associations

The first clinical studies of HLA and disease date from 1967 when associations with Hodgkin's disease were described (Amiel, HistocompTest, 1967; 79). Even though some exceptional early studies identified very strong associations accounting for more than 90 per cent of patients (Brewerton, Lancet, 1973; i:904), it was clear from the beginning that the diseases being studied were not HLA linked, with the notable exceptions of hereditary haemochromatosis (Simon, NouvPresseMed, 1975; 4:1432; Feder, NatureGen, 1996; 13:399) and congenital adrenal hyperplasia due to 21-hydroxylase deficiency (Dupont, Lancet, 1977; ii:1309). Although the general trend with HLA has been to seek ever stronger genetic associations, it is no surprise that associations accounting for 100 per cent of patients have not been described. Today, few authors expect to find disease genes on the short arm of chromosome 6. In fact, given the number and variety of diseases with documented HLA associations, this would be extraordinary. It is now generally realized that these genetic associations are in most instances only part of a more complex multifactorial/polygenic jigsaw (Todd, Diabetes, 1992; 41: 1029).

As a result of the X-ray crystallography data (referred to above) and subsequent developments in immunological theory there has been a radical change in our perspective on HLA–disease associations. The key to understanding the significance of HLA polymorphism in terms of disease susceptibility and resistance lies in the observation that the majority of the genetic variation between alleles is concentrated in that part of the gene which encodes the HLA class I α_1- and α_2-domains and the HLA class II α_1- and β_1-domains. Most of the resulting amino acid variation occurs in and around the antigen-binding groove. Substitution of one amino acid for another within this region may alter the antigen-binding characteristics of the molecule either directly through interaction with the antigenic peptide or through interaction with the peptide side chains. The resulting conformational changes to the MHC–peptide complex may result in more or less efficient interaction with the TCR. Different HLA alleles encode molecules with different peptide-binding characteristics and this alone may be sufficient to explain the great variety of diseases with HLA associations. Since we can now relate all disease association data, whether determined by serology or DNA-genotyping, to amino acid residues at specific positions in the antigen-binding groove, it has become fashionable to develop models of disease susceptibility/resistance based on particular amino acid sequences (i.e. motifs).

Linkage disequilibrium

Linkage disequilibrium describes the non-random association of two genes encoded at different loci. When HLA antigens/alleles occur together more often than predicted from the individual antigen/allele frequencies, they are said to be in linkage disequilibrium. The best example of this is the HLA A1-B8-DR3 haplotype which is present in 12 to 16 per cent of northern European populations but would occur in less than 2 to 3 per cent of the populations if these alleles were independently assorted. The physical basis of linkage disequilibrium is that two or more genes pass from generation to generation *en bloc*, preventing an equal assortment (i.e. equilibrium) being achieved. Linkage disequilibrium may result from strong selection effects, migration and admixture of populations, recent mutation, and genetic drift. Linkage patterns are usually specific to different racial groups, for example in Japan *DR8* is linked with *DQB1*0301* and *DPB1*0501*, whereas in northern Europe we find *DR8* with *DQB1*0402* and frequently with *DPB1*0301*. As we shall see, comparing different patterns of linkage disequilibrium between populations can be useful for defining the primary disease association.

HLA nomenclature

The current WHO nomenclature for the HLA region is reviewed by Bodmer *et al.*[5] The nomenclature of those HLA determinants referred to in the text of this chapter is summarized in Table 2.

Methods of HLA typing

As clinical transplantation developed in the late 1960s, so also did the need to group (type) the various HLA antigens for the purposes of matching organs. HLA phenotyping of populations with various diseases that required transplantation led to the serendipitous discovery of HLA–disease associations. Early work was based on the use of well-defined antibodies and leucocytes (i.e. serology) for the assignment of HLA 'types' (i.e. phenotyping). More recently, the widespread introduction of molecular genetics has permitted assignment of HLA types using genomic DNA (i.e. genotyping), which is not only more accurate and convenient, but also allows a

Table 2 Nomenclature for HLA antigens and genotypes used in this chapter

Serological determinant

Old name	Current name	Allele[c]
HL-A1	A1	A*0101, A*0102
HL-A8	B8	B*0801, B*0802
HL-A12	B12	B*4402 to B*4406
	Cw7	C*0701 to C*0704
Dw2/Dw12[a]	DR2	DRB1*1501, DRB1*1502
Dw3[a]	DR3[b]	DRB1*03011, DRB1*03012
Dw4[a]	DR4	DRB1*0401
Dw15[a]	DR4	DRB1*0405
DRw6	DR13	DRB1*1301 to DRB1*1319
DRw6	DR14	DRB1*1401 to DRB1*1418
DRw8	DR8	DRB1*0801 to DRB1*0811
DRw52a/Dw24	DR52	DRB3*0101
DRw52b/Dw25	DR52	DRB3*0201 to DRB3*0202
DQ2/Dw3	DQ2	DQB1*0201
DQ3/Dw4,5,8,13	DQ7	DQB1*0301
DQ3/Dw4,10,13,14	DQ8	DQB1*0302

[a] Specificities determined by mixed lymphocyte reaction. [b] The common split of DR3 was called DRw17, later DR17; however, this term was not widely used before it was replaced by the designation *DRB1*0301*. [c] Current nomenclature is based on DNA sequencing data and is reviewed by Bodmer *et al.* (ref. 19). In the current WHO nomenclature the first four letters represent the HLA locus (i.e. *DRB1*, *DQA1* etc.) and the first two numbers following the asterisk give the broad allelic group and are equivalent to the old antigen designations defined by serology, thus *DRB1*03* = DR3. The last two numbers represent the specific allele and are based on DNA sequencing data.

greater degree of discrimination between similar HLAs. Today, serology is being replaced by DNA genotyping and a range of methodologies can be applied. The most useful of the current methods is based on the polymerase chain reaction (**PCR**) using sequence-specific primers (**PCR-SSP**) to detect alleles, or PCR with locus-specific primers (i.e. *A*, *B*, *Cw*, *DRB*, *DQA*, *DQB*, or *DPB* primers) followed by allele detection with a series of sequence-specific oligonucleotide probes (**PCR-SSOP**). The earliest of the HLA-genotyping techniques, restriction fragment length polymorphism (**RFLP**) analysis, is more or less obsolete as a method for HLA genotyping, as is the more complex and cumbersome PCR–RFLP genotyping method which was widely used in Japan. However, PCR–RFLP may be used to detect polymorphism of non-MHC genes, such as interleukin 1 (IL-1).

Non-MHC genes

There are by definition many non-MHC genes with immune function. Here, however, we will describe briefly only those genes of current interest to the immunogenetics of liver disease.

The T-cell receptor (TCR)

The expressed TCR is a heterodimer of two polypeptide chains, either α/β or γ/δ. The γ/δ-heterodimer is the first TCR to appear in ontogeny and represents less than 10 per cent of peripheral T cells, the remainder have the α/β-heterodimer. The expressed TCR is non-covalently associated with the CD3 T-cell molecule. This stabilizes the TCR and may be important in signal transduction. The genetics of the TCR are very complex and are reviewed in depth by Davis and Bjorkman.[14] The majority of TCR variability is generated by somatic mutation and recombination and there is very little germ-line polymorphism. Each polypeptide chain is constructed from subunits for which the respective genetic regions are referred to as variable (*V*), constant (*C*), joining (*J*), and in the case of β- and δ-chains, diversity (*D*) regions. Within each genetic region there are numerous genes for each subunit. During the initial stages of T-cell differentiation in the thymus, prior to transcription, specific *V*, *J*, and *D* (for β- and δ-chains) gene segments undergo rearrangement and are fused with a particular *C* gene segment to form a complete *V*-coding domain (TCR variable domain). Peptide antigens are recognized by the TCR region encoded from a splicing of *V* and *J* (in TCR α or γ) or by *V*, *D*, and *J* (in TCR β or δ) segments. All of this recombination and mutation may generate as many as 10^{22} possible combinations.

Though there has been a considerable interest in TCR *Vβ* gene usage in autoimmune disease, the results obtained to date have been disappointing (Gold, CurrOpinImmunol, 1994; 6:907). Difficulties may arise from the fact that it is often impossible to determine which T cells are pathogenic. Though germ-line polymorphism is limited, recent studies have described associations with polymorphism of the TCR constant (*C*) region genes that may contribute to susceptibility to insulin-dependent diabetes mellitus, multiple sclerosis, rheumatoid arthritis, and autoimmune hepatitis.

The immunoglobulin genes

As with the TCR genes, most of the variability of immunoglobulin molecules is determined by gene rearrangements and somatic mutation. One particular germ-line polymorphism which has been studied in relation to autoimmune disease is that of the immunoglobulin heavy-chain constant region genes (*Gm*) which are encoded on chromosome 14 and are in linkage disequilibrium with the immunoglobulin heavy-chain variable genes (reviewed by Propert).[15] Gm allotypes arise through single amino acid substitutions and can be detected by a simple agglutination inhibition assay.

Cytokine genes

There is currently an increasing interest in the possible link between various cytokine genes and disease susceptibility. Key among these are IL-1 a proinflammatory cytokine and interleukin 10 (IL-10) an anti-inflammatory T_{H2} cytokine. The IL-1 gene family is located in the 2q13–14 bands on the long arm of chromosome 2 and includes genes encoding the two agonist forms of IL-1, *IL-1A* which encodes IL-1α and *IL-1B* which encodes IL-1β, and the IL1-receptor antagonist (*IL1-ra*) (Mansfield, Gastro, 1994; 106:1321; Lennard, CritRevImmunol, 1995, 15:77). All three genetic loci have limited polymorphism, currently there are thought to be two alleles of *IL-1A* (McDowell, ArthRheum, 1995; 38:221), two of *IL-1B* (Bioque, ClinExpImmun, 1995; 102:379), and five alleles of *IL1-ra* (Tarlow, HumGenet, 1993; 91:403). The IL-10 gene family is located on chromosome 1 and recent analysis has revealed three single base-pair substitutions in the IL-10 promotor gene which can be related to IL-10 protein production *in vivo* (Turner, EurJImmunogenet, 1997; 24:1). The *IL-1B2* allele and *IL1-ra2* allele have been associated with ulcerative colitis (Mansfield, Gastro, 1994; 106:1321;

Bioque, ClinExpImmul, 1995; 102:379), whilst *IL-1A* polymorphisms may be important susceptibility factors in juvenile rheumatoid arthritis (McDowell, ArthRheum, 1995; 38:221). As our interest in other areas of the human genome develops, no doubt other polymorphic cytokine genes will be added to this list.

Racial variations

In practice, immunogenetics involves the comparison of gene frequencies in populations. By comparing the frequencies of various polymorphic genes, usually HLA alleles, either between one group of patients and another, or more commonly between patients and healthy controls, it is possible to identify alleles which cause susceptibility or resistance to that disease. Alleles which are more common in the disease group are considered to be disease-susceptibility alleles, whilst those which are less common in the disease group are associated with disease resistance. The data derived from these studies may also be used to give information about disease severity and prognosis. However, as the genes of interest are highly polymorphic, it is essential that we compare like with like. Studies should be based on clear diagnostic criteria and controls should be drawn from the same racial group as the patients. There are marked differences in the distribution of HLA alleles between populations. These differences can be quite severe, for example the most common HLA haplotype in Britain and northern Europe (A1-B8-DR3) is almost absent in Japan, whereas DR8 is present in more than 30 per cent of Japanese but only 5 to 10 per cent of Britons. This is not unexpected between two such diverse racial groups. However, even within the same racial group, there are often significant variations in allele frequencies with geography; for example the DR4 antigen is found in 25 per cent of the French population and 40 per cent of Britons, and in the Republic of Ireland up to 40 per cent of individuals may have DR3 compared with 20 to 25 per cent in Britain. As a result there may be variation in the strength of genetic associations between populations. In addition, different genes may be associated with the same disease in different populations.

Statistics

The statistical analysis of immunogenetic data must be rigorous. HLA data are non-parametric and are analysed using univariate statistics. The statistics which are generally applied to HLA–disease association studies are the χ^2 test and Fisher's exact probability test. As studies usually involve multiple comparisons, probability values (*p*) must be corrected by multiplying *p* by the total number of antigen/alleles tested (*pc*) (i.e. Bonferroni correction). The only exception to this rule is when there is an *a priori* hypothesis (i.e. when previous data or trends are being confirmed in a second study). However, even in these circumstances, correction for the number of alleles identified in the *a priori* hypothesis should be applied. In practice, correction is rarely performed when data are being confirmed. Comparison at 'the phenotype level' (i.e. antigen frequencies or equivalent) is considered preferable to comparison of gene frequencies.[16] Counting genes effectively doubles the population without increasing the sample size and though this will increase the statistical power of the analysis it may also lead to type II statistical errors.

HLA association studies often quote a value referred to as relative risk, which gives a crude means of comparing data from different studies. The value quoted in most cases is calculated from the cross-products ratio of the two-by-two contingency table used in the χ^2 and Fisher's exact test and is in fact not the true relative risk, but a very crude approximation correctly referred to as the odds ratio. Calculation of true relative risk is more complex.

It is now becoming common to see studies where secondary associations have been sought. This can be done by reanalysing the distribution of the HLA alleles after eliminating all patients and controls who possessed the first identified susceptibility/resistance allele (primary association). This practice allows the investigator to take into account bias introduced by a strong positive or strong primary negative association, thereby identifying hidden associations.

When evaluating HLA associations care must be exercised over the interpretation of weak associations. Such associations are often difficult to explain as they usually account for only a small proportion of the patients studied. Investigators should consider subgroup analysis, taking into account disease heterogeneity and prognostic factors, and also the possibility that a disease with a weak genetic association in one population may have a much stronger genetic association in another population (e.g. see primary biliary cirrhosis below).

Clinical studies

Autoimmune liver disease

Autoimmune hepatitis

Early studies

Early studies identified HLA A1, B8, and Dw3 as susceptibility markers for autoimmune hepatitis.[1-3] This was most likely the result of an increased frequency of the A1-B8-DR3 haplotype in autoimmune hepatitis (Donaldson, Hepatol, 1991; 13:701). These studies also indicated that DR phenotypes may correlate with the age of onset of disease. Thus patients with DR4 tend to have late-onset autoimmune hepatitis (Williams, VoxSang, 1978, 35:366; Donaldson, Hepatol, 1991; 13:701) and those with DR3 have early-onset disease (Tait, HistocompTest, 1981:657; Donaldson, Hepatol, 1991; 13:701). In Japan the majority (90.3 per cent) of patients with autoimmune hepatitis were found to have DR4 (Seki, Hepatol, 1990; 12:1300). This was not surprising since the HLA A1-B8-DR3 haplotype is rare in Japan and the average age of onset for autoimmune hepatitis in Japanese patients is comparable with that of the older-onset subgroup in the United Kingdom.

Recent studies

There are presently four large series of patients with autoimmune hepatitis studied by HLA genotyping. Two of the four series were studied at King's College Hospital, London, one based on the local series of patients (Manabe, Hepatol, 1993; 18:1334; Doherty, Hepatol, 1994; 19:609; Doherty, Autoimmun, 1994; 18:243), and the other based on a collaboration with the Mayo Clinic (Rochester, USA) (Czaja, Hepatol, 1997; 25:317; Strettell, Gastro, 1997; 112:2028). The other two study groups are based in Japan (Ota, Immunogenet, 1992, 36:49; Seki, Gastro, 1992; 103:1041) and

Argentina (Fainboim, HumImmunol, 1994; 41:146; Marcos, Hepatol, 1994; 19:1371).

The findings of the King's and King's/Mayo Clinic series are summarized in Tables 3, 4, and 5. PCR genotyping for HLA DRB, DQA, and DQB revealed a three- to fourfold increase in the frequency of the extended HLA A1-B8-DR3 haplotype (*HLA DRB1*0301-DRB3*0101-DQA1*0501-DQB1*0201*) in patients compared with controls, a strong secondary association with one of the *DR4* alleles *DRB1*0401* and a weak negative association with the *B7-DRB1*1501-DRB5*0101-DQA1*0102-DQB1*0602* haplotype. The studies at King's failed to demonstrate associations with DQA, DQB, or DPB other than those expected by linkage with *DRB1*. The absence of a stronger genetic association with any of the other HLA class II loci was confirmed in both Japan and Argentina suggesting that the DRB region is the primary HLA class II susceptibility region in autoimmune hepatitis.

The King's data poses two questions: (i) Which of the two DRB alleles within the HLA *DRB1*0301-DRB3*0101* haplotype is the primary susceptibility allele? and (ii) Is there a common susceptibility determinant shared by either *DRB1*0301* or *DRB3*0101* and *DRB1*0401*?

Combining the two series, 53 per cent (109/205) of the patients were *DRB1*0301* positive and 58 per cent (118/205) had *DRB3*0101*. A 5 per cent difference with this number of patients is insufficient to discriminate between these two alleles. However, in Argentina, whilst adult-onset autoimmune hepatitis is associated with DR4 (Marcos, Hepatol, 1994; 19:1371), in children the disease has a strong association with *DRB1*1301* but no association with *DRB1*0301* (Fainboim, HumImmunol, 1994; 41:146). The difference between the Argentinian series and the series from the King's/Mayo Clinic group may be the key to determining which HLA DRB allele is the primary susceptibility allele in autoimmune hepatitis. As *DRB1*1301* is frequently found with *DRB3*0101*, this may indicate that *DRB3*0101* is the primary susceptibility allele for autoimmune hepatitis, and the association in northern Europeans with *DRB1*0301* may be simply due to linkage. However, this idea was discounted by Fainboim *et al.* (1994), but has not been rigorously tested in the Argentinian series.

Detailed analysis of the distribution of amino acid sequences resulting from HLA class II polymorphism documented by the King's/Mayo Clinic group revealed a particular motif Leu–Leu–Glu–Gln–Lys–Arg (single-letter code LLEQKR) at positions 67 to 72 of the DRβ polypeptide in all but 13 out of 205 (94 per cent) patients studied compared with 64 per cent of controls. This motif is shared by *DRB1*0301*, *DRB3*0101*, and *DRB1*0401* as well as a number of other alleles. The critical amino acid in this 'shared epitope' appears to be a lysine residue at position 71 (Table 5).

Whilst this model of susceptibility fits the northern European patients with autoimmune hepatitis, it does not hold in Japan. There are two principle differences: (i) the predominant DR4 allele associated with autoimmune hepatitis in Japan, *DRB1*0405*, has an arginine residue (R) at β71 and (ii) DR2 is thought to increase susceptibility to autoimmune hepatitis in Japan, whereas the most common DR2 allele in northern Europe, *DRB1*1501*, may confer resistance to autoimmune hepatitis. Consequently, susceptibility to autoimmune hepatitis in Japan is modelled on basic amino acids at position 13 of the DRβ-polypeptide, which are encoded by all of

Table 3 Summary of the King's College and Mayo Clinic autoimmune hepatitis data: percentage of HLA alleles encoded on haplotypes with primary HLA associations

Allele	King's series				Mayo Clinic series			
	Patients (N = 119)[a]	Controls (N = 177)[a]	Probability corrected	Relative risk	Patients (N = 86)	Controls (N = 102)	Probability corrected	Relative risk
A1	58.4	32.6	<0.0025	2.9	46.4[b]	24.5[c]	<0.05	2.67
B8	53.2	22	<0.00005	4.0	51.2[b]	20.4[c]	<0.00025	4.09
DRB1*0301	54.6	23.7	<0.00001	3.9	51.2	18.6	0.0005	4.58
DRB3*0101	58	24.9	<0.00005	4.2	57	28.4	0.001	3.33
DQA1*0501	67.2	38.4	<0.0005	3.3	55.8	34.3	0.05	2.42
DQB1*0201	63	41.8	<0.05	2.4	58.1	30.4	0.002	3.18
B7	18.5	23.4	ns	0.7	10.7	30.6	ns	
DRB1*1501	14.3	28.2	ns	0.4	11.6	30.4	<0.05	0.3
DRB5*0101	15.1	28.2	ns	0.5	11.6	30.4	<0.05	0.3
DQA1*0102	16	35	<0.05	0.4	17.4	38.2	<0.02	0.34
DQB1*0602	14.3	27.7	ns	0.4	12.8	29.4	ns	

[a] King's figures for HLA A and B totals = 125 patients and 141 controls; [b] N = 84; [c] N = 98; ns = not significant.

Table 4 Summary of the King's College and Mayo Clinic autoimmune hepatitis data: percentage of alleles encoded on haplotypes with secondary HLA associations

Allele	King's series				Mayo Clinic			
	Patients (N = 50)	Controls (N = 133)	Probability corrected	Relative risk	Patients (N = 42)	Controls (N = 83)	Probability corrected	Relative risk
DRB1*04	74	44	n/a	n/a	66.7	36.1	ns	
DRB1*0401	54	23.3	<0.01	3.9	54.8	16.9	<0.0002	5.97
DRB4*0103[a]	n/a	n/a	n/a	n/a	73.8	38.6	<0.03	4.49
DQA1*0301[b]	n/a	n/a	n/a	n/a	9.5	2.4	ns	
DQA1*0302[b]	n/a	n/a	n/a	n/a	61.9	34.9	ns	
DQB1*0301	52	32.3	ns	2.3	35.7	33.7	ns	
DQB1*0302	36	33.1	ns	1.1	40.5	22.9	ns	

[a] DRB4*0103 not determined in earlier analysis; [b] data presented for DQA1*0301 and DQA1*0302 combined only 66 per cent of patients compared with 43.6 per cent of controls, probability corrected = not significant, relative risk = 2.5.

Table 5 Pooled King's College/Mayo Clinic autoimmune hepatitis data: significant associations with amino acids of the DRβ-polypeptide

Amino acid residue	Position	Encoding alleles	Patients (N = 119 + 86 = 205)		Controls (N = 177 + 102 = 279)		χ^2	Probability corrected	Odds ratio
			n	%	n	%			
Tyrosine (Y)	β26	DRB1*0301 DRB1*0901 DRB3*0101	126	61.4	87	31.18	43.97	<0.000000001	3.52
Lysine (K)	β71	DRB1*0301[a] DRB1*0401 DRB1*0409 DRB1*0413 DRB1*0416 DRB1*1303 DRB3*[b]	192	93.6	175	62.7	61.69	<0.000000001	8.78
Arginine (R)	β74	DRB1*0301[a] DRB3*0101	124	60.48	81	29	47.89	<0.000000001	3.74

[a] Includes the DRB1*0301, DRB1*0302, and DRB1*0303 alleles but, although all three alleles were tested for, only DRB1*0301 was detected in this series.
[b] Lysine (K) at position 71 of the DRβ chain is encoded by all of the DRB3* alleles.

Table 6 Shared epitopes in autoimmune hepatitis: Japanese and King's College and King's College/Mayo Clinic data

Alleles DR		Position of amino acid			
		9 to 13	26	67 to 72	74
DRB1*					
0101		WQLLKF	L	LLEQRR	A
1501	DR2	WQLPKR	F	ILEQAR	A
1502		WQLPKR̲	F	ILEQAR	A
1601		WQLPKR̲	F	FLEDRR	A
1602		WQLPKR̲	F	LLEDRR	A
0301	DR3	LEYSTS	**Y**	LLE**Q**KR	**R**
0401	DR4	WELVKH	F	LLE**Q**KR	A
0402		WELVKH	F	ILEDER	A
0403		WELVKH	F	LLEQRR	E
0404		WELVKH	F	LLEQRR	A
0405		WELVKH̲	F	LLEQRR	A
0406		WELVKH̲	F	LLEQRR	E
0407		WELVKH̲	F	LLEQRR	E
0408		WELVKH̲	F	LLEQRR	A
DRB3*					
0101	DR52	LELRKS	**Y**	LLE**Q**KR	**R**
0201		LELLKS	F	LLE**Q**KR	Q
0202		LELLKS	F	LLE**Q**KR	Q
0301		LELLKS	F	LLE**Q**KR	

The standard WHO single-letter code for amino acids has been used. Amino acids in bold are those associated with autoimmune hepatitis in northern European and North American patients (Doherty, Hepatol, 1994; 19:609. Strettell, Gastro, 1997; 112: 2028). Amino acids underlined are associated with autoimmune hepatitis in Japanese patients (Ota, Immunogenet, 1992; 36:49).

the DR2 alleles and also by *DRB1*0405* (Ota, Immunogenet, 1992; 36:49) (Table 6). The idea that the basis of immunogenetic susceptibility to autoimmune hepatitis in northern Europe is different to that seen in Japan is not surprising as the two populations are genetically dissimilar.

HLA class III

Early research looking for a genetic explanation for persistently low levels of the complement proteins in autoimmune hepatitis led to the discovery that patients had both low C4A and C4B levels. The majority of children with autoimmune hepatitis have the null C4A (C4A*Q0) or C4B (C4B*Q0) phenotype (Vergani, Lancet, 1985; ii: 294). These data were confirmed later by studies of *C4* genotypes which can identify accurately the deleted C4 genes (Sculley, Gastro, 1993; 104:1478; Doherty, Autoimmun, 1994; 18:243). Analysis of the contribution which these complement genes make to susceptibility to autoimmune hepatitis is complicated by three facts: (i) the C4A null phenotype is in linkage disequilibrium with HLA DR3 and is almost always found on the *A1-B8-DRB3*0101-DRB1*0301-DQA1*0501-DQB1*0201* haplotype, (ii) the C4B null phenotype cosegregates with DR4, and (iii) null alleles are the product of non-functional genes, either non-expressed pseudogenes or deleted genes. Therefore, counting only those C4 nulls which arise as a result of gene deletions alone may significantly underrepresent the strength of this association. Studying the distribution of C4 genes in patients with autoimmune hepatitis from Japan, where the A1-B8-DR3 haplotype is not found, may offer a solution to one of these problems.

Non-MHC immunogenes

Studies of non-MHC genes in autoimmune hepatitis have sought susceptibility genes within the immunoglobulin and TCR regions but not with cytokine genes. Whittingham *et al.*[17] first investigated Gm allotypes in autoimmune hepatitis, reporting an increased frequency of the Gm ax allotype (G1m 1, 2) and evidence of interaction between HLA and Gm in determining susceptibility to autoimmune hepatitis. Thus patients who were both positive for HLA B8 and had the Gm ax allotype had a relative risk of autoimmune hepatitis 39 times greater than those who were HLA B8 negative but G1m ax positive. These data were based on a small number of cases, but raise the interesting possibility that the Gm ax allotype contributes to susceptibility to autoimmune hepatitis only in B8-positive individuals. A second study found the same Gm haplotype in HLA-B8/DR3-positive patients, but also found that many first degree relatives studied had the same Gm haplotype and HLA B8-DR3, though none had autoimmune hepatitis, reinforcing the idea of a polygenic susceptibility to autoimmune hepatitis (Krawitt, Hepatol, 1987; 7:1305).

Only one study has investigated the TCR genes in autoimmune hepatitis. Using RFLP analysis a 10-kb *Bgl* II fragment of the TCR constant-β (*C*β) gene was identified which may be particularly important in patients with early-onset disease (Manabe, Gastro, 1994; 106:1321).

Clinical correlates

Correlation between clinical features of a disease and HLA genotype may be of value in patient management. In rheumatoid arthritis it has been suggested that HLA may have 'more to do with disease severity than disease susceptibility' (Ollier, NatureMed, 1996; 2: 279). Genetic differences between early- and late-onset autoimmune hepatitis in adults and between autoimmune hepatitis in children and adults indicates that HLA may be an important determinant of disease severity and may have value in determining the prognosis.

In the series of adult patients with autoimmune hepatitis from King's and the Mayo Clinic, those with B8 or DR3 presented earlier and were more likely to relapse whilst on treatment (Donaldson, Hepatol, 1991; 13:701; Czaja, Hepatol, 1997; 25:317). In addition, in an analysis of 38 children with autoimmune hepatitis, only 2 (5 per cent) had DR4 compared with an expected frequency of 39 per cent in the general population (Gregorio, Hepatol, 1997; 25: 541). In addition, patients with autoimmune hepatitis with DR4 are more likely to have concurrent extrahepatic disease (Marcos, Hepatol, 1994; 19:1371; Czaja, Hepatol, 1997; 25:317).

It remains to be seen whether susceptibility and disease severity in autoimmune hepatitis are determined by the same or different HLA genes. In the study of Doherty *et al.* (Hepatol, 1994; 19:609), although there is a common susceptibility determinant (lysine β71), those with *DRB1*0301* had more severe disease than those with *DRB1*0401*. This may suggest genes in linkage with *DRB1*0401* and *DRB1*0301-DRB3*0101* determine severity and age of onset. Candidates for this role might include *HLA A1*, *Cw*0701*, *B8*, *C4* null alleles (see below), or *DQA1*0501* and *DQB1*0201* or other non-*HLA* genes encoded on these haplotypes.

An alternative possibility is that disease severity is determined by the number of lysine-DRβ71- encoding genes (i.e. a gene dosage effect). An individual may have from zero to a maximum of four (two per chromosome) expressed DRB genes encoding lysine DRβ71 depending on the *DRB1* allelic group (Table 1). When this possibility was investigated, those with one or fewer lysine DRβ71 alleles had a low risk of developing autoimmune hepatitis (one lysine β71, relative risk = 0.8; zero lysine β71, RR = 0.2), whilst those with two copies had a relative risk of 4.72 and those with four copies had a 14-fold risk of autoimmune hepatitis (Strettell, Gastro, 1997; 112:2028).

It should also be noted that in the analysis of amino acid sequences (Table 5), two other amino acid substitutions were significantly associated with susceptibility to autoimmune hepatitis after correction for multiple testing (probability corrected = $p \times 2000$). These were tyrosine (single letter code Y) at DRβ26 and an arginine (single letter code R) at DRβ74, both of which are encoded by the *DRB1*0301* and *DRB3*0101* alleles but not by *DRB1*0401*. Whether these substitutions enhance the susceptibility effect of lysine β71 is not known (Strettell, Gastro, 1997; 112:2028).

Subgroups of autoimmune hepatitis

There is a debate whether autoimmune hepatitis may be separated into different subgroups. The International Autoimmune Hepatitis Group (Johnson, Hepatol, 1993; 18:998) thought at present it is preliminary to distinguish separate subgroups of autoimmune hepatitis. However, there are several ways to distinguish subgroups of autoimmune hepatitis. The most common one is to establish serological subgroups by particular marker autoantibodies (Czaja, AmJGastr, 1995; 90:1206). Autoimmune hepatitis type 1 is characterized by antinuclear antibodies (**ANA**) with or without smooth muscle antibodies (**SMA**), autoimmune hepatitis type 2 is characterized by liver–kidney–microsomal antibodies type 1 (**LKM-1**), and autoimmune hepatitis type 3 is characterized by antibodies to cytosolic antigens (**SLA** and/or **LP**).

A separate way to distinguish subgroups is by immunogenetic background. As indicated above, autoimmune hepatitis type 1 has two peaks of age of manifestation. Patients with HLA DR3 are of younger age at onset, they relapse more frequently under and after immunosuppressive treatment, and the need for liver transplantation is more frequent. In contrast, patients with autoimmune hepatitis and HLA DR4 are of an older age at onset, disease activity is mild, and extrahepatic syndromes are more frequent.

Immunogenetic data on serological subgroups of autoimmune hepatitis based on autoantibody markers are limited and are mainly based on patients with autoimmune hepatitis type 1, that is, positive for ANA, SMA, or both. In their original paper on the characterization of autoimmune hepatitis type 2 (Homberg, Hepatol, 1987; 1:1333), the authors described HLA DR3 as increased with an incidence of 60 per cent. In Italy (Lenzi, JHepatol, 1991; 60 (Suppl 1):59), autoimmune hepatitis type 2 was also described as being associated with HLA DR3: 50 per cent in patients compared with 21 per cent in controls. Furthermore, HLA DQ2 was increased to 67 per cent compared with 41 per cent in controls. A German series (Manns, JHepatol, 1991; 60 (Suppl 1):16) found an increase in HLA DR3 with an incidence of 42 per cent in patients compared with 19 per cent in controls. However, this was not significant; in this small series of 19 German patients, 74 per cent had *C4A*Q0* alleles compared with 34 per cent in controls. These studies have to be extended using larger numbers of patients and with DNA-based

technology. In particular, hepatitis C virus infection has to be ruled out by all means. Patients with autoimmune hepatitis type 2 should not have serological markers of hepatitis C virus infection. Preliminary data on the MHC alleles determined by DNA-based technology in autoimmune hepatitis type 2 (Czaja, Hepatol, 1996; 24:231A) revealed that German patients with autoimmune hepatitis type 2 did not have the same susceptibility alleles as American patients with type 1 disease. However, extended studies are necessary in this area. There are no data on autoimmune hepatitis type 3.

Primary sclerosing cholangitis
Early studies

Early studies of primary sclerosing cholangitis described an increased frequency of HLA B8 and DR3 and not HLA A1, which appears to be associated with the disease through linkage with the B8-DR3 haplotype only.[1,2] Later reports based on 81 patients identified a strong secondary association with DR2 (Donaldson, Hepatol, 1991; 13:129).

Recent studies

There have been three large series of patients with primary sclerosing cholangitis in whom HLA PCR genotyping has been performed. These are from King's College Hospital, London (Farrant, Hepatol, 1992; 16:390; Underhill, Hepatol, 1995; 21:959), Oxford (Mehal, Gastro, 1994; 106:160), and Sweden (Olerup, Gastro, 1995; 108:870) and the findings of these three series are summarized in Table 7. The Oxford study sought only to confirm the associations described by the King's group and was not a full genotyping study. The two remaining studies both found a strong significant association with the *A1-B8-DRB3*0101-DRB1*0301-DQA1*0501-DQB1*0201* haplotype and an association with the *DRB1*1301-DRB3*0101-DQA1*0103-DQB1*0603* haplotype. The King's group and Oxford study also described a negative association with the *DRB1*04* alleles. As with autoimmune hepatitis, there were no significant associations with either DQA, DQB, or DPB other than those expected to occur as a result of linkage disequilibrium, indicating that DRB is the primary susceptibility locus in primary sclerosing cholangitis.

There is considerable controversy over the interpretation of the data from these three series. The King's group proposed that DRB3*0101 may be the primary susceptibility allele in primary sclerosing cholangitis as this allele is found on both susceptibility haplotypes. Further analysis revealed a possible link between susceptibility and HLA alleles which encode a leucine residue at position 38 of the DRβ polypeptide. The Oxford study agreed that *DRB3*0101* is the primary susceptibility allele in primary sclerosing cholangitis but not with the leucine-β38 hypothesis, and these ideas were not supported by the Swedish group who argued that the association with *DRB3*0101* is simply the result of linkage disequilibrium.

There is very little difference between these three studies and it is not possible to judge them on the basis of the raw data or statistics of each individual study. Analysis of the pooled data from these three studies appears to confirm the hypotheses generated from the King's study (Table 7). Thus there is a clear association with both *DRB1*0301* and *DRB3*0101* though the association appears to be

Table 7 HLA association with primary sclerosing cholangitis (recent PCR-based published studies only)

Series	Allele	Patients N	Patients %	Controls N	Controls %	p corrected
King's[a]	DR4	12	17	26	38	0.024
	DRB1*0301	31	44	16	24	0.06
	DRB1*1301	17	24	7	10	0.17
	DRB3*0101	39	55	15	22	0.00036
	Leu β38	56	79	32	47	0.0005
	Total No.	71		68		
Oxford[b]	DR4	17	20	27	42	0.022
	DRB1*0301	33	40	14	22	0.11
	DRB1*1301	—	—	—	—	—
	DRB3*0101	41	49	18	28	0.046
	Leu β38	65	78	32	50	0.0017
	Total No.	83		64		
Sweden[c]	DR4	11	15	92	37	0.0015
	DRB1*0301	25	33	43	17	0.013
	DRB1*1301	33	44	45	18	0.000019
	DRB3*0101	40	53	70	28	0.00024
	Leu β38	56	75	132	53	0.0039
	Total No.	75		250		
Pool	DR4	40	17	145	40	$<10^{-7}$
	DRB1*0301	89	38	73	19	$<10^{-7}$
	DRB1*1301	50[d]	22	52[d]	14	0.000001[d]
	DRB3*0101	120	52	103	27	$<10^{-8}$
	Leu β38	177	77	196	51	$<10^{-8}$
	Total No.	229		382		

Note that the statistical values in this table have all been recalculated. Probability is represented as pc with a correction factor of 5 based on the a priori hypothesis that DR4, DRB1*0301, DRB1*1301, DRB3*0101, and leucine at position 38 of the DRβ-polypeptide are associated with susceptibility or resistance to primary sclerosing cholangitis. [a] Farrant, Hepatol, 1992; 16:390; [b] Mehal, Gastro, 1994; 106:160; [c] Olerup, Gastro, 1995; 108:870; [d] Figures only available for Swedish and King's studies.

strongest with *DRB3*0101*. However, since data on *DRB1*1301* are only available for two out of the three studies, it is not possible to evaluate fully this question by considering *DRB1*1301* in comparison with *DRB3*0101*. In the pooled data analysis there is also a very significant association between alleles encoding leucine at DRβ38 and primary sclerosing cholangitis.

A second controversy exists regarding DR4. All groups observed a significant reduction in the frequency of DR4, but only the King's group interpreted this negative association as evidence of a protective effect of this allele. The Swedish group proposed that the lower frequency of DR4 may simply be a counterbalance for the two strong positive associations described (i.e. with *DRB1*0301* and *DRB1*1301*). The low frequency of DR4 observed by the Oxford group was explained by an apparent close relationship between DR4 and prognosis. When the basic data from all three series represented in Table 7 are considered (after adjustment of the probability values using a correction factor of 5), the frequency of DR4 was significantly lower in patients with primary sclerosing cholangitis in all three series, and by comparison *DRB1*0301* would not have been significant in the Oxford study had correction been applied and would have been borderline in the other series. Furthermore, the pooled data indicate a very strong negative association with *DR4*, which has been confirmed in a more recent

analysis of the King's series (Moloney, unpublished observations, 1996).

Non-MHC immunogenes

At present there are no studies of complement, Ig, or TCR genes in primary sclerosing cholangitis, though the King's group have recently investigated the *IL-1* gene family in this disease. The IL-1 genes are of particular interest in relation to primary sclerosing cholangitis because two-thirds of patients with this disease also have ulcerative colitis, and a link between *IL-1B* and *IL1-ra* and susceptibility to ulcerative colitis has been proposed (Mansfield, Gastro, 1994; 106:637; Bioque, ClinExpImmunol, 1995; 102:379). Preliminary analysis of more than 100 patients with primary sclerosing cholangitis indicates that neither *IL-1B* nor *IL1-ra* are associated with the disease and there is no difference in the distribution of the *IL-1B* and *IL1-ra* alleles comparing patients who have primary sclerosing cholangitis with and without ulcerative colitis (Donaldson P, unpublished observations, March 1997).

Clinical correlates

The correlation between HLA alleles and clinical outcome in primary sclerosing cholangitis reflects the controversy described in the previous paragraphs. Recent analysis reveals that neither DR4, *DRB1*0401*, *DRB1*0301*, nor *DRB3*0101* are associated with a poor prognosis in primary sclerosing cholangitis and there is no correlation between age of onset and HLA DR2 or DR3 (Olerup, Gastro, 1995; 108:870; Moloney M, unpublished observations, 1997), contrary to earlier reports.[1-3]

Primary biliary cirrhosis

In numerous studies describing HLA associations in primary biliary cirrhosis there are no reports of any significant association between this disease and the HLA class I A or B antigens; however, several investigations have described associations with HLA DR.[1-3] Of these only the association with DR8, originally described by Gores *et al.* (Hepatol, 1987; 7:889), has withstood the test of time.[1-3] Even this is disappointing since DR8 is relatively rare in northern Europeans and the frequency of patients with DR8 with primary biliary cirrhosis ranges from 11 to 36 per cent (Manns, Gastro, 1991; 101:1367; Underhill, Hepatol, 1992; 16:1404). Consequently, though several PCR genotyping studies have been performed in Europe and the United States, the common denominator is a weak association with DR8. Other associations such as the protective effect of the *DQA1*0102* allele (Begovitch, TissAnt, 1994; 43:71) and the susceptibility effect of *DPB1*0301* (Mella, Hepatol, 1995; 21:398) have not been confirmed in larger series (Underhill, Hepatol, 1995; 21:959; Underhill, unpublished data). These studies are summarized in Table 8.

The greatest interest in the immunogenetics of primary biliary cirrhosis has been in Japan, which has a more homogeneous population, and where up to 80 per cent of patients with this disease may have DR8 (Maeda, Gastro, 1992; 103:1118; Seki, Hepatol, 1993; 18:73). Recently, the association has been attributed to one particular DR8 allele, *DRB1*0803* (Oguri, IntHepatolComm, 1994; 2:263; Mukai, IntHepatolComm, 1995; 3:207). However, there is controversy over the precise HLA class II locus responsible for this association. Though studies so far have failed to find stronger

Table 8 Summary of European, North American and Japanese studies of HLA class II and class III in primary biliary cirrhosis

Author[a]	Year	Associated alleles/ haplotype	Susceptibility resistance	Method
Briggs	1987	C4B 2	S	Phenotyping
Gores	1987	DR8	S	Serology
		DR11	R	Serology
Manns	1991	DR8	S	Serology
		C4B*Q0/C4B*2	S	Phenotyping
Underhill	1992	DR8—DQB1*0402	S	RFLP/PCR-SSOP
Gregory	1993	DR8	S	RFLP/PCR-SSP
Begovitch	1994	*DRB1*0801*	S	PCR-SSOP
		*DQA1*0401/0601*		
		*DQB1*0402*		
		*DRB1*1501*	R	PCR-SSOP
		*DQA1*0102*		
		*DQB1*0602*		
		*DRB1*1302*	R	PCR-SSP
		*DQA1*0102*		
		*DQB1*0604*		
Mella	1995	*DPB1*0301*	S	PCR-SSOP
Maeda	1992	*DRB1*08*	S	Serology
Seki	1993	*DRB1*08*	S	PCR-SSO
		*DQB1*03*		Serology
		*DPB1*0501*		PCR–RFLP
Oguri	1994	*DRB1*0803*	S	PCR-SSO
Mukai	1995	*DRB1*0803*	S	PCR-SSO

[a] All references are given in the text.

associations at the DQ locus, one study suggested that the primary susceptibility allele may be *DPB1*0501*, which was found in 85 per cent of 47 patients studied (Seki, Hepatol, 1993; 18:73). Following an analysis of the distribution of amino acid residues for the *DPB1* locus, a model for disease susceptibility based on leucine residues at position 35 of the DPβ-polypeptide has been proposed by Seki *et al.* Leucine DPβ35 is shared by both *DPB1*0501* and *DPB1*0202*. However, this theory has not been confirmed and an alternative model with leucine at DRβ74 has been proposed by a rival group (Oguri, IntHepatolComm, 1994; 2:263). The second model is based on the observation that the DR locus is the primary susceptibility locus and the primary association is with *DRB1*0803*.

Polymorphism of the *HLA* class II subregion genes *TAP1* and *TAP2* has been studied in primary biliary cirrhosis in Europe (Gregory, QJMed, 1994; 87:23) and Japan (Maeda, Hepatol, 1994; 19:95I). Though the products of these genes, which are located in the class II region close to *HLA DR*, are required for processing and presentation of endogenous peptides, no association has been found in either European or Japanese patients with primary biliary cirrhosis.

HLA class III

The lack of a strong link with HLA in early studies of primary biliary cirrhosis shifted the search for immunogenetic associations towards the HLA class III region. Early studies identified a significant association with the *C4B*2* allele (Briggs, TissAnt, 1987; 29:141) and the C4A null (*C4A*Q0*) allele, with a relative risk of 183 for those with the combination DR8 and *C4A*Q0* (Manns, Gastro, 1991; 101:1367). A later study attempted to pinpoint the exact location of the susceptibility gene to the class III region using

a polymorphic class III gene *G91*, located midway between HLA DR and complement, but although they found an excess of a particular *G91A* fragment, this was simply due to linkage with DR8 and *C4B*2* (Mehal, Hepatol, 1994; 20:1213). An association has also been reported with the *TNF-α NcoI* fragment in primary biliary cirrhosis in Denmark (Fugger, ScaJImmunol, 1989; 30:185), but this was not confirmed by a similar study in Germany (Messer, ScaJImmunol, 1991; 34:735).

Non-MHC immunogenes

To date very few studies of primary biliary cirrhosis have looked outside the MHC for a genetic explanation for this disease. Studies of *TCRVβ* gene usage revealed an excess of *Vβ7* and *Vβ13.1* gene usage by T cells derived from the liver of patients with primary biliary cirrhosis, but similar trends were also seen in the control group (Mayo, Hepatol, 1996; 24:1148). In addition, early studies indicated a possible link between IL-1 gene polymorphism and primary biliary cirrhosis, but the data have not yet been published or confirmed.

Viral liver disease

There is currently a growing interest in the subject of HLA associations in relation to infectious diseases. This renewed interest is partly due to recent publications regarding resistance to malaria (Hill, Nature, 1991; 352:595) and an interest in whether HLA may determine the prognosis for AIDS patients (McNeil, QJMed, 1996; 89:177; Malkovsky, Nature, 1996; 348:142). The second reason for a renewed enthusiasm for studying HLA and infections relates to new technologies in the form of molecular genotyping and to a declining return from studies in autoimmune disease.

Hepatitis B virus infection

Early studies of HLA patients with hepatitis B virus (**HBV**) clearly showed that there was no association with either **HLA A** or B,[18] and more recent studies have failed to demonstrate an association with DR phenotypes (Verdon, JHepatol, 1994; 21:388; Zavaglia, JHepatol, 1996; 24:658). Two studies have re-examined this question with particular reference to the DR locus using genotyping techniques. The first used RFLP genotyping and described a reduced frequency of DR2 and increased frequency of DR7 in 34 patients with chronic persistent HBV infection from Qatar (Almarri and Batchelor, Lancet, 1994; 344:1194). The second described the protective effect of the DR6 allele *DRB1*1302* in 185 children with chronic persistent HBV infection from the Gambia (Thursz, NEJM, 1995; 332:1065). These associations may have practical consequences since DR7 has previously been linked with hypo-responsiveness to the HBV vaccine Hepatavax-B (Craven, AnnIntMed, 1986; 105:356; Weisman, JAMA, 1988; 260:1734) and DR6 with viral clearance (van Hattum, Hepatol, 1987; 7:11) and a favourable response to interferon therapy (Scully, Hepatol, 1990; 12:1111). However, both of the recent studies are limited to the DR locus and there is much work to be done before patients are selected for interferon therapy on the basis of their DR genotype.

The close association between HBV and hepatocellular carcinoma has also led to the search for host genes which may modulate the effect of virus infection and increase the risk of hepatocellular carcinoma developing. Early reports of HLA and hepatocellular carcinoma, mostly restricted to HLA A and B, found no such association.[18] A recent survey from the King's group in collaboration with the Chinese University of Hong Kong reported an extensive survey of HLA class II DRB, DQA, DQB, and DPB alleles in Hong Kong Chinese with hepatocellular carcinoma with and without HBV infection and though a number of associations were found in the preliminary analysis, none of the alleles tested were significant after correction for multiple testing (Underhill J, unpublished observations, March 1997). Because there is a risk that the statistical convention of correction may cause rejection of true genetic associations, the study should be considered as a preliminary analysis and a second study performed on a new cohort of patients. A similar strategy was applied in the Gambia study of HBV mentioned above (Thursz, NEJM, 1995; 332:1065).

Hepatitis C virus infection

The development of accurate diagnostic tests for detection of hepatitis C virus (**HCV**) is a relatively recent phenomenon and therefore there has been little chance to study the immunogenetics of this disease. Despite this there have been a surprising number of HLA studies, most of them negative, reflecting the world-wide incidence of HCV infection and the high incidence of persistent viraemia (up to 80 per cent). Many of the investigations of HLA and HCV have failed to find an association with HCV infection (Verdon, JHepatol, 1995; 45:356), others found a weak association with immunological complications and autoimmune features (Czaja, JHepatol, 1996; 24:666). Two Italian studies have identified an association with DR5 (Peano, ArchIntMed; 1994; 154:2733; Zavaglia, JHepatol, 1996; 24:658); though neither study performed *DQB1* PCR genotyping, both noted an increased frequency of the DQ3 phenotype in symptom-free patients with evidence of HCV infection. In contrast, a study in Sardinia reported that *DRB1*1601-DQB1*0502* is associated with a lower incidence of chronic HCV infection in at-risk patients with thalassaemia (Congia, Hepatol, 1996; 24:1338). This haplotype is rare outside of Sardinia. Studies in Japan have identified three associations: *DRB1*0405-DQB1*0401* appears to be associated with cirrhosis in HCV infection, while *DRB1*0901-DQB1*0303* confers resistance (Aikawa, JMedVirol, 1996; 49:274), and in a second study DR13 was associated with persistent viraemia and normal levels of alanine aminotransferase (Kuzushita, JMedVirol, 1996; 48:1).

Though these different HLA associations with HCV are confusing, a clear trend is beginning to emerge, at least in Europe. A recent survey of 104 patients with chronic HCV in Britain found that the *DRB1*04-DQA1*03-DQB1*0302* haplotype protects from chronic HCV infection; no other significant associations were described and the association appeared to be with the DQ alleles rather than DR (Tibbs, Hepatol, 1996; 24:1342). This explains why many of the studies based on HLA A, B, and DR alone have failed to demonstrate any association.

The story of HLA and HCV does not end there. In a follow-up to the first study, a fresh cohort of 104 patients were genotyped for HLA class II, including 55 with chronic infection and 49 without (Cramp, JHepatol, 1997; 26:81, abstract 103). In the second series, the overall protective effect of *DRB1*04-DQA1*0302* was confirmed and a second association between *DQB1*0301* and viral clearance noted. This association echoes the reports from Italy of a reduced incidence of DQ3 in those who exhibit symptom-free disease. These data indicate two effects in the patients: (i) overall resistance to HCV infection determined by the *DQB1*0302* allele, which is always found with *DRB1*04* in Britain, and (ii) an association of the *DQB1*0301* allele with viral clearance, which is linked with *DRB1*04* alleles but also *DRB1*13* alleles and is always found with the DR5 alleles. It is also generally agreed that there is no HLA class I association with HCV or chronic HCV infection.

Other liver diseases

Many different liver diseases have been the subject of immunogenetic investigations. Indeed wherever an immune, particularly autoimmune, pathogenesis has been suspected, HLA typing may have been performed. Most of these studies have been disappointing, but a few, including some of those described in this section, have given surprising results.

Alcoholic liver disease

The variable outcome for patients with liver disease following chronic alcohol consumption led investigators to consider the possibility that cirrhosis, fatty liver, and acute hepatitis may be determined to some degree by genetic factors. Though many HLA association studies were performed in the late 1970s and 1980s, the results were confusing and for the most part disappointing. However, it should be noted that the majority of these studies predate the introduction of molecular genotyping for HLA.

Cystic fibrosis

Approximately 4 per cent of children and up to 25 per cent of adults with cystic fibrosis develop features of chronic liver disease including hepatomegaly, portal hypertension, and cirrhosis. Liver disease may be severe at the time of diagnosis, and prognosis may be poor. Liver disease is not associated with any of the major cystic fibrosis gene mutations *ΔF508*, *G551D*, or *R553X* (Duthie, Hepatol, 1992; 15:660). Familial clustering of liver disease in cystic fibrosis and inappropriate immune responses to liver antigens indicate that immunogenetic factors may contribute to the development of liver disease. The King's group performed HLA A, B, DR, and DQB typing in a series of 247 children and adults with cystic fibrosis, 82 of whom had chronic liver disease. DQ6 was found in 66 per cent of those with liver disease compared with 33 per cent without. The study concluded that B7-DR15-DQ6 is associated with an increased risk of liver disease in patients with cystic fibrosis, particularly male patients and young adults (Duthie, JHepatol, 1995; 23:532).

α₁-Antitrypsin deficiency

As in cystic fibrosis, in α₁-antitrypsin deficiency a minority of patients (i.e. up to 20 per cent) may develop chronic liver disease. Familial occurrence of liver disease and immune responses to liver autoantigens suggested that genetically controlled autoimmune phenomena may lead to liver disease in α₁-antitrypsin deficiency. HLA A, B, DR, and DQ typing of 140 PiZZ individuals, of whom 92 had evidence of liver disease, and of a further 206 first-degree relatives identified a positive correlation between the presence of DR3, and in particular the DR3-Dw25 genotype (equivalent to the *DRB1*0301-DRB3*0201/0202* haplotype) and liver disease (Doherty, Hepatol, 1990; 12:218).

Biliary atresia

The aetiology of biliary atresia is unknown though there appear to be two forms of the disease. These have been called the embryonic/fetal form, which is associated with diverse congenital abnormalities, and the acquired form, where the congenital abnormalities are conspicuously absent. An immune pathogenesis for this condition has been suggested, but studies of HLA phenotypes have reported only weak associations with B12 and are not convincing (Silveira, JPediatGastrNut, 1993; 16:114). Since this disease probably develops during gestation and could involve a viral agent, maternal immunogenetics may be more important than those of the affected child. Recent studies suggest that maternal DRB genes may confer resistance to the development of schizophrenia in offspring (Wright, AmJPsychiat, 1996; 153:1530).

Interpretation of HLA associations in liver diseases

The strong HLA associations reviewed above (summarized in Table 9) suggest that these genes are not simply markers, by virtue of linkage disequilibrium, for an undiscovered disease gene or for a distant true susceptibility gene. Most of these diseases will have a multifactorial pathogenesis, perhaps involving multiple genes and environmental factors. The alternatives to the linked gene theory are that either the products of these susceptibility genes act directly in the development of the disease process, or these genes are markers of disease severity or both. These possibilities will be discussed below.

Mechanisms of HLA-encoded disease susceptibility

All autoimmune diseases involve failure to maintain tolerance to self. Complete self tolerance depends on the total absence of self-reactive T cells, and may be achieved either through deletion of self-reactive T cells during thymic development (clonal deletion) or through the active suppression of T cells recognizing self-antigens (peripheral tolerance). HLA gene polymorphisms which encode different amino acid residues and peptide motifs in the antigen-binding groove will dramatically affect the conformation and orientation with which the peptide is bound and presented to the TCR.

One hypothesis to explain HLA associations with autoimmune disease is that failure to induce tolerance is more likely to occur if there is weak binding of the self peptide to class II molecules (Nepom, Diabetes, 1990; 36:1153; Sheehy, Diabetes, 1992; 41:123). During thymic selection, weak binding of self peptides may result in failure to delete T-cell clones with TCRs that recognize autoantigens. Thus HLA class II molecules associated with an increased risk of a given disease may be simply those which bind an autoantigenic peptide with low affinity, while those class II molecules which are associated with a reduced risk of disease may bind the autoantigenic peptide with high affinity. This model can also apply to peripheral tolerance and accounts for those class II molecules which appear to confer resistance to autoimmune disease, since high-affinity binding will result in deletion or suppression of self-reactive T cells. It is possible that this is the basis of genetic susceptibility to autoimmune liver disease. Thus an HLA DR molecule bearing a lysine residue at position 71 or leucine at position 38 of the DRβ-polypeptide, or leucine at position 35 of the DPβ-polypeptide, may have low binding affinity for self peptides, rendering an individual susceptible to autoimmune hepatitis, primary sclerosing cholangitis, or primary biliary cirrhosis either through failure of clonal deletion or via failure of peripheral tolerance.

A similar hypothesis may account for HLA associations with infectious diseases, thus low-affinity binding of viral peptides may result in poor viral clearance and facilitate chronic infection, whilst high-affinity binding may lead to efficient viral clearance and protect the host from chronic infection. This may account for the protective effect of the *DRB1*1302* allele in HBV infection in the Gambia (Thursz, NEJM, 1995; 332:1065), the effect of the *DQB1*0301* in clearance of hepatitis C virus, and *DQB1*0302* in the general resistance to HCV infection (Tibbs, Hepatol, 1996; 24:1345. Cramp, JHepatol, 1997; 26:81, abstract 103).

An alternative to the forbidden clone theory for generation of autoimmune disease is the molecular mimicry hypothesis. The asialoglycoprotein receptor, a putative autoantigen in autoimmune hepatitis, and PDC-E2 peptide, a putative autoantigen in primary biliary cirrhosis, both share sequence homology with the DRα-polypeptide, which may act as a molecular mimic in these two diseases (Baum, ImmunolToday, 1996; 17:64). Mimicry does not necessarily involve the susceptibility alleles and the two theories are not exclusive, though caution should be the watchword when screening databases for sequence homology in search of potential mimics (Roudier, ImmunolToday, 1996; 1:357).

Table 9 Key HLA associations with autoimmune and chronic viral liver disease

Disease	Key haplotype or allele							Population[a]	Effect
	HLA.A	.... B	DRB3/4/5....	DRB1	DQA1	DQB1	DPB1		
AIH	A*01....	-B*08...	**DRB3*0101-**	**DRB1*0301**	-DQA1*0501	-DQB1*0201[b]		Caucasoid	S
	....	....	DRB4*0103-	**DRB1*0401**	....	....		Caucasoid	S
	....	....	DRB4*	**DRB1*0405**				Japanese	S
	....	B*07...	**-DRB5*0101**	**-DRB1*1501**	-DQA1*0102	-DQB1*0602		Caucasoid	R
PSC	A*01....	-B*08		**-DRB1*0301**	-DQA1*0501	-DQB1*0201[c]		Caucasoid	S
			DRB3*0101						
	....	....	**DRB3*0101**	-DRB1*1301	DQA1*0102	-DQB1*0603		Caucasoid	S
	....	....	DRB4*0103	**-DRB1*0401**	....	....		Caucasoid	R
PBC	....	....		**DRB1*0801**	-DQA1*0401	-DQB1*0402.	DPB1*0301	Caucasoid	S
	....	....		**DRB1*0803**	-DQA1*.	-DQB1*03........	**-DPB1*0501**[b]	Japanese	S
	....	....	DRB5*0101-	DRB1*1501-	**DQA1*0102**	DQB1*0602[c]		Caucasoid	R
	....	....	DRB3*........	-DRB1*1302-	**DQA1*0102**	DQB1*0604[c]		Caucasoid	R
HBV	....	....		**DRB1*1302**[c]	....	....		Gambia	R
HCV	....	....	DRB4*........	-DRB1*04.......	**-DQA1*03 ....**	[b]**DQB1*0302**		UK only	R
	....	....	DRB4*........	-DRB1*04.......	-DQA1*03.......	**-DQB1*0301**		Caucasoid	R[d]

Where there are incomplete genotypes the alleles at these loci have not been tested or are not associated with the disease (see text). The alleles in bold and underlined are those thought to be the key elements in each haplotype. [a] Caucasoid refers to populations from Europe and North Americans of European origin. [b] The key element in these haplotypes is currently controversial (see text). [c] This association is yet to be confirmed in independent series and is controversial. [d] The association between HCV and HLA DQB1*0301 is with viral clearance. AIH, autoimmune hepatitis; HBV, hepatitis B virus; HCV, hepatitis C virus; PBC, primary biliary sclerosis; PSC, primary sclerosing cholantitis.

HLA and disease severity

In a recent review of the immunogenetics of rheumatoid arthritis it was suggested that HLA may have 'more to do with disease severity than disease susceptibility' (Ollier, NatureMed, 1996; 2:279). The hypothesis that HLA associations are simply markers of more rapid disease progression and severity of symptoms is supported by the finding of an association of DR4 with late-onset autoimmune hepatitis and the observation that the patients with A1-B8-DR3 present earlier in life and relapse more frequently whilst receiving conventional therapies (Donaldson, Hepatol, 1991; 13:701; Czaja, Hepatol, 1997; 25:317). This is reinforced by the clear differences in the genetic background to autoimmune hepatitis in adults and children.

Susceptibility and severity are not exclusive, they may go together; for example, susceptibility to autoimmune hepatitis may be determined by the shared motif LLEQKR or the lysine residue at position 71 of the DRβ-polypeptide. This is a common (shared) feature of the HLA DRB alleles associated with both late-onset and early-onset disease. Severity of disease may be determined by the number of LLEQKR motifs or lysine β71 residues. By definition this will always be greater in those with the *DRB1*0301-DRB3*0101* haplotype, because both expressed DRB alleles encode the LLEQKR motif, whereas those with *DRB1*0401* have only one copy of LLEQKR per haplotype. In a similar way, other sites on same molecule may moderate the effect of the shared epitope; for example, tyrosine at DRβ26 and arginine at DRβ74, which are encoded by the *DRB1*0301* and *DRB3*0101* alleles but not by *DRB1*0401*, could enhance the effect of the lysine at DRβ71 resulting in a more rapid disease progression in patients with autoimmune hepatitis with the *DRB1*0301-DRB3*0101* haplotype compared with those with *DRB1*0401*.

The more or less universal association between the extended *HLA A1-B8-DRB1*0301* haplotype and autoimmune disease may be an indication that this haplotype encodes more than one susceptibility gene, and/or 'severity' gene. Candidates for this role could include any of the hundreds of genes located between the *DPB1* locus and *HLA A1* including many of those which we know, such as *A1*, *B8*, *Cw7*, and *C4A*Q0*. It is also possible that the gene products form novel α/β-heterodimers. The *trans*-pairing of DQα- and DQβ-chains encoded on different haplotypes has been identified as a susceptibility factor for insulin-dependent diabetes mellitus (Nepom, Diabetes, 1987; 36:114; Ronningen, Diabetes, 1991; 40:759). In addition, for each of these genes, polymorphism of the upstream promoters and regulatory transcription factors should also be considered.

Directions for future studies

In northern European patients with autoimmune hepatitis and primary sclerosing cholangitis, the DRB locus appears to encode the primary susceptibility alleles. However, not all patients are accounted for by the models reviewed above and the predominance of the extended *A1-B8-DR3* haplotype as a susceptibility marker in these and most other autoimmune diseases may indicate more than one susceptibility gene on this haplotype. Indeed, it is likely that there may be several genes, both within and outside the MHC region, that encode susceptibility to these diseases. Recent studies of insulin-dependent diabetes mellitus suggest that there may be as many as 18 susceptibility alleles (Todd, Diabetes, 1992; 41:1029). One or more of these genes may contribute to provide a permissive environment for the generation of the disease. Similarly, in autoimmune liver disease several genes may act, either individually or in concert, as a permissive gene pool for the generation of liver damage. A number of other MHC and non-MHC genes should be investigated as candidate susceptibility loci, in particular including the HLA class III genes, non-MHC genes involved in peptide recognition such as the T-cell receptor and the immunoglobulin genes, and also the genes which encode various cytokines.

Finally, let us for a moment consider the biological and evolutionary significance of HLA polymorphism. The high prevalence and conserved nature of some HLA haplotypes, especially *A1–B8–DR3*, suggests that these genes confer some selective advantage upon a population. It has been suggested that susceptibility to autoimmune disease may be the penalty acquired by a population for increased resistance to infectious diseases (Benacerraf, Science, 1981; 212:1229; de Vries, ClinInvestMed, 1992; 22:1). In this context it is interesting that one of the HLA haplotypes associated with HCV clearance is associated with susceptibility to autoimmune hepatitis.

References

1. Donaldson PT, Doherty DG, Underhill JA, and Williams R. Molecular genetics of autoimmune liver disease. *Hepatology*, 1994; **20**: 225–39.
2. Donaldson PT. Immunogenetics in liver disease. In Manns MP, ed. *Gastroenterology and liver immunology. Baillière's Clinical Gastroenterology*. London: Baillière Tindall, 1996: 533–49.
3. Manns MP and Kruger M. Immunogenetics of chronic liver disease. *Gastroenterology*, 1994; **106**: 1676–97.
4. Campbell RD and Trowsdale J. A map of the human major histocompatibility complex. *Immunology Today*, 1997; **18**: 43.
5. Bodmer JG *et al*. Nomenclature for factors of the HLA system, 1996. *Tissue Antigens*, 1997; **49**: 297–321.
6. Bjorkman PJ, Saper MA, Samraoui B, Bennett WS, Strominger JL, and Wiley DC. Structure of human class I histocompatibility antigen, HLA-A2. *Nature*, 1987; **329**: 506–12.
7. Bjorkman PJ, Saper MA, Samraoui B, Bennettt WS, Strominger JL, and Wiley DC. The foreign antigen binding site and T cell recognition regions of class I histocompatibility antigens. *Nature*, 1987; **329**: 512–18.
8. Doherty PC and Zinkernagel RM. A biological role for the major histocompatibility antigens. *Lancet*, 1975; **i**: 1406–9.
9. Brown JH *et al*. Three-dimensional structure of the human class II histocompatibility antigen HLA-DR1. *Nature*, 1993; **364**: 33–9.
10. Rammensee HG. Chemistry of peptides associated with MHC class I and class II molecules. *Current Opinion in Immunology*, 1995; **7**: 85–96.
11. Williams DB and Watts TH. Molecular chaperones in antigen presentation. *Current Opinion in Immunology*, 1995; **7**: 77–84.
12. Wilson AG, di Giovine FS, and Duff GW. Genetics of tumour necrosis factor-α in autoimmune, infectious and neoplastic diseases. *Journal of Inflammation*, 1995; **45**: 1–12.
13. Hill AVS. Genetics of infectious disease resistance. *Current Opinion in Genetics and Development*, 1996; **6**: 348–53.
14. Davis MM and Bjorkman PJ. T cell antigen receptor genes and T cell recognition. *Nature*, 1988; **334**: 395–402.
15. Propert ND. Detection of immunoglobulin polymorphisms. In Simons MJ and Tait BD eds. *Detection of immune associated genetic markers of human disease*. London: Churchill-Livingstone, 1984: 65–81.
16. Svejgaard A and Ryder LP. HLA and disease associations: detecting the strongest association. *Tissue Antigens*, 1994; **43**: 18–27.
17. Whittingham S, Mathews JD, Schanfield MS, Tait BD, and Mackay IR. Interaction of HLA and Gm in autoimmune chronic active hepatitis. *Clinical and Experimental Immunology*, 1981; **43**: 80–6.
18. Tiwari JL and Terasaki PI. *HLA and disease associations*. New York: Springer-Verlag, 1985.

2.8 Regulation of liver cell mass

2.8.1 Hepatic regeneration

Nelson Fausto

The liver has the unique capacity to regulate its growth and size. This biological property is particularly remarkable because hepatocytes, which constitute 90 to 95 per cent of the liver mass, are normally quiescent cells with low turnover and long lifespans. The liver mass of humans and laboratory animals has a relatively constant relationship to the body mass of the individual. The optimal ratio between liver functional mass and body mass is the set point for the adjustments in liver size that occur in adult individuals. Deviations from the optimal ratio are quickly corrected. Decreases in liver functional mass created by partial hepatectomy, 'small for size' transplants (Kawasaki, Lancet, 1992; 339:580; Francavilla, Hepatol, 1994; 19:210), or deficits created by hepatocyte death or injury are rapidly corrected by hepatic growth that involves hepatocyte replication (Yamanaka, Hepatol, 1993; 18:79). Similarly, excess hepatic functional capacity such as that encountered in 'large for size' transplants (Kam, Hepatol, 1987; 7:362), drug-induced hyperplasia, and in occasional cases of heterotopic hepatic transplantation (Willemse, Hepatol, 1992; 15:54), does not persist when the cause for the liver enlargement is eliminated (Bursch, ArchToxicol, 1986; 59:221). Excess capacity is corrected by a decrease in functional mass, believed to be effected by hepatocyte apoptosis, a process which persists until the optimal liver functional mass/body mass set point is reached (Bursch, Carcinogenesis, 1984; 5:453). In this chapter we will discuss the mechanisms of liver growth and focus on new information on the molecular mechanisms of liver regeneration. Most of the knowledge about this process has been obtained by detailed studies of hepatic regeneration after partial hepatectomy in rats and mice. This experimental system permits the study of the events that make quiescent hepatocytes replicate and then return to their normal non-proliferative state when the liver mass is restored. Although the molecular aspects of liver growth responses in humans have not been examined in detail, there is every reason to believe that the animal studies are entirely applicable for the understanding of the mechanisms that regulate the growth of human livers and provide relevant information for the management of liver disease.

Liver regeneration after partial hepatectomy has been studied for about one century (Turnbull, ArchPathInstLondonHosp, 1908; 2:35). In the past few years, reports about the expression of specific genes, growth factors, the activity of various enzymes, and many other biochemical, molecular, and morphological changes occurring during regeneration have reached overwhelming numbers. Hepatic regeneration is a classic 'black box' problem in which one knows both the cause of the process (partial hepatectomy) and its endpoints (DNA synthesis, restoration of liver mass). The major events of liver regeneration are well known and have been described in many comprehensive reviews.[1–21] The process is well synchronized and involves the replication of more than 95 per cent of hepatocytes in young rats and mice. After partial hepatectomy, hepatocytes enter a 'prereplicative phase' that lasts 12 to 14 h in rats and 24 to 30 h in mice. During this phase the level of hepatocyte DNA replication is not different from that of intact or sham-operated animals, but a major wave of DNA synthesis occurs with maximal levels 24 h and 40 h after partial hepatectomy in rats in mice, respectively, followed by mitosis (Grisham, CancerRes, 1962; 22:842). In young animals a second distinct peak of DNA replication can be detected (Bucher, IntRevCytol, 1963, 15:245). The liver mass returns to normal by 10 to 14 days without regrowth of the lobes removed at the operation. Instead, the lobes remaining after surgery greatly expand in size as a consequence of compensatory hyperplasia. After partial hepatectomy, there is a decrease in the amount of cell adhesion molecules and gap junction proteins (Traub, PNAS, 1983; 80:755; Odin, ExpCellRes, 1986; 164:63). Hepatocytes lose their interconnections (Meyer, JCellBiol, 1981; 91:505) and, on average, attach to only one other hepatocyte (in normal livers attachments are formed between 5 to 6 hepatocytes). Because the first wave of cell replication occurs before reformation of sinusoids, new cells are not immediately incorporated into an acinar structure. Reformation of normal acini occurs many hours later with the appearance of new sinusoids and laminin synthesis (Martinez-Hernandez, LabInvest, 1991; 64:157).

Recent studies of liver regeneration have been centred on identifying the linkages that may exist between partial hepatectomy and hepatocyte replication. A considerable amount of effort has been focused on proto-oncogenes, growth factors, and transcription factors as agents that may connect the early events after partial hepatectomy to DNA synthesis. From a basic biological perspective, liver regeneration represents the passage of cells from a quiescent state referred to as the G_0 phase into the cell cycle (Fig. 1). Cells entering the cell cycle (G_1 phase), progress through the cycle to undergo DNA synthesis (S phase) and mitosis (M phase). Between DNA synthesis and mitosis there is a gap period referred to as the G_2 phase. After partial hepatectomy hepatocytes replicate once or twice and then return to the G_0 (quiescent) state. It has been debated for many years whether the replicative capacity of hepatocytes in adult livers is limited only to very few rounds of replication. However, recent work demonstrates unequivocally that hepatocytes of adult animals have great replicative potential. Rhim and colleagues (Rhim, Science, 1994; 263:1149; Rhim, PNAS, 1995; 92: 4942) showed that a small number of hepatocytes, representing less than 10 per cent of the total number of cells, can reconstitute a whole liver, a process that required more than 10 rounds of hepatocyte replication. These experiments imply that hepatocytes return to quiescence during liver regeneration not because they have exhausted their replicative capacity. On the contrary, replication stops because rigid controls are imposed on the liver to prevent unrestrained proliferation. This chapter reviews some important aspects of liver regeneration after partial hepatectomy and places special emphasis on finding answers to five main questions:

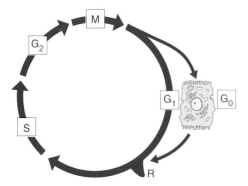

Fig. 1. The phases of the cell cycle. Hepatocytes in the liver *in vivo* are in a quiescent state referred to as 'G₀'. Before these cells can replicate their DNA (S phase) they need to enter the cell cycle (G₁ phase). To progress towards S the cells pass through various restriction points ('checkpoints', indicated by 'R' in the figure). Passage through these points requires that the cell overcomes the blocking effects of genes such as *p53* and retinoblastoma (*Rb*) which also act as tumour suppressors. After DNA replication, there is an interval referred to as 'G₂' (for gap 2) before the cells divide (M, mitosis). After division the daughter cells can continue to cycle or re-enter the G₀ quiescent state. (Modified and redrawn from Rubin and Farber, *Pathology*, (2nd edn), 1994, with permission from J.B. Lippincott, Philadelphia, USA.)

1. What factors regulate the passage of a quiescent hepatocyte into the G₁ phase of the cell cycle?
2. What factors regulate the progression of hepatocytes through the cell cycle leading to DNA synthesis?
3. Are the factors regulating these steps extrahepatic, intrahepatic, or both?
4. Are cytokines, particularly TNF and IL-6, required for triggering liver regeneration?
5. To what extent are non-parenchymal cells necessary for hepatocyte proliferation?

A brief summary about growth factors, proto-oncogenes, and transcription factors will be presented first. In the second part of this chapter this information will be used to explain how regeneration may be initiated and then progresses toward cell replication.

Growth factors: mitogens, adjuvants, and inhibitors

A relative large number of peptide growth factors can stimulate DNA synthesis of hepatocytes in primary culture (Table 1). Among these, hepatocyte growth factor, transforming growth factor-α, and epidermal growth factor have been shown to have a role in liver regeneration *in vivo*. These factors are considered to be 'complete' hepatocyte mitogens (Michalopoulos, FASEBJ, 1990; 4:176), that is, they can stimulate DNA synthesis in hepatocytes maintained in culture in serum-free media in the absence of any other growth factor. Other agents, variably referred to as co-mitogens, adjuvants, augmenters, or progression factors, have no mitogenic activity on their own but can enhance the stimulatory activity of growth factors on hepatocyte DNA synthesis. There are, however, peptides that inhibit hepatocyte DNA synthesis both in culture and during liver regeneration *in vivo*. The best studied of these inhibitory factors are transforming growth factor-β and activin, both of which can cause hepatocyte apoptosis (Oberhammer, PNAS, 1992; 89:5408; Schwall,

Table 1 Growth factors that induce DNA synthesis of hepatocytes in culture in the absence of serum or other factors
HGF, hepatocyte growth factor/scatter factor
TGF-α, transforming growth factor-α
EGF, epidermal growth factor
HB-EGF, heparin binding epidermal growth factor
KGF, keratinocyte growth factor
HGBF1, acidic fibroblast growth factor
Adjuvants, augmenters or co-mitogens for hepatocyte replication in culture
ALR, augmenter of liver regeneration
Insulin
IGF-2, insulin-like growth factor 2
Cyclosporin; FK506
Others

Hepatol, 1993; 18:347; Yasuda, JCI, 1993; 92:1491). Besides its antimitogenic activity on hepatocytes, transforming growth factor-β also has a strong fibrogenic effect through its effect on collagen production in hepatic stellate cells, a property not shared with activins (Fausto, CibaSymp, 1991; 157:165). Because of their inhibitory effect on hepatocyte proliferation (McMahon, CancerRes, 1986; 46:4665; Thoresen, CancerRes, 1992; 52:3598), it would be expected that the activity of both transforming growth factor-β and activin would be high in normal livers and decrease during liver regeneration. On the contrary, the expression of both of these factors is low in resting liver but increases during liver regeneration (Braun, PNAS, 1988; 85:1534). Although there is still no clear explanation for these observations, they suggest that liver regeneration may be a strictly regulated growth process because both stimulators and inhibitors of hepatocyte replication are activated during the process. Adjustments in the ratios between stimulators and inhibitors prevent uncontrolled hepatocyte proliferation and may signal the start and the end of the process.

Transforming growth factor-α

Expression of transforming growth factor-α (**TGFα**) in the liver is associated with hepatocyte proliferation (Fausto, ProgGrowthFactorRes, 1991; 3:219). It is high during the neonatal period and very low in the liver of adult humans and animals (Fausto, FASEBJ, 1996; 9:1527). TGFα increases transiently preceding DNA replication during liver regeneration in rats and mice. In humans, TGFα levels in the blood correlate well with the extent of regeneration in partially hepatectomized patients (Tomiya, Hepatol, 1992; 16:138; Tomiya, Hepatol, 1993; 18:304). TGFα is produced by hepatocytes and exerts its effects on these cells through an autocrine mechanism. TGFα has 35 per cent homology sequence to epidermal growth factor (**EGF**) and binds to the same receptor. The EGF receptor is very abundant in hepatocytes and is a component of an autocrine loop, that is, hepatocytes produce and secrete TGFα and can respond to it through binding of the factor to the EGF receptor at the cell membrane (Noguchi, Hepatol, 1992; 15: 88). Moreover, the TGFα autocrine loop can be enhanced by TGFα itself or EGF, creating an amplification effect for growth factor activity.

TGFα is synthesized as a 160 amino acid precursor that is anchored in the cell membrane and has extracellular, trans-membrane, and intracellular domains (Massague, JBC, 1990; 265: 21393). TGFα can act as a growth factor either as a diffusable factor or as a component of the membrane-bound precursor. The extracellular domain of the precursor contains the 50 amino acid processed (diffusable) form flanked by alanine/valine residues at each end, which are target sites for elastase cleavage (Brachmann, Cell, 1989; 56:691). The C-terminal valine residue of the in-tracellular domain transmits the signal for cleavage of the processed TGFα peptide from the precursor molecule (Bosenberg, Cell, 1992; 71:1157). Both TGFα and EGF contain three disulphide bridges which are located in identical positions in the two peptides.

During liver regeneration after partial hepatectomy in rats, TGFα mRNA increases, starting at about 4 h after partial hepa-tectomy, and reaches a maximum before the peak of DNA synthesis (Mead, PNAS, 1989; 86:1558). TGFα peptide levels are increased at 24 and 48 h after the operation (Webber, Hepatol, 1993; 18:1422). Interestingly, the 50 amino acid diffusable form of TGFα is detected only at 48 h, a time at which the major wave of hepatocyte replication has taken place (Russell, Endocrinol, 1993; 133:1731). Hepatic TGFα expression after partial hepatectomy and chemical injury, as well as during the early postnatal phase of liver development, coincides with DNA replication. In these situations the expression of TGFα is transient and returns to normal when the growth process terminates. On the other hand, transgenic animal models have been established in which TGFα expression in hepatocytes is constitutive. Analysis of liver growth in these animals demonstrated that constitutive expression of TGFα confers proliferative activity to hepatocytes in the liver of adult mice. These animals show major changes in liver growth which may be divided into three phases (Webber, AmJPathol, 1994; 145:398). During the first month of life, hepatocytes of TGFα transgenic mice have proliferative indices which are two to three times higher than normal and their livers are 25 to 40 per cent larger than normal. In transgenic mouse hepato-cytes, the shift to higher levels of ploidy, which is completed by 45 days of life in normal mice, is greatly delayed. At the second phase, which roughly encompasses the period between 3 and 8 months of life, labelling indices of hepatocytes of transgenic mice are six- to eightfold higher than normal. In both normal and transgenic mice there is a decrease in DNA replication after the first month of life but the decline is of much smaller magnitude in transgenic mice. At 3 to 5 months of age the hepatocyte labelling indices are 12 per cent and 2 per cent for transgenic and normal mice, respectively. Surprisingly, despite the higher levels of hepatocyte replication, livers of transgenic mice are not enlarged (Sandgren, Cell, 1990; 61:1121). The absence of enlargement in these highly proliferative livers occurs because the enhanced replication is com-pensated by high cell turnover. In the third phase (from 8 to 15 months of life) hepatocyte replication and high turnover continue but hepatocyte dysplasia becomes apparent (Lee, CancerRes, 1992; 52:5162). Liver morphology becomes progressively more abnormal and by 15 months of age approximately 85 per cent of mice develop hepatic tumours (Jhappan, Cell, 1990; 61:1137; Takagi, CancerRes, 1992; 52:5171). These observations demonstrate that overexpression of TGFα can make adult hepatocytes become replicating cells and that in this process the cells do not lose their differentiated traits.

The proliferative activity of adult hepatocytes under TGFα stimu-lation remains a regulated process that responds to ageing changes and is compensated by increased cell turnover. It is only after almost 12 months of continuous proliferation and high cell turnover that overt malignancy becomes apparent.

Because TGFα confers proliferative activity to hepatocytes which are normally quiescent non-replicating cells, hepatocytes that overexpress this growth factor can be maintained in primary culture for long periods of time (Wu, CancerRes, 1994; 54:5964; Wu, PNAS, 1994; 91:674). Most importantly, hepatocyte cell lines have been developed using these cells. Hepatocytes from these cell lines retained differentiated phenotypic traits and are non-transformed but can be easily propagated in culture.

Hepatocyte growth factor

Hepatocyte growth factor (**HGF**) is a heterodimeric glycoprotein consisting of a heavy (α) and a light (β) chain of approximate molecular weights of 6400 and 32 000, respectively (Nakamura, ProgGrowthFactorRes, 1991; 3:67; Matsumoto, CritRevOncogen, 1992; 3:27). The heterodimeric form is generated from a single-chain precursor with a molecular weight of 87 000 to 92 000. The α-chain has four kringle domains (double-loop structure with three disulphide bridges) with 40 per cent homology with plasminogen. The β-chain has homology with serine proteases but has no pro-teolytic activity of its own because of amino acid substitutions in the catalytic site.

Blood from a partially hepatectomized rat can stimulate hepa-tocyte DNA synthesis in the intact liver of a parabiotic partner (Moolten, Science, 1967; 158:272). Furthermore, hepatocytes trans-planted to ectopic sites also respond to partial hepatectomy with a wave of proliferation (Leong, CancerRes, 1964; 24:1496; Jirtle, CancerRes, 1982; 42:3000). Thus, it is unquestionable that the blood of partially hepatectomized rats contains agents that can induce hepatocyte DNA synthesis. The discovery of HGF was based on this premise, which culminated with the successful isol-ation and cloning of the factor (Michalopoulos, Hepatol, 1992; 15: 149). On a molar basis HGF is the most potent liver mitogen. After partial hepatectomy, blood levels of HGF increase within the first hour and remain high for 4 to 6 h (Lindroos, Hepatol, 1991; 13:743). In addition to its increase in blood, HGF expression, determined by mRNA analysis, increases in the liver at a later time and reaches a maximum 18 to 24 h after partial hepatectomy. Similar changes are also detected after liver injury (Webber, Hepatol, 1993; 18:1422). However, it is surprising that the HGF mRNA changes after partial hepatectomy and CCl4 injury have similar timing, because hepatocyte DNA synthesis after CCl4 injury occurs ap-proximately 1 day later than after partial hepatectomy. The highest level of blood HGF is found in patients with fulminant liver failure (Ghoda, JCI, 1988; 81:414; Tsubochi, Hepatol, 1989; 9:875; Hughes, JHepatol, 1994; 20:106; Shiota, Hepatol, 1995; 21:106). It has been proposed that HGF levels could be used to assess the prognosis of patients with fulminant liver failure because there is an inverse correlation between HGF levels in the blood and survival. HGF is produced by mesenchymal cells throughout the body. In the liver it is synthesized by stellate cells, Kupffer cells, and endothelial cells, but is not made by hepatocytes (Schirmacher, Hepatol, 1992; 15:5; Maher, JCI, 1993; 91:224). The factor is mitogenic for epithelial cells from various tissues, melanocytes, osteoblasts, osteoclasts, and endothelial cells, and has morphogenetic and motogenic effects (Naldini, EMBOJ, 1991; 10:2867; Bussolino, JCellBiol, 1992; 119:629; Zarnegar, JCellBiol, 1995; 129:1177; Grand, PNAS, 1996; 93:7644).

Despite its high mitogenic potency, it is still unclear whether HGF can trigger liver regeneration. HGF is produced in many different tissues and its accumulation in the blood in acute liver failure and probably also after partial hepatectomy appears to be caused by the decrease in liver functional mass that exists in these situations (Liu, AmJPhysiol, 1992; 26:G642; Appasamy, LabInvest, 1993; 68:270). Particularly in humans, it does not appear that a direct correlation exists between blood HGF levels and the extent of liver growth, as indicated from data obtained from partially hepatectomized patients and patients subjected to surgical procedures not affecting the liver (Tomiya, Gastro, 1992; 103:1621; Kimura, AmJGastr, 1996; 91:116). After partial hepatectomy in rats and mice there is an early increase in blood HGF and a later increase in HGF mRNA produced in liver non-parenchymal cells. Thus, HGF could act on hepatocytes by an endocrine mechanism (from blood) or have a paracrine effect (from hepatic non-parenchymal cells). It is uncertain whether one or both of these mechanisms are important in terms of the mitogenic effect of HGF after partial hepatectomy. One of the difficulties in establishing correlations between HGF blood levels and hepatocyte replication is that HGF is inactive in its precursor form that is present in variable amounts in the circulation. HGF requires proteolytic cleavage for activation and various enzymes have been shown to cleave the single-chain precursor (Gak, FEBSLett, 1992; 311:17). Cleavage may occur in the circulation, but it may also take place as a local event in tissues in which the factor becomes active (Naldini, EMBOJ, 1992; 11:4825; Miyazawa, JBC, 1993; 268:10024). Rapid proteolytic events have been found to occur after partial hepatectomy, involving activation of transcription factors as well as the enhanced expression of tissue plasminogen activator (urokinase) receptor (Mars, AmJPathol, 1993; 143:149). Increased hepatic protease activity at the start of liver regeneration could cause the conversion of single-chain inactive HGF to the heterodimeric active factor. If proteolytic cleavage of HGF after partial hepatectomy occurs only in the liver but not in other tissues, it would explain why circulating HGF in partially hepatectomized animals does not induce proliferation of cells in extrahepatic tissues. Regardless of the potential pathways for growth factor activation after partial hepatectomy, there is also compelling evidence to conclude that quiescent hepatocytes *in vivo* are relatively insensitive to the mitogenic effect of growth factors (Webber, Hepatol, 1994; 19:489; Liu, Hepatol, 1994; 19:1521). To respond to growth factors such as HGF, TGFα and EGF, quiescent hepatocytes *in vivo* need first to be 'primed' for the response (see below). Thus, liver regeneration after partial hepatectomy may start with changes in gene expression that make hepatocytes competent to respond to growth factors.

HGF transgenic and knockout mice

HGF overexpression in the liver has major effects on hepatic growth. Earlier observations indicated that transgenic mice which overexpress HGF had a large number of small diploid hepatocytes in the liver (Shiota, Hepatol, 1994; 19:962). After partial hepatectomy, the liver remnant of these animals regained normal weight faster than that of non-transgenic animals. More recent observations show that HGF overexpression causes major effects in liver cell composition and growth (Sakata, CellGrowthDiff, 1996; 7:1513). Livers of HGF transgenic mice are quite large and contain hepatocytes of small size which are mostly diploid. HGF overexpression also produces marked alterations in other organs, particularly the kidney. Two recent reports show that mice in which the HGF gene has been inactivated ('knockouts') die during embryonic development. Uehara (Nature, 1995; 373:702) attributed lethality to a placental defect but did not detect hepatic abnormalities in the embryos. Schmidt (Nature, 1995; 373:699) found that HGF knockouts had a major defect in liver development and that the embryonic livers of these mice were greatly reduced in size. These authors indicated that HGF may be essential for liver morphogenesis and considered the defect found in HGF knockouts to be similar to that described in mice with inactive c-*jun* (Hilberg, Nature, 1993; 365:179). Mice which lack c-*jun* also die during embryonic development with severe liver abnormalities (Table 2). A more detailed analysis of the variable phenotypes of HGF knockout mice is necessary before definitive conclusions are reached, but the results indicate that HGF has an essential role as a mediator of epithelial mesenchymal interactions in the liver and other organs, and that during embryonic liver development, this role cannot be taken over by other growth factors (Sonnenberg, FASEBJ, 1994; 8:420). Both *in vivo* and *in vitro*, hepatocyte gene expression is modulated by cellular matrix components (Bucher, SemLivDis, 1990; 10:11) and it is likely that HGF participates as a mediator of these interactions and in processes requiring branching morphogenesis during liver development.

Growth factor redundancy during liver regeneration

Although HGF and TGFα are potent liver mitogens, lack of activity of the respective genes in knockout animals has very different effects. In contrast to HGF knockouts which die during embryonic development, TGFα knockouts develop normally and grow into healthy adults which display only hair-growth abnormalities (Luetteke, Cell, 1993; 73:263; Mann, Cell, 1993; 73:249). Liver regeneration is not impaired in TGFα knockout mice (Russell, MolCarcinog, 1996; 15:183). The most likely explanation for these findings is that EGF may replace TGFα in most, if not of all, of its functions. Indeed, mice which are deficient in EGF receptor, the common receptor for EGF and TGFα, die either during embryonic development or during the first 2 postnatal weeks (Miettinen, Nature, 1995; 376:337; Sibilia, Science, 1995; 269:234; Threadgill, Science, 1995; 269:230).

Addition of TGFα to hepatocytes grown in primary culture induces DNA replication in approximately 45 per cent of the cells, but the combination of TGFα and HGF (that is, addition of HGF to medium containing optimal levels of TGFα) increases the percentage of proliferative cells to close to 80 per cent (Webber, Hepatol, 1993; 18:1422). The additive effect may be due to increased production of TGFα induced by HGF. Alternatively, hepatocytes might have differential sensitivity to individual growth factors, perhaps as a consequence of preferential distribution of receptors (EGF receptor and c-met) in cells located in different parts of the lobule (Gebhardt, PharmTher, 1992; 53:275). Redundancy of

Table 2 Embryonic lethality associated with defects of liver development in knockout mice

Gene	Defect	Reference
c-jun	Decreased number of hepatocytes and haemopoietic cells (E14–16)	Hilberg, Nature, 1993; 365:179
p65 (NF-κB)	Massive hepatocyte apoptosis (E15–16)	Beg, Nature, 1995; 376:167
HGF/SF	Placental defect (E14–16)	Uehara, Nature, 1995; 373:702
HGF/SF	Reduction of liver size (E14–16)	Schmidt, Nature, 1995; 373:699

hepatocyte mitogens may serve as a safety mechanism which evolved because liver regeneration is vital for life. Alternatively HGF and TGFα (or EGF) may not have redundant activities but may instead act at different stages of the cell cycle, although all three growth factors are complete mitogens for cultured hepatocytes. At this time there are no data indicating that EGF, TGFα, and HGF may activate different sets of genes which are specific for each factor. Analysis of growth factor induced gene expression in cultured hepatocytes is complicated by the observation that cells dissociated from the liver by collagenase digestion, even before they are plated into culture, express immediate early response genes (see below) which are not detectable in quiescent hepatocytes *in vivo*. This poses major difficulties in using cell cultures to determine whether growth factors can trigger liver regeneration because cultured cells are not strictly quiescent at the time of addition of the factors.

Augmenter of liver regeneration

This peptide was recently purified from the cytosol of weanling rat livers and its gene was cloned and sequenced from rats, mice, and humans (Hagiya, PNAS, 1993; 91:8142; Giorda, MolMed, 1996; 2: 97). The human gene is located on chromosome 16. Augmenter of liver regeneration (**ALR**) does not have mitogenic activity for hepatocytes in primary culture nor normal liver *in vivo* but it stimulates DNA synthesis *in vivo* in the livers of rats subjected to 40 per cent hepatectomy or in dogs with portocaval shunt. ALR has partial sequence homology with ERV-1, a gene which is essential for oxidative phosphorylation and vegetative growth in yeast. It is not known whether ALR may have an effect on oxidative phosphorylation in mammals. Although ALR is expressed in most tissues, the factor has immunosuppressive activities that are specific for the liver and are probably mediated by hepatic natural killer cells (Vujanovic, JImmunol, 1995; 154:6324). These cells lose their cytotoxicity during hepatic regeneration and it has been suggested that the immunosuppressive effect of ALR may enhance hepatocyte replication indirectly (Francavilla, Hepatol, 1994; 20:747). Levels of ALR mRNA do not increase after partial hepatectomy and the source of circulating ALR remains to be established.

Expression of proto-oncogenes and cell cycle genes during liver regeneration

Mesenchymal and epithelial cells in culture respond to the addition of serum and other mitogenic stimuli by rapidly increasing the expression of specific sets of genes (Herschman, AnnRevBiochem, 1991; 60:281). Because it occurs within minutes after the addition of the mitogenic agent, the reponse is referred to as the primary or immediate early gene response. An important characteristic of the response is that it occurs in the absence of new protein synthesis. The genes activated in the immediate early response do not share a common function and are not necessarily related to DNA synthesis. The first components of the immediate early gene response after partial hepatectomy to be identified were the proto-oncogenes c-*fos*, c-*jun*, and c-*myc*. The mRNAs for these genes were found to increase very rapidly after partial hepatectomy, reaching a peak at 1 to 3 h after the operation in rats or mice (Fausto, Hepatol, 1983; 3: 1016; Kruijer, JBC, 1986; 261:7929; Thompson, CancerRes, 1986; 46:3119; Brenner, DNA, 1989; 8:279; Fausto, LabInvest, 1989; 60: 4; Alcorn, Hepatol, 1990; 11:909; Morello, MolCellBiol, 1990; 10: 3185). Their expression is short lived and the mRNA levels return to normal by about 4 h after partial hepatectomy. Thus c-*fos*, c-*jun*, and c-*myc* show a rapid, sequential, and transient response to partial hepatectomy (Fig. 2). The mechanisms that regulate the expression of these proto-oncogenes in the immediate early gene response after partial hepatectomy are still not completely understood. Suffice to say that they involve both transcriptional and post-transcriptional mechanisms and that the events that control mRNA expression are particularly complicated in the case of c-*myc* (Morello, MolCellBiol, 1990; 10:3185; Morello, Oncogene, 1990; 5:1511; Morello, Oncogene, 1993; 8:1921). Transcriptional activation of c-*myc* after partial hepatectomy appears to be short lived and to last no more than 30 min. After that time, steady-state levels of the transcript are regulated by post-transcriptional mechanisms which may involve the protection of newly formed transcripts from degradation and stabilization of mature c-*myc* mRNA in the cytoplasm. Since the original description of proto-oncogenes as participants in the immediate early gene response after partial hepatectomy, it has been shown that as many as 70 genes may be involved in this response (Mohn, MolCellBiol, 1991; 11:381; Haber, JCI, 1993; 91:1319; Taub, FASEBJ, 1996; 10:413). In addition to proto-oncogenes, immediate early gene components may include genes for proteases, phosphatases, transcription factor inhibitors and stimulators, growth factor binding proteins, metabolic enzymes, etc., as well as a large number of genes that remain to be identified (Mohn, MolCellBiol, 1991; 11:1393; Diamond, MolCellBiol, 1994; 14: 3752). Animal models in which individual genes are either overexpressed (transgenic mice) or inactivated (knockout mice) have been of great value to determine which genes, among those involved

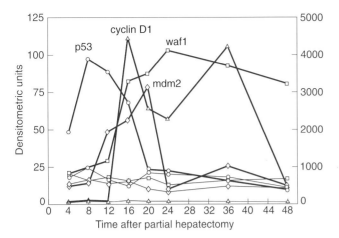

Fig. 2. Expression of cell cycle genes during liver regeneration. The figure shows the expression of mRNAs for cell cycle genes that are components of the secondary gene response after partial hepatectomy. Rats were partially hepatectomized and the livers removed at the times indicated on the abscissa. mRNA analyses were done by Northern blotting and mRNA levels are expressed in the ordinate as arbitrary densitometric units obtained by the scanning of the blots. Transcripts for the following genes are shown: *p53*, *mdm2*, *waf-1(p21)*, and *cyclin D1*. The flat curves at the bottom of the figure show corresponding mRNA measurements in sham-operated rats. Note that *p53* and *waf-1(p21)* are cell cycle blockers while *mdm2* and *cyclin D1* act as stimulators.

in the primary response, are required for DNA synthesis during liver regeneration.

Many of the genes involved in the primary response encode proteins which are transcription factors. Thus, the primary response itself sets in motion the transactivation of other sets of genes which establish a delayed gene activation phase referred to as the secondary gene response. This response involves the increased expression of cell cycle related genes, including cyclins and their associated kinases. Increased expression of such genes after partial hepatectomy takes place when hepatocytes progress through the G_1 phase of the cell cycle and reach the replicative stage (Lu, JBC, 1992; 267:2841; Albrecht, AmJPhysiol, 1993; 265:G857; Koch, BBResComm, 1994; 204:91; Loyer, JBC, 1994; 269:2491; Trembley, CellGrowthDiff, 1994; 5:99). The most salient components of the secondary response are represented by the expression of *p53*, *mdm2*, *waf-1* (also known as *p21*), and *cyclin D* (Fig. 2). All of these genes show transient increases of expression between 8 and 24 h after partial hepatectomy in rats, which generally precede by a few or several hours the major peak of DNA synthesis that occurs at 24 h. It is of interest that both *p53* and *p21* are cell cycle inhibitors and tumour suppressors, while *mdm2* and *cyclin D* are cell cycle activators. The transient and sequential increase of genes which are supposed to act as cell cycle blockers, suggests that the role of such genes during liver regeneration is to prevent the unregulated effect of cell cycle stimulators. In any event, it is doubtful that *p53* expression is essential for a single proliferative cycle of hepatocytes, because hepatocytes from *p53*-deficient mice are capable of replicating in culture. It is not known whether the genome of hepatocytes lacking *p53* becomes unstable and acquires tumorigenic properties after repeated rounds of cell division. The p21 protein is an inhibitor of the cyclin D1 dependent kinase, CDK4, in the liver.

Transgenic mice that overexpress p21 have small and abnormal livers and very deficient liver regeneration (Wu, GenesDevelop, 1996; 10:245). Thus, the transient increase in p21 mRNA during liver regeneration must be under strict regulatory controls, because overexpression of the gene can cause cell cycle arrest.

Kren and Steer (FASEBJ, 1996; 10:559) have studied in detail the mechanisms that regulate the expression of a large number of genes during liver regeneration. They showed that although the levels of many mRNAs are greatly increased after partial hepatectomy, the transcription rates for a majority of these mRNAs remain unchanged during liver regeneration. Instead, the regulation of mRNA levels depended on post-transcriptional mechanisms which served to increase the stability of cytoplasmic mRNA. Genes regulated by this mechanism after partial hepatectomy include *cyclins A*, *B1*, *D1*, *D3* and *E*, *cyclin dependent kinase 1*, *p53* and *mdm2*, among others. Thus, expression of most genes of the delayed response after partial hepatectomy depends predominantly, if not exclusively, on post-transcriptional controls that modulate mRNA stability ('half-life').

Transcription factor activation after partial hepatectomy

A very important aspect of the initiation of liver regeneration is the activation of several transcription factors which occurs shortly after partial hepatectomy. We will briefly review information on the activation of the transcription factors NF-κB, STAT3, AP1, and C/EBP.

NF-κB activation

NF-κB (nuclear factor for κ-chain in B cells) comprises a family of proteins that form homo- and heterodimers and are related to the *rel* oncogene and the Drosophila gene *dorsal*. Originally described in lymphocytes, NF-κB proteins have been detected in many different cell types and found to participate in gene activation related to defence mechanisms, immune reactions, and cell proliferation processes. NF-κB activation is a rapid process that involves post-translation modifications of proteins and is triggered by many different types of stimuli, such as endotoxins (lipopolysaccharide, **LPS**), tumour necrosis factor-α, interleukin-1, interleukin-2, ultra-violet light, and oxidants (Grilli, IntRevCytol, 1993; 143:1; Liou, CurrOpinCellBiol, 1993; 5:477). Its target genes include, among others, surface immunoglobulins, adhesion molecules, cytokines, acute-phase response genes, the c-*myc* proto-oncogene, and several viruses, including HIV. These genes contain NF-κB recognition sequences and are transcriptionally activated (transactivated) by NF-κB binding. NF-κB is present in the cytoplasm in an inactive form composed of two NF-κB subunits, designated as p50 and p65, bound to an inhibitor known as **IκB** (inhibitor of κB). Activation of NF-κB depends on the degradation of IκB and its dissociation from the complexes (Fig. 3). This is accomplished in at least two steps. The first step is the phosphorylation of IκB, through the activity of a phosphorylating enzyme whose activity is greatly enhanced by oxygen free-radicals. The second step involves the ubiquitination of phosphorylated IκB, a reaction that targets the molecule for digestion by proteases contained in large cytosol complexes known as proteasomes. Anderson *et al.* (PNAS, 1994; 91:11527) proposed

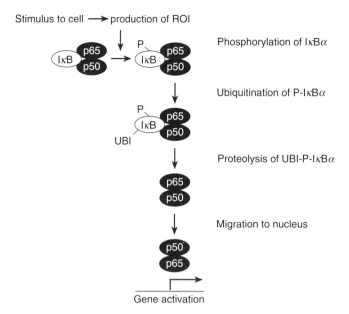

Stimulus to cell ⟶ production of ROI

Phosphorylation of IκBα

Ubiquitination of P-IκBα

Proteolysis of UBI-P-IκBα

Migration to nucleus

Gene activation

Fig. 3. Mechanisms of activation of NF-κB. The figure shows the activation of the transcription factor NF-κB. Various stimuli can initiate the process but tumour necrosis factor (TNF) is likely to be the major inducer of NF-κB after partial hepatectomy. NF-κB is composed of two subunits, p50 and p65, which are present in the cytoplasm bound to an inhibitor (IκB). When the cell receives the appropriate stimulus, activation of the transcription factor takes place by degradation of IκB and its release from the complex. NF-κB (p50/p65 heterodimer) then migrates into the nucleus where it initiates transcription of genes that contain NF-κB binding sequences. Degradation of IκB takes place through a series of steps which involve phosphorylation, ubiquitination of the phosphorylated molecule, and finally degradation by proteasome proteases of the ubiquitinated, phosphorylated molecule. The phosphorylation step is under control of a protein kinase that requires, or is enhanced by, reactive oxygen intermediates (ROI).

that, regardless of the nature of the stimulatory agent, NF-κB activation has a common pathway which involves the generation of mitochondrial oxidants followed by protein phosphorylation and degradation of IκB, leading to the production of active NF-κB (composed of the two subunits p50 and p65), which then migrates into the nucleus (Fig. 3). Blockage of NF-κB activity through induction of IκB synthesis has been shown to be a mechanism through which glucocorticoids cause immunosuppression and markedly inhibit cytokine secretion (Auphan, Science, 1995; 270: 286; Scheinman, Science, 1995; 270:283).

Tewari *et al.* (MolCellBiol, 1992; 12:2898) reported that a protein complex named **PHF** (post-hepatectomy factor) was activated and bound to DNA within minutes after partial hepatectomy. They also demonstrated the increased expression of an immediate early gene which was named **RL–IF1** (regenerating liver inhibitor factor 1). PHF was found to be a protein related to the transcription factor NF-κB, while RL–IF1 was identified as IκBα, a specific inhibitor of NF-κB activity. The authors proposed that PHF may act by competing with NF-κB for the same DNA binding sites. Because PHF binding was insensitive to RL–IF1 (IκBα) inhibition, Tewari *et al.* concluded that at the start of liver regeneration, IκBα gene activation would suppress NF-κB binding and enhance PHF activation. Further analysis by electrophoretic shift mobility assays of

the activation of NF-κB and related proteins after partial hepatectomy revealed that, on the contrary, authentic NF-κB itself, that is the p50/p65 heterodimer, is activated in the first hour after partial hepatectomy and binds to hepatocyte DNA (FitzGerald, CellGrowthDiff, 1995; 6:417). In addition to heterodimer binding, there is also increased binding of p50 homodimers as well as binding of a smaller component of lower molecular weight that corresponds to the PHF factor described by Tewari *et al.*

Increased NF-κB binding was detected in nuclear extracts from hepatocytes isolated 30 min after partial hepatectomy (FitzGerald, CellGrowthDiff, 1995; 6:417), indicating that this transcription factor is a component of the hepatocyte response to partial hepatectomy. These cells also contained p50 homodimers (which bind to DNA but lack transcriptional activity) and the minor complex which corresponded to PHF. Normal liver non-parenchymal cells also contain the three NF-κB complexes but no increase in NF-κB binding (that is, p50/p65 heterodimer) occurs in non-parenchymal cells at the start of liver regeneration. Thus, immediately after partial hepatectomy, there is activation of NF-κB in hepatocytes, leading to a dramatic increase in DNA binding. Presumably, increased NF-κB binding causes the transactivation of target genes that contain the NF-κB motifs (Cressman, JBC, 1994; 269:30429; FitzGerald, CellGrowthDiff, 1995; 6:417). Increased NF-κB binding to DNA was also detected after 30 per cent hepatectomy, but not in sham-operated rats, suggesting that NF-κB activation may be involved in the very early steps of the gene response after partial hepatectomy. NF-κB activation by itself is clearly not sufficient to cause DNA synthesis, because animals with 30 per cent hepatectomy do not undergo DNA synthesis. However hepatocytes from these animals become capable of responding to growth factors (Webber, Hepatol, 1994; 19:489) and are 'competent' to replicate.

The p65 component of NF-κB is essential for liver development (Table 2). Mice lacking this gene develop normally until day 14, but between days 14 and 16 of development, massive apoptosis occurs in the liver and causes 100 per cent embryonic lethality (Beg, Nature, 1995; 376:167). In contrast, mice that lack the p50 NF-κB component develop normally. Thus p65 NF-κB has an essential role in liver development which is not replaceable by other members of the NF-κB family of proteins. It may function as a stimulator of cell proliferation or as a 'survival factor' that prevents hepatocyte apoptosis.

The rapid activation of hepatocyte NF-κB after partial hepatectomy indicates that a signal for gene activation has been received in the nucleus of these cells almost immediately after the operation. It then becomes essential to identify the mechanisms and agents responsible for the activation. Moreover, because NF-κB is a transcription factor, its target genes (that is, genes that contain a NF-κB binding sequence and which may be transactivated by the factor after partial hepatectomy) need to be identified. Strong induction of NF-κB similar to that after partial hepatectomy can be produced 30 min after intraperitoneal injection of 5 μg of tumour necrosis factor in intact rats (FitzGerald, CellGrowthDiff, 1995; 6:417). Tumour necrosis factor stimulation of NF-κB DNA binding was also observed in liver cell cultures, in which tumour necrosis factor causes increases in NF-κB binding and c-*myc* mRNA levels similar to those induced by serum. Diehl and colleagues (Ackerman, AmJPhysiol, 1992; 263:G579; Diehl, AmJPhysiol, 1994; 267:G552; Diehl, Hepatol, 1995; 22:252) have concluded from experiments

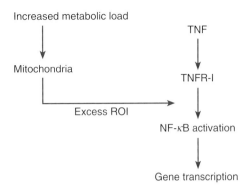

Fig. 4. Reactive oxygen and gene transcription. The figure shows how metabolic overload after partial hepatectomy may lead to gene transcription and initiation of the cascade that leads to DNA replication. The right side of the figure shows NF-κB activation after partial hepatectomy caused by the binding of tumour necrosis factor (TNF) to its type I receptor (TNFR-I). The left side indicates how increased metabolic load and enhanced oxidative phosphorylation in the mitochondria at the start of liver regeneration can produce excess reactive oxygen intermediates (ROI) which stimulate NF-κB activation (see Fig. 3).

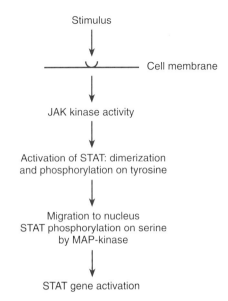

Fig. 5. STAT3 signal transduction and gene activation. The figure shows how the transcription factor STAT3 is activated. LPS, IL-6, and EGF are known stimuli that activate STAT3. Activation requires the activity of a JAK kinase and two phosphorylation steps. The active factor migrates into the nucleus where it initiates the transcription of genes that contain STAT3 binding sequences.

using tumour necrosis factor antibodies that tumour necrosis factor causes elevation of c-jun, jun-kinase, and AP1 after partial hepatectomy, and that blockage of tumour necrosis factor activity inhibits liver regeneration. It is thus possible that tumour necrosis factor contributes to the initiation of liver regeneration by being responsible for the activation of both NF-κB and AP1 (see below). On the other hand, NF-κB activation after partial hepatectomy may depend on factors that act directly on the phosphorylation and proteolytic degradation steps of the inhibitor IκB. The phosphorylation step is modulated by the redox state of the cell, while the proteolytic cleavage of IκB depends on proteasome activity (Pallombella, Cell, 1994; 78:773; Lin, PNAS, 1995; 92:552). Thus, NF-κB activation at the start of liver regeneration could be induced by extracellular stimuli such as tumour necrosis factor or by intracellular signals that activate a redox-sensitive protein kinase (IκB phosphorylation) or proteasome proteases (IκB degradation). Enhancement of the activation of NF-κB by changes in redox state or generation of excess oxygen free-radicals after partial hepatectomy is a particularly intriguing possibility. Changes in hepatocyte membrane potential occur within minutes after partial hepatectomy. It is also conceivable that there is excessive production of oxygen free-radicals generated by the high metabolic activity imposed on the small liver remnant after partial hepatectomy (Fig. 4). Reactive oxygen species are normal by-products of mitochondrial oxidative phosphorylation (Goossens, PNAS, 1995; 92: 8115). However, the amount produced in the first hours after partial hepatectomy may exceed the capacity of the liver to capture and eliminate these reactive molecules. Thus, the increased hepatocyte work load needed for metabolic adaptations after partial hepatectomy may cause an increase in reactive oxygen species which can enhance NF-κB activation and the transactivation of target genes.

STAT3 activation

STAT3 is a member of a family of transcription factors known as 'signal transducers and activators of transcription' (Zhong, Science,

1994; 264:95). As the name implies, these factors function as shuttles between stimuli received at the cell membrane and gene activation in the nucleus (Fig. 5). EGF, LPS, and interleukin-6 can activate STAT3 in the liver (Ruff-Jamison, JBC, 1994; 269:21933). The factor is present in the cytosol in an inactive form and requires two phosphorylation steps, one on tyrosine and the other on serine, for its activation (Fig. 5). Binding of STAT3 increases after partial hepatectomy with kinetics that are slightly slower than that of NF-κB. However, STAT3 activation is prolonged and remains high for 6 h or more (Cressman, Hepatol, 1995; 21:1443; Trautwein, Gastro, 1996; 110:1854). Thus, this transcription factor probably transactivates genes involved in the immediate early gene response as well as cell cycle genes which are components of the secondary response.

AP1 activation

The transcription factor AP1 is composed of heterodimers between c-Fos and a member of the Jun family or by dimers formed by Jun family members (Karin, JBC, 1995; 270:16483). In addition, a member of the Fos family that forms heterodimeric complexes with both Jun B and c-Jun in the regenerating liver has been identified by Taub and her colleagues (Hsu, PNAS, 1991, 88:3511) and is referred to as liver regeneration factor-1 (**LRF–1**). Growth factors are important AP1 activators in mesenchymal cells in culture and there is reason to believe that the same is true for the regenerating liver, although other types of agents can also activate this transcription factor. Activation of AP1 after partial hepatectomy occurs rapidly and transiently, and generally returns to normal at 6 h (Diehl, FASEBJ, 1996; 10:215; Taub, FASEBJ, 1996; 10:413). Binding activity of c-Jun in the AP1 complex increases within 1 h after partial hepatectomy. The binding activity is enhanced by a rapid increase in activity of Jun nuclear kinase. Different AP1

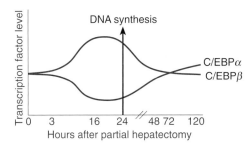

Fig. 6. Levels of C/EBPα and β after partial hepatectomy. The figure shows a representation of the levels of C/EBPα and C/EBPβ after partial hepatectomy in rats. Note the inverse relationship between these two isoforms of the C/EBP transcription factor. The changes start shortly after partial hepatectomy and persist after the major peak of DNA synthesis at 24 h has occurred. (Reprinted from Taub, FASEBJ, 1996; 10:413, with permission.)

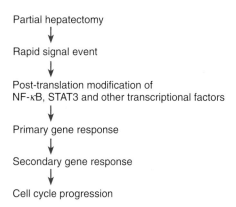

Fig. 7. Major steps of liver regeneration. See text for the description of each of the individual steps shown in the figure.

complexes, that is, c-Fos/c-Jun, c-Jun/c-Jun, LRF-1/c-Jun, etc. probably transactivate different but partially overlapping sets of genes. It has been suggested that the composition of the AP1 complexes changes progressively during the first few hours after partial hepatectomy (Hsu, MolCellBiol, 1992; 12:4654; Taub, FASEBJ, 1996; 10:413). In this manner immediate early as well as secondary response genes could be transactivated by various AP1 complexes during liver regeneration.

C/EBP activation

The transcription factor **C/EBP** (CAAT enhancer binding protein) is highly expressed in normal liver. As is the case for AP1, C/EBP is a member of the leucine zipper protein transcription factor family (**bZIP**). These proteins contain leucine residues that bind together two molecules by establishing a 'zipper' type of interaction. C/EBP monomers form a parallel, coiled structure containing a leucine zipper α-helix. C/EBP activates 'liver-specific' genes which are abundant in differentiated hepatocytes (Wang, Science, 1995; 269: 1108). Two important components of C/EBP in the liver are the isoforms known as C/EBPα and C/EBPβ. After partial hepatectomy there is no change in the overall binding of C/EBP. However, the relative proportions of C/EBPα and β are modified: C/EBPα decreases while C/EBPβ increases (Mischoulon, MolCellBiol, 1992; 12:2553; Diehl, Hepatol, 1994; 19:447; Greenbaum, JCI, 1995; 96:1351; Taub, FASEBJ, 1996; 10:413). These changes persist until the first wave of DNA synthesis in the regenerating liver is completed (Fig. 6). As C/EBPα has been shown to have antiproliferative effects in other cells, the increased ratio between C/EBPβ and C/EBPα after partial hepatectomy could permit hepatocyte replication without loss of differentiated traits (Soriano, InVitro, 1995; 31:703). It is of interest that hepatocytes of the AML12 cell line, which are replicative and differentiated, express a much larger proportion of C/EBPβ than C/EBPα.

Steps of the proliferative response during liver regeneration: priming and progression

The description of individual components of the hepatic regenerative response can not provide a complete picture of the process. This can only be done by placing these components into a framework in which the major events of liver regeneration are integrated into a series of sequential steps (Fig. 7). As already mentioned, many studies have shown that quiescent hepatocytes in the intact liver need to become 'primed' or competent before they enter the cell cycle. Thus, we consider that a crucial step in the triggering of liver regeneration is the passage of a quiescent hepatocyte (G_0 phase) into the G_1 phase of the cell cycle. The transition between G_0 and G_1 will be referred to as the priming or competence phase. The major events of this phase are transcription factor activation and the immediate early gene response. The secondary gene response and the expression of cell cycle genes that leads to DNA synthesis is grouped together under the term 'progression'.

The triggering of liver regeneration

A logical assumption from the data reviewed so far is that regeneration starts by the overexpression or activation of a growth factor or by activation of signalling from the receptor itself. Because HGF increases rapidly in the blood after partial hepatectomy or liver injury, it is a good candidate to be an initiator of liver regeneration. Although this is a plausible hypothesis, direct proof that this indeed is the case has not been obtained so far. The best way to test the notion that HGF initiates regeneration is to determine whether liver regeneration takes place in mice that lack a functional HGF gene. However, such animals, as mentioned above, die during embryonic development and thus can not be used for the study of liver regeneration.

The lack of tissue specificity of HGF mitogenic effects is an issue that needs to be considered in evaluating the role of this growth factor in triggering liver regeneration. HGF is a mitogenic agent for many different cell types in the organism and its concentration increases in the blood in both liver regeneration and kidney growth after unilateral nephrectomy. Yet, the mitogenic response is specific for each organ; that is, hepatic DNA synthesis but not renal cell replication occurs after partial hepatectomy, while kidney DNA synthesis but not hepatocyte proliferation takes place after uninephrectomy (Kono, BBResComm, 1992; 186:991). This suggests that the actual activity of the growth factor in the tissue depends more on local factors which may determine the capacity of the cell to respond to HGF stimulation than on HGF blood

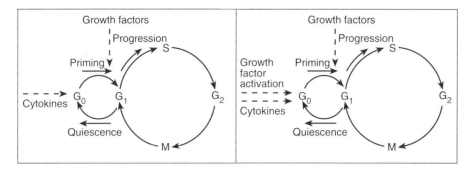

Fig. 8. Role of cytokines and growth factors in the initiation of liver regeneration after partial hepatectomy. The figure shows two models. The diagram on the left shows cytokines (TNF and IL-6) as the initiators of liver regeneration after partial hepatectomy while growth factors act on 'primed' cells to make them enter the G phase of the cycle and progress to DNA synthesis (S). The diagram on the right shows both cytokines and growth factors acting on quiescent hepatocytes through parallel pathways to initiate regeneration (see text). In both diagrams, two circles are shown. The small one represents the priming phase, which is reversible. The large circle represents the progression phase, in which primed hepatocytes enter the G_1 phase and progress to DNA synthesis.

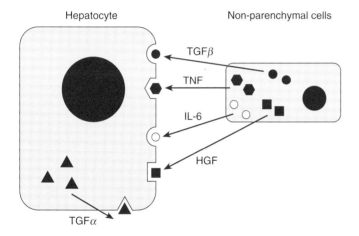

Fig. 9. Inter-relationships between hepatocytes and non-parenchymal cells in the production of cytokines and growth factors important in liver regeneration. Note that TGFα acts on hepatocytes through an autocrine circuit, while HGF has paracrine activity (HGF also has endocrine activity, not shown in the figure). Kupffer cells are considered to be the main producers of TNF and IL-6. HGF and TGFβ are produced by stelate (Ito) cells and also by other non-parenchymal cells. The cytokines and growth factors shown are only a subset of a much larger number of molecules that act as mediators in the interactions between hepatocytes and non-parenchymal cells.

concentration. The possibility that other growth factors besides HGF could initiate liver regeneration should also not be excluded. For instance, EGF appears to be required for liver regeneration in mice, as shown by the almost total inhibition of DNA synthesis after partial hepatectomy in animals in which the salivary glands have been surgically resected (Jones, AmJPhysiol, 1995; 268:G872). EGF has been reported to be produced by hepatocytes during a brief period of time shortly after partial hepatectomy, and can act both by endocrine and autocrine mechanisms (Noguchi, JEndocr, 1991; 128:425; Mullhaupt, JBC, 1994; 269:19667). Another interesting possibility is that growth factor precursors, such as pro-TGFα, which are anchored into the cell membrane become activated by partial proteolytic cleavage at the start of liver regeneration and have a strictly localized effect because they remain in the cell surface and are not released in a diffusable form.

HGF, TGFα, and other growth factors have a very potent effect on DNA synthesis of hepatocytes in primary culture. However, hepatocytes in the intact liver are not particularly sensitive to these factors. Although it is possible to induce hepatocyte replication in normal animals by repeated injection or prolonged infusion of growth factors such as HGF and keratinocyte growth factor (**KGF**) (Fujiwara, Hepatol, 1993; 18:1443; Housley, JCI, 1994; 94:1764; Roos, AmJPhysiol, 1995; 268:G380), hepatocytes of quiescent livers *in vivo* are relatively insensitive to mitogenic effects of 'complete' growth factors. Infusion of EGF, TGFα, or HGF directly into the portal vein of rats for 24 h had little effect on DNA replication (Webber, Hepatol, 1994; 19:489). Combinations of these factors infused directly into the liver also failed to induce substantial DNA replication. However, hepatocytes can be made to respond rapidly to growth factors *in vivo*. This has been accomplished by infusing the factors into 30 per cent partially hepatectomized rats or by administering the growth factors after perfusion of the liver with low concentrations of collagenase (Webber, Hepatol, 1994; 19:489). In contrast to the 70 per cent hepatectomy (the standard operation) which elicits a massive wave of hepatocyte replication, there is minimal change in DNA synthesis after a 30 per cent hepatectomy. Yet hepatocytes of rats with one-third hepatectomy respond vigorously to growth factor infusion. It is of interest that these animals, as well as rats with collagenase-perfused livers, respond equally well to HGF and TGFα, indicating that the effect of these procedures is not limited to a single growth factor and is unlikely to involve the activation of a specific growth factor receptor. However, since both c-Met (the HGF receptor) and the EGF receptor depend on tyrosine kinase activity for signalling, there might be common mechanisms of activation for the two receptors. In any event, the results of these experiments suggest that quiescent hepatocytes need to reach a general 'receptive' state before they can respond to the proliferative stimulus of partial hepatectomy. We suggest that this state, which we refer to as priming or competence, involves as its first step the increased binding of the transcription factors NF-κB and STAT3, which is followed shortly after by AP1 activation. The demonstration of a priming step in hepatocyte replication *in vivo* is not new. Moolten *et al.* (CancerRes, 1970; 30:2353) showed that pretreatment of rats with growth hormone or simple surgical stress accelerated the rise in DNA synthesis after partial hepatectomy,

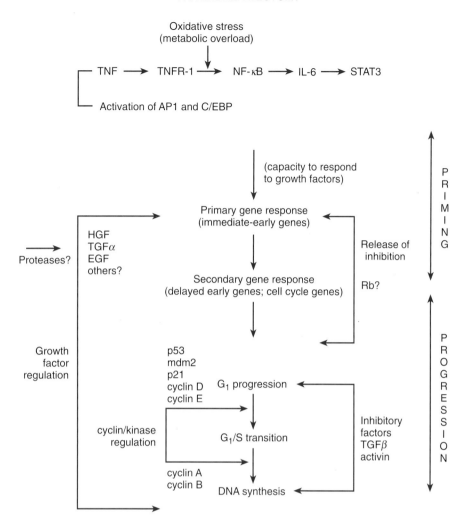

PARTIAL HEPATECTOMY

Fig. 10. Summary of the main events of liver regeneration after partial hepatectomy. The figure shows the main events of the process leading to DNA synthesis as described in the text. The initial event of the priming phase is the post-translation modification of transcription factors through TNF activity, involving signalling via the type-I receptor and IL-6. The left side of the diagram shows the stimulatory growth factors and some of the cell cycle genes involved. The right side indicates some peptide inhibitory factors which participate in liver regeneration.

although neither of these procedures had an effect on DNA synthesis in normal livers. These authors coined the term 'priming' and suggested that the regulation of liver regeneration can be divided into reversible events that prepare the liver for regeneration and regeneration-specific events which are irreversible and lead the cell into DNA synthesis. The acceleration of DNA synthesis described by Moolten *et al.* probably occurred because surgical stress or growth hormone injection primed quiescent hepatocytes to enter the cell cycle. Thus, the interval of time between partial hepatectomy and the peak of DNA synthesis was shortened because, at the time of the operation, hepatocytes were already in the cell cycle. A similar situation may occur when rats or mice are deprived of protein for 2 to 3 days. Refeeding protein to these animals causes a wave of hepatocyte DNA synthesis (Leduc, AmJAnat, 1949; 84: 397; Short, BBResComm, 1973; 50:430; Bucher, CibaSymp, 1978; 55:95; Horikawa, BBResComm, 1986; 140:574; Mead, CancerRes, 1990; 50:7023). The interval of time between refeeding and maximal DNA synthesis is short and is approximately 9 to 10 h less than the

time necessary for strictly quiescent hepatocytes to achieve DNA synthesis. Hepatocytes from these protein-deprived rats also show accelerated DNA synthesis when placed in culture, another indication that they have become competent to proliferate.

There is now considerable evidence that cytokines such as tumour necrosis factor and interleukin-6 may play essential roles in the initiation of liver regeneration after partial hepatectomy (see below). Based on these results, we constructed two possible overall schemes for the priming and progression phases of liver regeneration (Fig. 8). In both cases the priming phase is presented as a reversible process, while in the progression phase hepatocytes can no longer return to strict quiescence without DNA replication. The difference between the two diagrams is that, on the left, cytokines are presented as having an effect on quiescent hepatocytes to initiate liver regeneration while growth factors act in primed hepatocytes, whereas the diagram on the right shows both cytokines and growth factors acting simultaneously to initiate regeneration.

Recent evidence implicating tumour necrosis factor and interleukin-6 as required factors for the initiation of liver regeneration

Tumour necrosis factor (**TNF**) has a relatively weak mitogenic effect on hepatocytes (Shinozuka, Hepatol, 1996; 23:1572). Yet, DNA synthesis after partial hepatectomy in rats can be partially blocked by TNF antibodies (Akerman, AmJPhysiol, 1992; 263: G579). These antibodies also inhibit the activity of Jun kinase in the first few hours after partial hepatectomy (Westwick, JCI, 1995; 95:803). TNF is a strong inducer of NF-κB in hepatocytes both *in vivo* and in culture. Injection of TNF in rats leads to a very large increase in the binding of NF-κB in the liver within 30 min after the injection (FitzGerald, CellGrowthDiff, 1995; 6:417). All of this evidence is highly suggestive that TNF may be an important participant in the initiation of liver regeneration (Decker, JGast-Hepatol, 1995; 10:512).

The most direct way to determine whether a specific gene is required for a biological process is to establish mouse lines in which the gene under study has been inactivated. Gene inactivation is produced by the technique of homologous recombination, performed in mouse embryonic stem cells (ES cells) in culture. The cells with the inactive gene are then used to construct chimeric mice which are bred to produce mouse lines which are homozygous for the inactive gene ('knockout mice'). To determine whether TNF might be involved in triggering liver regeneration Yamada *et al.* used a mouse line which is deficient in one of the receptors for TNF. This cytokine acts by binding to two separate receptors (there are other minor receptors for TNF) known as TNFR-I and TNFR-II (Smith, Cell, 1994; 76:959). The mice used in these experiments lack TNFR-I but have intact TNFR-II. Yamada *et al.* found that DNA synthesis after partial hepatectomy is severely inhibited in TNFR-I-deficient mice. In addition, the increase in the binding of NF-κB and STAT3 transcription factors, which normally occurs shortly after partial hepatectomy, is almost completely abolished in these animals (Yamada, ProcNatlAcadSci, 1997; 94:1441). An injection of interleukin-6 (**IL-6**) 30 min before partial hepatectomy completely corrected the DNA synthesis defect in TNFR-I-deficient mice. In addition, IL-6 restored to normal the STAT3 binding response after partial hepatectomy but had no effect on NF-κB binding. Work with knockout mice that lack IL-6 (Cressman, Science, 1996; 274:1379) demonstrated that these animals have deficient liver regeneration and that a high proportion of IL-6 deficient mice die after partial hepatectomy. In IL-6 knockout mice, STAT3 binding fails to occur after partial hepatectomy and a single injection of IL-6 corrects the DNA synthesis deficiency and restores STAT3 binding. These results establish that TNF, acting through TNFR-I, is required for the start of liver regeneration utilizing a signalling pathway that involves IL-6 and STAT3 activation and follows the following sequence:

$$TNF \rightarrow TNFR\text{-}I \rightarrow NF\text{-}κB \rightarrow IL\text{-}6 \rightarrow STAT3 \ldots\ldots \ DNA \ synthesis$$

It is interesting to note that TNF and IL-6 can have harmful effects on the liver, and that both cytokines are major mediators of the acute phase response (Gauldie, ResImmunol, 1992; 143:755; Baumann, ImmunolToday, 1994; 15:74). IL-6 can actually inhibit DNA synthesis in primary cultures of hepatocytes (Satoh, JCellPhysiol, 1992;

150:134). After partial hepatectomy, TNF and IL-6 production is transient (Trautwein, Gastro, 1996; 110:1854; Yamada, Hepatol, 1998, in press) and must be very carefully balanced so that gene activation rather than cytotoxic effects occur. Nevertheless, the results suggest that liver regeneration and the acute phase response may be started by a similar set of mediators. The regenerative and acute phase responses would then differ by the activation of different sets of secondary genes. During regeneration, proliferation-related genes predominate, while in the acute phase response, cell adhesion proteins, coagulation factors, and other proteins related to the inflammatory response constitute the major component.

It remains to be determined whether TNF initiation of liver regeneration through its type I receptor is the only pathway by which the process is triggered or if this pathway is one of several events which are required but not in themselves sufficient to induce DNA synthesis. It has been shown that deficiency of TNF type II receptor in mice has no effect on the timing and DNA synthesis after partial hepatectomy, although it delays the activation of some early genes and AP1 and C/EBP binding (Yamada, Hepatol, 1998, in press). Moreover the TNFR-1 pathway activated after partial hepatectomy involving NF-κB, IL-6, and STAT3 is also involved in liver regeneration induced by CCl$_4$ injury (Yamada, AmJPathol, 1998, in press). If activation of TNFR-I is the sole mode of triggering the regenerative process, growth factor effects could take place at later steps. There are at least three points in the cascade at which growth factors may act:

$$TNF \rightarrow TNFR\text{-}I \rightarrow NF\text{-}κB \rightarrow IL\text{-}6 \rightarrow STAT3 \ldots\ldots DNA \ synthesis$$

The site of action of growth factors is indicated by numbers in the diagram. HGF could act at site 1 because it may have direct interactions with IL-6. Indeed, the HGF gene contains an IL-6-binding sequence (Liu, JBC, 1994; 269:4152). An example of a growth factor acting on site 2 is the stimulation of EGF on STAT3 binding (Ruff-Jamison, JBC, 1994; 269:21933). Site 3 target genes are the cyclins and cell cycle genes. TGFα could act at this stage as it has been shown that this growth factor increases cyclin D expression in cultured hepatocytes (Koch, BBResComm, 1994; 204:91).

An alternative possibility is that TNF and HGF (or other growth factors) act simultaneously through parallel but interactive pathways to initiate liver regeneration. In this case, one of the growth factors effects would be to activate the transcription factor AP1, which can also be induced by TNF. An example of how simultaneous parallel pathways may initiate liver regeneration is given below:

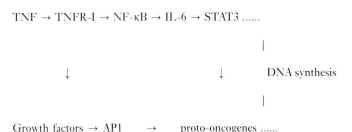

In any case, there is now strong evidence demonstrating that TNF is one of the factors that trigger liver regeneration and that its activation pathway involves TNFR-I, NF-κB, IL-6, and the transcription factor STAT3. In the presence of sufficient concentrations of IL-6, activation of NF-κB may not be required for hepatocyte DNA synthesis after partial hepatectomy.

LPS, TNF production, and the role of non-parenchymal cells

The liver produces both TNF and IL-6 in response to lipopolysaccharide (LPS or endotoxin), a structural component of the outer membrane of Gram-negative bacteria (Tran-Thi, EurCytokineNet, 1993; 4:363; Liao, AmJPhysiol, 1995; 37:R699; Colletti, Hepatol, 1996; 23:506). LPS is a mediator of toxicity in Gram-negative infections but it also has beneficial effects. It is normally produced by the bacterial flora of the gut, reaches the liver through the portal circulation and is cleared from the blood by Kupffer cells. Kupffer cells in primary culture produce TNF and IL-6 in response to LPS addition. In these cells LPS causes activation of both NF-κB and AP1 and blockage of NF-κB activation inhibits TNF production. The LPS effect on Kupffer cell NF-κB was quite rapid (starting at about 30 min after LPS addition) and persisted unchanged for 24 h. The AP1 response was biphasic with maximal levels at 30 min and 8 h after LPS addition. There are also data indicating that liver regeneration is delayed in mice which are resistant to LPS and in athymic and germ-free animals (Cornell, Hepatol, 1990; 11:923; Cornell, Hepatol, 1990; 11:916). Albrecht *et al.* (AmJPhysiol, 1993; 265:G857) recently demonstrated that in athymic nude mice, DNA synthesis as well as cyclin D activity is delayed after partial hepatectomy. Thus, it is plausible to assume that LPS carried in the portal vein could be the agent responsible for the increase in TNF immediately after partial hepatectomy and that Kupffer cells produce TNF and IL-6 to trigger regeneration. It is unlikely, however, that Kupffer cells constitute an exclusive site for the production of these cytokines in the liver. TNF can be produced by other non-parenchymal cells, while IL-6 may be synthesized by bile duct cells and hepatocytes. Nevertheless, these data strengthen the notion that hepatocyte proliferation *in vivo* requires close interaction between parenchymal and non-parenchymal cells. Indeed, the priming phase of liver regeneration after partial hepatectomy appears to depend primarily on cytokines produced by non-parenchymal cells. In addition to the production of cytokines, non-parenchymal cells are the source for HGF, TGFβ, and extracellular matrix components (Martinez-Hernandez, FASEBJ, 1995; 9:1401), molecules that may serve as signals for both the start and the termination of liver regeneration (Fig. 9).

Summarizing remarks

Despite the enormous complexity of the regenerative process, it is now possible to study it in an orderly fashion that fits into a sequential context. An outline of the major events of the process occurring during the priming and progression phases is presented in Fig. 10. There have been great advances in the understanding of the triggering mechanisms of liver regeneration after partial hepatectomy and of the role growth factors, proto-oncogenes, and transcription factors play in this process. This rapid progress should continue in the coming years and will be coupled to the application of these findings to clinical practice.

References

1. Fausto N and Webber EM. Liver regeneration. In Arias I, Boyer J, Fausto N, Jakoby W, Schachter D, and Shafritz D, eds. *The liver biology and pathobiology*. New York: Raven Press, 1994: 1059–84.
2. Bucher NLR. Liver regeneration then and now. In Jirtle RL, ed. *Liver regeneration and carcinogenesis: molecular and cellular mechanisms*. San Diego, CA: Academic Press, 1995: 1–25.
3. Fausto N. Hepatic regeneration. In Zakim D, and Boyer TD, eds. *Hepatology: a textbook of liver disease*, (3rd edn). Philadelphia: W.B. Saunders, 1996: 32–58.
4. Michalopoulos GK. Liver regeneration: molecular mechanisms of growth control. *FASEB Journal*, 1990; **4**: 176–87.
5. Fausto N and Mead JE. Regulation of liver growth: protooncogenes and transforming growth factors. *Laboratory Investigation*, 1989; **60**(1): 4–13.
6. Steer CJ. Liver regeneration. *FASEB Journal*, 1995; **9**: 1396–400.
7. Martinez-Hernandez A and Amenta PS. The extracellular matrix in hepatic regeneration. *FASEB Journal*, 1995; **9**: 1401–10.
8. Fausto N, Laird AD, and Webber EM. Role of growth factors and cytokines in hepatic regeneration. *FASEB Journal*, 1995; **9**: 1527–36.
9. Diehl AM and Rai RM. Regulation of signal transduction during liver regeneration. *FASEB Journal*, 1996; **10**: 215–27.
10. Taub R. Transcriptional control of liver regeneration. *FASEB Journal*, 1996; **10**: 413–27.
11. Taub R. Expression and function of growth-induced genes during liver regeneration. In Jirtle RL, ed. *Liver regeneration and carcinogenesis: molecular and cellular mechanisms*. New York: Academic Press, 1995: 71–97.
12. FitzGerald M, Webber E, Donovan J, and Fausto N. Rapid DNA binding by nuclear factor κB in hepatocytes at the start of liver regeneration. *Cell Growth and Differentiation*, 1995; **6**: 417–27.
13. Cressman DE, Greenbaum LE, Haber BA, and Taub R. Rapid activation of post-hepatectomy factor/nuclear factor κB in hepatocytes, a primary response in the regenerating liver. *Journal of Biological Chemistry*, 1994; **269**(48): 30429–35,
14. Webber EM, Godowski PJ, and Fausto N. *In vivo* response of hepatocytes to growth factors requires an initial priming stimulus. *Hepatology*, 1994; **19**(2): 489–97.
15. Akerman P, *et al.* Antibodies to tumor necrosis factor-α inhibit liver regeneration after partial hepatectomy. *American Journal of Physiology*, 1992; **263**(4): G579–G585,
16. Zarnegar R, DeFrances M, and Michalopoulos G. Hepatocyte growth factor: Its role in hepatic growth and pathobiology. In Arias L, Boyer J, Fausto N, Jakoby W, Schachter D, and Shafritz D, eds. *The liver: biology and pathobiology*. New York: Raven Press, 1994: 1047–57.
17. Mizuno K and Nakamura T. Molecular characteristics of HGF and the gene, and its biochemical aspects. In Goldberg ID and Rosen EM, eds. *Hepatocyte growth factor-scatter factor (HGF-SF) and the c-met receptor*. Basel: Birkhäuser Verlag, 1993: 1–29.
18. Matsumoto K and Nakamura T. Roles of HGF as a pleiotropic factor in organ regeneration. In Goldberg ID, and Rosen EM, eds. *Hepatocyte growth factor-scatter factor (HGF-SF) and the c-met receptor*. Basel: Birkhäuser Verlag, 1993: 226–49.
19. Grisham JW. A morphologic study of deoxyribonucleic acid synthesis and cell proliferation in regenerating rat liver; autoradiography with thymidine-H³. *Cancer Research*, 1962; **22**: 842–9.
20. Bucher NLR. Regeneration of mammalian liver. *International Review of Cytology*, 1963; **15**: 245–300.
21. Alison MR. Regulation of hepatic growth. *Physiological Reviews*, 1986; **66**: 500–41.

2.8.2 Apoptosis in the liver

Peter R. Galle and Martina Müller

Introduction

Apoptosis is a form of cell death which—in contrast to necrosis—is actively controlled. It serves as a mechanism to enable multicellular organisms to eliminate unwanted cells. The distinct morphological features of apoptosis were first described, in the early 1970s, as a form of cell death occurring in the liver after portal vein ligation (Kerr, JPath, 1971; 105:13). This biological phenomenon was suggested to be of general importance in the control of tissue kinetics and was termed apoptosis (Greek, meaning falling off).[3] However, it took about two decades before the importance of active cell death became generally accepted as a mechanism to control tissue and organ cellularity in concert with its functional counterpart, mitosis.

With the inclusion of apoptosis, as an active form of cell death, into the cell biological concepts of growth control and tissue kinetics, cell death is separated into two distinct processes: necrosis as the result of pathological stimuli leading to uncontrolled degradation and apoptosis as a gene-directed programme caused by physiological and pathological conditions.

The phenomenon of apoptosis

Morphological features, today recognized as being part of the apoptotic process, have been observed earlier in hepatopathology and terms such as shrinking necrosis, acidophil bodies, and Councilman bodies have been used to describe apoptotic hepatocytes before the term apoptosis was coined.[4]

Apoptosis is defined by distinct morphological changes which are, to various extents, accompanied by biochemical changes. Since the observed biochemical changes might not always be specific for apoptosis (Collins, IntJRadiatBiol, 1992; 61:451) morphological assessment still presents the 'gold standard' for the identification of apoptotic cell death.

Morphology of apoptosis

During the process of apoptosis[3] (Kerr, JPath, 1971; 105:13; Wyllie, Nature, 1980; 284:555) cells shrink and lose contact with their neighbouring cells. Chromatin condenses at the nuclear membrane and the nucleolus dissociates. At the same time the cytoplasm shows condensation and the formation of cytoplasmic blebs ('zeiosis'). Eventually fragmentation of cytoplasm and nucleus (Fig. 1) occurs resulting in membrane-bound, subcellular fragments, referred to as apoptotic bodies. Apoptotic bodies containing intact organelles are phagocytosed by neighbouring cells or specific macrophages.

An important feature of apoptosis is the maintainance of membrane integrity by the subcellular fragments, thus avoiding the liberation of potentially toxic intracellular contents, which explains the absence of an inflammatory response. In contrast, during necrosis as the result of severe trauma damaged cells swell, the membrane integrity is lost, and the resulting cytolysis elicits an

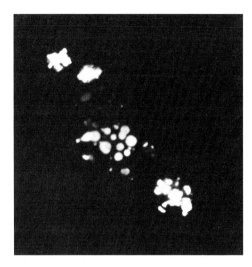

Fig. 1. Confocal laser scan microscopy of copper-treated HepG2 cells. TUNEL staining of the nuclei demonstrates typical features of apoptosis: intense nuclear staining due to DNA strand breaks and fragmentation of the nucleus into 'apoptotic bodies'.

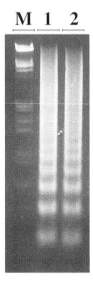

Fig. 2. Internucleosomal DNA fragmentation ('DNA laddering') of HepG2 cells after treatment with copper (1) or bleomycin (2). M = molecular weight; 1 = treatment of HepG2 cells with copper at a concentration of 100 µM; 2 = treatment of HepG2 cells with bleomycin at a concentration of 0.6 µg/ml.

inflammatory response.[5] It should be pointed out that both processes, apoptosis and necrosis, may occur in parallel, both contributing to cell death in liver diseases.

The extent of apoptotic cell death is frequently underestimated for the following reasons:

1. Apoptosis is a rapid event with an estimated duration of 2 to 3 h.[2]
2. Only scattered single cells may be affected and apoptotic bodies, which are readily eliminated, are small.

Biochemistry of apoptosis

Apoptotic cell death is accompanied by profound biochemical changes, including the degradation of cellular macromolecules.

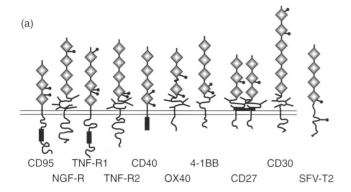

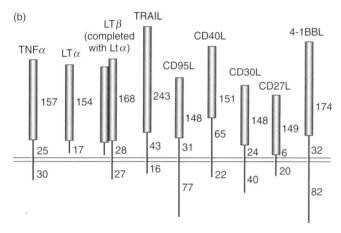

Fig. 3. The TNF/NGF receptor family and their respective ligands. (A) The TNF/NGF receptor family. Members include CD95, NGF receptor, TNF-R1, TNF-R2, B cell antigen CD40, T cell antigens OX40, 4-1BB, and CD27, Hodgkin's lymphoma antigen CD30, and the soluble protein coded by Shope fibroma virus (SFV-T2). The death domains (about 80 amino acids) in the cytoplasmic regions of CD95, TNF-R1, and CD40, which have some similarity are marked with the symbol ( ). The rectangles indicate cystein-rich subdomaines, the small symbols ° indicate N-glycosylation sites. (B) The TNF family. Members of the TNF family include TNF-α, CD95 ligand, TRAIL, the α and β subunit of lymphotoxin (LT), CD27 ligand, CD30 ligand, CD40 ligand, 4-1BB ligand, and OX40 ligand. The members of the TNF family are type II membrane proteins, except for the α subunit of lymphotoxin, which is a secretory protein. The shaded portion of each of the TNF family members is the extracellular region which shows significant similarity (25 to 30 per cent identity) among the members. The number of the amino acids in the homologous region and the cytoplasmic region are indicated.

Since these changes are not consistently observed, morphological assessment usually should be performed in parallel for identification and quantitation of apoptosis.

DNA degradation

Wyllie was the first to observe that glucocorticoid-induced apoptosis in lymphocytes was associated with endonuclease activity (Wyllie, Nature, 1980; 284:555), resulting in the fragmentation of genomic DNA into oligonucleosomes ('DNA ladder') (Fig. 2). This appears to take place in two steps:

1. DNA is cleaved into 300 and 50 kilo base (**kb**) fragments (Oberhammer, EMBOJ, 1993; 12:3679).

2. DNA is cleaved into 180 to 200 base pair (**bp**) fragments as the result of multiple single stranded nicks in the internucleosomal linker region (Hughes, CellDeathDiffer, 1994; 1:11).

The 300 and 50 kb fragments can be detected by pulse field electrophoresis (Walker, ExpCellRes, 1994; 351:150), whereas the small oligonucleosomal fragments can be detected by conventional agarose gel electrophoresis (Arends, AmJPathol, 1990; 136:593).

Interestingly, apoptosis can be induced in enucleated cells, suggesting that endonuclease activation, DNA degradation, or nuclear signalling are not necessary for the occurrence of programmed cell death (Schulze-Osthoff, JCellBiol, 1994, 127:15).

Transglutaminase

Tissue transglutaminase is a calcium-dependent enzyme which crosslinks lysine and glutamine residues. This enzyme seems to be specifically expressed in apoptotic cells (Fesus, FEBSLett, 1987; 224:104) and appears to be required for the formation of the rigid structure of the tightly sealed apoptotic bodies which contain extensively crosslinked proteins. An involucrin-like protein has been detected in liver (Tarcsa, JBC, 1992; 267:15648) which is crosslinked by transglutaminase, supporting the assumption of an involvement of transglutaminase in apoptosis of the liver. Cross-linking of involucrin and other proteins has been demonstrated during terminal differentiation of the skin and is believed to be important for mechanical stability.

Transglutaminase expression, which is not universally observed during apoptosis, is found in endothelial cells and smooth muscle cells of the liver and in hepatocytes only if they are undergoing apoptosis.[6] In endothelial cells, transglutaminase is capable of activating latent transforming growth factor-β, demonstrating an additional role of transglutaminase in the signalling of apoptosis (Kojima, JCellBiol, 1993; 121:439).

Changes at the cell surface

An inherent part of the apoptotic programme is the rapid phago-cytotic uptake of apoptotic bodies, a process which requires the recognition of these subcellular fragments. Several different membrane markers are expressed on the outer surface of apoptotic cells which are required for phagocytosis (Savill, ImmunolToday, 1993; 14:131).

Whereas in thymocytes outside exposure of phosphatidylserine, usually detectable only at the inner layer of the membrane, is a signal for removal, in liver cells the asialoglycoprotein receptor (Dini, FEBSLett, 1992; 296:174; Dini, EurJCellBiol, 1993; 61:329) mediates clearance of apoptotic cells.

Proteases

Apoptosis is accompanied by the proteolytic breakdown of structural proteins and proteins involved in signalling.[7] The respective enzymes involved, their substrate specificity, and their specific roles in the biochemical and morphological changes of apoptosis are complex and require further elucidation. Genetic studies in the nematode *Caenorhabditis elegans* resulted in the identification of a cysteine protease, cell death defective-3 (**Ced-3**), that is related to mammalian interleukin-1β-converting enzyme (**ICE**) (Miura, Cell, 1993; 75:563) which is essential for cell death. Among the identified

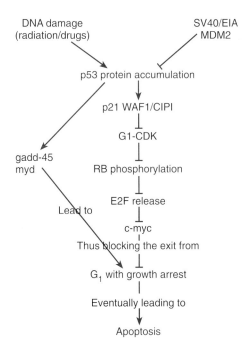

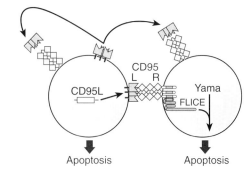

Fig. 5. A model of CD95-mediated apoptosis in toxic injury of hepatocytes. Toxic agents such as ethanol, copper, bleomycin, etc. turn on hepatocytic CD95 ligand (CD95L) expression inducing apoptosis via the CD95 receptor (CD95R) in an autocrine or paracrine fashion.

Fig. 4. Cell cycle arrest, DNA repair, and apoptosis induced by DNA damage. DNA damage induces p53 protein accumulation. p53 regulates genes involved in apoptosis, cell cycle arrest, and DNA synthesis and repair. Depending on the extent of DNA damage, p53 modulates G_1 growth arrest or apoptosis. (WAF-1, wild-type p53 activated factor; CDK, cyclin dependent kinases; gadd-45, growth arrest and DNA damage factor).

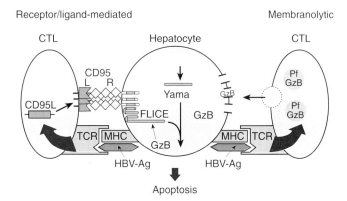

Fig. 6. A model of hepatocyte apoptosis in viral hepatitis B. This graph depicts elimination of hepatitis B virus positive hepatocytes by cytotoxic T lymphocytes via the CD95 or perforin (Pf)/granzyme B (GzB) systems.

substrates of ICE/Ced-3 proteases are poly-(ADP-ribose) polymerase (PARP), DNA-dependent protein kinase (DNA-PK), histone H1, lamins, fodrin, actins, delta isoform of protein kinase C (PKC δ), and the 70 kDa component of the U1 small nuclear ribonucleoprotein.

Overexpression in mammalian cells of ICE, the first of the ICE/Ced-3 proteases to be discovered, leads to apoptosis (Miura, Cell, 1993; 75:563). In humans, at least eight cysteine proteases homologous to Ced-3 have been identified so far.[8] Potent, specific inhibitors are available preventing apoptosis *in vitro* (Nicholson, Nature, 1995; 376:37) providing the potential for therapeutic intervention.

Mechanisms of suicidal cell death

Many different signals that may originate either from within or outside a cell have been shown to influence the decision between life and death. Various agents have been reported to stimulate (Table 1) or inhibit (Table 2) apoptosis.

Apoptosis allows the elimination of cells that have been produced in excess, developed improperly, or have sustained genetic damage. Molecular regulation of apoptosis can be classified as follows:

(1) signals initiating apoptosis (Table 1);
(2) receptor-mediated signal transduction;
(3) intracellular biochemical signalling pathways;
(4) genes involved in the regulation of apoptosis;
(5) genes that inhibit apoptosis.

However, it appears that the different signalling pathways ultimately converge to activate a common apoptotic programme.

The expression of antiapoptotic proteins, such as Bcl-2 and baculovirus p35, can inhibit apoptosis in response to many different death-inducing signals. This indicates that these proteins interact with components that are either shared among different signalling pathways or act downstream from the convergence point of these pathways.

Receptor-mediated signal transduction CD95 (Fas/APO-1)

Two cell surface cytokine receptors, CD95 (Fas/APO-1) and TNF-R1 (reviewed in references 1–10), have been shown to trigger apoptosis by their natural ligands or specific agonist antibodies. Both death receptors are members of the tumour necrosis factor (**TNF**)/nerve growth factor (**NGF**) receptor family, which also includes TNF-R2, low affinity NGFR, CD40, and CD30, among others. While family members are defined by the presence of cysteine-rich repeats in their extracellular domains, CD95 and TNF-R1 also share an intracellular region of homology, designated the 'death domain', required to signal apoptosis (Fig. 3).

Table 1 Inducers of apoptosis

Physiological inducers	Damage-related inducers	Autoimmune-related inducers	Therapy-associated agents	Toxins
1. Fas ligand	1. Viral infection (HBV, HCV)	1. Cytolic T cells	1. Gamma radiation	1. Alcohol-mediated liver injury
2. TNF	2. Bacterial toxins	2. Autoimmune hepatitis	2. UV radiation	2. Bile salt-induced hepatotoxicity during acute and chronic cholestasis
3. TGF-β	3. Oxygen radicals and oxydative stress	3. Primary biliary cirrhosis	3. Chemotherapeutic drugs bleomycin, doxorubicin, methotrexate, vincristine, topoisomerase inhibitors	3. β-Amyloid peptide
4. Calcium	4. Free radicals	4. Primary sclerosing cholangitis		4. Dimethylnitrosamine
5. Glucocorticoids	5. Nutrient deprivation	5. Allograft rejection after (liver) transplantation		5. *N*-nitrosomorpholine
6. Tissue hyperplasia	6. Cytolic T cells			6. Ethionine diet
7. Withdrawal of growth factors or trophic hormones	7. Tumour suppressors *P53*			7. Galactosamine
8. Cell damage	8. Oncogenes *C-FOS, JUN, MYC, REL, E1A*			8. Paracetamol (acetaminophen)
9. In embryogenesis: developmental programme	9. Interruption of the portal blood supply (liver)			
10. Loss of matric attachment	10. Heat shock			
11. Neurotransmitters glutamate dopamine *N*-methyl-D-aspartate				
12. Ceramide				
13. Activin				
14. cAMP				

Table 2 Inhibitors of apoptosis

Physiological inhibitors	Genes	Viral genes	Pharmacological agents
1. CD40 ligand	1. *BCL-2*	1. Adenovirus E1b	1. Tumour promoters—PMA, phenobarbital (PB), α-hexachlorocyclohexane (α-HCH)
2. Extracellular matrix	2. *PRB*	2. Herpesvirus γ1 34.5	2. Cysteine protease inhibitors
3. Growth factors		3. Epstein–Barr virus BHRF1, LMP-1	3. Calpain inhibitors
4. Oestrogens		4. Cowpox virus crmA	4. Hepatomitogens, nafe-nopin, PB, α-HCH, cyproterone acetate
5. Androgens		5. Baculovirus p35	
6. Zinc		6. Baculovirus IAP	
7. Neutral amino acids		7. African swine fever virus LMW5-HL	

Table 3 Methods for the detection of apoptosis

Characteristics of apoptosis	Experimental techniques
Morphological features	

Cytoplasmic blebs	Phase contrast microscopy
	  Bleb formation, cell shrinkage, and convolution of the cell membrane can be identified on phase
	  contrast microscopy.
	Scanning electron microscopy

Chromatin condensation and nuclear fragmentation	Light microscopy or phase contrast microscopy
	
	Fluorescence microscopy
	  DNA-binding dyes such as DAPI or DNA labelling by the TUNEL method can identify patterns of
	  chromatin condensation and nuclear fragmentation.
	Flow cytometry
	  Two distinct features of apoptotic cells (extensive DNA cleavage and preservation of the cell
	  membrane) provide the basis for the development of most flow cytometric assays to discriminate
	  between apoptosis and necrosis. Apoptotic cells show reduced DNA stainability. Alternatively, DNA
	  strand breaks in apoptotic cells can be labelled with biotinylated or digoxigenin-conjugated
	  nucleosides employing exogenous terminal deoxynucleotidyl transferase (TdT) or DNA polymerase
	  (nick translation).

Cellular ultrastructure	Transmission electron microscopy
	  Characteristic ultrastructural features of apoptosis such as intact organelles, cytoplasmic blebs,
	  chromatin condensation, and nuclear fragmentation can be identified.

Apoptotic bodies	Electron microscopy and all methods indicated above
	  Apoptotic bodies can be isolated on the basis of their insolubility in detergents, urea, and guanidine
	  hydrochloride and analysed by electron microscopy.

Molecular features	

DNA cleavage	Agarose gel electrophoresis
	  Identification of a ladder pattern indicative of internucleosomal cleavage is often detected during
	  apoptosis.
	Field inversion gel electrophoresis
	  Identification of 50-kb or 300-kb fragments
	Terminal deoxynucleotidyl transferase-mediated deoxyuridine triphosphate nick-end labelling
	  End labelling of 3-OH ends of cleaved DNA fragments using terminal deoxyribonucleotide transferase,
	  and biotin- or fluorescent-labelled nucleotides.
	In situ nick translation
	  Identification of DNA single strand breaks *in situ* using DNA polymerase-mediated incorporation of
	  labelled nucleotides.

Gene expression	Immunohistochemistry, PCR analysis, *in situ* hybridization, Western blotting
	  Detection of mRNA or protein of genes implicated during apoptosis, such as tissue transglutaminase,
	  TRPM-2, and RP-8.

Human CD95 consists of 325 amino acids with a signal sequence at the NH_2-terminus and a membrane-spanning region in the middle of the molecule, indicating that CD95 is a type I membrane protein. In humans, the *CD95* gene is located on the long arm of chromosome 10, whereas in the mouse the gene is on chromosome 19. CD95 is highly expressed in activated mature lymphocytes, or lymphocytes transformed with human T cell leukaemia virus, human immunodeficiency virus, or Epstein–Barr virus. Many non-lymphoid tissues, such as liver, are CD95 receptor positive (Galle, JExpMed, 1995; 182:1223; Ogasawara, Nature, 1993; 364:806; Owen-Schaub, CancerRes, 1994; 54:1580).

Triggering this pathway requires the crosslinking of CD95 either with agonistic antibodies, with cells expressing CD95L (see following section), or with purified CD95L.

CD95L

CD95L (Suda, Cell, 1993; 75:1169) is a 40 kDa, type II trans-membrane protein that mediates apoptosis in sensitive target cells. CD95L is expressed by activated T cells and has been shown to play a role in the maintenance of peripheral T and B cell homeo-stasis. CD95L can be proteolytically cleaved from the membrane

by a metalloprotease and occurs in a soluble form. Thus, CD95L may act as a cytotoxic effector molecule at a distance from the producer cell (Mariani, EurJImmun, 1995; 25:2303).

The CD95-mediated apoptotic cascade is initiated by the direct association of the death receptor CD95 with the adapter molecule, termed Fas-associated protein with death domain (**FADD**), and the effector protease, termed FADD homologous ICE/Ced-3-like protease = FADD-like ICE (**FLICE**), a novel member of the ICE/Ced-3 family (Muzio, Cell, 1996; 85:817). The assembly of this signalling complex occurs in a hierarchical manner upon receptor activation. The death domain of the receptor binds to the death domain of the adapter molecule FADD, which, in a manner that remains to be determined, binds and activates FLICE to generate the most apical enzymatic component of a death cascade composed of other ICE/Ced-3 family members.

TNF-R1, TNF-R2, and TNF

While the main activity of CD95 is to trigger cell death, TNF-R1 can signal a diverse range of activities, including fibroblast proliferation, resistance to intracellular pathogens including chlamydiae, synthesis of prostaglandin E2, inflammation, tumour necrosis, differentiation, and apoptosis (Liu, Cell, 1996; 87:565).

TNF is a cytokine produced by many cell types, including macrophages, monocytes, lymphoid cells, and fibroblasts, in response to inflammation, infection, and other environmental challenges. TNF elicits a wide spectrum of cellular responses, including fever, shock, tissue injury, tumour necrosis, anorexia, induction of other cytokines and immunoregulatory molecules, cell proliferation, differentiation, and apoptosis (Vandenabeele, TrendsCellBiol, 1995; 5:392).[11] These responses are mediated by TNF-induced trimerization of two distinct cell surface receptors, TNF-R1 (p55) and TNF-R2 (p75), at least one of which is present in almost every cell (Tartaglia, ImmunolToday, 1992; 13:151; Vandenabeele, Trends-CellBiol, 1995; 5:392).[12] The structural similarity between the two TNF receptors is limited to their extracellular domains (Tartaglia, ImmunolToday, 1992; 13:151). The TNFR ectodomains are related to those of CD30, CD40, CD27, and CD95, all of which belong to the TNF receptor superfamily. The ligands for these receptors are structurally related to TNF and many of them are cell-surface anchored.[12] Although most of the biological activities of TNF appear to be transduced by TNF-R1, many can also be mediated by TNF-R2 (Tartaglia, ImmunolToday, 1992; 13:151; Vandenabeele, TrendsCellBiol, 1995; 5:392).[12] TNF-R2, however, is a poor inducer of apoptosis.

Exposure to TNF results in activation of two transcription factors, AP-1 (Brenner, Nature, 1989; 337:661) and NF-κB (Osborn, PNAS, 1989; 86:2336). Following ligand-induced trimerization (Rothe, Cell, 1994; 78:681) TNF-R1, like CD95, recruits a multivalent adapter molecule, termed TNF-R1- associated death domain protein (**TRADD**), which, like FADD, contains a death domain required for receptor association. TRADD has been shown to bind a number of signalling molecules, including FADD, TNFR-associated protein 2 (**TRAF2**), and RIP. While activation of TNF-R1 results in recruitment of TRADD, triggering of TNF-R2 leads to recruitment of TRAF1 and TRAF2.

As the death domains of TNF-R1 and also CD95 are protein–protein interaction domains, they recruit the other signalling proteins (TRADD, FADD, and RIP) to the trimerized receptors. While FADD activates the apoptotic machinery, two other signals, TRAF2 and RIP, mediate NF-κB activation. In addition to its death domain, FADD has a death effector N-terminal domain, which recruits the ICE-like protease MACH/FLICE to activated receptor complexes. This seems to be the critical step in activation of the proapoptotic protease cascade.

The TNF-R1 signalling complex leads to activation of at least three effector functions: the protein kinase JNK, the transcription factor NF-κB, and induction of apoptosis. This multiplicity of effector functions may explain why TNF-R1 can transduce a large number of diverse biological functions. While TNF-induced apoptosis is most likely to be mediated via FADD-induced MACH/FLICE recruitment and activation of the proapoptotic protease cascade, JNK and NF-κB activation are mediated via TRAF2 and RIP recruitment. JNK activation probably induces AP-1. Together with NF-κB, AP-1 is likely to mediate induction of other cytokines and immunoregulatory molecules by TNF, leading to a variety of inflammatory responses.

As TRAF2 is also recruited to TNF-R2 and CD40, these receptors also lead to activation of NF-κB, JNK, and AP-1 mediated responses. Most importantly, NF-κB can protect against TNF-induced apoptosis. However, these receptors do not recruit FADD or other death domain proteins and therefore are unable to affect apoptosis as TNF-R1 and CD95 do. Indeed, a receptor such as CD95, which recruits FADD but not TRAF2, is unable to mediate inflammatory responses via JNK and NF-κB activation. As NF-κB activation protects cells against apoptosis, the inability of CD95 to induce NF-κB may explain why it is a more effective apoptosis inducer than TNF-R1 (Liu, Cell, 1996; 87:565; Beg, Science, 1996; 274:782; Wang, Science, 1996; 274:784; Van Antwerp, Science, 1996; 274:787).

TRAIL

The TNF-related apoptosis-inducing ligand (**TRAIL**) (Wiley, Immunity, 1995; 3:673; Pitti, JBC, 1996; 271:12687; Marsters, CurrBiol, 1996; 6:750), another member of the TNF family, was first cloned and characterized in 1995 (Wiley, Immunity, 1995; 3: 673). TRAIL consists of 281 and 291 amino acids in the human and murine forms, respectively, which share 65 per cent amino acid identity.

TRAIL is a type II membrane protein, whose C-terminal extracellular domain shows clear homology to other TNF family members. The *TRAIL* gene is located on chromosome 3 at position 3q26, which is not close to any other known TNF ligand family members. Both full length cell surface expressed TRAIL and picomolar concentrations of soluble TRAIL rapidly induce apoptosis in a wide variety of transformed cell lines of diverse origin. TRAIL transcripts are detected in a variety of human tissues, most predominantly in spleen, lung, and prostate. Trail has the characteristics of a type II membrane protein, that is no leader sequence and an internal transmembrane domain. Also, like other TNF family ligands, TRAIL has an N-terminal (cytoplasmic) domain which is not conserved across family members, while the C-terminal (extracellular) domains show significant conservation.[12] TRAIL has been shown to induce apoptosis in various cell lines characterized by blebbing of the cellular membrane, disruption of the cytoskeleton, fragmentation of DNA into 180 bp multimers, and decimation of metabolic activity.

TGF-β

Transforming growth factor-β1 (**TGF-β1**), a potent growth inhibitor, can induce growth arrest and apoptosis in many cell types (Fan, Oncogene, 1996; 12:1909; Oberhammer, PNAS, 1992; 89: 5408). TGF-β1 has been implicated in inducing cell death in hepatocytes (Oberhammer, Hepatol, 1993; 18:1238; Oberhammer, PNAS, 1992; 89:5408; Oberhammer, Hepatol, 1996; 23:329; Oberhammer, Carcinogenesis, 1995; 16:1363) and the Morris hepatoma cell line McA-RH7777 (Fukuda, Hepatol, 1993; 18:945). It has been shown that various epithelial and mesenchymal cell lines respond to TGF-β1 by slowing progression through the late G_1 phase of the cell cycle. Three isoformes, TGF-β1, TGF-β2, and TGF-β3, have been cloned from cDNA libraries derived from mammalian cells (Sanderson, PNAS, 1995; 92:2572). TGF-β1 is the best characterized of the three isoforms and is generally regarded as the prototype of the TGF-β family. TGF-β1 is biologically active as a 25-kDa homodimer linked by disulphide bonds and is a highly

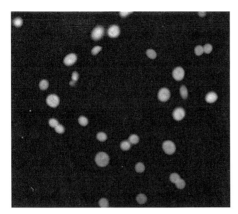

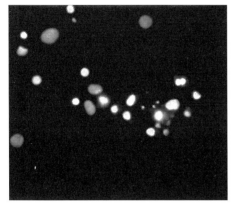

Fig. 7. Apoptosis in primary human hepatocytes after CD95 stimulation. DAPI (4′,6-diamidino-2-phenylindole) staining of DNA in untreated controls (A) and in primary human hepatocytes treated with 100 ng/ml anti-APO-1 (B) for 4.5 h. The CD95-stimulated hepatocytes in B show intense nuclear condensation and fragmentation.

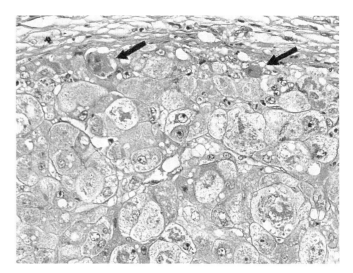

Fig. 8. Haematoxylin stain of a liver biopsy of a patient with chronic active hepatitis B virus infection. The arrows indicate hepatocytes undergoing apoptosis with condensation of the cytoplasm and formation of cytoplasmic blebs.

conserved molecule whose specific high-affinity receptors are present on essentially all cells. TGF-β1 is expressed in most tissues, with the highest concentrations found in bone and blood platelets. TGF-β1 is stored in, and secreted from, a variety of cell types as a biologically inactive, latent, high molecular weight complex incapable of binding to its receptors. Latent TGF-β1 remains inactive under neutral conditions but can be activated *in vitro* by acid, alkali, urea, heat, or proteases. The latent complex is activated extracellularly *in vivo* by a mechanism that is not fully characterized. This conversion into biologically active forms may constitute an important regulatory mechanism by which TGF-β1 activity is controlled *in vivo*.

The concentration of TGF-β1 is increased during carbon tetra-chloride-induced rat liver fibrosis and in other models of experimental liver fibrosis, such as murine schistosomiasis and following hepatic irradiation, and in cirrhotic human livers. These results suggest that TGF-β1 acts *in vivo* as a powerful stimulus for collagen formation during chronic tissue injury (Sanderson, PNAS, 1995; 92:2572).

Genes in apoptosis

Although diverse signals can induce apoptosis in a wide variety of cell types and tissues, a number of evolutionarily conserved genes regulate a final common cell death pathway that is conserved from worms to humans. Indeed, much of our current knowledge about

specific cell death genes has been derived from genetic studies in the nematode *Caenorhabditis elegans*.

Numerous overall similarities between apoptosis and the cell cycle have been noted, and it has been suggested that apoptosis and mitosis may be mechanistically related or even coupled. Support for a connection between apoptosis and mitosis has come from genes that play a role both in the regulation of cell proliferation and in the control of apoptosis, such as *P53*, *C-MYC*, *RB-1*, *E1A*, *CYCLIN D1*, *C-FOS*, and *P34*^{CDC2} kinase.

Proapoptotic genes (death genes)

p53

P53 mutations are the most common genetic alterations observed in human cancers. Of the approximately 6.5 million cancer cases worldwide each year, 2.4 million tumours are estimated to contain a *P53* mutation.[13,14] Inactivation of the wild-type *P53* gene through deletion or point mutation plays a critical role in the development of a large variety of human tumours, including hepatocellular carcinoma (e.g. Volkmann, Oncogene, 1994; 9:195). The principal function of *P53* appears to be in mediating the cellular response to DNA damage, thereby preventing accumulation of potentially oncogenic mutations and genomic instability.[15] This role of p53, as guardian of the genome (Lane, Nature, 1992; 358: 15), provides the basis for its tumour-suppressive activities. Both G_1 cell cycle arrest (Kastan, CancerRes, 1991; 51:6304; Kuerbitz, PNAS, 1992; 89:7491; Kastan, Cell, 1992; 71:587) and apoptosis[16, 17] (Clarke, Nature, 1993; 362:849; Lotem, Blood, 1993; 82:1092; Lowe, Nature, 1993; 362:847) were shown to depend on normal p53 function. The p53 protein senses genotoxic stress or DNA damage. This results in nuclear accumulation of p53. Subsequently, p53 activates the transcription of several genes whose products are involved in DNA repair or apoptosis (Fig. 4). Some of the genes regulated by p53 have been identified. These include genes coding for muscle creatinine kinase, gadd-45, waf-1/cip-1, Bcl-2/bax , cyclin G, mdm2, TGF-α, IGF-binding protein, and CD95[13]

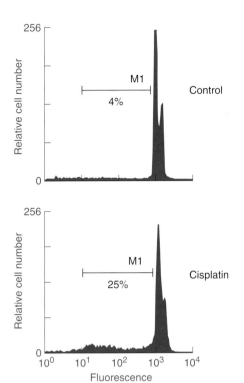

Fig. 9. Fluorescence-activated cell sorting (FACS) analysis of HepG2 cells treated with the anticancer agent cisplatin at 1 μg/ml for 24 h. The cells were washed with phosphate buffered saline, fixed in 70 per cent ethanol, and stained with propidium iodide (50 μg/ml phosphate buffered saline). DNA fluorescence was measured in a FACScan according to the method of Nicoletti (Nicoletti, JImmunolMethods, 1991; 139:271). The area M1 indicates less intensely stained apoptotic hepatocytes.

(Kastan, CancerRes, 1991; 51:6304; Kuerbitz, PNAS, 1992; 89: 7491; Kastan, Cell, 1992; 71:587; Barak, EMBOJ, 1993; 12:461; Chen, PNAS, 1994; 91:2684; El-Deiry, Cell, 1993; 75:817; Smith, Science, 1994; 266:1376; Müller, JCI, 1997; 99:403). The *WAF1/CIP1* gene, whose gene product, p21, blocks cyclin-dependent kinases, is activated by p53. p53 also activates *GADD45*, a gene whose product is involved in DNA repair.

MYC

Expression of c-myc has been associated with cell growth and proliferation.[18] Expression of c-myc is necessary for entry into the S phase of the cell cycle, and shutoff of c-myc expression is associated with cellular quiescence. Aberrant expression of c-myc has been implicated in carcinogenesis. C-myc expression has also been linked to apoptosis. Expression of c-myc in hepatoma cells results in cell death exhibiting apoptotic features. The molecular mechanisms mediating these opposite functions of the c-myc protein remain unclear. Myc dimerizes with its partner protein Max to bind DNA and dimerization is involved in both cell cycle progression as well as apoptosis.

Antiapoptotic genes
BCL-2

Bcl-2, a protein found on intracellular membranes, is a potent inhibitor of apoptosis.[19] Bcl-2 was first described in studies of

B-cell lymphoma located near to the breakpoint of t(14:18) (q32: q21) translocations (Tsujimoto, PNAS, 1986; 83:5214). Over-expression of Bcl-2 (or its homologue in *C. elegans*, Ced-9) leads to the survival of cells that would ordinarily die. Normally, cells need signalling molecules secreted by other cells to avoid apoptosis. Otherwise they die by default. This death-by-default mechanism can be blocked by Bcl-2. The precise mechanism by which it inhibits apoptosis remains unclear.

In the adult gastrointestinal tract,[20] Bcl-2 is predominantly expressed on cholangiocytes (bile duct epithelium), colonic epithelial cells, and pancreatic ductal epithelium (Krajewski, AmJPathol, 1994; 145:1323). *BCL-2* is regulated by the *BCL2* family of genes, including *BCLl-X*, *BAX*, *BAK*, and *BAD*. While Bcl-x also inhibits apoptosis, Bad, Bak, and Bax can dimerize with Bcl-2 or Bcl-x, inhibiting their function and thereby promoting apoptosis. Although the tissue-specific expression of Bak, Bad, and Bcl-x remains incompletely characterized, Bax has been identified in the liver, pancreas, stomach, and small and large intestine.

The tumour suppressor p53, implicated in the induction of both growth arrest and apoptosis following DNA damage, is a positive regulator of Bax expression and a negative regulator of Bcl-2 expression.

Regulation of apoptosis under physiological and pathological conditions

Programmed cell death seems to be a very old and basic process, since it has been observed in eukaryotic unicellular organisms and bacteria. It may have originated several times independently, with the basic function of removing virally infected cells in order to protect other cells from infection, and might have been included, at later stages, into developmental programmes. The diversification of programmed cell death into different functions could explain why so many different extracellular agents can trigger the same suicide programme.

In vertebrate tissues, the fate of a cell is determined by neighbouring cells. Cells kill themselves unless they are continuously signalled by other cells not to do so. If a vertebrate cell is taken out of its natural environment (e.g. for cell culture) and is not supplemented with growth and survival factors, it will die. Cells exert 'social control' over each other's death. In such a way, half of the vertebrate nerve cells die during development without nerve growth factor. Cells survive only where they are needed and behave in a co-ordinated fashion.

Regulation of apoptosis under physiological conditions

In normal liver apoptosis is a rare event. In rodents about one to five apoptotic cells per 10 000 hepatocytes are found (Bursch, VirchArchCP, 1985; 50:153) and these are preferentially located in zone 3 around the hepatic venules (Benedetti, JHepatol, 1988; 7: 319). It has been proposed that hepatocytes originate from the portal area and progress towards the perivenular region ('streaming liver') where they are eliminated via apoptosis.[21] It should be noted, however, that cell death is neither a prominent feature in the normal adult nor in developing embryonic liver[4] and the role of apoptosis in morphogenesis and homeostasis in the liver remains to be determined.

Adaptive liver growth

As an adaptive response to increased functional demand, rodent liver enlarges due to both hypertrophy and hyperplasia after treatment with a wide range of drugs or after contact with a variety of environmental pollutants.[2] A similar response is observed in overfeeding, pregnancy, or during severe protein loss. Once the stimulus (e.g. phenobarbital) is removed, the liver returns to its normal size by removing excessive hepatocytes via apoptotic cell death. TGF-β1 seems to be involved during liver involution (Oberhammer, ToxicolLett, 1992; 64:701).

Nutritional influence on apoptosis

The size of the liver and the degree of apoptotic cell death is also determined by the type and amount of food consumed (Grasl-Kraupp, PNAS, 1994; 91:9995). Food restriction causes reduction in liver mass and cell loss by apoptosis. In rodents, a higher rate of apoptosis is observed at the end of the daily light (fasting) period than at the end of the night (feeding) period, an observation which should be considered in experimental protocols.

Regulation of apoptosis under pathological conditions

Apoptosis not only occurs under physiological conditions but it is also an inherent part of liver disease. It should be noted (see 'Morphology of apoptosis' above) that apoptosis has been underestimated in the past and frequently the term necrosis has been used to describe cell death irrespective of the mechanism. Terms currently used such as 'piecemeal necrosis' and others to describe cell death might be inadequate and might actually describe apoptosis. It is also important to note that both apoptosis and necrosis may occur at the same time. The increasing interest in apoptosis has resulted in an increased appreciation of this phenomenon as a relevant factor in liver disease.[22]

Toxic and metabolic liver injury

Several drugs and toxins or their metabolites can cause liver injury both by necrosis and/or by apoptosis.[23] Hepatotoxic agents can be classified into type I agents, with predictable, dose dependent effects, and type II agents, where adverse reactions occur only in some subjects and in an unpredictable manner. For many hepatotoxic substances, evidence for induction of apoptosis has been obtained. This includes ethanol (Benedetti, JHepatol, 1988; 7: 319; Galle, JExpMed, 1995; 182:1223), acetaminophen (Tsukidate, AmJPathol, 1993; 143:918), bile salts (Patel, JCI, 1994; 94:2183), cytostatic drugs (Müller, JCI, 1997; 99:403), and many others.

Recent experimental data point to the possible involvement of the CD95 system in toxic liver damage. In alcoholic cirrhosis hepatocytes could be demonstrated to produce high levels of CD95 ligand mRNA. Since hepatocytes bear the CD95 receptor and are highly sensitive to CD95 stimulation (Ogasawara, Nature, 1993; 364:806; Galle, JExpMed, 1995; 182:1223), one CD95 ligand-expressing hepatocyte might kill another by induction of apoptosis (Fig. 5). Similar data have been obtained for cytostatic agents *in vitro* (Müller, JCI, 1997; 99:403) but also for copper-loaded hepatocytes in Wilson disease (Strand, in preparation). Thus, activation of the CD95 receptor and ligand system might represent a universal response of hepatocytes to toxic injury which eventually results in removal of damaged cells by apoptosis.

Viral liver disease and immune-mediated liver disease

Apoptosis in the liver has been observed during viral infection (Roberts, Gastro, 1993; 26:37).[24] Councilman bodies, a characteristic pathological feature in viral hepatitis, closely resemble apoptotic cells or fragments. Apoptosis as the result of viral infection is conceivable either as direct cytopathic effect or as a result of the host immune response. These two effects may not be easily differentiated and may be present at the same time. Since tissue culture systems for the cultivation of the hepatitis viruses A–G are not readily available, direct cytopathic effects are difficult to study.

Experimental data from hepatitis B virus transgenic animals demonstrated apoptosis as the result of cytotoxic T-lymphocyte activity (Ando, JExpMed, 1993; 178:1541). Cytotoxicity is mediated via the CD95 and the perforin systems and the CD95 ligand is expressed in T cells upon activation. The CD95 receptor is constitutively expressed in liver cells. Therefore, activated T cells might kill hepatitis B virus antigen-expressing hepatocytes by CD95 ligand/receptor interaction and, thus, clear hepatitis B virus from the liver. This is supported by experimental data from explanted livers of hepatitis B virus-infected patients showing colocalization of CD95 ligand mRNA and lymphocytic infiltration (Galle, JExpMed, 1995; 182:1223). It has been suggested that activated T killer cells may kill hepatitis B virus-infected hepatocytes using the CD95 system (Fig. 6). A different degree of CD95-mediated cytotoxicity may account for various disease stages. Such different levels of cytotoxicity may explain ineffective viral clearance in chronic hepatitis, regular clearance in acute, self-limiting hepatitis, or over-effective clearance in fulminant hepatitis. Indeed, in chronic hepatitis B virus-induced liver failure a poor response to hepatitis B virus antigens has been described for MHC class I and II restricted T cells.

Elimination of virus-infected cells by apoptosis may be counteracted by viral-encoded proteins which may permit ongoing viral replication and might even be required for the establishment of chronicity. Indeed, several viral proteins such as the Cowpox protein (CrmA) have been described which abrogate apoptotic programmes.[25]

The histopathological features of viral hepatitis B and autoimmune hepatitis are similar. As in viral hepatitis, autoimmune hepatitis shows lymphocytic infiltration and cell death by apoptosis with the pattern of 'piecemeal necrosis'. The precise mechanisms remain to be determined.

Another form of immune-mediated liver disease is the host-versus-graft reaction in allograft rejection. This is accompanied by lymphocytic infiltration, apoptotic cell death, and upregulation of apoptosis-associated factors such as TGF-β1 (Krams, Transpl, 1995; 59:621).

Hepatocarcinogenesis

Cancer results in excessive accumulation of cells. This may be the result of enhanced cell proliferation or of reduced cell death, or both. It is becoming increasingly recognized that the different stages of multistep carcionogenesis, from the initial genotoxic insult (initiation), through development from a premalignant population to a tumour (promotion), to further clonal expansion (progression), may involve genes regulating cell death.[2] This is supported by the observation that the actual growth rate of tumours is indeed slower than expected from the proliferation kinetics, suggesting a certain rate of ongoing apoptosis.

In hepatocarcinogenesis, initiated cells as well as preneoplastic and neoplastic cell populations show enhanced cell proliferation but also an increased rate of apoptosis.[26] Interestingly, tumour promoters, that is substances which shorten the time span between initiation and appearance of a tumour, shift the balance between birth and death by increasing the rate of proliferation and by decreasing the rate of apoptosis. Cessation of tumour promoter treatment results in enhanced apoptotic activity and in remodelling of preneoplastic foci. Thus, apoptosis might be a means of removal of preneoplastic cells and might thus protect from development of clinically detectable tumours.

We recently observed a frequent loss of CD95 in human hepatocellular carcinoma, possibly reducing the sensitivity of hepatoma cells to CD95-mediated apoptosis including cytotoxic T lymphocyte activity (Strand, NatureMed, 1996; 2:1361).

Methods for the investigation of apoptosis

There are a number of laboratory procedures available for detecting and quantifying levels of apoptosis. Current approaches to identifying apoptosis in cells and tissues are outlined in Table 3.

There is general agreement that the only current, universal features of apoptosis are the distinct morphological changes, such as chromatin condensation and nuclear fragmentation (Figs 1 and 7). The simplest method is to examine the morphology of cells stained with dyes such as haematoxylin (Fig. 8).

An alternative method that is widely used is extraction and analysis of DNA on agarose gels for internucleosomal DNA fragmentation, the hallmark ladder pattern (Fig. 2) being indicative of cell death via apoptosis. However, DNA fragmentation is not universally observed during apoptosis and furthermore may occur late during apoptosis. In addition, non-random DNA cleavage also occurs during cell necrosis. Thus, the sole reliance on demonstration of DNA fragmentation to indicate the presence of apoptosis is fraught with misinterpretation and complementary techniques should be used wherever possible.

Other methods that are widely used are the *in situ* demonstration of DNA cleavage using the terminal deoxynucleotidyl transferase-mediated deoxyuridine triphosphate nick-end labelling (TUNEL) (Fig. 1) or *in situ* nick translation techniques. Although these techniques appear to be promising methods to identifying apoptosis, they are not absolutely specific for apoptotic cell death (Grasl-Kraupp, Hepatol, 1995; 21:1465) and should be correlated with morphological evidence of apoptosis and non-random DNA cleavage on gel electrophoresis.

A flow cytometry method based on a reduction in DNA staining and cell shrinkage has many attractions for the routine detection of apoptosis. This method is based on the fact that the fragmentation of DNA seen during apoptosis is associated with a decrease in the DNA-binding of dyes such as propidium iodide, which can be readily detected by flow cytometry (Fig. 9). The shrinkage seen as cells undergo apoptosis can also be readily measured as a decline in forward light scatter in the flow cytometer (Li, BiotechHisto, 1995; 70:234; Li, ExpCellRes, 1996; 222:28).

Detection of specific mRNAs or proteins involved in the apoptotic process is an additional possibility although most candidate genes or proteins have not been proven to be absolutely specific for active cell death. Promising exceptions may be the expression of the precursor of TGF-β1 (pre-TGF-β1) in early apoptotic hepatocytes but not in necrotic hepatocytes or the detection of annexin V which is expressed on the surface of lymphocytes (Homburg, Blood, 1995; 85:532).

References

1. Steller H. Mechanisms and genes of cellular suicide. *Science*, 1995; **267**: 1445–9.
2. Schulte-Hermann R, Grasl-Kraupp B, and Bursch W. Apoptosis and hepatocarcinogenesis. In Jirtle RL, ed. *Liver regeneration and carcinogenesis*. San Diego, California: Academic Press, 1995.
3. Kerr JFR, Wyllie AH, and Curries AR. Apoptosis: a basic biological phenomenon with wide-ranging implications in tissue kinetics. *British Journal of Cancer*, 1972; **26**: 239–57.
4. Alison MR and Saraf CE. Liver cell death: patterns and mechanisms. *Gut*, 1994; **35**: 577–81.
5. Rosser B and Gores G. Liver cell necrosis: cellular mechanisms and clinical implications. *Gastroenterology*, 1995; **108**: 252–75.
6. Piacentini M, Davies P, and Fesus L. Tissue transglutaminase in cells undergoing apoptosis. In Tomei LD and Cope F, ed. *Apoptosis II: the molecular basis of apoptosis in disease*. New York: Cold Spring Harbor Press, 1994: 143–63.
7. Patel T, Gores GJ, and Kaufmann SH. The role of proteases during apoptosis. *FASEB Journal*, 1996; **10**: 587–97.
8. Henkart PA. ICE family proteases: mediators of all apoptotic cell death? *Immunity*, 1996; **4**: 195–201.
9. Nagata S and Golstein P. The Fas death factor. *Science*, 1995; **267**: 1449–56.
10. Thompson CB. Apoptosis in the pathogenesis and treatment of disease. *Science*, 1995; **267**: 1456–62.
11. Tracey KJ and Cerami A. Tumor necrosis factor, other cytokines and disease. *Annual Review of Cell Biology*, 1993; **9**: 317–43.
12. Smith CA, Farrah T, and Goodwin RG. The TNF receptor superfamily of cellular and viral proteins: activation, costimulation and death. *Cell*, 1994; **76**: 959–62.
13. Harris CC. p53 tumor suppressor gene: from the basic research laboratory to the clinic—an abridged historical perspective. *Carcinogenesis*, 1996; **17**: 1187–98.
14. Harris CC. Structure and function of the p53 tumor suppressor gene: clues for rational cancer therapeutic strategies. *Journal of the National Cancer Institute*, 1996; **88**: 1442–55.
15. Bates S and Vousden KH. p53 in signaling checkpoint arrest or apoptosis. *Current Opinions in Genetics and Development*, 1996; **6**: 12–19.
16. Liebermann DA, Hoffman B, and Steinman RA. Molecular controls of growth arrest and apoptosis: p53-dependent and independent pathways. *Oncogene*, 1995; **11**: 199–210.
17. Lee ML and Bernstein A. Apoptosis, cancer and the p53 tumour suppressor gene. *Cancer Metastasis Reviews*, 1995; **14**: 149–61.
18. Chiarugi V and Ruggiero M. Role of three cancer master genes p53, bcl-2 and c-myc on the apoptotic process. *Tumorigenesis*, 1996; **82**: 205–9.
19. Reed JC. Regulation of apoptosis by bcl-2 family proteins and its role in cancer chemoresistance. *Current Opinions in Oncology*, 1995; **7**: 541–6.
20. Que FG and Gores GJ. Cell death by apoptosis: basic concepts and disease relevance for the gastroenterologist. *Gastroenterology*, 1996; **110**: 1238–43.

21. Arber N, Zajicek G, and Ariel I. The streaming liver II. Hepatocyte life history. *Liver*, 1988; **7**: 319–24.
22. Patel T and Gores GJ. Apoptosis and hepatobiliary disease. *Hepatology*, 1995; **21**: 1725–41.
23. Kaplowitz N. Recent advances in drug metabolism and hepatotoxicity. *Seminars in Liver Disease*, 1990; **10**: 235–8.
24. Bursch W, Oberhammer F, and Schulte-Hermann R. Cell death by apoptosis and its protective role against disease. *Trends in Pharmacological Sciences*, 1992; **13**: 245–51.
25. Reed J. Bcl-2 and the regulation of programmed cell death. *Journal of Cell Biology*, 1994; **124**: 1–6.
26. Bursch W, Grasl-Kraupp B, Ellinger A, *et al.* Active cell death: role in hepatocarcinogenesis and subtypes. *Biochemistry and Cell Biology*, 1994; **72**: 669–75.
27. Cotter TG and Al-Rubeai M. Cell death (apoptosis) in cell culture systems. *Trends in Biotechnology*, 1995; **13**: 150–5.

2.9 Bilirubin metabolism

Johan Fevery and Norbert Blanckaert

Introduction

Disturbances of bilirubin metabolism are a frequent sign of hepatobiliary or haematological disorders. Some of these disorders can lead to brain damage (kernicterus) or to development of pigment gallstones. Bilirubin IXα is an endogenous compound which is very poorly water soluble at physiological pH values. It undergoes a series of metabolic steps; these sometimes stand as a model for the metabolism of other substances or drugs. The normal metabolism of bilirubin will be reviewed; more details can be found in *Bile Pigments and Jaundice*.[1]

Chemical characteristics[2]

Bilirubin is an open tetrapyrrole derived from haem (Fig. 1). Several natural isomers exist but the IXα pigment is by far the predominant fraction in adults. The non-α isomers dissolve readily in water and do not require esterification for effective hepatic removal and excretion in bile. In contrast, bilirubin IXα is poorly soluble in water (4–7 nmol at pH7.4) and requires esterification for efficient biliary excretion. At first glance, this is unexpected since the molecule contains two propionic acid side-chains and several polar NH and OH groups. However, a series of investigations initiated by Fog (Fog, Nature, 1963; 198:88) has led to the conclusion that these polar functions are not freely available for interaction with solvent. Bonnett *et al.* showed that the propionic acid groups are involved in hydrogen bonding with the two NH and one ketone group of the opposite dipyrrolic half of the molecule (Fig. 1).[3] This results in a chiral conformation with a ridge–tile structure. Such an H-bonded structure explains both the low hydrosolubility of bilirubin IXα and the poor accessibility for the central CH$_2$-bridge for reaction with diazoreagents. Intramolecular hydrogen bonds cannot form in the structural IXβ, IXγ, and IXδ isomers, which probably explains why these non-α isomers are freely soluble in water and readily excretable in bile in unconjugated form.

Light, whether natural or as part of phototherapy, can induce formation of geometrical 'photoisomers' of bilirubin IXα.[2,4] The photon energy induces disruption of the internal H bonds, which results in transformation of the Z configuration at the C-5 and/or at the C-15 methene bridges into an E configuration and formation of EZ, ZE, and EE photoisomers (Fig. 2). Polar functional groups are exposed to solvent in these photoisomers; therefore, they are more water soluble than the natural ZZ pigment and can be excreted in bile without prior esterification. This mechanism may explain excretion of small amounts of unconjugated bilirubin IXα in bile.

The photoisomers of bilirubin IXα are partially converted to an intramolecularly cyclized derivative, termed lumibilirubin. Such cyclized pigment seems to constitute the major part of the photoderivatives of bilirubin formed during phototherapy.

Bilirubin IXα is esterified enzymatically at one or both of its propionic acid side chains. A glycosyl moiety (glucuronosyl, glucosyl, or xylosyl) is attached in a β-D-ester linkage to the carboxylic acid function (Fig. 1). This esterification also disrupts intramolecular hydrogen bonds. Esterified bilirubins readily dissolve in water and are efficiently excreted in bile or, in some instances, in urine. When bilirubins esterified with sugars are kept for a prolonged period of time in a natural body fluid such as serum, bile, urine, or any other aqueous solution, 'hopping' of the bilirubin moiety along the sugar occurs, from C-1, to C-2 to C-3, then to C-4 (Fig. 3). Such acyl shifting involves a non-enzymatic mechanism and is accelerated when the pH is increased above 6 (Blanckaert, BiochemJ, 1978; 171:203; Compernolle, BiochemJ, 1978; 171:185). The non-C-1 positional isomers are resistant to the action of β-glycosidases from intestinal, leucocyte, or bacterial origin and thus seem more efficiently eliminated with the stools. Acyl shift has also been observed with glucuronides of some drugs including zomepirac (Caldwell, BiochemPharm, 1982; 36:953).

Another fraction of bilirubin conjugates has been detected in serum of patients with chronic liver disease (Lauff, ClinChem, 1982; 28:629; Weiss, NEJM, 1983; 309:147). The pigment seems irreversibly, and presumably covalently, bound to albumin (McDonagh, JCI, 1984; 74:763). Esterified bilirubins are the precursors of these albumin conjugates (Fig. 4) (Wu, ClinBioch, 1984; 17:221; Van Breemen, JChromatogr, 1986; 383:387). The non-enzymatic formation occurs during stagnation of mono- or di-esterified bilirubins in albumin-containing media *in vivo* and also occurs *in vitro*. The bilirubin–albumin conjugates can be measured by chromatographic separation, diffusion, or extraction procedures (Seligson, ClinChem, 1985; 31:1367; Blanckaert, JLabClinMed, 1986; 108:77; McKavanagh, BiomedChromatogr, 1987; 2:62; Sundberg, ClinChem, 1984; 30:1314). They are diazopositive. Due to their large size, these conjugates do not undergo glomerular filtration. Their plasma half-life is approximately 17 days and seems identical with that of albumin, suggesting that they are catabolized together with the conjugating albumin molecule. Covalent albumin linkage has been documented for anti-inflammatory agents such as zomepirac and oxaprozin (Smith, JCI, 1986; 77:934; Wells, Zenobiot, 1987; 17:1437).

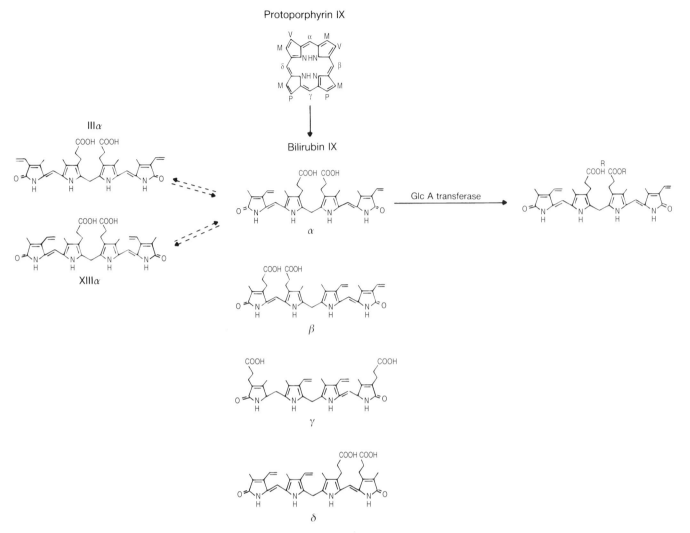

Fig. 1. Formation and structure of bile pigments.

Normal bilirubin metabolism

The metabolism of bilirubin can be subdivided schematically into several inter-related steps. They will be discussed consecutively.

Production

Bilirubin is formed by breakdown of the haem moiety of haemoglobin and other haem-containing proteins such as catalases and cytochromes. Two separate enzyme systems are involved in bilirubin formation.[6] The microsomal haem oxygenase (form I and II) converts haem to biliverdin. A cytosolic biliverdin IXα reductase subsequently reduces biliverdin IXα to bilirubin IXα (Maines, EurJBiochem, 1996; 235: 372).

Haem oxygenase activity is present in all tissues. The highest activity is found in spleen (Maines, FASEBJ, 1988; 2:2557). Haem oxygenase is localized in the endoplasmic reticulum and requires the concerted activity of microsomal NADPH-cytochrome P-450 reductase. The latter enzyme catalyses transfer of electrons from NADPH to convert or to retain iron in the reduced state and to activate molecular oxygen to oxidate the α-CH bridge of haem. Haem oxygenase has a high stereoselectivity for the α-meso bridge

of the haem substrate (Fig. 1); therefore, in adults virtually all natural bile pigment is of the IXα type. The β and in small amounts the δ isomer (Fig. 1), resulting from cleavage at the β or δ bridges, are present in fetal bile but only in trace amounts in adult bile. Haem oxygenase catalyses the degradation of cytochrome P-450 enzymes (Kutty, ArchBiochemBiophys, 1988; 260:638); the latter enzyme system plays a key role in the biotransformation of a majority of substrates. Biotransformation will thus indirectly be regulated by the haem oxygenase activity. In addition, haem oxygenase 1 is an important stress protein (Keyse, Nature, 1992; 359: 644). The nucleotide sequence of the gene encoding rat haem oxygenase has been characterized (Müller, JBC, 1987; 262:6802).

Tin and zinc protoporphyrin IX have been demonstrated to act as potent competitive inhibitors of haem oxygenase (Maines, BBActa, 1981; 67:339) and to prevent neonatal hyperbilirubinaemia in the rat (Drummond, PNAS, 1981; 78:6466; Drummond, JCI, 1984; 74:142). Further studies showed that tin mesoporphyrin was at least as potent. It has been given as a single dose of 6 μmol/kg intramuscularly in a large series of neonates; it produces a 25 per cent decrease of biliary bilirubin output, without any effect on bile flow or bile acid output but leading to a pronounced biliary excretion

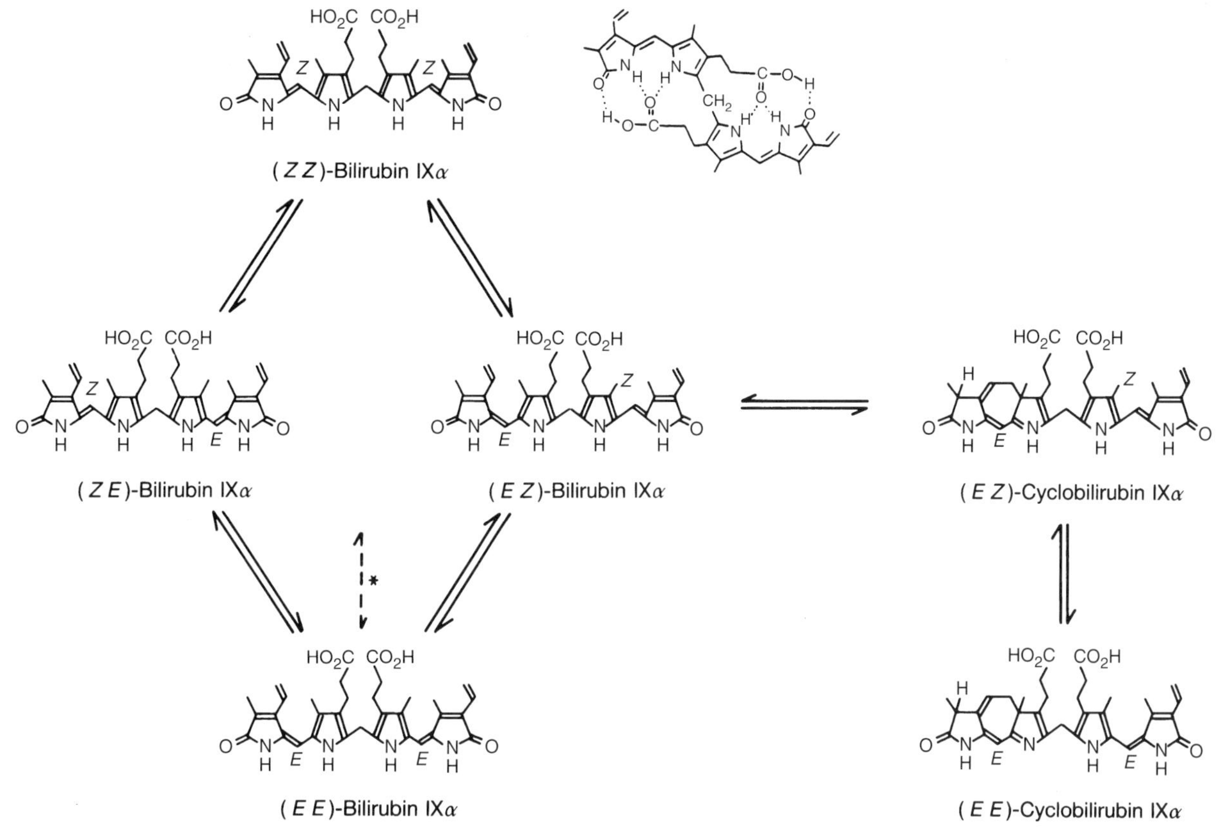

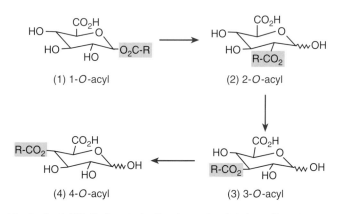

(Z Z)-Bilirubin IXα

(Z E)-Bilirubin IXα   (E Z)-Bilirubin IXα   (E Z)-Cyclobilirubin IXα

(E E)-Bilirubin IXα   (E E)-Cyclobilirubin IXα

Fig. 2. Photoderivatives of bilirubin IXα. Hydrogen bonds are represented by dotted lines (reproduced from Fevery, ClinGastroent, 1989; 3:283, with permission).

(1) 1-*O*-acyl   (2) 2-*O*-acyl

(4) 4-*O*-acyl   (3) 3-*O*-acyl

Fig. 3. Acyl shift. During stasis, the glycosyl moiety bound in ester linkage of bilirubin (represented by O_2C-R) shifts from linkage at C-1 to C-2, C-3, or C-4 of glucuronic acid (reproduced from Fevery, ClinGastroent, 1989; 3:283, with permission).

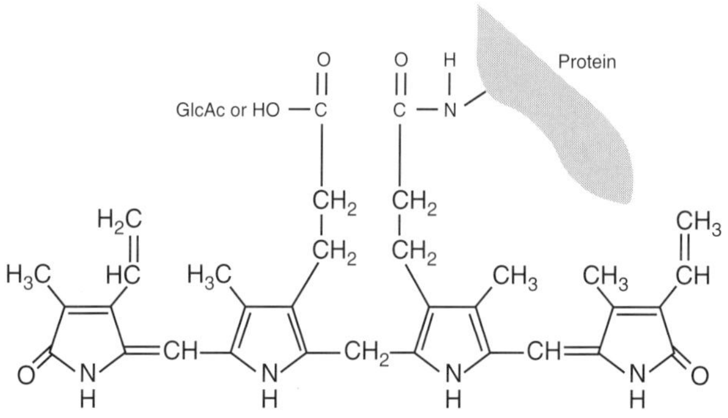

Fig. 4. Proposed structure of bilirubin–albumin conjugates.

of haem (Berglund, Hepatol, 1988; 84:1091) and markedly reduced the need for phototherapy (Kappas, Pediat, 1995; 95:468). Chronic administration of tin mesoporphyrin has been used successfully in two boys with Crigler–Najjar type I disease (Galbraith, Pediat, 1992; 89:175).

The human cytosolic biliverdin IXα reductase (39–42 kDa) is also a zinc protein (Yamaguchi, JBC, 1994; 269:24343; Maines, EurJBiochem, 1996; 235:372). It is present in almost all mammalian tissues, with highest activity in spleen, liver, and kidney. Its activity

is modulated by pronounced substrate inhibition and by intracellular biliverdin IXα binding proteins (Philips, BiochemPharm, 1994; 33: 1983). The enzyme has a high selectivity for biliverdin IXα. Recently, a separate biliverdin IXβ reductase has been isolated and shown to be identical to flavin reductase (Shalloe, BiochemJ, 1996; 316:385). It is present in hepatocytes, amongst other sites, and fetal haemoglobin might represent a possible substrate of this enzyme. Indeed, whereas adult bile contains mainly bilirubin IXα derivates, fetal, and less so neonatal bile, contain predominantly bilirubin IXβ (Blumenthal, BiochemJ, 1980; 186:693; Yamaguchi, EurJBiochem, 1995; 233:467) whereas Gunn rat bile contains small amounts of all non-α bilirubins (Blanckaert, BiochemJ, 1977; 164:237).

In agreement with these observations *in vivo*, activity of bi-liverdin IXβ reductase was higher than that of biliverdin IXα reductase in fetal liver and the converse was true in the adult (Yamaguchi, JBC, 1994; 289:24343). During development, meta-bolism is geared towards formation of the IXα bilirubin isomer. What would be the benefit of a shift from the IXβ to the IXα isomer since bilirubin IXβ is more hydrophilic and does not need conjugation before efficient biliary excretion in contrast to bilirubin IXα (Blanckaert, BiochemJ, 1977; 164:229)? Bilirubin IXα has important antioxidant activity (Stocker, Science, 1987; 235:1043) against, among others, oxidative stresses *in vivo* (Yamaguchi, BBRes-Comm, 1995; 214:11) possibly deriving from the higher oxygen pressure resulting from breathing after birth in contrast to placental respiration. This antioxidant activity seems to have other favourable effects since individuals with low plasma UCB-IXα (unconjugated bilirubin-IXα) presented with a higher incidence of coronary artery disease (Schwertner, Clin Chem 1994; 40:18) probably related to a lower inhibition by UCB-IXα of the oxidation of low density lipoprotein (Wu, Life Sci 1994; 54:477). Further studies confirmed that individuals with serum bilirubin levels below 7 μM had high density lipoprotein-cholesterol, lower serum albumin, lower forced expiratory volume, and higher cardiovascular risks especially when smoking (Breimer, ClinChem, 1995; 41:1504). The relationship between serum bilirubin and ischaemic heart disease was U-shaped since those with levels above 12 μM had an equal risk as those with values below 7 and higher than individuals with values between 7 and 12 (Breimer ClinChem, 1995; 41:1504). Whether this is directly related to the serum bilirubin level remains uncertified. Neonatal Gunn rats suffered less hyperoxia-induced lung oedema than heterozygous litter mates, again suggesting that unconjugated bili-rubin might have an antioxidant action (Demery; FreeR-adicBiolMet, 1995; 19:395).

Administration of the ^{3}H or ^{14}C-labelled haem precursors glycine or δ-aminolaevulinic acid allows the study of *in-vivo* production and catabolism of haem.[7] After pulse labelling with glycine, a major peak of radionuclide in biliary or faecal bile pigments can be demonstrated between 90 and 150 days. This period corresponds to the average life span of erythrocytes, and the labelled pigments stem from degradation of senescent red blood cells. In addition, 10 to 20 per cent of the radioactivity appears in faeces over the first days after injection. This 'early-labelled' bile pigment consists of two fractions; one peaking 1 to 3 h after injection and a second peaking after 1 to 3 days. The first peak is best observed after injection of labelled δ-aminolaevulinic acid. This precursor is efficiently taken up by the liver where it is incorporated in hepatic haem (mainly cytochrome P-450) which has a high turnover rate. The later phase of early-labelled pigment arises mainly from erythroid haem (produced but not released in circulation), from prematurely des-troyed erythrocyte precursors or abnormal erythrocytes in the bone marrow; this fraction greatly increases with dyserythropoiesis or 'ineffective erythropoiesis'. A minor part is also derived from haem proteins with slower turnover rates. One g of haemoglobin yields 36.2 mg of bilirubin. Daily production rate of bilirubin in adults, estimated from plasma turnover studies with radiolabelled bilirubin, averages 3.9 ± 0.7 mg/kg (mean ± 1 SEM) or 250 to 350 mg/day. Approximately two-thirds of the bilirubin derived from hepatic haem does not enter the plasma but passes directly from the hepatocytes into bile. The total bilirubin production is thus slightly higher than the estimates based on plasma bilirubin turnover stud-ies. Because one molecule of carbon monoxide is produced per molecule of degraded haem, total bilirubin production can also be determined by measurement of endogenous production of CO (Landow, JCI, 1970; 49:914); values obtained with this approach are 4.4 ± 0.7 mg/day of bilirubin produced per kg body weight.

Transport in plasma

Bilirubin formed in the monocytic macrophage cell system of liver, spleen, and bone marrow, and about 40 per cent of the pigment formed in hepatocytes from hepatic haem proteins, are released into plasma, where bilirubin is bound at a high affinity binding site (Ka 108/mol) of albumin. Secondary binding sites with lower affinity (Ka 105/mol) have been identified. *In vitro* numerous sub-stances interact with the bilirubin–albumin binding either because they can bind at the same site or at a different site but interacting with the bilirubin binding, for example by inducing conformational changes in the albumin molecule. Extensive studies by Brodersen have shown that, *in vivo*, only a small number of substances reach high enough concentrations or affinity constants to displace bilirubin effectively from albumin (Table 1).[8] The most important are sulphonamides and fatty acids. The latter are present at high concentrations in breast milk and can be part of fortified nutrition mixtures or of parenteral nutrition. Small fatty acid concentrations seem to induce conformational changes in the albumin molecule (Odell, JLabClinMed, 1977; 89:295) whereas high concentrations displace bilirubin, when the ratio of fatty acid to albumin exceeds four (Odell, AnnNYAcadSci, 1973; 226:255).[7]

Under normal conditions, only minute amounts of bilirubin are unbound in plasma. To date, exact, direct determination of the unbound bilirubin is not possible but extrapolation has led to calculated concentrations of 4 to 7 ng/l at pH7.4 (Brodersen, JBC, 1979; 254:2364). Enhanced amounts of free bilirubin will allow the pigment to enter tissue where it can exert toxic effects. This is especially important for the brain and can result in kernicterus. This abnormality can occur in neonates with a highly immature or defective conjugation and in Crigler–Najjar syndrome (see below). Titration studies have suggested that bilirubin is bound as a dianion to the high-affinity binding site of albumin. In the analbuminaemic rat, bilirubin binds to high density lipoprotein with an affinity of 108/mol (Suzuki, JBC, 1988; 263:5037); however, the patho-physiological relevance of this observation is not clear.

Albumin in the circulatory and extravascular intercellular space represents a vast binding reservoir and keeps the concentration of

Table 1 Compounds able to produce clinically significant displacement of bilirubin from its albumin binding site

Long-chain fatty acids in concentrations exceeding a 4:1 ratio
   of fatty acid–albumin
Cholangiographic contrast agents
Sulphonamides
Salicylates
Fusidic acid
Azapropazone
Sodium caprylate and *N*-acetyl tryptophan

Modified from Brodersen.[8]

unbound bilirubin very low in plasma and in tissues. Exchange transfusion combined with albumin administration, as used in newborns at risk for development of kernicterus, will produce a shift of bilirubin from tissues to plasma (Schmid, Nature, 1965; 204:1041; Sproul, JPediat, 1964; 65:12).

In unconjugated hyperbilirubinaemia, a minor fraction of bilirubin is attached to erythrocytes, probably by binding to membrane phospholipids.

Hepatocellular uptake and intracellular transport

Bilirubin is efficiently taken up by the liver parenchymal cells whereas the albumin remains in plasma. When a trace amount of bilirubin is injected intravenously in the rat, 40 per cent is recovered in the cytosol after 90 s (Brown, AmJPhysiol, 1964; 207:1237; Bernstein, JCI, 1966; 45:1194). The unbound unconjugated bilirubin is taken up by 'facilitated diffusion', that is via the interaction of a transport protein through the hepatocyte membrane. Indeed, the dissociation rate from the albumin is great enough (Weisiger, PNAS, 1985; 82:1563) to allow rapid dissociation. Three candidate transporters have been isolated from rat liver plasma membranes and their function studied by inhibition with antibodies: a bromosulphophthalein/bilirubin binding protein (Stremmel, JCI, 1983; 71:1796; Stremmel, JCI, 1986; 78:822); an organic anion binding protein (Wolkoff, JCI, 1985; 76:454); and bilitranslocase (Tiribelli, BBActa, 1978; 532:105; Torres, PNAS, 1993; 90:8136) but none of these has been unequivocally cloned. In contrast, a rat and human organic anion transporting polypeptide has been cloned and functionally expressed in *Xenopus laevis* oocytes. This transporter facilitates uptake of bromosulphophthalein, taurocholate, etc. but not of unconjugated bilirubin (Wolkoff, SemLivDis, 1996; 16:121).

Inside the hepatocyte, unconjugated bilirubin is bound to and/or transported by a variety of substances and organelles. Indeed, the cell is not a bag of solvents with floating organelles but has a complex structure (Gersham, PNAS, 1985; 82:5030). There is increasing evidence that transport from the liver plasma membrane to the endoplasmic reticulum (for conjugation) and to the biliary canaliculus (for secretion) of a large variety of molecules, including unconjugated bilirubin and bilirubin conjugates, involves cellular membranes and tubulovesicular movement (Crawford, AmJPhysiol, 1988; 255:G121) as well as cytoplasmic transport bound to transporter proteins (Zucker, SemLiverDis, 1996; 16:159). The role of the intracellular transport proteins, of which ligandin (or glutathion transferase B) is the most abundant, has been overemphasized; binding of unconjugated bilirubin to ligandin might in fact represent rather a protection of the organelles from too high (potentially toxic) concentrations of unconjugated bilirubin as is the case for albumin in plasma. The importance of binding to (intracellular) membranes has previously been underestimated on the basis of kinetic analysis. However, the binding of bilirubin to isolated membrane preparations is also saturable, and, when tested at high ligand concentrations, even a protein-free liposomal system will show apparent saturable binding or absorption kinetics, as the molar ligand to lipid ratio becomes unfavourable and the system starts deviating from ideal behaviour (Heirwegh, BiochemJ, 1988; 254:101).

Reflux back to plasma is also limited by the presence of cytosolic proteins (Wolkoff, AmJPhysiol, 1979; 236:638). Mathematical analysis of the plasma disappearance rate has demonstrated that up to 40 per cent of injected radiobilirubin can reflux back to plasma after initial uptake (Berk, AnnIntMed, 1981; 82:552). Part of the unconjugated pigment thus undergoes bidirectional transport across the sinusoidal membrane.

A fraction of the bilirubins found in the plasma are glucuronides (Muraca, Gastro, 1987; 92:309). It appears that these esters are also subject to bidirectional flux across the hepatocytic plasma membrane and that they may even share the transport system for bromosulphophthalein and unconjugated bilirubin (Shupeck, AmJGastro, 1978; 70:259). In infant monkeys, the concentration of ligandins increased to adult levels in parallel with the maturation of the transport mechanism for organic anions (Levi, NEJM, 1970; 283:1136).

In rat liver, ligandin is identical to glutathione S transferase B, and belongs to a group of enzymes that catalyse conjugation of glutathione with many different electrophilic substances (Wolkoff, ProgLivDis, 1979; 6:213). Some of them have been cloned and a new nomenclature was proposed (Jakoby, BiochemPharm, 1984; 33:2539). The transferases are dimers, some with identical and others with non-identical subunits. Two rat ligandins have been identified; a homodimer (1–1 or YaYa) and a heterodimer (1–2 or YaYc). The subunit 1 was thought to have a distinct, high affinity binding site for bilirubin, while a lower affinity constant was observed for the subunit 2(Yc), but the dimeric structure may be needed for high affinity binding (Boyer, JBC, 1986; 261:5363). The site for bilirubin binding is shared by lithocholic acid but not by other substances, nor by glutathione-acceptor substrates. Ligandins bind a variety of other compounds including bilirubin conjugates, haem, steroids, bromosulphophthalein, indocyanine green, and bile acids. They constitute 2 per cent of the cytosolic proteins in man and 5 per cent in the rat; smaller amounts are present in kidney and intestine.

Conjugation
Ester formation

This step involves enzymatic esterification or conjugation with a glycosyl group, derived from an activated sugar donor, produced in the cytosol. They comprise uridine diphosphate-xylose (**UDP-xylose**), UDP-glucose, and UDP-glucuronic acid. The last substance is formed in cytosol from UDP-glucose; the reaction is catalysed by UDP-glucose dehydrogenase. Decarboxylation of UDP-glucose yields UDP-xylose. In plants, conjugation with xylose is the predominant reaction; glucosidation predominates in bacteria and glucuronidation in mammals. In dogs, cats, and rabbits a major portion of bilirubin also undergoes xylosidation or glucosidation.

The sugars are bound in a β-d-ester linkage to either one or both carboxylic acid groups of the propionic acid side chains attached at C-8 and/or C-12 of bilirubin. The predominant natural diesters are diglucuronides, glucoglucuronides, and xyloglucuronides. Analysis of biliary bile pigments has demonstrated pronounced differences between species. Man, dog, cat, and rat excrete predominantly diesterified bilirubins whereas other animal species produce monoconjugates nearly exclusively (Fevery, BiochemJ, 1977; 164:737). Glucuronides are relatively more important in man, monkey, dog, cat, and rabbit bile than in other species. Monoconjugates at the C-8 side chain predominate in the rat, whereas monoesters at the C-12 side chain are more abundant in sheep.

Esterification is catalysed by an enzyme system located in the endoplasmic reticulum of the hepatocytes. In rat and human liver, and presumably also in cat and dog, a sequential conversion of bilirubin to monoglucuronide and diglucuronide is operative. Both steps are catalysed by the microsomal UDP-glucuronosyltransferase. It had previously been proposed that bilirubin diglucuronide is synthesized by a separate transglucuronidation enzyme—catalysing conversion of two molecules of monoglucuronide into one diglucuronide and one unconjugated bilirubin. This putative enzyme was thought to be located in the plasma membrane. However, it has been demonstrated that such transglucuronidation mechanism is not operative *in vivo* (Blanckaert, JCI, 1980; 65:1332) and that diglucuronide is formed by UDP-glucuronosyltransferase (Blanckaert, PNAS, 1979; 76:2037). It was ultimately demonstrated that the diglucuronide formed in the absence of UDP-glucuronosyltransferase had a IIIα or XIIIα composition and that it resulted from a non-enzymatic, non-physiological dipyrrole exchange with formation of IIIα and XIIIα compounds (Sieg, JCI,1982; 69:347; Adachi, ArchBiochemBiophys, 1985; 241:486) (Fig. 5). Indeed, cleavage of the asymmetrical bilirubin IXα molecule at the central methylene bridge can occur rapidly in strongly acidic conditions and more slowly at other pH values. The resulting dipyrrolic halves can recombine in a random fashion to reform the parent IXα compound (50 per cent) and the IIIα and XIIIα isomers (Fig. 5). Such dipyrrole exchange can lead to non-enzymatic formation of unconjugated and diglucuronidated bilirubin as a result of so-called scrambling of the IXα monoglucuronide (Fig. 5). However, the resulting diglucuronide and unconjugated bilirubin will have the symmetrical IIIα or XIIIα skeletal structure.

Microsomal UDP-glucuronosyltransferases

Bilirubin UDP-glucuronyltransferase belongs to a supergene family of isoenzymes, the UDP-glucuronosyltransferase (**UGT**),which are located primarily in the hepatic endoplasmic reticulum, where they are deeply embedded in the membrane. The mammalian ancestral *UGT1* (bilirubin/phenol UGTs) and *UGT2* (steroid/bile/odorant UGTs) gene families expanded in different ways on two different chromosomes. In man, the *UGT1* gene complex has been mapped to the long arm of chromosome 2 region q37 at 2937 (Moghrabi, AnnHumGen, 1992; 56:81), whereas the *UGT2* genes are present on chromosome 4 (Monaghan, Genomics, 1992; 13:908). The *UGT1* gene complex consists, at the 5′ end, of at least 10 unique exon 1s dispersed over approximately 85 kb and of four common exons, concentrated in a 6 kb region (Ritter, JBC, 1992; 267:3257). This complex encodes at least 10 mRNAs and results in formation of UDP-glucuronyltransferase isoforms. Exons 2 to 5 (at the 3′ end) encode respectively for 44, 29, 74, and 99 amino acids (246 in total) at the COOH-terminal region; this domain is identical for all glucuronyltransferases derived from *UGT1* and is responsible for the UDP-glycosyl binding (common to all isoforms) and also represents the membrane-spanning region. A unique exon 1 is derived by alternative splicing from the broad region and encodes for the specific NH$_2$-terminal (285 amino acid long) substrate-binding site (Fig. 6) (see Chapter 20.6).

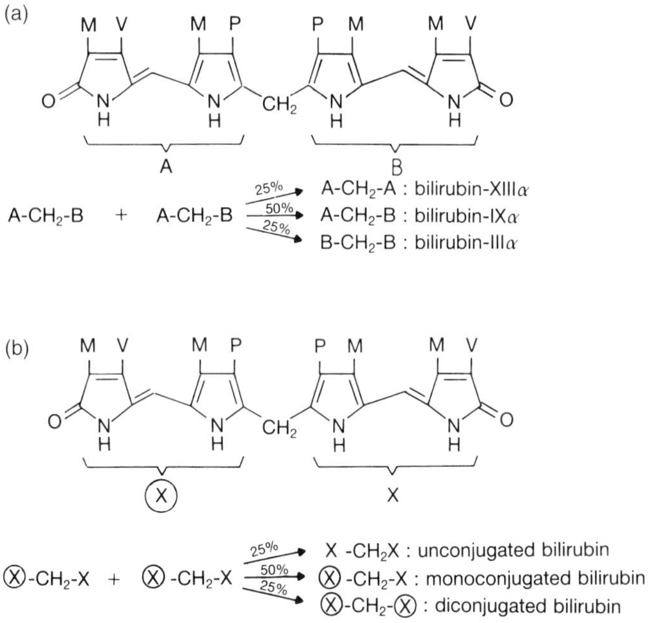

Fig. 5. Mechanism of dipyrrole exchange. The asymmetrical bilirubin IXα or its monoconjugate are represented by the association of two dipyrrole molecules linked by a central-CH$_2$ bridge (a). Cleavage and random reassembly will lead to reformation of the parent molecule (50 per cent) and to formation of symmetrical III and XIII isomers. In this way bilirubin diglucuronide IIIα or XIIIα can be formed non-enzymatically (b).

The UDP-glucuronyltransferases are integral membrane proteins. The xenobiotic binding domain and the sites involved in the UDP-glucuronic acid binding and catalysis project into the lumen of the endoplasmic reticulum. The protein is anchored in place by a membrane-spanning region near the C terminus of the protein, with the Lys-Lys stop transfer sequence at the C terminus exposed to the cytoplasm (Tephly, TrendsPharmacolSci, 1990; 2:277).

The UGT catalyse the glucuronidation of a wide variety of xenobiotic and endogenous compounds such as morphine, 4-methylumbelliferone, phenols and bilirubin, steroids, bile acids, thyroid hormone, and catecholamines. Separate isoenzyme classes had been predicted on the basis of differences in developmental and induction patterns observed in man and rat and on the observation that conjugation of *p*-nitrophenol, for example, was normal or near-normal in Gunn rats, Crigler–Najjar, or Gilbert patients who are characterized by a grossly deficient bilirubin conjugation rate. Glucuronidation of bilirubin in adult rat liver is preferentially induced by phenobarbital rather than by 3-methylcholantrene and is selectively induced by clofibric acid. Glucuronidation of *p*-nitrophenol, *o*-aminophenol, 2-naphthol, and 4-methylumbelliferone develops before birth in the rat fetal liver, and maturation can be triggered by glucocorticoid administration (Wishart, BiochemJ, 1978; 174:485). In contrast to this 'late fetal' group, transferases catalysing the glucuronidation of bilirubin, oestradiol, testosterone, and other substrates only develop in the early neonatal rat liver. A trigger for their development remains unknown. In man, however, a similar distinction between a 'late fetal' and an 'early neonatal' class of enzymes could not be made. Isoenzymes with distinct substrate selectivities (Falany, ArchBiochemBiophys, 1983; 227:

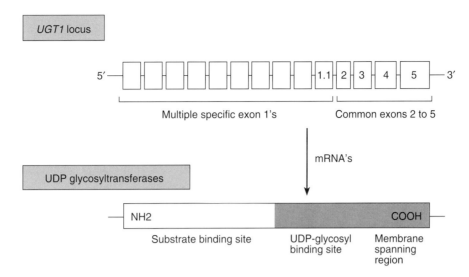

Fig. 6. The *UGT1* gene complex locus on chromosome 2 region q37 is composed of at least 10 unique exon 1s encoding the specific substrate binding site on the UDP-glucuronosyltransferase, whereas the common exons 2–5 encode the UDP-glycosyl binding and the membrane-spanning domain.

248) and specifically bilirubin selectivity (Scragg, FEBSLett, 1985; 183:37; Chowdhury, BiochemJ, 1986; 233:827) have been purified from rat liver. The purified enzyme forms both monoesters and the diester and displays glucuronosyl-, as well as glucosyl- and xylosyltransferase, activity. Competition between UDP-glucuronic acid, UDP-glucose, and UDP-xylose for conjugation of bilirubin suggests interaction with a common UDP-sugar binding site. Esterification of bilirubin is completely defective in the homozygous Gunn rat, whereas conjugation of other acceptor substrates is normal or only partially impaired. The Gunn rat cannot form bilirubin monoglucuronides, nor can it transform the mono-conjugates into diconjugates (Fevery, BiochemJ, 1972; 129:619). Recent investigations in the Gunn rat, documented the existence of a point mutation at codon 416 due to A to T transversion in a common exon (2 to 5) (Sato, BBResComm, 1991; 177:1161; Iyanagi, JBC, 1991; 266:24048) presumably leading to a truncated glucuronyltransferase involving reduced or absent activity with regard to several substrates. In humans, the bilirubin UDP-glucuronyltransferase seems to be encoded by the *UGT1A* gene (Bosma, JBiolChem, 1994; 269:17960) which shares exons 2 to 5 with the oestriol, *p*-nitrophenol etc. transferase genes, whereas they have a unique (specific) exon 1.

Microsomal UGTs are present in various tissues and most abundant in liver. Activities with several, mostly xenobiotic, compounds have been demonstrated in tissues such as kidney, lung, intestine, skin, and brain. However, in man bilirubin UDP-glucuronosyltransferase activity has only been documented in liver. Activity assessed *in vitro* was present in kidney tissue in most animal species analysed but not in man.

The purpose of diconjugate formation in rat, dog, cat, and man is also unclear. Most animal species excrete predominantly bilirubin monoglucuronide in bile. The Gunn rat also can excrete injected monoesters, which it cannot convert to diesters. Therefore, the formation of the monoesters appears to be the biologically essential step to allow rapid biliary excretion and disposal of bilirubins. It has been suggested that the concentration of bilirubin substrate

might bear directly on the proportion of mono- to diesters formed by microsomal enzyme systems. High loads of unconjugated bilirubin present in the incubation medium might effectively compete with monoesters formed *de novo* for glucuronidation, and thereby reduce the amount of diesters formed. This explanation assumes that the formation of mono- and diesters are competitive factors, for example because both types of products are formed at a single enzymatic site.

Some kinetic findings appear to support this hypothesis (Vanstapel, Biochem, 1987; 26:6074). The species-specific characteristic of producing preferentially the C-8 or C-12 conjugates is preserved by microsomal systems at non-saturating substrate concentrations and remains as good as at saturating bilirubin concentrations. Thus, both reactions display a single apparent Km value for bilirubin. Further, though a number of bilirubin analogues appear to be esterified by the bilirubin IXα conjugating transferase, none can selectively inhibit the formation of either conjugated isomer. These findings can be explained if both conjugation events at either the C-8 or C-12 side chain occur at a single enzymatic site. Therefore, the formation of the diester from either monoesterified isomer can also occur at this stage. Studies *in vitro* of the sequential formation of mono- and diesters suggest that the formation of the monoconjugate is a low-affinity, high-capacity step, whereas the ensuing diconjugate formation represents a high-affinity but low-capacity pathway (Cuypers, BBActa, 1983; 758:135).

Functional properties and latency of UGT

Two functional properties apply to each of the UGT isoenzymes, including the bilirubin-conjugating form, when assayed in native microsomal preparations. First, UGT activity is markedly latent in native, well-sealed microsomal vesicles. With normal human liver, bilirubin UDP-glucuronosyltransferase measured in digitonin-activated liver homogenate is about threefold higher than that measured in native, untreated preparations (Fevery, BiochemJ, 1977; 164:737), whereas addition of digitonin led to an 11- to

14-fold activation of rat liver glucuronosyltransferase (Heirwegh, BiochemJ, 1972; 129:605). Second, UDP-*N*-acetylglucosamine and to a lesser extent UDP-xylose enhance UGT activity in native microsomes (Bossuyt, BiochemJ, 1995; 305:321). There is evidence that both of these properties also apply to UGT in the intact hepatocyte (Banhegyi, FEBSLett, 1993; 328:149). The mechanisms responsible for these properties have for a long time been subjects of considerable debate.

Some investigators have postulated a 'conformational' model whereby the UGT enzyme faces the cytoplasmic side of the microsomal vesicle, with free access to extravesicular substrates.[11] These authors explain the limited expression of enzyme activity in untreated microsomes by postulating 'conformational constraint' of UGT activity when the enzyme is present in its native, unperturbed microsomal membrane. Disruption and perturbation of the microsomal membrane is thought to induce non-physiological conformational changes in the UGT protein and thereby to alter the catalytic properties of the enzyme, resulting in artificially enhanced UGT activity and loss of the stimulating effect of UDP-*N*-acetylglucosamine on transferase activity. The role of the lipids for the function of UDP-glucuronosyltransferases is indisputably evidenced by the necessity to reincorporate purified enzyme preparations into liposomal vesicles to restore enzyme activity (Erickson, BiochemJ, 1978; 17:3706). Changes in the composition and physicochemical properties of the phospholipids used in reconstitution experiments with purified enzyme appear to induce corresponding changes in the kinetic behaviour of the embedded enzyme. Thus, temperature-dependent changes in its co-operative characteristics and in its stimulation by the effector UDP-*N*-acetylglucosamine have been related to presumed phase transitions of the enzyme's lipid environment.

A second hypothesis proposes a 'compartmental' model suggesting that the latency of UGT is caused by a specific topological arrangement of the UGT protein in the microsomal membrane (Hallinan, HormCellReg, 1981; 5:73). The catalytic site of UGT seems to be oriented towards the lumen and is thus located within a membrane barrier which is almost impermeable to the hydrophilic UDP-sugar substrates. It is postulated that catalytic activity of UGT requires a transporter to carry the UDP-sugar across the endoplasmic reticulum membrane, from the cytosol where it is synthesized to the endoplasmic reticulum lumen where it is consumed in the conjugation reaction. Under these conditions, conjugation rate would depend on both the UDP-sugar carrier and the conjugation system. However, when the microsomal membrane permeability barrier is disrupted, hydrophilic UDP-sugars bypass the rate-limiting membrane translocation step and have unlimited access to the catalytic centre of UGT at the luminal face of the microsomal membrane. Hence, maximal catalytic expression of UGT is achieved and latency disappears in microsomes in which the membrane is either permeabilized or disrupted, for example by pretreatment with detergent or by sonication.

The primary sequences for cDNA encoding some UGT isoforms are now available; they indicate that these enzymes correspond to integral membrane proteins, with most of the protein, including the N-terminal, protruding within the lumen of the endoplasmic reticulum. There is as yet no direct evidence that this pertains to the catalytic domain of the enzyme. The proposed cysternal orientation of the glucuronosyltransferases (Shepherd, BiochemJ,

1989; 259:6171) is consistent with the fact that inactivation of the enzyme by membrane-impermeant reagent requires disruption of the membrane barrier (Vanstapel, ArchBiochemBiophys, 1988; 263: 216). Similarly, transferase-specific, although isoform-unspecific, antibodies react only with the enzyme after disruption of the microsomes. Furthermore, the reverse glucuronosyltransferase reaction demonstrated for several substrates seems also to be latent (Berry, FEBSLett, 1974; 42:73; Cuypers, Hepatol, 1984; 4:918). The UDP-glucuronic acid formed by the reverse reaction needs to accumulate within the microsomal lumen in order to drive the coupled, forward glucuronosyltransferase reaction.

Convincing evidence for carrier-mediated transport of intact UDP-glucuronic acid across the membrane into the lumen of the endoplasmic reticulum has now been reported (Bossuyt, BiochemJ, 1994; 302:261; Berg, Gastro, 1995; 108:183; Radominska, BBActa, 1994; 1195:63). It has also been demonstrated that UDP-*N*-acetylglucosamine and several other UDP-sugars are transported into the endoplasmic reticulum (Bossuyt, EurJBiochem, 1994; 223:981) and that UDP-glucuronic acid transport is markedly stimulated by UDP-*N*-acetylglucosamine (Bossuyt, BiochemJ, 1995; 305:321). This effect involves a *trans*-stimulation mechanism, whereby UDP-*N*-acetylglucosamine shuttles back and forth across the endoplasmic reticulum membrane. Furthermore, this hypothesis explains the stimulatory effect of UDP-*N*-acetylglucosamine on glucuronidation catalysed by the UGT isoenzymes by postulating that UDP-*N*-acetylglucosamine enhances transport of UDP-glucuronic acid into the endoplasmic reticulum. Thus, most recent experimental findings support the compartmentation theory initially proposed by Hallinan (Hallinan, HormCellReg, 1981; 5:73) and thereby account nicely for both the latency phenomenon and the stimulation of UGT in native microsomes by UDP-*N*-acetylglucosamine and by UDP-xylose.

Bilirubin oxidation

Since the Gunn rat cannot glucuronidate unconjugated bilirubin, much attention has been devoted to other pathways in this animal. Small amounts of mono- and dihydroxylated derivatives have been detected in Gunn rat bile (Berry, BBResComm, 1972; 49:1366; Blanckaert, BiochemJ, 1977; 164:237). The microsomal cytochrome P-450 Ia1 (previously P-448) and P-450 IA might be involved; it is higher in Gunn than in control rat liver (Kapitulunik, MolecPharmacol, 1993; 43:722) and induction of this isoenzyme by tetrachlordibenzo-*p*-dioxin led to a significant decrease of plasma bilirubin and the bilirubin pool and to an increase in bilirubin turnover (Kapitulunik, PNAS, 1977; 75:682). Proof that these changes are due to enhanced oxidation is, however, lacking and other pathways might be involved. Tetrachlordibenzo-*p*-dioxin is, however, too toxic to have a potential value in man.

Oxidation of bilirubin catalysed by a mitochondrial oxidase, present in rat intestine, kidney, and liver, has been documented *in vitro* (Cardenas-Vasquez, BiochemJ, 1986; 236:625; Yokosuka, BBActa, 1987; 923:268). Its role '*in vivo*' remains unclear; indeed, as an antioxidant, bilirubin itself is likely to at least partially undergo oxidation itself. *In vitro* studies demonstrated that microsomal lipid peroxidation caused concurrent degradation of added bilirubin but microsomal superoxide, hydrogen peroxide, or hydroxy radicles did not lead to bilirubin degradation. Injection of vitamin E into

Gunn rats completely inhibited microsomal lipid peroxidation and concurrent bilirubin degradation but this had no effect on plasma bilirubin (Joshi, BBActa, 1995; 1243:244).

Biliary secretion

It is not clear how the conjugates formed in the endoplasmic reticulum reach the bile. They might be linked to cytosolic proteins such as ligandin, stay in solution in cytosol, or be transported by vesicles. Indeed it has recently been suggested that bile acids (Dubin, Gastro, 1978; 75:450; Lamri, JCI, 1988; 82:1173) and bilirubin conjugates (Crawford, JLipRes, 1988; 29:144) may undergo vesicular transport in bile acid-depleted and bile acid-repleted rats or when high amounts of conjugates are injected. These conclusions were reached by using colchicine or related products as blocking agents of vesicular transport. In the case of bile acids, antibodies could localize bile acids in vesicular structures.

Biliary secretion *per se* represents a carrier-mediated transport characterized by saturation phenomena, competition, and selectivity. When infusing increasing amounts of so-called organic anions, a maximal secretory rate is obtained (usually denoted as hepatobiliary transport maximum or Tm). In analogy with enzyme kinetics, the hyperbolic relationship between biliary output and infusion rate has been viewed as representing saturation (Vmax) of a transport system. During infusion of sulphobromophthalein, a hyperbolic relationship was observed in the rat between biliary secretory rate and the 'free' concentration of unconjugated and conjugated sulphobromophthalein in liver tissue. However, the saturation level (Tm) can also be seen to represent an equilibrium state reached between enhancing secretion and toxicity as proposed for bile acids by Hardison et al.[12] Experiments showed that bilirubin diglucuronide administered during a maximal secretory rate of bilirubin induced a pronounced decrease of bile flow, bile acid, and bilirubin secretion (Sieg, Hepatol, 1989; 10:14). These results corroborate the view that high amounts of organic anions could 'intoxicate' the secretory process at the canalicular membrane. Such a negative effect is already reached at low infusion rates with indocyanine green, oestradiol, and dihydrotestosterone glucuronide (Vore, LifeSci, 1989; 44:2033) and occurs only at higher molar infusion rates with bilirubin glucuronides or ioglycamide (Mesa, JHepatol, 1985; 1:243). Similarly with bile acids, lithocholate rapidly exerts a cholestatic action whereas this is almost non-existent when ursodeoxycholate is given. As such, a 'cholestatic range' has been established for bile acids.

However, saturation does not necessarily represent the presence of a carrier transport mechanism, since binding of poorly water-soluble substrates to isolated membrane preparations is also saturable (Heirwegh, BiochemJ, 1988; 254:101). The discovery of a transport deficient mutant, Wistar rat (Janssen, Hepatol, 1985; 5: 573), has greatly added to our knowledge. Furthermore, a canalicular multispecific organic anion transporter has been isolated. This ATPase is regulated by protein kinase C and seems identical with the multidrug resistance associated protein (Oude Elferink, AmJPhysiol, 1990; 258:G699; Pikula, JBC, 1994; 269:27807). This transport protein is responsible for transport into the bile canaliculus of bilirubin and bile acid glycosides, cysteinyl-leuktrienes, glutathion conjugates, etc. Recent studies in the transport deficient (TR⁻) rats documented a single nucleotide deletion in the rat gene

encoding for the canalicular multispecific organic anion transporter; this results in reduced mRNA and absence of the carrier multispecific organic anion transporter protein (Paulusma, Science, 1966: 271:1126). It has recently been demonstrated that mutation in the human *cMOAT* gene which is homologous to the rat *cmoat* gene, is responsible for the transport defect in the Dubin-Johnson syndrome (Taulusma, Hepatol, 1997; 25:1539).

Biliary secretion of bilirubin conjugates undergoes competitive inhibition by several substances which do not need glucuronidation for biliary secretion, such as indocyanine green, bromosulphophthalein, or ioglycamide.

Biliary phospholipid and cholesterol secretion is markedly enhanced by bile acid administration (Wheeler, JCI, 1972; 51:1337). In contrast, infusion of bilirubin, ioglycamide, bromosulphophthalein, and biomocresol green at dosages resulting in their maximal secretory rates markedly decreased the biliary output of phospholipids and cholesterol in bile. Similarly ampicillin, or indocyanine green in the rat or hamster but not in dogs, decreased the phospholipid secretion. These effects also seem dose- and species-dependent and, as yet, a generalized mechanism cannot be proposed. Secretion of conjugated bilirubin, bromosulphophthalein, and other organic anions do not seem to exert a choleretic effect, in contrast to the bile flow elicited by bile acids. This led to the suggestion that their potential osmotic activity is masked due to possible incorporation in mixed micelles or other macromolecular aggregates (Scharschmidt, JCI, 1978; 62:1122). Obviously, at present, it is unclear whether biliary secretion is equilibrative or intrinsically concentrative.

Recently, the question of whether the maximal biliary secretion rate (Tm) reflects secretion alone or a combination of intrahepatic mechanisms including conjugation has been investigated. Indeed a remarkable relationship was obtained between the maximal biliary bilirubin secretion rate and the bilirubin UDP-glucuronosyltransferase activity assayed *in vitro* on liver homogenates of heterozygous Gunn and normal castrated or ovarectomized Wister rats, treated or untreated with testosterone or L-thyroxine (inhibitory effect) or with progesterone, secretin, glutethimide, phenobarbitone, clofibrate, or spironolactone (enhancing effect) (Muraca, ClinSci, 1983; 64:85; Van Steenbergen, Gastro, 1990; 99: 488). These data suggest that, *in vivo*, conjugation rather than the canalicular transport step itself may govern the overall biliary output.

The fate of bile pigments in the intestine

Esterified bilirubins undergo deconjugation and a series of reductive reactions catalysed predominantly by enzymes of bacterial origin and possibly to a small part by intestinal wall β-glucuronidase. *In vitro*, conjugates are more prone to reductive degradation than unconjugated bilirubin (Watson, BiochemMed, 1969; 2:461). If a similar situation holds *in vivo*, degradation would prevail above deconjugation. It should also be remembered that conditions in bile and intestine favour formation of non-C-1 glucuronides by the acyl shift. These are resistant to β-glucuronidase, and conditions are thus unfavourable for pronounced deconjugation.

In neonates whose bacterial flora have not yet developed, in germ-free rats, and in individuals submitted to broad-spectrum antibiotics, bilirubin and its conjugates are present in the stools, and reabsorption can lead to unconjugated hyperbilirubinaemia

(Poland, NEJM, 1971; 284:1). In normal conditions, the bulk of bilirubin is transformed to urobilinogens. The small amount of deconjugated bilirubin and part of the urobilinogen formed can undergo intestinal reabsorption for reconjugation and resecretion in bile. The enterohepatic circulation thus seems of minor importance, but nevertheless explains the presence of urobilinogen in urine of normal individuals and, even more so, in patients with haemolysis or liver disease (Bernstein, Gastro, 1971; 61:733). In the ileectomized rat, it has recently been shown that more unconjugated bilirubin is reabsorbed in the colon (Brink, Gastro, 1996; 110:1945); a similar situation might exist in patients with resections of the terminal ileum or even with severe Crohn's disease; this could explain the increased incidence of pigmented gallstones in these patients. In Gunn rats, more unconjugated bilirubin and urobilinogen are present in the intestine and are reabsorbed. During fasting, intestinal motility slows down, reabsorption is enhanced, and serum unconjugated bilirubin goes up (Kotal, Gastro, 1996; 111:217). A similar situation might exist in the neonate, where more unconjugated bilirubin is present in the intestine; delayed elimination of stools will lead to enhanced reabsorption and to increased serum unconjugated bilirubin levels.

References

1. Ostrow JD, ed. *Bile pigments and jaundice*. New York: Marcel Dekker, 1986.
2. McDonagh AF. Bile pigments: bilatrienes and 5, 15-biladienes. In Dolphin D, ed. *The Porphyrins*. New York: Academic Press, 1979.
3. Bonnett R, *et al.* The structure of bilirubin. *Proceedings of the Royal Society of London*, 1978; **202**: 249–68.
4. Lightner DA. Structure, photochemistry, and organic chemistry of bilirubin. In Heirwegh KPM and Brown SD, eds. *Bilirubin*. Vol. 1: Chemistry. Boca Raton, Florida: CRC Press, 1982: 1–58.
5. Hauser SC and Gollan J. Hepatic UDP-glucuronyltransferase and the conjugation of bile pigments. In Ostrow JD, ed. *Bile Pigments and Jaundice*. New York: Marcel Dekker, 1986: 211–42.
6. Bissell DM. Heme catabolism and bilirubin formation. In Ostrow JD, ed. *Bile Pigments and jaundice*. New York: Marcel Dekker, 1986: 133–56.
7. Robinson SH. Formation of bilirubin from erythroid and non-erythroid sources. *Seminars in Hematology*, 1972; **9**: 43–53.
8. Brodersen R. Aqueous solubility, albumin binding, and tissue distribution of bilirubin. In Ostrow JD, ed. *Bile pigments and jaundice*. New York: Marcel Dekker, 1986: 157–81.
9. Kotyk A and Janácek K. *Cell membrane transport principles and techniques*. New York: Plenum, 1970: 55–89.
10. Fevery J, De Groote J, and Heirwegh KPM. Properties of bilirubin UDP-glycosyltranstransferases. *Frontiers of Gastrointestinal Research*, 1976; **2**: 243–92.
11. Vessey DA and Zakim D. Are glucuronidation reactions compartmented? In Aitio A, ed. *Conjugation reactions in drug biotransformations*, Amsterdam: Elsevier/North-Holland Biomedical Press, 1978: 247–55.
12. Hardison WGM, *et al.* Nature of bile acid maximum secretory rate in the rat. *American Journal of Physiology*, 1982; **241**: G337–43.

2.10 Metabolism of bile acids

M. Fuchs and Eduard F. Stange

Introduction

The chemical structure of the major bile acids has been almost correctly defined for more than 70 years (Wieland, ZPhysiolChem, 1924; 140:186; Windaus, ZPhysiolChem, 1924; 140:177). The curative properties of ursodeoxycholic acid, present in bear bile, were appreciated long before the chemical structure of this bile acid was clarified (Iwasaki, ZPhysiolChem, 1936; 224:181). A few years later, the successful isolation of cholic acid from ox bile was reported and it was confirmed that bile acids are synthesized from cholesterol (Bloch, JBC, 1943; 149:511).

Bile acid metabolism has been studied in a variety of animals. Several reasons underline the importance of studying species differences. The elucidation of physiological and pathophysiological processes requires detailed knowledge of the participating biochemicals and their physicochemical properties. Bile acid chemistry plays an important role in the development of structure–activity relationship. Species differences in bile acids may not only provide valuable information in tracing evolutionary relationships between species, but are absolutely required for interpreting the results of toxicological studies in animals. For example, ursodeoxycholic acid, now widely applied to treat cholestatic liver diseases (see Chapter 23.3 'Intrahepatic cholestasis') without side-effects, is hepatotoxic in rabbits (Cohen, Gastro, 1986; 91:189).

Investigations on the chemical structure of bile acids provided useful information about the evolution of species and apparently support Haeckel's law of phylogeny recapitulating ontogeny: end products of bile acid synthesis in lower vertebrates are precursors of the end products of bile acids in higher vertebrates (Haslewood, PhysiolRev, 1955; 35:178; Haslewood, JLipRes, 1967; 8:535). The isolation of species-specific bile acids from bile has continued up to the present and new compounds have been reported during the last years.

This chapter highlights our current knowledge of bile acid metabolism in health and disease. We have witnessed substantial

The authors are grateful to the copyright owners and principal investigators who have allowed them to reproduce figures and tables from their articles. We wish to recognize important research contributions towards understanding the feedback regulation of bile acid synthesis carried out in our laboratory by Drs Jürgen Scheibner, Gisela Tauber, and Klaus Empen as well as by Erwin Hörmann and Michael Schiemann. Continual expert technical assistance was provided by Mrs Elke Preiss, Mrs Roswitha Rittelmann, and Ms Cornelia Engstler. This work was supported in part by the German Science Foundation through grants Sta 172 and the Falk Foundation, Freiburg, Germany.

progress since the early days of bile acid research. Powerful new technologies such as nuclear magnetic resonance and mass spectroscopy have pushed the field forward and have even allowed the design of bile acids with desired biological properties. The role of bile acids in the dissolution of cholesterol gallstones has been recognized and therapeutic effects of bile acids in chronic cholestatic liver disease are becoming one of the most exciting developments in hepatology. The immediate challenge in this field is built upon the modern techniques of molecular and cell biology that will open definitively a new area of research related to the hepatobiliary system. The authors are confident that future discoveries will be of great benefit for patients with hepatobiliary and intestinal diseases.

Physiological role of bile acids

Bile acids are the osmotic force for promoting water movement from the hepatocyte into bile.[1] In several ways these molecules represent key players in cholesterol homeostasis and provide a pathway to eliminate cholesterol quantitatively from the body. This is achieved by using cholesterol as a substrate for their own synthesis in the hepatocyte and by promoting biliary cholesterol secretion as unilamellar vesicles and mixed micelles (Carey, ArchIntMed, 1972; 130:506; Sömjen, FEBSLett, 1983; 156:265; Pattinson, Gastro, 1986; 91:697), eventually leading to their faecal loss. The formation of vesicles and micelles of cholesterol in the biliary tree and gallbladder prevents cholesterol crystallization and subsequent cholesterol gallstone formation.[2,3] By means of the enterohepatic circulation, bile acids continuously promote biliary cholesterol secretion and indirectly regulate cholesterol synthesis (Wilson, ArchIntMed, 1972; 130:493; Everson, SemLivDis, 1992; 12:420).

Within the intestine, bile acids participate in fat digestion and assimilation by serving as cofactors for digestive lipases, such as the pancreatic carboxyl ester hydrolase and the human milk lipase (Hamosh, AdvPediat, 1982; 29:33; Carey, SemGastroDis, 1992; 3:189). Full activity of these enzymes is obtained only in the presence of 7α-hydroxylated primary bile acids at concentrations below their critical micellar concentration (Hernell, EurJClinInv, 1975; 5:267). In addition, bile acids protect many lipolytic enzymes, such as gastric lipase and pancreatic phospholipase A_2, from proteolytic digestion and denaturation (Carey, SemGastroDis, 1992; 3:189).

Mixed micelles have been considered as sole vehicles for the solubilization and transport of lipolytic products (Hofmann, FedProc, 1962; 21:43; Hofmann, JCI, 1964; 43:247). However, even in the complete absence of intraluminal bile acids, more than 50 per cent of triacylglycerols are absorbed (Porter, Gastro, 1971; 60:997). This supports the view that non-micellar mechanisms for the dispersion of lipolytic products may contribute to the assimilation of lipids within the intestine. Indeed, recent studies suggest that micellar vesicles facilitate the dissolution of lipolytic products into unsaturated mixed micelles. Also, vesicles may be responsible for the efficient fat absorption from the small intestine under conditions where bile acids are deficient (Hernell, Biochem, 1990; 29:2041).

Having reached the intestine, bile acids are involved in the release of cholecystokinin and somatostatin during digestion (Riepl, Pancreas, 1994; 9:109). Thus it appears that gallbladder contraction is determined by the balance of the agonistic and antagonistic effects of cholecystokinin and somatostatin, respectively.

The role of bile acids in calcium absorption is related to the ability of micellar bile acids to enhance the absorption of vitamin D. However, recently it has been shown that bile acids in pre-micellar concentrations also may enhance calcium absorption, as evidenced by studies with isolated vesicles from the intestinal brush-border membrane (Sanyal, Gastro, 1994; 106:866). High-affinity binding may be essential for bile acid-induced enhancement of intestinal calcium uptake (Sanyal, Gastro, 1992; 102:1997) and, as shown for red cell membranes (Oehlberg, Hepatol, 1987; 7:245), bile acids may act as calcium ionophores. Nevertheless, recent studies investigating this hypothesis have shown that molecular mechanisms of bile acid-induced divalent cation transport apparently do not involve the creation of reverse micelles within the membrane. More likely, transmembrane transport of biologically relevant cations may underlie bile acid cytotoxic effects on cells (Albalak, Biochem, 1996; 35:7936). Ongoing studies should help to define the exact molecular basis of bile acid-mediated intestinal calcium uptake.

Almost 60 years ago, bile fistula experiments with iron-depleted dogs revealed the importance of bile in the absorption of orally administered iron (Hawkins, JExpMed, 1938; 67:89). Subsequently, it has been shown that bile diversion induced iron deficiency (Wheby, Gastro, 1962; 42:319). More recent *in vivo* studies in rats suggest that bile acids in pre-micellar concentrations also facilitate intestinal iron absorption (Sanyal, AmJPhysiol, 1994; 266:G318). This is in good agreement with earlier studies employing isolated intestinal apical brush-border membrane vesicles (Thompson, Hepatol, 1992; 16:261A). The molecular basis for this observation, however, requires further evaluation.

Studies with patients who have obstructive jaundice and T-tube drainage (Teo, BMJ, 1980; 281:831), as well as bile fistula experiments in rats (Bergesen, ScaJGastr, 1985; 20:589), have shown that bile acids may also be required for receptor-mediated internalization of the intrinsic factor–cobalamin complex (Robertson, Gastro, 1985; 88:908; Seetharam, AmJPhysiol, 1985; 248:G326; Ramasamy, AmJPhysiol, 1989; 257:G791). Mechanisms by which bile acids influence intestinal cobalamin absorption are not yet known. It has been proposed that luminal bile acids optimize ileal binding of the intrinsic factor–cobalamin complex via interaction with a putative ileal cytosolic factor (Seetharam, AmJPhysiol, 1992; 262:G210).

In summary, bile acids have multiple functions and may be involved in the pathogenesis of many hepatobiliary and intestinal diseases.

Bile acid analysis

To analyse bile acids that are abundant in many biological materials, their preliminary fractionation into bile acid classes is important. This can be done by liquid/liquid partition, ion-exchange chromatography, gel permeation chromatography, and liquid/solid phase adsorption.[4] Separation of individual bile acids[5] may be achieved by thin layer or column chromatography (adsorption chromatography), or high performance liquid or gel liquid chromatography (partition chromatography). Individual structure assignments require gas chromatography/mass spectrometry and nuclear magnetic resonance spectroscopy.[6]

The following example is a good illustration of the need for bile acid fractionation. In a series of patients with cholestasis, one patient apparently had large quantities of deoxycholic acid, at least as judged by gas liquid chromatography (Summerfield, ClinSci, 1977; 52:51). However, this seemed unlikely because the formation of deoxycholic acid is markedly reduced in cholestasis. Gas liquid chromatography combined with mass spectrometry subsequently revealed that the material was not deoxycholic acid, but ursocholic acid, the 7α-epimer of cholic acid. Reinvestigation of other samples also revealed the presence of ursocholic acid in several other patients.

Excellent reviews of the serum,[7] urine,[8] and faecal bile acids[9] of healthy subjects and patients with liver diseases have been published.

Bile acid structure and nomenclature

Bile acids consist of four fused rings (the cyclopentanophenanthrene or steroid nucleus), comprising three six-membered rings (A, B, and C) and one five-membered ring (D). Rules for numbering the carbon atoms of the steroid ring and the side chain are given in Fig. 1. Dependent on the orientation of the proton on C5 at the junction of rings A and B, bile acids may be divided into two groups. When the proton is *trans* with respect to the methyl group at C19, it is in the 5α-configuration (Fig. 2), with each of the A, B, C, and D rings being in the same plane. When the proton is *cis* to the methyl group at C19 (Fig. 2), it has the 5β-configuration, with ring A approximately at a right angle to the plane of the other rings. Although the 5α-cholanoic acids are chemically more stable than the 5β-cholanoic acids, the latter group is predominantly found in most creatures. In humans, most of the bile acids have 24 carbon atoms and are given the systematic root name of cholanoic acids (Table 1). For C24 bile acids, a five-carbon aliphatic side-chain, which ends in a carboxylic acid, is attached to the 17β-position in the D ring (Fig. 1). Bile acids are a family of molecules with side chains of variable length. They have a variable number of hydroxyl or keto groups either on the steroid nucleus or on the side chain.

The term primary bile acids refers to those bile acids synthesized *de novo* in the liver and the most common are cholic (3α,7α,12α-trihydroxy-5β-cholanoic acid) and chenodeoxycholic acid (3α,7α-dihydroxy-5β-cholanoic acid). Secondary bile acids are formed by bacterial degradation in the intestine and comprise deoxycholic (3α,12α-dihydroxy-5β-cholanoic acid) and lithocholic acid (3α-monohydroxy-5β-cholanoic acid). Bile acids that have undergone combined bacterial and hepatic modification are termed tertiary bile

Table 1 Systemic and trivial names of commonly found bile acids and their abbreviations

Systematic name[a]	Trivial name	Abbreviation
Monohydroxycholanoic acids		
3α-Hydroxy-	Lithocholic acid	LCA
Dihydroxycholanoic acids		
3α,6α-Dihydroxy-	Hyodeoxycholic acid	HDCA
3α,7α-Dihydroxy-	Chenodeoxycholic acid	CDCA
3α,7β-Dihydroxy-	Ursodeoxycholic acid	UDCA
3α,12α-Dihydroxy-	Deoxycholic acid	DCA
Trihydroxycholanoic acids		
3α,6α,7α-Trihydroxy	Hyocholic acid	HCA
3α,6β,7α-Trihydroxy	α-Muricholic acid	αMCA
3α,6β,7β-Trihydroxy	β-Muricholic acid	βMCA
3α,7α,12α-Trihydroxy	Cholic acid	CA
3α,7β,12α-Trihydroxy	Ursocholic acid	UCA
Other bile acids		
3α-Hydroxy-7-keto-	7-Ketolithocholic acid	KLCA
3α,7α,12α-Triketo-	Dehydrocholic acid	DHCA

[a] Except where stated, each bile acid is a derivative of 5β(H)-cholanoic acid. The full systematic name can be obtained by placing the substituent name in front of 5(α,β)-cholanoic acid.

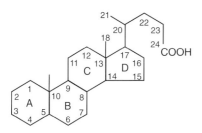

Fig. 1. Structure of common bile acids. The steroid nucleus is composed of three six-membered rings (A, B, and C) and a five-membered ring (D). The carbon atoms of the steroid ring and the side chain are given.

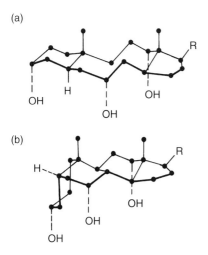

Fig. 2. Perspective drawing of bile acids. Bile acids with a 5α-hydrogen (a) and a 5β-hydrogen (b) at the AB ring junction. Whereas in the 5α-configuration the A, B, C, and D rings are in the same plane, in the 5β-configuration the A ring is approximately at a right angle to the plane of the other three rings.

acids and an example is ursodeoxycholic acid (3α,7β-dihydroxy-5β-cholanoic acid).

A summary of bile acid structures by Matschiner[10] is an additional source of information. In the following, bile acids are divided into their major classes for the purposes of discussion.

Monohydroxy bile acids

Lithocholic acid (3α-hydroxy-5β-cholanoic acid) and 3β-hydroxy-5-cholenoic acid are the major monohydroxy bile acids. They are largely found in the bile, blood, and urine of normal subjects and patients with liver diseases as sulphate esters or glucuronides of their amino acid conjugates. 3β-Hydroxy-5-cholenoic acid is one of the major bile acids of the meconium of newborn infants (Back, HoppeSeylerZPhysiolChem, 1973; 354:83). It retains the nuclear configuration of cholesterol from which it is thought to be formed by 27-hydroxylation and side-chain oxidation and cleavage (Anderson, JCI, 1972; 51:112). However, it could also arise from dehydroxylation of 3β,7α-dihydroxy-5-cholenoic acid. The 3β-hydroxy isomer (Danielsson, JBC, 1963; 238:2299), the 7β-hydroxy isomer (Ali, CanJBiochem, 1966; 44:957), and the *allo*-isomer of lithocholic acid (Makino, FEBSLett, 1971; 15:161) have also been reported. Two C27 monohydroxy bile acids, 3α-hydroxy-5β-cholestan-26-oic acid and 3β-hydroxy-5-cholesten-26-oic acid have been found in children with coprostanic acidaemia (Janssen, Steroids, 1981; 37:81). The latter bile acid is also present in the blood of both, healthy adults (Axelson, JLipRes, 1988; 29:629) and patients with liver diseases (Axelson, JLipRes, 1989; 30:1877,1883).

Monohydroxy bile acids have long been considered hepatotoxic and to have a role in the pathogenesis of certain hepatobiliary diseases. However, although they cause acute cholestasis in rats when administered intravenously (Kakis, Gastro, 1978; 75:595; Yousef, Gastro, 1981; 80:233) and portal inflammation as well as bile-duct proliferation in chronic animal models, direct evidence of their involvement in human hepatobiliary diseases remains elusive. Sulphate ester or glucuronide formation has been considered to reduce their toxicity; however, rather than reducing toxicity *per se*, these metabolic reactions may increase the rate of elimination of the monohydroxy bile acids and therefore prevent their accumulation.

Dihydroxy bile acids

The four most common bile acids are dihydroxy derivatives of 5β-cholanoic acid, hyodeoxycholic acid ($3\alpha,6\alpha$-dihydroxy-5β-cholanoic acid), chenodeoxycholic acid ($3\alpha,7\alpha$-dihydroxy-5β-cholanoic acid), ursodeoxycholic acid ($3\alpha,7\beta$-dihydroxy-5β-cholanoic acid), and deoxycholic acid ($3\alpha,12\alpha$-dihydroxy-5β-cholanoic acid). In bile, dihydroxy bile acids are almost exclusively found as glycine or taurine conjugates, whereas in urine they are excreted mostly as double conjugates. Chenodeoxycholic acid and deoxycholic acid appear as sulphates, glucuronides, and glucosides. Ursodeoxycholic acid, on the other hand, is the only bile acid known to undergo *N*-acetylglucosaminidation (Marshall, JCI, 1992; 89:1981). The identification of $3\alpha,7\beta$-dihydroxy-5β-chol-22-en-24-oic acid, Δ22-ursodeoxycholic acid, in the plasma, bile, liver, and intestinal content of rats following administration of ursodeoxycholic acid (Setchell, Biochem, 1995; 34:4169), suggests partial β-oxidation of this bile acid. The mechanism of formation as well as the physiological significance remains to be investigated. So far, this metabolite of ursodeoxycholic acid has not been found in humans (Colombo, JPediat, 1990; 117:482; Crosignani, Hepatol, 1991; 14:100). It thus remains possible that Δ22-ursodeoxycholic acid is specific to the rat. Hyodeoxycholic acid is extensively converted to its 6α-glucuronide.

Various isomers of these bile acids have been discovered with improved isolation techniques and analytical procedures. The C27 analogues (5β-cholestan-26-oic acids) of chenodeoxycholic acid and deoxycholic acid were first identified in alligators (Tint, Gastro, 1981; 80:114) before their detection in man.

Several unsaturated dihydroxy bile acids have been found in the blood of healthy subjects, namely $3\alpha,7\alpha$-dihydroxy-, $3\beta,7\alpha$-dihydroxy-, and $3\alpha,12\alpha$-dihydroxy-5-cholenoic acids (Ikeda, JBiochem, 1976; 83:799; Bremmelgaard, EurJClinInv, 1979; 9:341; Axelson, JLipRes, 1988; 29:629). They appear to arise from 7α- and 12α-hydroxylation of cholesterol when side-chain oxidation occurs before further modification to the steroid nucleus. These bile acids are excreted in the urine mainly as their sulphate esters and this is an important compensation process for children with a deficiency of 3β-hydroxy-ΔC27 steroid dehydrogenase/isomerase (Clayton, JCI, 1987; 79:1031).

Trihydroxy bile acids

Four common bile acids that have three hydroxy groups are hyocholic acid ($3\alpha,6\alpha,7\alpha$-trihydroxy-5β-cholanoic acid), α-muricholic acid ($3\alpha,6\beta,7\alpha$-trihydroxy-5β-cholanoic acid), β-muricholic acid ($3\alpha,6\beta,7\beta$-trihydroxy-5β-cholanoic), and cholic acid ($3\alpha,7\alpha,12\alpha$-trihydroxy-5β-cholanoic acid). Hyocholic acid, the principal bile acid of the pig (Hsia, JBC, 1957; 225:811), is found in patients with cholestasis (Summerfield, BiochemJ, 1976; 154:507; Shoda, JLipRes, 1988; 29:847) and in newborn infants, but not in healthy adults (Nakashima, CCActa, 1986; 160:47). α-Muricholic and β-muricholic acids are found in rats (Hsia, JBC, 1958; 230:573), and cholic acid is a primary bile acid in many species, including man. β-Muricholic acid is an important metabolite in experimental cholestasis in the rat (Greim, Gastro, 1972; 63:837), but not in man.

Trihydroxy bile acids are mostly found as their glycine or taurine conjugates in bile, blood, and urine. Sulphate, glucuronide, and glucoside conjugates are detected in urine, but in lesser amounts than mono- or dihydroxy bile acids.

Many other potential isomers of the 3,6,7- and 3,7,12-trihydroxy series exist. Ursocholic acid ($3\alpha,7\beta,12\alpha$-trihydroxy-5β-cholanoic acid) is present in most patients with cholestasis (Summerfield, ClinSci, 1977; 52:51) and in the urine of healthy adults of all ages (Nakashima, CCActa, 1986; 160:47). ω-Muricholic acid ($3\alpha,6\alpha,7\beta$-trihydroxy-5β-cholanoic acid), the 7β-epimer of hyocholic acid and now termed β-hyocholic acid (Hofmann, JLipRes, 1992; 33:599), is present in small amounts in the urine of healthy adults (Nakashima, CCActa, 1986; 160:47) and in patients with primary biliary cirrhosis (Batta, JLipRes, 1989; 30:1953). 1-Hydroxylated and 6-hydroxylated forms of deoxycholic acid have been discovered in patients with cholestasis (Bremmelgaard, EurJClinInv, 1979; 9:341; Thomassen, EurJClinInv, 1979; 9:425). However, 1β-hydroxylation is not restricted to cholestasis; these bile acids have been detected in the urine of healthy men and in patients with kidney disease (Tohma, ChemPharmBull, 1986; 34:2890). Chenodeoxycholic acid and ursodeoxycholic acid are also present as their 21-, 22-, and 23-hydroxylated forms in patients with cerebrotendinous xanthomatosis treated with these bile acids (Koopman, BBActa, 1987; 917: 238). The unsaturated bile acid, $3\alpha,7\alpha,12\alpha$-trihydroxy-5-cholenoic acid, was found in the urine of young twins with intrahepatic cholestasis (Clayton, JCI, 1987; 79:1031). The C27 analogue of cholic acid, $3\alpha,7\alpha,12\alpha$-trihydroxy-5β-cholestan-26-oic acid, a major bile acid of the alligator (Tint, JLipRes, 1980; 21:110), has been detected in children with certain cholestasis syndromes (Eyssen, BBActa, 1972; 273:212; Hanson, JCI, 1975; 56:577; Mathis, Gastro, 1980; 79:1311).

Tetrahydroxy bile acids

Tetrahydroxy bile acids have been reported in patients with cholestasis. Because of their polar nature, these bile acids are excreted into urine in the unconjugated form; only small amounts of tetrahydroxy bile acids appear in bile. As for dihydroxy bile acids, 1-hydroxylation and 6-hydroxylation of cholic acid occurs (Thomassen, EurJClinInv, 1979; 9:425; Bremmelgaard, JLipRes, 1980; 21: 1072). 23-Hydroxycholic acid, a bile acid thought to be restricted to snakes and seals (Bergstrom, ActaSocMedUppsal, 1959; 64: 160; Haslewood, BiochemJ, 1961; 78:352), has been found in man (Bremmelgaard, EurJClinInv, 1979; 9:341).

Keto bile acids and bile acid epimers

Keto bile acids, which are less soluble than their reduced hydroxy counterparts, are thought to originate from the action of bacteria on the hydroxy bile acids in the intestine. However, in the guinea pig it has been suggested that 3α-hydroxy-7-keto-5β-cholanoic acid, a major bile acid in this species, can be formed independently of intestinal bacteria (Peric-Golla, PSEBM, 1961; 106:177). Since 3- and 7-oxidoreductase activities have been demonstrated in rat liver (Ikeda, HoppeSeylerZPhysiolChem, 1984; 365:377; Amuro, BBActa, 1987; 917:101; Stolz, JCI, 1987; 79:427), conceivably circumstances may exist in which oxidation of hydroxy bile acids to keto bile acids occurs. However, the enzymatic properties of the purified oxidoreductases suggest that reduction of the keto groups, rather than formation of keto bile acids, is highly favoured (Amuro, BBActa, 1987; 917:101; Stolz, JCI, 1987; 79:427). It has recently been suggested that the altered redox state of the liver at the time of birth could account for the accumulation of unsaturated keto bile acids in the urine of newborns (Wahlen, JLipRes, 1989; 30:1847). The most abundant is 7α,12α-dihydroxy-3-oxo-5β-chol-1-enoic acid which may arise from elimination of water from 1β,3α,7α,12α-tetrahydroxy-5β-cholanoic acid. Another unsaturated keto bile acid is 7α-hydroxy-3-oxo-4-cholestenoic acid; this bile acid is formed when side-chain oxidation occurs before full reduction of the steroid nucleus. It is found in the blood of healthy subjects and those with liver diseases. Interestingly, it is elevated in patients receiving cholestyramine, or following an ileal resection, presumably due to an increase in the activity of 7α-hydroxylase (Axelson, JLipRes, 1989; 30:1883).

Since the keto bile acids which are absorbed from the intestine are mostly reduced to their hydroxy forms before excretion into bile, in liver diseases with reduced liver function an accumulation of keto bile acids should be anticipated.

Dehydrocholic acid, the 3,7,12-triketo derivative of cholic acid has been used clinically for 50 years as a choleretic agent. It was initially thought that the choleresis was due to excretion of unchanged dehydrocholic acid. However, it has been shown by many investigators that reduction of dehydrocholic acid to various hydroxylated bile acids (conjugated with glycine or taurine) occurs before excretion (Soloway, JCI, 1973; 52:715; Parkhill, PSEBM, 1979; 162:495).

Ursodeoxycholic acid may be formed from chenodeoxycholic acid by oxidation to 7-ketolithocholic acid and subsequent 7β-reduction of the keto bile acid in the liver (Mahowald, JBC, 1958; 230:581; Hellstrom, ActaPhysiolScand, 1961; 51:218; Salen, JCI, 1974; 53:612). However, this route has been disputed; it was suggested that a 6,7-monounsaturated intermediate was involved (Higashi, ActaHepatolJpn, 1978; 19:803; Fromm, AmJPhysiol, 1980; 239:G161) and such an unsaturated bile acid has since been isolated (Malavolti, JBC, 1985; 260:11011). On the other hand, bacteria have been identified which convert both cholic acid and deoxycholic acid to their 7β-epimers (ursocholic acid and ursodeoxycholic acid) in culture (Higashi, ActaHepatolJpn, 1978; 19:803; McDonald, JLipRes, 1981; 22:458).

Epimerization reactions account for many possible isomers of common bile acids discovered in faeces, although some of them occur in low amounts. The reduced amounts of bile acids entering the large bowel in patients with liver diseases may alter the bacterial flora and so affect the metabolism of bile acids. It is likely that each of these metabolites enters the enterohepatic circulation, but the extent of their occurrence has yet to be defined.

Allo-bile acids

Allo-bile acids are products isolated from some vertebrates[11] and from human biological fluids.[6,7,8,12] The synthesis of the 5α-cholanoic acids, given the prefix *allo*- to distinguish them from their 5β-isomers, is only occasionally reviewed. The term *allo* should only be used for C24 bile acids; for those bile acids with longer or shorter side chains, the systematic name should be used instead. The natural occurrence of the 5α-bile acids may be greater than is apparent from the literature as they are not commercially available and many investigators have simply not looked for them.

Allo-lithocholic acid was first characterized as a saturated monohydroxylated 5α-cholanoic acid in the urine of an infant with biliary atresia (Makino, FEBSLett, 1971; 15:161). Subsequently, *allo*-deoxycholic acid, *allo*-chenodeoxycholic acid, and *allo*-cholic acid and their epimers have been detected in patients with colon cancer or hepatobiliary diseases (Alme, JLipRes, 1977; 18:339; Thomassen, EurJClinInv, 1979; 9:425; Amuro, CCActa, 1983; 127:61; Setchell, BMJ, 1983; 286:1750).

In rabbits fed the *allo*-bile acid precursor, 5α-cholestanol, *allo*-glycodeoxycholic acid precipitates at concentrations found in bile (Hofmann, JBC, 1964; 239:2813).

Bile alcohols

Polyhydroxylated biliary sterols lacking a side chain or bile alcohols are major biliary compounds in lower vertebrates.[13] Several of the bile alcohols found in bile or urine are precursors of bile acids. Usually they are present in tiny amounts and probably have been lost during work-up procedures used for bile acids analysis. Bile alcohols are the major biliary components in amphibians and fish. Commonly they are in the form of sulphate esters, although sulphation of these compounds is usually on the side chain, rather than on the steroid nucleus, as occurs for mammalian bile acids.

Patients with cerebrotendinous xanthomatosis accumulate tetrols and pentols (Setoguchi, JCI, 1974; 53:1393; Shefer, JLipRes, 1975; 6:280; Yosuhara, Steroids, 1978; 31:333), and bile alcohols in bile are present as glucuronides and exceed the concentration of bile acids (Hoshita, JLipRes, 1980; 21:1015). The most abundant biliary bile alcohol in these patients is 5β-cholestane-3α,7α,12α,25-tetrol. In control patients without liver disease, bile alcohol (predominantly 5β-cholestane-3α,7α,12α,26- tetrol) sulphate ester conjugates substantially exceed the amounts of the glucuronide conjugates (Kuroki, JLipRes, 1985; 26:230).

In urine, 27-nor-5β-cholestane-3α,7α,12α,24,25-pentol is the major bile alcohol (as its glucuronide) in healthy control subjects and in patients with various liver diseases (Karlaganis, JSterBioch, 1981; 14:341; Ludwig-Kohn, EurJClinInv, 1983; 13:91; Weydert-Huijghebaert, JLipRes, 1989; 30:1673). Many other tetrols, pentols, and hexols are also present. Since the presence of hydroxyl group(s) in the side chain creates new asymmetric centres, it is important to determine which isomers are found physiologically (Batta, JLipRes, 1979; 20:935; Dayal, Steroids, 1979; 33:327).

Other bile alcohols could originate from the diet, particularly in those subjects consuming large amounts of fish, although normally the fish will have been gutted and so bile removed before ingestion. The appearance of oyster steroids in bile in humans has been reported (Connor, Gastro, 1981; 81:276).

Bile alcohols may undergo additional hydroxylations before being secreted into bile (Une, HiroshimaJMedSci, 1994; 43:37). C27 bile alcohols have been long known to occur in cyclostomes, cartilaginous fish, lobe-finned fish, and in amphibians such as salamanders and frogs.[14] These molecules have now been detected in the manatee, elephant, rhinoceros, hyrax, and horse.[15]

Physical chemistry of bile acids

Bile acids are amphiphilic biplanar molecules with two functionally different sides. The more hydrophobic or non-polar side of the

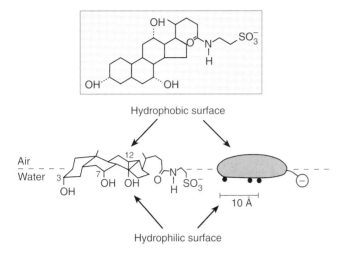

Fig. 3. Conventional (top), perspective (left), and space-filling (right) representations of the taurine conjugate of cholic acid. The molecule is depicted at an air–water interface, the hydrophilic groups oriented into the water and the hydrophobic portion exposed to the air. (Reprinted by copyright permission of the American Chemical Society from: Mazer NA, Carey MC, Kwasnick RF, and Benedek GB. Quasielastic light scattering studies of aqueous biliary lipid systems: size, shape and thermodynamics of bile salt micelles. *Biochemistry*, 1979; **18**: 3064–75).

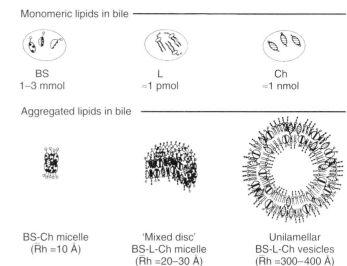

Fig. 4. Molecular models of the major biliary lipid molecules and the structure of lipid carriers in bile. Solubilities of monomeric bile acids (BS), phosphatidylcholine/lecithin (L), and cholesterol (Ch) in human bile are given as SI units. The average hydrodynamic radiuses (R_h) of aggregated lipids in bile are given in Ångstrom units (10^{-10} m). Cholesterol molecules are localized on the hydrophilic exterior of simple micelles. In mixed micelles, cholesterol is solubilized within the micelle. The unilamellar vesicles–micelles ratio depends on the bile acid and cholesterol content of bile. (Reproduced with kind permission of Raven Press Ltd, New York, from: Carey MC and Duane WC. Enterohepatic circulation. In Arias IM, Boyer JL, Fausto N, Jacoby WB, Schachter DA, and Shafritz DA, eds. The *liver: biology and pathobiology*, 3rd edn, 1994: 719–67).

molecule avoids contact with the aqueous phase. A conventional representation of the taurine conjugate of cholic acid is illustrated in Fig. 3, the hydrophilic surface facing the aqueous phase. Surface orientation of bile acid monomers may be verified employing a Langmuir–Pockel surface balance (Fahey, Biochem, 1995; 34: 10886). At a concentration defined as the critical micellar concentration, the maximum monomeric solubility is reached and molecular aggregation by means of micelle formation occurs.[16] In these simple micelles (Fig. 4), bile acid interaction most probably occurs via their hydrophobic sides and side chains.[17] The average number of bile acid molecules in a micelle is termed the aggregation number and may vary greatly. Because the less hydrophobic side of the bile acid monomer builds the external surface of the micelle, this side governs the growth of the micelle (Mazer, Biochem, 1979; 18:3064). This side also determines surface properties (Carey, Biochem, 1981; 20:637) and thin-layer as well as gas chromatographic properties of bile acids.[18] Simple micelles are composed principally of bile acid molecules, a few cholesterol molecules, but no phosphatidylcholines. The structure of such a simple micelle remains to be defined; however, the apparent size of its mean hydrodynamic radius is approximately 10 Å (10^{-10} m).[19]

Bile acid micelles can solubilize otherwise insoluble molecules, for example cholesterol in mixed micelles.[16,17,19] Mixed micelles (Fig. 4) are two to three times larger than simple micelles[19] and they consist mostly of phosphatidylcholine molecules, bile acids, and modest amounts of cholesterol. Knowledge of micellar size as determined by quasielastic light scattering, shape, and space-filling dimensions of the bile acid monomer is required for determination of the micellar structure. The last can be obtained from crystallographic measurements and space-filling molecular models of the bile acid molecule (Fig. 5). Small mixed micelles of globular shape may grow to larger 'rods' (Hjelm, ProgCollPolymerSci, 1990;

81:225; Long, BiophysJ, 1994; 67:1733) or 'worm-like' particles.[20] Although not yet visualized *in vivo*, these particles have been detected by *in vitro* systems designed to model physicochemical states of bile formation (Walter, BiophysJ, 1991; 60:1315). Interestingly, the more unsaturated phosphatidylcholines appear to partition into these micelles (Cohen, JLipRes, 1991; 32:1291; Booker, JLipRes, 1992; 33:1485). Mixed and simple micelles have been shown to coexist in human bile (Mazer, Biochem, 1983; 22: 425; Mazer, Biochem, 1984; 23:1994; Schurtenberger, Biochem, 1985; 24:7161; Cohen, JLipRes, 1990; 31:2103; Donovan, JLipRes, 1991; 32:1501). Cholesterol molecules may bind to the outside of a simple micelle, whereas they may be dissolved in the liquid hydrocarbon interiors of mixed micelles. Due to their thermodynamic stability, micelles never nucleate cholesterol molecules *in vivo* (Carey, AmJMed, 1970; 49:590).

Unilamellar vesicles (Fig. 4) are uniform in bile and their mean hydrodynamic radius has been reported to be about 300 to 400 Å, [19] thus representing particles that are much bigger than micelles. Their structure resembles a spherical lipid shell enclosing a water core in which bile electrolytes are dissolved.[19] These particles do exist transiently in unsaturated bile (Cohen, AmJPhysiol, 1989; 257:G1), however, their presence is a characteristic feature of supersaturated biles (Donovan, Hepatol, 1990; 12:94S). Persistent vesicles highly enriched with cholesterol (Mazer, Biochem, 1983; 22: 426) are thermodynamically unstable and responsible for initiating cholesterol crystal nucleation (Peled, BBActa, 1989; 1003:246).

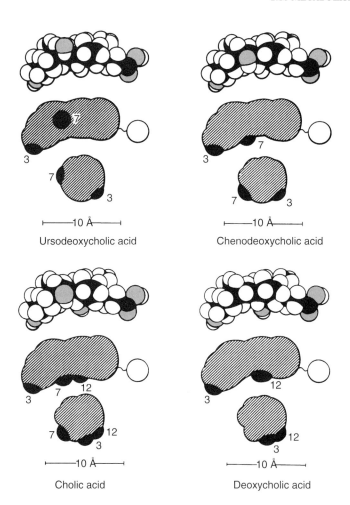

Ursodeoxycholic acid

Chenodeoxycholic acid

Cholic acid

Deoxycholic acid

Fig. 5. Schematic drawings of longitudinal and cross-sectional views of space-filling molecular models of common unconjugated bile acids. The Stuart–Briegleb molecular models represent four common bile acids: ursodeoxycholic, chenodeoxycholic, cholic, and deoxycholic. The cross-hatched areas represent hydrocarbon, whereas stippled atoms, closed circles, and ovals indicate positions and orientations of hydroxyl functions. (Reprinted by copyright permission of the American Chemical Society from: Carey MC, Montet JC, Phillips MC, Armstrong MJ, and Mazer NA. Thermodynamic and molecular basis for dissimilar cholesterol solubilizing capacities by micellar solutions of bile salts: cases of sodium chenodeoxycholate and sodium ursodeoxycholate and their glycine and taurine conjugates. *Biochemistry*, 1981; **20**: 3637–48).

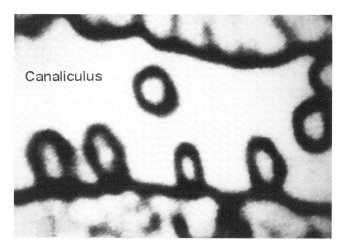

Fig. 6. Visualization of vesicles. Ultrarapid cryofixation of rat liver was employed to visualize the formation of lipid vesicles. Vesicles with an approximate diameter of 70 nm were observed in the bile canaliculus. As shown in this representative photomicrograph, five vesicles are attached to the canalicular membrane and two vesicles are within the canalicular space. (Reproduced with kind permission from: Crawford JM *et al*. Imaging biliary lipid secretion in the rat: ultrastructural evidence for vesiculation of the hepatocyte canalicular membrane. *Journal of Lipid Research*, 1995; **36**: 2147–63).

Quasielastic light scattering and electron microscopy techniques (Ulloa, Hepatol, 1987; 7:235; Cohen, AmJPhysiol, 1989; 257:G1; Cohen, AmJPhysiol, 1992; 263:G386) have shown conclusively the presence of unilamellar vesicles of cholesterol and phosphatidylcholines, which rapidly dissolve into micelles (Cohen, AmJPhysiol, 1989; 257:G1; Möckel, AmJPhysiol, 1995; 269:G73). Moreover, ultrarapid cryofixation techniques (Crawford, JLipRes, 1995; 36:2147) have visualized vesicles, for the first time, within the bile canaliculus (Fig. 6). The distribution of cholesterol between these aggregates depends on biliary lipid secretion rates: vesicles are predominant at low bile acid concentrations, whereas with increasing bile acid concentrations micelles play a more important carrier function (Pattinson, Gastro, 1986; 91:697). Lamellar structures that have been described in bile (Sömjen, BBActa, 1990; 1042:

28; Sömjen, FEBSLett, 1991; 289:163) seem spurious (Cohen, Hepatol, 1993; 18:1522).

The hydrophobic–hydrophilic balance of bile acids is influenced by several parameters, including (i) the state of ionization of the molecule, (ii) the number, orientation, and position of hydroxyl groups, and (iii) the presence and nature of ring or side-chain esters (Hofmann, JLipRes, 1984; 25:1477). Employing high-performance liquid chromatography with a stationary phase composed of octadecylsilane and a mobile phase containing methanol and water, the hydrophobic–hydrophilic balance of bile acids has been characterized (Armstrong, JLipRes, 1982; 23:70). The elution profile represents a function of the partition coefficients of monomers between the polar and non-polar phases. In other words, bile acids which spend more time in the polar phase will be eluted first. These investigations revealed that the hydrophobicity of bile acids increases in the order: ursodeoxycholic < cholic < chenodeoxycholic < deoxycholic < lithocholic acid with the taurine conjugates < the glycine conjugates (Armstrong, JLipRes, 1982; 23:70). Many, if not all, physicochemical and biological properties of individual bile acids may be a reflection of the hydrophobic–hydophilic balance.

Based on the weighted average of bile acid retention times as measured by high-performance liquid chromatography, the bile acid hydrophobicity index, a quantitative measure of the overall hydrophilicity of bile acid mixtures, has been developed (Heuman, JLipRes, 1989; 30:719). This descriptive tool has proven useful for the prediction of physicochemical properties of mixed bile acid solutions (Vlahcevic, JLipRes, 1990; 31:1063; Donovan, JLipRes, 1993; 34:1131). The novel method of immobilized artificial membrane chromatography represents another and probably more physiological approach to predict bile acid–membrane interactions (Cohen, JLipRes, 1995; 36:2251). Especially regarding molecular interactions of bile acids with the head groups of membrane phospholipids, this method should provide an optimal measure for

Table 2 Subcellular localization of enzymes involved in bile acid synthesis

Cholesterol	
Cholesterol 7α-hydroxylase	Endoplasmic reticulum
3β-hydroxy-Δ5-C27 steroid dehydrogenase/isomerase	Endoplasmic reticulum
Sterol 12α-hydroxylase	Endoplasmic reticulum
Δ4-3-oxosteroid 5β-reductase	Cytosol
3α-hydroxysteroid dehydrogenase	Cytosol
Sterol 27-hydroxylase	Mitochondria
Alcohol dehydrogenase	Cytosol
Acetataldehyde dehydrogenase	Cytosol
Bile acid CoA ligase	Endoplasmic reticulum
Bile acid CoA synthetase	Peroxisome
Bile acid acyl-CoA oxidase	Peroxisome
Bile acid hydratase/dehydrogenase	Peroxisome
Bile acid oxoacyl-CoA thiolase	Peroxisome
CoA/amino acid N-acyltransferase	Peroxisome
Bile acid conjugates	

predicting physiological processes depending on bile acid–membrane interactions.

The same physicochemical properties of bile acids that apparently determine their detergency also play an important role in determing their biological effects. The hydrophobic–hydrophilic balance of bile acids has been shown to influence phospholipid and cholesterol solubilization, cell integrity, biliary lipid secretion, and bile flow.[16,17] Because all these properties vary markedly among different bile acids, it is important to distinguish between bile salts and bile acids, the latter being virtually absent in bile. However, for reasons of simplification, we herein only use the term bile acid. A more detailed elaboration of physicochemical properties of bile acids is available elsewhere.[16,17,19,21]

Bile acid synthesis

Bile acid synthesis from cholesterol is complex and involves at least 14 reactions catalysed by a variety of enzymes found within different subcellular compartments of the liver cell (Table 2). Proposed pathways of bile acid synthesis have been derived mainly from kinetic enzyme studies or the administration of labelled putative intermediates. Identification of a variety of uncommon bile acids in bile, serum, urine, faeces, meconium, and amniotic fluid of patients with liver disease and of newborn infants has directed considerable attention to gain more insights into different pathways of bile acid synthesis. Concentrations of intermediates of bile acid synthesis

are extremely low, making it almost impossible to detect these compounds. Although the accumulation of bile acid intermediates in liver disease has added further information, one has always to consider that enzyme deficiencies may activate abnormal and not yet identified pathways of bile acid synthesis.

According to the 'neutral' and 'acidic' pathway, two different enzymes, cholesterol 7α-hydroxylase and sterol 27-hydroxylase respectively, initiate the conversion of cholesterol to bile acids. Two recent reviews describe in detail the bile acid synthesis pathways.[22, 23] Therefore, the following outline only features the major steps in the formation of bile acids.

In the 'neutral' pathway (Fig. 7), probably the one investigated better so far, microsomal 7α-hydroxylation of cholesterol (Step 1) is considered the rate-limiting step (Danielsson, EurJBioch, 1967; 2:44; Shefer, JLipRes, 1968; 9:328). 7α-Hydroxycholesterol is then oxidized to 7α-hydroxy-4-cholestene-3-one by a bifunctional microsomal NAD$^+$-dependent 3β-Δ5-C27-steroid oxidoreductase/isomerase enzyme (Step 2). The isoenzyme involved in bile acid synthesis shows absolute preference for C27 sterols (Wikval, JBC, 1981; 256:3376), thus being different from the isoenzymes which use C19 and C21 sterols as substrates. This is in line with the observation that an inborn deficiency of this enzyme has no impact on the endocrine function (Clayton, JCI, 1987; 79:1031). 7α-Hydroxy-4-cholestene-3-one can be further hydroxylated at the 12α-position by a microsomal sterol 12α-hydroxylase (Step 3) to yield 7α,12α-dihydroxy-4-cholesten-3-one. Purification of sterol 12α-hydroxylase to homogeneity (Ishida, JBC, 1992; 267:21319) has facilitated the cloning and sequencing of a complementary DNA coding for this enzyme (Eggertsen, JBC, 1996; 271:32269). Sterol 12α-hydroxylase is expressed only in liver (Eggertsen, JBC, 1996; 271:32269) and has a rather broad substrate specificity including 7α-hydroxylated C27 steroids. However, the substrate most efficiently hydroxylated appears to be 7α-hydroxy-4-cholestene-3-one (Einarsson, EurJBioch, 1968; 5:101). The availability of a complementary DNA for sterol 12α-hydroxylase will allow the study of its regulation by bile acids (Einarsson, JLipRes, 1992; 33:1591), thyroid hormones (Björkhem, FEBSLett, 1973; 31:20), and glucocorticoids on a molecular level.

The next step in bile acid synthesis is the reduction of 7α,12α-dihydroxy-4-cholesten-3-one (Step 4) by a recently cloned cytosolic Δ4-3-oxosteroid-5β-reductase (Onishi, FEBSLett, 1991; 283:215). It is noteworthy that the sequence does not appear to be related to the corresponding steroid 5α-reductase (Andersson, JBC, 1989; 264:16249). The latter enzyme catalyses the reduction with opposite stereospecificity of many sterols and is responsible for the formation of *allo*-bile acids. Subsequently, 3α,7α,12α-trihydroxy-5β-cholestanol is formed by the action of 3α-hydroxysteroid dehydrogenase (Step 5), which has been cloned by three groups of investigators (Cheng, MolEndocrin, 1991; 5:823; Pawlowski, JBC, 1991; 266:8820; Stolz, JBC, 1991; 266:15253). 3α-Hydroxysteroid dehydrogenase appears to be upregulated by thyroid hormones

Fig. 7. Pathways of bile acid synthesis—modifications to the sterol nucleus. Bile acid synthesis from cholesterol occurs via the 'neutral' pathway (reaction 1 to 5) and the 'acidic' pathway. For reasons of clarity, this flow chart can only represent a simplification of the rather complex pathways of bile acid synthesis. The enzymes depicted in this schematic may be active in both pathways as well as in the side-chain degradation of bile acid intermediates. (Adapted from ref. 22.)

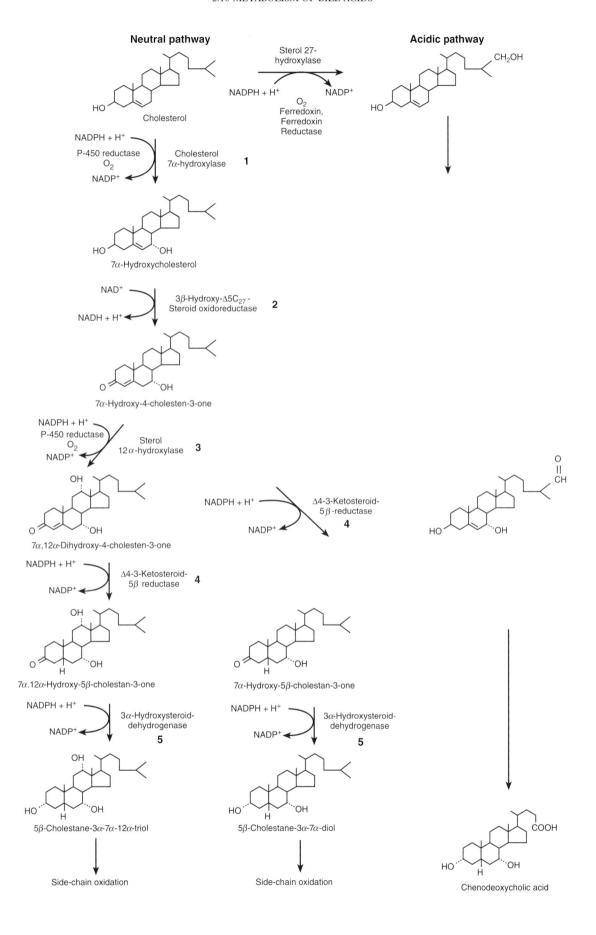

Fig. 7.

and glucocorticoids, but in contrast to cholesterol 7α-hydroxylase, hydrophobic bile acids apparently do not exhibit any inhibition (Stravitz, JLipRes, 1994; 35:239).

Before starting side-chain cleavage (Fig. 8), 27-hydroxylation (Step 6) occurs by a cytochrome P-450 mixed-function oxidase, sterol 27-hydroxylase, which is located in the inner membrane of mitochondria (Taniguchi, EurJBioch, 1973; 40:607). The enzyme has been purified and utilizes NADPH, ferredoxin, and ferredoxin reductase as well as molecular oxygen to oxidize different sterols (Wikval, JBC, 1984; 259:3800; Su, DNACellBiol, 1990; 9:657; Akiyoshi-Shibata, FEBSLett, 1991; 280:367). The enzyme often is referred to as sterol 26-hydroxylase, however, on the basis of the stereochemistry of the reaction catalysed (Danielsson, Acta-ChemScand, 1960; 14:348), it is now correctly named sterol 27-hydroxylase. In contrast to other cytochrome P-450 enzymes which exhibit restricted tissue expression (Gonzalez, PharmRev, 1989; 40:243), this enzyme is present in a variety of tissues, including fibroblasts and kidney (Skrede, JCI, 1986; 78:729; Andersson, JBC, 1989; 264:8222; Postlind, BBResComm, 1989; 159:1135; Su, DNA-CellBiol, 1990; 9:657). Upon reaction with sterol 27-hydroxylase, the resulting 3α,7α,12α-trihydroxy-5β-cholestanol-27-ol is oxidized by cytosolic NAD⁺-dependent 27-alcohol (Step 7) and 27-aldehyde dehydrogenase (Step 8) to form 3α,7α,12α-trihydroxy-5β-cholestanoic acid. Interestingly, 3α,7α,12α-trihydroxy-5β-cholestanoic acid may also be formed by the action of sterol 27-hydroxylase. This is due to the ability of this enzyme to catalyse multiple oxidation reactions at the C27 position of bile acid intermediates (Andersson, JBC, 1989; 264:8222; Dahlbäck, BBResComm, 1990; 167:391; Cali, JBC, 1991; 266:7774).

The final steps of side-chain oxidation occur in peroxisomes (Steps 9 to 14), a process similar to the β-oxidation of fatty acids. Coenzyme A (**CoA**) is linked to the 5β-cholestanoic acid by a microsomal steroid-CoA ligase, followed by oxidation that involves an oxidase and a bifunctional dehydrogenase/hydratase yielding a C24 hydroxylated bile acid intermediate. Following dehydrogenization, thiolytic cleavage results in the formation of propionyl-CoA and the CoA-linked 3α,7α,12α-trihydroxy-5β-cholanoic acid or cholic acid (Schram, PNAS, 1987; 84:2494). The generated bile acid CoA derivate then is conjugated with either glycine or taurine (Fig. 9).

An alternative pathway proposed for side-chain oxidation in the synthesis of cholic acid in humans and rats involves 25-hydroxylation of 3α,7α,12α-trihydroxy-5β-cholestane (Björkhem, JCI, 1975; 55:478; Shefer, JCI, 1975; 57:897). This pathway is believed to be specific for cholic acid but appears to contribute to only around 5 per cent of total cholic acid under normal conditions (Duane, JCI, 1981; 82:82; Duane, Hepatol, 1988; 8:613). It may be that the 25-hydroxylation pathway becomes important when the 27-hydroxylation is blocked.

In the neutral pathway, 7α-hydroxy-4-cholesten-3-one also can be reduced by the actions of Δ4-3-oxosteroid-5β-reductase (Step 4) and 3α-hydroxysteroid dehydrogenase (Step 5) to yield 3α,7α-dihydroxy-5β-cholestanol (Onishi, FEBSLett, 1991; 283:215). Subsequent hydroxylation by mitochondrial sterol 27-hydroxylase results in the formation of 3α,7α-dihydroxy-5β-cholestanol-27-ol. A series of enzymatic reactions finally yields 3α,7α,12α-trihydroxy-5β-cholanoic acid or chenodeoxycholic acid. It appears likely that

7α-hydroxy-4-cholesten-3-one represents a site of potential regulatory significance in determing the ratio of the two primary bile acids, cholic and chenodeoxycholic acid. However, there is no evident correlation between sterol 12α-hydroxylase and the ratio of these two bile acids (Björkhem, JLipRes, 1983; 24:1451). This implies that other steps in bile acid synthesis may influence the balance between the synthesis of cholic and chenodeoxycholic acid.

Bile acid synthesis initiated by 27-hydroxylation is the first step in the 'acidic' pathway (Fig. 7), followed by the formation of 3β-hydroxy-5-cholestenoic acid, which can be 7α-hydroxylated in microsomes (Shoda, Hepatol, 1993; 17:395). 27-Hydroxycholesterol is also a substrate for this microsomal 7α-hydroxylase, but this enzyme appears to be different from the 7α-hydroxylase involved in the 'neutral' pathway (Martin, JLipRes, 1993; 34:581). It thus may be concluded that at least two sterol 7α-hydroxylases exist in human liver and exhibit different substrate specificities and subcellular locations. Following a series of catalytic reactions, the predominantly formed bile acid in the 'acidic' pathway, namely chenodeoxycholic acid, is formed.

It is likely that the two pathways are regulated separately. Although generally believed to be of minor importance, the acidic pathway may actually contribute as much as 50 per cent of total bile acid synthesis (Axelson, JSterBioch, 1990; 36:631; Princen, BiochemJ, 1991; 275:501). The contribution of the 'acidic' pathway appears to be considerably small when bile acid synthesis is increased (Axelson, JSterBioch, 1990; 36:631). The relative importance of each pathway probably depends on the metabolic condition of the liver. This is in line with the formation of cholic and chenodeoxycholic acid from different cholesterol pools under normal conditions and from the same pool when the enterohepatic circulation is interrupted. Disruption of the cholesterol 7α-hydroxylase gene in mice (Ishibashi, JBC, 1996; 271:18017) revealed the importance of the first step in the neutral pathway for nutritional homeostasis in the neonate. These studies also showed that the 'acidic' pathway is not functionally active at the time of birth (Ishibashi, JBC, 1996; 271:18017; Schwarz, JBC, 1996; 271:18024).

Because conversion of cholesterol to bile acids is a major pathway to eliminate cholesterol from the body, overexpression of the cholesterol 7α-hydroxylase gene may lower cholesterol levels, thereby reducing the risk of developing atherosclerosis and cholesterol gallstones. This hypothesis was investigated in hamsters following adenovirus-mediated transfer of a cholesterol 7α-hydroxylase gene (Spady, JCI, 1995; 96:700). Transient overexpression of the gene increased the microsomal cholesterol 7α-hydroxylase activity and resulted in an expansion of the bile acid pool by almost 50 per cent. More importantly, plasma total and low density lipoprotein cholesterol levels were reduced significantly. This observation suggests that once sustained cholesterol 7α-hydroxylase gene overexpression can be achieved, this may become an attractive approach to reduce the cardiovascular risk. Whether the same strategy will be of benefit in terms of preventing the formation of cholesterol gallstones, deserves additional investigation.

Bile acids are rarely found in the unconjugated state in the body and only very recently, an inborn error of bile acid conjugation involving a deficiency in amidation has been discovered in a child.[24] Indeed, such a conjugation defect was proposed years ago (Hofmann, Lancet, 1988; ii:311). The formation of the various bile

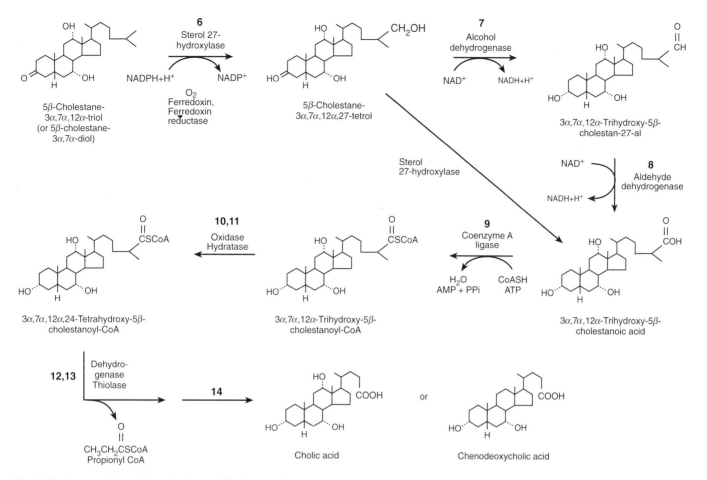

Fig. 8. Pathways of bile acid synthesis—modifications to the sterol side-chain. Bile acid synthesis via the 'neutral' pathway generates two bile acid intermediates, 3α,7α- dihydroxy-5β-cholestanol and 3α,7α,12α-trihydroxy-5β-cholestanol. These intermediates undergo modification of their side chains (step 6 to 14), resulting in the formation of cholic acid and chenodeoxycholic acid. (Adapted from ref. 22.)

Glycine NH_2CH_2COOH

Taurine $NH_2CH_2CH_2SO_3H$

FBAL $NH_2CH_2C(H)(F)COOH$

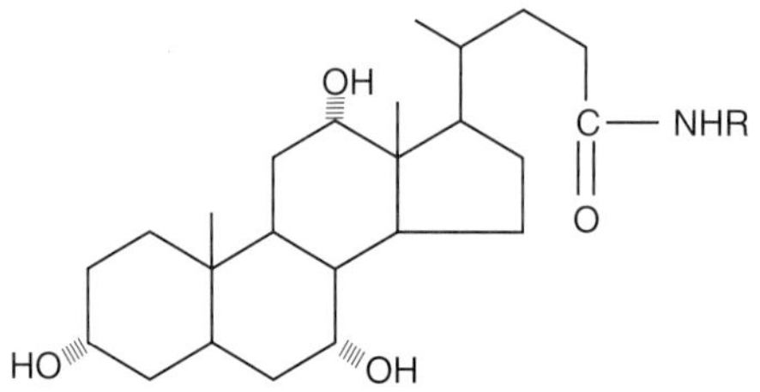

Fig. 9. General structure of common bile acid–amino acid conjugates. Amino acids are linked to the bile acid molecule via a peptide bond. Naturally occurring amino acids that are able to form bile acid conjugates are glycine and taurine and their chemical formulae are given.

acid conjugates serves to decrease their biological toxicity, to increase their solubility, and in several cases to have them more readily excreted from the body. For the most part, bile acids are secreted into bile as *N*-aminoacyl (glycine or taurine) conjugates (Fig. 9). Conjugation occurs between the amino group of the amino acid and the carboxyl group of the bile acid and involves two enzymes, a bile acid CoA synthetase and a bile acid CoA:amino acid *N*-acyltransferase. Bile acid CoA synthetase is localized in microsomes and forms bile acid CoA esters (Killenberg, JLipRes, 1978; 19:24; Prydz, JLipRes, 1988; 29:997). This enzyme has a lower affinity for C23 bile acids than their C24 counterparts (Kirkpatrick, Hepatol, 1988; 8:353). Consequently, C23 bile acids are largely excreted in bile as their glucuronides (see below), although other conjugates are present (Yoon, Gastro, 1986; 90:837). Bile acid CoA esters then react with the recently purified and cloned bile acid CoA:glycine/taurine *N*-acyltransferase (Johnson, JBC, 1991; 266:10227; Falany, JBC, 1994; 269:19375). This catalytic reaction may occur in microsomes as well as in the cytosol (Bremer, ActaChemScand, 1955; 9:689; Killenberg, JLipRes, 1978; 19:24; Lim, BiochemJ, 1981; 197: 611).

Substantial variation in the ratio of glycine- and taurine-conjugated bile acids occurs between species and between normal and cholestatic states. In humans, hamsters, guinea pigs, and rabbits, bile acids are mainly conjugated with glycine, whereas taurine conjugates are predominant in rats. In humans, significant amounts of taurine-conjugated bile acids may be observed in cholestatic liver disease. Because hepatocytes are not capable of synthesizing taurine

from other sulphur-containing amino acids (Lindstedt, JCI, 1965; 44:1754), the immediate dietary intake of this amino acid and its distribution dictates the amount of taurine-conjugated bile acids formed. This is evident in the case of intestinal malabsorption, where an increase in the proportion of glycine conjugates is noted.

Apart from glycine and taurine, the other naturally occurring amino acids are unable to form conjugates with bile acids. Rarely, bile acids are conjugated with taurine conjugates such as N-methyltaurine (Hagey, Hepatol, 1993; 18:305A) or the hydroxymethyl derivative of taurine, cysteinolic acid (Une, JLipRes, 1991; 32: 1619). It has been shown that 2-fluoro-β-alanine, an amino acid metabolite of 5-fluorouracil, is a substrate for the bile acid CoA: amino acid N-acyltransferase (Johnson, BiochemPharm, 1990; 40: 1241) (Fig. 9). This may explain its discovery as a conjugate with bile acids in human bile (Sweeny, PNAS, 1987; 84:5439; Malet-Martino, DrugMetDisp, 1988; 16:78).

Regulation of bile acid synthesis

Several methods for the determination of absolute and relative bile acid synthesis *in vivo* have been developed. In 1957, Lindstedt introduced the quantitative measurement of bile acid synthesis by the technique of isotope dilution (ActaPhysiolScand, 1957; 40:1). Bile acid synthesis is calculated as the product of bile acid pool size and fractional turnover rate. This method has been widely accepted and applied to studies in both animals and humans. The isotope dilution technique is based on the two assumptions that the bile acid pool is constant and behaves as a single compartment. The method involves repeated sampling of bile, serum, or intestinal content. However, a major disadvantage is the use of radioactive bile acids, although employed in trace amounts. Stable isotopes have now replaced radiolabelled bile acids and provide a suitable marker rendering this method attractive for human studies (Stellaard, JLipRes, 1984; 23:1313; Tauber, EurJGastroHepatol, 1996; 8:23). Another method has been described which requires a single collection of a serum or bile sample to calculate bile acid synthesis (Vantrappen, JLipRes, 1981; 22:528).

Under steady-state conditions, bile acid synthesis is essentially equal to the faecal bile acid excretion. Therefore, measurement of faecal bile acid excretion using balance techniques (Grundy, JLipRes, 1965; 6:397; Grundy, JCI, 1966; 45:1503) allows the determination of bile acid synthesis. However, there are two major limitations of this approach: (i) the difficulty in obtaining a complete faecal collection requires the use of faecal recovery markers, and (ii) the faecal bile acid measurement can be accurately performed only by the time-consuming technique of gas chromatography–mass spectrometry. Nevertheless, a fair agreement between bile acid synthesis rates obtained by isotope dilution and chemical measurement has been reported (Duane, Lipids, 1982; 17:345).

Plasma levels of 7α-hydroxycholesterol have been found to correlate with the activity of cholesterol 7α-hydroxylase (Björkhem, JLipRes, 1987; 28:889; Oda, JLipRes, 1990; 31:2209; Yoshida, JChromatogrB, 1993; 613:185) and also with bile acid synthesis (Okamoto, Hepatol, 1994; 20:95; Hahn, JLipRes, 1995; 36:2059). Although assessment of bile acid synthesis with this serum marker appears attractive, the possibility of auto-oxidation of cholesterol during sample handling and the elaborate analytical methodology limits its clinical application. A correlation has also been found

between serum levels of 7α-hydroxy-4-cholesten-3-one and cholesterol 7α-hydroxylase activity (Axelson, FEBSLett, 1991; 284: 216; Yoshida, JChromatogr, 1994; 655:179) as well as bile acid synthesis (Axelson, FEBSLett, 1988; 239:324; Eusufzai, Gut, 1993; 34:698). Recently, 7α-hydroxy-4-cholesten-3-one has been demonstrated to be a convenient marker for the semiquantitative assessment of bile acid synthesis in humans (Sauter, Hepatol, 1996; 24: 123).

Forty years ago, Eriksson demonstrated that the acute interruption of the enterohepatic circulation caused a dramatic rise in bile acid synthesis (PSEBM, 1957; 94:578). Subsequently, it was shown that this increase can be suppressed by bile acid infusion (Shefer, JLipRes, 1969; 10:646). This is in line with the concept that bile acids returning to the liver via the portal vein exhibit a negative feedback control on their own synthesis. More than 20 years ago it became evident that cholesterol 7α-hydroxylase plays a central role in the regulation of bile acid synthesis. This was based on the observation that taurocholic acid inhibited the conversion of acetate, mevalonate, and cholesterol, but not of 7α-hydroxycholesterol (Shefer, JLipRes, 1970; 11:404). Moreover, administration of the bile acid sequestrant cholestyramine or bile drainage increased cholesterol 7α-hydroxylase several-fold, while other enzymes involved in bile acid synthesis were affected to a much lesser extent (Danielsson, EurJBioch, 1967; 2:44; Johansson, EurJBioch, 1970; 17:292).

Traditionally it has been assumed that the feedback regulation is mediated by primary bile acids alone. However, this suppressive effect was not observed in cultured hepatocytes (Botham, BBActa, 1981; 666:238; Davis, JBC, 1983; 258:4079; Kubaska, JBC, 1985; 260:13459; Whiting, BBActa, 1989; 1005:137). Moreover, attempts to demonstrate an inhibitory effect of infused taurocholic acid in rats yielded positive (Pries, JLipRes, 1983; 24:141) and negative (Lee, PSEBM, 1965; 120:6; Singhal, BBActa, 1983; 752:214; Davis, JLipRes, 1988; 29:202; Duane, JLipRes, 1988; 29:212; Stange, JCI, 1989; 84:173; Pandak, Gastro, 1995; 108:533) results. These conflicting data most likely are related to the fact that the regulatory effect of bile acids is dose dependent (Heuman, Hepatol, 1988; 8: 358; Stange, JCI, 1989; 84:173; Scheibner, Hepatol, 1995; 21:529). However, these results also suggested that secondary bile acids may participate in the feedback regulation of bile acid synthesis. This concept was established by Stange and coworkers in animal studies and is in line with the enhanced bile acid synthesis following colectomy (Stange, Hepatol, 1988; 8:879), the major source of deoxycholic acid. Furthermore, bile duct-ligated rats deficient in secondary bile acids have an increased bile acid synthesis despite a dramatic increase in intracellular bile acid concentrations (Kinugasa, JLipRes, 1981; 22:201; Dueland, BiochemJ, 1991; 280:373), supporting a role of secondary bile acids in feedback regulation. Recent studies by Heuman (JLipRes, 1989; 30:1161) were in line with the concept that more hydrophobic bile acids (e.g. deoxycholic acid) are more potent suppressors of bile acid synthesis than more hydrophilic bile acids (e.g. cholic acid). Indeed, these observations obtained in animal studies have been confirmed in healthy humans (Fig. 10) who received a low dose of exogenous bile acids or a non-absorbable antibiotic (Tauber, EurJGastroHepatol, 1996; 8:23). This study also provided convincing evidence that the suppressive effect of cholic acid on bile acid synthesis most likely is mediated by the intestinal formation of deoxycholic acid (Fig. 11). Based on

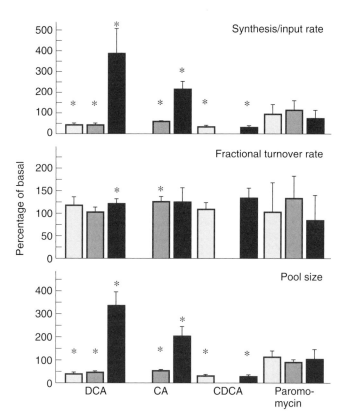

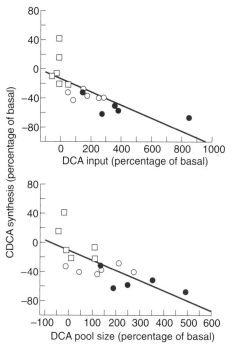

Fig. 10. Effect of oral bile acid administration and a non-absorbable antibiotic on bile acid kinetics in healthy humans. Cholic (light bar), chenodeoxycholic (purple bar), and deoxycholic acid (dark bar) kinetics were determined simultaneously with [^{13}C]-cholic, [^{13}C]-chenodeoxycholic, and [^{2}H]-deoxycholic acid before and during daily administration of 0.5 g of each bile acid for 4 weeks or 1 g of paromomycin sulphate for 2 weeks. Bile acid synthesis/input rate (upper panel), the fractional turnover rate (middle panel), and the bile acid pool size (lower panel) are given following challenge with bile acid or paromomycin administration. Data are expressed as the percentage of the respective control and represent the mean ± 1 SEM (* $p < 0.05$). (Adapted from: Tauber G, Empen K, Scheibner J, Fuchs M, and Stange EF. Feedback regulation of bile acid synthesis measured by stable isotope kinetics in humans. *European Journal of Gastroenterology and Hepatology*, 1996; **8**: 23–31).

Fig. 11. Bile acid kinetics in healthy humans. Bile acid kinetics were determined simultaneously with [^{13}C]-cholic, [^{13}C]-chenodeoxycholic, and [^{2}H]-deoxycholic acid before and during daily administration of 0.5 g of cholic (open circles) and deoxycholic acid (filled circles) for 4 weeks or 1 g of paromomycin sulphate (open squares) for 2 weeks. The relative change of deoxycholic acid (DCA) input (upper panel) and deoxycholic acid pool size (lower panel) is plotted against the degree of suppression of chenodeoxycholic acid synthesis. A negative linear correlation of the inhibition of chenodeoxycholic acid synthesis with the change of deoxycholic acid input ($r = -0.73$) and the deoxycholic acid pool size ($r = -0.72$) was observed. Data points represent the change of the parameter compared with the individual's control value before administration of the bile acid or antibiotic, respectively. (Adapted from: Tauber G, Empen K, Scheibner J, Fuchs M, and Stange EF. Feedback regulation of bile acid synthesis measured by stable isotope kinetics in humans. *European Journal of Gastroenterology and Hepatology*, 1996; **8**: 23–31).

these collective data it may be concluded that the bile acid composition in the portal vein is more relevant for the negative feedback regulation than the actual bile acid concentration.

A remarkable observation was made by Xu and coworkers (Gastro, 1992; 102:1717), demonstrating that glycine conjugates of cholic and deoxycholic acid exhibited different mechanisms in the feedback suppression of bile acid synthesis in the rabbit. Interestingly, cholic and deoxycholic acid may exert their feedback regulation of cholic acid by two different mechanisms (Scheibner, Hepatol, 1995; 21:529), at least in the rat.

Intestinal passage of cholic acid appears to be required for effective inhibition of cholesterol 7α-hydroxylase. The exact mechanism needs further experimentation, but so far three possibilities are considered (Fig. 12). First and most likely, regulation may involve a bile acid metabolite formed in the large bowel, for example deoxycholic acid which represents a major regulator of cholesterol 7α-hydroxylase (Stange, Hepatol, 1988; 8:879; Stange, JCI, 1989;

84:173). Second, bile acids in the intestine may induce the release of a neural or humoral factor which then may modulate either directly or indirectly the cholesterol 7α-hydroxylase. Potential candidates are glucagon (Hylemon, JBC, 1992; 267:16866), enteroglucagon or peptide YY (Adrian, Gut, 1993; 34:1219), or neurotensin (Dakka, Endocrinol, 1994; 134:603). A third possibility is the existence of a 'luminal factor' (Akerlund, JLipRes, 1990; 31:2159). However, this putative protein awaits identification (Heuman, Hepatol, 1996; 24:731A).

The major site of feedback regulation of bile acid synthesis occurs at the level of the microsomal cholesterol 7α-hydroxylase. Proposed mechanisms of regulation include alteration of (i) the enzyme synthesis or degradation and (ii) the enzyme catalytic activity by phosphorylation/dephosphorylation. The cloning and sequencing of the cholesterol 7α-hydroxylase gene in a variety of species such as the rat, hamster, mouse (Jelinik, Biochem, 1990; 29:7781; Nishimoto, JBC, 1991; 266:6467; Crestani, Arch-BiochemBiophys, 1993; 306:451; Tzung, Genomics, 1994; 21:244)

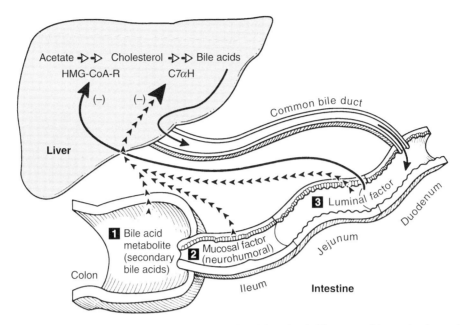

Fig. 12. Putative factors involved in the negative feedback regulation of bile acid synthesis. Three possible mechanisms whereby bile acids may affect bile acid synthesis are illustrated. First, and probably most likely, metabolites of primary bile acids such as deoxycholic acid (1), which are formed in the colon, appear to downregulate cholesterol 7α-hydroxylase. Second, bile acids could promote the release of a mucosal factor (2) that regulates bile acid synthesis at the level of cholesterol 7α-hydroxylase. Third, bile acids may release a luminal factor (3) that represses cholesterol 7α-hydroxylase and HMG-CoA reductase in a direct or indirect fashion. (Reproduced with kind permission of Kluwer Academic Publishers, Lancaster England, from: Vlahcevic ZR. Studies of cholesterol degradative pathways in the rat. In Hofmann AF, Paumgartner G, and Stiehl A, eds. *Bile acids in gastroenterology; basic and clinical advances*, 1995: 85–108).

and humans (Noshiro, FEBSLett, 1990; 268:137; Karam, BBResComm, 1992; 185:588; Cohen, Genomics, 1992; 14:153) has been achieved recently. In addition, the human gene has been mapped to chromosome 8q11–q12 (Cohen, Genomics, 1992; 14:153). These discoveries provided the opportunity to investigate the molecular basis of regulation of this important enzyme of bile acid synthesis.

Cholesterol 7α-hydroxylase enzyme expression of quantitative importance has been detected only in the liver, but minor enzyme expression has been detected also in the kidney, heart tissue, and lung (Chiang, JBC, 1990; 265:3889). However, cholesterol 7α-hydroxylase mRNA is present only in the liver and several sizes of a single transcript have been reported (Jelinik, JBC, 1990; 265:8190; Twisk, BiochemJ, 1993; 290:685). This is probably due to multiple polyadenylation sites present in the 3′-untranslated region. This region consists of sequence repeats that have been linked to rapid mRNA degradation (Shaw, Cell, 1986; 46:659; Binder, JBC, 1989; 264:16910). Along with this observation goes a half-life of less than 4 h for the mRNA (Twisk, BiochemJ, 1993; 290:685) as well as the enzyme (Einarsson, FEBSLett, 1968; 1:219; Danielsson, BBResComm, 1991; 103:46). The 5′-flanking region has been shown to harbour a number of sequences involved in the recognition by transcriptional factors (Fig. 13) (Molowa, Biochem, 1992; 3:2539; Nishimoto, BBActa, 1993; 1172:147).

Although post-transcriptional regulation of cholesterol 7α-hydroxylase has been proposed (Shefer, JLipRes, 1992; 33:1193), current concepts favour that the enzyme modulation occurs at the transcriptional level (Li, JBC, 1990; 265:12012; Noshiro, JBC, 1990; 265:10036; Jelinek, JBC, 1990; 265:8190; Sundseth, JBC, 1990; 265:15090; Pandak, JBC, 1991; 266:3416; Jones, JLipRes, 1993; 34:885). In this regard, two potential interactions of bile acids and the

cholesterol 7α-hydroxylase promoter region may occur. According to Chiang and coworkers (JBC, 1994; 269:17502), bile acids (e.g. bound to cytosolic receptors) enter the nucleus (Setchell, Gastro, 1997; 112:226) and may bind to a negative regulator bile acid-responsive protein, thereby preventing their interaction with liver-specific positive transcription factors. Consequently, positive regulators may not bind to a putative bile acid responsive element of the promoter (Hoekman, Gene, 1993; 130:217) and gene expression is repressed (Fig. 14). Stravitz and colleagues (JLipRes, 1995; 36: 1359) showed that bile acids appear to activate a protein kinase C-dependent signal transduction cascade. This may cause covalent modification of a transacting factor which interacts with the cholesterol 7α-hydroxylase promoter resulting in the repression of gene transcription.

A close linkage of cholesterol and bile acid synthesis reflected by parallel activities of HMG-CoA reductase and cholesterol 7α-hydroxylase under a variety of experimental conditions has been reported (Myant, JLipRes, 1961; 2:363; Mitropoulos, BBActa, 1973; 326:428; Takeuchi, Atheroscl, 1974; 20:481; Heuman, JLipRes, 1989; 30:1161; Pandak, JLipRes, 1990; 31:79). Also, the diurnal periodicity of cholesterol 7α-hydroxylase is synchronous with that of HMG-CoA reductase. In the case of nocturnal feeders such as the rat, the maximal protein mass, enzyme activity, and messenger RNA levels are apparently in the mid-dark phase (Danielsson, Steroids, 1972; 20:63; Mitropoulos, FEBSLett, 1972; 27:203; Chiang, JBC, 1990; 265:3889; Noshiro, JBC, 1990; 265:10036). Interestingly, diurnal variations persist under conditions where the enterohepatic circulation is interrupted, suggesting its independence from bile acid feedback mechanisms (Pooler, Hepatol, 1988; 8:1140). It has been proposed that glucocorticoids may play a

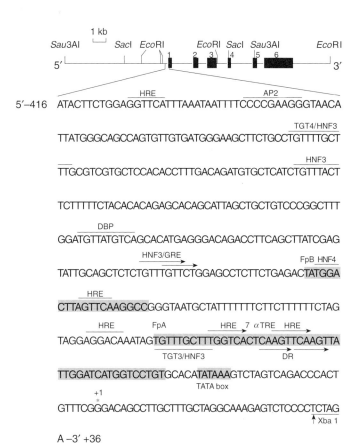

5'−416 ATACTTCTGGAGGTTCATTTAAATAATTTTCCCCGAAGGGTAACA

TTATGGGCAGCCAGTGTTGTGATGGGAAGCTTCTGCCTGTTTTGCT

TTGCGTCGTGCTCCACACCTTTGACAGATGTGCTCATCTGTTTACT

TCTTTTTCTACACACAGAGCACAGCATTAGCTGCTGTCCCGGCTTT

GGATGTTATGTCAGCACATGAGGGACAGACCTTCAGCTTATCGAG

TATTGCAGCTCTCTGTTTGTTCTGGAGCCTCTTCTGAGACTATGGA

CTTAGTTCAAGGCCGGGTAATGCTATTTTTTTCTTCTTTTTCTAG

TAGGAGGACAAATAGTGTTTGCTTTGGTCACTCAAGTTCAAGTTA

TTGGATCATGGTCCTGTGCACATATAAAGTCTAGTCAGACCCACT
+1
GTTTCGGGACAGCCTTGCTTTGCTAGGCAAAGAGTCTCCCCTCTAG
↑ Xba 1

A −3' +36

Fig. 13. Structure of the rat cholesterol 7α-hydroxylase gene. The rat cholesterol 7α-hydroxylase gene contains six exons (1 to 6) and five introns. Nucleotide sequences in the proximal promoter region (5'-flanking region from −416 to 36), DNAase I footprints, and proposed sequence motifs for liver-enriched transcription factors and nuclear receptors are shown. HRE, hormone responsive element; HNF, hepatocyte nuclear factors; 7α-TRE: thyroid hormone responsive element-like motif; GRE, glucocorticoid responsive element; DR, direct repeat sequence; FpA and FpB, DNAase I footprints A and B; DBP, albumin D site binding protein; TATA, TATAAA box; TGT3 and TGT4, TGTTT(T)GCTTT sequences. (Reproduced with kind permission of Kluwer Academic Publishers, Lancaster, England, from: Chiang JYL. Molecular mechanism of regulation of cholesterol 7α-hydroxylase gene. In: Hofmann AF, Paumgartner G, and Stiehl A, eds. *Bile acids in gastroenterology; basic and clinical advances*, 1995: 109–28).

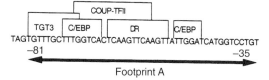

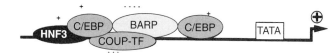

A. Basal transcriptional activation

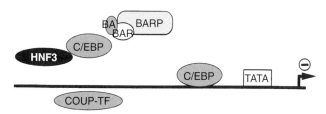

B. Bile acid feedback repression

Fig. 14. Proposed regulation of the cholesterol 7α-hydroxylase gene. Footprint A contains overlapping sequence motifs for positive transcription factors TGT3/HNF3, C/EBP, and COUP-TFII as well as a regulator bile acid response protein (BARP) which binds to a direct repeat (DR) sequence. (A). Basal transcriptional activation: a unit formed upon interactions of HNF3, C/EBP, COUP-TFII and BARP regulates the general transcriptional machinery TFIID complex. (B). Repression of bile acid synthesis: bile acids (BA) dependent on their relative hydrophobicity may bind to a bile acid receptor (BAR), thereby preventing interactions between BARP and other regulatory factors. Without interaction of BARP with the bile acid responsive element (BARE), binding of positive regulators to the promoter region of cholesterol 7α-hydroxylase may be prevented, thereby repressing gene expression. (Reproduced with kind permission of Kluwer Academic Publishers, Lancaster, England, from: Chiang JYL. Molecular mechanism of regulation of cholesterol 7α-hydroxylase gene. In Hofmann AF, Paumgartner G, and Stiehl A, eds. *Bile acids in gastroenterology; basic and clinical advances*, 1995: 109–28).

role in establishing the diurnal variation (Hutcher, BBActa, 1978; 529:409). However, evidence has been obtained that favours a role of liver-enriched transcription factors being involved in daily fluctuations of enzyme activity (Lee, JBC, 1994; 269:14681).

Traditionally it has been assumed that the majority of cholesterol substrate for bile acid synthesis is derived from newly synthesized cholesterol in the liver. Moreover, it has been hypothesized that the availability of newly synthesized cholesterol is of particular importance in the modulation of cholesterol 7α-hydroxylase (Balasubramaniam, EurJBioch, 1979; 34:77; Björkhem, JBC, 1979; 254:5252; Pandak, JLipRes, 1990; 31:79; Jones, JLipRes, 1993; 34:885; Vlahcevic, Hepatol, 1993; 18:660). However, the role of a continuous supply of cholesterol remains unclear and the substrate saturation of cholesterol 7α-hydroxylase remains controversial (Björkhem, JLipRes, 1988; 29:136; Straka, JBC, 1990; 265:7145). Recent studies

in the rat and hamster with tritiated water as a cholesterol precursor, in the presence or absence of an HMG-CoA reductase inhibitor, demonstrated only a minor contribution of *de novo* cholesterol for bile acid synthesis as well as biliary cholesterol secretion (Scheibner, Hepatol, 1993; 17:1095; Scheibner, JLipRes, 1994; 35:690). In the hamster, which has a bile acid, cholesterol, and lipoprotein metabolism similar to humans, only a minor portion of newly synthesized cholesterol was used as substrate for bile acid synthesis under near physiological conditions, such as the first hours following interruption of the enterohepatic circulation. A minor contribution of newly synthesized cholesterol to bile acid synthesis has also been shown for humans (Schwartz, JCI, 1993; 91:923).

Animal studies provided evidence for the existence of different cholesterol pools for bile acid synthesis and biliary cholesterol, whereas observations in humans (Schwartz, PSEBM, 1977; 156:261; Schwartz, JCI, 1993; 91:923) suggest a common cholesterol precursor pool. The basis for such a compartmentalization of hepatic cholesterol (Stange, BiochemSocTrans, 1987; 15:189) remains unclear, but one might speculate that bile acids direct hepatocellular cholesterol movement in a similar fashion as proposed for biliary phosphatidylcholine (Cohen, Biochem, 1994; 33:9975). Alternatively, an uneven distribution of enzymes involved in cholesterol and bile acid synthesis within the liver acinus (Singer, PNAS, 1984; 81:5556; Li, JLipRes, 1988; 29:781; Ugele, BiochemJ, 1991; 276:73) may give some clues regarding the utilization of cholesterol pools for bile acid synthesis. Under normal conditions, HMG-CoA reductase and HMG-CoA synthase are localized in the periportal zone (Singer, PNAS, 1984; 81:5556; Li, JLipRes, 1988; 29:781), whereas cholesterol 7α-hydroxylase and sterol 27-hydroxylase are found in the pericentral zone (Ugele, BiochemJ, 1991; 276:73; Twisk, JCI, 1995; 95:1235). In consideration of this separation of synthetic and catabolic routes of cholesterol, it is attractive to speculate that bile acids are synthesized predominantly from preformed cholesterol, at least under normal conditions. Moreover, utilization of certain cholesterol pools subserving bile acid synthesis appears to be dictated by the relative distribution of enzymes relevant for cholesterol and bile acid synthesis, rather than the preference of a cholesterol 7α-hydroxylase for a particular cholesterol pool. The alternative start of bile acid synthesis in two different compartments, cholesterol 7α-hydroxylase in microsomes and sterol 27-hydroxylase in mitochondria, raises the possibility that newly synthesized and preformed cholesterol may be channelled separately to cholic and chenodeoxycholic acid, respectively.

Hormones such as thyroxine (Mitropolous, FEBSLett, 1968; 1:13; Björkhem, FEBSLett, 1973; 31:20) and glucocorticoids (vanCantfort, Biochim, 1973; 55:1171; Princen, BiochemJ, 1989; 262:341) have been known to interfere with bile acid synthesis. However, only the recent cloning of the cholesterol 7α-hydroxylase gene has allowed more detailed studies on the mechanisms whereby hormones may influence bile acid synthesis. Physiological concentrations of both thyroxine and glucocorticoids appear to stimulate synergistically gene transcription activity. In contrast, glucagon apparently decreases transcriptional activity (Hylemon, JBC, 1992; 267:16886). The underlying molecular mechanism remains to be elucidated, but it may be linked to interactions of these hormones with putative thyroxine- and glucocorticoid-responsive elements present in the promoter region of the cholesterol 7α-hydroxylase gene. It is conceivable that cholesterol, thyroxine, and glucocorticoids are responsible for the basal level of cholesterol 7α-hydroxylase gene expression, while bile acid-mediated repression may modulate gene expression. Clearly, more detailed studies are required to pinpoint further the exact molecular mechanisms of regulation of the cholesterol 7α-hydroxylase gene.

Sterol 27-hydroxylase has not been studied as extensively as cholesterol 7α-hydroxylase, because it has not been considered important in the regulation of bile acid synthesis (Björkhem, JLipRes, 1992; 33:455). Complementary DNAs encoding the rabbit, rat, and human sterol 27-hydroxylase have been isolated (Andersson, JBC, 1989; 264:8222; Su, DNACellBiol, 1990; 9:657; Usui, FEBSLett, 1990; 262:135; Cali, JBC, 1991; 266:7774) and all encode a cleavable mitochondrial signal sequence. In contrast to the cholesterol 7α-hydroxylase sequence, sequences related to instability are virtually absent within the 3'-untranslated region (Andersson, JBC, 1989; 264:8222; Su, DNACellBiol, 1990; 9:657). This suggests that destabilization of mRNA apparently does not play a major role

in the regulation of this enzyme. An estimated half-life of 13 h for the messenger RNA (Twisk, BiochemJ, 1993; 290:685) is in good agreement with a much longer half-life of the enzyme compared with cholesterol 7α-hydroxylase. Because the enzyme activity and messenger RNA is detected in many tissues (Andersson, JBC, 1989; 264:8222; Su, DNACellBiol, 1990; 9:657), a functional restriction to bile acid synthesis appears unlikely. It has been shown that sterol 27-hydroxylase has much slower protein and mRNA turnover rates than cholesterol 7α-hydroxylase (Stravitz, JSterBioch, 1996; 57:337). However, as shown for cholesterol 7α-hydroxylase, the sterol 27-hydroxylase may be subject to negative feedback inhibition by hydrophobic bile acids (Vlahcevic, AmJPhysiol, 1996; 270:G646). Because both enzymes changed in tandem during diurnal variations (Vlahcevic, AmJPhysiol, 1996; 270:G646), sterol 27-hydroxylase also appears to be under the control of glucocorticoids.

Enterohepatic circulation

Molecules that are secreted into bile, absorbed from the intestine, and resecreted into the biliary tree are considered to undergo enterohepatic cycling (Fig. 15). Vectorial movement of bile acids from the portal blood into the bile canaliculus is mediated by coordinated interactions between bile acids and a variety of transport proteins, localized in the basolateral (sinusoidal) and canalicular membrane as well as cytosolic transport proteins and/or vesicular structures. In general, transport across the canalicular membrane appears to be rate limiting[25] and represents the anatomical site for many causes of intrahepatic cholestasis (see Chapter 23.3).

Hepatocellular bile acid transport

New concepts of intracellular bile acid transport have emerged in recent years. The rate of bile acid distribution within the hepatocyte has been shown to be in the order of minutes (Crawford, JLipRes, 1988; 29:144), suggesting the existence of specific intracellular transport mechanisms. The successful purification and cloning of a dihydrodiol dehydrogenase has shown that this protein appears to play a major role during intracellular bile acid trafficking in humans (Stolz, JBC, 1993; 268:10448). In contrast to the rat bile acid binder (Stolz, JBC, 1991; 266:15253), it does not exhibit 3α-hydroxysteroid dehydrogenase activity . Other putative bile acid-binding proteins such as the dimeric glutathione-S-transferases and fatty acid-binding proteins have higher bile acid dissociation constants, thereby providing little evidence for their physiological role in bile acid transport (Stolz, AnnRevPhysiol, 1989; 51:161).

Bile acids also interact with intracellular structures which may retard bile acid transit time. Most likely, these interactions promote the microtubular-dependent delivery of transport proteins and the delivery of phosphatidylcholine and cholesterol molecules via phosphatidylcholine transfer protein (Cohen, Biochem, 1994; 33:9975) and sterol carrier protein 2 (Puglielli, BiochemJ, 1996; 317:681; Fuchs, Gastro, 1997; 112:A1267) to the canalicular liver plasma membrane, respectively (Fig. 16).

Canalicular bile acid secretion

Canalicular bile acid secretion (Fig. 17) appears to be the major determinant of bile formation. Each day up to 30 g of bile acids are transported across the canalicular liver plasma membranes, making

Systems

Spaces

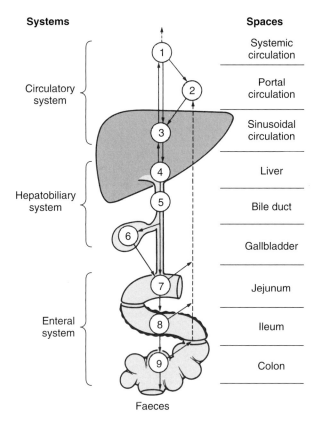

Fig. 15. Linear multicompartment model of the enterohepatic circulation of bile acids. The arrow connecting systemic circulation (space 1) with sinusoidal circulation (space 3) corresponds to hepatic arterial blood flow; the arrow connecting the systemic circulation to portal circulation (space 2) corresponds to the mesenteric circulation. (By copyright permission of the American Society for Clinical Investigation, from: Hofmann AF, Molino G, Milanese M, and Belforte G. Description and simulation of a physiological pharmacokinetic model for the metabolism and enterohepatic circulation of bile acids in man. Cholic acid in healthy man. *Journal of Clinical Investigation*, 1983; **71**: 1003–22).

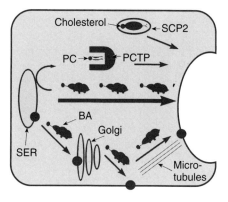

Fig. 16. Proposed hepatocellular bile acid trafficking and bile acid–membrane interactions. Once bile acids (BA) have been taken up across the basolateral liver plasma membrane, they bind to intracellular proteins. As indicated by the centre arrow, bile acid delivery to the canalicular liver plasma membrane occurs primarily via diffusion bound to proteins. Bile acids partition into membranes of intracellular organelles, such as the smooth endoplasmic reticulum (SER) and the Golgi apparatus. Interaction of bile acids with the smooth endoplasmic reticulum facilitates the release of phosphatidylcholine (PC) molecules for binding to phosphatidylcholine transfer protein (PCTP) and delivery to the canalicular liver plasma membrane for secretion. Cholesterol transport appears to be mediated by sterol carrier protein 2 (SCP2). The role of bile acids in promoting this pathway of cholesterol delivery to the canalicular liver plasma membrane remains to be elucidated. As indicated by the three bottom arrows, bile acids are also involved in the vesicular insertion of transport proteins (black circles) into the canalicular liver plasma membrane in a microtubule-dependent fashion.

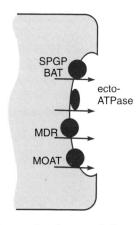

Fig. 17. Proposed transport systems mediating canalicular bile acid secretion. ATP-dependent bile acid transport activity by means of (a) bile acid transporter(s) (BAT) is present in the canalicular liver plasma. One such transporter appears to be the sister of P-glycoprotein (SPGP). Ecto-ATPase represents a putative bile acid transporter that is not dependent on the ecto-ATPase function. The multispecific organic anion transporter (MOAT/MRP2) appears to shuttle divalent bile acid sulphates and glucuronidates into bile. Multidrug resistance gene (MDR) products, P-glycoproteins, are involved in phosphatidylcholine and organic cation transport.

an efficient bile acid transport mechanism necessary. Several investigators have functionally characterized potential-dependent and ATP-dependent bile acid transport proteins (Adachi, Hepatol, 1991; 14:655; Müller, JBC, 1991; 266:18920; Nishida, JBC, 1991; 266: 13147; Stieger, BiochemJ, 1992; 284:67), but their molecular identity is still awaited. Upon fractionation of isolated canalicular membrane vesicles by free-flow electrophoresis, it became evident that a potential-dependent bile acid transport is probably restricted to the endoplasmic reticulum and not the canalicular membrane (Kast, JBC, 1994; 269:5179).

The canalicular glycoprotein ecto-ATPase may serve as a bile acid transporter (Sippel, JBC, 1993; 268:2083), but this remains controversial: the ATPase is oriented towards the exoplasmic rather than the endoplasmic membrane leaflet and the ATP hydrolytic domain may be functionally uncoupled from bile acid transport (Sippel, JBC, 1994; 269:19539). Moreover, on cellular fractionation this putative bile acid transporter appears to be separable from ATP-dependent bile acid transport (Sippel, JBC, 1994; 269:2820). Based on the complete nucleotide sequence of the ecto-ATPase

(Lin, JBC, 1989; 264:14403), the protein may have two membrane-spanning domains and appears homologous to members of the carcinoembryonic antigen gene family.

More recent studies provide evidence for novel ATP-binding cassette proteins involved in canalicular bile acid secretion (Lomri, SemLivDis, 1996, 16:211). One such protein may be encoded by a gene closely related to P-glycoprotein, which has been termed the sister of P-glycoprotein, *spgp* (Childs, CancerRes, 1995; 55:2029). Indeed, a more recent study identified SPGP as an ATP-dependent taurocholic acid transporter (Gerloff, Hepatol, 1997; 26:A919).

Canalicular secretion of divalent anionic bile acids, such as sulphates or glucuronides, appears to be via a separate, ATP-dependent transport protein termed canalicular multiorganic anion transporter (**MOAT**) (Kuipers, JCI, 1988; 81:1593; Kuipers, JLipRes, 1989; 30:1825; OudeElferink, BiochemJ, 1991; 274:281). The most prominent substrate for this transporter is conjugated bilirubin (Jansen, Hepatol, 1987; 7:71); however, as indicated by its name, the protein is capable of transporting a variety of organic compounds (OudeElferink, BBActa, 1995; 1241:215). Recent studies suggest that MOAT may be identical to the multidrug resistance-associated protein, (**MRP2**) (Jedlitschky, CancerRes, 1994; 54:4833; Müller, PNAS, 1994; 91:13033). The human gene has been cloned and mapped to chromosome 10q24 (Kartenbeck, Hepatol. 1996; 23: 1061; Taniguchi, CancerRes, 1996; 56:4124).

So far, the only mammalian tissue beside the canalicular liver plasma membrane found to exert ATP-dependent bile acid transport is the apical membrane of the human trophoblast (Marin, AmJPhysiol, 1995; 268:G685). Whether this protein with properties similar to the canalicular transporter is encoded by the same gene and the nature of its physiological role remain open for further investigations.

Following their monomeric secretion into bile, bile acids presumably accumulate in the exoplasmic canalicular membrane hemileaflet. Because bile acid uptake at the canalicular level appears to be excluded, lateral pressure may be generated in the canalicular membrane, thereby inducing vesiculation of biliary lipids (Crawford, JLipRes, 1995; 36:2147) (Fig. 6). During passage through the bile ducts, bile is modified by the secretory and absorptive activity of cholangiocytes. Bile acids are stored in the gallbladder and/or pass down through the ampulla of Vater into the lumen of the small bowel.

Intestinal bile acid absorption

Having reached the small intestine, bile acids are absorbed by active and passive mechanisms. Passive absorption may occur by ionic (bile salt) or non-ionic (bile acid) diffusion, the non-ionic diffusion being of greater importance (Dietschy, JLipRes, 1968; 9:297). The relative contributions of these transport processes greatly depend on the intraluminal pH, the dissociation constant of the individual bile acid, the maximum solubilizing capacity of bile acid micelles, and the partition coefficients of the ionic and non-ionic species into the absorptive membrane. Bile acids in their undissociated form traverse the intestinal membrane readily by spontaneous translocation ('flip-flop') to the inner membrane leaflet (Cabral, Biochem, 1987; 26:1801).

Whereas passive absorption may occur throughout the small intestine, active bile acid transport appears to be restricted to the ileum.[26] The Na$^+$-dependent transport protein responsible has been cloned and is located in the apical membrane of the ileocyte (Wong, JBC, 1994; 269:1340). More recently, the human gene has been mapped to chromosome 13q33 (Wong, Genomics, 1996; 33: 538). The ileal bile acid transporter may be regulated by intestinal bile acids by means of a positive feedback (Lillienau, Gastro, 1993; 104:38), but indirect evidence is in favour of a negative feedback (Redinger, JLipRes, 1984; 25:437). Additional studies are needed to straighten out these puzzling observations. Recently, it became evident that inherited mutations in the Na$^+$-dependent bile acid transporter gene may be responsible for some cases of familial hypertriglyceridaemia[27] and Crohn's disease (Wong, JBC, 1995; 270:27228). One may speculate that patients with primary bile acid malabsorption (Thaysen, Gut, 1976; 17:965; Popovic, Gastro, 1987; 92:1851) may have a Na$^+$-dependent bile acid transporter that is functionally inactive due to gene mutation (Oelkers, Gastro, 1996; 110:A56) or even not expressed at all. The sodium dependence of this transport mechanism highlights the importance of the electrochemical driving forces generated by the Na$^+$/K$^+$-ATPase on the basolateral membrane of the ileocyte (Schreiber, JPediatGastrNutr, 1983; 2:337). Following uptake into the cell, bile acids are transported to the basolateral membrane where they are secreted into the superior mesenteric vein via a Na$^+$-independent organic anion exchange system (Weinberg, JCI, 1986; 78:44). The overall efficiency of the small intestine with respect to bile acid absorption exceeds 95 per cent. The amount of bile acids ultimately lost in the faeces is, at least in the steady state, exactly balanced by the amount newly synthesized by the liver, keeping the bile acid pool size stable.[28,29]

Bile acids escaping absorption by the small intestine are exposed to a large number of bacteria present in the colon, where they will be further metabolized. Several different microbial biotransformations are known to occur.[30,31] Different bacterial strains are capable of bile acid deconjugation by hydrolysis of the amide bond yielding free bile acids. Oxidation of the hydroxy groups at positions C3, C7, and C12 occurs as well as reduction of the oxo groups yielding epimeric bile acids. Epimerization may be performed by different bacterial strains containing hydroxysteroid dehydrogenase activity.

However, the quantitatively most important biotransformation is 7α-dehydroxylation. In the case of cholic acid this results in the formation of deoxycholic acid (Fig. 18), a process which involves at least eight enzymatic reactions as previously demonstrated (Coleman, JBC, 1987; 262:4701; Hylemon, JLipRes, 1991; 32:89). As depicted, it is believed that most of the degradative steps occur with the bile acid being linked to CoA (Mallonee, JBacteriol, 1992; 174: 2065). The absorption efficiency for deoxycholic acid is in the range of 20 to 50 per cent (Hofmann, Gastro, 1987; 93:693), whereas the other secondary bile acid, lithocholic acid, is absorbed to a smaller extent (Allan, Gut, 1976; 17:413).

Another natural bile acid participating in the enterohepatic circulation, lagodeoxycholic acid (3α,7α,12β-trihydroxy-5β-cholanoic acid), is present in rabbit bile and in human faeces (Eneroth, JLipRes, 1966; 7:511) as well as in plasma of patients with bacterial overgrowth (Setchell, CCActa, 1985; 152:297). In the colon, this bile acid appears to be epimerized by bacterial 12β-dehydrogenases, presumably through a 12-oxo intermediate, to form deoxycholic acid (Edenharder, BBActa, 1988; 962:362).

Ursodeoxycholic acid may be directly 7β-dehydroxylated by intestinal bacteria. On the other hand, ursodeoxycholic acid may be

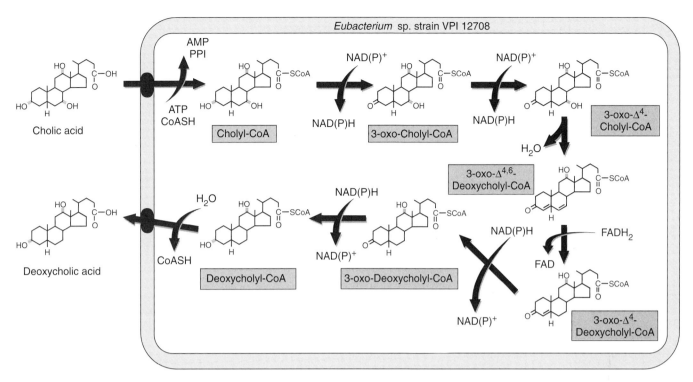

Fig. 18. Proposed pathways of bile acid 7α-dehydroxylation in a *Eubacterium* sp. VPI 12708 isolate. Metabolism of cholic acid in the colon results in the formation of deoxycholic acid. Names and molecular structures of bile acid intermediates that appear to be involved in bile acid 7α-dehydroxylation are shown in this illustration. (Reproduced with kind permission of WB Saunders Co., Philadelphia, from: Vlahcevic ZR, Heuman DM, and Hylemon PB. Physiology and pathophysiology of enterohepatic circulation of bile acids. In Zakim D and Boyer TD, eds. *Hepatology: a textbook of liver disease*, Vol. I, 3rd edn, 1996: 376–417).

formed from chenodeoxycholic acid by 7α-dehydroxylation with 7-oxo-lithocholic acid as intermediate, followed by bacterial reduction of the 7β-isomer of chenodeoxycholic acid (Fig. 19) (Hirano, JLipRes, 1981; 22:1060; MacDonald, ApplEnvironMicrobiol, 1982; 44: 1187). Recent studies in humans receiving ursodeoxycholic acid therapy suggest that iso-ursodeoxycholic acid is formed in the intestine via the intermediate 3-oxo-7β-hydroxy-5β-cholanoic acid (Beuers, JHepatol, 1991; 13:97).

Basolateral bile acid uptake

Bile acids absorbed from the small intestine and the right side of the colon are transported in the superior mesenteric vein, and those from the left side of the colon reach the portal vein via the inferior mesenteric vein. In the portal blood, bile acids are predominantly bound to albumin (Aldini, JLipRes, 1982; 23:1167; Roda, JLipRes, 1982; 23:490) and to a lesser extent to plasma lipoproteins, particularly high density lipoproteins followed by low density lipoproteins (Kramer, EurJBioch, 1979; 102:1; Salvioli, FEBSLett, 1985; 187:272). Unconjugated bile acids are probably bound more tightly than their conjugated counterparts. Fenestrae between the endothelial cells in the sinusoids permit access of album–bile acid complexes to the space of Disse and thus direct contact with the hepatocyte membrane. Hepatic uptake correlates well with the bile acid polarity (Aldini, JLipRes, 1982; 23:1167), thus being inversely related to the strength of binding to albumin and lipoproteins. In addition, bile acid conjugation greatly enhances basolateral uptake (Aldini, JLipRes, 1982; 23:1167).

Up to 98 per cent of bile acids are extracted from the portal blood during a single passage through the liver.[28] This highly efficient process is mediated by Na^+-dependent and Na^+-independent transport systems. The human sodium taurocholate-cotransporting polypeptide (**NTCP**), which was mapped to chromosome 14q24.1–24.2 (Hagenbuch, JCI, 1994; 93:1326), strictly mediates Na^+-dependent bile acid uptake (Hagenbuch, SemLivDis, 1996; 16:129). In the rat, this transport protein has been assigned to chromosome 6q24 (Cohn, MammGenome, 1995; 6:60). It appears to account for most, if not all, sodium-dependent bile acid uptake (Fig. 20). The reduced expression of this transporter in cholestasis (Gartung, Gastro, 1996; 110:199) may represent a protective mechanism to reduce uptake of potentially toxic bile acids. Another, but less well characterized, Na^+-dependent basolateral bile acid transporter may be *m*-epoxide hydrolase (vonDippe, AmJPhysiol, 1993; 264:G528). The availability of a complementary DNA for *m*-epoxide hydrolase (Porter, ArchBiochemBiophys, 1986; 248:121) should facilitate the expression of the protein, with subsequent functional studies to characterize further the bile acid-transporting capacity of this protein.

Na^+-independent bile acid uptake systems include: (i) the cloned organic anion-transporting polypeptide (**OATP**) mapped to chromosome 12 (Kullak-Ublick, Gastro, 1995; 189:1274); it not only transports bile acids but also a variety of non-bile acid amphipathic organic anions as well as anionic steroid conjugates (Jacquemin, PNAS, 1994; 91:133; Kullak-Ublick, Hepatol, 1994; 20:411; Bossuyt, JPharmExpTher, 1996; 276:891); (ii) a dicarboxylate/cholate anion exchange system (Zimmerli, PfluegersArchPhysiol, 1992; 421:

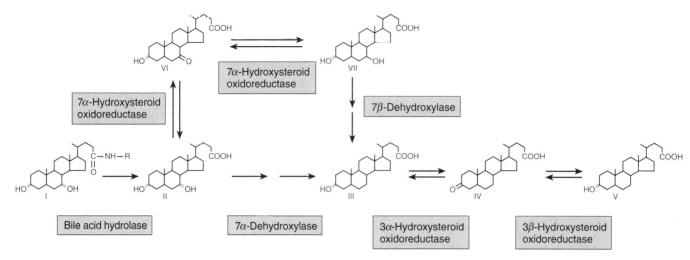

Fig. 19. Bile acid metabolism by intestinal bacteria. Enzymes and molecular structures of a variety of bile acid intermediates formed by intestinal micro-organisms are illustrated: (I) N-($3\alpha,7\alpha$-dihydroxy-5β-cholan-24-oyl)amino acid; (II) chenodeoxycholic acid; (III) lithocholic acid; (IV) 3-oxo-5β-cholanoic acid; (V) isolithocholic acid; (VI) 3α-hydroxy-7-oxo-5β-cholanoic acid; and (VII) ursodeoxycholic acid. (Reproduced with kind permission of WB Saunders Co., Philadelphia, from: Vlahcevic ZR, Heuman DM, and Hylemon PB. Physiology and pathophysiology of enterohepatic circulation of bile acids. In Zakim D and Boyer TD, eds. *Hepatology: a textbook of liver disease*, Vol. I, 3rd edn, 1996: 376–417).

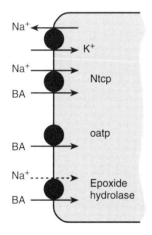

Fig. 20. Proposed basolateral transport systems mediating bile acid uptake in hepatocytes. Na^+-dependent bile acid uptake is mediated by the cloned Na^+-dependent taurocholic acid-cotransporting polypeptide (Ntcp). This transport is driven by the physiological outside–inside Na^+ gradient that is maintained by primary active ion pumping of the basolateral Na^+/K^+-ATPase. The organic anion-transporting polypeptide (oatp) transports bile acids and a variety of differently charged amphipathic compounds. The physiological driving force of this transport system is still unknown. Epoxide hydrolase may also be involved in bile acid uptake into the hepatocyte. As indicated by the stippled arrow, this transport does not display strict Na^+ dependency. Other putative transport systems involved in basolateral bile acid uptake are discussed in the text.

329; Boelsterli, AmJPhysiol, 1995; 268:G797); (iii) a non-ionic diffusion pathway for cholic acid (Blitzer, JBC, 1986; 261:12042; Veith, BBActa, 1992; 1103:51), probably influenced by the activity of a basolateral Na^+/H^+ exchange (Arias, JBC, 1984; 259:5406; Moseley, AmJPhysiol, 1986; 250:G35) and/or Na^+/HCO_3^- co-transport (Renner, JCI, 1989; 83:1225) and finally (iv) a multispecific sulphate anion exchanger (Hugentobler, AmJPhysiol, 1986; 251:

G656). It is noteworthy that the exact roles of the transporters beside OATP remain to be defined and their molecular characterization is still awaited.

Under normal conditions bile acid concentrations in the systemic blood circulation are low. Although serum bile acids may be an indicator of liver disease (Festi, Hepatol, 1983; 3:707), inefficient bile acid transport systems, especially in newborn babies and infants (Barnes, JCI, 1981; 68:775), and shunting of portal blood make interpretations difficult. Elevated serum bile acid levels in liver diseases are reflected by the presence of significant quantities of bile acids in urine (Makino, Gastro, 1975; 68:545). Bile acids not bound to proteins are filtered by glomeruli, enter the proximal tubules of the kidney, and may be secreted (Corbett, ClinSci, 1981; 61:773). However, the majority of bile acids will be reabsorbed in the proximal tubules (Barnes, BiochemJ, 1977; 166:65) and therefore the urinary bile acid composition reflects transport processes in the kidney as well as the circulating serum bile acid composition (Summerfield, ClinSci, 1977; 52:51).

Dynamic aspects of the enterohepatic circulation

Measurements of bile acid kinetics by a semidirect isotope-labelled bile acid dilution technique were introduced 40 years ago (Lindstedt, ActaPhysiolScand, 1957; 40:1). Improved techniques now permit the determination of bile acid pool size (Duane, JLipRes, 1975; 16:155) and both synthesis and turnover rate (Vantrappen, JLipRes, 1981; 22:528) from a single bile or serum sample (Table 3). The bile acid pool may be determined experimentally with an acute bile fistula (Fig. 21). Employing this technique, bile acid pool size is represented by the area under the washout curve; basal and derepressed bile acid synthesis rates may be obtained at the same time (Eriksson, PSEBM, 1957; 94:578). For obvious reasons this approach is usually impractical in humans. The model of an

Table 3 Kinetics of individual bile acids

Bile acid	Pool size (mg)	Fractional turnover rate (per day)	Bile acid synthesis (mg per day)	Bile acid input (mg per day)
Cholic acid	500–1500	0.2–0.5	180–360	—
Chenodoxycholic acid	500–1400	0.2–0.3	100–250	—
Deoxycholic acid	200–1000	0.2–0.3	—	40–200
Lithocholic acid	50–100	1.0	—	40–100
Total bile acids	1250–4000	—	280–610	80–300

extracorporeal bile duct allows the controlled interruption and restoration of the enterohepatic circulation and long-term bile collection for several days (Weis, JLipRes, 1978; 19:856; Stange, JCI, 1989; 84:173; Fuchs, JLipRes, 1992; 33:1383). This animal model demonstrated the diurnal variation in bile acid secretion as well as the derepression of bile acid synthesis (Fig. 22) in the rat (Stange, JCI, 1989; 84:173).

Other parameters of the enterohepatic circulation can be obtained and include the efficiency of intestinal bile acid absorption

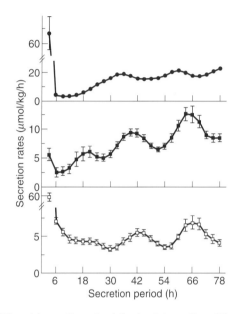

Fig. 22. Bile acid secretion rates following interruption of the enterohepatic circulation. Rats were fitted with an extracorporeal bile duct and allowed to recuperate for 1 week following surgery. Upon interruption of the exteriorized enterohepatic circulation, bile was collected at 3-h intervals for 78 h in the freely moving rat. The secretion rates are shown for taurocholic acid (upper panel), taurochenodeoxycholic acid (middle panel), and tauromuricholic acid (lower panel). Following 6 h of biliary drainage, bile acid secretion rates increased and demonstrated a clear diurnal variation. Each data point represents the mean ± 1 SEM (error bars are partly within symbols). (By copyright permission of the American Society for Clinical Investigation, from: Stange EF, Scheibner J, and Ditschuneit H. Role of primary and secondary bile acids as feedback inhibitors of bile acid synthesis in the rat *in vivo*. *Journal of Clinical Investigation*, 1989; **84**: 173–80).

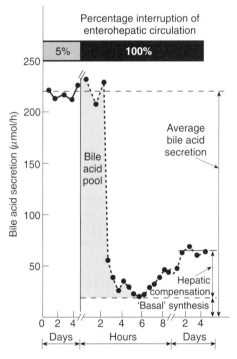

Fig. 21. Measurements of bile acid pool size, basal and derepressed bile acid synthesis rate in a rhesus monkey. Following complete interruption of the enterohepatic circulation by means of an acute bile fistula in a rhesus monkey, bile acid secretion rates decreased within 6 h to reach a plateau. The area under the curve represents the bile acid pool size of the animal. Following depletion of the bile acid pool after 6 h, bile acid secretion rates are a measure of the basal bile acid synthesis rate. The subsequent increase in bile acid secretion reflects hepatic compensation by derepression of bile acid synthesis. (Reproduced with kind permission of Raven Press Ltd, New York, from: Carey MC and Duane WC. Enterohepatic circulation. In Arias IM, Boyer JL, Fausto N, Jacoby WB, Schachter DA, and Shafritz DA, eds. *The liver: biology and pathobiology*, 3rd edn, 1994: 719–67).

and the recycling frequency of the bile acid pool (Mok, Gastro, 1977; 73:684). The latter varies between 4 and 14 per day in mammals. Plotting the recycling frequency of the bile acid pool against the bile acid pool size per kilogram of body weight (Fig. 23) revealed a curvilinear inverse relationship. Interestingly, this was not influenced by obesity, hyperlipidaemia, gallstone disease, and bile acid therapy.

Enterohepatic circulation of bile acids is important for their conservation, thereby limiting the amount of bile acids that have to be newly synthesized by the liver. More detailed information about the enterohepatic circulation is published regularly.[28,29]

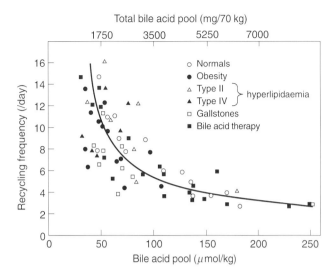

Fig. 23. Recycling frequency and bile acid pool size in relation to pathophysiological conditions. This figure illustrates a curvilinear inverse relationship between recycling frequency and bile acid pool size, standardized for body weight. This relationship appears to be constant, irrespective of the clinical status with regard to obesity (black circles), hyperlipidaemia (open and black triangles), gallstone disease (open square), or bile acid administration (black square). (Reproduced with kind permission of Raven Press Ltd., New York, from: Carey MC and Duane WC. Enterohepatic circulation. In Arias IM, Boyer JL, Fausto N, Jacoby WB, Schachter DA, and Shafritz DA, eds. *The liver: biology and pathobiology*, 3rd edn, 1994: 719–67).

Cholehepatic circulation

A decade ago, it was shown that the synthetic nor-chenodeoxycholic and nor-ursodeoxycholic acid induced hypercholeresis in rodents (Yoon, Gastro, 1986; 90:837; Palmer, AmJPhysiol, 1987; 252:G219). Combining the observation that these bile acids are present in bile partially in unconjugated form with the known capability of unconjugated bile acids to diffuse passively across epithelial cell membranes (Schiff, JCI, 1972; 51:1351; Wilson, JCI, 1972; 51:3015; Krag, JCI, 1974; 53:1686), a cholehepatic circulation of unconjugated bile acids was proposed. According to that hypothesis (Fig. 24), the unconjugated bile acid is secreted actively into the canalicular space and then absorbed passively in protonated form by cholangiocytes. Removal of the proton from ductular bile generates a bicarbonate anion, thereby keeping the luminal osmolality unchanged. The unconjugated bile acid molecule traverses the cholangiocyte and, following its excretion across the basolateral membrane, transport via the periductular capillary plexus to the terminal portal venule and then into the sinusoid may occur. Bile acids are then extracted by hepatocytes and resecreted into bile. Thus, cycling may continue until the molecule fails to be absorbed by the biliary epithelium, or is biotransformed by hydroxylation or conjugation to a metabolite that is not absorbed by cholangiocytes.

Cholehepatic circulation predicts that cycling should be terminated by hydroxylation or conjugation of the bile acid molecule. In the rat, which is known for its poor hydroxylation of deoxycholic acid, nor-deoxycholic acid is hypercholeretic. In the hamster, exhibiting efficient 7α-hydroxylation of deoxycholic acid, nor-deoxycholic acid shows only a modest hypercholeretic effect (Neoptolemos, Gastro, 1985; 88:1682). These observations provide

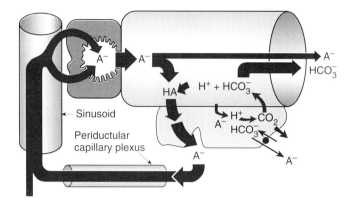

Fig. 24. Proposed cholehepatic circulation of unconjugated bile acids. Following secretion into the canalicular space and generating the bile acid-dependent flow, the unconjugated bile acid molecule is absorbed passively in protonated form by cholangiocytes. Because the removal of the proton from ductular bile generates a bicarbonate anion, luminal osmolality remains unchanged. The bile acid molecules then traverse the cholangiocyte and are transported across the basolateral membrane by mechanisms that await characterization. A proposed carrier mechanism may exchange the bile acid molecule for a bicarbonate anion, which may combine with a proton to form carbon dioxide and water, catalysed by carbonic anhydrase. Once the bile acid molecule has crossed the basolateral membrane of the cholangiocyte, it is transported into the sinusoid via the periductular capillary plexus. An efficient bile acid uptake occurs at the basolateral membrane of the hepatocyte and the bile acid molecule may be resecreted into bile. (Reproduced with kind permission of Kluwer Academic Publishers, Lancaster England, from: Hoffman AF, Yeh HZ, Schteingart CD, Bolder U, Ton-Nu HT, and Hagey LR. The cholehepatic circulation of organic anions: a decade of progress. In Alvaro D, Benedetti A, and Strazzabosco M, eds. *Vanishing bile duct syndrome. Pathophysiology and treatment*, 1996: 90–103).

strong support that cholehepatic cycling indeed occurs *in vivo*. Other bile acids for which cholehepatic circulation has been observed are summarized in Table 4.

If cholehepatic circulation also occurs in humans, its translation into therapeutic advances in the treatment of cholangiopathies will be the challenge for the future. Whether the development of drug targeting to the biliary epithelium may succeed remains to be seen.

Bile acid metabolism in hepatobiliary and intestinal diseases
Inborn errors of bile acid synthesis

Classic methods for measuring bile acids have proven unsuitable for the detection and identification of inborn errors of bile acid synthesis. However, recent advances in mass spectrometry such as fast atom bombardment ionization, gas chromatography, and liquid secondary ionization mass spectrometry have yielded unique and diagnostic bile acid profiles.[32] These tools provide screening tests that require only small amounts (microlitres) of a non-invasively obtained urine specimen and have excellent sensitivity and specificity. Unfortunately, these methods are very time-consuming owing to an intensive work-up of the samples. Importantly, the knowledge of bile acid synthesis disorders does not only provide insights into normal physiology, but may also offer potential treatment by means of bile acid therapy.

Table 4 Cholehepatic circulation of bile acids

Natural bile acids	Synthetic bile acids

Dihydroxy bile acids
    Ursodeoxycholic acid[1]
    12-Epi-deoxycholic acid[2]
    Hyodeoxycholic acid[3]
	C22 bile acids
	    Dinor-chenodeoxycholic acid[5]
	    11-Oxo-lithocholic acid[6]

Hydroxy-oxo bile acids
    7-Oxo lithocholic acid[1]
	C23 bile acids
	    Nor-chenodeoxycholic acid[7]
	    Nor-ursodeoxycholic acid[8]
	    Nor-deoxycholic acid[9]

Trihydroxy bile acids
    Cholic acid[4]
	C24 bile acids
	    7β-Methyl-chenodeoxycholic acid[10]

	C25 bile acids
	    Homo-ursodeoxycholic acid[11]
	    Homo-chenodeoxycholic acid[12]
	    α-Methyl-ursodeoxycholic acid[13]

The following list gives one representative that documents the choleretic potential of the individual bile acid.
[1] Gastro, 1980; 79:82; [2] Gastro, 1990; 99:1092; [3] JPhysiol, 1987; 386:106; [4] JPhysiol, 1977; 265:855; [5] Gastro, 1996; 110:1365; [6] JPhysiol, 1990; 424:68; [7] AmJPhysiol, 1987; 252:G219; [8] Gastro, 1986; 90:837; [9] Gastro, 1985; 88:1682; [10] JLipRes, 1991; 32:1729; [11] JLipRes, 1993; 34:915; [12] JLipRes, 1993; 34:915; [13] DigDisSci, 1992; 37:791.

In theory, each step during bile acid synthesis is a potential site of a primary inborn error in synthesis. Bile acid synthesis defects may arise from a primary enzyme defect/deficiency or may be secondary to organelle dysfunction (e.g. peroxisomes) and are summarized in Table 5. Progressive cholestatic liver disease is a common clinical manifestation of these inborn errors. Underlying pathophysiological mechanisms have been proposed and include low synthesis rates of primary bile acids possessing choleretic as well as trophic effects. In parallel, more 'toxic' bile acids accumulate in the hepatocyte, thereby causing cell damage. Because bile acid synthesis

Table 5 Inborn errors of bile acid synthesis

Enzyme defect
Defect in cholesterol side-chain degradation
    Cerebrotendinous xanthomatosis
Defect in steroid nucleus transformation
    3β-hydroxy-ΔC27 steroid dehydrogenase/isomerase deficiency
    Δ4-3-Oxosteroid 5β-reductase deficiency

Peroxisomal disorder
Complete loss of peroxisomal function
    Zellweger's syndrome (cerebrohepatorenal syndrome)
    Neonatal adrenoleukodystrophy
    Infantile Refsum's disease
    Hyperpipecolic acidaemia
    Leber's congenital amaurosis
Partial loss of peroxisomal function
    Rhizomelic chondrodysplasia punctata
    Zellweger-like syndrome
Loss of a single peroxisomal function
    X-linked adrenoleukodystrophy
    Thiolase deficiency (pseudo-Zellweger's syndrome)
    Bifunctional protein deficiency
    Acyl-CoA oxidase deficiency (pseudoneonatal adrenoleukodystrophy)
    Hyperoxaluria type I
    Acatalasaemia

Generalized dysfunction of the liver
Tyrosinaemia
Neonatal iron storage disease
Fulminant hepatic failure

Modified from: Balistreri WF and Schubert WK. Liver disease in infancy and childhood. In Schiff L and Schiff ER, eds. *Diseases of the liver*, 7th edn. Philadelphia: JB Lippincott, 1994: 1099–203.

is well developed in early gestation (Setchell, JBC, 1988; 263:16637), prenatal diagnosis by analysis of amniotic bile acids may offer the chance of early intervention and prevention of progressive disease.

Identified genetic defects involving reactions that result in changes to the steroid nucleus include deficiencies in the 3β-hydroxy-C27-steroid dehydrogenase/isomerase and the Δ4-3-oxosteroid 5β-reductase. In the first case, the second enzymatic reaction of the 'neutral' pathway is impaired, resulting in a dramatic reduction in the level, or complete loss, of primary bile acids. Characteristic for this enzyme deficiency is the occurrence of allylic 3β-hydroxy-Δ5 bile acids (Jacquemin, JPediat, 1994; 125:379), which not only lack transport across isolated canalicular membranes, but appear to inhibit the canalicular transport of taurine conjugates of cholic acid.[33] This underlying defect in bile acid transport may be the molecular mechanism responsible for the intrahepatic cholestasis in this disease. Conjugated hyperbilirubinaemia, elevated liver function tests, and malabsorption of fat-soluble vitamins are common in these patients (Jacquemin, JPediat, 1994; 125:379). Diagnostic features are the accumulation of 7α-hydroxycholesterol in serum and the detection of 3β,7α-dihydroxy-5-cholenoic acid and 3β,7α,12α-trihydroxy-5-cholenoic acid in urine (Clayton, JCI, 1987; 79:1031; Ichimiya, JLipRes, 1991; 32:829). Because the enzyme is expressed in fibroblasts (Buchmann, JCI, 1990; 86:2034), determination of its activity may provide confirmatory evidence. Clinical improvement has been observed following bile acid replacement therapy, using either chenodeoxycholic (Ichimiya, JLipRes, 1991; 32:829; Horslen, JInherMetDis, 1992; 15:38;) or ursodeoxycholic acid (Jacquemin, JPediat, 1994; 125:379); however, a combination of both bile acids may improve the outcome.

The second identified genetic defect that results in changes to the steroid nucleus is the deficiency of the cytosolic Δ4-3-oxosteroid 5β-reductase (Setchell, JCI, 1988; 82:2148), catalysing the fourth step in the 'neutral' pathway. Successful cloning has shown that the enzyme is expressed only in liver (Onishi, FEBSLett, 1991; 283: 215; Kendo, EurJBioch, 1994; 219:357). Its absence is reflected by low concentrations of primary bile acids and increased levels of 3-oxo-Δ4 bile acids such as 3-oxo-7α-hydroxy-4-cholenoic and 3-oxo-7α,12α-dihydroxy-4-cholenoic acid (Setchell, JCI, 1988; 82: 2148), which may not be secreted into bile.[33] Interestingly, patients with neonatal haemochromatosis have been found to exhibit similar biochemical profiles (Shneider, JPediat, 1994; 124:234). However, this presumably represents a secondary effect due to iron overload rather than a primary defect. Patients with this particular enzyme deficiency have clinical features of neonatal cholestasis and liver biopsy may reveal giant cell transformation (Daugherty, Hepatol, 1993; 18:1096). Oral administration of cholic acid and ursodeoxycholic acid has been demonstrated to improve liver function tests as well as liver histology (Setchell, SemLivDis, 1987; 7: 85; Daugherty, Hepatol, 1993; 18:1096).

A number of liver diseases are accompanied by a secondary deficiency of Δ4-3-oxosteroid 5β-reductase (Clayton, Lancet, 1988; ii:1283; Clayton, JInherMetDis, 1991; 14:478), which may be relevant for the progression of liver damage. In cases where this enzyme becomes rate limiting due to its low expression, 3-oxo-7α-hydroxy-4-cholenoic acid is formed and may inhibit canalicular bile acid secretion. This would result in an intracellular accumulation of potentially toxic bile acids, further damaging hepatocytes and concomitantly reducing the level of Δ4-3-oxosteroid 5β-reductase.

The observation of an aggravation of cholestasis in a patient with Δ4-3-oxosteroid 5β-reductase deficiency who received oral treatment with chenodeoxycholic acid, as well as its subsequent improvement following drug withdrawal, is in good agreement with the proposed concept.

Other inborn errors of bile acid synthesis involve the degradation of the cholesterol side-chain. A key discovery more than 20 years ago revealed a defective oxidation of the side chain during bile acid synthesis in patients with cerebrotendinous xanthomatosis, leading to the excretion of C27 bile alcohols in bile, faeces, and urine (Setoguchi, JCI, 1974; 531:1393). Cerebrotendinous xanthomatosis represents a lipid storage disease in which the metabolic defect is located to the mitochondrial 27-hydroxylase (Oftebro, JCI, 1980; 65:1418). Fibroblasts from homozygous patients do not express the enzyme activity, while the enzyme activity is reduced by approximately 50 per cent in heterozygotes (Skrede, JCI, 1986; 78: 729). Only very recently the underlying gene defect was discovered and revealed the existence of a variety of different mutations in the 27-hydroxylase gene (Cali, JBC, 1991; 266:7779; Leitersdorf, JCI, 1993; 91:2488; Kim, JLipRes, 1994; 35:1031; Garuti, JLipRes, 1996; 37:1459). A characteristic is the virtual absence of chenodeoxycholic acid and very low amounts of cholic and deoxycholic acid. Theoretically, no primary bile acid should have been formed, at least in homozygous patients. However, this is clearly not the case, indicating that alternative side-chain cleavage pathways may exist. It is believed that small amounts of cholic acid are probably formed via a 25-hydroxylation pathway. Chenodeoxycholic acid and ursodeoxycholic acid are also present as their 21-, 22-, and 23-hydroxylated forms in patients with cerebrotendinous xanthomatosis treated with these bile acids (Koopman, BBActa, 1986; 883:585; 1987; 917:238). Originally, 23-hydroxylation was thought not to occur in man, such derivatives being found only in certain snakes, the walrus, and seal. Accumulation of xanthomatous deposits in the tendon, brain, and lungs results in progressive neurological dysfunction, premature coronary heart disease, and pulmonary insufficiency ultimately causing death (Kuriyama, JNeurolSci, 1991; 102:225). Bile acid therapy with chenodeoxycholic acid appears to improve neurological function, whereas ursodeoxycholic acid may be less effective (Tint, JLipRes, 1989; 30:633). Long-term follow-up will demonstrate whether disabilities are potentially reversible.

Defective bile acid synthesis may also be secondary to peroxisomal dysfunction. In this case, polyhydroxylated cholestanoic acids are formed as bile acid intermediates and reflect deficiency in the final steps of bile acid synthesis. In the virtual absence of peroxisomes (Mooi, UltrastructPathol, 1983; 5:135), namely in Zellweger's syndrome or cerebrohepatorenal syndrome, failure of side-chain oxidation leads to excessive urinary excretion of 3α, 7α,12α-trihydroxy-5β-cholestanoic acid and 3α,7α-dihydroxy-5β-cholestanoic acid (Hanson, JCI, 1975; 56:577). Varanic acid, 3α,7α, 12α,24S-tetrahydroxy-5β-cholestan-26-oic acid, is another bile acid found in patients with Zellweger's syndrome (Kase, ScaJCLI, 1989; 49:1). It is thought to be an intermediate in the conversion of cholestan-26-oic acids to cholan-24-oic acids, although studies in man showed that it was poorly converted to cholic acid (Swell, JBC, 1981; 256:912), possibly because the inappropriate isomer was used, or perhaps because it is not part of the side-chain cleavage pathway in the synthesis of cholic acid. The primary defect is impaired assembly of peroxisomes induced by mutations in the peroxisome assembly factor-1 and -2 (Fukuda, AmJHumGen, 1996; 59:1210; Shimozawa, PediatRes, 1996; 39:812). Clinical features include psychomotor retardation, hypotonia, and kidney cysts (Smith, JPediat, 1965; 67:617; Passarge, JPediat, 1967; 71:691). The disease develops rapidly and patients usually die within months after birth. The future will show whether these patients benefit from oral bile acid therapy (Setchell, Hepatol, 1992; 15:198).

Other peroxisomal diseases have been characterized (Table 5) and more sophisticated technology will probably explain other defects in bile acid synthesis that occur in patients with still enigmatic liver diseases.

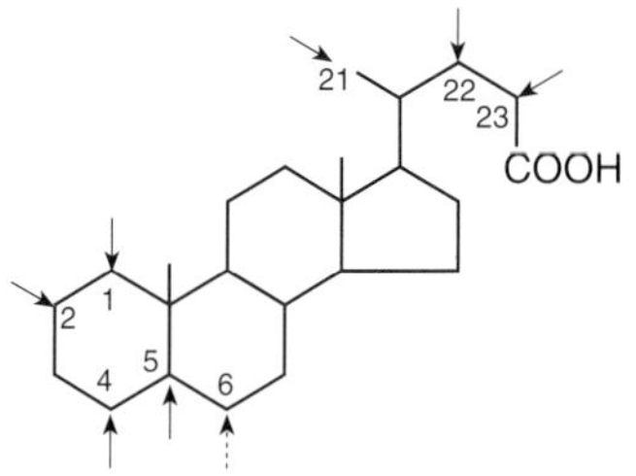

Bile acid metabolism in liver disease

It has been long appreciated that serum bile acids are elevated in liver disease (Rudman, JCI, 1957; 36:530; Carey, JCI, 1958; 37:1494; Makino, Gastro, 1969; 56:1033). Probably because total bile acid concentration in serum is extremely variable, their measurement as a sensitive parameter of liver function apparently has not provided any diagnostic value in liver disease and most likely remains an elusive goal.

Bile acid metabolism in chronic liver disease is disturbed in many ways. Contributive factors are the severity of parenchymal liver cell damage, portosystemic shunting, altered lipoprotein metabolism, and changes in the colonic microflora. In cholestatic liver disease, intermediates of bile acid synthesis accumulate intracellularly, thereby inducing reactions with enzymes that normally have other more avid substrates. In extreme human cholestasis, cholic acid synthesis substantially exceeds chenodeoxycholic acid synthesis, suggesting that minor pathways, not subject to negative feedback control, may contribute a significant proportion of newly synthesized bile acids. One such pathway leads to the formation of 3β-hydroxy-5-cholenoic acid (Anderson, JCI, 1972; 51:112), a bile acid found in human cholestasis (Minder, JLipRes, 1979; 20:986) and in large amounts in the meconium of newborn infants (Back, HoppeSeylerZPhysiolChem, 1973; 354:83). Further metabolism of 3β-hydroxy-5-cholenoic acid may yield lithocholic acid and chenodeoxycholic acid.

Other minor pathways involve 1-, 2-, 4-, 5-, 6-, and 7-hydroxylation of the steroid nucleus, and 21-, 22-, and 23-hydroxylation of the side chain (Fig. 25). 1β-Hydroxylated cholic, chenodeoxycholic, and deoxycholic acid have been detected in urine and faeces of patients with liver disease (Alme, JLipRes, 1977; 18:339; Bremmelgaard, EurJClinIinv, 1979; 9:341; Batta, JLipRes, 1989; 30:1953; Shoda, JChromatogr, 1989; 488:315; Miyara, BiomedChromatogr, 1990; 4:56; Shoda, JLipRes, 1990; 31:249; Jönsson, ScaJCLI, 1992; 52:555). 1β-Hydroxylated bile acids were also isolated from the urine, meconium, umbilical cord, and amniotic fluid of neonates and infants (Back, Gastro, 1980; 78:671; Strandvik, EurJClinInv, 1982; 12:301; Mahara, AnalSci, 1987; 3:449; Shoda, JLipRes, 1988; 29:847; Obinata, JPediatGastrNutr, 1992; 15:1; Wahlen, JPediatGastrNutr, 1994; 18:9), suggesting an important role of this bile acid pathway during early development, probably because of an immaturity of 12α-hydroxylation in the usual pathway of bile acid synthesis (Colombo, PediatRes, 1987; 21:197; Gustafsson, PediatRes, 1987; 21:99).

Phenobarbital stimulates 1β-hydroxylation yielding tetrahydroxylated bile acids excreted in the urine without conjugation

Fig. 25. Bile acid hydroxylation sites. Alternative bile acid synthesis pathways, in health and disease, may involve a variety of hydroxylation sites, either at the steroid nucleus or at the side chain. Alternative hydroxylation sites are indicated by the arrows.

(Back, KlinWschr, 1982; 60:541). These bile acids may be major metabolites being excreted into urine besides bile acid sulphates and glucuronides. The most abundant metabolites found in urine are 1β,3α,12α-trihydroxy-, 1β,3α,7α-trihydroxy-, 1β,3α,7α,12α-tetrahydroxy-, 3α,6α,7α-trihydroxy-, and 3α,6α,7α,12α-tetrahydroxy-5β-cholanoic acid (Shoda, JLipRes, 1990; 31:249). It has been suggested that the ratio ([1β,3α,7α,12α-tetrahydroxy-5β-cholanoic acid + 1β,3α,7α-trihydroxy-5β-cholanoic acid]/1β,3α,12α-trihydroxy-5β-cholanoic acid) may allow the distinction between mild and severe liver disease (Shoda, JLipRes, 1990; 31:249).

2β-Hydroxylated derivatives of cholic acid have been found in the urine of a patient with intrahepatic cholestasis (Bremmelgaard, JLipRes, 1980; 21:1072), as a component of gastric contents in neonates with intestinal obstruction (Clayton, BiochemJ, 1982; 206:489), and as a constituent of amniotic fluid (Nakagawa, JLipRes, 1990; 31:1089). 2β,3α,6α,7α-Tetrahydroxy-5β-cholanoic acid is frequently found in urine of healthy newborn infants (Strandvik, EurJClinInv, 1982; 12:301; Strandvik, ScaJCLI, 1994; 54:1).

4β-Hydroxylated bile acids have been found in appreciable quantities in fetal gallbladder bile, meconium, the faeces of healthy newborn infants (Colombo, PediatRes, 1987; 21:197; Setchell, JBC, 1988; 263:16637; Dumaswala, JLipRes, 1989; 30:847), and in the urine of neonates (Strandvik, ScaJCLI, 1994; 54:1). These bile acids could reflect a deficiency in 5β-reductase because the 3β-hydroxy group has been epimerized to the 3α-configuration—this might involve the addition of a molecule of water across the Δ4-5 double bond. Alternatively, they could arise from the action of a 4β-hydroxylase following the formation of the normal bile acids.

Hyocholic acid, 3α,6α,7α-trihydroxy-5β-cholanoic acid was first isolated by Haslewood from pig bile (BiochemJ, 1956; 62:637). It has also been found not only as a major urinary metabolite of chenodeoxycholic acid in patients with cholestatic liver disease (Bremmelgaard, JLipRes, 1980; 21:1072; Shoda, JLipRes, 1988; 29:847; Batta, JLipRes, 1989; 30:1953; Shoda, JChromatogr, 1989; 488:315; Nakagawa, Hepatol, 1990; 12:322; Shoda, JLipRes, 1990; 31:249), but also in the fetus and newborn infant (Back, Gastro, 1980; 78:671; Colombo, PediatRes, 1987; 21:197; Nakagawa, JLipRes, 1990; 31:1089; Strandvik, ScaJCLI, 1994; 54:1). The discovery of the 6α-hydroxy bile acids, however, was preceded by an *in vitro* demonstration of 6α-hydroxylation of lithocholic acid to hyodeoxycholic acid by human liver microsomes (Trulzsch, BiochemMed, 1974; 9:158).

Bile acids with a 6β-hydroxyl group are found in rats and mice (Hsia, JBC, 1958; 230:573) and are termed α-muricholic (3α,6β,7α-trihydroxy-5β-cholanoic acid) and β-muricholic acid (3α,6β,7β-trihydroxy-5β-cholanoic acid). These bile acids may be found also in patients with chronic liver disease (Huang, FedProc, 1979; 38:1118; Setchell, BMJ, 1983; 286:1750; Nakagawa, Hepatol, 1990; 12:322). In addition, another muricholic acid, β-hyocholic acid (3α,6α,7β-trihydroxy-5β-cholanoic acid), has been detected in humans with liver disease or cerebrotendinous xanthomatosis (Koopmann, BBActa, 1987; 917:238; Batta, JLipRes, 1989; 30:1953; Nakashima, Hepatol, 1990; 11:225).

Other 6-hydroxylated bile acids derived from deoxycholic and lithocholic acid and their epimers have been discovered in the urine of healthy infants or humans or in the urine under circumstances of chronic liver disease. These bile acids include: (i) hyodeoxycholic acid or 3α,6α-dihydroxy-5β-cholanoic acid (Summerfield, BiochemJ, 1976; 154:507; Gustafsson, PediatRes, 1987; 21:99); (ii) murideoxycholic acid or 3α,6β-dihydroxy-5β-cholanoic acid (Bremmelgaard, EurJClinInv, 1979; 9:341); (iii) 3α,6α,12α-trihydroxy-5β-cholanoic acid (Thomassen, EurJClinInv, 1979; 9:425; Alme, JSterBioch, 1980; 13:907; Bremmelgaard, JLipRes, 1980; 21:1072); and (iv) 3α,6β,12α-trihydroxy-5β-cholanoic acid (Alme, JLipRes, 1977; 18:339; Bremmelgaard, EurJClinInv, 1979; 9:341; Thomassen, EurJClinInv, 1979; 9:425).

7α-Hydroxylation of bile acids following side-chain oxidation is thought to be unlikely in man (Matern, MedBiol, 1975; 53:107), although such a pathway occurs in rat microsomes where deoxycholic acid is converted to cholic acid (Mahowald, JBC, 1957; 225:781; Murakami, JBC, 1981; 256:8658). Studies on the urine of patients with cholestasis have identified small amounts of 7β-hydroxylated bile acids (Summerfield, BiochemJ, 1976; 154:507; Bremmelgaard, EurJClinInv, 1979; 9:341). They may have arisen from the reduction of 7-keto bile acids, rather than from 7β-hydroxylation.

Bile acids with altered side chains have been described in cholestasis. The origin of the C20 and C21 bile acids, present in the meconium of human infants (Pyrek, JSterBioch, 1983; 18:341), is mysterious. These bile acids could arise from the oxidation of C21 steroids, such as pregnane derivatives, or could be formed following accumulation of 20- and 20,22-hydroxylated cholesterol, due to deficiencies in the synthesis of steroids in fetal life.

C23 bile acids found in patients with cholestasis, such as 23-norcholic acid (Bremmelgaard, EurJClinInv, 1979; 9:341; Thomassen, EurJClinInv, 1979; 9:425), suggest α-oxidation of C24 bile acids or β-oxidation of C25 bile acids. As noted earlier, C27 bile acids are found in large quantities in cholestatic liver diseases, particularly Zellweger's cerebrohepatorenal syndrome (Eyssen, BBActa, 1972; 273:212; Hanson, JCI, 1975; 56:577; Hanson, JBC, 1980; 255:1483; Mathis, Gastro, 1980; 79:1311). These bile acids arise from a failure to oxidize the side chain and may cause haemolysis at concentrations found in blood (Smith, JLabClinMed, 1979; 94:624).

The discovery of a C29 bile acid (Parmentier, EurJBioch, 1979; 102:173) raised serious questions whether cholesterol is the only precursor of bile acids in man. As shown for a patient with Zellweger's syndrome, the C29 bile acid may be derived from a C27 bile acid precursor (Kase, JCI, 1985; 76:2393), and probably does

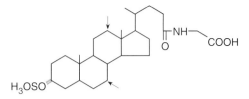

Fig. 26. Bile acid sulphation. Sulphate esters such as 3α-sulpholithocholylglycine are usually conjugated with glycine or taurine. Other sites of sulphation are indicated by the arrows.

represent a metabolite of β-sitosterol (Janssen, Steroids, 1981; 37:81).

In cholestatic liver disease, hepatic and systemic bile acid concentrations rise, resulting in modifications in bile acid metabolism, especially changes in the conjugation pattern. Thirty years ago, the formation and urinary excretion of bile acid sulphates was demonstrated for the first time (Palmer, PNAS, 1967; 58:1047). Sulphation by 3′-phosphoadenosine-5′-phosphosulphate sulphotransferases (**PAPS**), which occur in the liver and in extrahepatic tissue, is the dominant step for the elimination of lithocholic acid (Cowen, Gastro, 1975; 69:109). In addition, bile acid disulphates carrying more hydroxyl groups were minor components of the urine in cholestatic liver disease (Alme, JLipRes, 1977; 18:339). Although lithocholic acid is sulphated in the 3α-position (Fig. 26), several groups of investigators have reported for cholic and chenodeoxycholic acid that the 7α-monosulphate is the only isomer found for each bile acid (Summerfield, BiochemJ, 1976; 156:339; Chen, BBActa, 1978; 522:443; Barnes, JLipRes, 1979; 20:952). For deoxycholic acid, 12α-sulphation has been reported (Loof, BBActa, 1980; 617:192). Identification was based on co-chromatography with chemically synthesized bile acid sulphate standards. However, using high-pressure liquid chromatography, it was subsequently shown that it is the 3α-monosulphate of glycochenodeoxycholic acid which is formed by the liver in hamsters and rats (Kirkpatrick, JBC, 1980; 255:10157). In man, both 3α- and 7α-monosulphates have been detected using analysis of calcium–bile acid sulphate complexes by reversed phase thin-layer chromatography (Raedsch, JLipRes, 1979; 20:796).

Resolution of these disparate results requires methods that can produce derivatives whose structure can be unequivocally identified by mass spectrometry. Analytical methodology employing a solvolysis step to yield the parent bile acid loses information as to which hydroxyl group the sulphate ester is attached. Therefore, labelling of unoccupied hydroxyl groups on the bile acid sulphate with a moiety which can survive solvolysis has been suggested (Barnes, Gastro, 1979; 76:1095). Fast atom bombardment mass spectrometry, while being able to yield intact molecular ions of bile acids and their sulphates and other conjugates, cannot distinguish between different sites of attachment. The ideal arrangement would be a suitable combination of high–pressure liquid chromatography (to accomplish separation of different isomers) and mass spectrometry. It is possible that thermospray liquid chromatography–mass spectrometry may be the answer, but the problems of analysing doubly ionized sulphate conjugates have not been resolved (Setchell, JLipRes, 1989; 30:1459).

The composition of bile acids in urine is quite different from serum, the sulphate conjugates are in a greater proportion than in serum, for example their urinary clearance is much higher than that of their non-sulphated, non-glucuronidated analogues (Makino, Gastro, 1975; 68:545; Stiehl, Gastro, 1975; 68:534; van Berge Henegouwen, Gut, 1976; 17:861; Summerfield, ClinSci, 1977; 52: 51). This appears to be due to the properties of the transport mechanisms in the kidney (Barnes, BiochemJ, 1977; 166:65). Following glomerular filtration, tubular reabsorption of bile acids occurs in a manner and efficiency comparable with their transport in the distal small intestine (Weiner, AmJPhysiol, 1964; 207:964). In addition, proximal tubular secretion of the sulphate esters also occurs (Corbett, ClinSci, 1981; 61:773).

Studies with bile duct-ligated hamsters showed that the sharp rise in the serum bile acid concentration on the first day after ligation is followed by a steady decline as a result of substantial urinary excretion of bile acid sulphates. Because a decrease in the *in vitro* PAPS activity owing to a change in affinity of the enzyme for its bile acid substrate (Barnes, BiochemMed, 1979; 22:165) has been shown, the rise in urinary excretion of bile acid sulphates is probably not a result of induction of this enzyme.

Drugs affecting renal function could also alter urinary bile acid excretion in cholestasis, as could those affecting metabolic activity in the hepatocyte. Failure to form bile acid sulphates would cause bile acid accumulation in the blood. Although hepatic PAPS activity is inducible by oestradiol in oophorectomized rats (Hammerman, Gastro, 1978; 76:1021), this steroid hormone causes cholestasis, making it unsuitable for use in clinical applications. In any case, no sex difference in the activity of PAPS in human liver has been found (Loof, ScaJGastr, 1982; 17:69), although the marked ontogeny of PAPS activity in young rats (Balistreri, JLipRes, 1984; 25:228) could have a parallel in newborn infants. Indeed, only traces of bile acid sulphates are present in human fetal gallbladder bile (Setchell, JBC, 1988; 263:16637).

The enzymology of bile acid glucuronidation also has been studied in detail. Almost 25 years ago, Back established for the first time a glycosidic pathway for bile acid conjugation (Back, HoppeSeylerZPhysiolChem, 1974; 355:749). A major part of bile acid glucuronide in urine is hydroxylated at C6 (Alme, CCActa, 1978; 86:251; Alme, JSterBioch, 1980; 13:907). Multiple UDP-glucuronosyltransferases with distinct substrate specifities may evidently exist. Lithocholic acid may be converted to hyodeoxycholic acid via 6α-hydroxylation (Trülzsch, BiochemMed, 1974; 9:158) followed by glucuronidation at C6 (Parquet, FEBSLett, 1985; 189:183; Marschall, BBActa, 1987; 921:392; Radominska-Pyrek, JCI, 1987; 80:234). In this case, glucuronic acid is coupled via an ether glycosidic linkage (Fig. 27). Although the enzyme catalysing this reaction has not been purified so far, the cloning of three different human complementary DNAs (Fournel-Gigleux, FEBSLett, 1989; 243:119; Ritter, Biochem, 1992; 31:3409; Jin, JPharmExpTher, 1993; 264:475) and the functional expression of one of these genes (Fournel-Gigleux, MolPharm, 1991; 39:177) will allow the investigation of its regulation. As for the sulphate esters, bile acid ether glucuronides can also be conjugated with glycine or taurine (Goto, JChromatogr, 1985; 345:241). It was anticipated that the 3α-hydroxy group would be the favoured position for ether conjugation. Back synthesized the 3α-glucuronides of lithocholic and chenodeoxycholic acid (Back, HoppeSeylerZPhysiolChem, 1976; 357:219) and isolated a bile acid derivative from a patient with primary biliary cirrhosis which had an identical mass spectrum

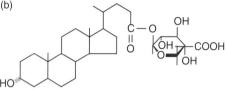

Fig. 27. Bile acid glucuronidation. The bile acid ether glucuronides are usually conjugated to glycine or taurine. The structures of lithocholic acid ether (top) and ester (bottom) β-glucuronides are given. In humans, hyodeoxycholate is glucuronidated in the 6α-position, as indicated by the arrow.

to that of authentic chenodeoxycholic acid-3α-glucuronide (Back, HoppeSeylerZPhysiolChem, 1976; 357:213). Although 3α-glucuronidation of cholic acid also occurs (Alme, JSterBioch, 1980; 13: 907), most of the bile acid glucuronides in urine are of hyodeoxycholic acid and an isomer of cholic acid, 3α,6α,12α-trihydroxy-5β-cholanoic acid; these bile acids are conjugated in the 6α-position (Alme, CCActa, 1978; 86:251). Preferential glucuronidation of the 6α-hydroxy group has been demonstrated in *in vitro* studies with human liver and kidney microsomes (Marschall, BBActa, 1987; 921:392; Radominska-Pyrek, JCI, 1987; 80:234; Parquet, EurJBioch, 1988; 171:329).

Interestingly, hyodeoxycholic acid may be a poor substrate for sulphation, suggesting that the affinity of bile acids for sulphation decreases as the degree of hydroxylation increases. As shown with human (Irshaid, DrugMetDisp, 1991; 19:173) and rat liver microsomes (Radominska-Pyrek, JLipRes, 1986; 27:89; Zimniak, JLipRes, 1988; 29:183), the formation of a glucuronide ester (Fig. 27) may also occur at the carboxyl group on the side chain of short-chain bile acids.

The proportion of bile acid glucuronides in bile of normal children is less than 1 per cent (Stiehl, EurJClinInv, 1980; 10:307) and is not significantly increased in adults with alcoholic cirrhosis (Stiehl, Hepatol, 1985; 5:492), or obstructive jaundice (Takikawa, Gut, 1985; 26:38). However, in children with intrahepatic cholestasis, this proportion is close to 5 per cent (Stiehl, EurJClinInv, 1980; 10:307).

In serum, bile acid glucuronides constitute up to 8 per cent of total bile acids in healthy controls and in patients with liver disease (Takikawa, Digestion, 1983; 27:189; Takikawa, DigDisSci, 1986; 31:487). In comparison, the proportion of bile acid glucuronides in serum is low in newborn infants with or without liver disease (Takikawa, BiochemMed, 1985; 33:381). This is attributed to the slow maturation of glucuronide formation following birth as is well described for bilirubin glucuronides. As with bile acid sulphates, bile acid glucuronides increase the urinary clearance rate, presumably due to poor tubular reabsorption following glomerular filtration. However, this increase is less pronounced than with bile acid sulphates. In patients with alcoholic cirrhosis, glucuronides represent less than 2 per cent of total urinary bile acids (Stiehl, Hepatol, 1985; 5:492), whereas they may account for up to 9 per cent in children with intrahepatic cholestasis (Stiehl, EurJClinInv, 1980; 10:307).

Bile acid glucuronidation has an advantage over bile acid sulphation in that the UDP-glucuronyltransferases are inducible by phenobarbital (Fröhling, BBActa, 1976; 444:525), as occurs for other UDP-glucuronyltransferases (Bock, BBActa, 1973; 327:46). Phenobarbital treatment of children with intrahepatic cholestasis reduces bile acids circulating in the blood and increases the proportion of bile acid glucuronides in bile, serum, and urine, all consistent with increased glucuronide formation (Stiehl, Pediat, 1973; 51:992). Increased faecal bile acid concentrations may also reflect impaired intestinal absorption of bile acid glucuronides (Oehlberg, DigDisSci, 1988; 33:1110). The proportion of bile acid glucuronides and sulphates may, however, depend on the type and dosage of drugs administered in the management of cholestasis.

Improved analytical techniques have allowed the identification of other bile acid conjugates in both healthy controls and in patients with liver disease. Usually these conjugates are present in smaller quantities than sulphate esters or glucuronides. Bile acid glucosidation at the hydroxyl group of C3 (Fig. 28) requires the microsomal enzyme glucosyltransferase, which has been localized to the liver (Gartung, JHepatol, 1994; 20:32), intestine, and kidney (Matern, BBActa, 1987; 921:1). The enzyme purified from human liver (Matern, PNAS, 1984; 81:7036) uses dolichol phosphoglucose as a glucose donor. The sugar donor is formed from UDP-glucose and dolichylphosphate via UDP-glucose dolichylphosphate glucosyltransferase purified from human liver (Matern, EurJBioch, 1990; 90:99). It appears to have a broad substrate specificity among various bile acids. Bile acid glucosides are constituents of urine of patients with liver disease, but also of urine of healthy adults (Marschall, FEBSLett, 1987; 213:411). Because excretion of total urinary bile acid glucosides only increased to a very small extent in patients with cholestasis compared with healthy humans and was much lower than that of bile acid glucuronides (Wietholtz, Hepatol, 1991; 13:656), bile acid glucosidation probably does not play an important role in detoxification of bile acids.

In contrast to glucuronidation and glucosidation, a third glycosidic conjugation pathway, N-acetylglucosaminidation (Fig. 28), appears to be selective for 7β-hydroxylated bile acids, such as ursodeoxycholic, iso-ursodeoxycholic, and allo-isoursodeoxycholic acid (Marshall, JBC, 1989; 264:12989; Marshall, JCI, 1992; 89:1981). The enzymatic reaction takes place in liver and kidney microsomes (Matern, FEBSLett, 1990; 270:11). Often these conjugates are present in very small quantities and so they may not play an important biological role.

Patients with liver cirrhosis have a normal chenodeoxycholic acid pool size, whereas the cholic and deoxycholic acid pool is small (Vlahcevic, Gastro, 1971; 60:491; Vlahcevic, Gastro, 1972; 62:1174; McCormick, Gut, 1973; 14:895). The latter is probably due to selective reduction in the 12α-hydroxylation, although other disturbances in the synthetic pathway may be present (Patterson, Gastro, 1980; 79:620). The decreased deoxycholic acid pool size

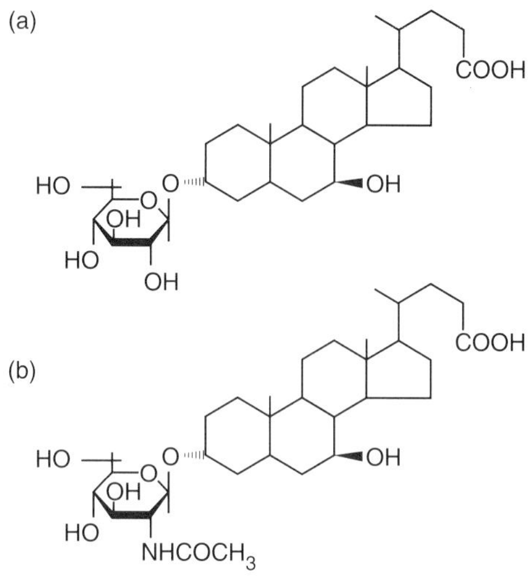

Fig. 28. Bile acid glucosidation and N-acetyl-β-glucosaminidation. The structures of the β-glucoside (top) and N-acetyl-β-glucosaminide (bottom) conjugates of ursodeoxycholic acid are given.

also observed in patients with liver cirrhosis is probably caused by a reduced bacterial conversion of cholic to deoxycholic acid (Knodell, Gastro, 1976; 71:196).

Increased plasma levels of 7α-hydroxy-4-cholesten-3-one and 7α-hydroxycholesterol have been reported hours after the ingestion of small amounts of alcohol (Axelson, FEBSLett, 1991; 281:155). This observation may be due to an increased bile acid synthesis (Axelson, FEBSLett, 1991; 284:216) and may explain the reduced risk of cardiovascular diseases and gallstone formation following small daily doses of alcohol.

Bile acid metabolism in cholesterol gallstone disease

Smaller bile acid pool sizes have commonly been observed in patients with cholesterol gallstone disease (Vlahcevic, Gastro, 1970; 59:165; Swell, Gastro, 1971; 61:716; Pomare, Gut, 1973; 14:885; Shaffer, JCI, 1977; 59:828). The most likely explanation of this observation is a gallbladder motility disorder, resulting in an increased diversion of hepatic bile into the small intestine (Jazrawi, Gastro, 1995; 109:582). To maintain homeostasis, a smaller bile acid pool attempts to keep secretory rates constant by enhanced circulation. A gradual expansion of the deoxycholic acid pool, resulting in inhibition of bile acid synthesis and with increasing impairment of the gallbladder motility (Marcus, Gut, 1986; 27:550; Berr, JCI, 1992; 90:859; Hussaini, Gastro, 1994; 107:1503; Shoda, Hepatol, 1995; 21:1291), is fully in line with this idea. Because cholecystectomy does not appear to change the deoxycholic acid pool size up to 8 years after surgery (Kullak-Ublick, Hepatol, 1995; 21:41), elevated levels of this bile acid before surgery (Marcus, Gut, 1986; 27:550; Hay, JLipRes, 1993; 34:759) clearly demonstrate increased conversion of cholic to deoxycholic acid prior to surgery (Marcus, Gut, 1986; 27:550; Berr, JCI, 1992; 90:859; Hay, JLipRes, 1993; 34:759; Kullak-Ublick, Hepatol, 1995; 21:41). The enhanced conversion of cholic to deoxycholic acid is caused by an increased 7α-hydroxylation activity of the intestinal microflora (Berr, Gastro, 1996; 111:1611).

Bile acid metabolism in hyperlipoproteinaemia

Anomalies in the metabolism of bile acids have been reported for patients with type II and type IV hyperlipoproteinaemia and are of particular relevance because cholesterol gallstones may occur in up to 50 per cent of these patients (Singh, CanMedAssJ, 1975; 113: 733; Ahlberg, AmJDigDis, 1979; 24:459).

Features observed in type II hyperlipoproteinaemia are decreased cholic acid synthesis rates and a diminished cholic acid pool size (Einarsson, EurJClinInv, 1972; 2:225; Einarsson, JCI, 1974; 54:1301). This anomaly may be corrected by administration of cholestyramine (Einarsson, EurJClinInv, 1974; 4:405).

In type IV hyperlipoproteinaemia, cholic acid synthesis is increased (Einarsson, EurJClinInv, 1972; 2:225; Einarsson, JCI, 1974; 54:1301; Angelin, JLipRes, 1978; 19:1004), which is reflected in an increase in total bile acid synthesis (Davidson, JLipRes, 1981; 22: 620; Davidson, JLipRes, 1986; 27:183). A more recent study revealed that altered bile acid synthesis is only present in type IV hyperlipoproteinaemia with familial hypertriglyceridaemia (Angelin, PNAS, 1987; 84:5434). In addition, based upon an inadequate postprandial rise in serum bile acid concentrations, a decreased intestinal bile acid absorption was suggested (Angelin, PNAS, 1987; 84:5434). The recent measurement of bile acid kinetics and bile acid absorption in familial hypertriglyceridaemia is fully consistent with this notion (Duane, JLipRes, 1995; 36:96). Indeed, an inherited mutation in the Na^+- dependent bile acid transporter gene has now been identified that could explain this finding.[27]

A relationship between bile acid metabolism and very low density lipoprotein synthesis has been appreciated for several years. Interruption of the enterohepatic circulation is associated with increased serum levels of triacylglycerols (Angelin, JLipRes, 1978; 19: 1017; Beil, Metabolism, 1982; 31:438; Akerlund, Gut, 1994; 35: 1116). Conversely, inhibition of bile acid synthesis decreases serum triacylglycerol levels in hyperlipidaemic patients (Miller, Lancet, 1974; ii:929). The molecular link between bile acid synthesis and hepatic triacylglycerol synthesis appears to be phosphatidic acid phosphatase (Shepherd, Cardiol, 1989; 76:65). This enzyme is activated by bile acids and promotes triacylglycerol synthesis in the liver with subsequent secretion of very low density lipoproteins.

Patients with primary dysbetalipoproteinaemia and the apoE-II homozygote phenotype are characterized by an enhanced chenodeoxycholic acid and total bile acid synthesis (Angelin, EurJClinInv, 1990; 20:143). Dependent on the existence of a single or different cholesterol precursor pools for bile acid synthesis, this may imply a disturbance of the normal precursor inflow of cholesterol to the liver, because apoE is involved in the hepatocellular uptake of triglyceride-rich lipoproteins.

Bile acid metabolism in coeliac sprue

Most patients with coeliac sprue have a defective emptying of the gallbladder. Kinetic studies revealed decreased cycling of the bile acid pool (Low-Beer, Gut, 1973; 14:204; Low-Beer, NEJM, 1975; 292:961), as evident by an increased cholic acid pool and a decrease in the formation of deoxycholic acid. An impaired propulsive intestinal motility represents another contributory factor (Low-Beer, Lancet, 1973; i:991; Spiller, ClinSci, 1987; 72:217) to the alterations in the dynamics of the enterohepatic circulation. A higher faecal bile acid excretion in patients with coeliac sprue compared with controls suggested that other disturbances in the intestinal absorption of bile acids may exist.

Bile acid metabolism in ileal dysfunction

Patients with ileal disease/resection (e.g. Crohn's disease, cystic fibrosis) or bypass surgery for morbid obesity have a greatly increased risk for the development of pigment stones (Carey, AmJSurg, 1993; 165:410). Gallbladder biles of patients with Crohn's disease involving the ileum have increased biliary levels of bilirubin (Dawes, SurgForum, 1991; 42:188; Brink, Gastro, 1996; 110:A24), but low levels of cholesterol (Lapidus, Gut, 1991; 32:1488). It has been hypothesized that increased bile acid malabsorption, for example during ursodeoxycholic acid administration (Stiehl, Gastro, 1990; 98:424), high carbohydrate diets (Meihoff, JCI, 1968; 47:261), or a high cholesterol diet via a cholestyramine-like effect (Björkhem, BBActa, 1991; 1085:329), may induce enterohepatic cycling of unconjugated bilirubin, similar to the concept underlying enteric hyperoxaluria in bile acid malabsorption (see below). Indeed, it has been shown recently that bile acid malabsorption can induce enterohepatic cycling of bilirubin (Brink, Gastro, 1996; 110:1945). This finding may explain not only persistent biliary sludge, frequent stone calcification, increased calcium levels in bile of patients receiving ursodeoxycholic acid (Gleeson, QJMed, 1990; 76:711; Roda, PharmTher, 1992; 53:167), and the epidemiological relationship between pigment gallstone disease and a high carbohydrate diet (Nagase, AmJSurg, 1978; 135:788), but also the interrelationship between cholesterol and calcium bilirubinate precipitation from bile such as in the gallstone nucleus.

Further studies may identify patients with pigment gallstones who have a mutation in the Na^+-dependent ileal bile acid transporter, which will be responsible for bile acid malabsorption (Wong, JBC, 1995; 270:27228) and therefore cause enterohepatic cycling of bilirubin. In addition, strategies to prevent this enteric hyperbilirubinobilia, for example dietary zinc (Mendez-Sanchez, Hepatol, 1996; 24:306A), which will precipitate bilirubin in the intestine, may prove a suitable approach to prevent pigment stones in ileal disease.

Cholerrhoeic enteropathy (bile acid diarrhoea)

Impaired intestinal bile acid absorption, in particular absorption from the ileum, may result in bile acid malabsorption. In this case, an increase in bile acid synthesis compensates for increased faecal bile acid loss, thereby maintaining bile acid concentrations in the small intestine within the normal range required for the digestion and absorption of dietary fat (Hofmann, Gastro, 1972; 62:918; Poley, Gastro, 1976; 71:38). Chenodeoxycholic and deoxycholic acid in concentrations above 3 mM in the colon cause fluid and electrolyte secretion (Mekhijian, Gastro, 1970; 59:120; Mekhijian, JCI, 1971; 50:1569; Poley, Gastro, 1976; 71:38; Chadwick, JLabClinMed, 1979; 94:661), being the pathophysiological correlate of watery diarrhoea with little fat malabsorption (cholerrhoeic diarrhoea). The exact molecular mechanisms inducing the watery diarrhoea await to be resolved, but a cyclic AMP-dependent mechanism appears to be involved (Binder, JCI, 1973; 52:1460; Binder, Gastro, 1975; 68:503). More recent data suggest that mast cells and histamine-mediated processes may contribute to the secretory effects of dihydroxy bile acids (Gelbmann, JCI, 1995; 95: 2831).

An elegant method to detect bile acid malabsorption is the SeHCAT test (Ferraris, Gastro, 1986; 90:1129) in which the taurine conjugate of selenium-75 homocholic aid is administered and γ-emission over the gallbladder monitored over time. Therapeutic efforts aim at the intraluminal binding of bile acids, which can be effectively achieved by bile acid sequestrants such as cholestyramine (Hofmann, NEJM, 1969; 281:397; Hofmann, Gastro, 1972; 62:918).

Under physiological conditions bile acids are conjugated preferentially with glycine. In patients with bile acid malabsorption due to ileal disease, a marked increase in glycine conjugation has been reported (McLeod, Lancet, 1968; i:873; Abaurre, Gastro, 1969; 57: 679; Garbutt, Gastro, 1969; 56:711). This occurs for both trihydroxy and dihydroxy bile acids (Abaurre, Gastro, 1969; 57:679). Because the capacity of bile acid conjugation with taurine is not impaired in these patients as evidenced by oral taurine supplementation of the diet (Garbutt, Gastro, 1969; 56:711), an increased demand on the conjugation system apparently depletes the taurine pool, resulting in an increase of the glycine to taurine ratio of conjugated bile acids.

Hyperoxaluria and an increased incidence of calcium oxalate kidney stones have been shown for patients with ileal disease (Dowling, Lancet, 1971; i:1103; Chadwick, NEJM, 1973; 289:172; Earnest, AmJClinNut, 1977; 30:72). The underlying pathophysiological mechanism involves preferential bile acid conjugation with glycine. Following bacterial deconjugation in the colon, glyoxalate forms, is absorbed, and is metabolized within the liver to oxalate, which then is excreted in the urine (Smith, NEJM, 1972; 286:1371). Normalization of urinary oxalate excretion with subsequent cessation of kidney stone formation following taurine administration (Admirand, TrAAP, 1971; 84:307; Admirand, NEJM, 1972; 286:1412) is in good agreement with this proposed mechanism.

Steatogenic enteropathy (fatty acid diarrhoea)

Steatorrhoea with or without fatty acid diarrhoea but almost no bile acid diarrhoea (Hofmann, Gastro, 1972; 62:918) is likely if patients with bile acid malabsorption do not benefit from cholestyramine therapy. If this is the case, the critical length of the diseased or resected ileum probably amounts to more than 100 cm (Hofmann, Gastro, 1972; 62:918; Poley, Gastro, 1976; 71:38). Under these conditions, hepatic bile acid synthesis cannot compensate for faecal bile acid loss and so the bile acid pool decreases. Consequently, impairment of micellar solubilization of lipids in the intestine and steatorrhoea occurs. Like bile acids, normal and hydroxylated fatty acids exert secretory effects on the colon (Ammon, Gastro, 1973; 65: 744; Bright-Astare, Gastro, 1973; 64:81). Under conditions where anaerobic colonization may be low[28] and a more acidic colonic pH predominates, unconjugated chenodeoxycholic and deoxycholic acid are precipitated (McJunkim, Gastro, 1981; 80:1454), a mechanism accounting for the relative unimportance of bile acid diarrhoea

in severely impaired ileal function. Importantly, a pathological [^{14}C]-glycocholic acid breath test requires the determination of faecal bile acids to distinguish between fatty acid diarrhoea and small bowel bacterial overgrowth. A novel therapeutic approach may be the oral administration of cholylsarcosine, a non-toxic synthetic bile acid which in humans does not appear to be metabolized in the intestine and liver (Schmasssmann, Gastro, 1993; 104:1171). This bile acid has already been proven to increase triglyceride absorption in a canine model of bile acid deficiency (Longmire-Cook, DigDisSci, 1992; 37:1217).

Small bowel bacterial overgrowth

Small bowel bacterial overgrowth or 'blind loop syndrome' may be a result of small bowel diverticulosis, scleroderma, diabetes, enteroenteral fistula, or surgical blind loops, such as in patients who have undergone Billroth II surgery. In these cases, large amounts of anaerobic colonic bacteria are found in the small intestine. Consequently, bile acid deconjugation and dehydroxylation lead to the formation of relatively insoluble deoxycholic and lithocholic acid within the small intestine (Rosenberg, NEJM, 1967; 276:1391; Tabaqchali, Lancet, 1968; ii:12; van Deest, JCI, 1968; 47:1314; Northfield, Gut, 1973; 14:341). Nevertheless, enteroliths do not form frequently (Fowweather, BiochemJ, 1949; 44:607), but more commonly bile acids are absorbed passively and subsequently enter the portal venous circulation. The increase in glycine conjugation of luminal bile acids in these patients (Tabaqchali, Lancet, 1968; ii: 12) may be a result of a relative taurine deficiency and an increased glycine–taurine ratio.

Because of the lower intraluminal bile acid concentration, intestinal micelle formation is compromised and causes malabsorption of fat and vitamins. A typical finding in small bowel overgrowth is an increase, in particular, of unconjugated bile acids in serum (Lewis, Lancet, 1969; i:219). The diagnosis may be obtained by employing a [^{14}C]-glycocholic acid breath test (Sher, NEJM, 1951; 285:656) or a [^{14}C]-xylose test (King, DigDisSci, 1980; 25:53). For a normal faecal bile acid excretion, an abnormal glycocholate breath test should enable the distinction between bile acid malabsorption and small bowel overgrowth (Thayssen, ClinGastroent, 1977; 6: 227). Alternatively, the non-radioactive H$_2$ glucose breath test may be used (Caspary, ZGastr, 1975; 13:704).

Bile acid metabolism in thyroid disease

Animal studies have demonstrated an increased ratio of cholic to chenodeoxycholic acid in hypothyroid states, whereas the reverse effect was observed for hyperthyroidism. This was attributed to an inhibitory effect of thyroid hormones on 12α-hydroxylase (Mitropoulos, FEBSLett, 1968; 1:13) and a stimulatory effect on sterol 27-hydroxylase (Björkhem, FEBSLett, 1973; 31:20). Hyperthyroidism in humans is characterized by a decreased cholic acid synthesis and an unchanged chenodeoxycholic acid synthesis (Pauletzki, Hepatol, 1989; 9:852), which is compatible with inhibition of 12α-hydroxylation by thyroid hormones. Because thyroid hormones are known to accelerate intestinal transit time (Thomas, AnnIntMed, 1973; 78:669), increased enterohepatic cycling of bile acids may be responsible for the inhibition of 12α-hydroxylase. Also, the cholesterol-lowering effect of thyroid hormones may not be related to an enhanced catabolism of cholesterol to bile acids (Angelin, EurJClinInv, 1983; 13:99; Pauletzki, Hepatol, 1989; 9:852).

Data on bile acid metabolism in hypothyroidism are conflicting. Cholic acid synthesis in patients with hypothyroidism is not significantly different from healthy humans (Hellström, JLabClinMed, 1964; 63:666; Angelin, EurJClinInv, 1983; 13:99). Therapy with L-thyroxine increases chenodeoxycholic acid synthesis, but total and cholic acid synthesis are not significantly changed (Angelin, EurJClinInv, 1983; 13:99). An unchanged net bile acid synthesis rate is supported by studies where L-thyroxine treatment was without effect on faecal bile acid excretion (Abrahms, JLipRes, 1981; 22:323).

Bile acids as therapeutic agents
Gallstone dissolution therapy

Oral bile acid administration aims at reversing conditions considered as a prerequisite for cholesterol gallstone formation, in particular the cholesterol supersaturation of bile. Gallstone dissolution may occur by either micellar solubilization of cholesterol and/or formation of a liquid crystalline phase (Salvioli, JLipRes, 1983; 24: 701). Chenodeoxycholic acid was the first naturally occurring bile acid employed for treatment and prevention of recurrence of radiolucent cholesterol gallstones. However, many patients experienced diarrhoea, hepatotoxicity, and modest hypercholesterolaemia, limiting the use of this bile acid for gallstone dissolution. Based on the observation of Japanese physicians that ursodeoxycholic acid dissolved gallstones without side-effects (Makino, JpnJGastroenterol, 1975; 72:690), this bile acid replaced chenodeoxycholic acid for gallstone dissolution therapy. To enhance the potency of ursodeoxycholic acid, both bile acids have been used in combination (Roehrkasse, DigDisSci, 1986; 31:1032; Podda, Gastro, 1989; 96: 222).

To date, gallstone dissolution therapy is restricted to a carefully selected small number of patients.[33] Because of the long duration of treatment requiring good patient compliance, oral gallstone dissolution is not considered as a first-line therapy (Strasberg, Hepatol, 1992, 16:820). Moreover, a general disadvantage of this kind of therapy is that gallstones may recur (Lanzini, JHepatol, 1986; 3:241; O'Donnell, Gut, 1988; 29:655) and there is no known measure of preventing this. In addition, the introduction of shockwave lithotripsy to disintegrate cholesterol gallstones (Sauerbruch, NEJM, 1986; 314:818) and of minimally invasive surgery (see Chapter 23.6) has further limited oral bile acid therapy to an adjunctive measure (Strasberg, Hepatol, 1992, 16:820). The role of bile acid therapy also has to be discussed in the context of cost-effectiveness. Oral bile acid therapy is competitive with surgery (Strasberg, Hepatol, 1992, 16:820) only in the limited number of patients where gallstone dissolution is expected to occur fast and with high efficacy.

In the search for a new generation of bile acids that are more potent in the treatment of cholesterol gallstone dissolution, other naturally occurring bile acids such as hyodeoxycholic (Singhal, JLipRes, 1984; 25:539,564; Cohen, Lipids, 1986; 21:575), hyocholic (Dusseree, CanJPhysPharm, 1988; 66:1028), and ursocholic acid (Howard, Gut, 1989; 30:97) appear to be either only effective in animals or even less effective than ursodeoxycholic acid.

Table 6 Putative mechanisms and sites of action of ursodeoxycholic acid in chronic liver disease

Restoration of impaired sorting of canalicular transport proteins

Stabilization of hepatocellular membranes

Change in composition of bile acid pool

Hypercholeresis

Immune modulation

Future research may be aimed at the design of optimal desaturating agents with similar safety to ursodeoxycholic acid. The availability of an effective and safe drug for the prevention of gallstone recurrence following dissolution or fragmentation will probably make oral bile acid therapy more attractive than cholecystectomy.

Cholestatic liver disease

The administration of ursodeoxycholic acid in the treatment of chronic cholestatic liver disease is aimed at retarding the rate of progression to endstage liver disease which ultimately requires liver transplantation, maintaining growth and development in children, and improving the quality of life, especially by improving refractory pruritus.

Knowledge of the mechanisms of action of ursodeoxycholic acid in liver disease remains incomplete. A number of potential mechanisms and sites of action have been proposed in the past decade (Table 6). It is beyond the scope of this chapter to give a detailed account of the vast amount of clinical trials on ursodeoxycholic acid. Therefore, we only briefly discuss five putative mechanisms by which this hydrophilic bile acid may be beneficial in the treatment of chronic cholestatic liver disease.

Restoration of impaired sorting of canalicular transport proteins

Under normal conditions, canalicular transport proteins are synthesized in the endoplasmic reticulum and are then shuttled to the basolateral membrane. From there, proteins are transcytosed as vesicles to the canalicular membrane (Bartles, JCellBiol, 1994; 105: 1241), a process which occurs after endocytotic vesicles fuse with, and then bud from, early endosomes. Vesicle movement is thought to occur via attachment to microtubules (Geuze, Cell, 1984; 37: 195). In good agreement with this view is the observation that taurocholic acid secretion into canaliculi of isolated hepatocyte couplets is related to the surface area of the canalicular plasma membrane (Gautam, JCI, 1989; 83:565). In addition, changes in the canalicular surface area obviously reflect an increase in the number of transport proteins in the membrane (Boyer, Gastro, 1995; 109: 1600).

When present in their correct topological location, canalicular transport proteins for biliary lipids and bile acids induce the formation of vesicles within the canalicular space (Crawford, JLipRes, 1995; 36:2147). In cholestasis, the bile acid transporter on the canalicular membrane is diminished, while being increased on the basolateral membrane (Fricker, JCI, 1989; 84:876). In addition, other canalicular membrane proteins involved in bile formation probably remain on the basolateral membrane (Barr, Gastro, 1993; 105:554; Stieger, JHepatol, 1996; 24:128; Oude Elferink, Hepatol, 1997; 26:964A). Being on the basolateral membrane, bile acid and phosphatidylcholine transporters form vesicles which enter the circulation. Vesicles are readily observed in the space of Disse under cholestatic conditions (Felker, PNAS, 1978; 75:3459) and become lipoprotein X following plasma modification with adsorbed apolipoproteins (Laggner, EurJBioch, 1977; 77:165; Sabesin, Gastro, 1982; 83:704). Being a unilamellar vesicle (Laggner, EurJBioch, 1977; 77:165), lipoprotein X is unique among lipoproteins. It is the major abnormal low density lipoprotein responsible for hypercholesterolaemia in cholestasis (Walli, JCI, 1984; 74:867) and consists of biliary-specific phosphatidylcholines (Picard, CCActa, 1972; 36:247), free cholesterol (Sabesin, Gastro, 1982; 83:704; Walli, JCI, 1984; 74:867), and traces of bile acids (Frison, Digestion, 1979; 19:411).

Administration of ursodeoxycholic acid will lead to a correct topological insertion of transport proteins in the canalicular membrane. This hypothesis is based on the following observations. First, ursodeoxycholic acid therapy causes a progressive decrease in lipoprotein-X serum levels (Poupon, Hepatol, 1993; 17:577). Second, following the relief of mechanical or chemical cholestasis, biliary lipid secretion rates dramatically rise, usually with overshoots for phosphatidylcholine and cholesterol (Hardison, JHepatol, 1986; 3:318; Tazuma, JGastHepatol, 1994; 9:35). Finally, consistent with a redirection of the multiorganic anion transporter from the basolateral to the canalicular membrane (Larkin, Gastro, 1993; 105:594), ursodeoxycholic acid treatment decreases serum levels of conjugated bilirubin (Poupon, ProgLivDis, 1992; 10:219) and of diconjugates of progesterone and its metabolites (Meng, JHepatol, 1997; 27:1029; Meng, Hepatol, 1997; 26:1573).

The exact molecular mechanisms by which ursodeoxycholic acid interacts with the intracellular sorting and trafficking of membrane proteins to reduce impaired hepatic bile acid secretion (Jazrawi, Gastro, 1994; 106:134) remains to be elucidated. A complex network of signals appears to be involved and putative key players are cytosolic free calcium (Beuers, Gastro, 1993; 104:604; Beuers, JCI, 1993; 92:2984), protein kinase C (Beuers, Gastro, 1996; 110:1553), and cell swelling (Häussinger, BiochemJ, 1993; 291:355; Noé, Gastro, 1996; 110:858).

Stabilization of hepatocellular membranes (cytoprotection)

Evidence for direct membrane-damaging effects of bile acids has been obtained *in vitro* (Leuschner, Gastro, 1989; 97:1268; Galle, Hepatol, 1990; 12:486; Heuman, Hepatol, 1991; 14:920; Güldütuna, Gastro, 1993; 104:1736) and *in vivo* (Barnwell, BiochemJ, 1983; 216:107; Kitani, AmJPhysiol, 1985; 248:G407). Hydrophobic bile acids appear to impair mitochondrial function, thereby inducing a signal pathway that ultimately causes apoptosis (Rosser, Gastro, 1995; 108:252). Apoptosis or cell death is characterized by nuclear and cellular fragmentation with subsequent break-up of the cell, but in contrast to cell necrosis, the plasma membrane remains intact during apoptosis. Postulated sequences of intracellular events during apoptosis by predominantly glycine-conjugated dihydroxy bile acids, such as chenodeoxycholic and deoxycholic acid, comprised an enhanced influx of Mg^{2+} into the cell followed by activation of Mg^{2+}-dependent endonucleases.[35] Because a clear

relationship between the hydrophobic–hydrophilic balance of bile acids and apoptosis was not evident, bile acid-mediated cell death appears to be unrelated to the structure and physicochemical properties of individual bile acids.[35]

In contrast to more hydrophobic bile acids such as chenodeoxycholic and deoxycholic acid, the relatively hydrophilic ursodeoxycholic acid shows little intrinsic toxicity. This observation led to the hypothesis that purely physicochemical properties of bile acids are responsible for the cytoprotective effect of ursodeoxycholic acid. More detailed investigations into the molecular mechanisms by which ursodeoxycholic acid protects membrane architecture make a direct membrane-stabilizing effect less likely (Heuman, Gastro, 1994; 106:1333). Instead, bile acids like tauro-ursodeoxycholic acid form simple micelles and sequester the more toxic bile acids, thereby reducing the mixed micellar solubilization of membrane lipids (Heuman, JLipRes, 1996; 37:562). In this regard, biliary secretion of vesicles enriched in phosphatidylcholines may have evolved as a mechanism to protect the biliary epithelium from potentially toxic bile acids. However, the protective effect of a bile acid does not appear to be purely a function of relative hydrophobicity, because the magnitude of protection does not correlate with the hydrophilicity of a given bile acid (Heuman, Gastro, 1994; 106:1333). So far there is no conclusive evidence that the described physicochemical membrane protection is relevant in patients with cholestatic liver diseases.

Changes in composition of the bile acid pool

Chronic administration of ursodeoxycholic acid causes significant changes in the composition of the bile acid pool, with conjugated ursodeoxycholic acid becoming the predominant bile acid (Stiehl, Hepatol, 1990; 12:492). Pool sizes of cholic, chenodeoxycholic and deoxycholic acids, were not affected in any significant way (Beuers, Hepatol, 1992; 15:603; Mazzella, DigDisSci, 1993; 38:896; Rudolph, Hepatol, 1993; 17:1028). However, increased fractional turnover and synthesis has been shown for cholic and chenodeoxycholic acid (Rudolph, Hepatol, 1993; 17:1028). This is in line with an impaired intestinal bile acid absorption during ursodeoxycholic acid therapy (Marteau, Hepatol, 1990; 12:1206; Stiehl, Gastro, 1990; 98:424; Eusufzai, Gut, 1991; 32:1044). These studies suggest that ursodeoxycholic acid does not simply replace the more hydrophobic bile acids, but induces a redistribution of bile acids within the enterohepatic circulation. This effect is probably due to an improved hepatic bile acid clearance (Jazrawi, Gastro, 1994; 106:134).

Hypercholeresis

The proposed cholehepatic circulation (described above) represents the most likely explanation for the hypercholeresis that may be induced with ursodeoxycholic acid in rodents. However, biliary levels of unconjugated ursodeoxycholic acid do not rise markedly during oral ursodeoxycholic acid administration in patients with primary biliary cirrhosis (Crosignani, Hepatol, 1991; 14:1000) and cystic fibrosis (Nakagawa, Hepatol, 1990; 2:322). Because hypercholeresis appears to be present only in rodents but not in humans (Knyrim, Hepatol, 1989; 10:134), the beneficial effect of ursodeoxycholic acid therapy may not be explained by such a mechanism.

Immune modulation

Primary biliary cirrhosis and primary sclerosing cholangitis are characterized by an aberrant expression of major histocompatibility complex class I antigen expression on hepatocellular membranes which is reduced by ursodeoxycholic acid treatment (Calmus, Hepatol, 1990; 11:12; Beuers, Hepatol, 1992; 16:707). Aberrant expression of these molecules, which renders cells more vulnerable to cytolytic T cells, can be induced in experimental cholestasis (Innes, Transpl, 1988; 45:749; Calmus, Gastro, 1992; 102:1371) and by incubating hepatocytes with bile acids at concentrations higher than the physiological range (Hillaire, Gastro, 1994; 107:781). It thus appears that the immune modulatory effect of ursodeoxycholic acid more likely represents some secondary phenomenon resulting from its anticholestatic effect.

Information about ursodeoxycholic acid treatment of a variety of chronic liver diseases may be found elsewhere in this book (see Chapter 23.3).

Drug delivery

Enterohepatic circulation of bile acids makes these molecules interesting as putative carriers to achieve a liver-specific drug delivery and to improve the intestinal absorption of otherwise poorly absorbed drugs. In principle, two different approaches for liver-specific drug delivery may be pursued: (i) a pharmacophore may be attached to the steroid nucleus substituting the bile acid side-chain and (ii) a pharmacophore may be covalently linked to modified bile acids creating a prodrug. Following internalization via specific receptors, this prodrug is further processed. Ongoing studies in this area certainly will enhance interest in bile acid research. More detailed information is available elsewhere in this book.

References

1. Boyer JL. Mechanism of bile secretion and hepatic transport. In Andreoli TA, Hoffmann JF, Fanestil DD, and Schulz SG, eds. *Physiology of Membrane Disorders*. 2nd edn. New York: Plenum Press, 1986: 609–36.

2. Carey MC and LaMont JT. Cholesterol gallstone formation. 1. Physical-chemistry of bile and biliary lipid secretion. *Progress in Liver Diseases*, 1992; **10**: 139–63.

3. LaMont JT and Carey MC. Cholesterol gallstone formation. 2. Pathobiology and pathomechanisms. *Progress in Liver Diseases*, 1992; **10**: 165–91.

4. Sjövall J and Setchell KDR. Techniques for extraction and group separation of bile acids. In Setchell KDR, Kritchevsky D, and Nair PP, eds. *The Bile Acids. Chemistry, Physiology, and Metabolism. Volume 4. Methods and Applications*. New York: Plenum Press, 1988: 1–42.

5. Nambara T and Goto J. High performance liquid chromatography of bile acids. In Setchell KDR, Kritchevsky D, and Nair PP, eds. *The Bile Acids. Chemistry, Physiology, and Metabolism. Volume 4. Methods and Applications*. New York: Plenum Press, 1988: 43–64.

6. Barnes S and Kirk DN. Nuclear magnetic resonance spectroscopy of bile acids. In Setchell KDR, Kritchevsky D, and Nair PP, eds. *The Bile Acids. Chemistry, Physiology, and Metabolism. Volume 4. Methods and Applications*. New York: Plenum Press, 1988: 65–136.

7. Murphy GM. Serum bile acids. In Setchell KDR, Kritchevsky D, and Nair PP, eds. *The Bile Acids. Chemistry, Physiology, and Metabolism. Volume 4. Methods and Applications*. New York: Plenum Press, 1988: 379–403.

8. Back P. Urinary bile acids. In Setchell KDR, Kritchevsky D, and Nair PP, eds. *The Bile Acids. Chemistry, Physiology, and Metabolism. Volume 4. Methods and Applications*. New York: Plenum Press, 1988: 405–41.

9. Setchell KDR, Street JM, and Sjövall J. Fecal bile acids. In Setchell KDR, Kritchevsky D, and Nair PP, eds. *The Bile Acids. Chemistry, Physiology, and Metabolism. Volume 4. Methods and Applications*. New York: Plenum Press, 1988: 441–70.

10. Matschiner J. Naturally occurring bile acids and alcohols and their origins. In Nair PP and Kritchevsky D, eds. *The Bile Acids. Chemistry, Physiology and Metabolism. Volume. 1, Chemistry*. New York: Plenum Press, 1971: 11–46.

11. Elliot WH. Allo bile acids. In Nair PP and Kritchevsky D, eds. *The Bile Acids. Chemistry, physiology and metabolism. Volume 1. Chemistry*. New York: Plenum Press, 1971: 47–93.

12. Elliot WH. Metabolism of bile acids in liver and extrahepatic tissues. In Danielsson H and Sjövall J, eds. *Sterols and Bile Acids, New Comprehensive Biochemistry*. Amsterdam: Elsevier, 1985: 303–29.

13. Hoshita T. Bile alcohols and primitive bile acids. In Danielsson H. and Sjövall J, eds. *Sterols and Bile Acids, New Comprehensive Biochemistry*. Amsterdam: Elsevier, 1985: 279–302.

14. Haslewood GAD. *The Biological Importance of Bile Salts*. Amsterdam: North-Holland, 1978.

15. Hagey LR. Bile acid biodiversity in vertebrates: chemistry and evolutionary implications. PhD thesis, University of California, San Diego, 1992.

16. Small DM. The physical chemistry of cholanic acids. In Nair PP and Kritchevsky D, eds. *The Bile Acids. Chemistry, Physiology and Metabolism. Volume 1. Chemistry*. New York: Plenum Press, 1971: 249–356.

17. Carey MC. Physical-chemical properties of bile acids and their salts. In Danielsson H and Sjövall J, eds. *Sterols and Bile Acids, New Comprehensive Biochemistry*. Amsterdam: Elsevier, 1985: 345–403.

18. Eneroth P and Sjövall J. Extraction, purification, and chromatographic analysis of bile acids in biological materials. In Nair PP and Kritchevsky D, eds. *The Bile Acids. Chemistry, Physiology and Metabolism. Volume 1. Chemistry*. New York: Plenum Press, 1971: 121–71.

19. Cabral DJ and Small DM. Physical chemistry of bile. In Schultz SG, Forte JG, and Rauner BB, eds. *Handbook of Physiology—the Gastrointestinal System*, Vol. 3, Section 6. Baltimore, MD: American Physiological Society, 1989: 621–62.

20. Cohen DE, Chamberlin RA, Thurston GM, Benedek GB, and Carey MC. Cylindrical 'worm-like' micelles in bile salt–lecithin solutions: implications for the earliest events in bile formation. In Paumgartner G, Stiehl A, and Gerok W, eds. *Bile Acids as Therapeutic Agents*. Dordrecht: Kluwer Academic Publishers, 1991: 147–50.

21. Carey MC and Cohen DE. Biliary transport of cholesterol in vesicles, micelles and liquid crystals. In Paumgartner G, Stiehl A, and Gerok W, eds. *Bile Acids and the Liver*. Lancaster: MTP Press, 1987: 287–300.

22. Russell DW and Setchell KDR. Bile acid biosynthesis. *Biochemistry*, 1992; **31**: 4737–49.

23. Vlahcevic ZR, Heuman DM, and Hylemon PB. Regulation of bile acid synthesis. *Hepatology*, 1991; **13**: 590–600.

24. Setchell KDR, Heubi JE, O'Connell NC, Hofmann AF, and Lavine JE. Identification of a unique inborn error in bile acid conjugation involving a deficiency in amidation. *International Bile Acid Meeting: Bile Acids in Hepatobiliary Diseases—Basic Research and Clinical Application*, 1996: 9 (Abstract booklet).

25. Erlinger S. Intracellular events in bile acid transport by the liver. In: Tavoloni N and Berk PD, eds. *Hepatic Transport and Bile Secretion. Physiology and Pathophysiology*. New York: Raven Press, 1993:467–75.

26. Wilson FA. Intestinal transport of bile acids. In: Schultz SG, ed. *Handbook of Physiology—The Gastrointestinal System*, Vol. IV. Bethesda: American Physiological Society, 1991: 389–404.

27. Love MW, Kirby LC, and Dawson PA. Identification of a mutant ileal bile acid and transporter gene in a patient with familial hyperglyceridemia. *International Bile Acid Meeting: Bile Acids in Hepatobiliary Diseases—Basic Research and Clinical Application*, 1996: A43 (Abstract booklet).

28. Carey MC and Duane WC. Enterohepatic circulation. In Arias IM, Boyer JL, Fausto N, Jacoby WB, Schachter DA, and Shafritz DA, eds. *The Liver: Biology and Pathobiology*. New York: Raven Press, 1994: 719–67.

29. Hofmann AF. Enterohepatic circulation of bile acids. In Schultz SG, ed. *Handbook of Physiology—The Gastrointestinal System*, Vol. III. Baltimore, MD: Bethesda: American Physiological Society, 1989: 567–96.

30. Hylemon PB. Metabolism of bile acids in intestinal microflora. In Danielsson H and Sjövall J, eds. *Sterols and Bile Acid, New Comprehensive Biochemistry*. Amsterdam: Elsevier, 1985: 331–43.

31. Hylemon PB and Glass TL. Biotransformation of bile acids and cholesterol by the intestinal microflora. In Hentges DJ, ed. *Human Intestinal Microflora in Health and Disease*. New York, Academic Press, 1983: 189.

32. Setchell KDR and O'Connell NC. Inborn errors of bile acid metabolism. In Suchy FJ, ed. *Liver Disease in Children*. Boston, MA: Mosby, 1994: 835–51.

33. Stieger B, Zhang J, O'Neill B, Sjövall J, and Meier PJ. Transport of taurine conjugates of 7α-hydroxy-3-oxo-4-cholenoic acid and 3β,7α-dihydroxy-5-cholenoic acid in rat liver plasma membrane vesicles. In van Berge Henegouwen GP, van Hoek B, de Groote J, Matern S, and Stockbrügger RW, eds. *Cholestatic Liver Disease*. Dordrecht: Kluwer Academic Publishers, 1994: 82–7.

34. Paumgartner G. Nonoperative management of gallstone disease. In Sleisenger KH and Fordtran JS, eds. *Gastrointestinal Disease: Pathophysiology, Diagnosis, Management*. Philadelphia: WB Saunders, 1994: 1844–57.

35. Patel T, Spivey J, Vadekekalam J, and Gores GJ. Apoptosis—an alternative mechanism of bile salt hepatotoxicity. In Paumgartner G and Beuers U, eds. *Bile Acids and Liver Disease*. Dordrecht: Kluwer Academic Publishers, 1995: 88–95.

2.11 Carbohydrate metabolism

Yolanta T. Kruszynska

Introduction

The liver plays a key role in carbohydrate metabolism. It helps to maintain blood glucose concentrations within relatively narrow limits: it takes up some of the glucose ingested in meals, and influences uptake of glucose by peripheral tissues; it releases glucose after the dietary sugar has been removed from the bloodstream. The liver thus ensures an even and predictable supply of glucose to extrahepatic tissues. The liver is also the major tissue responsible for uptake and metabolism of hexoses other than glucose, notably fructose and galactose, and of pentoses.

Carbohydrate metabolism in normal humans

Glucose metabolism in the fasted state

Some tissues have an obligatory requirement for glucose, which in normal overnight-fasted humans is about 160 to 180 g/day; the brain accounts for about 110 to 145 g of this, red and white blood cells and platelets for about 34 g, and renal medulla for about 2 g (Owen, ProgrBiochemPharm, 1971; 6:177). Other tissues, which also use glucose when available in large amounts after a meal, can satisfy their energy requirements between meals, and during an overnight fast, by oxidizing fatty acids and ketone bodies derived from the partial oxidation of fatty acids. Carbohydrate and fat oxidation each account for nearly 45 per cent of resting energy expenditure in overnight-fasted humans. With more prolonged fasting, the obligatory glucose requirement decreases, and ketone bodies become a major fuel of respiration in the brain. After a 3-day fast, the total body glucose requirement is approximately 80 g/day, falling to only 40 g/day after 5 to 6 weeks of starvation; at this time about 10 per cent of resting energy expenditure comes from carbohydrate oxidation and about 85 per cent from oxidation of fat.

Hepatic glucose production

Only the liver, and to a lesser extent the kidney, possesses glucose 6-phosphatase, which cleaves glucose 6-phosphate so releasing glucose for use by other tissues. Once the ingested glucose has been assimilated, the liver switches from glucose storage to glucose production, so that blood glucose falls only slightly with fasting. Glucose production rates after an overnight fast are 1.8 to 2.2 mg/min/kg, falling by about 20 per cent after a 2-day fast,[1] and by 50 to 60 per cent after 5 to 6 weeks (Owen, JCI, 1969; 48:574). After an overnight fast the liver accounts for about 90 per cent of glucose released into the circulation. However, with prolonged fasting (>1 week) renal gluconeogenesis increases and may account for up to 45 per cent of glucose production (Owen, JCI, 1969; 48:574). Early studies, employing hepatic vein catheterization techniques to allow calculation of net splanchnic uptake of gluconeogenic precursors (lactate, alanine, and glycerol), estimated that after an overnight fast 70 to 75 per cent of the glucose produced by the liver came from liver glycogen, the rest from hepatic gluconeogenesis (Wahren, JCI, 1972; 51:1870). More recent studies using ^{13}C-nuclear magnetic resonance (**NMR**) suggest that glycogen contributes only about one-third, and that gluconeogenesis accounts for about two-thirds of the glucose produced during the first 22 h of fasting.[1] Liver glycogen stores (70–80 g after an overnight fast),[1,2] fall to about 15 g after 40 h of fasting. With depletion of liver glycogen, gluconeogenesis accounts for essentially all of the glucose released by the liver.

The precursors for gluconeogenesis are lactate, pyruvate, glycerol, and the glucogenic amino acids (mainly alanine and glutamine)[3] (Consoli, AmJPhysiol, 1990; 259:E677). Lactate is quantitatively the most important, both after an overnight fast and after longer fasting. However, up to 80 per cent of lactate carbon comes from glucose metabolism in extrahepatic tissues, and much of the alanine released by extrahepatic tissues from transamination of pyruvate derived from glucose; carbon for net glucose synthesis must therefore come from protein breakdown, or from glycerol released from triglyceride hydrolysis. Protein, especially from skeletal muscle, supplies most of the carbon needed for net glucose synthesis, glycerol assuming a more important role during prolonged starvation. Amino acids from muscle protein are partially metabolized within muscle, and only alanine, glutamine, and glycine are released in significant amounts (see also Chapter 2.13.1). Alanine and glutamine make an equal contribution to glucose synthesis in overnight-fasted normal subjects; approximately 5 per cent of glucose carbon is derived from each of these precursors.[3] However, because more glutamine is released from muscle than alanine, and because a greater proportion of the glutamine released comes directly from protein and other amino acids (as much as 60–65 per cent of the alanine coming from plasma glucose directly or after its release from glycogen) (Chang, JBC, 1978; 253:3658; Simmons, JCI, 1984; 73:412), glutamine may be more important than alanine as a source of carbon for 'new' glucose synthesis.[3]

Glutamine is the major gluconeogenic precursor in the kidney (Schoolwerth, MinElecMetab, 1994; 14:347) but there is controversy as to whether it is used directly for hepatic gluconeogenesis.

Glutamine is a very good substrate for hepatic gluconeogenesis *in vitro* (Kaloyianni, JNutr, 1990; 120:116) but many consider glutamine's contribution to hepatic gluconeogenesis *in vivo* to be indirect. Support for this view comes from splanchnic balance studies in man (Felig, Diabetes, 1973; 22:573); animal studies (Windmueller, AdvEnzymReg, 1982; 53:202; Ardawi, JLab-ClinMed, 1990; 115:660) show that gut can convert a substantial amount of glutamine to alanine, which enters portal venous blood for extraction by the liver along with alanine coming from peripheral tissues. By contrast others have found that intestinal metabolism of glutamine accounts for a very small proportion of glutamine metabolism in overnight-fasted normal humans[3] (Dechelotte, AmJPhysiol, 1991; 260:G677), although it may assume importance with prolonged fasting.

Regulation of hepatic glucose production

Alterations in carbohydrate metabolism occurring with transition from the fed to the fasting state are largely explained by changes in circulating hormone concentrations, increased gluconeogenic substrate supply, changes in the activities of key hepatic enzymes, and by glucose autoregulation of hepatic glucose production.

Hormonal regulation

As blood glucose falls with fasting, insulin secretion decreases, glucagon secretion rises, and the plasma levels of glucocorticoids, catecholamines, and growth hormone are increased relative to insulin. Studies employing somatostatin[4] (Sacca, DiabetMetabRev, 1987; 3:207) to suppress endogenous insulin and glucagon secretion, with infusion of either hormone to produce normal or high arterial concentrations of the replaced hormone, have helped to define the roles of insulin and glucagon in regulating hepatic glucose production. The process is complicated.

The fall in plasma insulin from postprandial to basal concentrations is crucial for stimulation of hepatic glycogenolysis and gluconeogenesis. However, even basal insulin concentrations exert a sustained inhibitory action on hepatic glucose production (Insel, JCI, 1975; 55:1382) and prevent unrestrained mobilization of fatty acids and gluconeogenic precursors from extrahepatic tissues. They are essential for maintenance of normal fasting blood glucose concentrations; with insulin deficiency, as in type I diabetes, plasma glucose rises to high levels.

The role of glucagon in the regulation of hepatic glucose production during fasting was initially disputed, because of the brief response of hepatic glucose production to a sustained increase in plasma glucagon levels, even with constant plasma insulin concentrations (Fradkin, JClinEndoc, 1980; 50:698; Sacca, Diabet-MetabRev, 1987; 3:207). Using labelled precursors of glucose, it was shown that this decline in hepatic glucose production during glucagon infusion is due to attenuation of glycogenolysis; it does not reflect gluconeogenesis, which continues to increase[4] (Cherrington, Diabetes, 1981; 30:180). Basal amounts of glucagon are important for stimulating glucose output, in both the post-absorptive (Cherrington, JCI, 1976; 58:1407; Liljenquist, JCI, 1977; 59:369) and fasted states (Wahren, JCI, 1977; 59:299), when it accounts for about two-thirds of hepatic glucose production[3] (Liljenquist, JCI, 1977; 59:369).

Sustained physiological elevations of growth hormone (Rizza, Diabetes, 1982; 31:663), cortisol (Rizza, JClinEndoc, 1982; 54:131), and catecholamines (Lager, Diabetolog, 1986; 29:409) stimulate hepatic glucose production and help to maintain normal blood glucose levels during fasting. Decreased hepatic glucose production and fasting hypoglycaemia are features of growth hormone or cortisol deficiency. Both peripheral and hepatic actions of these hormones are important for stimulation of hepatic glucose production during fasting (McGuinness, AmJPhysiol, 1993; 265:E314).

Gluconeogenic substrate supply

The hormonal milieu of the fasted state decreases glucose oxidation by extrahepatic tissues, and enhances muscle protein breakdown, causing increased release of lactate, pyruvate, alanine, and glutamine into the circulation. Stimulation of adipose tissue lipolysis increases hepatic delivery of glycerol. With prolonged fasting plasma ketone body levels rise and the release of alanine and glutamine from muscle then falls, in parallel with a decrease in glucose production rates, as the brain derives much of its energy needs by oxidizing ketone bodies and glycerol.

The supply of substrates for gluconeogenesis during fasting is further enhanced by increased hepatic fractional extraction. For alanine and other glucogenic amino acids, carrier-mediated transport into hepatocytes is rate limiting for catabolism. The alanine transport system is markedly stimulated by glucagon and catecholamines; glucocorticoids play an important permissive role (Collarini, AnnRevNutr, 1987; 7:75; Christensen, PhysiolRev, 1990; 70:43;). The stimulation is such that blood alanine falls with fasting despite increased release from extrahepatic tissues (Pozefsky, JCI, 1976; 57:444). Hepatic fractional extraction of lactate, pyruvate, and glycerol is also enhanced when gluconeogenesis is increased (McGuinness, AmJPhysiol, 1993; 265:E314), even though their transport is not hormonally regulated; the intracellular concentration of these intermediates is probably decreased, thus facilitating their uptake. Since half-maximal rates of gluconeogenesis occur at concentrations of lactate, pyruvate, glycerol, and alanine that are greater than physiological concentrations, an increased supply of these precursors stimulates their incorporation into glucose 6-phosphate in the liver (Hue, DiabetMetabRev, 1987; 3:111). However, a substrate-driven increase in glucose 6-phosphate synthesis via gluconeogenesis does not result in increased hepatic glucose release unless there is a concomitant change in the hormonal environment and/or fall in plasma glucose levels. In normal, overnight-fasted subjects, substrate-stimulated gluconeogenesis does not increase hepatic glucose output or result in any change of plasma glucose, insulin, or glucagon levels (Jenssen, JCI, 1990; 86:489). The increased glucose 6-phosphate produced by gluconeogenesis when gluconeogenic precursor supply is increased may be channelled into glycogen (Fig. 1). Alternatively, since gluconeogenesis takes place mainly in periportal hepatocytes, it is possible that there may be increased release of glucose from periportal hepatocytes, but that the resulting increase in sinusoidal glucose concentration inhibits glucose output from more centrally located hepatocytes within the liver lobule. The net effect would be unchanged hepatic glucose output even though a much higher proportion of the glucose released was derived from gluconeogenesis (Diamond, Metabolism, 1988; 37:28; Jenssen, JCI, 1990; 86:489).

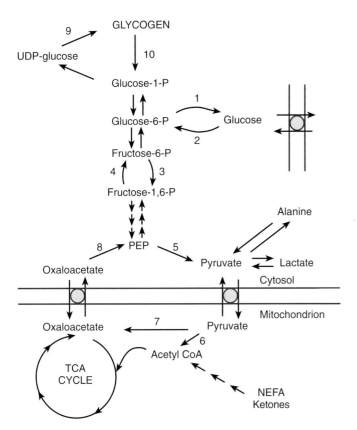

Fig. 1. Pathways of glycolysis, gluconeogenesis, and glycogen synthesis in liver. Glycolysis (metabolism of one molecule of glucose to two molecules of pyruvate) and gluconeogenesis (synthesis of glucose 6-phosphate from pyruvate) share many of the enzymes. The magnitude and direction of flux are determined by non-equilibrium reactions (steps 3, 4, 5, 7, and 8). Key to numbered enzymes: (1) glucose 6-phosphatase; (2) glucokinase; (3) phosphofructokinase-1; (4) fructose 1,6-bisphosphatase; (5) pyruvate kinase; (6) pyruvate dehydrogenase; (7) pyruvate carboxylase; (8) phosphoenolpyruvate carboxykinase (PEPCK); (9) glycogen synthase; (10) glycogen phosphorylase. (Reproduced with permission from Kruszynska YT. In Williams G, and Pickup J, eds. *Textbook of diabetes*, (2nd edn). Oxford: Blackwell Science, 1997:11.1–11.37.)

Fatty acid supply to the liver is important for gluconeogenesis during fasting and during recovery from insulin-induced hypoglycaemia (Fanelli, JCI, 1993; 92:1617). Non-esterified fatty acids provide a source of energy for gluconeogenesis, and increase intramitochondrial acetyl CoA, an obligatory positive allosteric effector of the key gluconeogenic enzyme, pyruvate carboxylase (Fig. 1) (Williamson, PNAS, 1966; 56:247). If fatty acid oxidation is inhibited, there is a marked decrease in gluconeogenesis.[5]

Regulation of hepatic enzymes

The hormonal regulation of intrahepatic enzymes determines the direction and magnitude of carbon flux (Exton, DiabetMetabRev, 1987; 3:163; Hue, DiabetMetabRev, 1987; 3:111; Pilkis, AnnRevNutr, 1990; 11:465). Net glycolytic or gluconeogenic flux depends on the activities of certain key enzymes, unique to glycolysis or gluconeogenesis, that catalyse non-equilibrium reactions. The major

regulatory sites are the fructose 6-phosphate/fructose 1,6-bisphosphate cycle, which controls the first committed step of glycolysis, and the pyruvate/phosphoenolpyruvate cycle, which controls that of gluconeogenesis (Fig. 1). Periportal hepatocytes contain higher levels of rate-limiting enzymes involved in glycogen breakdown and gluconeogenesis, whereas hepatocytes around the hepatic venules have higher levels of enzymes involved in glycolysis, glycogen synthesis, and lipogenesis (Jungermann, PhysiolRev, 1989; 69:708). The glucose/glucose 6-phosphate cycle is a further site for regulation of hepatic glucose production.

Acute hormonal regulation of liver carbohydrate metabolism mainly involves changes in cytosolic levels of cyclic AMP and calcium. Agents that increase cytosolic calcium (for example, adrenaline and noradrenaline via α_1-receptors) primarily affect hepatic glycogenolysis, and have a smaller effect on hepatic gluconeogenesis and glycolysis.

An increase in cyclic AMP is important for both glycogenolysis and gluconeogenesis; it activates cyclic AMP-dependent protein kinase, which in turn inactivates pyruvate kinase and phosphofructokinase-2, and activates fructose 2,6-bisphosphatase. Insulin opposes these actions in part by stimulating phosphodiesterase, thus decreasing hepatic cyclic AMP concentrations and increasing fructose 2,6-bisphosphate levels (Assimacopoulos-Jeannet, JBC, 1990; 265:7202).

With fasting, the fall in insulin, and the relative increase in glucagon, decreases the activity of pyruvate kinase, which converts phosphoenolpyruvate to pyruvate (Fig. 1). Pyruvate, derived from lactate and the transamination of alanine, is transported into mitochondria; there it is carboxylated to oxaloacetate, which is subsequently decarboxylated and phosphorylated by phosphoenolpyruvate carboxykinase to give phosphoenolpyruvate; both reactions are increased by fasting. The channelling of pyruvate to phosphoenolpyruvate, with the decrease in pyruvate kinase activity, explains the accumulation of phosphoenolpyruvate and its increased conversion to glucose 6-phosphate, as well as decreased lactate and pyruvate production.

Regulation of the fructose 6-phosphate/fructose 1,6-bisphosphate cycle (Fig. 1) results mainly from allosteric control by fructose 2,6-bisphosphate and AMP (Pilkis, AnnRevNutr, 1990; 11: 465). Fructose 2,6-bisphosphate stimulates phosphofructokinase-1, which converts fructose 6-phosphate into fructose 1,6-bisphosphate, and inhibits fructose 1,6-bisphosphatase. These effects are synergistic with those of AMP. An increase in fructose 2,6-bisphosphate therefore favours glycolysis, while a decrease stimulates gluconeogenesis. The inhibition of phosphofructokinase-2, and stimulation of fructose 2,6-bisphosphatase by cyclic AMP-dependent protein kinase, both lead to depletion of fructose 2,6-bisphosphate and hence decreased glycolysis, thus explaining the action of glucagon on this cycle. Glycerol at physiological concentrations also decreases hepatic fructose 2,6-bisphosphate concentration. This effect is mediated by glycerol 3-phosphate, an inhibitor of phosphofructokinase-2 and an activator of fructose 2,6-bisphosphatase. Insulin increases fructose 2,6-bisphosphate levels. However, the timing of the rise in fructose 2,6-bisphosphate levels in response to insulin depends on nutritional state; the increase occurs within minutes when insulin is infused into postabsorptive rats but is delayed for 5 to 6 h in rats fasted for 24 to 48 h, even though the effect of insulin to suppress hepatic glucose production and promote glycogen synthesis occurs promptly (Sugden, BiochemJ, 1989; 263:313; Holness, BiochemJ, 1988; 252:357). The delayed rise in fructose 2,6-bisphosphate levels may be important for ensuring that gluconeogenesis continues after meals until liver glycogen stores are replete. A subsequent increase in glycolysis would favour the use of glucose carbon for lipogenesis.

Flux through the glucose/glucose 6-phosphate cycle (Fig. 1) is increased in insulin-deficient states and during fasting, and the equilibrium is shifted towards glucose production. However, the regulation of this cycle is poorly understood, partly because of the complexity of glucose 6-phosphatase, a multienzyme complex located in the endoplasmic reticulum (Burchell, MolMembrBiol, 1994; 11:217). The active site of glucose 6-phosphatase is within the lumen of the endoplasmic reticulum whereas glucose 6-phosphate is generated in the cytosol; transport proteins for glucose 6-phosphate, phosphate, glucose, and pyrophosphate are needed and are potential sites of regulation. Glucose 6-phosphatase activity decreases promptly with feeding without any change in the concentration of glucose 6-phosphate (Newgard, Diabetes, 1984; 33:192). Whether this is due to changes in activity of the phosphatase *per se* or one of the associated transporters (for example, impaired transport of glucose 6-phosphate into the lumen of the endoplasmic reticulum) has yet to be elucidated. Glucokinase activity (determined by the cell content of this enzyme (see below)) will also affect flux through this cycle.

Decreased plasma insulin concentrations promote glycogen breakdown, which is also enhanced by glucagon and catecholamines acting via cyclic AMP-dependent protein kinase, and by hormones that increase intracellular calcium. Glycogen phosphorylase activity is increased, that of glycogen synthase inhibited. A relative increase in glucose 6-phosphatase to glucokinase activity promotes the dephosphorylation of glucose 6-phosphate (coming from glycogen or gluconeogenesis) to free glucose that can be released into the circulation.

As well as short-term regulation by substrates and hormones, liver carbohydrate metabolism is affected by long-term adaptive changes in the concentration of pathway enzymes. These alterations are due to changes in enzyme synthesis and correspond to changes in the levels of mRNA for these enzymes. Enzymes such as glucokinase and phosphoenolpyruvate carboxykinase undergo rapid changes in their hepatic levels due to effects of hormones on gene transcription. Induction of glucokinase mRNA is apparent within minutes of treatment of diabetic animals with insulin or refeeding of fasted animals (Iynedjian, JBC, 1987; 262:6032). The increased phosphoenolpyruvate carboxykinase activity during fasting is entirely due to increased synthesis of this enzyme; insulin inhibits transcription of this gene and decreases the hepatic content of phosphoenolpyruvate carboxykinase (O'Brien, DiabetCare, 1990; 13:327). Long-term adaptive changes in hepatic enzymes are also important for the conversion of carbohydrate into fat. High carbohydrate diets increase the synthesis of some enzymes important for *de novo* lipogenesis, including fatty acid synthase, ATP citrate lyase, acetyl CoA carboxylase, malic enzyme, and glucose 6-phosphate dehydrogenase. Glucokinase and pyruvate kinase activities are decreased by high-protein or high-fat diets, and increased by carbohydrate-rich diets.

Autoregulation of hepatic glucose production

Superimposed on the hormonal regulation of hepatic carbohydrate metabolism is the effect of blood glucose concentration *per se*. The glucose transporter of hepatocytes, unlike that of peripheral tissues, is not regulated by insulin and it has a high capacity (Table 1). Transport of glucose across the liver cell membrane is rapid. Since physiological glucose concentrations are below the K_M of glucokinase for glucose, a low blood glucose with fasting will decrease glucose 6-phosphate production, and the rate of cycling between glucose and glucose 6-phosphate, so that net flux is towards glucose production. Glucose also regulates glycogen phosphorylase and glycogen synthase (Stalmans, DiabetMetabRev, 1987; 3:127); it binds to and inhibits phosphorylase *a*, which releases glucose 1-phosphate from glycogen. The glucose–phosphorylase *a* complex is a better substrate for phosphorylase phosphatase, which converts phosphorylase to its inactive *b* form. When the proportion of phosphorylase *a* falls below about 10 per cent, bound phosphatase is released and is free to remove phosphate from, and so activate, glycogen synthase, which stimulates glycogen synthesis from UDP-glucose. Inactivation of hepatic glycogen phosphorylase explains in part the inhibition of hepatic glucose production by increased glucose concentrations (Yki-Jarvinen, JCI, 1987; 79:1713; Pagliassotti, JCI, 1996; 97:81). The intracellular glucose and glucose 6-phosphate concentrations also influence production of the allosteric effector, fructose 2,6-bisphosphate, and hence the direction of carbon flux through glycolysis/gluconeogenesis.

Glucose utilization in the fasted state

In the fasted state when insulin levels are low, most glucose uptake (75–85 per cent) is non-insulin mediated (Gottesman, AmJPhysiol, 1983; 244:E632; Baron, JCI, 1985; 76:1782). Peripheral insulin-dependent tissues, namely skeletal muscle and adipocytes, have very low glucose extraction ratios at basal insulin concentrations. Insulin-independent glucose uptake by the brain accounts for 50 to 60 per cent of basal glucose disposal; skeletal muscle accounts for only 15 to 20 per cent[11] (Andres, JCI, 1956; 35:671; Gerich, Diabetes, 1990; 39:211). Brain fractional glucose extraction falls with increasing blood glucose concentration so that its uptake remains relatively constant (Brooks, JCerebBloodFlowMetab, 1986; 6:240). In tissues other than brain, non-insulin-mediated glucose uptake increases linearly with increasing glucose concentrations by a mass action effect. However, if glucose 6-phosphate accumulates because of more rapid glucose entry than required for cell metabolism, it will inhibit hexokinase and hence phosphorylation of incoming glucose. Intracellular free glucose will rise and net glucose entry will then decrease.

Much of the glucose taken up by tissues such as the gut and red cells is metabolized to lactate, pyruvate, and alanine, which are then released into the circulation and taken up by the liver for reincorporation into glucose (the Cori cycle). By contrast, more than 90 per cent of glucose taken up by the brain is oxidized, and brain accounts for 70 to 90 per cent of total glucose oxidation after an overnight fast. In muscle about 60 per cent of the glucose entering glycolysis is metabolized to lactate and about 40 per cent is oxidized (Andres, JCI, 1956; 35:671), so that muscle (which accounts for <20 per cent of basal glucose uptake) accounts for less than 10 per cent of whole-body basal plasma glucose oxidation. The

Table 1 Tissue distribution of facilitative glucose transporters

Glucose transporter	Distribution	Comments
Glut 1	Erythrocytes, endothelial cells, brain, adipocytes	Location, mainly in plasma membrane K_M for glucose, ~ 2 mM Mediates basal glucose transport in insulin-dependent (adipocytes) and non-insulin-dependent tissues
Glut 2	Hepatocytes, islet β-cells, intestine (basolateral membranes)	Location, plasma membrane High K_M, ~ 66 mM, allows cells to act as 'glucose sensors' Downregulated by hyperglycaemia in islet β-cells
Glut 3	Brain, intestine, placenta	K_M ~ 9 mM Upregulated in brain by hypoglycaemia
Glut 4	Skeletal muscle, adipocytes, heart	K_M ~ 5 mM Mainly intracellular in basal state Insulin (and muscle contraction) recruit Glut 4 to plasma membrane
Glut 5	Skeletal muscle, intestine (apical membrane)	Transports fructose K_M for fructose, ~ 6 mM

increased supply of non-esterified fatty acids and ketone bodies during fasting plays an important role in limiting skeletal muscle glucose oxidation and glucose uptake (Randle, Lancet, 1963; i:785; Kruszynska, DiabetAnn, 1995; 9:107).

Glucose metabolism in the fed state

Factors determining blood glucose concentrations after oral glucose

The shape of the blood glucose concentration curve following oral glucose depends on the size of the glucose load, the rate of absorption from the gut, the proportion retained by the splanchnic tissues (especially liver), the degree of associated suppression of hepatic glucose production, and the amount of glucose taken up by peripheral tissues. The responses of the liver and peripheral tissues are modulated by endocrine, neural, and metabolic signals.

Tissue distribution of ingested glucose

Although the liver plays a central role in glucose homeostasis, there is still uncertainty about the metabolic fate of ingested glucose and the relative importance of liver and peripheral tissues in removing it from the blood. Blood glucose levels are much lower when glucose is given orally, rather than intravenously, and it was assumed that the liver, because of its anatomical position, removes large amounts of ingested glucose during its first passage through the portal circulation (Scow, AmJPhysiol, 1954; 179:435; Janes, JPhysiol, 1965; 181:59). However, intraportally and peripherally administered glucose result in identical peripheral arterial glucose and insulin concentrations.[6] Furthermore, studies with radiolabelled ingested glucose showed that first-pass uptake by the liver is less than 15 per cent.[7-9] Thus first-pass hepatic uptake of ingested glucose does not explain the better tolerance to oral glucose.

Hepatic vein catheterization techniques allow calculation of net splanchnic balance of glucose, by multiplying the concentration difference between arterial and hepatic venous blood by the estimated hepatic blood flow. Using this method Felig *et al.* (Diabetes, 1975; 24:468) calculated that after 100 g of oral glucose only 40 g

appeared in the hepatic vein during the following 3 h; later studies in humans (Waldhausl, Diabetolog, 1983; 25:489) and dogs found a lower splanchnic retention of glucose following an oral glucose load. Ferrannini *et al.*,[8] using hepatic vein catheterization and a dual-label radio-isotope approach to trace total glucose turnover and glucose derived from the gut, showed that after ingestion of 68 g of glucose about one-third was taken up by splanchnic tissues. Similar conclusions were reached by investigators quantifying glucose uptake across the forearm[10,11] or leg (Katz, Diabetes, 1983; 32:675).

The term 'splanchnic glucose retention' does not imply that all the glucose retained by the splanchnic bed is taken up by the liver. Apparent splanchnic glucose retention also depends on the extent of intestinal glucose absorption, direct utilization of absorbed glucose by the gut, and extrahepatic splanchnic uptake of absorbed, recirculated glucose. Calculation of splanchnic uptake must also take into account suppression of hepatic glucose production. Studies using radioactive glucose to quantify glucose flux rates have shown that after a 70 to 100 g oral glucose load, hepatic glucose production decreases by 50 to 60 per cent over the 3 to 5 h absorptive period.[7-11] Earlier studies may therefore have overestimated the role of the liver in the disposal of an oral glucose load; first, by assuming unchanged hepatic glucose production following glucose ingestion and, secondly, by assuming complete intestinal absorption of glucose by 3 h. Studies in man (Bjorkman, Diabetes, 1990; 39: 747) and dogs (Abumrad, AmJPhysiol, 1982; 242:E398) suggest that only 85 per cent of a glucose load may be absorbed within this period. Furthermore, the hepatic vein catheter technique is highly dependent on the accuracy of hepatic blood flow measurements, a major source of error in these studies. However, studies with oral glucose labelled with ^{14}C may underestimate hepatic uptake of glucose because of recycling from liver glycogen. Thus, some of the [^{14}C]glucose appearing in the systemic circulation late in the study may be derived from glycogen labelled with ^{14}C early in the absorptive period. However, studies by Radziuk suggest this error to be small.[7]

The general consensus is that 25 to 40 per cent of an oral glucose load is taken up by the liver; the proportion may increase with increasing size of the glucose load (Bratusch-Marrain, Metabolism,

1980; 29:289). These estimates of total hepatic glucose uptake are not inconsistent with glucose kinetic studies, which show that first-pass uptake is less than 15 per cent.[7-9] If we assume that a 100 g glucose load is completely absorbed in 3 h, we can estimate that the portal blood glucose concentration will be, on average, only about 3.1 mmol/l greater than that in arterial blood, and this assumes no uptake of glucose by the extrahepatic splanchnic bed in response to an increase in blood glucose and insulin. Glucose coming directly from the gut is therefore a small proportion (about one-third) of glucose delivered to the liver. Thus, if 8 g of a 100 g load is taken up on first pass,[7] uptake of recirculating glucose will be approximately 15 to 25 g, implying a total glucose uptake of 20 to 35 g. A 50 to 60 per cent suppression of hepatic glucose output over a 3 h period would represent about 10 to 15 g of glucose, and if this is not taken into account, net hepatic glucose uptake would be underestimated by this amount.

First-pass and total hepatic glucose uptake after glucose ingestion are not constant during the 3 to 4 h absorptive period; they are highest early after glucose ingestion.[8] During this early period sinusoidal blood is maximally enriched with ingested glucose, and the portal–arterial glucose gradient (see below) maximal, because absorption is at its highest while the arterial glucose level is still relatively low. The combination of high net uptake of sinusoidal glucose and its enrichment with newly absorbed glucose during the first 30 min or so after glucose ingestion causes a disproportionate increase in the amount of ingested glucose taken up by the liver on first pass during this early period. Thus, although first-pass hepatic uptake is quantitatively unimportant in terms of overall glucose disposal, it may be important in limiting the rate of entry of ingested glucose into the systemic circulation before there is an adequate rise in insulin levels, and distribution of this insulin to peripheral tissues.

Our understanding of glucose metabolism is derived mainly from studies using glucose alone as the test meal. After a mixed meal, plasma glucose concentrations tend to be lower, and insulin levels higher, than after glucose alone (Rabinowitz, Lancet, 1966; ii: 454). Furthermore, glucagon concentrations decrease after oral glucose but not after a meal containing protein (Ahmed, AmJClin-Nutr, 1980; 33:1917). The pattern of postprandial hepatic and extrahepatic responses might differ when glucose is administered as part of a mixed meal. However, McMahon et al. (JClinEndoc, 1989; 68:647) found that, apart from a slight delay in the initial systemic appearance of glucose contained in a mixed meal, the postprandial pattern of glucose metabolism was virtually identical to that found when the same quantity of glucose was ingested as a drink. Thus splanchnic uptake of ingested glucose, suppression of hepatic glucose output, incorporation of labelled bicarbonate into glucose (a measure of gluconeogenesis), and the oxidation of glucose and lipid (determined by indirect calorimetry) were all comparable.

Hepatic glucose metabolism

The quantitative aspects of hepatic glucose metabolism in the fed state have been the subject of much controversy. When liver glycogen is depleted, most of the glucose taken up by liver appears to be used for glycogen synthesis; very little is converted to triglyceride (Acheson, Metabolism, 1982; 31:1234). Taylor et al. (JCI, 1996; 97:126) using ^{13}C-NMR spectroscopy to quantitate liver glycogen in normal subjects, found that 19 per cent of the carbohydrate content

of a liquid meal consumed after an overnight fast was incoporated into liver glycogen. Similar results were obtained in dogs: liver glycogen deposition accounted for 22 per cent of an intraduodenal glucose load and 60 per cent of the net cumulative hepatic glucose uptake (Moore, JCI, 1991; 88:578). Glycogen synthesis and breakdown can occur concurrently. Liver glycogen concentration is an important determinant of its net rate of synthesis. Net glycogen deposition slows as liver glycogen accumulates (Friedmann, JBC, 1963; 238:2899; Magnusson, AmJPhysiol, 1994; 266:E796), in part because glycogen inhibits the inactivation of phosphorylase a (Stalmans, EurJBioch, 1974; 41:127), with a secondary impairment of glycogen synthase activation (Stalmans, IntJBiochem, 1974; 41:127). The rate of glycogenolysis increases with increasing liver glycogen content, even in the presence of high insulin and glucose levels (Magnusson, AmJPhysiol, 1994; 266:E796), thus limiting hepatic glycogen accumulation.

Some of the glycogen synthesized is not derived directly from glucose, but from three-carbon intermediates such as lactate and alanine. Evidence for this indirect mechanism of glycogen synthesis was provided many years ago by Boxer and Stetten (JBC, 1944; 155:237) who found incorporation of D_2O into liver glycogen. However, subsequent studies (Cook, JBC, 1952; 199:1; Hers, JBC, 1955; 214:373), using unphysiologically high glucose concentrations, suggested that most liver glycogen was synthesized directly from glucose; this became accepted dogma. Observations on glycogen synthesis in isolated hepatocytes (Seglen, BBActa, 1974; 338:317) and perfused rat liver (Hems, BiochemJ, 1972; 129:529) prompted a re-evaluation of the pathways of liver glycogen formation. These studies showed that glucose at physiological concentrations (5–10 mM) was a poor substrate for net glycogen synthesis. By contrast, glycogen synthesis was high when gluconeogenic precursors such as lactate, alanine, and glycerol were present in addition to glucose. Although glucose itself was not used efficiently, it prompted the conversion of gluconeogenic substrates into glycogen.

Further in vivo studies in rats using labelled gluconeogenic precursors, or tracer $NaH^{14}CO_3$ along with an unlabelled glucose load, demonstrated that gluconeogenesis continues after a meal or glucose load, and that the glucose 6-phosphate formed by gluconeogenesis was diverted into glycogen[12] (Shikama, AmJPhysiol, 1978; 235:E354). When gluconeogenesis was inhibited by 3-mercaptopicolinic acid (an inhibitor of phosphoenolpyruvate carboxykinase), postprandial glycogen formation was markedly impaired, but could be restored by infusion of glycerol, which enters the gluconeogenic pathway distal to the block (Newgard, JBC, 1984; 259:6958).

The contribution of the direct and indirect pathways to liver glycogen synthesis was quantified, by giving glucose specifically labelled with ^{14}C and by determining the distribution of label in the carbons of the glucose units in liver glycogen. Shulman et al. (JCI, 1987; 80:387), using NMR spectroscopy to assess the distribution of ^{13}C following 1-^{13}C-glucose administration to fasted rats, estimated that less than a third of glycogen was synthesized via the direct pathway, most of the remainder coming from three-carbon intermediates. Similar results were obtained by McGarry et al. (AnnRevNutr, 1987; 7:51). However, exact quantitation was not possible because of the dilution of label in pyruvate as it traverses the pool of oxaloacetate, a common intermediate in both the gluconeogenic pathway and the tricarboxylic acid cycle.

Studies in man have confirmed the importance of gluconeogenesis for repletion of liver glycogen after a fast. Radziuk (FedProc, 1982; 41:110) estimated that after 100 g of oral glucose direct incorporation of gut-derived glucose into liver glycogen accounted for only 10 g, equivalent to 25 per cent of the liver glycogen synthesized. The best evidence comes from direct measurement of hepatic 1-^{13}C-glycogen accumulation by NMR following ingestion of a glucose load or meal enriched with 1-^{13}C-glucose, in combination with radio-isotopic determination of systemic glucose flux rates. These studies have shown that after an overnight fast about 50 per cent of hepatic glycogen is synthesized by gluconeogenesis, the remainder coming directly from glucose (Shulman, AmJPhysiol, 1990; 259:E335; Taylor, JCI, 1996; 97:126).

The source of the lactate for hepatic glycogen synthesis remains unclear. Forearm studies have shown that skeletal muscle takes up lactate during the first 2 h after an oral glucose load (Radziuk, Diabetes, 1983; 32:977), and it appears that most of the lactate is of splanchnic origin. Lactate formation and glycogen synthesis may proceed simultaneously in different zones of the liver (Pilkis, BioEssays, 1985; 2:273; Chapter 2.18). The implication is that much of the glucose taken up by liver is metabolized via glycolysis to lactate, and that recirculating lactate is the major substrate for hepatic glycogen synthesis via the gluconeogenic pathway (Moore, JCI, 1991; 88:578).

Most studies have been performed on rats fasted for 24 to 48 h, and on humans after a 12 to 14 h fast. Eating during the day may increase the proportion of glycogen synthesized directly from glucose (Boxer, JBC, 1944; 155:237; Magnusson, Metabolism, 1989; 38:583; Shulman, AmJPhysiol, 1990; 259:E335). Taylor et al. (JCI, 1996; 97:126) found that the contribution of the direct pathway to hepatic glycogen synthesis increased with time following a liquid meal. Eating might also alter the distribution of glucose carbon between the pathways of glycogen and lipid synthesis. When liver glycogen is replenished, more of the glucose taken up will enter glycolysis and gluconeogenetic flux will be limited. In the presence of replenished glycogen stores the lactate produced by glycolysis, together with lactate taken up from plasma, will be more readily used for de novo triglyceride synthesis. Since glycogenolysis increases with increasing liver glycogen content, even in the presence of high insulin and glucose levels (Magnusson, AmJPhysiol, 1994; 266:E796), hepatic glycogen may also provide carbon for hepatic lipogenesis.

Muscle glucose metabolism

Assuming that endogenous glucose production is decreased by 15 g during the 3 h after 100 g of oral glucose, then delivery of 50 to 70 g of glucose to peripheral tissues would represent an increment of 35 to 55 g above basal requirements. Skeletal muscle accounts for about 85 per cent of this enhanced disposal[11] (Katz, Diabetes, 1983; 32: 675); the glucose taken up by muscle will be incorporated into glycogen, or metabolized via the glycolytic and Krebs cycle pathways. Much of the enhanced glucose utilization after oral glucose represents glucose oxidized to provide energy that in the basal state was provided by lipid oxidation. Additional energy is needed to support synthetic processes such as glycogen and lipid storage.

Indirect calorimetry has been used to assess the relative importance of Krebs cycle oxidation and glycogen synthesis for the enhanced glucose disposal. Estimates vary widely. However, it is clear that following glucose ingestion whole-body oxidation of glucose is stimulated, and reaches saturation at approximately 4 mg/kg/min. We found that in normal subjects glucose oxidation accounted for 55 per cent of the increased glucose disposal after a 75 g glucose load[9] consistent with findings that 50 per cent of the glucose taken up by skeletal muscle was oxidized during 5 h after glucose ingestion.[10,11] The proportion of glucose stored as muscle glycogen increases with the size of the glucose load (Moeri, DiabeteMetab, 1988; 14:1).

Regulation of tissue response to glucose ingestion

The metabolic response of the liver and peripheral tissues to oral glucose will be determined by a variety of endocrine, neural, and metabolic factors.

Role of insulin

Insulin normally reaches the liver from the pancreas via the portal vein. Portal vein insulin concentrations are 1.5- to tenfold higher than in systemic blood, because the liver extracts 30 to 50 per cent of the insulin presented to it, and because portal blood flow is a relatively small proportion of cardiac output. Both the timing and the magnitude of the insulin secretory response are important for normal glucose tolerance. The importance of an early insulin response is suggested by numerous studies, in diabetic humans and dogs, employing pre-programmed insulin infusion systems to control the blood glucose response. The preabsorptive insulin secretory response is mediated by the vagus. Delay in onset of insulin secretion, and the associated deterioration in glucose tolerance, after truncal vagotomy in humans and animals attests to the importance of an early insulin response, which ensures prompt suppression of hepatic glucose production to about 10 to 20 per cent of basal, thus limiting the rise in plasma glucose[9] (Taylor, JCI, 1996; 97:126).

Plasma insulin levels are much higher after oral glucose than after the same amount of intravenous glucose (McIntyre, JClinEndoc, 1965; 25:1317). The most likely explanation is glucose-induced release of an intestinal hormone which stimulates insulin secretion. Glucose-dependent insulinotropic peptide and glucagon-like peptide 1 [7–36 amide] are the main hormones potentiating insulin secretion after glucose ingestion (Kreymann, Lancet, 1987; ii:1300; Creutzfeldt, DiabetMetabRev, 1992; 8:149). Vagal enhancement of insulin secretion, and decreased hepatic extraction of insulin during glucose absorption (Gibby, BMJ, 1983; 286:921; Shapiro, Diabetes, 1987; 36:1365) may also contribute to the higher systemic insulin concentrations seen when glucose is given orally.

Insulin is of prime importance for glucose uptake by skeletal muscle and adipocytes. Skeletal muscle is the main site of enhanced glucose disposal after oral or intravenous glucose. In skeletal muscle and adipocytes glucose transport is normally rate limiting for glucose disposal by these tissues (Fink, Metabolism, 1992; 41:897). Glucose uptake is mediated by a family of at least five facilitated glucose transporters with tissue-specific distribution (Gould, BiochemJ, 1993; 295:329; Stephens, EndocrRev, 1995; 16:529) (Table 1). One of these species, Glut 4, is very responsive to an acute rise in insulin levels. Glut 4 is present only in skeletal muscle, adipocytes, and heart muscle, and this largely explains the ability of insulin to stimulate glucose uptake in these tissues. By contrast with other isoforms of the glucose transporter family, Glut 4 is mainly intracellular under basal conditions. Insulin increases glucose transport by stimulating the translocation of Glut 4 from the intracellular pool to the plasma membrane with which it fuses, and may also increase the intrinsic activity of Glut 4 (Simpson, AnnRevBiochem, 1986; 55:1059; Guma, AmJPhysiol, 1995; 268:E613; Stephens, EndocrRev, 1995; 16:529; Kelley, JCI, 1996; 97:2705). Efficient glucose uptake requires that glucose that has entered the cell is rapidly phosphorylated to glucose 6-phosphate in order to maintain the transmembrane glucose gradient. Insulin helps to maintain the transmembrane glucose gradient by its stimulatory effects on the enzymes of glycogen synthesis and glucose oxidation that use the glucose 6-phosphate formed. This combined action of insulin on intracellular enzymes and Glut 4 accounts for the large increase in glucose uptake in skeletal muscle. The suppression of lipolysis by insulin, and hence decreased fatty acid oxidation, enhances the direct action of insulin on skeletal muscle glucose uptake (Randle, BiochemSocSymp, 1978; 43:47; Kruszynska, DiabetAnn, 1995; 9: 107). Insulin promotes glycogen deposition by activating glycogen synthase; it also stimulates glucose oxidation by increasing the activity of pyruvate dehydrogenase (which converts pyruvate to acetyl CoA), indirectly via suppression of non-esterified fatty acid flux, and possibly by a direct action on skeletal muscle which may, however, depend on muscle type and nutritional state (Kruszynska, BiochemJ, 1989; 258:699).

Hepatic glucose output is almost completely suppressed at peripheral plasma insulin concentrations of approximately 40 mU/l (Rizza, AmJPhysiol, 1981; 240:E630). Insulin's ability to suppress hepatic glucose output is due to both direct hepatic effects and extrahepatic actions (Rebrin, Diabetes, 1995; 44:1038; Lewis, Diabetes, 1996; 45:454). Bergman and colleagues (Diabetes, 1995; 44: 1038) found that in dogs infused with insulin, suppression of hepatic glucose output correlated better with arterial insulin levels than with calculated portal venous insulin concentrations. They suggested that insulin's effect on glucose ouput may in part be mediated by suppression of adipose tissue lipolysis, because they found a very strong relationship between the effects of insulin on plasma nonesterified fatty acid levels and hepatic glucose output. Normally the insulin level necessary for half-maximal suppression of nonesterified fatty acid release is around 13 mU/l (Bonadonna, AmJPhysiol, 1990; 259:E736). Peak peripheral plasma insulin levels after oral glucose are between 40 and 100 mU/l. Thus, both peripheral insulin levels (assuming suppression of lipolysis is the important peripheral action of insulin in this context) and insulin concentrations at the liver, with portal insulin delivery, are supramaximal for inhibition of hepatic glucose output.

Plasma insulin concentrations necessary for half-maximal stimulation of muscle glucose uptake are about three times those required for half-maximal inhibition of hepatic glucose production (Rizza, AmJPhysiol, 1981; 240:E630; DeFronzo, Diabetes, 1983; 32:35). Peak peripheral plasma insulin concentrations after an oral glucose load, or a carbohydrate-containing meal, are well within the straightline part of the dose–response curve for peripheral glucose disposal in man, but near maximal for inhibition of hepatic glucose output. Therefore it is the skeletal muscle response which is more dependent

on the size of the insulin secretory response. The different sensitivity to insulin of liver and skeletal muscle, and the increased insulin levels after oral glucose compared to intravenously administered glucose, suggest that peripheral tissues may play a major role in the better tolerance observed with the oral route of glucose administration. Some support for this explanation comes from the finding of larger peripheral arteriovenous differences when glucose is given orally rather than intravenously (Perley, JCI, 1967; 46: 1954). Although glucose uptake by the liver is also enhanced by administration of glucose orally[13] (Ishida, JCI, 1983; 72:590), this appears not to be mediated by the augmented insulin response, but possibly by a signal resulting from the portal–arterial glucose gradient during portal glucose delivery.[13,14]

In view of the sensitivity of hepatic glucose production to insulin, the delivery of insulin via the portal route may be less important for normal glucose homeostasis than hitherto thought. In diabetic dogs less insulin was required to achieve normal blood glucose concentrations with intraduodenal (Stevenson, AmJPhysiol, 1983; 244:E190) or intraportal (Botz, Diabetes, 1976; 25:691) glucose infusion, if it was given via a peripheral vein rather than into the portal vein. In severely diabetic rats, peripheral insulin delivery, from islets transplanted under the renal capsule, resulted in consistent normoglycaemia and normal peripheral insulin concentrations, both in the fasting state and in response to an oral glucose load (Kruszynska, Diabetolog, 1985;28:167). As there was no first-pass hepatic extraction of insulin in these animals, the normal plasma insulin levels implied a decreased rate of insulin secretion. In normal dogs with peripheral insulin delivery achieved by pancreatic venous diversion into the inferior ven cava, postprandial hepatic and extrahepatic carbohydrate metabolism were similar to those of dogs with portal insulin delivery (Kryshak, Diabetes, 1990; 39:142). These studies suggest that portal insulin delivery is not necessary for normal glucose tolerance; indeed glucose homeostasis may be achieved more economically in terms of the supply of insulin when it is given peripherally.

Autoregulation by glucose

Although insulin suppresses hepatic glucose production, it does not cause net hepatic glucose uptake, or stimulation of liver glycogen deposition, without an increased portal venous glucose concentration[12-15] (Niewoehner, Diabetes, 1988; 37:1559). When hormonal responses to hyperglycaemia are prevented, hyperglycaemia alone suppresses hepatic glucose output, but basal insulin levels are a prerequisite (Wahren, JCI, 1972; 51:1870; Cherrington, JCI, 1978; 62:664). The extent of direct hepatic glucose uptake after a glucose load is believed to depend on the portal vein glucose concentration[12] (Lang, AmJPhysiol, 1986; 251:E584). Studies in the rat showed that the intracellular glucose concentration determines the direction of glucose flux (Niewoehner, Diabetes, 1988; 37:1559; Wals, Metabolism, 1993; 42:1492). When glucose is being released from the liver the intracellular glucose concentration must be higher than that in the sinusoidal blood. For rapid net glucose uptake to take place following an oral glucose load a gradient must be established in the other direction; furthermore, the sinusoidal glucose concentration must not only reach a higher level than that found intracellularly but this gradient must be maintained even in the face of an increase in the intracellular glucose concentration. As the increase in portal vein glucose levels after a glucose load is relatively small this may explain the limited hepatic glucose uptake following oral glucose.

Insulin is essential for activation of glycogen synthase after feeding or glucose administration[14] (Miller, AmJPhysiol, 1978; 234:E13; Langdon, Diabetes, 1984;32:134), but this role may be permissive, the immediate effector of changes in hepatic glycogen synthase activity, and of the switch from net hepatic glucose output to net glucose uptake, being glucose itself[12,15] (Bergman, AmJPhysiol, 1974; 227:1314; Davidson, Metabolism, 1981; 30:279). As stated above, this effect of glucose is explained by its inhibition of phosphorylase a. Activation of glycogen synthase may reduce the concentration of glucose 6-phosphate and thus facilitate hepatic uptake of glucose.

Although glucose has no effect on skeletal muscle glycogen phosphorylase or synthase, increased blood glucose levels promote skeletal muscle glucose uptake and glycogen deposition by a mass action effect[15] (Yki-Jarvinen, JCI, 1987; 80:95).

Role of enterohepatic and neural factors

Both insulin and the blood glucose concentration are important determinants of the metabolic response of the liver and peripheral tissues to oral glucose. That other factors are also important was suggested by human studies showing that increases in plasma glucose and insulin achieved by infusing glucose into a systemic vein result in only a small net uptake of glucose by the liver, even though portal venous concentrations of glucose and insulin should have been similar to, or greater than, those occurring during oral absorption of glucose; in these studies net splanchnic glucose uptake accounted for less than 15 per cent of the glucose infused (De-Fronzo, PNAS, 1978; 75:5173). This led to the idea that a 'gut factor', released during absorption of oral glucose, may promote hepatic uptake of glucose. However, doubts about this factor were raised by dog studies which demonstrated that rates of hepatic glucose uptake similar to those found during oral glucose absorption could be obtained with hyperglycaemia achieved by infusing glucose directly into the portal vein (Bergman, Diabetes, 1982; 31:27; Ishida, JCI, 1983; 72:590). As in man, these rates were significantly greater than those found during peripheral intravenous infusion of glucose. When portal delivery of insulin, glucagon, and glucose was carefully controlled, Cherrington et al. demonstrated convincingly that net hepatic glucose uptake in dogs depends on the portal route of glucose administration, and is strongly correlated with the arterial–portal glucose gradient.[13,14] Furthermore, stimulation of hepatic glucose uptake by portal glucose delivery in the presence of hyperglycaemia and basal insulin levels is rapid, reaching a maximal effect within 15 min. Although a fourfold rise in insulin, together with a similar degree of hyperglycaemia achieved by peripheral glucose infusion, produced an equivalent maximal net hepatic glucose uptake, this was attained only after 90 min.[14] Cherrington et al. suggested that the arterial–portal glucose gradient, or some other 'portal signal' associated with portal glucose delivery, triggers net hepatic glucose uptake and thus is an important determinant of the distribution of glucose between liver and peripheral tissues. The rapidity with which the 'portal signal' can trigger net hepatic glucose uptake is in keeping with the promptness with which the liver switches from glucose output to net glucose uptake after glucose ingestion (Abumrad, AmJPhysiol, 1982; 242:E398).

One mechanism by which portal vein glucose delivery may modulate hepatic glucose handling is through a neural reflex arc. The liver is richly innervated by autonomic nerve fibres from the splanchnic and vagus nerves; their central connections are believed to be in the ventromedial hypothalamic nucleus and the lateral hypothalamic nucleus, respectively. Enhancement of net hepatic glucose uptake by the 'portal signal' is abolished in dogs that have undergone complete hepatic surgical denervation (Adkins-Marshall, AmJPhysiol, 1992; 262:E679).

Electrical stimulation of the hepatic splanchnic nerve in rabbits results in marked increases in the activities of glycogen phosphorylase and glucose 6-phosphatase, and a concomitant depletion of liver glycogen. Peripheral stimulation of the vagus results in activation of glycogen synthase and enhanced liver glycogen deposition (Shimazu, BBActa, 1971; 252:28). This effect is not eliminated by prior pancreatectomy, indicating that it is not due to vagal enhancement of insulin secretion, but mainly to direct neural control. These effects are rapid, maximal effects on enzyme activities occurring within 30 s of stimulation. Further evidence for autonomic nervous system involvement in the control of hepatic carbohydrate metabolism comes from studies in which the ventromedial hypothalamic nucleus or lateral hypothalamic nucleus have been stimulated electrically or by neurotransmitter microinjection techniques.

This is good evidence for an effector limb of a neural reflex arc that could modulate hepatic glucose metabolism after portal glucose delivery. Evidence for an afferent limb is also available. When Niijima (JAutonNervSyst, 1983; 9:207) introduced glucose into the portal vein, afferent nerve fibres in the hepatic branch of the vagus nerve decreased their discharge rate in a concentration-dependent manner. Furthermore, the discharge rate of the efferent pancreatic branch of the vagus nerve increased, while that of the hepatic branch of the splanchnic nerve decreased. These effects of intraportal glucose were abolished by sectioning the hepatic branch of the vagus. The effect of these changes in autonomic nervous system activity would be to inhibit glycogenolysis and hepatic glucose production, and to stimulate hepatic glycogen synthesis and net hepatic glucose uptake.

Carbohydrate metabolism during physical activity

Fuels used by skeletal muscle during physical activity

Exercise enhances fuel utilization, necessitating a number of metabolic changes to ensure adequate substrate delivery to both exercising muscle and other tissues. The proportions of carbohydrate and fat used, and the relative importance of stored muscle glycogen and triglyceride versus blood-borne substrates to meet energy demands, depend on the intensity and duration of exercise, and on the nutritional state, fitness level, and muscle fibre type. During the first few minutes of sustained exercise, muscle glycogen is the main source of energy. As exercise continues, plasma non-esterified fatty acids and glucose become increasingly important. Mobilization of non-esterified fatty acids from adipose tissue is maximally enhanced during low-intensity exercise and is the major energy substrate (Fig. 2). With increasing exercise intensity, the additional energy is

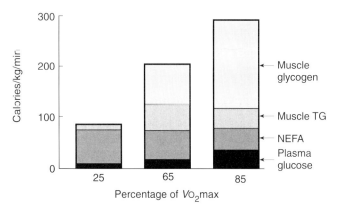

Fig. 2. Fuels utilized to meet energy needs after 30 min of exercise at 25, 65, or 85 per cent of maximal oxygen consumption. Values for energy expenditure from plasma glucose and non-esterified fatty acids represent maximal estimates; those for muscle glycogen and triglyceride are minimal estimates. Note the increased dependence on carbohydrate with increasing intensity of physical activity. (Reproduced from ref. 16, with permission.)

provided by fatty acids from intramuscular triglyceride stores, from muscle glycogen, and increased muscle glucose uptake.[16] As work rates are increased above the anaerobic threshold (~50 per cent of maximum oxygen consumption) carbohydrate (from muscle glycogen and plasma glucose) is the predominant fuel (Fig. 2)[16] (Ragusio, Diabetes, 1995; 44:1066). Carbohydrate is also the preferred substrate when oxygen availability is limited, since by comparison with fat, less oxygen is required for its oxidation. Glycogen depletion during exercise leads to decreased ATP regeneration, an increase in the degradation of ATP to AMP, which is further degraded to inosine monophosphate (**IMP**) and ammonia. Glycogen depletion and an increase in IMP are both associated with the onset of fatigue (Norman, ClinPhysiol, 1987; 7:503).

Glucose uptake by an exercising limb may increase up to twenty-fold above resting levels, and whole-body glucose uptake increases severalfold during intensive exercise. Even moderate-intensity exercise results in a two- to threefold increase in the rate of whole-body glucose utilization[16,17] (Ragusio, Diabetes, 1995; 44:1066). This enhancement of glucose uptake involves both an increase in muscle blood flow (with an opening-up of previously non-perfused capillaries), and an enhancement of muscle glucose transport. Muscle contraction, like insulin (see above) induces the translocation of glucose transporters (Glut 4) from within the muscle to their site of action in the sarcolemmal membrane. Muscle contraction and insulin appear to recruit Glut 4 from distinct intracellular pools (Douen, JBC, 1990; 265:13427; Coderre, JBC, 1995; 270:27584), so that their action on muscle glucose transport is additive. Muscle glucose uptake is also enhanced in the postexercise period. The glucose taken up is used to replenish glycogen stores. Insulin is important for repletion of glycogen stores after exercise; the exercised muscles show increased sensitivity to insulin for 16 to 20 h (Annuzzi, EurJClinInv, 1991; 21:6), and this ensures that glucose is directed to glycogen-depleted muscles (Richter, AmJPhysiol, 1984; 246:E476).

Plasma glucose homeostasis during exercise

Increased glucose utilization by working muscle is matched by a prompt increase in hepatic glucose output with the onset of exercise

so that plasma glucose levels are maintained within narrow limits[16, 17] (Kjaer, AmJPhysiol, 1995; 268:E636). Blood glucose levels remain essentially unchanged for the first 1 to 2 h of low- and moderate-intensity exercise; they may increase with strenuous exercise.[16] Blood glucose may fall after 2 to 3 h of continuous exercise without caloric intake if hepatic glucose production is unable to match the increased rate of glucose utilization (Felig, NEJM, 1982; 306:895). In overnight-fasted subjects the initial increase in hepatic glucose output is due almost entirely to an increase in glycogenolysis; gluconeogenesis does not contribute significantly during the first 40 min or so, irrespective of exercise intensity, but becomes increasingly important with prolonged exercise as liver glycogen stores are depleted (Wasserman, AmJPhysiol, 1991; 260:E811). Exercise increases the hepatic delivery of gluconeogenic precursors; the hepatic extraction of gluconeogenic amino acids and the efficiency with which they are converted to glucose are also enhanced (Wasserman, AmJPhysiol, 1988; 254: E518). Stimulation of lipolysis increases glycerol delivery to the liver. Increased breakdown of glycogen to lactate, in exercising and non-exercising muscle, increases the provision of lactate (Ahlborg, JCI, 1982; 69:45), while increased peripheral tissue and gut proteolysis result in increased hepatic delivery of gluconeogenic amino acids (Eriksson, ClinPhysiol, 1985; 5:325; Wagenmakers, AmJPhysiol, 1991; 260:E883; Wasserman, Metabolism, 1991; 40:307). Hepatic proteolysis may also provide amino acids for gluconeogenesis during prolonged exercise (Kasperek, BiochemJ, 1982; 202:281).

Regulation of fuel fluxes and maintenance of normoglycaemia during exercise is dependent on changes in plasma insulin, glucagon, and catecholamine levels, and to a lesser extent cortisol and growth hormone. Insulin levels decrease, while glucagon, adrenaline, noradrenaline, cortisol, and growth hormone increase. The fall in insulin and rise in glucagon levels is important for stimulating hepatic glucose production (Wolfe, JCI, 1986; 77:900); the increase in sympathetic activity and plasma catecholamine levels increase lipolysis, and reduce plasma glucose utilization, as well as enhancing hepatic glucose production[17] (Sigal, Diabetes, 1996; 45:148). Inhibition of one or other of these hormonal responses may have little effect on the plasma glucose response to exercise. However, if insulin levels are prevented from falling, then adrenergic blockade results in a marked impairment of the glucoregulatory response to exercise and hypoglycaemia ensues.[17] Administration of propranolol to patients with insulin-treated diabetes greatly increases the risk of exercise-induced hypoglycaemia (Simonson, JCI, 1984; 73:1648).

Sympathetic hepatic innervation does not appear to be important for the increase in hepatic glucose production during exercise since the response is normal after surgical denervation in dogs (Wasserman, AmJPhysiol, 1990; 259:E195) and in liver transplant patients (Kjaer, AmJPhysiol, 1995; 268:E636).

Influence of nutritional state on metabolic response to exercise

The metabolic response to exercise is influenced by nutritional state. After a fast sufficient to deplete liver glycogen stores, increased glucose production by the liver is entirely due to an enhancement of gluconeogenesis. The hepatic response is facilitated under these circumstances by several factors (Bjorkman, AmJPhysiol, 1983; 245:

E443). First, insulin levels are very low as a result of the prolonged fast, and the counter-regulatory hormone response to exercise tends to be exaggerated. Secondly, the delivery of gluconeogenic precursors to the liver is exaggerated. Thirdly, adipose tissue lipolysis and ketogenesis are enhanced and muscle fat oxidation is increased; the exercise-induced increase in muscle glucose utilization is diminished, thereby decreasing the demand on the liver. The proteolytic response and rise in plasma ammonia levels during exercise are enhanced when glycogen stores are depleted by fasting (Knapik, JApplPhsyiol, 1991; 70:43; Wagenmakers, AmJPhysiol, 1991; 260:E883).

Carbohydrate (glucose) ingestion before or during exercise increases the plasma glucose and insulin levels, and attenuates the glucagon response. The increase in hepatic glucose production is blunted, and the lipolytic response smaller. The rise in insulin and glucose levels augment the exercise-induced increase in muscle glucose uptake. During low-intensity activity after carbohydrate ingestion, circulating glucose may suffice to meet the increased energy needs of muscle contraction, providing there is sufficient enhancement of muscle glucose transport, and the rate of entry of ingested glucose into the circulation is sufficient to balance the increased rate of muscle glucose uptake so that plasma glucose does not fall. However, with increasing intensity of physical activity, circulating glucose will not suffice to meet muscle energy needs; the shortfall must be met by muscle glycogen or fatty acids. In the presence of hyperinsulinaemia, fatty acid mobilization (from adipose tissue and from intramuscular triglyceride stores) will be impaired, and muscle glycogen utilization is enhanced. The hyperinsulinaemia that follows the ingestion of glucose prior to exercise, often results in a fall in plasma glucose levels during exercise, and often results in more rapid depletion of muscle glycogen stores (Costill, JApplPhysiol, 1977; 43:695; Levine, JApplPhysiol, 1983; 55:1767).

Fructose induces a much smaller insulin response, and the hypoglycaemic effect seen after glucose ingestion is often avoided. Depletion of muscle glycogen during exercise is slower after fructose than after glucose ingestion (Levine, JApplPhysiol, 1983; 55:1767).

Metabolism of fructose

Fructose is a major component of a typical Western diet as it is a component of sucrose, a disaccharide containing equimolar amounts of glucose and fructose. An average Western diet contains about 300 g of carbohydrate; about 80 to 120 g of this is sucrose and so the daily fructose intake is about 40 to 60 g, or about 7 to 10 per cent of energy intake.

Within the body phosphorylated forms of fructose are important intracellular intermediates in the metabolism of glucose. Free fructose is not produced in tissues, except in the prostate and possibly in the brain and blood vessels, and it is not found in fasting plasma in any significant amount.

Dietary sucrose is hydrolysed by sucrase, present in the brush border of the epithelial cells of the upper small intestine. The glucose and fructose released by hydrolysis traverse the epithelial cells and enter the portal vein. Fructose is transported by a specific fructose transporter, Glut 5 (Table 1) (Rand, AmJPhysiol, 1993; 264: G1169). After meals containing sucrose the increase in peripheral arterial blood glucose concentration is much higher than the increase in fructose; this is hardly surprising as fructose normally constitutes

only about one-sixth of the total carbohydrate of the meal, the rest is mainly glucose (in polysaccharides, sucrose, and lactose). Even if pure sucrose is fed, the glucose increment is still much greater than that of fructose. The intestine may metabolize some absorbed fructose, with production of lactate, and it has been claimed that a small amount of fructose is converted into glucose by the gut wall. These factors, together with a relatively slow rate of absorption, may help to explain the low blood levels seen after oral fructose, but a major factor is its removal from portal vein blood during its first passage through the liver.

Over 60 years ago Cori and Cori (JBC, 1927; 72:597) found, in rats, that when fructose was infused into a mesenteric vein the amount needed to produce fructosuria was much greater than when it was infused into a systemic vein; in dogs arterial fructose levels were much lower with intraportal than with peripheral venous infusions of fructose.[6] Animal studies have also shown a portal–hepatic venous fructose gradient during intestinal absorption of fructose (Weinstein, JLabClinMed, 1952; 40:39). These studies suggest a large first-pass uptake of fructose by the liver, the major site of metabolism of orally administered fructose. Even when fructose is infused into a systemic vein, splanchnic balance studies suggest that the liver removes about 40 to 50 per cent of the fructose infused (Weichselbaum, Metabolism, 1953; 2:434; Wolfe, JCI, 1975; 56:970; Bjorkman, JCI, 1989; 83:52). Tissue fructose uptake is proportional to the plasma fructose level[18] and independent of insulin (DeKalbermatten, Metabolism, 1980; 29:62). Clearance is rapid; the normal plasma half-life being about 18 min (Smith, JCI, 1953; 32:273).

The high capacity of the liver for fructose uptake and metabolism is a consequence of the presence of the enzyme fructokinase which has a capacity three to five times that of glucokinase and hexokinase combined. Fructose within the hepatocyte is rapidly phosphorylated by fructokinase to fructose 1-phosphate; this helps to maintain a gradient which facilitates fructose entry into the cell. Unlike hexokinase, which phosphorylates glucose, fructokinase is not inhibited by the phosphorylated hexose and it has a much higher affinity than that of the facilitated transport system. Some tissues other than liver, notably kidney and small intestinal mucosa, also contain fructokinase and can use fructose as a source of energy.

Intracellular fructose 1-phosphate is cleaved by aldolase type B into glyceraldehyde and dihydroxyacetonephosphate (deficiency of aldolase type B results in hereditary fructose intolerance which is a cause of cirrhosis in children). Thus fructose is converted to trioses by a different pathway to that of glucose and so escapes the controlling influences in the early stages of the glycolytic pathway. Triokinase converts glyceraldehyde to glyceraldehyde 3-phosphate which is interconvertible with dihydroxyacetonephosphate. Both of these trioses may be converted to pyruvate (via glycolysis) or to glucose (via gluconeogenesis).

About 30 per cent of a fructose load is metabolized directly to pyruvate and lactate; the rise in blood pyruvate and lactate concentrations is more marked than after an equivalent glucose load[9,19] (Martines, Nutrition, 1994; 10:521). The conversion of fructose to glucose (Anundi, JBC, 1987; 262:9529) explains the small increase in blood glucose which occurs when fructose is given either orally or intravenously[18,19] (Bjorkman, JCI, 1989; 83:52). This rise in blood glucose is associated with a small increase in plasma insulin levels,[18,19] which helps to divert glucose 6-phosphate within the hepatocyte into glycogen and so limit the rise in glucose production; fructose is a good precursor for glycogen formation (Nilsson, ScaJCLI, 1974; 33:5).

Adipose tissue and skeletal muscle can also use fructose even though they lack fructokinase. Several investigators have demonstrated a peripheral arterial–venous fructose gradient during intravenous fructose administration in man (van Itallie, PSEBM, 1953; 84:713; Weichselbaum, Metabolism, 1953; 2:434); studies *in vitro* with isolated fat cells and muscle preparations have shown uptake of fructose, incorporation of fructose carbon into glycogen and lipids, and oxidation to CO_2 (Zierath, BiochemJ, 1995; 311: 517). Fructose uptake by skeletal muscle is mediated by Glut 5 (Table 1). Skeletal muscle glycogen content increases after intravenous fructose administration (Nilsson, ScaJCLI, 1974; 33:5).

In tissues that lack fructokinase, fructose is phosphorylated by hexokinase to fructose 6-phosphate. Its subsequent metabolism is thus similar to that of glucose, and is subject to similar controls at the beginning of the glycolytic pathway. However, the affinity of hexokinase for glucose is much higher than for fructose and glucose acts as a competitive inhibitor of fructose phosphorylation. This will be important in tissues in which free glucose is present in the cytoplasm, namely non-insulin-dependent tissues, and skeletal muscle exposed to elevated glucose concentrations. In adipose tissue and skeletal muscle glucose transport is rate limiting for glucose utilization at basal plasma glucose and insulin concentrations. Under these conditions the intracellular free glucose concentration is not high enough to compete for phosphorylation and fructose can be utilized efficiently. In adipose tissue some fructose is metabolized to glycerol 3-phosphate which is used to esterify fatty acids, and this is the main mechanism by which fructose leads to a reduction in adipocyte non-esterified fatty acid release.[18]

The ability of tissues such as muscle and adipose tissue to use fructose via the hexokinase pathway probably explains the relatively low urinary excretion of fructose (10 to 20 per cent of an intravenously administered dose) in patients with hereditary fructose intolerance and essential fructosuria (fructokinase deficiency).

One feature of the metabolic response to the administration of fructose (and sucrose) is a relatively rapid increase in plasma triglyceride which is carried in very low density lipoproteins (**VLDL**). Several animal studies have shown that fructose is a more potent stimulus to hepatic fatty acid synthesis than glucose, with greater incorporation of fructose carbon into fatty acid molecules; this would increase the intrahepatic availability of fatty acids. Most VLDL-triglyceride produced on a fructose-rich diet is, however, derived from circulating fatty acids rather than fatty acids synthesized *de novo* (Schonfeld, JLipRes, 1971; 12:614), and it is estimated that only a small proportion of fructose carbon is incorporated into fatty acids (Nikkila, AdvLipRes, 1969; 7:63). When fructose is fed, the fall in plasma free fatty acids is less than that observed after glucose; the suppression of whole-body lipid oxidation is, however, more marked than after an equivalent glucose load[9,19] (Tappy, AmJPhysiol, 1986; 250:E718). Thus, the greater triglyceride response to fructose, by comparison with glucose, is due, first, to a smaller fall in plasma non-esterified fatty acid levels and, secondly, to more of the fatty acids taken up by the liver being re-esterified to triglyceride instead of being oxidized. Glycerol 3-phosphate produced from dihydroxyacetonephosphate (derived

from the cleavage of fructose 1-phosphate) provides the glycerol for re-esterification of these fatty acids.

Galactose metabolism

Galactose is a component of lactose, a disaccharide containing equimolar amounts of glucose and galactose. It is an important nutrient in infancy, and sometimes in later life depending on the amount of milk in the diet. Dietary lactose is hydrolysed by lactase present in the brush border of the upper small intestinal epithelium. Absorption of the released glucose and galactose is associated with a relatively small rise in blood galactose because of first-pass hepatic uptake.

Galactose is phosphorylated in liver by galactokinase to galactose 1-phosphate. This is the rate-limiting step for galactose uptake in the liver. In normal human liver the V_{max} for galactokinase-mediated phosphorylation of galactose, and thus the elimination capacity, is about 2 mmol/min/kg liver (Tygstrup, ActaMedScand, 1964; 175: 281). Galactose 1-phosphate is converted to glucose 1-phosphate by a uridyl transferase and an epimerase. Glucose 1-phosphate can then be used directly for glycogen synthesis, or after conversion to glucose 6-phosphate by phosphoglucomutase, it can enter the glycolytic pathway or give rise to glucose that can be released into the circulation.

Carbohydrate metabolism in patients with liver disease
Glucose metabolism in the fasted state

As the liver is the major source of blood glucose, except for a few h after a meal, one might expect patients with liver disease to develop hypoglycaemia during the night or after more prolonged fasting. However, significant hypoglycaemia is uncommon in liver disease and is rarely symptomatic. Indeed, fasting blood glucose levels are usually normal or elevated. This may be due, in part, to the large reserve capacity of the liver for glucose production; as little as 20 per cent of the functional hepatocyte mass may be needed to maintain glucose output at normal fasting levels.

When hypoglycaemia occurs, it is generally due to severe hepatocellular failure occurring as a terminal event in patients with chronic liver disease, or in acute fulminant disease. Symptomatic hypoglycaemia may be associated with severe liver damage, due to toxins such as paracetamol or chloroform or acute viral hepatitis; asymptomatic hypoglycaemia is more common[20] (Record, ClinSci, 1975; 49:473). Hypoglycaemia complicating hepatocellular carcinoma is discussed in Chapter 25.2.

Hypoglycaemia is common in fulminant hepatic failure, particularly in children, and can develop rapidly. Apart from a reduction in functional hepatocyte mass and depletion of glycogen stores with fasting, hepatic lactate extraction and gluconeogenesis may be inhibited if acidosis develops (Arieff, DiabetMetabRev, 1989; 5:637). Increased glucose utilization also contributes to the development of hypoglycaemia in these patients. Normally, glucose requirements fall with prolonged fasting as the brain derives more of its energy from the oxidation of ketone bodies. However, in liver failure ketogenesis is impaired and glucose requirements remain high. Anaerobic glycolysis and basal glucose requirements may be further increased by cytokines, such as tumour necrosis factor-α (Evans, AmJPhysiol, 1989; 257:R1182; Lang, Endocrinol, 1992; 130:43), and by tissue hypoxia, which is common in fulminant hepatic failure (Bihari, CritCareMed, 1985; 13:1034). The glucose requirement may also be increased as a result of alkalosis which can stimulate glycolysis and impair oxygen utilization in certain tissues, notably the gut (Arieff, DiabetMetabRev, 1989; 5:637; Bersin, AmJMed, 1989; 87:7; Buchalter, DiabetMetabRev, 1989; 4:379).

Hypoglycaemia should be managed by infusion of glucose intravenously at a rate that ensures adequate delivery to tissues with an obligatory glucose requirement. As discussed above this is about 160 to 200 g over a 24 h period, which may be given as 10 per cent glucose (dextrose) (1.6–2.0 l/day), or 20 per cent glucose via a central vein if fluid restriction is necessary. In some patients glucose requirements may be greater due to an increased metabolic rate (for example, due to sepsis) or a switch from lipid to glucose metabolism, and increased anaerobic glycolysis secondary to hypoxia, the effects of cytokines, or acid–base disturbance. In these patients a higher glucose delivery rate will be necessary as indicated by the blood glucose response. Excessive amounts of glucose should be avoided. These patients are extremely insulin resistant (Vilstrup, EurJClin-Inv, 1986; 16:193), and hyperglycaemia and hyperosmolality can develop rapidly; the resulting osmotic diuresis can lead to hypernatraemia and other electrolyte disturbances (Wilkinson, BMJ, 1974; 1:186).

Hepatic glucose production

The fasting blood glucose concentration reflects the balance between hepatic glucose production and tissue glucose utilization. If these processes increase or decrease concurrently, there may be a marked change in turnover without much effect on the blood glucose level. That fasting blood glucose levels in patients with liver disease are normal or high does not, therefore, imply normal hepatic glucose production. Several groups, using radio-isotopic methods[21] (Piniewska, HormMetRes, 1986; 18:834) or hepatic vein catheterization[22] (Myers, JCI, 1950; 29:1421), have found hepatic glucose production in cirrhotics to be 20 to 40 per cent lower than in normals following an overnight fast. Others have reported normal values[9,19,23–25] (Perez, JClinEndoc, 1978; 46:778; Keller, JClinEndoc, 1982; 54:961). Differences in patient selection or methodology may partly account for these differences. Diabetic cirrhotics with fasting hyperglycaemia have increased rates of hepatic glucose production after an overnight fast.[26]

Keller et al. (JClinEndoc, 1982; 54:961) claimed that relatively normal rates of hepatic glucose production were maintained by increased glucagon stimulation in alcoholic cirrhotics studied in the basal state. When somatostatin was infused to suppress glucagon secretion, a much greater fall in net splanchnic glucose output and blood glucose concentration occurred in patients than in normal subjects. When glucagon was replaced by infusion into a peripheral vein the rise in net splanchnic glucose production, and in blood glucose concentration, was significantly less in cirrhotics than in controls, despite similar plasma glucagon concentrations.

Other studies also suggest a diminished hyperglycaemic response to the administration of glucagon in liver disease, whether it is given alone[20] (Feruglio, ClinSci, 1966; 30:43; Yeung, Gut, 1974; 15:907; Petrides, Metabolism, 1994; 43:85) or with adrenaline (Van Itallie, JCI, 1955; 34:1730). Possible explanations are:

(1) hepatic resistance to glucagon;
(2) decreased hepatic delivery of glucagon and gluconeogenic substrates as a result of portosystemic shunting; and
(3) decreased liver glycogen content.

In view of the primary importance of glycogenolysis for the initial rise in glucose production following glucagon in overnight-fasted normal human (Magnusson, Diabetes, 1995; 44:185), and the short duration (30–60 min) of the glucagon stimulus in the above studies, decreased liver glycogen content in cirrhotic patients might account for the poor hyperglycaemic response. There are few data on liver glycogen content in patients with liver disease. Owen et al., [22] in alcoholic cirrhotics (Child's B and C) fasted overnight, found values of 25.8 $\pm$ 3.6 mg/g wet weight, which were lower than those found in two normal subjects (32.0–48.0 mg/g wet weight), and lower than liver glycogen concentrations reported by Nilsson (ScaJCLI, 1973; 32:317) for 58 normal subjects (43.7 $\pm$ 1.81 mg/g). Liver volume was not reported, and it is therefore unclear whether total liver glycogen stores were reduced in the alcoholic cirrhotics studied by Owen.[22] Decreased liver glycogen concentration was also found in patients with acute viral hepatitis;[20] in this study, however, liver biopsies were performed 2 to 3 h after breakfast and it is not clear whether the nutritional state of patients and controls was comparable. While low liver glycogen stores would seem a likely explanation for the poor glycaemic response to glucagon, it is likely that hepatic glucagon resistance, possibly due to chronically elevated plasma glucagon levels (Chapter 25.2) is also important. Support for this notion comes from the finding that other metabolic responses to glucagon, including stimulation of gluconeogenesis (Sherwin, Gastro, 1978; 74:1224) are also impaired in cirrhosis.

Contributions of glycogenolysis and gluconeogenesis to hepatic glucose production

Animal studies have suggested a close correlation between liver glycogen content and the direction of carbon flux through glycolysis/gluconeogenesis. The mechanisms are unclear but are probably related to hepatic concentrations of fructose 2,6-bisphosphate (Foster, Diabetes, 1984; 33:1188; Holness, BiochemJ, 1988; 252:357; Sugden, BiochemJ, 1989; 263:313). Impaired synthesis of glycogen after meals, and hence more rapid depletion of glycogen stores on fasting, might mean that fasted patients with liver disease will more rapidly develop the profile of hepatic enzyme activities characteristic of starvation, with earlier activation of gluconeogenesis and ketogenesis. Some support for this hypothesis came from measurement of transhepatic balances of intermediary metabolites and glucose.[22] In overnight-fasted alcoholic cirrhotics hepatic glucose production was decreased 38 per cent, but uptake of gluconeogenic precursors was twice that found by Wahren et al. in younger normal subjects (JCI, 1972; 51:1870). It was estimated that gluconeogenesis accounted for two-thirds of hepatic glucose production, the remainder coming from glycogen.[22] By contrast, in the normal overnight-fasted subjects studied by Wahren (JCI, 1972; 51:1870) 70 to 80 per cent of glucose was estimated to come from glycogen and approximately 20 per cent from gluconeogenesis. After a 3 day fast gluconeogenesis accounted for the entire hepatic glucose output in cirrhotics but only for two-thirds in normal subjects. Increased gluconeogenesis in the cirrhotics was associated with increased hepatic ketone body production. There is some doubt over the interpretation of the above studies. First, the contribution of glycogenolysis to hepatic glucose production in the normal subjects may have been overestimated. As discussed earlier, studies following the decline in liver glycogen concentration by ^{13}C-NMR suggest that in normal subjects only one-third of the glucose produced by the liver during the first 22 h of fasting comes from liver glycogen.[1] Secondly, other investigators could not show increased splanchnic uptake of gluconeogenic precursors in cirrhotics.[23,27]

The reasons for the disparate findings are unclear. Severity of liver disease, nutritional state, and preceding dietary intake could all be important. Owen *et al.*[22] studied patients shortly after a major bleed from oesophageal varices. Many were malnourished and had evidence of hepatic decompensation. By contrast, the alcoholic cirrhotics studied by Nosadini *et al.*[23] had better liver function and were better nourished. Splanchnic balance studies depend on accurate measurement of hepatic blood flow—a particular problem in cirrhotics with intra- and extrahepatic portosystemic shunting. Errors inherent in measurement of hepatic blood flow in patients with cirrhosis are probably the main reason for the discrepancy between the two studies. Owen *et al.* found hepatic blood flow to be increased by 36 per cent in their cirrhotics compared with normal controls, while Nosadini's patients had significantly lower effective hepatic blood flow and there was a strong correlation between blood flow and uptake of gluconeogenic precursors. Thus, while cirrhotic patients with normal blood flow had normal or increased uptake, those with decreased blood flow, as a result of portosystemic shunting, had impaired uptake of lactate, alanine, pyruvate, and glycerol. Portosystemic shunting was also associated with decreased hepatic clearance of fatty acids, decreased output of triglycerides, but increased ketone body production. Increased ketone body production was also found in these patients by radio-isotopic turnover methods.

Further evidence that gluconeogenesis is not enhanced in overnight-fasted cirrhotics comes from studies showing normal rates of incorporation of radioactive glycerol into glucose, and a similar percentage of the glycerol released from adipose tissue being used for gluconeogenesis in cirrhotics and matched normal subjects.[25] Behaviour of the other gluconeogenic substrates would be expected to parallel that of glycerol. The finding of normal glucose carbon recycling (a measure of Cori cycle activity) in compensated cirrhotics (Piniewska, HormMetRes, 1986; 18:834) suggests that gluconeogenesis from lactate and alanine are not enhanced. Further indirect evidence that gluconeogenesis from amino acids is not increased comes from the finding of either normal,[9] (Muller, Hepatol, 1992; 15:782) or lower[22,25] (Merli, Hepatol, 1990; 12:106) urinary nitrogen excretion and protein oxidation rates in overnight-fasted cirrhotics; approximately 1 g nitrogen is excreted in the urine for every 3.6 g of glucose produced by gluconeogenesis from amino acids (Schulz, JNutr, 1975; 105:200).

Activities of the key gluconeogenic enzymes (pyruvate carboxylase, phosphoenolpyruvate carboxykinase, and fructose 1,6-bisphosphatase) in overnight-fasted alcoholic cirrhotics were within the normal range when expressed per unit weight of liver.[22] Glucose 6-phosphatase activity was decreased. Reduced glucose 6-phosphatase activity was also found by others (Sotaniemi, JHepatol, 1985; 1:277). Since fibrous tissue accounted for approximately 40 per cent of liver tissue, 'normal' values might indicate enhanced gluconeogenic enzyme activity in remaining viable hepatocytes.

There is little information on peripheral production of gluconeogenic precursors in cirrhosis. One group found a small decrease in fasting forearm lactate production,[28] whereas Nosadini[23] reported normal leg fluxes of lactate and pyruvate, but decreased alanine production, in cirrhotic patients. In patients with alcoholic liver disease and elevated plasma glycerol concentrations, glycerol production rates were found to be normal[18,25] (Johnston, Gut, 1982; 23:257). Available evidence thus suggests that hepatic gluconeogenic substrate supply is not increased. Decreased hepatic clearance appears the major determinant of the elevated blood lactate, pyruvate, and glycerol concentrations found in many patients with cirrhosis of varying aetiology (Stewart, EurJClinInv, 1983; 13:397), and in patients with viral hepatitis (Record, ClinSci, 1973; 45:677).

Taken together, these studies suggest that when cirrhotics are fasted, there may indeed be a more rapid transition to a pattern of hepatic metabolism characteristic of starvation, with a more rapid switch to utilization of fatty acids and ketones thus decreasing glucose requirements. The physiological reduction in hepatic glucose production that occurs during fasting (see earlier) may occur sooner in cirrhosis, accounting for the lower hepatic glucose production rates found in some studies. Decreased delivery of gluconeogenic substrates may limit the capacity for gluconeogenesis.

Glucose utilization

In the postabsorptive state, whole-body glucose utilization is equal to glucose production (1.8–2.4 mg/kg/min). Non-insulin-dependent tissues such as nervous tissue, blood cells, and extrahepatic splanchnic tissues, account for the greater part of glucose utilization; skeletal muscle accounts for less than 20 per cent of basal glucose uptake. Whole-body glucose oxidation rates are less than glucose utilization rates (Fig. 3) because in non-neuronal tissues much of the glucose is metabolized to lactate and pyruvate which are released into the plasma for resynthesis of glucose in the liver. Brain accounts for 70 to 90 per cent of total glucose oxidation after an overnight fast, whereas skeletal muscle accounts for less than 10 per cent.

Both normal and decreased rates of glucose utilization are reported in overnight-fasted cirrhotic patients. Glucose metabolic clearance rate (glucose utilization rate/plasma glucose concentration) is usually decreased by 25 to 40 per cent, so that fasting plasma glucose levels are similar to, or higher than, those of controls. The reduction in glucose metabolic clearance rate is found despite plasma insulin levels that are two to six times normal.

The reason for the decreased efficiency of glucose removal from plasma in the fasted state is unclear. It could result from increased oxidation of fatty acids and ketone bodies by peripheral tissues. Plasma non-esterified fatty acid levels are increased in many patients with liver disease. Whether plasma non-esterified fatty acids increase from decreased hepatic clearance[23] or increased adipose tissue lipolysis,[18,24] the net effect will be an increase in their availability to peripheral tissues for oxidation. Hepatic ketone body production is increased in some cirrhotic patients[22,23] and increased uptake across the leg has been found[23] (Merli, JHepatol, 1986; 3:348).

The idea that basal glucose uptake by peripheral tissues might be impaired because of increased utilization of these lipid fuels is

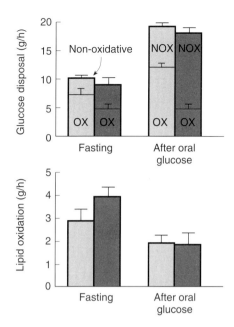

Fig. 3. Glucose utilization (upper panel) and lipid oxidation (lower panel) after an overnight fast and during a 4 h period after a 75 g oral glucose load in eight control subjects ▦ and eight alcoholic cirrhotics ▪. Mean ± SEM. Whole-body glucose disposal is similar in cirrhotics and controls in the basal state. Note that it increases normally in cirrhotics after oral glucose despite glucose intolerance. Glucose disposal comprises oxidative (OX) and non-oxidative glucose disposal (NOX). In the basal state glucose oxidation tends to be reduced and lipid oxidation enhanced in cirrhotics; after oral glucose, glucose and lipid oxidation rates are similar to those of controls. In the basal state NOX is due to metabolism of glucose by glycolysis to lactate; glycogen synthesis accounts for much of the increase in NOX after oral glucose. Although non-oxidative glucose disposal may be similar to that of controls, there is evidence that glycolysis accounts for a larger proportion of this in cirrhotics, and NOX may underestimate the defect in glycogen deposition. (Based on data in ref. 9, with permission.)

supported by studies using indirect calorimetry, which found that overnight-fasted cirrhotics derive more of their energy requirements from the oxidation of fat and less from carbohydrate[29] (Merli, Hepatol, 1990; 12:106) (Fig. 3). Owen *et al.*,[29] in a study of a small group of overnight-fasted alcoholic cirrhotics with poor liver function, many of whom were malnourished, found that only 13 per cent of energy requirements were met by oxidation of carbohydrate compared to 39 per cent in normal subjects. Lipid oxidation accounted for 69 per cent of energy expenditure in cirrhotics compared to 40 per cent in controls. The pattern of fuel utilization in overnight-fasted cirrhotics was similar to that of normal subjects fasted for 3 days. Not all studies have found increased lipid oxidation rates in overnight-fasted cirrhotics[18,19,24],[27] (Muller, AmJPhysiol, 1991; 260:E338). Different subject characteristics may explain the conflicting reports. Muller (AmJPhysiol, 1991; 260: E338)[30] found that basal fat oxidation rates were increased in cirrhotics with advanced liver disease (Child's C) but not in well-compensated Child's class A cirrhotics.

Since fatty acids are normally the main oxidative substrate for skeletal muscle after an overnight fast, inhibition of plasma glucose utilization by muscle will decrease whole-body glucose utilization by only 10 to 15 per cent. The most likely explanation for the more

marked reduction in circulating glucose utilization, and in glucose oxidation found in some studies,[22,29] is enhanced utilization of ketone bodies by the brain.

Glucose metabolism in the fed state

After glucose ingestion many patients with liver disease have abnormally elevated blood glucose concentrations. This glucose intolerance was first described by Naunyn[31] who coined the term 'hepatogenous diabetes'. The fall in blood glucose after an intravenous glucose bolus is somewhat slower in cirrhotics than in controls,[32] and correlates well with their intolerance to oral glucose.[32] The prevalence of glucose intolerance in cirrhosis varies, depending on the criteria used for defining glucose intolerance and the type of patient studied. Using WHO criteria, more than 60 to 80 per cent of patients with cirrhosis are glucose intolerant (Chapter 25.2). Glucose intolerance is also frequently found in patients with acute viral hepatitis (Record, ClinSci, 1973; 45:677; Chupin, Diabetes, 1978; 27:661), fatty liver (Rehfeld, Gastro, 1973; 64:445), autoimmune chronic active hepatitis (Alberti, ClinSci, 1972; 42:591), and toxic liver damage (Record, ClinSci, 1975; 49:473).

Overt diabetes mellitus (with elevated fasting glucose levels) occurs two to four times more frequently in cirrhotics than in the general population (see Chapter 25.2). Diabetic cirrhotics have a much lower rate of fall of plasma glucose after an intravenous glucose bolus (see Chapter 25.2, Fig. 2). As discussed below, peripheral tissue insulin insensitivity is a major factor in the aetiology of glucose intolerance in cirrhosis. Insulin insensitivity is a feature of both diabetic and non-diabetic cirrhotic patients. However, fasting hyperglycaemia is not explicable on the basis of peripheral tissue insulin insensitivity because most basal glucose utilization is non-insulin-mediated. Overtly diabetic cirrhotics, in addition to insulin resistance, have a marked impairment of insulin secretion (Chapter 25.2). The insulin secretory defect results in increased basal rates of hepatic glucose production (accounting for fasting hyperglycaemia) and impaired suppression of hepatic glucose output after meals or glucose administration, which contributes to their greater glucose intolerance. Available data suggest that diabetes develops in those cirrhotics who have an underlying tendency to develop diabetes, probably on a genetic basis, and that the insulin resistance that characterizes cirrhotic patients results in the expression of the disease and the higher prevalence than in non-cirrhotic patients. For this reason it is important to consider diabetic and non-diabetic cirrhotics separately. This chapter focuses on the glucose intolerance of liver disease with reference to abnormalities in diabetic cirrhotics where appropriate; the pathogenesis and management of overt diabetes in patients with cirrhosis is discussed in detail in Chapter 25.2.

Blood glucose and intermediary metabolite responses to meals

Blood glucose levels are higher after meals in patients with liver disease than in matched normal subjects[33] (Marchesini, Hepatol, 1981; 1:294; Stewart, EurJClinInv, 1983; 13:397). Whereas normal subjects show a postprandial blood glucose increment of 1 to 2 mmol/l, patients with alcoholic cirrhosis or alcoholic hepatitis/ fatty liver have an exaggerated rise of 4 to 8 mmol/l (Fig. 4).

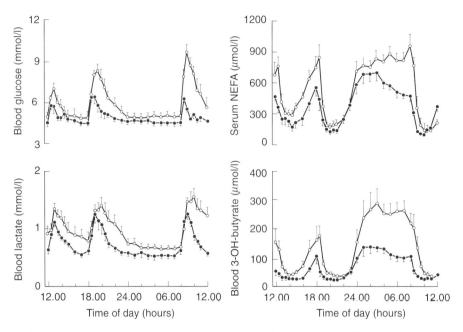

Fig. 4. Twenty-four-hour profiles of blood glucose, lactate, 3-hydroxybutyrate, and serum non-esterified fatty acid concentrations in 9 cirrhotic patients (○—○) and 10 normal control subjects (●—-●) on a standard diet. Mean ± SEM. (Reproduced from ref. 33, with permission.)

This is accompanied by increases in the concentrations of lactate, pyruvate, and insulin, particularly in patients with established cirrhosis[33] (Stewart, EurJClinInv, 1983; 13:397). The greater initial rise in lactate levels after meals in cirrhotics (Fig. 4), suggests increased lactate production. Since postprandial lactate levels correlate with plasma glucose levels in cirrhotic and normal subjects, [33] non-insulin-dependent tissues (for example, intestine and skin) are a likely source; hyperglycaemia increases glycolysis and lactate production in these tissues (Yki-Jarvinen, Metabolism, 1990; 39: 859). Decreased hepatic clearance of lactate in cirrhosis (Connor, ClinSci, 1978; 54:33) is also thought to be important for the hyperlactataemia after oral glucose or mixed meals. Decreased skeletal muscle lactate uptake might also contribute as muscle takes up lactate during the first 2 to 3 h following a meal or oral glucose load (Jackson, Diabetes, 1973; 22:442; Radziuk, Diabetes, 1983; 32: 977). Decreased muscle lactate clearance might be expected in alcoholic cirrhotics as a consequence of the decreased muscle mitochondrial volume fraction (Kiessling, ScaJCLI, 1975; 35:601). The forearm data of Leatherdale[28] support this view.

After meals, plasma non-esterified fatty acids and 3-hydroxybutyrate levels are suppressed in cirrhotic patients to low levels similar to those found in control subjects (Fig. 4). Thus, although cirrhotics may derive more energy from the oxidation of lipid fuels in the fasting state, when exogenous carbohydrate is made available it is the preferred oxidative substrate.

Mechanisms of glucose intolerance in liver disease

Possible explanations for glucose intolerance in liver disease are:

(1) a reduced rate of glucose removal from the systemic circulation;
(2) an increase in the amount of glucose entering the systemic circulation, because of

(a) a lesser inhibition of hepatic glucose output following oral or intravenous glucose; or
(b) in the case of oral glucose, shunting of glucose past the liver, even though first-pass hepatic uptake of glucose is normally relatively small;

(3) a combination of (1) and (2).

These abnormalities of glucose metabolism could in turn be due to:

(1) insensitivity of the liver and peripheral tissues to insulin;
(2) an impairment of insulin secretion;
(3) a decrease in the ability of hyperglycaemia *per se* to enhance tissue glucose uptake and inhibit hepatic glucose output (i.e. diminished 'glucose effectiveness'); or
(4) portosystemic shunting.

Response to intravenous glucose in cirrhosis

The fall in blood glucose after an intravenous glucose bolus is somewhat slower in cirrhotics than in controls.[32,34,35] However, the abnormality in terms of plasma glucose levels after an intravenous glucose bolus is quite small (see Chapter 25.2, Fig. 2) by comparison with the response to oral glucose, even though there is a good correlation between intolerance to intravenous and oral glucose. The plasma insulin response to intravenous glucose is prompt and exaggerated in cirrhotics with normal (Megyesi, Lancet, 1967; ii:1051) or mild impairment of intravenous glucose tolerance.[32] However, because there is a delay between a rise in plasma insulin levels and the effect of this rise on the promotion of tissue glucose uptake, insulin-mediated glucose uptake plays a smaller role in determining the plasma glucose response to intravenous glucose than to oral glucose. More important are the suppression of hepatic glucose output by insulin and enhancement of glucose uptake by the mass action effect of glucose. Both of these are normal in cirrhosis. The small role of insulin-mediated glucose uptake in determining the plasma glucose response to an intravenous glucose bolus explains the relatively good intravenous glucose tolerance of cirrhotic patients despite peripheral tissue insulin resistance. Diabetic cirrhotics have a much lower rate of fall of blood glucose after an intravenous glucose bolus (see Chapter 25.2, Fig. 2). In diabetic cirrhotics the absence of a first-phase insulin response to intravenous glucose (Chapter 25.2) results in impaired suppression of hepatic glucose output, and partly explains their greater intolerance to IV glucose. One would expect peripheral tissues to play a greater role in determining glucose tolerance during a continuous infusion of glucose (and prolonged stimulation of insulin secretion) than in response to an intravenous glucose bolus, and that insulin-resistant non-diabetic cirrhotics would either have a higher plasma glucose level at a given glucose infusion rate, or require less glucose to maintain plasma glucose levels at a target level. However, this is not so. There are two reasons for this. First, the pattern of insulin secretion in response to a sustained glucose stimulus (for example a 10 mmol/l clamp) is biphasic. After the initial peak, plasma insulin levels in normal subjects are quite low (Fig. 5), a reflection of the fact that intravenous glucose is normally a relatively poor stimulus to insulin secretion. These insulin levels would be expected to have a relatively small effect on skeletal muscle glucose uptake, and insulin sensitivity will play only a small part in determining overall tissue glucose uptake. The plasma glucose level, and the ability of glucose to promote its own uptake by a mass action effect, are major determinants of tissue glucose uptake under these conditions. As discussed below, the mass action effect of glucose appears to be normal in cirrhosis. The second reason for the normal glucose response to a continuous intravenous glucose infusion in cirrhotics is their much greater insulin response[26,36] (Fig. 5). Even if this has little effect on peripheral tissue glucose uptake, it will ensure sustained suppression of hepatic glucose output. In diabetic cirrhotics the glucose requirement during a hyperglycaemic clamp is reduced.[26] This is primarily due to a marked impairment of insulin secretion and failure to inhibit hepatic glucose output.[26]

Response to an oral glucose load in cirrhosis

To determine the contributions of diminished glucose removal and increased input of glucose into the systemic circulation (due to diminished first-pass hepatic uptake of glucose or impaired suppression of hepatic glucose output) after a 75 g oral glucose load, Kruszynska et al.[9] used oral 1-^{14}C-glucose and intravenous 6-^{3}H-glucose to quantify glucose appearance and disappearance rates. Fasting plasma glucose was similar in cirrhotics and controls, but the plasma glucose curves diverged after glucose ingestion, and continued to do so for 80 min (Fig. 6). For the first 20 min the divergence was due to a higher rate of appearance of the oral 1-^{14}C-glucose in the systemic circulation, suggesting less first-pass hepatic uptake of portal venous glucose. From 30 to 80 min the divergence was due to a lower rate of glucose disappearance in cirrhotics (Fig. 6), despite insulin levels that were three to six times higher in cirrhotics. There was no evidence that there was a lesser inhibition of hepatic glucose output following oral glucose in cirrhotics (Fig. 6). Reduced first-pass uptake of ingested glucose accounted for about

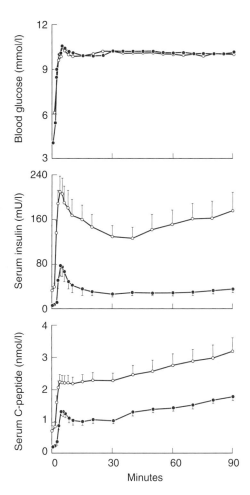

Fig. 5. Blood glucose, serum insulin, and C-peptide levels during a 10 mmol/l hyperglycaemic clamp in 10 cirrhotic patients (○) and 9 normal controls (●). Mean ± SEM. (Reproduced from ref. 36, with permission.)

one-third, and reduced glucose removal for about two-thirds, of the difference in the plasma glucose responses between cirrhotics and controls.

Glucose removal over the entire 4 h period after the glucose load was similar in cirrhotic (73 ± 4 g/4 h) and control patients (77 ± 2 g/4 h). This is in keeping with the forearm studies of Leatherdale and colleagues[28] who found normal forearm glucose uptake in cirrhotic patients following an oral glucose load (albeit at higher plasma glucose and insulin levels, both of which would promote tissue glucose utilization, thus compensating to some extent for tissue insulin resistance). The rise in glucose metabolic clearance rate after oral glucose reflects the enhancing effect of insulin on glucose uptake, and is largely independent of plasma glucose levels within the physiological range (Gottesman, Diabetes, 1984; 33:184). The much lower glucose metabolic clearance rate after oral glucose in cirrhotics (Fig. 6), despite three- to sixfold higher insulin levels, suggests marked insulin resistance; the relatively small difference in glucose utilization rates by comparison with glucose metabolic clearance rate, and the normal overall glucose utilization after oral glucose in cirrhotics, emphasizes the importance of hyperglycaemia in compensating for insulin resistance. As muscle is the main tissue to increase its rate of glucose uptake after

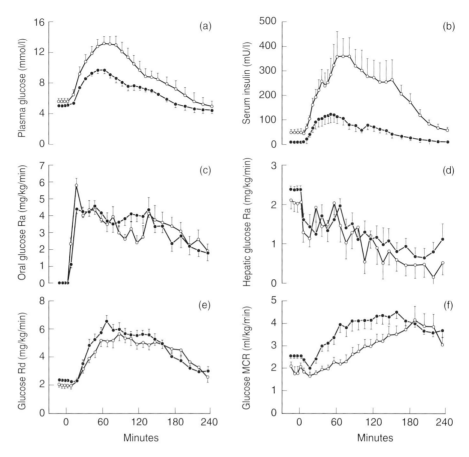

Fig. 6. Plasma glucose (a), serum insulin concentrations (b) and glucose kinetics (c to f) after ingestion of a 75 g glucose load in 8 cirrhotic patients (○) and 8 normal control subjects (●). Mean $\pm$ SEM. 6-3H-glucose was given as a constant intravenous infusion for 2 h before glucose ingestion and continued until the end of the study. The oral glucose load was labelled with 1-^{14}C-glucose so that its rate of appearance (Ra) in the systemic circulation (c) and the Ra of glucose coming from the liver (d) could be calculated. Rd = total rate of glucose disappearance from plasma (e). (f) Glucose metabolic clearance rate (MCR). (Reproduced from ref. 9, with permission.)

glucose ingestion, the findings indicate that skeletal muscle insulin resistance plays a key role in the oral glucose intolerance of cirrhosis.

Much of the enhanced glucose utilization after oral glucose is accounted for by increased glucose oxidation to provide energy that in the basal state was provided by lipid fuels. Additional energy is needed to support synthetic processes such as glycogen storage. Stimulation of glucose oxidation after oral glucose is normal in cirrhosis (Fig. 3). By contrast, enhancement of non-oxidative glucose disposal is impaired. This is particularly apparent when this is at a maximum after glucose ingestion (during the half-hour or so after peak plasma insulin and glucose levels); in our study, peak rates of non-oxidative glucose disposal were 37 per cent lower in cirrhotics than in controls.[9] Non-oxidative glucose disposal comprises glycogen synthesis and metabolism of glucose via glycolysis to lactate. During a euglycaemic clamp (see below) defects of non-oxidative glucose disposal are essentially due to impaired skeletal muscle glycogen deposition. However, after oral glucose, hyperglycaemia in cirrhosis results in increased lactate production by non-insulin-dependent tissues such as the gut, and defects of non-oxidative glucose disposal therefore underestimate the defect of muscle glycogen synthesis. Thus, although the overall impairment of non-oxidative glucose disposal after oral glucose may

be relatively small (Fig. 3), one would expect a larger defect of muscle glycogen deposition.

Insulin insensitivity

Tissue insensitivity to insulin is a major factor in the glucose intolerance of patients with acute and chronic forms of liver disease. Several points support this conclusion. First, impaired glucose tolerance is found despite elevated serum insulin levels, and forearm glucose uptake after oral glucose is no higher than in controls, despite hyperinsulinaemia and hyperglycaemia.[28] Secondly, the dual label studies of the disposition of a glucose load in cirrhosis,[9] discussed above, indicate that while both hepatic and peripheral tissue abnormalities contribute to the glucose intolerance in liver disease, peripheral tissue insulin insensitivity is quantitatively more important. Early studies showed that the hypoglycaemic response to exogenous insulin is diminished in cirrhotic patients (West, ClinEndoc, 1975; 4:573). The most convincing evidence of insulin insensitivity comes from studies using the hyperinsulinaemic glucose clamp technique, in which insulin sensitivity is defined in terms of the amount of glucose which must be infused to maintain a constant blood glucose level during a constant intravenous infusion of insulin. The near steady state achieved allows more detailed

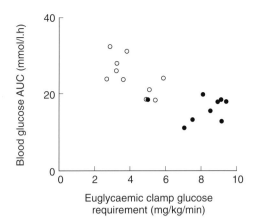

Fig. 7. Relationship between the area under the 3 h blood glucose concentration curve after 75 g oral glucose and the glucose requirement to maintain blood glucose levels at 4.0 mmol/l during a 0.1 U/kg/h hyperinsulinaemic glucose clamp (insulin sensitivity) in 10 cirrhotic patients (○) and 9 normal controls (●). For cirrhotic patients $r = -0.64$, $p < 0.05$. (Reproduced from ref. 36, with permission.)

glucose turnover and tissue studies to be performed at the same time. In most studies using this technique, insulin-mediated glucose disposal at high physiological insulin concentrations (50–150 mU/l) is 20 to 60 per cent lower in cirrhotic patients compared with normal controls;[21,24,26,36–39] at supraphysiological insulin levels (~1000 mU/l) some (Proietto, ClinEndoc, 1984; 21:677; Barzilai, JEndocrInv, 1991; 14:727) but not all[24] (Iversen, Gastro, 1984; 87:1138; Cavallo-Perin, JCI, 1985; 75:1659; Muller, AmJPhysiol, 1991; 260:E338) investigators have found normal rates of glucose disposal. The degree of oral glucose intolerance in non-diabetic cirrhotics is inversely related to their whole-body insulin sensitivity (Fig. 7).[36]

After an overnight fast, blood glucose levels and the rate of hepatic glucose output are normal in most cirrhotics, despite high fasting insulin levels[9,19,24–26] (Kaye, JHepatol, 1994; 20:782). This suggests hepatic insensitivity to insulin. However, because of capillarization of hepatic sinusoids and portosystemic shunting, it is not known whether the concentration of insulin at the hepatocyte surface is also increased. Petrides *et al.*[24] found hepatic sensitivity to insulin to be normal in non-diabetic cirrhotics with modestly raised fasting insulin levels; an increment of only 10 mU/l caused 50 per cent suppression of hepatic glucose output during a glucose clamp. The insulin levels generally used during a glucose clamp (50–150 mU/l) completely suppress hepatic glucose output in normal subjects and cirrhotics[24–26] (Kaye, JHepatol, 1994; 20:782). Diabetic cirrhotics, like patients with type II diabetes mellitus, show impaired suppression of hepatic glucose production during a glucose clamp.[26]

As hepatic glucose output is effectively suppressed during a hyperinsulinaemic euglycaemic clamp in normal and cirrhotic subjects, and as the liver takes up less than 10 per cent of the infused glucose (DeFronzo, Diabetes, 1983; 32:35), peripheral tissues (essentially skeletal muscle) must be responsible for the lower glucose utilization rate (i.e. insulin resistance) in cirrhotics; adipose tissue accounts for only a small proportion of glucose metabolism. Skeletal muscle has been confirmed to be the main site of insulin resistance during a glucose clamp in cirrhotics by dynamic positron emission

tomography (**PET**) scanning, which showed impaired accumulation in skeletal muscle of the glucose analogue 18-fluorodeoxyglucose.[39]

Most investigators have studied patients with alcoholic cirrhosis, many of whom will have continued to consume alcohol up to the time of investigation. Since alcohol itself decreases peripheral tissue sensitivity to insulin (Yki-Jarvinen, JClinEndoc, 1985; 61:941), continuing alcohol consumption might exacerbate any defect in peripheral tissue sensitivity resulting from liver disease *per se*. Furthermore, since muscle mass correlates with insulin sensitivity in normal subjects (Yki-Jarvinen, Diabetes, 1983; 32:965), the atrophy of type 2 muscle fibres found in two-thirds of chronic alcoholics (Martin, QJMed, 1985; 55:233) might contribute to insulin insensitivity. This atrophy is reversible with abstention from alcohol (Slavin, JClinPath, 1983; 36:772), which may explain why the impairment of insulin sensitivity (20 per cent decrease in clamp glucose disposal) in a small group of Child's A alcoholic cirrhotics who had abstained for 6 months or more was relatively mild.[38]

A more profound decrease in insulin sensitivity in alcoholic cirrhotics compared with patients with primary biliary cirrhosis[37] also suggests that additional factors operate in the alcoholic patient. Increased tissue iron deposition (Merkel, NEJM, 1988; 318:809) and malnutrition might be important. None the less, although the abnormalities may be more pronounced in the non-abstaining alcoholic cirrhotic, patients with other forms of cirrhosis in good nutritional state are undoubtedly insensitive to insulin[21,24,32,37] (Cavallo-Perin, JCI, 1985; 75:1659; Kaye, JHepatol, 1994; 20:782).

Oxidative and non-oxidative glucose disposal

Glucose taken up by muscle can either be stored as glycogen or converted to pyruvate, which in turn can be oxidized via the tricarboxylic acid cycle. The distribution of glucose between oxidative and non-oxidative pathways depends on glucose flux and hence on insulin concentration. At the insulin concentrations used for assessing *in vivo* insulin sensitivity, whole-body glucose oxidation represents the smaller part of intravenous glucose disposal in normal subjects (Thiebaud, Diabetes, 1982; 31:957; Lillioja, JCI, 1986; 62:922); in cirrhotics, however, who have a lower glucose flux, oxidation may be relatively more important. Direct measurement of skeletal muscle glycogen concentration in needle biopsy samples, taken from a group of well-nourished alcoholic cirrhotic patients before and after a glucose clamp, revealed a 29 per cent decrease in glycogen deposition compared to normal controls, and impaired activation of skeletal muscle glycogen synthase.[38] The clamp glucose requirement in these patients showed a strong relationship with both muscle glycogen deposition ($r = 0.78$) and glycogen synthase activity ($r = 0.82$). Assuming skeletal muscle to be 35 per cent of body mass, muscle glycogen appears to account for around 50 per cent of the glucose infused. As non-insulin-dependent glucose disposal would account for much of the remainder, the data suggest that under glucose clamp conditions peripheral insensitivity to insulin in alcoholic cirrhotics is determined predominantly by the pathway between plasma glucose and muscle glycogen. These conclusions are consistent with the findings of normal oxidative glucose disposal as measured by indirect calorimetry[24,26,39] (Muller, AmJPhysiol, 1991; 260:E338), and of normal skeletal muscle pyruvate dehydrogenase activity,[38] which is rate limiting for pyruvate oxidation.

At lower insulin infusion rates and in patients with more severe cirrhosis a defect in oxidative glucose metabolism might be apparent. However, it may be difficult to ascertain whether this represents an abnormality intrinsic to skeletal muscle, or whether it merely reflects differences in availability of non-esterified fatty acids. Suppression of plasma non-esterified fatty acids is impaired in cirrhotics at low insulin infusion rates, even though complete suppression is achieved at high physiological insulin levels[24] (Kaye, JHepatol, 1994; 20: 782). Increased availability of lipid fuels during low-dose hyper-insulinaemic glucose clamps could impair glucose oxidation (Robinson, PhysiolRev, 1980; 60:143; Lillioja, JCI, 1985; 75:1106; Kruszynska, DiabetAnn, 1995; 9:107), particularly in cirrhotics who derive more of their basal energy needs from the oxidation of non-esterified fatty acids and ketone bodies (see above). Continuing alcohol consumption might be associated with abnormalities of glucose oxidation as chronic alcohol abuse decreases mitochondrial volume fraction, and the activities of several glycolytic enzymes in skeletal muscle (Kiessling, ScaJCLI, 1975; 35:601).

Possible mechanisms for insulin insensitivity

The mechanism for insulin insensitivity in cirrhosis is unknown. It could be due to an abnormality at one or more levels:

1. It could be due to an abnormality of insulin transport from plasma into the interstitial space.
2. There could be an abnormality of insulin receptor function, of glucose transporters, and/or intracellular enzymes important for glucose metabolism.
3. The effect of insulin might be antagonized by increased circulating levels of hormones, metabolites (for example, non-esterified fatty acids), or cytokines that inhibit glucose uptake and metabolism.

Insulin distribution

For plasma insulin to stimulate peripheral tissue glucose uptake, insulin must first be transported across the capillary wall into the interstitial fluid in order to reach the receptors at the cell surface of target tissues. Changes in lymph (and hence interstitial fluid) insulin concentration lag behind those of plasma, and clamp glucose disposal rates correlate best with lymph insulin concentration, which is much lower than that of plasma, both in the basal state and during steady-state hyperinsulinaemia (Yang, JCI, 1989; 84:1620; Poulin, Diabetes, 1994; 43:180). These findings indicate that the transport step is rate limiting for insulin action during glucose clamps, and accounts for the delay in the peripheral action of insulin after intravenous injection. The gradient for insulin between plasma and the interstitial space implies that insulin is removed by the peripheral tissues on which it acts (as well as by the liver and kidneys).

Cirrhotic patients show a slower rise in the amount of glucose needed to keep blood glucose levels constant during a euglycaemic clamp; they take longer to reach a steady-state glucose requirement than control subjects.[32,36] Furthermore, after glucose ingestion there is a markedly delayed rise in glucose metabolic clearance rate, which cannot be explained by a delayed rise in the plasma insulin levels (Fig. 6).[9] Both peripheral tissue insensitivity to insulin and impaired insulin transport into the interstitial fluid would explain the plasma glucose and insulin responses of non-diabetic cirrhotics in response to oral and intravenous glucose, and also their reduced glucose disposal rates during a hyperinsulinaemic euglycaemic clamp. However, it is difficult to explain the marked delay in the apparent effect of insulin solely on the basis of peripheral tissue insensitivity to insulin, but it is easily explained if, in cirrhotics, there is impaired transport of insulin into the interstitial fluid; there would then be a slower rise in the interstitial fluid insulin concentration, particularly if insulin was also being removed from the interstitial space.

Whether the transfer of insulin from plasma to the interstitial fluid is governed solely by physical factors (blood flow, capillary density, molecular size, etc.) or whether endothelial insulin receptors (Bar, JClinEndoc, 1978; 47:699) also play a role is unclear. King and Johnson (Science, 1985; 227:1583) found that transport of insulin across cultured endothelial monolayers was saturable and unidirectional, and concluded that transendothelial insulin transport was mediated by endothelial insulin receptors. However, the transport of insulin across the capillary *in vivo* is not saturable; it is actually enhanced by pharmacological insulin levels, with a reduction in the steady-state plasma–interstitial fluid insulin gradient (Steil, JCI, 1996; 97:1497). This is strong evidence that transcapillary insulin transport is by diffusion, and not receptor mediated. Enhanced diffusionary transport at high insulin levels could be due to dilatation of capillaries or recruitment of new capillaries (Steil, JCI, 1996; 97:1497); muscle capillary density correlates with *in vivo* insulin sensitivity in normal subjects (Lillioja, JCI, 1987; 80:415). Insulin may augment muscle glucose uptake in part by increasing skeletal muscle blood flow (Laasko, JCI, 1990; 85:1844; Baron, AmJPhysiol, 1994; 266:E248), although not all investigators (Yki-Jarvinen, JCI, 1987; 79:1713; Natali, Diabetes, 1990; 39:490) support this view. An impairment of muscle microcirculatory regulation by insulin in cirrhosis could impair insulin transfer into the interstitium, resulting in a delayed and reduced effect of insulin on tissue glucose uptake.

Insulin receptors, glucose transporters, and intracellular enzymes

Most *in vitro* studies on the action of insulin have been performed on adipose tissue on the assumption that any abnormalities would also be found in skeletal muscle, and would be relevant to the insulin insensitivity of cirrhosis. In so far as the two tissues are exposed to similar regulatory signals, this may be a valid assumption. However, animal studies have demonstrated the heterogeneity of the effect of insulin on different tissues (Kraegen, Diabetolog, 1986; 29:192; Kraegen, AmJPhysiol, 1985; 248:E353), and regulation of glucose transporters differs in muscle and adipocytes (Garvey, Diabetes, 1992; 41:465; Fryer, DiabetNutrMetab, 1993; 6:241); abnormalities in adipocytes should be extrapolated to skeletal muscle with caution. Adipocyte studies have shown decreased sensitivity to insulin of glucose transport (Cavallo-Perin, JCI, 1985; 75:1659), and of lipogenesis[37] (Harewood, Metabolism, 1982; 31:1241). Skeletal muscle proteolysis may also be resistant to insulin (Marchesini, Hepatol, 1981; 1:294; McCullough, Gastro, 1992; 102:1325), although conclusions reached by various investigators depend on the denominator (body weight, lean body mass, etc.) used to express the data (McCullough, Gastro, 1992; 102:1325); interpretation is further complicated by the low plasma insulin-like growth factor-1 levels in cirrhosis (Chapter 25.2), which is an important determinant of muscle proteolytic rates (Chapter 2.13.1).

The finding of defects in insulin action in several biochemical pathways in muscle and adipocytes of cirrhotics suggests that an early step in the action of insulin is involved. Insulin initiates its action in target tissues by binding to its cell surface receptor—composed of two α-subunits (135 kDa) and two β-subunits (95 kDa) linked by disulphide bonds. The α-subunits are extracellular while the β-subunits span the membrane and have a large cytoplasmic domain. The α-subunits contain the insulin binding domain while the β-subunit contains the insulin-regulated tyrosine protein kinase activity which is essential both for transduction of the insulin signal and for internalization of the receptor and its bound insulin (McClain, JBC, 1987; 262:14663; Wilden, JBC, 1992; 267:13719; Cheatham, EndocrRev, 1995; 16:117). Only a fraction of surface receptors need be occupied by insulin to achieve a maximal effect. This fraction varies according to cell type, and the particular action of insulin. In muscle and adipocytes only 10 to 20 per cent of cell surface receptors need be occupied for maximal activation of glucose transport (Kolterman, ClinEndMetab, 1982; 11:363).

The binding of insulin to its receptor causes a conformational change in the receptor, and rapidly induces a cascade of tyrosine phosphorylation in the β-subunit; autophosphorylation of the insulin receptor β-subunit leads to full activation of the tyrosine kinase so that it can then phosphorylate tyrosine residues on intracellular phosphoprotein substrates such as insulin receptor substrate-1 (Sun, Nature, 1991; 352:73) that are involved in insulin signalling. Much still remains to be learnt before a clear picture emerges of how the early insulin signalling events are coupled to the various insulin-regulated enzymes, membrane transport systems, and insulin-responsive genes that mediate the metabolic and mitogenic effects of insulin. Different signalling pathways may mediate the different effects of insulin (for example, on glucose transport versus glycogen synthesis). Theoretically, insulin insensitivity could result from an abnormality of insulin binding due to decreased affinity of the receptor for insulin or to fewer receptors on target tissues. It could also result from alterations in signal transduction by the insulin–receptor complex, or alterations in any one of the post-receptor steps in insulin action.

Insulin binding to adipocytes from cirrhotic patients has been reported to be normal (Harewood, Metabolism, 1982; 31:1241) or decreased.[37] Taylor et al.[37] found a 16 per cent decrease in insulin binding to receptors at tracer insulin concentration (15 pmol/l, 3 mU/l) but not at the insulin concentration (300 pmol/l, 60 mU/l) used to measure in vivo insulin-mediated glucose disposal; their data suggested a decrease in receptor number but normal affinity for insulin. Although insulin binding at tracer insulin concentrations in these cirrhotic patients correlated with in vivo insulin sensitivity ($r = 0.63$), this was largely accounted for by patients with alcoholic cirrhosis. Patients with primary biliary cirrhosis and cryptogenic cirrhosis had normal insulin binding but marked peripheral tissue insensitivity to insulin under glucose clamp conditions. These findings and the lack of correlation between insulin binding to adipocyte receptors and abnormalities of insulin-stimulated lipogenesis in these cells, suggest that abnormalities of insulin binding to receptors do not play a major role in the tissue insensitivity to insulin in cirrhotics. Post-binding insulin receptor functions (tyrosine kinase activity, endocytosis, phosphorylation of

intermediate signalling molecules) have not been studied in cirrhosis. Normal insulin binding does not exclude defects in these functions which could clearly impair insulin signal transduction.

Glucose transporter abnormalities could explain insulin resistance as glucose transport is normally rate-limiting for glucose utilization in skeletal muscle and adipocytes. Selberg,[39] using PET scanning, found that the impairment of skeletal muscle, and hence whole-body, glucose disposal during a hyperinsulinaemic glucose clamp in cirrhotics was associated with an impairment of glucose transport; phosphorylation of incoming glucose appeared to be normal. An important determinant of insulin's effect on glucose transport is its ability to recruit glucose transporters (specifically Glut 4) from an intracellular pool to their site of action in the plasma membrane. Normal Glut 4 levels were found in skeletal muscle and adipose tissue from cirrhotics undergoing transplantation or an elective shunt for prevention of variceal bleeding (Kruszynska, JHepatol, 1993; 18:S12); insulin-stimulated Glut 4 translocation in adipocytes was also normal but there have been no studies on their function in muscle.

The function of insulin receptors and of glucose transporters is influenced by their membrane lipid environment (Gould, JBC, 1982; 257:477; Sweet, FASEB, 1987; 1:55). Cirrhotic patients have abnormalities of membrane lipid composition due to disturbed metabolism of polyunsaturated fatty acids and plasma lipoproteins (Chapter 2.12). Characteristically, there is an increase in cholesterol/phospholipid and phosphatidylcholine/sphingomyelin ratios, and in the proportion of saturated long-chain fatty acids. Membrane fluidity is decreased (Owen, JLipRes, 1982; 23:124). These changes might be expected to influence tissue insulin sensitivity. The observation that ethanol increases the cholesterol/phospholipid ratio in membranes, and decreases synthesis of polyunsaturated fatty acids by inhibiting liver microsomal δ-5 and δ-6 desaturase activities (Nervi, Lipids, 1980; 15:263), might explain the more marked insulin insensitivity in patients with alcoholic liver disease, including those with fatty liver. In non-alcoholic liver disease, and in abstinent alcoholic cirrhotics, there is little support for the hypothesis that the membrane lipid changes are causally related to insulin insensitivity. The membrane lipid abnormalities do not correlate with in vivo insulin sensitivity (Barzilai, JEndocrInv, 1991; 14:727); they tend to be more pronounced in cholestatic liver disease, and in patients with decompensated hepatocellular disease (Child–Pugh classes B and C), whereas insulin resistance is more marked in patients with hepatocellular disease and is unrelated to severity of liver disease (Muller, Gastro, 1992; 102:2033).

There is no evidence for a primary abnormality of insulin-regulated enzymes in cirrhosis Glycogen synthase and pyruvate dehydrogenase are the two key insulin-regulated enzymes controlling glycogen synthesis and glucose oxidation. Muscle pyruvate dehydrogenase is normal.[38] Activation of glycogen synthase by insulin is impaired, but this is not due to an abnormality of the enzyme because full activation by glucose 6-phosphate can be achieved in vitro.[38]

Insulin antagonists

The effect of insulin might be expected to be antagonized by increased circulating levels of hormones and metabolites (for example, non-esterified fatty acids) or cytokines (for example, tumour necrosis factor-α) that inhibit glucose uptake and metabolism.

Serum concentrations of glucagon[21,25] (Dudley, Gut, 1979; 20:817; Marchesini, Hepatol, 1981; 1:294), growth hormone[21,40] (Stewart, EurJClinInv, 1983; 13:397; Donaghy, Hepatol, 1995; 21: 680), and catecholamines (Ring-Larsen, Hepatol, 1982; 2:304; Silva, JHepatol, 1988; 6:325) are increased in patients with cirrhosis. Levels are similar to those shown to inhibit the suppression of hepatic glucose production by insulin and to reduce peripheral glucose uptake in normal humans (Rizza, Diabetes, 1982; 31:663; Lager, Diabetolog, 1986; 29:409; Del Prato, JCI, 1987; 79:547; Orskov, JClinEndoc, 1989; 68:276; Moller, Metabolism, 1992; 41: 172). These hormones might therefore contribute to insulin resistance and glucose intolerance in cirrhosis. However, there is little direct evidence to support this hypothesis. Increased fasting glucagon concentrations are not associated with increased hepatic glucose production, or elevated fasting blood glucose concentrations, suggesting hepatic insensitivity to glucagon. Resistance to glucagon in cirrhosis is also suggested by the impaired stimulation of hepatic glucose output during intravenous infusions of glucagon[21] (Keller, JClinEndoc, 1982; 54:961; Petrides, Metabolism, 1994; 43:85). Hypersecretion of glucagon in cirrhosis (Sherwin, Gastro, 1978; 74:1224; Greco, Diabetolog, 1979; 17:23; Kruszynska, Hepatol, 1995; 22:441A) thus seems an unlikely cause of the glucose intolerance.

Growth hormone shifts fuel utilization from glucose to lipid. High physiological concentrations of growth hormone increase lipolysis and serum non-esterified fatty acids and ketone body levels. Lipid oxidation is increased at the expense of glucose oxidation, and insulin-stimulated muscle glucose uptake and glycogen synthesis are impaired (Moller, AmJPhysiol, 1990; 258:E86; Moller, JClinEndoc, 1990; 70:1179; Bak, AmJPhysiol, 1991; 260:E736). These effects of growth hormone bear some resemblance to the abnormalities in cirrhotic patients. Because the abnormalities of carbohydrate metabolism in cirrhosis do not correlate with basal serum growth hormone concentrations, growth hormone has been considered to be unimportant as a cause of insulin resistance in cirrhosis. However, it is important to note that growth hormone secretion is pulsatile (Chapter 25.2), that the metabolic effects are seen 2 to 4 h after a rise in growth hormone levels, and that they persist for several hours after growth hormone levels return to basal. Thus, even if there were a relationship, it would be difficult to demonstrate it in studies measuring a single basal growth hormone level. Shmueli et al.[40] found that suppression of plasma growth hormone levels for 5 h had no effect on whole-body insulin sensitivity or forearm glucose uptake during a hyperinsulinaemic euglycaemic clamp. Furthermore, suppression of growth hormone with somatostatin did not lower the elevated fasting non-esterified fatty acid levels in cirrhotic patients. Petrides (Hepatol, 1995; 22:238A) found that a 4-day subcutaneous infusion of octreotide increased insulin sensitivity in cirrhotics. He suggested that suppression of insulin secretion and systemic insulin levels explained the improvement. However, suppression of growth hormone secretion may be a more likely explanation.

The role of catecholamines in the glucose intolerance of liver disease has not been addressed. However, the observation of tissue resistance to catecholamines suggests that they do not play a major role.

Increased availability of non-esterified fatty acids has been suggested to play a role in the insulin resistance of cirrhosis by competing with glucose for oxidative metabolism (Randle, Lancet, 1963; i:785; Kruszynska, DiabetAnn, 1995; 9:107). Adipose tissue lipolysis is less sensitive to insulin in cirrhotics than in normal subjects.[24] However, after oral glucose, plasma non-esterified fatty acid levels usually show normal suppression, albeit at higher plasma glucose and insulin levels (Collins, ArchIntMed, 1970; 126: 608).[9] Moreover, at the insulin infusion rates used to measure insulin sensitivity during a glucose clamp there is normal suppression of plasma non-esterified fatty acids in cirrhosis, and there is no correlation between non-esterified fatty acid turnover or lipid oxidation and the glucose requirement during the clamp (Kaye, JHepatol, 1994; 20:782). These findings suggest that increased availability of fatty acids does not explain the insulin insensitivity of cirrhosis.

A number of cytokines, particularly tumour necrosis factor-α can cause insulin resistance and glucose intolerance (Lang, Endocrinol, 1992; 130:430; Hotamsligil, Science, 1996; 271:665). Production of tumour necrosis factor-α is increased in patients with cirrhosis due to alcohol or viral infection (Yoshioka, Hepatol, 1989; 10:769). Although serum levels are usually normal, local tissue production of tumour necrosis factor-α could impair tissue sensitivity to insulin (Hotamsligil, JCI, 1995; 95:2409; Saghizadeh, JCI, 1996; 97:1111).

Effect of hyperglycaemia on glucose disposal in cirrhosis

During a hyperglycaemic clamp the ability of hyperglycaemia to promote whole-body and forearm glucose uptake, in the presence of fasting insulin concentrations, is normal in non-diabetic cirrhotics[27] (Vetter, GastrClinBiol, 1990; 14:483; Petrides, Hepatol, 1993; 18:284). Petrides et al. (Hepatol, 1993; 18:284) suggested that it might be impaired in cirrhotics with overt diabetes. However, interpretation of their data is difficult because they clamped blood glucose at a higher level in the diabetic cirrhotics (15.9 mmol/l) than in controls (11.9 mmol/l) or non-diabetic cirrhotics (11.8 mmol/l). The effect of a 6.9 mmol/l increment in the blood glucose level on glucose uptake would be expected to be less at higher glucose levels (i.e. in the diabetic patients) because of the curvilinear relationship between glucose uptake and plasma glucose concentration (Gottesman, Diabetes, 1984; 33:184). Furthermore, insulin levels were maintained at basal levels in the controls but reduced by half in the diabetic cirrhotics. The effects of these hormonal peturbations on glucose kinetics were not assessed independently of hyperglycaemia. The reduction in insulin levels might have impaired glucose utilization (Baron, JCI, 1985; 76:1782) and contributed to the lower enhancement of glucose uptake by hyperglycaemia in the diabetic cirrhotics (Petrides, Hepatol, 1993; 18:284).

In the presence of basal insulin levels, hyperglycaemia will also suppress hepatic glucose production. The ability of hyperglycaemia to inhibit hepatic glucose output and to promote glucose uptake has been termed 'glucose effectiveness' (S_G). It can be assessed by Bergman's 'minimal model' of plasma insulin and glucose kinetics during a frequently sampled, 3-hour-long intravenous glucose tolerance test (Bergman, Diabetes, 1989, 38.1512). S_G takes into account the effect of hyperglycaemia on hepatic glucose output, and not just its ability to promote tissue uptake of glucose (Cobelli,

AmJPhysiol, 1986; 250:E591). Thus, in subjects in whom suppression of hepatic glucose output by insulin (+ hyperglycaemia) is normal, S_G may be a reasonable index of the ability of glucose to promote tissue uptake by a mass action effect; this is not true in diabetic patients (with or without cirrhosis) because basal hepatic glucose output is increased and its suppression impaired.[26]

Cirrhotics with normal fasting blood glucose levels (but postprandial hyperglycaemia) have a normal S_G.[32] In diabetic cirrhotics we found S_G to be reduced by 29 per cent.[32] Most of our non-diabetic cirrhotics had a K_G greater than 1.0 while seven out of eight of our diabetic cirrhotics had a K_G below 1.0. A K_G below 1.0 is usually taken to indicate the presence of diabetes (Brunzell, JClinEndoc, 1976; 42:222; Chapter 25.2). Two of our cirrhotic patients had a fasting blood glucose less than 6.7 mmol/l but a K_G below 1.0; these patients also had a very low S_G.[32] Two other studies used Bergman's minimal model to measure S_G in cirrhosis.[34,35] Marchesini et al.[34] reported a reduction in S_G in 'non-diabetic cirrhotics'. However, four of their nine cirrhotics had a K_G below 1.0. Regression analysis of their data showed a strong relationship between S_G and K_G ($r = 0.8$, $p < 0.01$), and S_G in the five subjects with a K_G above 1.0 was similar to that of controls. In the study of Letiehxe et al.[35] S_G in cirrhotics with normal fasting glucose levels tended to be lower than in controls but the difference was not significant. K_G in their cirrhotics was about 50 per cent of that of controls; on the basis of the K_G value some were probably diabetic. As in the other studies, S_G was related to K_G ($r = 0.07$, $p < 0.05$).

The three studies using the minimal model are consistent in that non-diabetic cirrhotics have a normal S_G; diabetic cirrhotics with elevated fasting blood glucose and a K_G below 1.0 have a reduced S_G.[32,34,35] A reduced S_G is also found in cirrhotics with normal fasting blood glucose but a K_G below 1.0, a group that is probably diabetic. The reduced S_G in diabetic cirrhotics is likely to be due to impaired suppression of hepatic glucose output. Hyperglycaemia suppresses hepatic glucose output only if there is adequate basal hepatic insulinization; complete suppression requires an accompanying increase in insulin delivery. Fasting hyperglycaemia in diabetic cirrhotics is due mainly to an increase in hepatic glucose output implying inadequate basal hepatic insulin delivery. In addition they lose their acute insulin response to intravenous glucose (see Chapter 25.2) which is important for the suppression of hepatic glucose output after an intravenous glucose bolus (Luzi, AmJPhysiol, 1989; 257:E241). One would therefore expect less suppression of hepatic glucose output in the diabetic cirrhotics, and hence a lower S_G. It remains to be seen whether a defect in the ability of glucose to promote peripheral tissue uptake also contributes to their reduction in S_G. It is relevant that the ability of hyperglycaemia to promote whole-body or forearm glucose uptake in patients with type II diabetes without liver disease is normal (Baron, JCI, 1985; 76:1782), yet they have a reduced S_G (Bergman, Diabetes, 1989; 38: 1512).

Since both glucose effectiveness (from the minimal model) and the ability of hyperglycaemia to promote glucose uptake at near basal insulin levels are normal in non-diabetic cirrhotics, one would expect their higher plasma glucose levels after glucose ingestion to compensate for tissue insulin resistance, so that the overall glucose use may be near normal, at least in quantitative terms (Fig. 6).[9, 28]

Hepatic factors and portosystemic shunting

There is little evidence that decreased hepatic parenchymal mass per se is an important cause of glucose intolerance, although it might be important in the presence of other factors. Architectural disorganization, pericellular collagen deposition, decreased hepatic blood flow, and decreased portal blood flow may all limit access of substrates and hormones to hepatocytes. The importance of sinusoidal and intracellular glucose concentrations, in regulating the enzymes of glycogen synthesis and breakdown, and in determining the net direction of glucose carbon flux, was discussed earlier. Clearly, decreased portal delivery of glucose might impair glycogen synthesis,[14] a defect that would be compounded by the decreased capacity to phosphorylate glucose to glucose 6-phosphate because of decreased hepatic glucokinase activity in cirrhosis (Sotaniemi, JHepatol, 1985; 1:277). The effect on hepatic metabolism of distortion of normal oxygen, substrate, and hormonal gradients within the liver lobule is discussed in Chapter 2.18.

Portosystemic shunting in chronic liver disease might be expected to contribute to glucose intolerance because of shunting of either glucose or insulin directly into the systemic circulation. With portal hypertension, the liver receives more of its blood flow from the hepatic artery, and is thus exposed to lower concentrations of both insulin and glucose. However, portal insulin delivery may be less important for normal glucose tolerance than previously thought; animals with peripheral insulin delivery have normal glucose tolerance (Waddell, JApplPhysiol, 1967; 22:808; Kruszynska, Diabetolog, 1985; 28:167; Kryshak, Diabetes, 1990; 39:142).

Shunting of glucose appears to be more important. The concentration of glucose in the portal vein is an important determinant of the direction of hepatic glucose flux and the extent of uptake of glucose by the liver.[13,14] However, first-pass hepatic uptake of glucose is normally relatively small ($\sim$10 per cent of an oral glucose load) so that shunting of glucose has been considered to be unimportant in the glucose intolerance of cirrhosis. However, portosystemic shunting does explain the faster rise in blood glucose levels in cirrhotics after oral glucose because first-pass uptake is relatively more important early after glucose ingestion (see earlier); decreased first-pass hepatic uptake of ingested glucose accounted for one-third of the greater rise in plasma glucose levels in cirrhotic patients compared to normal control subjects (see above) (Fig. 6).[9] The lower first-pass hepatic uptake of glucose in cirrhotics was apparent only during the first 20 min, corresponding to the period of maximal first-pass uptake in normal subjects; the total amount of ingested glucose removed on first pass over 4 h was not different from that of controls (8.3–13.2 per cent versus 7.7–12.8 per cent, respectively). These results are not inconsistent with earlier studies showing normal glucose tolerance (but somewhat higher glucose levels compared with normal subjects) in patients with portacaval shunts but without liver disease[41] (Smith-Laing, Gastro, 1979; 76:685), and normal glucose tolerance after portacaval anastomosis in rats (Assal, Metabolism, 1971; 20:850). If insulin sensitivity is normal, the peripheral hyperinsulinaemia associated with portosystemic shunting will enhance peripheral glucose disposal and minimize the effect of reduced first-pass uptake on plasma glucose levels. It is likely that in the presence of peripheral tissue insulin resistance in cirrhotics, impaired first-pass hepatic uptake of ingested glucose becomes quantitatively more important in terms of the plasma glucose response. Portosystemic shunting may alter the distribution of glucose between liver and peripheral tissues. Cherrington et al.[13, 14] found that in dogs although portal glucose delivery stimulated direct uptake of glucose by the liver, it did not increase whole-body glucose disposal. This implies a redistribution of glucose away from peripheral tissues toward the liver. Portosystemic shunting in liver disease might thus be an important mechanism of the impaired hepatic synthesis and storage of glycogen.[22]

The lack of deterioration of glucose tolerance in cirrhotic patients after portacaval anastomosis might be explained by the fact that they were already glucose intolerant with a degree of shunting preoperatively (Conn, DigDis, 1971; 16:227; Holdsworth, Gut, 1972; 13:58; Shurberg, Gastro, 1977; 72:301; Dudley, Gut, 1979; 20:817). Studies in dogs have given conflicting results. Lickley et al. (Metabolism, 1975; 24:1157) observed a deterioration in oral glucose tolerance after end to side portacaval anastomosis, whereas Waddell and Sussman (JApplPhysiol, 1967; 22:808) found blood glucose levels after shunting to be lower than in control dogs. In view of the marked species variation in the response to portacaval shunting, animal experiments should be interpreted with caution. The dog often shows marked anorexia and wasting after portacaval shunting, which may cause some of the ensuing metabolic abnormalities and liver glycogen depletion (Sexton, SurgForum, 1964; 15:120).

Portosystemic shunting may influence plasma levels of substrates and hormones that have been implicated in insulin resistance, and thus indirectly impair peripheral tissue sensitivity to insulin. Portosystemic shunting decreases hepatic clearance of non-esterified fatty acids and may thus increase arterial non-esterified fatty acid levels but there is little support for a role of non-esterified fatty acids in the glucose intolerance of cirrhosis. Perhaps of greater significance is the effect of portosystemic shunting on hepatic production of insulin-like growth factor-1 and hence growth hormone (Chapter 25.2), which may play a role in the insulin resistance and glucose intolerance. Portosystemic shunting may result in hepatic underinsulinization despite high systemic insulin levels, and this could impair hepatic insulin-like growth factor-1 production in cirrhosis (Chapter 25.2); low insulin-like growth factor-1 may increase growth hormone levels indirectly (Chapter 25.2). Glucagon hypersecretion correlates with the extent of portosystemic shunting (Sherwin, Gastro, 1978; 74:1224) but, as discussed above, is not thought to play a role in the glucose intolerance of cirrhosis. However, the very high glucagon levels found in some overtly diabetic cirrhotic patients (Chapter 25.2) could contribute to the increased basal rates of hepatic glucose production, and their impaired suppression of hepatic glucose output after glucose ingestion or intravenous insulin.[26]

Available data suggest that portosystemic shunting in cirrhosis may play a role in the presence of decreased peripheral tissue sensitivity to insulin or impaired insulin secretion.

Insulin secretion (see Chapter 25.2)

Impaired insulin secretion is central to the development of overt diabetes, and is also important in those with pancreatic damage due to alcohol or haemochromatosis (Chapter 25.2). Decreased insulin secretion has also been suggested to contribute to the glucose intolerance seen in chronic active hepatitis (Alberti, ClinSci, 1972;

42:591) and in some patients with viral hepatitis (Chupin, Diabetes, 1978; 27:661). However, insulin secretory abnormalities have not been considered important in most cirrhotics with normal fasting glucose levels, because their fasting and postprandial insulin levels are increased two- to sixfold. Recent studies indicate that this view is incorrect. Peripheral insulin concentrations are a poor index of insulin secretion because the liver removes a large (about 60 per cent) and variable amount of the insulin secreted into the portal vein (Blackard, Diabetes, 1970; 19:302). Furthermore, hepatic extraction of insulin falls in cirrhosis due to portosystemic shunting or hepatocellular dysfunction (Chapter 25.2). Thus, peripheral hyperinsulinaemia in cirrhosis does not necessarily imply increased insulin secretion. Since C-peptide is co-secreted from the islet β-cell in equimolar amounts with insulin, but not significantly extracted by the liver, insulin secretion rates can be estimated from peripheral C-peptide concentrations and clearance. Studies employing serum C-peptide measurements indicate that insulin secretion is an important determinant of the presence of normal or impaired glucose tolerance in cirrhotics with normal fasting blood glucose levels. Cirrhotics with overt diabetes have striking abnormalities of insulin secretion. These are discussed in Chapter 25.2.

Fasting

Fasting peripheral plasma insulin concentrations are generally increased in cirrhotics,[9,32-41] with either normal or increased C-peptide concentrations. The C-peptide/insulin molar ratio is, however, decreased even in patients with increased plasma C-peptide levels. indicating that fasting insulin secretion is generally normal or increased, and that decreased hepatic extraction of insulin contributes to fasting hyperinsulinaemia. Early suggestions that the hyperinsulinaemia is partly due to increased concentrations of proinsulin in cirrhosis (Kasperska-Czyzykowa, Diabetolog, 1983; 25:506) have not been confirmed by studies employing proinsulin-specific antibodies (Ballmann, ClinEndoc, 1986; 25:351; Kruszynska, Metabolism, 1995; 44:254).

Insulin secretion in response to intravenous glucose and non-glucose secretagogues

Insulin secretion is usually increased in non-diabetic cirrhotics in response to intravenous glucose given as a bolus or as a constant infusion.[26,32,34-36] During a 10 mmol/l hyperglycaemic clamp, which has the advantage that the plasma glucose level can be precisely controlled, insulin secretion rates are approximately twice those of normal control subjects (Fig. 6).[36] Insulin secretory capacity measured at maximally stimulating glucose concentrations (25–30 mmol/l) is also increased (Kruszynska, Hepatol, 1995; 22: 238A). Insulin secretion to non-glucose secretagogues such as tolbutamide and arginine increases with the prevailing plasma glucose level. The acute (incremental) insulin secretory response to arginine or tolbutamide measured at basal plasma glucose levels is usually normal in non-diabetic cirrhotics, although decreased responses have also been found. Two studies found subnormal portal vein insulin concentrations in cirrhotics given intravenous glucose, arginine, or tolbutamide, suggesting impaired insulin secretion (Greco, Diabetolog, 1979; 17:23; Pelkonen, ActaEnd, 1981; 97:496). Fasting blood glucose levels were normal in both studies. However, the patients studied by Greco (Diabetolog, 1979; 17:23) had a

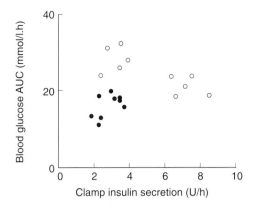

Fig. 8. Relationship between the area under the 3 h blood glucose concentration curve after 75 g oral glucose and the amount of insulin secreted between $+30$ and $+90$ min of a 10 mmol/l hyperglycaemic clamp (see Fig.5) in 10 cirrhotic patients ($\bigcirc$) and 9 normal controls ($\bullet$). For cirrhotic patients, $r = -0.76$, $p < 0.02$. (Reproduced from ref. 36, with permission.)

K_G of only 0.67 ± 0.2 per cent/min after intravenous glucose, suggesting that they were probably diabetic (see Chapter 25.2). The cirrhotics studied by Pelkonen (ActaEnd, 1981; 97:496) were somewhat unusual in that their fasting plasma insulin and C-peptide levels were not increased.

Cirrhotic patients with increased insulin secretion to glucose *per se* also have a greater insulin secretory response to intravenous tolbutamide or arginine when this is measured at elevated glucose levels, implying a greater enhancement of the response by glucose in cirrhotics (Kruszynska, Hepatol, 1995; 22:238A).

Insulin secretion in response to intravenous glucose and non-glucose secretagogues varies widely. Some patients have insulin secretion rates to intravenous glucose similar to those of control subjects while others have secretion rates three to four times higher.[36] Those patients with 'normal' insulin secretion rates have a greater degree of oral glucose intolerance (Fig. 8).

Insulin secretion after oral glucose

Peripheral plasma insulin levels are increased in cirrhotic patients after oral glucose; however, plasma C-peptide concentrations and insulin secretion increase more slowly in cirrhotics, and during the first hour, despite higher glucose levels, are similar to those of normal subjects (Fig. 9).[36,37,41,42] The early hyperinsulinaemia after glucose ingestion is essentially due to decreased hepatic extraction of insulin. By contrast with the increased maximal insulin secretion rates seen with intravenous glucose, peak insulin secretion rates after oral glucose are similar in cirrhotics and normal subjects (Fig. 9).[42] The greater overall insulin output after glucose ingestion in cirrhotics is essentially due to insulin secretion remaining elevated for longer, because of the greater and more prolonged elevation in plasma glucose levels. The slow increase in insulin secretion after oral glucose is similar to that seen in patients with mild type II diabetes.

As with intravenous glucose, insulin secretion rates after glucose ingestion vary widely. The blunting of the initial C-peptide response after oral glucose is due mainly to those cirrhotics with 'normal' insulin secretion rates to intravenous glucose (during a hyperglycaemic clamp). These cirrhotics have a greater degree of oral

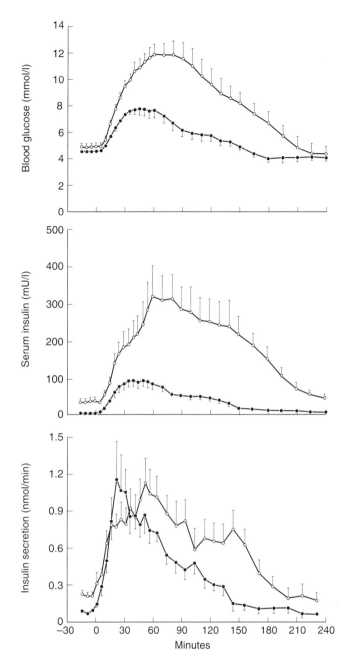

Fig. 9. Blood glucose, serum insulin, and insulin secretion rates after a 75 g oral glucose load in 10 cirrhotic patients ($\bigcirc$—$\bigcirc$) and 10 normal controls ($\bullet$—$\bullet$). Mean $\pm$ SEM. Insulin secretion rates were calculated from serum C-peptide levels by a two-compartment model[42] using C-peptide kinetic parameters that had been determined in each individual on a separate day by bolus intravenous injection of human C-peptide. Note that despite the higher glucose levels, insulin secretion rates were not increased in cirrhotics during the first hour after glucose ingestion. (Reproduced from ref. 42, with permission.)

glucose intolerance, suggesting that the blunted early response is important. Possible explanations for the blunted early insulin response to oral glucose are: diminished islet β-cell response to gut hormones (glucose-dependent insulinotropic peptide and glucagon-like peptide-1 [7–36 amide]) that enhance insulin secretion after glucose ingestion (see Chapter 25.2) or a parasympathetic autonomic neuropathy.

There seems little doubt that abnormalities of insulin secretion contribute to oral glucose intolerance in some cirrhotic patients. Whether these patients will, in the long-term, go on to develop more marked abnormalities of insulin secretion and overt diabetes is unclear. It is also unclear whether the abnormalities are primary or secondary to hyperglycaemia, alcohol, malnutrition, or other factors. Chronic hyperglycaemia may cause a reversible impairment of glucose-stimulated insulin secretion (Leahy, JCI, 1986; 77:908; Rossetti, JCI, 1987; 80:1037). Elevated fatty acid levels have also been implicated in the deterioration of islet β-cell function in insulin-resistant states (Unger, Diabetes, 1995; 44:863).

Most studies have contained many alcoholic cirrhotics and numbers have generally been too small for adequate analysis of subgroups. Since chronic alcohol abuse may itself be associated with a reversible impairment of insulin secretion (Sereny, Metabolism, 1978; 27:1041), continuing alcohol consumption may contribute to the insulin secretory defect and glucose intolerance. However, the insulin secretory abnormality is not confined to alcoholic cirrhotics.

Glucose intolerance after energy deprivation is well recognized and is due primarily to impaired insulin secretion. Poor nutrition is common in patients with liver disease; particularly in those with alcohol-related disease (Chapter 29.2), and in those with complications (ascites, recurrent infections, bleeding) requiring dietary restrictions or repeated hospital admission. Malnutrition may thus contribute to impaired insulin secretion and glucose intolerance in some patients. Pezarossa and colleagues (Metabolism, 1986; 35:984) reported improved insulin secretion and glucose tolerance after calorie supplementation in alcoholics without liver disease, irrespective of continued alcohol consumption. Inadequate dietary intake may also contribute to potassium depletion which is found in many patients with alcoholic cirrhosis, and which might also impair insulin secretion and glucose tolerance. Conn (AmJMedSci, 1970; 259:394) and Podolsky (NEJM, 1973; 288:644) found that dietary potassium supplementation (120–180 mmol/day) improved glucose tolerance in approximately 50 per cent of alcoholic cirrhotics with glucose intolerance. As glucose intolerance is also found in patients with liver disease in good nutritional state, and who are not potassium depleted, other factors must also be involved.

Insulin resistance is the main cause of oral glucose intolerance in cirrhotics with normal fasting blood glucose levels. However, because many normal subjects show a degree of peripheral tissue insulin resistance comparable to that found in cirrhotic patients, other factors must also play a role (Reaven, Diabetes, 1988; 37: 1595). Insulin-resistant normal subjects maintain normal glucose tolerance by hypersecretion of insulin. Some cirrhotics compensate for insulin resistance by secreting more insulin. Those cirrhotics who cannot augment their insulin response to intravenous glucose and have a blunted early insulin response to oral glucose develop impaired glucose tolerance. It is unclear whether they are at risk of developing overt diabetes. Further studies are needed to clarify the relationship of glucose intolerance to abnormalities of tissue insulin sensitivity and impaired insulin secretion. Portosystemic shunting explains the faster rise in blood glucose levels in cirrhotics during the first 20 min after glucose ingestion. Poor nutrition, although unlikely to be of primary importance in the pathogenesis of glucose intolerance, may compound the metabolic disturbance.

Metabolic response to exercise in liver disease

Relatively little work has been done on the metabolic response to physical activity in liver disease. Fatigue and asthenia are common symptoms, and exercise endurance is decreased. The maximal work capacity is reduced and is inversely related to severity of liver disease as assessed by the Child–Pugh score (Campillo, JHepatol, 1990; 10:163). The anaerobic threshold is lower implying a decreased capacity for oxidative metabolism. Possible aetiological factors include bed rest, muscle disuse, acute illness, anaemia, and malnutrition (Barac-Nieto, AmJClinNutr, 1980; 33:2268). Impaired oxygen delivery to working muscles due to impaired cardiovascular responses to exercise (Grose, JHepatol, 1995; 22:326; Iwao, AmJGastr, 1994; 89:1043) may be important in some patients. In addition, some cirrhotics have arterial hypoxaemia (Chapter 25.1), with a further drop in arterial Pao_2 during physical activity (Kennedy, Chest, 1977; 72:305; Agusti, AmRevRespDis, 1989; 139:485; Thorens, EurRespJ, 1992; 5:754). However, in most patients the reduced aerobic capacity seems to be due primarily to alterations of muscle metabolism and/or substrate supply.

Moller (ScaJGastr, 1984; 19:267) found a reduction in skeletal muscle ATP levels and an increased ADP/ATP ratio in overnight-fasted, resting cirrhotics despite normal glycogen levels and modestly reduced phosphocreatine levels. These changes suggest a defect in muscle oxidative metabolism. Maintenance of a higher cytosolic ADP concentration, at rest and during exercise in cirrhotics, may be important for maintaining normal rates of ATP synthesis in the presence of an oxidative defect (Brindle, Biochem, 1989; 28:4887; Radda, FASEBJ, 1992; 6:3032).

Hepatic glycogen stores and an appropriate increase in hepatic glucose output are important determinants of exercise endurance and aerobic capacity (Zinker, JApplPhysiol, 1990; 69:1849). Impaired hepatic release of glucose in response to increased physical activity is likely to contribute to the poor exercise tolerance and reduced aerobic capacity of cirrhotic patients. In the fasted state this may be due to reduced liver glycogen stores and/or impaired glycogenolytic response to glucagon and catecholamines (see above). In the postprandial state, high plasma insulin levels may further impair the hepatic response to exercise.

One would expect the metabolic response of overnight-fasted cirrhotics to resemble that of normal subjects after a prolonged fast (Zinker, JApplPhysiol, 1990; 69:1849). The data of DeLissio and colleagues[43] support this hypothesis. They studied four overnight-fasted cirrhotic patients during a 90 min period on a treadmill at 50 per cent of each individual's predetermined Vo_{2max}. Maximal work capacity (Vo_{2max}) was 34 per cent lower in the cirrhotics than controls. Cirrhotic patients showed no enhancement of glucose uptake from plasma and no increase in hepatic glucose production (even after 90 min). By contrast, circulating glucose utilization and hepatic glucose output increased by two- to 2.5-fold in the normal control subjects. Plasma glucose levels remained constant during exercise in both groups. Plasma non-esterified fatty acids and ketone body levels were higher in the cirrhotic patients before and during exercise, and they derived a greater proportion of their total energy needs from the oxidation of fat. Since the proportion of energy derived from carbohydrate increases with increasing intensity of physical activity (Fig. 2), limitation in circulating glucose supply could contribute to the reduction in $V_{O_{2max}}$ and decreased endurance of cirrhotics.

Campillo *et al.*[44] studied 10 cirrhotics 3 h after breakfast. 'Fed' cirrhotic patients, in contrast to fasted cirrhotics,[43] used carbohydrate almost exclusively, and to a greater extent than normal subjects, during a 32 min period on a treadmill that increased oxygen uptake three- to fourfold over that at rest. Plasma glucose fell from 5.2 ± 0.2 to 4.0 ± 0.4 mmol/l in cirrhotics, but was unchanged in controls,[44] and cirrhotics had a greater lactate response. While decreased hepatic lactate clearance probably contributed to the hyperlactataemia (Almenoff, CritCareMed, 1989; 17:870), the observation that lactate levels subsequently fell, in parallel with the fall in plasma glucose,[44] suggests that increased muscle glycolysis also contributed to the hyperlactataemia. The greater reliance on carbohydrate in these 'fed' cirrhotic patients is readily explained by the much higher postprandial insulin levels. These high insulin levels resulted in the cirrhotics having lower pre-exercise plasma non-esterified fatty acid levels. The fall in plasma glucose suggests that the elevated insulin levels also prevented the normal rise in hepatic glucose output. In cirrhotic patients the fall in insulin levels may be crucial for enhancement of hepatic glucose output during exercise (Wolfe, JCI, 1986; 77:900; Wasserman, AmJPhysiol, 1989; 19:E500) because of the impaired glycogenolytic response to glucagon. Postprandial hyperinsulinaemia and delayed insulin clearance in cirrhotics could play a major role in limiting fuel supply to working muscles (non-esterified fatty acids from adipose tissue and glucose from the liver) and thereby lead to early fatigue and decreased maximal aerobic capacity (Wolfe, JCI, 1986; 77:900).

Skeletal muscle glycogen stores also determine aerobic capacity and endurance (Wagenmakers, AmJPhysiol, 1991; 260:E883). Muscle glycogen content after an overnight fast is normal in most patients with cirrhosis (Moller, ScaJGastr, 1984; 19:267; Selberg, Hepatol, 1994; 20:135),[38] and although insulin-stimulated muscle glucose uptake and glycogen synthesis are impaired, the defect in muscle glycogen deposition after meals is likely to be much smaller since the higher postprandial blood glucose levels and hyperinsulinaemia can compensate to some extent for skeletal muscle insulin resistance; after meals containing fructose (see below) cirrhotics may synthesize more muscle glycogen from fructose because their postprandial plasma fructose levels are much higher (Avgerinos, JHepatol, 1992; 14:78).[19] Reduced muscle glycogen content is thus an unlikely explanation for the poor exercise tolerance and reduced maximal aerobic capacity. Muscle glycogen content may, however, influence the fuel mix used to meet energy needs; Selberg (Hepatol, 1994; 20:135) reported a good correlation between the exercise-induced respiratory quotient and muscle glycogen content in 14 cirrhotics studied 6 h after breakfast. Furthermore, if the release of glucose from the liver is impaired during exercise, depletion of muscle glycogen may occur sooner, particularly if lipolysis is suppressed by high plasma insulin levels in the postprandial state. β-Adrenergic receptor blockade has a similar effect. It suppresses lipolysis and impairs hepatic glucose production; the decreased availability of non-esterified fatty acids leads to earlier depletion of muscle glycogen and enhances muscle glucose uptake during exercise (Issekutz, JApplPhysiol, 1978; 44: 869).[17]

Reduced availability of carbohydrate to meet the energy needs of contracting muscle results in increased protein catabolism to supply amino acids for gluconeogenesis, and increased oxidation of amino acids, particularly the branched chain amino acids (Knapik, JApplPhysiol, 1991; 70:43; Wagenmakers, AmJPhysiol, 1991; 260: E883). In an attempt to maintain a high ATP/ADP ratio when ATP regeneration is impaired by carbohydrate deficiency, degradation of ATP to AMP, and of AMP to IMP and ammonia is enhanced. The greater release of ammonia from muscle of cirrhotics during exercise (Allen, YaleJBiolMed, 1960; 33:133) may be due to increased oxidation of branched chain amino acids (Knapik, JApplPhysiol, 1991; 70:43; Wagenmakers, AmJPhysiol, 1991; 260:E883) and/or degradation of AMP to IMP and ammonia (Graham, AdvExpMedBiol, 1994; 368:181).

Nuclear magnetic resonance studies of muscle during exercise would further our understanding of the pathophysiological basis of fatigue and the diminished aerobic capacity of cirrhotic patients.

Fructose metabolism in liver disease

After oral fructose, patients with cirrhosis have much higher plasma fructose levels than matched normal subjects[19] (Grace, ArchIntMed, 1969; 124:330; Martines, Nutrition, 1994; 10:521) (Fig. 10). By contrast, when fructose is infused intravenously, plasma fructose levels are no higher in cirrhotics than in normal subjects, even when fructose is infused more rapidly than estimated peak rates of intestinal fructose absorption[18] (Smith, JCI, 1953; 32: 273). The metabolic clearance rate of systemically infused fructose is normal in cirrhosis,[18] and the plasma half-life either normal, or prolonged by less than 20 per cent[18] (Smith, JCI, 1953; 32:273). Since normal subjects have a large first-pass hepatic uptake of oral fructose,[6] the most likely explanation for the oral fructose intolerance in cirrhosis is reduced first-pass hepatic uptake of fructose. This can be explained either by shunting of blood past hepatocytes or by impaired hepatocellular uptake of fructose.

Martin *et al.* (ArchSurg, 1962; 85:104) suggested that the higher blood fructose levels in cirrhosis were due to spontaneous porto-systemic shunting; they found higher urinary fructose excretion after a surgical portosystemic anastomosis than before the operation, and suggested that this criterion could be used to test the patency of a shunt. Holdsworth *et al.* (Gut, 1972; 13:58) also noted worse fructose tolerance in cirrhotics following end-to-side portacaval anastomosis, but only in subjects with relatively good liver function and normal fructose tolerance preoperatively.

Grace *et al.* (ArchIntMed, 1969; 124:330) showed a relationship between the blood fructose response to 1 g/kg of oral fructose and the severity of liver disease. With severe cirrhosis, there was a twofold increase in peak levels (2.3 ± 0.2 mmol/l), while in patients with mild cirrhosis peak fructose concentrations were not significantly different from controls (1.1 ± 0.1 mmol/l); a further small increase was noted in subjects following a portacaval shunt. Peak plasma fructose levels showed a strong correlation with arterial ammonia levels after oral administration of ammonium acetate. These results are explicable either by spontaneous portosystemic shunting or by impaired hepatocellular uptake of fructose. That portosystemic shunting may be the major determinant of oral fructose intolerance in cirrhosis is strongly suggested by the finding of normal intravenous fructose tolerance, because the liver is a

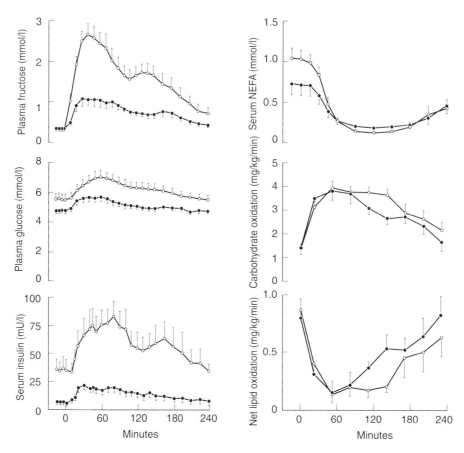

Fig. 10. Plasma fructose, glucose, serum insulin, and non-esterified fatty acid concentrations and whole-body carbohydrate and lipid oxidation rates measured by indirect calorimetry in the basal state and after a 75 g oral fructose load at t = 0 min in 8 cirrhotics (○—○) and 6 normal control subjects (●—●). Mean ± SEM. (Reproduced from ref. 19, with permission.)

major site of uptake of intravenous as well as oral fructose; splanchnic tissues account for 40 to 50 per cent of fructose removal during systemic intravenous fructose administration (Weichselbaum, PSEBM, 1950; 75:816; Bjorkman, JCI, 1989; 83:52).

Fructose ingestion elicits a small rise in plasma glucose and insulin levels, a rise in lactate levels, and a prompt increase in carbohydrate oxidation; plasma non-esterified fatty acids and lipid oxidation are rapidly suppressed (Fig. 10).[19] The increase in plasma glucose is due to a transient increase in the rate of glucose production, which is assumed to be due to conversion of fructose to glucose via hepatic gluconeogenesis. One might expect that with reduced first-pass hepatic uptake of fructose, and much higher plasma fructose levels in cirrhosis, the glucose response would be impaired. However, the rise in plasma glucose after oral fructose is actually greater in cirrhotics than controls.[19] There are two possible reasons. First, even with a reduced hepatic extraction ratio for fructose, the liver may still take up large amounts of fructose in cirrhotics because of their higher plasma fructose levels. Secondly, renal gluconeogenesis from fructose (Bjorkman, JCI, 1989; 83: 52) might be enhanced by the higher systemic fructose levels in cirrhotics.

The stimulation of carbohydrate oxidation and suppression of lipid oxidation after fructose ingestion are normal in patients with cirrhosis[19] (Martines, Nutrition; 1994; 10:521). Most fructose which is absorbed but not oxidized is used for glycogen synthesis

in liver and skeletal muscle (Nilsson, ScaJCLI, 1974; 33:5); a small amount may be used for triglyceride synthesis. Our studies suggested that the amount of fructose stored as glycogen after a 75 g oral fructose load was normal in cirrhotics.[19] However, we found a much smaller increase in energy expenditure after fructose ingestion. Glycogen synthesis is a major determinant of the increase in energy expenditure after fructose, as it is after oral glucose, and during a hyperinsulinaemic euglycaemic clamp. During a euglycaemic clamp the reduced thermogenic response in cirrhotics correlates with the defect in non-oxidative glucose disposal, which is mainly accounted for by glycogen synthesis. Because the energy cost of muscle glycogen synthesis from fructose is only about half that in liver,[19] an altered distribution of fructose between liver and peripheral tissues in cirrhotics could readily explain the lower energy expenditure with normal overall disposal of fructose; the higher plasma fructose levels would enhance muscle fructose uptake and incorporation into glycogen, and less would be used for hepatic glycogen and fatty acid synthesis.

It would seem that dietary fructose is a good source of energy in cirrhosis. Muscle fructose uptake is insulin-independent and fructose, at plasma levels similar to those found in cirrhotic patients after fructose ingestion, is a good substrate for glycogen synthesis (Nilsson, ScaJCLI, 1974, 33:5; Zicrath, BiochemJ, 1995; 311:517); in patients with cirrhosis, fructose may be a better substrate than glucose for muscle glycogen synthesis.

Potential hazards of fructose administration

The superiority of fructose over glucose as a substrate for hepatic glycogen synthesis, and its independence of insulin for metabolism, led to its use in parenteral nutrition. However, in the late 1960s deleterious effects of high doses of intravenous fructose were reported, namely hyperuricaemia, lactic acidosis, hypoglycaemia, hypophosphataemia, and impaired hepatic protein synthesis. These effects can be explained by the very rapid rate of fructose metabolism when it is given intravenously. The rate-limiting step in the metabolism of oral fructose is its absorption from the gut. If this is bypassed by intravenous administration, rapid hepatic uptake and phosphorylation of fructose to fructose 1-phosphate exceeds the capacity of aldolase type B, and fructose 1-phosphate accumulates. Hepatic ATP concentration falls as it is consumed in the fructokinase reaction (Oberhaensli, Lancet, 1987; ii:931; Terrier, Radiol, 1989; 171:557); because inorganic phosphate is trapped in fructose 1-phosphate it is unavailable for regeneration of ATP. Other high-energy phosphate compounds, such as GTP, UTP, and UDP-glucose, are also depleted.

The fall in phosphate and high-energy phosphate compounds causes further metabolic changes. Depletion of ATP inhibits protein and RNA synthesis; detoxification of ammonia is impaired and there is interference with energy-dependent membrane transport processes. Adenine nucleotide breakdown is stimulated, and AMP deaminase, the rate limiting enzyme, is activated by the fall in phosphate and GTP. Stimulation of adenine nucleotide breakdown leads to accumulation of IMP and increased uric acid production. IMP is an inhibitor of aldolase and may thus aggravate the build up of fructose 1-phosphate.

Compensated cirrhotics show less marked changes in liver phosphate and ATP levels in response to intravenous fructose than normal control subjects (Dufour, Hepatol, 1992; 15:835) consistent with an impairment in the capacity for hepatic fructose metabolism. Physiological doses of fructose given intravenously (35–50 g over 2 h) have no effect on plasma uric acid or phosphate levels;[18] however, with high rates of infusion (35 g in 10 min), even well-compensated cirrhotic patients (Child's grade A) may be more susceptible to hyperuricaemia than normal subjects (Budillon, ItalJGastr, 1992; 24:373).

The depletion of ATP inhibits gluconeogenesis and stimulates glycolysis, resulting in the accumulation of lactic acid. The entry of fructose metabolites into the glycolytic pathway distal to the non-equilibrium phosphofructokinase reaction (the main regulatory step of glycolysis), and the allosteric activation of pyruvate kinase by fructose 1-phosphate, are also major determinants of the increased lactate production in response to fructose administration. Normally liver and kidneys take up lactate and thus contribute to the maintenance of blood pH. The daily uptake of lactate by the liver and kidneys corresponds to the removal of approximately 500 mmol/day of H^+. This compares with about 100 mmol/day of H^+ that is excreted in combination with urinary buffers. Thus the transition from a situation in which the liver and kidneys remove lactate, to one in which they are net lactate producers at high rates of fructose delivery means that lactic acidosis can develop very rapidly. This risk will be exaggerated in patients with disturbed acid–base balance, in those who are hypotensive and hypoxic, and in patients with decompensated liver disease (Craig, BMJ, 1971; 4:211; Woods, Lancet, 1972; i:1354).

Compensated cirrhotic patients do not have a greater lactate response to oral or physiological doses of fructose given intravenously[18,19] (Smith, JCI, 1953; 32:273). Since it is a good energy substrate, is oxidized in preference to lipid,[18] and does not produce excessive lactate or uric acid levels, a moderate intake of fructose in the diet is likely to be beneficial in these patients. However, fructose should not be administered intravenously in a clinical setting because of the risks of lactic acidosis and other adverse metabolic effects.

References

1. Rothman DL, Magnusson I, Katz LD, Shulman RG, and Shulman GI. Quantitation of hepatic glycogenolysis and gluconeogenesis in fasting humans with ^{13}C NMR. *Science*, 1991; **254**: 573–6.
2. Nilsson LH. Liver glycogen content in man in the postabsorptive state. *Scandinavian Journal of Clinical Laboratory Investigation*, 1973; **32**: 317–23.
3. Nurjhan N, *et al.* Glutamine: a major gluconeogenic precursor and vehicle for interorgan carbon transport in man. *Journal of Clinical Investigation*, 1995; **95**: 272–7.
4. Cherrington AD, *et al.* Insulin, glucagon, and glucose as regulators of hepatic glucose uptake and production *in vivo*. *Diabetes Metabolism Reviews*, 1987; **3**: 307–32.
5. Sherratt HSA. In Hue L, and van der Werve G, eds. *Short-term regulation of liver metabolism*. Amsterdam: Elsevier/North Holland Biomedical Press, 1981: 199–227.
6. McIntyre N, Turner DS, and Holdsworth CD. The role of the portal circulation in glucose and fructose tolerance. *Diabetologia*, 1970; **6**: 593–6.
7. Radziuk J, McDonald TJ, Rubenstein D, and Dupre J. Initial splanchnic extraction of ingested glucose in normal man. *Metabolism*, 1978; **27**: 657–79.
8. Ferrannini E, *et al.* The disposal of an oral glucose load in healthy subjects: a quantitative study. *Diabetes*, 1985; **34**: 580–8.
9. Kruszynska YT, Meyer-Alber A, Darakhshan F, Home PD, and McIntyre N. Metabolic handling of orally administered glucose in cirrhosis. *Journal of Clinical Investigation*, 1993; **91**: 1057–66.
10. Kelley D, *et al.* Skeletal muscle glycolysis, oxidation, and storage of an oral glucose load. *Journal of Clinical Investigation*, 1988; **81**: 1563–71.
11. Mitrakou A, *et al.* Contribution of abnormal muscle and liver glucose metabolism to postprandial hyperglycaemia in NIDDM. *Diabetes*, 1990; **39**: 1381–90.
12. Newgard CB, Hirsch LJ, Foster DW, and McGarry JD. Studies on the mechanism by which exogenous glucose is converted into liver glycogen in the rat. *Journal of Biological Chemistry*, 1983; **258**: 8046–52.
13. Adkins BA, *et al.* Importance of the route of intravenous glucose delivery to hepatic glucose balance in the conscious dog. *Journal of Clinical Investigation*, 1987; **79**: 557–65.
14. Pagliassotti MJ, Holste LC, Moore MC, Neal DW, and Cherrington AD. Comparison of the time courses of insulin and the portal signal on hepatic glucose and glycogen metabolism in the conscious dog. *Journal of Clinical Investigation*, 1996; **97**: 81–91.
15. Kruszynska YT, Home PD, and Alberti KGMM. *In vivo* regulation of liver and skeletal muscle glycogen synthase activity by glucose and insulin. *Diabetes*, 1986; **35**: 662–7.
16. Romijn JA, *et al.* Regulation of endogenous fat and carbohydrate metabolism in relation to exercise intensity and duration. *American Journal of Physiology*, 1993; **265**: E380–E391.
17. Hoelzer DR, Dalsky GP, Clutter WE, Shah SD, Holloszy JO, and Cryer PE. Glucoregulation during exercise: hypoglycaemia is prevented by redundant glucoregulatory systems, sympathochromaffin activation, and changes in islet hormone secretion. *Journal of Clinical Investigation*, 1986; **77**: 212–21.
18. Kruszynska YT, Harry DS, Fryer LG, and McIntyre N. Lipid metabolism during intravenous fructose administration in cirrhosis. *Metabolism*, 1994; **43**: 1171–81.

19. Kruszynska YT, Meyer-Alber A, Wollen N, and McIntyre N. Energy expenditure and substrate metabolism after oral fructose in patients with cirrhosis. *Journal of Hepatology*, 1993; **19**: 241–51.

20. Felig P, Brown V, Levine R, and Klatskin G. Glucose homeostasis in viral hepatitis. *New England Journal of Medicine*, 1970; **283**: 1436–40.

21. Proietto J, Alford FP, and Dudley FJ. The mechanism of carbohydrate intolerance of cirrhosis. *Journal of Clinical Endocrinology and Metabolism*, 1980; **51**: 1030–6.

22. Owen OE, *et al.* Hepatic and renal substrate flux rates in patients with hepatic cirrhosis. *Journal of Clinical Investigation*, 1981; **68**: 240–52.

23. Nosadini R, *et al.* Carbohydrate and lipid metabolism in cirrhosis. Evidence that hepatic uptake of gluconeogenic precursors and of free fatty acids depends on effective hepatic blood flow. *Journal of Clinical Endocrinology and Metabolism*, 1984; **58**: 1125–32.

24. Petrides AS, Groop LC, Riely CA, and DeFronzo RA. Effect of physiologic hyperinsulinaemia on glucose and lipid metabolism in cirrhosis. *Journal of Clinical Investigation*, 1991; **88**: 561–70.

25. Kruszynska YT and McIntyre N. Hepatic glucose production from glycerol is not increased in overnight fasted cirrhotic patients. *Endocrinology and Metabolism*, 1994; **1**: 23–31.

26. Petrides AS, Vogt C, Schulze-Berg D, Matthews DE, and Strohmeyer G. Pathogenesis of glucose intolerance and diabetes mellitus in cirrhosis. *Hepatology*, 1994; **19**: 616–27.

27. Shmueli E, Walker M, Alberti KGMM, and Record CO. Normal splanchnic but impaired peripheral insulin-stimulated glucose uptake in cirrhosis. *Hepatology*, 1993; **18**: 86–95.

28. Leatherdale BA, *et al.* Forearm glucose uptake in cirrhosis. *Clinical Science*, 1980; **59**: 191–8.

29. Owen OE, *et al.* Nature and quantity of fuels consumed in patients with alcoholic cirrhosis. *Journal of Clinical Investigation*, 1983; **72**: 1821–32.

30. Muller MJ, *et al.* Energy expenditure and substrate oxidation in patients with cirrhosis: The impact of cause, clinical staging and nutritional state. *Hepatology*, 1992; **15**: 782–94.

31. Naunyn B. Der diabetes mellitus. In Holder A, ed. *Nothnagels Handbuch-Spez Path Ther.*, (1st edn). Vienna, 1898: 7.

32. Kruszynska YT, Harry DS, Bergman RN, and McIntyre N. Insulin sensitivity, insulin secretion and glucose effectiveness in diabetic and non-diabetic cirrhotics. *Diabetologia*, 1993; **36**: 121–8.

33. Kruszynska YT, Munro J, Home PD, and McIntyre N. Twenty-four hour C peptide and insulin secretion rates and diurnal profiles of glucose, lipids and intermediary metabolites in cirrhosis. *Clinical Science*, 1992; **83**: 597–605.

34. Marchesini G, Pacini G, Bianchi G, Patrono D, and Cobelli C. Glucose disposal, B-cell secretion, and hepatic insulin extraction in cirrhosis: a minimal model assessment. *Gastroenterology*, 1990; **99**: 1715–22.

35. Letiexhe MR, *et al.* Insulin secretion, clearance, and action on glucose metabolism in cirrhotic patients. *Journal of Clinical Endocrinology and Metabolism*, 1993; **77**: 1263–8.

36. Kruszynska YT, Home PD, and McIntyre N. The relationship between insulin sensitivity, insulin secretion and glucose tolerance in cirrhosis. *Hepatology*, 1991; **14**: 103–11.

37. Taylor R, *et al.* Insulin action in cirrhosis: *in vivo* and *in vitro* studies. *Hepatology*, 1985; **5**: 64–71.

38. Kruszynska YT, Williams N, Perry M, and Home PD. The relationship between insulin sensitivity and skeletal muscle enzyme activities in hepatic cirrhosis. *Hepatology*, 1988; 8: 1615–19.

39. Selberg O, *et al.* Insulin resistance in liver cirrhosis. A PET scan analysis of skeletal muscle glucose metabolism. *Journal of Clinical Investigation*, 1993; **91**: 1897–902.

40. Shmueli E, Stewart M, Alberti KGMM, and Record CO. Growth hormone, insulin-like growth factor-1 and insulin resistance in cirrhosis. *Hepatology*, 1994; **19**: 322–8.

41. Johnston DG, *et al.* C-peptide and insulin in liver disease. *Diabetes*, 1978; **27** (Suppl. 1): 201–6.

42. Kruszynska YT, Ghatei MA, Bloom SR, and McIntyre N. Insulin secretion and plasma levels of glucose-dependent insulinotropic peptide and glucagon-like peptide 1 [7–36 amide] after oral glucose in cirrhosis. *Hepatology*, 1995; **21**: 933–41.

43. DeLissio M, Goodyear LJ, Fuller S, Krawitt EL, and Devlin JT. Effects of treadmill exercise on fuel metabolism in hepatic cirrhosis. *Journal of Applied Physiology*, 1991; **70**: 210.

44. Campillo B, *et al.* Hormonal and metabolic changes during exercise in cirrhotic patients. *Metabolism*, 1990; **39**: 18–24.

2.12 Plasma lipids and lipoproteins

D. S. Harry and Neil McIntyre

Plasma lipids

Several types of lipid are carried in plasma in relatively large amounts—cholesterol and cholesteryl esters, triglycerides, and phospholipids. Insoluble in water, they are present in plasma in the form of lipoproteins. From their ultracentrifugal behaviour lipoproteins are classified as very low density lipoprotein (**VLDL**), low density lipoprotein (**LDL**) and high density lipoprotein (**HDL**). Chylomicrons, a fourth major class of lipoprotein, are found after meals and are large enough to be recognized by dark-ground microscopy.

Cholesterol

Cholesterol is present in all cellular membranes and is a precursor of bile acids and steroid hormones. Apart from the hydroxyl group at C3, and the double bond between C5 and C6, cholesterol is a fully saturated, non-polar hydrocarbon; it is insoluble in water and chemically unreactive, and thus admirably suited to its role as a structural component of membranes. Cholesterol in membranes and bile is present almost exclusively as free sterol. In plasma, and tissues such as the liver, adrenal glands, and skin, cholesteryl esters are also found; in these the 3β-hydroxyl group of cholesterol is esterified with the carboxyl group of a long-chain fatty acid, and they are even less soluble in water than cholesterol.

Cholesterol is synthesized by nearly all cells, a process controlled by the intracellular cholesterol content; cells also obtain it by taking up cholesterol-containing lipoproteins from plasma. The amount synthesized each day has been estimated to be at least twice that ingested in the average Western diet (which contains 250 to 750 mg/day); about 50 per cent of dietary cholesterol is absorbed by the small intestine and the rest is excreted.

Cholesterol is lost from the body either as faecal neutral sterols (cholesterol, or other sterols produced within the intestine), which are derived from dietary cholesterol or from cholesterol entering the intestine in bile or shed epithelial cells, or as bile acids, which are synthesized from cholesterol in the liver. About 600 to 750 mg of cholesterol is lost each day in bile acids, and about 500 to 600 mg in faecal neutral sterols; 75 to 100 mg is shed by the skin and 35 to 50 mg is converted into steroid hormones.

Triglycerides

Triglycerides have a backbone of glycerol, the three hydroxyl groups of which are esterified with fatty acids. Naturally occurring triglycerides contain a variety of fatty acids. Dietary fat, which is an important energy source, is mainly present as triglyceride. Within the body, triglyceride is used to store energy (particularly in adipose tissue), or to transport it in plasma either as chylomicrons, which are produced by the intestine, or as VLDL of hepatic origin. The body's capacity for the storage of energy as glycogen is limited, but enormous quantities can be stored as triglyceride in adipose tissue. The triglyceride fatty acids stored in this way may come from the diet, or they may be synthesized *de novo* from carbohydrate or other precursors.

Phospholipids

Phospholipids are a heterogeneous group of compounds, containing one or more phosphoric acid groups, another polar group (a nitrogenous base such as choline, ethanolamine, or sphingosine; the amino acid serine; or the polyalcohol inositol), and one or more long-chain fatty acid residues. The phospholipids are much more complex in terms of their chemical reactivity than cholesterol and cholesteryl esters. With cholesterol, they are important constituents of cellular membranes and take part in a large number of chemical reactions. The most abundant phospholipid in plasma, and in most cellular membranes, is phosphatidyl choline or lecithin; because different fatty acids may be attached to the glycerol backbone, there are in fact a family of phosphatidyl cholines which have different physicochemical characteristics.

Fatty acids

Fatty acids are hydrocarbon chains with a terminal carboxyl group. Naturally occurring fatty acids, which have an even number of carbon atoms, are short-chain (C 4 to 8), medium-chain (C 10 to 14), or long-chain fatty acids (C 16 or longer). 'Saturated' fatty acids (e.g. palmitic and stearic) lack double bonds; as a result their hydrocarbon chains are flexible because each –CH2–CH2-link is free to act as a hinge. 'Unsaturated' fatty acids have one or more double bonds. Oleic (C 18:1) and palmitoleic (C 16:1) have one double bond; linoleic (C 18:2), linolenic (C 18:3), and arachidonic (C 20:4) have more than one and are called polyunsaturated fatty acids. The double bonds may be *cis* or *trans* in their orientation; naturally occurring fatty acids have predominantly *cis* double bonds which impart a distinct bend to the fatty acid chain. This, together with the absence of movement around a double bond, means that polyunsaturated fatty acid chains are much less flexible than their saturated counterparts and do not pack together as well. For this reason membranes which contain polyunsaturated fatty acids have greater 'fluidity'. Unsaturated fatty acids are chemically more re-active than saturated fatty acids and are prone to alteration by processes such as lipid peroxidation.

Within the body, fatty acids may have their chains elongated, and additional double bonds can be inserted into the molecule. Oleic acid has its double bond between C9 and C10 (counting from the carboxyl end of the molecule). Additional double bonds can be inserted into the molecule between the double bond and the carboxyl group, but not between the double bond and the terminal methyl group. The extra double bonds in linoleic (C18:2 d 9,12) and α-linolenic (C18:3 d 9,12,15) acids are in the latter region of the molecule; for this reason they are 'essential' fatty acids and must be provided in the diet. They are present in large amounts in many plant fats, such as soya bean, corn, and safflower oils.

Essential fatty acids are sometimes classified by the position of the first double bond numbered from the methyl (or ω) end of the fatty acid chain; linoleic acid is an example of an ω-6, and α-linolenic acid of an ω-3 fatty acid. Both types are important as they are converted into many biologically active compounds. Arachidonic acid (C20:4 d 5,8,11,14), an ω-6 fatty acid, is synthesized from linoleic acid; it is a precursor of the 2-series prostaglandins and thromboxanes, and the 4-series leukotrienes. α-Linolenic acid is converted in the body to eicosapentaenoic (20:5) and docoso-hexanoic (22:6) acids. Eicosapentaenoic acid is a precursor of the 3-series prostaglandins and thromboxanes, and of the 5-series leu-kotrienes.

Most of the body's fatty acids are esterified in triglycerides or phospholipids, which act as storage or transport vehicles for fatty acids. In plasma there is also a relatively small amount of 'free' or non-esterified fatty acids (**NEFA**), which constitute about 5 per cent of the total fatty acid of plasma. Plasma NEFA come mainly from adipose tissue, which releases them by hydrolysing storage triglyceride, but some enter plasma during the intraplasmatic hy-drolysis of the triglyceride of chylomicrons and VLDL. Although their plasma concentration is low, NEFA have a very rapid turnover (a half-life of only minutes) and they are an important energy source for body tissues. They have limited water solubility and are mainly bound to plasma albumin, which has specific binding sites for NEFA.

Plasma lipoproteins[1-3]

The plasma lipoproteins are complex particles that carry plasma lipids in association with proteins known as apoproteins (see later). Their surface is made up of cholesterol, phospholipid, and apo-proteins, and their core contains the more hydrophobic lipids—cholesteryl ester and triglyceride. There are several classes of lipoproteins; their structural and biochemical characteristics, and their concentrations in normal fasting plasma, are presented in Tables 1 and 2.

Chylomicrons

Chylomicrons are very large particles (more than 70 nm) secreted into the intestinal lymphatics by small intestinal mucosal cells following a fatty meal. About 90 per cent by mass is triglyceride which, with cholesteryl ester and some fat-soluble vitamins, forms a hydrophobic core. Circulating chylomicrons are a mixture of particles at various stages of their natural history. When secreted the particles contain apoB-48, apoA-I and apoA-IV but, after entering plasma via the thoracic duct, they lose apoA-I and apoA-IV and acquire apoE and C apoproteins (including apoC-II which activates lipoprotein lipase). As triglyceride is removed their surface components, including the C apoproteins, are transferred to HDL. Eventually chylomicron remnants remain which retain apoB-48 and apoE; these particles are removed by hepatocytes which have a chylomicron remnant receptor that binds the apoE.

Very low density lipoproteins (VLDL)

VLDL are also large particles (25 to 70 nm); they are secreted by hepatocytes, and probably by intestinal mucosal cells. About 50 to 60 per cent of their mass is triglyceride and a greater proportion of their cholesterol is present as cholesteryl ester than is the case with chylomicrons. As their triglyceride is removed, surface components, including the C apoproteins, are transferred back to HDL. Plasma VLDL, like chylomicrons, are a heterogeneous mixture of particles of varying composition and physical characteristics. Eventually they are transformed to IDL (LDL1) and then to LDL (LDL2).

Intermediate density lipoproteins (LDL1)

Low density lipoprotein was originally defined as the lipoprotein fraction having a density range 1.006 to 1.063 g/ml, but this fraction contains at least two types of particle. The minor subfraction (density range 1.006 to 1.019 g/ml) is now usually referred to as 'intermediate density lipoprotein' or IDL, and sometimes as LDL1. IDL are derived from intraplasmatic catabolism of VLDL, and their lipid composition is intermediate between that of VLDL and LDL (Table 2). The major apoproteins of IDL are the C apoproteins and apoE, and there is one molecule per particle of apoB-100—the key structural component. IDL is either removed by the liver (about 50 per cent in man) or converted to LDL2. During conversion to LDL2, triglyceride is removed and cholesteryl ester added from HDL. IDL may be present in appreciable amounts in plasma because apoC-II, the activator of lipoprotein lipase, is lost from the surface of VLDL particles as their triglyceride is removed, thus slowing or preventing further triglyceride hydrolysis. Subsequently, triglyceride may be lost via the action of transfer proteins.

Low density lipoproteins (LDL2)

In fasting plasma the major subfraction of 'classical' LDL is in the density range 1.019 to 1.063 g/ml. It is called LDL2 or simply LDL (therefore you must check the meaning when you come across the term LDL; we will use it to mean LDL2). The composition of LDL is given in Table 2. The only apoprotein is a single molecule of apoB-100. Normally, cholesteryl ester forms 80 per cent of the core lipids (on a molar basis). LDL2 carries about 75 per cent of the total cholesterol in human plasma; its major functions appear to be the provision of cholesterol for many extrahepatic tissues and for the transport of excess cholesterol from tissues to the liver, where it can be excreted in the bile either as cholesterol or bile acids.

High density lipoproteins (HDL)

The normal plasma HDL fraction is heterogeneous. It is commonly separated into two major classes, HDL2 (density range 1.063 to

Table 1 Human lipoproteins

(a) Physical chemistry of human serum lipoproteins

	Chylomicrons	VLDL	LDL$_1$	LDL$_2$	HDL$_2$	HDL$_3$
Molecular weight	$>0.4 \times 10^9$	$5-10 \times 10^6$	$4-4.8 \times 10^6$	2.8×10^6	3.6×10^5	1.8×10^5
Diameter (mm)	>70	24–80	22–25	18–22	7–10	4–7
Density (g/ml)	<1.006	<1.006	1.006–1.019	1.019–1.063	1.063–1.125	1.125–1.21
Flotation rate:						
Sf (1.063)[1]	>400	20–400	12–20	0–12	—	
Sf (1.21)[2]	—	—	—	—	3.6–9.0	0–3.5
Electrophoretic mobility:						
Paper, agarose	Origin	Prebeta	(Fast beta)	Beta	Alpha	Alpha

(b) Protein and lipid composition of human lipoproteins (% w/w)

Composition	Chylomicrons	VLDL	LDL$_1$	LDL$_2$	HDL$_2$	HDL$_3$
Free cholesterol	1–3	5–10	7–8	7–10	5	3–4
Cholesteryl ester*	2–4	10–15	18–22	35–40	12–18	10–12
Triglycerides	85–90	50–65	25–30	6–10	4–6	3–5
Phospholipids	8–10	16–20	18–22	20–24	25–30	22–25
Protein	2–4	8–12	15–20	20–25	42–45	50–55
Concentration in fasting plasma (mg %)	None	20–300	10–20	200–400	40–100† 60–150‡	120–300† 200–350‡

* Calculated as cholesteryl esters, i.e. mass of cholesterol + fatty acid (assuming average molecular weight of fatty acid is 270).
† Males, ‡ females. Sf = Svedberg unit, at the indicated solvent density.

Table 2 Plasma apoprotein concentrations (mg/dl)

A-I	A-II	A-IV	B	C-II	C-III	D	E
110–140	30–35	10–15	60–80	5–10	10–20	5–10	5–10

1.125 g/ml) and HDL3 (density range 1.125 to 1.21 g/ml) (Table 1); a minor subclass, HDLI, which floats largely within the HDL2 density range, is rich in apoE. There may be greater heterogeneity of HDL when special techniques are used. The apoprotein composition of HDL is complex (see Table 1).

The spectrum of mature, spherical (i.e. core-containing) HDL particles of normal plasma appears to be produced in plasma from core-deficient precursors. These 'nascent' HDL particles, which are rich in cholesterol and phospholipid and contain apoE or apoA-I (both activators of lecithin cholesterol acyltransferase, **LCAT**), appear to be secreted by both liver and intestine; they may also be derived from surface remnants of triglyceride-rich VLDL and chylomicrons following lipolysis. Their remodelling to mature plasma HDL is complex; it involves the actions of LCAT, hepatic lipase, and various lipid transfer proteins. Although not usually found in normal plasma, 'nascent' HDL are present in relatively large amounts in familial LCAT deficiency and in many patients with liver disease; they are heterogeneous in size and shape, and small spherical and large discoidal particles are present on electron microscopy (Fig. 1).

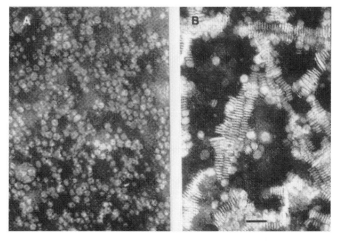

Fig. 1. A. Normal high density lipoproteins (× 220 000). B. Abnormal disc-shaped ('nascent') high density lipoproteins (× 121 000) which are found in patients with obstructive jaundice and in parenchymal liver disease when LCAT activity is low. (Bar marker = 50 nm.)

Apoproteins[4]

The plasma apoproteins are the polypeptide chains found in the various plasma lipoprotein subfractions. They appear to be structural components of lipoprotein particles, but they also have other important functions. In 1966 Gustafson *et al.* (ScaJCLI, 1966; 39: 377) proposed the existence of three major groups of apoproteins: apoA in HDL, apoB in LDL, and apoC in VLDL. This is now known to be a gross oversimplification. The ABC nomenclature has survived, however, although there have been additions to it. The

Table 3 Apoproteins of plasma lipoproteins

Apoprotein	Major component	Minor component
AI	HDL*	† CM, VLDL
AII	HDL*	CM, VLDL
AIV		CM, VLDL, HDL
B$_{100}$	LDL$_1$, LDL$_2$, VLDL, CM	
B$_{48}$	CM	VLDL
CI	VLDL, CM	HDL, LDL$_1$
CII	VLDL, CM	HDL
CIII	VLDL, CM	HDL
D		HDL, VLDL
E		CM, VLDL, HDL

* Apo-AI is the major apoprotein of HDL but the ratio of apo-AI to apo-AII is different in HDL$_2$ compared to HDL$_3$. Ratio AI:AII; HDL$_2$ 2.5:1, HDL$_3$ 2:1.
† CM = chylomicrons.

main apoprotein groups are described by capital letters, non-identical polypeptides by Roman numerals, and polymorphic forms by arabic numbers. Some characteristics of the plasma apoproteins are presented in Table 3.

ApoA-I[5]

Mature apoA-I is a single polypeptide chain of 243 amino acids. Its gene is on chromosome 11 close to those for apoC-III and apoA-IV. ApoA-I mRNA has been sequenced; it codes for a precursor polypeptide, prepro-apoA-I, which has 24 amino acids attached to the N-terminal of the mature apoprotein. Eighteen of these form a hydrophobic prepeptide, which is removed intracellularly during translation. A propeptide is secreted into the plasma and lymph; the other six amino acids are removed in the plasma to leave mature apoA-I. ApoA-I is synthesized by the liver and intestine. It has a lipid- binding domain and also a segment which appears to activate LCAT.

ApoA-II[5]

Plasma apoA-II is a protein of 154 amino acids, made up of two identical polypeptide chains linked by a single disulphide bond at position 6 of their sequences. The gene is on chromosome 1; its mRNA encodes a polypeptide chain of 100 amino acids, prepro-apoA-II, of which 18 form a hydrophobic prepeptide which, like that of apoA-I, is removed intracellularly; another 5 amino acids are removed from the propeptide in plasma to leave mature apoA-II. ApoA-II appears to activate hepatic triglyceride lipase.

ApoA-IV[6]

Mature apoA-IV is an apoprotein of 377 amino acids with a molecular weight between 44 000 and 46 000. It contains about 6 per cent carbohydrate and is present in plasma as a number of isoforms. The gene for apoA-IV is on chromosome 11; its mRNA codes for a polypeptide of 397 amino acids, 20 of which form a signal prepeptide which is cleaved to give the final polypeptide chain. There is no propeptide.

ApoA-IV is synthesized in the intestine; during fat feeding most newly synthesized apoA-IV in intestinal lymph is in chylomicrons

and VLDL, with some in HDL. ApoA-IV is probably transferred from chylomicrons to HDL in plasma; LCAT may be involved in this transfer, and apoA-IV appears to activate LCAT. Patients with cirrhosis appeared to have a low level of apoA-IV mRNA in the intestinal mucosa, even though serum apoA-IV levels were normal, suggesting either an increased translational rate or delayed clearance of serum apoA-IV (Seishima, IntHepatolComm, 1995; 4:153).

ApoB-100 and apoB-48 (Knott, Science, 1985; 230:37; Scott, JRoyCollPhys, 1990; 24:101)

Plasma apoB-100 and apoB-48 are two apoproteins, sharing a number of features, which are found in plasma lipoproteins. ApoB-100, which is produced in the liver, is one of several apoproteins present in VLDL and IDL, and in LDL2 it is the only protein found. These lipoproteins contain only one apoB molecule per particle. ApoB-48 is produced in the intestine and is found in plasma chylomicrons and chylomicron remnants; its molecular weight is 48 per cent of that of B-100 and it is essentially the N-terminal end of the B-100 molecule.

There is only one gene for apoB, which is found on chromosome 2. In the liver it codes for apoB-100 which has a polypeptide chain of 4536 amino acids (with a molecular weight of 549 000); apoB-100 is the largest monomeric protein yet identified and the most hydrophobic of the apoproteins. In the intestine the same gene codes for the much smaller apoB-48, which has 2152 amino-acid residues. The production of these two different polypeptides from the same gene appears to be due to a novel and poorly understood mechanism (Chen, Science, 1987; 238:363; Powell, Cell, 1987; 50: 831). A stop codon (UAA) is introduced into the intestinal mRNA instead of the CAA which normally encodes Gln-2153 in apoB-100, a change not dictated by the gene sequence at that point. ApoB-100 binds to the LDL receptor; apoB-48 does not because the section of apoB-100 responsible for binding is not present in apoB-48.

ApoC-I[6,7]

ApoC-I is a small peptide of 57 amino acids which, like apoA-I, is an activator of LCAT. Its gene is on chromosome 19 within 4 kilobases of the gene for apoE and the gene for apoC-II is also on this chromosome.

ApoC-II[5]

Mature apoC-II is a single chain of 73 amino acids; it activates lipoprotein lipase. Its gene is on chromosome 19 and shows close genetic linkage with that of apoE. Its mRNA codes for a precursor polypeptide, prepro-apoC-II; of the 22 amino acids attached originally to the N-terminal of the mature apoprotein, 16 form a hydrophobic prepeptide which is removed intracellularly; the other 6 amino acids are removed later as a propeptide.

ApoC-III[6,7]

ApoC-III contains 79 amino-acid residues; a carbohydrate chain is attached to a threonine at position 74. The gene is on chromosome 11. The oligosaccharide chain contains one galactose and one galactosamine and zero, one, or two residues of sialic acid, thus accounting for three forms in plasma, each having the same polypeptide chain but a different content of sialic acid; these can be separated on polyacrylamide gel electrophoresis, giving bands designated as apoC-III0, apoC-III1 and apoC-III2.

ApoD (Albers, Atheroscl, 1981; 39:395)[6]

ApoD has a molecular weight of about 33 000; its gene is on chromosome 3. It appears to be a glycosylated polypeptide chain of 169 amino acids. In plasma it is found mainly in HDL in association with LCAT and apoA-I. Three isoforms are present on isoelectric focusing. Its function is unknown.

ApoE (Breslow, JBC, 1982; 257:14639; Davignon, Arterioscl, 1988; 8:1)

The gene for apoE is found on chromosome 19; it encodes for a single polypeptide chain of 299 amino acids which is subsequently glycosylated. There are three common alleles of apoE—E2, E3, and E4—of which E3 is the commonest. ApoE4 differs from apoE3 because there is an arginine instead of a cysteine at residue 112, while in apoE2 cysteine replaces the arginine-158 of apoE3. The latter substitution affects the ability of apoE2 to bind to the LDL and chylomicron remnant receptors, and this causes type III hyperlipoproteinaemia; a number of other apoE variants have been described. There are six common genotypes E2/E2, E3/E3, E4/E4, E2/E3, E2/E4, and E3/E4.

ApoE is synthesized primarily in the liver but also in a number of other tissues including the spleen, kidney, adrenal glands, gonads, brain, and macrophages.

ApoJ (de Silva, JBC, 1990; 265:13240; JBC, 1990; 265:14292)

ApoJ is a 70-kDa glycoprotein circulating as a disulphide-linked heterodimer component of lipid-poor HDL and VHDL. The liver has a relatively high level of ApoJ mRNA, which is also found in the brain, ovaries, and testes. Its function is not clear but it may be involved in lipid transport, regulation of complement function, sperm maturation, and membrane recycling.

Lp(a) (McLean, Nature, 1987; 300:132)[6]

A lipoprotein fraction called Lp(a) is present in human plasma; its concentration is very variable. It resembles LDL2 in terms of its lipid composition but migrates between the normal β- and preβ-bands. Lp(a) results from covalent binding of a carbohydrate-rich apoprotein, apo(a), to apoB-100 via disulphide bridges. At least six molecular weight isoforms of apo(a) result from different alleles at the same locus. The type of isoform present seems to determine the level of Lp(a) present in plasma. Sequencing of apo(a) has revealed considerable homology with plasminogen. The function of Lp(a) is not clear, but the variation in plasma levels within individuals suggests that it behaves like an acute- phase reactant. The presence of large amounts of Lp(a) appears to increase the risk of coronary artery disease.

Enzymes, transport proteins, and receptors

Lecithin cholesterol acyltransferase[8]

Lecithin cholesterol acyltransferase (EC 2.3.1.43) or LCAT is a plasma enzyme. It is synthesized and glycosylated in the liver, then enters the plasma where it catalyses the transfer of a fatty acid from the 2-position of lecithin to the 3β-OH group of free cholesterol to produce cholesteryl ester and lysolecithin. The high reaction rate suggests a key role for LCAT in the turnover of plasma cholesterol and lecithin. High density lipoproteins (HDL) form the substrate and LCAT plays an important role in the metabolism of the HDL subclasses.

The LCAT gene is present on chromosome 16, and the amino-acid sequence of mature LCAT is known.[9,10] It has 416 amino acids with several stretches of hydrophobic residues, and a sequence homologous to the interfacial active site of several lipases (which is assumed to be the active site of the enzyme); it is heavily glycosylated, carbohydrate making up about 25 per cent of its mass. The 1550-base LCAT mRNA has been detected in the liver and in HepG2 cells but not in the small intestine, spleen, pancreas, placenta, or adrenal tissue.

Lipoprotein lipase (EC 3.1.1.34)[6,11]

Lipoprotein lipase (**LPL**) is an enzyme present on the luminal surface of capillary endothelial cells, where it is bound to a heparin-like glycosaminoglycan. It is displaced from this site by heparin which remains bound to the enzyme; an association with either heparin or the glycosaminoglycan seems essential for lipolytic activity. LPL also has binding sites for lipid and for apoC-II (which activates LPL), and a separate site is responsible for triglyceride hydrolysis. The natural substrate for LPL is the triglyceride in the core of chylomicrons and VLDL.

The gene for lipoprotein lipase is on chromosome 8. It codes for a protein of 448 amino acids showing similarities to hepatic triglyceride lipase and pancreatic lipase.

LPL activity is found in many tissues including adipose tissue, skeletal muscle, myocardium, mammary gland, placenta, brain, and lung, but it is not clear whether the LPL in these sites results from products of a single gene. Different proteins appear to be present showing different substrate affinities. Rat heart LPL, for example, has a much higher affinity than adipose tissue LPL; it therefore seems likely that heart could obtain energy from circulating triglycerides even during fasting, when these are at low levels; at this time the adipose tissue would hydrolyse little circulating triglyceride, although it would hydrolyse its own fat stores thus releasing free fatty acids into the bloodstream. After fat feeding, or during carbohydrate-induced hypertriglyceridaemia, adipose tissue LPL would hydrolyse more circulating triglyceride and store the released fatty acids; the high affinity LPLs would already be saturated and would play little part in disposing of the excess triglyceride. The LPLs in different tissues also respond differently to various hormonal stimuli. The LPL activity of adipose tissue rises with fat or carbohydrate feeding, and falls with fasting, probably in response to circulating levels of insulin and other hormones; breast LPL is responsive to prolactin and rises markedly during lactation.

Hepatic triglyceride lipase[6]

Hepatic triglyceride lipase is an enzyme which is synthesized and secreted by hepatocytes and then bound to the endothelial cells of the liver. Its cDNA has been isolated and sequenced, and the gene has been located on chromosome 15. Like lipoprotein lipase it is released from its binding site by heparin and then its plasma activity can be measured. In animal studies it appears to play a role in the intraplasmatic metabolism of VLDL and IDL. In man, hepatic lipase deficiency is associated with an accumulation of smaller VLDL particles, suggesting impaired conversion to IDL; even so, IDL accumulates and there is a marked reduction in LDL concentration, which suggests that the conversion of IDL to LDL is profoundly impaired (Demant, JLipRes, 1988; 29:1603).

Lipid transfer proteins[6,7]

There are several transfer proteins in plasma which appear to facilitate transfer of lipids between lipoproteins, and between lipoproteins and cell membranes. One is cholesteryl ester transfer protein (CETP), or triglyceride transfer protein, a hydrophobic glycoprotein with a molecular weight between 63 000 and 69 000; its gene is on chromosome 16. Its major function appears to be the transfer of cholesteryl ester (formed in HDL by the action of LCAT) from HDL to VLDL and IDL, and thus to LDL. It may also transport triglyceride from VLDL to the other lipoprotein fractions. It may be produced by the liver although, as there was no significant difference between plasma transfer protein activity in controls and patients with decompensated cirrhosis, the liver may not be the main site of synthesis in man (Tahara, Metabolism, 1993; 42:19).

There is rapid phospholipid exchange between lipoprotein fractions and between lipoproteins and cell membranes. This appears to be facilitated by a phospholipid transfer protein with a molecular weight over 100 000. It may supply phospholipids and their polyunsaturated fatty acids to tissues.

Low density lipoprotein receptor[12]

A low density lipoprotein receptor is present on fibroblasts, hepatocytes, and many other cell types, and promotes the delivery of LDL cholesterol to these cells. Defects in the functioning of this receptor cause familial type II hypercholesterolaemia.

LDL receptors are clustered, with receptors for other ligands, in clathrin-coated pits on the cell surface. These pits are internalized, lose their clathrin coat, and become small vesicles called endosomes; the receptors are separated off from the other contents and congregate in small vesicles which return them to the cell surface. LDL particles, and other ligands, remain in vesicles which fuse with lysosomes and their constituents are degraded by lysosomal enzymes.

The LDL receptor, whose gene is on chromosome 19, is a dimer of two identical polypeptide chains each of 839 amino acids. Fifty amino acids at the carboxyl end are within the cytoplasm, and a sequence of 22 hydrophobic amino acids spans the cell membrane. Just outside the cell there is a sequence of 48 amino acids, rich in serine and threonine residues to which carbohydrate chains are attached; it is connected to a long sequence showing considerable homology to the epidermal growth factor precursor. The N-terminal end is a sequence of 322 amino acids that is extremely rich in cysteine residues which form disulphide bonds; it contains eight repeats of 40 amino acids which are thought to be the ligand-binding sites.

Chylomicron remnant receptor (Hui, JBC, 1986; 261:4256)

There is another receptor on hepatocytes which binds apoE-containing lipoproteins, but not lipoproteins in which only apoB is present. This is the chylomicron remnant receptor, which removes chylomicron remnants rapidly from plasma after a fat meal. It also recognizes VLDL remnants and HDL subspecies which are rich in apoE. Newly secreted chylomicrons were also recognized by this receptor in *in vitro* studies using isolated human hepatocyte membranes (Floren, ScaJGastr, 1984; 19:473). However, only remnants are recognized *in vivo* because chylomicrons are too large to traverse the fenestrations in the sinusoidal membranes and so gain access to the space of Disse and the surface of hepatocytes (Fraser, Hepatol, 1995; 21:863).

HDL receptors[13]

High affinity binding sites for HDL are present on both parenchymal and non-parenchymal cells of the liver, but parenchymal cells appear to be more active in HDL uptake. Only some of the bound HDL is degraded, suggesting that not all of it is internalized. In the rat, HDL binding is inhibited competitively by VLDL, LDL, and HDL but not by heparin or apoE; binding does not seem to be inhibited by chemical modification of HDL proteins. This suggests that there is a hepatic HDL receptor distinct from both the LDL receptor and the apoE receptor. HDL receptors have been found on adrenal cells; their numbers are increased by ACTH which promotes an increase in the uptake and hydrolysis of cholesteryl esters without an increase in HDL protein degradation. The intestine, kidney, and fibroblasts also appear to have receptors for HDL.

Lipid and lipoprotein metabolism

Only a simplified version of lipid and lipoprotein metabolism will be presented here. For further details readers are referred to a number of excellent reviews.[1,13]

Cholesterol, phospholipids, triglycerides, and most fatty acids can be synthesized in the body. Free cholesterol and phospholipids may be incorporated into the membranes of the cell of origin, or be exported from cells either by transfer to circulating lipoproteins or by incorporation into lipoproteins. Cholesteryl ester and triglyceride are stored or exported, and triglyceride is particularly important for storing energy and for transporting it between tissues.

Dietary fat is present mainly as triglyceride of animal or plant origin. Within the intestinal lumen this is hydrolysed by pancreatic lipases and the resulting monoglyceride and fatty acids are incorporated, with bile acids, into mixed micelles. These are taken up by small intestinal mucosal cells, in which most of the monoglyceride and fatty acid are re-esterified into triglyceride. This newly synthesized triglyceride enters plasma, via lymphatics, in triglyceride-rich chylomicrons and possibly in VLDL of intestinal origin. Some dietary fat may be absorbed directly into the portal vein as non-esterified fatty acids (NEFA); the physiological importance of this is unclear (see later). Lipoprotein lipases in peripheral tissues hydrolyse the triglyceride of circulating chylomicrons and VLDL; the fatty acids released are largely removed by tissues where they are metabolized or, particularly in adipose tissue, re-esterified and stored as triglyceride; a small amount of released fatty acids enters the circulation and contributes directly to the plasma NEFA pool.

After removal of triglyceride, chylomicron remnants remain in the plasma; they bind to the apoE receptors on hepatocytes, are then internalized, and their lipid, including cholesteryl ester, can be utilized or stored intracellularly.

Triglycerides are also made in the liver, either from fatty acids synthesized *de novo*, or from NEFA removed from the blood; these triglycerides are either stored or incorporated into hepatic VLDL prior to secretion into plasma. After secretion into plasma the triglyceride of hepatic VLDL, like that of chylomicrons, is hydrolysed by lipoprotein lipase, and the fatty acids are taken up by peripheral tissues. With the loss of their triglyceride, VLDL are converted into IDL (VLDL remnants). IDL are either removed by the liver, or are converted further to circulating LDL. During the process of conversion to mature LDL particles, surface lipids and apoproteins (other than the one molecule of apoB-100 present in VLDL) are removed from VLDL, as they are from chylomicrons, and are incorporated into HDL. Cholesteryl ester, which is synthesized in plasma as a result of the action of LCAT on the free cholesterol and lecithin of HDL particles, is transferred from HDL to VLDL and IDL particles via cholesteryl ester transfer protein.

Mature LDL particles rich in cholesteryl ester are able, because of their apoB-100 molecule, to bind to high affinity LDL receptors in liver and many other tissues. The number of these receptors is regulated by the cholesterol content of the cells, which also controls synthesis of cholesterol via the activity of hydroxymethylglutaryl CoA reductase—the rate-limiting enzyme in cholesterol biosynthesis. The ability of tissues to take up LDL may depend on the transcapillary transport rate as well as the number of receptors. Liver and adrenal tissue have a fenestrated endothelium (and many receptors) and may therefore take up LDL rapidly, while muscle and adipose tissue, which lack a fenestrated epithelium (and have few LDL receptors), take up LDL more slowly.

After binding to the LDL receptor, LDL particles are internalized by receptor-mediated endocytosis, and transferred to lysosomes for degradation. Their cholesteryl esters are hydrolysed to free cholesterol, which is used for membrane synthesis or conversion to steroid hormones or bile acids. Excess cholesterol is re-esterified by acyl cholesterol acyltransferase and stored as cholesteryl ester.

In humans, 70 to 80 per cent of LDL is removed via LDL receptors, the rest by non-specific endocytosis and the so-called 'scavenger' pathway—a receptor-mediated process involving phagocytic cells of the reticuloendothelial system.[12] The scavenger pathway is thought to remove lipoproteins which have been chemically altered or complexed with other molecules, and to remove LDL when it is present in high concentration. In the absence of LDL receptors, scavenger cells are a major mechanism for removing plasma cholesterol, and these cells, particularly macrophages, become lipid-rich foam cells which accumulate in xanthomas and atherosclerotic plaques.

The metabolism of HDL is more complex. HDL is secreted as a precursor lipoprotein which is very different from circulating 'normal' HDL. Secretory or 'nascent' HDL is discoidal in shape and composed of apoproteins (A and E), phospholipid (lecithin), and free cholesterol (Fig. 1). Nascent HDL is secreted mainly by the liver, with an unquantified amount coming from the intestine. Similar particles form within plasma from the phospholipid and free cholesterol of the surface coat of chylomicrons and VLDL, which becomes redundant as their core triglyceride is hydrolysed and removed.

During the hydrolysis of chylomicron and VLDL triglyceride, there is transfer of apoproteins (particularly C apoproteins), and of phospholipid and free cholesterol, to the nascent HDL, and of apoE to the triglyceride-rich particles. At the same time, lipid transfers occur; cholesteryl esters, which are produced in HDL by the action of LCAT, shift to VLDL and IDL (and subsequently to LDL), and some triglyceride moves in the opposite direction.

The formation of spherical HDL particles depends largely on the action of LCAT, and in primary and secondary deficiencies of this enzyme 'nascent' HDL can be found in plasma. HDL3 is probably produced first, and is then converted to the larger HDL2 particles by the further action of LCAT; this generates cholesteryl esters which enter the core to form less dense HDL2. HDL also acquires free cholesterol from cell membranes and this is probably an important mechanism for removing excess cholesterol from peripheral tissues. It is HDL2 that is finally catabolized by a variety of tissues.

Our understanding of the mechanisms of removal and catabolism of HDL2 is still incomplete. HDL probably interacts with cells in a variety of ways. The liver seems the major site of removal of HDL cholesterol and apoproteins, and in hepatic lipase deficiency there is an increase in the amount of HDL2 relative to that of HDL3. About 10 to 12 mg of HDL apoA-I plus ApoA-II per kilogram of body weight appear to be degraded daily by the liver; this would account for the removal of only about 250 to 300 mg of cholesterol if whole HDL particles are taken up. However, there is evidence that HDL particles may serve as a shuttle, and that their cholesteryl ester may be removed by hepatocytes without simultaneous removal of the apoproteins.

The effects of liver disease on plasma lipids and lipoproteins

There are important plasma lipid and lipoprotein abnormalities in liver disease. Total cholesterol tends to rise in obstructive jaundice (large duct obstruction or intrahepatic cholestasis) and to fall in severe parenchymal liver disease. The high serum cholesterol of obstructive jaundice is due mainly to increased free cholesterol (Widal, SemaineMed, 1912; 32:529); cholesteryl ester may be high, normal, or low. In severe parenchymal liver disease, cholesteryl ester is reduced (Epstein, ArchIntMed, 1932; 50:203) and free cholesterol normal or high. Serum triglyceride is often elevated, both in obstructive jaundice and, less often, in parenchymal liver disease, but the serum is rarely turbid which accords with the fact that the excess triglyceride is not usually carried in VLDL.

In obstructive jaundice, total phospholipid rises and there is a linear relationship between lecithin and free cholesterol. In parenchymal liver disease, total phospholipid is usually normal, but lecithin is increased (Phillips, JCI, 1960; 39:1639). Lysolecithin falls with severe liver damage, and is often low in obstructive jaundice even when lecithin is markedly elevated (Gjone, ScaJCLI, 1966; 18: 209). Unfortunately, simple lipid measurements on whole plasma provide an inadequate picture of the lipid abnormalities in liver disease, which can be understood only by detailed analysis of individual plasma lipoproteins.

Lecithin cholesterol acyltransferase (LCAT) and lipoprotein lipases in liver disease

It was thought originally that plasma cholesteryl esters were of hepatic origin, thus explaining their fall in severe liver disease. However, most cholesteryl ester of plasma results from the action of LCAT (Glomset, BBActa, 1962; 65:128; JLipRes, 1968; 9:155). Reduced LCAT activity is a key pathogenetic factor for the lipid and lipoprotein changes of liver disease, which resemble those seen in familial LCAT deficiency (Norum, ScaJCLI, 1967; 20:231). LCAT is synthesized by the liver, and its mRNA may be confined to the liver.[9,10]

Low plasma LCAT activity is found in many patients with liver disease, and correlates closely with plasma cholesteryl ester levels (Takahashi, JapJGastr, 1968; 65:1139; Gjone, ActaMedScand, 1970; 187:153; Simon, NEJM, 1970; 283:841; Calandra, EurJCI, 1971; 1: 352). The low activity is primarily a consequence of low LCAT protein (Floren, ScaJCLI, 1987; 47:613),[14] presumably due to reduced synthesis or impaired release of the enzyme by damaged liver. LCAT has a short plasma half-life and its activity falls quickly when there is significant reduction in hepatocellular function; indeed some groups have claimed that plasma LCAT activity is the best single prognostic indicator in patients with liver disease (De Marties, JIntMedRes, 1983; 11:232; Simko, JIntMedRes, 1985; 13: 249).

Plasma triglycerides are normally cleared by the action of peripheral lipases (LPL) and hepatic triglyceride lipases (**HTGL**). As one might expect, the activity of HTGL in postheparin plasma is reduced in patients with obstructive and parenchymal liver disease (Sauar, CCActa, 1978; 87:327; Baldo-Enzi, DigDisSci, 1988; 33: 1201).[15,16] A relatively high level of plasma triglyceride may be found in acute and chronic hepatitis, and in obstructive jaundice (Muller, EurJCI, 1974; 4:419; Pearson, Digestion, 1974; 10:322); in patients with severe liver disease, normal-sized LDL particles are triglyceride rich,[17,18] and in some cases, large triglyceride-rich particles resembling IDL are also present. It has been suggested that the high level of triglyceride is due to decreased HTGL activity, but this probably accounts only for the occasional presence of the large IDL particles, as one would expect LDL levels to fall with HTGL deficiency (Demant, JLipRes, 1988; 29:1603). Reduced HTGL activity may cause the elevated HDL2:HDL3 ratio seen in both obstructive jaundice and hepatocellular liver disease (see later). Peripheral lipase activity may also be reduced in liver disease,[15, 16] and low LCAT activity and peripheral lipase activity correlate best with the increase of triglyceride in the LDL fraction 1.019 to 1.063 g/ml (Sauar, CCActa, 1978; 87:327).[11,12]

Lipoproteins in obstructive jaundice[17]

There are many old studies on lipoprotein changes in obstructive jaundice, particularly in primary biliary cirrhosis in which

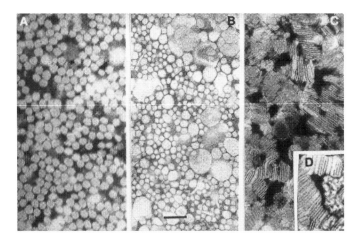

Fig. 2. A. Normal low density lipoproteins ($\times$ 182 000). B. Low density lipoproteins containing large triglyceride-rich particles ($\times$ 182 000). C. Low density lipoproteins containing LP-X ($\times$ 182 000). Inset, a picture of purified LP-X, demonstrating the bilamellar nature of the particles.(Bar marker = 50 nm.)

cholesterol and phospholipid levels may be far higher than in extrahepatic biliary obstruction. An increased LDL was found with a marked reduction in HDL (Gofman, Plasma, 1954; 2:413), and several lipoproteins of abnormal composition were thought to be present in the LDL fraction (Russ, JCI, 1956; 35:133; Furman, JCI, 1957; 36:713).

Very low density lipoproteins

In obstructive jaundice increased plasma triglyceride is not usually due to increased VLDL. When LCAT activity is high, plasma lipoprotein electrophoresis is normal, a preβ-band is seen, and VLDL is of normal composition. With low LCAT activity only a broad, densely staining β-band is seen. VLDL runs in this broad band (Seidel, EurJCI, 1972; 2:359) because of its altered apoprotein content; its lipid composition is abnormal, with a high phospholipid and free cholesterol and a low cholesteryl ester and triglyceride.

Low density lipoproteins

A key observation was the finding of an abnormal lipoprotein in patients with biliary obstruction. Switzer (JCI, 1967; 46:1855) found an abnormal LDL in primary biliary cirrhosis, which was rich in phospholipid and free cholesterol; triglyceride and cholesteryl esters were virtually absent and its protein had an amino-acid composition like that of VLDL. Seidel et al.[19,20] confirmed these findings and called the abnormal lipoprotein LP-X, believing it contained a specific apoprotein, apoX; in fact it contained the apoC peptides of VLDL. LP-X is also found in familial LCAT deficiency.

On electron microscopy, plasma LP-X appears as disc-shaped particles (40 to 60 nm wide by 10 nm thick), tending to form rouleaux (Hamilton, Science, 1971; 172:475) in which free cholesterol and lecithin are present in a 1:1 molar ratio (Fig. 2).

LP-X has been claimed to be of diagnostic use in 'cholestasis', but is of little practical value because cholestasis, and LP-X, is sometimes found in hepatitis and cirrhosis, and not simply with extrahepatic obstruction and classic types of intrahepatic cholestasis. Furthermore, LP-X may be undetectable in patients with either primary biliary cirrhosis, or with clear evidence of surgical or other forms of obstruction to the biliary tree (Ross, Gut, 1970; 11:1035; Ritland, CCActa, 1973; 49:251; Vergani, CCActa, 1973; 48:243; Magnani, Gastro, 1976; 71:87).[21] This limits the value of LP-X even for screening.

There are other abnormal particles in LDL (density 1.006 to 1.063 g/ml) in obstructive jaundice, depending on plasma LCAT activity (Fig. 2).[17] When LCAT is high, only 20-nm LDL particles are seen (as in normal LDL) and these have a normal composition. When LCAT activity is low, however, the picture is complex; LP-X accounts for most of the increase in free cholesterol and phospholipid, but a large (30 to 70 nm) triglyceride-rich particle may also be present which contains apoB and apoC (Muller, EurJCI, 1974; 4:419; Kostner, BiochemJ, 1976; 157:401).

With low LCAT activity the normal-sized 20-nm particles have an abnormal composition; they are triglyceride rich and cholesteryl ester poor. These non-polar lipids form the core of spherical LDL; if particle size is unchanged then increase in one must be accompanied by decrease in the other. As normal-sized LDL is also triglyceride rich in familial LCAT deficiency, in which lipase activities are normal, it seems likely that in obstructive jaundice the primary cause of this abnormality is reduced LCAT activity, a hypothesis supported by the correlation existing between plasma LCAT activity and the triglyceride–cholesteryl ester ratio of the 20-nm particles.

High density lipoproteins

α-Lipoprotein is often absent on plasma electrophoresis in patients with obstructive jaundice; this appears to be related to low plasma LCAT activity. When LCAT activity is high, a prominent α-band is visible and the HDL concentration may be greater than normal.[14,17] Even when LCAT activity is low, HDL can be isolated by ultracentrifugation; its concentration is low and uptake of electrophoretic stains is further impaired by its low cholesteryl ester content.

The composition and physicochemical characteristics of HDL particles in obstructive jaundice are still relatively poorly documented. This reflects, in part, the heterogeneity of normal plasma HDL. When serum LCAT activity was normal or elevated, high levels of virtually normal HDL were present; with low LCAT, HDL in obstructive jaundice contained at least three distinct particles on agarose column chromatography.[17] Of the two major peaks, one was like normal HDL, but with a high triglyceride and free cholesterol, and a low cholesteryl ester and phospholipid; the other was rich in free cholesterol and phospholipid, with a low cholesteryl ester and protein; this fraction contained 'stacked discs', or 'nascent' HDL, resembling those found in familial LCAT deficiency (Norum, JCI, 1971; 50:1131; Fig. 1a). In some patients with a low level of LCAT there was a third HDL peak in which there were tiny, spherical particles, rich in triglyceride and phospholipid, seen also in familial LCAT deficiency and thought to be of intestinal origin.

Reduced serum apoA-I and apoA-II levels were found in cholestasis, with a disproportionate reduction of apoA-II. As HDL3 has a lower apoA-I:apoA-II ratio than HDL2, Fujii et al. (CCActa, 1981; 115:321) suggested a more profound decrease in HDL3, which has been confirmed by several methods. Because conversion of HDL3 to HDL2 is catalysed by LCAT, while the transformation

of HDL2 to HDL3 requires hepatic lipase, it was argued that the elevated HDL2:HDL3 ratio in obstructive jaundice may result from low HTGL activity (Baldo-Enzi, DigDisSci, 1988; 33:1201), perhaps in combination with normal or intermediate LCAT activity (Sabesin, Gastro, 1985; 89:1426). In severe advanced liver disease, HDL concentrations and LCAT activity are very low, and the increased HDL2:HDL3 ratio is less apparent.[14] There may be a heat-labile plasma inhibitor of hepatic lipase in patients with primary biliary cirrhosis;[14] this still awaits confirmation.

Hiraoka et al. (Hepatol, 1993; 18:103) studied the mechanism of the high HDL cholesterol sometimes found with primary biliary cirrhosis. In five patients with this condition, HDL cholesterol was greater than 90 mg/dl; in another five it was lower. In both groups lipoprotein particles in HDL2 (density 1.063 to 1.125 g/ml) were apoE rich and larger in size than those of normal controls, HTGL activity was reduced (due to reduced protein mass), LPL activity and mass were normal, but there were increases in CETP activity and mass which were greater in those with hypera-α-lipoproteinaemia. The authors suggested that decreased HTGL levels at least partly explain the appearance of apoE-rich large HDL particles in primary biliary cirrhosis.

The most striking HDL apoprotein abnormality in obstructive jaundice is an elevation in apoE (Koga, GastrJap, 1983; 18:32; Owen, JLipRes, 1984; 25:919; Coulhoun, CCActa, 1985; 145:163; Floren, ScaJCLI, 1985; 45:103), with normal apoE allele frequencies (Butler, Hepatol, 1996; 24:313A). There may be two subclasses of apoE-rich particles, one containing only apoE and another in which apoA-I is present (Danielsson, ScaJCLI, 1978; 38(S15o):214).

Recently, Tallet et al. (CCActa, 1996; 244:1) reported detailed studies on the composition of HDL in patients with cholestasis, using a variety of analytical techniques. They confirmed many of the observations reported above. By isotachophoresis, they found six fractions (a to f) in HDL from normal subjects and patients with cholestasis. In healthy subjects fractions c, d, and e were predominant; in the patients the main fractions were a and f. HDLa contained apoE and apo(E:A-II) complexes; the apoprotein in HDLf was almost exclusively apoA-I. Bidimensional electroimmunodiffusion showed complexes containing only apoA-I, A-II, or E, or a combination of apoA-I plus A-II or of apoE plus A-II. These authors suggested that binding of bile acids to plasma lipoproteins might account for some of the observed changes.

The hyperlipidaemia of obstructive jaundice

Hyperlipidaemia occurs in obstructive jaundice even when the individual lipoprotein fractions appear to have a normal composition.[17] The reason for this is not entirely clear.[22]

It was argued that the hypercholesterolaemia of obstructive jaundice results from regurgitation of free cholesterol-rich bile into the bloodstream. When the bile duct was obstructed in dogs on which a cholecystectomy had been performed, free cholesterol and lecithin levels in plasma increased, but the concentration in the stagnant bile fell. The amount of lecithin normally excreted in bile appeared to account for the increase in plasma lecithin.[23] However, regurgitation of biliary cholesterol does not appear to account for the rise in plasma cholesterol; in rats only about one-third of the extra cholesterol found in plasma after 24 h of biliary obstruction could come from biliary cholesterol.

Where then does the extra plasma cholesterol come from, if bile is not the only source? Electron microscopy studies of the liver in obstructive jaundice do not show LP-X awaiting secretion, and there is no evidence of greater cholesterol secretion in normal lipoproteins (Stein, LabInvest, 1973; 29:166; Cooper, Gastro, 1974; 66:584). Hepatic cholesterol synthesis increases after bile duct ligation (Fredrickson, JExpMed, 1954; 99:43), but plasma free cholesterol rises markedly even if increased hepatic cholesterol synthesis is prevented by cycloheximide (Harry, BBActa, 1973; 296: 209).

The hypercholesterolaemia of obstructive jaundice is probably secondary to the accumulation in plasma of biliary lecithin. When lecithin alone was infused into the obstructed biliary tree in dogs, almost all appeared in plasma; as plasma lecithin increased so did plasma cholesterol.[23] Hypercholesterolaemia was also found when phospholipid was infused into animals after hepatectomy (Byers, JBC, 1962; 237:3375; Lipids, 1969; 4:123) suggesting that cholesterol came, at least partly, from pre-existing tissue cholesterol. Increased hepatic cholesterol synthesis occurring with infusion of lecithin did not take place when an equimolar amount of cholesterol was also given (Quarfordt, Gastro, 1973; 65:566). Presumably with infusion of lecithin alone, cholesterol is removed from the liver and cholesterol synthesis increases as a compensatory mechanism.

Regurgitation of phospholipid, and secondary accumulation of free cholesterol, could account for the appearance of plasma LP-X (in which they are in a 1:1 molar ratio). But why should phospholipid regurgitation increase the concentration of apparently normal lipoproteins (as in obstructed patients with high LCAT levels)? When lecithin was infused intravenously into normal human volunteers, plasma cholesteryl ester and LDL increased (Thompson, EurJCI, 1976; 6:241), suggesting that normal lipoproteins might accumulate if plasma LCAT could cope with the extra substrate. There was transient accumulation of phospholipid initially, presumably because LCAT was temporarily overloaded. Rapid biliary regurgitation of phospholipid might similarly exceed LCAT's ability to cope in obstructed patients with normal or high LCAT levels; this could explain why LP-X is sometimes found in such patients (Blomhoff, CCActa, 1974; 53:197).

With severe and prolonged obstruction, however, liver function becomes impaired; LCAT activity falls, and is inversely related to the plasma bilirubin. Free cholesterol, lecithin, and LP-X then accumulate in plasma as they do in familial LCAT deficiency. However, the amount of lipid present would not depend only on LCAT activity. With a large amount of biliary regurgitation, plasma lecithin and free cholesterol could reach very high levels (as they do in some patients with chronic obstruction). However, if liver cells fail then bile flow, and presumably regurgitation of phospholipid and cholesterol, would fall; this could account for the fall in plasma lecithin and cholesterol seen with en-stage biliary obstruction.

The lipoproteins of parenchymal liver disease[18]

In early studies, minor changes were found in plasma LDL concentration in cirrhosis (Pierce, Circul, 1951; 4:25), while in acute hepatitis there were abnormal lipoproteins, with a low cholesteryl ester:free cholesterol ratio and an abnormal electrophoretic mobility.[24] In acute viral hepatitis, α- and preβ-bands tend to be absent with agarose gel electrophoresis of serum; the β-band is broader, stains more densely, and migrates slightly faster than normal. In mild to moderate cases the α-lipoprotein band returns quickly with recovery; in severe fulminant cases it is absent for a longer period and may not reappear before death (Thalassinos, AmJDigDis, 1975; 20:148).

The lipoprotein changes in parenchymal liver disease appear to be related to LCAT activity.[18] With normal or high LCAT, the electrophoretic pattern is normal; with moderate reduction of LCAT activity, the preβ-band is lost; and with severe reduction, the preβ- and α-bands disappear. Both VLDL and HDL can be isolated by ultracentrifugation, even when preβ- and α-bands are absent.

Low density lipoproteins

In acute viral hepatitis a high level of plasma triglyceride may be found, due not to an increase in VLDL but to the presence of LDL with a low cholesteryl ester and high triglyceride content (Pearson, Digestion, 1974; 10:322); with recovery, LDL cholesteryl ester rises and its triglyceride falls. Hypertriglyceridaemia and LDL abnormalities were also found, and associated with decreased plasma LCAT activity, in patients with acute alcoholic liver disease (Sabesin, Gastro, 1977; 72:510): the predominant lipoprotein was a 30 to 70-nm particle, but the triglyceride content of normal-sized (20-nm) LDL was not measured; LP-X was present as a minor component. Unfortunately, these patients also had massive fatty liver and intrahepatic cholestasis, both of which may affect plasma lipoproteins.

We studied plasma lipoproteins in parenchymal liver disease of varying severity, and with a wide range of plasma LCAT activity, [18] but without evidence of intra- or extrahepatic cholestasis. When LCAT activity was normal or high, lipoproteins were of normal structure, electrophoretic mobility, and composition. When LCAT activity was low, there was only one LDL peak on gel filtration, as in normal controls; the particles were the same size as normal LDL, but they were cholesteryl ester poor and triglyceride rich. The finding of triglyceride-rich LDL of normal size in parenchymal liver disease, 'low LCAT' obstructive jaundice, and familial LCAT deficiency suggests that it results from low LCAT activity, less cholesteryl ester being produced to replace triglyceride in the particle core during catabolism of VLDL to LDL.

Patients with parenchymal liver disease may have a low level of total plasma lipids but a normal mean plasma LDL concentration. As the plasma level of VLDL, the precursor of LDL, is usually very low in these patients, it seems likely that they have a reduced rate of removal of LDL. Lower levels of hepatic apoB mRNA were found in patients with alcoholic cirrhosis than in normal subjects; but as there was little difference in serum apoB levels, it would appear that post-transcriptional regulation of apoB production and/ or control of apoB catabolism are more important factors in explaining serum apoB concentrations than apoB mRNA levels (Mathurin, Hepatol, 1996; 23:44).

High density lipoproteins

In acute alcoholic liver disease with markedly reduced plasma LCAT activity, Sabesin et al. (Gastro, 1977; 72:510) found on electron microscopy that the HDL fraction was composed largely of long chains of bilamellar discs. However, their results are difficult to interpret because of the accompanying cholestasis and fatty liver. We studied HDL in parenchymal liver disease of varying severity and with a wide range of plasma LCAT activity, but without cholestasis.[18] When LCAT activity was normal or high, HDL were of normal structure, electrophoretic mobility, and composition. When LCAT activity was low, the concentration of HDL was reduced; they were of abnormal composition and consisted largely of stacked discs on electron microscopy, like those found in obstructive jaundice with low LCAT activity, and in familial LCAT deficiency (Fig. 1). The protein content of the HDL was reduced. The similarity of the HDL changes in obstructive and parenchymal liver disease, and in familial LCAT deficiency, again suggests that they are due to LCAT deficiency *per se*, with reduced action of LCAT on 'nascent' HDL.

As in obstructive jaundice, the apoA-I:apoA-II ratio is elevated in parenchymal liver disease (Fuji, CCActa, 1981; 115:321), although apoA-I levels *per se* are also reduced, as they are in cholestatic liver disease (Floren, ScaJGastr, 1987; 22:454); this probably results from a reduction in hepatic apoA-I mRNA levels as these appear to be related to the severity of liver disease at least in alcoholic patients (Mathurin, Hepatol, 1996; 23:44). The low apoA-I:apoA-II ratio reflects a preferential reduction of HDL3 levels compared with HDL2 (Koga, GastrJap, 1983; 18:32). The HDL fraction is apoE rich (Tada, BBActa, 1981; 664:207; Weidman, JLipRes, 1982; 23: 556), as in cholestatic liver disease, and the apoE-containing particles may be devoid of apoA-II (Marcel, PNAS, 1980; 77:2969). This apoE-rich HDL appears to influence cellular metabolism in a number of ways (see below).

Very low density lipids and non-esterified fatty acids (NEFA)

In patients with severe parenchymal liver disease the fasting plasma VLDL concentration is low, probably because the production of VLDL of hepatic origin is impaired; the total level of plasma triglyceride remains relatively normal because the LDL in such patients is triglyceride rich.[18] Plasma NEFA are a major precursor for the triglyceride of circulating VLDL, and in normal subjects high NEFA levels tend to be associated with high plasma VLDL levels. In patients with cirrhosis, however, VLDL levels are low even though fasting NEFA are increased[15,25] and there is increased flux of NEFA (Mortiaux, Gut, 1961; 2:304). The increased flux is to be expected, as basal hepatic glucose output is low in people with cirrhosis and more NEFA are presumably required to meet the fasting energy requirements of peripheral tissues. It would appear, however, that hepatic handling of NEFA is disturbed in patients with cirrhosis; there is less incorporation of circulating NEFA into plasma triglyceride, and this appears to correlate with the severity of the liver disease (Santos, ArchIntMed, 1974; 134: 457).

In normal subjects, plasma triglyceride levels rise with a carbohydrate-rich diet, even if total caloric intake is not increased. There is fasting hypertriglyceridaemia after several days and the excess triglyceride is carried in VLDL; it seems likely that the increased triglyceride results from increased hepatic synthesis of fatty acids, as plasma NEFA fall. The plasma lipid and lipoprotein response to carbohydrate feeding is abnormal in patients with cirrhosis; the increase in fasting plasma triglyceride is less than in

normal subjects, particularly when the patients sre sick.[16] In normal subjects, and in people with cirrhosis with good liver function, most of the triglyceride increment is in VLDL; however, in patients with cirrhosis who are sick, most of it is in triglyceride-rich LDL. The most likely explanation for the poor triglyceride and VLDL response to carbohydrate feeding in patients with cirrhosis is impaired hepatic fatty acid synthesis and VLDL production.

There are also changes in the NEFA, VLDL, and chylomicron response of people with cirrhosis to fat feeding. The products of intestinal triglyceride hydrolysis (i.e. fatty acid and monoglyceride) are absorbed from the small intestine and re-esterified in the mucosa; the resulting triglyceride enters chylomicrons, and possibly VLDL of intestinal origin, and these large particles go directly to the systemic circulation via lymphatics, thus bypassing the liver and portal circulation even in normal subjects. Postprandial hypertriglyceridaemia results. Transport of dietary fatty acids as NEFA via the portal vein is usually considered to be quantitatively unimportant. Normal subjects show a small increase in plasma NEFA after fat feeding (Heimberg, JLabClinMed, 1974; 83:393; Nicholls, IrJMedSci, 1985; 154:348), which has been attributed to release of NEFA during the lipolysis, in peripheral tissues, of the triglyceride of chylomicrons and VLDL. However, this small rise in NEFA may mask a much greater relative contribution of dietary fatty acids to the plasma NEFA pool, as dietary fat appears to inhibit the release of NEFA from adipose tissue (Munckner, ScaJCLI, 1959; 11:394; Paluszak, AnnMedSectPolAcadSci, 1975; 20:201).

We found that people with cirrhosis with good liver function had a normal total plasma triglyceride response to fat feeding, although they carried less of the triglyceride increment in VLDL. People with cirrhosis who were sick had a poor plasma triglyceride response, and there was a smaller rise in both chylomicrons and VLDL.[15] Neither group had steatorrhoea, as assessed by measurement of 3-day faecal fat. We found subsequently that sick patients with cirrhosis have a striking postprandial rise in plasma NEFA, and even people with cirrhosis with good liver function have a much greater NEFA rise than controls (Avgerinos, Hepatol, 1986; 6:1152). There seem to be three explanations, not mutually exclusive, for the marked increase in NEFA found after fat feeding in the sick patients with cirrhosis:

1. More NEFA may have been released by the action of LPL on the triglyceride of chylomicrons and VLDL in the patients with cirrhosis. This seems unlikely given the low plasma chylomicron and VLDL concentrations in the patients who were sick, who also had a low postheparin plasma LPL activity. Alternatively, release of a normal or reduced amount of NEFA might have caused high levels if there was impaired NEFA removal from systemic blood; this also seems unlikely in view of the high NEFA flux which has been found in people with cirrhosis who were fasting (Mortiaux, Gut, 1961; 2:304).[25]

2. There may be portal transport of NEFA from the intestine in people with and without cirrhosis. While NEFA may be avidly removed from portal blood by normal livers, cirrhotic livers may show impaired uptake of portal NEFA due to hepatocyte dysfunction and/or portal–systemic shunting of blood; this would increase the amount of absorbed NEFA entering the

systemic circulation and so account for the high NEFA levels after fat feeding in people with cirrhosis.

3. People with cirrhosis may transport more dietary fat as NEFA via the portal vein than normal subjects. Increased portal vein carriage of NEFA was thought to occur in patients with biliary obstruction (Blomstrand, ActaChirScand, 1969; 135:329), and in animals following bile diversion (Saunders, Gut, 1963; 4:254); it has been attributed to a low intraluminal bile salt concentration, which is known to occur in cirrhosis (Badley, Gastro, 1970; 58: 781).

Others have suggested, on the basis of animal experiments, that portal vein transport of NEFA accounts for incomplete recovery of absorbed, labelled, long-chain fatty acids in intestinal lymph (Blomstrand, ActaPhysiolScand, 1954; 32:99; Gallagher, ClinSci, 1965; 29:73), and that the portal transport of polyunsaturated fatty acids is greater than that of saturated fatty acids (McDonald, AmJPhysiol, 1980; 239:G141). Selective portal transport of essential polyunsaturated fatty acids would make physiological sense as it would allow their preferential utilization by the liver for a variety of metabolic processes, including phospholipid synthesis.

It has been claimed that the increase in VLDL which occurs with alimentary lipaemia is due to intestinal VLDL (Lewis, Atheroscl, 1973; 17:455). However, if large amounts of dietary fatty acids are normally transported by the portal vein, and are removed by the liver during their first portal passage, they could be converted to triglyceride, and be secreted as hepatic VLDL which might then make a significant contribution to circulating VLDL after fat feeding. Two observations in man support this hypothesis, and suggest that the intestine's role in the plasma VLDL response to fat feeding may have been overemphasized. One is that enrichment of chylomicrons with dietary fatty acids appeared to occur well before that of VLDL (Edelin, Metabolism, 1968; 17:544). The other is that a biphasic serum triglyceride response was seen following a low fat load (Olefsky, AmJClinNut, 1976; 29:535); 90 per cent of the first peak, at 1 h, was due to chylomicrons, more than 80 per cent of the second peak, at 5 h, due to VLDL. One would expect later release of hepatic VLDL than of chylomicrons. The NEFA might have come directly to the liver via the portal vein, or indirectly from the systemic circulation following chylomicron triglyceride hydrolysis. However, Cohn et al. (Metabolism, 1989; 38:484) found that when there was a biphasic rise in the serum triglyceride after fat feeding, the second peak was rich in apoB-48 and retinyl ester, both of which are markers of lipoproteins of intestinal origin. This suggests that the later part of the increase in triglyceride cannot be be due solely to hepatic output of VLDL, but it does not not mean that it is due only to the presence of intestinal lipoproteins.

These observations may still account for our finding that, after fat feeding, people with cirrhosis carry less plasma triglyceride in VLDL than controls. In people with cirrhosis, incorporation of systemic plasma NEFA into circulating triglyceride is impaired (Santos, ArchIntMed, 1974; 134:457), due either to reduced hepatic uptake of NEFA, to impaired incorporation of intracellular fatty acids into triglyceride, or to impaired synthesis of VLDL particles. While all three mechanisms would explain the small VLDL/triglyceride increment seen after fat feeding in our patients with cirrhosis, only the first would explain the elevated postprandial levels of plasma NEFA (if impaired hepatic uptake of portal vein

NEFA allowed more dietary fatty acid to enter the systemic circulation).

If portal transit of NEFA increases when intestinal bile acid levels are low, as suggested above, we would expect increased hepatic uptake of dietary fatty acids, and increased VLDL secretion, in bile- diverted animals with otherwise normal livers. Increased hepatic uptake of dietary fatty acids was shown to occur in rats with bile fistulas (Saunders, Gut, 1963; 4:254), and an increased (and unexplained) output of VLDL, presumed to be of hepatic origin, was found after partial biliary diversion in the rhesus monkey (Adler, Metabolism, 1978; 27:607).

Energy handling and cirrhosis

In the period following a meal, tissues can obtain energy directly from plasma nutrients, such as glucose, fructose, and triglyceride. The carbohydrate and fat absorbed in excess of immediate tissue requirements is stored; carbohydrate is deposited as glycogen in liver and muscle, and fat and some carbohydrate is stored as triglyceride in adipose tissue. NEFA are subsequently released from adipose tissue and, with glucose secreted by the liver, they help to meet the continuing energy demands of tissues. Before adipose tissue can store triglyceride, however, it must receive the necessary precursors. The major carriers of dietary energy to adipose tissue are the triglyceride-rich lipoproteins, chylomicrons, which carry dietary fat and VLDL; human adipose tissue appears to have a limited capability for the synthesis of fatty acids directly from glucose and fructose (Patel, Metabolism, 1975; 24:161; Shrago, AmJClinNut, 1976; 29:540; Pearce, ProcNutrSoc, 1983; 42:263), and so carbohydrate energy must be converted into fatty acids by the liver, and carried to the adipose tissue in VLDL triglyceride, before it can be stored there as triglyceride.

As sick patients with cirrhosis have low plasma VLDL after carbohydrate feeding, and low chylomicrons and VLDL after fat feeding, their ability to transfer dietary energy to adipose tissue in such triglyceride-rich particles may be impaired, whether they result from fat or carbohydrate feeding. However, if this is the case, what happens to the carbohydrate and fat which would normally be stored in adipose tissue? After carbohydrate feeding, plasma levels of glucose (Stewart, EurJClinInv, 1983; 13:397) and fructose (Grace, ArchIntMed, 1969; 124:330) are higher in people with cirrhosis than in controls and the increases are more sustained (Avgerinos, JHepatol, 1992; 14:78). Therefore, in people with cirrhosis, the tissues may utilize these sugars directly from the bloodstream for a longer period of time. Similarly, dietary fat may be directly available from the increased plasma NEFA levels seen after fat feeding in people with cirrhosis.

If, in subjects who are in a steady state from day to day, more dietary nutrients are utilized directly from the blood then, over a 24-h period, less energy will be available for storage in adipose tissue and subsequent release as NEFA. Although fasting levels of plasma NEFA are high in people with cirrhosis, and more fat than carbohydrate is used during fasting,[25] this might not hold over a 24-h period; after a glucose load there is a fall in plasma NEFA in people with cirrhosis, as in normal subjects (Riggio, Metabolism, 1982; 31:627). Indeed, we showed that on a high carbohydrate diet, NEFA levels during the day were significantly lower in people with cirrhosis than in controls (Avgerinos, JHepatol, 1992; 14:78); this suggests less adipose tissue lipolysis. If people with cirrhosis continued to release large amounts of NEFA from adipose tissue, then large amounts of triglyceride would also have to be deposited in adipose tissue if rapid weight loss were not to ensue. This deposition would presumably necessitate initial transport of the fatty acids to the adipose tissue in triglyceride-rich lipoproteins. Our results suggest that sick patients with cirrhosis may be incapable of transporting the large amounts of triglyceride required for this purpose, and it may be this, rather than excessive breakdown, that accounts for the loss of adipose tissue in these patients.

The clinical implications of the plasma lipoprotein abnormalities of liver disease

There are few overt clinical consequences of the plasma lipoprotein abnormalities found with liver disease. Cutaneous xanthomas may appear in chronic obstructive jaundice when plasma lipids are very high (Ahrens, JCI, 1949; 28:1565); they may be scanty or widespread, and characteristically occur in palmar and plantar creases, around the eyes, over the elbows, buttocks, and knees, and in areas of pressure or trauma. The cholesterol in xanthomas is mainly cholesteryl ester. We believe that cholesterol accumulates in these tissues because of unrestricted 'diffusion' of free cholesterol from the abnormal plasma lipoproteins—esterification within cells maintaining a gradient for the continued transfer of free cholesterol (Owen, BiochemSocTrans, 1983; 11:336). Xanthomatous deposits in peripheral nerves may be associated with palmar and plantar skin tenderness, due to a mild sensory neuropathy (Thomas, Brain, 1965; 88:1079). One patient with primary biliary cirrhosis suffered from a hyperviscosity syndrome, which responded to plasma exchange; the viscosity of the serum was directly related to its concentration of cholesterol (Rosenson, Gastro, 1990; 98:1351).

Because a broad, densely staining β-band is found, together with a high total serum cholesterol and triglyceride in obstructive jaundice, a diagnosis of type IIa or type III hyperlipoproteinaemia may be made (Beaumont, BullWHO, 1970; 43:891); inappropriate dietary or other advice may be given on this basis. Dietary measures do not reduce the hypercholesterolaemia of obstructive jaundice, and steroids are of no value (Schaffner, Gastro, 1969; 57:253). Cholestyramine, which binds bile acids in the gut and is useful for pruritus, lowers serum cholesterol and may cause clearing of xanthomas (Van Itallie, NEJM, 1961; 265:469). Total plasma cholesterol also falls when ursodeoxycholic acid is given orally to patients with primary biliary cirrhosis. Poupon et al. (Hepatol, 1993; 17:577) noted a fall in the mean value from 7.5 to 4.4 mmol/l, due mainly to a reduction in LDL cholesterol although VLDL cholesterol also fell. Total HDL levels did not change, but there was a reduction in the HDL2:HDL3 ratio.

Clofibrate caused an increase in serum cholesterol in patients with primary biliary cirrhosis, and xanthomas increased in size (Schaffner, Gastro, 1969; 57:253). Clofibrate given to rats with ligated bile ducts caused a greater increase in free cholesterol and phospholipid than biliary ligation alone,[26] but until recently there was no good explanation for this effect. We now realize that the excretion of phospholipid in bile depends on the presence in biliary canaliculi of a phospholipid transport protein thought to act as a

'flippase' (Smit, Cell, 1993; 75:451). This transfers lecithin, and possibly other phospholipids, from the inner to the outer layer of the canalicular membrane. It was thought to be one of the P-glycoproteins present in excess in cancer cells which are resistant to many hydrophobic drugs—the so-called 'multidrug resistant (MDR) cells'. In man it is coded for by the MDR3 gene, which is closely related to the mouse mdr2 gene; neither gene product confers resistance to any antitumour drug. MDR3 and mdr2 gene products are expressed in several tissues, and particularly in biliary canicular membranes. In homozygous mdr2 knockout mice (–/–) no mdr2 gene product is found in biliary canaliculi or other tissues, and the animals show a striking reduction in the biliary output of phospholipid and cholesterol.

In rats clofibrate, and other fibrates, caused a significant rise in biliary phospholipid, together with an increase in the amount of P-glycoprotein in canalicular membrane proteins and in hepatic mdr2 mRNA levels (Chianale, BiochemJ, 1996; 314:781). Biliary phospholipid output correlated significantly with relative levels of mdr2 mRNA. It thus appears that the paradoxical effect of clofibrate on serum cholesterol levels in primary biliary cirrhosis, and on cholesterol and phospholipid levels in rats with biliary obstruction, is due to enhanced secretion of lecithin into bile, leading to the regurgitation of a larger amount of lecithin into serum, which in turn increases serum cholesterol levels (see earlier).

Severe xanthomatous neuropathy has been successfully treated with plasmapheresis or plasma exchange; the plasma cholesterol fell, symptoms improved, and the xanthomas regressed (Turnberg, Gut, 1972; 13:976). Unfortunately, these methods are costly, time-consuming, and inconvenient for the patient as they have to be repeated many times. Plasma exchange combined with mevinolin (which inhibits cholesterol biosynthesis) has also been used to reduce hypercholesterolaemia (Thompson, ApheresisBull, 1983; 1: 26).

Ahrens (BullNYAcadMed, 1950; 26:151) found aortic atheroma in hyperlipidaemic patients with primary biliary cirrhosis, but paradoxically the extent of atheroma seemed inversely related to plasma lipid levels. Four patients with marked cutaneous xanthomatosis had minimal atheroma; three patients without xanthomas had arterial lesions which were disproportionately severe in relation to the patients' age and sex. It is generally believed that ischaemic heart disease is uncommon in primary biliary cirrhosis, but Schaffner (Gastro, 1969; 57:253) quoted three series in which it was present in some patients; in his own series of over 50 patients, four had had a myocardial infarct and two had severe angina. More recently, Crippin et al. (Hepatol, 1992; 15:858) followed 312 patients with primary biliary cirrhosis for a median period of 7.4 years. The incidence of atherosclerotic death was a little higher in patients with primary biliary cirrhosis than would have been expected in the white population of the United States generally, but the difference was not statistically significant and the authors concluded that the hyperlipidaemia of primary biliary cirrhosis does not increase the risk of atherosclerosis.

Gregory et al. (Atheroscl, 1994; 105:43) tried to explain this anomaly by measuring the levels of Lp(a), a lipoprotein incriminated in premature development of atherosclerosis. Lp(a) levels were lower in primary biliary cirrhosis than in other forms of liver disease and in healthy controls; it was argued that this exerted a protective effect despite elevated levels of LDL. Others found that Lp(a) levels reflect the severity of liver disease, not the cause (Cimminiello, BiomedPharmacoth, 1995; 49:364; Selvais, PressMed, 1995; 24: 382), and that Lp(a) increases as liver function improves (Malaguarnera, ClinTher, 1995; 17:721). Lp(a) seems unlikely to be an important factor in liver disease.

Effects on cellular metabolism
Cell membrane lipid composition

The surface composition of plasma lipoproteins changes in severe liver disease. There is an excess of free cholesterol and lecithin, less arachidonate in phospholipid fatty acyl chains, and the apoprotein composition of lipoproteins, particularly HDL, is abnormal. Because free cholesterol and phospholipid molecules on the surface of lipoproteins exchange and equilibrate with those on cell surface membranes, similar lipid abnormalities are found in red cell and platelet membranes in liver disease. Changes in the fatty acids of the red cell surface in patients with alcoholic cirrhosis may enable the cells to resist lipid peroxidation (Punchard, Gut, 1994; 35:1753).

Cell surface lipid changes may also affect membrane function by changing membrane fluidity, by altering binding of charged substances to phospholipid head groups, by affecting interaction of hydrophobic substances with the membrane interior, by changing the state of water at both surfaces of the membrane, and by reducing the level of arachidonic acid which is a precursor of prostaglandins and thromboxanes.

Membrane fluidity affects many membrane properties and functions, including membrane permeability; it alters the activity of membrane proteins acting as receptors, transport proteins, or enzymes. Membrane fluidity falls with an increase in the free cholesterol–phospholipid (**C–PL**) ratio and/or a reduction in the proportion of polyunsaturated fatty acids in membrane phospholipids; it increases with elevation of the lecithin:sphingomyelin ratio.

In liver disease the bulk membrane fluidity of red cells is reduced, reflecting the increased C–PL ratio (Owen, JLipRes, 1982; 23:124). An increased C–PL ratio reduced ouabain-insensitive sodium efflux (Owen, BBActa, 1978; 510:168) by inhibiting the frusemide-sensitive component (Jackson, ClinSci, 1982; 62:101). Further enrichment of red cell membranes with cholesterol inhibited Na^+-K^+-ATPase-mediated sodium transport (the Na^+ pump). Anion exchange (pyruvate influx with either chloride or hydroxyl efflux) was similarly reduced when the C–PL ratio increased, and its sensitivity to frusemide is almost identical to that of sodium transport. It seems likely that both processes are mediated via the band 3 intramembrane protein (Jackson, BBActa, 1982; 693:99). Recently, Kakimoto et al. (Metabolism, 1995; 44:825) found that the decreased membrane fluidity found with cirrhosis was associated with a fall in the activity of the red cell membrane proteins, Mg^{2+}-ATPase and acetylcholinesterase, but there was little or no effect on Na^+-K^+-ATPase activity.

When normal platelets are enriched with cholesterol they show increased sensitivity to aggregation by ADP and adrenaline (Shattil, JCI, 1975; 55:636). Platelets in liver disease are cholesterol rich, but their aggregability is diminished. This hypoaggregability is associated with reduced arachidonic acid in platelet phospholipids; [27] our suggestion that this may result in diminished production of the proaggregatory thromboxane A_2 has been confirmed (Laffi,

Gastro, 1986; 90:274; Hepatol, 1988; 8:1620). The possible implications of these findings, and of the ability of HDL from jaundiced patients to impair platelet aggregation (see below), are obvious but further work is needed to establish their significance for the disturbances of haemostasis seen in severe liver disease.

In liver disease the red cell membrane contains more free cholesterol, or more free cholesterol and phospholipid, than that of normal cells. The surface area expands without corresponding change in volume and so the shape of the red cells changes. In wet films they are 'bowl' shaped, but drying before staining distorts them and in conventional blood films they appear as 'target' cells (Barrett, JPatholBacteriol, 1938; 46:603; see Chapter 25.3), which are also present in familial LCAT deficiency;[8] their formation would seem, therefore, to be the consequence of low LCAT activity and the subsequent acquisition of cholesterol (and possibly lecithin) molecules from abnormal lipoprotein particles.

It seems likely that membranes of other tissues and organs are similarly affected by the lipoprotein abnormalities found in liver disease. Renal failure occurs in familial LCAT deficiency. Large amounts of cholesterol and phospholipid accumulate in the renal cortex and there is histological evidence of lipid deposition in glomeruli. Progressive renal failure, and similar histological changes, have been seen in advanced liver disease when plasma LCAT activity is low (Gjone, AdvNephrol, 1981; 10:167). We have shown by direct measurements that membrane lipid abnormalities occur in the kidney in experimental liver disease (Kawata, BBActa, 1987; 896:26); there is an increase in the C–PL ratio and a reduction in the arachidonic acid content. We also showed that the change in the C–PL ratio found in the renal cortical brush border of rats with a ligated bile duct is associated with an increase in Na^+-dependent glucose transport by these membranes (Imai, Hepatol, 1989; 10: 618), so it seems likely that renal lipid changes might affect other aspects of renal function.

In patients with chronic liver disease there are complex effects on the polyunsaturated fatty acid content of the plasma lipids. The major deficiency is of arachidonic acid (Johnson, PNAS, 1985; 82: 1815), a minor component of the diet which can be synthesized in the body from linolenic acid. Red cell (Owen, JLipRes, 1982; 23: 124) and platelet[27] arachidonic acid is also reduced in liver disease. Arachidonic acid is the precursor of the 2 series prostaglandins, of thromboxane A_2 and prostacyclin, and of hydroxy acids such as the leukotrienes. Although we know a good deal about the conversion of arachidonic acid to these compounds, we know little about the conversion of linoleate to arachidonate or about the transport and tissue uptake of arachidonic acid.

Prostaglandin E_2 appears to play an important role in renal function in liver disease. Patients with ascites, but without functional failure and with reasonable free water clearance, have high urinary prostaglandin E_2 levels, which may protect the kidney against the vasoconstrictor influences which are present in such patients (Section 9); a low urinary prostaglandin E_2 is found when renal failure develops or when there is a marked reduction in free water clearance (Arroyo, EurJClinInv, 1983; 13:271; Perez-Ayuso, KidneyInt, 1984; 26:72). The fall in urinary prostaglandin E_2 levels may be an important factor in the worsening of renal function, as functional renal failure often develops in patients with ascites when they are given prostaglandin synthetase inhibitors such as the nonsteroidal anti-inflammatory drugs (Zipser, JClinEndoc, 1979; 48:

885). The low urinary prostaglandin E_2 which occurs spontaneously may be due to a reduced renal supply of arachidonic acid at a time when demand for it is high; plasma phospholipids have a reduced amount of arachidonate in liver disease,[27] and the plasma arachidonic acid level was found to be lowest in patients with cirrhosis with functional renal failure (Parelon, GastrClinBiol, 1985; 9:290). Cabre *et al.* (AmJGastr, 1993; 88:718) followed 101 patients with cirrhosis over a mean period of 14.8 months; in a univariate analysis, mortality was significantly associated with arachidonic acid deficiency.

In a recent review on 'cirrhotic cardiomyopathy', Ma and Lee (Hepatol, 1996; 24:451) suggested that changes in the membrane fluidity of myocardial cells might affect cardiac function; in experimental cirrhosis the response to β-adrenergic stimuli is blunted, and this appears to be due, at least in part, to reduced membrane fluidity. They also suggested that an alteration in the physical properties of the membrane may cause ECG abnormalities in cirrhosis (see also Chapter 25.1).

Apoprotein-mediated effects on cells

Changes in the apoprotein composition of lipoproteins also have important functional effects. HDL from patients with severe liver disease are rich in apoE, which competes with apoB of LDL for binding to the B,E receptor present on many cell surfaces. This receptor controls cellular uptake of LDL, the major carrier of plasma cholesterol, and therefore the supply of this essential nutrient to cells. The HDL of liver disease interferes with LDL uptake by cells *in vitro* (Owen, JLipRes, 1984; 25:919); this may help to explain the relatively normal levels of LDL found *in vivo* in severe parenchymal liver disease,[16] despite the low plasma levels of its precursor particle, VLDL. Reduced cellular uptake of LDL may have important implications for cellular cholesterol metabolism; even though the abnormal HDL particles are ingested following binding, they have a low cholesteryl ester content. The clinical significance of these phenomena is unclear.

The abnormal HDL of liver disease also appear to be important in the conversion of normal erythrocytes to spiculated cells called echinocytes (see Chapter 25.3); there was a close correlation between the number of echinocytes found in wet film preparations from many patients with cirrhosis and the ability of the HDL from those patients to transform normal red cells into echinocytes *in vivo*.[28] Other lipoprotein classes and plasma proteins were non-echinocytogenic. HDL-induced echinocytosis was not accompanied by enrichment with cholesterol or phospholipid; the important factor seemed to be reversible, saturable binding of the abnormal HDL particles by the erythrocyte surface. It seems likely that the presence of large numbers of echinocytes is an important factor in the production of acanthocytes; these are bizarrely shaped cells, like those seen in abetalipoproteinaemia, which are found in the peripheral blood of the very small number of patients with cirrhosis who develop 'spur-cell' anaemia (Smith, NEJM, 1964; 271:396). Most of the red blood cells in these patients are echinocytes, and their HDL has a powerful echinocytogenic effect on normal erythrocytes. It has been suggested that 'spur-cell' anaemia is caused by marked elevation of the membrane C–PL ratio (Cooper, SemHemat, 1970; 7:296), but this seems an unlikely explanation as the C–PL ratio is just as high in familial LCAT deficiency in which target cells, but not acanthocytes, are seen.

The abnormal HDL of liver disease has other biological effects. HDL isolated from patients with cirrhosis inhibits ADP-induced platelet aggregation (Desai, Lancet, 1989; i:625). This anti-aggregatory effect of cirrhotic HDL appears to be related to its high apoE content, as apoE-enriched HDL1 from normal plasma also impairs the reactivity of platelets to a variety of agonists, apparently by binding to saturable sites on the cell surface (Desai, JLipRes, 1989; 30:831). ApoE-rich HDL from patients with jaundice also inhibits mitogen-induced lymphocyte transformation (Owen, TrendsBiochemSci, 1984; 9:238) and this may account, in part, for the increased susceptibility to infection in liver disease.

Because lipoprotein research, using adequate methods, is difficult and time-consuming, few have studied lipoprotein abnormalities in liver disease in any depth. There has been even less interest in the cellular changes which may result. However, it seems likely that many metabolic disturbances in patients with liver disease may result from changes in the composition and function of cell membranes. Further studies seem justified as it may be possible to reverse some of the lipoprotein abnormalities, at least on a temporary basis; this may help in the management of severe hepatitis and in the preparation of jaundiced patients for surgery.

References

1. Havel RJ and Kane JP. Introduction: structure and metabolism of plasma lipoproteins. In Scriver CR, Beaudet AL, Sly WS, and Valle D, eds. *The Metabolic bases of inherited disease.* 7th edn. New York: McGraw-Hill, 1995: 1841–51.

2. Segrest JP and Albers JJ, eds. *Plasma lipoproteins—Part A: preparation, structure and molecular biology*, Vol. 128 of *Colowick and Kaplan's methods in enzymology.* Orlando, Florida: Academic Press, 1986.

3. McIntyre N and Harry DS. *Lipids and lipoproteins in clinical practice.* London: Wolfe Publishing, 1991.

4. Li W-H, Tanimura M, Luo C-C, Datta S, and Chan L. The apolipoprotein multigene family: biosynthesis, structure, structure–function relationships, and evolution. *Journal of Lipid Research*, 1988; **29**: 245–71.

5. Law SW, Lackner KJ, Fojo SS, Hospattankar A, Monge JC, and Brewer HB. The molecular biology of human apoA-I, apoA-II, apoC-II and apoB. In Angel A and Frohlich J, eds. *Lipoprotein deficiency syndromes*, Vol. 201 of *Advances in experimental medicine and biology.* New York: Plenum Press, 1986.

6. Lusis AJ. Genetic factors affecting blood lipoproteins: the candidate gene approach. *Journal of Lipid Research*, 1988; **29**: 397–429.

7. Calvert GD and Abbey M. Plasma lipoproteins, apolipoproteins, and proteins concerned with lipid metabolism. *Advances in Clinical Chemistry*, 1985; **24**: 217–98.

8. Glomset JA, Assmann G, Gjone E, and Norum KR. Lecithin:cholesterol acyltransferase deficiency and fish eye disease. In Scriver CR, Beaudet AL, Sly WS, and Valle D, eds. *The Metabolic bases of inherited disease.* 7th edn. New York: McGraw-Hill, 1995: 1933–51.

9. McLean J, Wion K, Drayna D, Fielding C, and Lawn R. Human lecithin-cholesterol acyltransferase gene: complete gene sequence and sites of expression. *Nucleic Acids Research*, 1986; **14**: 9387–406.

10. Tata F, *et al.* The isolation and characterisation of cDNA and genomic clones for human lecithin:cholesterol acyltransferase. *Biochimica et Biophysica Acta*, 1987; **910**: 142–8.

11. Quinn D, Shirai K, and Jackson RL. Lipoprotein lipase: mechanism of action and role in lipoprotein metabolism. *Progress in Lipid Research*, 1983; **22**: 5–78.

12. Brown MS and Goldstein JL. A receptor mediated pathway for cholesterol homeostasis. *Science*, 1986; **232**: 34–47.

13. Breslow JL. Familial disorders of high-density lipoprotein metabolism. In Scriver CR, Beaudet AL, Sly WS, and Valle D, eds. *The metabolic bases of inherited disease*. 7th edn. New York: McGraw-Hill, 1995: 2031–52.

14. Jahn CE, *et al.* Lipoprotein abnormalities in primary biliary cirrhosis. *Gastroenterology*, 1985; **89**: 1266–78.

15. Avgerinos A, *et al.* Plasma lipid and lipoprotein responses to fat feeding in alcoholic liver disease. *Hepatology*, 1983; **31**: 349–55.

16. Avgerinos A, Kourti A, Chu P, Harry DS, Raptis S, and McIntyre N. plasma lipid and lipoprotein response to carbohydrate feeding in cirrhotic patients. *Journal of Hepatology*, 1988; **6**: 315–24.

17. Agorastos J, Fox D, Harry DS, and McIntyre N. Lecithin:cholesterol acyltansferase and the lipoprotein abnormalities of obstructive jaundice. *Clinical Science and Molecular Medicine*, 1978; **54**: 369–79.

18. Day RC, Harry DS, Owen JS, and McIntyre N. Plasma lecithin-cholesterol acyltransferase and the lipoprotein abnormalities of parenchymal liver disease. *Clinical Science*, 1979; **56**: 575–83.

19. Seidel D, Alaupovic P, and Furman RH. A lipoprotein characterizing obstructive jaundice. I. Method for quantitative separation and identification of lipoproteins in jaundiced subjects. *Journal of Clinical Investigation*, 1969; **48**: 1211–23.

20. Seidel D, Alaupovic P, Furman RH, and McConathy WJ. A lipoprotein characterizing obstructive jaundice. II. Isolation and partial characterization of the protein moieties of low density lipoproteins. *Journal of Clinical Investigation*, 1969; **49**: 2396–407.

21. Eder G, *et al.* Conclusions of LP-X determinations in more than 2500 patients. In Peeters H, ed. *Proteides of biological fluids*, Vol 25. Oxford: Pergamon Press, 1977: 341–7.

22. McIntyre N, Harry DS, and Pearson AJG. The hypercholesterolaemia of obstructive jaundice. *Gut*, 1975; **16**: 379–91.

23. Quarfordt SH, Oelschlager H, and Krigbaum WR. Effect of biliary lipids obstruction on canine plasma and biliary lipids. *Lipids*, 1973; **8**: 522–30.

24. Eder HA, *et al.* Protein–lipid relationship in human plasma; in biliary cirrhosis, obstructive jaundice and acute hepatitis. *Journal of Clinical Investigation*, 1955; **34**: 1147–62.

25. Owen OE, *et al.* Nature and quantity of fuels consumed in patients with alcoholic cirrhosis. *Journal of Clinical Investigation*, 1983; **72**: 1821–32.

26. Pyrovolakis J, *et al.* Elevation of plasma cholesterol by clofibrate in rats with biliary obstruction. In Gerok W and Sickinger K, eds. *Drugs and the liver.* Stuttgart: Schattauer Verlag, 1975: 381–6.

27. Owen JS, Hutton RA, Day RC, Bruckdorfer KR, and McIntyre N. Platelet lipid composition and platelet aggregation in human liver disease. *Journal of Lipid Research*, 1981; **22**: 423–30.

28. Owen JS, *et al.* Erythrocyte echinocytosis in liver disease. Role of abnormal plasma high density lipoproteins. *Journal of Clinical Investigation*, 1985; **76**: 2275–85.

2.13 Amino acid metabolism, urea production, and pH regulation

2.13.1 Amino acid metabolism

Yolanta T. Kruszynska and Neil McIntyre

Amino acid metabolism in normal humans

Amino acids are important biological compounds; they are building blocks of proteins, precursors of many other molecules, and a major source of energy in the diet. Amino acids have the same basic structure; they differ in the nature of their side-group, –R, which may be non-polar, uncharged but polar, acidic, or basic. Although only 20 amino acids are incorporated into polypeptide chains during the translation of messenger RNA (i.e. the 'protein' amino acids, Table 1), more than 20 can be found in proteins, because several amino acids may undergo post-translational modification. In proteins and peptides an amide linkage, the 'peptide bond', joins the amino group of one amino acid to the carboxyl group of the next. There are many other amino acids, not found in proteins, which have important functions.

Amino acids having a carbon skeleton which can be synthesized within the body are not essential dietary constituents. 'Essential amino acids' (Table 1) cannot be synthesized *de novo* and must be present in adequate amounts in the diet in order to sustain growth or nitrogen balance.[1,2] Although tyrosine and cysteine are not strictly essential, they can only be synthesized from phenylalanine and methionine, which are essential. Arginine and histidine are essential in infants, who cannot synthesize enough of them to meet the demands for rapid growth; histidine is also an essential amino acid in adults during periods of physiological stress.[1,3] Dietary protein can be fully utilized only if it contains the required amount of each essential amino acid. If, for example, the diet contains only 50 per cent of the required leucine then only 50 per cent of its protein could be used for tissue protein synthesis; the rest would be used to provide energy, and its nitrogen wasted. Therefore, the requirements for essential amino acids are often expressed as grams of amino acid per kg of dietary protein (Table 1).[1]

Dietary protein is hydrolysed within the intestinal lumen and the resulting amino acids and oligopeptides are taken up by the small intestinal mucosa; further hydrolysis of oligopeptides occurs in the mucosa. There may be some metabolism of dietary amino acids within the mucosa, but the bulk of them are transported from the intestine via the portal vein. After a meal amino acids reach the liver in a relatively high concentration. They may be removed by the liver on the first portal circulation, or they may pass into the systemic circulation where they are available for uptake by peripheral tissues.

In normal subjects in steady state the dietary intake of amino acids must be fully utilized each day, and their carbon skeletons metabolized. The initial step in the catabolism of most amino acids is the removal of the amino group, either by deamination, or by transamination, which transfers the amino-group to a ketoacid with the formation of another amino acid and a different ketoacid from the first amino acid. Pyridoxal 5-phosphate is the prosthetic group for all the aminotransferases. Transamination is involved in the synthesis of non-essential amino acids and the reamination of essential ones. The carbon skeletons of amino acids are involved in a large number of reactions. Those that can give rise to pyruvate or intermediates of the tricarboxylic acid cycle can be converted into glucose (thus their amino acids are glucogenic). Amino acids whose carbon skeletons are metabolized to acetyl CoA are ketogenic. Some are both glucogenic and ketogenic.

The liver plays a key role in the metabolism of amino acids. It removes them from plasma for protein synthesis and gluconeogenesis; it is the major site for the synthesis and interconversion of non-essential amino acids, and in the reamination of the carbon skeleton of most essential amino acids; it releases amino acids into blood for utilization by peripheral tissues, particularly skeletal muscle; it plays a major role in the breakdown of amino acids, removing their nitrogen as urea. Skeletal muscle is the major source of plasma amino acids during periods of dietary protein deprivation, and the interchange of amino acids between the liver and skeletal muscle plays a key role in nitrogen metabolism.

The individual protein amino acids[4]

The metabolism of the different amino acids varies widely. The 'normal' dietary intake of amino acids depends on the amount and nature of the proteins in the diet,[2] and the figures given in Table 1 are therefore an approximation. The plasma levels of amino acids vary in relation to meals, and some show a diurnal variation. However, the intraindividual variation is less than the interindividual variation for all amino acids, except for aspartate and taurine. For many amino acids the concentration in intracellular water is severalfold higher than that of plasma[5,6] (Ryan, Nature, 1966; 212:292; Bergstrom, JApplPhysiol, 1974; 36:693). These transmembrane amino acid concentration gradients are maintained by specific transporters (see below).

Table 1 The individual amino acids

	Side chain	Essential/ non-essential	Recommended daily intake (g/kg protein)	Average intake (g/day)	Plasma level (μmol/l)
Glycine	$-H$	NE		3–5	232 ± 44
Alanine	$-CH_3$	NE	4–8	360 ± 69	
Leucine	$-CH_2-CH(CH_3)CH_3$	E	40–50	7–10	133 ± 39
Valine	$-CH(CH_3)CH_3$	E	40–50	4–7	264 ± 79
Isoleucine	$-CH(CH_3)CH_2-CH_3$	E	40–50	4–7	64 ± 23
Proline	$H_2C-CH_2, H_2C-CH-COO^-, N-H_2$ (ring)	NE		5–8	100–450
Phenylalanine	$-CH_2-C_6H_5$	E	28	4–6	58 ± 15
Tryptophan	$-CH_2-$ indole	E	14	1–2	
Methionine	$-CH_2-CH_2-S-CH_3$	E	22	2–5	24 ± 8
Cysteine (and cystine)[a]	$-CH_2-SH$	NE	20	1–2	61 ± 13
Asparagine	$-CH_2-C(=O)NH_2$	NE		6–9	62 ± 19
Glutamine	$-CH_2-CH_2-C(=O)NH_2$	NE		10	650 ± 146
Serine	$-CH_2-OH$	NE		3–6	113 ± 30
Threonine	$-CH(CH_3)OH$	E	28	3–5	145 ± 39
Tyrosine	$-CH_2-C_6H_4-OH$	NE		2–4	64 ± 19
Aspartic acid	$-CH_2-C(=O)O^-$	NE		6–10	7 ± 4
Glutamic acid	$-CH_2-CH_2-C(=O)O^-$	NE		15–20	34 ± 13
Lysine	$-CH_2-CH_2-CH_2-CH_2-NH_3^+$	E	16[b]	4–8	192 ± 44
Arginine	$-CH_2-CH_2-CH_2-NH-C(=NH_2^+)NH_2$	NE	14	4–8	94 ± 20
Histidine	$-CH_2-C$ (imidazole)	E	22	2–5	94 ± 14

The plasma levels are not fasting levels, but the means ($\pm$SD) of results in normal males and females taken at different times throughout the day (Scriver, *Metabolism*, 1985; 34:868; see also Milsom, *Metabolism*, 1979; 28:313).
[a] See text.
[b] Based on Technical Report Series No. 724, WHO 1985, Geneva. Recent studies suggest a requirement of 50 g/kg protein intake. See ref. 2.

Amino acids with non-polar side-chains

Glycine[7]

Glycine is abundant in most animal proteins. Its tissue concentration is much higher than in plasma.[5,6] As well as being used for protein synthesis, it participates in many biochemical reactions.[1] There is rapid interconversion with serine;[5] 10-N-methylene tetrahydrofolate, an intermediate in this interconversion, is an important donor of methyl groups in biosynthetic reactions. Glycine, via serine which, in turn, can be converted to pyruvate, can enter gluconeogenesis, and when carbon-labelled glycine is fed, the label appears in glycogen. Much of the nitrogen of glycine also appears in glutamate and glutamine (Matthews, Metabolism, 1981; 30:886). Excess dietary glycine intake may rapidly stimulate its hepatic catabolism (Ewart, BiochemJ, 1992; 283:441).

Glycine is an important precursor of purines, hippuric acid, ethanolamine and choline, and of creatine and glutathione. δ-Aminolaevulinic acid, formed by the condensation of glycine and succinyl CoA, is on the biosynthetic pathway of porphyrins and haem. The conjugation of glycine with bile salts enhances their ability to form micelles in the gut. Glycine is an inhibitory neurotransmitter in the central nevous system.

Alanine

Alanine is abundant in most animal proteins. The main fate of alanine is its incorporation into protein, and its participation in transamination reactions, particularly with α-ketoglutarate (by alanine aminotransferase) to form pyruvate and glutamate (Fig. 1). It is an important gluconeogenic substrate (Chapter 2.11). Alanine turnover is between 0.25 and 0.35 mmol/kg/h[8] (Fanelli, JCI, 1993; 92:1617). Skeletal muscle releases large amounts of alanine. Around 60 to 65 per cent of the alanine released is synthesized in muscle from pyruvate derived from plasma glucose (directly or after its release from glycogen) (Chang, JBC, 1978; 253:3685; Simmons, JCI, 1984; 73:412). The liver avidly removes the alanine, and converts it to pyruvate, a major precursor for hepatic glucose synthesis. Glucose generated from alanine can enter the blood, return to the periphery, and be converted to pyruvate, which can then be transaminated with other amino acids derived from proteolysis, to give alanine. This is the glucose–alanine cycle.[9] It does not, of course, provide net substrate for gluconeogenesis, unless pyruvate is formed from non-carbohydrate precursors in muscle, as would happen in starvation. It is, however, effective in transporting nitrogen to the liver from skeletal muscle (see below).

Branched-chain amino acids: leucine, valine, and isoleucine[10]

The essential amino acids leucine, valine, and isoleucine are branched-chain amino acids (BCAAs) (see Table 1). There is some dispute about the daily requirements, but about 40 to 50 g of each are required per kg of dietary protein. Valine is the most abundant BCAA in plasma, and the leucine concentration is higher than that of isoleucine (Table 1).

Unlike other essential amino acids, BCAAs are taken up mainly by extrahepatic tissues, especially muscle and gut, and to a lesser extent by the kidney and adipose tissue;[11] there is relatively little hepatic uptake of BCAAs[12] (Gelfand, AmJPhysiol, 1986; 250:

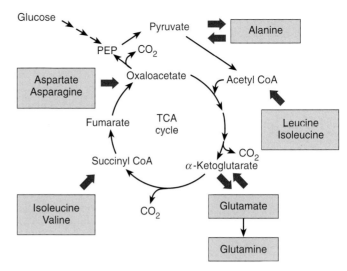

Fig. 1. Synthesis of alanine and glutamine in muscle. Only acetyl CoA can be oxidized by the tricarboxylic acid (TCA) cycle. Complete oxidation of the carbon chains that give rise to TCA cycle intermediates requires their conversion to oxaloacetate which is removed from the cycle, converted to pyruvate, and finally to acetyl CoA. Glucose is the main source of pyruvate for alanine sythesis. Glutamate is synthesized from α-ketoglutarate. The carbon skeleton of glutamate may thus be derived from amino acids that can enter the TCA cycle, e.g. proline, arginine, or histidine entering at α-ketoglutarate, phenylalanine and tyrosine entering at fumarate, and methionine at succinyl CoA, in addition to those shown; their nitrogen will be available for incorporation into glutamate or alanine by transamination. The second amino group of glutamine could come from leucine or other nitrogenous compounds (e.g. AMP). (Reproduced from Kruszynska YT. In Williams G, and Pickup J, eds. *Textbook of diabetes,* (2nd edn). Oxford: Blackwell Science, 1996: 11.1–11.37.)

E407). BCAAs therefore account for about 70 per cent of the dietary amino acids reaching the systemic circulation after passage through the liver, although they constitute only about 20 per cent of the amino acids of dietary protein.[13] The α-amino nitrogen of BCAAs catabolized in extrahepatic tissues (primarily muscle) eventually reaches the liver, after transamination into other amino acids, especially alanine and glutamine.

The first step in metabolism of the BCAAs is deamination by BCAA aminotransferase. α-Ketoglutarate, the main acceptor, is converted to glutamate and one of three branched-chain ketoacids (BCKAs) is formed (Fig. 2). The BCKAs may be reaminated to their BCAAs, or may undergo oxidative decarboxylation by the mitochondrial BCKA dehydrogenase complex (Fig. 2). The end products of leucine metabolism are acetoacetate and acetyl CoA, making it ketogenic; isoleucine yields propionyl CoA and acetyl CoA, and is thus glucogenic and ketogenic; valine yields succinyl CoA and is glucogenic.[1,4]

There is marked tissue variation in the activities of the BCAA aminotransferase and the BCKA dehydrogenase. Deamination is most active in muscle, but also takes place in kidney, brain, adipose tissue, and ovary. In rodents and primates the activity of the aminotransferase is lower in liver than in any other organ studied, [12] and this may explain the limited hepatic uptake of BCAA, although expression of the liver enzyme is increased after glucocorticoid administration.[12] By contrast, BCKA dehydrogenase

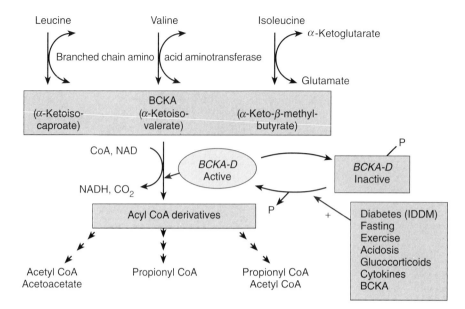

Fig. 2. Metabolism of branched-chain amino acids (BCAA). Oxidative decarboxylation, catalysed by branched-chain ketoacid dehydrogenase (BCKA-D), is the rate-limiting step. BCKA-D is a multienzyme complex regulated by phosphorylation, and also inhibited by the reaction products (NADH, acyl CoA derivatives). Valine and isoleucine give rise to propionyl CoA and can therefore be used for pyruvate and glucose synthesis; leucine cannot. (Reproduced from Kruszynska YT. In Williams G, and Pickup J, eds. *Textbook of diabetes*, (2nd edn). Oxford: Blackwell Science, 1996: 11.1–11.37.)

activity is highest in the liver, heart, and kidney, and relatively low in muscle.[14] In sheep both enzymes are concentrated in liver rather than muscle (Goodwin, BiochemJ, 1987; 242:305). In humans, 30 per cent of BCKA dehydrogenase is in the liver and 60 per cent in muscle (Khatra, JCI, 1977; 59:558); however, this does not take into account the degree of activity of the enzyme in the tissues.[14] If any one of the BCAAs is fed, its concentration in systemic blood rises quickly; so does that of the corresponding BCKA, which suggests rapid deamination. If a BCKA is fed, there is an early and pronounced rise in the plasma level of the corresponding BCAA, suggesting that reamination of BCKA is also rapid. The speed of these interconversions has been confirmed by the infusion of labelled BCAA and BCKA; the label disappears rapidly from plasma and appears in the corresponding BCAA or BCKA within minutes. Reamination of BCKA is important as it preserves the carbon skeleton of the essential BCAA following deamination. The cycling of BCAA carbons via deamination–reamination is quantitatively much more important than the subsequent decarboxylation of the BCKA (Matthews, Science, 1981; 214:1129).

Oxidative decarboxylation of BCKA by BCKA dehydrogenase is irreversible and rate limiting for BCAA metabolism in peripheral tissues (Fig. 2) (Odessey, BiochemJ, 1979; 178:475). BCKA dehydrogenase may also be involved in the catabolism of threonine and methionine (Paxton, BiochemJ, 1986; 234:295). The BCKA dehydrogenase is subject to complex regulatory mechanisms, including phosphorylation and feedback inhibition by NADH and its acyl CoA products (Fig. 2); substrates which produce intramitochondrial NADH (fatty acids and ketone bodies) compete for oxidation (Nair, JCI, 1988; 82:198). Dephosphorylation of the enzyme results in activation (Yeaman, BiochemJ, 1989; 257:625). The kinase that phosphorylates and inactivates the enzyme is

inhibited by the BCKA, particularly that of leucine (ketoisocaproic acid, **KICA**), such that administration of leucine or its ketoacid results in a marked acceleration of whole-body BCAA oxidation, and decreased tissue and plasma levels of valine, isoleucine, and their ketoacids (May, DiabetesMetabRev, 1989; 5:227). The BCKA dehydrogenase in muscle is activated by glucocorticoids. Surprisingly, insulin does not stimulate the enzyme in muscle (Aftring, AmJPhysiol, 1988; 254:E292). With fasting, trauma, injury, sepsis, exercise, or poorly controlled diabetes, flux through decarboxylation in muscle increases, thus increasing BCAA catabolism (Fig. 2). The activity of the BCKA dehydrogenase in rat liver is increased by glucagon and adrenaline, particularly in animals fed a low-protein diet in whom the activity is low (Block, BiochemJ, 1985; 232:593).

Dietary protein intake is an important regulator of both the hepatic and muscle BCKA dehydrogenase. Most of our information on the regulation of this enzyme comes from studies in rats. The liver enzyme complex is mainly in the active form in chow-fed rats, and is not further activated by administering BCAA. By contrast only 5 to 10 per cent of muscle BCKA dehydrogenase is in the active form in rats fed *ad libitum*, or in fed, resting normal subjects (Rush, JApplPhysiol, 1995; 78:2193); activity falls further with fasting but is restored following a protein-containing meal (Block, JCI, 1987; 79:1349). Protein deprivation decreases the activity of the enzyme in liver and muscle (Harris, AdvEnzymReg, 1986; 25: 219; Beggs, BiochemJ, 1988; 256:929), which helps to conserve BCAAs for protein synthesis; following amino acid administration the activity increases in both tissues. Activation of the liver BCKA dehydrogenase is not specific to leucine, whereas the muscle enzyme is specifically activated by leucine and its ketoacid (KICA). Prolonged feeding of a high-protein diet increases both the postabsorptive activity of muscle BCKA dehydrogenase level and the extent of activation of the enzyme in response to a protein-containing meal (Block, JCI, 1987; 79:1349). The activity of liver BCKA dehydrogenase may also increase in rats fed diets rich in BCAAs or BCKAs (Wohlheuter, JBC, 1970; 245:2391). The oxidation rate of [^{13}C]leucine and [^{13}C]valine rises with increasing dietary intake of leucine and valine, respectively (Meguid, AmJClinNutr, 1986; 43:770 and 781; Cortiella, AmJClinNutr, 1988; 48:998). These diet-induced adaptive changes in BCKA dehydrogenase activity are partly due to alterations in the synthesis and amounts of the kinase that phosphorylates the enzyme (Harris, JNutr, 1995; 125:1758S) and, to a lesser extent, to changes in the amount of the BCKA dehydrogenase enzyme complex (Zhao, ArchBiochemBiophys, 1994; 308:446).

The liver has a high capacity for BCKA uptake and metabolism. In the dog about 35 per cent of an oral KICA load is taken up by the liver; approximately two-thirds of this is metabolized to ketone bodies and CO_2, and one-third is reaminated to leucine (Abumrad, AmJPhysiol, 1982; 243:E123). Some of the KICA is reaminated to leucine during intestinal absorption so that net splanchnic output of KICA may amount to only 27 per cent; most of the KICA carbon skeleton reaches the periphery as ketone bodies or leucine. In the rat, because of the low capacity of muscle BCKA dehydrogenase, the liver may also play an important role in metabolism of BCKAs produced by muscle in the postabsorptive state.[12,14] A significant proportion of ketoacids produced by deamination in rat muscle may be released along with alanine and glutamine; BCKAs are then transported to the liver and other tissues for decarboxylation or reamination. Most of the BCKAs taken up by the liver in the rat are probably oxidized, since in rat hepatocytes the reamination rate of KICA to leucine was found to be less than 10 per cent of the degradation rate of KICA (Williamson, JBC, 1979; 254:11511). Such BCAA/BCKA cycling between liver and skeletal muscle could play a major role in providing nitrogen for the cycling of other compounds, for example alanine/glucose, glutamine/glutamate[11, 14] (Aoki, JCI, 1981; 68:1522), and it would allow the liver to control the rate of degradation of BCAAs via the BCKAs. There is, however, little evidence for such a cycle in humans; the arteriovenous difference for BCKAs across the leg is minimal under basal conditions, and muscle efflux of BCKAs is low during an infusion of leucine or after protein ingestion, despite a large increase in BCAA uptake (Abumrad, JSurgRes, 1982; 32:453; Elia, ClinSci, 1983; 64:517).

When arterial KICA concentrations are raised by an intravenous infusion of KICA in normal subjects, there is a marked enhancement of the net uptake of KICA by the leg and brain, as well as by splanchnic tissues. The arterial concentration of leucine also increases rapidly (Eriksson, ClinSci, 1982; 62:285). The tissue contribution to the marked elevation of plasma leucine when KICA is infused is unclear; Eriksson (ClinSci, 1982; 92:285) found little or no change in the arteriohepatic and arteriofemoral differences for leucine, while the arteriojugular venous leucine difference increased. Increased splanchnic output of ketone bodies could account for more than two-thirds of the KICA taken up by the splanchnic bed, suggesting that peripheral tissues were the main site of KICA reamination and release of leucine into plasma.

A high leucine intake depresses the valine and isoleucine levels in blood and muscle, and the plasma concentrations of their respective BCKAs[12] (Hagenfeldt, ClinSci, 1980; 59:173; Schauder, JLabClinMed, 1985; 106:701); the plasma concentrations of phenylalanine, tyrosine, and methionine are also reduced. These effects of leucine are unique; infusions of either isoleucine or valine do not change the levels of the other two BCAAs (Eriksson, ClinSci, 1981; 60:95). The leucine-induced reduction in concentration of valine and isoleucine, and of methionine and aromatic amino acids, is probably due to a combination of increased BCAA oxidation, via stimulation of BCKA dehydrogenase activity, and of increased net protein synthesis (May, DiabetesMetabRev, 1989; 5:227). Both leucine and KICA may directly affect protein turnover, leucine stimulating protein synthesis and KICA inhibiting protein degradation. A balanced amino acid intake is therefore important in maintaining BCAA homeostasis.

Proline (and hydroxyproline) [15]

Proline and hydroxyproline are imino acids because the nitrogen in the pyrrolidine ring has only one hydrogen attached (Table 1). The absence of a primary amino group excludes proline and hydroxyproline from the decarboxylation and transamination reactions, using pyridoxal 5-phosphate as a coenzyme, which are so important in the metabolism of the other amino acids.

Proline is synthesized mainly from ornithine, but glutamate is also a precursor; production is inhibited by high proline levels. The first step in proline degradation is the production, by proline oxidase, of pyrroline 5-carboxylate, which is also the immediate precursor in proline synthesis; pyrroline 5-carboxylate is then converted to glutamate. Although proline can give rise to α-ketoglutarate, it is not a major gluconeogenic precursor in normal postabsorptive humans (Jaksic, Metabolism, 1987; 36:1040). Hydroxyproline is derived from the post-translational hydroxylation of proline in nascent polypeptide chains, particularly those of collagen; it does not appear to come from any other source.

Phenylalanine [16]

Phenylalanine is an essential aromatic amino acid derived from the diet and from protein breakdown. In the renal and intestinal brush borders there is a Na^+-dependent carrier; in hepatocytes, and other cells, there is a Na^+-independent carrier for entry, which is shared by other aromatic amino acids and by branched-chain amino acids, while phenylalanine leaves cells by a system shared with many neutral amino acids (Table 2).

Most of the phenylalanine leaving plasma is hydroxylated to tyrosine (by phenylalanine hydroxylase), some enters protein, and a small amount is transaminated to phenylpyruvic acid which is metabolized via several pathways. In humans phenylalanine hydroxylase is present and active only in hepatocytes, but incorporation into protein occurs in all tissues. The phenylalanine hydroxylase reaction is an obligatory and rate-limiting step in the oxidation of phenylalanine to CO_2 and water.

Tryptophan [4]

Tryptophan in plasma is bound non-covalently to albumin, and only about 10 per cent is in the free form. This may be important in controlling its uptake into the brain. Bound tryptophan can be displaced by non-esterified fatty acids, and by a number of drugs, including salicylates, indomethacin, and clofibrate.

Table 2 Neutrol amino acid transport systems

	System				
	A	**ASC**	**L**	**N^m**	**N**
Tissue distribution	Ubiquitous	Ubiquitous	Ubiquitous	Muscle	Liver
Preferred substrates	Ala, Gly, Pro, Ser, Met	Ala, Ser, Cys Pro, Thr	Leu, Ile, Val Met, Phe	Gln	Gln, His, Asn
Affinity (K_M) (mM)	High (<1)	Medium ($\sim$3)	Low ($\sim$20)	Low ($\sim$8)	High (<1)
Na$^+$ dependent	+	+	−	+	+
Hormonal regulation					
Insulin	+[a]	−	−	+[b]	−
Glucagon	+[a]	−	−	−	−
Glucocorticoids	−	−	−	+[c]	+[d]

[a] Glucagon (in hepatocytes) and insulin increase the V_{max} for transport. Insulin increases synthesis of transporter protein and also inhibits its degradation.[23]
[b] Insulin stimulates inward transport (Rennie, JNutr, 1996; 126:1142S).
[c,d] Glucocorticoids stimulate glutamine efflux in muscle by N^m and uptake in hepatocytes by N.[24]

Tryptophan is oxidized to formylkynurenine, by tryptophan oxygenase, and is then converted to acroleylaminofumarate which, by separate pathways, is a precursor of acetyl CoA and of nicotinamide adenine dinucleotide (**NAD**) and nicotinamide adenine dinucleotide phosphate (**NADP**). NADH is important in the respiratory chain for the generation of ATP, while the major role of NADPH is as an electron donor in reductive biosyntheses. Tryptophan is also converted to quinolinic acid, tryptamine, and 5-hydroxytryptamine (serotonin).

Methionine[17]

Methionine is a sulphur-containing essential amino acid, the side-group containing a thio-ether linkage. The first step in methionine metabolism is its essentially irreversible conversion to *S*-adenosylmethionine (Fig. 3); an adenosyl group is transferred from ATP to form a sulphonium bond between the ribose and the sulphur of methionine. *S*-Adenosylmethionine is a precursor of the polyamines spermidine and spermine, but its major role is as a donor of methyl groups, for example in the conversion of creatine to creatinine, of phosphatidylethanolamine to phosphatidylcholine, and of noradrenaline to adrenaline. It also inactivates catecholamine neurotransmitters by methylation. *S*-Adenosylmethionine synthesis increases after a methionine load. It is converted to *S*-adenosylhomocysteine by loss of its methyl group, and then to homocysteine, which can be converted back to methionine by interaction with 5-methyltetrahydrofolate in the activated methyl cycle (in which vitamin B$_{12}$ is involved) (Fig. 3). The main route for the disposal of dietary methionine is the 'transsulphuration pathway' in which homocysteine condenses with serine to produce cystathionine and then cysteine and inorganic sulphate (Fig. 3). Indeed, *S*-adenosylmethionine inhibits the conversion of homocysteine to methionine. Methionine may also undergo 'transamination' to α-ketomethiolbutyrate, which is further catabolized to formate. The major site for all of these reactions appears to be the liver.

Cysteine and cystine[17]

The side-chain of cysteine contains a thiol group. It is not essential if enough methionine is present in the diet. Cysteine exists in

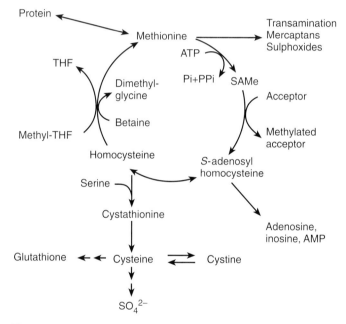

Fig. 3. Hepatic methionine metabolism. SAME, *S*-adenosylmethionine.

plasma in three forms: as 'free cysteine' with its free thiol group; as 'cystine'—a disulphide formed by two molecules of cysteine; and as a mixed disulphide in which it is linked to the cysteinyl residues of albumin and other plasma proteins (Chawla, Gastro, 1984; 87:770). The plasma concentration of cystine is much higher than that of free cysteine. Cysteine is synthesized from methionine (Fig. 3), and it may be catabolized via a number of pathways. The major pathway appears to be via direct oxidation to cysteine sulphinate, followed by conversion to pyruvate and SO_4^{2-}, or to taurine. It may also be transaminated to 3-mercaptopyruvate, which is also converted to pyruvate. It is a component of glutathione (γ-glutamyl-cysteinylglycine), which is important as a reducing agent, as a scavenger of peroxides and free radicals, in the detoxification of certain compounds, and as a means of getting amino acids into cells. Sulphate is also important for detoxification of many compounds. It forms conjugates with steroids, bile acids, and a large number of other compounds, thereby enhancing their solubility and excretion. Cysteine residues in proteins play an important role in determining the conformation of proteins, by forming disulphide bridges with cysteine molecules in other parts of the protein.

Uncharged polar side-chains

Asparagine

Asparagine is an amino acid amide, formed from aspartate by amide transfer from glutamine. Asparagine is hydrolysed by asparaginase to NH_4^+ and to aspartate, which can be transaminated to give oxaloacetate. Asparagine residues within proteins are sites for the addition of N-linked oligosaccharide side-chains in the synthesis of glycoproteins.

Glutamine (see also glutamate, below)

Glutamine, like asparagine, has an amide group in its side-chain. Although a great deal is known about the reactions in which it takes part, its physiology is difficult to study because for isotopic studies its nitrogen must be labelled with the stable isotope ^{15}N; furthermore, its carbon skeleton is shared with glutamate and α-ketoglutarate—a component of the Krebs' cycle so it is easily lost into the metabolic pool.

Glutamine accounts for more than 60 per cent of the free α-amino acids in the body and is the most abundant amino acid in plasma (Table 1). It is produced in large amounts in skeletal muscle (Curthoys, AnnRevNutr, 1995; 15:133), and to a lesser extent in adipose tissue (Frayn, ClinSci, 1991; 80:471), by the addition of NH_4^+ to glutamate, glutamine synthetase being the enzyme responsible. Under some conditions the lung may also be an important source of glutamine (Curthoys, AnnRevNutr, 1995; 15:133). The glutamine production rate in overnight-fasted humans is 20 to 25 mmol/h[8] (Matthews, AmJPhysiol, 1993; 264:E848); skeletal muscle may account for about 70 per cent of this.[8] The concentration of glutamine in skeletal muscle is about 20 mmol/l, some 30 times that of plasma. This large glutamine concentration gradient favours the release of glutamine from muscle into the circulation. The main sites of glutamine removal are the splanchnic bed and kidney. Glutamine is an important substrate for renal and hepatic gluconeogenesis (Chapter 2.11). It is also an important fuel for intestinal mucosa (Windmueller, JBC, 1978; 253:69), and hence maintenance of the intestinal permeability barrier.

The relative contributions of the intestine and liver to splanchnic glutamine uptake vary between species (Welbourne, AmJPhysiol, 1987; 253:F1069). In the rat the gut accounts for about two-thirds of splanchnic glutamine uptake and a large proportion of the glutamine is metabolized by the gut to alanine, citrulline, proline, ornithine, and ammonia, which are then released into the portal vein for transport to the liver. Early studies in humans suggested a relatively low splanchnic uptake of glutamine; in overnight-fasted man, net splanchnic glutamine uptake was only around 17 to 23 per cent.[18] (Marliss, JCI, 1971; 50:814), and because the intestine removed about 13 per cent of the glutamine delivered to it,[18]

hepatic glutamine uptake was considered to be quantitatively unimportant. Contrary to *in vitro* studies showing that glutamine was a good substrate for hepatic gluconeogenesis (Ross, BiochemJ, 1967; 105:869; Kaloyianni, JNutr, 1990, 120:116), it was believed that much of the glutamine used for gluconeogenesis was first metabolized to alanine in the gut (as in the rat) before its carbon skeleton could be used for synthesis of glucose, and its nitrogen incorporated into urea. Studies employing labelled glutamine indicate a much higher splanchnic extraction of glutamine in man (Matthews, AmJPhysiol, 1993; 264:E848). The explanation is that glutamine uptake and production occur in different zones of the liver. Thus glutamine is taken up by periportal hepatocytes and used for gluconeogenesis and urea synthesis, while perivenous hepatocytes synthesize glutamine from glutamate and ammonia that has escaped uptake by periportal hepatocytes (see later). Thus, significant amounts of glutamine may be taken up by the liver and used for gluconeogenesis even though net splanchnic uptake may be relatively small. Glutamine is the main source of 'new' carbon for synthesis of glucose[8] (see Chapter 2.11).

In the fed state, glutamine promotes hepatic glycogen synthesis from glucose and may itself be a substrate (Katz, PNAS, 1976; 73: 3433; Baquet, BiochemJ, 1991; 273:57). A significant proportion of an oral glutamine load would be expected to be taken up by the liver (Cersosimo, AmJPhysiol, 1986; 250:E248). Matthews *et al.* (AmJPhysiol, 1993; 264:E848) estimated that in normal, overnight-fasted subjects first-pass splanchnic uptake of nasogastrically administered glutamine was 55 per cent.

Proteolysis and gluconeogenesis decline with prolonged fasting as the brain derives much of its energy needs from the oxidation of ketone bodies and glucose requirements fall. The reduction in amino acid catabolism decreases the need for urea synthesis. Under these conditions periportal glutamine uptake and urea synthesis fall, and the potentially toxic ammonia is largely taken up by perivenous hepatocytes and incorporated into glutamine;[19] the liver may then become a net producer of glutamine (Cersosimo, AmJPhysiol, 1986; 250:E248) which must be delivered to the kidney for excretion of nitrogen as NH_4^+. The implications of the acinar heterogeneity of glutamine metabolism in acid–base control are discussed later.

In overnight-fasted subjects net glutamine uptake by the kidney (2.5 mmol/h)[20] accounts for about 12 per cent of glutamine production rate. It increases twofold after an 84-h fast[20] and with chronic acidosis (Owen, JCI, 1963; 42:263; Welbourne, AmJPhysiol, 1987; 253:F1069). In dogs infused with glutamine to produce a moderate increase in arterial glutamine levels, 20 per cent of the infused load was removed by the kidneys (Cersosimo, AmJPhysiol, 1986; 250:E248). The glutamine removed by the kidney is the major source of urinary ammonium ions (see later). However, urinary excretion of NH_4^+ accounts for only 1 to 2 per cent of the glutamine amide nitrogen turnover (Golden, ClinSci, 1982; 62:299). There are two reasons for the discrepancy between net renal glutamine uptake and the urinary excretion of ammonium ions:

(1) only 30 to 50 per cent of the ammonia produced by the kidney from glutamine is normally excreted, the rest is released into the renal vein (Owen, JCI, 1963; 42:263; Dejong, JCI, 1993; 92: 2834);

(2) some of the glutamine nitrogen is used to transaminate other amino acids that are then released from the kidney, notably

serine and arginine[20] (Tizianello, ContribNephrol, 1985; 47: 44).

The fraction of ammonia generated by the kidneys that is excreted increases when plasma ammonia levels increase, and also with acidosis, along with the enhanced renal glutamine extraction.

Glutamine is a precursor of purines and pyrimidines, glucosamine, and other amino acids. Like enterocytes, rapidly dividing cells of the immune system and many tumour cells have a very high rate of glutamine utilization which is used for biosynthetic purposes and to meet the energy needs of these cells. Some of the glutamine is oxidized completely to CO_2 but a greater proportion undergoes partial oxidation to produce lactate, aspartate, and ammonia. The aspartate and ammonia together with glutamine are used for nucleotide synthesis. Under conditions of stress associated with injury, sepsis, and inflammation there is a marked increase in glutamine consumption by the gut, immune cells, inflammatory tissue, and kidneys. Large amounts of glutamine are released from muscle, and muscle concentrations of glutamine fall despite a marked increase in glutamine synthesis. Glucocorticoids, and to a lesser extent adrenaline, increase muscle glutamine efflux and reduce the glutamine concentration gradient across the muscle cell membrane (Rennie, JNutr, 1996; 126:1142S). Muscle glutamine may decrease by 50 per cent whereas plasma glutamine concentrations may be maintained or show a smaller decline. The increased requirements for glutamine and associated increased efflux of glutamine from muscle in sick patients contributes to muscle wasting and negative nitrogen balance. Many consider glutamine to be an essential amino acid during critical illness and there is much interest in whether glutamine supplementation of enteral and parenteral nutrition regimens may help to preserve muscle protein, improve immune function, and maintain intestinal integrity.

Serine

Serine has an alcohol group in its polar side-chain. In addition to dietary intake, serine is formed from glycine and, more importantly, from phosphoglycerate. Serine is deaminated by serine dehydratase to give pyruvate, and is thus a glucogenic amino acid; it can also be converted to glycine and N-5,10-methylenetetrahydrofolate (see above), and to cysteine by condensing with homocysteine (Fig. 3). Serine residues in proteins are sites for addition of O-linked oligosaccharide side-chains in the synthesis of glycoproteins; they are also sites for reversible phosphorylation, which causes activation and inactivation of key regulatory enzymes.

Threonine

Threonine is an essential amino acid, which also has an alcohol in its polar side-group. The first step in the major route of catabolism of threonine is its conversion, by threonine dehydrogenase, to 2-amino-3-oxobutyrate and then to amino-acetone; it may also be converted to oxo-butyrate by threonine deaminase. Threonine residues in proteins, like those of serine, are sites for addition of O-linked oligosaccharide side-chains to glycoproteins and for reversible phosphorylation of key regulatory enzymes.

Tyrosine[4,21]

Tyrosine can be produced in the body from the essential amino acid phenylalanine (Fig. 4). Tyrosine aminotransferase is rate limiting

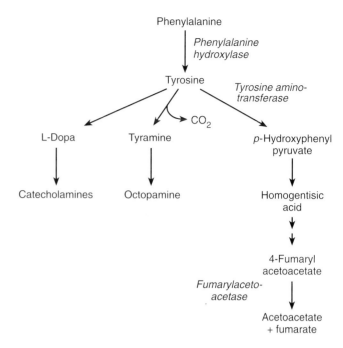

Fig. 4. Pathway for metabolism of phenylalanine via tyrosine and the homogentisic acid pathway in liver. Phenylalanine hydroxylase and tyrosine aminotransferase are rate limiting for the oxidation of phenylalanine and tyrosine, respectively, to CO_2. Impaired metabolism of tyrosine via the homogentisic acid pathway in liver disease increases the production of tyramine and octopamine in extrahepatic tissues with increases in their plasma levels.

for tyrosine metabolism. It converts tyrosine, mainly in the liver, to p-hydroxyphenylpyruvic acid. This in turn is converted, via homogentisic acid, to fumarylacetoacetic acid which is cleaved to fumaric and acetoacetic acids by fumarylacetoacetic acid hydrolase (the enzyme deficient in tyrosinaemia I, which is associated with chronic active hepatitis, cirrhosis, and hepatocellular carcinoma); it is thus glucogenic and ketogenic. Tyrosine is also converted, in sequence, to dopa, dopamine, noradrenaline, and adrenaline. The post-translational iodination of tyrosine in proteins in the thyroid gland is a key step in the production of thyroid hormones.

Acidic side-chains

Aspartic acid (aspartate)

Aspartic acid has a carboxyl group in its side-chain. It is formed by transamination of oxaloacetic acid, a key intermediate in the Krebs' cycle (Fig. 1). Aspartate is converted into the amino acid amide, asparagine, by amide transfer from glutamine. Aspartate can condense with carbamyl phosphate, and the resulting carbamyl aspartate can be converted, via orotic acid, to the pyrimidine bases uridine and cytidine. Aspartate is also an excitatory neurotransmitter.

Glutamic acid (glutamate)

Glutamate, like aspartate, has a carboxyl group in its side-chain. Glutamate is produced in large amounts in metabolic reactions, because its ketoacid, α-ketoglutarate—a component of the Krebs' cycle (Fig. 1)—is the major acceptor of amino groups from other amino acids in transamination reactions. Glutamate is also the key donor of amino groups in the production of other amino acids from their corresponding ketoacids; for example, alanine from pyruvate and aspartic acid from oxaloacetate, via alanine and aspartate aminotransferases, respectively. Proline and arginine can be produced from glutamate, but by a different series of reactions.

Glutamate can also be produced from α-ketoglutarate and NH_4^+ by the action of glutamate dehydrogenase. NH_4^+ can be added to glutamate, by the action of glutamine synthetase, to form glutamine; this reaction plays a crucial role in nitrogen metabolism, and in interorgan amino acid transport (see below).

Glutamate is a precursor of γ-aminobutyric acid (**GABA**), an important inhibitory neurotransmitter, and is a constituent of glutathione. The post-translational γ-carboxylation of glutamate, in which vitamin K plays a key role, is important in the synthesis of calcium-binding proteins, such as the clotting factors II, VII, IX and X, and osteocalcin.

Basic side-chains

Lysine[4,22]

Lysine is an essential six-carbon dibasic amino acid, which cannot be replaced in the diet by its ketoacid. The major pathway of lysine degradation involves the transfer of the ε-amino group (at the end of its side-chain) to α-ketoglutarate through the stable intermediate saccharopine. This is converted to α-aminoadipic semialdehyde and then to α-aminoadipic acid, which is eventually converted to acetyl CoA via glutaryl CoA and crotonyl CoA. It is thus a ketogenic amino acid. An alternative pathway of degradation is removal of the α-amino group by oxidative deamination to form pipecolic acid, which is converted to α-aminoadipic semialdehyde, thus joining the saccharopine pathway. In many proteins some of the ε-amino groups of lysine are methylated to mono-, di-, or tri-methyllysine; this may be important in the functioning of histones. Trimethyllysine is important because in mammals it is an obligatory precursor in the biosynthesis of carnitine, a key compound in the transport of fatty acids across the inner mitochondrial membrane.

Arginine

Arginine (Table 1) shares a transport system with lysine, ornithine, and cysteine in the gut, brain, and red cells. The liver has a very high clearance rate for arginine, which is an intermediate in the urea cycle (see later), and the pathway for its synthesis is the same as that for urea. Urea and ornithine are produced from arginine by the action of arginase; ornithine can then be converted to glutamate semialdehyde which is converted to glutamate. The kidney is an important site of arginine synthesis from gut-derived citrulline (Cynober, NutrBioch, 1995; 6:402). Apart from its role in urea and protein synthesis, it is associated with a variety of other reactions. It is a precursor of nitric oxide (Chapter 25.1), and of creatine (which is important in cell energy metabolism), and it plays an important role in regulating T-cell function. Increased levels of arginine stimulate secretion of a nuimber of hormones, including insulin, glucagon, growth hormone, and prolactin (Barbul, JPEN, 1986; 10:227).

Histidine[3,4]

Histidine, a basic amino acid, is an essential amino acid in young children, but there is debate about its essential nature later in life;

it is possible that the histidine requirements of adults can be met for a time by histidine released from the breakdown of haemoglobin, which is rich in histidine, or from muscle carnosine (alanylhistidine). The major pathway of histidine degradation is through urocanic acid and formaminoglutamic acid to glutamate, the last step requiring tetrahydrofolate as a cofactor. Histidine is also decarboxylated to histamine, and it can be transaminated to imidazolepyruvic acid.

Amino acid transport[23]

Because amino acids are charged molecules, they do not cross cell membranes freely. They are transported into cells, and absorbed from the gut and renal tubule, by active transport systems, some of which require co-transport of sodium ions. Some handle particular types of amino acid (e.g. neutral, acidic, or basic) (Table 2). Similar systems are present in different tissues, but there are also organ-specific transporters. Some of the systems are antiporters which can transport two different amino acids in opposite directions at the same time.[1] Regulation of amino acid transport is important in regulating cell protein balance and the fluxes of amino acids between tissues. Alanine is transported by systems A and ASC. System A is increased by glucagon in hepatocytes and to a lesser extent by insulin in skeletal muscle, heart, adipocytes, and liver. Glutamine transport is mediated by a very high activity transporter (N^m) that allows muscle to maintain very high intracellular glutamine concentrations (~20 mmol/l compared to plasma levels of ~0.5 mmol/l). Activity is modulated by the membrane potential, the transmembrane sodium gradient, and hormones. Insulin stimulates glutamine transport into muscle (Rennie, JNutr, 1996; 126:1142S) while glucocorticoids (Muhlbacher, AmJPhysiol, 1984; 247:E75) or fasting (Jepson, AmJPhysiol, 1988; 255:E166) enhance glutamine efflux, reducing the gradient across the plasma membrane. Hepatic glutamine transport by a transporter distinct from that in muscle (Table 2) is rate limiting for glutamine utilization. Corticosteroids increase the hepatic fractional extraction of glutamine by increasing the activity of the transporter in parallel with that of the glutamine metabolizing enzymes.[24] Regulation of glutamine and alanine membrane transport plays an important role in interorgan nitrogen exchange (see below).

Protein and amino acid turnover

The average protein turnover of a 70 kg man is 250 to 300 g/day—much higher than the average daily protein intake of about 70 to 100 g.[25-27] There is clearly an extensive turnover of endogenous proteins, with release and reutilization of their amino acids. Protein turnover may account for 15 to 20 per cent of resting energy expenditure[26] (Welle, AmJPhysiol, 1990; 258:E990). Most of the amino acids released from endogenous protein breakdown re-enter the protein pool, either directly or following incorporation of their nitrogen into other newly synthesized amino acids. However, about 30 g of the endogenous pool of amino acids is fully catabolized each day, and must be replaced by amino acids from dietary protein; to maintain nitrogen balance a minimum of 56 g of dietary protein is needed.[2] When amino acids are fully catabolized their nitrogen can be removed in various ways, but the major route is via urea synthesis and excretion. Excess dietary amino acids are also broken down, as they cannot be stored.

Muscle protein synthesis and degradation accounts for 25 to 35 per cent of total body protein turnover (Rennie, ClinSci, 1989; 76:447). This estimate of the contribution of skeletal muscle to total body protein synthesis, from stable isotope studies, agrees with calculations based on the excretion of urinary 3-methylhistidine, which results mainly from myofibrillar protein breakdown (Young, FedProc, 1987;37:2291). Hepatic protein synthesis (Chapter 2.14.2) accounts for about 15 per cent of total body protein turnover, and the average daily synthesis of albumin, the major secretory protein, is about 15 g (Rothschild, Hepatol, 1988; 8:385). The total amount of protein synthesized in the human liver is about half that made by the total musculature, a ratio consistent with the relative amounts of mRNA in these tissues. The splanchnic region contributes up to 50 per cent of whole-body protein turnover (Gelfand, Diabetes, 1988; 37:1365).

Inadequate dietary intake of protein and/or energy, or catabolic illness, result in protein breakdown exceeding protein synthesis and a negative nitrogen balance. With protein restriction (Hoerr, AmJPhysiol, 1993; 264:E567) or prolonged fasting[25] negative nitrogen balance is associated with reduced protein turnover. During the first 24 to 48 h of fasting, the liver protein content falls, but there is little change in that of muscle. After 48 h, muscle proteolysis is enhanced to provide amino acids for gluconeogenesis; it subsequently falls as glucose requirements fall (Chapter 2.11). The reduction in proteolysis and gluconeogenesis with prolonged fasting is associated with a fall in urinary nitrogen excretion and excretion of NH_4^+ rather than urea (Owen, JCI, 1969; 48:574). In catabolic illness, such as sepsis and after surgery or trauma, protein breakdown and synthesis are both increased, with breakdown predominating[28,29] (Wolfe, DiabetMetabRev, 1989; 5:149; Carli, ClinSci, 1990; 78:621; Arnold, ClinSci, 1993; 84:655). The magnitude of the response in protein turnover, and the gap between synthesis and breakdown, increases with the severity of injury or illness. Amino acids not reincorporated into protein are oxidized; hepatic uptake of amino acids, urea synthesis, and utilization of amino acids for gluconeogenesis are all enhanced. Most of the elevation of protein breakdown occurs in skeletal muscle, while the increase in whole-body protein synthesis is largely accounted for by increased synthesis of acute-phase proteins by the liver,[28] the enhanced immune response (white cell proliferation and cytokine production), and tissue repair.

Methods of assessing protein turnover

The main methods of assessing whole body protein turnover are: (1) nitrogen balance; (2) nitrogen turnover methods; and (3) measurement of the plasma flux of an essential amino acid (such as leucine or phenylalanine) from which body protein turnover rates are extrapolated. All of these are associated with methodological problems and an awareness of these is required in interpreting the various studies.

Much of our information comes from nitrogen balance studies but the method has severe limitations.[30] These include overestimation of nitrogen intake and underestimation of nitrogen losses due to incomplete urine and faecal collections, and unmeasured losses from skin, sweat, and other sources. Because nitrogen balance represents the difference between intake and output, relatively small errors in their measurement can produce large errors in calculated

balance. Moreover, since these errors are not random, their propagation results in a large error in estimated cumulative balance in studies conducted over prolonged periods. At protein intakes above basal requirements there is an 'apparent' retention of approximately 20 per cent of the extra nitrogen intake, raising questions as to its use as the 'gold standard' for determining the balance between protein synthesis and breakdown at the whole-body level.

Nitrogen turnover methods involve the injection of a ^{15}N-labelled amino acid tracer (usually glycine) which mixes with the 'active body amino nitrogen' pool by various nitrogen exchange processes. After a sufficient mixing period, the extent of dilution of the label in the pool by unlabelled nitrogen (assumed to come solely from amino acids from dietary or body protein) is estimated by measuring the ^{15}N enrichment of urinary urea and/or ammonia. Because of the slow turnover of the urea pool and hence the delay in reaching a plateau of ^{15}N enrichment in urea, the studies take 24 h or more. The most important assumption underlying the method is that for all amino acids, ^{15}N and unlabelled nitrogen are incorporated into proteins and into urea in the same ratio. However, this and many other assumptions have been shown to be incorrect.[26,30] None the less, under many conditions, results obtained with the [^{15}N]glycine method agree with those derived from the measurement of the flux rates of a suitable essential amino acid[30] (Ang, AmJClinNutr, 1995; 61:1062).

The rate of appearance of an essential amino acid in plasma in the postabsorptive state should provide a measure of tissue protein breakdown since essential amino acids cannot be synthesized de novo. The finding that the plasma rates of appearance of the essential amino acids are directly proportional to their relative contents in muscle protein lends support to the use of their flux rates to estimate protein turnover.[30] Labelled leucine or phenylalanine are most commonly used. The advantage of this method of estimating protein turnover is that, unlike the nitrogen balance and turnover techniques, it can be used to study acute changes in protein turnover (e.g. in response to infused hormones); if combined with the arteriovenous balance technique, it provides information about the contribution of individual organs to nitrogen balance. The method is not without problems,[30] and estimates of protein turnover may differ depending on choice of tracer (Bennet, AmJPhysiol, 1990; 259:E185; Newman, Metabolism, 1994; 43:70). An important problem is that amino acid specific activity is determined by sampling plasma, whereas tracer dilution occurs intracellularly. As these are not in equilibrium, and tracer is being infused into the plasma, dilution of the intracellular labelled amino acid as a result of proteolysis will be underestimated.[31] Biolo et al.[31] found that during infusions of ring-^{13}C6-phenylalanine, 1-^{13}C-leucine, and 2-^{15}N-lysine, the enrichments of phenylalanine, leucine, and lysine in quadriceps skeletal muscle were approximately 75 per cent, 62 per cent, and 42 per cent of their respective enrichments in femoral venous plasma. Overestimation of the intracellular amino acid specific activity will lead to errors in calculated rates of amino acid oxidation or incorporation into protein. Since some of the intracellular amino acids resulting from protein breakdown are directly reincorporated into protein without entering plasma, protein synthesis tends to be underestimated when plasma amino acid specific activities are used to estimate those in the intracellular compartment.

A reduction in the plasma appearance rate of an essential amino acid is generally interpreted as indicating a reduction in proteolysis. However, Biolo et al.[31] using arteriovenous sampling across the leg together with serial muscle biopsies to determine the intracellular free amino acid enrichment, and incremental enrichment of muscle protein during infusion of labelled phenylalanine, lysine, and leucine, found that stimulation of muscle protein synthesis decreased the plasma appearance rate of these essential amino acids without any change in muscle proteolysis. This is because the rate of appearance of the amino acid in plasma is dependent on the relative rates of outward transport of the amino acid and protein synthesis. In the case of $[^{13}C]$- or $[^{14}C]$leucine an increase in oxidation due to enhanced activity of the branched-chain ketoacid dehydrogenase (BCKA dehydrogenase) could similarly decrease the plasma appearance rate of unlabelled leucine.

A major problem in studies using $[^{13}C]$- or $[^{14}C]$BCAAs, is that when the α-amino group is removed by transamination the carbon label remains in the branched chain ketoacid (BCKA) and returns rapidly to the amino acid pool with reamination of the BCKA. Similarly, if a carbon-labelled BCKA is infused, the label enters the BCAA pool and returns to the BCKA pool following deamination. Although leucine transamination is about 12 times faster than leucine oxidation in the fasted state, and about five times faster in the fed state (Matthews, Science, 1981; 14:1129), the rate of label recycling between carbon-labelled leucine and α-ketoisocaproic acid (α-KICA) is not sufficient to achieve equilibration of their intracellular specific activities. In general, the specific activity of α-KICA is about 0.75 to 0.85 times that of the infused leucine tracer,[30] but may deviate from this with changes in the BCKA dehydrogenase activity (Fig. 2)—hence the distribution of intracellular α-KICA between reamination or irreversible decarboxylation by BCKA dehydrogenase, for example during exercise (Wolfe, JApplPhysiol, 1982; 52:458) or insulin deprivation of type I diabetic patients (Nair, JCI, 1995; 95:2926). Use of plasma α-KICA specific activity rather than that of leucine provides a more accurate estimate of intracellular leucine and KICA-specific activities when $[^{13}C]$- or $[^{14}C]$leucine is infused (Watt, PNAS, 1991; 88:5892).

In studies using $[^{13}C]$- or $[^{14}C]$leucine (and other BCAAs), protein synthesis is estimated by subtracting the rate of amino acid oxidation from the total amino acid disposal rate. Oxidation of $[^{13}C]$- or $[^{14}C]$leucine is estimated from the specific activity and quantity of exhaled CO_2 after correction for bicarbonate fixation and exchange of label in the TCA cycle. In overnight-fasted normal subjects, oxidation accounts for 10 to 35 per cent of leucine flux, increasing two- to threefold after a protein meal or leucine load (Matthews, Science, 1981; 14:1129; Nissen, AmJPhysiol, 1986; 250: E695; Beaufrere, AmJPhysiol, 1989; 257:E712). Errors in estimating leucine oxidation (e.g. use of an inappropriate correction factor for label fixation) (Sidossis, JCI, 1995; 95:278) will lead to errors in estimated rates of protein synthesis.

Amino acid response to meals

After a protein-containing meal, the plasma amino acid profile does not reflect that of the ingested protein. Although the portal venous concentrations of various amino acids may be high after a meal, there is relatively little change in peripheral venous amino acid concentrations, other than for the BCAAs.[9] This is due partly to removal of absorbed amino acids by the liver, and partly to the dilution of dietary amino acids by the large amounts of amino acids released by endogenous protein turnover. However, the liver has only a limited capacity to remove and metabolize BCAAs; the amino acid mixture presented to peripheral tissues after a meal is therefore relatively enriched in BCAAs. However, even in the case of leucine, the first-pass hepatic uptake of which is only about 20 per cent (Matthews, AmJPhysiol, 1993; 264:E109), only about one-third entering systemic plasma after a protein meal comes from the meal, the rest comes from endogenous protein (Tessari, Diabetes, 1988; 37:512).

A protein meal affects the rate of hepatic protein synthesis, and also the activity of liver enzymes involved in amino acid catabolism (Fishman, PNAS, 1969; 64:677). The hepatic metabolism of most essential amino acids increases only when intake exceeds requirements, but the changes are large and rapid; tyrosine aminotransferase and tryptophan oxidase activities increase severalfold within 4 to 6 h. These mechanisms may have a protective role, as in the case of tryptophan (which is potentially neurotoxic because it can be transformed into the inhibitory neurotransmitter serotonin). The amount of tryptophan entering the peripheral circulation after a meal appears to be limited by the induction of hepatic tryptophan oxidase (Young, JNutr, 1973; 103:1756).

The plasma amino acid response to a meal will be influenced by the hormonal response, which in turn depends on the composition of the meal. Protein ingestion elicits a small rise in insulin and glucagon levels (Wahren, JCI, 1976; 57:987) and a delayed rise in growth hormone (Rabinowitz, Lancet, 1966; ii:454). Leucine is likely to be the amino acid responsible for these hormonal responses (Adibi, JLabClinMed, 1980; 95:475). The opposing actions of insulin and glucagon on liver metabolism ensure that plasma glucose levels remain unchanged even though hepatic amino acid uptake and conversion to glucose 6-phosphate are enhanced. After a mixed meal, the rise in plasma glucose levels results in a much greater insulin response; the rise in insulin inhibits proteolysis by about 25 per cent (Tessari, Diabetes, 1988; 37:512) and may augment protein synthesis[31] (see above) but this remains controversial[32] (Ljungqvist, Diabetes, 1996; 45:103A). In insulin-deficient type I diabetic patients, the increased basal rates of proteolysis, and a failure to suppress proteolysis after a meal, account for the higher fasting plasma BCAA levels and greater and more sustained postprandial rise in BCAA levels (Tessari, Diabetes; 1988; 37:512). Insulin does not stimulate BCAA uptake[11,32] (Eriksson, ClinSci, 1983; 65:491).

When carbohydrate is ingested alone, the stimulation of insulin secretion and resulting inhibition of whole-body proteolysis results in a reduction in the plasma levels of most amino acids, especially the BCAAs.

Interorgan amino acid exchange

Skeletal muscle, liver, and the kidneys play a major role in determining the plasma levels of amino acids and their turnover. Muscle contains more than 50 per cent of the total body pool of free amino acids, while the urea cycle enzymes necessary for the disposal of surplus nitrogen are in the liver;[9] the kidneys must eventually dispose of ammonia that has not been incorporated into urea. These tissues participate in the interconversion of amino acids and their re-entry into plasma. Extensive interorgan exchange occurs with only minor changes in the plasma concentration of amino acids[9, 11,20] (Elwyn, AmJPhysiol, 1972; 222:1333; Scriver, Metabolism, 1985; 34:868). Erythrocytes contribute significantly to the interorgan transport of amino acids (Felig, PNAS, 1973; 70:1775), and the concentration of some amino acids in whole blood is quite different from that found in the plasma (Hagenfeldt, CCActa 1980; 100:133).

Skeletal muscle is the main source of amino acids for synthesis of essential proteins and for gluconeogenesis during fasting. Glutamine and alanine each account for about 30 to 40 per cent of the total amino acids released from the leg in the postabsorptive state. There is a small but consistent peripheral uptake of serine, citrulline, cysteine, and glutamate.[9,20,23] Alanine and glutamine are released from muscle in amounts much greater than would be expected from their relative abundance in intracellular protein—together they constitute about 15 per cent of the amino acids in muscle protein (Felig, Science, 1970; 167:1003). Around 60 to 65 per cent of the alanine released (>90 per cent of that synthesized *de novo* in muscle) comes from plasma glucose (directly or after its release from glycogen) (Chang, JBC, 1978; 253:3685; Simmons, JCI, 1984; 73:412). Glutamine is synthesized from amino acids that give rise to intermediates of the tricarboxylic acid cycle (Fig. 1). The BCAAs, particularly leucine, are an important source of amino nitrogen for the synthesis of alanine and glutamine (Fig. 1) (Haymond, Diabetes, 1982; 31:86; Darmaun, AmJPhysiol, 1991; 260:E326). Arterial ammonia is not an important source of muscle glutamine nitrogen; net muscle uptake of ammonia may increase with elevated plasma ammonia levels but it could account for only about 10 per cent of the glutamine nitrogen production rate (Hod, EurJClinInv, 1982; 12:445; Fine, ContribNephrol, 1985; 47:1; Dejong, Gastro, 1992; 102:936).

Net splanchnic uptake of alanine, can essentially account for the alanine released by muscle.[13,20] Glutamine is consumed by the small intestine, liver, and kidneys (see above). Intestinal glutamine metabolism releases the amino nitrogen into the portal vein as alanine, citrulline, and ammonia.[33] The alanine is taken up by the liver, together with the alanine coming directly from muscle and adipose tissue. Renal uptake of glutamine and citrulline is associated with the release of significant amounts of glutamate, serine, and arginine, which may in turn be recycled back to the liver and peripheral tissues.[20]

Skeletal muscles are a major recipient of nutrients from the gut and liver. Replenishment of amino nitrogen in muscle is achieved primarily by the transfer from gut to muscle of the BCAAs. After protein ingestion, skeletal muscle uptake of BCAAs accounts for more than 50 per cent of the total amino acid uptake[13], and greatly exceeds the requirement for protein synthesis; some of the BCAAs must be catabolized. After a mixed meal, whole-body leucine oxidation increases twofold or more[34] (Nissen, AmJPhysiol, 1986; 250:E695; Beaufrere, AmJPhysiol, 1989; 257:E712). Much of this enhanced oxidation occurs in muscle. The nitrogen from BCAAs that are oxidized is used to transaminate other amino acids (Odessey, JBC, 1974; 249:7623). However, muscle alanine output falls after protein feeding while muscle glutamine release shows little change[13] (Elia, ClinSci, 1983; 64:517). Since muscle remains in

positive nitrogen balance during the postprandial period of enhanced BCAA uptake, it is likely that some of the amino nitrogen derived from the BCAAs is used to synthesize those non-essential amino acids required for the burst of protein synthesis that are not released in sufficient amounts by the liver. After an oral leucine load or during an intravenous leucine infusion, by contrast with the response to a mixed meal, the marked enhancement of leucine uptake across the forearm is associated with an increased output of glutamine and a failure to suppress alanine output (Aoki, JCI, 1981; 68:1522; Elia, ClinSci, 1983; 64:517); there is little enhancement of protein synthesis, and nitrogen balance across the forearm remains negative. A similar impairment of the anabolic response is seen if a protein meal lacking BCAAs is fed (Nissen, AmJPhysiol, 1986; 250: E695). These studies emphasize the importance of an appropriate mix of amino acids if nitrogen balance is to become positive. Increased delivery of BCAAs to muscle without a concomitant increase in delivery of other essential amino acids results in increased catabolism of BCAAs, their nitrogen being carried in alanine and glutamine to the liver and kidneys for elimination.

BCAAs may account for as much as 25 per cent of the total amino acids extracted by the kidney after a meal, even though there is no net uptake of BCAAs by the kidneys in the basal state (Tizianello, ContribNephrol, 1985; 47:44). Their renal metabolism contributes to the enhanced renal ammonia production and excretion after a protein-containing meal.

Hormonal and substrate control of amino acid metabolism

Amino acid levels play an important role in regulating protein turnover. They are probably the prime regulators of hepatic proteolysis with insulin, glucagon, and other hormones playing a secondary role. Inhibition of hepatic proteolysis requires the combined action of eight amino acids (Leu, Gln, Phe, Tyr/Pro, Met, His, Trp) with leucine being the most important (Mortimore, DiabetMetabRev, 1989; 5:49); leucine's effect may be mediated by a plasma membrane receptor (Miotto, JBC, 1992; 267:22066). Insulin and alanine may play a permissive role at normal basal levels of these amino acids, but do not appear to be important when the levels of these amino acids are increased two- to fourfold. In skeletal muscle and heart only leucine and α-KICA inhibit proteolysis; leucine (but not α-KICA) also stimulates protein synthesis in both tissues. Muscle glutamine concentrations may also regulate muscle protein turnover. In rats muscle protein synthetic rates correlated strongly with muscle glutamine levels (Jepson, AmJPhysiol, 1988; 255:E166); non-myofibrillar protein breakdown was inversely related to muscle glutamine levels (MacLennan, FEBSLett, 1988; 237:133); the decline in muscle glutamine levels in sick patients (see above) would favour net muscle protein breakdown.

Infusion of a balanced amino acid solution into normal postabsorptive subjects, to raise plasma amino acid levels two- to threefold, reduces whole-body proteolysis, increases protein synthesis, and stimulates leucine oxidation (Castellino, JCI, 1987; 80: 1784; Gelfand, Diabetes, 1988; 37:1365). Splanchnic and peripheral tissues contribute about equally to these metabolic changes (Gelfand, Diabetes, 1988; 37:1365). Giordano *et al.* (Diabetes, 1996; 45: 393), using graded amino acid infusions, found that protein synthesis did not increase significantly until total amino acid levels

Table 3 Effects of hormones on plasma amino acid (AA) levels and protein turnover

Hormone	AA levels	Proteolysis	Protein synthesis	Comments
Insulin	↓ (except Ala)	↓	↑	Inhibits gluconeogenesis
Glucagon	↓ glucogenic AA (Ala, Gly, Ser, Thr, Pro, Lys) ↓ urea cycle AA (ornithine, citrulline) No effect on BCAA	↑→[a]	→	↑ hepatic Ala uptake, AA oxidation, gluconeogenesis, and urea synthesis Effects delayed (2–3 h) but persistent
Growth hormone	↓ total AA	→	↑	Delayed effect (3–6 h)
IGF-1	↓ total AA	↓	→	
Glucocorticoids	↑ BCAA, Phe, Tyr, His, Ala	↑	↓	In the short term glucocorticoids increase protein turnover but AA levels (except Ala) and protein turnover are normal with chronic glucocorticoid excess
Adrenaline	↓ total AA, especially BCAAs	↓	→	↑ muscle Ala production and release ↑ splanchnic uptake of Ala and other glucogenic AA ↑ clearance of BCAA
Thyroxine	↑ BCAA, Phe, Thy ↓ Ala	↑	→	↑ splanchnic uptake of Ala, Gln Stimulates gluconeogenesis

[a] Glucagon has no effect on proteolysis if normal basal insulin levels are maintained.
IGF-1, insulin-like growth factor 1.

were twice those in the basal state, whereas a 25 to 50 per cent increase (similar to that seen after meals) was sufficient to inhibit proteolysis and stimulate leucine oxidation. Their study, and that of others using leucine turnover, suggests that proteolysis and leucine oxidation are more sensitive to amino acid supply than protein synthesis. However, one must be cautious in accepting this conclusion because of the underestimation of changes in protein synthetic rates when plasma rather than intracellular amino acid specific activities are used to measure the turnover of an essential amino acid (see above).

Other nutrients may also influence protein turnover. Glucose *per se* has little effect (Heiling, JClinEndoc, 1993; 76:203), but elevated plasma non-esterified fatty acid and ketone body levels during fasting may limit proteolysis and spare muscle protein. Elevation of plasma non-esterified fatty acids lowers the levels of alanine and other glucogenic amino acids, decreases urinary nitrogen excretion, and may produce a small fall in BCAA levels (Ferrannini, AmJPhysiol, 1986; 250:E686; Walker, AmJPhysiol, 1993; 265:E357). An increase in plasma non-esterified fatty acid levels decreased leucine flux and oxidation in dogs (Tessari, JCI, 1986; 77:575) but Walker *et al.* (AmJPhysiol, 1993; 265:E357) found no effect of raised fatty acid levels in normal subjects on forearm balance of phenylalanine or whole-body phenylalanine turnover. Infusion of 3-hydroxybutyrate in normal subjects had no effect on proteolysis but it decreased leucine oxidation and had a small stimulatory effect on leucine incorporation into protein (Nair, JCI, 1988; 82:198).

The effects of hormones on plasma amino acid levels and protein turnover are summarized in Table 3. Since amino acid levels *per se* influence protein turnover, it is important to control their plasma levels when assessing the effects of a hormone on protein metabolism.

Insulin lowers the plasma concentrations of all amino acids except alanine. Forearm studies in which insulin has been infused into the brachial artery, and changes in systemic insulin and amino acid levels avoided, suggest that muscle proteolysis is very sensitive to insulin; in overnight-fasted normal subjects the forearm deep venous insulin concentration required for half-maximal inhibition of forearm leucine release was only 13 mU/l, with a maximal effect at about 50 mU/l (Louard, JCI, 1992; 90:2348). These insulin concentrations were much lower than those required for half-maximal and maximal stimulation of muscle glucose uptake in the same subjects. Inhibition of proteolysis explains the reduction of plasma amino acid levels when insulin is infused systemically. Alanine is not decreased, because insulin increases production of alanine via pyruvate from glucose[31] and may also inhibit gluconeogenesis and hepatic alanine uptake. In poorly controlled type I diabetic patients hepatic alanine uptake is increased and this may result in low plasma alanine levels.[13] Insulin augments the effects of hyperaminoacidaemia to suppress proteolysis after a meal; the greater postprandial rise in BCAAs in insulin-deficient type I diabetic patients is due to a failure to suppress protein breakdown (see above).

Insulin enhances protein synthesis in isolated muscle and in hepatocytes, provided sufficient amino acids are present. However, *in vivo* studies of insulin's effect on protein synthesis have yielded conflicting results. Studies using phenylalanine suggest a stimulatory effect of insulin on phenylalanine disposal and incorporation into protein at normal or increased plasma amino acid levels (Bennet, AmJPhysiol, 1990; 259:E185; Newman, Metabolism, 1994; 43:70), but leucine turnover studies have failed to show any enhancement of non-oxidative leucine disposal (an index of protein synthesis) by insulin, even when basal amino acid levels are maintained

(Castellino, JCI, 1987; 80:1784; Newman, Metabolism, 1994; 43: 70). Use of plasma rather than intracellular amino acid specific activities (see above), may partly explain these conflicting findings. Biolo et al.[31] performed serial quadriceps muscle biopsies during infusions of ring-^{13}C6-phenylalanine, in the basal state and during an infusion of insulin into the femoral artery which did not perturb arterial amino acid levels. From the intracellular free phenylalanine enrichment, and incremental [^{13}C]phenylalanine enrichment in muscle protein during the study, they showed a 65 per cent increase in protein synthesis in response to insulin, despite a reduction in muscle amino acid levels during the insulin infusion.

Although insulin enhances the transport of some amino acids, notably alanine and possibly glutamine (Rennie, JPhysiol, 1987; 393:283; King, AmJPhysiol, 1994; 35:C524), regulation of transmembrane amino acid transport does not appear to mediate insulin's effects on muscle protein synthesis or the reduction in plasma amino acid levels.[31]

Growth hormone and insulin-like growth factor-1 are the other main hormones that promote protein anabolism and positive nitrogen balance. Although many of growth hormone's actions are mediated via insulin-like growth factor-1, growth hormone also has direct effects, and the actions of growth hormone and insulin-like growth factor-1 are complementary (Table 3). Thus insulin-like growth factor-1 decreases whole-body and skeletal muscle protein breakdown but has not been found to stimulate protein synthesis, whereas growth hormone stimulates protein synthesis and decreases the oxidation of BCAAs but does not suppress proteolysis,[34] it may even antagonize insulin's antiproteolytic action (Fryburg, Diabetes, 1992; 41:424). Growth hormone and insulin-like growth factor-1 have been used to promote anabolism in critically ill patients (for example, after major surgery or burns) and in patients with chronic diseases that lead to wasting and loss of lean body mass, such as liver disease, chronic renal failure, and the acquired immune deficiency syndrome. Growth hormone improves nitrogen balance in subjects maintained on hypocaloric diets and after elective surgery. However, in severely catabolic patients (for example, after major trauma) it fails to induce a positive nitrogen balance. This appears to be due to an impaired hepatic insulin-like growth factor-1 response to growth hormone. Despite the anabolic effects of infused insulin-like growth factor-1 in short-term studies, clinical trials with insulin-like growth factor-1 in sick patients have mostly been negative (Lieberman, JClinEndoc, 1994; 78:404; Goeters, AnnSurg, 1995; 222:646). This may be due to an inhibitory effect on growth hormone secretion (see Chapter 24.2), an inhibition of insulin secretion (Mauras, JClinEndoc, 1992; 75:1192), and a progressive decline in plasma insulin-like growth factor-1 levels with chronic treatment (Goeters, AnnSurg, 1995; 222:646). The fall in insulin-like growth factor-1 levels may be due in part to alterations in the plasma binding proteins for insulin-like growth factor-1 (**IGFBP**) with a decline in IGFBP-3 and increased levels of IGFBP-1 (see Chapter 24.2); a redistribution of insulin-like growth factor-1 from the high molecular weight IGFBP-3-containing complex to lower molecular weight complexes markedly increases the plasma clearance of insulin-like growth factor-1. Kupfer et al. (JCI, 1993; 91:391) found that in normal subjects maintained on a hypocaloric diet insulin-like growth factor-1 alone failed to induce a positive nitrogen balance but the combination of growth hormone and insulin-like growth factor-1 resulted in postive nitrogen balance,

and insulin-like growth factor[1]induced hypoglycaemia was less of a problem. It remains to be seen whether this combination will also be able to prevent nitrogen losses and promote protein anabolism in 'sick' patients.

Glucocorticoids are essential for the enhanced muscle proteolysis during fasting and in response to stress, by increasing the activity of an ATP–ubiquitin-dependent pathway in muscle that degrades myofibrillar proteins, proteins with short half-lives, and abnormal proteins (Wing, AmJPhysiol, 1993; 264:E668). Glucocorticoids promote muscle BCAA oxidation by increasing the activity of BCKA dehydrogenase (Jaspers, Metabolism, 1989; 38:109)(see above). They increase the *de novo* synthesis of alanine and glutamine severalfold, much of the nitrogen coming from the enhanced oxidation of the BCAAs (Darmaun, AmJPhysiol, 1988; 255:E366). Plasma total amino acid levels are increased (Table 3),[34] but the total amino nitrogen in muscle falls due to a marked decrease in muscle glutamine levels resulting from increased glutamine efflux (Muhlbacher, AmJPhysiol, 1984; 247:E75). Glucocorticoids are a major determinant of the fall in muscle glutamine levels in critically ill patients (Askanazi, AnnSurg, 1980; 192:78). Plasma glutamine levels may show little change, or a even a fall, despite increased muscle glutamine release. This is because glucocorticoids also markedly enhance hepatic, gut, and renal glutamine uptake and metabolism;[24] intestinal alanine and NH_4^+ production and release into the portal vein are increased[24] (Souba, Metabolism, 1985; 34: 450). Thus glucocorticoids induce a marked transfer of amino nitrogen in the form of alanine and glutamine from muscle to liver to support enhanced rates of gluconeogenesis, urea synthesis, and glutathione production.[24]

Glucagon's main site of action is the liver. Glucagon levels increase with fasting, after protein ingestion, or in response to stress. Glucagon stimulates gluconeogenesis (Stevenson, Diabetes, 1987; 36:382) and urea synthesis (Boden, AmJPhysiol, 1990; 259: E225) and increases the uptake of alanine and other glucogenic amino acids by the liver. It enhances the hepatic catabolism of amino acids by increasing the synthesis and activities of several amino acid catabolizing enzymes, including alanine, tyrosine, ornithine, and asparagine aminotransferases and serine dehydratase. It also increases the activities of all of the urea cycle enzymes. As a result it lowers the plasma levels of glucogenic amino acids and those of the urea cycle (Table 3). Glucagon promotes protein catabolism in the insulin-deficient state (Nair, AmJPhysiol, 1987; 253:E208) but not in the presence of normal basal insulin levels. This proteolytic effect is probably due to its action on splanchnic tissues since glucagon has no direct effect on muscle amino acid metabolism (Pozefsky, Diabetes, 1976; 25:128). Although glucagon does not influence BCAA levels (Couet, AmJPhysiol, 1990; 258:E78), it does increase their oxidation by activating hepatic BCKA dehydrogenase (Block, BiochemJ, 1985; 232:593). This occurs at the expense of their incorporation into protein (Ostaszewski, AmJPhysiol, 1988; 254: E372) and contributes to a less positive nitrogen balance.

Thyroxine causes an increases in muscle release of most amino acids and increases gluconeogenesis and the splanchnic uptake of alanine and glutamine. Plasma levels of most amino acids, with the exception of alanine and glutamine, are increased in thyrotoxicosis (Morrison, EurJClinInv, 1988; 18:62).

Amino acid degradation in liver and muscle

The non-essential amino acids are readily oxidized in both liver and muscle. The essential amino acids arginine, histidine, lysine, methionine, phenylalanine, tryptophan, and threonine are oxidized primarily in the liver.[35] The ketoacids of the BCAAs are readily oxidized in liver and peripheral tissues but deamination occurs primarily in extrahepatic tissues (see above). Amino acid clearances *in vivo* vary greatly from one amino acid to another. Essential amino acids have a relatively low clearance.[36] The hepatic enzymes which degrade them have high K_M values, and are thus quantitatively important only at high amino acid concentrations; this may help to conserve essential amino acids. The enzymes degrading non-essential amino acids tend to have low K_M values; these amino acids are easily reconstituted from their metabolic intermediates.[37] Arginine, a urea cycle intermediate, has a very high clearance rate, probably related to the high hepatic concentration of arginase. Excess dietary protein, or starvation, results in an adaptive increase in the amount of the first enzyme of the catabolic pathways of at least 16 amino acids (Krebs, AdvEnzymReg, 1972; 10:397).

Amino acid metabolism in liver disease

Plasma amino acid concentrations are often disturbed in patients with liver disease. In fulminant hepatic failure plasma concentrations of all amino acids, except BCAAs, are high, with striking elevations of methionine and the aromatic amino acids (Record, EurJClinInv, 1976; 6:387; Rosen, Gastro, 1977; 72:483). These changes are most likely due to a markedly increased protein turnover (O'Keefe, Gastro, 1981; 81:1017) (as in other critically ill patients), together with impaired amino acid uptake by the diseased liver. Degradation of protein and release of amino acids from the necrosing liver may contribute but cannot be a major factor; since the total liver protein amounts to only about 300 g, the entire liver protein content would have to be degraded within 6 to 8 h to account for the increased protein turnover rates found (O'Keefe, Gastro, 1981; 81:1017). Some 15 to 20 times more protein is present in skeletal muscle because of its greater mass, and muscle is probably the main source of amino acids, as it is in other severely catabolic patients. BCAA concentrations are low or normal in fulminant hepatic failure because they undergo predominantly peripheral metabolism, and because their oxidation in peripheral tissues is markedly enhanced in 'sick' patients, possibly by the effects of tumour necrosis factor-α and other cytokines.

In cirrhotic patients with poor liver function the fasting blood α-amino nitrogen concentration is high, due to reduced clearance of total α-amino nitrogen, and urea synthesis is lower than in control subjects.[36,37] The plasma profile of amino acids in cirrhosis (Table 4) typically shows an increase in the aromatic amino acids, phenylalanine and tyrosine, and in free tryptophan and methionine, thought to be related to impaired hepatic utilization of these amino acids and to portosystemic shunting. There is a consistent reduction in fasting plasma levels of BCAAs in cirrhosis and in other types of liver disease; the mechanism underlying these changes is not clear (see below).

Estimations of the levels of other amino acids in fasting plasma, have been quite variable (Table 4). The results of studies on plasma amino acids must be interpreted with caution, because of technical difficulties in their measurement and differences in the clinical status of the patients studied. Most of the free amino acid pool of the body is present in the intracellular fluid, and changes seen in the plasma levels of amino acids do not necessarily reflect their overall metabolic availability. In patients with cirrhosis the concentration of tyrosine and phenylalanine in skeletal muscle water was high in proportion to the increase in plasma levels.[6] The valine concentration in muscle water was lower, as in plasma; but muscle leucine was the same as in controls, while muscle isoleucine showed an increase, despite the lower levels of these two amino acids in plasma.

Both the elevation of aromatic amino acids and the reduction in BCAAs have been incriminated in the genesis of hepatic encephalopathy (Fischer, Surgery, 1976; 80:77); however, some workers have found no correlation between amino acid levels and either the presence or degree of hepatic encephalopathy (Morgan, Gut, 1978; 19:1068; Marchesini, DigDisSci, 1980; 25:763; Weber, DigDisSci, 1982; 27:103). This topic is discussed in Section 9.

Amino acid response to protein and amino acid loads in cirrhotics

Vilstrup *et al.*[36] infused a balanced amino acid mixture for 12 h in a small group of cirrhotics and controls at a rate sufficient to raise plasma amino nitrogen concentration four- to fivefold over that in the basal state. The plasma amino nitrogen concentration achieved during the infusion was higher in patients with cirrhosis than in controls, even though the cirrhotics received a smaller amount of the mixture. The apparent clearance of most amino acids, assuming inhibition of protein catabolism as a result of the administration of the amino acid load, was lower than in controls, and this difference was significant for glycine, proline, lysine, threonine, and arginine. There was little or no difference in the clearance of the BCAAs nor, surprisingly, in that of phenylalanine and tryptophan. Tyrosine clearance in 32 patients with endstage liver disease studied by Shanbhogue (Metabolism, 1987; 36:1047) was only 49 per cent of that in matched normal subjects; a smaller impairment of phenylalanine clearance was also found but this did not reach statistical significance. As discussed below, others have found decreased clearance of the aromatic amino acids (tryptophan, phenylalanine, and tyrosine), and of methionine and cysteine. BCAA clearance is normal when measured during an infusion of the BCAAs.[38] As might be expected from the importance of the liver for alanine disposal, reduced alanine clearance has also been found in cirrhosis (Elia, ClinSci, 1980; 58:301; Hamberg, Hepatol, 1994; 19:45).

Iob and his colleagues (JSurgRes, 1966; 6:233) fed a protein meal to cirrhotic patients and found a smaller increase in the BCAAs than in control subjects; there was also a smaller increase in lysine, methionine, and threonine, but this difference was not significant. The increment in phenylalanine and tryptophan was similar in the two groups. A similar result was obtained in a study in which 40 g of protein was fed; there was a much smaller increase in total BCAAs in cirrhotics than in controls, and although there was a greater increase in the total concentration of aromatic amino acids + methionine in cirrhotics, this difference was not significant (Ibrahim, SurgForum, 1983; 34:36). Marchesini *et al.* (Gastro, 1983; 85:283) fed a protein meal (approximately 40 g) to cirrhotics, who

Table 4 Changes in fasting amino acid levels in patients with cirrhosis

	Ref. 1 1977	Ref. 2 1982	Ref. 3 1982	Ref. 4 1982	Ref. 5 1983	Ref. 6 1984	Ref. 7 1984	Ref. 8 1984	Ref. 9 1987	Ref. 10 1988	Ref. 11 1989	Ref. 12 1990	Ref. 13 1990	Ref. 14 1991
Glycine	=	↓a	=	=	=	=	↑c	↑	=	=	=	↓	nd	=
Alanine	↓	↓a	↓	↓	=	=	=	=	=	L	=	↓	↓	=
Serine	=	↑b	=	=	H	↑	H	=	=	=	↑	↓	nd	=
Threonine	↓	↑b	=	=	=	=	=	=	=	=	=	↓	nd	=
Proline	L	=	=	nd	=	H	↑	=	=	↓	nd	nd	nd	nd
Leucine	↓	↓	↓	↓	↓	↓	=	↓	=	↓	↓	↓	↓	↓
Isoleucine	↓	↓	↓	↓	↓	↓	=	↓	↓	↓	↓	↓	↓	↓
Valine	↓	↓	↓	↓	↓	↓	↓	↓	↓	↓	nd	↓	↓	↓
Phenylalanine	↑		↑	=	↑	↑	↑	↑	↑	↑	↑	=	↑	↑
Tyrosine	↑	↑c	↑	↑	↑	H	↑b	↑	↑	↑	↑	↑	↑	↑
Tryptophan			nd		nd		nd	nd	nd	nd	nd	nd	nd	nd
Free			↑		↑									
Total	H		↓		=		↑b							
Methionine	↑	↑	nd	↑	↑	↑	↑b	↑	↑	↑	↑	↑	nd	H
Total cysteine	nd	H	nd	nd	nd	=	nd	nd	nd	nd	↑	nd	nd	=
Free cysteine		nd	nd	nd	nd	↓	nd	nd	nd		nd		nd	
Cystine			nd	nd	H	=	nd	nd	↑		nd		nd	
Taurine	=	nd	nd	=	nd	↓	nd	=	=	=	↓	nd	nd	=
Asparagine	nd	H	nd	nd	nd	nd	nd	nd	=	=	nd	=	nd	H
Glutamine	nd	nd	nd	=	=	nd	nd	nd	=	nd	=	↓	↓	=
Aspartic acid	↑	↑c	nd	↓	nd	nd	↑	nd	=	=	nd	↓	nd	nd
Glutamic acid	↑	nd	nd	H	H	nd	nd	↑	=	nd	nd	↓	↑	=
Histidine	L	=	=	=	=	nd	=	=	=	↓	nd	L	nd	nd
Lysine	=	=	=	↓	=	nd	=	=	=	↓	nd	↓	nd	nd
Arginine	L	↑c	=	↑	H	nd	=	↑	=	=	nd	H	nd	nd
Ornithine	=	=	=	=	↑	nd	Hb	↑	=	=	nd	↓	nd	nd
Total AA	nd		nd	nd	nd	nd		nd	=	nd	nd	↓	nd	=

a Decreased in alcoholic cirrhotics; normal in non-alcoholic cirrhotics.
b High in alcoholic cirrhotics but normal or increased to a lesser extent in non-alcoholic cirrhotics.
c Increased in non-alcoholic cirrhotics only.

Ref. 1   Rosen, Gastro, 1977; 72:483
Ref. 2   Morgan, Gut, 1982; 23:362
Ref. 3   Marchesini, Hepatol, 1982; 2:420
Ref. 4   Eriksson, ClinSci, 1982, 62:285
Ref. 5   Marchesini, Gastro, 1983; 85:283
Ref. 6   Chawla, Gastro, 1984; 87:770
Ref. 7   Joelsson, ScaJGastr, 1984; 19:547
Ref. 8   Horst, Hepatol, 1984; 2:279
Ref. 9   Marchesini, JHepatol, 1987; 4:108
Ref. 10   Montanari, Hepatol, 1988; 8:1034
Ref. 11   Tribble, AmJClinNutr, 1989; 50:1401
Ref. 12   Plauth, Hepatogast, 1990; 37:135
Ref. 13   Morrison, ClinSci, 1990; 78:613
Ref. 14   Petrides, Hepatol, 1991; 14:431

showed a greater increase in plasma levels of BCAAs, and of phenylalanine and total tryptophan, than normal controls; alanine increased significantly in controls but not in cirrhotics, and the other amino acids behaved similarly in the two groups. Morgan *et al.* (AlimPharmTher, 1990; 4:183) fed a 30 g meal of either protein or amino acids to control subjects and to patients with well-compensated cirrhosis. The plasma level of all amino acids rose after the meals but, although there were greater increases of some amino acids in the cirrhotics, they did not differ significantly from those seen in the controls; it was concluded that there was no fundamental difference in the handling of the protein and amino acid loads in these well-compensated cirrhotics.

Protein turnover in cirrhosis

The muscle wasting seen in patients with advanced liver disease could be due to increased rates of protein degradation, impaired protein synthesis, or both. These abnormalities could, in turn, be due to inadequate dietary intake of nutrients or impaired nutrient utilization for anabolic purposes. Various methods have been used to assess protein metabolism in cirrhotics, with little consensus

between investigators. Many factors contribute to the discordant findings, including heterogeneity of the patients studied and failure to take into account preceding calorie and protein intake,[25,39] or preceding episodes of acute illness in inpatients.

Urinary excretion of 3-methylhistidine derived from the catabolism of muscle actin and myosin has been found to be increased in cirrhotics without evident muscle wasting (Marchesini, Hepatol, 1981; 1:294) suggesting increased turnover of myofibrillar protein. In cirrhotics with muscle wasting excretion of 3-methylhistidine was similar to that in normal subjects but inappropriately high for their reduced muscle mass (Zoli, ClinSci, 1982; 62:683).

Most studies employing labelled leucine have found no difference in whole-body protein turnover rates between cirrhotic and normal subjects studied after an overnight fast.[40-43] However, both lower and increased protein turnover rates have been reported. McCullough *et al.* (Gastro, 1992; 103:571) reported normal leucine turnover and lower leucine oxidation in fasted cirrhotics when this was calculated from the plasma [^{13}C]leucine enrichment, but increased turnover and leucine oxidation if they used the plasma [^{13}C]KICA, enrichment which provides a better estimate of the intracellular leucine enrichment during infusion of labelled leucine; surprisingly urinary nitrogen excretion was significantly lower in their cirrhotics. To account for this discrepancy they postulated that protein breakdown and amino acid oxidation was increased in cirrhotics but that the excess nitrogen was eliminated by some extrarenal route. Tessari et al. (Gastro, 1993; 104:1712), using simultaneous infusions of labelled leucine and phenylalanine, found that protein turnover rates were reduced in cirrhotics (11 Child's A; 4 Child's B) if they used the leucine data, but increased by 28 per cent when turnover was calculated from the phenylalanine data. Surprisingly, the plasma BCAA levels were not reduced in their cirrhotics. Hirsch et al. (JAmCollNutr, 1995; 14:99) reported increased leucine (hence protein) turnover in actively drinking alcoholic cirrhotics but not in abstinent patients, while Pacy et al. (AlcAlc, 1991; 26:505) found normal leucine appearance rates in alcoholics but a decrease in muscle protein synthetic rate.

Morrison et al.[42], in malnourished cirrhotics who were losing weight at the time of the study, found a lower net efflux of leucine, alanine, and glutamine from the leg but increased efflux of tyrosine and phenylalanine by comparison with normal subjects. Clearly, these studies are difficult to interpret, but since tyrosine and phenylalanine cannot be oxidized by muscle, their increased release suggests increased muscle proteolysis. 3-Methylhistidine efflux (i.e. myofibrillar protein breakdown) was not increased.

Swart et al. (ClinSci, 1988; 75:101) used the [^{15}N]glycine method[44] to measure protein turnover in a group of cirrhotics in hospital shortly after recovery from complications of their cirrhosis. They found that in the fasting state protein turnover and nitrogen balance were similar to those in normal subjects but protein turnover was increased when the subjects were fed either an adequate diet or a protein-restricted diet (0.5 g/kg body weight); nitrogen balance was actually more positive in the cirrhotics. These authors suggested that the nitrogen requirements in cirrhotics are increased. The efficient nitrogen retention in the cirrhotics may be a reflection of the preceding period of poor calorie/protein intake[25] or acute illness.[28] The high protein turnover rates found could also have a methodological basis; the [^{15}N]glycine technique may not be valid in liver disease because of differing enrichment of the precursor pool for urea synthesis compared to that for protein synthesis throughout the body.[44]

Increased protein turnover would be expected to be accompanied by increased urinary nitrogen excretion, but this is normal or low in most cirrhotics in both fasting and fed states, suggesting diminished amino acid catabolism. Decreased protein turnover in cirrhotics could reflect a lower intake of energy and/or protein in the weeks before study, since in normal subjects restriction of either is followed by a reduction in protein turnover.[25] It could also be a consequence of malnutrition. An important question is whether cirrhotics are able to reduce their protein turnover and amino acid catabolism appropriately when energy and or protein intake are reduced.

Studies on individual amino acids in liver disease

Branched-chain amino acids: leucine, valine, and isoleucine

The reduced plasma BCAAs found in overnight-fasted cirrhotic patients have long been a puzzle. Merli (ClinNutr, 1985; 4:249)

suggested that the reduced plasma BCAA levels in cirrhosis may, in part, be secondary to malnutrition, often present in severe liver disease. However, low BCAA levels are also found in well-nourished cirrhotics. Catecholamines might reduce muscle efflux of BCAAs and lower their plasma levels (Table 3); BCAA levels in cirrhotics increase promptly following an oral 40 to 80 mg dose of propranolol (Eriksson, Hepatogast, 1992; 39:451). Fasting hyperinsulinaemia in cirrhosis as a cause of the low plasma BCAA levels has received the most attention; insulin lowers plasma BCAAs (Table 3), and BCAA levels are increased in insulin-deprived type I diabetic patients. Some support for a role of insulin as a cause of lowered BCAA levels comes from the finding that plasma BCAA concentrations increase in cirrhotics when insulin levels are reduced by infusion of somatostatin (Limberg, Gut, 1984; 25:1291). However, such a rise would be expected irrespective of the primary cause of the lowered BCAA levels. In general, plasma BCAA levels do not correlate with plasma insulin levels (Marchesini, DigDis, 1979; 24:594).

If insulin or catecholamines were responsible for the lowered plasma BCAA levels in cirrhosis, there must either be a reduced rate of leucine delivery into the plasma compartment, enhanced removal of leucine from plasma, or both. Contrary to popular belief, insulin does not stimulate muscle or splanchnic BCAA uptake in humans[32] (Abumrad, Metabolism, 1982; 31:463; Eriksson, ClinSci, 1983; 65:491); it lowers plasma BCAA levels by decreasing splanchnic and peripheral tissue BCAA release. Several groups have used [^{14}C]- or [^{13}C]leucine to estimate leucine turnover in cirrhotic patients with low fasting plasma BCAA levels. Bearing in mind the methodological issues discussed earlier, most studies have found normal leucine turnover;[40–43] none of the studies reported reduced rates of plasma leucine appearance, as might be expected if insulin played a major role. McCullough et al. (Gastro, 1992; 103: 571) also found normal rates of leucine appearance when this was calculated using the plasma [^{13}C]leucine enrichment but increased rates using the plasma [^{13}C]KICA enrichment (see above). By contrast, Petrides et al.[40] found that leucine turnover was similar in cirrhotics and controls irrespective of whether plasma leucine or KICA specific activity was used. Normal whole-body leucine flux rates were also found by Morrison et al.[42] using the plasma [^{13}C]KICA enrichment. While most of these studies included well-nourished cirrhotics with good liver function, Morrison[42] studied malnourished patients who were losing weight and had relatively poor liver function.

Because BCAAs are poorly removed by the liver, but removed by other tissues, it has been suggested that their peripheral uptake must be enhanced in cirrhosis. Clearly, the leucine turnover studies do not support this. In the fasting state the rate of leucine disposal equals its rate of release from tissue protein. Furthermore, insulin has little acute effect on the muscle BCKA dehydrogenase (see above), and the reduction in BCAA and other amino acid levels induced by insulin is associated with a reduction in leucine oxidation. The higher clearance of leucine in the basal state in cirrhotics (measured with labelled leucine) is explained by their lower plasma leucine levels; the relationship between leucine clearance and plasma leucine levels is curvilinear and not influenced by insulin[32] (Fukagawa, JCI, 1985; 76:2306). Most studies have found normal rates of whole-body leucine oxidation rates in cirrhosis using either the plasma KICA enrichment,[40] (McCullough, Gastro, 1992; 103:571) or leucine enrichment[40,41] during infusion of labelled leucine. One study[42] found increased leucine oxidation in cirrhotics but this was offset by a reduction in protein synthesis, so that total leucine disposal was normal.

Thus, most cirrhotics with low plasma BCAA levels have normal fasting leucine turnover despite insulin levels that are usually 3 to 6 times higher (15–40 mU/l) than those in control subjects (see Chapter 2.11). Clearly, hyperinsulinaemia cannot explain the low BCAA levels. Moreover, the data imply that cirrhotics are resistant to insulin, not only in terms of glucose metabolism but also in terms of whole-body leucine metabolism, since the insulin concentration necessary for half-maximal suppression of leucine appearance (proteolysis) in normal subjects is about 13 to 20 mU/l.

A possible explanation for the lowered fasting plasma BCAA levels is an altered distribution of BCAAs between intracellular and extracellular compartments. Petrides found that not only were the leucine turnover rates virtually identical in cirrhotics and controls, but that the plasma KICA and leucine-specific activities achieved when 1-^{14}C-leucine was infused at the same rate were also the same in the two groups. This implies that the leucine and KICA pool sizes must have been the same, even though plasma leucine and KICA levels were lower in the cirrhotic patients. This could be explained by an increase in the extracellular volume as suggested by McCullough *et al.*[41] and/or altered partitioning of leucine and KICA between intracellular and extracellular compartments so that a greater proportion of the pool is intracellular. Two studies found normal leucine levels in muscle water in cirrhotics despite low plasma leucine levels, resulting in a threefold gradient for leucine across the plasma membrane by comparison with a 1.4- to 1.8-fold gradient in controls.[5,6] In one of these the intracellular isoleucine concentration was actually higher in the cirrhotics.[6] Increased plasma and tissue levels of phenylalanine might explain this altered BCAA partitioning in some cirrhotics. Phenylalanine has a very high affinity for the amino acid transport system L that transports the BCAAs (Table 2).[23] In hepatocytes, skeletal muscle, and other tissues, phenylalanine inhibits the exit of neutral amino acids, including the BCAAs, by system L (DeCespides, JInherMetDis, 1989; 12:166), resulting in an increase in their intracellular concentration. In the case of leucine, the resulting increase in its gradient across the plasma membrane would eventually enhance the leucine efflux rate, establishing a new steady state.

Another postulated mechanism for the low fasting BCAA concentrations in liver disease is increased glutamine production secondary to hyperammonaemia. BCAAs are consumed during ammonia detoxification, donating their amino group to α-ketoglutarate. In rats an infusion of ammonia rapidly reduces the plasma concentrations of BCAAs, a change preceded by an increase in plasma glutamine. *In vitro*, ammonia increases leucine oxidation in both rat muscle and adipose tissue.[45] Ganda and Ruderman (Metabolism, 1976; 25:427) found a large arteriovenous difference across the forearm for glutamine in cirrhotics with poor liver function maintained on a low-protein diet (0–40 g/day) and suggested that cirrhotics might release more glutamine from muscle than healthy controls. However, they neither studied control subjects nor did they measure forearm blood flow. Others found a much lower net efflux of glutamine across the leg in cirrhotics than controls.[42] Clearly further studies are needed to determine whether increased glutamine production by skeletal muscle and possibly other tissues (for example, brain) contributes to the low

plasma BCAA concentrations. Given the normal whole-body rates of leucine production and disposal, and normal leucine oxidation rates found in most studies, increased utilization of BCAAs for glutamine synthesis is an unlikely explanation for the low BCAAs. Furthermore, many patients with low plasma BCAA levels do not have increased plasma ammonia levels.

The handling of an intravenous BCAA (or corresponding ketoacid) load appears to be normal in cirrhosis. Similar steady-state plasma BCAA levels are attained in cirrhotic and normal subjects when BCAAs are infused intravenously, and the calculated clearance of BCAAs (infusion rate/plasma concentration) is normal[36,38] (Shanbhogue, Metabolism, 1987; 36:1047). The plasma half-life of leucine is also normal in cirrhotics (Elia, ClinSci, 1980; 59:275). Leucine clearance is independent of insulin (Fukagawa, JCI, 1985; 76:2306), and thus it is not surprising that despite the marked insulin resistance of cirrhotics,[40] BCAA levels, and hence clearance rates, are similar in cirrhotics and controls when insulin is co-infused with an amino acid mixture. When, in another study, KICA was infused intravenously, the plasma level of KICA rose less in cirrhotics than in control subjects; the plasma leucine levels achieved were similar in both groups, but there was a greater rise in cirrhotics because of the lower initial levels (Eriksson, ClinSci, 1982; 62:285). The lower rise in plasma KICA in cirrhotics could be due to more rapid KICA disposal, but it could also be due to their lower plasma albumin or increased fasting non-esterified fatty acids, which compete with KICA for binding to plasma albumin (Nissen, AmJPhysiol, 1982; 242:E67).

The plasma BCAA levels achieved during the intravenous infusion of BCAAs or an amino acid mixture reflects not only the ability of the tissues to take up and metabolize the infused amino acids but also the extent of suppression of amino acid release from endogenous protein. During an amino acid infusion, there is often a small rise in insulin levels. Both insulin and the rise in plasma amino acid levels are important in suppressing proteolysis. The response to amino acids *per se* is likely to be of greater importance in determining the overall response to an amino acid load, but insulin may assume greater importance after a mixed meal or with a large intravenous or oral leucine load, because of the greater insulin response. The effects of amino acids *per se* on suppression of proteolysis in cirrhosis have not been examined. When insulin is infused intravenously during a hyperinsulinaemic euglycaemic clamp (Chapter 2.11) to produce plasma insulin levels in the high physiological range, suppression of leucine appearance is normal, and similar low plasma BCAA levels are attained in cirrhotics and controls[40] (Marchesini, Hepatol, 1983; 3:184), although the relative fall in plasma BCAA levels tends to be less in cirrhotics (because of their lower baseline levels). This has been interpreted as indicating normal sensitivity of amino acid metabolism to insulin in cirrhosis.[40] However, the insulin levels achieved in these studies were greater than those necessary for maximal inhibition of leucine turnover, particularly when amino acid levels were prevented from falling;[40] the leucine turnover rates in the basal state may be a better reflection of the sensitivity of amino acid metabolism to insulin.

Delivery of dietary BCAAs into the systemic circulation after a protein meal or BCAA load ought to be similar in cirrhotics and controls since only about 20 per cent of an oral leucine load is taken up by splanchnic tissues on first pass (Matthews, AmJPhysiol, 1993;

264:E109). Thus, given the normal handling of an intravenous BCAA load, one would expect that cirrhotics would have a normal plasma BCAA response to an oral BCAA load. After a protein meal or oral BCAA load most investigators have found similar (Morgan, AlimPharmTher, 1990; 4:183) or somewhat lower plasma BCAA responses in cirrhotics compared with normal subjects[43] (Ibrahim, SurgForum, 1983;34:36), although a greater rise, resulting in increased postprandial BCAA levels, has also been reported (Marchesini, Gastro, 1983; 85:283). Schauder (Hepatol, 1984; 4:667) found that following the oral administration of valine to overtly jaundiced cirrhotics the serum levels of both valine and its corresponding ketoacid (**KIVA**) reached higher levels than in control subjects; the same was true when KIVA was fed. However, when leucine was fed, the increase in serum leucine and KICA were similar in the two groups; after oral KICA, serum leucine reached thc same level in both groups, but from a lower baseline in the cirrhotics, and there was a significantly greater rise in serum KICA. The different handling of valine and leucine and their respective ketoacids in this study is difficult to understand given that the same transaminase and BCKA dehydrogenase enzymes are responsible for their metabolism. Some of their cirrhotics had elevated fasting blood glucose levels and were probably diabetic.[46] This might explain their valine intolerance. Tessari *et al.* (AmJPhysiol, 1994; 267:E140) found that in poorly controlled diabetic cirrhotics given a mixed meal containing a mixture of crystalline amino acids there was a greater increase in valine and isoleucine than in controls or three non-diabetic cirrhotics, while basal and post-meal leucine levels did not differ. The greater rise in plasma BCAA levels after BCAA ingestion found in some studies is likely to be due to impaired suppression of BCAA release from endogenous protein during the postprandial period rather than impaired BCAA removal (Tessari, AmJPhysiol, 1994; 267:E140).

In keeping with the normal plasma BCAA response to protein ingestion in most cirrhotics, Millikan *et al.*[43] using an infusion of doubly labelled leucine (^{15}N,^{13}C) found no difference in leucine kinetics between cirrhotics and normal individuals during the enteral infusion of a standard meal, in terms of either leucine nitrogen or carbon flux, leucine oxidation (based on leucine enrichment), or deamination and reamination rates. When a meal enriched in BCAAs was fed, the additional BCAAs were oxidized and there was no further suppression of endogenous proteolysis or enhancement of non-oxidative leucine disposal ('protein synthesis').[43]

Proline (and hydroxyproline)

In patients with fulminant hepatic failure plasma proline levels are increased approximately threefold (Record, EurJClinInv, 1976; 6: 387; Rosen, Gastro, 1977; 72:483). Most cirrhotics have normal fasting plasma proline levels, but they may be increased in those with decompensated liver disease, in patients with alcoholic hepatitis (Mata, Gastro, 1975; 68:1265), and in alcoholic cirrhotics during the acute phase of alcohol withdrawal (Shaw, Hepatol, 1984; 4:295). Low plasma proline levels have been found in patients with fatty liver or viral hepatitis (Morgan, Gut, 1982; 23:362) and also in some cirrhotic patients (Table 4); low proline levels are often found in sick patients without liver disease (Mata, Gastro, 1975; 68:1265). In one study, proline levels were normal in patients with non-alcoholic

chronic liver disease, but increased in alcoholic cirrhosis (Mata, Gastro, 1975; 68:1265). However, in other studies elevated proline levels were no more common in patients with alcoholic than in other forms of liver disease (Morgan, Gut, 1982; 23:362; Shaw, Hepatol, 1984; 4:295). In the study of Mata *et al.* (Gastro, 1975; 68:1265) proline levels fell in several of the alcoholic patients with alcohol abstention, suggesting that the elevation was largely due to the acute effects of alcohol.

In some studies a strong correlation was found between plasma proline and lactate levels (Cerra, AnnSurg, 1979; 190:577; Kershenobich, Gastro, 1981; 80:1012). As lactate is an inhibitor of proline oxidase (Kowaloff, PNAS, 1977; 74:5368), and high proline levels are found in lactic acidosis, it has been suggested that the high proline levels may be a consequence of hyperlactataemia. Hyperlactataemia may play a role in patients with fulminant liver failure, in whom lactic acidosis is common. It could also contribute to increased proline levels during alcohol withdrawal and in patients with decompensated cirrhosis irrespective of aetiology (Shaw, Hepatol, 1984; 4:295).

The liver fluke, *Fasciola hepatica*, secretes relatively large amounts of proline, which may play a role in the hyperplasia of the biliary epithelium and fibrosis. In addition, it secretes an inhibitor of hepatic proline oxidase[1] so that infection with this parasite is associated with very high biliary concentrations of proline and may lead to an increase in plasma proline levels and increased urinary excretion of this amino acid (Isseroff, Science, 1977; 198;1157; Chi, JNutr, 1979; 109:1299).

Phenylalanine and tyrosine

Most phenylalanine leaving plasma is hydroxylated to tyrosine (Fig. 4), a reaction occurring mainly in the liver. Patients with cirrhosis have higher phenylalanine levels in plasma than normal subjects (Table 4). When patients with acute hepatitis or cirrhosis were fed phenylalanine, plasma phenylalanine levels rose more than in normal subjects and there was a smaller increase in plasma tyrosine levels (Heberer, KlinWschr, 1980; 58:1189). The activity of phenylalanine hydroxylase, measured in liver biopsies from patients with cirrhosis and alcoholic hepatitis, was lower than in normal subjects, but there was no correlation between phenylalanine hydroxylase activity and either the phenylalanine elimination rate or the tyrosine production rate.

When phenylalanine was administered intravenously, and the kinetics analysed as a two compartment model, the volume of the central compartment was reduced in cirrhotics, reflecting a diminished liver pool size (Jagenburg, CCActa, 1977; 78:453). Total phenylalanine clearance was reduced in cirrhotics, probably due to a reduced liver cell mass or to changes in hepatic membrane permeability. In another study, on patients with endstage liver disease of various types, phenylalanine clearance, although reduced, was not significantly different from that in controls (Shanbhogue, Metabolism, 1987; 36:1047). Because phenylalanine has a low extraction ratio (about 0.15), changes in hepatic blood flow are unlikely to play a significant role in the reduction of phenylalanine clearance.

Plasma tyrosine levels tend to be slightly increased in patients with hepatitis and biliary obstruction, and more markedly increased in patients with cirrhosis (Table 4) or fulminant hepatic failure (Rosen, Gastro, 1977; 72:483; O'Keefe, Gastro, 1981; 81:1017).

Portacaval anastomosis (Joelsson, ScaJGastr, 1984; 19:547) and distal spleno-renal shunting (Trevisani, Hepatol, 1994; 19:329) in cirrhotics is associated with a further rise in tyrosine levels, but in patients with idiopathic portal hypertension without significant liver disease fasting tyrosine levels were not significantly increased (Iwasaki, Gastro, 1980; 78:677). After protein or tyrosine ingestion, plasma tyrosine levels increase to a greater extent in cirrhotics than matched normal subjects, and there is a delayed return to fasting levels (Levine, JCI, 1967; 46:2012).

In patients with fulminant hepatic failure, both increased tissue protein breakdown and impaired tyrosine metabolism contribute to their markedly elevated plasma tyrosine levels. However, in most patients with cirrhosis protein turnover is normal (see above) and impaired tyrosine metabolism, and hence decreased clearance, is the main mechanism for their increased fasting and postprandial tyrosine levels. Impaired suppression of body protein breakdown in response to increased amino acid delivery may make a small contribution to the higher plasma tyrosine levels after protein ingestion; tyrosine flux in patients with decompensated endstage liver disease during infusion of an amino acid mixture (FreAmine, which contains very little tyrosine) was increased by only 11 per cent, while tyrosine clearance was decreased by 51 per cent (Shanbhogue, Metabolism, 1987; 36:1047). O'Keefe (Gastro, 1981; 81:1017) measured tyrosine flux rates during the infusion of glucose and an amino acid mixture (2.5 g/h) in patients with varying severity and aetiology of cirrhosis; tyrosine flux rates in seven cirrhotics with encephalopathy were similar to those found by other workers in six normal subjects studied in the fed state (James, ClinSci, 1976; 50: 525), but increased in four cirrhotics without encephalopathy who had lower plasma tyrosine levels than the patients with encephalopathy. These data suggest that increased tyrosine flux (i.e. increased protein breakdown) is not an important determinant of increased plasma tyrosine levels in most cirrhotics.

With increasing severity of liver disease a smaller proportion of whole-body tyrosine flux appears to be accounted for by oxidation to CO_2 (O'Keefe, Gastro, 1981; 81:1017). This fits with data of Nordlinger et al. (JLabClinMed, 1979; 94:832) showing that oral tyrosine intolerance in cirrhotics is associated with decreased catabolism of tyrosine through the homogentisic acid pathway (Fig. 4). Fasting plasma tyramine levels were increased in their cirrhotics, suggesting increased diversion of tyrosine to tyramine (Fig. 4). They suggested that impaired tyrosine catabolism was due to decreased tyrosine aminotransferase activity which catalyzes the first rate-limiting step in this pathway, but that in some patients there were additional defects resulting in impaired clearance of the downstream intermediates, p-hydroxyphenylpyruvic acid and homogentisic acid (Fig. 4). Low tyrosine aminotransferase activity was found in liver biposies from decompensated alcoholic cirrhotics, and from alcoholics with advanced fatty liver with fibrosis and/or alcoholic hepatitis (Anderson, Gastro, 1982; 82:554). However, tyrosine aminotransferase activity was not decreased in cirrhotic liver in another study (Henderson, DigDisSci, 1981; 26:124), nor was it decreased in dogs with a portacaval shunt, in which plasma tyrosine levels were increased (Farouk, JPharmExpTher, 1980; 214: 516).

During parenteral nutrition with tyrosine-free amino acid mixtures, in cirrhotics with poor liver function plasma tyrosine levels may fall below fasting levels despite a greater rise in phenylalanine (Rudman, Gastro, 1981; 81:1025). This fall in tyrosine levels is due to suppression of endogenous proteolysis and to inadequate conversion of phenylalanine to tyrosine to meet the needs of protein synthesis. The fall in tyrosine levels is associated with an impaired anabolic response to parenteral nutrition; oral supplementation with tyrosine increases plasma tyrosine levels and may improve nitrogen balance (Rudman, Gastro, 1981; 81:1025). Plasma tyrosine levels should be measured in cirrhotic patients who have a poor anabolic response to parenteral nutrition.

Tryptophan

Tryptophan is oxidized mainly in the liver, and tryptophan clearance has been found to be reduced in patients with cirrhosis (Rossle, BrJClinPharm, 1986; 22:633). Total plasma tryptophan levels are usually normal but plasma free tryptophan levels may be increased, particularly in those with poor liver function (Rossle, BrJClinPharm, 1986; 22:633; Moja, LifeSci, 1991; 48:409). There appears to be a correlation between the fasting plasma levels of tryptophan and the total amino nitrogen and plasma ammonia levels. In one study, free tryptophan levels appeared to correlate with the degree of encephalopathy present (Cascino, DigDis, 1978; 23:591). When tryptophan was fed to cirrhotics the plasma level rose more in cirrhotics than in controls, and more cirrhotics complained of drowsiness, dizziness, and disturbance of gait (Hirayama, CCActa, 1971; 32:185).

Methionine

Patients with cirrhosis show hypermethioninaemia, and the plasma clearance of this amino acid after intravenous administration is delayed (Kinsell, JCI, 1948; 27:677; Marchesini, Hepatol, 1992; 16: 149). Marchesini et al. found a good inverse relationship between fasting plasma methionine levels and methionine clearance ($r = -0.84$); methionine clearance correlated with galactose elimination capacity ($r = 0.82$) and Child–Pugh score ($r = -0.80$). When methionine was fed to cirrhotic patients, there was rapid absorption; after the peak, plasma methionine levels remained high for a longer period than in controls, the apparent half-life being 458 ± 81 min compared to 146 ± 10 min in controls (Horowitz, Gastro, 1981; 81: 668). Urine SO_4^{2-} excretion was significantly lower in cirrhotics for the 12 h period following the methionine load. The block in the metabolism of methionine appeared to be before the production of homocysteine, possibly at the level of S-adenosylmethionine formation or disposal (Fig. 3).

Hepatic S-adenosylmethionine synthase activity is decreased in cirrhosis (Martin-Duce, Hepatol, 1988; 8:65) due to a specific loss of the high molecular weight form of the enzyme (Cabrero, Hepatol, 1988; 8:1530). However, plasma and liver S-adenosylmethionine levels were found to be normal in cirrhotics, despite the large reduction in S-adenosylmethionine synthase activity (Cabrero, Hepatol, 1988; 8:1530), implying diminished S-adenosylmethionine utilization. Thus, the reduced sulphate excretion, and diminished glutathione and cysteine production following a methionine load in cirrhosis may be due to both an impairment of S-adenosylmethionine formation and an impairment of its subsequent metabolism. S-Adenosylmethionine is an important donor of methyl groups, and patients with cirrhosis show impaired synthesis of phosphatidylcholine by transmethylation (Martin-Duce, Hepatol,

1988; 8:65). Reduced glutathione levels in cirrhosis may impair the elimination of toxic substances and increase the susceptibility of SH-groups in proteins to oxidation. Oxidation of SH-groups in *S*-adenosylmethionine synthase could explain the lower activity of this enzyme in cirrhosis (Corrales, Hepatol, 1990; 11:216). Administration of *S*-adenosylmethionine to cirrhotics increases hepatic glutathione levels (Vendemiale, ScaJGastr, 1989; 24:407). Impairment of the trans-sulphuration pathway for methionine metabolism probably leads to an increase in the transaminative pathway (Cooper, AnnRevBiochem, 1983; 52:187; Martensson, ScaJGastr, 1992; 27:405).

Cysteine

In cirrhotics on a mixed diet, the fasting levels of free cysteine, taurine, and glutathione were lower than in normal subjects; there was no significant difference in the level of cystine, or of total plasma cyst[e]ine (Chawla, Gastro, 1984; 87:770). The low cysteine, taurine, and glutathione were attributed to reduced conversion of methionine to cysteine (see above) (Fig. 3). With feeding of cysteine, the increase in plasma cyst[e]ine in cirrhotics was twice as large as in controls, due mainly to an elevation of cystine (Tribble, AmJClinNutr, 1989; 50:1401). The subsequent elimination of the cyst[e]ine from plasma was slower in the cirrhotics, and the appearance of sulphur in the urine was delayed, although the amount excreted over 24 h was the same. The greater and more prolonged elevation of plasma cyst[e]ine after oral cysteine may be due to impaired hepatic uptake, either immediately after absorption or as a result of reduced plasma glutathione, as glutathione potentiates hepatic cysteine uptake by liberating cysteine from cystine.

Because of the impaired conversion of methionine to cysteine and taurine, parenteral nutrition with commercial amino acid mixtures that do not contain these 'non-essential' amino acids may result in low plasma cysteine and taurine levels in cirrhotics with poor liver function; relative deficiency of these amino acids may limit the anabolic response, which may be improved by oral cysteine supplements (Rudman, Gastro, 1981; 81:1025).

Glutamine

Plasma glutamine levels are usually normal in cirrhosis but may be decreased in malnourished patients[42] and those with decompensated liver disease or complications such as sepsis; somewhat elevated levels have also been found (Table 4). Glutamine is an important gluconeogenic precursor in the kidney, and possibly liver (see above), and plays an important role in acid–base homeostasis (see later). As discussed earlier, large increases in glutamine flux occur in critically ill patients, with little change, or a fall, in plasma glutamine levels. In fasted cirrhotics net splanchnic uptake of glutamine was twice that in normal control subjects; the liver appeared to account for about 60 per cent of net splanchnic glutamine uptake in the cirrhotics (Owen, JCI, 1981; 68:240; Owen, JCI, 1985; 76:1209). Increased splanchnic (probably hepatic) glutamine uptake in cirrhotics is consistent with the four- to sixfold increase in glutamine uptake by liver slices from cirrhotic patients, [19] and the increased glutaminase (Matsuno, CancerRes, 1992; 52: 1192) and diminished glutamine synthase activities in cirrhotic liver (Kaiser, EurJClinInv, 1988; 18:535). Net renal glutamine uptake in the cirrhotics studied by Owen *et al.* (JCI, 1981; 68:240; JCI, 1985;

76:1209) was much higher than that found in normal subjects in another study.[20] This contrasts with the reduction in renal glutamine extraction, despite increased arterial glutamine levels, in rats following a portacaval shunt (Dejong, JCI, 1993; 92:2834).

If glutamine utilization is increased in cirrhotics, production must also be increased. Enhanced glutamine production by muscle (and its subsequent renal metabolism) has been suggested as a means of removing ammonia in patients with a diminished capacity for urea synthesis; cirrhotics with muscle wasting would then be more susceptible to increases in plasma ammonia levels with hepatic decompensation (Ganda, Metabolism, 1976; 25:427). While muscle ammonia uptake increases linearly with plasma ammonia levels (Bessman, NEJM, 1955; 253:1143), there are conflicting data on muscle glutamine release in cirrhotics. Morrison *et al.*[42] found diminished glutamine efflux rates across the leg in malnourished cirrhotics. Ganda (Metabolism, 1976; 25:427), by contrast, found that the arteriovenous difference for glutamine across the forearm in malnourished, decompensated alcoholic cirrhotics was similar to that found by Aoki (AmJClinNutr, 1976; 29:340) in normal subjects; assuming increased muscle blood flow in their cirrhotics they concluded that muscle glutamine production was increased. Enhanced release of glutamine from muscle is usually accompanied by a reduction in muscle glutamine levels; Plauth *et al.*[5] found normal muscle glutamine levels in cirrhotics. Although glutamine release by the rat hindquarter was increased following a portacaval shunt, net ammonia uptake by muscle was not observed and circulating ammonia did not appear to be an important donor of nitrogen to the glutamine released from muscle (Dejong, Gastro, 1992; 102: 936). In dogs infused with ammonium chloride, elevations of arterial ammonia within the range likely to be encountered in patients with encephalopathy or acute liver failure (<3 mmol/l) did not enhance muscle glutamine production (Fine, ContribNephrol, 1985; 47:1). An alternative site of enhanced glutamine production in cirrhosis and liver failure is the brain. Normally the arteriovenous difference for glutamine across the brain is close to zero, but brain glutamine production and efflux may be markedly enhanced when ammonia levels increase (Cooper, PhysiolRev, 1987; 67:440; Dejong, JNeuroch, 1992; 59:1071).

Enhanced glutamine flux and hepatic glutamine uptake in cirrhosis may be essential for upregulating urea synthesis in the face of diminished urea synthetic capacity (see Chapter 2.13.2); it may be less important for increasing urinary ammonia excretion—this may be largely achieved by decreasing the release of ammonia generated from renal glutamine metabolism into the renal vein, and increasing the proportion that is excreted in the urine (Dejong, JCI, 1993; 92:2834).

In view of the importance of glutamine as a fuel for enterocytes and cells of the immune system, and its possible role as a regulator of muscle protein synthesis (Jepson, AmJPhysiol, 1988; 255:E166), it has been suggested that the demands for glutamine in cirrhosis may exceed the glutamine synthetic capacity of skeletal muscle, and that an increased intake of glutamine may reduce intestinal endotoxin absorption and help to conserve lean body mass (Teran, AmJClinNutr, 1995; 62:897). However, when cirrhotics awaiting liver transplantation were fed an oral 10 to 20 g glutamine load, plasma ammonia increased more than twofold within 1 h and there was an associated deterioration in performance on psychometric testing (Oppong, Gastro, 1995; 108:A1138).

References

1. Bender DA. *Amino acid metabolism*, (2nd edn). Chichester: John Wiley and Sons, 1985.

2. Young VR and El-Khoury AE. The notion of the nutritional essentiality of amino acids, revisited, with a note on the indespensable amino acid requirements in adults. In Cynober LA, ed. *Amino acid metabolism and therapy in health and nutritional disease*. London: CRC Press, 1995: 191–232.

3. Levy HL, Taylor RG, and McInnes RR. Disorders of histidine metabolism. In Scriver CR, Beaudet AL, Sly WS, and Valle D, eds. *The metabolic basis of inherited disease*, (7th edn). New York: McGraw Hill, 1995: 1107–23.

4. Mehler AH. Metabolism of the individual amino acids. In Devlin TM, ed. *Textbook of biochemistry*, (3rd edn). New York: John Wiley and Sons, 1992: 491–528.

5. Plauth M, Egberts EH, Abele R, Muller PH, and Furst P. Characteristic pattern of free amino acids in plasma and skeletal muscle in stable hepatic cirrhosis. *Hepato-gastroenterology*, 1990; **37**: 135–9.

6. Montanari A, *et al.* Free amino acids in plasma and skeletal muscle of patients with liver cirrhosis. *Hepatology*, 1988; **8**: 1034–9.

7. Hamosh A, Johnston MV, and Valle D. Nonketotic hyperglycinaemia. In Scriver CR, Beaudet AL, Sly WS, and Valle D, eds. *The metabolic basis of inherited disease*, (7th edn). New York: McGraw Hill, 1995: 1337–48.

8. Nurjhan N, *et al.* Glutamine: a major gluconeogenic precursor and vehicle for interorgan carbon transport in man. *Journal of Clinical Investigation*, 1995; **95**: 272–7.

9. Felig P. Amino acid metabolism in man. *Annual Review of Biochemistry*, 1975; **44**: 933–55.

10. Chuang DT and Shih VE. Disorders of branched chain amino acid and keto acid metabolism. In Scriver CR, Beaudet AL, Sly WS, and Valle D, eds. *The metabolic basis of inherited disease*, (7th edn). New York: McGraw Hill, 1995: 1239–78.

11. Abumrad NN, *et al.* Inter-organ metabolism of amino acids *in vivo*. *Diabetes Metabolism Reviews*, 1989; **5**: 213–26.

12. Harper AE, Miller RH, and Block KP. Branched-chain amino acid metabolism. *Annual Review of Nutrition*, 1984; **4**: 409–54.

13. Wahren J, Felig P, and Hagenfeldt L. Effect of protein ingestion on splanchnic and leg metabolism in normal man and in patients with diabetes mellitus. *Journal of Clinical Investigation*, 1976; **57**: 987–99.

14. Wagenmakers AJM, and Soeters PB. Metabolism of branched-chain amino acids. In Cynober LA, ed. *Amino acid metabolism and therapy in health and nutritional disease*. London: CRC Press, 1995: 67–87.

15. Phang JM, Yeh GC, and Scriver CR. Disorders of proline and hydroxyproline metabolism. In Scriver CR, Beaudet AL, Sly WS, and Valle D, eds. *The metabolic basis of inherited disease*, (7th edn). New York: McGraw Hill, 1995: 1125–46.

16. Scriver CR, Kaufman S, Eisensmith RC, and Woo SLC. The hyperphenylalaninemias. In Scriver CR, Beaudet AL, Sly WS, and Valle D, eds. *The metabolic basis of inherited disease*, (7th edn). New York: McGraw Hill, 1995: 1015–75.

17. Mudd SH, Levy HL, and Skovby F. Disorders of transsulfuration. In Scriver CR, Beaudet AL, Sly WS, and Valle D, eds. *The metabolic basis of inherited disease*, (7th edn). New York: McGraw Hill, 1995; 1279–328.

18. Felig P, Wahren J, Karl I, Cerasi E, Luft R, and Kipnis DM. Glutamine and glutamate metabolism in normal and diabetic subjects. *Diabetes*, 1973; 22: 573–6.

19. Kaiser S, Gerok W, and Haussinger D. Ammonia and glutamine metabolism in human liver slices: new aspects on the pathogenesis of hyperammonaemia in chronic liver disease. *European Journal of Clinical Investigation*, 1988; **18**: 535–42.

20. Lochs H, Hubl W, Gasic S, Roth E, Morse EL, and Adibi SA. Glycylglutamine: metabolism and effects on organ balances of amino acids in postabsorptive and starved subjects. *American Journal of Physiology*, 1992; **262**: E155–E160.

21. Mitchell GA, Lambert M, and Tanguay RM. Hypertyrosinaemia. In Scriver CR, Beaudet AL, Sly WS, and Valle D, eds. *The metabolic basis of inherited disease*, (7th edn). New York: McGraw Hill, 1995: 1077–106.

22. Cox RP, and Dancis J. Errors of lysine metabolism. In Scriver CR, Beaudet AL, Sly WS, and Valle D, eds. *The metabolic basis of inherited disease*, (7th edn). New York: McGraw Hill, 1995: 1233–8.

23. Christensen HN. Role of amino acid transport and countertransport in nutrition and metabolism. *Physiological Reviews*, 1990; **70**: 43–77.

24. Tamarappoo BK, Nam M, Kilberg MS, and Welbourne TC. Glucocorticoid regulation of splanchnic glutamine, alanine, glutamate, ammonia, and glutathione fluxes. *American Journal of Physiology*, 1993; **264**: E526–E533.

25. McNurlan MA and Garlick PJ. Influence of nutrient intake on protein turnover. *Diabetes Metabolism Reviews*, 1989; **5**: 165–89.

26. Waterlow JC. Whole-body protein turnover in humans—past, present and future. *Annual Review of Nutrition*, 1995; **15**: 57–92.

27. Hellerstein HK and Munro HN. Interaction of liver, muscle, and adipose tissue in the regulation of metabolism in response to nutritional and other factors. In Arias IM, Jakoby WB, Popper H, Schachter D, and Shafritz D, eds. *The liver: biology and pathobiology*, (3rd edn). New York: Raven Press, 1994: 1169–91.

28. Burns HJG. The metabolic and nutritional effects of injury and sepsis. *Baillère's Clinical Gastroenterology*, 1988; **2**: 849–67.

29. Hasselgran P-O, Pedersen P, Sax HC, Warner BW, and Fischer JE. Current concepts of protein turnover and amino acid transport in liver and skeletal muscle during sepsis. *Archives of Surgery*, 1988; **123**: 992–9.

30. Bier DM. Intrinsically difficult problems: the kinetics of body proteins and amino acids in man. *Diabetes Metabolism Reviews*, 1989; **5**: 111–32.

31. Biolo G, Declan Fleming RY, and Wolfe RR. Physiologic hyperinsulinaemia stimulates protein synthesis and enhances transport of selected amino acids in human skeletal muscle. *Journal of Clinical Investigation*, 1995; **95**: 811–19.

32. Tessari P. Effects of insulin on whole-body and regional amino acid metabolism. *Diabetes Metabolism Reviews*, 1994; **10**: 253–85.

33. Windmueller HG. Glutamine utilization by the small intestine. *Advances in Enzymology*, 1982; **53**: 201–37.

34. Horber FF and Haymond MW. Human growth hormone prevents the protein catabolic side effects of prednisone in humans. *Journal of Clinical Investigation*, 1990; **86**: 265–72.

35. Elwyn D. The role of the liver in regulation of amino acid and protein metabolism. In Munro HN, ed. *Mammalian protein metabolism*. New York: Academic Press, 1970: 523–71.

36. Vilstrup H, Bucher D, Krog B, and Damgard SE. Elimination of infused amino acids from plasma of control subjects and of patients with cirrhosis of the liver. *European Journal of Clinical Investigation*, 1982; **12**: 197–201.

37. Vilstrup H. On urea synthesis—regulation *in vivo*. *Danish Medical Bulletin*, 1989; **36**: 415–29.

38. Marchesini G, Bianchi GP, Vilstrup H, Checchia GA, Patrono D, and Zoli M. Plasma clearances of branched-chain amino acids in control subjects and in patients with cirrhosis. *Journal of Hepatology*, 1987; **4**: 108–17.

39. Hoerr RA, Matthews DE, Bier DM, and Young VR. Effects of protein restriction and acute refeeding on leucine and lysine kinetics in young men. *American Journal of Physiology*, 1993; **264**: E567–E575.

40. Petrides AS, Luzi L, Reuben A, Riely C, and DeFronzo RA. Effect of insulin and plasma amino acid concentration on leucine metabolism in cirrhosis. *Hepatology*, 1991; **14**: 432–41.

41. McCullough AJ, Mullen KD, and Kalhan SC. Body cell mass and leucine metabolism in cirrhosis. *Gastroenterology*, 1992; **102**: 1325–33.

42. Morrison WL, Bouchier IAD, Gibson JNA, and Rennie MJ. Skeletal muscle and whole body protein turnover in cirrhosis. *Clinical Science*, 1990; **78**: 613–19.

43. Millikan WJ, *et al.* *In vivo* measurement of leucine metabolism with stable isotopes in normal subjects and in those with cirrhosis fed conventional and branched-chain amino acid enriched diets. *Surgery*, 1985; **98**: 405–12.

44. Wolfe RR. *Radioactive and stable isotope tracers in biomedicine. Principles and practice of kinetic analysis*. New York: Wiley-Liss, 1992: 377–416.

45. Riggio O, James JH, Peters JC, and Fischer JE. Influence of ammonia on leucine utilization in muscle and adipose tissue *in vitro*. In Kleinberger G, Ferenci P, Riederer P, and Thaler H, eds. *Advances in hepatic encephalopathy and urea cycle diseases*. Basel: Karger, 1984: 519–26.

46. WHO. *Diabetes mellitus*. Technical Report Series, No. 727, 1985; 9–20.

2.13.2 Ammonia, urea production, and pH regulation

D. Häussinger

Ammonia plays a central role in nitrogen metabolism. It is a major by-product of protein and nucleic-acid catabolism, and its nitrogen can be incorporated into urea, amino acids, nucleic acids, and many other nitrogenous compounds. Ammonia is present in body fluids as both NH_3 and NH_4^+, and these are in equilibrium according to the equation:

$$NH_3 + H^+ \rightleftharpoons NH_4^+$$

The pK_a of this reaction is 9.25, so that at physiological pH there is a great excess of the ionized form. NH_3 can diffuse freely across membranes, while NH_4^+ is probably carried by an active transport system. When the pH increases more ammonia is present as NH_3.

The blood ammonia concentration is normally very low (less than 35 µmol/l); this is important as ammonia is toxic at higher concentrations and causes neurological problems. Excessive uptake of ammonia is thought to deplete the brain of glutamate, itself a neurotransmitter, by its conversion to glutamine, an important reaction for the removal of excess ammonia in many tissues. Increased cerebral glutamine may on the one hand induce brain cell swelling (Hawkins, JNeuroch, 1993; 60:1000; Häussinger, Gastro, 1994; 107:1475) and on the other increase brain uptake of tryptophan (a precursor of 5-hydroxytryptamine) via a glutamine/tryptophan countertransport system.

The liver is the most important site of ammonia metabolism; it removes much of the toxic ammonia presented to it to form the non-toxic product urea and depending on the metabolic conditions by glutamine synthesis. By doing so the liver may also play a major role in the metabolic regulation of systemic pH, because hydrogen ions released from NH_4^+ during the synthesis of urea neutralize the excess bicarbonate produced by the breakdown of amino acids (see below).

Urea is electroneutral and is transported across biological membranes by facilitated diffusion. A phloretin-sensitive urea transporter has been cloned which is present also in liver (You, Nature, 1993; 365:844; vom Dahl, BiolChemHS, 1996; 377:25). Although urea is not further metabolized by mammalian enzymes, it interferes with the activity of K^+ channels in the plasma membrane (Hallbrucker, PfluegersArchPhysiol, 1994; 428:552) and can cause liver cell shrinkage at concentrations found in uraemia. Urea is excreted by the kidney, and it appears in the urine in relatively high concentration despite back-diffusion of filtered urea in the renal tubules (Knepper, AmJPhysiol, 1989; 256:F610).[1] It is normally present in plasma and body fluids at a concentration of about 3.0 to 6.5 mmol/l.

Sources of ammonia

Whereas urea production takes place largely within the liver, much of the ammonia used in urea synthesis is derived, directly or indirectly, from extrahepatic tissues. The intestine and kidney release some nitrogen into the blood as ammonia, and liver, resting muscle, and brain remove ammonia from the blood; 25 per cent of the nitrogen utilized in urea synthesis reaches the liver via the portal vein, from ammonia formed in the small intestine and colon (see below).[2,3] Most of the nitrogen transported to the liver for incorporation into urea is carried not as ammonia, but as amino acids, such as alanine or glutamine; these are converted into ammonia in the liver by amino acid degradation.

Within the liver, glutamate and glutamine are major sources of ammonia (Krebs, BiochemJ, 1978; 176:733). Glutamate is released directly from protein, but more importantly it is formed from the other amino acids released from protein breakdown; all of them, except lysine and threonine, can be transaminated, and their amino group can combine with α-ketoglutarate to form glutamate. Glutamate is formed by deamidation of glutamine, and from the carbon skeletons of proline, histidine, and glutamine.[4] Ammonia is released from glutamate by its oxidative deamination by glutamate dehydrogenase, an enzyme present in the mitochondrial matrix. Glutamate dehydrogenase activity is highest in the liver, but the enzyme is also present in muscle, brain, and kidney.

Amino acids can also be transaminated with glyoxalate to form glycine, which is deaminated by glycine oxidase to yield ammonia; this pathway is thought to be quantitatively important in mammalian ammonia production. Several other amino acids, including serine, threonine, cysteine, cystathione, and homoserine, are metabolized in pyridoxal phosphate-dependent deamination reactions which produce ammonia, and these occur mainly in the liver. Ammonia can be released from histidine, a reaction catalysed by histidine lyase, which does not use pyridoxal phosphate. Ammonia is generated by the deamidation of glutamine (Addae, AmJPhysiol, 1968; 215:269) and asparagine.

Ammonia is also produced by amine oxidases, which deaminate several monoamines and diamines including adrenaline, noradrenaline, and serotonin, but the amounts involved are small.

In addition, endogenous ammonia used in urea synthesis can be generated from the metabolism of purines and pyrimidines. Most of the ammonia produced from purine nucleotides is derived from adenosine monophosphate, in a reaction catalysed by adenylate deaminase.[5] This pathway becomes particularly important during exercise when ammonia formation and release from muscle is increased.[6] The pyrimidine, cytosine, is also deaminated to ammonia. In the complete degradation of the pyrimidine ring, one of the two nitrogen atoms is converted to ammonia.

Ammonia from the intestine

The intestine is a major site of ammonia production. Some 15 to 30 per cent of the urea synthesized by the liver is degraded by bacterial ureases in the gut with the liberation of ammonia and carbon dioxide (Jones, ClinSci, 1969; 37:825).[7] Urea is hydrolysed in the mucosa or the juxtamucosal area of the colon, and to a lesser extent in the small intestine (Wolpert, Lancet, 1971; ii:1387). The ammonia generated in these reactions is completely absorbed, enters the portal circulation, and returns to the liver to be converted back to urea;[7] faeces do not contain urea (Wrong, ClinSci, 1965; 28: 357) or any ammonia originating from urea hydrolysis (Wrong, ClinSci, 1985; 68:193). The oral administration of antibiotics, such as neomycin, reduces the bacterial degradation of urea in the intestine (Wolpert, NEJM, 1970; 283:159).

A second source of ammonia from the gut, quantitatively of equal importance, is the intestinal mucosa itself. The intestine of germ-free animals, mainly the small intestine, produces a significant quantity of ammonia, which comes primarily from the metabolism of glutamine removed from arterial blood. The small intestine is a major site of glutamine metabolism, and it also produces ammonia from the intraluminal amino acids, alanine, leucine, and glutamine, but not from threonine, serine, and glycine (Weber, AmJPhysiol, 1988; 254:G264). Most of the ammonia produced in the colon comes from bacterial degradation of urea and other nitrogenous substances; non-bacterial production accounts for only 10 per cent of the ammonia produced in the colon; in the dog, ammonia produced by the small intestine is approximately equal to that produced in the uncleansed colon (Weber, Gastro, 1979; 77:235).

The ammonia from the intestine enters the portal circulation and is taken up by the liver (Windmueller, JBC, 1974; 2149:5070). The ammonia concentration in the portal vein is up to 10-fold higher than elsewhere in the circulation, and it is estimated that several grams of ammonia enter the portal venous circulation daily from the intestine in well-nourished adults (Summerskill, AmJClinNut, 1970; 23:633).

Ammonia detoxication by the liver

There are two major pathways for ammonia detoxication by the liver: urea and glutamine synthesis. Both pathways are embedded into a sophisticated structural and functional organization in the liver acinus.

Urea production

Approximately 90 per cent of surplus nitrogen in man enters the urea cycle for irreversible conversion to urea, which is excreted by the kidneys. Approximately 30 g of urea is excreted daily in healthy adults, and it results mainly from the breakdown of amino acids. Using tracer techniques it has been observed that calculated urea production exceeds urinary urea excretion by about 20 to 30 per cent.[7] This difference is attributed to extrarenal losses, largely accounted for by the intestinal hydrolysis of urea.

When urea is hydrolysed its nitrogen atoms are rapidly incorporated into newly synthesized urea. It is generally assumed that the carbon atom of urea is not preferentially reincorporated into urea because of its dilution in the large bicarbonate pool. However, in comparative studies in the same subjects, using urea labelled with isotopes of both carbon and nitrogen, similar calculated urea production rates were observed. It was therefore suggested that the urea carbon may be preferentially utilized for urea synthesis by its recycling via carbamate, a potential intermediate in the intestinal hydrolysis of urea (Long, AmJClinNut, 1978; 31:1367). Carbamate could serve as a precursor for carbamoyl phosphate which directly enters the urea cycle. Reincorporation of the carbon atom of urea would cause the rate of intestinal urea hydrolysis to be underestimated in studies using a carbon label (Fig. 1.)

The urea cycle and its enzymes

Urea is formed from ammonia and bicarbonate. The initial reaction is the formation of carbamoyl phosphate, a reaction catalysed by

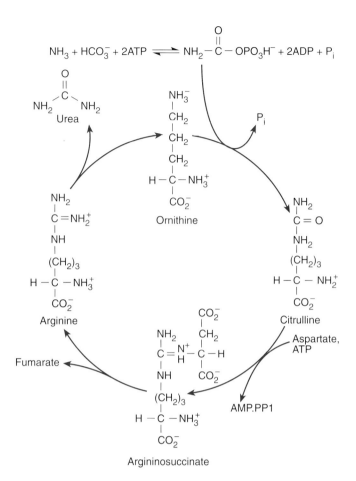

Fig. 1. The urea cycle.

carbamoyl phosphate synthetase I, a major protein of hepatic mitochondria (Clarke, JBC, 1976; 251:950). It accepts only ammonia as the nitrogen donor and requires N-acetylglutamate as an allosteric cofactor.[2,4] Bicarbonate ions, not carbon dioxide, provide the required carbon. As two molecules of ATP are cleaved during the reaction, it is essentially irreversible.

The carbamoyl phosphate is condensed with ornithine to form citrulline (by ornithine transcarbamylase); this in turn condenses with aspartate to give argininosuccinate (by argininosuccinate synthetase), a reaction which requires the cleavage of two further high-energy phosphate bonds.

Argininosuccinate is hydrolysed to fumarate and arginine (by argininosuccinase). Arginine is cleaved by arginase to give urea and ornithine. This series of reactions, returning to ornithine, is known as the 'urea cycle'. Its role not only resides in the removal of potentially toxic ammonia, but also in the irreversible removal of bicarbonate (Atkinson, TrendsBiochemSci, 1984; 9:297; Häussinger, TrendsBiochemSci, 1984; 9:300).

Ornithine transcarbamylase, like carbamoyl phosphate synthetase I, is also a major mitochondrial protein (Clarke, BBResComm, 1976; 71:1118); the remaining enzymes are in the cytoplasm of hepatocytes. This necessitates the entry of ornithine into mitochondria and the exit of citrulline, and these processes occur via a cotransporter (LaNoue, AnnRevBiochem, 1979; 48:871). The condensation of citrulline and aspartate by argininosuccinate synthetase is a freely reversible reaction, but cleavage of one of the products, pyrophosphate, ensures that the reaction favours the formation of argininosuccinate. The reaction is inhibited by various amino acids (Takada, JBioch, 1979; 85:1309). Some citrulline is probably transported from the liver to other tissues for conversion to arginine and subsequent protein synthesis.

Of the two nitrogen atoms in urea, one comes from the ammonia used for the synthesis of carbamoyl phosphate, the other from aspartate. Aspartate is formed by transamination of oxaloacetate—an intermediate in the citric acid cycle; the fumarate released from argininosuccinate enters the citric acid (Krebs) cycle for conversion to oxaloacetate. These two steps provide a link between urea synthesis, the citric acid cycle, and gluconeogenesis.

The liver is quantitatively the major organ involved in urea synthesis as the first two enzymes of urea synthesis, carbamoyl phosphate synthetase I and ornithine transcarbamylase, are largely confined to the liver. They are present, to a much lesser extent, in the small intestine (Raijman, BiochemJ, 1974; 138:225). The kidney contains all five urea-cycle enzymes, and can produce urea, but the levels of the enzymes involved in citrulline synthesis are less than 1/10 000 of those present in the liver and so the contribution of the kidney to urea synthesis is of little significance. Minor amounts of urea are formed by enterocytes from developing pigs, which contain all urea cycle enzymes (Wu, BiochemJ, 1995; 312:717). Within the liver the urea cycle enzymes are located primarily in the periportal zone (Häussinger, AdvEnzymReg, 1986; 25:159).

Regulation of urea synthesis

Ammonia production is very variable and it is essential that the activity of the urea cycle be regulated, not only to prevent the accumulation of ammonia, which is toxic when present in excess, but to provide ammonia for the synthesis of other nitrogenous compounds.

Short-term regulation of the rate of urea production is achieved via alterations of ammonia and bicarbonate provision for mitochondrial carbamoyl phosphate synthetase and the activity of the urea-cycle enzymes, whereas long-term control is effected by changes in enzyme concentrations. Substrate provision for the urea cycle depends on amino acid delivery, the activity of amino acid transport systems, and amino acid metabolizing enzymes and these factors are therefore important determinants of urea synthesis *in vivo*. Studies in man using stable isotopes have shown that the hepatic ureagenic response is acutely sensitive to the plasma amino-nitrogen concentration. Indeed, the increase in urea production resulting from an exogenous amino acid load is directly related to the corresponding elevation of plasma amino-nitrogen concentration, up to at least a concentration of 15 mmol/l (Vilstrup, Gut, 1980; 21:990). Urea synthesis cannot therefore be saturated at realistic substrate concentrations.

In vitro, argininosuccinate synthetase seems to be the rate-limiting enzyme of the urea cycle at saturating ammonia concentrations. At physiologically low ammonia concentrations, however, carbamoyl phosphate synthesis is the rate-controlling step in urea synthesis (Meijer, EurJBioch, 1985; 148:189). Also *in vivo*, the intermediates (citrulline, argininosuccinate, and arginine) are present in such low concentrations that carbamoyl phosphate synthetase I is probably the rate-limiting enzyme (Stewart, JBC, 1980;

255:5270), and it is the primary regulatory site for changes in substrate concentrations.

Short-term regulation of urea synthesis primarily takes place at the level of ammonia and bicarbonate provision for mitochondrial carbamoyl phosphate synthetase I, which presumably is the rate-controlling enzyme for the cycle at physiological substrate concentrations.[2,8] The Km (NH_4^+) of carbamoyl phosphate synthetase I is 1 to 2 mmol/l; that is, by far higher than the portal NH_4^+ concentration of 0.2 to 0.3 mmol/l. Thus, the urea cycle has a low affinity for ammonia. This low affinity is in part compensated for by mitochondrial glutaminase which is activated by its own product ammonia in the physiological concentration range (Häussinger, EurJBioch, 1979; 101:179): ammonia activates glutaminase, which in turn liberates additional ammonia from glutamine. Liver glutaminase therefore acts as a mitochondrial amplification system for ammonia and the activity of this enzyme becomes an important determinant of urea cycle flux.[2,3,8,9] All factors known to increase urea synthesis, such as glucagon, ammonia, or alkalosis, activate glutaminase and accordingly, via amplification, ammonia provision for carbamoyl phosphate synthetase. Urea synthesis is also controlled at the level of mitochondrial bicarbonate supply, which is determined by pH, the CO_2 concentration, and the activity of mitochondrial carbonic anhydrase V. This enzyme is required for the fast conversion of CO_2 into HCO_3^-, which is the substrate for carbamoyl phosphate synthetase I. Its inhibition by acetazolamide blocks urea synthesis (Häussinger, EurJBioch, 1985; 152:381, Dodgson, JApplPhysiol, 1986; 60:646).

Short-term increases in ureagenesis, within 10 to 30 min, are also thought to be mediated via N-acetylglutamate, a cofactor which stimulates carbamoyl phosphate synthetase I activity (Shigesada, EurJBioch, 1978; 85:385), although its role as a short-term regulator of overall flux through the urea cycle has been disputed (Lund, BiochemJ, 1984; 218:991). An intraperitoneal injection of a complete amino acid mixture causes rapid activation of ureagenesis. N-Acetylglutamate increases fivefold, causing a fivefold increase in the activity of carbamoyl phosphate synthetase I (Stewart, JBC, 1980; 255:5270). Since the half-life of N-acetylglutamate in the liver is about 20 min, there is also a rapid response to a reduced protein intake.[2,5] The concentration of ornithine may also play a role in the regulation of carbamoyl phosphate synthetase I activity, and of flux through the urea cycle (Lund, BiochemJ, 1986; 239:773).

The activities of carbamoyl phosphate synthetase I, argininosuccinate synthetase, and argininosuccinase are subject to immediate allosteric regulation. MgATP and free Mg^{2+} are both positive effectors of carbamoyl phosphate synthetase I, while argininosuccinase is also subject to negative allosteric regulation.[5] All three substrates for argininosuccinate synthetase—citrulline, aspartate, and MgATP—are negative allosteric effectors for this enzyme, which is also regulated via product inhibition by AMP, argininosuccinate, and inorganic phosphate. There is no feedback inhibition of the urea cycle by urea within the physiological concentration range. Only at very high urea concentrations is there some inhibition of argininosuccinate lyase (Menyhart, EurJBiochem, 1977; 75:405).

In the longer term, there are changes in the urea-cycle enzymes which occur within 4 to 8 days following an alteration in dietary protein or amino acid content (Schimke, JBC, 1962; 237:1921; JBC, 1963; 238:1012; Snodgrass, JNutr, 1981; 111:586). When protein intake is increased there is a proportional increase in the total hepatic content of all five urea-cycle enzymes, resulting in increased urea production and increased urinary urea excretion. Comparable results (two- to fivefold increase) are obtained when mRNA levels for the five enzymes are measured (Morris, ArchBiochemBiophys, 1987; 256:343). mRNA levels for carbamoyl phosphate synthetase and argininosuccinate synthetase increase immediately following partial hepatectomy (Tygstrup, JHepatol, 1995; 22:349). Reduction in protein intake decreases urea synthesis, making urea nitrogen available for reutilization in protein synthesis (Picou, AmJClinNut, 1972; 25:1261).

Urea synthesis is subject to hormonal influence. Glucagon, which increases during starvation, and glucocorticoids, which increase protein breakdown, are both associated with increased enzyme levels (Sigsaard, Liver, 1988; 8:193). Glucagon increases urea excretion in humans (Wolfe, Surgery, 1979; 86:248). It is thought to regulate urea synthesis by rapid mechanisms, by activation of mitochondrial glutaminase (Häussinger, BBActa, 1983; 755:272), possibly by increasing the synthesis of N-acetylglutamate (Staddon, BiochemJ, 1984; 217:855), by enhancing hepatocyte amino-acid transport (Fehlmann, JBC, 1979; 254:10431), and by stimulating hepatic proteolysis due to hepatocyte shrinkage (vom Dahl, BiochemJ, 1991; 278:771). A longer-term effect is mediated by increased synthesis of urea-cycle enzymes (Snodgrass, JBC, 1978; 253:2748). Insulin probably has no direct effect on urea synthesis, but is a powerful modulator of other known hormonal regulators such as glucagon and a potent inhibitor of liver proteolysis (Hallbrucker, EurJBioch, 1991; 199:467), and is therefore still a major regulator of urea synthesis *in vivo*. Hypothyroidism is associated with increased activity of the urea-cycle enzymes and urea production in rat liver. There is no change in urea-cycle activity with hyperthyroidism (Marti, Endocrinol, 1988; 123:2167). However, urea synthesis from infused amino acids is increased in hyperthyroidism (Marchesini, Metabolism, 1994; 43:1023); this may be explained by an increased amino acid transport into the liver. Interleukin 1 increases urea synthesis from amino acids *in vivo* (Heindorff, EurJClinInv, 1994; 24:388). Growth hormone lowers urea production, possibly by reducing the supply of nitrogen to the liver (Dahms, Metabolism, 1989; 38:197; Wothers, JClinEndoc, 1994; 78:1220). Pregnancy and ageing are also associated with reduced urea synthesis (Kalhan, Metabolism, 1982; 31:824; Fabbri, Liver, 1994; 14:288).

The availability of arginine affects the levels of urea-cycle enzymes, the level of arginase being altered in an opposite direction to the other enzymes. Excess arginine decreases the activity of the first four enzymes and increases the activity of arginase, suggesting that arginine synthesis can be increased at the expense of urea synthesis. Reducing the supply of arginine has the opposite effect. In endotoxaemia, arginase and nitric oxide synthetase can compete for arginine (Wettstein, Hepatol, 1994; 19:641; Stadler, AmJPhysiol, 1995; 268:G183). A short circuit of the urea cycle occurs under these conditions, because arginine is converted directly to citrulline by inducible nitric oxide synthase; however, compared with total urea-cycle flux, this pathway of arginine metabolism is small in the hepatocyte. Glucose suppresses urea production, probably due to a combination of a direct reduction in urea-cycle activity and inhibition of hepatic gluconeogenesis from amino acids (Jahoor, AmJPhysiol, 1987; 253:E543). It is not related to a reduction in substrate nitrogen supply.

Sepsis, surgery, and trauma are associated with increased levels of glucagon and cortisol. Both these hormones increase urea synthesis, contributing to the negative nitrogen balance often observed in these conditions.[10]

Carnitine reduces plasma ammonia and protects against acute ammonia intoxication, when potentially lethal doses are given to mice or rats, by increasing urea synthesis (Costell, BBResComm, 1984; 120:726). The mechanism is not known, but may be due to increased mitochondrial ATP as there is no increase in N-acetylglutamate levels. Arginine also protects against ammonia intoxication by stimulating N-acetylglutamate synthetase (Kim, PNAS, 1972; 69:3530).

Drugs may influence urea synthesis. The antiepileptic agent, sodium valproate, increases plasma ammonia concentrations and reduces urea synthesis by 30 per cent (Hjelm, Lancet, 1986; ii:859). This is due largely to a reduction in the activity of carbamoyl phosphate synthetase I in the hepatic mitochondria, although renal ammonia production is also affected (Marini, Neurology, 1988; 38:365). There is a dose-dependent inhibition of urea synthesis by acetylsalicylic acid in perfused rat livers and by hypokalaemia.

Studies using isolated perfused liver preparations have shown that the pH of the perfusate influences the rate of urea production (Lueck, JBC, 1970; 245:5491; Häussinger, EurJBiochem, 1985; 152:381; Häussinger, BiochemJ, 1986; 236:261). Such observations are consistent with the hypothesis that the liver plays a central role in the metabolic regulation of systemic pH (see later). Acetazolamide and loop diuretics containing a sulphonamide moiety inhibit the activity of mitochondrial carbonic anhydrase V and act as inhibitors of urea synthesis by impairing bicarbonate supply for carbamoyl phosphate synthesis (Häussinger, BiochemPharm, 1986; 35:3317).

Ammonia detoxication by glutamine synthesis

The other major pathway for ammonia fixation in liver is glutamine synthesis. Liver glutamine synthetase is a cytosolic enzyme (Deuel, JBC, 1978; 253:6111) and its gene has been cloned (van de Zande, Gene, 1990; 87:225).

As shown by metabolic flux measurements, immunohistochemistry, and *in situ* hybridization, glutamine synthetase is restricted to a small hepatocyte subpopulation at the perivenous end of the liver acinus (Gebhardt, EMBOJ, 1983; 2:567; Häussinger, EurJBioch, 1983; 133:269; Gebhardt, FEBSLett, 1988; 241:89), which is free of urea-cycle enzymes.[2,3,8] Thus, following the direction of sinusoidal blood flow, the two ammonia detoxication systems, urea and glutamine synthesis, are anatomically switched behind each other and present the sequence of a low- and high-affinity system for ammonia detoxication, respectively.[8,9] The cells, which contain glutamine synthetase, have been termed perivenous scavenger cells (Häussinger, EurJBioch, 1988; 175:395), because they eliminate with high affinity the ammonia which was not used by the upstream urea-synthesizing compartment. They are of crucial importance for the maintenance of non-toxic ammonia levels in the hepatic vein: selective damage of perivenous scavenger cells does not impair upstream urea synthesis, but leads to hyperammonaemia due to a failure of scavenger function (Häussinger, ChemBiolInteract, 1984; 48:191). *In vivo* and *in vitro* 7 to 25 per cent of the ammonia delivered via the portal vein escapes periportal urea synthesis and is used for glutamine synthesis (Häussinger, EurJBioch, 1983; 133:269; Cooper, JBC, 1987; 262:1073). Perivenous scavenger cells have a high capacity to synthesize glutamine and this pathway is augmented by the presence of high-affinity transport systems in their plasma membrane for α-ketoglutarate, malate, and other dicarboxylates (Stoll, EurJBioch, 1989; 181:709; Stoll, Hepatol, 1991; 13:247), which are taken up from the blood and serve as carbon precursors for glutamine synthesis.

Like urea synthesis, glutamine synthetase is subject to short- and long-term regulation. Due to the exclusive downstream localization of glutamine synthetase in the liver acinus, flux through the urea cycle in the periportal compartment will determine the amount of ammonia reaching the perivenous scavenger cells. Accordingly, all factors that regulate urea synthesis will indirectly exert control on the glutamine synthesis located more downstream. Also, the availability of carbon skeletons can control the rate of glutamine synthesis (Stoll, Hepatol, 1991; 13:247).

In vivo, glutamine synthetase activity is down-regulated by hypophysectomy (Wong, Endocrinol, 1980; 106:268) and following portocaval anastomosis (Girard, DigSurg, 1992; 37:1121; Häussinger, Enzyme, 1993; 46:72). Glutamine and cell swelling decrease, whereas insulin and dexamethasone increase, the levels of glutamine synthetase mRNA (Abcouwer, JSurgRes, 1995; 59:59; Warskulat, BiolChemHS, 1996; 377:57). The age-related increase in oxidized protein in the liver and brain is accompanied by a loss of glutamine synthetase activity (Stadtman, EXS, 1992; 62:64) and acetaminophen inhibits its catalytic activity (Bulera, Tox-ApplPharmacol, 1995; 134:313).

The intercellular glutamine cycle and ammonia detoxication[2,3,8,9]

Whereas glutamine synthetase, which acts as a high-affinity ammonia scavenger, is localized in perivenous hepatocytes, glutaminase is located in periportal hepatocytes and in the mitochondria together with carbamoyl phosphate synthetase. As mentioned above, glutaminase acts as a pH- and hormone-modulated ammonia amplifier. Its activity is an important determinant of urea-cycle flux in view of the physiologically low ammonia concentrations, which are about one order of magnitude lower than the *Km* (ammonia) of carbamoyl phosphate synthetase. Periportal glutaminase and perivenous glutamine synthetase are simultaneously active, resulting in a periportal breakdown and perivenous resynthesis of glutamine. This intercellular glutamine cycle[8,9] also operates *in vivo*[11] (Welbourne, HoppeSeylerZPhysiolChem, 1986; 367:301) and allows the maintenance of a high urea-cycle flux, despite the low affinity of carbamoyl phosphate synthetase for ammonia and the presence of physiologically low ammonia concentrations: glutamine utilized for ammonia amplification in periportal hepatocytes is resynthesized in perivenous scavenger cells from the ammonia which escaped upstream urea synthesis (Fig. 2). However, the regulatory properties of the intercellular glutamine cycle allow the liver to become a net producer or net consumer of glutamine depending on the nutritional and hormonal conditions[3,8] (Häussinger, BBActa, 1983; 755:272; Cooper, JBC, 1988; 263:12268). Intercellular glutamine cycling also provides an effective means to shift hepatic ammonia detoxication from urea to net glutamine synthesis in acidosis (see below).

Urea and ammonia metabolism in liver disease

In patients with severe decompensated liver disease, acute or chronic, the plasma urea level tends to fall and there is reduction in the amount of urea excreted in the urine (Hansen, ScaJGastr, 1985; 20:346). Urea synthesis is reduced in severe liver disease (Rudman, JCI, 1973: 52:2241) in parallel with glutamine synthesis (Kaiser, EurJClinInv, 1988; 18:535), and this tends to be correlated with deterioration in other markers of hepatocellular function (Vilstrup, EurJClinInv, 1982; 12:197; Vilstrup, EurJClinInv, 1986; 16:193). The metabolic zonation in the human hepatic lobules with respect to urea and glutamine metabolism is preserved in fibrotic lesions, but is lost in cirrhotic nodules (Racine-Samson, Hepatol, 1996; 24: 104).

In patients with well-compensated cirrhosis, urea production rates are similar to those of healthy controls under basal conditions, but the maximal urea production capacity in response to a protein or amino acid load is significantly reduced (Rypins, Gastro, 1980; 78:1419; Vilstrup, Gut, 1980; 21:990). In these patients, as in controls, there is a linear relationship between urea production and the plasma amino-nitrogen concentration, but the rate of urea synthesis increases less steeply with increasing plasma amino-acid concentrations (Rafoth, JCI, 1975; 56:1170). Such patients are therefore able to achieve a normal urea synthesis rate, but at the price of a higher amino-nitrogen concentration. In line with this, glutaminase activity is increased four- to fivefold in cirrhosis (Kaiser, EurJClinInv, 1988; 18:535; Häussinger, KlinWschr, 1990; 68:175; Matsuno, CancerRes, 1992; 52:1192), which augments urea synthesis by increased ammonia amplification. Zinc supplementation speeds up the kinetics of nitrogen conversion from amino acids into urea in those with cirrhosis, but not in healthy individuals (Marchesini, Hepatol, 1996; 23:1084). This can be explained by the zinc dependence of several urea-cycle enzymes and carbonic anhydrase V and a zinc deficiency, which is frequently found in cirrhosis.

Reduction in the maximal capacity for urea production in patients with cirrhosis is associated with a decrease, in liver biopsies, in the activity of all five urea-cycle enzymes, especially the rate-controlling enzymes, argininosuccinate synthetase and carbamoyl phosphate synthetase I (Khatra, JLabClinMed, 1974; 84:708; Maier, KlinWschr, 1979; 57:661). The decreased capacity for urea production in cirrhosis is not related to the loss of hepatic mass *per se* (Kekomaki, ScaJGastr, 1970; 5:375), but rather to the reduction of 'functional liver mass' (Vilstrup, Gut, 1980; 21:990). Standardized measurement of the daily urea synthesis rate might allow prediction of the amount of protein that patients with liver disease could tolerate. It correlates with Child's criteria, electroencephalogram scores, and neuropsychological tests (Rikkers, Gastro, 1978; 75: 462), and with the stage of chronic active hepatitis. In patients with advanced cirrhosis and encephalopathy, fasting urinary urea is a predictor for 'wake-up' or death (Vilstrup, JHepatol, 1985; Suppl. 2:347), and in fulminant hepatitis it distinguishes survivors from those that die (Nusinovici, GastrClinBiol, 1977; 1:875).

In patients with liver disease there is a tendency for blood ammonia levels to rise. The main reason for this is presumably the failure of the liver, due to portosystemic shunting and hepatocellular dysfunction, to remove ammonia from the portal venous blood, in

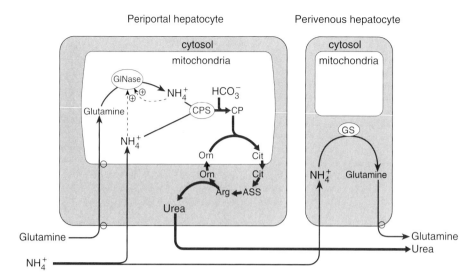

Fig. 2. Structural and functional organization of hepatic ammonia and glutamine metabolism. Periportal hepatocytes contain urea-cycle enzymes and glutaminase, but no glutamine synthetase. The latter enzyme is restricted to a small perivenous hepatocyte population near the outflow of the sinusoidal bed, which is virtually free of urea-cycle enzymes. Urea and glutamine synthesis are anatomically switched behind each other and represent functionally the sequence of a periportal high capacity, but low-affinity, system and a perivenous high-affinity system for ammonia detoxication. Periportal glutaminase is activated by its product ammonia and is highly sensitive to changes of the extracellular pH. Glutaminase acts as a pH-modulated amplifier of the mitochondrial ammonia concentration and is an important determinant of urea-cycle flux. Ammonia which escaped periportal urea synthesis ('low-affinity system') is disposed of by the perivenous scavenger glutamine synthetase ('high-affinity system'). This guarantees the effective detoxication of ammonia, even when urea-cycle flux is inhibited in acidosis. At normal extracellular pH, glutaminase flux equals glutamine synthetase flux (so-called 'intercellular glutamine cycle'): portal ammonia is completely converted into urea. In acidosis, glutaminase flux und urea synthesis decrease, whereas glutamine synthetase flux increases due to an increased ammonia delivery to perivenous hepatocytes: the liver switches ammonia detoxication from urea to net glutamine synthesis. From ref. 8.

which the concentration is always much higher than in other parts of the circulation. In line with this, liver cirrhosis is characterized by a severe scavenger cell defect (Kaiser, EurJClinInv, 1988; 18: 535), which also occurs after portocaval shunting (Girard, Dig-DisSurg, 1992; 37:1121; Häussinger, Enzyme, 1992; 46:72). The amount of ammonia entering the portal vein may also be increased in those with cirrhosis, as they show an increase of approximately 50 per cent in the amount of urea hydrolysed in the gut (Hansen, ScaJGastr, 1985; 20:346) due, possibly, to the overgrowth of urease-containing bacteria (Lal, Gastro, 1972; 62:275). This can be reduced by inhibiting bacterial ureolysis with antibiotics, and there is a resulting fall in urea production from gut ammonia. Agents which increase nitrogen incorporation into the intestinal microflora, such as lactulose (Weber, Gastro, 1979; 77:518) and pectin (Herrmann, Gastro, 1987; 92:1795), also decrease urea synthesis in subjects with cirrhosis by reducing the amount of nitrogen made available from the gut to the liver for urea synthesis.

In the presence of severe liver impairment and portosystemic shunting, skeletal muscle becomes an important organ in ammonia homeostasis (Lockwood, JCI, 1979; 63:449). In patients with chronic liver failure, muscle takes up more ammonia and releases much more glutamine than in controls (Bessman, JCI, 1955; 34:622; Fazekas, AmJMedSci, 1957; 234:145). The extraction of ammonia from the circulation is significantly less in patients with cirrhosis and muscle wasting, and this may contribute to the hyperammonaemia often found in these patients (Ganda, Metabolism, 1975; 25:427). Exercise causes a greater release of ammonia from

muscle in patients with cirrhosis than in controls (Allen, Yale-JBiolMed, 1960; 33:133).

In patients with cirrhosis the blood ammonia, which is already high, may occasionally rise further as a result of gastrointestinal bleeding, renal failure, acid–base disturbances, or the administration of diuretics, and the patient may develop hepatic encephalopathy.

Urea-cycle disorders[12,13]

Deficiencies of all five urea-cycle enzymes, and of *N*-acetyl-glutamate, have been described. The hyperammonaemia and coma with which they are associated makes them of interest to hepatologists. They are uncommon disorders, with ornithine transcarbamylase deficiency the most frequently reported. Their clinical features are discussed in Section 26.

pH regulation and the liver[2,8,14-16]

The regulation of the acidity of the extracellular fluid is due primarily to the control of plasma CO_2 and HCO_3^- by the lungs, the liver, and the kidneys. Multiple buffer systems, such as proteins, $H_2PO_4^-/HPO_4^{2-}$, and the bicarbonate buffer, are in chemical equilibrium in the extracellular fluid. Despite its modest buffer capacity at physiological pH, the bicarbonate buffer is of special interest because the concentrations of its constituents HCO_3^- and CO_2 can be regulated very effectively. The Henderson–Hasselbalch equation describes the relationship between pH and the concentrations of CO_2 and HCO_3^- in extracellular fluids:

$$pH = 6.1 + \log [HCO_3^-]/[CO_2]$$

This equation predicts that mechanisms for the maintenance of extracellular pH must keep the $[HCO_3^-]/[CO_2]$ ratio constant and CO_2 and HCO_3^-, which are continuously generated during the oxidation of energy fuels, need to be eliminated from the body at the same velocity as they are generated metabolically. The complete oxidation of fat and carbohydrates yields CO_2 and water as the only products and the lungs fulfil the role to regulate P_{CO_2}.[16] However, the hydrolysis of proteins yields bipolar amino acids, whose complete oxidation generates not only CO_2 and water, but also HCO_3^- and NH_4^+, which are derived from the carboxylic and amino/amido moieties of amino acids, respectively. During oxidation of neutral amino acids, such as alanine, HCO_3^- formation equals that of NH_4^+, whereas the dicarboxylic amino acids, glutamate and aspartate, give rise to another HCO_3^- ion, which is derived from their second carboxylate group. The dibasic amino acids, arginine and lysine, have a second NH_3 group, and give rise to another NH_4^+ ion. Although dietary protein usually contains a slight excess of dibasic over dicarboxylic amino acids, the amounts of NH_4^+ and HCO_3^- produced during protein oxidation are almost equal and high: the daily oxidation of 100 g of protein produces about 1 mol HCO_3^- and 1 mol NH_4^+. Thus, protein oxidation creates a strong alkali burden for the body. Only about 5 per cent of this bicarbonate is neutralized by H^+, which is generated during the metabolism of sulphur-containing amino acids. The major pathway for removal of HCO_3^- is hepatic urea synthesis, which consumes 2 mol of HCO_3^- per 1 mol urea produced.

$$2NH_4^+ + HCO_3^- \rightarrow NH_2CONH_2 + H^+ + 2H_2O$$

$$HCO_3^- + H^+ \rightleftharpoons CO_2 + H_2O$$

Summary: $2NH_4^+ + 2HCO_3^- \rightarrow NH_2CONH_2 + CO_2 + 3H_2O$

In chemical terms, urea synthesis is an irreversible, energy-driven neutralization of the strong base HCO_3^- by the weak acid NH_4^+ and the average daily excretion of 30 g of urea is equivalent to the disposal of about 1 mol of HCO_3 per day. Thus, a major function of hepatic urea synthesis is to effect this neutralization, without which the body would otherwise be confronted by a major load of alkali. This important role of ureogenesis has been overlooked in the past, when the role of urea synthesis was identified exclusively with that of ammonia detoxication.

Apart from the liver-specific presence of a quantitatively important pathway for irreversible HCO_3^- removal—urea synthesis—the important role of the liver in bicarbonate homeostasis is based on two further features. First, a sensitive control of urea formation by extracellular pH, which establishes a homeostatic feedback control loop between bicarbonate-consuming urea synthesis and the actual acid–base status. Second, a structural and functional organization of the pathways of ammonia detoxication in the liver acinus, which uncouples urea synthesis from the vital need to detoxify ammonia.[8] Whenever the pH and/or the HCO_3^- concentration drop in the extracellular space, the liver responds with a decrease of urea synthesis relative to the rate of protein catabolism and oxidation. Consequently, a fraction of the bicarbonate generated

during protein breakdown is retained in the body and can be used to correct the underlying acidosis. The efficiency of such a mechanism is high: a 10 per cent inhibition of ureogenesis relative to protein breakdown in acidosis will retain about 100 mmol HCO_3^- per day. In a well-balanced acid–base situation, however, the rate of bicarbonate removal (urea synthesis) from the organism must match the rate of bicarbonate production (protein catabolism) and the regulation of urea-cycle flux appears to be controlled by the rate of protein breakdown only.

In general, pH control of urea synthesis occurs at the level of provision of substrates for carbamoyl phosphate synthetase, but not within the urea cycle itself. The mechanisms involved include pH-dependent changes in the NH_3/NH_4^+ ratio, the pH dependence of amino acid transport across the hepatocyte membrane, and the regulatory properties of mitochondrial glutaminase and carbonic anhydrase V. These latter enzymes adjust the input of the substrates ammonia and HCO_3^- into the carbamoyl phosphate synthetase reaction, which is *in vivo* the rate-controlling step of urea synthesis. Mitochondrial glutaminase is activated by its own product ammonia and acts as an amplifier of the mitochondrial ammonia concentration, whose activity is sensitively controlled by pH: lowering the extracellular pH from 7.4 to 7.3 already inhibits flux through the enzyme by 70 per cent (Häussinger, TIBS, 1984; 9:300). Due to the low affinity of carbamoyl phosphate synthetase for ammonia, inhibition of ammonia amplification in acidosis diminishes urea-cycle flux. Inhibition of flux through glutaminase at low pH is only in part due to an inhibition of enzyme activity, but more importantly due to an inhibition of glutamine transporters in the plasma and the mitochondrial membrane (Lenzen, EurJBioch, 1987; 16:483). Although the physiological glutamine concentration in plasma is only about 0.6 mmol/l, the concentrative action of these two transport systems normally creates intramitochondrial glutamine concentrations close to the *Km* of 28 mmol/l of mitochondrial glutaminase (Häussinger, EurJBioch, 1985; 152:597). Inhibition of these transporters in acidosis therefore inhibits intramitochondrial glutamine hydrolysis by decreasing the intramitochondrial glutamine concentration. Also the uptake of other amino acids into the liver is inhibited in acidosis. This shifts the site of amino acid catabolism from the liver to non-hepatic tissues (Fafournoux, BiochemJ, 1983; 216:401; Boon, AmJPhysiol, 1994; 267:F1015; Christensen, NutrRev, 1995; 53:74). The other enzyme, mitochondrial carbonic anhydrase V, is also sensitively controlled by pH and plays an important role in providing HCO_3^- inside the mitochondria for carbamoyl phosphate synthetase (Häussinger, EurJBioch, 1985; 152: 381). This is explained by the fact that the mitochondrial membrane is impermeable to HCO_3^- but not to CO_2 (Balboni, JBC, 1986; 261: 3563) and that the rate of spontaneous (uncatalysed) conversion of CO_2 into HCO_3^- (or more exactly to H_2CO_3) is by far not fast enough to meet the bicarbonate requirements for intramitochondrial biosynthetic pathways (Häussinger, EurJBioch, 1985; 152:381). This is why carbonic anhydrase inhibitors, such as acetazolamide, are potent inhibitors of urea synthesis in the liver. In acidosis, both carbonic anhydrase and glutaminase are inhibited and, consequently, also irreversible bicarbonate consumption and urea synthesis. Discrimination of respiratory from metabolic acidosis is brought into this regulatory system by the fact that the spontaneous (uncatalysed) CO_2 conversion to HCO_3^- inside the mitochondria is pH insensitive, whereas the carbonic anhydrase-catalysed conversion is inhibited at low pH. Thus, at high CO_2 concentrations, pH control exerted by carbonic anhydrase is bypassed through an augmentation of the spontaneous formation of HCO_3^-, and urea synthesis is inhibited much more strongly in metabolic than in respiratory acidosis. This seems well designed because sparing of bicarbonate can correct metabolic acidosis, whereas in respiratory acidosis it can only achieve a compensation but not abolish the hyperkapnia. Urea synthesis is also controlled by the extracellular CO_2 and HCO_3^- concentrations, independent of the pH. Even at a normal extracellular pH *in vitro*, the liver can respond to a decrease in buffer capacity of the extracellular HCO_3^-/CO_2 system with an inhibition of urea synthesis and a sparing of bicarbonate.

A sophisticated structural and functional organization of the pathways of nitrogen metabolism in the liver acinus has evolved which uncouples urea synthesis from the need to maintain NH_4^+ homeostasis, despite the ultimate link of HCO_3^- and NH_4^+ generation during protein catabolism. It provides the other basis for a pH-stat function of the liver and eliminates the threat of hyperammonaemia, which would otherwise result from an acidosis-induced inhibition of urea synthesis. Due to the sequential organization of urea and glutamine synthesis in the liver acinus, perivenous scavenger cells maintain ammonia homeostasis by glutamine synthesis, even when upstream urea synthesis is switched off (Fig. 2). Here, acidosis shifts hepatic ammonia detoxication from bicarbonate-consuming urea synthesis to net glutamine synthesis, which is the result of both an increased glutamine formation by perivenous scavenger cells and a reduced glutamine consumption at periportal glutaminase. Thus, intercellular glutamine cycling in the liver is an elegant means to adjust ammonia flux into either urea or glutamine depending on the acid–base situation.

Of course, enhanced glutamine formation by the liver and other organs in acidosis may prevent hyperammonaemia but does not provide a final sink for ammonia elimination. This is achieved by the kidneys, where NH_4^+ is liberated again from glutamine and is excreted as such into the urine. This process of so-called renal ammoniagenesis is long known to be stimulated in acidosis[16] and involves the action of kidney glutaminase, which is regulated by pH in an opposite way to the liver enzyme.[17] It functions as a spill-over for surplus NH_4^+, which cannot be disposed of by urea synthesis. Thus, when urea synthesis is switched off in acidosis in order to spare bicarbonate, the kidneys take over the task of final NH_4^+ elimination and glutamine serves as a non-toxic transport form of ammonia to the kidney (Fig. 3). This spill-over function of the kidney is critical for the pH-stat function of the liver, because otherwise accumulation of surplus NH_4^+ in the organism, albeit in the form of glutamine, would override the acid–base control of hepatic HCO_3^- elimination by an inadaequate NH_4^+- (or glutamine-) driven stimulation of urea synthesis. With respect to ammonia and HCO_3^- homeostasis, the liver and kidney act as a team and impairment of one organ's function will give rise to acid–base disturbances. Fig. 3 summarizes this concept of acid–base regulation: in acidosis, bicarbonate is spared in the liver by switching off urea synthesis relative to the rate of protein breakdown, whereby ammonia homeostasis is maintained by renal ammoniagenesis. In line with this, urea excretion decreases at the expense of urinary NH_4^+ excretion in acidosis (Oliver, ClinSci, 1975; 48:515). It is important to stress that it is the change of urea synthesis relative

to protein breakdown which affects the bicarbonate pool in the body, whereas absolute changes of urea synthesis do not allow conclusions on bicarbonate homeostasis unless the rate of protein oxidation is assessed simultaneously. Failure to do so has led in the past to erroneous conclusions.[14]

The pH in urine normally varies between 5 and 8, and the net amount of protons excreted or retained by the kidney can be assessed by titrating the urine pH back to plasma pH. This 'titratable acid excretion' is normally about 30 to 50 mmol/day and largely reflects protons bound to urinary buffers such as phosphate. Using Bronstedt's acid/base definition, titratable acid excretion is the net effect of the kidneys on pH_e homeostasis. This contribution seems small, especially when comparison is made with CO_2 excretion by the lungs (10 to 20 mol/day) or with HCO_3^- disposal during hepatic urea synthesis (about 1 mol/day). The historical term 'non-titratable acid' reflects the quantity of NH_4^+ in the urine. NH_4^+ excretion into urine is normally about 40 mmol/day and represents the small 'physiological' gap between the daily formation of HCO_3^- (about 960 mmol) and NH_4^+ (about 1000 mmol) resulting from the oxidation of about 100 g of protein.

There is controversy about the role of the liver in acid–base homeostasis. The elimination of the two nitrogens of glutamine, as urinary NH_4^+, leaves behind an α-ketoglutarate ion which, when it is metabolized in the kidney, consumes two H^+ ions; on this basis it has been argued that measurement of NH_4^+ excretion can still be used to quantify the elimination of H^+ by the kidney (Halperin, KidneyInt, 1983; 24:709). However, the α-ketoglutarate can be regarded (correctly) as just another of the amino acid skeletons released from protein breakdown, which would generate two bicarbonate ions that have to be neutralized if the nitrogen of the amino acid escapes incorporation into urea (Häussinger, BiochemJ, 1986; 236:261). Also, the repeatedly asked question of whether urea synthesis is regulated primarily by the acid–base status or whether the prime determinant is the need for nitrogen disposal cannot be answered because ammonia and bicarbonate homeostasis are closely interlinked and involve a co-ordination of liver and kidney function.[8,14,16] Clearly, it is the rate of urea synthesis relative to protein breakdown which underlies a homeostatic feedback control by the acid–base status, but the absolute rate of protein breakdown may vary considerably and this calls simultaneously for mechanisms which adapt urea synthesis to this parameter.

Lactate metabolism

The liver has another role in the regulation of the acidity of the extracellular fluid because of its role in the metabolism of lactate. In a resting 70-kg person, about 1.3 mol of 'lactic acid' is produced daily in peripheral tissues and enters the circulation.[18] Because of its low pK_a (3.8), the lactic acid is almost all dissociated, and approximately 1.3 mol of H^+ ions are therefore available to titrate extracellular bicarbonate. However, lactate is converted either to glucose, or to carbon dioxide and water, and the bicarbonate concentration remains normal because a hydrogen ion is consumed in these processes and bicarbonate is regenerated. The liver removes 50 to 70 per cent of the lactate produced each day.

An efficient homeostatic system should have control mechanisms which speed it up when it is under pressure, but lactate conversion to glucose in perfused rat liver is markedly inhibited by acidosis

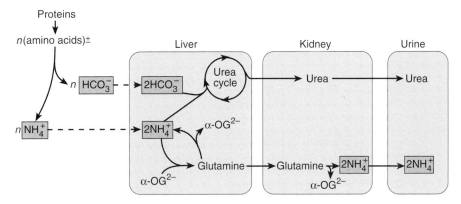

Fig. 3. Co-ordinate regulation of HCO_3^- and NH_4^+ homeostasis by the liver and kidneys. NH_4^+ and HCO_3^- arise in almost equimolar amounts during protein oxidation. Whereas urea synthesis irreversibly consumes HCO_3^- and NH_4^+ in a 1:1 stoichiometry, $HCO_3[-]$ is spared when urea synthesis is switched off in acidosis ('bicarbonate homeostatic response' of the liver). Under these conditions, NH_4^+ homeostasis is maintained by NH_4^+ excretion into urine ('ammonium homeostatic response' of the kidney). A feedback control loop between bicarbonate-consuming urea synthesis and the extracellular pH, $[CO_2]$, and $[HCO_3[-]]$ adjusts hepatic HCO_3^- consumption to the needs of acid–base homeostasis. In metabolic acidosis, flux through the urea cycle and hepatic glutaminase is decreased, whereas flux through hepatic glutamine synthetase and renal glutaminase is increased. The co-ordination of these processes results in NH_4^+ disposal from the organism without concomitant HCO_3^- removal from the organism in acidosis. When NH_4^+ is excreted into urine, there is no net production or consumption of α-oxoglutarate (α-OG) in the organism. From Häussinger, BiochemJ, 1986; 236:261.

(Iles, BiochemJ, 1977; 164:185). This could explain the fulminating lactic acidosis seen in some patients with diabetes treated with phenformin—but it does not explain how stability is maintained in health. Lactate entry across the plasma membrane of the hepatocyte occurs through two distinct mechanisms; one is a saturable stereospecific transporter (Monson, ClinSci, 1982; 62:411; Fafournoux, JBC, 1985; 260:292) and is energy dependent, and the other has not yet been fully characterized. Recently the proton/monocarboxylate (lactate) transporters MCT1 and MCT2 have been cloned (Garcia, Genomics, 1994; 23:520; JBC, 1995; 270:1843). MCT2 is found in liver and has been characterized (Jackson, JBC, 1996; 271:861). Its Km for lactate is 4.7 mmol/l. The kinetics of the transporter suggest that it might be of major importance when the blood lactate is less than 2 mmol/l, that is, within the normal or slightly elevated range of blood lactate. The transporter mechanism is stimulated by extracellular acidosis (Sestoft, ClinSci, 1986; 70: 19), and is therefore homeostatic for acid–base balance as it operates best at low blood lactate levels, when it is thought to be rate-limiting for lactate removal. At higher levels of blood lactate, the second mechanism (which might be non-ionic diffusion) is the major route of lactate entry into the liver cell and, in studies demonstrating inhibition of lactate removal by acidosis, the lactate concentrations employed were always 2 mmol/l or above. At these levels the transporter becomes saturated, and the major site of flux control lies in the chemical reactions of gluconeogenesis, at a step between pyruvate and oxaloacetate.

Clinical consequences

It is clear that the liver may play an important role in the regulation of the acidity of the extracellular fluids, and that impairment of the relevant mechanisms may account for some of the acid–base disturbances seen in liver disease. Further, important consequences arise from the relationship between urea synthesis and ammonia homeostasis.

Metabolic alkalosis is commonly seen in fulminant hepatic failure and in decompensated cirrhosis,[19,20] and is often attributed to potassium deficiency and hyperaldosteronism, particularly as a result of diuretic therapy (Oster, JHepatol, 1986; 2:299). However, metabolic alkalosis may be found without these factors, and it may be due, in part, to impairment of urea synthesis in liver disease; indeed the alkalosis caused by some diuretics may be produced by this mechanism (Guder, JClinChemClinBioch, 1986; 24:2070). There is an inverse relationship between plasma bicarbonate concentration in man *in vivo* and the capacity for hepatic urea synthesis *in vitro* (Kaiser, EurJClinInv, 1988; 18:535; Häussinger, KlinWschr, 1989; 68:175; Häussinger, KlinWschr, 1990; 68:1096). Although the *in vitro* capacity of human liver for urea synthesis is decreased by about 80 per cent in compensated cirrhosis, there is only a minor decrease in urinary urea excretion (Häussinger, ClinInvest, 1992; 70:411), indicating some compensation of the urea-cycle defect. This compensation is in part brought about by a four- to fivefold increase in the activity of glutaminase in cirrhosis, which augments mitochondrial ammonia amplification (see above) and thereby allows the maintenance of near normal flux through the urea cycle in compensated liver cirrhosis. Metabolic alkalosis is one factor which mediates this activation of glutaminase and must be viewed as an important driving force for residual urea synthesis in cirrhosis: it helps to maintain a life-compatible urea-cycle flux, despite a reduction of the urea-synthesizing capacity (Fig. 4). This may explain why acidotic episodes can provoke hyperammonaemia in cirrhosis. In view of this, careful attention has to be paid to the acid–base status and metabolic acidosis requires treatment (Häussinger, ClinInvest, 1992; 70:411).

The view previously held that metabolic alkalosis is a precipitating factor of hepatic encephalopathy has to be reconsidered

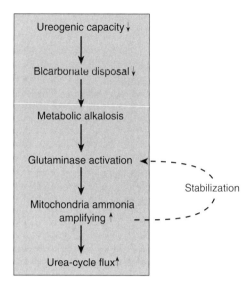

Fig. 4. Metabolic alkalosis as a driving force for urea synthesis in cirrhosis.

because both hyperammonaemia and hyperbicarbonataemia are the result of an impaired urea synthesis in cirrhosis. Thus, metabolic alkalosis is an epiphenomenon rather than a cause of hyperammonaemia in cirrhosis. Increased ammonia amplification in cirrhosis maintains a near-normal urea-cycle flux, but also produces periportal hyperammonaemia, which strongly inhibits lysosomal acidification in Kupffer cells (Schreiber, BiochemJ, 1996; 315:385). It is not clear whether this impairs the clearence function of liver macrophages; such a mechanism was hypothesized to provide a link between hyperammonaemia, endotoxaemia, and renal dysfunction.

Severe liver disease may also prevent the production of glutamine from ammonia by the pericentral cells, and this may exacerbate the hyperammonaemia seen in liver disease, particularly in conditions in which the liver damage is predominantly centrilobular, such as viral hepatitis and carbon tetrachloride poisoning (Häussinger, ChemBiolInteract, 1984; 48:191). Hepatic glutamine synthetase activity in cirrhosis is diminished by about 80 per cent, reflecting a defect of perivenous 'ammonia-scavenging cells'.[3,8] This defect is, besides portosystemic blood shunting, of importance for the development of hyperammonaemia in cirrhosis. This scavenger defect may also explain why loop diuretics can cause hyperammonaemia in patients with cirrhosis but not those without liver disease. Such diuretics slightly inhibit urea synthesis at therapeutic concentrations and increase by that means the ammonia load to downstream scavenger hepatocytes. Normally, ammonia is converted here to glutamine, but in patients with cirrhosis, hyperammonaemia may ensue when the scavenger cells are severely injured.

Respiratory alkalosis is more common in liver disease than metabolic alkalosis.[19] The cause is unknown, but hyperammonaemia has been considered as a possible factor (Wichser, RespirPhysiol, 1974; 20:393); similarly, this might be linked to a reduction in urea synthesis.

Although the liver plays a key role in lactate metabolism and lactate levels tend to be moderately elevated, overt lactic acidosis is relatively uncommon in liver disease and is usually found only when there are other factors which would increase lactate production, or

further decreases in hepatic uptake of lactate, such as shock, sepsis, and bleeding (Oster, JHepatol, 1986; 2:299). In fulminant hepatitis the development of lactic acidosis is associated with an uniformly high mortality; it has been attributed to tissue hypoxia resulting from arteriovenous shunting, as it occurred in patients with an apparently adequate systemic blood pressure, blood flow, and arterial oxygen tension (Bihari, JHepatol, 1985; 1:405).

The liver may also be involved in other types of acid–base disorder.[14] In patients with chronic renal failure the ability to acidify the urine and to excrete titratable acid is often well preserved (Relman, AmJMed, 1968; 44:706), whereas ammonium ion excretion into urine is diminished (Welbourne, JCI, 1972; 51:1852, Tizianello, JCI, 1980; 65:1162). Acidosis was assumed to occur because of the failure of the kidney to excrete appropriate quantities of H^+ in the urine as NH_4^+; however, since NH_4^+ excretion does not represent H^+ excretion, this explanation cannot be correct. It would appear that the unexcreted nitrogen is diverted to the liver, where extra urea may be synthesized because substrate pressure predominates over the control of urea synthesis by pH; this would generate H^+ ions and consume HCO_3^- ions (Häussinger, BiochemJ, 1986; 236:261). Thus, metabolic acidosis is the price paid for maintenance of ammonia homeostasis in renal insufficiency.

Urea-nitrogen production may be increased in chronic renal failure in man (Blondeel, PSEBM, 1966; 122:156), and an increased rate of urea synthesis has been found experimentally both *in vivo* (Persike, AmJPhysiol, 1949; 158:149) and in perfused livers or isolated hepatocytes in animals with acute (Lacy, AmJPhysiol, 1969; 216:1300) or chronic renal failure (Klim, ClinSci, 1986; 70:627). Such an increase in urea synthesis would not necessarily have a striking effect on the level of blood urea. If a subject taking 100 g of protein per day were suddenly to suffer a renal insult reducing NH_4^+ excretion by 50 per cent, the nitrogen diverted to the liver would cause an increase of only about 4 per cent in urea synthesis, but the increase in H^+ production would be enough to produce a substantial systemic acidosis in 1 to 2 weeks.

Finally, the liver may be involved in the increase of plasma bicarbonate which compensates for CO_2 retention as a result of chronic airway obstruction. This is usually attributed to increased renal reabsorption of bicarbonate, but if, before the exacerbation, the urine pH is around 6.5, there is little or no bicarbonate in the urine to reabsorb, and so it could not readily account for the rise in extracellular bicarbonate commonly seen. A respiratory acidosis may transiently suppress urea synthesis, and so depress hepatic HCO_3^- removal. This would lead to a rise in plasma bicarbonate allowing urea synthesis to return to normal after compensation of the respiratory acidosis.

References

1. Knepper MA, Packer R, and Good DW. Ammonium transport in the kidney. *Physiological Reviews*, 1989; **69**: 179–249.

2. Meijer AJ, Lamers WH, and Chamuleau RAFM. Nitrogen metabolism and ornithine cycle function. *Physiological Reviews*, 1990; **70**: 701–48.

3. Häussinger D, Lamers WH, and Moorman AFM. Metabolism of amino acids and ammonia. *Enzyme*, 1993; **46**: 72–93.

4. Powers-Lee SG and Meister A. Urea synthesis and ammonia metabolism. In Arias IM, Jakoby WB, Popper H, Schachter D, and Shafritz DA, eds. *The liver: biology and pathobiology.* New York: Raven Press, 1988: 317–29.

5. Krebs HA, Hems R, Lund P, Halliday D, and Read WWC. Sources of ammonia for mammalian urea synthesis. *Biochemical Journal*, 1978; **176**: 733–7.

6. Lowenstein JM. Ammonia production in muscle and other tissues: the purine nucleotide cycle. *Physiological Reviews*, 1972; **52**: 382–414.

7. Walser M and Bodenlos LJ. Urea metabolism in man. *Journal of Clinical Investigation*, 1959; **38**: 1617–26.

8. Häussinger D. Nitrogen metabolism in liver: structural and functional organization and physiological relevance. *Biochemical Journal*, 1990; **267**: 281–90.

9. Häussinger D. Hepatocyte heterogeneity in glutamine and ammonia metabolism and the role of an intercellular glutamine cycle during ureogenesis in perfused rat liver. *European Journal of Biochemistry*, 1983; **133**: 269–73.

10. Hasselgren P-O, Pedersen P, Sax HC, Warner BW, and Fischer JE. Current concepts of protein turnover and amino acid transport in liver and skeletal muscle during sepsis. *Archives of Surgery*, 1988; **123**: 992–9.

11. Cooper AL. Ammonia metabolism in normal and portocaval-shunted rats. In Grisolia S and Felipo V, eds. *Cirrhosis, hepatic encephalopathy and ammonium toxicity*. New York: Plenum Press, 1990: 24–46.

12. Brusilow SW and Horwich AL. Urea cycle enzymes. In Scriver CR, Beaudet AL, Sly WS, and Valle D, eds. *The metabolic basis of inherited disease*. 7th edn. New York: McGraw Hill, 1995: 1187–232.

13. Batshaw ML. Inborn errors of urea synthesis. *Annals of Neurology*, 1994; **35**: 133–41.

14. Bourke E and Häussinger D. pH homeostasis: the conceptual change. *Contributions to Nephrology*, 1992; **100**: 58–88.

15. Atkinson DE and Camien MN. The role of urea synthesis in the removal of metabolic bicarbonate and the regulation of blood pH. *Current Topics in Cellular Regulation*, 1982; **21**: 261–302.

16. Häussinger D, ed. *pH homeostasis*. London: Academic Press, 1988.

17. Curthoys NP and Watford M. Regulation of glutaminase activity and glutamine metabolism. *Annual Review of Nutrition*, 1995; **15**: 133–59.

18. Cohen RD and Woods HF. *Clinical and biochemical aspects of lactic acidosis*. Oxford: Blackwell Scientific, 1976.

19. Oster JR and Perez GO. Acid–base homeostasis and pathophysiology in liver disease. In Epstein M, ed. *The kidney in liver disease*. 3rd edn. Baltimore: Williams & Wilkins, 1988: 119–31.

20. Record CO, Iles RA, Cohen RD, and Williams R. Acid–base and metabolic disturbances in fulminant hepatic failure. *Gut*, 1975; **16**: 144–9.

2.14 Secretory proteins

2.14.1 Transcription, RNA processing, liver specific factors, RNA translocation, translation, protein co-translocation, secretion

Ellen Carmichael and George Y. Wu

One of the primary characteristics of the adult mammalian liver is its ability to synthesize a large number of proteins, many of which are specific for the liver, and some of which are produced in vast amounts (Table 1). The predominant means by which this tissue-specific distribution of proteins is achieved is at the level of the synthesis of messenger RNA (**mRNA**) molecules within the nuclei of liver cells. Cell-specific regulation of gene expression is achieved through an immensely complex interplay of interactions of cellular proteins not

---

Table 1 Examples of hepatospecific proteins

1. Secretory proteins
   Albumin
   Transthyretin
2. Transport proteins
   Lipoproteins
   Transferrin
   Caeruloplasmin
   Steroid hormone-binding proteins
   Thyroid hormone-binding proteins
   Vitamin A-binding proteins (retinol-binding protein)
   Vitamin D-binding proteins (transcalciferin)
3. Coagulation and fibrinolysis proteins
   Coagulation factors
   Complement system
   Protease inhibitors
   α_1-Antitrypsin
   α_1-Antichymotrypsin
   α_2-Macroglobulin
   Inter-α-trypsin inhibitor
   Antithrombin III
   α_2-Antiplasmin
   Heparin cofactor II
   Activated protein C inhibitor
   C1 inhibitor
4. Other proteins
   α_1-Acid glycoprotein
   C-Reactive protein
   Serum amyloid A
   Tyrosine aminotransferase
   Phosphoenol pyruvate carboxykinase
   Vitellogenin
   α-Fetoprotein

---

only with the DNA genome, but also with nascent RNA molecules themselves. Because RNA synthesis and processing are of such importance to liver-specific gene expression, it is necessary at the outset to summarize the processes of transcription initiation and pre-mRNA splicing.

Transcription

The vast majority of protein-coding genes within mammalian cells are differentially expressed, in various cell types, at differing stages of development, at different times in the cell cycle, and in response to extracellular environmental signals. The process by which RNA transcripts are synthesized from a DNA template is, therefore, often highly regulated. Control of the transcriptional process occurs at DNA sequences located in particular regions of the gene, usually upstream of the transcription start site. Two types of regulatory DNA sequences exist:

(1) general control elements (promoters), common to many genes; [1] and
(2) control elements (enhancers), that can be specific for certain cell types.[2]

The promoters are necessary, but usually not sufficient for efficient transcription of a gene. There are several general components of a transcriptional promoter. The first is the TATA box (consensus TATAAA), located 20 to 30 base pairs upstream of the transcription start site. The TATA box is responsible for determining precisely where RNA synthesis begins, and mutations within this core promoter element cause a significant reduction in transcriptional initiation.[3] Many genes have other general control elements such as the CAAT box and the GC box[1] usually located between -40 and -110 bases. In many promoters there is, in addition, an 'initiator' element that spans the start site and which influences transcriptional efficiency. The TATA and initiator elements usually constitute the core, or basal promoter, which contains sufficient information to recruit RNA polymerase II, resulting in a basal level of RNA synthesis. RNA polymerase II is the enzyme responsible for recognizing promoter elements and initiating transcription of messenger RNAs (Fig. 1). The basal transcription machinery consists not only of RNA polymerase II, but also of the basal transcription factors. These transcription factors are highly conserved and are ubiquitously expressed in cells and tissues. TFIID is the only one of these factors that has specific DNA binding activity. This activity is conferred by one of its subunits, the TATA-box binding protein (**TBP**). The key to promoter recognition and transcription initiation is the interaction of TFIID with the TATA element, followed by the recruitment of RNA polymerase II and the other basal factors, to form a transcription-competent initiation complex (Fig. 2).

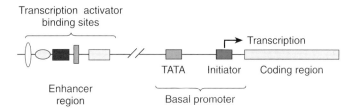

Fig. 1. The typical structural organization of DNA sequences controlling an RNA polymerase II promoter. Multiple sites are usually present for binding transcription activators in the enhancer region. The basal promoter contains the TATA box and an initiator sequence.

However, high levels and regulated expression require additional DNA elements, termed enhancers, which can lie upstream or downstream of the core promoter (Fig. 1). Enhancers are regulatory DNA sequences, which have no promoter activity of their own, but increase the rate of transcription of a certain gene in specific cells. In contrast to promoters, enhancers have no fixed location in a gene, and are, to a first approximation, both distance and orientation independent in their ability to affect transcription. Thus, some promoters contain enhancer elements close to the core elements, while others can lie thousands of bases upstream or downstream of the transcription start sites. Frequently more than one enhancer is involved in the tissue-specific expression of a gene. Enhancer elements are composed of many short motifs (usually 6–8 base pairs long) that serve as specific recognition sites for non-histone nuclear proteins—the transcription activator proteins. Recent work has shown that these proteins have the ability to interact with one or more components of the basal transcription machinery, usually the TBP-associated proteins (**TAFs**), which are components of TFIID (Fig. 2). Distant DNA regions can be wound into loops by the binding of specific proteins. In this way, sites distant in the linear sequence can be brought close together. These interactions frequently allow initiation of transcription to proceed much more efficiently, leading to higher RNA levels, and multiple interactions appear to be synergistic in their effects. Thus, the primary regulation of expression of many genes occurs through the availability and abundance of factors that bind to DNA sequences in the enhancer regions of their promoters.

Transcription activator proteins

There are hundreds, perhaps thousands, of distinct transcription activator proteins, which are expressed in different amounts, in different tissues, and at different times in development. Each has the ability to interact with specific DNA sequences. When bound to their target DNA sequences, most stimulate transcription, while some inhibit. Some of these factors are ubiquitously expressed in cells, while others are found only in a limited number of cell types. Thus, the regulation of transcription is a complicated interplay of *cis*-acting DNA sequences with many *trans*-acting factors that enhance or retard transcription.

In the past decade it has become apparent that transcription activators are generally modular in structure (Fig. 3). Most contain distinct structural domains that confer specific DNA activity and transcription activation potential. In addition, some possess domains that allow regulation of activity. These domains can be sites of protein modification, such as phosphorylation, or can be capable of binding effectors such as hormones. Numerous DNA-binding polypeptide domains have been described.

RNA processing

In mammalian cells, several steps are involved in the conversion of primary transcripts into mature mRNA molecules. These include the addition of a cap structure at the 5′ end of the message, addition of a poly(A) tail to the 3′ end, and removal of internal sequences by the process of RNA splicing.

Cap formation is a co-transcriptional event (Shatkin, Cell, 1976; 9:645; Venkatesan, JBC, 1980; 255:2835; Coppola, PNAS, 1983; 80: 1251). Before the primary transcript has been elongated past 20 to 30 bases, a phosphate is released from the 5′-triphosphate end of the nascent RNA molecule. The 5′-diphosphate end then attacks the α-phosphorus atom of guanosine triphosphate (**GTP**) and an unusual 5′-5′-triphosphate linkage is formed, the so-called cap. The 5′ end is further modified by methylation of N7 of the terminal guanine (cap 0), and additional methylation of the first adjacent riboses (cap 1 and cap 2). The cap structure has three functions:

1. It is important because RNA splicing is often used by cells to regulate gene expression to create different protein products from a single gene.
2. It protects the 5′ end from phosphatases and nucleases.
3. It enhances the efficiency of mRNA translation.

Polyadenylation of the 3′ end of the primary transcript is a post-transcriptional event (Birnstiel, Cell, 1985; 41:349). Some eukaryotic genes contain a hairpin structure followed by a series of U residues as termination signal. Transcription proceeds and terminates beyond the site of polyadenylation (Nevins, Cell, 1978; 15:1477). The primary transcript is cleaved by an endonuclease at a distinct site up to several hundred bases away from its 3′ end, forming a new 3′ end. An important recognition signal for DNA cleavage is the sequence AAUAAA, found 10 to 30 nucleotides upstream from the poly(A) addition site for most transcripts (Fitzgerald, Cell, 1981; 24:251; Montell, Nature, 1983; 305:600). However, this signal alone is not sufficient for cleavage; its context is also important (McDevitt, Cell, 1984; 37:993). Once a new 3′ end is formed, 200 to 250 adenylate residues are added by the enzyme polyadenylate polymerase.[4] The poly(A) tail is not important for RNA splicing or RNA translation, but it stabilizes mRNA and prolongs its survival in the cytoplasm (Zeevi, MolCellBiol, 1982; 2: 517).

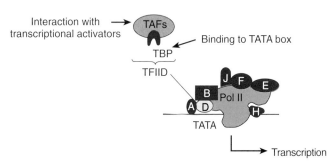

Fig. 2. A typical transcription initiation complex. TAF, transpiration activating factors; TBP, TATA-box binding protein; TFIID, transcription factor IID, Pol II, RNA polymerase II; A, B, D, E, F, J, H, accessory proteins involved in transcription initation.

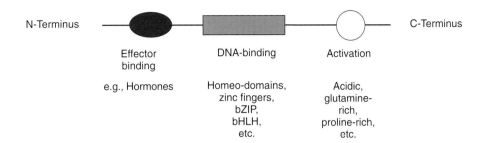

N-Terminus — Effector binding — DNA-binding — Activation — C-Terminus

Effector binding
e.g., Hormones

DNA-binding
Homeo-domains, zinc fingers, bZIP, bHLH, etc.

Activation
Acidic, glutamine-rich, proline-rich, etc.

Fig. 3. A typical modular arrangement of functional domains of transcriptional activators.

Most mammalian genes are interrupted by intervening sequences called introns (Fig. 4). Introns must be removed before functional mRNA molecules are formed, because only the exon sequences encode proteins. Splicing is the process by which intervening intron sequences are removed from pre-mRNAs (formerly termed heterogeneous RNA), and exons are linked together resulting in mature mRNAs. Exons are flanked by 5′ splice sites and 3′ splice sites that are recognized by the splicing machinery. Splicing is a complex process involving multiple *cis* sequences and multiple *trans* factors. The *cis* signals include the 5′ splice site, the 3′ splice site, and the branch point sequence. The consensus sequences for these sites are shown in Fig. 5. Primary RNA transcripts are not found as naked RNA in the nucleus, but are associated with a variety of different proteins (Choi, JCellBiol, 1984; 99:1997), and a certain number of small nuclear RNAs (snRNAs), called U1 to U6. This complex, called a spliceosome, is composed of 50 to 100 proteins, and is the site of RNA splicing. Assembly of this entity requires numerous specific protein–RNA and protein–protein interactions (Lamond, BioEssays, 1993; 15:595; Newman, CurrOpinCellBiol, 1994; 6:360). U1snRNA recognizes the 5′ splice site (Mount, Cell, 1983; 33:509), U2snRNA binds to the branch site and to the polypyrimidine track close to the 3′ splice site (Chabot, Science, 1985; 230:1344). Thus, like transcription initiation, the splicing process can be regulated by the availability or abundance of specific factors that interact with particular splicing signals.

Alternative splicing is a process in which a single pre-mRNA can be spliced into several alternative mRNAs (Rio, CurrOpinGenetDevelop, 1993; 3:574). This process is commonly used to regulate cellular gene expression and to generate diversity, as graphically depicted in Fig. 4. In constitutive (normal) splicing, all introns are removed in sequence, resulting in the joining of all exons. In alternative splicing, one or more splicing signal is ignored by the splicing machinery, giving rise to a new message, which can encode a variant protein with an important biological activity. Although many of the molecular details of constitutive splicing have been described, relatively little is known about most cases of regulation of alternative splice site selection at the molecular level. Three sites are important for proper RNA splicing: (1) the 5′ splice site of an intron; (2) the 3′ splice site of an intron; and (3) the internal branch site of an intron. The 5′ end of an intron always begins with the base sequence GU, the 3′ end always ends with the sequence AG. The consensus sequence at the 5′ end of vertebrate introns is AG/GUAAGU, the consensus sequence at the 3′-end is (Py)10NCAG/G (Py = any pyrimidine, N = any nucleotide). The branch site is located 20 to 50 bases upstream of the 3′ splice site. In mammals, a variety of sequences is found at this site. By alternate splicing, multiple protein isoforms can be generated from single genes.[7]

Transcription factors important for liver-specific gene expression

The expression of genes in the liver is mostly controlled at the transcriptional level, and depends on the regulatory interactions between *cis*-acting sequences and *trans*-acting molecules. Proximal promoters and distant enhancers in combination with a number of ubiquitous transcription factors, hepatocyte-enriched DNA-binding proteins, and general transcription factors interact specifically with these elements and control the expression of liver-specific genes. Liver-specific expression appears to be a consequence of the combinatorial action of these factors in the hepatocyte (Lai, TrendsBiochemSci, 1991; 16:427). The transcription factors that act in hepatocyte-specific gene expression include proteins that are present primarily in liver cells (members of the C/EBP, HNF-1, HNF-3, HNF-4 families) (Table 2), and factors that are widely distributed among tissues (AP-1, NF-1, Sp1, Oct-1, NF-Y/ACF). The genes encoding each of the liver-enriched factors exhibit different patterns of transcriptional regulation in different tissues (Xanthopoulos, PNAS, 1991; 88:3807). The majority of the genes encoding these proteins are themselves regulated at the transcriptional level, although both transcriptional and post-transcriptional events modulate their expression during development, hepatocyte differentiation, and disease. These observations have suggested that a transcriptional cascade may play a critical role in mammalian liver development and differentiation (Xanthopoulos, EurJBioch, 1993; 216:353).

C/EBPα, C/EBPβ (LAP, NF-IL6, IL6-DBP), and DBP

The CCAAT/enhancer-binding protein (C/EBPα) is a bZIP protein that is preferentially expressed in certain cell types, such as adipocytes and hepatocytes. This factor was originally purified as the CCAAT-binding protein (Landschulz, Science, 1988: 240:1759) from non-liver cells. However, it does have a limited tissue and cell distribution, and is relatively abundant in the liver (Maire, Science, 1989; 244:343). It is now known to exist as a family of bZIP proteins, and has been shown to be important for transcription of the albumin, transthyretin, and α1-antitrypsin genes, among others. C/EBP family members appear to be conserved in vertebrate evolution.

The gene encoding the liver-enriched transcriptional-activator protein C/EBPβ (LAP, NF-IL6) has also been shown to produce

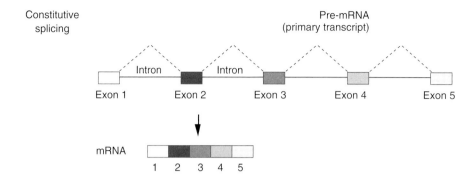

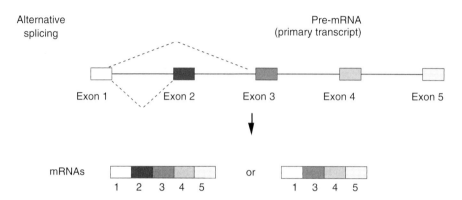

Fig. 4. Two RNA splicing mechanisms involved in the processing of pre-mRNA to mature mRNA; constitutive (normal) and alternative splicing. In constitutive splicing, all introns are removed and all exons are joined together. In alternative splicing, exon skipping occurs, resulting in a truncated message.

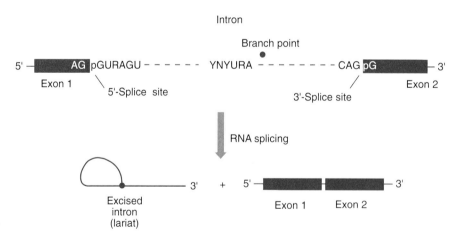

Fig. 5. A typical donor and acceptor site for RNA splicing to produce an excised intron and ligated sequential exons.

two proteins, LAP and the liver-enriched transcriptional-inhibitory protein, LIP (Descombes, Cell, 1991: 67:569). These two factors have different transcription-activation potentials. Recently it has been reported that LAP can inhibit hepatoma cell proliferation (Buck, EMBOJ, 1994; 13:851).

DBP, the albumin promoter D-site binding protein, belongs to the same family of related transcription factors that includes Fos, Jun, CREB, and C/EBP. Among several rat tissues tested, significant levels of this protein were only observed in liver.[8] DBP accumulates to significant levels only in adult animals (Roesler, JBiolChem, 1992; 267:21235). During chemically induced liver regeneration, DBP expression is rapidly downregulated, suggesting that DBP may be involved in the proliferation control of hepatocytes.[8] DBP accumulates according to a very strong circadian

Table 2 Examples of factors important for liver-specific transcription

1. C/EBP (CCAAT/enhancer-binding protein) family
   C/EBPα
   C/EBPβ (NF-IL6, LAP/LIP, IL-6DBP)
   C/EBPδ
2. DBP (albumin promoter D-site binding protein)
3. HNF-1 (hepatic nuclear factor-1) family
   HNF-1α (LFB-1, APF)
   HNF-1β (vHNF-1)
4. HNF-3 (hepatic nuclear factor-3) family
   HNF-3α
   HNF-3β
   HNF-3γ
5. HNF-4 (hepatic nuclear factor-4; steroid receptor) superfamily
   ARP-1 (apolipoprotein AI regulatory protein 1) EAR2
   EAR3/COUP-TF (chicken ovalbumin upstream promoter-transcription factor)

rhythm (Wuarin, JCellSci(Suppl.), 1992; 16:123). In rat parenchymal hepatocytes, the protein is barely detectable during the morning hours. At about 2 tp.m., DBP levels begin to rise, reach maximal levels at 8 tp.m. and decline sharply during the night.

HNF-1

HNF-1α (previously referred to as HNF-1, LFB-1, and APF) contains a divergent homeodomain and is required for transcription of many liver-specific genes, including albumin. The related protein HNF-1β (vHNF-1, LFB-3) interacts with the same regulatory DNA element, and like HNF-1α is expressed primarily in liver, kidney, and intestine. HNF-1α is unique among the vertebrate homeodomain-containing proteins in that it dimerizes in the absence of its DNA recognition sequence, suggesting the possibility that its function may be modulated by forming heterodimers with other related proteins (Mendel, GenesDevelop, 1991; 5:1042). The importance of HNF-1α for liver-specific gene expression is underscored by the observation that a minimal promoter, consisting of an HNF-1α binding-site and a TATA box, is highly active only in hepatoma cell lines (Blumenfeld, Development, 1991; 113:589).

The hepatitis B virus preS1 promoter shows hepatocyte specificity, which has been ascribed to binding of HNF-1 to a cognate DNA sequence upstream of the TATA box. There is an adjacent site that binds the ubiquitous transcription factor, Oct-1. Both the Oct-1 and HNF-1 sites are necessary for liver-specific transcription of the preS1 promoter, but neither can activate transcription alone (Zhou, MolCellBiol, 1991; 11:1353). These results demonstrate an important fact about liver-specific transcription factors: they may require the assistance of other transcription factors that are not restricted to hepatocytes.

Recent work has demonstrated that human liver encodes several isoforms of HNF-1α and HNF-1β generated by the differential use of polyadenylation signals and alternative splicing.[9] As a result of alternative RNA processing, the new isoforms all contain different C-terminal domains. For HNF-1α it has been shown that its C-terminal region is responsible for the activation of transcription. The transactivation potential of HNF-1β is modified by alternative splicing. Two forms of HNF-1β have been described, derived by

alternative splicing from a common pre-mRNA (Ringeisen, JBC, 1993; 268:25706). A third, new isoform of HNF-1β, vHNF1-C, is unable to transactivate and behaves as a transdominant repressor when introduced into cells along with HNF-1α isoforms, HNF1-A, -B or -C.[9] All of the different isoforms of HNF-1α and HNF-1β can form homo- and heterodimers and are differentially expressed in fetal and adult human liver, kidney, and intestine, suggesting distinct roles during development.[9]

Although relatively little is known about how liver-specific transcription factors are themselves restricted to the liver, there is some available data concerning the regulation of HNF-1α activity. There is some evidence that serum colloid osmotic pressure can control the hepatic output of plasma proteins, including albumin. Activity of HNF-1α is modulated by a fluctuation in the level of osmotically active macromolecules (Pietrangelo, PNAS, 1994; 91: 182). Further, HNF-1α has recently been shown to act as a repressor of its own transcription (Piaggio, NucAcidRes, 1994; 22, 4284). The promoter region of the rat HNF-1α gene contains two positive cis-elements: site A, to which the transcription factor HNF-4 protein can bind, and site B, to which HNF-1α itself can bind (Miura, NucAcidRes, 1993; 21:3731).

HNF-3

Three distinct hepatic nuclear factor 3 (HNF-3) proteins (HNF-3α, HNF-3β, and HNF-3γ) help to regulate the transcription of many liver-specific genes. The regulatory regions of numerous hepatocyte-specific genes contain HNF-3 binding sites. The HNF-3 proteins bind to DNA as monomers through a 'winged-helix' motif (Qian, MolCellBiol, 1995; 15:1364). The HNF-3/fkh DNA-binding domain recognizes its cognate DNA binding site as a monomer. HNF-3 may, therefore, be a member of a large gene family of transcription factors that plays a role in tissue-specific gene regulation and development. HNF-3 proteins are needed for the proper expression of some liver-specific genes, but not for expression of the transcription factors found in hepatocytes (Vallet, MolCellBiol, 1995; 15:5453). There is evidence that the extracellular matrix promotes tissue morphogenesis, cell migration, and the differentiation of a variety of cell types. However, the mechanisms by which the extracellular matrix causes differentiated gene expression are largely unknown. Interestingly, the extracellular matrix has been shown to induce an increase in the levels of HNF-3α (DiPersio, MolCellBiol, 1991; 11:4405). Also, the enhancer region of HNF-3β, a binding site for the HNF-3 protein, was found within its own promoter, suggesting that HNF-3β may regulate its own expression (Pani, MolCellBiol, 1992; 12:552).

HNF-4

HNF-4 was first detected as a factor that bound to the transthyretin promoter, and was shown to be a member of the nuclear steroid–thyroid receptor family whose ligands are unknown (orphan receptors). Binding sites for this factor have now been found in many liver-specific promoters (Sladek, Receptor, 1994; 4:64). For example, hepatic cytochrome P450 genes, including members of CYP1 to CYP4 families, comprise the majority of the CYP gene superfamily. HNF-4 appears to act as a common regulator for the liver-specific expression of many of these genes (Chen, JBC, 1994;

269:5420). Other orphan members of the steroid receptor super-family, ARP-1, EAR-2, EAR-3/COUP-TF, have also been implicated in liver-specific transcription (Legraverend, Biochem, 1994; 33:9889).

HNF-4 family members have been implicated both in activation and in repression of gene expression. Their conflicting transcriptional effects may be mediated by direct competition for DNA binding, suggesting that the transcription is dependent, at least in part, upon the intracellular balance of these positive and negative regulatory factors (Mietus, MolCellBiol, 1992; 12:1708). An example of HNF-4 regulation of gene expression is in the synthesis of ornithine transcarbamylase, which is expressed primarily in the liver. Two sites in its promoter/enhancer region are recognized by both HNF-4 and COUP-TF, indicating that these factors have similar DNA binding specificities. Interestingly, HNF-4 activates expression from the ornithine transcarbamylase promoter, while COUP-TF represses expression, even though it is considered a ubiquitous transcriptional activator (Kimura, JBC, 1993; 268: 11125). These results suggest that repression of a tissue-specific promoter by a ubiquitous factor and derepression by a related tissue-enriched activator may be an important mechanism for tissue-specific gene activation.

Recent studies have directly implicated HNF-4 in disease states. HNF-4 has been shown to be involved in the regulation of several blood protease genes as well as genes involved in lipid metabolism. A T-to-A transversion in the HNF-4 binding site of factor IX causes a severe bleeding disorder, and a corresponding mutation in the HNF-4-binding site of factor VII reduced promoter activity by 20 to 50 per cent (Erdmann, JBC, 1995; 270:22988).

Some examples of liver-specific enhancer regions

Figure 6 is a graphic illustration of the DNA elements essential for liver-specific transcription of the apolipoprotein B, α1-antitrypsin, and transthyretin genes. In the apolipoprotein B promoter, there are binding sites for C/EBP and HNF-4 between about 50 and 80 base pairs upstream of the transcription start site. In the α1-antitrypsin promoter, important transcription factor binding sites extend further upstream, to about 500 base pairs before the start site. In addition, this promoter is more complex in that it contains binding sites for HNF-1, C/EBP, HNF-3 and the ubiquitous nuclear factor AP-1. Finally, the transthyretin promoter is much larger, extending almost 2000 base pairs upstream of the transcription start site. Here, there are important binding sites for C/EBP, HNF-1, HNF-3, and HNF-4 between 80 and 200 base pairs upstream of the start site, as well as important sites for AP-1, C/EBP, and HNF-4 between 1860 and 1960 base pairs upstream.

An example of liver-specific transcription—the α-fetoprotein gene

Expression of α-fetoprotein, carbamoylphosphate synthase, and albumin, characteristic of the hepatocytic phenotype, are regulated by a distinct set of transcription factors. α-Fetoprotein is normally expressed in fetal liver and is transcriptionally silent in adult liver, but can be reactivated in hepatocellular carcinoma. The high level of α-fetoprotein expression in hepatocellular carcinoma is transcriptionally controlled by the 5′ flanking sequence of the α-fetoprotein gene. The positive and negative transcriptional regulatory elements of the human α-fetoprotein gene, which play an important role in its developmental regulation, extend over about 4000 base pairs. Transcription factors of the C/EBP, HNF-1, and nuclear factor-1 (NF-1) families can bind to the promoter of the rat (Ido, CancerRes, 1995; 55:3105) and human[10] α-fetoprotein genes. C/EBPα, C/EBPβ, and DBP have been found to activate the α-fetoprotein promoter, while LIP was found to be a potent negative regulator. Both HNF-1α and HNF-1β allowed expression of the α-fetoprotein promoter in cells of non-hepatic origin.[10] There is evidence that changing combinations of trans-acting factors may tightly modulate the α-fetoprotein promoter activity in the course of liver development and carcinogenesis.[10]

RNA translocation

The fully processed RNA exits the nucleus and enters the cytoplasm. It is assumed that the nucleocytoplasmic transport is through nuclear pores. There is evidence that RNAs exchange the proteins with which they are associated in the nucleus during transport to the cytoplasm (Kumar, JMolBiol, 1975; 96:353). However, little is known about the mechanism of this transport. Cytoplasmic mRNAs associated with specific proteins form messenger ribonucleoprotein particles (mRNPs). Untranslated (non-polysomal) RNAs thus form so-called cytoplasmic ribonucleoprotein particles.[11]

Translation

Protein synthesis on ribosomes can be divided into three steps:[12] initiation, elongation, and termination. Initiation is the rate-limiting process in protein biosynthesis. The first step in initiation is the binding of methionine to $tRNA_i^{met}$ by the specific methionyl-tRNA synthetase.[13] $tRNA_i^{met}$ (i standing for initiation) differs from $tRNA^{met}$ by its ability to bind to a small ribosomal subunit once it is activated (acylated) by methionine. In contrast to methionyl $tRNA_i^{met}$, methionyl $tRNA^{met}$ can be used to incorporate methionine within the polypeptide chain.

Methionyl $tRNA_i^{met}$ is brought to the small (40S) ribosomes subunit by the GPT form of the eukaryotic initiation factor eIF2.[14] The complex of methionyl $tRNA_i^{met}$–GPT–eIF2–40S ribosomal subunit is attached to the cap structure at the 5′ end of mRNA by a specific cap-binding protein (Sonenberg, JBC, 1987; 253:6630). Cap-binding protein is a 24 kDa protein which is part of a larger macromolecular aggregate. The 40S ribosomal subunit then moves stepwise down the mRNA in the 5′ to 3′ direction in search of the start codon, AUG (Kozak, NucAcidRes, 1987; 15:8125), which is usually 50 to 200 nucleotides away from the 5′ end of mRNA. The oligonucleotide sequence of mRNA between the 5′ end and the starting codon is called the leader region. Once the AUG start codon is found, the anticodon of methionyl $tRNA_i^{met}$ pairs with the AUG codon, and the ribosomal 60S subunit joins the complex of methionyl $tRNA_i^{met}$, mRNA, and 40S subunit to form the 80S initiation complex. Besides eIF2 and cap-binding protein, additional proteins (initiation factors) are needed for the formation of the initiation complex.

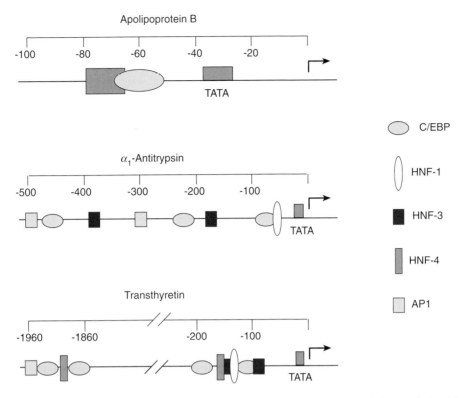

Fig. 6. The DNA elements and factors known to bind to the respective elements for liver-specific control of transcription. The scale indicates the distance upstream from the translational start site. The transcription factors are shown on the right.

Methionyl tRNA$_i^{met}$ is positioned at the 80S ribosome at the P site (P indicates peptidyl). For peptide bond formation another aminoacyl-tRNA must be brought into proper position on the ribosome. This is on the A site (A indicates aminoacyl). The peptide bond between the carboxyl group of the starter methionine and the amino group of the second amino acid is then formed by the peptidyl transferase site of the ribosome (Skogerson, JBC, 1968; 243:5354).

Once the peptide bond is formed, the ribosome plus its attached peptidyl-tRNA moves one codon, i.e. three nucleotides closer to the 3′ end of the mRNA. During this movement tRNAimet is released, the newly formed peptidyl tRNA moves from the A site to the P site of the ribosome, and the aminoacyl-tRNA can be attached to the A site. The cycle is repeated for the addition of each amino acid. Thus, proteins are synthesized in the amino to carboxyl direction.

Certain proteins (elongation factors) are needed for the attachment of aminoacyl-tRNAs to the ribosome, and for the movement of the ribosome down the mRNA chain. In eukaryotes elongation factor eF1a delivers aminoacyl-tRNA to the A site of the ribosome.

The energy for this process is yielded by hydrolysis of GTP to GDP catalysed by eF1b (Ejiri, FEBSLett, 1977; 82:111). Translocation reaction is mediated by eF2, also using energy from the hydrolysis of GTP (Skogerson, ArchBiochBiophys, 1978; 125:497).

Because the formation of a peptide bond between a peptidyl-tRNA and an aminoacyl-tRNA is a thermodynamically favourable reaction, a major role of the ribosome is to select the proper aminoacyl-tRNA before it is brought close to the peptidyl-tRNA.

This selection is based on a correct codon–anticodon match. The selection of the proper aminoacyl-tRNA is the slowest process in protein elongation. On the average about five peptide bonds are formed per second.[15]

Protein elongation is terminated when the ribosome arrives at a stop codon on the mRNA: UAA, AGA, or UAG. Normal cells do not have tRNAs with anticodons to these stop codons. Instead, these codons are recognized by the eukaryotic release factor eRF, which cleaves the peptidyl-tRNA complex, and releases the newly synthesized protein and the uncharged tRNA (Goldstein, PNAS, 1970; 67:99). After release of the tRNA the ribosome disengages from the mRNA and divides into its two subunits, when the whole cycle can start again.

Co-translational translocation of secretory proteins across the endoplasmic reticulum membrane

Cytosolic proteins, and proteins which are incorporated into mitochondria or into peroxisomes, are synthesized by ribosomes that are free in the cytosol. Secretory proteins, integral membrane proteins, and lysosomal proteins are synthesized by ribosomes attached to the endoplasmic reticulum and are co-translationally transported across the endoplasmic reticulum membrane (Fig. 7). This targeting is mediated by signal sequences common to all these proteins (Blobel, JCellBiol, 1975; 67:835). Signal sequences of different proteins are not identical, but have several common features (Leader, TrendsBiochemSci, 1979; 4:205). They are generally located at the amino

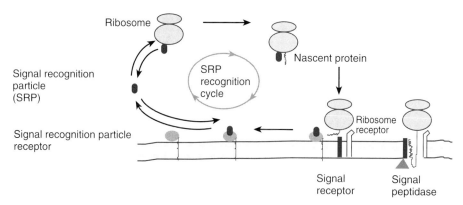

Fig. 7. The signal recognition particle cycle. The signal sequence of a nascent peptide is recognized by a signal recognition particle (SRP). Binding of the signal recognition particle to the signal sequence of nascent proteins inhibits further elongation of the polypeptide chain. The signal recognition particle is then bound by its receptor on the endoplasmic reticulum, and polypeptide chain elongation is resumed. The nascent polypeptide chain is delivered to the translocation machinery of the endoplasmic reticulum membrane, and signal recognition particle is released into the cytosol.

terminus of the protein and range in length from 13 to 36 amino acids. Characteristically, these signal sequences contain 4 to 12 hydrophobic amino acids in the centre. There are some exceptions to this general rule, e.g. ovalbumin has no amino-terminal but does have an internal signal sequence.

When a secretory protein carrying an amino-terminal signal sequence is synthesized, the signal sequence is recognized by a signal recognition particle.[16] This happens as soon as the amino-terminal sequence of the newly synthesized protein emerges from the ribosome; that is, after about 70 amino acids. The signal recognition particle is a complex consisting of a 300-nucleotide RNA molecule (7S RNA) and six different proteins. Binding of the signal recognition particle to the signal sequence of nascent proteins inhibits further elongation of the polypeptide chain.[17] A receptor for signal recognition particle exists on the endoplasmic reticulum membrane.[17] Once the signal recognition particle is bound to its receptor on the endoplasmic reticulum, polypeptide chain elongation is resumed, the nascent polypeptide chain is delivered to the translocation machinery of the endoplasmic reticulum membrane, and the signal recognition particle is released into the cytosol. Binding of ribosomes to the endoplasmic reticulum further involves a ribosome receptor, which includes two integral membrane proteins called ribophorin I and II (Kreibich, JCellBiol, 1978; 77:488).

The mechanism of translocation of the newly synthesized secretory protein into the lumen of the endoplasmic reticulum is poorly understood. There is evidence that the translocation machinery can function independently of protein synthesis (Walter, Cell, 1984; 38:5). However, it can be presumed that the co-translational transport of newly synthesized proteins has the advantage that the protein is still unfolded, because it has just emerged from the ribosome.

Once the secretory protein has entered the lumen of the endoplasmic reticulum, the signal peptide is rapidly cleaved by a specific protease, the signal peptidase (Evans, PNAS, 1986; 83:581). Therefore, proteins still carrying their signal sequences (preproteins) cannot be isolated *in vivo*, but only in *in vitro* translation systems devoid of signal recognition particle and endoplasmic reticulum membranes.

Protein secretion

Once newly synthesized secretory proteins have been introduced into the lumen of the endoplasmic reticulum, they must be matured and transported to their ultimate destination. Maturation includes a number of post-translational modifications; for example, formation of disulphide bonds, glycosylation, limited proteolytic cleavage, assembly of single polypeptide chains to form complex aggregates, sulphation, γ-carboxylation, and hydroxylation. Different secretory proteins undergo different post-translational modifications. The modification reactions occur in distinct organelles of the secretory pathway.

The secretory pathway

Secretory proteins are never found as free soluble proteins in the cytoplasm, but are always located within the lumen of the structures of the secretory pathway.[18] As described above, they are co-translationally imported into the lumen of the endoplasmic reticulum. They are transported from the endoplasmic reticulum to the Golgi complex by transitional vesicles, travelling from *cis*- to *trans*-Golgi and leaving the Golgi complex, packaged in secretory vesicles. They are exocytosed by fusion of secretory vesicles with the plasma membrane (Fig. 8).

Aberration in these very complex interactions can result in liver disease. For example, many patients with hepatocellular carcinoma have elevated concentrations of serum α-fetoprotein. The serum α-fetoprotein levels in the patients appear to be regulated by α-fetoprotein expression in the tumour cells, but not in surrounding normal liver. Understanding the transcriptional regulation of α-fetoprotein has led to use of the promoters and regulatory sequences in gene therapy protocols to target these aberrations (Ido, CancerRes, 1995; 55:5283).

Endoplasmic reticulum

The endoplasmic reticulum is a network of cisternae, tubules, and lamellae, which spans the cytoplasm of the hepatocyte.[19] It occupies about 15 per cent of the liver cell volume; its surface area

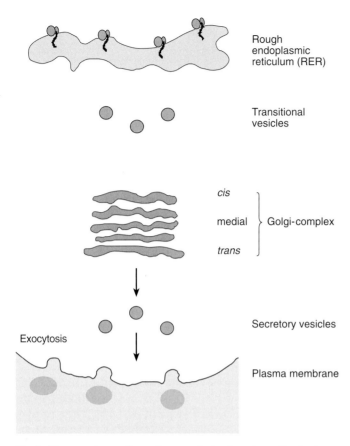

Fig. 8. The secretory pathway for exocytosis of newly synthesized proteins. Secretory proteins are co-translationally imported into the lumen of the endoplasmic reticulum. They are transported from the endoplasmic reticulum to the Golgi complex by transitional vesicles, travelling from *cis*- to *trans*-Golgi and leaving the Golgi complex, packaged in secretory vesicles. Then they are exocytosed by fusion of secretory vesicles with the plasma membrane.

is about 10 m²/g liver. About 60 per cent of the endoplasmic reticulum is dotted with ribosomes (rough endoplasmic reticulum) and 40 per cent is not (smooth endoplasmic reticulum). The rough endoplasmic reticulum is generally arranged in parallel cisternae. Its lumen is 200 to 300 Å wide. The smooth endoplasmic reticulum consists of widely dispersed tubules and vesicles. The lumen of the smooth endoplasmic reticulum is 300 to 600 Å wide.

Newly synthesized secretory proteins are commonly free in the lumen of the endoplasmic reticulum, but they may be attached to the luminal site of the endoplasmic reticulum membrane during certain phases of their maturation, when they are modified and bound to enzymes in the endoplasmic reticulum membrane. Various secretory proteins exhibit different residence times in the endoplasmic reticulum, ranging from 25 to 120 min, before they reach the Golgi complex (Lodish, Nature, 1983; 304:80; Yeo, JBC, 1985; 260:7896). The reason for this is unclear. It is likely that specific receptors are involved, which recognize secretory proteins and trigger their transport to the Golgi complex (Wieland, Cell, 1987; 50:289). Protein mutations, for example replacement of Glu342 to Lys in Z-type α1-antitrypsin (Jeppson, FEBSLett, 1976; 65:195), and modifications of the carbohydrate moieties of secretory hepatocyte proteins (Gross, JBC, 1983; 258:12203; Lodish, JCellBiol,

1984; 98:1720) impair the transport of certain of these proteins from the endoplasmic reticulum to the Golgi complex. However, these results cannot be generalized. Presumably the three-dimensional structure of each protein, determined by its amino acid sequence, and its specific post-translational modifications are important for proper secretion.

Proteins are transported from the endoplasmic reticulum to the Golgi complex in transitional vesicles.[20] These vesicles have a diameter of 20 to 30 nm and possess a coat different from the clathrin coat of endocytotic vesicles. Transport from the endoplasmic reticulum to the Golgi complex requires energy. Lowering of cellular ATP levels blocks the exit of certain proteins from the endoplasmic reticulum (Kabcenell, JCellBiol, 1985; 101:1270). However, the exact transport mechanisms are still not well understood.

References

1. Corden J, Wasylyk B, Buckwalder D, Sassone-Cors D, Kedinger D, and Chambon P. Promotor sequences of eukaryotic protein coding genes. *Science*, 1980; **209**: 1406–13.
2. Atchison ML. Enhancers: mechanisms of action and cell specificity. *Annual Review of Cell Biology*, 1988; 4: 127–53.
3. Breathnach R, and Chambon P. Organization and expression of eukaryotic split genes coding for proteins. *Annual Review of Biochemistry*, 1981; **50**: 349–83.
4. Nevins JR. The pathway of eukaryotic mRNA formation. *Annual Review of Biochemistry*, 1983; 52: 441–66.
5. Heinrich PC, Gross V, Northemann W, and Scheurlen M. Structure and function of nuclear ribonucleoprotein complexes. *Reviews of Physiology, Biochemistry and Pharmacology*, 1978; **81**: 101–34.
6. Busch H, Reddy R, Rothblum L, and Choi YC. SnRNAs, snRNPs, and RNA processing. *Annual Review of Biochemistry*, 1982; **51**: 617–54.
7. Breitbart RE, Andreadis A, and Nadal GB. Alternative splicing: a ubiquitous mechanism for the generation of multiple protein isoforms from single genes. *Annual Review of Biochemistry*, 1987; 56: 467–95.
8. Mueller CR, Maire P, and Schibler U. DBP, a liver-enriched transcriptional activator, is expressed late in ontogeny and its tissue specificity is determined posttranscriptionally. *Cell*, 1990; **61**: 279–91 [published erratum appears in *Cell*, 1991; 65(5): following 914].
9. Bach I and Yaniv M. More potent transcriptional activators or a transdominant inhibitor of the HNF1 homeoprotein family are generated by alternative RNA processing. *EMBO Journal*, 1993; **12**: 4229–42.
10. Bois JB and Danan JL. Members of the CAAT/enhancer-binding protein, hepatocyte nuclear factor-1 and nuclear factor-1 families can differentially modulate the activities of the rat alpha-fetoprotein promoter and enhancer. *Biochemistry Journal*, 1994; **301**: 49–55.
11. Dreyfuss G. Structure and function of nuclear and cytoplasmic ribonucleoprotein particles. *Annual Review of Cell Biology*, 1986; **2**: 459–98.
12. Moldave K. Eukaryotic protein synthesis. *Annual Review of Biochemistry*, 1985; **54**: 1109–49.
13. Schimmel P. Aminoacyl tRNA synthetase: general scheme of structure–function relationships in the polypeptides and recognition of transfer RNAs. *Annual Review of Biochemistry*, 1987; **56**: 125–58.
14. Maitra U, Stringer EA, and Chaudhuri A. Initiation factors in protein biosynthesis. *Annual Review of Biochemistry*, 1982; 51: 869–900.
15. Darnell JE, Lodish H, and Baltimore D. *Molecular cell biology*. Scientific American Books, 1986: 1986.
16. Walter P and Lingappa VR. Mechanism of protein translocation across the endoplasmic reticulum membrane. *Annual Review of Cell Biology*, 1986; **2**: 499–516.

17. Walter P and Blobel G. Translocation of proteins across the endoplasmic reticulum. III. Signal recognition protein (SRP) causes signal sequence-dependent and site-specific arrest of chain elongation that is released by microsomal membranes. *Journal of Cell Biology*, 1981; **91**: 557–61.
18. Pfeffer SR and Rothman JE. Biosynthetic protein transport and sorting by the endoplasmic reticulum and Golgi. *Annual Review of Biochemistry*, 1987; **56**: 829–852.
19. DePierre JW, Andersson G, and Dallner G. Endoplasmic reticulum and Golgi complex. In Arias JM, Jakoby WB, Popper H, Schacter D, and Shafritz DA, eds. Book. New York: Raven Press, 1988: 165–87.
20. Rose JK and Dorns RW. Regulation of protein export from the endoplasmic reticulum. *Annual Review of Cell Biology*, 1988; **4**: 257–88.

2.14.2 Protein secretion, degradation, and function

Wolfgang Gerok and Volker Gross

Protein secretion

Once newly synthesized secretory proteins have been introduced into the lumen of the endoplasmic reticulum, they must be matured and transported. Maturation includes a number of post-translational modifications, for example the formation of disulphide bonds, glycosylation, limited proteolytic cleavage, the assembly of single polypeptide chains to form complex aggregates, sulphation, γ-carboxylation, and hydroxylation. Different secretory proteins undergo different post-translational modifications. Modifications frequently found in secretory liver proteins are the formation of disulphide bonds and glycosylation. The modification reactions occur in distinct organelles of the secretory pathway.

The secretory pathway

Secretory proteins are not found, with only few exceptions (see below), as free soluble proteins in the cytoplasm, but are always located within the lumen of the structures of the secretory pathway.[1-3] They are cotranslationally imported into the lumen of the endoplasmic reticulum. They are transported from the endoplasmic reticulum to the Golgi complex by transitional vesicles, travelling from *cis-* to *trans-*Golgi and leaving the Golgi complex packaged in secretory vesicles. They are exocytosed by fusion of secretory vesicles with the plasma membrane (Fig. 1).

Some proteins, such as basic fibroblast growth factor or interleukin 1, are transported to the cell surface without entering the classical secretory pathway, moving directly to and across the membrane without vesicles. The mechanism of this unconventional secretion is unknown. It is supposed that 'private' transport systems, for example ATP-driven pumps, each specialized for the transport of a polypeptide or small protein, provide the secretion of these proteins.[4-6]

Endoplasmic reticulum

The endoplasmic reticulum is a network of cisternae, tubules, and lamellae that spans the cytoplasm of the hepatocyte.[4,7] It occupies about 15 per cent of the liver cell volume; its surface area is about 10 m^2/g liver. About 60 per cent of the endoplasmic reticulum is dotted with ribosomes (rough endoplasmic reticulum), and 40 per cent is not (smooth endoplasmic reticulum). The rough endoplasmic reticulum is generally arranged in parallel cisternae; its lumen is 200 to 300 Å wide. The smooth endoplasmic reticulum consists of widely dispersed tubules and vesicles; its lumen is 300 to 600 Å wide.

Newly synthesized secretory proteins are commonly free in the lumen of the endoplasmic reticulum, but they may be attached to the luminal side of its membrane during certain phases of their maturation, when they are modified and bound to enzymes in that membrane. Various secretory proteins exhibit different residence times in the endoplasmic reticulum, ranging from 25 to 120 min, before they reach the Golgi complex (Lodish, Nature, 1983; 304: 80; Yeo, JBC, 1985; 260:7896). The reason for this is unclear. It is likely that specific receptors are involved that recognize secretory proteins and trigger their transport to the Golgi complex (Wieland, Cell, 1987; 50:289). Protein mutations, for example replacement of Glu342 to Lys in Z-type α_1-antitrypsin (Jeppson, FEBSLett, 1976; 65:195), and modifications of the carbohydrate moieties of secretory hepatocyte proteins (Gross, JBC, 1983; 258: 12203; Lodish, JCellBiol, 1984; 98:1720), impair the transport of certain of these proteins from the endoplasmic reticulum to the Golgi complex.

The three-dimensional structure of each protein determined by its amino-acid sequence and its specific post-translational modifications is presumably decisive for proper secretion. This structure, for example the folding of the polypeptide chain, is controlled by the transient interactions of the secretory proteins with specific proteins, the chaperones, within the endoplasmic reticulum. Two families of chaperones are identified in the endoplasmic reticulum: the heat-shock protein family (Rothman, Nature, 1994; 372:55) and several calcium-binding phosphoproteins, most notably calnexin and calreticulin (Ou, Nature, 1993; 364:77). As trimming of the oligosaccharide side-chains progresses the secretory glycoprotein α_1-antitrypsin interacts with calnexin, a 88-kDa transmembrane endoplasmic reticulum-resident phosphoprotein (Fig. 2). First, the outermost glucose is removed by glucosidase I, and then the two remaining glucose residues are removed sequentially by glucosidase II. Calnexin binds only glycoproteins with oligosaccharide side-chains trimmed to the innermost glucose residue (Herbert, Cell, 1995; 81:425). Binding to calnexin retains the monoglucosylated glycoprotein in the endoplasmic reticulum until it is correctly folded. Once folding is correct, the protein is free to leave the endoplasmic reticulum. A reglucosylating enzyme, the UDP–glucose: glycoprotein glucosyltransferase, can transfer glucose on to incorrectly folded or denatured, deglucosylated proteins in the endoplasmic reticulum. Thus, the incorrectly folded proteins bind again to calnexin until folding is correct. Then, the innermost glucose residue is again removed by the action of glucosidase II and the deglucosylated protein can leave the endoplasmic reticulum.[8]

Proteins are transported from the endoplasmic reticulum to the Golgi complex in transitional vesicles. These vesicles have a diameter of 20 to 30 nm and possess a coat different from the clathrin coat of endocytic vesicles. Transport from the endoplasmic reticulum to the Golgi requires energy. Lowering of cellular ATP levels blocks the exit of certain proteins from the endoplasmic reticulum (Kabcenell, JCellBiol, 1985; 101:1270). The exact transport mechanisms, however, are still not understood.

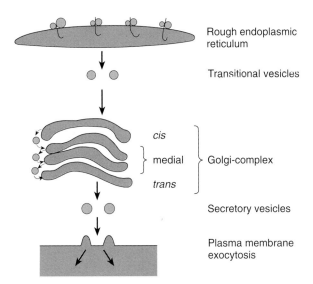

Fig. 1. The secretory pathway.

Golgi complex

The Golgi complex of hepatocytes consists of a stack of four to six cisternae.[9-11] Each cisterna is about 1 nm long and 30 nm wide.

The rims of the cisternae are slightly dilated. The Golgi complex has a typical convex–concave shape; the convex surface faces the nucleus and parts of the endoplasmic reticulum. The convex face of the Golgi complex is called proximal, since this is where secretory proteins arrive from the endoplasmic reticulum. The next one or two stacks belong to the medial Golgi; the one or two distal cisternae at the concave surface constitute the *trans*-Golgi. These different Golgi regions are not only defined morphologically, but also functionally. They have a different enzyme repertoire (Farquahr, JCellBiol, 1981; 91:77) and thus exert different functions in the post-translational modification reactions. This is well understood for protein glycosylation (see below).

The unidirectional vectorial transit of proteins from endoplasmic reticulum through the *cis*- and *trans*-Golgi cisternae to the plasma membrane is due to repeated rounds of budding and fusion of transport vesicles. The mechanisms of these processes are energy-dependent protein–protein interactions (Fig. 3).

For budding 'coat proteins' (cops), which are not identical with clathrin, small GTP-binding proteins and an ADP-ribosylation factor (**ARF**), another small specific GTP-binding protein, assemble at the membrane of the 'donor' compartment. The assembly is presumably mediated by myristyl-CoA. For assembly and budding, ATP is required. The resulting vesicle is coated on its outer (cytoplasmic) surface with proteins forming an electron-dense layer.

For fusion the coated vesicles must lose their coats in a reaction that probably requires or is linked to GTP hydrolysis. The fusion of the uncoated vesicle with the target membrane is mediated by the interaction of specific proteins: A *N*-ethylmaleimide-sensitive fusion protein (**NSF**), several small soluble NSF attachment proteins (**SNAPs**), and the SNAP-receptor protein are integrated within the target membrane. ATP hydrolysis by NSF is needed to fuse membranes; at the same time NSF dissociates from the target membrane. The biophysical mechanisms of fusion are unknown, as yet. It is an interesting speculation that fusion is promoted by the creation of a protein bridge between adjacent bilayered surfaces, forming a kind of 'gap junction' with an internal aqueous channel and thus destabilizing the bilayers of the membranes.[12,13]

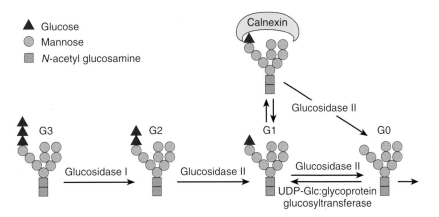

Fig. 2. Model of trimming of the carbohydrate side-chains and reglucosylation of α_1-antitrypsin in relation to interaction with calnexin as chaperone in the endoplasmic reticulum (from reference 8).

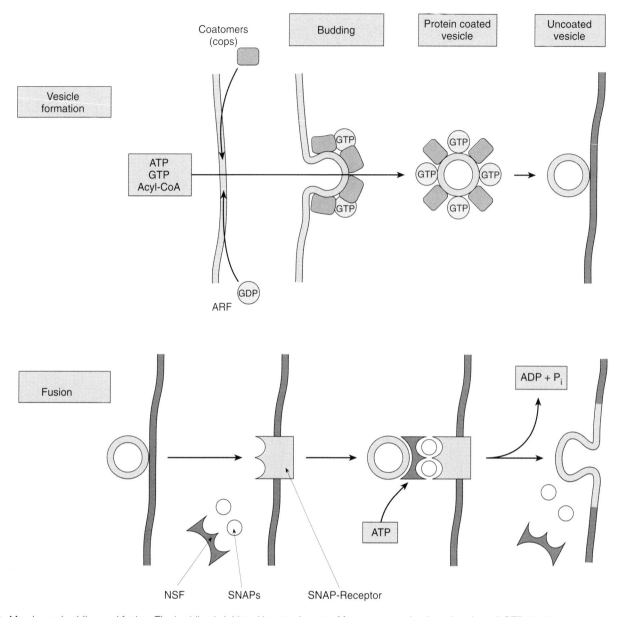

Fig. 3. Membrane budding and fusion. The budding is initiated by attachment of four coat proteins (cops) and small GTP-binding proteins to the membrane. The attachment is mediated by the CoA-derivatives of higher fatty acids. Hydrolytic cleavage of ATP is necessary for the budding and forming the 'cop'-coated vesicle as well for its uncoating. The fusion involves the interactions of the uncoated vesicle with several proteins (NSF, SNAPs; see text) and with a receptor protein for SNAPs in the target membrane. Also, the process of fusion is energy-dependent (modified from reference 13).

A system of membranes, called the *trans*-Golgi network,[14] is interconnected with the furthest *trans*-Golgi cisternae. This membrane system seems to be the cross-roads for sorting of both exocytic and endocytic proteins. Cisternae and vesicles in the *trans*-Golgi have an acidic interior.[15,16] This is maintained by a proton-translocating ATPase (Glickman, JCellBiol, 1983; 97:1303). The acidic interior plays an essential part in the proper function of these structures, since inhibitors of acidification, for example weak bases such as chloroquine (De Duve, EurJBioch, 1983; 137:391) or carb-oxylic ionophores such as monensin, inhibit both the modification reactions located in this compartment and protein secretion.[17]

The proteins that are synthesized in the endoplasmic reticulum and pass through the Golgi apparatus are sorted in the *trans*-Golgi network according to their final destination.[4,18] The mechanism of sorting is well understood for lysosomal proteins: lysosomal hydrolases are modified by forming mannose-6-phosphate in the *cis*-Golgi-network. In the *trans*-Golgi network a mannose-6-phosphate receptor binds the modified protein. Vesicles budding from the *trans*-Golgi-network with this receptor concentrate and transport the lysosomal hydrolases to endosomes, where after fusion the hydrolases dissociate from the receptors at a low pH. The receptors are recycled to the Golgi apparatus. In late endosomes the phosphate is removed from mannose. By fusion of late endosomes with lysosomes the enzymes arrive at their definitive destination.[19,20]

Secretory vesicles

Secretory proteins are transported from the *trans*-Golgi region to the cell surface by secretory vesicles.[18] There are at least two types of secretory vesicles, constitutive and regulated. Constitutive secretion is continuous. Proteins are not stored in constitutive secretory vesicles, but are rapidly transported to the cell surface and exocytosed. The rate of protein secretion is thus proportional to the rate of protein synthesis. In regulated vesicles, proteins are stored and concentrated, and secreted only upon a specific signal.

In polarized cells such as the hepatocyte the plasma membrane has two distinct domains: the basolateral (sinusoidal) and the apical (canicular). The two domains are separated by tight junctions and have different types and amounts of proteins.

The differences between plasma membrane domains may be realized by two mechanisms. (1) The membrane components could be delivered to all regions of the plasma membrane but then be selectively stabilized or removed in specific domains. (2) Transport vesicles loaded with specific proteins for distinct domains mediate a targeted delivery of the appropriate membrane components. If different proteins are secreted through the sinusoidal and canicular membrane, this second mechanism must be used. The sorting of proteins for distinct membrane domains and their arrival in different transport vesicles occurs in the *trans*-Golgi network. It is supposed that, in some cases, vesicles with proteins for both basolateral and canicular membranes have distinct sorting signals that direct them to the appropriate domain, whereas in other cases only vesicles with proteins destined for one of the two domains have a sorting signal, while the other domain is reached by random delivery without a sorting signal. However, the signals responsible for these sorting processes in the liver are not known.

Proteins that have the characteristics of sorting carriers have been purified from canine pancreas (Chung, Science, 1989; 243: 192).

Microtubules are involved in the movement of secretory vesicles from the Golgi to the cell surface. Inhibition of microtubule polymerization, e.g. by colchicine, impairs the secretion of most plasma proteins synthesized by the liver (Gross, EurJBioch, 1982; 129:317). Proteins are exocytosed by fusion of secretory vesicles with the plasma membrane.[21]

Post-translational modifications of secretory proteins

Formation of disulphide bonds

Disulphide bonds[22] are formed between two cysteine residues. They are an important stabilizing force in the secondary structure of a protein. In general, disulphide bonds are found in secretory proteins (but not all) and in certain membrane proteins, but not in cytoplasmic proteins. The formation of disulphide bonds occurs in the lumen of the endoplasmic reticulum while the polypeptide chain is still growing. Disulphide bonds can either be formed sequentially, i.e., the first cysteine reacts with the second, the third with the fourth, etc., or unsequentially, when cysteine residues that are not neighbours are brought together due to the three-dimensional structure of the protein. Similarly, disulphide bonds can be formed between different polypeptide chains of a multimeric protein.

Glycosylation

There are two basic types of protein glycosylation:[23]

(1) *N*-glycosylation, i.e., attachment of oligosaccharides to certain asparagine residues of the protein backbone;
(2) *O*-glycosylation, i.e., attachment of oligosaccharides to certain serine or threonine residues.

Except for albumin, most secretory liver proteins are glycoproteins. Many of them are *N*-glycosylated; only a few carry *O*-linked oligosaccharides.

N-glycosylation

N-glycosylated proteins carry oligosaccharide side-chains attached to asparagine.[24-28] Only asparagine residues in the sequence Asn-*x*-Ser or Asn-*x*-Thr (*x* represents any amino acid, except possibly proline and aspartic acid) can be glycosylated (Marshall, AnnRevBiochem, 1972; 41:673). However, not every asparagine in such a sequence is glycosylated. Obviously, besides the primary structure, the tertiary structure of the protein determines which asparagine residues are glycosylated.

There are three major types of *N*-linked oligosaccharides:

(1) complex-type oligosaccharides,
(2) high-mannose-type oligosaccharides,
(3) hybrid-type oligosaccharides.

Their structures are shown in Fig. 4. Almost without exception, secretory liver glycoproteins carry oligosaccharides of the complex type.

The three types of *N*-linked oligosaccharides share a common precursor and are synthesized by the same pathway. The common precursor is a Glc3Man9GlcNAc2-oligosaccharide, which is synthesized lipid-bound in the endoplasmic reticulum (Fig. 5) and is cotranslationally transferred to nascent glycoproteins in the lumen of the endoplasmic reticulum.[24,29] The lipid carrier of the precursor oligosaccharide is dolichol (**Dol**), a long lipid containing 15 to 19 isoprene (C5) units. The topography of glycosylation reactions in the endoplasmic reticulum has been extensively studied.[30] Two activated (UDP-)GlcNAc and five activated (GDP-)Man are sequentially added to dolichol phosphate. This occurs at the cytoplasmic site of the endoplasmic reticulum. The intermediate Dol-P-P-GlcNAc2-Man5 is then translocated to the luminal site of the endoplasmic reticulum. The subsequent four mannose and three glucose residues are transferred to the dolichol pyrophosphate-bound oligosaccharide, not directly from sugar nucleotides, but from their respective lipid intermediates Dol-P-Man and Dol-P-Glc. This requires transport of mannose and glucose from cytoplasmic nucleotide sugars across the membrane of the endoplasmic reticulum. The three terminal glucose residues of the precursor oligosaccharide are a signal for the transfer of the carbohydrate chain from dolichol to protein.

Once the oligosaccharide chain (GlcNAc2Man9Glc3) has been transferred to a protein (step 1), oligosaccharide processing occurs (Fig. 6). The three terminal glucose residues are rapidly cleaved off in the endoplasmic reticulum. Two glucosidases are involved in this

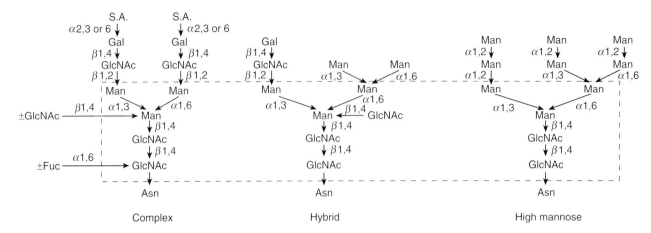

Fig. 4. Structure of the major types of *N*-linked oligosaccharides (from Kornfeld, AnnRevBiochem, 1985; 54:631).

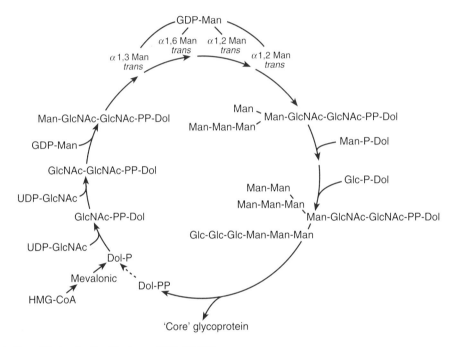

Fig. 5. The dolichol cycle (from Elbein, AnnRevBiochem, 1987; 56:497).

reaction (Kornfeld, JBC, 1978; 253:7771; Burns, JBC, 1982; 257: 9991). Glucosidase I removes the outermost glucose (step 2), which is linked $\alpha1$–2, and glucosidase II the two inner glucoses linked $\alpha1$–3 (step 3). The resulting deglucosylated oligosaccharide GlcNAc2Man9 represents a high-mannose type structure.

When complex-type oligosaccharides are to be synthesized, further trimming occurs. The four ($\alpha1$–2)-linked mannose residues are removed by mannosidase I. Two different enzymes with mannosidase I activity exist. One is located in the endoplasmic reticulum (Bischoff, JBC, 1983; 258:7907), and cleaves not more than two mannose residues (step 4); the other is found in the *cis*-Golgi region. Golgi mannosidase I (Tabas, JBC, 1979; 254: 11 655) leads to the formation of GlcNAc2Man5 intermediates (step 5). Thereafter, GlcNAc can be transferred from the mannose-linked $\alpha1$–3 to the β-linked mannose by GlcNAc transferase I (step 6) (Oppenheimer, JBC, 1981; 256:799). The resulting GlcNAc2Man5GlcNAc is a suitable substrate for mannosidase II (Tulsiani, JBC, 1983; 258:

7578), which cleaves the peripheral $\alpha1$–3- and $\alpha1$–6-linked mannose residues (step 7). These reactions are localized to the medial Golgi.

The compound formed by mannosidase II is a substrate for GlcNAc transferase II (Harpaz, JBC, 1980; 255:4885), which transfers GlcNAc from the mannose-linked $\alpha1$–6 to the β-linked mannose (step 8). In addition, a fucose residue can be transferred $\alpha1$–6 to the proximal GlcNAc by the action of a fucosyl transferase (step 9) (Wilson, BBResComm, 1976; 72:909). The assembly of biantennary complex-type oligosaccharides is then completed by the stepwise addition of galactose (step 10) (Rao, Biochem, 1978; 17:5632) and sialic acid residues (step 11) (Weinstein, JBC, 1982; 257: 13835). This transfer is located in the *trans*-Golgi region. The formation of triantennary and tetra-antennary oligosaccharides requires the addition of more than one GlcNAc residue to each α-linked mannose.

When mannosidase II activity is impaired, only one antenna [that linked to the ($\alpha1$–3)-linked mannose] can be processed to a

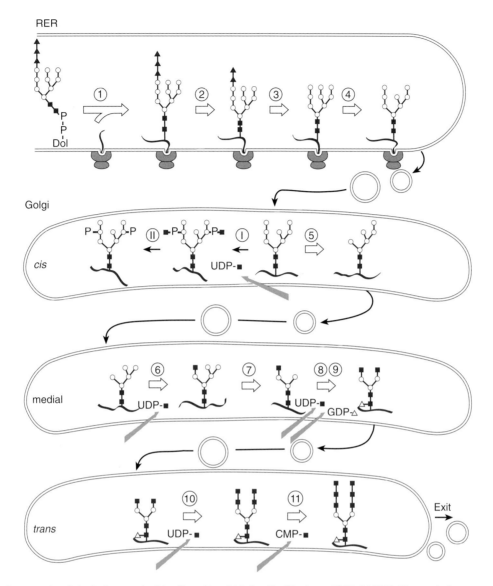

Fig. 6. Processing of asparagine-linked oligosaccharides (from Kornfeld, AnnRevBiochem, 1985; 54:631). The symbols represent ■ *N*-acetylglucosamine; ○, mannose; ▲, glucose; △, fucose; ●, galactose; ◆, sialic acid.

complex-type structure, while the other remains in a high-mannose type form. The resulting oligosaccharide has a hybrid structure (Gross, JBC, 1983; 258:4032).

As discussed above, most plasma proteins are *N*-glycosylated. One to six *N*-linked carbohydrate side-chains can be found per polypeptide chain. It is important to understand the function of *N*-linked complex-type oligosaccharides of secretory proteins. In many, but not all, cases, glycosylation is needed for a normal rate of secretion. Inhibition of *de novo* glycosylation or even inhibition of the processing glucosidases in the endoplasmic reticulum leads to impaired secretion of a number of hepatic proteins. The respective proteins accumulate in the endoplasmic reticulum (Gross, EurJ-Bioch, 1982; 129:317; Gross, JBC, 1983; 258: 12 203; Lodish, JCellBiol, 1984; 98:1720).[31]

With respect to the stability of secretory proteins, there is evidence that carbohydrate side-chains protect the proteins from proteolytic breakdown (Andus, EurJBioch, 1983; 136:253).[31]

The circulatory lifetime of secretory liver glycoproteins is greatly determined by their carbohydrate side-chains. Complete lack of their complex-type oligosaccharide side-chains leads to a rapid clearance of lower molecular-weight glycoproteins by the kidney.[32,33] Glycoproteins not properly processed to the sialylated complex type are removed from the circulation by specific receptors. High-mannose-type and hybrid-type glycoproteins are removed by a Man/GlcNAc receptor localized on macrophages and macrophage-derived cells.[34] Carbohydrates lacking their terminal sialic acid residues are bound by the galactose receptor of hepatocytes.[35]

The glycosylation pattern of liver proteins can be changed by various diseases.[36] During acute inflammatory processes a relative decrease of the branching of complex-type oligosaccharides linked to acute-phase proteins is observed (Mackiewicz, Electrophoresis, 1989; 10:830). A number of cytokines that also regulate the synthesis of these proteins, for example, interleukin (**IL**) 6, leukaemia inhibitory factor, interferon-γ, transforming growth factor-β,

IL-11, oncostatin M, and ciliary neurotrophic factor (**CNTF**) are involved in these processes (Gryska, AnnNYAcadSci 1995; 762: 413).

Chronic liver diseases are in general accompanied by reduced sialylation and increased glycan branching, whereas cancer is accompanied by increased sialylation and increased fucosylation. In patients with hepatocellular carcinoma, transferrin with increased biantennary complex-type oligosaccharides with core fucose was found (Matsumoto, CCActa, 1994; 224:1).

In alcoholics the sialic acid content of transferrin is reduced (Stibler, ClinExpRes, 1981; 5:545), but a reduction in galactose and N-acetyl-glucosamine has been reported as well (Stibler, ClinExpRes, 1986; 10:61). The appearance of carbohydrate-deficient transferrin is related to the amount of alcohol consumed rather than the degree of alcoholic liver disease (Stibler, ClinExpRes, 1987; 11: 468).

O-glycosylation

O-linked oligosaccharides are typical of epithelial mucins and are only rarely found on secretory liver proteins, e.g. haemopexin (Takahashi, PNAS, 1984; 81:2021), fetuin (Gejyo, JBC, 1983; 258: 4966), α_2-heat-stable glycoprotein (Bergh, JBC, 1983; 258:7430). In contrast to N-linked oligosaccharides, O-linked oligosaccharides are not synthesized as a lipid-linked precursor in the endoplasmic reticulum. O-glycosylation is localized in the Golgi complex. O-linked oligosaccharides are formed by the sequential transfer of activated monosaccharides to the protein backbone by specific glycosyl transferases. Activated nucleoside diphosphate or nucleoside monophosphate sugars are transported into the lumen of the Golgi by special transport antiports.[27] The glycosyl transferases have a high specificity, both for the sugar to be transferred and for the sugar or amino-acid acceptor.

Generally the O-linked oligosaccharides of secretory liver proteins have a Gal(β1–3)GalNAc core linked to serine or threonine residues of the protein backbone. To this core at least one sialic acid residue is bound [frequently in an (α2–3-linkage to galactose].[37]

Limited proteolysis

With a few exceptions all secretory proteins have an N-terminal signal sequence that targets them to the endoplasmic reticulum.[38, 39] Since the signal sequence is rapidly cleaved off by the signal peptidase,[40] once the protein has entered the lumen of the endoplasmic reticulum those secretory proteins still carrying their signal sequences (preproteins) cannot be detected *in vivo*. However, some secretory proteins are synthesized as longer precursors, which can be found intracellularly. These longer precursors are called proproteins. The additional amino acids in the pro form can either be located at the N-terminus (e.g. prealbumin), at both ends (e.g. proglucagon), or in the middle of a polypeptide chain (e.g. proinsulin). In the case of albumin the proprotein differs from the mature protein by an aminoterminal extension of six amino acids.[41] Proalbumin is converted into albumin with a single cleavage by an endoprotease found in secretory vesicles.[42] Similarly, conversion of other proproteins, for example the vitamin K-dependent coagulation factors prothrombin, factor VII, factor IX, factor X, and protein C and protein S,[43] to mature proteins is a late step in the secretory pathway.

Other post-translational modifications

Other post-translational modifications occurring in secretory liver proteins are sulphation, γ-carboxylation, and hydroxylation.

Glycoproteins carrying asparagine-linked oligosaccharides can be further modified by sulphation of mannose and N-acetyl-hexosamine residues.[26] The topography of sulphation reactions appears to be very similar to that of the terminal glycosylation in the Golgi apparatus.[27]

Vitamin K-dependent blood coagulation proteins, which are synthesized in the liver, contain γ-carboxyglutamic acid residues in their aminoterminal domain.[43,44] With the exception of prothrombin, they contain another modified amino acid, β-hydroxyaspartic acid (Drakenberg, PNAS, 1983; 80:1802). The biological function of this hydroxylation is still unknown.

Regulation of secretory proteins

Sites of regulation

The amount of a specific protein secreted by the liver can be controlled on different levels: control of transcription, control of translation, and control of degradation. For the majority of proteins the initiation of transcription is the most important point of control. Also, the regulatory effects of exogenous factors are predominantly mediated by stimulation or inhibition of the transcriptional process. The transcription of eukaryotic genes is controlled by regulatory proteins, which bind to regulatory sequences of genes. Some of the regulatory proteins are transcriptional activators, while others are repressors. With regard to the interaction of protein and DNA, several types of regulatory proteins are described. The regulatory sequences are extremely variable with regard to their position in relation to the regulated gene.

The translation can be controlled by specific proteins, which bind either to a specific sequence in the 5′-untranslated region of distinct mRNA, blocking its translation, or to a binding site in the 3′-untranslated region, stimulating translation by protection of the distinct mRNA against degradation. An example is the regulation of the synthesis of ferritin and the transferrin receptor protein.[45]

The degradation of proteins is performed by lysosomal proteases by the ubiquitine–proteasomal system or by cytosolic proteases, the calpains. The lysosomal degradative pathway is unselective. The protein is coated with a membrane, forming an autophagosome that can fuse with a lysosome. For degradation by the ubiquitine–proteasomal system the misfolded, damaged, or denatured protein is marked by covalent binding of a small protein, called ubiquitin. The first ubiquitin molecule adds to a lysine residue of the target protein; thereafter additional ubiquitin moieties are covalently attached, forming a multiubiquitine chain. This structure is recognized by a receptor in the proteasome (Fig. 7). These large protein complexes are present in many copies in the cell. Each proteasome consists of multiple proteins forming a cylinder (20s complex), and a 'stopper'. The proteins of the cylindrical structure are proteases with active sites on the inner site of the cylinder. Some stopper proteins can hydrolyse ATP. The ubiquitin-marked protein is taken up in the lumen of the cylinder. After closure by the stopper-protein complex the enclosed protein is degraded by the proteases to short peptides, which are then released.[46-48]

The significance of calpains is not well understood. They are a group of proteases in the cytosol that are activated by increase of

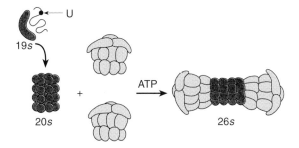

Fig. 7. Protein degradation by the ubiquitin–proteasome system. The damaged or misfolded protein is marked for degradation by ubiquitin, which is covalently bound to lysyl residues of the protein. One component of the proteasome (19s complex) recognizes the ubiquitin-marked protein and transports it in the lumen of the 20s complex. This complex consists of four rings, each formed by seven different proteins. Their proteolytic activity is localized at the luminal side of the cylindrical complex. After enclosure of the ubiquitin-marked protein into the lumen, the ubiquitin residue is cleaved off and the 20s complex is 'stoppered' by two protein complexes. Within this 26s complex the protein is degraded (modified after[46]).

the intracellular Ca^{2+}-concentration.[49] It is supposed that calpains are involved in the process of apoptosis.

Factors in regulation

Factors that influence the hepatic synthesis and secretion of secretory proteins are: nutritional (inclusive of ethanol), hormonal, and cytokines. The influence of nutrients and hormones on hepatic protein synthesis and secretion has been well known for many years. Recent investigations have demonstrated that nutrients and hormones exert their effects on metabolism and gene expression, at least in part, by modification of the cellular hydration state, with consequent alterations of cell volume such as swelling or shrinkage.[50,51] Therefore, in the following, the general effects of the cell hydration state on the protein metabolism of the liver is first described, followed by special aspects of nutrition (inclusive of ethanol) and various hormones. The last part deals with the role of cytokines for the synthesis of acute-phase proteins by the liver.

Effect of hepatic cellular hydration state

The cellular hydration state depends on the intra-/extracellular concentration gradients of several ions, especially K^+, Na^+, and Cl^-, and of the intracellular concentration of organic osmolytes. An intracellular increase of ions and/or osmolytes induces a swelling, an intracellular decrease a shrinkage of the cell.

Cellular hydration state and cell volume are dynamic and change within minutes under the influence of aniso-osmolarity, nutrients, and hormones. Most importantly, small fluctuations of cell hydration, i.e. cell volume, act as a separate and potent signal for cellular metabolism and gene expression.

Aniso-osmotic exposure may primarily be seen under experimental conditions, although, during intestinal absorption of water, portal venous blood may become slightly hypotonic, and under pathological conditions relevant severe aniso-osmolarities have been documented (Lee, NEJM, 1994; 331:439; Häussinger, Gastro, 1994; 107:1475). Physiologically more important, however, are cell volume changes due to the uptake of nutritients, especially amino acids, and under the influence of hormones. Amino acids are taken up from the hepatocyte by cotransport with Na^+, which is extracted in exchange for K^+ by the electrogenic Na^+/K^+-ATPase.

The result is an intracellular accumulation of amino acids and K^+, leading to hepatocyte swelling (Häussinger, EurJBioch, 1990; 188:689; Wettstein, BiolChemHS, 1990; 371:493). A regulatory

mechanism with K^+ efflux prevents cell swelling from becoming excessive, but the hepatocytes remain in a swollen state as long as the amino acid load continues. Importantly, amino acid-induced cell swelling and volume-regulatory responses occur upon exposure to amino acids in the physiological concentration range (Wettstein, BiolChemHS, 1990; 371:493), and physiological fluctuations in the portal amino-acid concentration are accompanied by parallel alterations of liver-cell volume. The degree of amino acid-induced swelling seems to be related largely to the steady-state intra-/extracellular amino acid concentration gradient.

Hormones are potent modulators of liver-cell volume by affecting the activity of volume-regulatory ion-transport systems (Hallbrucker, EurJBioch, 1991; 199:467; Vom Dahl, BiochemJ, 1991; 280:105; Al-Habori, BiochemJ, 1992; 282:789). In liver, insulin stimulates Na^+/H^+ exchange, Na^+, K^+ and Cl^- cotransport, and the Na^+/K^+-ATPase. The concerted activation of these transporters leads to cellular accumulation of K^+, Na^+ and Cl^-, and consequently cell swelling. This effect is strengthened by the increased uptake of amino acids under the influence of insulin. In contrast, glucagon activates Na^+/K^+-ATPase, but simultaneously depletes cellular K^+, probably due to opening of K^+ channels. As a result of the cellular Na^+ and K^+ depletion, hepatocytes shrink (vom Dahl, BiochemJ, 1991; 280:105; Hallbrucker, PflügersArch, 1991; 418:519). The physiological relevance is underlined by the finding that half-maximal effects of insulin and glucagon on liver-cell hydration are found at hormone concentrations normally present in portal venous blood *in vivo* (vom Dahl, BiochemJ, 1991; 278: 771). Thus, transmembrane ion movements under the influence of hormones are an integral part of hormonal signal-transduction mechanisms, with alterations of cellular hydration acting as another second messenger of hormone action.

Recent evidence suggests that the cellular hydration state is an important determinant of cell function. Nutrients and hormones exert their effects on metabolism and gene expression in part by a modification of cell volume.[51] The alterations of metabolism occur within minutes in response to cell-volume changes and are fully reversible upon restoration of the resting cell volume. There is a dose response relation between the extent of hydration change that remains after the completion of volume-regulatory ion fluxes and the metabolic response. Several metabolic effects of hormones or amino acids can be mimicked by equipotent aniso-osmotic cell swelling or shrinkage. Also, some hormone-induced changes in cell

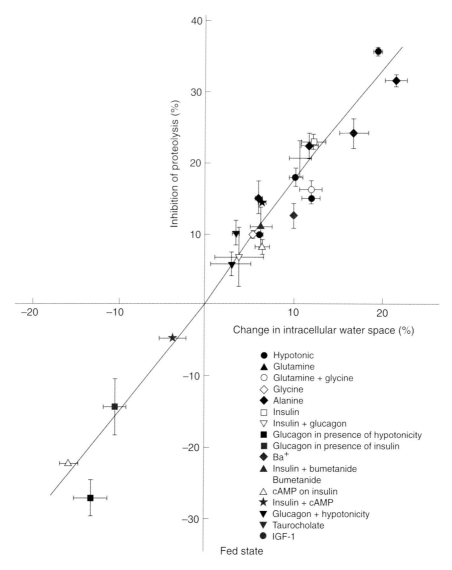

Fig. 8. Relation between cell hydration state and proteolysis in the liver. Changes in cell hydration state (abscissa) alter proteolysis in liver cells: cell shrinkage stimulates proteolysis; cell swelling inhibits it. The relation is independent of the mode by which the changes of cellular hydration are induced (from reference 51).

volume are prevented. Thus, changes in cellular hydration in response to physiological stimuli by nutrients and hormones are an important and until recently unrecognized signal that helps to adapt cellular metabolism to environmental alterations.

In the hepatic metabolism of proteins, hepatocellular hydration state is a major control point of proteolysis (Häussinger, FEBSLett, 1991; 283:70). Cell swelling inhibits, and conversely cell shrinkage stimulates, protein degradation under conditions when proteolysis is not already fully activated. There is a close relation between proteolytic activity and hepatocellular hydration regardless of whether the latter is modified by hormones, amino acids, K^+-channel blockers or anisotonic exposure (Fig. 8), indicating that the hydration changes are the common mechanism underlying proteolysis control by these heterogeneous effectors.

Apparently the known antiproteolytic effect of insulin and several (but not all) amino acids is mediated in large part by cell swelling, whereas stimulation of proteolysis by glucagon is apparently mediated by cell shrinkage (Häussinger, FEBSLett, 1991; 283:70). The

nutritional state exerts its control on proteolysis by determining the swelling potencies of hormones and amino acids.

Liver-cell hydration also affects protein synthesis in the opposite direction to proteolysis: cell shrinkage inhibits, whereas cell swelling stimulates protein synthesis (Meijer, EurJBioch, 1993; 215:494). The cAMP-induced inhibition of protein synthesis in liver may, at least in part, be ascribed to cell shrinkage, because equipotent hyperosmotic cell shrinkage decreases protein synthesis to a comparable extent. A close relation exists between cell shrinkage and the inhibition of protein synthesis under the influence of hyperosmotic exposure, cAMP, and vasopressin. On the other hand, insulin has no significant effect on protein synthesis associated with cell swelling. So changes in cell volume may be only one factor among several mediating the hormonal control of protein synthesis.

The mechanisms by which cellular hydration exerts control on proteolysis are not clear. Intact microtubular structures are required. Recent evidence suggests a role for protein phosphorylation in mediating the relation between cell volume and proteolysis. This

Table 1 Molecular mechanisms for the effect of fasting or protein–caloric-deficient diet on hepatic protein synthesis

Decreased availability of amino acids
Decreased RNA content (increased RNAse activity)
Disaggregation of membrane-bound polysomes
Decrease of cellular hydration state
Alteration of subcellular mRNA distribution

could reside at the level of ribosomal protein phosphorylation (Luiken, BiochemSocTrans, 1994; 22:458), acidification of pre-lysosomal vesicular compartments (Schreiber, BiochemJ, 1994; 303: 113), and possibly at the level of microtubule-associated proteins. On a long-term scale, cellular hydration affects celluar metabolism by modifying gene expression. This involves not only osmo-regulatory genes, such as genes for osmolyte transporters, but also genes coding for proteins that are not linked to volume regulation (for review, see[51]).

Fasting, protein–caloric-deficient diet

All studies have demonstrated that under fasting or protein-deficient diet conditions, hepatic protein synthesis decreases. Refeeding with a diet containing all amino acids results in an increase of protein synthesis.[52–55] Possible molecular mechanisms for the effect of fasting on hepatic protein synthesis are summarized in Table 1. These mechanisms are induced at least in part by the cellular hydration state.

Decreased availability of nutritional amino acids may reduce hepatic protein synthesis. During short periods (fewer than 2 days) of fasting the reduced supply of nutritional amino acids to the liver is compensated for by degradation of proteins in extrahepatic organs, especially muscle, with transport of the resulting amino acids to the liver, or by degradation of liver proteins. Tryptophan probably plays a crucial part (see below). The limitation of activated amino acids (aminoacyl tRNAs) decreases the rate of elongation in protein synthesis.

The RNA content of the liver is decreased by starvation for at least 48 h. Since the decreased RNA content precedes the decrease in protein synthesis, the latter was thought to be secondary. The reduced RNA content in starvation might be due to the activation or release of ribonucleases. Increased ribonuclease activity is demonstrable in malnutrition.

Disaggregation of membrane-bound polysomes in the liver under fasting may be followed by a reduction of protein synthesis and secretion by the liver. The molecular mechanism of the disaggregation is unknown. In contrast to the membrane-bound polysomes the free cytoplasmic polysomes are not disaggregated.

An alteration of the subcellular distribution of albumin mRNA under the influence of fasting was demonstrated with RNA–cDNA hybridization. After starvation for 18 h, total cytoplasmic albumin mRNA was decreased and disaggregation of membrane-bound polysomes was demonstrated.

ATP and GTP as high-energy phosphate compounds are essential at many steps in protein synthesis and secretion (see above). GDP competes with GTP and therefore inhibits initial steps and elongation processes in protein synthesis. Depletion of ATP and GTP is generally followed by inhibition of translation.

The effect of refeeding with a diet containing all amino acids depends on whether protein deficiency has been long- or short-term. In long-term deficiency, protein synthesis is reduced at the transcriptional as well as translational level. This defect is less rapidly reversible by refeeding than after short-term deficiency with a defect only at the translational level, in line with the observation that the content of RNA is rate-limiting in the refeeding condition (Conde, BiochemJ, 1980; 192:935).

Tryptophan has a special and crucial role. This amino acid alone can correct many of the abnormalities in hepatic protein synthesis under starvation. Increased RNA content, reaggregation of membrane-bound polysomes, increased transcription rates, and increased transport of mRNAs from the nucleus to the cytoplasm were demonstrated after refeeding of tryptophan and are viewed as possible mechanisms for the effect of tryptophan on protein synthesis. In addition, under tryptophan refeeding the re-utilization of mRNAs, which are stored as mRNPs, has been suggested.[54,55]

The question of whether a disproportionate or proportionate reduction of the synthesis and secretion of various proteins takes place under starvation is controversial. In the majority of studies the synthesis of all proteins is similarly reduced under starvation.[55] However, there may be a disproportionate reduction of protein synthesis under the influence of fasting, which may be explained by differences in the quantity or quality of mRNAs for specific proteins, or by different affinities of various mRNAs for initiation factors. Such differences of affinity have not yet been demonstrated in hepatocytes, but have been found in other cell types with starvation, e.g. myeloma cells and reticulocytes.

Effect of alcohol

There are many studies on the influence of alcohol on hepatic protein synthesis and secretion (for reviews, see[53,56–58]). The reasons for their conflicting results are the various experimental models, the different effects of alcohol on protein synthesis or secretion under various conditions, and the types of proteins investigated.

Acute alcohol administration *in vitro* inhibits the synthesis of secretory proteins. This effect is associated with disaggregation of membrane-bound polysomes. However, when alcohol metabolism is blocked with 4-methyl-pyrazole, protein synthesis is still depressed, but the polysomes are not disaggregated. Therefore, disaggregation of polysomes is a concomitant phenomenon, but probably not the reason for the inhibition of protein synthesis by alcohol.[58] Experimental evidence exists for the inhibition of aminoacyl-tRNA synthetases by acute alcohol administration followed by blockage of polypeptide chain elongation (David, JBC, 1983; 258:7702). In contrast, acute alcohol administration *in vivo* inhibits only the secretion of proteins, whereas the synthesis of hepatic proteins is unchanged.[57]

Studies with chronic alcohol administration are more relevant to alcoholic liver disease in man. A diet with more than 36 per cent of the caloric content as alcohol induces an increased synthesis of albumin and constituent hepatic proteins associated with a decreased protein secretion (Zern, Hepatol, 1983; 313:7). This defect in the secretory process has been demonstrated for albumin and for glycoproteins. Glycoproteins are retained in the endoplasmic reticulum (Tuma, Gastro, 1981; 80:273; Sorrel, Gastro, 1983; 84:

580). Alcohol inhibits the secretion step after incorporation of the terminal sugars in the carbohydrate chains (Volentine, Gastro, 1984; 86:228). A consequence of the secretory defect is swelling of hepatocytes by retention of protein and water. The secretory defect does not involve all secretory proteins uniformly. Synthesis and secretion of lipoproteins are enhanced after alcohol administration.

Acetaldehyde is probably an important mediator of the defect in hepatic protein synthesis and secretion after alcohol administration.[58] Inhibition of alcohol oxidation to acetaldehyde protects against the alcohol effects (Volentine, Gastro, 1984; 86: 225).Covalent binding of acetaldehyde to hepatic proteins or to albumin may lead to metabolic and structural derangement and ultimately to cell death in the liver (Donohke, ArchBiochBiophys, 1983; 222:239).

Effect of hormones

Alterations of hepatic protein synthesis by hormones are well-known phenomena through observations in endocrine disorders with hyper- or hypoproduction of a particular hormone (for review, see[55]). However, the effect of a single hormone on hepatic protein synthesis in vivo is difficult to delineate. The reason is that several hormones frequently interact in producing a metabolic or another functional effect. Moreover, hormones may influence the nutritional state and vice versa, and it is therefore often hard to decide whether the effect is caused by the hormone or by the nutritional state or both. Finally, a specific hormone can affect protein synthesis in various organs in a different and often controversial manner, so that the exchange of metabolites between the organs can modify the original hormone effect in the particular organ. Protein biosynthesis in the liver can be affected by a particular hormone at several molecular levels.

Insulin

Insulin has an anabolic effect: it stimulates protein synthesis (Clark, BiochemJ, 1980; 190:615) and RNA synthesis in the liver (Horvat, Nature, 1980; 286:906), and inhibits proteolysis (Häussinger, FEBSLett, 1991; 283:70). Studies with hepatocytes and with isolated, perfused livers of diabetic animals have demonstrated that hepatic protein biosynthesis is diminished in insulin deficiency (Jefferson, JBC, 1983; 258:1369). Synthesis of secretory proteins is more reduced than synthesis of constituent proteins. Albumin synthesis and secretion is greatly reduced. Studies of protein biosynthesis in cell-free systems, and with cDNA hybridization, showed a significant reduction of the albumin mRNA content with insulin deficiency, and normalization of albumin mRNA and albumin biosynthesis with the addition of insulin (Jefferson, JBC, 1983; 258:1369). However, the reason for the reduced albumin mRNA content and diminished protein biosynthesis might also be the reduced nutritional state or structural disorganization, for example disorganization of the rough endoplasmic reticulum in insulin-deficient diabetes.

Glucagon

Glucagon diminishes hepatic protein biosynthesis. This was shown in vivo, in isolated hepatocytes, and in liver slices. The effect is mediated by cAMP, which activates protein kinases in the liver. The result is phosphorylation, and therefore inactivation, of the initiation factor eIF2. Excess of eIF2 in the experimental system overcomes the inhibitory effect of glucagon. Thus, the cAMP-dependent phosphorylation–dephosphorylation of eIF2 is proposed as a means for the regulation of protein biosynthesis (Ranu, FEBSLett, 1980; 112:211).

Thyroid hormones

Thyroxine and tri-iodothyronine increase hepatic protein synthesis (Hertzberg, JBC, 1981; 256:563; Peavy, AmJPhysiol, 1981; 240: E19). This was shown in human and animal studies in vivo and in vitro.

The effect of thyroid hormones is primarily the induction of RNA synthesis. In animals without thyroids, the liver mRNA and rRNA content is diminished. Tri-iodothyronine induces a rise in nuclear RNA synthesis. A direct stimulation of transcription of specific genes by thyroid hormones has also been demonstrated (Sul, JBC, 1983; 259:555).

Growth hormone

The effect of growth hormone on hepatic protein synthesis was shown by hypophysectomy, which is followed by decreased protein and albumin synthesis, a significant reduction of albumin mRNA, and an increased RNAse activity in the liver. These effects could be reversed by growth hormone. They are at least in part mediated by somatomedins. However, the weight loss after hypophysectomy, and the weight gain after administration of growth hormone, demonstrate that nutritional factors play an additional part and may explain (at least partly) the alterations in protein synthesis, mRNA content, and RNAse activity. There is also evidence for a combined action of growth hormone, tri-iodothyronine, and nutritional factors in the regulation of hepatic mRNA (Liaw, Biochem, 1983; 22:213).

Glucocorticoids

In extrahepatic organs, especially in skeletal muscle, glucocorticoids induce protein degradation, which supplies the liver with amino acids for gluconeogenesis. The effect of glucocorticoids on hepatic protein metabolism cannot be generalized. Glucocorticoids increase the mRNA content for specific proteins (tyrosine aminotransferase (Scherer, PNAS, 1982; 79:7205), tryptophan oxygenase (Danesch, JBC, 1983; 258:4753), and metallothionein (Karin, Nature, 1984; 308:513)). Glucocorticoid administration in man is followed by increased synthesis and degradation of albumin (Rotschild, JCI, 1961; 40:545). The effect of glucocorticoids on the synthesis of acute-phase proteins is a permissive one.

Effect of cytokines (acute-phase reaction)

Tissue injury, chemical or physical insults, neoplastic growth, and viral, bacterial or parasitic infections lead to an acute-phase response.[59] This includes immediate local responses such as vaso-dilatation and the release of cellular contents (such as lysosomal enzymes, histamine, serotonin, and prostaglandins), secondary responses (neutrophil chemotaxis, respiratory burst, release of prostaglandins and leukotrienes), and, subsequently, systemic reactions including fever, pain, and an alteration in plasma protein composition. The concentrations of some plasma proteins, called acute-phase proteins, are increased under these conditions, while those of others are decreased. The first acute-phase protein to be described was C-reactive protein (Tillet, JExpMed, 1930; 52:561; MacLeod, JExpMed, 1941; 73:191). The hepatocyte is the main site of synthesis of acute-phase proteins, but secondary sites of synthesis exist, e.g. monocytes and macrophages.[60]

According to their rate of synthesis during the acute-phase response, plasma proteins can be divided into four groups:[61]

group I: several hundred-fold increase, e.g. C-reactive protein, serum amyloid A;
group II: I two- to four-fold increase, e.g. α_1-antitrypsin, α_1-acid glycoprotein, α_1-antichymotrypsin, fibrinogen, haptoglobin;
group III: about 50 per cent increase, e.g. complement C3, caeruloplasmin;
group IV: decrease, e.g. albumin, prealbumin.

It should be noted, however, that species differences exist. α_2-Macroglobulin, for example, is one of the major acute-phase proteins in the rat, increasing several hundred-fold during the acute-phase reaction (Northemann, EurJBioch, 1983; 137:257), but in man its plasma concentration is not increased during inflammation. α_1-Acid glycoprotein increases two- to four-fold in man, but 90-fold in the rat (Ricca, JBC, 1981; 256: 10 362).

The factors that lead to a change in hepatic protein synthesis during the acute-phase response are considered below. It has been shown that corticosteroids are necessary for the increased synthesis of acute-phase proteins. In rats with hypophysectomy or adrenalectomy, inflammation does not lead to increased synthesis of α_2-macroglobulin (Heim, Nature, 1965; 208:1330; Heim, Nature, 1967; 213:1260; Thompson, BiochemJ, 1976; 156:25). The stimulation of acute-phase protein synthesis in hepatocytes in primary culture and in hepatoma cell cultures requires the presence of corticosteroids (Baumann, JBC, 1981; 256: 10145; Gross, ExpCellRes, 1984; 151:46; Andus, EurJImmunol, 1988; 18:739). Corticosteroids, however, have only a permissive role, and are not sufficient to induce the alterations in protein synthesis observed during inflammation *in vivo*.

Cytokines secreted by inflammatory cells mediate the induction of acute-phase protein synthesis in the liver. There are three major groups of acute-phase regulatory cytokines:[62]

1. IL-6-type[63] cytokines (IL-6, IL-11, leukaemia inhibitory factor, oncostatin M, and CNTF (Gauldie, PNAS, 1987; 84:7251; Andus, FEBSLett, 1987; 221:18; Baumann, MolBiolMed, 1990; 7:147; Scholtink, FEBSLett, 1992; 314:280). IL-6 is the principal regulator of most acute-phase protein genes. It enhances the production of IL-6-specific acute-phase proteins. These include in most species the fibrinogen chains, haptoglobin, and at least one of the major protease inhibitors (α_1-antitrypsin, α_1-antichymotrypsin, thiostatin, and α_2-macroglobulin). In IL-6-deficient mice the acute-phase response to tissue damage or infection is severely compromised, yet it is only moderately affected after challenge with lipopolysaccharide. Although IL-11, oncostatin M, leukaemia inhibitory factor, and ciliary neurotrophic factor are structurally distinct from IL-6, they stimulate a similar pattern of acute-phase proteins, since they use the same signal-transduction pathway as IL-6.[64,65]
2. IL-1 and tumour necrosis factor regulate a distinct set of acute-phase proteins. They can enhance the expression of C-reactive

protein, serum amyloid A, α_1-acid glycoprotein, complement C3, and haptoglobin, depending on the species. IL-1- and tumour necrosis factor-mediated stimulation of acute-phase-proteins is in most cases synergistically enhanced by IL-6-type cytokines. On the other hand, IL-1 and tumour necrosis factor do not enhance the synthesis of IL-6-type acute-phase proteins.
3. The growth factors transforming growth factor-β, insulin-like growth factor, hepatocyte growth factor, and insulin can modulate the response of the liver to IL-6-type cytokines, IL-1 or tumour necrosis factor. Transforming growth factor-β enhances the effects of IL-6 on acute-phase protein genes but suppresses IL-1 stimulation (Mackiewitz, PNAS, 1990; 87:1491). Insulin attenuates the stimulation of most acute-phase protein genes (Campos, MolCellBiol, 1992; 12:1789).

Cloning of several rodent and human acute-phase protein genes has allowed the definition of their principal regulatory elements. Nuclear factor (**NF**)-κB-related factors are involved in the enhanced expression of IL-1-induced acute-phase proteins including serum amyloid A (Ray, JBC,1995; 270:7365), and α_1 acid glycoprotein. CCAAT/enhancer activated protein (C/EBP) isoforms (Baumann, JBC, 1992; 267: 19744; Ramji, NucAcidRes, 1993; 21:289; Ray, JBC, 1995; 270:7365) are involved in the synthesis of acute-phase proteins induced by the IL-6 family or IL-1.

NF–IL-6 and acute-phase response factor are important for signalling of IL-6 and related proteins.

Considerable progress has recently been made in understanding the signal-transduction pathway of the IL-6 family of cytokines (Fig. 9).[64,65] The IL-6 receptor consists of an IL-6-binding subunit (gp80) (Taga, Cell, 1989; 58:573) and a signal-transducing protein (gp130) (Hibi, Cell, 1990; 63:1149). Binding of IL-6 to its receptor induces homodimerization of gp130. Gp130 also functions as a cytokine signal transducer for leukaemia inhibitory factor, oncostatin M, CNTF, and IL-11. While the IL-11/IL-11 receptor complex also induces a gp130 homodimer, the CNTF/CNTF receptor complex induces heterodimerization of gp130 and leukaemia inhibitory factor-receptor (Davis, Science, 1993; 260:1805). Leukaemia inhibitory factor-receptor is highly homologous with gp130 (Gearing, EMBOJ, 1991; 10:2839). Leukaemia inhibitory factor induces heterodimerization of its receptor/gp130 complex (Gearing, Science, 1992; 255:1434). Oncostatin M presumably also induces heterodimerization of that complex and the complex of its own receptor with gp130 (Lin, JBC, 1992; 267: 16763; Thoma, JBC, 1994; 269:6215).

Homodimers or heterodimers of gp130 activate JAK kinases associated with gp130 (Lütticken, Science, 1994; 263:89; Stahl, Science, 1994; 263:92). This leads to tyrosine phosphorylation of the distal part of the cytoplasmic region of gp130, which attracts STAT3 (identical with acute-phase response factor). STAT3 is then tyrosine phosphorylated by JAK kinases, resulting in a STAT3 dimer, which is translocated into nuclei.

Another pathway from gp130 to acute-phase protein gene expression involves NF-IL-6. NF–IL-6 was originally identified as a nuclear factor that binds to a 14-bp palindromic sequence within an IL-1-responsive element in the human IL-6 gene (Isshiki, MolCellBiol, 1990; 10:2757), but various acute-phase genes also contain the recognition sequence of NF–IL-6 (Poli, Cell, 1990; 63:643).

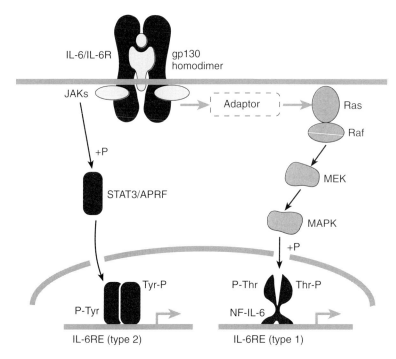

Fig. 9. IL-6 signal-transduction pathway. Two pathways lead from gp130 to acute-phase protein gene expression. Homodimerization of gp130 activates the STAT3/acute-phase response factor (APRF) pathway as well as the MAP (mitogen activated protein) kinase (K) cascade. An adaptor molecule not yet identified is postulated to link gp130 homodimer to ras, leading to the critical threonine phosphorylation of nuclear factor (NF)-IL-6 through MAPK activation. The STAT3 dimer and the NF–IL-6 dimer bind to type 1 and type 2 IL-6RE, respectively, of the acute-phase protein genes.

NF–IL-6 is serine/threonine phosphorylated. It shows a ras-dependent activation that is mediated through phosphorylation of Thr235 by MAP kinases (Nakajima, PNAS, 1993; 90:2207). An adaptor molecule linking the gp130 homodimer to ras is, however, still hypothetical.

Properties and function of secretory liver proteins

Albumin

Albumin, the most abundant plasma protein, is a polypeptide of 573 amino acids. In contrast to most other plasma proteins it contains no carbohydrate moiety. The liver is the exclusive site of albumin biosynthesis. In a normal adult the liver synthesizes and secretes about 120 mg albumin per kg body wt daily. The total exchangeable pool amounts to 3.5 to 5.0 g/kg; 38 to 45 per cent of this pool is located intravascularly. In the steady state, albumin synthesis is in equilibrium with degradation. In contrast to albumin synthesis there is no exclusive site of degradation; all cells can degrade albumin by lysosomal proteases. Liver, muscle, kidney, and skin are the main organs (Yedgar, AmJPhysiol, 1983; 244:E101). In the liver, albumin degradation is favoured by the fenestrated endothelium of the sinusoids, which allows direct access of plasma proteins to the hepatocytes.

Albumin is primarily synthesized as preproalbumin with an *N*-terminal extension of 24 amino acids. From this polypeptide chain, 18 amino acids are cleaved off after completion of the polypeptide chain in the rough endoplasmic reticulum. The resulting pro-albumin is converted to albumin in secretory vesicles. The putative cleavage protease for this step resembles cathepsin B (Oda, BBResComm, 1981; 105:766). The hexapeptide released in the cytoplasmic compartment probably has a regulatory function for the synthesis and secretion of albumin (Weigand, Biochem, 1982; 21:6053). An important predisposition for regulation is the existence of a free and uncommitted pool of albumin mRNA in the cytoplasmic compartment. This pool is used when albumin synthesis must be increased rapidly. In addition to the non-specific regulatory mechanisms in protein synthesis and secretion there are some more specific regulatory factors. Ornithine, which is not incorporated into proteins, has a stimulatory effect on albumin synthesis. This effect is mediated by increased polyamine synthesis (Oratz, Hepatol, 1983; 3:567). Furthermore, albumin synthesis and secretion is regulated by extracellular oncotic pressure; the liver responds to a decreased oncotic pressure with an increased rate of albumin synthesis and secretion.

Albumin has two functions in the circulation. It is the most important regulator of the plasma oncotic (colloid osmotic) pressure, and it is the principal transport protein for many endogenous and exogenous substances.

The concentration of albumin in the plasma is the net result of three processes: synthesis, degradation, and distribution. Thus, the serum albumin is not indicative of hepatic malfunction in terms of albumin synthesis alone.[66] Using methods that allow differentiation between the three possibilities leading to hypalbuminaemia, it was shown that a combination of them frequently exists. Rates of albumin synthesis, measured by incorporation of [^{13}C]leucine, were decreased in alcoholic and non-alcoholic cirrhosis. There was a significant correlation between the rate of albumin synthesis and the Child score (Ballmer, Hepatol, 1993; 18: 292). Newly synthesized albumin is released not only into the plasma, but also directly into ascites and lymph fluid. The cause of hypoalbuminaemia in patients with ascites may be an abnormal intra-/extravascular distribution and intravascular dilution.

Transport proteins

Lipoproteins

Lipids are transported in plasma predominantly in large macromolecular complexes, the lipoproteins. Very low-density lipoproteins are produced in the liver. High-density lipoproteins arise as a 'nascent' form in the liver. The enzymes for the intravascular metabolism of lipoproteins (LCAT: lecithine–cholesterol-acyltransferase; H–TGL: hepatic triglyceride lipase) are also synthesized and secreted by the liver. Biosynthesis, degradation, metabolism, and function under normal conditions and in liver diseases are described in Chapter 2.12.

Free fatty acids, bile salts, and lysolecithin as relatively polar lipids are transported bound to albumin. For lipids with particular function (e.g. cortisol, retinol) specific binding proteins exist (see below).

Transferrin

This transport protein for iron in plasma consists of a single polypeptide chain with two similar, but not identical, iron-binding sites. The liver is the principal but not exclusive site of transferrin synthesis. The gene for human transferrin, which is located on chromosome 3 with the gene for the transferrin receptor (Yang, PNAS, 1984; 81:2752), has been cloned (Park, PNAS, 1985; 82: 3149).

Transferrin biosynthesis in the liver is probably regulated by the iron content (McKnight, JBC, 1980; 255:144). An inverse correlation exists between intrahepatic ferritin and transferrin synthesis. The regulation of the synthesis of transferrin by the iron pool is different from that of ferritin. Control of transferrin synthesis is performed on a transcriptional level, with increase of transferrin mRNA in iron deficiency. Ferritin synthesis is regulated translationally.

The first step in transferrin degradation is the binding of the iron-bearing transport protein to a specific receptor (Cole, BBActa, 1983; 762:102; Young, BBActa, 1980; 633:145). The receptor protein has been located in the membrane of various cells, especially in haemopoietic cells with the capacity for haemoglobin synthesis, and in hepatocytes. The synthesis of the receptor in hepatocytes is regulated by the iron content of the cell. The receptor is a disulphide-linked dimeric glycoprotein consisting of two identical subunits. As the second step in transferrin degradation the transferrin–iron–receptor complex enters the hepatocyte by endocytosis. In a third step a non-lysosomal endocytic vesicle is formed, in which iron is released from the protein by lowering pH. The transferrin–receptor complex is degraded by proteases, or can be recycled to the plasma membrane of the cell (Young, Hepatol, 1981; 1:114; Young, JBC, 1983; 258:492).[67]

Caeruloplasmin

This glycoprotein, with electropheretic migration within the α_2 fraction, is the specific binding protein for copper. About 98 per cent of the serum copper is bound to this glycoprotein, the rest to albumin. The protein is named from its blue colour, caused by the bound copper (for review, see[68]). It has a molecular mass of 130-kDa and contains approx. 7.5 to 8.0 per cent carbohydrates. Each molecule binds six atoms of copper, of which half are in the cupric form. The protein moiety can be cleaved to form two different subunits. Two different polypeptide chains have been isolated. The carbohydrate moiety consists of 8 to 10 oligosaccharide chains terminated by sialic acid residues. Human caeruloplasmin, from which the terminal sialic acid residues have been cleaved by neuraminidase, disappears from the circulation within minutes, whereas native caeruloplasmin has been shown to have a half-life of 56 h. If the preterminal galactosyl residue exposed by neuraminidase is removed by galactosidase, the half-life of ceruloplasmin returns to normal.

Caeruloplasmin is synthesized in the liver and secreted into the blood. The gene coding for caeruloplasmin is located on chromosome 3 (Yang, PNAS, 1986; 83:3257). There is partial homology between this gene and the genes of clotting factors V and VIII (Kane, PNAS, 1986; 83:6800). The level of caeruloplasmin gene expression is regulated on a transcriptional level (Githin, JBC, 1988; 263:6281).

The main function of caeruloplasmin is the transport and storage of copper. Half of the copper atoms of each caeruloplasmin molecule can exchange with ionic copper under appropriate conditions. An apocaeruloplasmin, a low copper-containing protein, constitutes between 10 and 20 per cent of the total caeruloplasmin in human serum. Caeruloplasmin exhibits oxidase activity towards polyphenols, catecholamines, polyamines, and ascorbic acid. Histaminase activity has also been attributed to caeruloplasmin. The physiological significance of these activities is unclear. The oxidation of Fe^{2+} to Fe^{3+}, catalysed by caeruloplasmin, is possibly important for the binding of iron to transferrin.

Steroid hormone-binding proteins

In the blood plasma steroid hormones are reversibly bound to proteins. Only a very small amount circulates in the free form. The function of protein binding is not the solubilization of the steroids. At their low concentration in serum, steroid hormones would be soluble. Protein binding has three functional aspects.

1. It protects steroid hormones from rapid enzymatic inactivation and renal excretion. Therefore the protein binding influences the half-life of the hormones in serum.
2. It has a buffering effect that prevents rapid variations of active hormone levels. Only in the free, unbound form are the hormones in the active state.
3. It mediates the vectorial transport of the hormones to their target organs by competition of the extracellular binding protein and the intracellular receptor protein with the hormone.

All binding proteins for steroid hormones have a low, overlapping specificity. The following proteins synthesized and secreted by the liver are involved in the binding and transport of steroid hormones (for review, see[69]): corticoid-binding globulin ('transcortin'), sex-hormone binding globulin (SBG), orosomucoid, and albumin.

Transcortin is the most important binding protein for corticosteroids. It has a high affinity for the physiological hormones of the adrenal cortex (cortisol, corticosterone, deoxycorticosterone) as well as for the pharmacological derivative prednisone. The protein shows also a high affinity for progesterone and a moderate affinity for testosterone and oestradiol. In contrast, the affinity of transcortin for cortisol metabolites, aldosterone and dexamethasone is low or negligible (Dunn, JClinEndoc, 1981; 53:58). About 90 per cent of plasma cortisol is bound to transcortin and 10 per cent is free under normal conditions. However, the binding sites of transcortin are fully saturated at a plasma cortisol concentration of 30 µg/100 ml. At higher concentrations the free plasma concentration increases to between 20 and 30 per cent, and an increasing amount of the hormone is bound to albumin.

Transcortin is a glycoprotein with a molecular mass of about 52 kDa and a carbohydrate content of 26 to 29 per cent. Little is known about the regulation of its synthesis and secretion by the liver. A striking increase of the serum transcortin is induced by oestrogens. However, this effect is only produced with high oestrogen concentrations, which do not exist during the normal menstrual cycle but only in pregnancy or during administration of oral contraceptives.

Sex hormone-binding globulin (**SBG**) binds predominantly testosterone and oestradiol. The binding is mediated for both male and female sex hormones by the same binding sites, but testosterone has a higher affinity than oestradiol. There is competition by the two hormones for the binding sites of SBG. In contrast, there is no affinity to the synthetic oestrogen diethylstilboestrol.

SBG is a glycoprotein with a molecular mass of 52 kDa. It migrates with the β-globulins. Its synthesis and/or secretion by the liver is induced by oestrogen. The mechanism of regulation of its synthesis and secretion require further investigation.

Orosomucoid, also known as α_1-acid glycoprotein, binds progesterone and, with lower affinity, also testosterone and oestradiol. The protein concentration and therefore the binding capacity is higher than that of SBG and transcortin, but its affinity to the steroid hormones is lower. Synthetic oestrogens are predominantly bound by orosomucoid. The protein migrates with the α_1-globulins. Its carbohydrate content is extremely high (42 per cent). Its molecular mass is about 40 kDa.

Albumin has a high binding capacity for steroids because of its high serum concentration, but its affinity to steroid hormones is very low. Therefore the binding of the native hormones is only relevant when the more specific binding proteins (transcortin, SBG) are saturated. However, the conjugates of steroids (glucuronides, sulphates) are predominantly bound to albumin. Furthermore, albumin is the most important transport protein for aldosterone.

Thyroid hormone-binding proteins

In plasma over 99 per cent of thyroxine (**T4**) and of tri-iodo-thyronine (**T3**) circulate bound to protein (for reviews, see[70,71]). The binding between protein and hormones is non-covalent, in contrast to the covalent binding of the hormones to thyroglobulin within the thyroid gland. The small free-hormone fraction is in dynamic equilibrium with the protein-bound hormone. Only the free fraction of hormone is active in regard to the hormonal effects. The functions of the binding proteins are identical to those of the steroid-binding proteins (see above).

Three proteins synthesized and secreted by the liver are involved in the binding of thyroid hormones in blood plasma: thyroxine-binding globulin, thyroxine-binding prealbumin, also known as transthyretin, and albumin.

Thyroxine-binding globulin is an α-globulin that binds 60 per cent of the circulating T4. At a normal plasma concentration of the protein (12–34 mg/l) and at full saturation of the binding sites, thyroxine-binding globulin binds approx 20 µg T4/100 ml. T3 binds less strongly to thyroxine-binding globulin than T4. The molecular mass of thyroxine-binding globulin is about 58 kDa.

Thyroxine-binding prealbumin (transthyretin) binds about 30 per cent of circulating T4 through electrostatic interactions and hydrogen bridges in a central trough of the molecule. At full saturation, 200 µg T4/100 ml plasma can be bound. T3 does not bind, or only to a limited extent. Thyroxine-binding prealbumin is a tetramer with molecular mass of 54 kDa (Andrea, Biochem, 1980; 19:55).

Albumin binds about 10 per cent of the circulating T4. Because of its high concentration in plasma the binding capacity is very high, but its affinity is low. Therefore, albumin plays a significant part in binding and transport of thyroid hormones only when the more specific binding proteins are saturated.

Since thyroid hormone function correlates much more closely with the tiny fraction of free hormones than with the total plasma concentration of the hormones (free + protein-bound hormones), the liver as source of the binding proteins influences the hormonal status. Little is known about the regulation of hepatic synthesis and secretion of these specific transport proteins. Oestrogens induce the synthesis and secretion of thyroxine-binding globulin and cause misleadingly high values of the total hormone concentration, with little or no change in the functional free-hormone level.

Vitamin A-binding protein (retinol-binding protein)

The liver is the most important storage site of vitamin A. Ninety per cent of the vitamin is stored as retinyl ester in the Ito cells of the liver (Hill, AnticancerRes, 1983; 3:171; Glover, ProcNutrSoc, 1983; 42:19). A prerequisite for mobilization of the vitamin is the hydrolytic cleavage of the retinyl ester and the binding of retinol to retinol-binding protein in the Golgi apparatus. The retinol–retinol-binding protein complex is secreted by the liver. In plasma, retinol-binding protein forms a further complex with thyroxine-binding prealbumin. Less than 5 per cent of retinol circulating in the blood is in the free unbound form. Only the complex of retinol, retinol-binding protein, and thyroxine-binding prealbumin reacts with the specific receptor in the target organs. The hepatic secretion of the retinol–retinol-binding protein complex is regulated by vitamin A. In vitamin A deficiency the release of the retinol–retinol-binding protein complex is reduced and the apo-retinol-binding protein accumulates in the liver. Readministration of vitamin A induces the release of the complex. With high-dose vitamin A administration, and saturation of the specific-binding protein, retinol is also taken up and transported by lipoproteins (for reviews, see[72-74]).

Vitamin D-binding proteins (transcalciferin)

Vitamin D₃ (cholecalciferol) and its active metabolites 25-hydroxy-cholecalciferol (calcidiol) and 1,25-dihydroxycholecalciferol (calcitriol) are bound in plasma to a specific protein (D-binding protein, transcalciferin) (for review, see[75]). D-binding protein binds with high-affinity calcidiol, the main vitamin D metabolite circulating in plasma. Calcidiol and cholecalciferol are bound with stepwise lowered affinity.

Transcalciferin is synthesized exclusively in the liver. It consists of a single polypeptide chain with post-translationally added carbohydrate chains. A genetic polymorphism arises from variations of the primary structure of the protein backbone, as well as from variations of the carbohydrate moiety. The molecular mass is about 58 kDa. One molecule of D-binding protein binds one molecule of calcidiol. Vitamin D-binding protein is structurally homologous to albumin and to α-fetoprotein, at both the protein level and the genomic DNA level (Gibbs, MolBiolEvol, 1987; 4:364). The mechanisms by which its hepatic synthesis and secretion are regulated are unknown. In contrast to the regulation of retinol-binding protein the serum concentration of D-binding protein is not influenced by the level of calcidiol.

There are several functions of the specific binding protein, D-binding protein:

1. Vectorial transport of vitamin D and its active metabolites to their target organs (within the systemic and enterohepatic circulations);
2. Interaction with a specific receptor located in the cell membrane or in the intracellular compartment of the target organs. An interaction of D-binding protein with actin was described; its significance is unknown (Emerson, Electrophoresis, 1984; 5:22);
3. 'Buffering' of high vitamin D concentrations by its binding to D-binding protein with subsequent inactivation;
4. Storage of vitamin D and its metabolites.

Vitamin D and its metabolites are also transported in the plasma by binding to albumin and to lipoproteins. D-binding protein, however, has the highest affinity for vitamin D and its active metabolites. D-binding protein is therefore quantitatively and qualitatively the most important transport protein. For a further discussion of vitamin D metabolism and D-binding protein in liver diseases, see Chapter 25.10.

Proteins of coagulation and fibrinolysis (see Chapter 2.14.3)

Complement system

The complement system plays an important part in host defence against infectious agents[76] and during inflammation. The system is composed of 13 glycoproteins, which are part of the classical and alternative activation pathways, with the major component C3 having a central role in each. In addition seven plasma proteins and about 15 membrane-bound proteins and receptors are involved in the control of the system.[77] Figure 10 shows a schematic representation of the complement system. The plasma proteins of the complement system are mainly synthesized in liver[78] but several are also produced at extrahepatic sites, for example peripheral blood monocytes (Hetland, ScaJImmunol, 1986; 24:241),

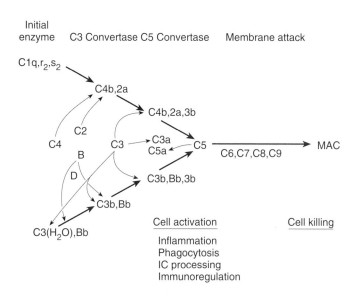

Fig. 10. Schematic representation of the complement system (from Müller-Eberhardt, AnnRevBiochem, 1988; 57:321).

macrophages (Falus, Immunol, 1987; 60:547), endothelial cells (Ueki, Immunol, 1987; 61:11), fibroblasts (Miura, JBC, 1987; 25:262). In addition to the complement proteins circulating in the plasma, local production of complement components by immunological cells accumulated at sites of inflammation may be an important component of the inflammatory response.[79]

The assumption that liver is the primary site of synthesis of complement components is based on studies in patients who have received liver transplants. After transplantation the allotypes of C3, C6, C8, and factor B in these patients became those of the donor. The primary structure of most complement components was derived from the sequence of cDNA clones obtained from liver, e.g. C1q (Reid, BiochemJ, 1985; 231:729), C1r and C1s (Journet, BiochemJ, 1986; 240:738), C2 (Bentley, BiochemJ, 1986; 239:339), C3 (deBruijn, PNAS, 1985; 82:708), C4 (Belt, Cell, 1984; 36:907), C5 (Lundwall, JBC, 1985; 260:2108), C7 (Di Scipio, JBC, 1988; 263:549), C8a (Rao, Biochem, 1987; 26:3556), C4bp (Chung, BiochemJ, 1985; 230:133), factor H (Kristensen, JImmunol, 1986; 136:3407), factor B (Sackstein, JBC, 1983; 258: 14693), factor I (Goldberger, JBC, 1987; 262: 10065). Furthermore, *de novo* synthesis of complement factors has been demonstrated in liver cells and hepatoma cells: for example, of C2, C4, C3, and factor B in rat hepatocytes (Anthony, BiochemJ, 1985; 232:93), of C1q, C1r, C1s, C3, C8, C9 in guinea-pig hepatocytes (Ramadori, EurJImmun, 1986; 16:1137; Ramadori, Immunobiology, 1985; 170:203), of C9 in rat hepatoma cells, of C1r, C1s, C2, C3, C4, C5, C6, and factor B in human hepatoma cells (Morris, JCI, 1982; 70:906).

The classical complement pathway is initiated by the binding of C1 to an antigen–antibody complex and activation of antibody-bound C1.[80-82] C1 is a metalloprotein complex of two reversibly interacting subunits, C1q and C1r2s2.[83] C1q is the subunit that binds to antigen–antibody complexes. It has a molecular mass of 460 kDa and is composed of 18 polypeptide chains—three chain types (A, B, C) with six copies of each per molecule. C1q has a central core and six radiating arms, which end in carboxyterminal globular regions. The arms have a triple helical, collagen-like structure. Binding of C1q to Fc regions of antibodies occurs through the globular structures at the end of the arms. For the binding of C1q to a pentameric IgM antibody, a conformational change in the structure of the antibody appears to be essential. This conformational change is produced by the attachment of IgM to antigen. In the case of IgG, a structural change in the antibody molecule seems to be unnecessary for binding of C1q. It has been shown that native C1 interacts with IgG monomers, albeit weakly. Evidently, a cluster of closely associated IgG molecules, for example on the surface of a cell, provides multiple points of C1q attachment and thus allows binding of C1q.

Besides IgG- and IgM-containing immune complexes, lipopolysaccharide and porins from Gram-negative bacteria (Zohair, BiochemJ, 1989; 257:865), and ligand-bound C-reactive protein (Jiang, JImmunol, 1991; 146:2324) bind C1q. The classical complement pathway may also be activated by tissue-damage products, including, for example, mitochondrial cardiolipin, mitochondrial proteins or other highly charged polymers.[84]

C1r and C1s are homologous single-chain zymogens of serine proteases, of 95 and 87 kDa, respectively. These chains form a tetrameric structure (C1r2s2), which is inserted between the collagenous strands of C1q. Activation of C1 is associated with cleavage of each of the C1r chains and each of the C1s chains into a heavy chain and a light chain, with the exposure of an active site on each of the smaller subunits. In the absence of serum, spontaneous activation of C1 proceeds rapidly (Ziccardi, JImmunol, 1982; 128:2500). This spontaneous activation is normally inhibited by C1 inactivator. However, binding of C1 to an immune complex releases it from the inhibitory influence of C1 inhibitor. Under these conditions the two C1r chains are cleaved reciprocally; activated C1r then cleaves and activates C1s.[85]

The natural substrates of activated C1s are C4 and C2. C4 is composed of three disulphide-linked chains termed α (93 kDa), β (78 kDa), and γ (33 kDa). C4 is synthesized as a single-chain precursor. The formation of the three-chain structure is a post-translational event (Fey, FedProc, 1980; 40:2099). C4 possesses an internal thioester in its α-chain (Tack, SpringerSemImmunopathol, 1983; 6:259). Activated C1s cleaves a 10-kDa aminoterminal peptide (C4a) from the α-chain of C4 and thus generates C4b, thereby enabling the internal thioester to form amide or ester bonds with amino or carboxyl groups on the target surface. An active C1 molecule cleaves multiple C4 molecules (about 35) (Ziccardi, JImmunol, 1981; 126:1769). Some C4b molecules bind to the region surrounding the antibody–C1 site, while others react with water and remain unbound in the fluid phase.

C2 is a single-chain polypeptide of 102 kDa. It binds reversibly to C4b in the presence of magnesium ions. When C2 is cleaved by activated C1s, two fragments are formed—a small N-terminal fragment (C2b) and a large C-terminal fragment (C2a). C2b is released into the fluid phase, while C2a becomes firmly associated with C4b. The C4b2a complex is the C3 convertase of the classical pathway. The C4b2a complex has a half-life of 3 min.

The classical pathway of complement activation is under regulatory control. C4b can be cleaved by factor I, a serum protease of high substrate specificity, which occurs in serum as an active enzyme. For cleavage of C4b, factor I needs C4-binding protein as a cofactor. C4-binding protein is composed of seven identical polypeptide chains of 70 kDa each linked by disulphide bonds.

The alternative pathway of complement activation can operate without the participation of antibody. Phylogenetic data indicate that the alternative pathway is the older and that the classical pathway evolved from it.[86] It can be activated by certain particulate polysaccharides, fungi, bacteria, viruses, mammalian cells, and aggregates of immunoglobulins.[83] Recognition of these structures involves C3b (Pangburn, JImmunol, 1980; 124:977). The details of this recognition process are not fully understood. The microenvironment of bound C3b determines whether C3b prefers binding of factor B, which leads to activation of the alternative pathway, or of factor H, which abrogates the pathway.

Factor B is a 93-kDa single-chain polypeptide (Christie, BiochemJ, 1983; 209:61). It is the zymogen of a serine protease. Binding of factor B in the presence of magnesium ions to C3b exposes a site in the factor B molecule, which can be cleaved by factor D.

Factor D is a 23-kDa single-chain glycoprotein. It is found in trace amounts in the circulation as active protease. Its natural substrate is factor B, which can only be cleaved when it is bound to C3b. When factor B is cleaved by factor D, two fragments are formed: a smaller fragment (Ba) and a larger fragment (Bb). Ba is released. Bb, which is a serine protease, forms a complex with C3b. The C3bBb complex is the C3 convertase of the alternative pathway. C3b binds native C3, which is then cleaved by Bb. The C3bBb complex dissociates rapidly. Its dissociation rate is decreased by properdin, which binds to C3bBb and thus promotes activation of the alternative pathway.

Enzymatic activity of the alternative-pathway C3 convertase is controlled by factors H and I. Factor H has C3b-binding activity (Alsenz, BiochemJ, 1985; 232:841). It can displace factor B from the C3 convertase and in addition can function as a cofactor in the cleavage of C3b by factor I. Factors I and H are required to prevent spontaneous fluid-phase assembly of the alternative-pathway C3 convertase. There are several factor H-related proteins that display significant homology to factor H but that do not show factor H-like complement regulatory activities.[87]

C3 has the central role in both the classical and alternative complement pathways. Human C3 is a 190-kDa glycoprotein composed of two chains; an α-chain (about 110 kDa) and a β-chain (about 75 kDa) linked by a disulphide bond. C3 is synthesized as a single-chain precursor, which is cleaved post-translationally. C3 has an internal thioester in its α-chain. When C3 is cleaved by C3 convertase of either the classical (C4b2a) or alternative (C3bBb) pathway, the α-chain dissociates into two fragments. The smaller fragment is termed C3a. It consists of the N-terminal part of the α-chain and is released. The larger C-terminal fragment remains bound to the β-chain. This complex is termed C3b. Cleavage of the α-chain of C3 leads to a conformational change of the protein and the exposure of the internal thioester, which then can react with appropriate substrates, e.g. aldehydes, carboxyl groups, nitrogen nucleophiles, or water. This is the mechanism by which C3b is bound covalently to surfaces.

When C3b is produced by activation of the classical pathway, it can be used for the activation of the alternative pathway, which in turn leads to the formation of more C3b. In this situation the alternative pathway amplifies complement activation initiated by the classical pathway. However, the alternative pathway can also be initiated without prior activation of the classical pathway.[88] Since the thioester bond in C3 is not completely stable, it is subject to slow hydrolysis, even when C3b is not cleaved by C3 convertase. C3 with a hydrolysed thioester shares some properties with C3b, including its ability to bind factor B, factor H, and native C3. Thus, an alternative-pathway convertase is formed, leading to a baseline C3 turnover in serum, called 'C3 tickover'. This turnover is under control of factors H and I, and occurs at a slow rate. However, it may provide the initial C3b, which can bind to certain surfaces and start the activation of the alternative pathway.

The terminal complement components C5 to 9 form the membrane-attack complex.[83,89] The complex forms transmembrane pores or channels and thereby damages biological and artificial membranes causing cell lysis.

C5 is composed of two disulphide-linked chains: α (about 115 kDa) and β (about 75 kDa). C5 must be cleaved to become biologically active. C5 can be cleaved either by the C5 convertase of the classical pathway (C4b2a3b) or of the alternative pathway (P(C3b)2Bb). Cleavage of C5 yields fragments C5a and C5b. Fragment C5a is released. It has potent independent biological activity. C5a is the classical complement anaphylatoxin. It promotes chemotaxis of neutrophils and monocytes, and enhances immunoglobulin secretion by lymphocytes.[79,90,91] C5b combines sequentially with C6, C7, C8, and C9 to form the membrane-attack complex. Besides cleavage by C5 convertase, C5 can also be cleaved into biologically active peptides by non-complement proteinases, such as trypsin, plasmin, granulocyte elastase, or cathepsin G.[92]

C6 and C7 are both single-chain glycoproteins of about 100 kDa each.[89] Once C5b is formed, it binds C6. The C5b6 complex remains loosely bound to C3b on the target-cell surface until it reacts with C7. The C5b–7 complex then undergoes hydrophilic–amphiphilic transition (Preissner, JImmunol, 1985; 135:445) and anchors itself firmly in the membrane.

Whereas C5b–7 penetrates only slightly into the hydrophobic region of the lipid bilayer, the C5b–8 complex penetrates the hydrophobic phase more deeply. C8 is composed of three non-identical chains: α (64 kDa), β (64 kDa), and γ (22 kDa). The α- and γ-chains are disulphide-linked and the β-chain is bound non-covalently. The β-chain possesses a recognition site for C5 (Stewart, Complement, 1985; 2:76), the α-chain for C9 (Stewart, Biochem, 1985; 24:4598).

Creation of the membrane-attack complex is accomplished by the binding of multiple C9 molecules, leading to the formation of a $C5b_1C6_1C7_1C8_1C9_n$ complex, where n can vary from 1 to 18. C9 is a single-chain glycoprotein of 71 kDa, with an amphiphilic organization of its primary structure (Di Scipio, PNAS, 1984; 81: 7298). Whereas the aminoterminal part of the molecule is predominantly hydrophilic, the carboxyterminal part is considerably more hydrophobic. Whereas C5b–8 forms a small functional channel of about 30 Å diameter, the channel site increases to about 100 Å when increasing numbers of C9 molecules are incorporated.

As in other steps of complement activation, channel formation by the terminal complement components is under the control of soluble and membrane regulatory proteins[83] such as S-protein and homologous restriction factor.

Protease inhibitors

Liver is not only the site of synthesis of the inactive precursors of plasma proteases of the coagulation and complement system, but also the major site of synthesis of protease inhibitors. These protease inhibitors are not only directed towards the active forms of proteases normally circulating in the plasma, but also towards proteases released from different cells and tissues under pathological conditions, such as tissue necrosis or inflammation.

Protease inhibitors constitute about 10 per cent of the plasma proteins. Under normal conditions the protease inhibitory capacity of plasma is much higher than the proteolytic activity. Only under specific conditions is there a local predominance of proteases, for example at the site of vascular injury, where the proteases of the coagulation cascade are activated.

The major plasma protease inhibitors,[93,94] synthesized in the liver are α_1-antitrypsin, α_1-antichymotrypsin, inter-α-trypsin inhibitor, α_2-macroglobulin, antithrombin III, α_2-antiplasmin, heparin cofactor II, activated protein C inhibitor, and C1 inhibitor.

α_1-Antitrypsin

α_1-Antitrypsin,[95] also known as α_1-proteinase inhibitor, is the protease inhibitor with the highest plasma concentration (2–4 g/l). Its concentration is increased to about 7 g/l during an acute-phase reaction. α_1-Antitrypsin is an inhibitor of serine proteases. Its primary biological function is the inhibition of granulocyte elastase (Beatty, JBC, 1980; 255:3931). It is less effective in the inhibition of chymotrypsin, cathepsin G, trypsin, plasmin and thrombin. α_1-Antitrypsin is a single-chain glycoprotein of 54 kDa. It carries three N-linked oligosaccharide chains of the complex type. It has a methionine in its reactive centre. Oxidation of this active site methionine, for example by cigarette smoke or by oxygen radicals produced by leucocytes, impairs the protease inhibitory capacity of α_1-antitrypsin. There is a vast genetic polymorphism of α_1-antitrypsin phenotypes. The common phenotype is PiMM. About 4 per cent of northern Europeans are heterozygotes for the Z-deficiency mutant. The phenotype PiZZ is of major clinical importance, because it leads to greatly reduced concentrations of α_1-antitrypsin in plasma. Z-type α_1-antitrypsin differs from M-type α_1-antitrypsin by a single amino-acid substitution (Glu342–Lys) (Jeppson, FEBSLett, 1976; 65:195). The secretion of Z-type α_1-antitrypsin is impaired, leading to the accumulation of the incompletely processed protein in the endoplasmic reticulum of the hepatocyte. α_1-Antitrypsin deficiency is accompanied by early onset of degenerative lung disease and, in some instances, liver disease. Lung disease is due to increased proteolytic breakdown of lung parenchyma as a consequence of a protease–antiprotease imbalance in α_1-antitrypsin deficiency (Pierce, JAMA, 1988; 259:2890). Liver disease is caused by the accumulation of unsecreted Z-type α_1-antitrypsin in the hepatocytes.[96]

α_1-Antichymotrypsin

α_1-Antichymotrypsin is an inhibitor of serine proteases. It is a single-chain, 69-kDa glycoprotein with a carbohydrate content of about 25 per cent. Its normal plasma concentration is 250 mg/l, but this increases rapidly and dramatically during an acute-phase reaction, for example in major surgery or burn injuries. The target substrates of α_1-antichymotrypsin are cathepsin G, a granulocyte protease, and mast-cell chymase (Gaffer, JBC, 1980; 255:8334). α_1-Antichymotrypsin is not only synthesized by the liver, but also by alveolar macrophages (Burnett, AmRevRespDis, 1984; 129:473).

Familial α_1-antichymotrypsin deficiency has been described. It is assumed that deficiency of this protease inhibitor may predispose to liver and lung disease (Erikson, ActaMedScand, 1986; 220:447).

Inter-α-trypsin inhibitor

Inter-α-trypsin inhibitor is a plasma proteinase inhibitor that can act as an extracellular matrix stabilizing factor (Chen, JBC, 1992; 267: 12380; Castillo, FEBSLett, 1993; 318:292). It is the major form of a family of proteins synthesized in the liver from four genes located on three different chromosomes (Diarra-Mehrpour, BBActa, 1992; 1132:114). Three of them code for the heavy-chain polypeptides H1, H2 and H3, the last one for a hybrid polypeptide chain that is cleaved into α_1-microglobulin and bikunin (Bourguignon, BiochemJ, 1989; 261:305; Odum, IntJBiochem 1992; 24:215; Sjöberg, BBActa, 1992; 295:217). Mature inter-α-trypsin inhibitor is composed of three chains, HC1, HC2 and bikunin, cross-linked by chondroitin sulphate bridges (Héron, BiochemJ, 1994; 302:573). Other plasma proteins related to inter-α-trypsin inhibitor have also been described: pre-α-trypsin inhibitor (Enghold, JBC, 1989; 264: 15975), and H2c–bikunin complex (Enghild, JBC, 1993; 268:8711).

α_2-Macroglobulin

α_2-Macroglobulin is the plasma protease inhibitor with the widest spectrum of protease inhibitory activity. It inhibits proteases of all four catalytic classes: serine, cysteine, aspartic, and metallo-proteases. α_2-Macroglobulin is a high molecular-weight (750 kDa) glycoprotein containing about 10 per cent carbohydrate.[97] It is composed of four identical chains. Pairs of subunit chains are held together by disulphide bridges and the two pairs are joined by non-covalent bonding. Each α_2-macroglobulin chain has, near its centre, a region where different peptide bonds can be cleaved by different proteases (bait region) (Sottrup-Jenson, FEBSLett, 1981; 127:167). Cleavage in the bait region leads to the exposure of an internal thiol ester (Sottrup-Jenson, FEBSLett, 1980; 121:275), which thereby becomes available for nucleophilic attack by water or by amino groups on the protease (Eccleston, JBC, 1985; 260: 10 196). Thiol ester hydrolysis results in a conformational change in the α_2-macroglobulin molecule with a resultant entrapment of the protease (trap hypothesis). The trapped protease is still active towards small substrates, but proteins are protected from it.[97] Once α_2-macroglobulin–protease complexes are formed, they are rapidly cleared from the circulation. This clearance is mediated by specific receptors on macrophages and on fibroblasts. Rare cases of α_2-macroglobulin deficiency have been described, which presented no specific clinical symptoms.

C1 inhibitor

C1 inhibitor[98] inhibits the first component of human complement. C1 inhibitor is a single-chain glycoprotein of about 100 kDa. Its carbohydrate content is 35 per cent. C1 inhibitor inhibits C1 by the formation of a 1:1 molar complex. Besides C1 it inhibits activated factor XII, factor XII fragments, kallikrein, activated factor XI, and plasmin. C1 inhibitor contributes about 75 per cent to the plasma inhibitory activity towards factor XII fragments and about 50 per cent to the inhibitory activity towards kallikrein (de Agostini, JCI, 1984; 73:1542; Schapira, JCI, 1982; 69:462). C1 inhibitor deficiency

leads to angioneurotic oedema but not to coagulation abnormalities, perhaps because of the overlapping activities of other protease inhibitors.[99]

Protease inhibitors of coagulation and fibrinolysis

These inhibitors are discussed in Chapter 2.14.3.

Other proteins
α_1-Acid glycoprotein

α1-Acid glycoprotein[100] is a single-chain glycoprotein of 40 kDa. Its carbohydrate content is 42 per cent. Human α_1-acid glycoprotein carries five N-linked oligosaccharide chains of the complex type. Both the protein and carbohydrate contents of α_1-acid glycoprotein are microheterogenous, i.e., there are differences in individual amino acids or carbohydrate residues from molecule to molecule. The 181 amino acids bear some resemblance in their sequence to that of the immunoglobulins (Schwick, AngewChemIntEdEngl, 1980; 19:87). The normal plasma concentration of α_1-acid glycoprotein is 0.6 to 1.2 g/l; during acute-phase conditions its plasma concentration is elevated to between 1.5 and 2.5 g/l. Several functions have been attributed to α_1-acid glycoprotein.

1. Immunomodulation: *in vitro* α_1-acid glycoprotein inhibits the proliferation of lymphocytes stimulated by mitogens or by allo-genic cells (Cheresh, Immunol, 1984; 51:541). α_1-Acid glyco-protein added to cultured mouse spleen cells was also found to inhibit antibody formation, the mitogenic responses to con-canavalin A and lipopolysaccharide, the mixed lymphocyte re-action, and the induction of cytolytic lymphocytes reactive to alloantigens (Bennett, PNAS, 1980; 77:6109).
2. Inhibition of platelet aggregation (Costello, Nature, 1981; 281: 667). This may be the mechanism by which α_1-acid glycoprotein protects against tumour necrosis factor-induced lethality (Libert, JExpMed, 1994; 180:1571).
3. Control of malaria virulence: α_1-acid glycoprotein has been shown to block the binding of the merozoite of the falciparum malaria parasite to the human erythrocyte (Friedman, PNAS, 1983; 80:5421).
4. Drug binding: it has been shown that α_1-acid glycoprotein binds progesterone (Ganguly, JBC, 1968; 243:6130), pteridine (Ziegler, CancerRes, 1982; 42:1567), phenothiazine neuroleptics, and vari-ous basic drugs (Javaid, BiochemPharm, 1983; 32:1149; Müller, JPharmPharmacol, 1983; 35:684). Thus, changes in the plasma concentration of α_1-acid glycoprotein during acute-phase con-ditions may alter the kinetics and efficacy of those drugs (Ab-ramson, ClinPharmTher, 1982; 32:659).

C-reactive protein

C-reactive protein together with serum amyloid P protein is a member of a unique plasma protein family named 'pentraxins'.[101-104] These proteins are composed of five subunits of 20 kDa each arranged in a cyclic pentameric symmetry. C-reactive protein was the first acute-phase protein to be identified. Its primary physio-logical function is the removal of 'foreign' material from the organ-ism.[104] C-reactive protein binds phosphorylcholine residues with high affinity in the presence of calcium ions. Materials containing phosphorylcholine are widely distributed in nature, both in mammalian cell membranes and in polysaccharides of bacterial, fungal, and parasitic origin. C-reactive protein is selectively deposited on necrotic cells that have phospholipids exposed on damaged membranes. It binds to bacterial cells and can thereby mediate precipitation, agglutination, capsular swelling of bacteria or activation of the classical complement pathway (Pepys, ClinImmunAllergy, 1981; 1:77). Inflammatory cells, such as neutrophils, appear to have a specific surface receptor for C-reactive protein (Müller, JImmunol, 1986; 136:2202), whose expression is increased upon cell stimulation. Ingestion of several types of bacteria by neutrophils is greatly enhanced by C-reactive protein either in the presence or absence of complement (Mold, JExpMed, 1981; 154: 1703; Mold, InfectImmun, 1982; 37:987; Holzer, JImmunol, 1984; 133:1424).

Serum amyloid A

Serum amyloid A[103,104] is an acute-phase protein whose serum concentration rises from 0.01 g/l in normal plasma to between 1 and 2 g/l in acute-phase plasma. Serum amyloid A is detected in serum fractions of 80 to 200 kDa, but can be isolated under dissociating conditions as a 12.5-kDa protein. It is assumed that proteolytic cleavage of serum amyloid A, near the carboxyterminus, leads to the generation of protein Aa, which is the main constituent of the fibrillar protein material found in systemic secondary amyloidosis (Gorevic, JCI, 1979; 63:254). Serum amyloid A enhances the binding of high-density lipoprotein 3 to macrophages during inflammation, concomitant with a decrease in the binding capacity of high-density lipoprotein 3 to hepatocytes (Kisilevsky, LabInvest, 1992; 66:778). These data support the hypothesis that serum amyloid A may remodel high-density lipoprotein 3 and redirect it from hepatocytes to macrophages, which can then engulf cholesterol and lipid debris at sites of necrosis.

References

1. Pfeffer SR and Rothman JE. Biosynthetic protein transport and sorting by the endoplasmic reticulum and Golgi. *Annual Review of Biochemistry*, 1987; **56**: 829–52.
2. Burgess TL and Kelly RB. Constitutive and regulated secretion of proteins. *Annual Review of Cell Biology*, 1987; **3**: 243–93.
3. Rose JK and Dorns RW. Regulation of protein export from the endoplasmic reticulum. *Annual Review of Cell Biology*, 1988; **4**: 257–88.
4. Alberts B, Bray D, Lewis J, Raff M, Roberts K, and Watson JD. *Molecular biology of the cell*, 3rd edn. New York: Garland, 1994.
5. Hong W and Tang BL. Protein trafficking along exocytotic pathway. *Bioessay*, 1993; **15**: 231–8.
6. Burgoyne RD and Morgan A. Regulated exocytosis. *Biochemical Journal*, 1993; **293**: 305–316.
7. De Pierre JW, Andersson G, and Dallner G. Endoplasmic reticulum and Golgi complex. In Arias JM, Jakoby WB, Popper H, Schachter D, and Shafritz DA, eds. *The liver: biology and pathobiology*. New York: Raven, 1988: 165–87.
8. Perlmutter DH. Molecular pathogenesis of α_1-antitrypsin deficiency. In Schmid R et al., eds. *Acute and chronic liver diseases. Molecular biology and clinics*. Dordrecht: Kluwer, 1996: 216–30.
9. Farquhar MG and Palade GE. The Golgi apparatus (complex)—1954–1981—from artifact to center stage. *Journal of Cell Biology*, 1981; **91**: 77–106.
10. Farquhar MG. Progress in unraveling pathways of Golgi traffic. *Annual Review of Cell Biology*, 1985; **1**: 447–88.
11. Dunphy W and Rothman JE. Compartmental organization of the Golgi stack. *Cell*, 1985; **42**: 13–21.
12. Rothman JE. The reconstitution of intracellular protein transport on cell-free systems. *Harvey Lectures*, 1992; **86**: 65–85.
13. Rothman JE and Orci L. Molecular dissection of the secretory pathway. *Nature*, 1992; **355**: 409–15.
14. Griffiths G and Simons K. The trans Golgi network: sorting at the exit site of the Golgi complex. *Science*, 1986; **234**: 438–43.
15. Mellman I, Fuchs R, and Helenius A. Acidification of the endocytic and exocytic pathways. *Annual Review of Biochemistry*, 1986; **55**: 663–700.
16. Saraste J and Kuismanen E. Pathways of protein sorting and membrane traffic between the rough endoplasmic reticulum and the Golgi complex. *Seminars in Cell Biology*, 1992; **3**: 343–55.
17. Tartakoff AM. Perturbation of vesicular traffic with the carboxylic ionophore monensin. *Cell*, 1983; **32**: 1026–8.
18. Pryer NR, Wuesthube LJ, and Schekman R. Vesicle mediated protein sorting. *Annual Review of Biochemistry*, 1992; **61**: 471–516.
19. Dahms NM, Lobel P, and Kornfeld S. Mannose-6-phosphate receptors and lysosomal enzyme targeting. *Journal of Biological Chemistry*, 1989; **264**: 12 115–18.
20. von Figura K. Molecular recognition and targeting of lysosomal proteins. *Current Opinions in Cell Biology*, 1991; **3**: 642–6.
21. De Lisle RC and Williams JA. Regulations of membrane fusion in secretory exocytosis. *Annual Review of Physiology*, 1986; **48**: 225–38.
22. Darnell J, Lodish H, and Baltimore D. *Molecular cell biology*. New York: Scientific American Books, 1986: 953–4.
23. Hanover JA and Lennarz WJ. Transmembrane assembly of membrane and secretory glycoproteins. *Archives of Biochemistry and Biophysics*, 1981; **211**: 1–19.
24. Hubbard SC and Ivatt RJ. Synthesis and processing of asparagine-linked oligosaccharides. *Annual Review of Biochemistry*, 1981; **50**: 555–83.
25. Snider MD and Robbins PW. Synthesis and processing of asparagine-linked oligosaccharides of glycoproteins. *Methods in Cell Biology*, 1981; **23**: 89–100.
26. Kornfeld R and Kornfeld S. Assembly of asparagine-linked oligosaccharides. *Annual Review of Biochemistry*, 1985; **54**: 631–64.
27. Hirschberg CB and Snider MD. Topography of glycosylation in the rough endoplasmic reticulum and Golgi apparatus. *Annual Review of Biochemistry*, 1987; **56**: 63–87.
28. Rademacher TW, Parekh RB, and Dwek RA. Glycobiology. *Annual Review of Biochemistry*, 1988; **57**: 785–838.
29. Parodi AJ and Leloir LF. The role of lipid intermediates in the glycosylation of proteins in the eukaryotic cell. *Biochimica et Biophysica Acta*, 1979; **599**: 1–37.
30. Abeijon C and Hirschberg CB. Topography of glycosylation reactions in the endoplasmic reticulum. *Trends in Biochemical Sciences*, 1992; **17**: 32–6.
31. Olden K, Parent JB, and White SL. Carbohydrate moieties of glycoproteins. A re-evaluation of their function. *Biochimica et Biophysica Acta*, 1982; **650**: 209–32.
32. Gross V, *et al.* The role of N-glycosylation for the plasma clearance of rat liver secretory glycoproteins. *European Journal of Biochemistry*, 1987; **162**: 83–8.
33. Gross V, *et al.* Involvement of various organs in the initial plasma clearance of differently glycosylated rat liver secretory proteins. *European Journal of Biochemistry*, 1988; **173**: 653–9.
34. Stahl PD, Rodman JS, Miller MJ, and Schlesinger PH. Evidence for receptor mediated binding of glycoproteins, glycoconjugates, and lysosomal glycosidases by alveolar macrophages. *Proceedings of the National Academy of Sciences (USA)*, 1978; **75**: 1399–403.
35. Ashwell G and Morell AG. The role of surface carbohydrates in the hepatic recognition and transport of circulating glycoproteins. *Advances in Enzymology*, 1974; **41**: 99–128.
36. Turner GA. N-glycosylation of serum proteins in disease and its investigation using lectins. *Clinica Chimica Acta*, 1992; **208**: 149–71.
37. Beyer TA and Hill RL. Glycosylation pathways in the biosynthesis of nonreducing terminal sequences in oligosaccharides of glycoproteins. In Horowitz MI, ed. *The glycoconjugates*. New York: Academic, 1982: 25–45.

38. Blobel G and Dobberstein B. Transfer of proteins across membranes I. Presence of proteolytically processed and unprocessed nascent immunoglobulin light chains on membrane-bound ribosomes of murine myeloma. *Journal of Cell Biology*, 1975; **67**: 835–51.

39. Walter P, Gilmore R, and Blobel G. Protein translocation across the endoplasmic reticulum. *Cell*, 1984; **38**: 5–8.

40. Evans EA, Gilmore R, and Blobel G. Purification of ribosomal signal peptidase as a complex. *Proceedings of the National Academy of Sciences (USA)*, 1986; **83**: 581–5.

41. Russell JH and Geller DM. The structure of rat proalbumin. *Journal of Biological Chemistry*, 1975; **250**: 3409–13.

42. Judah JD. Synthesis and secretion of serum albumin. In Glaumann H, Peters TJr, and Redman C, eds. *Plasma protein secretion by the liver*. London: Academic, 1983: 311–30.

43. Jorgensen, MJ, Furie BC, and Furie B. Vitamin K-dependent blood coagulation proteins. In Arias IM, Jakoby WB, Popper H, Schachter D, and Shafritz DA, eds. *The liver: biology and pathobiology*. New York: Raven, 1988: 495–503.

44. Suttie JW. Vitamin K-dependent carboxylase. *Annual Review of Biochemistry*, 1985; **54**: 459–77.

45. Melefors Ö and Hentze MW. Iron regulatory factor—the conductor of cellular iron regulation. *Blood Reviews*, 1993; **7**: 251–8.

46. Rechsteiner M, Hoffman L, and Dubiel W. The multicatalytic and 26S proteases. *Journal of Biological Chemistry*, 1993; **268**: 6065–8.

47. Rivett AJ. Proteasomes: multicatalytic proteinase complexes. *Biochemical Journal*, 1993; **291**: 1–10.

48. Peters JM. Proteasomes: protein degradation machines of the cell. *Trends in Biochemical Sciences*, 1994; **19**: 377–82.

49. Sorimachi H, Saido TC, and Suzuki K. New era of calpain research. Discovery of tissue-specific calpains. *FEBS Letters*, 1994; **343**: 1–5.

50. Häussinger D, Gerok W, and Lang F. Regulation of cell function by the cellular hydration state. *American Journal of Physiology*, 1994; **267**: E343–55.

51. Häussinger D. The role of cellular hydration in the regulation of cell function. *Biochemical Journal*, 1996; **313**: 697–710.

52. Quartey-Papafio P, Garlick PJ, and Pain VM. Effects of dietary protein on liver protein synthesis. *Biochemical Society Transactions*, 1980; **15**: 357.

53. Rotschild, MA, Oratz M, and Schreiber SS. Effect of nutrition and alcohol on albumin synthesis. *Alcoholism: Clinical and Experimental Research*, 1983; **7**: 28–30.

54. Tavill AS. Hepatic protein metabolism: basic and applied biochemical and clinical aspects. In Arias IM, Frenkel M, and Wilson JHP, eds. *Liver annual 4*. Amsterdam: Elsevier, 1983: 53–96.

55. Shafritz DA and Panduro A. Protein synthesis and gene control in pathophysiologic states. In Arias IM, Jakoby WB, Popper H, Schachter D, and Shafritz DA, eds. *The liver: biology and pathobiology*, 2nd edn. New York: Raven, 1988: 83–101.

56. Baroana E and Lieber CS. Effect of alcohol on hepatic transport of proteins. *Annual Review of Medicine*, 1982; **33**: 281–92.

57. Lieber CS. Alcohol, protein metabolism and liver injury. *Gastroenterology*, 1980; **79**: 373–90.

58. Rothschild MA, Oratz M, and Morland L. Effects of ethanol on protein synthesis and secretion. *Pharmacology, Biochemistry and Behavior*, 1980; **13** (Suppl. 1): 31–6.

59. Gordon AH and Koj A. The acute phase response to injury and infection. *Research monographs in cell and tissue physiology*. Amsterdam: Elsevier, 1985; 10.

60. Fey GH and Fuller GM. Regulation of acute phase gene expression by inflammatory mediators. *Molecular Biology and Medicine*, 1987; **4**: 323–38.

61. Kushner I. The phenomenon of the acute phase response. *Annals of the New York Academy of Sciences*, 1982; **389**: 39–48.

62. Baumann H and Gauldie J. The acute phase response. *Immunology Today*, 1994; **15**: 74–80.

63. Akira S, Taga T, and Kiohimoto T. Interleukin-6 in biology and medicine. *Advances in Immunology*, 1993; **54**: 1–78.

64. Kishimoto T, Akira S, Narazaki M, and Taga T. Interleukin-6 family of cytokines and gp130. *Blood*, 1995; **86**: 1243–54.

65. Taga T and Kiohimoto T. Signaling mechanisms through cytokine receptors that share signal transducing receptor components. *Current Opinions in Immunology*, 1995; **7**: 17–23.

66. Rotschild MA, Oratz M, and Schreiber SS. Serum albumin in liver disease. In Bianchi L, *et al.*, eds. *Liver in metabolic diseases*. Lancaster: MTP, 1983; 137–44.

67. Young StP and Aisen P. The liver and iron. In Arias IM, Boyer JL, Fausto N, Jakoby WB, Schachter DA, and Shafritz DA, eds. *The liver: biology and pathobiology*. New York: Raven, 1994: 597–617.

68. Sternlieb I. Copper and zinc. In Arias IM, Boyer JL, Fausto N, Jakoby WB, Schachter DA, and Shafritz DA, eds. *The liver: biology and pathobiology*. New York: Raven Press, 1994: 585–96.

69. Labhart A, ed. *Clinical endocrinology*. Berlin: Springer, 1986.

70. Bürgi H. The thyroid gland. In Labhardt A, ed. *Clinical endocrinology*. Berlin: Springer, 1986; 189.

71. Cody V. Thyroid hormone interactions: molecular conformation, protein binding and hormone action. *Endocrinology Review*, 1980; **1**: 140–66.

72. Friedrich W. *Handbuch der Vitamine*. München: Urban and Schwarzenberg, 1987.

73. Blomhoff R, Green MH, Berg T, and Norum KR. Transport and storage of vitamin A. *Science*, 1990; **250**: 399–403.

74. Blaner WS. Retinoid (vitamin A) metabolism and the liver. In Arias IM, Boyer JL, Jakoby WB, Fausto N, Schachter DA, and Shafritz DA, eds. *The liver: biology and pathobiology*. New York: Raven, 1994; 529–541.

75. De Luca HF and Schoes HK. Vitamin D: recent advances. *Annual Review of Biochemistry*, 1983; **52**: 411–39.

76. Joiner KA, Brown EJ, and Frank MM. Complement and bacteria: chemistry and biology in host defense. *Annual Review of Immunology*, 1984; **2**: 461–91.

77. Campbell RD, Law SKA, Reid KBM, and Sim RB. Structure, organization, and regulation of the complement genes. *Annual Review of Immunology*, 1988; **6**: 161–95.

78. Perlmutter DH and Colten HR. Molecular immunobiology of complement biosynthesis: a model of single-cell control of effector-inhibitor balance. *Annual Review of Immunology*, 1986; **4**: 231–51.

79. Brown EJ, Joiner KA, and Frank MM. Complement. In Paul WE, ed. *Fundamental immunology*. New York: Raven Press, 1984: 645–8.

80. Cooper NR. The classical complement pathway: activation and regulation of the first complement component. *Advances in Immunology*, 1985; **37**: 151–216.

81. Schumaker VN, Hanson DC, Kilchherr E, Phillips ML, and Poon PH. A molecular mechanism for the activation of the first component of complement by immune complexes. *Molecular Immunology*, 1986; **23**: 557–65.

82. Schumaker VN, Zavodszky P, and Poon PH. Activation of the first component of complement. *Annual Review of Immunology*, 1987; **5**: 21–42.

83. Müller-Eberhard H. Molecular organization and function of the complement system. *Annual Review of Biochemistry*, 1988; **57**: 321–47.

84. Sim RB and Reid KBM. C1: molecular interactions with activating systems. *Immunology Today*, 1991; **12**: 307–11.

85. Reid KBM and Porter RR. The proteolytic activation systems of complement. *Annual Review of Biochemistry*, 1981; **50**: 433–64.

86. Farries TC, Knutzen Steuer KL, and Atkinson JP. Evolutionary implications of a new bypass activation pathway of the complement system. *Immunology Today*, 1990; **11**: 78–80.

87. Zipfel PF and Skerka C. Complement factor H and related proteins: an expanding family of complement—regulatory proteins? *Immunology Today*, 1994; **15**: 121–6.

88. Pangburn MK and Müller-Eberhard HJ. Relation of a putative thioester bond in C3 to activation of the alternative pathway and the binding of C3b to biological targets of complement. *Journal of Experimental Medicine*, 1980; **152**: 1102–14.

89. Müller-Eberhard HJ. The membrane attack complex of complement. *Annual Review of Immunology*, 1986; **4**: 503–28.

90. Fearon DT and Wong WW. Complement ligand–receptor interactions that mediate biological responses. *Annual Review of Immunology*, 1983; **1**: 243–71.

91. Gerard C and Gerard NP. C5a anaphylatoxin and its seven transmembrane–segment receptor. *Annual Review of Immunology*, 1994; **12**: 775–808.

92. Goldstein IM and Perez HD. Biologically active peptides derived from the fifth component of complement. *Progress in Hemostasis and Thrombosis*, 1980; **5**: 41–79.

93. Travis J and Salvesen GS. Human plasma proteinase inhibitors. *Annual Review of Biochemistry*, 1983; **52**: 655–700.

94. Harpel PC. Blood proteolytic enzyme inhibitors: their role in modulating blood coagulation and fibrinolytic enzyme pathways. In Colman RW, Hirsh J, Marder VJ, and Salzman EW, eds. *Hemostasis and thrombosis*. Philadelphia: Lippincott, 1987: 219–34.

95. Carrell RW, *et al*. Structure and variation of human α_1-antitrypsin. *Nature*, 1982; **298**: 329–34.

96. Lomas DA and Carell RW. A protein structural approach to the solution of biological problems: α_1-antitrypsin as a recent example. *American Journal of Physiology*, 1993; **265**: L211–19.

97. Barrett AJ. α_2-Macroglobulin. *Methods in Enzymology*, 1981; **80**: 737–53.

98. Sim RB and Reboul A. Preparation and properties of human C1 inhibitor. *Methods in Enzymology*, 1981; **80**: 43–53.

99. Davis AE. C1 Inhibitor and hereditary angioneurotic edema. *Annual Review of Immunology* 1988; **6**: 595–628.

100. Koj A. Definition and classification of acute-phase proteins. In Gordon AH and Koj A, eds. *The acute-phase response to injury and infection*. Amsterdam: Elsevier Science, 1985: 139–45.

101. Pepys MB. C-reactive protein. A review of its structure and function. *European Journal of Rheumatology and Inflammation*, 1982; **5**: 386–97.

102. Pepys MB. C-reactive protein fifty years on. *Lancet*, 1981: i ; 653–7.

103. Koj A. Phylogenetic aspects of the acute-phase response and evolution of some acute-phase proteins. In Gordon AH and Koj A, eds. *The acute-phase response to injury and infection*. Amsterdam: Elsevier Science, 1985: 161–72.

104. Steel DM and Whitehead AS. The major acute phase reactants: C-reactive protein, serum amyloid P component and serum amyloid A protein. *Immunology Today*, 1994; **15**: 81–8.

2.14.3 The liver and coagulation

Marie-Helene Denninger

Physiology of coagulation

Blood coagulation is a defence system that participates in maintaining the integrity of circulatory system after injury to blood vessels. Coagulation is a complex physiological process resulting in the formation of a fibrin–platelet thrombus that plugs the hole in the vessel, preventing excessive bleeding. This process involves the initiation of blood clotting and its localization to the site of vascular injury.

In the absence of vascular injury, circulating blood is in contact with endothelial cells that line the inner wall of blood vessels. These cells are unique in their capacity, in resting conditions, to inhibit the activation of blood coagulation and the adhesion of circulating platelets. By the expression of anticoagulant, heparin-like substances on the membrane surface, by the presence of protein complexes that lead to the production of anticoagulant (such as activated protein C), and by the synthesis of an antiaggregant substance, prostacyclin, the vascular endothelium is a non-thrombogenic surface that contributes to blood flow. Damage to this surface exposes extracellular matrix proteins that promote platelet adhesion and aggregation (Fressinaud, BloodCoagFibrinol, 1991; 2:333), and subendothelium tissue factor that activates blood clotting.

Platelet adhesion and aggregation

Platelets are anucleated cytoplasmic fragments of megakaryocytes 'uniquely programmed to seal any breaks in the continuity of vascular endothelium'.[1] Under normal circumstances they circulate in the blood in a resting form, without adhering to endothelium. When vascular injury, and thus alteration of the endothelium, occurs, they rapidly attach to exposed subendothelial structures. Two possible mechanisms might explain how the site of vascular lesion is recognized as different from normal endothelium by resting, circulating platelets. The first is that platelets could be 'activated' by substances produced as a consequence of the lesion, and that activated platelets could then interact with adhesive proteins at the site of injury. The second is that 'resting' platelets could interact with those adhesive proteins exposed exclusively at the site of endothelium injury. Both events are indeed likely to occur during the formation of a platelet plug. The initial event is probably the creation by the lesion of a local adhesive site to which resting platelets attach. Thus platelet adhesion is probably the first event preceding, and responsible for, platelet activation.[2] The interaction of platelets with injured vessels requires von Willebrand factor, a large, multimeric plasma protein that binds to a specific platelet membrane receptor, glycoprotein Ib, as well as to collagen exposed on subendothelium. Thus, von Willebrand factor acts as a link between platelets and subendothelium and plays a critical part in the adhesion of platelets to the injured vessel wall. Von Willebrand factor is synthesized in endothelial cells as a single chain of 225 kDa that dimerizes and is packaged in the Weibel–Palade bodies (Wagner, JCellBiol, 1982; 95:355) prior to the secretion in circulating blood. The secretion regulated pathway releases polymerized multimeric von Willebrand factor whose molecular weight can approach 10^7 kDa. The high molecular-weight species exhibit the highest platelet adherence activity (Wagner, PNAS, 1987; 84:1955). Von Willebrand factor circulates in the blood in a non-covalent complex with factor VIII. Von Willebrand factor binding to glycoprotein Ib generates platelet intracellular signalling towards secretory granules and the cytoskeleton, and exposes glycoprotein IIb-IIIa, the receptor for fibrinogen on the platelet membrane.[1] Platelets are then activated, undergo shape change, and are transformed to a 'spiculate sphere'.[1] In resting conditions, phospholipids of the platelet membrane are asymmetrically arranged, with neutral phospholipids on the outer surface, and negatively charged phospholipids on the inner. This asymmetrical order is maintained by a membrane translocase (Devaux, Biochem, 1991; 30:1163) and by the internal cytoskeleton proteins (Schroit, BBActa, 1991; 1071:313). When platelets are activated, there is a reversal in the order of their membrane phospholipids. Negatively charged phospholipids, among which is phosphatidylserine, move from the inner to the outer surface of the platelet membrane. This movement could be due to the inhibition of translocase and to the rearrangement of proteins of the cytoskeleton. It provides the negatively charged surface necessary for the assembly of clotting factors. Although platelets are anucleated 'cells', they are capable of complex metabolic processes. Thus activated platelets synthesize and secrete thromboxane A_2, an aggregation agonist, and secrete from their α-granules the proteins synthesized by their parent cell, the megakaryocyte, that is, fibrinogen, von Willebrand factor, factor V, platelet factor 4, β-thromboglobulin, and other proteins involved in haemostasis.

From their dense granules they secrete serotonin and ADP, another aggregating substance. Whereas the process of adhesion brings the first layer of platelets into contact with the thrombogenic surface, the subsequent growth of the haemostatic plug, necessary to build a thrombus capable of stopping haemorrhage, depends essentially on platelet-to-platelet interactions, that is, on platelet aggregation. This process is mediated by interaction between fibrinogen and its receptor, glycoprotein IIb–IIIa, exposed at the surface of activated platelets. One fibrinogen molecule can interact with two different glycoprotein IIb–IIIa complexes (Weisel, JBiolChem, 1992; 267: 16637) by two recognition sites located on the carboxyterminal ends of its two γ-chains, thus providing a molecular bridge between two adjacent platelets. This interaction plays a pivotal part in the formation of platelet thrombi. However, in high-shear stress conditions, von Willebrand factor is the required glycoprotein IIb–IIIa ligand to support aggregation,[2] and platelet cohesion. It has been suggested that high-shear forces could give multimers of von Willebrand factor the shape of extended filaments, such as are observed with electron microscopy. A filamentous structure would offer a great number of binding sites for platelet receptors, providing multivalent interaction and increasing the strength of interaction. At lower shear, other adhesive proteins such as fibrinogen or thrombospondin, a platelet protein, may provide sufficient force of interaction.[2] Circulating platelets are then activated by thromboxane A_2 and ADP secreted by the previously activated platelets, and are recruited to participate in growth of the platelet aggregate. Newly formed thrombin is also able to activate platelets through binding to its own receptor on platelet membranes.

Coagulation
Introduction

At the beginning of the twentieth century, in 1905, it had been recognized that the initiating event in blood coagulation was the exposure of blood to damaged tissues (Morawitz, ErgebPhysiol, 1905; 4:207). The substance present in tissues, responsible for the induction of coagulation, and initially termed tissue thromboplastin, is now known as tissue factor. This process, which is recognized to constitute the essential mechanism for the initiation of blood clotting, had been formerly termed the 'extrinsic pathway' of blood coagulation.[3,4] A second mechanism, which did not require tissue factor, had been proposed, and termed the 'intrinsic pathway', the initiating event being the contact between blood and a negatively charged surface. These two pathways constitute the coagulation 'cascade' and 'waterfall' hypotheses described in 1964.[3,4] Through the extrinsic and intrinsic pathways, blood clotting involves sequential activation of plasma proteins to their enzyme forms by limited proteolysis, and complex interactions between those proenzymes, enzymes, and cofactors. This process leads to the generation of thrombin, the major enzyme for clotting. Thrombin initiates the proteolytic conversion of soluble plasma fibrinogen to solid fibrin, which is the major structural support for the blood clot. Clot is also made of activated platelets and retains red and white blood cells as well as some plasma. Once the primary function of the clot, that is the prevention of blood loss, has been accomplished, it is progressively degraded by enzymes of the fibrinolytic system and wound healing ensues.

Coagulation proteins

The plasma proteins involved in haemostasis belong to three systems with different physiological roles. The first system involves procoagulation factors and promotes clot formation. It comprises proenzymes, cofactors, and structural proteins. A second system includes regulatory proteins that modulate clot formation and localize it to the site of vessel injury. These proteins are plasma protease inhibitors, and enzymes that specifically inactivate procoagulant factors. The third system consists of the fibrinolytic proteins, enzymes, and protease inhibitors, which proceed to the degradation of the fibrin clot during the healing process (Table 1). Although proteins belonging to these three different systems have opposite physiological roles, they nevertheless share common functional features. One group of proteins, including procoagulant factors, inhibitors, and fibrinolytic activator, are zymogens of serine proteases. They share a common catalytic site constituted by a characteristic triad of amino acids, serine, histidine, aspartic acid, critical to their mechanism of action. Some of them bear marked structural and functional homology to the digestive enzymes trypsin and chymotrypsin; these include factors XII, XI, X, VII, and II. Like trypsin and chymotrypsin, the serine proteases of blood coagulation cleave peptide bonds involving Arg or Lys residues. They have, however, a much higher degree of specificity, with a limited number of substrates and possible cleavage sites, restricted to one or two (Furie, JBiolChem, 1982; 257:3875).[5] Another group of proteins including procoagulant factors and inhibitors is synthesized in a vitamin K-dependent reaction, providing them with γ-carboxyglutamic (**GLA**) residues. These GLA residues are responsible for the unique membrane-binding properties of this group. Proteins of the haemostatic system also share common features in their three-dimensional structure. Thus, many of them contain one or more regions homologous with a region of the epidermal growth factor and known as epidermal growth-factor domains. These domains may play a part in the high-affinity interaction of proteins with cell surfaces, receptors, or other proteins. The kringle domain, so-called by analogy with a Scandinavian pastry, is another structure commonly encountered in these proteins, and one which is likely to contain recognition elements essential for macromolecular assembly. Finger domains play a part as binding sites. Thus, the coagulation and fibrinolytic proteins constitute a family of proteins made of the assembly of common structural domains with functional autonomy. The unique specificity of each of these proteins is, however, assured by different molecular surfaces surrounding the common enzyme catalytic sites or structural domains. Coagulation proteins thus have a number of common structural features devoted to molecular assembly (Fig. 1).

The assembly of blood-clotting enzymes and of their substrates in complexes with cofactors on membrane surfaces is critical to the process of coagulation and to its control. These surfaces provide distinct binding sites for enzymes and substrates, and the assembly occurs with a high degree of specificity and with high affinity. This results in conformational changes that make the substrate more accessible to limited proteolytic cleavage by the active enzyme. The assembly process thus enhances the activity of the enzymes. They exhibit a very low Michaelis constant (K_m) and a high catalytic rate (k_{cat}). Moreover, the active enzymes generated by limited proteolysis of the substrates remain bound to the surface through the particular

Table 1 Properties of the haemostatic components

Component	Name or synonym	Synthesis	Mol. wt	Half-life	Function
Proteins of the coagulation system					
Tissue factor		Membrane glycoprotein	37 000		Cofactor/initiator
Factor I	Fibrinogen	Hepatocyte	340 000	4–6 days	Substrate—structural protein
Factor II*	Prothrombin	Hepatocyte	72 000	2–5 days	Serine protease—zymogen
Factor V	Proaccelerin	Hepatocyte, Megakaryocyte	330 000	12–36 h	Cofactor
Factor VII*	Proconvertin	Hepatocyte	50 000		Serine protease—zymogen
Factor VIII	A-antihaemophilic factor	Hepatocyte, Spleen, Other tissues	300 000	10–16 h	Cofactor
Factor IX*	B-antihaemophilic factor, Christmas factor	Hepatocyte	57 000	24 h	Serine protease—zymogen
Factor X*	Stuart factor	Hepatocyte	59 000	36–48 h	Serine protease—zymogen
Factor XI	Plasma thromboplastin antecedent, Rosenthal factor	Hepatocyte	160 000	2–3 days	Serine protease—zymogen
Factor XII	Hageman factor	Hepatocyte	80 000	2–3 days	Serine protease—zymogen
Factor XIII	Fibrin-stabilizing factor		300 000	6–12 days	A-chain: transglutaminase Zymogen
Prekallikrein	Fletcher factor		85 000	35 h	Serine protease—zymogen
Height molecular-weight kininogen	Fitzgerald, Flaujeac or Williams factor		110 000	6 days	Cofactor
von Willebrand factor	Ristocetin agglutination cofactor	Endothelial cell	225 000 × n**	6–20 h	Platelet adhesion
Antithrombin III		Hepatocyte	65 000	2–3 days	Serpin
Protein C*		Endothelial cell, Hepatocyte	62 000	6–8 h	Serine protease—zymogen
Protein S*		Hepatocyte, Megakaryocyte	70 000	ND	Cofactor
Heparin cofactor II		Hepatocyte	65 000	2.5 days	Serpin
Tissue-factor pathway inhibitor	Extrinsic pathway inhibitor (EPI), Lipoprotein-associated coagulation Inhibitor (LACI)	Endothelial cell	42 000	ND	Kunitz inhibitor
Proteins of the fibrinolytic system					
Tissue-type plasminogen activator		Endothelial cell	72 000	2–10 min	Serine protease
Platelet activator inhibitor 1		Hepatocyte, Megakaryocyte, Smooth muscle cell, Endothelial cell	52 000	1–3 min	Serpin
Platelet activator inhibitor 2		Placenta			
α_2-antiplasmin		Hepatocyte	70 000	2.6 days	Serpin
Plasminogen		Hepatocyte	92 000	2.2 days	Serine protease—zymogen

* Vitamin K-dependent proteins; **n, denotes number of subunits whose mol. wt is 225 000; ND, not determined.

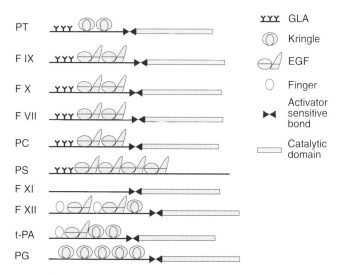

Fig. 1. Structural domains of the proteins involved in haemostasis. Schematic structure of coagulation factors prothrombin (PT), factor IX (FIX), factor X(FX), factor VII (FVII), factor XI (FXI); factor XII (FXII), of coagulation inhibitors protein C (PC) and protein S (PS), of fibrinolytic activator, tissue-type plasminogen activator (t-PA), and of plasminogen (PG). The different structural domains described in the text are: GLA, kringle, epidermal growth factor (EGF), finger.

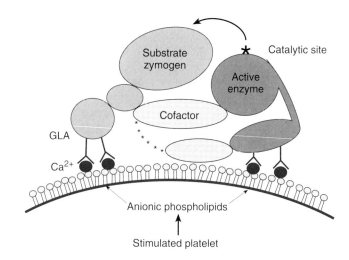

Fig. 2. Schematic representation of molecular complex associated with zymogen activation. Each reaction complex involves an active enzyme (a serine protease), a cofactor protein, and a cell-membrane surface composed of anionic phospholipids. The combination on the cell membrane of enzyme, cofactor, and substrate gives rise to maximum activity. The vitamin K-dependent proteins, enzyme, and substrate are bound to the phospholipid surface through γ-carboxyglutamyl (GLA) residues in the presence of calcium ions. The cofactor is bound to the phospholipid surface through hydrophobic bonds. The cofactor also binds both enzyme and substrate, bringing them into close proximity and thus favouring proteolytic cleavage of the substrate by the active enzyme.

domains involved in their inactivation by specific proteases inhibitors. Thus, the activation of coagulation is enhanced and accelerated at the membrane surface, which moreover prevents local inhibition of the newly formed clotting enzymes. An example of such an assembly in given in Fig. 2. By contrast, active enzymes not bound to this membrane surface expose their catalytic site to circulating protease inhibitors that prevent intravascular dissemination of clotting. The membrane surface thus has a modulatory role that favours the coagulation process at the site of vessel injury and restricts it to this site.

Tissue factor and factor VII activation

Blood coagulation is primarily triggered by exposure of blood to tissue factor after tissue injury. Tissue factor expressed at the cell surface forms a complex with factor VII, a plasma single-chain zymogen, in the presence of calcium ions. Tissue factor is an integral membrane glycoprotein tightly associated with phospholipids. The molecule is located on the outer surface of the cell membrane except for a transmembrane domain and a cytoplasmic tail (Edgington, ThrombHaem, 1991; 66:87). Cells that express tissue factor are strategically located to create a protective haemostatic barrier when tissue injury occurs. Among them are cells of the outer layers of the skin, fibroblasts in the capsule of many organs, cells of the nervous system, cells within the placenta (Wilcox, PNAS, 1989; 86:2838; Fleck, ThrombRes, 1990; 57:765; Callander, Cancer, 1992; 70: 1194).[6] To possess optimal functional activity, tissue factor must be associated with anionic phospholipid (Pitlick, Biochem, 1970; 9: 5105; Bjorklid, BiochemJ, 1977; 165:89; Wijngaards. BBActa, 1977; 488:161), particularly phosphatidylserine. Native factor VII/tissue factor complexes are still physiologically inactive. Nevertheless, binding of tissue factor to factor VII markedly enhances its ability to be activated by proteolytic enzymes (Rao, PNAS, 1988; 85:6687),

such as trace amounts of factor Xa.[7] However, the question is: how could factor Xa be formed in the absence of the functional factor VIIa/tissue factor complex? There is now evidence (Macik, Blood, 1991; 78 Suppl.1:61a; Altieri, PNAS, 1988; 85:7462) that trace amounts of factor VIIa are normally present in circulating blood and trigger tissue factor-dependent coagulation. Factor VIIa can autocatalytically activate factor VII after it is bound to tissue factor (Nakagaki, Biochem, 1991; 30: 10819). The conversion of factor VII to the enzyme factor VIIa occurs through cleavage of a single peptide bond (Arg152–Ile), which unmasks the serine protease catalytic site. Factor VIIa must remain bound to tissue factor to exert its enzymatic activity[8] towards its two substrates, factor X (Nemerson, Biochem, 1966; 5:601) and factor IX (Osterud, PNAS, 1977; 74:5260). Tissue factor serves as a cofactor to factor VIIa in increasing its catalytic activity (Pedersen, JBiolChem, 1990; 265: 16 786; Lawson, JBiolChem; 1992; 267:4834) and in enhancing its ability to associate with its substrates.

Factor X activation

When the concentration of tissue factor is high, the factor VIIa/tissue factor complex preferentially converts factor X to factor Xa, another serine protease, through the proteolytic cleavage of one single peptide bond (Arg52–Ile) on the heavy chain of factor X, removing a 52-amino acid activation peptide. The factor VIIa/tissue factor complex activates factor X many times faster than it activates factor IX (Almus, ThrombHaem, 1989; 62:1067; Komiyama, Biochem, 1990; 29:9418; Bom, ThrombHaem, 1991; 66:283). Activation of factor IX by the factor VIIa/tissue factor is due to proteolytic cleavage of the two peptide bonds, Arg145–Ala and Arg180–Val, on factor IX, with removal of a 35-amino acid activation peptide, leading to the formation of the serine protease, factor IXa. Factor IXa engaged in an equimolecular complex with factor VIIIa at the negatively charged phospholipid surface of activated platelets is able to activate factor X in the same way as factor VIIa/tissue factor complex, thus reinforcing its action. The enzyme, factor IXa, and its substrate, factor X, both vitamin K-dependent proteins, bind to the phospholipid surface through their GLA residues in the presence of calcium ions. Factor VIIIa binds to the same surface through hydrophobic bonds. Factor VIIIa behaves as a cofactor bringing the enzyme and the substrate close together in an optimal conformation for interaction after binding to each other (Fig. 2). In the form in which it circulates in the plasma, factor VIII, as well as factor V, is incapable of serving as a cofactor in the clotting mechanism. It has to undergo a limited proteolysis that removes the central region of the molecule and leads to the formation of factor VIIIa, which comprises two subunits covalently linked by calcium ions (Eaton, Biochem, 1986; 25:505). This proteolysis, catalysed by the first traces of newly formed factor Xa or thrombin, shifts the affinity of factor VIIIa from von Willebrand factor towards procoagulant phospholipid.[9] The role of the cofactor is to increase about 1000-fold the number of substrate molecules that one molecule of enzyme can transform per unit time, that is, to increase the velocity of the reaction.[9]

Prothrombin activation

Similarly, the serine protease factor Xa forms an equimolecular complex with a cofactor, factor Va, on the platelet phospholipid surface in the presence of calcium ions. This catalytic unit is known as 'prothrombinase' (Mann, BiophysJ, 1982; 37:106). Its substrate prothrombin, factor II, is, as factor Xa, a vitamin K-dependent protein bound to phospholipid through GLA residues in the presence of calcium ions. Prothrombinase, built in the same way (Fig. 2) as the complex of factor IXa/cofactor VIIIa/phospholipids, activates prothrombin through the cleavage of two peptide bonds (Arg271–Thr and Arg320–Ile). An aminoterminal activation peptide containing the GLA domain and the kringle domains, and called fragment 1 + 2, is removed, leading to the generation of the two-chain serine protease, thrombin. Due to the loss of the phospholipid-binding GLA domain, thrombin is released from the membrane phase into solution. Like factor VIII, factor V has to be proteolysed by factor Xa or thrombin itself to be effective. Factor V and factor VIII have homologous structures and, like factor VIIIa, factor Va comprises two subunits covalently linked by calcium ions.

Pathological expression of tissue factor

In the absence of vascular injury, blood is not exposed to tissue factor and activation of coagulation is negligible. However, monocytes and endothelial cells in contact with circulating blood can express tissue-factor activity at the surface membrane when stimulated by endotoxin (Rivers, BrJHaemat, 1975; 30:311 ; Colucci, JClinInvest, 1983; 71:1893) or cytokines (Bevilacqua, JExpMed, 1984; 160:618) (Fig. 3). Thus, in pathological conditions such as Gram-negative endotoxaemia, substantial tissue-factor activity may be expressed (Rivers, BrJHaemat, 1975; 30:311), and disseminated intravascular coagulation may occur. Similarly, tumour cells whose surface membranes continuously expose tissue factor to the circulating blood may induce persistent, low-grade, disseminated intravascular coagulation.

Intrinsic pathway

Initiation of the intrinsic pathway of blood coagulation involves the activation of factor XII to factor XIIa. This reaction is promoted by electronegative surfaces such as glass, or collagen exposed in the subendothelium after vessel damage. Factor XII and high molecular-weight kininogen bind to these surfaces. Factor XI and prekallikrein also bind to such surfaces through high molecular-weight kininogen (Colman, JClinInvest, 1984, 73:1249). The physiological mechanism of factor XII activation is unknown, but it follows the binding of factor XII to the surface. Factor XIIa, with high molecular-weight kininogen as cofactor, converts factor XI to factor XIa and prekallikrein to kallikrein. Kallikrein activates factor XII and, thus, enhances the formation of factor XIIa. Kallikrein also activates complement, inflammation, and the kinin system. Factor XIa is an unusual serine protease with two catalytic systems. In the presence of calcium ions, factor XIa converts factor IX to factor IXa in the same way as the complex factor VIIa/tissue factor (Fig. 3). Although this intrinsic pathway is important for blood clotting in vitro, especially in the absence of tissue factor, its physiological importance is questioned by the absence of abnormal bleeding in patients lacking factor XII, prekallikrein, or high molecular-weight kininogen, which do not seem to be required for haemostasis. By contrast, patients with factor XI deficiency have a variable, usually mild but sometimes severe, bleeding diathesis. This implies that, in certain conditions, the amount of factor IXa produced by factor VIIa/tissue factor is insufficient and that additional factor IXa produced by factor XIa is necessary. It was recently shown that thrombin could activate factor XI in the presence of negatively charged surfaces (Naito, JBiolChem, 1991, 266:7353; Gailani, Science, 1991, 253:909). The reinforcement of factor XI activity by this retroactive activation could thus indicate that the production of factor IXa by factor XIa has some physiological importance.

Thus, the 'cascade' and 'waterfall' hypotheses for blood clotting, segregating coagulation factors into the intrinsic and extrinsic pathways, fail to reflect physiological haemostasis. In the revised theory of coagulation, the factor VIIa/tissue factor pathway, with direct activation of factor X reinforced by the bypassing action of factor IXa, has a predominant role, and the formation of additional factor IXa by the intrinsic pathway is thus ancillary. This theory seems to fit better with the reality of haemorrhagic diseases. Patients with trace amounts of plasma factor XI activity withstand the traumatic events of daily life without abnormal musculoskeletal bleeding, unlike patients with severe haemophilia. This could also explain why haemophiliacs A or B (factor VIII or IX deficiency) usually bleed into organs poor in tissue factor, such as joints and muscles, rather than into those rich in tissue factor, such as the brain.

Thrombin

Unlike other factors in blood coagulation, thrombin has several functions in haemostasis, from tissue injury to tissue repair. Thus, thrombin not only converts fibrinogen into fibrin, the visible step of the clotting process, but has a number of other functions.

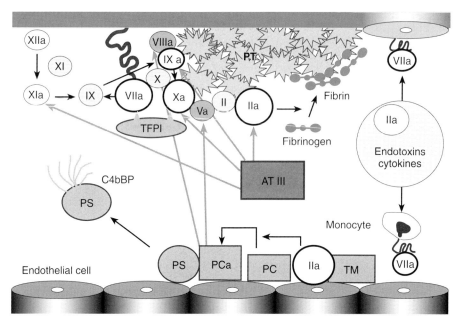

Fig. 3. Schematic representation of coagulation activation. Blood clotting is initiated by the contact of blood with tissue factor (TF) present on the subendothelium at the lesion site. The complex TF/factor VIIa activates factor X to factor Xa in the presence of calcium ions. On the phospholipid surface of aggregated platelets (PT), factor Xa activates factor II to factor IIa (thrombin) in the presence of a cofactor, factor Va, and of calcium ions. Thrombin then converts soluble fibrinogen to solid fibrin that constitutes on to PT the structural support of the clot. TF/factor VIIa complex is also able to activate factor IX to factor IXa. Factor IXa, in the presence of a cofactor, factor VIIIa, and of calcium ions, also activates factor X, thus reinforcing factor Xa formation. Activation of factor XII by contact with the subendothelium is responsible for subsequent factor XI activation. Factor XIa activates factor IX through a secondary coagulation-activation pathway that sustains factor Xa production. The clotting process is controlled and limited to the lesional site by physiological inhibitors. Tissue-factor pathway inhibitor (TFPI) forms a quaternary complex with TF/factor VIIa and factor Xa, thus inhibiting TF/factor VIIa and factor Xa. Antithrombin III (AT III) inhibits serine proteases: factors XIIa, XIa, Xa, IXa, and thrombin (IIa). Activated protein C (PCa), with its cofactor protein S, inhibits cofactors Va and VIIIa. Protein C is activated to PCa by thrombin (IIa) complexed with thrombomodulin (TM) at the phospholipid surface of endothelial cell. A major part of protein S circulates in blood complexed with C4b binding protein (C4bBP) and only free protein S is active as a cofactor for protein C. In pathological conditions, endotoxins and cytokines as well as thrombin are able to induce TF expression on monocytes and endothelial cells, which physiologically do not express TF, and thereby induce intravascular coagulation activation.

Thrombin stimulates platelet activation and secretion, and subsequent aggregation. It can accelerate and amplify its own generation through the activation of factors V and VIII in a positive feedback, but can also down-regulate its own formation by activating protein C in a negative feedback. Native α-thrombin is a unique proteinase in that it has a very steep and narrow active site, and exosites between which substrates are bridge-bound. The structure of the anion exosite I is highly defined and is involved in the recognition of fibrinogen and binding of fibrin, allowing thrombin to be incorporated in the clot. There, thrombin is available to activate factor XIII, the fibrin-stabilizing factor. Native α-thrombin is also the most potent stimulator of the release by endothelial cells of the tissue plasminogen activator, a profibrinolytic enzyme. Thus, most probably, thrombin initiates thrombolysis in the endstage of thrombus evolution. Ultimately, degraded forms of thrombin, produced by proteases generated inside the clot, promote wound healing.[10] Apart from haemostasis, thrombin is capable of cell interaction through a specific receptor, and is thus implicated in inflammation, chemotaxis, cellular proliferation, angiogenesis, atherosclerosis, and the metastatic process.[10]

Fibrin formation

Clot forms when fibrinogen is converted by thrombin to fibrin, the structural protein that assembles into the fibrin polymer providing scaffolding for the other elements of the thrombus. Fibrinogen, the soluble plasma precursor of fibrin, is a tridomainal disulphide-bridged molecule, composed of two symmetrical half-molecules, each consisting of three different polypeptide chains termed Aα, Bβ, and γ (Doolittle, AnnNYAcadSci, 1983; 408:13; Henschen, AnnNYAcadSci, 1983; 408:28; Mosesson, ProgHaemThromb, 1976; 3:61).[11] The N-terminal regions of these three chains are joined in a central domain, the E-domain. The N-terminal ends of the Aα- and Bβ-chains are composed of the fibrinopeptides A (Aα 1–16) and B (Bβ 1–14), which are exposed on this E-domain. The two half-molecules are oriented in an antiparallel manner, and exhibit a loose, interdomainal structure between this central E-domain and two outer D-domains, where the Aα-, Bβ- and γ-chains are tightly assembled and from which emerge the Aα C-terminal ends (Fig. 4). Binding of thrombin to fibrinogen through the thrombin exosite 1 and the fibrinogen substrate site leads to proteolytic cleavage of an Arg–Gly peptide bond in the Aα- (Aα 16/17) and in the Bβ- (Bβ 14/15) chain, releasing fibrinopeptides A and B. This cleavage of fibrinopeptides A and B by thrombin initiates the process of fibrin assembly (Blomback, ArkivKemi, 1958; 12:321; Laurent, ActaChemScand, 1958; 12:1875).[12] The release of fibrinopeptides A and B generates fibrin monomer units where two types of binding sites are exposed in the E-domain of the molecule (Kudryk, JBiolChem, 1974; 249:3322). These polymerization sites subsequently align with complementary sites in the D-domain of other fibrin monomers, whose E-domain polymerization sites align in turn with the D-domain complementary sites of other molecules, and so on. Fibrin molecules are thus arranged in a staggered, overlapping manner by non-covalent intermolecular interactions between outer (D) and central (E) domains (Budzynski, AnnNYAcadSci, 1983; 408:301), forming double-stranded polymerized fibrils (Fig. 4). The release of fibrinopeptide B is slower than that of fibrinopeptide A, and is accelerated by fibrin polymerization.[12] Fibrils then undergo lateral association, resulting in increased fibre thickness (Carr, Biopolymers, 1977; 16:1), as well as branching, allowing the formation of a three-dimensional fibrin network. This clot, held together by non-covalent interactions, is, however, prone to irreversible deformation when subjected to stress and strain,[11] and is unable to resist blood flow. The incorporation of covalent bonds between the fibrin monomers results in a cross-linked clot with almost perfect elastic properties, [11] more rigid, highly resistant to deformation (Ferry, in BioSynthPolymNetworks, Elsevier, 1988:41), and with a very stable structure. Interchain cross-linking between fibrin monomers results from the formation of covalent ε- (γ-glutamyl) lysyl bonds by factor XIIIa, the activated fibrin-stabilizing factor, in the presence of calcium ions (Pisano, Science, 1968; 160:892). Cross-linking occurs within fibrils between the C-terminal regions of the γ-chains of two different fibrin monomers, forming γ-dimers.[13] Reciprocal bridges occur between Lys406 of one γ-chain and Glu399 of another γ-chain (Doolittle, BBResComm, 1971; 44:94) (Fig. 4). Intermolecular cross-linking also occurs at a slower rate between α-chains, creating oligomers and larger α-chain polymers (McDonagh, FEBSLett, 1971; 14:33). Other plasma proteins, among which are α_2-antiplasmin and fibronectin, become cross-linked to α-chains by the same way (Tamaki, BBActa, 1981; 661:280). Cross-linking of α_2-antiplasmin, the plasmin inhibitor, to fibrin clot, prevents too rapid degradation of the clot. Fibronectin, an adhesive protein synthesized by the liver (Tamkun, JBiolChem, 1983; 258:4641) is cross-linked both to the γ-chain of fibrin and to collagen, and thus allows anchoring of fibrin clots to subendothelial tissues. Factor XIII binds to fibrinogen during the clotting process. This plasma proenzyme comprises two α and two β subunits. The α-chains, which possess catalytic potential, are cleaved by thrombin. This cleavage is promoted by the presence of calcium ions as well as the dissociation of β-chains from α-chains (Takagi, Biochem, 1974; 13: 750), which is necessary for the expression of factor XIIIa catalytic activity.[13] Activation of factor XIII is enhanced in the presence of fibrin(ogen),[13] and this effect seems to depend on the formation of a ternary complex between α-thrombin, factor XIII, and fibrin (Greenberg, Blood, 1987; 69:867). Thus fibrin itself plays a critical part in regulating the cross-linking that reinforces the structure of the thrombus. Cross-linking of the fibrin clot is an absolute requirement for it to be haemostatically effective. The total lack of factor XIII is thus responsible for severe haemorrhagic manifestations, such as intracranial bleeding in the neonatal period.

The process of fibrin formation is thus designed to regulate the rate and extent of clotting, as well as the rate and extent of cross-linking and fibrinolysis. The ability of fibrin to bind thrombin at a non-catalytic site prevents release of thrombin into the circulation while locally maintaining its catalytic potential (Liu, JBiolChem, 1979; 254:421). Similarly, fibrin binding to factor XIII regulates

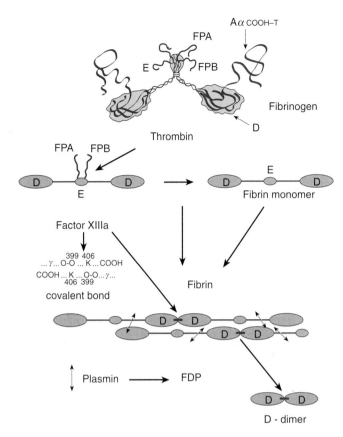

Fig. 4. Schematic model of fibrinogen, fibrin assembly, and fibrinolysis. Fibrinogen is a domainal molecule constituted of two sets of three different polypeptide chains, Aα, Bβ and γ, joined by their aminoterminal regions in a central E-domain linked by loose-coiled coils to the two outer D-domains. Fibrinopeptides A and B (FPA, FPB) are represented on the E-domain. The carboxyterminal ends of the Aα-chains emerge from the D-domains. The proteolytic cleavage of FPA and FPB by thrombin leads to the formation of fibrin monomeric units that assemble in a staggered, overlapping manner by non-covalent interactions between the E- and D-domains, producing fibrin fibrils. Fibrin is then cross-linked by activated factor XIII that forms covalent bonds between γ- and Aα-chains. The reciprocal bonds formed between γ 406-lysyl and γ 399-glutaminyl residues of two different γ-chains are indicated. When fibrin undergoes fibrinolysis under proteolytic action of plasmin the peptides joining the D- and E-domains are cleaved, leading to generation of fibrin degradation products (FDP) among which D-dimers (D-D) uncleaved by plasmin are fibrin specific.

and limits the activation of factor XIII to factor XIIIa, whereas fibrin binding to α_2-plasmin inhibitor, tissue plasminogen activator, and plasminogen (see below) regulates the fibrinolytic process.[11]

Regulation of the clotting process

Clotting must remain a localized process confined to the site of vessel injury; it is thus physiologically limited by antithrombotic mechanisms. These mechanisms are involved in the inhibition of platelet deposition, the limitation of fibrin accumulation, and the destruction of fibrin. Most of them are triggered by, and depend on, a normally functioning endothelium. They include: signal transduction pathways mediated by nitric oxide and prostacyclin that produce vascular relaxation and inhibition of platelet aggregation

(Knowles, TIBS, 1992; 17:399); the limitation of thrombin generation and thus of fibrin deposition by inhibition and clearance of activated coagulation factors; and the elimination of excess fibrin by the fibrinolytic system.

Inhibition of factor VIIa/tissue factor catalytic activity

The neutralization of factor VIIa/tissue factor activity differs from that of other enzyme/cofactor complexes of the clotting process in that it requires a feedback reaction, in which one of the reaction products, factor Xa, participates.[14] In other words, the inhibition can only occur once the product of the reaction has been formed and is effective. By contrast, the enzymes factors IXa and Xa are more effectively neutralized by antithrombin III before they form complexes (Marciniak, BrJHaemat, 1973; 24:391), as are the cofactors VIIIa and Va by their inhibitor, activated protein C. Factor VIIa cannot be rapidly cleared from the blood (Seligsohn, Blood, 1979; 53:828) nor inhibited in the absence of tissue factor. The inhibitor responsible for inactivating factor VIIa/tissue factor catalytic activity is the plasma tissue-factor pathway inhibitor (**TFPI**), formerly referred to as either extrinsic pathway inhibitor[14] or lipoprotein-associated coagulation inhibitor.[15] The major intravascular pool of TFPI has been found on the luminal surface of vascular endothelium and a small amount is present in the platelets (Novotny, Blood, 1988; 72:2020). The primary site of synthesis of plasma TFPI appears to be vascular endothelium (Bajaj, PNAS, 1990; 87:8869). TFPI is a Kunitz-type protease inhibitor with multiple Kunitz-type domains, a fact consistent with its dual inhibitory activity towards factor Xa and factor VIIa/tissue factor. The inhibition of factor VIIa/tissue factor by TFPI is dependent on factor Xa and involves the formation of a quaternary complex consisting of factor Xa, TFPI, and factor VIIa/tissue factor. In this complex, the first Kunitz domain of TFPI binds factor VIIa, while the second binds factor Xa (Girard, Nature, 1989; 338: 518) (Fig. 3).[15] This complex results from the initial binding of a reactive-centre arginine in the second Kunitz domain of TFPI to the active site of factor Xa,[15] with formation of a factor Xa/TFPI complex and loss of factor Xa activity. In a second step, this factor Xa/TFPI complex binds to factor VIIa engaged in the factor VIIa/tissue factor complex through the first Kunitz domain of TFPI. Heparin, through simultaneous binding to factor Xa and TFPI, increases their interaction, and thus enhances the inhibition of factor Xa by TFPI (Wesselschmidt, Blood, 1992; 79:2004). Moreover, injection of heparin releases TFPI from endothelial pool, raising plasma TFPI by from two- to tenfold (Sandset, ThrombRes, 1988; 50:803).

Thus, in physiological conditions, TFPI does not inhibit the activity of factor VIIa/tissue factor until some factor Xa has been produced, but exerts only feedback inhibition of the factor VIIa/tissue factor complex through factor Xa. Moreover, factor Xa is most effectively recognized by TFPI when part of the prothrombinase complex, with factor Va, calcium ions, and phospholipids (Huang, JBiolChem, 1993; 268: 26950) is already formed. Thus, the inhibitory effect of TFPI can only appear with the generation of factor Xa, but prevents further generation of factor Xa and factor IXa by factor VIIa/tissue factor. If the initial generation of factor Xa is sufficient to produce amounts of thrombin able to induce local platelet aggregation and the activation of cofactors V and VIII, it is insufficient due to the inhibitory effect of TFPI, to sustain haemostasis. The production of factor Xa must then been enhanced by factors IXa and VIIIa, through the alternative pathway, and ultimately by factor XIa for persistent haemostasis. Thus, the particular mode of action of TFPI seems to favour, in an initial step, the burst of coagulation, allowing the generation of a first wave of factor Xa, and, in a second step, to slow down the clotting process by limiting this production of factor Xa, leaving the activation of factor X dependent on the factor IXa/factor VIIIa/phospholipid complex.

Inhibition of serine proteases: serpins

Most of the inhibitors that control the proteinases involved in coagulation and fibrinolysis, as well as in inflammation and complement activation, are members of the serine protease inhibitor superfamily of serpins.[16] Although their mechanism of action is poorly understood (Enghild, JBiolChem, 1994; 269: 20159), these inhibitors are thought to trap a serine protease by presenting their reactive site as an ideal substrate. The association between enzyme and inhibitor is rapid, with the formation of a tightly bound, 1:1 enzyme–inhibitor complex with negligible dissociation, the reactive site of the inhibitor acting as a bait.[16] The specificity of serpins is defined by a single amino acid at the reactive centre so that a particular serpin targets a particular proteinase. Thus, in the clotting and fibrinolytic processes, antithrombin III, plasminogen activator inhibitor 1, and α_2-antiplasmin are responsible for thrombin, tissue plasminogen activator, and plasmin inhibition, respectively. During the coagulation process antithrombin III reacts through its reactive centre exhibiting an arginyl residue with clotting serine proteases, chiefly thrombin, but also factors Xa, IXa, XIa, and XIIa.[17] Due to its broad inhibitory action, antithrombin III is the principal physiological inhibitor of coagulation and plays a central part in the regulation of haemostasis *in vivo*. The ability of antithrombin III to inhibit serine proteases is greatly increased by heparan sulphate present at the surface of endothelial cells, and heparin,[17] whose anticoagulant activity occurs through antithrombin III. The interaction of heparin with antithrombin leads to a conformational change in antithrombin that increases the reactivity of the inhibitor. Acquired or genetic reduction in the amount of antithrombin III results in an increased risk of early development of venous thrombotic disease (Egeberg, ThrombDiathHaemorrh, 1965; 13:516; Lane, BloodCoagFibrinol, 1992; 3:315). Hereditary deficiency of antithrombin III is a rare disorder characterized by recurrent deep-vein thrombosis and pulmonary embolism. The prevalence of antithrombin III deficiency in recurrent venous thromboembolism is 2 to 3 per cent. The other serpins that interfere with the clotting process are heparin cofactor II, α_1-antitrypsin, C1 inhibitor, and protease nexin I. Heparin cofactor II and protease nexin I are thrombin inhibitors whose activity is increased by heparin; α_1-antitrypsin is able slowly to inhibit thrombin and also the contact phase of coagulation, as is C1 inhibitor. The importance of their physiological role is uncertain.

Protein C system

The protein C inhibitory pathway modulates, on demand, the activation of the coagulation process,[18] playing a part only when thrombin is generated. Protein C, a vitamin K-dependent protein, is the precursor of a serine proteinase, activated protein C (Clouse, NEJM, 1986; 314:1298). The anticoagulant effect of activated protein C is due to the inactivation of the two cofactors, factor Va and factor VIIIa (Fig. 3).[19] Activated protein C cleaves the two Arg506–Gly and Arg306–Ser peptide bonds on factor Va. Factor Va thus loses its capacity to bind prothrombin and factor Xa, whilst its affinity for phospholipids decreases (Odegaard, JBiolChem, 1987; 262: 11 233). On factor VIIIa, activated protein C cleaves the Arg562–Gly peptide bond, and seems thus, to decrease the affinity of factor VIIIa for factors IXa and X (Fay, JBiolChem, 1991; 266: 20 139). This proteolytic inactivation requires calcium ions and occurs in some minutes.[19] Protein C is activated on the surface of endothelium by a complex consisting of thrombomodulin and thrombin. Thrombomodulin is an integral membrane protein of the endothelial cell that binds circulating thrombin in the presence of calcium ions. When bound to thrombomodulin, thrombin loses its ability to clot fibrinogen and to activate factor V (Esmon, JBiolChem, 1982; 257:7944) as well as to activate platelets, whilst it acquires the capacity to activate protein C. Thus, binding of thrombin to thrombomodulin changes the substrate specificity of thrombin. This represents a unique example of reversal of total enzyme specificity, switching the procoagulant enzymatic activity to an anticoagulant activity (Esmon, FASEBJ, 1995; 9:946). Thrombomodulin exerts its specificity both by interacting directly with the fibrinogen-binding site and by modifying the conformation of the thrombin active site.[18] The formation of the thrombomodulin–thrombin complex increases 30 000 fold the rate of generation of activated protein C, and, as for clotting complexes, phospholipid membranes accelerate the activation of protein C. The thrombomodulin–thrombin complex proteolytically activates protein C, releasing a dodecapeptide from the N-terminal part of its heavy chain. Once formed, activated protein C binds to protein S, another vitamin K-dependent protein, on the phospholipid membrane surface (Walker, JBiolChem, 1981; 256:11128). In circulating blood, 60 per cent of the protein S is complexed with a component of the complement system, the C4b binding protein, and only the free form of protein S is capable of enhancing the anticoagulant activity of activated protein C. The presence of protein S and phospholipids enhances the anticoagulant effect of activated protein C (Fig. 3).

Activated protein C is also capable of neutralizing a circulating inhibitor of tissue plasminogen activator (Van Hinsbergh, Blood, 1985; 65:444), increasing the activity of circulating tissue plasminogen activator. Activated protein C thus accelerates the conversion of plasminogen to plasmin and facilitates fibrinolysis.

Inhibition and clearance of activated protein C are mediated by two serpins, α_1-antitrypsin and protein C inhibitor, and by α_2-macroglobulin (Heeb, Blood, 1989; 73:446; Scully, ThrombHaem, 1993; 69:448). Protein C inhibitor has been isolated and was found to slowly form a 1:1 complex with activated protein C (Suzuki, JBiolChem, 1983; 258:163).

Clinically, abnormalities of this pathway, such as genetic deficiencies of proteins C or S, account for recurrent thrombotic disease in early adulthood. Particularly common (approximately 5 per cent of the general population and 20 per cent of patients with recurrent thrombotic disease) is a mutated factor V with Arg506–Gln substitution on one of the two activated protein C cleavage sites. This abnormality, termed factor V Leiden, is responsible for resistance to activated protein C and predisposition to thrombosis (Bertina, Nature, 1994; 369:64; Dahlback, PNAS, 1993; 90:1004).

Fibrinolysis

The haemostatic clot has a temporary role. When wound healing occurs and normal tissue structure and function is restored, the clot must disappear. The fibrin clot is thus gradually removed through the action of the fibrinolytic system (Astrup, SemThrombHaemost, 1991; 17:161). The specificity of fibrinolysis and the extent of the control of fibrin degradation are assured by solid-phase activation and liquid-phase inhibition. Fibrin, the solid phase that constitutes the physical support of the haemostatic clot, functions as a 'suicide cofactor' (Fears, BiochemJ, 1989; 261:313) by virtue of its capacity to bind specifically both plasminogen and plasminogen activator, the promoters of fibrinolysis. Tissue plasminogen activator has affinity for fibrin (Hoylaerts, JBiolChem, 1982; 257:2912) while urokinase plasminogen activator has not. Thus intravascular fibrinolysis is essentially induced by tissue plasminogen activator, whereas urokinase is the most important extravascular inducer of extracellular proteolysis.[20] Binding sites for tissue plasminogen activator and plasminogen are buried in fibrinogen and unveiled by cleavage of fibrinopeptides A and B and the polymerization of fibrin monomers.[11] Binding of plasminogen to fibrin is mediated by interactions between lysine-binding sites of kringle 1 and 4 on plasminogen and lysine residues of fibrin. Similarly, one kringle domain of tissue plasminogen activator mediates its binding to lysine fibrin residues, whereas its finger domain mediates its binding to fibrin fragment D. Binding of tissue plasminogen activator and plasminogen to fibrin results in a trimolecular complex. This assembly leads to a considerable enhancement of the reaction rate between tissue plasminogen activator and plasminogen since within the complex, tissue plasminogen activator activity is increased 100-fold. The formation of this trimolecular complex thus constitutes the most important mechanism for the acceleration and amplification of fibrinolysis. Plasminogen is transformed by tissue plasminogen activator into the double-chain active enzyme plasmin by cleavage of the Arg561–Val562 peptide bond. The catalytic site of this serine protease is located in the carboxyterminal region. Plasmin generated at the surface specifically degrades fibrin, producing fibrin degradation products by cleaving lysyl and arginyl bonds. The critical step in degradation involves cleavage of the coiled coils between D- and E-domains, which liberates cross-linked derivatives from particulate fibrin. Factor XIIIa-induced intermolecular covalent bonds result in unique degradation products, such as D-dimer consisting of two-fragment D-moieties from adjacent fibrin monomers, covalently bound by γ-chain cross-links (Fig. 4).[21] The plasma concentration of D-dimers reflects the formation of fibrin together with its fibrinolytic degradation, and it is now widely accepted that when plasma D-dimer is normal, deep venous thromboembolism or pulmonary embolism can be excluded (Bounameaux, AmJClinPath, 1989; 91:82; Demers, ThrombHaem, 1992; 67:408). The fibrin network that binds the platelets to each other and to the vessel wall is thus progressively digested. Moreover, the binding of plasminogen to carboxyterminal lysine residues unveiled by cleavage of plasmin increases progressively with the degradation of the fibrin surface (Fleury, Biochem, 1991; 30:7630). Localization of fibrinolysis activation at the clot surface ensures that the generation and activity of plasmin are directed and restricted to fibrin. In addition to specifically degrading fibrin, free circulating plasmin may cleave other proteins, especially fibrinogen and clotting factors such as factors V, VIII, XIIIa, and von Willebrand. In addition, plasmin is capable of lysing a variety of proteins on cell surfaces and matrix constituents. Plasmin thus catalyses pericellular proteolysis and participates in physiological processes such as ovulation, embryonic development, wound healing, angiogenesis, as well as in pathological processes such as tumour cell invasion.[20]

The inhibition of fibrinolytic enzymes, plasmin and tissue plasminogen activator, proceeds only in the fluid phase, that is in the circulating blood where inhibitors are present. These inhibitors belong to the serpin family and are α_2-antiplasmin, the specific inhibitor of plasmin, and plasminogen activator inhibitor 1, the major inhibitor of plasminogen activator in plasma. The interaction between plasmin and α_2-antiplasmin in plasma is one of the fastest known interactions between proteins (Wiman, EurJBioch, 1978; 84:573); it occurs through the reactive site of the inhibitor and the catalytic site of the enzyme, and also through the lysine-binding sites of plasmin when they are not involved in binding with fibrin, that is, when plasmin is free in the circulation. Thus α_2-antiplasmin can only inhibit free plasmin not bound to fibrin by its lysine-binding site. Inhibition of plasmin in solution by α_2-antiplasmin impairs further degradation of the fibrin surface and controls the extent of fibrinolysis (Angles-Cano, BBActa, 1992; 1156:34). Similarly, plasminogen activator inhibitor 1 is unable to inhibit fibrin-bound tissue plasminogen activator. Plasminogen activator inhibitor circulates in plasma complexed to tissue plasminogen activator or reversibly bound to vitronectin, a protein that stabilizes its activity (Angles-Cano, ChemPhysLip, 1994; 67/68:353). Plasminogen activator inhibitor is present in platelet α-granules; the platelet is the main reservoir of plasminogen activator inhibitor 1 in blood (Erickson, JClinInvest, 1984; 74:1465) and is, through platelet aggregation, highly concentrated in the clot, where it may prevent premature lysis. When α_2-antiplasmin is decreased or depleted, α_2-macroglobulin, capable of complexing proteases of any type, may act as a secondary inhibitor. Therapeutic inhibition of fibrinolysis by ϵ-aminocaproic acid and tranexamic acid is based on the capacity of these lysine analogues to bind to lysine-binding sites, preventing the binding of tissue plasminogen activator and plasminogen to fibrin.

In the absence of a fibrin clot, tissue plasminogen activator has a low capacity to transform plasminogen. Plasmin is not generated in circulating blood in resting conditions. Fibrinolysis is essentially triggered by the presence of fibrin.

Factor XIIa also plays a part in the activation of the fibrinolytic system. It is capable of activating tissue plasminogen activator directly or through the generation of kallikrein (Kluft, SemThrombHaemost, 1987; 13:50).

Functions of the liver

The liver plays a major part in the control of haemostasis by producing proteins of the clotting and fibrinolytic systems, clearing from the circulating blood the corresponding active enzymes, and thus regulating these two systems.

Synthesis of the coagulation proteins
Proteins of coagulation

All clotting proteins, coagulation factors, and inhibitors, and most of the components of the fibrinolytic system, are synthesized by hepatocytes, except for von Willebrand factor produced by endothelial cells and megakaryocytes (Jaffe, JClinInvest, 1973; 52:2757) and tissue plasminogen activator (Levin, PNAS, 1983; 80:6804) produced by endothelial cells, as well as urokinase-type plasminogen activator produced by kidney cells.[22] Hepatic synthesis of coagulation proteins has been demonstrated by different experimental methods: for example, by induced hepatic necrosis for coagulation factors II, VII, IX, X, XI, and XII (Cornillon, CompBiochPhys, 1985; 80c:277), and by isolated liver perfusion for coagulation factors II (Owens, BBActa, 1981; 676:365), V,[23] VIII, X (Dodds BrJHaemat, 1974; 26:497), and antithrombin III (Koj, BBActa, 1978; 539:496). Secretion of factors II (Munns, FedProc, 1983; 42:1010; Anderson, AmJPhysiol, 1964; 206:929), VII (Prydz, ScaJCLI, 1964; 16:540), V (Mazzorana, ThrombRes, 1989; 54:655), fibrinogen (Barnhardt, VoxSang, 1963; 8:461; Rugstad, ExpCellRes, 1972; 71:41), factor XIII (Nagy, Blood, 1986; 68:1272; Nagy, ThrombHaem, 1985; 54:274),[23] protein C and protein S[24] has been detected in cultures of hepatocytes and hepatocyte cell lines, such as HepG2 continuous human tumour cell lines retaining representative phenotypic characteristics of the normal human liver. The site of synthesis of fibrinogen, factor II (Chung, in *Proteins in biology and medicine*, NY: Acad. Press, 1982:309), and factor VIII[25] has been confirmed by demonstration of mRNA. Fibrinogen synthesis is directly stimulated by interleukin 6 (**IL-6**, hepatocyte-stimulating factor) by increasing transcriptional activity in liver parenchymal cells (Fuller, JCellBiol, 1985; 101:1481). It has also been shown that the endstage degradation product of the plasmin-mediated digestion of fibrinogen, fragment D or FDP-D, binding to the hepatocyte, might act as a direct regulator of the synthesis of fibrinogen by that cell, though to a lesser extent than IL-6. This could play a regulatory part (Laduca, PNAS, 1989, 86:8788), favouring fibrinogen synthesis when degradation of fibrinogen molecules occurs in circulating blood. The degradation of fibrinogen also controls the replacement of antithrombin III. Macrophages treated with fragment D appear to secrete IL-6, which promotes the synthesis of antithrombin III by hepatocytes (Hoffman, ThrombHaem, 1986; 41:707) as well as that of fibrinogen.

The α-, β-, and γ-chains of fibrinogen are encoded by three independent genes. Their assembly does not seem to need hepatocyte-specific engineering but essentially information inherent in the fibrinogen chains themselves, and it has been proposed that $\alpha\gamma$ and $\beta\gamma$ dimers, as well as $\alpha\beta\gamma$ half-molecules, are intermediates in the assembly of mature fibrinogen molecules (Huang, JBiolChem, 1993; 268:8919).

Fibrinogen, factor II, factor VII, and protein C are exclusively synthesized in the liver. Although fibrinogen is present in the α-granules of platelets, it is not synthesized in megakaryocytes (Louache, Blood, 1991; 77:311; Lange, Blood, 1991; 78:20) and the presence of fibrinogen in platelets is probably due to endocytosis of the molecule from plasma. Conversely, factor V present in plasma and in the α-granules of platelets is not only synthesized by the liver but also by megakaryocytes (Chiu, JClinInvest, 1985; 75:339;

Gewirtz, Blood, 1986; 67:1639). The same also applies to protein S (Schwarz, Blood, 1985; 66:353a; Ogura, Blood, 1987; 70:301). Protein S, antithrombin III, and plasminogen activator inhibitor 1 are also synthesized in the vascular endothelial cell (Chan, Thromb-Haem, 1981; 46:504).[24,26] Factor VIII is mainly synthesized by the hepatocyte and the spleen (Kelly, BrJHaemat, 1984; 56:535)[25] but also to a lesser extent in a variety of other tissues[25] and in the reticuloendothelial system.

Hepatocytes are thought not to synthesize plasma tissue factor-pathway inhibitor (Bajaj, PNAS, 1990; 87:8869), and a normal plasma tissue factor-pathway inhibitor has been reported in patients with severe hepatocellular disease (Bajaj, JClinInvest, 1987; 79:1874; Novotny, Blood, 1991; 78:387; Sandset, Haemostasis, 1991; 21:219).

Vitamin K-dependent proteins

The clotting factors II, VII, IX, X, and the protein C and S of the protein C anticoagulant system, are vitamin K-dependent proteins. These proteins are defined by an NH$_2$-terminal peptide of approx. 40 aminoacids that contains 10 to 12 glutamic residues that are carboxylated to γ-carboxyglutamic acid (GLA) by a vitamin K-dependent liver carboxylase (Suttie, AnnRevBiochem, 1985; 54:459; Vermeer, Haematol, 1985; 18:71).[27] Those GLA residues have the essential function of binding calcium ions, allowing vitamin K-dependent proteins to undergo a conformational change that leads to the expression of binding properties to negatively charged phospholipid surfaces. This binding is necessary for the assembly of clotting proteins on activated platelet surfaces, which favours rapid generation of thrombin (Suttie, Hepatol, 1987; 7:367) (see above: Physiology of coagulation). γ-Carboxylation occurs during the post-translational modification of proteins. A propeptide, NH$_2$-terminal to the Glu-rich domain, is required for recognition by the vitamin K-dependent carboxylase and removed by proteolytic cleavage before secretion of the protein. The cofactor necessary to the reaction catalysed by carboxylase is the reduced form of vitamin K. Metabolic transformation of vitamin K occurs in liver microsomes, where it is reduced to the vitamin K hydroquinone by vitamin K reductase. As well as the reduced form of vitamin K, the carboxylation reaction requires molecular oxygen, carbon dioxide, and the precursor form of the vitamin K-dependent protein as substrate. During the carboxylation, vitamin K hydroquinone is converted to vitamin K epoxide. This epoxide is then cycled back to vitamin K by the vitamin K epoxide reductase (Fig. 5).[27] In human adults the requirement for vitamin K is low and about half of the daily requirement is from dietary intake, mainly phyllokinone, and the remainder from synthesis by gut micro-organisms. A major source of vitamin K is dark-green leafy vegetables. Naturally occurring vitamin K is fat-soluble, and thus bile salts are required for its absorption in the upper part of the small bowel. Vitamin K is then incorporated into chylomicrons, and appears in the lymph and then in plasma, until it is transferred to the liver where it is stored.[28]

In deficiency or absence of vitamin K, vitamin K-dependent coagulation factors are synthesized at a normal rate, but lack all or part of the GLA residues necessary for calcium binding to phospholipids and thus lack their procoagulant function. Inhibition

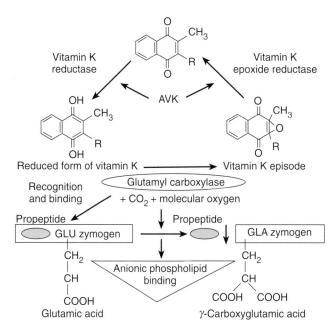

Fig. 5. Schematic representation of vitamin K cycle and carboxylation of vitamin K-dependent proteins during protein synthesis. Vitamin K is converted to the vitamin K hydroquinone by a vitamin K reductase. The reduced form of vitamin K is the substrate for the vitamin K-dependent glutamyl carboxylase that carboxylates glutamic acids (Glu) to γ-carboxyglutamic acids (GLA), while vitamin K epoxide is formed. CO$_2$ and molecular oxygen are also required. Then, through the action of vitamin K epoxide reductase, vitamin K is generated. The major site of vitamin K antagonist (AVK) action is the vitamin K epoxide reductase, but vitamin K reductase is also inhibited. The vitamin K-dependent carboxylase binds to a recognition site on the propeptide of the precursor form of the vitamin K-dependent protein (propeptide GLU zymogen). When GLU have been converted to GLA, the propeptide is cleaved and the fully processed protein, able to bind to anionic phospholipids, is secreted into the circulation.

of γ-carboxylation by vitamin K antagonists is the basis of current oral anticoagulant therapy. The precursors of vitamin K-dependent coagulation factors have been termed proteins induced by vitamin K antagonists or absence (PIVKA).

In new-born infants, the two major sources of vitamin K are decreased or suppressed. First, intake of lipid-soluble vitamin K is reduced due to a relatively poor transport of lipids by the placenta, and secondly the endogenous synthesis of vitamin K by micro-organisms is absent because the gut is sterile for a few days after birth. Thus, in normal infants, plasma vitamin K-dependent factors may fall to a low concentration on the second and the third days of life. If these fall to below 10 per cent of normal (<10 U/dl), haemorrhagic disease of the new-born appears.[28] With food intake the concentrations reach normal adult values over weeks. Nevertheless, human milk is a poor source of vitamin K, and breast-fed infants are specially at risk of haemorrhagic disease if not supplemented with exogenous vitamin K.

Vitamin K has no effect on the synthesis of the vitamin K-dependent proteins, and in hepatocellular insufficiency there is no increase in vitamin K-dependent protein antigen or activity after vitamin K therapy (Corrigan, JAMA, 1982; 248:1736; Feldsohn, Hepatol, 1983; 3:858).

Proteins of fibrinolysis

Hepatic synthesis of plasminogen has been demonstrated by experiments using isolated liver perfusion (Owens, JLabClinMed, 1985; 105:368), and hepatic parenchymal cells have been shown to secrete α_2-plasmin inhibitor (Aoki, ClinChimActa, 1978; 84:99; Saito, Blood, 1981; 58:225a; Fair, JLabClinMed, 1983; 101:372). Type 1 plasminogen activator inhibitor is synthesized by the liver (Cwickel, JBiolChem, 1984; 259:6847; Sprengers, JLabClinMed, 1985; 105:751) and by endothelial cells (Pyke, CancerRes, 1991; 51:4067; Whawell, JPath, 1993; 169:67; Schneiderman, PNAS, 1992; 89:6998; Philips, BBA, 1984; 802:99; Bartha, JBiolChem, 1991; 266:792).[26] Hepatocytes express the plasminogen activator inhibitor 1 gene (Thornton, Fibrinolysis, 1995; 9:9), and the liver is probably a major source of plasma plasminogen activator inhibitor 1, which is also synthesized by vascular smooth-muscle cells (Knudsen, JClinInvest, 1987; 80:1082) and is present in the platelet α-granules and synthesized by megakaryocytes (Konkle, ArtSclerThromb, 1993; 13:669). The platelets, however, probably do not contribute to the plasma plasminogen activator inhibitor 1 under physiological conditions.[29] Production of plasminogen activator inhibitor 1 is highly regulated. It is induced by a variety of growth factors, such as transforming growth factor-β, by cytokines such as tumour necrosis factor-α, and by inflammatory mediators such as endotoxin.[30]

Clearance

Enzyme–inhibitor complexes and free enzymes are cleared by cells of the reticuloendothelial system, especially in the liver, where the system comprises Kupffer and endothelial cells that clear particulate and soluble matter, respectively. The clearance of tissue plasminogen activator is very rapid since its half-life in the circulation is estimated to be 4 min in man (Tanswell, Fibrinolysis, 1989; 3:79); [31] the liver is the major site of removal and catabolism of tissue plasminogen activator.[31] The human hepatoma cell line HepG2 has a high-capacity, high-affinity cell-surface receptor capable of specific catabolism of tissue plasminogen activator.[32] Uptake of tissue plasminogen activator by the liver is mediated by two recognition systems: a high-affinity system, specific for tissue plasminogen activator, on the parenchymal cells; and a mannose receptor on the endothelial cells, which takes up tissue plasminogen activator by recognizing carbohydrate groups on the molecule (Narita, JClinInvest, 1995; 96:1164).[31]

The mannose-receptor cycle between the cell surface and an intracellular compartment proceeds at a very high speed, the half-life of the receptors located on the surface being about 10 s. This is the reason why the ligands for the receptor, among which is tissue plasminogen activator, are so efficiently cleared from the circulation (Smedsrod, BiochemJ, 1990; 266:313). Extracellular matrix-associated plasminogen activator inhibitor 1 appears to modulate the binding of tissue plasminogen activator to the high-affinity binding site and thus to participate in the clearance of the activator by hepatocytes. Specific binding of preformed tissue plasminogen activator–inhibitor complexes was demonstrated in HepG2 cells; in the rat these complexes are cleared significantly more rapidly by the liver than either free tissue plasminogen activator or free inhibitor 1 (Wing, JLabClinMed, 1991; 117:109). Thus, circulating tissue plasminogen activator may interact with inhibitor 1 in the extracellular matrix of the hepatocyte, where the inhibitor accumulates in its active form, to form a complex, which is subsequently bound, internalized, and degraded by hepatocytes through lysosomal processing. Fragments of degraded tissue plasminogen activator are then released by the cells (Owensby, JBiolChem, 1989; 264: 18180; Morton, JBiolChem, 1989; 264:7228). Similarly, exogenous tissue plasminogen activator delivered intravenously for thrombolytic therapy accumulates in the liver and is then degraded. Plasminogen activator inhibitory activity is also very rapidly cleared from the circulation, and a half-life as short as 3.5 min is reported in animals; experimental findings suggest that its clearance takes place primarily in the liver.[29] The amount of plasmin potentially produced by activation of total plasma plasminogen overwhelms the inhibitory capacity of plasma for plasmin; in other words, if all the plasminogen in plasma were to be converted to plasmin, inhibitors such as α_2-plasmin inhibitor and others would be able to inhibit only half the circulating plasmin. Consequently, in the case of an acute increase in tissue plasminogen activator in circulating blood, rapid hepatic clearance is essential to maintain normal haemostasis.

The reticuloendothelial system of the liver is also closely involved in the clearance of activated clotting factors (Deykin, JClinInvest, 1966; 45:256) and activation complexes. The complexes resulting from the interaction of antithrombin III or other serpins with their target serine proteinases are recognized by one or two hepatocyte membrane receptors termed serpin receptors 1 and 2 (Pizzo, AmJMed, 1989; 87 Suppl. 3B: 14S; Pratt, ArchBiochemBiophys, 1988, 262:111). [33–35]The receptor recognition sites possibly are exposed by a conformational change of the serpin while binding to the proteinase during complex formation. The serpin receptor 1 recognizes proteinase complexes of antithrombin III and heparin cofactor II (Pratt, ArchBiochemBiophys, 1988; 262:111),[33–37] and the serpin receptor 2 the α_2-antiplasmin–plasmin complex.[34] The clearance of complexes involving antithrombin III is very rapid, with half-lives of some minutes only. After their uptake in hepatocytes, those complexes are localized in the lysosomes where they are degraded (Shifman, JBiolChem, 1982; 257:3243).[36,37] Thus the clearance by the liver of products of the activation of coagulation is as rapid as the clearance of the profibrinolytic enzyme, tissue plasminogen activator. Clearance of intermediate products of fibrin conversion as well as fibrinogen/fibrin degradation products occurs in the liver (Gans, Blood, 1967; 29:526). Kupffer's cells are also considered important in clearing microthrombi in the hepatic sinusoids (Oka, ArchPathLabMed, 1983; 107:570). Moreover, the hepatic reticuloendothelial system is able to clear altered platelets or blood-borne microaggregates rapidly.[38]

Regulatory function

The liver has a major role in the regulation of the fibrinolytic system, protecting the organism from bleeding complications, as well as in the regulation of the coagulation activation, protecting the organism from intravascular coagulation. Impairment of liver function results in a decrease in clearance of tissue plasminogen activator, which accumulates in the circulation. It is also responsible for a decrease in the synthesis of the naturally occurring inhibitors, plasminogen activator inhibitor 1 and α_2-antiplasmin, thereby leading to a global increase in the circulating fibrinolytic activity.

Similarly, when the liver reticuloendothelial system is impaired or overloaded, extrahepatic localization and microembolization of particulate material as microthrombi or microaggregates occurs, and may induce tissue injury. The integrity of this clearance mechanism probably represents a major determinant of organ function during conditions of intravascular coagulation and shock.[38]

In summary, liver impairment favours bleeding due to impaired synthesis of coagulation factors and increased fibrinolytic activity, yet it also increases susceptibility to intravascular coagulation resulting from impaired clearance of procoagulant material.

References

1. Hawiger J. Mechanisms involved in platelet vessel wall interaction. *Thrombosis and Haemostasis*, 1995; **74**: 369–72.
2. Ruggeri ZM. New insights into the mechanisms of platelet adhesion and aggregation. *Seminars in Hematology*, 1994; **31**: 229–39.
3. Davie EW and Ratnoff OD. Waterfall sequence for intrinsic blood clotting. *Science*, 1964; **145**: 1310–12.
4. MacFarlane RG. An enzyme cascade in the blood clotting mechanism and its function as a biochemical amplifier. *Nature*, 1964; **202**: 498–9.
5. Furie B and Furie BC. The molecular basis of blood coagulation. *Cell*, 1988; **53**: 505–18.
6. Drake IA, Morrissey JH, and Edgington TS. Selective cellular expression of tissue factor in human tissues: implications for disorders of hemostasis and thrombosis. *American Journal of Pathology*, 1989; **134**: 1087–97.
7. Nemerson Y and Repke D. Tissue factor accelerates the activation of coagulation factor VII: the role of a bifunctional coagulation cofactor. *Thrombosis and Research*, 1985; **40**: 351–8.
8. Rapaport SI and Rao LVM. Initiation and regulation of tissue factor-dependent blood coagulation. *Arteriosclerosis and Thrombosis*, 1992; **12**: 1111–21.
9. Hemker HC and Kessels H. Feedback mechanisms in coagulation. *Haemostasis*, 1991; **21**: 189–96.
10. Fenton II JW, Ofosu FA, Brezniak DV, and Hassouna HI. Understanding thrombin and hemostasis. *Hematology/Oncology Clinics of North America*, 1993; **7**: 1107–19.
11. Mosesson MW. Fibrin polymerization and its regulatory role in hemostasis. *Journal of Laboratory and Clinical Medicine*, 1990; **116**: 8–17.
12. Blomback B, Hessel B, Hogg D, and Therkildsen L. A two-step fibrinogen–fibrin transition in blood coagulation. *Nature*, 1978; **275**: 501–5.
13. Chung SI, Lewis MS, and Folk JE. Relationships of the catalytic properties of human plasma and platelet transglutaminases (activated blood coagulation factor XIII) to their subunit structures. *Journal of Biological Chemistry*, 1974; **249**: 940–50.
14. Rao LVM and Rapaport SI. Studies of a mechanism inhibiting the initiation of the extrinsic pathway of coagulation. *Blood*, 1987; **69**: 645–51.
15. Broze GJ Jr, Warren LA, Novotny WF, Higuchi DA, Girard TJ, and Miletich J. The lipoprotein-associated coagulation inhibitor that inhibits factor VII–tissue complex also inhibits Xa: insight into its possible mechanism of action. *Blood*, 1988; **71**: 335–43.
16. Carrell R and Travis J. α_1-antitrypsin and the serpins: variation and counter-variation. *Trends in Biochemical Sciences*, 1985; **10**: 20–4.
17. Rosenberg RD and Damus PS. The purification and mechanism of action of human antithrombin-heparin cofactor. *Journal of Biological Chemistry*, 1973; **248**: 6490–505.
18. Esmon CT. The roles of protein C and thrombomodulin in the regulation of blood coagulation. *Journal of Biological Chemistry*, 1989; **264**: 4743–6.
19. Marlar RA, Kleiss AJ, and Griffin JH. Mechanism of action of human activated protein C, a thrombin-dependent anticoagulant enzyme. *Blood*, 1982; **59**: 1067–72.
20. Scully MF. Plasminogen activator-dependent pericellular proteolysis. *British Journal of Haematology*, 1991, **79**: 537–43.
21. Francis CW and Marder VJ. Mechanisms of fibrinolysis. In Williams WJ et al. eds. *Hematology*, 3rd edn. New York: McGraw-Hill, 1983: 1206–76.
22. Mammen EF. Coagulation abnormalities in liver disease. *Hematology/Oncology Clinics of North America*, 1992; **6**: 1247–57.
23. Giddings JC, Shaw E, Tiddenhaus EGD, and Bloom AL. The synthesis of factor V in tissue culture and isolated organ perfusion. *Thrombosis et Diathesis Haemorrhagica*, 1975; **34**: 321.
24. Fair DS and Marlar SA. Biosynthesis and secretion of factor VII, protein C, protein S, and the protein C inhibitor from a human hepatoma cell line. *Blood*, 1986; **67**: 64–70.
25. Wion K, Kelly DA, Summerfield JAS, Tuddenham EGD, and Lawn D. Distribution of factor VIII mRNA and antigen in human liver and other tissues. *Nature*, 1985; **317**: 726–9.
26. Loskutoff DJ, Van Mourik JA, Erickson LA, and Laurence D. Detection of an unusually stable fibrinolytic inhibitor produced by bovine endothelial cells. *Proceedings of the National Academy of Sciences (USA)*, 1983; **80**: 2956–60.
27. Furie B and Furie BC. Molecular basis of vitamin K-dependent γ-carboxylation. *Blood*, 1990; **75**: 1753–62.
28. Olson RE. The function and metabolism of vitamin K. *Annual Review of Nutrition*, 1984; **4**: 281–337.
29. Sprengers ED and Kluft C. Plasminogen activator inhibitors. *Blood*, 1987; **69**: 381–7.
30. Loskutoff DJ, Sawdey M, Keeton M, and Schneiderman J. Regulation of PAI-1 gene expression *in vivo*. In Aznar J, Estelles A, and Gilabert J, eds. *Fibrinolytic inhibitors, cellular, biological and clinical aspects*. Madrid: Editorial Garsi, 1994.
31. Kuiper J, Otter M, Rijken DC, and Van Berkel TJC. Characterization of the interaction *in vivo* of tissue-type plasminogen activator with liver cells. *Journal of Biological Chemistry*, 1988; **263**: 18220–4.
32. Owensby DA, Sobel BE, and Schwartz AL. Receptor-mediated endocytosis of tissue-type plasminogen activator by the human hepatoma cell line Hep G2. *Journal of Biological Chemistry*, 1988; **263**: 10587–94.
33. Fuchs HE, Shifman MA, and Pizzo SV. *In vivo* catabolism of 1-proteinase inhibitor-trypsin, antithrombin III-thrombin and 2-macroglobulin-methylamine. *Biochimica et Biophysica Acta*, 1982; **716**: 151–7.
34. Gonias SL, Fuchs HE, and Pizzo SV. A unique pathway for the plasma elimination of α_2-antiplasmin-protease complexes in mice. *Thrombosis and Haemostasis*, 1982; **48**: 208–10.
35. Pizzo SV, et al. *In vivo* catabolism of α_1-proteinase inhibitor, antithrombin III and heparin cofactor II. *Biochimica et Biophysica Acta*, 1988; **964**: 158–62.
36. Fuchs HE, et al. Hepatocyte receptors for antithrombin III-proteinase complexes. *Journal of Cellular Biochemistry*, 1984; **24**: 197–206.
37. Fuchs HE, Michalopoulos G, and Pizzo SV. Hepatocyte uptake of α_1-proteinase inhibitor-trypsin complexes *in vitro*. Evidence for shared uptake mechanisms for proteinase complexes of α_1-proteinase inhibitor and antithrombin III. *Journal of Cellular Biochemistry*, 1985; **25**: 231–43.
38. Kaplan JE and Saba TM. Platelet removal from the circulation by the liver and spleen. *American Journal of Physiology*, 1978; **235**: H314–20.

2.15 Function and metabolism of collagens and other extracellular matrix proteins

Detlef Schuppan and A. M. Gressner

Introduction

Abnormal deposition of extracellular matrix is the hallmark of liver fibrosis and cirrhosis. In fibrosis both the quantity of most extracellular matrix molecules, especially the fibrillar collagens, and their local composition change dramatically. Even in a terminally cirrhotic and shrunken liver, the total collagen content may be increased six- to tenfold. Fibrosis results from an imbalance of the extracellular matrix that is removed by proteolysis (fibrolysis) in favour of the extracellular matrix that is synthesized and laid down (fibrogenesis). Accelerated fibrogenesis is not unique to the liver. It is the body's general response to injury, where it is aimed at wound closure and protection from further damage. An example is the necessity for rapid closure of skin wounds to prevent the invasion of pathogens. However, the wound healing response may go astray in chronic diseases when injury becomes repetitive, resulting in scar formation with concomitant distortion of the regular architecture and loss of organ function. The consequences are particularly obvious in chronic liver diseases, where the abnormal and excessive extracellular matrix deposition leads to vascular obstruction, architectural distortion and formation of novel diffusion barriers, and the well-known consequences of portal hypertension and liver cell insufficiency. Whereas portal fibrosis decreases sinusoidal blood supply by shunting portal blood via porto-portal and porto-venous collaterals, perisinusoidal fibrosis may severely compromise diffusion of nutrients between hepatocytes and sinusoidal blood or diminish detoxification of gut-derived toxins. Perisinusoidal fibrosis is the main cause of portal hypertension. Its histological basis is the 'capillarization of the sinusoids' (Schaffner, Gastro, 1963; 44:239; Hahn, Gut, 1980; 21:63) which is characterized by formation of a complete instead of a discontinuous basement membrane, accompanied by massive deposition of interstitial extracellular matrix in the space of Disse and loss of the membrane pores (fenestrations) that characterize the sinusoidal endothelial cells. Figure 1 illustrates the process of sinusoidal capillarization in which hepatic stellate cells and the endothelium are the major producers of the abnormal extracellular matrix (for a detailed discussion of the cells involved in liver fibrosis refer to Chapter 6.2).

Much work has been done to develop methods that target fibrogenic effector cells, mainly the hepatic stellate cell (synonymous with Ito cell, perisinusoidal lipocyte), with agents that halt their proliferation or that downregulate synthesis and deposition of the most abundant extracellular matrix protein in fibrosis, collagen type I, either by interfering with transcription of its mRNA from the gene or by inhibiting the formation of collagen fibrils (see below).

Apart from its mere abundance, the altered extracellular matrix environment of fibrosis modifies the behaviour of the cells embedded in it. Most extracellular matrix molecules elicit signals that are transferred to the cellular interior via specific receptors such as the integrins. Importantly, the presence of signals from the extracellular matrix may up- or downregulate classical signal transduction initiated by, for example, growth factors and hormones. Signals from the extracellular matrix converge with classical signal transduction pathways and modulate the cell's receptiveness for various stimuli. Furthermore, certain growth factors bind to extracellular matrix molecules which can serve as their extracellular storage sites and release them upon tissue damage, further accelerating the healing process. Taken together, the cells can condition their own environment or that of neighbouring cells by the deposition, or the proteolytic removal, of a specific extracellular matrix, combined with secretion of classical mediators. This interplay results in numerous interactions and levels of feedback regulation that control cell proliferation and the biosynthetic pattern in a given tissue and are finely tuned for maintenance or restoration of tissue homeostasis (Fig. 2).

Signalling properties of the abnormal extracellular matrix often reside in small structural domains or even oligopeptide sequences, making research into the functional properties of extracellular matrix molecules, their receptors, and the signal transduction pathways involved an attractive topic in current cell and molecular biology. Since there are essentially no differences between certain extracellular matrix molecules of liver and non-hepatic organs such as kidney, lung, and skin, most findings obtained with the latter tissues and cells can be applied to the liver and vice versa. In fact, liver fibrosis research has profited from the other areas, and many of the data shown below are justified extrapolations from these systems. This applies equally well to the molecules that are involved in proteolysis of the extracellular matrix, namely the matrix

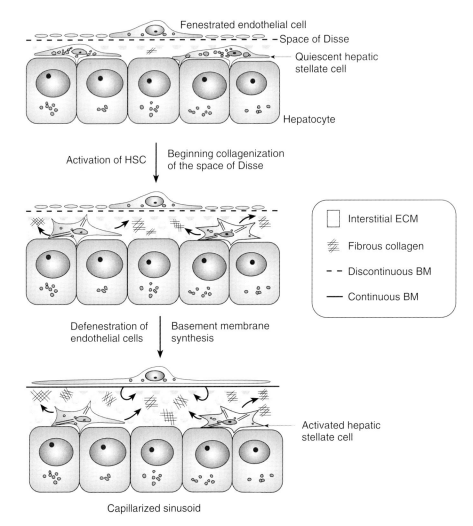

Fig. 1. Capillarization of the sinusoids. The sinusoids of normal liver are enveloped in a sheath of fenestrated endothelial cells that rest on a delicate layer of connective tissue which consists of a basement membrane as well as interstitial matrix. Quiescent hepatic stellate cells (synonymous with Ito/vitamin A storing cells, lipocytes) are embedded in this loose perivascular connective tissue (the space of Disse) where their membrane processes contact the hepatocytes. When activated by fibrogenic stimuli, hepatic stellate cells acquire actin stress fibres and a biosynthetically active rough endoplasmic reticulum, and lose the vitamin A-containing lipid droplets. The resultant cell (activated stellate cell, myofibroblast-like cell) starts to proliferate and to synthesize a vast excess of extracellular matrix, including fibrillar collagens and basement membrane proteins. Endothelial cells become altered, losing their fenestrations and producing basement membrane material. The result is a sinusoid that resembles a capillary, where the previously free exchange between the blood and hepatocytes becomes severely impeded.

metalloproteinases and their inhibitors, which, in spite of their complex regulation, are attractive effectors for antifibrotic therapies.

The liver extracellular matrix

The extracellular matrix is a complex assembly of macromolecules that rapidly undergo remodelling during growth and after injury, in order to re-establish cellular functions and tissue homeostasis. As in other epithelial–mesenchymal organs, the hepatic extracellular matrix does not simply serve as a mechanical scaffold, but rather provides the resident (hepatic) and incoming (e.g. inflammatory) cells with signals that are indispensable for cell polarity, migration, proliferation, quiescence, and differentiation.[1] The constituents of the normal, as well as the fibrotic, hepatic extracellular matrix include collagens, non-collagenous glycoproteins, and proteoglycans/glycosaminoglycans.[2,3] However, a clear-cut sub-division of extracellular matrix molecules into distinct classes is no longer possible, since evolution has produced hybrid molecules by genetic interchange of specialized interactive domains, a process termed exon shuffling, finally creating multi-domain molecules with multiple functions.[1] Indeed, most extracellular matrix proteins have such a multi-domain structure (see below). In addition, the extracellular matrix also encompasses certain growth factors, matrix metalloproteinases (to which the collagenases belong), and their inhibitors that associate with the extracellular matrix, as well as some transmembrane proteoglycans that are shed into and immobilized in the extracellular matrix. Figure 3 gives an idea of the diversity of extracellular matrix molecules that have been found in the liver, exploiting techniques such as immunohistology, *in situ* hybridization, and protein (Western) and RNA (Northern) blotting in the analysis of liver tissue or cultured liver cells. The structure of some of these molecules has been analysed in detail and knowledge

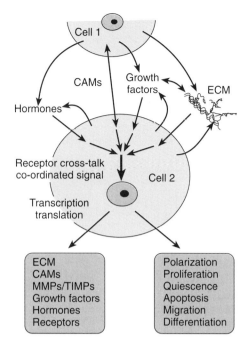

Fig. 2. Cellular activities are regulated by integration of many signals. The cell receives different receptor-mediated stimuli that are derived from hormones, growth factors/cytokines, the extracellular matrix (ECM) or from cell–cell contacts (cell adhesion molecules, CAMs). These stimuli signal the cell to adapt the appropriate social behaviour in a multicellular organism. The cross-talk between the different signals that reach the cellular interior generates a delicately balanced response that affects the synthesis of molecules that act in an auto- or paracrine way to modify the cellular environment or to initiate biological programmes such as proliferation, migration, differentiation, or apoptosis. This establishes an autoregulatory loop aimed at tissue homeostasis, the disruption of which may lead to autonomous growth and malignant transformation.

about the regulation of their synthesis, proteolytic removal, and signalling properties is growing fast. Due to limited space, only selected examples can be discussed which illustrate the progress that has been made in dissection of the functional architecture of extracellular matrix molecules and their receptors. These molecules form the basis for most of the current research in the area of liver fibrosis.

Collagens

To date, 19 different types of collagens are known.[1,4,5] They are defined as extracellular matrix proteins that contain domains of repeating tripeptide units with the amino acid sequence glycine (Gly)–Xaa–Yaa, where Xaa and Yaa may be any amino acid, but preferentially proline (Pro) in the Xaa or Yaa position, or hydroxyproline (Hyp) in the Yaa position. Consequently, classical collagens contain about 33 per cent of the amino acid glycine, 10 to 13 per cent of hydroxyproline, and 10 to 15 per cent of proline. This unique composition allows the formation of the rigid collagen triple helix, in which three identical or similar polypeptide chains are coiled into a left-handed helix, with the small Gly residues positioned in the centre of the helix and the Pro residues limiting rotation of the individual protein chains. Further stabilization via

hydrogen bonds is achieved by post-translational hydroxylation of Pro to Hyp in the Yaa position. Variation of amino acids in the Xaa and Yaa position, interruptions of the (Gly–Xaa–Yaa)$_n$ sequence, or specialized terminal domains dictate the supramolecular organization of individual triple helices to lateral aggregates (fibrils), chain-like molecules, networks, or other structures. In addition, they may form specific recognition sites for other molecules, such as proteoglycans, non-collagenous extracellular matrix proteins, growth factors, and extracellular matrix receptors. The collagens can be subdivided into several groups based on similar structural features and their supramolecular assemblies:

(1) the classical fibril-forming collagens (types I, II, III, V, and XI);
(2) the network-forming collagens (types IV, VIII, and X);
(3) the collagen that assembles to beaded microfilaments (type VI);
(4) the collagen that forms anchoring filaments (type VII);
(5) the group of fibril-associated collagens with interrupted triple helices (FACITs) (types IX, XII, XIV, XVI, and XIX);
(6) the transmembrane collagen, type XVII; and
(7) collagens with yet unknown function (types XIII, XV, and XVIII).

Ten of these collagens (types I, III, IV, V, VI, VIII, XIV, and XVIII) have been found in the liver (Table 1), and others may still be detected once suitable reagents are available. The structural diversity of the known collagens is depicted in Fig. 4.

Fibril-forming collagens

These are the most abundant collagens in most connective tissues, with types I and III representing between 80 and 90 per cent of collagens, both in normal and fibrotic liver (Fig. 4(a)). The fibril-forming collagens are of similar size (roughly 1050 amino acids per chain) and the Gly–Xaa–Yaa triplets of their constituent chains are not interrupted by non-collagenous sequences, rendering them stiff and rod-like molecules that can assemble spontaneously to the characteristic cross-striated collagen fibrils observed by electron microscopy. Fibril growth occurs by lateral alignment along the fibril axis in a regular stagger of about a quarter of the length of one collagen molecule. The fibril-forming collagens are synthesized as precursors that contain amino-terminal and carboxy-terminal propeptides (N- and C-propeptides, respectively) which are completely (C-propeptide) or mainly (N-propeptide) devoid of collagenous sequences. The presence of the C-propeptide is necessary for the selection of the appropriate collagen chains and for the initiation of triple helix formation in the endoplasmic reticulum of the cell. It is removed by a C-propeptidase before assembly into fibrils occurs. The N-propeptide, for which an extracellular N-propeptidase exists, can be retained much longer, and incompletely processed collagen molecules, so-called pN-collagens, may coat the surface of fibrils, where they appear to regulate fibril diameter (usually 30 to 60 nm in soft connective tissues such as the liver), since fibril growth cannot proceed by lateral association when the bulky N-propeptide is still present. Accordingly, most hepatic collagen fibrils can be visualized with an antibody to the N-propeptide of type III collagen which labels the pNIII collagen that covers their surface.

Collagen types I, III, and V do not form separate structures, but are rather incorporated into composite fibrils, where the relative

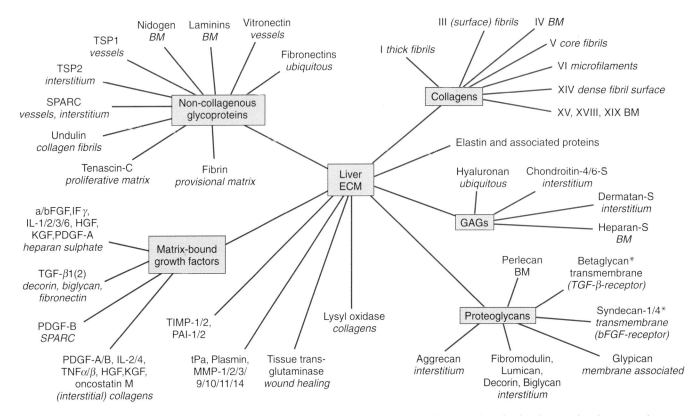

Fig. 3. The hepatic extracellular matrix. Composite view of the collagens, non-collagenous glycoproteins, elastin, glycosaminoglycans, and proteoglycans that have been found in the liver extracellular matrix. Other proteins that are specifically bound to the extracellular matrix, such as fibrin, plasmin and tissue plasminogen activator (tpa), tissue transglutaminase, lysyl oxidase, growth factors/cytokines, metalloproteinases (MMPs), tissue inhibitors of metalloproteinases (TIMPs), and plasminogen activator inhibitor (PAI) are included. Some transmembrane proteoglycans (*) that serve as receptors may be shed from the cell and sequestered in the extracellular matrix after proteolytic cleavage. TSP, thrombospondin; SPARC, secreted protein acidic and rich in cysteine (synonymous with osteonectin or BM-40); a/bFGF, acidic/basic fibroblast growth factor; IF, interferon; IL, interleukin; HGF, hepatocyte growth factor; KGF, keratinocyte growth factor; PDGF, platelet-derived growth factor; TGF, transforming growth factor; BM, basement membrane; S, sulphate.

Table 1 Hepatic collagens. Chain composition, localization and estimated relative percentages of the collagen found in the liver (from refs 1, 4, 5, and Rojkind, Gastro, 1979; 76:710)

Collagen type	Chain composition	Localization	Relative % (normal liver)	Relative % (cirrhotic liver)
I	$[\alpha1(I)]_2\ \alpha2(I)$	Major fibrils	40–50	60–70
III	$[\alpha1(III)]_3$	Major fibrils	40–50	20–30
IV	$[\alpha1(IV)]_2\ \alpha2(IV)$	Basement membranes	1	1–2
V	$[\alpha1(V)]_2\ \alpha2(V)$	Interstitial core fibrils	2–3	3–5
VI	$\alpha1(VI)\ \alpha2(VI)\ \alpha3(VI)$	Interstitial microfilaments	0.1	0.2
VIII	$[\alpha1(VIII)]_2\ \alpha2(VIII)$	Elastin associated?	?	?
XIV	$[\alpha1(XIV)]_3$	Fibril associated	0.1 (?)	?
XV, XVIII, XIX	$[\alpha1(XV)]_3$? $[\alpha1(XVIII)]_3$? $[\alpha1(XIX)]_3$?	Basement membranes	?	?

Collagen XIV and undulin are identical molecules. It is not known whether collagens XV, XVIII and XIX consist of a single α-chain.

contribution of the collagen types seems to determine diameter and mechanical properties of the fibrils (Romanic, JBC, 1991; 266: 12703). In systems other than the liver, type V has been found in pericellular fibrils of small diameter and in the centre of larger fibrils (Birk, JCellBiol, 1988; 106:999; Becker, JHistochemCytochem, 1991; 39:103), suggesting that it may form a nidus for fibril growth.

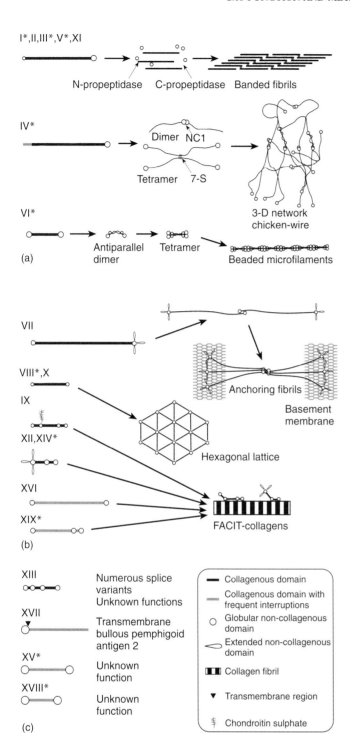

Fig. 4. Structure and supramolecular assembly of the collagens. Collagens are now subdivided into subfamilies according to their structure and function: the collagens that (a) form fibrils (types I, II, III, V, and XI), (b) establish networks (types IV, VIII, and X), (c) assemble to beaded microfilaments (type VI), (d) constitute anchoring filaments (type VII), (e) belong to the fibril-associated collagens with interrupted triple helices (FACITs) (types IX, XII, XIV, XVI, and XIX), (f) have a transmembrane domain (type XVII), and (g) collagens with yet unknown function (types XIII, XV, and XVIII). The ten collagens that have been found in the liver are marked by an asterisk (see also Table 1). The amino-terminal end of the molecules is located at the left side.

Composite fibrils of collagens I and III have also been demonstrated in the liver by immunoelectron microscopy (Geerts, Hepatol, 1990; 12:233). An interesting but still unproven hypothesis is the differential sensitivity of fibrils of mixed composition to proteolytic attack by collagenases, since these enzymes show selectivity for a given collagen type (e.g. matrix metalloproteinase-1 for collagen type I>III but not type V, whereas matrix metalloproteinase-9 degrades collagen type V>II but not type I, see also Chapter 2.15.12).

Network-forming collagens

Type IV (basement membrane) collagen is the prominent representative of this group (Fig. 4(a)). Unlike the fibril-forming collagens, triple-helical collagen IV does not undergo extracellular processing by removal of the propeptides. These propeptides rather serve as crosslinking domains that, via generation of tetramers at the amino-terminal and dimers at the carboxy-terminal end, assemble to a three-dimensional network. This network becomes further intertwined by lateral alignment of individual triple-helical and carboxy-terminal domains to form a 'chicken-wire' structure (Yurchenco, JCellBiol, 1987; 105:2559; Hudson, JBC, 1993; 268:26033). Apart from a molecule of the chain composition $[(\alpha1(IV)]_2\alpha2(IV)$, which predominates in most tissues and which appears to be the only variant that is expressed in the liver (Miner, JCellBiol, 1994; 127:879), other more rare basement membrane collagens with chains $\alpha3(IV)$, $\alpha4(IV)$, $\alpha5(IV)$ and $\alpha6(IV)$ are found in kidney, lung, and in membranes of the inner ear. The carboxy-terminal propeptide domain of $\alpha3(IV)$ has been identified as the autoantigen of Goodpasture's syndrome, which is characterized by haemoptysis, haematuria, and rapid progressive glomerulonephritis (Saus, JBC, 1988; 263:13374), whereas genetic defects in the carboxy-terminal domain of the $\alpha5(IV)$ and $\alpha6(IV)$ chains are responsible for the X chromosome-linked forms of Alport syndrome, a heritable disease characterized by early onset deafness, renal failure, and splitting of the glomerular basement membrane (Tryggvason, KidneyInt, 1993; 43: 38; Oohashi, JBC; 1994; 269:7520). Due to frequent short interruptions of its triple helix by non-collagenous sequences, type IV collagen forms a flexible backbone on which supramolecular complexes with the other basement membrane molecules assemble (see below). In the liver, immunostaining for this collagen is not only found in the vascular basal lamina and underneath biliary epithelia, but also around portal fibroblasts and in the non-fibrotic perisinusoidal space which lacks an electron microscopically detectable basement membrane (Schaffner, Gastro, 1963, 44:239; Hahn, Gut, 1980; 21:63).

The other two collagens of this group, types VIII and X (Fig. 4(b)), form hexagonal lattices. They are expressed in Descemet's membrane of the eye and underneath various endothelia (type VIII) or, as the product of hypertrophied chondrocytes, in the calcifying zone of cartilage (type X). Type VIII has been found in the liver, where it is associated with elastic fibres of portal triads and of the capsule (Sawada, CellStructFunct, 1991; 16:455). The function of these collagens is not known.[3,4]

The microfilament-forming collagen

To date type VI is the only representative of this subgroup. This collagen is made up of three different chains that form a short triple helix, approximately one-third the length of the fibril-forming collagens, with two large terminal globular domains. The uncleaved globular domains serve to cross-link two monomers to an antiparallel dimer and two dimers to a tetramer. The tetramer constitutes a member of a chain-like molecule (Fig. 4(a)) which can be visualized by immunoelectron microscopy as a beaded filament that runs between large collagen fibrils (Keene, JCellBiol, 1988; 107:1995; Becker, JHistochemCytochem, 1991; 39:103). It is found ubiquitously in soft tissues and in association with loosely packed fibrils of collagens type I and III, where it may play a role in anchoring vascular structures to the interstitium. In the liver, collagen type VI is detectable in the portal tract interstitium and in the perisinusoidal space of Disse, with an increased expression from the periportal towards the pericentral zone (Griffiths, Histopath, 1992; 21:335). The large globular domains of collagen VI contain repetitive domains, each of nearly 200 amino acids length, that bear similarity to the A domains of von Willebrand factor (Bonaldo, JBC, 1990; 264:20235; Zhang, BiochemJ, 1993; 291:787). These A domains appear to mediate interactions with the collagen triple helices, either for oligomerization of collagen VI or for interaction with fibrillar collagens. A most recent finding has been a potent growth-promoting effect of soluble collagen VI on various adherent mesenchymal and epithelial cells, including hepatic stellate cells (Atkinson, ExpCellRes, 1996; 228:283). This growth stimulation, which is seen at nanomolar concentrations (comparable to one of the most potent growth factors for mesenchymal cells, platelet-derived growth factor) could be part of a feedback loop that induces rapid wound closure once degradation of the easily accessible collagen VI filaments occurs. Interestingly, the growth signal resides in the triple helix of collagen VI and can be inhibited by single chains of collagen VI, presenting the possibility of a peptide-derived approach to inhibit liver fibrosis.

The collagen of anchoring filaments

Collagen type VII forms this unique structure that appears to be limited to the epidermal basement membranes (Burgeson, JInvDermatol, 1993; 101:252). Type VII has the longest known triple helix, 1530 amino acids long, with numerous non-collagenous interruptions (Christiano, JBC, 1994; 269:20256). The small carboxy-terminal propeptides overlap in an antiparallel fashion to generate a dimer, and several of these dimers align by lateral association to form the anchoring fibril. The crosslink region interacts with humps of collagen IV and laminin that are dispersed in the subepithelial connective tissue. The amino-terminal globular domain of collagen VII is unusually large and contains nine type III homologies of fibronectin and one A domain of von Willebrand factor per chain (see below). This is the region that anchors the fibril to yet unidentified molecules in the basement membrane. The loop thus formed firmly connects the basement membrane to the underlying stroma which is necessary in a mechanically strained organ like skin (Fig. 4(b)).

The FACIT collagens

The fibril associated collagens with interrupted triple helices (FACITs), collagens IX, XII, XIV, XVI, and XIX, represent a growing subfamily with apparently related functions and considerable structural diversity. They do not form fibrils on their own but associate with the surface of pre-existing fibrils of the fibril-forming collagens.

They have a few or multiple short collagenous sequences that are separated from each other by more extended non-collagenous domains. The function of type IX collagen, the triple helix of which contains three different α-chains (α1(IX), α2(IX), and α3(IX)) and which is only expressed in cartilage and the vitreous body of the eye, is the most studied. Its carboxy-terminal triple helix aligns with the surface of mature fibrils of type II collagen, whereas its carboxy-terminal end extends into the extracellular space where it appears to regulate the distance between the type II fibrils and their supramolecular arrangement. This function appears to be supported by a side-chain of chondroitin sulphate that is attached to the α2(IX) chain. Interestingly, the chondroitin sulphate chain that serves as a repellent for other macromolecules is much larger in the vitreous body of the eye than in cartilage. In the former it helps to maintain the collagen in a wide spatial arrangement that allows light transmission (Yada, JBC, 1990; 265:6992).

The similar collagens XII and XIV bear only two short collagenous domains, each between 110 and 130 amino acids long, and a large non-collagenous amino-terminal domain that is composed of a mosaic of fibronectin type III repeats and A domains of von Willebrand factor (Fig. 4(c)). This non-collagenous domain represents more than 80 per cent of the molecular mass (Yamagata, JCellBiol, 1991; 115:209; Wälchli, EurJBioch, 1993; 212:483; Bauer, BBActa, 1997; 1354:183). Both proteins are composed of a single α-chain, which undergoes complex alternative splicing in the case of type XII. Contrary to type XII, type XIV, which appears to derive from the same gene as undulin (Just, JBC, 1991; 266:17326; Wälchli, EurJBioch, 1993; 212:483; Ehnis, JBC, 1997; 272:20414), is widely expressed in the liver. It is found predominantly in the portal tract stroma and is located on the surface of densely packed, mature (diameter of approximately 60 nm), and remarkably regular fibrils of collagens I and III, whereas it is absent or decreased in the unorganized connective tissue of active liver fibrogenesis (Schuppan, JBC, 1990; 265:8823). In line with this observation, freshly isolated (quiescent) hepatic stellate cells, which produce only minor amounts of other extracellular matrix molecules, express considerable quantities of undulin/collagen XIV mRNA and protein (Knittel, ExpCellRes, 1992; 203:312). Furthermore, acetaldehyde downregulates its expression, whereas that of collagen and fibronectin is upregulated (Casini, 1994; BBResComm; 199:1019). But its expression by hepatic stellate cells does not cease in liver fibrosis (Milani, Hepatol, 1994; 20:908), perhaps as a result of upregulation by the fibrogenic cytokine transforming growth factor-β1 (Casini, 1994; BBResComm; 199:1019), although the molecule might escape incorporation into the unorganized fibrillar matrix. The exact functions of undulin/collagen XIV are still incompletely defined. It interacts with interstitial collagens *in vitro* (Schuppan, JCellBiol, 1991; 115:106a), with the proteoglycan decorin (Ehnis, JBC, 1997; 272:20414), and a chondroitin–dermatan sulphate variant of CD44 (the hyaluronic acid receptor) that is highly expressed on haematopoietic cells, but it is not recognized by an integrin (the classical extracellular matrix receptors, see below) (Ehnis, ExpCellRes, 1996; 229:388). Interestingly, the active form of the *N*-propeptidase that allows collagen fibrils to grow (by cleaving the N-terminal propeptide from the fibril-forming collagens) is specifically bound to collagen XIV, pointing to novel mechanisms in fibril formation (Colege, JBC, 1995; 270:16724).

Collagens XVI and XIX have been obtained by homology cloning from cDNA derived from human placenta and human fibroblasts (type XVI: Te-Cheng, PNAS, 1992; 89:6565; Yamaguchi, JBioch, 1992; 112:856) or from rhabdomyosarcoma cells (type XIX; Myers, JBC, 1994; 269:18549). Using a peptide antibody, collagen XVI was found in association with dense fibrils in placental membranes. Although the overall domain structure of these collagens as derived from cDNA has been well delineated, little is known about their functions, or their tissue- and cell-specific expression.

The transmembrane collagen

Type XVII (Fig. 4(c)) is one of the two autoantigens of the dermal disorder bullous pemphigoid. This disease is characterized by tense subcutaneous blisters due to splitting of the dermo-epidermal basement membrane, accompanied by an inflammatory infiltrate. This collagen, which is synthesized by basal keratinocytes, is unusual in that it possesses a large intracellular non-collagenous domain of more than 500 amino acids per chain (1500 amino acids per triple-helical molecule), a single transmembrane segment, and a collagen tail extending into the extracellular space (Giudice; JInvDermatol, 1992; 99:243; Li, JBC, 1993; 268:8825). As a component of hemidesmosomes it has not been found in the liver.

Yet unclassified collagens

The most remarkable feature of type XIII, a small collagen with four globular and three triple-helical domains (Fig. 4(c)), is a complex pattern of alternative splicing that involves the amino-terminal half of the molecule and theoretically generates more than 100 isoforms, some of which have been identified in several mesenchymal and epithelial cell lines and tissues (Juvonen, JBC, 1992; 267:24693 and 24700). In situ hybridization demonstrated expression of this collagen in dermal appendages, bone, cartilage, striated muscle, and the intestinal mucosa, but apparently not in liver (Sandberg, JCellBiol, 1989; 109:1371).

Collagens XV and XVIII (Fig. 4(c)) show significant sequence similarities to each other but, as with collagen XIII, their function is unclear. They consist of a large N-terminal and a smaller C-terminal globular domain and a highly interrupted triple helix (Muragaki, JBC, 1994; 269:4042; Oh, PNAS, 1994; 91:4229; Rehn, PNAS, 1994; 91:4234). Inspection of the cDNA sequence indicates that these collagens should have glycosaminoglycan side-chains and a high degree of glycosylation. In situ hybridization for collagen XV showed mRNA expression over fibroblasts and endothelial cells in a variety of tissues studied (Kivirikko, AmJPathol, 1995; 147:1500). Collagen XVIII RNA, as detected by Northern blot analysis, is primarily expressed in liver, followed by lung and kidney. It appears to be localized in basement membranes (Muragaki, PNAS, 1995; 92:8763; Myers, CellTissRes, 1996; 286:493). Quite in contrast to the other collagens, hepatocytes and bile duct epithelia could be identified as the main source of this collagen type in the liver (Cramer, Gastro, 1997; 112:A1587). This is of interest, since a 20 kDa fragment of the C-terminal propeptide of collagen XVIII (endostatin) has been identified as a potent circulating inhibitor of tumour angiogenesis (O'Reilly, Cell, 1997; 88:277; Boehm, Nature, 1997; 390:404). There exist three splice variants of collagen XVIII in the N-terminal globular domain. The largest form contains a 110

amino acid cysteine-rich sequence with homology to G protein-coupled membrane receptors (Rehn, JBC, 1995; 270:4705).

Collagen synthesis and novel prospects for antifibrotic treatment

As mentioned above, collagens type I and III represent the bulk of the extracellular matrix in most connective tissues, including the liver. For obvious reasons inhibition of their synthesis and deposition, or stimulation of their removal is considered the key to antifibrotic treatment. Therefore, being well aware of potentially important contributions of minor extracellular matrix molecules to the evolution of fibrosis, major effort has focused on elucidation of the molecular steps that lead to the accumulation of collagen I in tissues. Figure 5 illustrates the steps of collagen (type I) biosynthesis and deposition, and the possibilities of interfering specifically with these processes, as discussed below. Collagen mRNA is transcribed from its gene and transported to the rough endoplasmic reticulum, where the trimmed mRNA is translated into protein. During translation the nascent collagen chains undergo extensive hydroxylation at proline residues, catalysed by prolyl-4-hydroxylase, and at lysine residues, catalysed by lysyl hydroxylase, followed by addition of galactose or galactose plus glucose to some of the hydroxylysine residues, and N-glycosylation of the propeptides. After and during completion of protein synthesis and chain processing, the C-pro-peptide directs chain selection and correct folding of the triple helix. The collagen is then transported to the Golgi apparatus and secreted into a cell-membrane-protected extracellular space, where cleavage by the N- and C-propeptidase allows fibril growth. The enzyme lysyl oxidase, which is immobilized in the extracellular matrix, converts some of the lysyl and hydroxylysl residues to aldehydes. These aldehydes undergo firm covalent linkages with the same aldehydes or lysins of neigbouring triple helices (Fig. 5). This last step of covalent crosslinking is believed to confer resistance towards proteolysis in advanced fibrosis, as has been shown in echinococcal liver disease (Reiser, FASEBJ, 1992; 6:2439; Ricard-Blum, Hepatol, 1992; 15:599). The activities of prolyl and lysyl hydroxylase and of the hydroxylysyl-glucosyl and -galactosyl transferases are increased in rat liver fibrosis (Risteli, BiochemJ, 1974; 144:115). Whereas the degree of hydroxylation and glycosylation of lysyl residues may be important for fibril packing, extensive hydroxylation of proline residues at the Yaa position is crucial for the stability of triple-helical collagen. Thus triple helices of collagen that is underhydroxylated in proline cannot associate at body temperature and are rapidly degraded by intracellular proteases. Prolyl-4-hydroxylase is a tetramer of two α- and two β-chains. The catalytic activity resides in the α-chains, whereas the β-chains are required to keep the α-chains in a catalytically active conformation (Helaakoski, PNAS, 1995; 92:4427). Interestingly, the β-chain has many other functions: it is identical with protein disulphide isomerase that catalyses intracellular disulphide exchange and folding in many proteins (Pihlajaniemi, EMBOJ, 1987; 6:643); it serves as the major cellular thyroid hormone-binding protein and as the small subunit of the microsomal triglyceride transfer protein (Freedman, TrendsBiochemSci, 1994; 19:331); it may, furthermore, act as a dehydroascorbate reductase (Wells, JBC, 1990; 265:15361) and play a role as

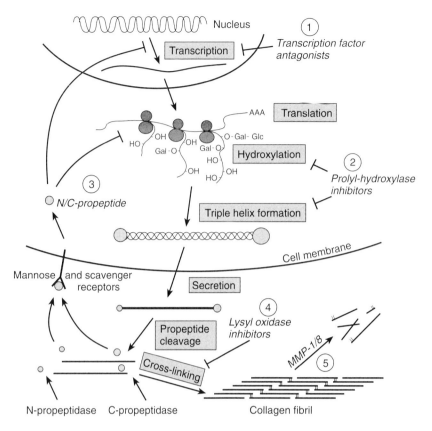

Fig. 5. Steps of collagen biosynthesis. The scheme applies to the well-studied fibril-forming collagens. Collagen mRNA is transcribed from the gene and translated into protein in the rough endoplasmic reticulum. During translation, the nascent polypeptide chains are hydroxylated on lysine and proline residues, glycosylated, and assembled to form the triple helix, starting from the C-terminal end. After secretion, N- and C-terminal propeptides are cleaved off by specific proteases and fibril growth occurs by quarter-staggered lateral assembly. Fibrils are then stabilized by formation of covalent crosslinks. Antifibrotic approaches that target either collagen biosynthesis (1–3), stabilization of the fibrils by crosslinking (4), or that activate collagenases (5) are discussed elsewhere.

the developmentally regulated retinal protein r-cognin (Krishna Rao, PNAS, 1993; 90:2950).

Inhibition of collagen-modifying enzymes

Prolyl-4-hydroxylase has been a preferred target for the development of antifibrotic drugs, and natural as well as synthetic agents have been developed that mimic and competitively inhibit 2-oxoglutarate, which, together with molecular oxygen, ascorbic acid, and Fe^{2+}, is a central cofactor in the active centre of the enzyme (Kivirikko, AnnMed, 1993; 25:113). Such an agent is pyridine-2,4-dicarboxylic acid which has to be derivatized to a prodrug, a hydrophobic ester-amide, in order to penetrate the plasma membrane.[6] The active acid is generated from the prodrug by a lidocaine metabolizing cytoplasmic enzyme and carried to the endoplasmic reticulum by the oxoglutarate transporter. This leads to a generalized uptake in numerous cell types, but activation almost exclusively in hepatocytes and kidney epithelia (Kellner, JHepatol, 1991; 13:S48). Since hepatocytes appear to play only a minor role in collagen synthesis, prodrugs that are preferentially hydrolysed in activated stellate cells are required.

Lysyl hydroxylase, a copper-dependent enzyme that covalently crosslinks fibrillar collagen and elastin, can be inhibited by β-aminopropionitrile, D–penicillamine (an agent that is used for long-term treatment of the copper overload of Wilson's disease), and

related compounds, resulting in fibrils that may be more easily accessible to interstitial collagenase (Kagan, AmJRespCellMolBiol, 1991, 5:206). There are, however, no convincing studies showing inhibition of fibrosis by these drugs. A reason for this may be that lysyl oxidase displays not only a highly stimulated but also a high constitutive expression in liver (Wakasaki, BBResComm, 1990; 166: 1201; Sommer, LabInvest, 1993; 90:460), and that much of the enzyme is deposited in the extracellular matrix, with up to 150 μg/g of dry liver tissue (Rucker, JNutr, 1996; 126:51).

Feedback inhibition by procollagen propeptides

It was shown that addition of the N-terminal propeptides of procollagens I or III could inhibit collagen synthesis by cultured human and bovine dermal fibroblasts (Wiestner, JBC, 1979; 254:7016). Later studies provided evidence that this effect is due to receptor-mediated endocytosis of the propeptides, which block the translation of the procollagen mRNAs into protein (Hörlein, PNAS, 1981; 78: 6163; Schlumberger, EurJCellBiol, 1988; 46:244). Furthermore, transfection of fibroblasts with an inducible minigene that directs expression of the N-propeptide of the α1(I) chain to the cytosol suppresses procollagen I translation, whereas other extracellular matrix proteins remain unaffected (Fouser, PNAS, 1991; 88:10158).

Similar inhibition has also been observed with the C-terminal propeptide of procollagen I (Wu, JBC, 1986; 261:10482; Wu, JBC, 1991; 266:2983) which is mainly taken up by the mannose receptor of endothelial cells (Smedsrød, BiochemJ, 1990; 271:345). Recent findings identified the transforming growth factor-β (TGF-β) family member bone morphogenetic protein 1 (BMP-1) as the C-propeptidase that removes the C-progestols from the procollagen molecule (Li, PNAS, 1996; 93:5127; Kessler, Science, 1996; 271: 360).

Modulation of collagen synthesis by mediators and transcription factors

Many external factors influence synthesis of type I collagen (which appears to be co-regulated with that of type III in most cells), including cytokines and growth factors, hormones, and the matrix environment (Fig. 2). Since the cell biology of fibrogenesis is dicussed in Chapter 6.1, this section will focus on the mechanisms of collagen gene expression.

Transcription of the constituent chains of collagen type I, α1(I), and α2(I), is tightly regulated. Most data as to transcriptional regulation of their genes have been obtained under artificial *in vitro* conditions of cell culture.[7] Cytokines, however, exert their influence in concert with many other mediators, such as various soluble factors, produced in an autocrine or paracrine fashion, and insoluble factors, such as extracellular matrix molecules, as well as contact with neighbouring cells. Furthermore, the local concentration, and especially the sequence of exposure to these factors, may determine whether a fibrogenic or an antifibrogenic response is induced in the target cell. This is exemplified in Fig. 6, where interferon-γ activates macrophages to release fibrogenic factors in the early stages of wound healing, but inhibits proliferation of fibroblasts (Rosenbloom, BBResComm, 1984; 123:365) and hepatic stellate cells (Rockey, Hepatol, 1992; 16:776) that start to populate the wound in later stages. The opposite is true for transforming growth factor-β (TGF-β), which suppresses the activation of mononuclear cells in the early stage of the wound-healing response, but is the most potent fibrogenic mediator for activated fibroblastic cells (Border, JCI, 1992; 90:1). The isoforms of TGF-β, namely TGF-β1/2/3, are expressed by all hepatic cell populations during regeneration and fibrosis, with the highest mRNA levels in stellate cells, but significant quantities also in Kupffer cells, sinusoidal endothelia, hepatocytes, and bile duct epithelia (Milani, AmJPathol, 1991; 139:1221; Bissell, JCI, 1995; 96:447). All TGF-β isoforms have to be proteolytically activated by a protease, especially plasmin, which localizes to the surface of, for example, endothelial cells (Flaumenhauft, JCellBiol, 1992; 118:901; Rieder, Hepatol, 1993; 18:937) and by tissue transglutaminase (Kojima, JCellBiol, 1993; 121:439), in order to become biologically active. In primary culture of purified cells much of the stellate cell-derived TGF-β is activated, whereas that of the liver epithelia is released mainly as inactive precursors (Bissell, JCI, 1995; 96:447). This may be important, since active TGF-β, which is fibrogenic for stellate cells, induces growth inhibition and apoptosis of hepatocytes (Schwall, Hepatol, 1993; 18:347).

The activation of collagen gene transcription by TGF-β1 is at least partly mediated by collagen transcription factor/nuclear factor-1. TGF-β1 binds to its ubiquitous cell surface receptor type II

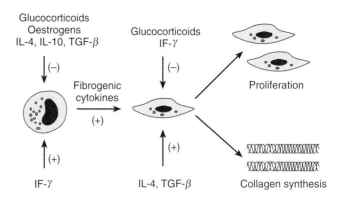

Fig. 6. A single mediator may exhibit fibrogenic or antifibrogenic properties. By activating macrophages (monocytes, lymphocytes) interferon-γ (IF-γ) may be proinflammatory and potentially profibrogenic in early phases of wound healing, whereas it inhibits fibroblast collagen synthesis and proliferation in later (chronic) phases. The opposite is true for interleukin-4 (IL-4) and transforming growth factor-β (TGF-β) which can inhibit mononuclear cell activation, but are stimulators of fibroblast collagen synthesis. Although glucocorticoids block inflammation as well as fibroblast collagen synthesis, they may also suppress collagenase expression which is necessary to dissolve excess connective tissue.

(TβR-II) which is a constitutively active transmembrane threonine/serine kinase. With TGF-β (TGR-β) bound, TβR-II then undergoes a conformational change that enables it to recruit and transphosphorylate another transmembrane serine/threonine kinase, receptor type I (TβR-I) which is the proper signal transducing receptor, although it necessitates the presence of TβR-II to sense extracellular TGF-β (Carcamo, MolCellBiol, 1995; 15:1573). Furthermore, a transmembrane proteoglycan (betaglycan, TβR-III) serves to concentrate extracellular TGF-β on the cell surface, thus potentiating the biological response.[8] These receptors appear to be upregulated on activated hepatic stellate cells (Friedman, JBC, 1994; 269:10551). The recombinant extracellular domains of TβR-I and TβR-II or other modulators of TGF-β activities are attractive agents for fibrosuppressive therapy, and many researchers and pharmaceutical companies are active in this field.

Whereas little is known about the cytoplasmic events downstream of receptor activation, researchers have been able to elucidate some of the nuclear events that follow TGF-β signal transduction. These signals activate collagen transcription factor/nuclear factor-1, which binds to sequences at positions -316 to -285 base pairs (bp) in the mouse α2(I) promoter and at around position -1600 bp in the rat α1(I) promoter (Rossi, Cell, 1988, 52:405; Ritzenthaler, JBC, 1993; 268:13625). Collagen transcription factor/nuclear factor-1 protein and its binding to the α2(I) promoter are increased after exposure of human hepatic stellate cells to acetaldehyde, the major toxic metabolite of ethanol (Anania, Hepatol, 1995; 21:1640), explaining in part the observed stimulation of collagen synthesis by acetaldehyde *in vitro* (Casini, Hepatol, 1991; 13:758). Alternatively, TGF-β1 activates a signalling cascade that, via tyrosine dephosphorylation of a nuclear protein, leads to assembly of a complex of transcription factors, including SP-1 (see below). This complex binds between positions -378 and -108 of the collagen α2(I) promoter to start transcription of the gene (Inagaki, JBC, 1994; 269: 14828; Greenwel, MolCellBiol, 1995; 15:6813).

When fibroblasts are cultivated with tumour necrosis factor-α in the presence of serum, collagen production is suppressed (Diaz, JBC, 1993; 268:10364), whereas it is enhanced under serum-free conditions (Elias, JInvDermatol, 1989; 92:699) and in an experimental model of silica-induced pulmonary fibrosis (Piguet, Nature, 1990; 344:245). A major regulatory DNA element appears to reside in a so-called AP-1 site (AP-1 is a transcription factor that is activated by tumour necrosis factor-α) in the first intron of the α1(I) procollagen gene (Katai, MolCellBiochem, 1992; 118:119; Määttä, BiochemJ, 1993; 264:365). This AP-1 site may activate or inhibit gene transcription from the promoter, depending on other transcription factors that are present, for example those in fetal calf serum that is often used in cell culture. It is not possible to judge the fibrogenic potential of a factor by considering just one side of the picture, that is collagen production, since molecules such tumour necrosis factor-α and interleukin-1 are also potent stimulators of the genes of collagenases, most of which have AP-1 responsive elements in their promoters (Brenner, Nature, 1989; 337:661). This may tilt the balance in favour of fibrolysis despite the concomitant induction of collagen genes. Consequently, final proof of the usefulness of a factor or its antagonist for antifibrotic therapy can only come from *in vivo* experiments with suitable animal models of liver fibrosis, followed by clinical studies using appropriate surrogate markers to monitor the antifibrotic effect (see also Chapter 6.2). Being aware of the above mentioned caveats, Table 2 summarizes the prevailing effects of some major cytokines, growth factors, and hormones on collagen synthesis, collagenase (mostly matrix metalloproteinase-1) expression, and cell proliferation.

An attractive future strategy to treat liver fibrosis could be based on findings that collagen gene expression depends on different transcription mechanisms that are aimed at different promoter elements in different cell types (so-called lineage-specific gene expression). Mice that harbour a transgene with 900 bp of the α1(I) proximal promoter coupled to a lacZ or luciferase reporter gene show expression of this transgene exclusively in skin fibroblasts, whereas a construct containing 3500 bp of the promoter also directed collagen I gene expression in osteoblasts and tendon fibroblasts, but not in vascular smooth muscle cells. The latter depended on the presence of additional intronic sequences in the proximal and distal region of the gene (Bedalov, JBC, 1994; 269:4903). Dermal fibroblasts, in particular, appear to require the first intron of the α1(I) gene for efficient transcription (Liska, JCellBiol, 1994; 125: 695). An osteoblast-activating promoter region was localized to a 117 bp segment at position -1656 to -1540 of the collagen α1(I) gene (Rossert, PNAS, 1996; 93:1027). These remote promoter regions do not appear to stimulate collagen synthesis in hepatic stellate cells, since high transcriptional activity is obtained with a promoter construct covering only 440 bp of the 5′-flanking region (Houglum, JCI, 1995; 96:2269). However, promoter studies have to be interpreted with care, since in liver of mice transgenic for the 3500 bp α1(I) promoter, expression of the transgene is stimulated 21-fold by chronic ethanol administration, whereas the original collagen α1(I) gene is not activated. This indicates repressor elements further up- or downstream of this already large promoter (Walton, Hepatol, 1996; 23:310). Thus collagen gene transcription is more complex, as exemplified by distant gene regulatory elements such as an enhancer region located between 13 000 and 20 000 bp upstream of the pro-α2(I) gene (Bou-Gharios, JCellBiol, 1996; 134:1333). It is

Table 2 Effect of cytokines/growth factors and hormones on fibroblastic/stellate cell proliferation, collagen synthesis, and collagenase expression

Factor	Proliferation	Collagen synthesis	Collagenase expression
IL-1	↑	↑↓	↑
IL-4	O	↑	O
TNF-α	↑↓	↑↓	↑
TNF-β	↑↓	↑↓	↑
TGF-β1/2	↑↓	↑↑	↑
PDGF	↑	↑	↑
EGF/TGF-α	↑	O	↑
b-FGF	↑	O	↑
IF-α/β/γ	↑	↓	↑
Relaxin	↓	O	↑
Gro-α	O	↓	O
IGF-1	↑	↑	O
PGE₂	↓	↓	↑
RA	↓	↑	↓
GC	O	↓*	↓

Data are extrapolated from studies predominantly of fibroblastic cells of liver, lung, kidney, and skin. They represent a cross-section of occasionally conflicting results depending on the experimental conditions. IL, interleukin; TNF, tumour necrosis factor; TGF, transforming growth factor; PDGF, platelet-derived growth factor (dimers BB>AB>AA); EGF, epidermal growth factor; b-FGF, basic fibroblast growth factor; IF, interferon (γ>α/β); IGF, insulin-like growth factor; PGE, prostaglandins E; RA, retinoic acid; GC, glucocorticosteroids; (O), no effect; (↑), enhanced; (↓), decreased; (↑↓), decreased or enhanced depending on factor concentration and the presence of serum.
*Has not been shown in stellate cell cultures (Niki, Hepatol, 1996; 23: 1673).

quite probable that such remote elements regulate accessibility of the proximal promoter to the ubiquitously expressed transcription factors in a cell-specific manner.

None the less, efforts are under way to identify transcription factors or a combination of them that may be unique for directing collagen synthesis in hepatic stellate cells. Such work may finally lead to tools for a targeted inhibition of liver fibrogenesis (Rippe, Hepatol, 1995; 22:241; Jensen, Hepatol, 1995; 22:293A).

Non-collagenous glycoproteins

As mentioned before, functions as well as structures of collagens and non-collagenous proteins often overlap. Figure 7 illustrates the domain structures of fibronectin, tenascin, and collagen XIV. Comparison between these molecules shows that each is composed of a set of distinct domains. Such domains, which display a high degree of sequence homology and fold into similar three-dimensional structures, may exert similar but not necessarily identical functions. Examples are binding to fibrillar collagens (A domains of von Willebrand factor) or to heparan sulphate and cellular receptors (fibronectin type III repeats). Some of these domains appear to have lost a specific function and to serve merely as spacers that position other, functional domains correctly.

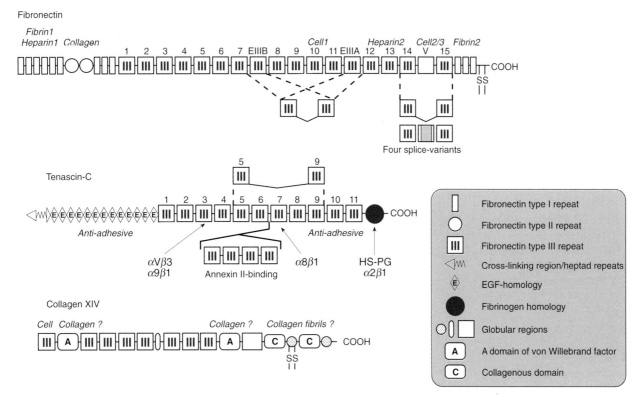

Fig. 7. Domain structure and assigned functions of fibronectin, tenascin-C, and collagen type XIV (undulin). Note the presence of several of the homologous fibronectin type III repeats (each composed of approximately 95 amino acids) in each molecule. These repeats harbour regions that interact with cellular receptors ('cell'), part of them integrins (such as αVβ3, α8β1, and α9β1 in tenascin), heparin, or heparan sulphate. Fibronectin forms a disulphide-linked (SS) dimer; tenascin-C, a hexamer; and collagen XIV (undulin), a trimer. EIIIA/B, extradomain A or B; V, variable region of fibronectin; HS-PG, heparan sulphate proteoglycan. Differential splicing may generate up to 20 different isoforms per fibronectin chain and at least four different forms of tenascin-C.

Fibronectin

Most cell types are able to synthesize one or more forms of fibronectin. Consequently, the dimeric molecule is found in all connective tissues, including the hepatic stroma and the more or less complete basement membranes of blood vessels, bile ducts, and sinusoids. The modular structure of fibronectin, with different functional domains (Fig. 7), allows interactions with many other molecules of the extracellular matrix, with extracellular matrix receptors (among them at least eight integrins and several transmembrane heparan sulphate proteoglycans, see below), and even with staphylococcal cell walls, facilitating phagocytosis by macrophages (Kupffer cells) that express fibronectin (Armbrust, BBRes-Comm, 1995; 213:750) as well as its receptors.[9] Fibronectin binds to fibrin, and both molecules constitute the primordial extracellular matrix during early phases of wound healing in the liver (Neubauer, Gastro, 1995; 108:1124; Martinez-Hernandez, FASEBJ, 1995; 9: 1401). Crosslinking of fibronectin with fibrinogen and other extracellular matrix molecules occurs by a fibronectin-bound enzyme, tissue transglutaminase, which is released from hepatocytes, endothelial, and fibroblastic cells upon wounding (Jeong, JBC, 1995; 270:5654).

Remarkable functional diversity of fibronectin is generated by differential splicing of a single precursor mRNA that yields a theoretical maximum of 20 isoforms per chain (Fig. 7). Two of the 17 type III repeats are subject to alternative splicing, namely

extradomains A and B (**EIIIA** and **EIIIB**). Whereas plasma fibronectin that is secreted by hepatocytes and amounts to approximately 400 mg/l is devoid of these extradomains, cellular fibronectin, mainly the product of mesenchymal cells, contains EIIIA (Schwarzbauer, EMBOJ, 1987; 6:2573), which is important for polymerization and incorporation of fibronectin into the extracellular matrix. EIIIB is absent from fibronectin of normal and regenerating liver (Caputi, NucAcidRes, 1995; 23:238), but is expressed in liver cell carcinoma and in the surrounding, apparently normal, tissue (Taviari, IntJCanc, 1994; 56:820). EIIIB represents an oncofetal variant and plays a yet unknown role in carcinogenesis (Carnemolla, JBC, 1992; 267:24689).

Major integrin-binding regions of fibronectin have been identified in the tenth type III repeat and in the 'variable region' localized between the sixteenth and seventeenth type III repeat (Ruoslahti, Science, 1987; 238:491; Mould, JBC, 1991; 266:3569). The tenth type III repeat harbours the classical 'adhesive recognition sequence' RGD (Arg–Gly–Asp) that is necessary for binding fibronectin to the integrin receptor α5β1 and for binding of some extracellular matrix molecules to several other integrins. The variable region of fibronectin contains the recognition sequences REDV (Arg–Glu–Asp–Val) and LDV (Leu–Asp–Val) for integrin α4β1. These oligopeptide sequences and their more stable cyclical variants can modulate fibronectin-dependent cell behaviour, including growth and the spread of tumour cells (Humphries, JCI, 1988; 81: 782; Nowlin, JBC, 1993; 268:20352).

Tenascins

The tenascin family consists of three members that are derived from different genes. The originally described tenascin-C has been studied extensively, whereas little is known about tenascin-R and tenascin-X.[11,12] The constituent chain of human tenascin-C is composed of 14.5 epidermal growth factor repeats, 8 to 15 type III repeats, and a domain with homology to the β- and γ-chains of fibrinogen (Nies, JBC, 1991; 266:2818). The variable number of type III repeats arises from alternative splicing (Fig. 7). The N-termini of the tenascin-C monomers associate to a hexamer, thus allowing for multivalent interactions with cells and other extracellular matrix molecules.

Tenascin-C is widely expressed during embryogenesis, but shows a restricted distribution in adult tissues in areas of active epithelial–mesenchymal interplay. Whereas in normal liver it is found exclusively in the perisinusoidal space, it is highly expressed in the periportal mesenchyme of active fibrogenesis, bile duct proliferation, and neovascularization (Van Eyken, JHepatol, 1990; 11:45). This corresponds to the stromal induction of tenascin-C expression in dermal wound healing and in the desmoplastic extracellular matrix of invasive tumours (Mackie, PNAS, 1987; 84: 4621; Mackie, JCellBiol, 1988; 107:2757; Whithby, JCellSci, 1991; 99:583). Synthesis of tenascin-C is upregulated if fibroblasts are strained mechanically (Chiquet-Ehrismann, BioEssays, 1995; 17: 873) or exposed to the cytokine interleukin-1 (McCachren; Arth-Rheum, 1992; 35:1185), and serum levels may rise in parallel to the acute-phase response in inflammatory conditions (Schienk, IntJCanc, 1995; 63:665). In the liver, tenascin-C is mainly produced by activated stellate and myofibroblast-like cells (Ramadori, Virch-ArchCP, 1991; 60:145; Knittel, ExpCellRes, 1992; 203:312). The protein is an adhesive as well as an anti-adhesive substrate, depending on the cell-type, its receptor equipment, and the splicing variant. Experiments with recombinant fragments of the molecule have demonstrated the presence of both adhesion-promoting domains, e.g. the third type III repeat that contains an RGD sequence (which is a major receptor-binding sequence in fibronectin, see above) and the fibrinogen-like C-terminal knob, and anti-adhesive regions, e.g. the EGF repeats (Spring, Cell, 1989; 59:325; Prieto, JCellBiol, 1992; 119:663; Aukhil, JBC, 1993; 268:2542; Joshi, JCellSci, 1993; 106:389). The cell-migration-promoting effect of tenascin-C resides in the highly glycosylated, alternatively spliced type III repeats (Kaplony, Development, 1991; 112:605). Whereas in laminin-1 the approximately 30 amino acid long EGF repeats were shown to stimulate cell proliferation (Engel, FEBSLett, 1989; 251:1; Panayotou, Cell, 1989; 56:93), this has not yet been demonstrated for tenascin-C. Since tenascin-C loosens but does not break cell–substrate interactions, it can facilitate processes such as cell migration and division. Furthermore, its fragments, released during the proteolysis that always accompanies its enhanced expression during tissue remodelling, may exert multiple and even contrary effects on cells.

Whereas all these functions suggest an important biological role for the molecule, it came as a surprise that mice in which the gene had been deleted by homologous recombination (tenascin 'knockout'; Saga, GenesDevelop, 1992; 6:1821) do not exhibit a pathological phenotype, even after wounding (Forsberg, PNAS, 1996; 93:6594). This indicates that other molecules can substitute for tenascin-C under normal conditions, but does not exclude a vital role for tenascin-C in wound healing or under conditions of stress.

Thrombospondins and SPARC

The extracellular matrix molecules thrombospondin-1 and **SPARC** (secreted protein acidic and rich in cysteine, synonymous with osteonectin and BM40) also have adhesive as well as anti-adhesive properties.[12]

Three thrombospondins, TSP-1, TSP-2, and TSP-3, encoded by different genes, are known to date.[13] They form homotrimers in which three arms extend from a central crosslinking domain, each terminating in a large terminal nodule. From the N- to the C-terminus, TSP-1 and TSP-2 contain the crosslinking region, followed by domains with homology to the N-propeptide of $\alpha 1(I)$ procollagen, to properdin, and to epidermal growth factor, and finally repetitive calcium-binding domains that form the C-terminal nodule. TSP-3 lacks the properdin-like domains, which harbour the sequence Cys–Ser–Val–Thr–Cys–Gly that is an adhesive recognition sequence (see above) for TSP-1 and TSP-2 and also for the circumsporozoite protein of *Plasmodium malariae* (Tuszynski, JCellBiol, 1992; 116:209), indicating that the parasites use molecular mimicry to TSP for entry into cells.

TSP-1 is released from platelets during degranulation, where it stabilizes the haemostatic plug by interacting with molecules such as fibronectin, fibrinogen, laminin, collagen types I and V, heparan sulphate, and plasmin. It is furthermore synthesized by endothelial and other mesenchymal cells (Mosher, JCellBiol, 1982; 93:343; Raugi, JCellBiol, 1982; 95:351) and appears to inhibit endothelial proliferation during certain stages of angiogenesis.[14] Since it is expressed rapidly after exposure of cells to serum and mitogens, TSP-1 qualifies as an immediate early gene (Majack, JBC, 1987; 262:8821; Donoviel, JCellPhysiol, 1990; 145:16). Much less is known about the role and functions of TSP-2 and TSP-3. After carbon tetrachloride intoxication, which causes centrolobular damage in the rat liver, TSP-1 mRNA is induced rapidly in vascular endothelial and some mesenchymal cells, whereas TSP-2 shows a temporospatial expression resembling that of a constitutive extracellular matrix protein like collagen I (Herbst, Gastro, 1996; 112: A431).

SPARC is a glycosylated 40 kDa protein with four distinct domains: I and IV with calcium-binding sites, II with homology to the the serpin protease inhibitor follistatin, and III with an α-helical structure.[15] It can interact with various collagens, albumin, and thrombospondin-1, and plays a role in binding the mitogens platelet-derived growth factor-BB or –AB (Raines, PNAS, 1993; 89: 1281). SPARC contacts yet unidentified receptors on endothelial cells (Yost, JBC, 1993; 268:25790). Exogenous SPARC upregulates the expression of the plasminogen antagonist PAI-1, of thrombospondin-1 and fibronectin, later followed by that of the matrix metalloproteinases-1/3/9 (see Chapter 2.16.2) in endothelial cells and fibroblasts (Lane, JBC, 1992; 267:16736; Tremble, JCellBiol, 1993; 115:1127). The intact protein seems to inhibit endothelial proliferation (Sage, BiochemCellBiol, 1992; 70:579), whereas the copper-binding peptide, Lys–Gly–His–Lys, that derives from plasmin cleavage of SPARC, is a potent angiogenic factor, previously identified in serum (Pickart, MethodsEnz, 1987; 147:314; Funk, JCellPhysiol, 1993; 154:53). Since it is released from endothelial

Table 3 Laminin isoforms and their chain composition

New denomination	Chain composition	Previous denomination
Laminin-1	α1β1γ1	EHS laminin
Laminin-2	α2β1γ1	Merosin
Laminin-3	α1β2γ1	s-Laminin
Laminin-4	α2β2γ1	s-Merosin
Laminin-5	α3β3γ1	Kalinin/nicein
Laminin-6	α3β1γ1	k-Laminin
Laminin-7	α3β2γ1	ks-Laminin

Laminins are trimers composed of α-, β- and γ-chains. The prototype laminin variant α1β1γ1 has been isolated from the murine EHS (Engelbreth–Holm–Swarm) tumour. Several chains were subsequently discovered that bear homology to chains of the EHS laminin and that assemble to different trimeric molecules showing unique patterns of tissue expression. Chains α1, α2, β1, β2, γ1, and α4 have been found in the liver. The composition of the laminin variant that contains α4 is not yet defined. Four more laminins have been described recently, extending the nomenclature to laminin-11.

cells during angiogenesis, SPARC, like TSP-1, appears to be an auto- and paracrine regulator of this process (Iruela-Arispe, Lab-Invest, 1991; 64:174). In the liver after acute or chronic injury, SPARC mRNA is expressed by stellate cells in a pattern resembling the expression of collagen type 1 (Frizell, Hepatol, 1995; 21:847; Herbst, Gastro, 1996; 110:A1209).

Laminins

The laminins are a family of at least eleven heterotrimeric glycoproteins encoded by at least nine different genes.[15,16] The individual laminin chains show a tissue- and cell-specific, as well as a developmentally regulated, expression in basement membranes. The laminins are assembled from variants of one α-, one β-, and one γ-chain (Table 3). The chains A, B1, and B2 of the first described and most thoroughly studied Engelbreth–Holm–Swarm (**EHS**) tumour laminin have been given the designation α1β1γ1. Laminin chain variants show significant sequence similarity, with 46 per cent identical amino acids between, for example, α1 and α2 (Bernier, MatrixBiol, 1995; 14:447). Most laminins can be visualized in the electron microscope as an asymmetric cross with three short arms derived from the amino termini and a long arm derived from the supercoiled carboxy termini of the three constituent chains (Fig. 8). All laminins exhibit a complex repertoire of biological functions, modulating cellular adhesion, proliferation, polarization, differentiation, and phenotype.[16] When epithelial cells, including hepatocytes, are plated on laminin or a laminin-rich gel, they maintain their differentiated, secretory properties for extended periods of time (Bissell, EurJCellBiol, 1986; 40:72). Several laminin chains have been found in fetal or adult liver, namely α1, α2 (Bernier, MatrixBiol, 1995; 14:447; Ponce, Hepatol, 1995; 22:620), α4 (Tivanainen, FEBSLett, 1995; 365:183), β1 (Milani, AmJPathol, 1989; 134:1175), β2 (Tivanainen, MatrixBiol, 1995; 14:489), and γ1, but little is known about the cell types involved in their synthesis or about their functions, since previous cell culture studies used laminin-1 which is only a minor variant in liver. In this line, a liver

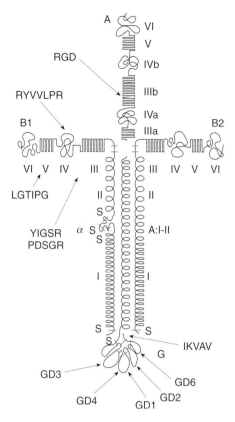

Fig. 8. Structure and adhesive recognition sequences of laminin-1. Laminin-1, the prototype of the cross-shaped laminins, is composed of the three chains A (α1), B1 (β1), and B2 (γ1), with the C-termini of all three chains forming a coiled coil structure. The arms can be subdivided into domains I–VI, α, and G. Domains III and V encompass repetitive epidermal growth factor (EGF)-like repeats, which can transmit growth stimulatory signals to cells in a similar way to EGF (Panayotou, Cell, 1989; 56:93). Domains III, IV of chain β1, and domains VI and G of chain α1 bear several 'adhesive recognition sequences' that are recognized by cellular matrix receptors (active peptides in the one-letter code: A, Ala; D, Asp; G, Gly; I, Ile; K, Lys; L, Leu; P, Pro; S, Ser; T, Thr; R, Arg; Y, Tyr; V, Val). Binding sites for heparan sulphate and integrins have been localized to subdomains GD1–GD6. (See also Table 3; for details refer to the text.) Modified from ref.[16].

biomatrix enriched in the α2-chain variant (a component of either laminin-2 or -4) is a much better adhesive substrate for hepatocytes than laminin-1 (Ponce, Hepatol, 1995; 22:620).

Laminins (and other basement membrane constituents such as collagen type IV) are also primary matrix anchors for metastasizing cells that have to penetrate basement membranes in order to enter the vascular system and to form distant colonies. Like fibronectin (see above), several biologically active oligopeptide sequences that mediate cell adhesion and spreading, as well as differentiation and metastasis, have been identified in laminin-1 (Fig. 8). These 'adhesive recognition sequences'[17], that interact with integrin or non-integrin receptors, include YIGSR (Tyr–Ile–Gly–Ser–Arg) and RYVVLPR (Arg–Tyr–Val–Val–Leu–Pro–Arg), both of the laminin β1 chain that inhibit metastasis of melanoma cells (Graf, Biochem, 1987; 26:6896; Skubitz, CancerRes, 1990; 50:7612), but also IKVAV (Ile–Lys–Val–Ala–Val) of the laminin α1 chain that stimulates the secretion of type IV collagenase and promotes tumour spread (Kanemoto, PNAS, 1990; 87:2279). IKVAV has recently been shown to promote experimental colon cancer metastasis to the liver (Bresalier, CancerRes, 1995; 55:2476). Additional domains in the terminal globule of the long arm (GD1–GD6 in the C-terminus of the α1-chain, Fig. 8) mediate binding to heparin and (trans-membrane) heparan sulphate proteoglycans (Skubitz, JCellBiol, 1991; 115:1137), and to the integrins α3β1 (Gehlsen, JCellBiol, 1992; 117:449), α2β1 and α6β1 (Nomizu, JBC, 1995; 270:20583). Binding sites for the integrin α1β1 have been localized in the N-terminal domain VI of the α1-chain (Colognato-Pyke, JBC, 1995; 270:939) and in the centre of the laminin-1 molecule (Forsberg, ExpCellRes, 1994; 215:33). The hepatotropism of *Entamoeba histolytica* may be due to a specific interaction of the amoebic 27 kDa protease with laminin (Li, InfectImmun, 1995; 63:4150).

Elastin and associated proteins

Elastin is synthesized as a 72 kDa precursor (tropoelastin) which becomes highly crosslinked to a rubber-like polymer once secreted into the extracellular space.[18] The crosslinking is carried out by lysyl oxidase, an enzyme that also acts on fibrillar collagen (see above). Tropoelastin that undergoes alternative splicing (Pierce, Biochem, 1990; 29:9677) possesses a unique chemical composition, with high amounts of hydrophobic amino acids, glycine, proline, and alanine, being the basis for the elastic properties of the polymer.

Elastin may comprise up to 4 per cent of the extracellular matrix in skin and up to 50 per cent of the extracellular matrix of large arteries. Due to its insolubility it may have a long biological half-life. *In vitro* elastin synthesis by fibroblasts is upregulated by insulin-like growth factor and downregulated by tumour necrosis factor-α (Kahari, JBC, 1992; 267:26134; Rich, AmJPhysiol, 1992; 263:L276). In the liver, elastin is found in arteries, surrounding bile ducts, and in the portal tract stroma, where it appears as amorphous patches or as a fibrous network (Porto, AnatRec, 1990; 228:392).

Elastin polymers are accompanied by microfibrils of 10 to 12 nm diameter. A major constituent of these structures is fibrillin, a 350 kDa glycoprotein with multiple epidermal growth factor-like domains (Maslen, Nature, 1991; 352:334). Defects of fibrillin and a smaller variant that arises from a different gene are implicated in Marfan's syndrome, a heritable disease that affects the elastic fibre system and is characterized by aortic dissection, mitral valve prolapse, and ectopia lentis (Dietz, Nature, 1991; 352:337; Lee, Nature, 1991; 352:330; Sykes, NatureGen, 1993; 3:99). Nothing is known about the elastin-associated microfibrillar proteins in liver.

Proteoglycans

Proteoglycans consist of a core protein that is substituted with a variable number of glycosaminoglycans, unbranched, sulphated, and acidic carbohydrate polymers that contain a high proportion of sugar acids (uronic acids).

The glycosaminoglycan chains that are either O-linked to serine or N-linked to aspartate residues of the protein backbone are classified into heparan sulphate, dermatan sulphate, chondroitin sulphate, and keratan sulphate. They usually have 15 to 25 chain members, whereas the unsulphated hyaluronic acid, which is not covalently linked to protein, may be much larger (see below). The glycosaminoglycan content of normal human liver is low, with approximately 100 µg uronic acid/g of dry, defatted liver tissue (compared to the amount of collagen: approximately 5 mg/g). However, in cirrhosis the amount of dermatan sulphate, chondroitin sulphate and hyaluronic acid, which are found mainly in the interstitial extracellular matrix may increase up to tenfold, while heparan sulphate, which is expressed on the surface of cells and in basement membranes, is only moderately elevated.[19]

A prominent function of the highly negatively charged and space-occupying glycosaminoglycans is the creation of water-filled compartments that are protected from other macromolecules while allowing passage of small molecular weight solutes. In addition, due to their charge but also to specific features of the substituted sugar moieties, they may undergo interactions with proteins, including certain growth factors (see below).

Biochemical work with proteoglycans in the past was hampered by the diversity of their glycosaminoglycan chains, but unravelling of the protein structures has allowed a novel classification based on common features of the core proteins. These are composed of interactive domains with functions comparable to those of the other extracellular matrix proteins.[19-21] Figure 9 illustrates the domain structure of some proteoglycans.

Cell culture studies have identified activated stellate cells as the primary producers of most liver proteoglycans in fibrogenesis (Schäfer, Hepatol, 1987; 7:680; Arenson, Gastro, 1988; 95:441). This has been corroborated by mRNA analysis from cultured cells and by *in situ* hybridization studies on rat liver demonstrating the expression of the core proteins of fibromodulin, lumican, and aggrecan (Krull, FEBSLett, 1992; 312:47), and of decorin and biglycan (Meyer, Hepatol, 1992; 16:204; Krull, Hepatol, 1993; 18:581). Although not yet detected, other proteoglycans, such as versican, may well be present in liver.

Aggrecan may contain roughly 100 chondroitin sulphate and several keratan sulphate side-chains, resulting in a molecular mass of approximately 3000 kDa per molecule. Together with a small adaptor protein (link protein), many molecules of aggrecan can bind via the N-terminus to the glycosaminoglycan polymer hyaluronic acid, forming expanded, highly hydrated aggregates that absorb compressive forces in cartilage (Vertel, TrendsCellBiol, 1995; 5:458). The glycosaminoglycan component of aggrecan in the liver, an organ that contains no keratan sulphate, is different from the cartilage form. Interestingly, the C-terminal tridomain structure of the aggrecan core protein bears a region with homology to epidermal growth factor (this may be spliced out), to lectins, and to complement regulatory proteins (Fig. 9), identifying it as a member of the selectin family, cellular receptors that mediate cell–cell recognition in inflammation.[20]

The small dermatan/chondroitin sulphate proteoglycans decorin and biglycan (synonymous with PGI and PGII, respectively) have core proteins of 42 to 43 kDa and a single (decorin) or two (biglycan) chondroitin/dermatan sulphate side-chains. They harbour an N-terminal glycosaminoglycan attachment domain, a central region with up to 12 leucine-rich repeats, and a C-terminal disulphide loop.[21] Fibromodulin and lumican, which are predominantly keratan sulphate proteoglycans, exhibit similar structures, although the glycosaminoglycan attachment sites differ.

The core proteins of decorin and fibromodulin bind to fibrillar collagens, an interaction that is modulated by the length and

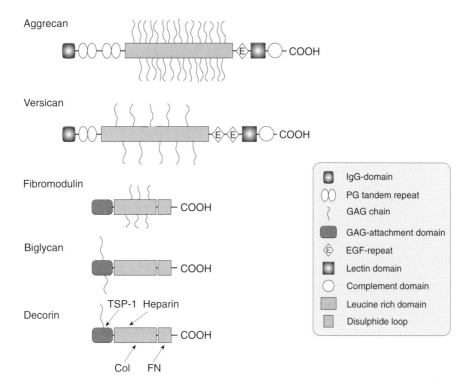

Fig. 9. Domain organization of proteoglycans. As found in other extracellular matrix proteins, the core proteins of proteoglycans are composed of different functional domains. Major diversity is introduced by the attachment of a variant number of glycosaminoglycan (GAG) chains of different length and composition. Approximately 100 GAG chains, mainly chondroitin sulphate, render aggrecan an extended molecule that creates a huge solute compartment and provides mechanical resistance in tissues such as cartilage. With the aid of link protein chains of the GAG, hyaluronic acid can bind numerous aggrecan monomers via their N-terminal domains, thus forming aggregates with a mass of several hundred kilodaltons. An apparently less glycosylated variant of aggrecan is expressed in liver. The small dermatan/chondroitin sulphate proteoglycan, decorin, has been studied in more detail, and its interactive sites with thrombospondin-1 (TSP-1), heparin/heparan sulphate, collagen I (col), and fibronectin (FN) have been mapped. For further details refer to the text.

composition of the glycosaminoglycan chains (Scott, BiochemJ, 1988; 52:313; Oldberg, EMBOJ, 1989; 8:2601; Hedbom, JBC, 1993; 268:27307). Decorin apparently plays a role in the supramolecular assembly of the extracellular matrix, and binding sites for thrombospondin-1, heparin/heparan sulphate, and fibronectin have been mapped (Fig. 9). Contrary to decorin, biglycan does not interact with collagens. The core proteins of both molecules bind and thus modulate the activities of the fibrogenic cytokine transforming growth factor-β1 (see below). In primary cultures of hepatic stellate cells, decorin and biglycan mRNA levels increase three- to fourfold, whereas they decrease in stellate cells that have made the transition to myofibroblast-like cells (Meyer, Hepatol, 1992; 16:204). This study also shows that, contrary to primary stellate cells, myofibroblast-like cells upregulate their decorin and biglycan mRNA expression in response to transforming growth factor-α, but are unresponsive to transforming growth factor-β1, underlining the dependence of growth factor responsiveness and extracellular matrix (proteoglycan) synthesis on the cellular activation state.

Perlecan, the large heparan sulphate proteoglycan of basement membranes, has a molecular mass of up to 1600 kDa and a core protein of 396 kDa. It is found in all liver basement membranes, including those of the perisinusoidal space, of portal vessels and, to a minor degree, of bile ducts (Rescan, AmJPathol, 1993; 142:199; Takahashi, JHepatol, 1994; 21:500). Being the product mainly of endothelial cells, it influences the transport of solutes between the sinusoidal blood and the hepatocytes. The core protein of perlecan encompasses (from N- to C-terminal) the following domains: I, heparan sulphate attachment; II, homology to the low density lipoprotein (**LDL**) receptor; III, homology to the N-terminus of the laminin α1-chain; IV, repetitive immunoglobulin repeats similar to those of the cell–cell adhesion molecule, N-CAM; V, homology to the C-terminal G-domain of the laminin α1 and α2 chains; and interspersed epidermal growth factor-like repeats (Doege, Genomics, 1991; 10:673; Kallunki, JCellBiol, 1992; 116:559). Perlecan interacts with fibronectin and various of the other basement membranes components (Fig.10), but little is known about the specific function of its various domains.

The transmembrane and membrane-associated proteoglycans will be mentioned here, since they can be cleaved close to their membrane insertion by trypsin-like protease, allowing their release into the extracellular matrix. Furthermore, they form a functional continuum with the proteoglycans of the extracellular matrix, e.g. by immobilizing and modulating the activities of growth factors (see below).

The syndecans are a family of four related heparan/chondroitin sulphate proteoglycans with core proteins of molecular mass 30 to 40 kDa that have divergent extracellular but highly conserved transmembrane and cytoplasmic domains. The extracellular domain may be substituted with two to four glycosaminoglycan chains. [22,23] Syndecan 1, the major variant in liver (Kato, JBC, 1994;

269:18881; Lyon, JBC, 1994; 269:11208) has been studied in most detail. Its glycosaminoglycan chains mediate preferential interactions with fibrillar collagens type I, III, and V (Koda, JBC, 1984; 259:11763), fibronectin (Saunders, JCellBiol, 1988; 106:423), thrombospondin-1 (Sun, JBC, 1989; 264:2885), and tenascin-C (Salmivirta, JBC, 1991; 266:7733). Exposure of cells to transforming growth factor-β1 upregulates the chondroitin sulphate but downregulates the heparan sulphate content of the syndecans, which appears to alter their affinity to collagen (Rapraeger, JCellBiol, 1989; 109:2509). Syndecan-1, and probably other members of the syndecan family, are necessary co-receptors for the mitogen basic fibroblast growth factor (Yayon, Cell, 1991; 64:841; see below) and, in addition to the integrins, appear to transmit signals from the extracellular membrane to the interior of the cell (Leppä; PNAS, 1992; 89:932). Interestingly, syndecans serve as receptors for herpes simplex virus (Shieh, JCellBiol, 1992; 116:1273).

A more recent study has investigated the distribution of syndecans 1 to 4 in normal human liver (Roskams, Hepatol, 1995; 21: 950). The authors localized syndecan-1 to sinusoidal endothelial cells, bile duct epithelia, and hepatocytes; syndecan-2 and -3 to mesenchymal (including stellate) cells and vessel endothelia; and syndecan-4 to the bile canalicular site of hepatocytes. In addition, the peripheral (glycosyl-phosphatidyl-inositol-anchored) proteoglycan, glypican, was found in the portal tract mesenchyme and in nerve bundles.

Betaglycan, a co-receptor for the transforming growth factors β1, β2, and β3, carries either heparan or chondroitin sulphate side-chains. It bears only a short cytoplasmic tail and has no signalling properties *per se*. However, betaglycan concentrates biologically active transforming growth factor-β on the cell surface and potentiates signal transduction mediated by the serine/threonine kinase receptors TβR-I and TβR-II (see above).

CD44, synonymous with hyaluronic acid receptor, extracellular matrix receptor type III, and hermes antigen, is a widely distributed transmembrane protein that interacts with hyaluronic acid via the N-terminal extracellular domain.[20,23,24] This domain shares homology with cartilage link protein. Binding has also been described to collagen types I and VI (Carter, JBC, 1988; 263:4193), to fibronectin, and to laminin-1 (Jalkanen, JCellBiol, 1992; 116:817). Binding to fibronectin and collagen XIV (Ehnis, ExpCellRes, 1996; 229:388) appears to be mediated by chondroitin sulphate variants that represent a minor fraction of the CD44 molecules on haematopoietic and mesenchymal cells. Furthermore, CD44 mediates homing of lymphocytes to mucosal lymphoid tissue. The CD44 gene may undergo complex alternative splicing, and some cells express combinations of additional exons, the so-called variable domains v1 to v10. Expression of the CD44 variant that contains just the additional domain v6 confers metastatic behaviour to pancreatic, colonic, and gastric carcinoma cells (Rudy, CancerRes, 1993; 53: 1262; Wielenga, CancerRes, 1993; 53:4754; Dämmrich, JMolMed, 1995; 73:395). Heparan sulphate is found exclusively on the variant domain v3 of CD44, where it serves as a co-receptor for heparin-binding epidermal growth factor and basic fibroblast growth factor (Bennett, JCellBiol, 1995; 128:687). The role of CD44-v3 in binding these growth factors could underlie its expression by epithelial tissues, especially in association with inflammation and tumour growth (Fox, CancerRes, 1994; 54:4540), processes that require both angiogenesis induced by basic fibroblast growth factor and

epithelial cell proliferation mediated by heparin-binding epidermal growth factor.

In the liver CD44 is expressed on portal and perisinusoidal mesenchymal, on bile duct, and on Kupffer cells (Picker, JCellBiol, 1989; 109:927), whereas hepatocytes are negative. Hepatocellular carcinoma cells that grow in the peritoneal cavity begin to express CD44 which, together with hyaluronic acid, provides a growth advantage in suspension (Haramaki, Hepatol, 1995; 21:1276), and the splice variant containing variable domains v8 to v10 has been demonstrated in all of 60 colon cancers metastatic to the liver (Takeuchi, JpnJCancerRes, 1995; 86:292).

CD44 has a relatively large cytoplasmic domain. This domain can be phosphorylated on several serine residues (Neame, EMBOJ, 1992; 11:4733), displays some GTPase activity (Lokeshwar, JBC, 1992; 267:22073), and interacts with various components of the actin-based cytoskeleton (Tsukita, JCellBiol, 1994; 126:391), suggesting a direct role of CD44 in signal transduction.

Hyaluronic acid

This is the only non-sulphated glycosaminoglycan and it is not linked to a protein core. Hyaluronic acid is a highly hydrated linear polymer with the repetitive disaccharide [D-glucuronic acid (1-β-3) N-acetyl-D-glucosamine (1-β-4)]n with a chain length of 10 up to 1000 sugar units.[25] Hyaluronic acid is mainly synthesized by mesenchymal cells and distributed ubiquitously. The highest amounts are found in gelly-like tissues such as umbilical cord, synovial fluid, vitreous of the eye, and cartilage. Unlike the other glycosaminoglycans that are produced in the Golgi, hyaluronic acid synthesis occurs in the cytoplasm by a membrane-bound hyaluronic acid synthase. Hyaluronic acid synthesis is upregulated by several growth factors, including epidermal growth factor, platelet-derived growth factor, insulin-like growth factor-1, and transforming growth factor-β (Heldin, BiochemJ, 1989; 258:919). Accordingly, enhanced pericellular expression of hyaluronic acid is observed during cell proliferation (Brecht, BiochemJ, 1986; 239:445) and locomotion (Turley, JCellBiol, 1991; 112:1041). These events are mediated by specific transmembrane receptors, mainly CD44 (mentioned above), but also by the intercellular adhesion molecule, ICAM-1 (McCourt, JBC, 1994; 269:30081). ICAM-1 appears to be the major hyaluronic acid receptor on liver sinusoidal endothelial cells, which are highly active in removing hyaluronic acid from the circulation (Erikson, ExpCellRes, 1983; 144:223; Smedsrød, 1990; BiochemJ; 266:313). Circulating hyaluronic acid (usually below 100 μg/l) comes from peripheral tissues via the lymph and, due to the rapid uptake by the liver, has a half-life of only 3 to 5 min (Smedsrød, BiochemJ, 1984; 223:617). The turnover of hyaluronic acid in most tissues is high, with a half-life of 12 h in skin and joints (Laurent, AdvDrugDelivRev, 1991; 7:237). High serum levels are found in advanced liver disease, probably a result of compromised uptake by the sinusoidal endothelium (Bramley, JHepatol, 1991; 13:8; Ueno, Gastro, 1993; 105:475). Hyaluronic acid also offers therapeutic potential. Thus its injection into rabbits prevents homing and activation of natural killer cells in a model of acute (sinusoidal) liver injury induced by *Propionibacterium* sp. and lipopolysaccharide (Nakayama, CellImmunol, 1995; 166:275).

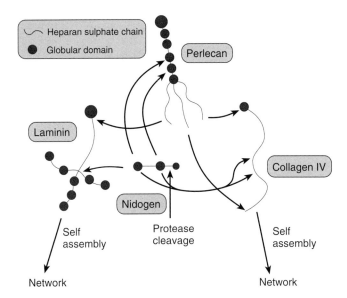

Fig. 10. Formation of supramolecular complexes in basement membranes. By virtue of its multiple interactions, nidogen (entactin) serves as an organizer of basement membranes. The protease-sensitive region in the C-terminal rod-like domain of nidogen allows for rapid local dissolution of basement membranes. Such local dissolution may allow penetration of, for example, inflammatory cells from the vessel lumen into the subepithelial connective tissue. This scheme neglects many of the minor and not yet characterized components of basement membranes that may, nonetheless, fulfil important roles. (Modified after ref.[26].)

Supramolecular complexes

Extracellular matrices are complex assemblies of covalently and non-covalently associated macromolecules. The complexity and plasticity of these assemblies can be easily understood when considering the multiple but specific interactions of extracellular matrix molecules such as those mentioned above. A simplified example showing the major components that assemble to basement membranes is shown in Fig. 10. Here the non-collagenous glycoprotein nidogen (entactin) binds to collagen 4, laminin, and perlecan. Both laminin and collagen IV can self-assemble to network structures, and interact individually with the heparan sulphate chains of perlecan. Nidogen contains an extremely protease-sensitive region, the cleavage of which leads to local disassembly of basement membranes. This defect, which may be repaired rapidly, could allow penetration of, for example, granulocytes or metastasizing tumour cells through basement membranes. Therefore, nidogen has been assigned a central role in the organization of these supramolecular structures.[26] In the liver nidogen is synthesized by hepatic stellate cells, sinusoidal endothelia, and portal fibroblasts (Schwoegler, LabInvest, 1994; 70:525). Viability and the differentiated phenotype of hepatocyte cultures is maintained for longer periods on complex extracellular matrices such as a gel-like basement membrane extract (EHS-matrix) (Bissell, EurJCellBiol, 1986; 40:72) or even on a combination of laminin-1 and nidogen (Levavasseur, JCellPhysiol, 1994; 161:257), than on the single basement membrane components.

Other assemblies include the already mentioned collagen fibrils with fibril-associated collagens (Fig. 4), non-collagenous glycoproteins and proteoglycans, and the complexes of hyaluronic acid, link protein, and aggrecan.

Modulation of growth factor activities by extracellular matrix

An important function of the extracellular matrix that has only been recognized recently is the retention and specific binding of cytokines (used here synonymously with growth factors). These interactions involve a limited set of extracellular matrix molecules and cytokines. The affinity of a given factor to its extracellular matrix ligand is between 10- and 1000-fold lower than to its transmembrane signalling receptor (usually a tyrosine or serine/threonine kinase). Nonetheless, apart from regulating the availability of certain cytokines by imposing on them a temporal and spatial pattern, the extracellular matrix may modify their biological activity.

This is exemplified by the extensively studied group of heparin (heparan sulphate) binding growth factors[1,20,27,28] which play important roles in wound healing and angiogenesis, processes that are associated with the proliferation and the biosynthetic and migratory activation of mesenchymal, epithelial, and endothelial cells. Binding to matrix heparan sulphate prevents diffusion of these factors and offers protection from proteolytic degradation. However, the matrix-bound factors can be released rapidly when the extracellular matrix becomes proteolytically degraded during organ growth or after injury. The family of heparin-binding growth factors includes interferon-γ (Lortat-Jacob, JCI, 1991; 87:878), acidic and basic fibroblast growth factor (FGF-1 and FGF-2), Int-2 (FGF-3) (Folkman, AmJPathol, 1988; 130:393; Vlodavsky, TIBS, 1991; 16: 268), keratinocyte growth factor (KGF or FGF-7) (Rubin, PNAS, 1989; 86:802), hepatocyte growth factor/scatter factor (**HGF**) (Masumoto, BBResComm, 1991; 174:90), vascular endothelial growth factor (VEGF) (Gitay-Goren, JBC, 1992; 267:6093), the interleukins IL-1α/β, IL-2, IL-3, and IL-6 (Roberts, Nature, 1989; 332:376; Ramsden, EurJImmun, 1992; 22:3027), and the long form of platelet-derived growth factor-AA (Raines, JCellBiol, 1992; 116: 533). Notably, not all heparan sulphates bind these factors equally well. An example is the interaction of HGF, the most potent hepatocyte mitogen during liver regeneration (Zarnegar, JCellBiol, 1995; 129:1177), where binding is found for heparan sulphate proteoglycans derived from liver but not for those from a murine basement membrane producing tumour (Ashikari, JBC, 1995; 270: 29586).

Transforming growth factor-β1 (TGF-β1), the strongest known inducer of desmoplasia and fibrosis (see above and Chapter 6.1) is bound and modulated by a variety of matrix molecules, including fibronectin (Mooradian; JCellBiochem, 1989; 41:189), the core proteins of the proteoglycans decorin, biglycan (Yamaguchi, Nature, 1990; 346:281), and betaglycan (Fukushima, JBC, 1989; 268:22710), and by thrombospondin which catalyses its conversion from the latent to the active form (Schultz-Cherry, JCellBiol, 1993; 122:923). TGF-β1, which speeds up rapid wound closure and scar formation by stimulating excessive matrix deposition, may be considered a first-line defence factor, protecting the organism from disassembly and fatal infection. However, once out of control, TGF-β1 is a major culprit during the development of atherosclerosis and endstage fibrosis of parenchymal–mesenchymal organs such as liver, lungs, and kidneys (Border, JCI, 1992; 90:1; Friedman, NEJM, 1993; 328:1828; Ross, Nature, 1993; 362:801; Border, NEJM, 1994; 331:1286). In fibroblastic cells, TGF-β1 increases the expression of collagens, of other extracellular matrix components, and of integrin receptors, but decreases interstitial collagenase (matrix metal-loproteinase-1) while upregulating its specific inhibitor, **TIMP-1** (tissue inhibitor of metalloproteinase-1). A surplus of the small core protein of the small proteoglycan decorin can compete with the binding of TGF-β1 to its signalling receptor (Yamaguchi, Nature, 1990; 346:281), and it was shown that injection of recombinant decorin or the decorin gene suppressed early fibrogenesis in a rat model of glomerular sclerosis, representing a novel approach to the treatment of fibrosis (Border, Nature, 1992; 360:361; Isaka, NatureMed, 1996; 2:418).

In addition to heparin/heparan sulphate, proteoglycans, and non-collagenous glycoproteins, collagens have recently emerged as extracellular ligands for growth factors and cytokines. This is exemplified by the binding of the isoforms of platelet-derived growth factor (PDGF-AA, -BB, and -AB) to collagens type I, II, III, IV, V, and VI (Somasundaram, JBC, 1996; 271:26884), a finding that explains the previous detection of matrix-bound platelet-de-rived growth factor in collagen-rich fibrotic and wound tissues (Gay, JInvDermatol, 1989; 92:301; Whitby, DevBiol, 1991; 147:207). Binding is mediated by one or two short peptides that are found in all of these major collagen types and that can be used as inhibitors of the interaction. Excess platelet-derived growth factor, which is a major mitogen for mesenchymal cells (Ross, Nature, 1993; 362:801) including hepatic stellate cells (Pinzani, JCI, 1989; 84:1786), can thus become immobilized on the newly synthesized collagen of fibrotic lesions, further stimulating mesenchymal cell influx and proliferation. Biologically stable analogues may therefore be de-signed from the identified collagenous consensus peptides that remove collagen-bound platelet-derived growth factor, allowing a 'lesion-targeted' antifibrotic therapy.

Other factors that bind via consensus peptides to collagens are interleukin-2 and -4, tumour necrosis factor-α and -β, hepatocyte growth factor, keratinocyte growth factor, and oncostatin M (Schup-pan, AnnNYAcadSci, 1994; 733:87; Schuppan, Gastro, 1998; 114: 1), all of which play a role in liver inflammation, regeneration, and fibrogenesis.

Figure 11 illustrates how cytokines (growth factors) adhere to molecules of the extracellular matrix and to cell surface pro-teoglycans, where they are stored in a latent form or their biological activity is modified. The term crinopexy (secreted and adherent) has been coined for this phenomenon (Feige, KidneyInt, 1995; 47: S15).

Integrins and signal transduction

The understanding of the receptors for extracellular matrix molecules, especially the integrins, has made tremendous progress, as reflected by the number of recent reviews on this topic.[29-38] Integrins do not simply tether cells to the extracellular matrix, but also transmit many signals to the cellular interior that operate in concert with cytokine or hormone signalling (Fig. 2). The integrins are membrane-spanning heterodimers of a non-covalently as-sociated α-chain and a β-chain. Presently 16 different α- and eight β-chains are known, which can occur in various combinations. These combinations determine the binding specificity of the integrin for certain collagens, non-collagenous extracellular matrix glyco-proteins, or membrane proteins. All integrins possess a large extra-cellular domain, a single transmembrane segment, and, except for

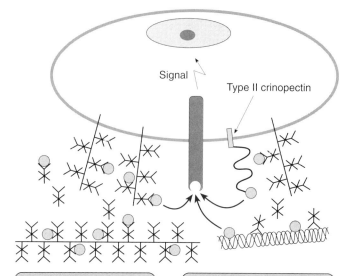

ECM-bound growth factors (type I crinopectins):	Transmembrane growth factor precursors (type II crinopectins): –
heparin-binding: fibroblast growth factors (FGF-1/2/3/7) granulocyte macrophage colony stimulating factor (GM-CSF) interleukins (IL-1/2/3/6) hepatocyte growth factor (HGF) vascular endothelial growth factor (VEGF), PDGF-AA	epidermal growth factor (EGF) heparin binding EGF GM-CSF-isoform colony stimulating factor (CSF-1) mast cell growth factor stem cell factor (c-kit ligand)
collagen-binding: platelet-derived growth factors (PDGF-A/B) IL-2/4, HGF, KGF (FGF-7) TNF-α/β, oncostatin M	**Coreceptors for presentation:**
multiple binding: transforming growth factors (TGF-β1/2/3) bone morphogenetic proteins (BMP-1/2/3)	*for FGF-receptors-1(flg)/2 (bek)/3/4, VEGF-receptor:* syndecans *for activin/TGF-receptors I/II:* betaglycan

Fig. 11. The extracellular matrix as a modulator of cytokine activities. The extracellular matrix can localize and store certain growth factors (cytokines), the so-called type I crinopectins. In addition, it may modulate their biological activities and provide protection from proteolysis. The heparin/heparan sulphate binding growth factors are further concentrated on the cell surface by membrane-associated heparan sulphate proteoglycans (for example the syndecans) which, in the case of the fibroblast growth factors and vascular endothelial growth factor, are necessary co-receptors for signal transduction via their tyrosine kinase receptors. Type II crinopectins are growth factors that are cell-associated due to a membrane anchor. They act predominantly on neighbouring, receptor-bearing cells, where they may also function as a cell–cell adhesion molecule. (Modified and updated from Feige, KidneyInt, 1995; 47;S15.)

the large β4-chain, a short cytoplasmic domain of less than 50 amino acids (Fig. 12). The β-chain intracellular domain can associate with the cytoskeletal proteins talin and α-actinin. Talin and α-actinin then couple the integrin to a variety of other cytoskeletal proteins, notably filamentous α-actin, the major component of stress fibres. The extracellular N-terminal domain forms the ligand-binding pocket, the affinity of which is positively modulated by the divalent cations Mg^{2+} and Mn^{2+}, and downregulated by Ca^{2+}. These cations

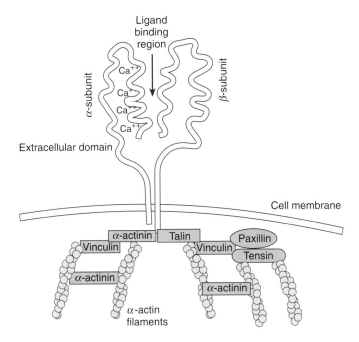

Fig. 12. Cytoskeletal associations of integrins. The heterodimeric integrins are dimers of a non-covalently linked α-subunit and a β-subunit. Integrins have a large extracellular and a small cytoplasmic domain. Affinity of the ligand-binding region is modulated by divalent cations. Once activated by ligand binding, the integrin cytoplasmic domain interacts with the focal adhesion proteins α-actinin and talin, which are partly involved in the formation of actin stress fibres. There are indirect links with vinculin, tensin, paxillin, and numerous cytoskeleton-associated proteins that are not shown here. Stress fibre formation and reorganization of the cytoskeleton is linked intricately to the activation of classical signal transduction pathways, with consequent changes in gene expression and cellular phenotype. See also Fig. 15.

co-ordinate 3 to 4 so-called EF-hand loops in the α-chain, structures that bear repetitive aspartate residues. The co-ordination centre is complemented by an aspartate that is found in most 'adhesive recognition sequences' contributed by integrin ligands, such as RGD (Arg–Gly–Asp) and LDV (Leu–Asp–Val) in fibronectin (see above).

Engagement of integrins by extracellular ligands can modify or elicit classical signal transduction pathways. However, this signalling is linked intricately with reorganization of the cytoskeleton. Ligand binding induces a conformational change in the integrin cytoplasmic domain that alters the cytoskeletal organization and modifies classical pathways of signal transduction.[29–32,34–37]

Figure 13 illustrates the possible combinations of integrin α- and β-chains that result in different ligand specificities. Thus α5β1 only recognizes the RGD (Arg–Gly–Asp) motif in fibronectin, whereas the promiscuous vitronectin receptor αVβ3 binds to vitronectin, von Willebrand factor, denatured collagens, fibrinogen, tenascin, thrombospondin-1, and osteopontin. The β2 and β7 integrins predominantly mediate cell–cell binding, whereas the β1, β3 to β6, and β8 integrins are mainly involved in cell–matrix interactions. However, overlaps occur frequently. Furthermore, integrins may serve as entry port for pathogenic organisms and viruses. Examples are α2β1 for echovirus type 1 (Bergelsen, Science, 1992; 255:1718), αVβ3 for HIV Tat protein (Barillari, PNAS, 1993; 90:7941), αVβ3

and αVβ5 for adenovirus (Wickham, Cell, 1993; 73:309), αIIbβ3 for *Borrelia burgdorferi*, which causes Lyme disease (Coburn, PNAS, 1993; 90:7059), and αMβ2 for *Bordetella pertussis* (Relman, Cell, 1990; 61:1375).

There is a growing number of cytoplasmic molecules that, having undergone tyrosine phosphorylation, can be recruited to the newly formed membrane complex of adhesion (termed focal adhesion) or that can become otherwise activated after ligand binding. A central feature of such activation is the tyrosine phosphorylation of the focal adhesion kinase, a cytoplasmic molecule of molecular mass 125 kDa,[39] and of the cytoskeletal proteins paxillin (Weng, JBC, 1993; 268:14956) and tensin (Bockholt, JBC, 1993; 268:14565). Tyrosine-phosphorylated paxillin and tensin are more efficiently recruited to focal adhesions and, by engaging vinculin and α-actinin, allow the formation of actin stress fibres (Fig. 12). Autophosphorylation and activation of focal adhesion kinase is a relatively late event in integrin signalling and rather serves as a point of convergence for signals that originate from the extracellular matrix as well as from classical mediators (Zachary, JBC, 1992; 267:19031; Huang, JCellBiol, 1993; 122:473; Zachary, JBC, 1993; 268:22060), since tyrosine phosphorylation of focal adhesion kinase and of paxillin is induced much earlier after fibroblasts have been exposed to bombesin, vasopressin, or endothelin-1 than after integrin activation (within 1 min, compared to 20 min).

Initiation of cellular and biochemical responses by integrins has been demonstrated in numerous studies. Activation of α5β1, the most widely expressed of the nine integrin fibronectin receptors, increases intracellular pH via stimulation of the Na^+/H^+-antiporter in fibroblasts and endothelial cells (Schwartz, PNAS, 1991; 88:7849) and increases the transcription factor AP-1 in T-helper cells (Yamada, JImmunol, 1992; 146:53). Both these events are associated with cellular proliferation. Adhesion of melanoma cells to collagen type IV, probably through integrin α1β1, opens Ca^{2+}-channels (Savarese, JBC, 1992; 267:21928), and that of neuroblastoma cells to fibronectin through integrins αVβ1 and α5β1 elicits an inward K^+-current that is dependent on a pertussis toxin-sensitive G protein (Arcangeli, JCellBiol, 1993; 122:1131). After cell adhesion to fibronectin, laminin, and collagen type IV, a G protein, Giα2, stimulates motility and metastatic potential in melanoma cells (Aznavoorian, JCellBiol, 1990; 110:1427; Lester, IntJCancer, 1991; 48:, 113). Most importantly, integrins like α5β1 support survival of cells on extracellular matrix proteins such as fibronectin by upregulating the expression of the anti-apoptosis gene *Bcl-2* (Zhang, PNAS, 1995; 92:6161), rendering a molecular explanation for the anchorage-dependent growth of most normal cells. In this context, signals elicited by binding of a polymeric ligand to integrins can be dissected into those that are caused by receptor occupation, for example by a monomeric ligand, and those elicited by receptor clustering, for example as induced by anti-integrin antibodies (Yamada, Science, 1995; 267:883).

The small G protein, rho, appears to be a crucial link between integrin and growth factor, as well as between classical growth factor and actin cytoskeleton-based signal transduction. Rho acts upstream of tyrosine phosphorylation of focal adhesion kinase (Seufferlein, JBC, 1995; 270:24343), regulates actin stress fibre formation (Ridley, Cell, 1992; 70:389; Bussey, Science, 1996; 272:224), and stimulates phosphatidylinositol phosphate kinase (Chong, Cell, 1994; 79:507). Phosphatidylinositol-phosphate kinase provides an enhanced supply

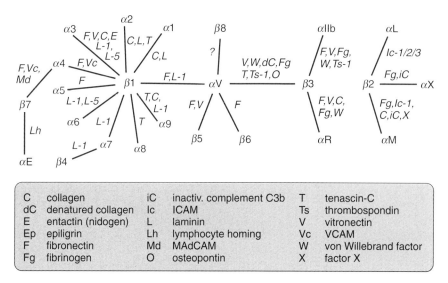

C	collagen	iC	inactiv. complement C3b	T	tenascin-C
dC	denatured collagen	Ic	ICAM	Ts	thrombospondin
E	entactin (nidogen)	L	laminin	V	vitronectin
Ep	epiligrin	Lh	lymphocyte homing	Vc	VCAM
F	fibronectin	Md	MAdCAM	W	von Willebrand factor
Fg	fibrinogen	O	osteopontin	X	factor X

Fig. 13. Integrins and their extracellular ligands. Associations of the heterodimeric integrins and known integrin ligands. Note that some integrins only have a single or few ligands, whereas others are promiscuous. A given cell type expresses only a limited spectrum of integrins that may change during activation or differentiation. Furthermore, their quantity and affinity can be altered by, for example, cytokines and intracellular mediators.

of phosphatidylinositol bisphosphate, which is the substrate of phospholipase Cγ (McNamee, JCellBiol; 121:673). Phospholipase Cγ is recruited to the cytoplasmic domain of ligand-activated tyrosine kinase receptors (e.g. the receptors for platelet-derived growth factor or epidermal growth factor) and serves as the key enzyme for generation of the second messengers inositol trisphosphate and diacylglycerol from phosphatidylinositol bisphosphate.[30] These findings start to provide the molecular basis for the cross-talk between integrin and growth factor receptors (Fig. 14), and explain the unresponsiveness of cells in relaxed collagen lattices, where integrins are not activated, to growth factors such as platelet-derived growth factor (Lin, JCellBiol, 1993; 122:663; Marx, KidneyInt, 1993, 43:1027).

Also, the events further upstream of rho are becoming clearer. Thus the small G (GTP-binding) protein rac (Ridley, Cell, 1992; 70:401) is either activated via tyrosine kinase receptors (for example, by those for epidermal growth factor and platelet-derived growth factor) and ras, or via the so-called 7-membrane receptors (for example, via those for endothelin and vasopressin) and Cdc42.[40] Also ras and Cdc42 are G proteins. Ras is recruited to tyrosine phosphates of the activated (autophosphorylated) cytoplasmic domains of tyrosine kinase receptors by the aid of molecular adaptors such as Grb2. These adaptors are cytoplasmic proteins that contain both phosphotyrosine-binding SH2 (src-homology 2) domains and G protein-binding SH3 (src-homology 3) domains[37] (Pawson, Cell, 1992; 71:359). The prototype of these molecular adaptors, p-src, also binds to molecules such as paxillin and to integrins (Burridge, JCellBiol, 1992; 119:893; Cooper, Cell, 1993; 73:1050). Recent data show that focal adhesion kinase that can associate with the β-chain of integrins may also recruit and activate ras via the mentioned molecular adaptors.[36,37,40] In this context, integrin activation may stimulate mitogen-activated protein kinase (Chen, JBC, 1994; 269:26602). Since ras is a key activator of the mitogenic

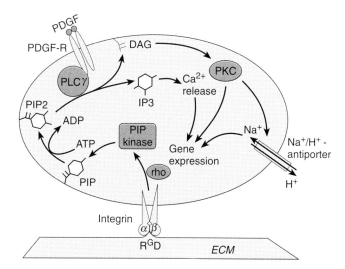

Fig. 14. Cross-talk between integrin and growth factor signalling. Simplified scheme with the dimeric platelet-derived growth factor receptor (PDGF-R), a member of the tyrosine kinase receptors, the cytoplasmic domains of which autophosphorylate each other after ligand binding. The phosphorylated PDGF-R recruits and activates phospholipase Cγ (PLCγ) via a phosphotyrosine–SH2 interaction (see text). PLCγ cleaves membrane-bound phosphatidylinositol bisphosphate (PIP$_2$) into the second messengers diacylglycerol (DAG) and inositol trisphosphate (IP$_3$). DAG and IP$_3$ activate protein kinase C (PKC) and liberate calcium from intracellular stores, respectively. Both pathways finally influence the expression of many genes, including activation of the Na$^+$/H$^+$-antiporter which causes cytoplasmic alkalinization and promotes cell division. Ligand-activated integrins can stimulate phosphatidylinositol phosphate kinase (PIPK), an enzyme that enhances the supply of PIP$_2$ that is utilized by the growth factor receptor dependent signal transduction via PLCγ. Recent data implicate the small G protein rho as a key activator of PIPK (see Fig.15).

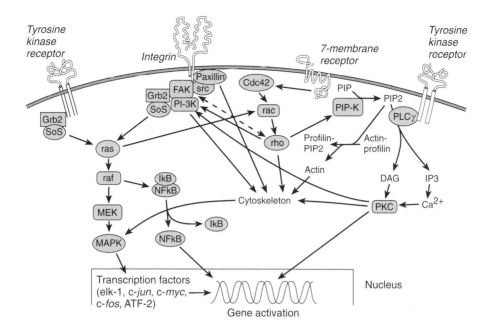

Fig. 15. Signal transduction by integrins. Ligand-activated integrins recruit a number of signalling molecules in complexes called focal adhesions. Once phosphorylated on tyrosines, paxillin and the focal adhesion kinase (FAK) can bind to the β-chain cytoplasmic domain of the dimeric integrin. Paxillin then associates with the tyrosine kinase src and the cytoskeleton, whereas FAK binds phosphatidylinositol-3-kinase (PI3K), an enzyme that generates a set of 3-phosphorylated inositols, which play a yet ill-defined role in vesicle formation and proliferation, and the molecular adaptor Grb2 (growth factor receptor binding protein 2) that via SoS (the *Drosophila* protein 'son of sevenless') activates the small G protein, ras. Ras is linked to 'classical' signal transduction from tyrosine kinase growth factor receptors (e.g. the receptors for epidermal growth factor and platelet-derived growth factor) and propagates the downstream phosphorylation cascade that, via the kinases raf and MEK, activates mitogen-activated protein kinase (MAPK). Activated MAPK translocates into the nucleus where it phosphorylates and thus activates various nuclear transcription factors. Phosphorylated raf (and signals of oxidative stress) also cause nuclear translocation of the transcription factor, nuclear factor kappa B (NFκB) after dissociation from its cytoplasmic inhibitor (inhibitor kappa B, IκB). Ras, as well as signalling by 7-membrane receptors (with, for example, endothelin and vasopressin as ligands), can also activate the small G protein rho via Cdc42 and the small G protein rac. Rho stimulates phosphatidylinositol phosphate kinase (PIPK), but also modulates the cytoskeleton and the focal adhesion complex. An increased level of phosphatidylinositol bisphosphate (PIP2), apart from representing the substrate of PLCγ, sequesters profilin from monomeric actin, allowing actin polymerization and stress fibre formation.

cascade that involves raf and mitogen-activated protein kinase, this provides a second pathway for the comitogenic effect of integrin activation. Figure 15 summarizes the complex events of integrin and growth factor signalling.

The cellular distribution of β1 integrins in human liver was studied in normal and pathological liver biopsies (Volpes, Gastro, 1991; 101:206). The authors found α1, α2, α3, α5, and α6 on endothelia, α1 and α2 on portal fibroblasts, α1, α2, and α5 on sinusoidal lining (stellate) cells, α1 and α5 on hepatocytes, and α2, α3, α5, and α6 on bile duct epithelium. Another report describes the expression of integrins α1β1, α2β1, αVβ1, and α6β4 by cultured human stellate cells (Carloni, Gastro, 1996; 110:1127). In hepatitis, hepatocytes expressed additional chains α3 and α6. The expression of integrins α3β1 and α6β1, which are the major laminin receptors, is in line with the enhanced deposition of laminins during inflammation and sinusoidal capillarization. In cholestasis, hepatocytes adopted the bile ductular phenotype with chains α1, α2, α3, α5, and α6. Apart from supporting the observation of the ductular metaplasia of hepatocytes during chronic cholestasis, the *de novo* expression of α2β1, which serves as major (interstitial) collagen receptor, parallels the observed periductular collagen accumulation around proliferating bile ducts. The integrin pattern was not much altered in poorly differentiated hepatocellular carcinoma, where the neoplastic cells expressed the set of bile duct-type α-chains, whereas

a decrease in the bile duct-type integrin α-chains was found on poorly differentiated cholangiocarcinoma cells (Volpes, AmJPathol, 1993; 142:1483). Cholangiocarcinomas could be clearly differentiated from hepatocarcinoma, since they expressed the laminin receptor α6β4 and the vitronectin receptor αVβ3. When searching for hepatocarcinoma-specific genes by the method of differential display, researchers identified the integrin chain α6 as a tumour-specific marker (Begum, Hepatol, 1995; 22:1447). An integrin that is predominantly expressed in liver is the recently discovered α9β1 (Forsberg, ExpCellRes, 1994; 213:183). It mediates binding to the long arm of laminin-1 and to a peptide in the α1 chain of collagen I. Its cell-specific expression has not been defined.

Integrins and matrix peptides as modulators of cell activation and growth

As mentioned above, the extracellular matrix profoundly influences cellular behaviour. With the dissection of the molecular architecture of extracellular matrix molecules and their receptors, and with the analysis of the signalling processes involved, strategies are emerging that exploit these findings in the design of novel extracellular matrix-derived therapeutics for fibrosis and cancer.

Tumour angiogenesis, a process of neo-vessel formation that is necessary for neoplastic growth beyond 1 mm[41,42] is mediated by the the integrins αVβ3 and αVβ5 (both are vitronectin receptors) on endothelial cells that populate the tumour[43] (Friedlander, Science, 1995: 270:1500). αVβ3 is upregulated by the tumour-derived cytokines basic fibroblast growth factor and tumour necrosis factor-α, whereas αVβ5 expression is increased by vascular endothelial growth factor, transforming growth factor-α and protein kinase C activation through phorbol esters. Both integrins recognize Arg–Gly–Asp (RGD) motifs in their extracellular matrix ligands vitronectin and denatured collagens. The RGD sequence is commonly found in extracellular matrix proteins. It is a basic recognition sequence for various integrins that nonetheless display high substrate specificity (see above). Since simple synthetic RGD peptides inhibit all RGD-dependent integrins, with expected undesirable side-effects, receptor-specific RGD-analogues had to be developed. This has been accomplished with the cyclic peptide Arg–Gly–Asp–D–Phe–Val (cyclo-[RGDDFV]) which specifically blocks both vitronectin receptors, but not, for example, the RGD-dependent integrins fibronectin receptor α5β1 and platelet receptor αIIbβ3 (Pfaff, JBC, 1994; 269:20233). Cyclo-[RGDDFV]), by depriving the (anchorage-dependent) angiogenic endothelial cells of their extracellular matrix contact, effectively induces apoptosis and tumour regression in experimental models (Brooks, Science, 1994; 264:569; Brooks, Cell, 1994; 79:1157). Also, certain integrins that mediate invasion and metastasis of the tumour cells themselves might be targets for specific integrin-antagonists. Examples are α3β1, a broad-spectrum receptor for laminins, fibronectin, and vitronectin (Melchiori, ExpCellRes, 1995; 219:233), and α4β1, a receptor for fibronectin (Qian, Cell, 1994; 77:335).

The finding that the fibroblast's synthetic capacity is tightly linked to changes of its extracellular matix environment offers attractive approaches for a targeted antifibrotic therapy. Fibroblasts and other mesenchymal cells are highly activated when cultivated in the conventional two-dimensional tissue culture system, a situation that resembles the stimulus induced by a wound *in vivo*. Such activated cells are characterized by a high rate of proliferation, a low expression of matrix metalloproteinase-1 (interstitial collagenase) and a high expression of collagens and the tissue inhibitor of matrix metalloproteinase (TIMP-1), resulting in a fibrogenic, i.e. stressed, phenotype. Transfer of the stressed cells into a three-dimensional collagen matrix that allows stress-relaxation reverses the activated fibrogenic to a quiescent phenotype that is characterized by little proliferation, a low production of collagen and TIMP-1, and an enhanced expression of matrix metalloproteinase-1[44,45] (Mauch, ExpCellRes, 1988; 178:1508; Mauch, FEBSLett, 1989; 250:301) (Fig. 16). Signalling events that appear to be derived primarily from integrins, particularly the collagen receptors α1β1 and α2β1, mediate the fibrogenic response in this system. Once stressed, α1β1 upregulates collagen I production and α2β1 downregulates matrix metalloproteinase-1, a process reversed by stress relaxation expression (Eckes, JCellBiol, 1995; 131:1903). Furthermore, stress relaxation induces downregulation of, or unresponsiveness to, growth factor receptors, for example that for platelet-derived growth factor (Lin, JCellBiol, 1993; 122:663; Marx, KidneyInt, 1993; 43: 1027; Figs 14 and 15).

Another interesting observation is that nanomolar concentrations of soluble collagen VI further stimulate proliferation of cells that are already activated by culture in a two-dimensional environment (Atkinson, ExpCellRes, 1996; 228:283). Collagen VI, a microfilamentous structure that interconnects collagen fibrils (see above), may thus serve as a molecular sensor of tissue destruction. This is reflected by an almost 100% sensitivity and specificity of elevated circulating levels of collagen VI to detect liver fibrosis in a large group of children (Oerling, NEJM, 1997; 336:1611). Once released by proteolysis it could trigger mesenchymal cell proliferation in an autocrine manner. The responsible receptor does not appear to be a known integrin, but collagen VI primary structures can effectively inhibit activation.

Blocking the non-RGD-dependent integrins α1β1 and α2β1 or the proliferation-promoting receptor for collagen VI should not affect mesenchymal cells in normal tissues, but rather in wounded, actively fibrosing tissues. Work is under way to develop such agents, an approach that is based on identification of the collagen structures involved (Vandenberg, JCellBiol, 1991; 113:1475; Eble, EMBOJ, 1993; 12:4795; Kern, EurJCellBiol, 1994; 215:151), *in vitro* binding studies (Pfaff, EurJCellBiol, 1994; 225:975), and the search for potent and specific antagonists exploiting stabilized synthetic peptides (Nowlin, JBC, 1993; 268:20352; Pfaff, JBC, 1994; 269:20233; Greenspoon, 1993, Biochem; 32:1001) or sequences derived from phage display libraries (Koivunen, JBC, 1993; 268:20205).

Metalloproteinases and matrix degradation

The amount and quality of extracellular matrix is determined both by the production and by the removal of its constituents. Accordingly, fibrosis is always the result of a disbalance of fibrolysis in favour of fibrogenesis. Consequently, the importance of understanding the mechanisms of matrix degradation is increasingly recognized, since a once-established fibrosis can only be reversed by a stimulated fibrolysis. Fibrolytic enzymes are: the lysosomal cathepsins, which act mainly intracellularly; some players in the blood coagulation and fibrinolytic cascade, such as thrombin and plasmin; and the matrix metalloproteinases (**MMPs**) that act exclusively in the extracellular space. Due to their central role in extracellular matrix degradation, only the MMPs will be discussed in more detail.

The MMPs comprise a growing family (currently 15) of zinc-dependent enzymes that bear common structural and functional characteristics.[46-51] Eight of the MMPs have been found in liver, and they cover a broad range of substrate specificities, ranging from the native, triple-helical collagens I, II, and III, to denatured collagens, elastin, proteoglycan core proteins, laminin, and fibronectin (Table 4). As shown in Fig. 17, all MMPs consist of an N-terminal propeptide of roughly 80 amino acids, followed by the catalytic domain and a hinge region that allows the C-terminal hemopexin repeats to fold back on the catalytic domain. This hemopexin domain, which also binds the MMP inhibitors (TIMPs, see below), is absent from matrilysin (MMP-7), whereas the basement membrane collagen-degrading MMP-2 and MMP-9 contain an extra 175 amino acid stretch with three collagen-binding fibronectin type II repeats that precede the zinc-binding region of the catalytic domain. These type II repeats appear to further define substrate specificity. The function of the short procollagen V-like

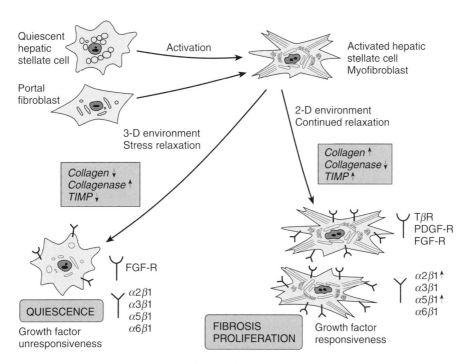

Fig. 16. Stress relaxation and induction of cellular quiescence. Continued mechanical stress maintains the fibrogenic phenotype. The fibrogenic phenotype is characterized by a responsive (stressed) conformation of certain extracellular matrix receptors, such as the integrins $\alpha1\beta1$, $\alpha2\beta1$, and $\alpha5\beta1$ that serve as extracellular matrix-directed environmental sensors. Furthermore, it may be accompanied by an enhanced expression of the cellular receptors for fibrogenic growth factors (TβR for transforming growth factor-β, FGF-R for basic fibroblast growth factor and PDGF-R for platelet-derived growth factor), the effect of which is increased by the activated integrins (see also Figs 14 and 15). Independently of growth factors, stressed integrins enhance the expression of collagens and the tissue inhibitor of metalloproteinases (TIMP-1), and downregulate collagenase (MMP-1). The whole process is aimed at rapid wound closure. It is usually self-limited and subsides once the wound is filled with an appropriate extracellular matrix. However, it remains continuously operative in active liver fibrosis. Novel therapies can be designed that utilize so-called adhesive recogniton sequences from extracellular matrix molecules to compete with the integrins, inducing a relaxed mesenchymal phenotype, with subsequent upregulation of collagenases and downregulation of collagens and TIMPs.

Table 4 Matrix metalliproteinases and their substrates		
MMP	**Synonym**	**Extracellular matrix substrate**
MMP-1*	Interstitial collagenase	CI, II, III, VII, VIII, X; dC; PG
MMP-2*	Gelatinase A, BM-collagenase	dC; CIV, V, VII, X, XI; EI; FN
MMP-3*	Stromelysin-1	dC; CIV, V, IX, X; FN; LN; pro-MMP-1
MMP-7	PUMP-1, matrilysin	FN, LN; PG; CIV; dC
MMP-8*	Granulocyte-collagenase	Similar to MMP-1
MMP-9*	Gelatinase B	dC; CIII, IV, V, XIV; PG
MMP-10*	Stromelysin-2	Similar to MMP-3
MMP-11*	Stromelysin-3	Similar to MMP-3?
MMP-12	Metalloelastase	EI; similar to MMP-9?
MMP-13	Collagenase 3	Similar to MMP-1
MMP-14*	Membrane type MMP	Pro-MMP-2

Summary of the 11 best-characterized matrix metalloproteinases (MMPs), most of which are expressed in the liver (designated*). Their substrates include diverse collagen types (C), denatured collagens ('gelatins', dC), core proteins of proteoglycans (PG), elastin (EI), fibronectin (FN), and laminins (LN). Homology cloning revealed at least three more membrane-type MMPs (MMP-15-16, and -17).

region that is only found in MMP-9 is yet unknown. The freshly synthesized pro-matrix metalloproteinases (**pro-MMPs**) are proteolytically inactive, since the propeptide folds back on the catalytic domain. The underlying molecular mechanism of latency of the pro-MMPs is complexation of the catalytic zinc by a Cys-containing region, the so-called cysteine-switch in the propeptide.[4,49,50]

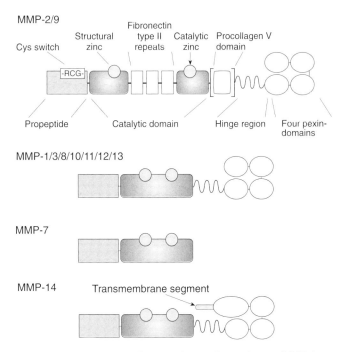

Fig. 17. Domain structure of the matrix metalloproteinases (MMPs). The MMPs consist (from N- to C-terminal) of the 77–87 amino acid long propeptide region; the catalytic domain, with both a structural and a catalytic zinc-binding site; a hinge region; and, except for MMP-7 (matrilysin), a hemopexin domain. MMP-2 and -9 harbour an additional set of three collagen-binding fibronectin type II repeats close to the catalytic zinc, and MMP-9 a 53 amino acid region with homology to procollagen V, the function of which is unknown. Proteolytic activation by plasmin or furin-type membrane proteases leads to removal of the cysteine switch (complexation and blockage of the catalytic zinc atom by the cysteine in the propeptide sequence Arg–Cys–Gly). The tissue inhibitors of metalloproteinases (TIMP-1 and TIMP-2) bind to the the hemopexin domains via their C-terminus, while their free N-terminus can block the catalytic domain of the MMPs. (Modified from ref.[49]; see also Table 4.)

The activity of MMPs is controlled at many levels. First, their gene expression can be upregulated by the cytokines epidermal growth factor, fibroblast growth factor, interleukin-1, transforming growth factor-α, tumour necrosis factor, and platelet-derived growth factor, and downregulated by transforming growth factor-β, interleukin-4, retinoic acid, and glucocorticoids[52] (Clark, JCI, 1987; 80:1280), factors that at the same time have distinct and often divergent effects on cell proliferation and extracellular matrix synthesis (see Table 2 and Chapter 6.1). An exception is the basement membrane collagen degrading MMP-2 which is up-regulated by transforming growth factor-β1 (Overall, JBC, 1989; 264:1860). All matrix metalloproteinase genes analysed so far have at least one AP-1 site in their promoters, and the dimeric AP-1 transcription factor appears to play an important role in the stimulation of MMP gene expression.[53] However, collagen type I gene expression may also be activated by AP-1, as mentioned above.

In addition, soluble fragments of fibronectin have been shown to increase MMP-1 and MMP-3 expression via the fibronectin receptor α5β1, an effect not observed with polymeric fibronectin offered as the adhesion substrate (Werb, JCellBiol, 1989; 109:887). Stimulation of the integrin αVβ3 (vitronectin receptor), which

also mediates endothelial cell angiogenesis during tumour growth, enhances melanoma cell invasion via an increase in MMP-2 expression (Seftor, PNAS, 1992; 89:1557), and the laminin α1 chain peptide IKVAV (see above) increases MMP-2 expression in melanoma and fibrosarcoma cells (Kanemoto, PNAS, 1990; 87:2279) and supports colon cancer metastasis to the liver (Bresalier, CancerRes, 1995; 55:2476), a mechanism that does not appear to involve an integrin. The induction of MMP-1 by stress–relaxation through the integrin α1β1 (mainly a collagen IV receptor) has been mentioned above.

A second level of control is the proteolytic activation of the latent pro-MMP to the active enzyme. This step involves cleavage of the propeptide domain (approximately 80 amino acids long), leading to a release of the cysteine switch from its complexation with the zinc atom in the catalytic domain (see above and Fig. 17). Plasmin and its activators **uPA** and to a lesser degree **tPA** (urokinase and tissue plasminogen activators, respectively) have been implicated in this cleavage reaction, which would assign them a key role in extracellular matrix degradation (Murphy, JBC, 1992; 267:9612). Accordingly, melanoma invasion and metastasis is closely linked to the activation of uPA, which is regulated by uPA binding to its membrane receptor (**uPA-R**). Interestingly, expression of the vitronectin receptor, αVβ3, and the uPA-R are co-ordinately regulated in these melanoma cells (Nip, JCI, 1995; 95:2096). Furthermore, uPA also appears to play a role in the proteolytic activation of single–chain hepatocyte growth factor to the dimeric, biologically active form. Thus after partial hepatectomy, hepatocyte uPA-R is highly up-regulated within 1 h (Mars, Hepatol, 1995; 21:1695). However, other proteases, such as the membrane-bound furins, are suspected activators of both MMPs and pre-hepatocyte growth factor. Once in the active form, MMP-3 and MMP-10 (stromelysin-1 and -2) may remove only one or two more N-terminal amino acids from active MMP-1 to enhance its *in vitro* activity five- to twelvefold, a process termed 'superactivation' (Windsor, JBC, 1993; 268:17341). A simplified scheme of MMP and hepatocyte growth factor activation is shown in Fig. 18. However, MMP-2, a product of predominantly mesenchymal cells, is proteolytically activated by a distinct pathway. It is bound to and activated by a recently cloned membrane-type metalloproteinase (MMP-14), forming a ternary complex with the MMP-2 inhibitor TIMP-2 (Sato, Nature, 1994; 370:61; Strongin, JBC, 1995; 270:5331). MMP-14 expression correlates both with MMP-2 activation and with invasiveness of human tumours (Gilles, IntJCanc, 1996; 65:209; Yamamoto, CancerRes, 1996; 56:384). Since MMP-2 is secreted by mesenchymal cells and MMP-14 is produced by mesenchymal as well as epithelial cells, MMP-2 activation is a co-operative event during tissue restructuring and invasion.

A third level of control is introduced with the tissue inhibitors of metalloproteinases, TIMP-1, TIMP-2, and the recently cloned TIMP-3.[52] These proteins with molecular masses between 21 and 29 kDa are either produced by the same cells that secrete the MMPs they are destined to inhibit, or by neighbouring cells, indicating a tight spatial regulation of MMP activity. The TIMPs share approximately 40 per cent sequence homology and a high structural similarity. TIMP-1 and TIMP-2 can inhibit all MMPs, with their C-terminus anchored to the C-terminus of the MMPs, and with their N-terminus folding back on the MMP catalytic site. TIMP-2 preferentially inhibits MMP-2, and TIMP-1 can block the

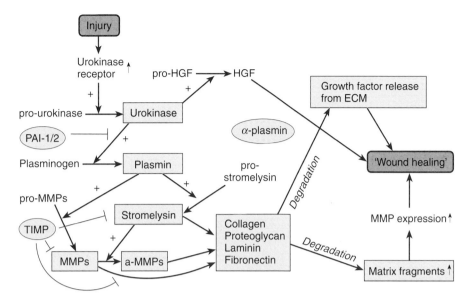

Fig. 18. Activation of matrix metalloproteinases (MMPs) and hepatocyte growth factor (HGF). Injury leads to upregulation of the cell-bound urokinase plasminogen activator receptor that converts inactive to active urokinase. Urokinase (as well as tissue plasminogen) activator triggers a cascade of proteolytic MMP activation via generation of plasmin. Plasmin (and most probably other, membrane-bound proteases) removes the inhibitory propeptides from the pro-MMPs, including pro-stromelysins-1 and -2 (pro-MMP-3 and -10). MMP-3 and -10 can 'superactivate' other MMPs by proteolytic removal of one or two additional N-terminal amino acids. The active MMPs degrade extracellular matrix proteins, generating fragments that, via integrin and non-integrin receptors, can further upregulate cellular MMP expression. During matrix degradation, extracellular matrix-bound growth factors are also liberated, accelerating wound healing by enhancing angiogenesis and extracellular matrix deposition. In addition, urokinase can generate the active dimeric hepatocyte growth factor from its inactive single-chain precursor. Activation of MMP-2 follows a different pathway, with proteolytic cleavage by membrane-bound MMP-14.

activity of the other MMPs. Most studies of TIMP-1 have been performed on interstitial collagenase (MMP-1), stromelysin (MMP-3), and basement membrane collagenase/gelatinase B (MMP-9).

Often the genes for TIMP-1 and MMP-1 are co-ordinately upregulated by factors such as platelet-derived growth factor, epidermal growth factor, basic fibroblast growth factor, interleukin-1, and phorbol esters (Murphy, JBC, 1985; 260:3079; Edwards, EMBOJ, 1987; 6:1899) and downregulated by, for example, corticosteroids (Clark, JCI, 1987; 80:1280). Inverse regulation, i.e. downregulation of MMP-1 and upregulation of TIMP-1, has been reported for retinoic acid (Bailly, JInvDermatol, 1990; 94:47) and transforming growth factor-β1 (Overall, JBC, 1989; 264:1860). However, the effects of the factors may vary considerably depending on culture conditions and the tissues from which the cells are derived. Thus, retinoic acid can increase the expression of MMP-1 and MMP-3, and decrease that of TIMP-1 in osteoblastic cell cultures. In contrast, the overt profibrogenic effect of transforming growth factor-β1, i.e. lowering MMP-1 and increasing TIMP-1 (Border, JCI, 1992; 90:1), is an apparently ubiquitous phenomenon. Transforming growth factor-β1 downregulates TIMP-2 (Stetler-Stevenson, JBC, 1990; 265:13933) and increases MMP-2 (see above), suggesting that it induces fibrolysis of basement membrane collagen, whereas it accelerates the accumulation of interstitial extracellular matrix. A peculiar inhibitor is formed by the complex of MMP-2 and TIMP-2 ('large inhibitor of metalloproteinases', LIMP). This complex has properties similar to TIMP-1, blocking the activities of MMP-1 and MMP-3 (Kolkenbrock, EurJBioch, 1991; 198:775; Curry, BiochemJ, 1992; 285:143).

A general inhibitor of all secreted proteases, including MMP-1 and MMP-3, is α₂-macroglobulin, a homotetramer of 724 kDa

(Enghild, JBC, 1989; 264:8779). It is produced mainly by hepatocytes and constitutes a significant fraction of the plasma proteins. Due to its large molecular size, penetration from plasma into the extracellular matrix should be low. However, an autocrine or paracrine action on MMPs is possible.

Furthermore, plasminogen activator inhibitors (PAI-1 and PAI-2), both molecules of approximately 50 kDa, apparently interfere with the early phase of MMP activation by blocking plasmin (He, PNAS, 1989; 86:2632; Cajot, PNAS, 1990; 87:6939) (see Fig. 18). PAI-1 is not expressed by colon carcinoma cells but in the surrounding stroma where it may support the desmoplastic reaction (Koretz, EurJCan, 1993; 27A:1194). In normal liver, low-level expression of PAI-1 is observed by hepatocytes, endothelium, and Kupffer cells. Whereas lipopolysaccharide induces mainly endothelial and Kupffer cell PAI-1 (Podor, JImmunol, 1993; 150:225), partial hepatectomy in rats leads to its ninefold upregulation in hepatocytes, with maximal expression reached after 2 to 8 h (Schneiderman, AmJPathol, 1993; 143:753; Thornton, CancerRes, 1994; 54:1337), qualifying it as an immediate early response gene. *In vitro*, hepatic stellate as well as sinusoidal endothelial cells secrete PAI-1 (Knittel, Gastro, 1996; 111:745). Whereas normal human livers show only little PAI-1 expression as detected by *in situ* hybridization, PAI-1 mRNA is particularly upregulated in hepatocytes in areas of increased inflammatory or fibrogenic activity (Herbst, Gastro, 1996; 110:A1210), underscoring the importance of parenchymal cells for the control of fibrosis. PAI-1 that is specifically bound by vitronectin in the extracellular matrix can be induced by the mitogen hepatocyte growth factor, which is also immobilized in the extracellular matrix by heparan sulphate and collagen (see above). Since hepatocyte growth factor activation depends on proteolytic cleavage by plasmin (which is blocked by PAI-1), this indicates that hepatocyte growth factor may regulate its biological activity by a PAI-1-mediated loop of feedback inhibition (Wojta, Blood, 1994; 84:151). Although mice in which the PAI-1 gene has been deleted by homologue recombination develop normally (Carmeliet, JCI, 1993; 92:2746), this does not exclude the emergence of a pathological phenotype after injury.

Earlier studies suggested that collagenase activity is an important determinant of collagen accumulation in the liver. Thus collagenolysis attributable to MMP-1 (MMP-8) progressively decreases in late stages of carbon tetrachloride-induced liver fibrosis in rats (Perez-Tamayo, ExpMolPath, 1987; 47:300), and increases again when the toxin is withdrawn (Rojkind, Gastro, 1978; 75: A984), which may underlie the steady disappearance of hepatic collagen under these conditions. Similarly, collagenolytic activity is suppressed in advanced murine schistosomiasis that produces a portal fibrosis around the trapped eggs (Takahashi, BiochemJ, 1984; 220:157), and the quantity of MMP-1 protein is reduced in human alcoholic cirrhosis (Maruyama, LifeSci, 1982; 30:1379).

An investigation that used specific antisera to recombinant MMPs showed that MMP-1, -2, -3, -9, -10, and -11 may be expressed in human liver (Lichtinghagen, EurJClinChemClinBioch, 1995; 33:65) (Table 4). Cell culture studies have demonstrated that several hepatic cell types can synthesize MMP-1, -2, -3 and -9. *In vitro* hepatic stellate cells express the mRNA for MMP-1 (Milani, AmJPathol, 1994; 144:528), MMP-2 (Arthur, JCI, 1989; 84:1076), and MMP-3 (Herbst, VirchArchCP, 1991; 60:295). Stellate cell MMP-2 is biologically active in degrading denatured as well as native basement membrane collagen (Arthur, BiochemJ, 1992; 287:701). Its mRNA content may increase 20- to 30-fold during stellate cell activation *in vitro* (Benyon, Gastro, 1996; 110: 821). Since the membrane-type MMP (MMP-14) which activates MMP-2 (see above) is also expressed by cultured hepatic stellate cells, MMP-2 activity may be further upregulated in these cells, which suggests an autocrine activation (Hovell, Hepatol, 1995; 22: A1052). Bioactive MMP-9 (also a basement membrane collagenase) is primarily secreted by isolated Kupffer cells, well in line with its predominant expression by monocytes and macrophages in other systems (Winwood, Hepatol, 1995; 22:304).

However, *in vitro* data using artificial cell culture conditions have to be interpreted with care, and studies using *in situ* hybridization showed that, quite in contrast to cell culture, MMP-1 transcripts were essentially absent both from normal and fibrotic human liver, whereas MMP-2 expression was co-localized with vimentin-positive, probably stellate cells (Milani, AmJPathol, 1994; 144:528). After acute carbon tetrachloride intoxication in rats, MMP-3 mRNA was highly expressed in 10 to 15 per cent of pericentral hepatocytes as early as 6 h after the injury, reaching a maximum after 24 h, and later appeared in mesenchymal cells, with a maximum at 48 h (Herbst, VirchArchCP, 1991; 60:295), underlining the importance of the temporospatial pattern of MMP expression *in vivo*. However, even in *in situ* hybridization studies, MMP expression at the mRNA level is not necessarily linked to protein synthesis, and protein levels of MMPs may not reflect enzyme activity, as has been outlined above.

Less is known about the expression of the TIMPs in the liver. Cell culture shows that hepatic stellate cells express bioactive TIMP-1 which increases with transition to the myofibroblastic phenotype (Iredale, JCI, 1992; 90:282). TIMP-1 and -2 are also synthesized by hepatoma cells and hepatocytes (Roeb, FEBSLett, 1994; 349:45; Roeb, FEBSLett, 1995; 357:33). *In situ* hybridization showed that in fibrotic rat and human livers TIMP-1 and TIMP-2 mRNAs are expressed predominantly by stellate cells (Herbst, AmJPathol, 1997; 150:1647). TIMP-mRNA appears as early as 3 h after acute injury, pointing to a role in protecting the liver from accidental proteolysis. Since TIMP-2 expression is essentially unchanged, whereas MMP-2 increases, the degradation of basement membrane collagen (the major substrate for MMP-2) relative to that of interstitial collagen appears to prevail during fibrogenesis.

Ideally, the effect of certain MMPs on the removal of excess collagen in chronic liver disease could be tested using specific activators of a given MMP in an appropriate experimental model such as rat secondary biliary fibrosis. Such agents are not yet available. Furthermore, they could threaten to deprive cells of their matrix environment, thus selecting for anchorage-independent growth and finally neoplasia, especially in the context of ongoing injury.

On the other hand, fairly specific non-peptidic inhibitors of MMPs, such as batimastat, have the potential for the treatment of primary and metastatic cancers (Wang, CancerRes, 1994; 54:4726; Watson, CancerRes, 1995; 55:3629). In nude mice with malignant ascites due to ovarian cancer, survival was increased fivefold (Davies, CancerRes, 1993; 53:2087). In particular MMP-2 has been correlated with the progression of breast, colorectal, and gastric cancers (D'Errico, ModPathol, 1991; 4:239) and, as might be expected, tumours treated with batimastat have a more pronounced connective tissue capsule.[54] The drug has no obvious acute toxicity. It blocks MMP-1, -2, -7, and -9 to a similar degree, and MMP-3 slightly less efficiently, whereas other zinc-proteases, like the angiotensin- or endothelin-converting enzymes remain unaffected.[54] The crystal structure of the batimastat–MMP-8 complex has been resolved, paving the way for the development of even more specific MMP inhibitors (Grams, Biochem, 1995; 34:14012). The better, soluble marimastat is currently in phase II clinical trials for the adjuvant treatment of gastric, pancreatic, and ovarian cancer. Such agents may aid to further elucidate the role of MMPs and their inhibitors during the evolution of liver fibrosis.

References

1. Schuppan D, Herbst H, and Milani S. Matrix, matrix synthesis and molecular networks in hepatic fibrosis. In Zern MA and Reid L, eds. *Extracellular matrix. Chemistry, biology and pathobiology with emphasis on the liver.* New York: Marcel Dekker, 1993: 201–54.

2. Schuppan D. Structure of the extracellular matrix in normal and fibrotic liver: collagens and glycoproteins. *Seminars in Liver Diseases*, 1990; **10**: 1–10.

3. Gressner AM. Activation of proteoglycan synthesis in injured liver – a brief review of molecular and cellular aspects. *European Journal of Clinical Chemistry and Clinical Biochemistry*, 1994; **32**: 225–37.

4. Van der Rest M and Garrone MR. Collagen family of proteins. *FASEB Journal*, 1991; **5**: 2814–23.

5. Prockop DJ and Kivirikko KI. Collagens: molecular biology, diseases and potentials for therapy. *Annual Review of Biochemistry*, 1995; **64**: 403–34.

6. Hanauske-Abel HM. Prolyl 4-hydroxylase, a target enzyme for drug development. Design of suppressive agents and the *in vitro* effects of inhibitors and proinhibitors. *Journal of Hepatology*, 1991; **13** (Suppl. 3): S8–S16.

7. Slack JL, Liska DA, and Bornstein P. Regulation of expression of the type I collagen gene. *American Journal of Medical Genetics*, 1993; **45**: 140–51.

8. Attisano L, Wrana JL, Lopez-Casillas F, and Massague J. TGF-β receptors and actions. *Biochimica Biophysica Acta*, 1994; **1222**: 71–80.

9. Ruoslahti E. Fibronectin and its receptors. *Annual Review of Biochemistry*, 1988; **57**: 375–413.

10. Erickson HP. Tenascin-C, tenascin-R, and tenascin-X – a family of talented proteins in search of functions. *Current Opinion in Cell Biology*, 1993; **5**: 869–76.

11. Lightner VA. Tenascin: does it play a role in epidermal morphogenesis and homeostasis? *Journal of Investigative Dermatology*, 1994; **102**: 273–7.

12. Sage H and Bornstein P. Extracellular proteins that modulate cell–matrix interactions. *Journal of Biological Chemistry*, 1991; **266**: 14831–4.

13. Bornstein P. Thrombospondins: structure and regulation of expression. *FASEB Journal*, 1992; **6**: 3290–9.

14. Lane TF and Sage EH. The biology of SPARC, a protein that modulates cell–matrix interactions. *FASEB Journal*, 1994; **8**: 163–73.

15. Timpl R. Structure and function of basement membrane proteins. *European Journal of Biochemistry*, 1989; **180**: 487–502.

16. Burgeson RE *et al*. A new nomenclature for the laminins. *Matrix Biology*, 1994; **14**: 209–11.

17. Yamada K. Adhesive recognition sequences. *Journal of Biological Chemistry*, 1991; **266**: 12809–12.

18. Rosenbloom J, Abrams W, and Mecham R. The elastic fiber. *FASEB Journal*, 1993; **7**: 1115–23.

19. Gressner AM. Activation of proteoglycan synthesis in injured liver—a brief review of molecular and cellular aspects. *European Journal of Clinical Chemistry and Clinical Biochemistry*, 1994; **32**: 225–37.

20. Hardingham TE and Fosang AJ. Proteoglycans: many forms and many functions. *FASEB Journal*, 1992; **6**: 861–70.

21. Kresse H, Hausser H, and Schönherr E. Small proteoglycans. *Experientia*, 1993; **49**: 403–16.

22. Bernfield M, *et al*. Biology of the syndecans, a family of transmembrane heparan sulfate proteoglycans. *Annual Review of Cell Biology*, 1992; **8**: 365–93.

23. David G. Integral membrane heparan sulfate proteoglycans. *FASEB Journal*, 1993; **7**: 1023–30.

24. Lesley J, Hyman R, and Kincade PW. CD44 and its interaction with extracellular matrices. *Advances in Immunology*, 1993; **54**: 271–335.

25. Laurent TC and Fraser JRE. Hyaluronan. *FASEB Journal*, 1992; **6**: 2397–404.

26. Aumailley M, *et al*. Nidogen mediates the formation of ternary complexes of basement membranes. *Kidney International*, 1993; **43**: 7–12.

27. Nathan C and Sporn M. Cytokines in context. *Journal of Cell Biology*, 1991; **113**: 981–6.

28. Ruoslahti E and Yamaguchi Y. Proteoglycans as modulators of growth factor activities. *Cell*, 1991; **64**: 867–9.

29. Hynes RO. Integrins: versatility, modulation and signaling in cell adhesion. *Cell*, 1992; **69**: 11–25.

30. Schwartz MA. Transmembrane signalling by integrins. *Trends in Cell Biology*, 1992; **2**: 304–8.

31. Juliano RL and Haskill S. Signal transduction from the extracellular matrix. *Journal of Cell Biology*, 1993; **120**: 577–85.

32. Williams MJ, Hughes PE, O'Toole TE, and Ginsberg MH. The inner world of cell adhesion: integrin cytoplasmic domains. *Trends in Cell Biology*, 1994; **4**: 109–12.

33. Kühn K and Eble J. The structural basis of integrin–ligand interactions. *Trends in Cell Biology*, 1994; **4**: 256–61.

34. Haas TA and Plow EF. Integrin–ligand interactions: a year in review. *Current Opinion in Cell Biology*, 1994; **6**: 656–62.

35. Shattil S, Ginsberg MH, and Brugge JS. Adhesive signaling in platelets. *Current Opinion in Cell Biology*, 1994; **6**: 695–704.

36. Rosales C, O'Brien V, Kornberg L, Juliano R. Signal transduction by cell adhesion receptors. *Biochimica et Biophysica Acta*, 1995; **1242**: 77–98.

37. Clark EA and Brugge JS. Integrins and signal transduction pathways: the road taken. *Science*, 1995; **268**: 233–9.

38. Gumbiner BM. Cell adhesion: the molecular basis of tissue architecture and morphogenesis. *Cell*, 1996; **83**: 957–68.

39. Schaller MD and Parsons JT. Focal adhesion kinase: and associated proteins. *Current Opinion in Cell Biology*, 1994; **6**: 705–10.

40. Simons M. Rho family GTPases: the cytoskeleton and beyond. *Trends in Biochemical Sciences*, 1996, **21**: 178–85.

41. Weinstat-Saslow D and Steeg PS. Angiogenesis and colonization in the tumour metastatic process. *FASEB Journal*, 1994; **8**: 401–7.

42. Folkman J. Angiogenesis in cancer, vascular, rheumatoid and other diseases. *Nature Medicine*, 1995; **1**: 27–31.

43. Nip J and Brodt P. The role of the vitronectin receptor, αVβ3 in melanoma metastasis. *Cancer and Metastasis Reviews*, 1995; **14**: 241–52.

44. Grinnell F. Fibroblasts, myofibroblasts and wound contraction. *Journal of Cell Biology*, 1994; **124**: 401–4.

45. Gailit J and Clark RAF. Wound repair in the context of extracellular matrix. *Current Opinion in Cell Biology*, 1994; **6**: 717–25.

46. Krane S. Clinical importance of metalloproteinases and their inhibitors. *Annals of the New York Academy of Sciences*, 1994; **732**: 1–10.

47. Woessner JF. Matrix metalloproteinases and their inhibitors in connective tissue remodeling. *FASEB Journal*, 1991; **5**: 2145–54.

48. Stetler-Stevenson WG, Liotta L, and Kleiner DE. Role of matrix metalloproteinases in tumor invasion and metastasis. *FASEB Journal*, 1993; **7**: 1434–41.

49. Woessner JF. The family of matrix metalloproteinases. *Annals of the New York Academy of Sciences*, 1994; **732**: 11–21.

50. Birkedahl-Hansen H. Proteolytic remodeling of the extracellular matrix. *Current Opinion in Cell Biology*, 1995; **7**: 728–35.

51. Arthur MJP. Collagenases and liver fibrosis. *Journal of Hepatology*, 1995; **22**: 43–8.

52. Murphy G, *et al*. Regulation of matrix metalloproteinase activity. *Annals of the New York Academy of Sciences*, 1994; **732**: 51–61.

53. Matrisian LM. Matrix metalloproteinase gene expression. *Annals of the New York Academy of Sciences*, 1994; **732**: 42–50.

54. Brown PD. Matrix metalloproteinase inhibitors: a novel class of anticancer agents. *Advances in Enzyme Regulation*, 1995; **35**: 293–301.

2.16 Iron, copper, and trace elements

2.16.1 Normal iron metabolism

Pierre Brissot and Yves Deugnier

Iron is an essential element in human metabolism, carrying out a wide range of biological functions. It is especially involved in oxygen transport (haemoglobin, myoglobin) and in electron transport (cytochromes). Iron is also an integral part, or a cofactor, of many enzymes implicated in reactions such as hydroxylations (associated with drug biotransformation), DNA synthesis, and collagen formation. Due to its high propensity for hydrolysis in aqueous solutions, iron needs special molecules to remain in a soluble form at physiological pH, both for its transport (transferrin) and for its storage (ferritin). The biological importance of iron accounts for the highly conservative nature of iron metabolism in man; the normal daily loss of iron, balanced by an equivalent intestinal absorption, is limited to about 1 mg, representing only 0.02 per cent of total body iron.

Iron distribution and balance[1,2] (Fig. 1)

The total iron content of the human body is normally about 4 g, mainly located in erythrocyte haemoglobin (60 per cent) and in body stores (25 per cent for liver, spleen, and bone marrow); about 10 per cent is present in skeletal muscle (myoglobin). The remaining amount, quantitatively small but functionally important, corresponds to circulating transferrin iron and to intracellular enzyme iron.

The total body iron content is normally kept constant by a balance between the amount absorbed and the amount lost (1 mg/day). Iron losses occur mainly through exfoliated intestinal epithelial cells; smaller amounts are lost via the bile (0.5 mg/day), skin (desquamated cells and sweat), or urine (0.1 mg/day). In addition, there is minimal intestinal blood loss (0.3 mg/day). In normal adults these losses are balanced by the absorption of dietary iron (1–2 mg/day), corresponding to about 10 per cent of a normal diet containing 10 to 20 mg of iron.

Iron absorption[3] (Fig. 2)

Iron absorption occurs essentially in the proximal small intestine (duodenum and upper jejunum), consisting of the mucosal uptake of food iron from the gut lumen followed by the transfer of this iron from the enterocyte into the blood. Luminal and cellular factors of iron absorption will be considered before discussing its overall regulatory process.

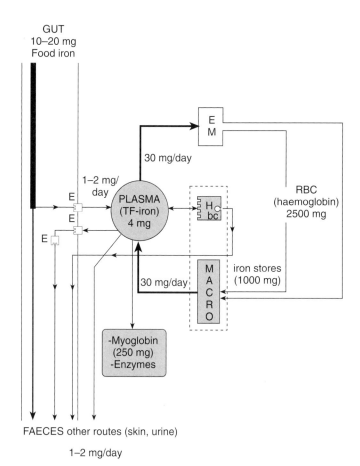

Fig. 1. Schematic pathways of iron metabolism: bc = bile canaliculus, E = enterocyte, EM = erythroid marrow, H = hepatocyte, MACRO = macrophage, RBC = red blood cell, TF = transferrin.

Luminal factors

Several factors influence intestinal absorption of iron.

The dietary iron content

Iron absorption increases with the amount of food iron but the percentage absorbed decreases with increasing quantities of iron.

The physicochemical form of iron

1. Inorganic iron (= non-haem iron) is present in vegetables and fruits. Its absorption is enhanced by dietary constituents such as sugars, amino acids, and amines which render it soluble at the alkaline pH of the small intestine. The stimulation of iron absorption by ascorbic acid is partly due to reduction of iron and

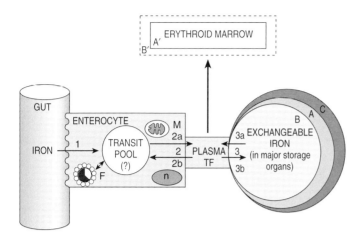

Fig. 2. Regulation of iron absorption: 1 = mucosal uptake (membrane carrier?), 2 = mucosal transfer, 3 = exchange between transferrin iron and body stores, F = ferritin, m = mitochondrion, n = nucleus, A = 'normal' exchangeable iron, B = reduced exchangeable iron leading to ↑2a and ↑1, C = increased exchangeable iron leading to ↑2b and ↓1, A' = normal erythropoietic activity, B' = increased erythropoietic activity leading to ↑3a, ↑2a, and ↑1. TF = transferrin.

partly to the formation of soluble iron-ascorbate chelates. Non-haem iron absorption is also promoted by haem iron. Inorganic iron absorption is decreased by calcium and by compounds which lead to molecular aggregation or precipitation, including phytates (bran, vegetables), polyphenols (tea, coffee), and dietary fibres.

2. Organic iron (= haem iron) is present in meat and fish. It behaves as a stable chelate, and enters the enterocyte as an intact metalloporphyrin. It is absorbed more efficiently (~25 per cent) than inorganic iron (<5 per cent). Being soluble in alkaline solutions, haem iron absorption is not affected by the various compounds which modify the absorption of inorganic iron. Despite these differences, organic iron (once the iron has been released from the porphyrin ring within the enterocyte) shares a common absorptive pathway with inorganic iron.

Gastrointestinal secretions

Gastric hydrochloric acid dissolves ferric iron; bile salts may favour iron absorption (Sanyal, AmJPhysiol, 1994; 266:G318); pancreatic bicarbonate decreases iron absorption; intestinal enzymes, by releasing sugars and amino acids from food, increase the absorption of iron.

Cellular factors

Iron absorption by the enterocytes involves classically a two-step process; iron uptake from the gut lumen by the cell ('mucosal uptake') and iron release from the enterocyte into the blood stream ('mucosal transfer'). The molecular processes whereby iron is absorbed are incompletely understood.

The role of the mucosal iron-binding proteins is diverse. The relationship of mucosal ferritin with iron absorption is demonstrated in normal subjects by the finding (Whittaker, JCI, 1989; 83:261) of a significant negative correlation between mucosal L (and at a lesser degree H) ferritin and non-haem (and to a lesser degree haem) iron absorption. Moreover, in the human duodenum, ferritin H and L

subunit mRNA is increased in iron deficiency and decreased in secondary iron overload (Pietrangelo, Gastro, 1992; 102:802). Whether human mucosal ferritin functions exclusively as a storage protein or has other functions, remains to be established. Mucosal transferrin plays no significant role in iron absorption (Peters, AnnNYAcadSci, 1988; 526:141):

1. Only trace levels of transferrin are present in the gut lumen.
2. Neither transferrin nor transferrin receptors could be significantly detected in the brush border of human intestinal absorptive cells (Parmley, BrJHaemat, 1985; 60:81; Banerjee, Gastro, 1986; 91:861).
3. No transferrin synthesis has been found in rat enterocytes (Osterloh, Blut, 1985; 51:41) and no transferrin mRNA could be demonstrated in rat or human mucosal extracts (Idzerda, PNAS, 1986; 83:3723; Pietrangelo, Gastro, 1992; 102:802).
4. No significant correlation was observed, in normal subjects, between the concentration of mucosal transferrin and iron absorption (Whittaker, JCI, 1989; 83:261).

The role in iron absorption of newly identified iron-binding proteins within human duodenal mucosa (Teichmann, JCI, 1990; 86:2145; Conrad, Blood, 1992; 79:244) awaits further investigation.

Free fatty acids, which enhance iron uptake in microvillous membrane vesicles, may play a role (Peters, AnnNYAcadSci, 1988; 526:141).

The existence of an intramucosal chelatable iron pool, analogous to that proposed for hepatocytes, has been suggested following the observation that, in rats and in man, parenteral desferrioxamine blocks the absorption of iron presented to the small intestinal mucosa either as inorganic or as haem iron (Levine, Gastro, 1988; 95:1242).

Overall regulation

Intestinal iron absorption is the key process ensuring the iron homeostasis of the body. Two main factors—the body iron status and the erythropoiesis rate—regulate iron absorption. An inverse relationship exists between the body iron stores and absorption of iron, and hepatocyte iron stores are a major determining factor controlling iron absorption (Adams, Transpl, 1989; 48:19). Increased erythropoietic activity (by bleeding or haemolysis) is linked to enhanced iron absorption. However, the mechanisms involved in regulation remain poorly defined. An attractive hypothesis (Cavill, Nature, 1975; 256:328) is that mucosal transfer of iron may be considered as part of the equilibrium between plasma iron and exchangeable (or labile) iron in the body (exchangeable iron corresponds to intracellular iron, whatever the cells, which is available for binding to transferrin; the iron pool, within the enterocyte, is a small part of this exchangeable iron). In the steady state, the number of iron atoms delivered from the exchangeable iron to transferrin is equal to the number cleared from the plasma, which corresponds to the plasma iron turnover. Generally, the total exchangeable iron reflects the level of storage iron. Any decrease in exchangeable iron within the main storage organs must be counteracted by an increased transfer of iron from the intestinal epithelium in order to maintain the equilibrium (and inversely in the case of increased exchangeable iron). Enhanced erythropoiesis leads to increased iron shift out of the various labile iron pools, including the absorptive enterocytes.

The increase in total transferrin receptor mass in the erythroid marrow is likely to be a key factor influencing the removal of iron from the intestinal mucosa (Finch, Blood, 1982; 59:364).

Hence, it may be seen that iron absorption is the major regulatory process of iron balance in the body. Increasing evidence, however, suggests that iron excretion, especially biliary excretion in animals (Lesage, JCI, 1986; 77:90; Brissot, DigDisSci, 1985; 28:616) as well as in man (Cleton, Hepatol, 1986; 6:30), but also postabsorption excretion (Bjorn-Rasmussen, Lancet, 1983; 1:914) and iron excretion from goblet cells (Refsum, ScaJGastr, 1980; 15:1013) may play a significant role in iron homeostasis of the body.

Extracellular iron transport and utilization[1,3,4]

Transferrin-iron transport

Iron is transported in the plasma predominantly bound to transferrin. The normal iron level is about 20 μmol/l. Transferrin is a betaglobulin of molecular weight 80 000 Da. This glycoprotein consists of (a) two-branched carbohydrate chains (glycans) and (b) a single polypeptide chain with two separate binding sites each capable of binding one atom of ferric iron. Therefore, four molecular forms can exist in the plasma; diferric, monoferric A, monoferric B, and apotransferrin. Physiologically, however, transferrin can be considered as a single homogeneous pool. The average plasma concentration of transferrin is 30 μmol/l so that the transferrin is about 30 per cent saturated with iron. The plasma pool of transport iron is turned over more than 10 times per day. Iron entering this pool comes essentially from mononuclear macrophages, following the breakdown of senescent red blood cells; a small part comes from the intestine and from hepatocytes. The uptake of iron by transferrin is likely to require a plasma ferrous oxidase such as caeruloplasmin. Over 80 per cent of the iron leaving the plasma pool is delivered to erythroid precursors in the bone marrow in order to form haemoglobin; a small amount can be delivered to the hepatocytes or the intestine. Therefore, the major movement of body iron is unidirectional, in the following cycle:

transferrin → erythroid marrow → red blood cells →

mononuclear phagocytic system → transferrin

A limited flow (located at the hepatic and intestinal levels) is bidirectional. In transferrin-bound iron uptake by erythroid cells, which forms the bulk of iron leaving the plasma pool, a major role is played by transferrin receptors. The transferrin receptor (TfR) is a transmembrane protein consisting of two identical subunits, each of 95 000 Da. The TfR is absent in mature red cells so that transferrin-bound iron is not taken up by these cells. The mechanism of iron–transferrin receptor dissociation remains somewhat controversial. It is possible that the release of some iron into the cell interior occurs at the level of the cell membrane; however, receptor-mediated endocytosis of transferrin is the only uptake mechanism of quantitative significance—it consists of the endocytosis of the entire complex, with release of iron intracellularly, followed by externalization of the receptor and return of the apotransferrin to the extracellular space. TfR numbers are the main regulator of iron

uptake rate by the erythroid cells (Morgan, AnnNYAcadSci, 1988; 526:65). With regard to transferrin-bound iron uptake by the hepatocytes, at least two mechanisms may be involved (Morgan, AnnNYAcadSci, 1988; 526:65); receptor mediated endocytosis, which is most important at low concentrations of transferrin iron, and fluid-phase endocytosis. A third mechanism, consisting of a redox-mediated plasma membrane process (Thorstensen, JBC, 1988; 263:8844), remains controversial (Thorstensen, BBActa, 1990; 1052:29; Oshiro, JBC, 1993; 268:21586).

Non-transferrin iron transport

Normal plasma contains a small amount (<1 μmol) of non-transferrin-bound iron. Non-transferrin bound iron is thought to circulate complexed to low molecular weight molecules. Non-transferrin-bound iron uptake has been shown to occur both in the liver (Brissot, JCI, 1985; 76:1463) and to a lesser extent in reticulocytes (Morgan, BBActa, 1988; 943:428).

Plasma ferritin is selectively taken up by hepatocytes, probably through specific ferritin receptors (Adams, Hepatol, 1988; 8:719; Adams, Hepatol, 1990; 11:805), but, unlike transferrin, ferritin is thereafter degraded within the cell. In normal individuals, however, ferritin is unlikely to provide a significant route for iron transport due to its low iron content.

Haem iron is carried as haemoglobin bound to haptoglobin or as haem bound to haemopexin. In normal humans about 10 per cent of erythrocyte destruction is handled by the haptoglobin and haemopexin systems; these iron forms are delivered only to the hepatocytes.

Transmembrane iron transport

Iron must cross a cellular membrane before entering the hepatocyte cytosol. This applies to the penetration of non-transferrin-bound iron through the outer (plasma) membrane of the hepatocyte as well as to the egress of iron out of the endosome (after iron has been released from transferrin).

The main characteristics of the transferrin-independent iron transport system appear to be the following:

1. Its efficiency is very high (Brissot, JCI, 1985; 76:1463), with not only absence of down regulation when cellular iron load is increased (Wright, JBC, 1986; 261:10909) but also increased activity under cell iron exposure (Kaplan, JBC, 1991; 26:2997; Randell, JBC, 1994; 269:16046).
2. It involves a surface ferrireductase activity, to provide iron in a soluble form which allows its transport through the cell membrane (Jordan, BiochemJ, 1994; 302:875). Study of this process has benefited from work with the yeast *Saccharomyces cerevisiae*, in which several genes responsible for iron transport have been identified. Some of them are ferrireductase genes, but others are related to copper metabolism, illustrating the increasingly recognized connection between iron and copper (Dancis, Cell, 1994; 76:393; Askwith, Cell, 1994; 76:403).
3. The nature of the putative iron transporter remains unknown. The human melanotransferrin (also known as p97) has been identified as a cell surface iron binding protein involved in the transferrin-independent uptake of iron in mammals (Kennard, EMBOJ, 1995; 14:4178). A new divalent cation transporter,

DCT1, has been identified in the rat. DCT1 is upregulated by iron deficiency, and may represent a key mediator of intestinal iron absorption (Gunshin, Nature, 1997; 388:482).

Intracellular iron metabolism

Liver cell iron metabolism

The main characteristics of iron metabolism within liver cells will be considered before evoking some aspects of human cellular iron metabolism.

Hepatocyte iron metabolism (Fig. 3)

Iron can be distributed schematically into three main pools:

1. The 'transit pool'. Its biochemical composition, not yet precisely determined, is likely to involve low molecular weight compounds. The transit pool functions as a reservoir capable of expanding or contracting at the interface between the hepatocyte plasma membrane and the other intracellular iron pools (i.e. the functional and storage pools).

2. The 'functional iron pool' comprises:

   (a) mitochondrial iron, which participates in haem formation and thus in the synthesis of haemoproteins such as the cytochromes involved in the respiratory process;

   (b) extra-mitochondrial iron, which is present in various proteins such as microsomal haemoproteins including: cytochrome P-450 which is involved in xenobiotic biotransformation; peroxisomal haemoproteins such as catalases and peroxidases which act as free radical scavengers; iron-dependent enzymes such as prolylhydroxylase, which catalyses a critical step of collagen biosynthesis, ribonucleotide reductase which catalyses the reduction of ribo- to deoxyribonucleotides, and xanthine oxidase which catalyses the oxidation of purines to uric acid and the incorporation of copper into caeruloplasmin.

3. The 'storage iron pool' includes:

   (a) Ferritin-iron (holoferritin)—this is the principal form of iron storage under physiological conditions. The iron is localized within the hollow central part of apoferritin which is a soluble macromolecule (with a molecular weight of approximately 450 000 Da) forming a shell consisting of 24 subunits. There are two types of ferritin subunits, designated H (heavier) and L (lighter). These can be differentiated by molecular weight and also by amino-acid content and immunological reactivity. The isoferritin profiles found in individual tissues are, at least partly, related to the respective proportions of H and L subunits. L Ferritin (which predominates in the liver) appears to function primarily as an iron storage protein, whereas H ferritin can exert additional roles, for example in immuno-suppression and in haem synthesis. Each apoferritin molecule can store up to 4500 atoms of iron in the ferric form. Iron enters the ferritin molecule through channels formed between the subunits; ferrous iron is the predominant form of iron incorporated into ferritin and is

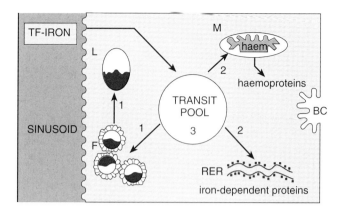

Fig. 3. Hepatocyte iron metabolism: 1 = storage iron, 2 = functional iron, 3 = transit iron, BC = bile canaliculus, F = ferritin, L = lysosome, M = mitochondrion, RER = rough endoplasmic reticulum, TF = transferrin, ■ = iron deposit.

probably oxidized through these channels. Once inside the protein shell, iron forms 'clusters' of ferric oxyhydroxide phosphate. The release of iron from ferritin is facilitated by reducing agents such as ascorbate or flavoproteins. Thus, the main functions of ferritin are to sequester potentially toxic iron inside the protein shell and to provide a readily accessible store of the metal.

   (b) Haemosiderin is an amorphous, insoluble, and biochemically ill-defined storage compound. It corresponds to a degradation product of ferritin, produced by the partial digestion of the protein and the release of iron leading to the formation of insoluble aggregates.

Kupffer cell iron metabolism

The iron traffic within the erythrophagocytosing macrophage is intense, the Kupffer cell being able to process more than 10^7 iron atoms/min (Aisen, AnnNYAcadSci, 1988; 526:93). Following phagocytosis, senescent erythrocytes are degraded within secondary lysosomes and their iron is liberated from haem by the action of microsomal haem oxygenase. The Kupffer cell synthesizes ferritin in response to erythrophagocytosis (Kondo, Hepatol, 1988; 8:32). Iron is released by Kupffer cells to apotransferrin without internalization of the protein. It has also been proposed that ferritin plays a role in the transfer of iron from Kupffer cells to the hepatocytes (Sibille, Hepatol, 1988; 8:296).

Endothelial cell iron metabolism

Liver endothelium has been shown to take up transferrin iron complexes through a specific receptor-mediated mechanism which is different from the endosomal system of other cells in that transferrin and iron remain associated; moreover, in this process, transferrin becomes partially desialylated. After externalization into the space of Disse, the uptake of this endothelium-processed transferrin occurs via asialoglycoprotein receptors of hepatocytes (Tavassoli, AnnNYAcadSci, 1988; 526:83; Irie, JCI, 1988; 82:508). It is, however, unlikely that this process plays an important role in transferrin iron uptake by the hepatocytes, as exogenous transferrin

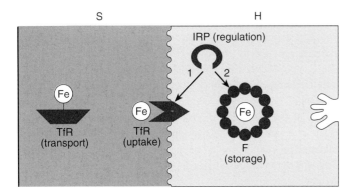

Fig. 4. Major proteins of iron metabolism. Tf = transferrin, TfR = = transferrin receptor, F = ferritin, IRP = iron regulatory protein (when intracellular iron ↑: 1 ↓ (uptake) and 2 ↑ (storage); when intracellular iron ↓: 1 ↑ (uptake) and 2 ↓ (storage)), S = sinusoid, H = hepatocyte.

is taken up by the liver in its fully sialylated form (Goldenberg, BBActa, 1988; 968:331).

Regulation of human cellular iron metabolism (Fig. 4)

The need for the cell to ensure its metabolic requirement for iron, and also to protect itself from potentially toxic iron, forms the basis of the regulation process. There is regulation of both the uptake and sequestration of iron, accomplished by the iron regulatory protein (IRP, formerly called IRF or IRE-BP) which modulates the expression of both the transferrin receptor (**TfR**) and ferritin. The isolation of the genes encoding the human TfR, ferritins, and iron regulatory protein have led to a major improvement in our understanding of these mechanisms.

Iron-dependent regulation of the ferritin gene

Genes coding for H and L subunits have been assigned to chromosomes 11 and 19, respectively. Iron stimulates ferritin synthesis at the translational level. A critical region, termed the iron regulatory element, is responsible for this iron-dependent translational regulation. The iron regulatory element is a stem–loop structure located in the 5′-untranslated region of the human ferritin mRNAs. This iron regulatory element serves as a recognition site for a cytoplasmic protein, the iron regulatory protein, which binds to it and represses translation when intracellular iron is low (Rouault, Science, 1988; 241:1207). Iron regulatory protein, which is the cytosolic aconitase (Kennedy, PNAS, 1992; 89:11730), is an iron–sulphur cluster protein whose gene is located on chromosome 9 (Hentze, NucAcidRes, 1991; 19:1739). Beside this translational regulation, there is also a transcriptional control of ferritin synthesis. L ferritin mRNA is preferentially increased after iron administration (White, JBC, 1988; 263:8938), leading to the production of ferritins enriched in L subunits, that are known to be implicated in iron storage (Munro, NutrRev, 1993; 51:65).

Iron-dependent regulation of the *TfR* gene

The *TfR* gene has been assigned to chromosome 3. Synthesis of TfR is highly regulated by iron (much more than transferrin itself)—an increase in cellular iron decreasing receptor synthesis

and vice versa. The expression of *TfR* is regulated at the level of transcription. Five iron regulatory element copies have been identified within the 3′-untranslated region of human *TfR* mRNA (Casey, Science, 1988; 240:924). Similar to its function in the 5′-untranslated region, the iron regulatory element in the 3′-untranslated region binds iron regulatory protein when iron concentration is low. This binding stabilizes *TfR* mRNA and, by preventing its degradation, enhances expression of *TfR*.

Clinical aspects
Clinical investigations of iron metabolism

Iron status evaluation is a major aspect of clinical investigation. From a biochemical viewpoint it is based on the measurement of various serum parameters:

1. Serum iron. Its concentration (~ 20 μmol/l) fluctuates physiologically over a twofold range during the day (values are maximal in the morning, minimal in the evening). Various factors (besides variations in iron load) may influence serum iron levels; thus, serum iron is increased with haemolysis or liver cytolysis and decreased in inflammatory conditions.
2. Transferrin saturation. It is determined by the ratio of serum iron to total iron-binding capacity. Total iron-binding capacity varies, in normal subjects, from 50 to 70 μmol/l, corresponding to a transferrin saturation of 0.30 (30 per cent).
3. Serum ferritin. Normally less than 300 μg/l in men and 200 μg/l in women, it shows little or no circadian variations. Serum ferritin is a sensitive index of total body iron stores, provided that there is neither hepatic cytolysis nor inflammation, both conditions known to increase ferritinaemia.

Iron kinetics in the body can be explored by injecting radioactive iron (^{59}Fe) firmly bound to transferrin. ^{59}Fe is an easily counted, gamma-emitting nuclide with a half-life of 45 days. By following its fate one can obtain valuable information on the plasma iron pool, marrow utilization for erythropoiesis, and the tissue distribution of iron.

Clinical iron disorders

They consist of two main situations:

(1) iron deficiency, which is one of the most prevalent nutritional disorders in the world;
(2) iron overload, which is especially related to two genetic disorders, haemochromatosis and thalassaemia, both representing major health burdens on a worldwide scale.

References

1. Brock JH, Halliday JW, Pippard MJ, and Powell LW, eds. *Iron metabolism in health and disease*. London: WB Saunders, 1994.
2. Young SP and Aisen P. The liver and iron. In Arias IM, Boyer JL, Fausto N, Jakoby WB, Jakoby WB, Schachter DA, and Shafritz DA, eds. *The liver: biology and pathobiology*. New York: Raven Press, 1994: 597–617.
3. De Silva DM, Askwith CC, and Kaplan J. Molecular mechanisms of iron uptake in eukaryotes. *Physiological Reviews*, 1996; **76**: 31–47.
4. Klausner RD, Rouault TA, and Harford JB. Regulating the fate of mRNA: the control of cellular iron metabolism. *Cell*, 1994; **72**: 19–28.

2.16.2 Normal copper metabolism

Irene Hung and Jonathan D. Gitlin

Copper homeostasis

Copper is a ubiquitous element in nature that plays a fundamental part in the biochemistry of all living organisms. The electron structure of this metal permits a direct interaction with spin-restricted dioxygen, enabling copper to serve as a facile cofactor in key redox reactions of diverse metabolic pathways. In humans, copper is essential for cellular respiration, antioxidant defence, pigmentation, neurotransmitter and peptide production, connective tissue biosynthesis, and iron metabolism. The liver is the central organ of copper homeostasis, and the hepatocyte serves as both the primary site of copper storage and the major determinant of copper excretion (Fig. 1).

The normal adult maintains a total body balance of about 100 mg of copper entirely through the regulation of gastrointestinal uptake and excretion. The specific sites of copper uptake in the gastrointestinal tract have not been defined but data from surgical patients suggest that both the gastric mucosa and constituents of gastric juice modify the amount of copper absorbed. The normal diet contains about 5 mg copper/day and kinetic studies indicate a 50 per cent efficiency of absorption at a site consistent with duodenal uptake. The mechanisms of gastrointestinal copper uptake are unknown but data from patients with Menkes disease indicate that the Menkes ATPase is essential to this process. Zinc intake can inhibit copper absorption by increasing the metallothionein content of enteric mucosal cells, resulting in increased copper binding by this protein with subsequent loss during villous shedding. Consistent with this, zinc is used as a treatment to prevent copper overload in Wilson disease and copper deficiency has been reported following the long-term ingestion of excessive amounts of zinc.

Kinetic studies demonstrate the rapid uptake of an absorbed copper dose into the portal venous circulation with near complete first-pass removal by the liver (Fig. 1). Copper is found in the plasma complexed with histidine and bound to albumin, which contains a single high-affinity site for this metal, suggesting a role for ternary complexes of copper, albumin, and histidine in the process of copper transport. Albumin is not essential for copper transport as patients with a complete absence of this serum protein (analbuminaemia) do not have abnormalities of copper metabolism. Although the mechanisms of copper uptake by the hepatocyte are unknown, recent studies in yeast and plants have identified specific plasma-membrane copper transporters and it is likely that homologous proteins exist on the surface of hepatocytes and other cell types involved in copper uptake (Dancis, Cell, 1994; 76:393; Culotta, JBC, 1995; 270: 28 479).

The hepatocyte is the central storage site of copper and mediates copper delivery into the bile, which is the only physiological site of copper excretion in man. Upon entry into the hepatocyte, copper is bound to and transported by a 67-amino acid protein termed HAH1. This protein delivers copper to the Wilson ATPase, which is essential for entry of copper into the secretory pathway of the hepatocyte (Fig. 2). Once in this pathway, copper is available both for incorporation into caeruloplasmin and excretion into the bile. The liver has an enormous capacity for storage and excretion and under normal circumstances the amount of copper in bile is directly proportional to the size of the hepatic copper pool. The balancing of this process by the liver serves to prevent states of copper deficiency or overload. Although the molecular nature of copper in bile is unknown, little or no copper is reabsorbed from this compartment and there is no enterohepatic circulation of this metal. The liver of the newborn human infant is notable for a marked accumulation of copper with little or no holocaeruloplasmin biosynthesis or biliary copper excretion until after birth. This suggests a developmental block at the site of delivery of copper into the secretory pathway but the role of the Wilson ATPase in this process has not been explored. This difference results in a marked decrease

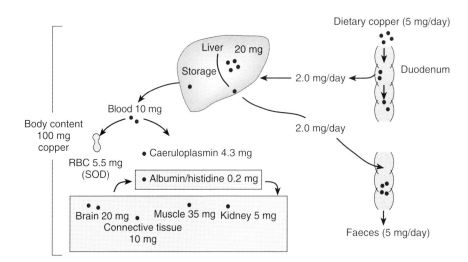

Fig. 1. Diagram of copper metabolism in the adult indicating the sites of absorption and excretion. The central role of the liver in this process is indicated.

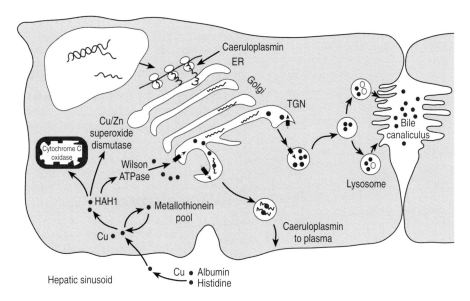

Fig. 2. Pathways of copper transport in the hepatocyte. The central role of the Wilson ATPase in determining copper transport into the secretory pathway and thus holocaeruloplasmin secretion and biliary copper excretion is shown.

in serum caeruloplasmin concentration in the new-born infant, eliminating this as a useful screening tool for Wilson disease in the neonatal period.

Hepatic copper proteins

More than 30 copper proteins have been identified in man, several of which are now recognized as essential by virtue of the diseases associated with their inherited defects. Nevertheless this current discussion will be limited to those proteins with a defined role in copper metabolism or liver disease.

Metallothionein

The metallothioneins (**MT**) constitute a multigene family of low molecular-weight, metal-binding proteins characterized by an abundant cysteine content. The *MT-I* and *MT-II* genes are expressed in almost all tissues and cell types, including hepatocytes. The metallothionein genes are induced by heavy metals such as zinc, cobalt and copper and have been proposed to play an essential part in metal storage and detoxification in cells. Studies in transgenic mice indicate that MT-I and MT-II are not essential for normal growth and development. Copper metabolism is normal in these mice, indicating that, if these proteins are a site of intracellular copper storage in the hepatocyte, this function can be replaced by other cellular proteins (Masters, PNAS, 1994; 91:584). Nevertheless, breeding these mice with a Menkes mouse model has recently revealed an essential role for MT-I and MT-II in preventing tissue damage from copper overload, suggesting that this may be the normal function of these proteins in copper metabolism (Kelly, NatureGen, 1996; 13:219).

HAH1

Human atx1 homologue (**HAH1**) is an abundant, 67-amino acid protein expressed in all tissues. This protein contains a single copper-binding site identical in sequence to that observed in the Wilson and Menkes ATPases. HAH1 has been highly conserved in evolution and was characterized as a homologue of a yeast protein identified as a copper-dependent antioxidant (atx1). Recent studies in yeast indicate that this protein functions in the cytosol to bind copper and to deliver this metal for transport into the secretory pathway. These studies suggest that HAH1 may serve as the predominant intracellular copper storage and transport protein in the cytosol of hepatocytes (Lin, PNAS, 1995; 92:3784).

Caeruloplasmin

Greater than 95 per cent of plasma copper is contained in the serum α_2-glycoprotein caeruloplasmin. This protein is synthesized in hepatocytes and secreted into the plasma as a single-chain protein with six atoms of copper per molecule. Within 6 h of a tracer dose of oral radioactive copper this isotope begins to appear in newly synthesized caeruloplasmin. Copper does not affect the rate of synthesis or secretion of apocaeruloplasmin but failure to incorporate copper during biosynthesis results in secretion of an unstable apoprotein lacking oxidase activity (Sato, JBC, 1991; 266: 5128). This metabolic detail explains the decrease in serum caeruloplasmin observed in patients with Wilson disease, where copper fails to enter the secretory pathway and is thus unavailable for incorporation into apocaeruloplasmin before secretion. Clinical studies have revealed the acute-phase nature of this protein and the serum concentration is increased during inflammation as well as after administration of oestrogen, during pregnancy, and in certain malignancies.

The precise function of caeruloplasmin has recently been clarified by the identification of patients with diabetes, retinal degeneration, and neurological disease in association with a complete absence of serum caeruloplasmin and excess parenchymal iron accumulation (Harris, PNAS, 1995; 92:2539; Yoshida, NatureGen, 1995; 4:267). Molecular genetic analysis of these patients revealed mutations in the caeruloplasmin gene, thus indicating an essential role for caeruloplasmin in human biology and identifying acaeruloplasminaemia as a novel autosomal-recessive disorder of iron metabolism. Affected patients accumulate hepatic iron within both hepatocytes and Kuppfer cells in amounts equivalent to that observed in primary haemochromatosis. These findings are consistent with recent studies on the role of an homologous copper oxidase in iron metabolism in yeast and reveal an essential role for caeruloplasmin as a plasma ferroxidase functioning to facilitate the oxidation and transfer of iron into transferrin (Dancis, Cell, 1994; 76:393). Copper metabolism is entirely normal in patients with acaeruloplasminaemia, indicating that caeruloplasmin has no essential role in copper transport or metabolism in man. Nevertheless, patients with acaeruloplasminaemia have a marked reduction in serum copper, owing to the absence of circulating caeruloplasmin, and awareness of this disorder is important in the differential diagnosis of Wilson disease.

Hepatic copper toxicity

The chemical properties that make copper biologically useful are also potentially toxic if copper homeostasis is perturbed. Excess copper accumulation has been reported in most species and always results in toxicosis. Given the central role of the liver in copper storage and excretion, copper toxicosis in humans almost inevitably results in hepatic cirrhosis. Although Wilson disease accounts for the majority of patients with liver disease due to copper accumulation, other clinical conditions have been reported, mostly in clusters of cases occurring in children. Pedigree analysis in such cases suggests that in addition to consumption of diets rich in copper an underlying autosomal-recessive gene is essential for the development of hepatic copper accumulation and liver injury. These cases were originally brought to attention in Indian children but have subsequently been recognized in Tyrolean pedigrees and sporadically elsewhere, and are now referred to as idiopathic copper toxicosis (Müller, Lancet, 1996; 347:877). Tanner first suggested a combination of genetic and dietary factors as underlying this disorder and this is supported by evidence that excess dietary copper in normal individuals does not lead to hepatic copper accumulation (Scheinberg, Lancet, 1994; 344:1002).

The mechanisms of hepatic injury in copper toxicosis are largely unknown. As any process that interrupts biliary flow will result in hepatic copper accumulation, the specific role of copper in most forms of hepatic cirrhosis is unclear. Nevertheless, free copper can result in free radical-mediated tissue injury and it seems likely that this process is involved in cellular injury from copper accumulation once the mechanisms for copper sequestration are surpassed. In support of this concept, increased lipid peroxidation and mitochondrial injury has been reported in experimental and clinical states of hepatic copper overload (Sokol, Gastro, 1994; 107:1788). These and subsequent studies report depletion of α-tocopherol and other hepatic antioxidants following copper-related injury, suggesting a potential role for such compounds in ameliorating liver injury in clinical conditions leading to excess hepatic copper.

Further reading

Danks DM. Disorders of copper transport. In *The metabolic and molecular basis of inherited disease*. New York: McGraw-Hill, 1995: 2211–35.
Vulpe CD and Packman S. Cellular copper transport. *Annual Review of Nutrition*, 1995; **15**: 293–322.
Harris LH and Gitlin JD. Genetic and molecular basis for copper toxicity. *American Journal of Clinical Nutrition*, 1996; **63**: 836–41S.

2.16.3 Trace elements

Andreas Ochs and J. Schölmerich

Trace elements
Definition

The term 'trace elements' is used for elements that are found in the body in similar or smaller amounts compared with iron and could only be detected in traces when only chemical analytical methods were available.[1–3] With sophisticated tools, determination of trace element concentrations in fluid and tissue became feasible.[4–9] The term trace element does not necessarily mean that the element is essential for body homeostasis.[10–16] If the estimated dietary requirement for laboratory animals is between 1 µg/g and 50 ng/g or less of the diet, the term 'ultratrace element' is used.[11] In addition to copper and iron, arsenic, bromine, chromium, cobalt, fluorine, iodine, lead, molybdenum, nickel,[7–11] selenium,[17] silicon,[1] tin,[1] vanadium,[11] and zinc[18–22] are considered 'essential' in humans and higher organisms. Concentrations and proportions are probably similar in all vertebrates.

Introduction

Iron and copper are discussed in Chapters 2.16.1 and 2.16.2. The 'macroelement' magnesium is included in this chapter.

Most trace elements are enzyme activators and/or part of proteins (structural or functional) such as membranes, hormones, and metalloenzymes.[1–3] When the trace element is deficient, enzyme activity is reduced or lost, for example glutathione peroxidase activity (EC 1.11.1.9) in selenium deficiency.[2,3]

Analytical techniques

Sampling and analytical techniques are of paramount importance in the interpretation and comparison of data regarding trace elements in body fluids and tissues.[1–6] Contamination from blood sampling cannulas can significantly affect serum concentrations of nickel, cobalt, or chromium. Laboratory dust contains copper, zinc, lead, aluminium, and iron. While in 1961 the upper reference limit for serum manganese concentration was considered to be 45 nmol/l, today it is 10 nmol/l due to better contamination control and analytical techniques.[5] Diurnal variations must also be considered.[5]

Table 1 gives an overview for commonly used analytical methods with their advantages and limitations.[4] The most commonly used analytical technique is atomic absorption spectroscopy using different means of ashing. The flame-free technique (i.e. with electrothermal ashing) is more sensitive than flame atomic absorption spectroscopy. Loss of elements, resulting from excessive temperatures and open systems, can lead to incorrect results. X-ray fluorescence spectroscopy makes use of ion-induced secondary

Table 1 Properties, detection limits, and special features of different analytical methods (modified from ref. 4)

Method	Sample size (diameter, μm)	Sample mass	Detection limit μg/g	Destruction of sample	Spatial resolution	Availability	Comments
AAS Atomic absorption spectrophotometry	—	mg	10^{-1}–10^{-5}	Yes	No	Good	Widely available, best for routine diagnostic
Micro-PIXE Proton-induced X-ray emission	1–5	10^{-11} g	<5–10	Locally carbonized at beam impact	Yes	Rare	Simultaneous analysis possible even in histological tissue sections. Time-consuming, expensive
EIXE Electron-induced X-ray emission	0.2–1	10^{-12} g	10^2–10^3	No	Yes	Must be attached to an electron microscope	Ideal for simultaneous subcellular analysis of elements
NAA Neutron activation analysis	—	mg to g	10^{-3}–10^{-6}	No	No	Rare	Lowest detection limit, time-consuming, determination of zinc only possible after a 12-day decay of copper
LAMMA Laser microprobe mass analysis	2–5	10^{-11} g	10^{-1}–10^{-2}	Local evaporation of 3–5 μm	Yes	Rare	Absolute quantification difficult

radiation and is suitable for multielement analysis.[6–8] Only concentrations more than five times the detection limit of the different techniques can be used with certainty.[7] Neutron activation analysis is a very sensitive but laborious technique. Depending on the element in question it is used in a destructive or non-destructive mode.[2]

Only methods with spatial resolution such as particle-induced X-ray emission (**PIXE**) can differentiate the amount of trace elements in various liver cell types, different parts of hepatic parenchyma, and/or the biliary tree with high resolution. Scarce availibility and high costs restrict these methods to experimental work. Particle induced X-ray emission uses electrons, photons, or protons, the best detection limit with the last of these being about 1 mg/g dry weight (Dyson, JRadioanalChem, 1978; 46:309).[6] With laser microprobe mass analysis, topical resolution is also possible and with the use of internal standards, quantitative analysis is feasible (Schmidt, TraceElemMed, 1984; 1:13).

Concentrations in serum or blood are given in SI units (mol/l), with tissue concentrations as μg/g. Wet weight can be converted into dry weight using a factor of 0.234 for normal liver.[7,8] This factor varies in abnormal tissue (Okuno, TraceElemMed, 1988; 5: 130). Blood in the vascular compartments results in an error of up to 18 per cent with respect to iron concentration. No such errors have been reported for other trace elements (Milman, ScaJCLI, 1983; 43:691) although they are to be expected. As a rule, tissue concentrations should be used with caution.

Metallothioneins

Metallothioneins represent an important class of proteins that bind to trace metals providing protection against heavy metals (Cd, Cu, Hg) (Bhave, Toxicology, 1988; 50:231). Metallothioneins are proteins of low molecular weight containing cadmium and other metals.[9] These proteins are found in plants, lower animals, vertebrates, and mammals.

Metallothioneins play a role in metal detoxification (ref. 9, p.25). In mammals, metallothioneins contain 60 or 61 amino acids (about 30 per cent cysteine). Human kidney contains more cadmium-copper-metallothionein, while in the liver, zinc-metallothionein dominates. Through orientation of S-groups a tetrahedral arrangement of ligands occurs, and an α- and a β-domain can be distinguished (clusters A and B). Both clusters form metal–thiolate complexes and have different affinities with different metals. Cadmium has an affinity 10 000 times higher than that of zinc. Affinity to cluster A is 30 times higher than to cluster B. This explains the variable distribution of different metals in metallothioneins, i.e. in a zinc/cadmium-metallothionein cadmium is more related to cluster A, and zinc more to B. Cluster A usually contains four atoms and cluster B three atoms, with metal release usually occurring from the latter. Genes are located on chromosome 16 and transcription is regulated through metals, glucocorticoids, and other hormones. Stimuli are metals, phorbol esters, iodoacetate, steroids, interferons, and acute-phase inducers (Sato, ChemBiolInteract, 1995; 98:15). Metallothioneins probably have a role as free hydroxyl radical scavengers (ref. 9, p.63).

Individual trace elements

In this section the individual trace elements are discussed according to the following sequence:

1. Analytical techniques
2. Reference values
3. Uptake, distribution, and excretion
4. Function

5. Toxicity
6. Abnormalities in liver disease
7. Treatment and/or substitution in liver disease

A complete range of information is not available for some elements.

Aluminium (Al, atomic weight 26.98)

Analytical techniques

Electrothermal atomic absorption spectroscopy is used for urine and bile (Williams, AnnIntMed, 1986; 104:782). Neutron absorption spectroscopy is less suitable since phosphorus and aluminium are transformed to the isotope ^{28}Al (van de Vyver, TraceElemMed, 1986; 3:52; Blotcky, AnalChem, 1992; 64:2910). In rat liver, micro-PIXE has been used (Horino, ScanMicrosc, 1993; 7:1215).

Reference values

Body content: 50–150 mg.[1] Blood concentration: 0.4–1.5 μmol/l.[2] Serum concentration: 0.06–0.13 mmol/l (van de Vyver, Trace-ElemMed, 1986; 3:52) up to 0.37 mmol/l (Williams, AnnIntMed, 1986; 104:782). Liver tissue concentration: <1.0 μg/g wet weight (van de Vyver, 1986).

Uptake, distribution, and excretion

Absorption from nutrients is poor (less than 0.1 per cent).[1] Aluminium hydroxide is better absorbed at acid pH in the stomach. Aluminium is bound to plasma proteins, in particular transferrin (van de Vyver, TraceElemMed, 1986; 3:52). The highest concentrations are found in bone, muscle, and brain. Excretion is in bile and urine. Oral administration of aluminium hydroxide increases aluminium excretion in bile (Williams, AnnIntMed, 1986; 104:782).

Function

Aluminium increases biliary excretion of iron (Allain, PSEBM, 1988; 188:471).

Toxicity

No intoxication is known with normal renal function. Bone abnormalities have been found with bone concentrations of 30 μg/g or more. Microcytic anaemia, encephalopathy, and myopathy have been observed (van de Vyver, TraceElemMed, 1986; 3:52).[2] Intravenous desferrioxamine allows aluminium to be dialysed at a clearance rate of 65 ml/min and eliminated by haemoperfusion (Chang, IntJArtifOrg, 1986; 9:285; ref. 3, p.45). Intravenous aluminum application led to the appearance of periportal aluminium-positive multinucleated cells in rabbits (Wills, AnnClinLabSci, 1993; 23:1).

Abnormalities in liver disease

Hepatic abnormalities are rarely found with aluminium overload. Two patients with autoimmune hepatitis and primary sclerosing cholangitis developed aluminium osteopathy in spite of normal renal function (Williams, AnnIntMed, 1986; 104:782). Liver concentration of aluminium in patients on chronic haemodialysis increases (2.9–45.1 mg/g wet weight) (van de Vyver, TraceElemMed, 1986; 3:52). Occasional observations of periportal liver cell necrosis and aluminium-containing phagolysosomes (Al content 0.1–1.0 per

cent) have been reported in man and reproduced in rats with aluminium overload (Galle, NouvPresseMed, 1982; 11:1123). Increased urinary excretion and liver tissue concentration has been found in a patient with Wilson's disease (Yasui, FolPsych-NeurolJapon, 1979; 33:547). In rats, intravenous aluminum administration led to cholestasis, with higher serum bile acid concentrations and reduction of bile flow by 33 per cent. Transferrin proved to be the major aluminum-binding protein. Within days, biliary transferrin excretion increased (Klein, PharmacolToxicol, 1993; 72:373). Induction of cholestasis through aluminum contamination may contribute to parenteral nutrition-induced hepatobiliary dysfunction (Klein, PediatRes, 1988; 23:275). Concurrent iron deficiency may enhance both aluminum absorption and accumulation in liver and spleen (Brown, BiolTraceElemRes, 1992; 34:1). In rats, hepatocarcinomas induced by 3'-dimethyl-aminoazobenzene showed an aluminum concentration more than three times higher than in normal liver tissue. The role of aluminum in hepatocarcinogenesis is unknown, but may be explained by reduced protective selenium concentrations in cancerous tissue (Ogoshi, JTraceElemElectrolHlthDis, 1994; 8:27).

Arsenic (As, atomic weight 74.92)

Analytical techniques

Neutron activation analysis has a detection limit around 1 ng, and atomic absorption spectroscopy around 10 ng (Calmus, GastrClinBiol, 1982; 6:910).

Reference values

Body content: 8–20 mg.[1] Blood concentration: 0.027–0.31 μmol/l up to 8.5 μmol/l.[1,10,11] Serum concentration: 0.022–0.20 μmol/l. Liver tissue concentrations vary in the literature between 0.01–0.02 μg/g wet weight,[1] and 0.05–0.28 μg/g wet weight (Calmus, GastrClinBiol, 1982; 6:910). Geographical variations have been reported (New Zealand: 0.05 μg/g compared with Japan: 0.19 μg/g wet weight).

Uptake, distribution, and excretion

Uptake is better from organic compounds of arsenic (As^{3+} and As^{5+}). In blood, arsenic is bound mainly to cellular components.[1, 11] Active accumulation occurs in the liver of animals. In man there may be an enterohepatic circulation which can be interrupted by chelating agents (Calmus, GastrClinBiol, 1982; 6:910). Arsenic is excreted in urine and bile,[1] and is not bound to proteins in bile. Biliary excretion has not been definitively proved. It is probable that organic arsenic is excreted unchanged in urine while inorganic arsenic is excreted into bile after hepatic accumulation. Concentrations of less than 20 μg/l urine are physiological, more than 200 μg/l should be investigated, and more than 500 μg/l must be considered as toxic (Calmus, 1982; Dhawan, ToxicolLett, 1983; 15: 105).

Function

In four animal species it has been shown that arsenic is an essential element. Arsenic deprivation led to depressed growth and disturbed reproduction (Anke, TraceSubEnvirHlth, 1987; 21:533). It may play an important role in methionine and labile methyl metabolism;

[11] arsenic deprivation depressed the activity of *S*-adenosylmethionine decarboxylase and ornithine decarboxylase.[11] In the rat, sodium arsenite can induce both ornithine decarboxylase and haem oxygenase activity, suggesting a role as a promoter rather than an initiator of carcinogenesis (Brown, CancerLett, 1996; 98:227).

Toxicity

Both chronic and acute toxicity are known. Only As^{3+} and As^{5+} are toxic. A large number of toxic effects have been described in animals. As^{3+} binds to disulphydryl groups present in several enzymes of intermediary metabolism (involved in the Krebs–Henseleit cycle, β-oxidation of fatty acids, cholesterol biosynthesis, detoxification systems). Abnormalities of peroxisomes and mitochondria have been found. **BAL** (2,3-dimercaptopropanol) forms cyclic dithioarsenate, which can be eliminated. Arsenic administration induces hepatic zinc-metallothionein, an effect which does not depend on the chemical form administered (Maitani, ToxicolLett, 1987; 39:63).

Abnormalities in liver disease

Chronic exposure to arsenic has been considered a cause of Indian childhood cirrhosis. A metabolic defect common for arsenic and copper has been proposed. The disease only occurs when both elements are present in the environment in high concentrations. In France increased concentrations of arsenic have been found in several liver diseases (alcoholic cirrhosis: 0.6–2.7 µg/g wet weight, chronic active hepatitis: 1.1–2.7 µg/g, primary biliary cirrhosis: 2.6–3.3 µg/g) (Calmus, GastrClinBiol, 1982; 6:910). In India values of 4.9 ± 1.4 µg/g dry weight have been found in alcoholic cirrhosis. This is probably due to 'home-made brew' including arsenic-containing animal parts (Dhawan, ToxicolLett, 1983; 15:105). There have been case reports of 'idiopathic' portal hypertension due to chronic ingestion of medicines containing arsenic. Increased concentrations have also been found in hair and liver (5.2 µg/g wet weight) (Chainuvati, DigDisSci, 1979; 24:70). Alcohol, hepatitis B, and preceding treatment with arsenic are considered as inducers of incomplete septal cirrhosis, which bears a three times higher risk of variceal bleeding when compared with classic macronodular cirrhosis (Nevens, Gastro, 1994; 106:459). In rats, arsenic-contaminated drinking water induced hepatocyte proliferation, particularly around larger hepatic veins (Constan, Carcinogenesis, 1995; 16:303).

Arsenic is a known carcinogen, most commonly associated with basal cell and squamous cell carcinomas of the skin, as well as with angiosarcomas of the liver. These tumours normally occur after a long exposure time (30 years or more) to arsenic. However, single cases of angiosarcoma of the liver have been reported after only 6 months of ingestion of arsenic (Roat, AmJMed, 1982; 73:933). The risk of developing liver cancers is closely related to the daily ingested dose of arsenic compounds (Chen, BrJCanc, 1992; 66:888).

Bromine (Br, atomic weight 79.90)
Analytical techniques

Both X-ray fluorescence spectroscopy and particle-induced X-ray emission are used.[4,11]

Reference values

Body content: approximately 200 mg.[1] Serum concentration: 38–68 µmol/l.[1] Reported liver tissue concentrations vary considerably: 0.3[1]–38 µg/g dry weight.[4,8]

Uptake, distribution, and excretion

Excretion is probably in urine[1] and bile, where bile flow correlates with the amount of excreted bromium (Dijkstra, JHepatol, 1991; 13:112).

Function

Bromine deficiency in goats results in reduced growth, infertility, anaemia, and reduced lifespan (ref. 10, p.618).

Toxicity

Inhaled bromine can cause toxic pulmonary oedema. Urea derivates containing bromine are used as hypnotics. An overdose of these drugs results in acute renal and respiratory failure, and sudden myocardial arrest. Furthermore, bromureide poisoning leads to somnolence or coma depending on the amount ingested and can cause disseminated intravascular coagulation. Neurological findings are very variable and the severity of intoxication cannot be established.

Abnormalities in liver disease

An increased concentration has been found in cirrhotic livers.[8] Accumulation in fibrous tissue has been suggested and demonstrated with particle-induced X-ray emission.[4] In rats with ligated bile ducts, bromine, like copper, accumulates in the liver, the amount correlating with the duration of cholestasis.[4] The importance of this finding is unknown.

Cadmium (Cd, atomic weight 121.41)
Analytical techniques

Atomic absorption spectroscopy is used (Kido, JTraceElemElectrolHlthDis, 1988; 2:101).

Reference values

Body content: 30–38 mg, depending on the environment. Blood concentration: 2.6–57 nmol/l (ref.[12], p.229). Serum concentration: 87–614 nmol/l.[1] Reported liver tissue concentrations: 2–3 µg/g wet weight,[1] 0.3–4.1 µg/g wet weight (ref. 12, p.229). A higher concentration is seen in Japanese people (up to 12 µg/g wet weight) (Kido, JTraceElemElectrolHlthDis, 1988; 2:101). In Spain, in livers of patients not exposed to heavy metal contamination, cadmium concentrations of 0.98 ± 0.5 µg/g wet weight were found that correlated with liver zinc concentrations (Torra, SciTotalEnv, 1995; 170:53). Liver and kidney concentrations reflect cadmium status better than blood and serum levels (ref. 12, p.607).

Uptake, distribution, and excretion

Cadmium is taken up by inhalation (smoking) and via the intestinal tract. In blood, cadmium is bound to erythrocytes and in particular to haemoglobin. In the body the main deposits are in the kidney and liver and to a lesser extent in the brain, pancreas, bone, and skin.[1] The cadmium content of liver is 30 per cent of that in the kidney (ref. 12, p.607). Cadmium in tissue is mainly bound to metallothionein.[9] In the liver, cadmium-induced metallothionein was demonstrated predominantly in hepatocytes and sinusoidal endothelial cells (Leyshon-Sorland, HistochemJ, 1993; 25:857). In rats, ethanol intake can enhance the excretion of cadmium bound to glutathione into bile (Arizono, TraceElemElectrol, 1994; 11:125).

Function

Metallothionein is the only known naturally occurring protein containing cadmium. Other functions are not known (ref. 9, p.25).

Toxicity

Acute cadmium exposure in mice induces hepatic and renal injury by damaging hepatocytes and sinusoidal endothelial cells. Injury is mediated by cytokines, in particular by tumour necrosis factor-α (Kayama, ToxApplPharmacol, 1995; 131:224). Cadmium exposure to rats before partial hepatectomy suppressed hepatic regeneration, probably due to the inhibition of thymidine kinase (Margeli, Arch-Toxicol, 1994; 68:85). Chronic exposure results in bone disorders, renal dysfunction, and enteropathy. Renal abnormalities are due to tubular damage with moderate proteinuria (Kido, JTrace-ElemElectrolHlthDis, 1988; 2:101). Cadmium accumulates in the liver to a lesser extent than in the kidneys. In livers of exposed women, levels up to 60 μg/g wet weight have been found. Concomitantly, zinc content increases and copper decreases. In animals, hepatic necrosis has been produced by the acute administration of cadmium, probably due to increased lipid peroxidation. Animals chronically exposed to cadmium have had lower acute mortality, and less lipid peroxidation, probably due to induction of metallothionein binding (Anderson, PharmacolToxicol, 1988; 63:173). Data on lipid peroxidation are controversial (Siegers, ToxicolLett, 1986; 34:185; Raun, PharmacolToxicol, 1988; 63:173). The inhibition of superoxide dismutase activity is due to competition with other trace elements (zinc and copper) (Hussain, PharmacolToxicol, 1987; 606: 355). Cadmium content in liver can be reduced by chelating agents (CaNa$_3$DTPA, Na$_2$CDTA, NaDDC, and triethylene tetramine hydrochloride) in animals. These agents increase metallothionein synthesis and the amount of metallothionein-bound zinc in the liver (Tewari, ClinExpPharmPhys, 1988; 15:71).

Chromium (Cr, atomic weight 51.99)
Analytical techniques

Only electrothermal atomic absorption spectroscopy[2] or atomic absorption spectroscopy with graphite furnace attachment (Brown, DigDisSci, 1986; 31:661) are suitable. Contamination from cannulas may increase the apparent concentration several fold. Thus, deficiency is difficult to prove (Kruse-Jarres, DiabetStoffw, 1995; 4: 291).

Reference values

Body content: 1–5 mg,[1] 10–20 mg.[2] Blood concentration: 53–865 nmol/l. Serum concentration: 2.3–40 nmol/l. Liver tissue concentration: 8–72 ng/g wet weight (ref. 12, p.229).[1]

Uptake, distribution, and excretion

Daily uptake is between 60 and 90 μg/day; only 1 per cent of inorganic chromium salts (Cr^{3+}), but 15 to 20 per cent of organic chromium in food is absorbed. Uptake is by the proximal small bowel,[2] probably through complex formation with transferrin and transport to the liver. Chromium accumulates in the spleen and heart and is excreted in urine (normal range 0.5–1.0 μg/day) and faeces.[1]

Function

Chromium is found in high concentrations in bovine liver, in nucleoproteins involved in the protection of nucleic acids against thermal denaturation. It has a stimulating effect on RNA synthesis and is important for the action of insulin (Anderson, AmJClinNutr, 1985; 41:1177).

Toxicity

Chromium can induce diarrhoea, coagulation abnormalities, and renal dysfunction.[2]

Abnormalities in liver disease

Chromium deficiency due to long-term parenteral nutrition results in a decreased availability of the glucose tolerance factor.[2] This is a complex of Cr^{3+}, nicotinic acid, and amino acids (or glutathione) and is produced in the liver. The factor is necessary for the binding and effects of insulin (Mertz, JNutr, 1993; 123:626).

Chromium deficiency is known to produce insulin-resistant hyperglycaemia despite adequate insulin concentrations in serum. Substitution with chromium led to improvement without measurable increases of serum levels (Brown, DigDisSci, 1986; 31: 661). Other symptoms of deficiency are polyneuropathy, abnormal nitrogen metabolism, and increased fatty acids in serum.

Chromium substitution improves these abnormalities and leads to reduced low-density lipoprotein cholesterol and an increased high-density lipoprotein fraction in addition to a higher insulin sensitivity. Patients with diabetes type I have increased excretion which could be stimulated by insulin. In a randomized controlled trial, chromium supplementation increased levels of high-density lipoprotein cholesterol in men taking β-blockers (Roeback, Ann-IntMed, 1991; 115:917). Using the model of the regenerating rat liver after hemihepatectomy, a 70-kDa protein with five or six chromium atoms has been found to stimulate RNA synthesis.

Treatment and/or substitution in liver disease

With suspected chromium deficiency, 200 μg/day chromium chloride (= 26 μg chromium) is used; standard infusions contain only 6 μg/day (Brown, DigDisSci, 1986; 31:661).

Cobalt (Co, atomic weight 58.93)
Analytical techniques

Neutron activation analysis is useful (Okuno, TraceElemMed, 1988; 5:130). Deficiency cannot be proved.[2] Contamination is a major problem.[5]

Reference values

Body content: 1–3 mg.[1,2] Blood concentration: 0.3–5.0 nmol/l;[2] there is poor reproducibility. Serum concentration: 1.9–7.6 nmol/l.[10] Liver tissue concentration: 6–151 ng/g wet weight; other workers have found similar values: 30–62 ng/g (Okuno, TraceElemMed, 1988; 5:130). A biopsy cannula can add up to 230 ng/g to the apparent concentration.

Uptake, distribution, and excretion

Cobalt is absorbed in the stomach and duodenum. Two uptake systems are known. In plasma, cobalt is bound to albumin,[1] and accumulates in liver and fat cells.[1] The absorption of cobalt bound to vitamin B_{12} is dependent on intrinsic factor. Transport to the liver depends on transcobalamin II.[1] Inorganic cobalt is rapidly excreted in urine (ref.[13], p.363); vitamin B_{12} is, in part, excreted in bile bound to transcobalamin II and undergoes partial enterohepatic circulation.[1]

Function

Cobalt is an enzyme activator. However, activation is not specific: Zn^{2+}, Mn^{2+}, Fe^{2+}, Ni^{2+}, and Cd^{2+} have similar effects. This 'exchangeability' has been used to study metalloenzymes with spectroscopy (nuclear magnetic resonance) (ref. 13, p.363). Enzymes activated are hydrolases, carnosinase (EC 3.4.13.3), arginase (EC 3.5.3.1), phosphatase, and glucokinase (EC 2.7.1.2). Cobalt is part of carboxypeptidase A (EC 3.4.17.1) and B (EC 3.4.17.2).[2] Cobalt (like cadmium) stimulates the activity of ornithine decarboxylase (EC 4.1.1.17) and haemoxygenase (EC 1.14.99.3). This activation is abolished by inhibitors of protein synthesis (Yoshida, BiochemJ, 1986; 233:577). Furthermore, cobalt is necessary for methylmalonyl CoA mutase activity in fatty acid biosynthesis (EC 5.4.99.2) and for methyltetrahydrofolate-homocysteine transmethylase, which catalyses methionine formation from homocysteine. Thus, it is involved in erythropoiesis and cell proliferation.[1]

Toxicity

Little is known about toxicity; abdominal cramps, rheumatoid symptoms, and toxic pulmonary oedema have occasionally been described.[2]

Abnormalities in liver disease

Cobalt deficiency has not yet been found except as the deficiency of vitamin B_{12} in gastric and ileal diseases. The uptake of cobalt and iron is increased in patients with haemochromatosis as a result of the shared transport system (ref. 13, p.363). In hepatoma tissue, decreased concentrations of cobalt were found compared with surrounding liver tissue (23 ± 19 compared with 46 ± 16 ng/g wet weight) (Okuno, TraceElemMed, 1988; 5:130). Increased serum vitamin B_{12} concentrations have been described in acute hepatitis as a sign of cell necrosis. In inactive liver cirrhosis, increased vitamin B_{12} is explained by decreased extraction. With hepatocellular carcinoma (particularly the fibrolamellar type), increased vitamin B_{12} and transcobolamin concentrations are explained by a high level of synthesis of an abnormal transcobolamin.[1]

Lead (Pb, atomic weight 207.20)

Analytical techniques

Electrothermal atomic absorption spectroscopy and X-ray fluorescence spectroscopy[7] are used.

Reference values

Body content: approximately 120 mg. Plasma concentration: 0.7–1.9 µmol/l.[10] Liver tissue concentration: 0.3–2.3 µg/g wet weight (ref. 12, p.229).[1] In 13 of 74 normal livers lead was found at a concentration of 0.4 to 11 µg/g dry weight.[7] A mean of 11 µg/l (range 6.3–13) has been described in urine.[10]

Uptake, distribution, and excretion

Five per cent is absorbed from nutrients. Lead is probably protein bound in erythrocytes; it accumulates in bone and is excreted in bile.[1] By contrast, 40 per cent is absorbed if lead is inhaled (Spaedy, AmJGastr, 1988; 83:581).

Toxicity

Toxic hepatitis may be found even with low serum concentrations (5 µmol/l). At such concentrations 50 per cent of patients have signs of liver damage. Lead concentration in serum correlates with aminotransferases (Cartón Sánchez, GastroHepato, 1985; 8:24). Increased urinary excretion of δ-aminolaevulinic acid and coproporphyrin has been found due to inhibition of δ-aminolaevulinic acid dehydratase. Chelating agents (EDTA, BAL, DMSA, or penicillamine) and the combined application of zinc and thiamine have been used in lead intoxication (Spaedy, AmJGastr, 1988; 83:581; Flora, JIntMedRes, 1989; 17:68). In rats, lead poisoning decreased peripheral hepatic benzodiazepine receptors (Fonia, EJPTox, 1995; 293:335).

Abnormalities in liver disease

In patients with alcoholic liver disease lead concentrations in the liver and in serum are increased, correlating with iron concentration. This is probably due to increased uptake or dietary consumption.[7] In experimental hepatocarcinogenesis, lead nitrate induced liver cell proliferation and hyperplastic foci without liver cell necrosis, probably regulated by tumour necrosis factor-α (Kubo, Hepatol, 1996; 23:104). A specific pattern of regression of initiated hepatocytes was observed, due to apoptosis (Nakajima, JGastro, 1995; 30:725, Columbano, Carcinogenesis, 1996; 17:395).

Magnesium (Mg, atomic weight 24.30)

Analytical techniques

Atomic absorption spectroscopy is used (Al-Jurf, MagnesBull, 1981; 2:104; Heaton, Magnesium, 1984; 3:21).

Reference values

Body content: 35 g (magnesium is a 'macroelement').[2] Serum concentration: 0.9 ± 0.1 mmol/l. Liver tissue concentration: in infants and children 1.5 ± 0.4 µg/g dry weight (Göksu, JPediatGastrNutr, 1986; 5:459).

Uptake, distribution, and excretion

Enteral absorption is decreased by aldosterone and fat malabsorption. In blood, 25 per cent is bound to proteins and 75 per cent is free as ionized magnesium. Mg^{2+} and H^+ ions compete for protein binding (Cohen, Magnesium, 1985; 4:1).

Function

Magnesium is an activator of hydrolases, for aminopeptidases and pantethine kinase in association with manganese, and for alkaline phosphatase with manganese, zinc, cobalt, and calcium. Magnesium is necessary for the activation of the zinc metalloenzyme alkaline phosphatase (EC 3.1.3.1). In the rat, seven forms of alkaline phosphatase may be separated by polyacrylamide gel electrophoresis from several tissues such as liver, kidney, small intestine, and bone. Each form separates into two bands. Magnesium and zinc deficiency have different effects on the activity of individual bands of the enzyme (Heaton, MagnesBull, 1981; 2:101).

Toxicity

Intoxication is unlikely with normal renal function. After oral ingestion, concentrated solutions can cause gastrointestinal symptoms. Intoxication produces neurological symptoms.

Abnormalities in liver disease

In serum of patients with liver cirrhosis the level of magnesium was 0.75 ± 0.13 mmol/l (Sullivan, AmJClinNutr, 1963; 13:297; Burch, ArchIntMed, 1979; 139:680). In another study, five patients with untreated non-alcoholic cirrhosis were investigated. They were without hypoalbuminaemia. Low magnesium concentrations within the cortex of bones correlated with decreased plasma ionized magnesium concentrations; by contrast, total plasma and trabecular bone magnesium were normal (Cohen, IsrJMedSci, 1982; 18:679). However, in children with non-alcoholic cirrhosis, magnesium concentrations in the liver were about 50 per cent decreased compared with normal subjects. Alcohol and diuretics may contribute to magnesium deficiency (Cohen, Magnesium, 1985; 4:1). Metabolic alkalosis and vitamin D deficiency, hyperaldosteronism, and fat malabsorption are further causes of hypomagnesaemia (Cohen, 1982). An association between low serum magnesium and enhanced toxic effects of nitrogenous compounds has been described in cirrhosis (Flink, JLabClinMed, 1995; 46:814). In rats, magnesium deficiency enhanced hepatic iron accumulation and may serve as a model of experimental haemochromatosis (Kimura, BiolTraceElemRes, 1996; 51:177).

Secondary hyperaldosteronism leads to continuous loss of magnesium and potassium and to retention of sodium. The effect is aggravated by thiazide or loop diuretics. In patients with cirrhosis, the intolerance for ammonia and ammonium salts is greatly increased in magnesium deficiency. Hepatic encephalopathy is multifactorial, but magnesium deficiency may contribute to tremor and somnolence. Magnesium deficiency and the alcohol withdrawal syndrome display some overlapping symptoms such as delirium and tremulousness. Alcohol itself increases urinary excretion of magnesium. After alcohol withdrawal, serum free fatty acids rise and magnesium concentration decreases. There is some evidence that free fatty acids can block Mg ATP-dependent reactions, particularly in the presence of magnesium deficiency (Flink, MagnesBull, 1981; 1a:209).

Magnesium deficiency leads to loss of potassium, accumulation of sodium and calcium, and a reduced rate of protein synthesis; mitochondria seem to play an important role, since swelling of mitochondria has been observed histologically in magnesium-deficient rats. Heaton showed a partial uncoupling of oxidative phosphorylation in whole mitochondria and a complete uncoupling with inner membrane preparations of magnesium-deficient rats. Magnesium deficiency probably increases the permeability of the mitochondrial inner membrane, weakening the coupling between oxidation and phosphorylation (Heaton, Magnesium, 1984; 3:21). In rats, the induction of hepatocyte injury after glycodeoxycholate led to hepatocyte apoptosis, mediated by an increase of free cytosolic Mg^{2+} and enhanced activity of magnesium-dependent endonucleases. Mg^{2+}-free medium could prevent this rise in cytosolic magnesium, resulting in a reduced DNA fragmentation (Patel, JCI, 1994; 94:2183).

The incomplete form of distal renal tubular acidosis sometimes seen in patients with cirrhosis may be caused by magnesium deficiency. Distal renal tubular acidosis was demonstrated by the $CaCl_2$ loading test in four patients with non-alcoholic cirrhosis and was corrected by administration of magnesium (Cohen, Magnesium, 1986; 5:39).

Portocaval shunting corrected the decreased magnesium and calcium serum levels and decreased intestinal absorption found after parathyroidectomy in rats. Hypophosphataemia produced by portocaval shunting may have stimulated production of 1,25-dihydroxycholecalciferol (Al-Jurf, MagnesBull, 1981; 2:104). In liver disease without concurrent renal failure, pseudohypomagnesaemia may be detected by direct determination of ionized magnesium (Kulpmann, EurJClinChemClinBioch, 1996; 34:257). On the other hand, high levels of citrate administered during orthotopic liver transplantation may reduce ionized magnesium (Kimura, Transpl, 1996; 61:835).

Treatment and/or substitution in liver disease

Spironolactone has improved hypomagnesaemia in children with cirrhosis (Cohen, JPediat, 1970; 76:453).

Administration of magnesium may improve complications of alcohol withdrawal, or magnesium deficiency not induced by alcohol, including hypocalcaemia, hypokalaemia refractory to K^+ replacement, and serious ventricular arrhythmias. A positive magnesium balance was observed for up to 4 weeks after alcohol withdrawal and infusion of magnesium. Determination of urinary excretion after a parenteral dose of magnesium was shown to be a suitable method to detect magnesium deficiency. In patients with the alcohol withdrawal syndrome, treatment with a solution containing glucose and magnesium sulphate lowered levels of free fatty acids, and in some cases dramatically improved the clinical course and outcome. Careful correction of hypomagnesaemia can reduce the myocardial and renal toxicity of cyclosporin in patients after organ transplantation (Rob, TransplProc, 1994; 26:1736).

Manganese (Mn, atomic weight 54.94)

Analytical techniques

X-ray fluorescence spectroscopy has been used.[7] Sampling may produce errors of up to 150 per cent by contamination from rubber stoppers (vacutainers). Concentrations in tissue (liver, kidney, and heart) as well as in hair have been used to estimate manganese status in goats with manganese deficiency. In contrast, hair concentration is not useful in man (ref. 12, p.607).

Reference values

Body content: 12–20 mg.[1,2] Blood concentration: 145–340 nmol/l. In the rat lower concentrations have been found (<100 nmol/l, free Mn <20 nmol/l). Serum concentration: 20 $\pm$ 37 nmol/l (Zarski, GastrClinBiol, 1985; 9:664); 9–32 nmol/l (ref. 12, p.229). Data for liver tissue concentration vary greatly: 1–1.3 µg/g wet weight, with increased excretion at higher levels (ref. 12, p.140); 1.2–5.0 µg/g wet weight;[1,7] 13–21 µg/g protein (Zarski, 1985); 1.8 $\pm$ 0.7 µg/g wet weight (Okuno, TraceElemMed, 1988; 5:130). Isolated rat hepatocytes contain approximately 30 nmol Mn^{2+}/ml of cell water, which is comparable with the concentration in fresh liver tissue (Schramm, FedProc, 1986; 45:2805).

Uptake, distribution, and excretion

Only 3 to 4 per cent is absorbed from nutrients, by the duodenum and small bowel.[1,2] Manganese is absorbed and transported through the mucosa as a complex with nucleic acids.[2] Manganese and iron show a competitive uptake. In the blood, manganese is bound to transferrin.[1]

Uptake into rat hepatocytes is mainly in the ionized form ($K_m =$ 1.2 µmol/l; $V_{max} =$ 54 nmol/min per g cells), probably as 'facilitated diffusion'. The Co^{2+} ion is a competitive inhibitor while Ca^{2+}, Mg^{2+}, and Fe^{2+} ions are weak inhibitors. There is active transport of Mn^{2+} ions into mitochondria (Schramm, FedProc, 1986; 45: 2805).

Manganese accumulates mainly in cells rich in mitochondria (liver, bone, pancreas, kidney, and hair).[1,8] Rat hepatocytes contain between 1 and 2 per cent of free Mn^{2+} ions, probably in mitochondria (determined by electron paramagnetic resonance); the remainder are bound to ligands (proteins and phosphorylated compounds) (Schramm, FedProc, 1986; 45:2817).

Excretion is in bile with binding to bile acids (Dijkstra, JHepatol, 1991; 13:112). Renal elimination is minimal. In rats, rapid biliary excretion of oral and intravenous manganese occurs without signs of accumulation. No hormonal influence has been found (Schramm, FedProc, 1986; 45:2817).

Function

Manganese is a cofactor for arginase, alkaline phosphatase, and other enzymes (Table 2). Succinate dehydrogenase and prolidase are activated by manganese as are other enzymes of the muco-polysaccharide metabolism.

Toxicity

After inhalation of manganese (e.g. in mine workers), hepatic abnormalities (increased aminotransferases and bilirubin) can precede neurological symptoms.[2] Treatment of rare cases of acute or chronic poisoning is non-specific. Manganese-induced pneumonia due to inhalation requires antibiotic treatment. A beneficial effect of manganese administration has been described in hydralazine-induced lupus erythematosus, bronchial asthma, and neuroleptic-induced dyskinesia (ref. 3, p.140).

Abnormalities in liver disease

In rats, sequential administration of manganese and bilirubin induces a decrease of bile flow (up to 75 per cent) but not of bile salt secretion (Ayotte, Hepatol, 1988; 8:1069). Accordingly, manganese concentration in liver has been found by some to increase in liver cirrhosis, particularly in alcoholic cirrhosis and in infants with extrahepatic biliary atresia (Bayliss, JTraceElemMedBiol, 1995; 9: 40).[8] In contrast, other authors have found lower liver concentrations, similar to those in normal subjects.

Urinary excretion was found to decrease while serum concentrations were increased (Zarski, GastrClinBiol, 1985; 9:664); similar results were reported earlier (Sullivan, JNutr, 1979; 109: 1432). In contrast, decreased serum and urine concentrations have also been reported (Vai, MinDietGastro, 1983; 29:219).

Several recent reports described MRI hyperintensity of T_1-weighted signals in basal ganglia of individuals with cirrhosis and children with chronic liver disease (Barron, PediatrNeurol, 1994; 10:145; Deveny, Gastro, 1994; 106:1068). These bright ganglia are caused by increased manganese concentrations, as shown by direct measurement of manganese in the brain of patients with cirrhosis at autopsy (Hauser, AnnNeurol, 1994; 36:871; Krieger, Lancet, 1995; 346:270; Pomier-Layrargues, Lancet, 1995; 345:735). Manganese concentrations in the blood were correlated with pallidal hyperintensity and extrapyramidal symptoms (Mirowitz, Radiol, 1991; 181:117; Spahr, Hepatol, 1996; 24:1116) . Similar alterations were found in humans and primates after manganese intoxication (Nelson, BrJIndMed, 1993; 50:510; Shinotoh, Neurology, 1995; 45: 1199) and patients receiving manganese supplementation during long-term parenteral nutrition (Mirowitz, 1991).

In a study of 57 patients with cirrhosis, 38 showed pallidal hyperintensity and extrapyramidal symptoms resembling Parkinson's disease (Spahr, Hepatol, 1996; 24:1116). Manganese seems to exert a toxic effect on basal ganglia leading to dopaminergic dysfunction (Butterworth, MetBrainRes, 1995; 10:259).

A correlation of blood manganese concentrations with the Child–Pugh score, indocyanin green clearance, or ammonia levels was demonstrated in four studies (Inoue, Radiol, 1991; 179:551; Kulisevsky, Hepatol, 1992; 16:1382; Pujol, Neurology, 1993; 43:65; Taylor-Robinson, MetabolBrainDis, 1995; 10:175). This view was challenged in a recent study, where pallidal hyperintensity and increased manganese concentrations in the blood were predominantly found in patients with surgical shunts or transjugular intrahepatic portosystemic stent shunts (TIPS), suggesting shunting rather than impaired liver function being the major cause (Spahr, Hepatol, 1996; 24:1116). After liver transplantation, manganese concentrations in the blood returned to normal, and symptoms and bright basal ganglia improved (Geissler, Hepatol, 1997; 25:48).

Similar findings with severe neurological symptoms were obtained in patient with Alagille's syndrome, which were corrected within 2 months after liver transplantation (Devenyi, Gastro, 1994; 106:1068). Future studies will show whether chelating agents can improve manganese depositions and neurological symptoms.

Table 2 Manganese-dependent enzymes (examples)

Glucokinase (with Zn, Mg, Co, Ca) (EC 2.7.1.2)

Panthethine kinase (with Mg) (EC 2.7.1.34)

Alkaline phosphatase (EC 3.1.3.1)

Leucine aminopeptidase (with Mg) (EC 3.4.11.1)

Amino-acid-histidine-dipeptidase (with Zn and Co) (EC 3.4.13.3)

Prolyldipeptidase (EC 3.4.13.8)

Proline dipeptidase (EC 3.4.13.9)

Arginase (EC 3.5.3.1)

Enolase (with Zn, Fe, K) (EC 4.2.1.11)

Pyruvate carboxylase (EC 6.4.1.1)

Glycyl-glycine dipeptidase

Glycine leucine dipeptidase (with Zn)

Phosphatases (with Mg, Co, Fe, Zn)

A manganese-containing constrast dye has been used to differentiate between normal and cirrhotic liver tissue during magnetic resonance imaging (Murakami, Radiol, 1996; 198:567). Concentrations of manganese are lower (50 per cent) in hepatoma than in surrounding hepatic tissue (Okuno, TraceElemMed, 1988; 5: 130). Manganese concentration in liver is not influenced by parenteral nutrition, in contrast to zinc and copper (Tolikoura, ScaJGastr, 1986; 21:421). In Long–Evans cinnamon rats, which have a genetic defect of copper metabolism similar to that of Wilson's disease, the disturbed function of Cu,Zn-superoxide-dismutase was found to be compensated for by increased activity of Mn-superoxide-dismutase (Suzuki, Carcinogenesis, 1993; 14:1881).

Molybdenum (Mo, atomic weight 94.94)
Analytical techniques

Neutron activation analysis and particle-induced X-ray emission are used.

Reference values

Body content: approximately 20 mg. Blood concentration: 3–13 nmol/l.[2] Serum concentration: 5.7 ± 2.1 nmol/l. Liver tissue concentration: 0.16–0.72 mg/g wet weight (Versieck, JLabClinMed, 1981; 97:535) or 0.36–0.800 µg/g dry weight.[10] There are lower concentrations in infants and children.

Uptake, distribution, and excretion

Molybdenum is easily absorbed (60 to 100 per cent). Binding proteins are unknown. Labelled molybdenum is almost completely found in the liver.[2] Excretion is mainly in urine.[1] In icteric states an increase of molybdenum is found in serum, suggesting biliary excretion (Versieck, JLabClinMed, 1981; 97:535).

Function

Molybdenum is part of the flavine-containing enzymes xanthinoxidase (EC 1.2.3.2), aldehyde oxidase (EC 1.2.3.1), and sulphite oxidase (EC 1.8.3.1).[2]

Toxicity

Hyperuricaemia, diarrhoea, and general fatigue can be caused by high doses.[2] After exposure to dust containing molybdenum, patients may present a slight increase of uric acid and a pronounced increase in serum caeruloplasmin. No treatment has been reported.

Abnormalities in liver disease

In acute viral hepatitis, liver cirrhosis, and chronic active hepatitis, increased serum concentrations have been found (up to 72 nmol/l). The increase correlates with that of bilirubin, alkaline phosphatase, and serum aminotransferases. Decreased hepatic uptake or impaired excretion due to cellular damage have been suggested mechanisms, as extrahepatic obstruction does not result in increased levels of molybdenum in serum (Versieck, JLabClinMed, 1981; 97:535). In rats, oral administration of Na_2MoO_4 improved carbohydrate and lipid metabolism (Ozcelikay, AmJPhysiol, 1996; 33:E344). In rodent experiments, molybdenum could prevent the hepatocarcinogenesis of N-nitroso compounds by preservation of normal calcium metabolism and stimulation of nitroso compound metabolism via a nontoxic pathway (Koizumi, BiolPharmBull, 1995; 18:460).

No deficiency is known. Only a few cases of molybdenum cofactor deficiency have been reported, leading to a sulphite oxidase defect, resulting in early death due to cerebral atrophy and dysfunction. Molybdenum in the form of ammonium tetrathiomolybdate binds copper in a tripartite complex with protein and is used for the initial treatment of patients with Wilson's disease presenting with neurological symptoms (Brewer, Nutrition, 1995; 11:114). This copper-chelating effect was shown in copper-loaded LEC rats. Ammonium tetrathiomolybdate was taken up by the liver according to the amount of copper, and the complexes were mainly excreted via faeces (Ogra, JTraceElemMedBiol, 1995; 9:165).

Nickel (Ni, atomic weight 58.69)
Analytical techniques

Electrothermal atomic absorption spectroscopy is suitable. Neutron activation analysis is not useful.[2]

Reference values

Body content: 5–10 mg.[1,2] Serum concentration: 0.34–0.68 µmol/l.[1] Liver tissue concentration: 1.8 ± 0.95 µg/g wet weight (Bona, HumExpToxicol, 1992; 11:311) or 0.12–1.0 µg/g wet weight.[1,10]

Uptake, distribution, and excretion

Between 3 and 5 per cent of dietary nickel is taken up from nutrients.[1] Nickel is bound to albumin,[2] accumulates in liver, kidney, whole blood, testis, skin, and muscle,[1] and is excreted in urine (Severa, HumExpToxicol, 1995; 14:955).[2]

Function

Nickel is an enzyme activator (hydrolases, arginase (EC 3.5.3.1), and part of carboxypeptidase A (EC 3.4.1.7.1)) which acts exchangeably with, or together with, cobalt, iron, manganese, and zinc. A deficient diet leads to reduced growth, infertility, and decreased enzyme activity (amylase in rats, sorbitol dehydrogenase in goats). In goats, low concentrations of liver nickel reflect deficiency.[10]

Toxicity

Inhalation of nickel compounds leads to vomiting, nausea, and chest pain. Pulmonary oedema can cause death. Concentrations of nickel of more than 500 µg/l in urine are considered to be indicative of severe intoxication. Chelators, particularly sodium diethyldithiocarbonate, are used in treatment.

Abnormalities in liver disease

Decreased serum concentration has been found in liver cirrhosis. No deficiency symptoms are known (Nielsen, FASEBJ, 1991; 5: 2661). Nickel has been used as an agent for investigating the relation between hormone-induced Ca^{2+} influx and bile flow in the perfused rat liver (Karjalainen, CellCalcium, 1995; 18:214).

Selenium (Se, atomic weight 78.96)

Analytical techniques

Neutron activation analysis and electrothermal atomic absorption spectroscopy are suitable (Aeseth, ClinBioch, 1982; 15:281; Okuno, TraceElemMed, 1988; 5:130). Serum selenium levels are a good indicator of body status (ref. 10, p.607).

Reference values

Body content: 6–21 mg.[1] Blood concentration: 0.5–1.5 µmol/l;[2] 0.7–2.9 µmol/l (ref.[10], p.229). Serum concentration: 0.9–3.7 µmol/l;[1] 0.8–1.2 µmol/l (Välimäki, CCActa, 1983; 130: 291). Plasma concentration: 0.7–1.3 µmol/l.[17] Liver tissue concentration: 0.2–0.7 µg/g wet weight.[1,2,4] Selenium was detected in 59 of 74 normal livers by X-ray fluorescence spectroscopy (mean: 1.9 µg/g dry weight).[7] In another study, normal liver concentration was found to be slightly lower (1.23 ± 0.3 µg/g dry weight).[17]

Uptake, distribution, and excretion

Between 35 and 85 per cent is absorbed from the diet.[1] There may be deficient uptake in the normal subject: activity of glutathione peroxidase in platelets could be increased by oral substitution of selenium (ref. 10, p.371). Selenium is absorbed in the distal ileum. Amino acids are ligands.[17] Inorganic selenium is transported by very low-density and low-density lipids. In serum, selenium is bound to proteins (e.g. selenoenzymes) and a postulated transport protein. Accumulation takes place in liver, spleen, heart, and nails.

Selenium is mainly excreted in urine and also in bile and sweat.[1]

Function

Selenium is incorporated into selenium-dependent proteins via selenocysteine. Genetic control of selenocysteine insertion is exerted uniquely by the codon U(T)GA, normally used as a stop codon (Chesters, NutrRev, 1992, 50:217). The resulting tRNA is charged with L-serine, which is then converted into selenocysteine by at least two steps (Burk, FASEBJ, 1991; 5:2274). Glutathione peroxidases (EC 1.11.1.9) are well-characterized selenoenzymes (Chesters, NutrResRev, 1988; 1:39) and contain the most selenium. With vitamin E, superoxide dismutase (zinc, copper), and glutathione, this enzyme belongs to the defence system against oxidative stress and lipid peroxidation.[1,15] In rats, a selenium-deficient diet reduces activity and synthesis of glutathione peroxidase (Arthur, BiochemJ, 1987; 248:539; Knight, JNutr, 1987; 117:732). In humans, high concentrations of a gastrointestinal glutathione peroxidase have been found in hepatocytes and colonic enterocytes (Chu, JBC, 1993; 268:2571). An endemic selenium-deficiency disease is known in China (Keshan disease), but selenium deficiency causes no particular liver disease in this area. Reduced glutathione peroxidase activity results in increased methaemoglobin leading to myofibrillar dystrophy (heart and muscle).[1–3] Hepatic and thyroidal 5′-deiodinase (type 1) activity is also selenium dependent (Berry, Nature, 1991; 349:438; Vadhanavikit, JNutr, 1993; 123:1124) and inhibition of hepatic deiodination of thyroxine is caused by selenium deficiency (Beckett, BiochemJ, 1987; 248:443; Behne, AmJClinNutr, 1993; 57:310S). Selenoprotein P, with multiple selenocysteines, contains the most selenium in rat plasma (Burk, JNutr, 1994; 124:1891). Selenoprotein P may serve as selenium transporter and may protect mitochondrial membranes from oxidative stress (Read, JBC, 1990; 265:17899).

Toxicity

Only a few cases of selenium intoxication have been reported. The symptoms were alopecia and emotional lability. The toxicity, metabolism, and absorption of selenite was investigated using isolated rat hepatocytes. An LD_{50} of 500 µmol for selenite was found (Park, Toxicology, 1995; 100:151). The intraperitoneal application of 1.6 mg/kg sodium selenite caused deterioration of rat hepatic mitochondrial matrices (Earla, ToxicolLett, 1992; 62:73). With oral administration of selenium to rats, nodular regenerative hyperplasia can be induced with capillarization of adjacent sinusoids and the deposition of laminin and type IV collagen (Dubuisson, Hepatol, 1995; 21:805).

Abnormalities in liver disease

In alcoholic cirrhosis, liver selenium is decreased by about 65 per cent.[15,17] Liver selenium was found to be significantly lower in non-alcoholic cirrhosis (0.57 ± 0.6 µg/g dry weight) compared with alcoholic cirrhosis (0.86 ± 0.3 µg/g dry weight) or in normal subjects

(1.23 ± 0.3 µg/g dry weight).[17] In patients with alcoholic cirrhosis, serum selenium was lowered to 0.64 ± 0.2 µmol/l compared with 1.53 ± 0.25 µmol/l in normal subjects (Aaseth, NEJM, 1980; 303: 944), but this was not due to increased urinary selenium excretion.[17] In chronic liver disease, regardless of aetiology, serum selenium concentrations are significantly correlated with serum albumin and zinc concentrations and nutritional status.[17] Data are not consistent (Sullivan, JNutr, 1979; 109:1432; Aeseth, ClinBioch, 1982; 15:281; Johansson, BrJNutr, 1986; 55:227). Platelet glutathione peroxidase (EC 1.11.1.9), but not blood glutathione peroxidase activity, was decreased in alcoholic cirrhosis with low serum selenium (Johansson, 1986). In primary biliary cirrhosis, serum selenium is decreased as in alcoholic cirrhosis. Acute alcohol intake in healthy subjects or abstinence and selenium-rich food in alcoholics have no significant influence on serum concentrations (Valimäki, CCActa, 1983; 130:291).

In another study, liver selenium in alcoholic cirrhosis was lower (0.7 ± 0.1 µg/g dry weight) than in controls (1.4 ± 0.2 µg/g) and was inversely correlated with prothrombin time, but not with serum albumin and aminotransferases (Dworkin, DigDisSci, 1988; 33:1213). Serum selenium and vitamin E were decreased in alcoholics with and without liver disease (Tanner, DigDisSci, 1986; 31:1307). Serum selenium concentrations correlated inversely with the aminoterminal peptide of type III procollagen, a marker of fibrotic activity, suggesting a protective role of selenium against fibrosis (Casaril, CCActa, 1989; 182:221).

In patients with intrahepatic cholestasis of pregnancy, decreased serum selenium has been found in combination with reduced glutathione peroxidase activity (Kaupilla, BMJ, 1987; 294:150; Ribalta, GastroHepato, 1995; 18:114). Interestingly, patients with primary sclerosing cholangitis showed increased hepatic selenium concentrations of 2.2 ± 0.7 µg/g dry weight compared with 1.3 ± 0.3 µg/g dry weight in controls; selenium-dependent proteins were normal (Aaseth, ScaJGastr, 1995; 30:1200). Selenoproteins other than glutathione peroxidase are reduced or absent in serum in alcoholic cirrhosis.[15] In patients with hepatocellular carcinoma, there was reduced liver selenium in tumour tissue (0.34 ± 0.09 µg/g wet weight) compared with surrounding normal tissue (0.46 ± 0.11 µg/g wet weight) (Okuno, TraceElemMed, 1988; 5:130).

Treatment and/or substitution in liver diseases

Selenium alone is not effective in preventing azaserine-induced liver carcinogenesis. In contrast, a combination of selenium with retinoids has a better effect than retinoids alone (Curphey, Pancreas, 1988; 3: 36). Sodium selenite was able to protect rats from acetaminophen-induced hepatotoxicity (Schnell, ToxApplPharmacol, 1988; 95:1). Selenium-deficient rats but not controls developed liver and kidney necrosis after phorone administration, a substance known to deplete glutathione. Selenium restitution was able to prevent phorone toxicity. Protection from lipid perioxidation and diquat-induced liver necrosis may be exerted by increased selenoprotein P concentrations but not by glutathione peroxidase (Burk, LabInvest, 1995; 72:723, Burk, Hepatol, 1995; 21:561). Selenium depletion alone, without inducers, is not able to increase lipid peroxidation and malondialdehyde formation (Lee, Lipids, 1994; 29:345). Selenium, given prior to exposure to endotoxin, could not prevent hepatotoxicity in the form of focal coagulative necrosis in the rat (Shibayama, ExpToxPath, 1994; 46:101). In the isolated perfused rat

liver, low-dose selenite exerted a potent insulin-like effect and counteracted glucagon action, whereas high-dose selenite may severely impair liver function (Roden, Hepatol, 1995; 22:169). No systematic attempt has been made to substitute selenium in human liver diseases.

Vanadium (V, atomic weight 50.94)
Analytical technique

Neutron activation analysis preferably without preirradiation is sufficiently sensitive.[10]

Reference values

Body content: 10 mg;. Blood concentration: 0.4–16 nmol/l. Serum concentration: 98–450 nmol/l. Liver tissue concentration: approximately 6 ng/g wet weight.

Uptake, distribution, and excretion

Only 0.1–1.5 per cent of vanadium is absorbed from nutrition. Vanadium binds to transferrin and accumulates in fat tissue. It is excreted in urine.[1]

Function

Low doses are necessary for bone formation.

Toxicity

Vanadium may be hepatotoxic (Younes, ResCommChemPath-Pharm, 1984; 43:487). Zinc can prevent the toxic effect of higher doses (Yamaguchi, ResExpMed, 1989; 189:47).

Abnormalities in liver disease

In streptozotocin-induced diabetes in rats, sodium orthovanadate may mimic an insulin effect and restore glucokinase activity (Gil, JBC, 1988; 263:1868). In primary cultures of rat hepatocytes both insulin and vanadate enhance intracellular glycogen accumulation. It is probable that a differential affinity of vanadate for the insulin receptor is responsible for its different effects when compared with insulin (e.g. on ApoB secretion) (Jackson, Diabetes, 1988; 37:1234). The insulin-like effect of vanadate administration on an isolated perfused rat liver was not exerted by inhibition of hepatocellular insulin extraction (Bruck, HormMetRes, 1994; 26:360). Vanadium had a strong inhibitory effect on rat liver carcinogenesis by unknown mechanisms (Bishayee, BrJCanc, 1995; 71:1214).

Zinc (Zn, atomic weight 65.38)
Analytical techniques

Atomic absorption spectroscopy, X-ray fluorescence spectroscopy, and particle-induced X-ray emission are all used (Prasad, JAm-CollNutr, 1985; 4:591; ref. 12, p.367).[7] With Zinquin (ethyl (2-methyl-8-p-toluenesulphonamido-6-quinolyl-oxyacetate) a semi-quantitative fluorescent probe is available allowing 'staining' of zinc in living cells (Coyle, BiochemJ, 1994; 303:781). Assessment of zinc status is difficult (Sandstead, JLabClinMed, 1994; 124:322). Serum concentrations give inconsistent information and can be affected by several factors (nutrition, diurnal rhythm, haemolysis, trauma, surgery) (Prasad, 1985).[2] Determination of serum metallothionein concentrations may more reliably reflect the body zinc status (Pluhator, CanJGastr, 1996; 10:37). Serum ferritin concentrations in the upper normal range usually reflect diets rich in meat and may serve as an indirect parameter of sufficient zinc intake (Yadrick, AmJClinNutr, 1989; 49:145).

Reference values

Body content: 1600–4000 mg. Serum concentration: $16.6 \pm 3.0 \,\mu$mol/l (Zarski, GastrClinBiol, 1985; 9:664); $14.8 \pm 1.9 \,\mu$mol/l (Sullivan, JNutr, 1979; 109:1432) (erythrocyte concentration: $190 \pm 28 \,\mu$mol/l, thus haemolysis has to be avoided). Liver tissue concentration: 40–$50 \,\mu$g/g wet weight,[1] and 100–$300 \,\mu$g/g dry weight.[4] In fetal and newborn human liver, zinc concentrations of 10 to $300 \,\mu$g/g wet weight have been found (Dorea, JAmCollNutr, 1987; 6:491). In the rat, zinc concentrations increase rapidly prior to term within the fetal liver and are accompanied by increased metallothionein concentrations. The rate-limiting step of maternal/fetal zinc transfer is unknown, since during pregnancy zinc uptake rates measured in placental microvillar vesicles and fetal liver plasma membrane vesicles did not change (Lindsay, BiolRepro, 1994; 51: 358). In the first year of life, human liver tissue concentration is $455 \pm 88 \,\mu$g/g dry weight, later decreasing (Göksu, JPediatGastrNutr, 1986; 5:459). No sex and adult age variations have been found ($75 \pm \,\mu$g/g wet weight using particle-induced X-ray emission) (Bode, Hepatol, 1988; 8:1605). Zinc concentrations may vary widely in different areas in healthy liver (Schölmerich, LebMagDarm, 1984; 14:288). These data have not been confirmed by other studies (König, JClinChemClinBiochem, 1979; 17:23).

Uptake, distribution, and excretion

Between 10 and 50 per cent is absorbed from the diet (dependent on composition) (Fairweather-Tait, NutrResRev, 1988; 1:23).[1,2] Zinc is taken up in the duodenum and jejunum. With binding to a mucosal protein, uptake is regulated by metallothionein (Cousins, NutrRev, 1979; 37:97). A newly described cysteine-rich intestinal protein may play an important role as an additional zinc transport protein (Hempe, JNutr, 1992; 122:89, O'dell, NutrRev, 1993; 50: 232). Zinc–amino acid complexes are better absorbed than zinc sulphate (Schölmerich, AmJClinNutr, 1987; 45:1480). In blood, zinc is bound to albumin, α_2-macroglobulin, transferrin, and amino acids.[1,2] Over 80 per cent of zinc is bound in bone and muscle. With increased intake, five sites of regulation of zinc metabolism have been defined: absorption from the gut, excretion in urine, exchange with erythrocytes, release from muscle, and secretion into the gut (Wastney, AmJPhysiol, 1986; 251:R398).

Hepatocyte zinc is in dynamic equilibrium with plasma zinc. Two intracellular pools have been identified using isolated rat hepatocytes. In one there is weak binding of zinc and rapid interaction with the medium. This represents a labile pool accounting for net accumulation. In the other pool, zinc is bound tightly and interacts slowly with the medium, representing an exchange process with the bulk of total cell zinc. This slow pool is related to the metallothionein content of hepatocytes (Pattison, FedProc, 1986; 45:2805), which parallels the hepatocyte zinc concentration (Saito, ResCommMolPathPharm, 1995; 88:99). Hepatocytes are able to retain zinc and to maintain the function of zinc-dependent enzymes

and proteins even in the virtual absence of zinc in the basal medium (Schroeder, JNutr, 1991; 121:844). Glucagon, adrenalin, and corticoids increase uptake or exchange and induce gene expression for metallothionein (Schroeder, PNAS, 1990; 87:313; Taylor, BBActa, 1994; 1193:240). Interleukins 1 and 6 and tumor necrosis factor (Hunter, JNutr, 1994; 124:2319) also increase gene expression (Huber, JNutr, 1988; 118:1570), which seems to be part of the acute-phase response as demonstrated in an experimental model of inflammation-induced wasting syndrome (Rofe, AgentsActions, 1994; 42:60). The increased concentration of the radical scavenger metallothionein provides more binding sites for zinc and may, in addition to the decrease in α_2-macroglobulin, lead to the hypozincaemia seen in acute inflammation. Endotoxin leads to zinc accumulation in liver cells (Fukushima, BBResComm, 1988; 152: 874). This accumulation cannot take place in mice lacking the metallothionein gene (Philcox, BiochemJ, 1995; 308:543). Zinc is excreted in pancreatic juice, bile, skin and hair sloughing, and urine.[1] Biliary zinc secretion poorly correlates with bile flow (Dijkstra, JLabClinMed, 1993; 121:751).

Function

More than 200 zinc metalloenzymes and zinc proteins have been found in man and animals (Sandstead, JLabClinMed, 1994; 124: 322). Zinc-containing enzymes are present in all six classes of 'enzyme nomenclature' (Table 3). Furthermore, zinc is important as a part of metal–protein complexes, in particular metallothionein.[1–3] Zinc enzymes are involved in the replication, transcription, and translation of the genetic material of all species.[1–3, 9] Zinc has been found to be of importance for membrane protection (Bettger, LifeSci, 1981; 28:1425) as an antioxidant (Dittmer, BiochemJ, 1992; 285:113), for epithelial differentiation, immune response, anticarcinogenic effects, RNA and DNA synthesis and repair, testicular function, prostaglandin metabolism, fatty acid metabolism, sensory functions, cerebral function, growth, platelet aggregation, insulin secretion, and wound healing. So-called zinc-finger proteins function as highly specific DNA-transciption factors.[16] A genetic defect of zinc absorption leads to acrodermatitis enteropathica (Moynahan, Lancet, 1974; ii:399) that can be treated successfully by oral zinc supplementation (Neldner, NEJM, 1975; 292:879).

Zinc is involved in vitamin A homeostasis. This may be due to its influence on synthesis of the retinol-binding protein (Smith, JLabClinMed, 1974; 84:692). In zinc deficiency, the concentration of vitamin A in liver tissue is increased.[19] Furthermore, the activity of enzymes regulating vitamin A metabolism in the liver is modified; in particular the irreversible reaction from retinal to retinoic acid is increased. In addition, biliary excretion of vitamin A is altered.[19] In rats with portocaval shunts, vitamin A in the liver increases and correlates with a decreased concentration of zinc (Schölmerich, Gastro, 1991; 100:1054). In rats, dogs, and in patients with portocaval shunts, very low concentrations of zinc and vitamin A have been found in the blood circulation (Schölmerich, Hepatogast, 1983; 30:143; Ming, ChinMedJ, 1988; 101:267).[20,21]

Toxicity

At very high doses, abdominal cramps, pulmonary oedema, and necrotizing pancreatitis have been described.[2] Oral application of

Table 3 Zinc metalloenzymes (examples)

Name	EC number	Reference
Class I: Oxidoreductases		
Alcohol dehydrogenase	(EC 1.1.1.1)	Fairweather-Tait, NutrResRev, 1988; 1:23
Superoxide dismutase	(EC 1.15.1.1)	Chesters, NutrResRev, 1988; 1:39
Lactic acid dehydrogenase	(EC 1.1.1.27)	Chesters, NutrResRev, 1988; 1:39
Class II: Transferases		
Reverse transcriptase (oncogenic viruses)		Prasad, JLabClinMed, 1973; 82:461
Nuclear poly(A) polymerase		
Ornithine transcarbamoylase	(EC 2.1.3.3)	Fairweather-Tait, NutrResREv, 1988; 1:23
DNA polymerase	(EC 2.7.7.7)	Fairweather-Tait, NutrResRev, 1988; 1:23
Class III: Hydrolases		
Alkaline phosphatase	(EC 3.1.3.1)	Chesters, NutrResRev, 1988; 1:39
Fructose 1,6-biphosphatase	(EC 3.2.3.4)	Chesters, NutrResRev, 1988; 1:39
Aminopeptidase	(EC 3.4.1.1.14)	Chesters, NutrResRev, 1988; 1:39
Angiotensin-converting enzyme	(EC 3.4.15.1)	Chesters, NutrResRev, 1988; 1:39
Carboxypeptidase A and B	(EC 3.4.17.1/2)	Chesters, NutrResRev, 1988; 1:39
Collagenase	(EC 3.4.24.3)	Rabbani, AmJPhysiol, 1978; 235:E203
Aminoacyclase	(EC 3.5.1.14)	
Class IV: Lyases		
δ-Aminolaevulinic acid dehydratase	(EC 4.2.1.24)	Guzelian, LifeSci, 1982; 31:1111
Carbonic anhydrase	(EC 4.2.1.1)	
Glyoxalase I	(EC 4.4.1.5)	
Class V: Isomerases		
Phosphomannose isomerase (yeast)	(EC 5.3.1.8)	
Class VI: Ligases		
tRNA synthetase (*Escherichia coli*)		
Pyruvate carboxylase (yeast)	(EC 6.4.1.1)	

zinc leads to gastric abnormalities, nausea, and vomiting, particularly when zinc sulphate is used.[18,20]

In Japanese individuals with high exposure to cadmium, the liver tissue concentration of zinc is increased (112 µg/g wet weight), which may be due to induced metallothionein (Kido, JTraceElemElectrolHlthDis, 1988; 2:101).

Abnormalities in liver disease

Vallee and coworkers first showed abnormalities of zinc metabolism in liver cirrhosis.[18] Decreased serum zinc and increased urinary excretion of zinc were observed. These findings have been reproduced by several groups. The mean serum zinc concentration of 100 patients with cirrhosis was significantly lower than that of 153 normal subjects (9.0 ± 2.4 compared with 11.9 ± 0.6 µmol/l) (Poo, DigDisSci, 1995; 13:136). Liver tissue concentration is decreased in cirrhosis (Dyson, JRadioanalChem, 1978; 46:309; Mills, ClinSci, 1983; 64:527; Göksu, JPediatGastrNutr, 1986; 5:459).[7,15] Lower concentrations of zinc in cirrhotic liver are not due to increased collagen content (Boyett, DigDis, 1970; 15:797), but zinc concentrations are lower within fibrous septa.[4]

Data on uptake of zinc in liver cirrhosis are inconsistent. Increased uptake has been found using ^{65}Zn (Mills, ClinSci, 1983; 64:527). No significant alteration (Milman, ScaJGastr, 1983; 18:871), decreased uptake (Dinsmore, Digestion, 1985; 32:238), or 'hepatointestinal extraction' (Keeling, ClinSci, 1981; 61:441) have been described. In subcellular fractions of cirrhotic livers, zinc deficiency is most pronounced in fractions containing cell nuclei, membranes, and mitochondria (Bode, Hepatol, 1988; 8:1605).

Decreased serum concentrations of zinc have been found in non-alcoholic liver diseases such as haemochromatosis (Brissot, Digestion, 1978; 17:469), Indian childhood cirrhosis (Bhandari, JAssocPhysInd, 1981; 29:641), schistosomiasis (Mikhail, HumNutrCN, 1982; 36:289), acute hepatitis (Kahn, AmJClinPath, 1965; 44:426), and fulminant liver failure (Canalese, AustNZJMed, 1985; 15:7). In addition, reduced erythrocyte (Prasad, JLabClinMed, 1965; 66:508) and leucocyte zinc content (Keeling, ClinSci, 1982; 62:109) have been found in liver disease. Malabsorption of zinc has been described in non-alcoholic cirrhosis (Karayalcin, DigDisSci, 1988; 33:1096; Gohshi, Hepatogast, 1995; 42:487). Thus, alcohol intake *per se* does not account for the observed deficiency of zinc. In addition to other factors, portosystemic shunting seems to be of importance for the development of zinc deficiency in cirrhosis (Schölmerich, Hepatogast, 1983; 30:143; Ming, ChinMedJ, 1988; 101:267). However, the hepatic zinc concentration of 26 patients with portocaval shunts did not differ significantly from that of 37 control subjects (164 ± 12 compared with 166 ± 12 µg/g dry weight) (Adams, Hepatol, 1994; 19:101). A shift to non-protein ligands (Schlechter, EurJClinInv, 1976; 6:147) with resulting hyperzincuria (Srivastava, JAssocPhysInd, 1981; 28:303) has been described.

Symptoms of zinc deficiency occur in liver cirrhosis; in particular, dark-adaption abnormalities, abnormal sense of taste and smell, and skin abnormalities have been studied.[21,22] Lower serum zinc has been found in patients with hypogonadism in liver cirrhosis (Abdu-Gusau, EurJClinNutr, 1989; 43:53). An association of zinc deficiency with hepatic encephalopathy has been postulated

Table 4 Other trace elements in man

Element in order of abundance	Atom weight	Total in adult-man (average mg)	Ease of dietary absorption (%)	Plasma concentration (µg/dl)	Binding to plasma components	Main organ of accumulation	Liver concentration (µg/g wet weight)	Main route of excretion
Fluorine (F)[a]	18.90	2500–4000	40–100	20–100	Albumin	Bone, teeth	0.05–0.9[b]	Urine
Silicon (Si)[a]	28.06	(1100)[c]	(1–4)	500	Monosilicic acid	Skin	10–15	Urine?
Zirconium (Zr)	91.22	250–420	0.01		Transferrin (?)	Fat?	6.3	?
Strontium (Sr)	87.63	340	<20		5% bound, 50% chelated	Bone	0.02	Urine?
Rubidium (Rb)	85.48	320	90	20	Free ions (like K$^+$)	None	25–50[b]	Urine?
Boron (B)[a]	10.82	48	99	2,2 ± 0.5		Bone	0.1–0.2	Urine
Barium (Ba)	137.36	22	1–15	2.0–10.0		Skin?		Urine
Germanium (Ge)	76.60	(20)	Easy			Spleen	(0.2)	Urine
Iodine (I)[a]	126.92	10–20	100	2.4	Mainly as T_3, T_4	Thyroid	0.01–0.02	Urine
Tin (Sn)[a]	118.70	14	2			Liver, spleen	0.35–1	Urine?
Mercury (Hg)	200.61	13	5–10	0.06 (?) 0.5–1.0[b]	Complex	Kidney	0.5	Urine
Titanium (Ti)	47.90	9	1–2			(Lung), hair[d]	0.08–0.15	Bile?
Tellurium (Te)	127.61	7	20–50			Bone		Urine
Antimony (Sb)[a]	121.76	6	Poor			Spleen, liver, kidney		Bile, sweat glands

[a] Determined as essential (at least for animals).
[b] Value for various animal species.
[c] Values in parentheses uncertain.
[d] Accumulation from airborne sources and from Ti-screw tapes or fixtures.
(Table modified from Linder MC, SemLivDis, 1984; 4:264–76, with permission; part of data from ref. 10.)

(Reding, Lancet, 1984; ii:493; Grüngreiff, ZGastr, 1988; 26:409; Garcia-Compean, GastrClinBiol, 1994; 18:295), since an inverse relationship has been found between zinc and ammonia concentration. Serum zinc concentrations were significantly lower in patients with hepatic encephalopathy and correlated inversely with serum bilirubin concentrations and prothrombin time (Loomba, IndJGastro, 1995; 14:51). In zinc deficiency, abnormalities of urea-cycle enzymes have been described (Rabbani, AmJPhysiol, 1978; 235:E203; Rahmatullah, Experientia, 1980; 36:1281; Schölmerich, Gastro, 1989; 96:A657). Concentrations of zinc in the brain were decreased in animals with hepatic encephalopathy (Baraldi, BrainRes, 1983; 258:170).

Finally, zinc deficiency has been implicated in the pathogenesis of alcoholic liver disease (Moussavian, Hepatol, 1981; 1:533). Collagen formation was decreased with oral zinc after tetrachloride injury (Antinen, Gastro, 1984; 86:532). Zinc deficiency favoured fibrogenesis in alcoholic liver disease (Panés, JHepatol, 1985; 2:300), and zinc supplementation decreased fibrogenesis in rats with portocaval shunts (Alie, JHepatol, 1988; 7:S3). Furthermore, it has been proposed that alcoholic hepatitis occurs only in the subgroup of alcoholics with zinc deficiency (ref. 13, p.333). Liver alcohol dehydrogenase is decreased in cirrhotic liver and is correlated with liver zinc (Mills, ClinSci, 1983; 64:527). In hepatoma, zinc concentration is 60 per cent lower than in surrounding hepatic tissue

(Okuno, TraceElemMed, 1988; 5:130). Low plasma zinc concentrations and elevated oestradiol levels have been found in patients with chronic liver disease and hepatocellular carcinoma (Frezza, Hepatogast, 1994; 41:367). Zinc deficiency may also contribute to the development of oesophageal carcinoma often observed in alcoholics (Narang, TraceElemMed, 1994; 11:109). Seemingly excessive hepatic zinc concentrations have been described in association with severe progressive cholestasis in childhood. The reported zinc concentration within the liver, however, was not particularly high, and the meaning of the results remains unclear (Phillips, Lancet, 1996; 347:866).

Treatment and/or substitution in liver disease

Oral supplementation of zinc is possible in patients with cirrhosis, although uptake is reduced (Schölmerich, AmJClinNutr, 1987; 45:1487). Zinc must be taken 1 h before a meal in order to be sufficiently absorbed. Zinc–amino acid complexes are better tolerated and lower doses may be used (Schölmerich, AmJClinNutr, 1987; 45:1480, 1487).

Oral substitution with zinc in cirrhosis leads to improvement of dark adaption (Morrison, AmJClinNutr, 1978; 31:276; Herlong, Hepatol, 1981; 1:348), taste abnormalities (Weismann, ActaMedScand, 1979; 205:361), hyperkeratosis (Weismann, ArchDermatol, 1978; 114:1509), and immune function (Solis Herruzo, GastroHepato, 1984; 7:33; Verneau, GastrClinBiol, 1984; 8:121). Only two of these studies have been placebo controlled. In contrast, controlled trials have failed to show any effect upon hypogonadism (Goldiner, JAmCollNutr, 1983; 2:157) or hypogeusia and hyposmia (Sturniolo, JHepatol, 1985; 1:136).

Zinc has been used to treat hepatic encephalopathy in animal studies and clinical trials in man. In experimental cirrhosis of the rat, zinc supplementation reduced the blood ammonia concentration significantly, and increased liver ornithine transcarbamylase activity (Riggio, Hepatol, 1992; 16:785). In humans, beneficial effects on hepatic encephalopathy were found in two placebo-controlled trials (Reding, Lancet, 1984; ii:493, Bresci, EurJMed, 1993; 2:414) and in single case reports (Antoniello, ItalJGastr, 1986; 18:27, van der Rijt, Gastro, 1991; 100:1114). A controlled study showed that 3 months of zinc histidine and zinc sulphate improved hepatic encephalopathy, dark adaption, and hypogeusia when compared with placebo.[21] Another placebo-controlled crossover study showed no improvement of hepatic encephalopathy after short-term oral zinc supplementation (Riggio, DigDisSci, 1991; 36:1204). In a controlled study, zinc supplementation was not able to increase the seroconversion rate after hepatitis B vaccination in patients with chronic uraemia and proven zinc deficiency who were undergoing haemodialysis (Holtkamp, TraceElemElectrol, 1995; 12:32).

The role of zinc substitution in chronic liver disease, and its potential in the prevention of fibrosis, warrants further studies.

Competition for absorption between zinc and copper (Festa, AmJClinNutr, 1985; 41:285) is the basis for the treatment of Wilson's disease with zinc (Brewer, Drugs, 1995; 50:240). The zinc-induced increase of metallothionein concentrations is not paralleled by increased copper concentrations within the intestinal endothelial cells, suggesting a direct luminal effect of zinc on copper transport into the epithelial cell (Reeves, NutrRes, 1994; 14:897). A high body content of zinc is necessary to achieve this effect (Cossack, JPediatGastrNutr, 1987; 6:296). The antagonistic effect of zinc therapy is maintained after the cessation of zinc supplementation (van den Hamer, TraceElemMed, 1984; 1:88). With high doses of zinc, copper deficiency may occur leading to anaemia and leucopenia (Hoffman, Gastro, 1988; 94:508, Sohler, TraceElemMed, 1987; 4:173).

Other trace elements

Several trace elements have been little, or not at all, studied in relation to the liver or its diseases. Basic data, as far as they are available, are given in Table 4.[1,9,10]

References

1. Linder MC. Other trace elements and the liver. *Seminars in Liver Disease*, 1984; **4**: 264–76.
2. Kruse-Jarres JD. Clinical indications for trace element analyses. *Journal of Trace Elements, Electrolytes, and Health Diseases*, 1987; **1**: 5–19.
3. McClain CJ, Marsano L, Burk RF, and Bacon B. Trace metals in liver disease. *Seminars in Liver Disease*, 1991; **11**: 321–39.
4. Ochs A, Heck D, Schaefer HE, and Gerok W. Toxic elements in tissue sections detected by proton induced X-ray emission (Micro-PIXE). *Progress in Histochemistry and Cytochemistry*, 1991; **23**: 164–77.
5. Knapp G. Sample preparation techniques—an important part in trace element analysis for environmental research and monitoring. *International Journal of Environmental Analytical Chemistry*, 1985; **22**: 71–83.
6. Folkmann F. Analytical use of ion-induced X-rays. *Journal of Physics E. Experimental: Science Instruments*, 1975; **8**: 429–44.
7. Milman N, Laursen J, Podenphant J, and Asnaes S. Trace elements in normal and cirrhotic human liver tissue I. Iron, copper, zinc, selenium, manganese, titanium, and lead measured by X-ray fluorescence spectrometry. *Liver*, 1986; **6**: 111–17.
8. Milman N, Laursen J, Asnaes S, and Podenphant J. Elements in normal and cirrhotic human liver tissue II. Potassium, sulphur, chlorine and bromine measured by X-ray fluorescence spectrometry. *Liver*, 1987; **7**: 206–10.
9. Kägi JHR and Kojima Y, eds. *Metallothionein II*. Basel: Birkhäuser, 1987.
10. Iyengar V and Woittiez J. Trace elements in human clinical specimens: evaluation of literature data to identify reference values. *Clinical Chemistry*, 1988; **34**: 474–81.
11. Nielsen FH. Ultratrace elements of possible importance for human health: an update. *Progress in Clinical and Biological Research*, 1993; **380**: 355–76.
12. Brätter P and Schramel P, eds. *Trace element analytical chemistry in medicine and biology*, Vol. 5. Berlin: de Gruyter, 1988.
13. Powell LW, ed. *Metals and the Liver*. New York: Marcel Dekker, 1978.
14. Mertz W. Essential trace metals: new definitions based on new paradigms. *Nutrition Reviews*, 1993; **51**: 287–95.
15. Ritland S and Aeseth J. Trace elements and the liver. *Journal of Hepatology*, 1987; **5**: 118–22.
16. Chesters JK. Trace element–gene interactions with particular reference to zinc. *Proceedings of the Nutrition Society*, 1991; **50**: 123–9.
17. Thuluvath PJ and Triger DR. Selenium in chronic liver disease. *Journal of Hepatology*, 1992; **14**: 176–82.
18. Vallee BL, Wacker WEC, Bartholomay AF, and Robin ED. Zinc metabolism in hepatic dysfunction. I. Serum zinc concentrations in Laennec's cirrhosis and their validation by sequential analysis. *New England Journal of Medicine*, 1956; **255**: 403–8.
19. Boron B, *et al.* Effect of zinc deficiency on hepatic enzymes regulating vitamin A status. *Journal of Nutrition*, 1988; **118**: 995–1001.
20. Turnland JR. Future directions for establishing mineral/trace element requirements. *Journal of Nutrition*, 1995; **124**: 1765S–1770S.
21. Schölmerich J, Löhle E, Köttgen E, and Gerok W. Zinc and vitamin A deficiency in liver cirrhosis. *Hepato-Gastroenterology*, 1983; **30**: 119–25.
22. Schölmerich J. Zinc and vitamin A in liver cirrhosis. In Boyer JL and Bianchi L, eds. *Liver cirrhosis*. Lancaster: MTP Press, 1987: 421–32.

Haem biosynthesis and excretion of porphyrins

Yves Nordmann

Introduction

Porphyrins are molecules that are precursors of haem in the animal kingdom and of chlorophyll in the vegetable kingdom. Synthesis of porphyrins occurs in nearly all mammalian cells, mostly in liver and in erythropoietic tissues. Haemoproteins such as haemoglobin or myoglobin, mitochondrial or microsomal cytochromes, catalase, peroxidase or tryptophan pyrrolase are very important in electron and oxygen transport, in activation of oxygen or hydrogen peroxide, and finally in hydrogen peroxide decomposition.

Haem biosynthesis

Structure of porphyrins

Porphyrins are cyclic tetrapyrroles in which the pyrrole rings, conventionally designated as A, B, C, and D, are linked through their α-carbon atoms by methene (—CH=) bridges (Fig. 1).

The naturally occurring porphyrins all have side-chains on the carbon atoms of the pyrrole rings. The type of side-chain allows us to distinguish between several types of porphyrins (e.g. acetyl and propionyl in uroporphyrins; methyl and propionyl in co-proporphyrins). There are four isomers of each of these porphyrins; only the I and III isomers occur in nature. In isomer I, the side-chains are arranged symmetrically around the ring; in isomer III the substituents on ring D are reversed. In animals the complex between ferrous iron and protoporphyrin is usually called haem. Haem functions as the prosthetic group of haemoproteins.

Biosynthesis

The two types of cells in the body that are responsible for synthesizing most of the haem are the erythropoietic cells (80 per cent) and the liver parenchymal cells (20 per cent). The steps in the pathway are outlined in Fig. 2. The workers most commonly associated with elucidating this pathway are Shemin, Rittenberg, and Neuberger (between 1946 and 1955).

Biosynthesis of δ-aminolaevulinic acid (Fig. 3)

Condensation of glycine and succinyl-CoA to form δ-amino-laevulinic (after decarboxylation of a precursor, α-amino-β-keto adipic acid) is catalysed by δ-aminolaevulinic synthase, a mito-chondrial protein that requires pyridoxal phosphate as a cofactor.

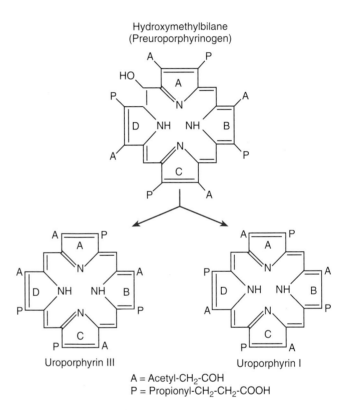

Fig. 1. Structure of porphyrins.

Hydroxymethylbilane
(Preuroporphyrinogen)

Uroporphyrin III   Uroporphyrin I

A = Acetyl-CH$_2$-COH
P = Propionyl-CH$_2$-CH$_2$-COOH

Precursors of this enzyme are newly synthesized in the cytoplasm (on ribosomes) and translocated to the mitochondrion.

Synthesis of porphobilinogen

δ-Aminolaevulinic then passes into the cytoplasm where δ-amino-laevulinic dehydratase catalyses the condensation of two molecules of δ-aminolaevulinic to form the pyrrole porphobilinogen (Fig. 4).

Synthesis of uroporphyrinogen III

Two cytoplasmic enzymes, porphobilinogen deaminase and uro-porphyrinogen III cosynthetase (cosynthetase), convert four molecules of porphobilinogen to uroporphyrinogen III (with lib-eration of four molecules of ammonia).

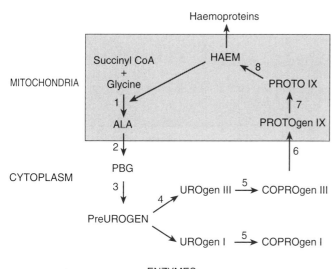

Fig. 2. Biosynthesis of haem.

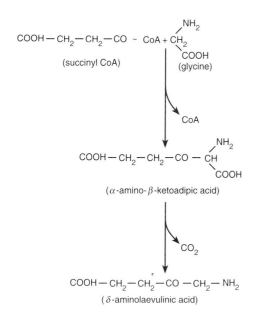

Fig. 3. Biosynthesis of δ-aminolaevulinic acid.

Porphobilinogen deaminase catalyses the condensation of four molecules of porphobilinogen to form a linear tetrapyrrole (pre-uroporphyrinogen or hydroxymethylbilane) (Fig. 1). In the absence of cosynthetase, spontaneous cyclization of preuroporphyrinogen gives uroporphyrinogen I. Cosynthetase catalyses the intramolecular rearrangement yielding uroporphyrinogen III. Only isomer III can be used in the remaining steps.

Synthesis of coproporphyrinogen

Another cytoplasmic enzyme, uroporphyrinogen decarboxylase, converts the four acetic acid side-chains to methyl groups to give

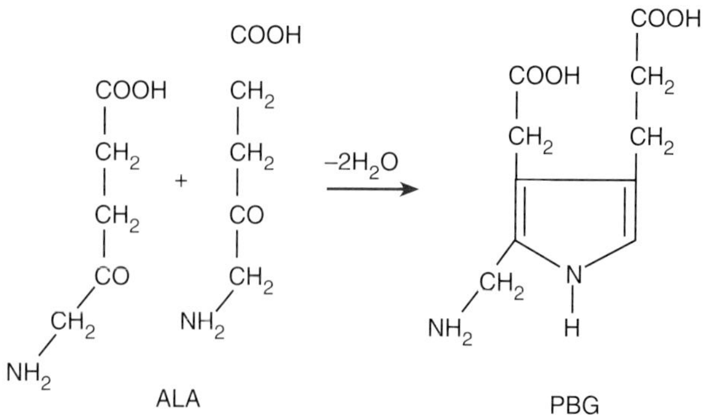

Fig. 4. Biosynthesis of porphobilinogen (PBG) from δ-aminolaevulinic (ALA).

coproporphyrinogen III (Fig. 5). The remaining steps in haem biosynthesis occur in the mitochondrion.

Synthesis of protoporphyrinogen (Fig. 6)

Coproporphyrinogen oxidase oxidatively decarboxylates two propionic acid chains to vinyl groups, giving protoporphyrinogen IX.

Synthesis of protoporphyrin (Fig. 7)

Protoporphyrinogen IX is oxidized to protoporphyrin IX: six hydrogen atoms are removed (four from methylene bridges and two from pyrrole rings). Only oxidized molecules (porphyrins) are brightly coloured, whereas reduced porphyrins (porphyrinogens) are colourless. This oxidation may occur spontaneously; in fact, protoporphyrinogen oxidase, a mitochondrial enzyme, catalyses this step.

Synthesis of haem

Iron (Fe^{2+}) is then inserted by ferrochelatase (or haem synthetase), forming haem. The biosynthesis of haem requires 8 moles of glycine and 8 moles of succinic acid.

Location of steps (Fig. 2)

The biosynthetic pathway starts in the mitochondrion and, after passing through three cytoplasmic stages, re-enters the

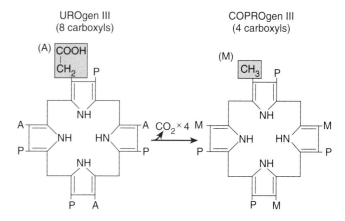

Fig. 5. Biosynthesis of coproporphyrinogen III from uroporphyrinogen III. A, acetyl; M, methyl; P, propionyl.

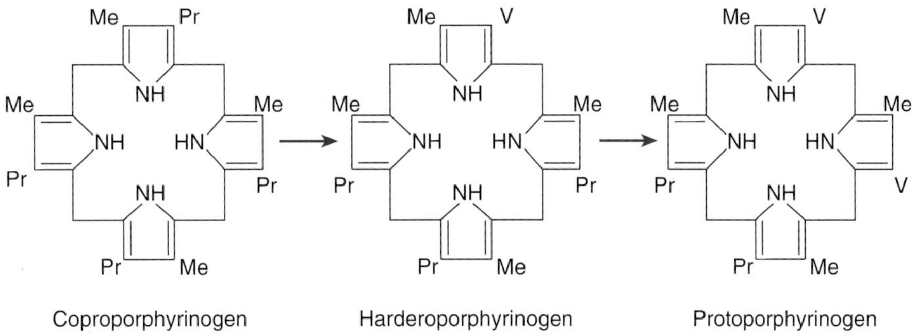

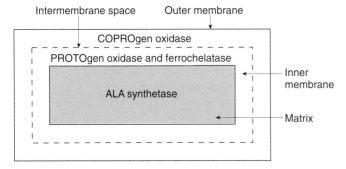

Fig. 6. Biosynthesis of protoporphyrinogen IX. Me, methyl (—CH₃); Pr, propionyl (—CH₂—CH₂—COOH); V, vinyl (—CH=CH₂).

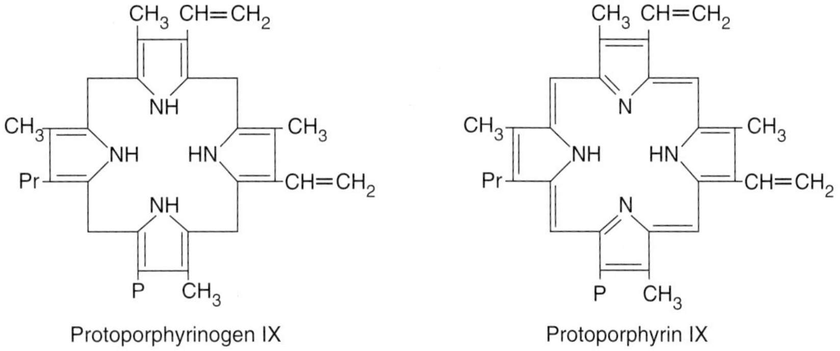

Fig. 7. Biosynthesis of protoporphyrin IX.

Fig. 8. Mitochondrion: location of some enzymes of the haem biosynthesis pathway.

Table 1 Enzymes of haem biosynthesis in human liver: activity	
Enzyme	**Activity (nmol/h/g)**
ALA synthetase	22
ALA dehydrase	2250
PBG deaminase	21
Uroporphyrinogen decarboxylase	1900
Coproporphyrinogen oxidase	1600
Ferrochelatase	2800

mitochondrion for the final steps of haem formation. Location of the enzymes into the mitochondrion is shown in Fig. 8.

Regulation of haem synthesis

In vitro, there are two limiting enzymes in the haem biosynthetic pathway: δ-aminolaevulinic synthase and porphobilinogen deaminase (Table 1). However, *in vivo*, porphobilinogen deaminase does not become rate-limiting when the rate of formation of δ-aminolaevulinic is not increased; therefore only the regulation of δ-aminolaevulinic synthase activity will be described.

The role of haem in liver

There is negative feedback regulation of δ-aminolaevulinic synthase activity by intracellular levels of the end-product of the pathway,

haem. Inhibition of the enzyme occurs *in vitro* at haem concentrations as high as 10^{-5} M, and therefore does not appear to be a physiologically important process. On the other hand, there is strong experimental evidence that haem regulates δ-aminolaevulinic synthase in liver through repression of its synthesis: for example, repression of synthesis of δ-aminolaevulinic synthase under inducing chemicals occurs at a haem concentration of 10^{-7} M. Three potential targets for regulating the formation of δ-aminolaevulinic synthase by haem may be considered: at either (i) the transcriptional or (ii) the translational levels; and (iii) by modulation of the rate of entry of the enzyme into the mitochondria. It has already been shown clearly (Ades, ArchBiochemBiophys, 1987; 253:297) that haem inhibits the production of the mRNA at the transcriptional level; it has also been shown (Hayashi, BBResComm, 1983; 115: 700) that haem blocks the transfer of a precursor form of the enzyme from cytoplasm into mitochondria. There is still controversy about other post-transcriptional effects such as the possibility that haem causes a block in the translation of δ-aminolaevulinic synthase

Table 2 Porphyrin and precursor levels in urine, faeces, and erythrocytes from healthy controls

	Urine (/mmol creatinine)		Faeces (/g dry weight)		Erythrocyte (/l)	
	Mean	SD	Mean	SD	Mean	SD
δ-Aminolaevulinic acid (μmol)	1.60	0.60				
Porphobilinogen (μmol)	0.35	0.15				
Uroporphyrin (nmol)	<20		Traces		Traces	
Coproporphyrin (nmol)	10	6	24	17	76	46
Protoporphyrin (nmol)			48	32	760	275

SD = standard deviation.

mRNA; however this post-transcriptional effect can be explained entirely by the effect of haem on the maturation of the enzyme.

The role of haem in erythroid cells

Recent studies suggest that there are distinct regulatory features of haem biosynthesis in erythroid cells (for example, erythroid δ-aminolaevulinic synthase is not inducible by drugs that induce hepatic porphyrias, except 5-β-H steroids). It is not clear from the current literature how δ-aminolaevulinic synthase is controlled by haem. One finding (Granick, JBC, 1978; 253:5402) was that haem could induce haem-pathway enzyme activities, including δ-aminolaevulinic synthase; this led to the belief that the control of erythroid δ-aminolaevulinic synthase differs from that of the liver and is under positive haem control. In contrast, another finding (Beaumont, ExpCellRes, 1984; 154:474) was that in erythroid cells haem suppresses the induction of δ-aminolaevulinic synthase by dimethyl sulphoxide. There is clearly a need for further work to clear up these contradictions.

However, it is now known that δ-aminolaevulinic synthase is coded for by two genes, one erythroid-specific and one liver-specific: there are two distinct isozymes (Yamamoto, PNAS, 1985; 82:3702).

Excretion of porphyrins and of porphyrin precursors

Porphyrins and porphyrin precursors are excreted in urine and/or in bile. In relation to the total rate of haem synthesis, excretion of porphyrins is very small; in other words, few porphyrins (and porphyrin precursors) 'escape' during haem formation and therefore are not transformed in bilirubin. Each day, bone marrow and liver synthesize about 375 mg of haem. In humans the mean level of δ-aminolaevulinic excreted in urine is approx. 3 mg/day; this means that less than 0.5 per cent of δ-aminolaevulinic synthesized each day has not been used for haem synthesis.

Urine (Table 2)

Porphyrin precursors (δ-aminolaevulinic and porphobilinogen) are excreted only in the urine

After injection, a large fraction of labelled δ-aminolaevulinic is excreted unaltered in urine; a small fraction is much more efficiently incorporated into hepatic haem than into haemoglobin of erythropoietic cells, probably because of the relative impermeability of the erythropoietic cell membrane to δ-aminolaevulinic.

Injected labelled porphobilinogen cannot be demonstrated in the liver, probably also because it does not pass the liver-cell membrane; the impermeability of the cell membrane is only relative, since in instances where the amount of endogenous porphobilinogen is considerably increased (for instance, acute porphyrias), huge amounts of porphobilinogen are found in urine. Moderately increased excretion of precursors is also observed in patients with hepatic diseases.

Porphyrins

Coproporphyrin is the predominant porphyrin in normal human urine (Table 2). However, urine contains only 30 to 35 per cent of the total coproporphyrin; the remainder is found in bile. The type III isomer predominates (70 per cent) over the type I in urine, whereas the reverse is found in bile. It is now widely accepted that the unequal excretion rates of the isomers can be attributed to a hepatic carrier that favours the excretion of the I isomer (Kaplowitz, JCI, 1972; 51:2895). In several human liver diseases with impaired hepatic excretory mechanisms there is an increase in the total urinary excretion of coproporphyrin with a concomitant shift in the isomer ratio towards a predominance of the type I compound.

Other porphyrins present in normal human urine include uroorphyrin and traces of porphyrins with seven, six, and five carboxyl groups. A large fraction of the porphyrins present in urine is excreted in the form of reduced, colourless precursors (porphyrinogens). Freshly voided urine of patients with acute porphyria may have little if any increase in concentrations of preformed porphyrin; this probably explains why urine is frequently of normal colour when freshly passed, but darkens gradually on exposure to light and air. Porphobilinogen can also be converted non-enzymatically to porphyrins (mostly uroporphyrin type I) by exposure to light and air: it is therefore very important to protect urine from light and to store it between 4 and 10°C if precursors have to be measured.

Faeces (Table 2)

Significant amounts of porphyrins are excreted in faeces (mostly the whole protoporphyrin and 70 per cent of coproporphyrin). They may represent pigments that have reached the intestinal tract with the bile; however, they may be derived from chlorophyll and haem proteins of ingested food or intestinal haemorrhages; they may also be formed by intestinal micro-organisms. Because of this, faecal porphyrins should be measured only if the patient's food has been devoid of green vegetables and bleeding meat over the past 3 days.

The mechanism by which protoporphyrin is excreted into bile has been studied mostly after description(s) of fatal liver disease in erythropoietic protoporphyria (see Chapter 20.5). Among haem-forming tissues, the bone marrow is the major source of proto-orphyrin, a very poorly water-soluble compound: in the plasma, over 90 per cent of protoporphyrin is bound to albumin (Bloomer, Hepatol, 1988; 8:402) with some bound to haemopexin (Lamola, BiochemJ, 1981; 196:693). Within the hepatocyte, protoporphyrin is associated with several proteins, among them one of the Z class of liver cytosolic proteins (Vincent, JBC, 1985; 260:14521).

The mechanism by which the liver clears protoporphyrin from the plasma has not been clearly demonstrated. Since most of the protoporphyrin in plasma is bound to albumin, hepatic uptake may occur through a process similar to that for other organic anions (such as bilirubin or bromosulphonephthalein) that are bound to albumin. This involves a receptor protein for protoporphyrin in the plasma membrane (Bloomer, Hepatol, 1988; 8:402). In the isolated, *in situ*-perfused rat liver the overall disappearance of protoporphyrin followed first-order kinetics; the rate-limiting step for the overall transport of protoporphyrin from plasma to bile appeared to be canalicular secretion, since less than 5 per cent of the protoporphyrin extracted by liver was secreted into bile (Avner, JLabClinMed, 1982; 99:885). The basal rates of bile secretion of porphyrins have also been studied in healthy humans (McCormack, EurJClinInv, 1982; 12:257): the flow of protoporphyrin (mean value, 39 nmol/h) is slightly higher than the flow of coproporphyrin (mean, 27 nmol/h); the flow of uroporphyrin is lower (mean, 5 nmol/h).

Hepatic conjugation with glucuronic acid does not occur for protoporphyrin and coproporphyrin. Approximately 85 per cent of hepatic protoporphyrin remains metabolically unaltered before being eliminated by bile secretion; 15 per cent of protoporphyrin extracted by the liver may be converted to bilirubin, with non-haemoglobin haem species as intermediary, and is also excreted in bile.

Hepatic infusion of micelle-forming bile acids facilitates canalicular protoporphyrin secretion (Ibrahim, PSEBM, 1968; 127:890): the micelle-forming taurocholate increased biliary protoporphyrin concentration (by more than six times) and secretion (by more than 12 times), considerably more than dehydrocholate (a non-micelle-forming bile acid). Some bile acids (taurocholate and glycocholate) increase protoporphyrin metabolism 1.7- to 2.7-fold over control values. There are a number of direct and indirect ways in which bile acids might alter the metabolism of protoporphyrin, including either the stimulation of the activity of enzymes such as ferro-chelatase and haem oxygenase or the solubilization of proto-porphyrin (Berenson, Gastro, 1987; 93:1086). Before its final faecal excretion a significant proportion of protoporphyrin is reabsorbed in the intestine and may circulate through the enterohepatic system (Ibrahim, PSEBM, 1968; 127:890). However, it is not yet known how much intestinal micro-organisms or food contribute to the total faecal porphyrin excretion.

Further reading

1. Kappas A., Sassa S, Galbraith RA, and Nordmann Y. The porphyrias. In: Scruver CR, Beaudet AL, Sly WS, and Valle D, eds. *The metabolic basis of inherited disease*, 2, 7th edn. New York: McGraw-Hill, 1995: 2103–59.
2. Meyer UA and Schmid R. The porphyrias. In: Stanbury JB, Wyngaarden JB, and Fredrickson DS, eds. *The metabolic basis of inherited disease*, 4th edn. New York: McGraw-Hill, 1978: 1166–220.
3. Sassa S and Kappas A. Genetic, metabolic and biochemical aspects of the porphyrias. In: Harris H and Hirschhorn K, eds. *Advances in human genetics*, 11. New York: Plenum Press, 1981: 121–231.
4. Moore MR, McColl KE, Rimington C, and Goldberg A. *Disorders of porphyrin metabolism*. New York: Plenum Medical, 1987.
5. Tait GH. The biosynthesis and degradation of heme. In: De Matteis F and Aldridge WN, eds. *Heme and hemoproteins*. Berlin: Springer, 1978: 1–48.
6. Elder GH. Haem synthesis and breakdown. In: Jacobs A and Worwood M, eds. *Iron and biochemistry and medicine*, II. London: Academic Press, 1980: 245–92.

2.18 Functional organization of the liver

Jorge J. Gumucio

The liver is an excellent example of the relation between structure and function. In the last 25 years, considerable progress has been made in our understanding of the compartmentalized nature of liver function. Here, we review present knowledge of liver structure, gene regulation, and the resultant compartmentalized function. Clearly this field has now moved from a descriptive to a mechanistic mode in attempting to define the molecular mechanisms responsible for the compartmentalized expression of genes. The sequences responsible for the expression of some genes in selected hepatocytes have been partially defined. It is conceivable that in the near future we may be in a position, through molecular interventions, to manipulate physiological and pathophysiological liver conditions. This would represent a major change in the way we practise hepatology. This chapter describes the present state of knowledge on the functional organization of the liver and emphasizes the progress made in the elucidation of the molecular mechanisms involved in regulating its function.

The functional unit of hepatic parenchyma

Anatomists have debated for years whether the traditional hexagonal hepatic lobule described by Kiernan,[1] the hepatic acinus of Rappaport,[2] or a more recent version of the lobule,[3] represents the microvascular unit of hepatic parenchyma. A microvascular unit has been defined as that area of tissue in which all liver cells receive blood from a common final vessel. The most recent version describes the microvascular unit as a triangular territory, the base of which is the final septal branch of the portal vein and the vertex, the hepatic venule.[3] However, to date, there is no clear evidence that all cells within that vascular territory or in any other version of a microvascular unit have a co-ordinated function as a unit. What we do know is that liver function occurs at the level of the liver cell plate. Here, we propose that the liver cell plate is the functional unit of the hepatic parenchyma. This view does not preclude the possibility that various cell plates may act in a co-ordinated fashion, but this remains to be defined.

The liver cells

Hepatocytes and bile-duct cells are derived from epithelial cells while the non-parenchymal cells, the endothelial and stellate (Ito, perisinusoidal or fat-storing) cells, are derived from mesenchymal cells. The rest of the non-parenchymal cells, the Kupffer and Pit cells, are derived from haemopoietic cells. The epithelial-derived bile-duct cells are assembled as bile ducts inside portal tracts and the hepatocytes as liver cell plates extending from the portal tract into the hepatic venules. These two types of structures are connected by the bile ductules, located in the portal tract and carrying bile originating in hepatocytes into the bile ducts. The bile ductules or canals of Hering, contain transitional cells and are the proposed site of the liver cell precursors (thought to be ductular or periductular in location).[4]

The hepatocytes are the liver cells in which most of the physiological processes traditionally comprising liver function are performed. The non-parenchymal cells can be visualized as a system encompassing sensors, an extensive communicating network (among non-parenchymal cells, and between non-parenchymal and parenchymal cells) in which cytokines seem to play a predominant part, as well as defensive mechanisms (phagocytosis). The Kupffer and Pit cells are located inside the sinusoids and presumably sense and adapt to intravascular events. The stellate cells are located in the space of Disse, that is, between the sinusoidal domain of the hepatocytes and the external side of the endothelial cells forming the sinusoids. The endothelial cells form the walls of the sinusoids and possess pores or fenestrations that allow the passage into the space of Disse of all molecules with the exception of large chylomicrons, but not of cells. Non-parenchymal liver cells are detailed elsewhere. Therefore, the subsequent description will focus exclusively on the configuration of hepatocytes.

The liver cell plates

The first row of hepatocytes, or limiting plate, surrounds a small portal tract and is in contact with the bile ductules. The limiting plate represents a landmark used by pathologists to define the inflammatory disruption of the hepatic parenchyma. As shown in Fig. 1, the liver cell plate is formed by 15 to 25 hepatocytes that extend from the limiting plate to the hepatic venule. Hepatocytes are assembled in columns one cell thick, surrounded by the space of Disse and the hepatic sinusoids. The space of Disse separates the last hepatocyte in the plate from the endothelium of the hepatic venules. While bile moves from the hepatic venules towards the portal tract, blood moves from portal to hepatic venule. At the entry into the sinusoid, blood is a mixture from the hepatic artery (oxygen tension 146 mmHg) and portal vein (oxygen tension 48 mmHg) (Tygstrup, JClinInvest, 1962; 41:447). We do not know the proportions contributed by each system and therefore we do not know the exact oxygen tension at the sinusoidal entry. The hepatic venules

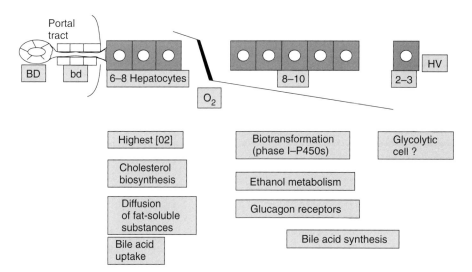

Fig. 1. The liver cell plate, the functional unit of liver. At the intersection of the initial 'periportal' 6–8 hepatocytes and the rest of hepatocytes, we propose that there is a significant oxygen gradient. Also, we propose that the last 1–2 hepatocytes in the plate, contiguous with the hepatic venule, represent 'centrilobular' hepatocytes that are different from the rest of the upstream 'centrilobular' hepatocytes. BD, bile duct; bd, bile ductule; HV, hepatic venule.

have an oxygen tension of approx. 33 mmHg. Therefore, there is a significant oxygen gradient across the sinusoid, although the shape of this gradient inside the sinusoid has not been directly assessed. Blood perfuses hepatocytes in the plate sequentially. There seems to be no significant recirculation of blood. As hepatocytes in the plate are perfused, the composition of the blood changes. Substances such as oxygen are removed, others such as albumin and glucose are secreted. Hence, hepatocytes located in different parts of the liver cell plate are exposed to different microenvironments. This, as discussed below, may have an important influence on the functional compartmentalization of the cell plates.

There has been no three-dimensional characterization of the cell plates, but hepatic sinusoids have been described morphometrically; 'periportal' sinusoids showed a larger surface:volume ratio and a smaller volume fraction than in sinusoids near the hepatic venules (Miller, Gastro, 1979; 76:965). These findings suggest that sinusoids near the portal tracts are narrow, interconnecting, and tortuous, as actually observed by two-dimensional light microscopy as well as by scanning electron microscopy. Although, as mentioned, the three-dimensional configuration of cell plates has not been defined, it is most probable that it is a 'mirror image' of the sinusoids. Light- and scanning-microscopic findings suggest that near portal tracts the cell plates are characteristically interconnected; this configuration is depicted in Fig. 2. Interconnecting plates comprise approximately the initial six to eight hepatocytes. Hepatocytes in this segment do not belong to a distinct plate. Closer to hepatic venules, approximately at the level of hepatocytes 9–10 in the plate, sinusoids change into wider, parallel conduits radially oriented towards the hepatic venules (Miller, Gastro, 1979; 76:965). Concomitantly, at least by simple light-microscopic inspection, the configuration seems also to change into that of well-defined, parallel cell plates, which, as the sinusoids, are more radially oriented towards the hepatic venule. At this level, each hepatocyte has a well-defined location in a distinct cell plate. We propose and discuss below that these differences in the configuration of 'periportal' sinusoids play

a major part in the development, within the initial eight to nine hepatocytes, of a functionally significant oxygen gradient.

Gene expression in the cell plate

As shown in Fig. 3, some genes such as for albumin and C/EBP, are expressed by all hepatocytes, although that for albumin seems to be expressed at a higher level closer to portal tracts (Bernuau, CellBiolIntRep, 1985; 9:31). Some genes, such as for 3-hydroxy-3-methylglutaryl coenzyme-A reductase, the rate-limiting enzyme in cholesterol biosynthesis, are expressed in a few hepatocytes surrounding the portal tracts (Singer, ProcNatlAcadSciUSA, 1984; 81:5556). Therefore, it seems that cholesterol biosynthesis takes place in a few 'periportal' hepatocytes. In contrast, the basal expression of cholesterol 7α-hydroxylase (*CYP7A* gene), the rate-limiting enzyme in bile acid synthesis from cholesterol, is located in a few 'centrilobular' hepatocytes.[5] Circadian variation in expression of the *CYP7A* gene results in the diurnal recruitment of other hepatocytes for expression.[5] Therefore, basal bile-acid synthesis occurs predominantly or exclusively in a few 'centrilobular' hepatocytes. Glutamine synthetase and the expression of the erythroid/brain or GLUT-1 (see below) glucose transporter represent two examples of gene expression restricted to one or two hepatocytes surrounding the hepatic venules.[6,7] The expression of specific genes in the last hepatocytes in the plate has raised the possibility that these last two hepatocytes may be different from other 'centrilobular' hepatocytes.

Regulation of the compartmentalized expression of genes in the cell plate

There are at least two levels at which regulation of gene expression in the cell plate can be analysed. First, gene expression in selected hepatocytes can be the consequence of a transcriptional or post-transcriptional turning on or off of a gene in a hepatocyte, and

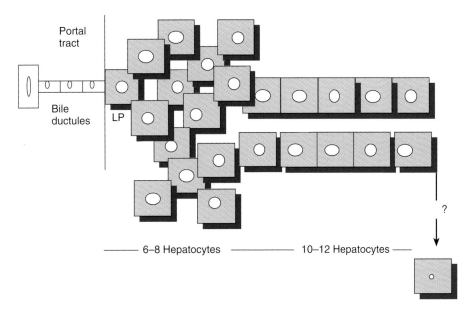

Fig. 2. Hypothetical configuration of cell plates derived from the measured configuration of sinusoids: two types of liver cell plates are depicted. Hepatocyte at the bottom right is apoptotic. LP, limiting plate.

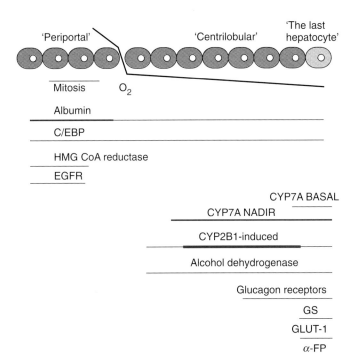

Fig. 3. Gene expression in the adult liver cell plate. *CYP7A* basal, basal expression of cholesterol 7α-hydroxylase gene at the time of minimal diurnal expression. *CYP2B1*, phenobarbital-inducible P450b in the rat. GS, glutamine synthetase; *a-FP*, α-fetoprotein gene; EGFR, epidermal growth factor receptor.

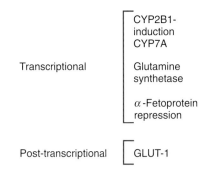

Fig. 4. Mechanisms by which the expression of genes in selected hepatocytes is regulated.

second, there have to be factors which determine that a gene is turned on or off at certain levels in the cell plates. Figure 4 illustrates the level of regulation for the few genes studied. As shown, some are, most probably, transcriptionally regulated, that is, gene transcription is turned on at a specific level in the cell plate, while the

GLUT-1 gene is most probably regulated post-transcriptionally.[7]

An interesting example is provided by the α-fetoprotein gene. This gene is expressed at high levels in fetal liver and is turned off during the first month after delivery. The shut-off is transcriptionally regulated (Vacher, Science, 1990; 250:1732). Three recent studies have shed light on the mechanisms involved in α-fetoprotein expression in the newborn and adult livers. Analysis by *in situ* hybridization in rat liver showed that the α-fetoprotein gene was turned off at different times in different segments of the cell plate; hepatocytes near the hepatic venules turned off the gene the latest (Poliard, JCellBiol, 1986; 103:777). Transgenic mice were later prepared containing an α-fetoprotein construct comprising the known regulators, three enhancers and a repressor, the α-fetoprotein promoter, and a minigene consisting of 5 of the 11 exons: deletion of sequences located between −838 bp and −250 bp in the 5′-flanking region resulted in high levels of expression of the α-fetoprotein transgene in adult mouse liver, predominantly in a few 'centrilobular' hepatocytes (Emerson, DevDyn, 1992; 195:55). Finally, transgenic mice were prepared containing the three enhancers linked to a β-globin promoter and the *H-2Dd* gene (mouse major histocompatibility complex-encoded class I structural gene) used here as a reporter gene (Ramesh, MolCellBiol, 1995; 15:4947). Antibodies were available to recognize the location of the protein. Enhancer 3 located between −7.6 and −5.3 kb determined expression of the transgene in a single hepatocyte surrounding the hepatic venule, similar to the reported expression of the *GLUT-1* and glutamine synthetase genes.[6,7] In contrast, enhancer 2 resulted in expression of the transgene in about one-half of the centrilobular hepatocytes. These studies reveal that hepatocytes in different locations in the cell plate seem to synthesize different transcription factors, which interact, as in the case of the α-fetoprotein gene, with either repressors or enhancers determining expression of the transgenes in selected hepatocytes in the cell plate.

This example suggests that the expression of transcriptionally regulated genes in selected hepatocytes very probably implies the synthesis at specific levels in the cell plate of proteins acting as transcriptional regulators. These proteins are ultimately responsible for the compartmentalized expression of genes and, thus, of function in the cell plate.

We do not know what triggers the synthesis of transcription factors at specific levels of the cell plate. Within the last 10 years there have been two main lines of thought. One, known as the streaming liver hypothesis,[8] proposed that hepatocytes are generated from precursors and move along the plate between portal tracts and hepatic venules. As the cells move, they age and attain states of progressive differentiation. This concept was expanded to explain the generation of hepatomas with different degrees of differentiation.[9] Both aspects of this streaming hypothesis, hepatocyte movement and the age-dependent, progressive, irreversible differentiation, have lost support.[10,11] The second proposal centred on regulation within the sinusoidal microenvironment: substrates, hormones or oxygen concentration at specific sites trigger regulatory events in hepatocytes resulting in changes in gene expression.

Two interesting examples from experiments *in vivo* point toward the sinusoidal microenvironment playing an important part in gene regulation. In the first, the human erythropoietin gene was used to prepare transgenic mice (Koury, Blood, 1991; 77:2497). These mice were made anaemic by bleeding and changes in expression of erythropoietin mRNA in liver were assessed by *in situ* hybridization. Interestingly, expression of the erythropoietin mRNA became apparent only in hepatocytes located distal to the 'periportal' third of the cell plate. This observation indicates that a functionally significant oxygen gradient develops between the initial hepatocytes and those in the distal two-thirds in the plate. This is the first indication of the 'shape' of the oxygen gradient inside the sinusoids. It is of interest that expression of the erythropoietin mRNA was turned on approximately at the level of hepatocyte 8–10, roughly corresponding to the site at which the sinusoidal configuration changes. It is our hypothesis that the narrow and tortuous 'periportal' sinusoids favour contact between hepatocytes and solutes.[6] It is plausible that the transit time of red blood cells in this segment of sinusoids is slower than near hepatic venules, but this needs to be determined. Regardless, transit through this sinusoidal area results in a significant decrease in the oxygen tension of blood, capable, in this experiment, of stimulating erythropoietin expression in downstream hepatocytes. Expression of the erythropoietin mRNA decreased in hepatocytes surrounding hepatic venules even though these cells should be subjected to an even lower oxygen

—— HRE ——

ccc TACGTGCT gtc	Human epo 3′FR
gca GACGTGCG tgt	Human epo 5″FR
gcg TACGTGCT gca	Mouse phosphofructokinase IVS-1
tga GACGTGCG gct	Human phosphoglycerate kinase 1-5′FR
gcg GACGTGCG gga	Mouse lactate dehydrogenase A
ggc CACGTGCG ccg	Human enolase 1-5′FR
ctt CACGTGCG ggg	Human aldolase IVS-4

The HRE acts as an enhancer

Fig. 5. Genes inducible by hypoxia: the hypoxia-responsive element (HRE).

tension than those upstream. This finding suggests, as mentioned above, that hepatocytes in the vicinity of hepatic venules are regulated differently from other 'centrilobular' hepatocytes located upstream in the plate.

Is it possible that oxygen tension in sinusoids may be a major regulator of the compartmentalized expression of genes in the cell plate? Present evidence supports the concept that hypoxia can induce a series of oxygen-sensitive genes,[12–16] as listed in Fig. 5. The mechanisms by which these genes are induced by hypoxia have been best studied with the erythropoietin gene, although, presumably, they are similar to mechanisms operating in other hypoxia-sensitive genes. Induction by hypoxia involves sequences that have received the name of hypoxia-responsive elements, as detailed in Fig. 5. Hypoxia seems to first increase the content of a hypoxia-inducer factor, a protein recently characterized as a basic helix–loop helix–PAS heterodimer transcription factor (Wang, ProcNatlAcadSciUSA, 1995; 92:5510). This protein would interact with the sequences of hypoxia-responsive elements present in these hypoxia-responsive genes, stimulating transcriptional activity. Therefore, the amount of hypoxia-inducer factor has to increase in hepatocytes located in position 8–10 from the portal tract to explain the induction of the erythropoietin mRNA seen in the transgenic experiments detailed above. Therefore, for transcriptionally regulated genes, the crux of gene regulation in liver involves, in addition to general transcription factors needed for liver-specific expression, [17,18] additional transcription factors synthesized by hepatocytes at certain positions in the cell plate. As discussed, one of the microenvironmental regulators triggering the appearance of a zonal transcription factor seems to be oxygen tension. Most probably, there are several other regulators acting on other transcription factors specific for different genes.

The second example which indicates that the sinusoidal microenvironment plays an important part in gene regulation in the cell plate is that of the *CYP7A* gene.[5] As mentioned above, expression of this gene in the cell plate follows a diurnal cycle. At the time of minimal expression, few 'centrilobular' hepatocytes express mRNA for cholesterol 7α-hydroxylase. At the time of maximal diurnal expression, hepatocytes located farther from the hepatic venule are recruited for expression. This suggests that factors triggered by the circadian clock and, most probably, present in sinusoidal blood, act on hepatocytes at specific locations in the plate. It is of interest that the expression of glucagon receptors, one of the few hormonal receptors studied, is compartmentalized. Glucagon receptors seem to predominate in the distal or 'centrilobular' half of the cell plate (Berthoud, AmJPhysiol, 1992; 263:G650). Hormonal effects exerted on selected hepatocytes because these target cells contain specific receptors may have a major influence on zonal gene expression. Similarly, other potential regulators, such as the epidermal growth factor receptor, are also compartmentalized; they are found predominantly in 'periportal' hepatocytes (Marti, EurJCellBiol, 1991; 55:158).

Physiological and pathophysiological hepatocyte renewal in the cell plate

Injection of [³H]thymidine results in incorporation of this DNA precursor predominantly in hepatocytes located in positions 3–5 in the liver cell plate (Blikkendaal-Lieftinck, ExpMolPath, 1977; 26: 184). This finding indicates that these two or three hepatocytes have the fastest turnover rate. Still, the turnover rate of hepatocytes is very slow, estimated at between 148 and 400 days, a range that reveals how difficult it is to measure cell turnover at such a slow rate. Since hepatocytes can divide, the assumption is that cell replication originating in these areas of fastest relative turnover maintains the population of hepatocytes under physiological conditions. It is also assumed that apoptosis occurs at the end of the cell plate (Benedetti, JHepatol, 1988; 6:137). Again, apoptosis has been difficult to determine given the slow cell turnover.

A recent attempt to establish the nature of hepatocyte movement in the cell plate involved the labelling of hepatocytes by *in vivo* transfection with recombinant retroviral vectors. These vectors contained the β-galactosidase gene of *Escherichia coli* coupled to a nuclear localization signal and under the control of the viral long terminal repeat.[10] The nuclear localization signal assured that hepatocytes containing the construct would have a blue nucleus on incubation with the substrate X-Gal. There were three rats per group, followed for 3 days, 15 days or 15 months. The location of hepatocytes expressing β-galactosidase was quantified, and two important observations made. First, the rate of replication, as assessed by the size of cluster formation, was faster in hepatocytes near portal tracts than in intermediate hepatocytes near hepatic venules. Clusters grew from the original labelled hepatocytes, increasing its diameter as more cells were formed. Second, the percentage of clusters in each of the three positions analysed, 'periportal' 'intermediate' and 'centrilobular', remained constant throughout 15 months. Although the number of observations was rather low, these findings have been interpreted as indicating that hepatocytes do not traverse from portal to hepatic venules as stated by the streaming liver theory.[8,9]

These observations and proposals raise the issue of how is physiological renewal of hepatocytes accomplished. Are hepatocytes renewed by replication of contiguous hepatocytes? This would imply that to maintain constant liver size, given the differences in replication rate in 'periportal' and 'centrilobular' hepatocytes, apoptosis should occur at multiple sites and at the zonal rate of cell replication. To date, this has not been observed (Benedetti, JHepatol, 1988; 6:137). If hepatocytes are renewed only or mainly from cells of faster turnover located in the 'periportal' area, then the cells have to move, albeit slowly. Following 'centrilobular' damage by

carbon tetrachloride, hepatocytes seemed to move from a 'periportal' localization to the zone of cell damage (Rajvanshi, Hepatol, 1994; 20:266A).

After experimental partial hepatectomy, most hepatocytes are engaged in mitosis (Rabes, CellTissKinet, 1976; 9:517); this is an artificial situation in which normal hepatocytes are called to restore liver size and is not liver regeneration. In humans, a similar condition exists after liver transplantation. The size of the donor liver has to adjust to the size of the recipient to keep the ratio liver–body size constant (Van Thiel, Gastroenterol, 1987; 93:1414). In most pathological conditions, hepatocytes are initially damaged and cell restoration is initiated from a damaged parenchyma. Cell renewal, under these conditions, occurs by replication of hepatocytes. However, recent findings obtained by damaging 'periportal' hepatocytes with allyl alcohol suggest that liver cell precursors are turned on before any hepatocyte replication is observed (Yavorkovsky, Hepatol, 1995; 21:1702). In humans, electron-microscopic studies have revealed that liver cell precursors appear at the periphery of portal tracts under various pathological conditions (De Vos, AmJPathol, 1992; 140:1441). Therefore, the mechanisms of physiological hepatocyte renewal in the cell plate and the roles of liver cell precursors and hepatocyte replication under pathological situations still need to be defined.

Liver function and compartmentalization of physiological processes

The liver is strategically located between the splanchnic and the systemic circulation, interacting with both circulatory systems. It receives blood from the splanchnic territory via the portal vein and from the systemic circulation via the hepatic artery. The liver modifies the composition of the incoming blood and returns it to the systemic circulation via the hepatic veins. Portal-vein blood carries solutes into the liver that have been absorbed from the intestine (mesenteric veins), solutes that have been modified in the spleen (splenic vein), as well as peptides, the products of pancreatic and intestinal endocrine secretion into the portal vein. The liver has a large surface for interaction with these solutes and several mechanisms operate to modify the quantity and quality of solutes that will pass the liver 'filter' into the systemic circulation. Uptake, biotransformation, synthesis, and secretion of *de novo* synthesized or biotransformed products, either back into sinusoidal blood or into bile, are the major mechanisms responsible for these modifications. The hepatic artery allows solutes already in systemic blood to establish contact with the liver on a 'second pass'. This may serve as a feedback loop for events occurring in the territory of the systemic circulation. It can be proposed, as an integrated view of liver function, that the major role of the liver is to provide an adequate concentration of solutes to organs located in the systemic territory—the brain, the muscles, the heart, the endocrine system, and the kidneys. The entire functional organization of the liver is designed to receive and remove raw materials from the intestine, and to biotransform, synthesize, and secrete manufactured products to be delivered into the systemic circulation and intestine via the hepatic venules and bile, respectively. A slow cell turnover, a compartmentalized expression of genes, and the resultant compartmentalized function—a large capacity for synthesis and biotransformation in addition to a unidirectional perfusion of cells with blood coming from both the splanchnic and systemic territories—is the design that has evolved to accomplish these purposes.

Having described the major characteristics of the functional organization of the liver, it seems appropriate to review how complex metabolic processes are performed within this organization. This subject has been the topic of several reviews and will therefore be discussed here mainly as an illustration of the relation between structure and function.

Carbohydrates

One of the metabolic challenges for the liver is the shift from glycogen synthesis and glycolysis, processes predominant during the absorptive state, to the glycogenolysis and gluconeogenesis that predominate during the postabsorptive state.[19] Several factors seem to be involved in the regulation of this metabolic shift: substrate availability, the concentration of glucagon, insulin and other hormones, the activity of hepatic nerves, and finally, the compartmentalization of these processes in different hepatocytes. Hepatocytes located in the 'periportal' area contain higher activities of rate-limiting enzymes involved in glycogenolysis and gluconeogenesis. Those located in the 'centrilobular' area have higher activities of rate-limiting enzymes involved in glycogen synthesis and glycolysis. In addition, receptors for hormones such as glucagon are predominantly located in 'centrilobular' hepatocytes. During the absorptive state, it is proposed, glucose will be taken up by most hepatocytes and converted into glycogen or degraded via the glycolytic pathway. During the late postabsorptive state, 'periportal' hepatocytes will secrete glucose into the sinusoidal blood to supply glucose needed by peripheral organs while 'centrilobular' hepatocytes are seen as mainly glucose-removing cells.

As shown in Fig. 6, hepatocytes have two glucose-transport systems. The liver glucose transporter or GLUT-2 system and the erythroid/brain or GLUT-1 system. While the GLUT-2 transporter seems to be expressed in every hepatocyte (Tal, JClinInvest, 1990; 86:986), the GLUT-1 transporter is expressed by most hepatocytes but inserted in the sinusoidal domain of the plasma membrane, thus becoming functional only in the last one or two hepatocytes contiguous with the hepatic venules.[7] The GLUT-2 transporter has a K_m for glucose of 15 to 20 mmol and is responsible for the bidirectional transport of glucose by hepatocytes. These concentrations of glucose can be attained during the immediate absorptive state. The question is, why do we need a second transporter? The GLUT-1 transporter has a K_m for glucose of 1 to 2 mmol. As mentioned, it is functional only in hepatocytes at the end of the cell plate; those are the hepatocytes subjected to the lowest oxygen concentration. Given both the location and K_m for glucose of GLUT-1, this transporter is most probably not a regulator of glucose concentration in sinusoidal blood (the transporter should be saturated constantly). We have proposed[7] that GLUT-1 is functional at the end of the plate because those hepatocytes, most probably, live off glycolysis. GLUT-1 assures that glycolytic hepatocytes at the end of the plate will receive adequate amounts of glucose even during the late postabsorptive state. This working hypothesis needs to be further tested. It is of interest that several

of the genes controlling carbohydrate metabolism, and especially glycolysis, are induced by hypoxia, as described in Fig. 5 and discussed above.

Lipids

There is still uncertainty as to the metabolic zonation for lipid metabolism. From the zonal localization of key enzymes it was proposed that fatty acid synthesis may occur predominantly in perivenous hepatocytes (Katz, JHepatol, 1985; Suppl.1:S74), which may also be predominantly involved in ketogenesis. It has also been proposed made that energy in 'periportal' hepatocytes is supplied by β-oxidation. However, there is controversy about this proposal, since in some studies the key enzyme 3-hydroxyacyl-coenzyme A-dehydrogenase was distributed almost homogeneously throughout the cell plate. Immunohistochemical studies have shown that the cytosolic fatty acid-binding protein (L-FAB or Z protein), a 14.2-kDa protein, was predominantly localized in periportal hepatocytes of control male rats and inducible by clofibrate in the same hepatocytes; interestingly there was a much more homogeneous distribution of this protein throughout the cell plate in female rats.[20]

Proteins

All hepatocytes seem to synthesize albumin,[7] which is secreted by them into sinusoidal blood and is not taken up by hepatocytes located downstream in the cell plate. To this extent, all albumin molecules synthesized reach the systemic circulation. Among the various functions of albumin, its capacity for binding to various compounds is pertinent to this discussion. Due to the anatomy of the liver sinusoids, solutes in portal blood or hepatic artery blood will first contact 'periportal' hepatocytes. If that solute is taken up by simple diffusion, the first few hepatocytes in the cell plate may remove most of the load.[21] How do solutes with these characteristics reach hepatocytes located in intermediate and 'centrilobular' areas of the cell plate, or reach the systemic circulation?

One of the mechanisms involves solute binding to plasma proteins. Some of these solutes have a great affinity for albumin or other plasma proteins. Binding to albumin decreases the uptake of solutes on first passage, thus allowing a more homogeneous distribution of solutes throughout cell-plate hepatocytes, and, consequently, a higher concentration of these solutes in hepatic vein. This has been shown using substances that can be visualized during hepatic transport such as various fluorescent compounds and bromosulphophthalein.[22]

Bile acid transport and bile secretion

Autoradiographic studies have shown that taurocholate is first taken up by those hepatocytes in contact with the incoming load. Therefore, at low concentrations, taurocholate is taken up predominantly by 'periportal' hepatocytes, with a gradient of decreasing concentrations in intermediate and 'centrilobular' hepatocytes. At higher concentrations, those more distal hepatocytes are progressively recruited to the task of transport (Groothuis, AmJPhysiol, 1981; 243:G455). It has been established that the uptake of taurocholate involves a carrier-mediated, sodium-coupled mechanism deriving its energy from the hydrolysis of ATP by a Na^+–K^+ATPase located in the basolateral domain of the hepatic plasma membrane.

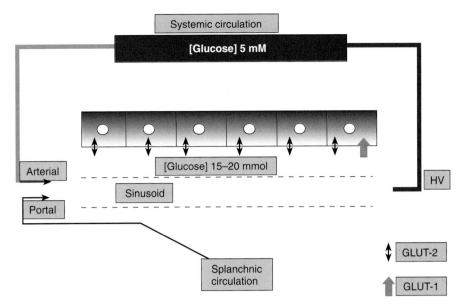

Fig. 6. Distribution of glucose transporters in the liver cell plate. GLUT-1, the erythroid/brain glucose transporter (K_m for glucose of 1–2 mmol) GLUT-2, liver glucose transporter. This is the main transporter of glucose in liver (K_m for glucose 10–15 mmol).

Other bile acids such as glycocholate, cholate, and glycochenodeoxycholate, although taken up by a saturable, sodium-coupled mechanism, are extracted less efficiently than taurocholate on first pass by the liver (Van Dyke, AmJPhysiol, 1982; 243:G484). In general, the higher the extraction rate on first pass, the steeper should be the difference in the cellular concentration of bile acids between hepatocytes located in the 'periportal' and 'centrilobular' areas. Conjugation, the number of hydroxyl groups on the bile acid molecule, and the binding affinity of the bile acid species to albumin also modulate the efficiency of bile acid extraction by the liver. There are also differences in the biliary secretion of bile acids depending on whether the bile acid is transported by a 'periportal' or by a 'centrilobular' hepatocyte. For taurocholate, the rate of biliary secretion is apparently slower in hepatocytes in the 'centrilobular' area than in those in the 'periportal' area. Moreover, studies using taurodeoxycholate showed that the apparent intracellular transit time of this bile acid was slower when perfused in a retrograde fashion (presumably representing transit through 'centrilobular' hepatocytes); concomitant with the slower transit there was a greater degree of biotransformation (Baumgartner, AmJPhysiol, 1986; 251:G431). In summary, there seem to be differences in the relative rates of uptake, intracellular transit time, and biliary secretion of bile acids by 'periportal' and 'centrilobular' hepatocytes, differences that vary with the characteristics of the bile acid molecule to be transported.

Bile acids are main contributors to canalicular bile formation, that is, bile formed in hepatocytes. About 60 to 70 per cent of canalicular bile is secreted as a consequence of the movement of bile acids from hepatocytes into the biliary space across the bile canalicular membrane. The remainder, 30 to 40 per cent of canalicular bile, is called the 'bile salt non-dependent or independent fraction'. The origin of this 'independent' fraction is unknown, although it has been proposed that bicarbonate secretion and, more recently, glutathione excretion (Ballatori, AmJPhysiol, 1988; 254:

G1) play an important part in its formation. Under physiological conditions in the rat, an animal without a gallbladder, 'periportal' and 'intermediate' hepatocytes take up most of the bile acid load. Therefore, these hepatocytes would be mainly responsible for the generation of the 'bile salt-dependent fraction' of canalicular bile. It is possible that in man, during the interdigestive period, 'periportal' hepatocytes are also mainly involved in bile acid transport. However, after a meal, and following the contraction of the gallbladder, large amounts of bile acids are released into the intestine. These will be reabsorbed and presented to the liver. The increased load will probably result in the recruitment of most hepatocytes in the cell plate for bile acid transport.

The *CYP7A* gene seems to be predominantly regulated at the level of transcription; in agreement with this, the activity of this rate-limiting enzyme in bile acid synthesis was found to be several-fold higher in perivenous than in periportal hepatocytes (Ugele, BiochemJ, 1991; 276:73). Since cholesterol 7α-hydroxylase activity seems to be under the negative feedback control of bile acids, it is conceivable that the higher enzyme activity in 'centrilobular' hepatocytes may be explained by a lower concentration of bile acids in these cells. According to this proposal, during the immediate postabsorptive state (7–9 p.m.) in the rat, hepatocytes located in the 'periportal' and 'intermediate' areas of the plate are subject to the highest concentrations of inhibitory bile acids. During this time, expression of the cholesterol 7α-hydroxylase mRNA occurs in a few hepatocytes surrounding the hepatic venules.[5] Thus, 'centrilobular' hepatocytes seem to be predominantly involved in basal bile-acid synthesis. This may be explained, in part, by the low concentration of bile acids in these hepatocytes. However, as discussed above, other factors also regulate the expression of the *CYP7A* gene in liver.[5] Therefore, transcriptional regulation of the *CYP7A* gene in the cell plate most probably involves bile salts, circadian regulators, and hormones.

The removal of ammonia by the liver: urea and glutamine synthesis

The concentration of arterial ammonia (about 30 mmol/l) is maintained by the balance between ammonia generated in various tissues (intestines, kidney) and ammonia removed by the liver. Urea synthesis and glutamine synthesis are the two major pathways used by the liver in this process. Of these, urea synthesis is responsible for 95 per cent of the ammonia removed. Immunohistochemical studies have shown that the enzymes involved in the synthesis of urea, such as carbamylphosphate synthetase, are predominantly localized in 'periportal' and 'intermediate' hepatocytes (Moorman, JHistochemCytochem, 1988; 36:751). In contrast, glutamine synthetase is exclusively localized in one or two rows of hepatocytes surrounding the hepatic venules.[6] In addition to this zonal compartmentalization of crucial enzymes, studies involving perfusion of the liver from either the portal to the hepatic vein (anterograde) or vice versa (retrograde) have also shown this metabolic compartmentalization. Thus, when these perfusions were performed under conditions in which ammonia supply was rate-limiting, urea synthesis occurred predominantly in 'periportal' hepatocytes while glutamine was synthesized by 'centrilobular' hepatocytes (Haussinger, EurJBioch, 1983; 133:269). Of interest, the affinity for ammonia of these two processes is different. The periportal carbamylphosphate synthetase has a relatively high K_m for ammonia (above 50 mmol/l) while the perivenular glutamine synthetase has a lower K_m. Based on these kinetic differences as well as on the localization of the two enzymes, it has been proposed that the removal of ammonia by the liver cell plate is organized in a zonal manner. Urea synthesis, a process with a low affinity but a high capacity for processing of ammonia, is localized at the entry to the cell plate. Here, it should encounter the highest concentrations of ammonia. As the concentration of ammonia in sinusoidal blood decreases, another system, glutamine synthetase with a higher affinity for ammonia but lower capacity for processing, takes over, providing a final adjustment in ammonia concentration immediately before sinusoidal blood reaches the systemic circulation.

Biotransformation

Biotransformation has been divided into two phases: initial modifications resulting in a more polar compound or phase I, and conjugation or phase II. Of these two phases, the distribution of the mixed-function oxidase system in the cell plate has been more extensively studied. The product of the interaction between a drug and the phase I system may be a less active metabolite, a more active metabolite, or a toxic metabolite that needs to be removed by conjugation (phase II) to avoid the initiation of intracellular damage. The NADPH–cytochrome P450 reductase and various cytochromes P450 play a major part in phase I of drug biotransformation. Immunofluorescence studies have shown that the NADPH–cytochrome P450 reductase is predominantly localized in 'intermediate' and 'centrilobular' hepatocytes. In contrast to the reductase, of which only one form is known, the cytochromes P450 are members of a multigene superfamily (known as *CYP* genes). Several families of cytochrome P450, each with various members, have been described. These multiple isoenzymes encoded by different genes provide the versatility that the liver needs for the biotransformation of multiple compounds with very different chemical structures. The cytochromes P450 can be induced by several compounds, but the induction is compartmentalized. For instance, the phenobarbital-inducible and the methylcholanthrene-inducible forms of P450 predominate in 'intermediate' and 'centrilobular' hepatocytes (Baron, JBiolChem, 1981; 256:5931). Also, the induction of the ethanol-inducible form of P450 occurs mainly in 'centrilobular' hepatocytes (Ingelman-Sandberg, Biochem-BiophysResComm, 1988; 157:55). The present concept is that hepatocytes located distal to hepatocytes 6–8 in the cell plate are responsible for the metabolism of drugs involving the P450 system.

The process of conjugation in the cell plate has been only partially studied. It seems that 'centrilobular' hepatocytes participate very actively in conjugation involving glucuronic acid, while 'periportal' hepatocytes are involved in sulphation (Pang, JPharmExpTher, 1983; 224:647). The physiological advantage of the location of the drug-metabolizing enzyme system not at the entry but more distally in the cell plate is still poorly understood. However, as mentioned above, some of these genes, such as the phenobarbital-inducible *CYP2B1* gene (P450b) seem to be modulated by hypoxia (Webster, Hepatol, 1995; 22:221A). It is therefore conceivable that oxygen and hormonal gradients within hepatic sinusoids may play a part in determining the location of the drug-metabolizing system in the cell plate.

Hepatocyte damage: centrilobular cells, the 'Achilles heel' of liver organization?

Most of the liver pathology secondary to drugs, toxicants, and hypoxia, as well as following liver transplantation, involves approximately four to six hepatocytes surrounding the hepatic venules or distal 'centrilobular' hepatocytes. In contrast, it is difficult to damage 'periportal' hepatocytes unless by inflammation. Is it possible that the distal 'centrilobular' area represents the 'Achilles heel' of this structural–functional organization? Given the sequential perfusion of hepatocytes and the oxygen gradient already discussed, the damage-susceptible 'centrilobular' hepatocytes are perfused with blood of the lowest oxygen content. The critical oxygen concentration, if altered further by low-perfusion states such as heart failure, results in damage to the hepatocyte and cell death. Actually, any change in sinusoidal flow slowing sinusoidal transit time will increase hypoxia at the end of the cell plate.

As discussed, most drugs metabolized in liver involve the P450 phase I system. The *P450* genes are expressed and induced by drugs predominantly in the last 8–10 hepatocytes. The *CYP2B1* (P450b) mRNA content after phenobarbital administration is highest in hepatocytes in position 12–14 from the portal tract (Wojcik, JClin-Invest, 1988; 82:658). As a product of drug–P450 interactions, toxic metabolites may be generated in hepatocytes; these will be 'centrilobular' hepatocytes. However, it is predominantly the last four to six hepatocytes that are, most frequently, involved in cell damage, so there must be another factor to explain the location of cell damage at the end of the cell plate. These distal 'centrilobular' hepatocytes are the cells that may derive energy predominantly from glycolysis, possibly a relatively limited source of energy. It is plausible, although not yet well studied, that the capacity of distal 'centrilobular' hepatocytes to either conjugate potentially toxic compounds, to excrete toxic compounds, and/or to repair partial cell damage may be lower than the corresponding capacities of 'periportal' hepatocytes or of 'centrilobular' hepatocytes located upstream from the susceptible area. Finally, distal centrilobular hepatocytes are the first to receive the impact of pathology affecting distal sinusoidal endothelial cells and hepatic venules. For instance, the loss of sinusoidal fenestrations in chronic alcoholics, an event known to affect solute exchange between blood and hepatocytes (Horn, Liver, 1981; 5:301), occurs predominantly in distal 'centrilobular' hepatocytes. Similarly, centrilobular necrosis of the last four to six hepatocytes is a frequent finding after liver transplantation, although its pathogenesis is still undetermined (Turlin, LiverTransplSurgery, 1995; 1:285).

References

1. Kiernan F. The anatomy and physiology of the liver. *Philosophical Transactions of the Royal Society, London,* 1833; **123**: 711–70.
2. Rappaport AM, Borowy ZJ, Longheed WM, Lotto, WN. Subdivision of the hexagonal liver lobules into a structural and functional unit: role in hepatic physiology and pathology. *Anatomical Record* 1954; **119**: 11–34.
3. Ekataksin W, Wake K, McCuskey RS. Liver unit in three dimensions: *in vivo* microscopy and computer-aided reconstruction of microvascular zonation in mammalian liver. *Hepatology,* 1992; **16**: 135–40.
4. Sell S. Is there a liver stem cell? *Cancer Research,* 1990; **50**: 3811–15.
5. Berkowitz CM, Shen CS, Bilir BM, Guibert E, Gumucio JJ. Different hepatocytes express the cholesterol 7a-hydroxylase gene during its circadian modulation *in vivo. Hepatology,* 1995; **21**: 1658–67.
6. Gebhardt R, Mecke D. Heterogeneous distribution of glutamine synthetase among rat liver parenchymal cells *in situ* and in primary culture. *EMBO Journal,* 1983; **2**: 567–70.
7. Bilir BM, *et al.* Novel control of the position-dependent expression of genes in hepatocytes: the GLUT-1 transporter. *Journal of Biological Chemistry,* 1993; **268**: 19776–84.
8. Zajicek G, Oren J, Weinreb M. The streaming liver. *Liver,* 1985; **5**: 293–300.
9. Reid LM. Stem cell biology, hormone/matrix synergies and liver differentiation. *Current Opinion in Cell Biology,* 1990; **2**: 121–30.
10. Bralet MP, Branchereau S, Brechot C, Ferry N. Cell lineage study in the liver using retroviral mediated gene transfer. Evidence against the streaming of hepatocytes in normal liver. *American Journal of Pathology,* 1994; **144**: 896–905.
11. Grisham JW. Migration of hepatocytes along the hepatic plates and stem cell-fed hepatocyte lineages. *American Journal of Pathology,* 1994; **144**: 849–54.
12. Semenza GL, Roth PH, Fang H-M, Wang GL. Transcriptional regulation of genes encoding glycolytic enzymes by hypoxia-inducible factor 1. *Journal of Biological Chemistry,* 1994; **269**: 23757–63.
13. Kourembanas S, Hannan RL, Faller DV. Oxygen tension regulates the expression of the platelet-derived growth factor-B-chain gene in human endothelial cells. *Journal of Clinical Investigation,* 1990; **86**: 670–4.
14. Cowan DB, Weisel RD, Williams WG, Mickle DAG. Identification of oxygen responsive elements in the 5′-flanking region of the human glutathione peroxidase gene. *Journal of Biological Chemistry,* 1993; **268**: 26904–10.
15. Wang GL, Semenza GL. General involvement of hypoxia-inducible factor 1 in transcriptional response to hypoxia. *Proceedings of the National Academy of Sciences (USA),* 1993; **90**: 4304–8.
16. Goldberg MA, Schneider TJ. Similarities between the oxygen-sensing mechanisms regulating the expression of vascular endothelial growth factor and erythropoietin. *Journal of Biological Chemistry,* 1994; **269**: 4355–9.
17. De Simone V, Cortese R. Transcription factors and liver-specific genes. *Biochimica et Biophysica Acta,* 1992; **1132**: 119–26.
18. Zaret KS. Genetic control of hepatocyte differentiation. In Arias IM *et al.* eds. *The liver: biology and pathobiology,* 3rd edn. New York; Raven Press, 1994: 53–68.
19. Jungermann K. Metabolic zonation in liver parenchyma: significance for the regulation of glycogen metabolism, gluconeogenesis and glycolysis. *Diabetes Metabolism Reviews,* 1987; **3**: 269–93.
20. Bass N. Organization and zonation of hepatic lipid metabolism. *Cell Biology Reviews,* 1989; **19**: 61–86.
21. Gumucio JJ. Functional and anatomical heterogeneity in the liver acinus: impact on transport. *American Journal of Physiology,* 1983; **244**: G578–82.
22. Gumucio DL, *et al.* Albumin influences sulfobromophthalein transport by hepatocytes of each acinar zone. *American Journal of Physiology,* 1984; **246**: G86–95.

2.19 *In vitro* techniques: isolated organ perfusion, slices, cells, and subcellular elements

Thomas T. Luther and Nathan M. Bass

Introduction

Much of the fundamental understanding of hepatic pathophysiology has come from the ingenious application of powerful *in vitro* techniques to a variety of research questions. Understanding these techniques provides insight not only into their possibilities as research tools, but also into the limitations of current *in vitro* approaches to the study of liver physiology and disease.

In vitro study enables the dissection of the living organism and its organs into progressively smaller components, yielding information about the function of each (Fig. 1). Once a particular component (e.g. liver, cell, peroxisome) is isolated in a relatively homogeneous state, it can be studied through the systematic manipulation of experimental conditions. As the organism is dissected into increasingly smaller components, many aspects of the investigation of the molecular basis of its physiology and pathophysiology become easier to control and understand. On the other hand, the enthusiasm for these investigative techniques must be tempered by the awareness of the inescapable fact that conclusions based upon data derived from such simplified model systems may not always be validly extrapolated to the biological function of the intact organ or whole organism.

In this chapter, different approaches to the *in vitro* study and 'fractionation' of the liver will be described. Methodological approaches of the major *in vitro* techniques are reviewed, as well as their current applications and limitations. The morphology of most of the cellular entities and subcellular structures described in this chapter is illustrated in Chapters 1.2 and 1.3.

Liver perfusion

Ex vivo perfusion of the liver was one of the earliest *in vitro* techniques to be developed. It allows the study of the liver as an isolated but intact organ, independent of uncontrolled influences resulting from its connection to the organism as a whole: for example, variations in neural afferent input, circulating substrates, hormones, blood-flow rates, and temperature.

Claude Bernard first described a method for perfusion of the isolated rat liver over 100 years ago. It remains a very popular and eminently useful technique. Other *in vitro* techniques, including liver slices, cultured cells and subcellular fractionation, which are of greater value in cell biological research, cannot provide the structural context inherent in the isolated perfused liver, which preserves the overall architecture of the organ. Cell–cell interaction and epithelial polarity are maintained while the physiology of the hepatic microcirculation and the formation and flow of bile remain intact. This technique allows conclusions of a broad, organ-based, physiological significance to be drawn, in addition to inferences regarding function at the cellular level.

Low cost, easy maintenance, and convenient size are the main reasons for the rat being the standard choice of animal for the performance of isolated liver perfusion. Other animals have been used, but far less frequently.

Technique

The organ is prepared according to the following steps.[1] The animal is anaesthetized, and the liver is exposed by transverse subcostal and longitudinal midline incisions and dissected free from the surrounding ligaments. The bile duct is cannulated with fine polyethylene tubing and the liver is heparinized by portal-vein injection. An oxygenated buffer maintained at 37°C is next perfused into the portal vein. The chest cavity is then opened and the superior vena cava is cannulated, while the abdominal inferior vena cava is ligated above the kidneys. The perfusion can be done either with the liver remaining in the carcass of the animal (*in situ*) or the liver can be transferred into a perfusion chamber, where constant temperature and humidity are more readily maintained.

The basic liver-perfusion system consists of three components connected in series: a perfusate reservoir, a pump, and an oxygenator (Fig. 2). The perfusate needs to conform to several criteria: it has to have appropriate buffering properties, it must provide the liver with an energy source and oxygen, and it must maintain oncotic pressure. Krebs' bicarbonate buffer with 10 mM glucose and 1 to 2 per cent bovine serum albumin is most commonly used. The buffer is oxygenated with 95 per cent oxygen/5 per cent CO_2, which also maintains the pH within the physiological range. Addition of red blood cells increases the oxygen-carrying capacity of the perfusate, but the release and metabolism of compounds by the

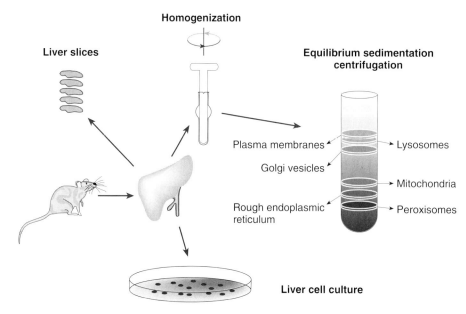

Fig. 1. Overview of *in vitro* techniques. The isolated liver can be perfused or processed into liver slices. Cells isolated from the liver can be maintained in culture. Following homogenization, liver tissue can be used to isolate subcellular elements using techniques that include equilibrium sedimentation centrifugation.

circulating cells may influence experimental results. The oxygen-carrying capacity of the perfusate is more conveniently increased by the incorporation of a fluorocarbon emulsion (Fluosol®) into the perfusate, which is then oxygenated via a gas-permeable tubing 'lung' (Lutz, PfleugersArch-Physiol, 1978; 376:1). Depending on the purpose of the experiment, other compounds (e.g. amino acids, lipoproteins) can be added to the perfusate. Continuous infusion of bile acids in the perfusate is physiological in the rat as this species lacks a gallbladder. In studies of bile formation and biliary excretion, supplementation of bile acids is essential for maintaining bile flow and transcellular transport at normal levels.

Liver perfusion lends itself to a variety of experimental variations. Simultaneous perfusion of the portal vein and hepatic artery has been used in some experimental settings to increase the viability of bile-duct epithelial cells, to examine the contribution of hepatic arterial flow, and for the delivery of hormones and substrates via the arterial circulation (Watanabe, Hepatol, 1994; 19:1198; Miura, Hepatol, 1993; 18:1410). The direction of flow can be reversed from the normal, or physiological, anterograde (portal-to-central) to retrograde (central-to-portal) directions. Changing the direction of flow in this manner has proved useful in the study of zonal differences in hepatocellular functions including extraction of bile acids, the metabolism of amino acids and glucose, and the bio-transformation of pharmacological agents.

Recirculating perfusate is often used in experiments where metabolites or compounds that are synthesized *de novo* by the liver are the subject of interest. Over time, the accumulation of products (e.g. proteins, lipoproteins) or metabolites in the per-fusate permits their detection in measurable concentrations. By the same token, the progressive accumulation of toxic metabolites in the perfusate may also limit the viability of the perfused organ. Once-through, or non-recirculating, perfusion of the liver is used most often for measuring the first-pass extraction of drugs and other compounds.

Applications

The isolated, perfused rat liver has proved a valuable tool in many different areas of hepatobiliary research (Table 1). The perfused liver lends itself particularly well to the study of transport kinetics. Pharmacological variables for a given compound, such as first-pass hepatic extraction and clearance, can be measured as well as substrate interactions and competition for transport. The hepatic extraction and transport of many compounds ranging from small anions and cations to more complex organic ions, including DNA, has been studied with this technique, employing models of varying sophistication and complexity. These have ranged from the simple measurement of first-pass extraction to the modelling of transport in several hepatic compartments using the multiple-indicator dilution technique. In this technique, different radiolabelled markers (e.g. red blood cells, albumin, sucrose, and H_2O) for several distribution spaces in the liver (e.g. sinusoidal, Disse space, and total water space) are perfused simultaneously with the compound of interest.[2]

Since the isolated perfused rat liver can sustain bile flow over several hours and the global architecture and cell polarity of the organ is preserved, the physiology of transcellular transport mech-anisms can be studied in great detail and with considerable validity. This includes the characterization of inhibitors of hepatocellular transport from blood to bile as well as the action of choleretic agents. Indeed, much of the knowledge of the physiology of bile formation has come from studies on the isolated perfused rat liver.

Newer techniques are readily applied to the isolated perfused liver and have further enhanced it as a research tool. Magnetic resonance and microfluorometric techniques have been used to

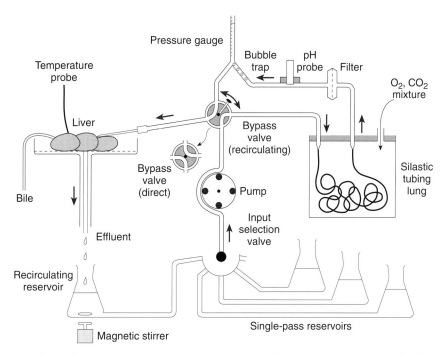

Fig. 2. The isolated perfused rat liver. In the recirculating mode, the perfusate originating from the liver is channelled through the reservoir, pump, membrane lung, filter, pH probe, and bubble trap. In the single-pass mode, a series of samples can be collected at the outflow cannula. The bypass valve is used to exclude system components that are not required for single-pass perfusion. (Reproduced, with permission, from the American Society for Clinical Investigation, Inc., The Rockefeller University Press, and the authors).

obtain direct, dynamic measurements of the concentration of intracellular metabolites. Microfluorometry has been to measure the concentrations of NADH selectively in the periportal and perivenous hepatocytes in the perfused liver. When this has been coupled with switching between anterograde and retrograde directions of perfusate flow, it has allowed the selective probing of zonal differences in the uptake, metabolism, and regulatory influences of different substances. This approach has been valuable in demonstrating important differences in the properties of periportal as compared with pericentral hepatocytes in drug and amino acid metabolism, and the hepatocellular response to extracellular signalling molecules (Haussinger, EurJBioch; 1989; 185:189).

Almost all of the metabolic pathways in the liver that involve the uptake of substrate or release of products have been studied in the isolated, perfused rat liver. These include oxidative phosphorylation, gluconeogenesis, glycogenolysis, ureagenesis, ketogenesis, and conjugation mechanisms (Assimacopoulos-Jeannet, JBC, 1986; 261:8799; Deaciuc, BiochemPharm, 1992; 44:1617; Martin-Requero, BBActa, 1993; 1158:166; Constantin, FEBSLett, 1994; 352:24; Eriksson, BiochemJ, 1994; 298:17).

Among its many versatile experimental uses, the perfused liver has been of fundamental value in the study of the synthesis and secretion of proteins (e.g. tumour necrosis factor-α, interleukin 6, transferrin, coagulation factors, albumin, and lipoproteins) as well as other biologically important molecules (e.g. glutathione, gangliosides, and nitric oxide), and also in the assessment of hepatic responses to noxious stimuli, including hypoxia, hypo- and hyperthermia and cytotoxic drugs (Akerboom, JBC, 1982; 257:4248;

Zimmerman, Hepatol, 1982; 2:255; Lemasters, JCellBiol, 1983; 97: 778; Liao, AmJPhysiol, 1995; 268:R896).

The perfused rat liver has also provided an increasingly important means for studying the physiology and pathophysiology of the intrahepatic microcirculation and its role in the regulation of portal haemodynamics. For example, recent work comparing perfused normal and cirrhotic livers has illuminated a potential role for contractile cellular elements (myofibroblasts) present in the hepatic sinusoids in the modulation of intrahepatic resistance to portal flow. These studies have further indicated a role for endothelin and other vasoactive mediators in the contractile response of these cells (Rockey, Hepatol, 1996; 24:233).

Shortcomings

The isolated perfused rat liver has contributed significantly to knowledge in the basic science of hepatology, but this useful tool has considerable limitations. Not least of these is that the perfused liver is removed from all its normal afferent connections with the intact animal. These include its physiological blood supply and innervation; the perfused liver does not receive autonomic neural stimuli that clearly influence many of the haemodynamic and cellular functions of the organ *in vivo*.

However carefully it is maintained in a perfusion chamber, the liver, once removed, is essentially a dying organ. Even with the best available techniques, the viability of the isolated perfused liver is limited to only several hours. Furthermore, for practical purposes, only livers from small animals such as rats, mice or rabbits can be

Table 1 Research applications of the isolated perfused rat liver

Major applications	Examples
Extraction	First-pass hepatic extraction of organic anions and cations
	Hepatic clearance ($T_\frac{1}{2}$)
	Receptor-mediated endocytosis
	Ion transport
Excretion	Transcellular transport
	Bile formation
	Biliary excretion
Metabolism	Effect of hormones
	Oxidative phosphorylation
	Glucogenolysis
	Glycogenolysis
	Ureagenesis
	Ketogenesis
	Conjunction
Lobular heterogeneity	Localization of hepatic extraction
	Localization of drug-metabolizing enzymes
	Response to adenosine and extracellular ATP
	Metabolism/uptake of amino acids and ammonia
Toxicity	Drugs
	Hypoxia
	Temperature
	Free radicals
	Heavy metals
	Endotoxin
Synthesis and release	Coagulation factors
	Lipoproteins
	Albumin
	Glutathione and glutathione disulphide
	Cytokines
	Gangliosides
	Taurine
	Nitric oxide
Miscellaneous	Neural stimulation
	Intrahepatic haemodynamics

Adapted from reference 1.

studied. Larger organs, and most notably human livers, are very cumbersome to study by perfusion techniques and only a few attempts have been made to perfuse human organs *in vitro* (Burwen, Hepatol, 1982; 2:426).

Liver-slice tissue culture

Liver slices have a long history of use in the study of liver physiology and clinical pharmacology. They have played a particularly important part in the study of the biotransformation and toxicity of drugs and other compounds in the liver. A major advance in this technique was the development of methods for preparing precision-cut liver slices in the mid-1980s. This technique reproducibly yields slices with precisely determined volumes and readily allows the comparative study of livers from different species, including humans (Dogterom, DrugMetDisp, 1993; 21:705; Fisher, HumExpToxicol, 1995; 14:414; Vickers, DrugMetDisp, 1995; 23:327).

Technique

Although manual slicing was the first method used, new cutting techniques have greatly improved the preparation of liver slices.

For precision-cut liver slices, the organ is removed and tissue cylinders are rapidly cored out with a sharpened, rotating steel tube. The tissue cylinders are then sliced with a Krumdieck® or a Brendel-Vitron® tissue slicer by means of either oscillating or rotating razor blades submerged in oxygenated iso-osmotic buffer. The ideal slice thickness is about 200 to 250 μm. This is not easily achieved by manual slicing but is reproducibly obtained with precision cutting equipment. This thin slicing ensures cell viability through the entire width of the slice. On the other hand, necrosis commonly occurs with manually cut slices, which tend to be greater than 0.3 mm thick.[3]

Different incubation systems have been described. In submersion culture, slices are placed in 12-well plates in Krebs–Henseleit buffer with monosaccharides as the carbohydrate source. The viability of slices with this method is usually less than a day. A roller culture method, on the other hand, has maintained viable hepatocytes for up to 120 h. With this method, slices are fixed to a mesh surface and rotated in the tubes containing medium and exposed to an incubator atmosphere.

Cell viability during the course of an experiment is usually determined from the release of intracellular potassium or lactate

Table 2 Research applications of liver slices

Major applications	Examples
Toxicity	Paracetamol
	Aflatoxin B_1
	Halogenated hydrocarbons
	Endotoxin
	Cocaine
	Ethanol
	Cyanobacteria
	Ischaemia
Carcinogenesis	Nitrosamines
Metabolism	Caffeine
	Steroids (including cholesterol)
	Gluconeogenesis
	Lipogenesis
	Ureagenesis
Cytoprotection	Zinc
	Antioxidants
	Fructose
Organ preservation	Cryopreservation

dehydrogenase, and from the maintenance of normal cellular bio-chemical functions such as protein synthesis or gluconeogenesis. Histology is used to evaluate the morphological integrity of cells.

Perfusion systems using liver slices have also been developed; these have been employed to emulate, in principle, the once-through, non-circulating flow of medium of the isolated perfused rat liver.

Applications

Liver slices have been used at least since the 1920s to study the metabolic functions of the liver as well as drug biotransformation and toxicity. More recently, mechanisms of carcinogenesis and hepatic cytoprotection by antioxidants have been studied using this research tool (Chen, FreeRadicBiolMed, 1993; 14:473; Lakshmi, Carcinogenesis, 1995; 16:1565; Martin, Toxicology, 1996; 107:177). It is noteworthy that, in liver slices, the era of liver transplantation has found a convenient model for research into organ preservation. In contrast to isolated hepatocyte cultures, tissue slices offer an *in vitro* system that more closely approximates the *in vivo* context because of the relatively well-preserved microarchitecture, cellular and functional heterogeneity of the slice.

Liver slices have emerged as a potentially useful tool for studying the effects of cryopreservation and cold ischaemia for two important reasons. First, slices can be stored for prolonged periods of time; secondly, this approach dramatically reduces the number of animals usually needed for this type of research in which the results from whole livers are usually compared. The precision-cut liver slice thus offers a convenient, simplified model for the study of whole-organ preservation and, ultimately, for improving results of liver transplantation.

Liver slices have been used in the study of the toxicology of many compounds in the liver (see Table 2), including halogenated hydrocarbons, aflatoxin B_1, endotoxin, cyanobacteria, and ethanol. Recent studies in this field have included the characterization of DNA adduct formation and metabolism of hepatocarcinogens such as nitrosamines (Connors, ChemBiolInteract, 1995; 96:185).

Comparison of the results of liver-slice tissue culture with data from other *in vitro* models, as well as with data from *in vivo* experiments, has generally supported the validity of this technique as a research tool, but this requires further evaluation (Miller, ToxApplPharmacol, 1993; 122:108).

Shortcomings

Although the technique of liver-slice culture has gained increasing attention over last decade—mainly because of methodological improvements—it remains a less popular system for *in vitro* liver research, and its major use has been in the investigation of drug biotransformation and toxicity. Although cell viability has been greatly increased, it has still not achieved the time scale needed to study the full range of cell growth characteristics or long-term drug effects. A two-dimensional aspect of organ architecture is maintained to a degree in the slice, but the physiological, three-dimensional acinar structure, necessary for the study of key aspects of liver physiology such as bile formation, is lost. Indeed, liver slices more closely approximate primary cell culture, but with a heterogeneous cell population embedded in native extracellular matrix, and grown in suspension. Precision tissue slicers also tend to be expensive items of equipment, a potentially important consideration in the decision of whether or not to use this technique.

Cell culture

The understanding of cell biology has been greatly advanced by the ability to isolate homogeneous populations of cells and grow these in significant quantities for extended periods of time.

The earliest attempts at culturing liver cells *in vitro* made use of the liver-slice technique, in which a piece of tissue was transferred to defined medium in a culture dish and successfully maintained for a finite period of time. Shortly after the Second World War, the first cell lines were developed. Since that time, a rapid evolution in the applications of cell culture has occurred. Substantial advances have been made over the past few decades in the technology for the isolation of homogeneous cell populations from the liver and in the culture techniques required to maintain these cells in a differentiated state *in vitro*. Originally, culturing cells literally meant growing them *in vitro* (on glass). We now use the term *in vitro* in a much broader sense to imply the study of a biological system outside its natural or physiological context. In the case of liver-cell culture, glass has long since been replaced by plastic and, more recently, by sophisticated extracellular matrix supports upon which maintenance of many aspects of cell function clearly depends.

Advances in the technology of hepatocyte culture have also promoted the development of new therapeutic applications including hepatocyte transplantation, artificial extracorporeal liver devices, and gene therapy through genetically engineered cells. This is now one of the most exciting areas of technological development in liver research. From a standpoint of developing technologies, the field of liver-cell culture is extremely dynamic, continuing to make important progress on several fronts. For example, the recent introduction of differentiated cholangiocyte lines (Yamada, BrJ-Canc, 1995; 71:543; Vroman, LabInvest, 1996; 74:303) has opened new fields and possibilities in basic liver research.

Table 3 Cell populations in the liver

Cell type	Number (% of total)	Volume (% of total)	Protein content (% of total)
Hepatocytes	60	92	>90
Kupffer cells	15	3	
Endothelial cells	20	3	
Stellate cells	5–8	2	

Technique

Release of cells from the extracellular matrix

Every cell in the liver is tightly connected by molecular interactions to the extracellular matrix and by intercellular junctions to other cells. The first step in the isolation of cells is the disruption of these cell–cell connections, which are strongly dependent on calcium (Berry, JCellBiol, 1969; 43:506).[4] The organ is therefore first perfused with Ca^{2+}-free medium. This step also removes blood from the liver. With rat liver, the entire organ is usually perfused *in situ*; the isolation of cells from human livers has also been successfully achieved through the perfusion of tissue wedges. The liver is next perfused with buffer containing collagenase to digest the polypeptide structure of the extracellular matrix. When dissolution of the structure of the liver first becomes evident, the organ is carefully removed and placed in a glass dish. The fibrous capsule is removed and the liver is gently agitated in buffer to yield a crude cell suspension that can be separated from residual cell clumps and debris by passage through gauze. Intact cells are subsequently sedimented by low-speed centrifugation. The cells are next re-suspended in medium and viability is tested by trypan-blue staining; intact cells retain the ability to exclude the dye. Cells directly prepared from the organ in this manner are called primary cells.

Separation according to cell type

The ratios of the different cell types that constitute the intact liver are listed in Table 3. Several approaches have been developed to separate these different cell types from a mixed cell suspension. These exploit a variety of different physical and biological properties of these cells. Centrifugation and elutriation techniques are based on differences in physical density or size of the different cell types. Differential adherence of cell types present in the liver to glass or plastic has also been exploited for their separation. Finally, cell-specific expression of proteins such as receptors expressed on the plasma membrane can be recognized by specific, fluorescent-tagged antibodies, and has enabled the development of cell separation based on fluorescence-activated cell-sorter (**FACS**) technology.

Centrifugal separation is based on the principle of applying a strong gravitational field to a cell mixture, which then separates according to differences in the size and density of the different cell types. This technique, in modified form, was first developed for the fractionation of subcellular elements. It is described in more detail in the next subsection.

Preparative ultracentrifuges are used to create the large centrifugal forces needed for cell separation. The success of simple preparative ultracentrifugation is dependent mainly on the presence of large differences in cell size. To prevent the separated cell bands from convective mixing, the solution in the centrifuge tube in which the cells are separated can be modified. Density-gradient centrifugation makes use of non-linear, stepwise, or linear continuous-density gradients created using a solution of macromolecules such as Percoll, Nycodenz, arabinogalactan, and Ficoll-Hypaque. This technique exploits differences in the buoyant density of cells, which is independent of cell shape and size. Under the gravitational force generated by centrifugation, each cell moves down the density gradient and eventually reaches a position where its density equals the density of the solution: the isopycnic point.

One major drawback of density-gradient centrifugation for cell preparation is the potential toxicity of the density solution used to form the gradient. Osmotic as well as toxic effects may occur. In this regard, centrifugal elutriation has distinct advantages. The principle of centrifugal elutriation is the separation of particles (cells) according to their rate of sedimentation through two forces, centrifugal force and the flow of a liquid in the opposite direction to the centrifugal force. Particles with sedimentation rates less than that of the flow velocity of the counterflowing liquid stream are washed away from the larger, heavier particles. The liquid used in centrifugal elutriation can be of any suitable composition, so that a physiological solution rather than potentially toxic gradient-forming agents can be used (see Fig. 3).

Cell-specific expression of cell-surface antigenic structures, such as receptors, or the presence of fluorescent intracellular substances (e.g. vitamin A) have been used very elegantly to achieve the separation of different cell types isolated from the liver using the FACS. Antibodies tagged with a fluorescent dye are used to recognize and label cell-specific proteins. The cells then flow essentially in single file in a fine stream through a laser beam and the fluorescence of each cell is determined. Further downstream, a vibrating nozzle forms minute droplets, each of which, for the most part, contains only one cell. Depending on whether the cell has been determined to be fluorescent or not, a positive or negative charge is imparted to the droplet. An electrical field is applied to the cell-containing droplets, which are by this means separated into two streams (fluorescent and non-fluorescent) that are collected in separate containers.

FACS has the disadvantage in that it cannot be used to generate pure cellular fractions in large quantities. It is nonetheless an important analytical tool that has been used to detect differences among subpopulations of liver cells. This approach has also been used to harvest enriched, perivenous and periportal hepatocyte fractions after selectively labelling zones in the liver acinus with fluorescent markers by anterograde and retrograde perfusion (Gumucio, Gastro, 1981; 80:639). Another method successfully used to produce a zonally enriched population of liver cells is a brief

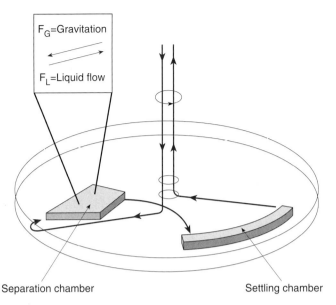

F_G=Gravitation

F_L=Liquid flow

Separation chamber   Settling chamber

Fig. 3. The principle of centrifugal elutriation. The elutriator consists of a rotor with two sets of chambers. One set is functional, the other set is included for symmetry. The separation solution is introduced at the centre of the rotor, from where it is channelled to the bottom of the separation. In this chamber, the solution is pumped towards the centre of the rotor and against the centrifugal field. Fluid emerging from the top of the separation chamber flows next into a settling chamber in which flow is perpendicular to the centrifugal force field and there is no elutriation effect. The purpose of the settling chamber is to allow cells emerging from the separation chamber to be selectively sedimented and hence retrieved. The fluid leaving the settling chamber flows inward to the outlet chamber, where it is removed from the system (McEwen, AnalBioch, 1968; 23:369).

perfusion with digitonin either in the anterograde direction, via the portal vein, or in the retrograde direction into the hepatic vein, to destroy periportal and pericentral cells, respectively, before cell isolation. This allows the harvest of an enriched, zone-specific, hepatocyte subfraction (Quistorff, BBResComm, 1986; 139:1055; Quistorff, BiochemJ, 1987; 243:87).

Pronase digestion, which preferentially destroys parenchymal liver cells, has been used with collagenase treatment to enrich the yield of stellate, Kupffer, and endothelial cells. Often, a combination of the techniques described above may be used to improve the purity of the preparation.

Cell lines

Most mammalian primary cells die after a finite number of cell cycles in culture. Some may survive for several months in culture, but usually die after 50 to 100 divisions. It was speculated that this limitation in lifespan is related to the finite lifespan of the animal from which the cells were derived. In the case of hepatocytes, the primary cells are terminally differentiated, and do not divide further in culture. They also rapidly lose many of their differentiated, cell-specific features once plated *in vitro*.

There are several ways, however, to transform these cells into a cell line, which proliferates indefinitely. Some cell lines (such as HH02, HH09, and HH25) have been developed from normal liver tissue by subjecting cocultures of human hepatocytes with rat liver epithelial cells to frequent subculturing in a highly enriched

medium. The addition of conditioned medium from hepatoma cell lines or treatment of cells with mutagens or carcinogens to propagate spontaneous mutations have also yielded cell lines with indefinite growth. These lines display many of the characteristics of differentiated hepatocytes and exhibit hepatocyte-specific protein expression, including albumin, prothrombin, fibrinogen, α_1-antitrypsin, α_1-acid glycoprotein, and P450 isoenzymes.

Certain viruses induce tumour growth by activation of oncogenes. One such virus, simian virus 40, is able to transform normal primary cells into immortalized clones, which can subsequently be propagated as a cell line. This approach has been used with some success with primary hepatocytes (Fang, CancerRes, 1992; 52: 173; Miyazaki, ExpCellRes, 1993; 206:27).[5] For the most part, however, most hepatocyte cell lines have been derived from spontaneously arising tumours. Hep 3B, Hep G2, SK-HEP-1 and Huh-6 and 7, PLC/PRF/5, and KYN-3 are among the more commonly used human hepatoma/hepatoblastoma-derived cell lines, whereas HTC, Morris hepatoma, RL-PR-C, and H4II EC3 are derived from rat tumours.[6] Recently, cholangiocytes were successfully transformed into several different cell lines (e.g. NRC-1, NRC-2, MZ-ChA-1) (Vroman, LabInvest, 1996; 74:303).

The utility of these cell lines as models for physiological and pathophysiological hepatobiliary research is dependent on the extent to which they share cell biological and biochemical similarity with the primary cell type from which they arose. Unfortunately, a major disadvantage of cell lines is that, almost invariably, they are substantially dedifferentiated from their cell of origin. This is, in part, a consequence of their major advantage: their ability to sustain indefinite growth.

Ideally, primary cells could be used for all experiments requiring isolated cells. However, cell lines are much easier and less expensive to prepare and maintain. Cell lines typically grow rapidly and thus produce considerable material for study without the expense and inconvenience of having to harvest cells from living animals as is necessary for the preparation of primary hepatocytes. Therefore, from a practical standpoint, many more experiments are performed on cell lines these days.

Culturing techniques
Media

In classic cell culture, the cells are plated on to an inflexible, plastic substratum and are suspended in or covered with a liquid medium. The broad array of media employed for liver cell-line culture suggests that no one formulation is dramatically superior to another. The basal media that are commonly used (e.g. RPMI, DME, Ham's F12, Waymouths) were originally developed for culturing fibroblasts. They contain a defined mixture of salts, amino acids, vitamins, trace elements, and carbohydrates. Basal media are usually enriched with 5 to 25 per cent of a biological fluid, usually serum, to supply more poorly defined, but necessary, requirements for cell growth, including hormones (e.g. insulin), other growth factors, and transferrin. The serum is usually obtained from animals that are routinely slaughtered in large numbers, such as cows, horses, sheep or pigs. Calf serum and fetal bovine serum are the most commonly used. Serum-supplemented media appear to serve many of the physiological needs of primary cells in culture, but it must be remembered that serum is not the same as whole blood. The preparation of serum requires a clotting process, which physiologically occurs only under circumstances of acute or chronic injury and which liberates various polypeptides that may affect the growth of cells in culture. It has therefore been speculated that culturing liver cells in serum-supplemented media may produce conditions more representative of the cellular milieu in which fibrosis or cirrhosis occurs.[7]

To overcome this problem and to more clearly define the exact needs of liver cells beyond the 'black box' of serum, chemically defined, serum-free media have been developed. Media for hepatoma cell lines as well as primary hepatocytes are currently available, with defined quantities of hormones, lipids, growth factors and trace elements that permit optimal tissue-specific gene expression.

Cell culture in suspension

Hepatocytes in suspension culture lose viability rapidly, usually over a period of hours. However, for brief experiments, for example studies of initial uptake rates, short-term metabolic processes, or assays of drug biotransformation, primary cells can be studied while suspended in simple media (Schwarz, BiochemPharm, 1992; 43: 1195; Zhou, AntiCancerRes, 1994; 14:1017; Sorrentino, AmJPhysiol 1996; 270:G385).

Substrates

When primary hepatocytes are cultured on glass or untreated plastic dishes, their ability to attach to the support and to migrate outward is greatly impeded, and cell-specific characteristics are lost within hours. These cell-specific characteristics are highly dependent on cell–matrix and cell–cell contact. Irradiation of polystyrene induces negative charges on the surface of the plastic, which allows the cells to attach by charge binding. Synthesis of albumin by cells cultured on plastic ceases after 2 to 3 days, basically paralleling the decline in albumin mRNA. This decline occurs mainly because of a drastic reduction in transcription.

To overcome the rapid dedifferentiation of primary cells in culture, attempts have been made to reproduce their physiological environment *in vitro* as closely as possible. Hepatocytes *in vivo* are in contact with type IV collagen, laminin, heparan sulphate proteoglycan, and fibronectin, the components of a typical basement membrane. The existence of a true basement membrane in the liver has been a matter of some debate, but recent sophisticated immunohistochemical techniques have localized this structure in liver to the space of Disse.[8]

When primary cells were plated on top of various substrates consisting of fibroblasts, type IV collagen, type I collagen from rat-tail tendon, laminin, and fibronectin, none was able to sustain albumin synthesis at normal levels for prolonged periods of time. The introduction of the Engelbreth–Holm–Swarm murine sarcoma gel (**EHS** matrix, now commercially available as Matrigel®), produced in the Swiss–Webster mouse, greatly improved tissue-specific gene expression of cultured primary hepatocytes. EHS matrix is a laminin-rich gel that contains many of the fundamental components of extracellular matrix. Its complex composition of matrix proteins stimulates cell-specific growth characteristics. Marker proteins specific to the differentiated hepatocyte phenotype, such as albumin or cytochromes P_{450}, are expressed for up to a month in hepatocytes grown on EHS gel. Hepatocytes grown on EHS gel may also exhibit a columnar growth pattern similar to that observed in the liver sinusoids *in vivo* (Bissell, JCI, 1987; 79:801).

The ability to reconstitute the liver *in vitro* with all relevant cell types, cell–cell and cell–matrix interactions would prove of immense value in the understanding of the requirements for maintenance of differentiated liver-cell phenotypes, and would also serve the purpose of development of an artificial-liver support device. With these goals in mind, there have been encouraging recent advances towards the prospect of 'three-dimensional' liver-cell culture. These techniques have utilized alginate manuronic–guluronic acid polymer beads and the culture of hepatocytes between two layers of hydrated collagen (collagen gel sandwich). In the latter, structures resembling bile canaliculi have been observed. Coculturing parenchymal and stromal liver cells in a three-dimensional mesh on nylon screens or bioresorbable polyglycolic acid has also permitted their subsequent transplantation into the peritoneal cavity and subcutaneous tissues of adult rats where they have shown sustained growth over a period of 30 days (Naughton, ApplBiochemBiotechnol, 1995; 54:65).

Applications

Today, many laboratories engaged in basic hepatological research use cell-culture techniques to some extent. It is an affordable system, generally easy to maintain in the laboratory, and applicable to a very broad array of research questions.

Cell culture has been used to define growth-regulation and signalling pathways; it has contributed to understanding in the areas of transport, drug metabolism and cellular toxicity, and permitted the subcellular localization of certain functions. Many of the major characteristics of the individual cell types present in liver tissue (hepatocytes, Kupffer, stellate, and endothelial cells) as well as the properties of the extracellular matrix have been defined using cell-culture techniques. In the important field of viral hepatitis, the mechanisms of liver cell infection by hepatitis viruses and viral replication have been elucidated using a variety of cell-culture methods. Finally, the clinical application of hepatocyte transplantation, gene transfer, and artificial liver systems, although still in its infancy, would not even have been feasible without the basic knowledge derived from cell-culture techniques.

Much has been learned from cell culture concerning the impact on the cell of fundamental environmental factors such as the composition of the medium and substratum and the spatial configuration of the culture. From these fundamental considerations, in turn, much has been learned about the requirements and physiological determinants of tissue-specific cell growth and the process of dedifferentiation, including the relation of the latter to tumour-cell growth. Coculture of different cell types has elucidated other determinants of differentiation and dedifferentiation. The production of, and reaction to, cytokines and other signalling molecules has been extensively studied in cell culture. Signal transduction pathways, from the characterization of receptors to downstream events, have been the subject of research in hepatocyte culture. Both cultured primary hepatocytes and hepatocyte cell lines have been used exhaustively to study the dynamics of proliferation and apoptosis.

Transport and metabolism of various drugs, glucose, amino acids, bilirubin, bile acids, and many other substances have been extensively assessed in cultured liver cells both in short-term suspension culture and in long-term attached monolayer cultures.

Movement of electrolytes through the cell membranes can be studied in individual cells. Hepatocyte couplets, which result from incomplete digestion with collagenase, have the particular advantage of preserving the structure and intact physiological function of the bile canaliculus between the two cells. Couplets have been successfully cultured for studies on bile formation and membrane-protein targeting.[9] (Nathanson, AmJPhysiol, 1992; 262:G1079; Weinman, AmJPhysiol, 1993; 264:G220; Benedetti, PNAS, 1994; 91:792). Characteristics of transport mechanisms effecting electrolyte movement have been investigated by sophisticated electrophysiological techniques such as patch clamping. Using this technique, a single channel or transporter can be isolated and electronically recorded while the current of a single type of ion can be monitored. Other ingenious approaches to the study of molecular transport in hepatocyte culture include confocal microscopy (Elsing, AmJPhysiol, 1995; 269:G842) and photobleaching techniques, whereby the intracellular transport and movement of fluorescent molecules can be measured and even visualized (Luxon, AmJPhysiol, 1993; 265:G831).

Highly differentiated liver-cell lines have been used to study the infectivity and replication of hepatitis viruses. For example, recent work has used HuH7 cells to identify specific viral-binding sites or receptors. Species differences in susceptibility to infection with hepatitis B were assayed by studies of the affinity between the virus and hepatocytes isolated from different species. Although infection of hepatocytes *in vitro* with human hepatitis viruses has been difficult to accomplish reproducibly, the viral genome can be introduced into hepatocytes by means of transfection techniques, with subsequent autonomous replication *in vitro* (Liang, JCI, 1993; 91:1241; Yoo, JVirol, 1995; 69:32; Walter, Hepatol, 1996; 24:1). By selectively introducing only parts of the viral DNA or RNA, the functions of specific regions of the viral genome have been determined.

Most of the applications discussed above have been confined to research on hepatocytes. With recent advances in the techniques for separating the individual cell types in the liver, the possibilities for better characterization of the biology of non-parenchymal liver cells, including stellate, Kupffer, pit, and endothelial cells as well as small and large cholangiocytes, in terms of their gene expression, morphological attributes in culture, and functional characteristics and involvement in human disease, have become enormous.

Transfection has become one of the most common uses of cultured cells in laboratories involved in research in the molecular and cell biology of liver cells. In this technique, the DNA of a gene or genes of interest inserted into a suitable expression vector is introduced into the host cell, which then expresses the corresponding protein. A variety of methods for achieving transfection of DNA into cultured cells has been described, including introduction by electroporation or complexed with calcium phosphate, DEAE–dextran or liposomes, or incorporated in viral vectors such as adenoviruses and retroviruses. Following its expression, the function of the gene product can be studied. A similar strategy can be employed to transfect antisense sequences to hybridize with the mRNA of specific genes normally expressed in the cell, and in this manner, inhibit their expression. Usually, non–liver-derived cell lines such as 3T3, COS, CHO or MDCK lineages, originating from fibroblasts, kidney or ovary, are employed to express transfected genes. Primary hepatocytes are amenable to transfection (Watanabe, JBiochem (Tokyo), 1994; 116:1220; Holmen, Invitro, 1995; 31:347;

Hilliard, IntJBiochemCellBiol, 1996; 28:639) but have proved more challenging in this respect. The advantage of being able to perform transfection studies in primary cells is that they contain the entire array of tissue-specific proteins that may potentially interact with the gene product of interest. On the other hand, cell lines offer the advantage of having a low background expression of differentiated cell-specific genes, which in turn facilitates the study of the function of these genes.

Shortcomings

The most important drawback in culturing liver cells is their tendency towards dedifferentiation with loss of their characteristic morphology and tissue-specific gene expression. Beginning with the earliest steps of the isolation process and progressing through the duration of the experiment, many of the characteristics of a specific type of cell—often the original object of interest—can be lost. For example, loss of cell polarity soon after isolation will lead to the loss of vectorial transport processes, such as targeting of specific proteins and vesicles to basolateral and apical membranes. For reasons that remain poorly understood, the processing of cells for culture usually leads to the loss of those surface macromolecules necessary for viral entry. The defining properties of a particular cell type are usually incompletely understood and are thus the subject of *in vitro* study. These properties are often further obscured by the artificial culture environment, and it may become extremely difficult to discriminate between findings that are representative and real and those that are artefacts resulting from the *in vitro* approach.

However sophisticated the development of 'physiological' culturing conditions may become, it remains unphysiological for a cell to divide indefinitely. In this regard, despite their ease of use, cell lines will never replace primary cells as the most valid model for the study of liver-cell biology. Even data obtained from the study of primary liver cells must often be interpreted with caution, and the results validated by appropriate means using alternative approaches and *in vivo* observations.

Subcellular elements

From the perspective of this chapter, subcellular organelles represent the smallest components of the liver yielded through the progressive fractionation of the organ. Dissection of cellular function beyond this point lies within the realms of biochemistry and molecular cell biology. The term organelle is used to describe the membranous entities that comprise not only the structural architecture of the cell but also the functional subunits that fulfil specialized tasks inside the cell.

The complex subcellular structures first visualized in detail in eukaryotes by electron microscopy proved more challenging to separate and purify. Currently, methods exist to study the characteristics and functions of all the major cell organelles, which include the plasma membrane (and its specialized polar domains), endoplasmic reticulum, Golgi apparatus, endosomal vesicles, lysosomes, mitochondria, peroxisomes, and nuclei.

The liver parenchyma is comprised predominantly of hepatocytes, which are easy to disrupt or isolate and which, due to the diverse functions of this cell type, contain almost every organelle found in the animal kingdom. Thus the hepatocyte has established its place as an excellent model for the study of cell biology in general. Indeed, much of the available knowledge concerning cell biology is based on studies in hepatocytes.

Technique

Subcellular fractions are prepared following either the disruption of the whole liver or of specific cells after their isolation from the liver. Whole liver is usually disrupted in a glass or Teflon–glass homogenizer, in which manual or mechanically powered rotation and up-and-down movement of a closely fitting plunger generates shear forces that lead to disruption of cells. This homogenization procedure is usually done in an isotonic, physiologically buffered salt solution at 4°C. The resultant homogenate contains all the components of the cell in a particulate suspension. Isolated or cultured cells are more often disrupted by exposure to high-frequency sound (sonication). Available methods have even been successfully used to isolate organelles from small pieces of human liver biopsy material (Eaton, BiochemSocTrans, 1995; 23:497).

As briefly described in the preceding subsection on the preparation of isolated cells, several properties of subcellular structures may be exploited in order to isolate them from the crude cellular homogenate as relatively pure preparations. These properties include size, shape, density, surface charge, surface structures, and the differential uptake of substrates.

In preparative ultracentrifugation, the homogenate is subjected sequentially to different centrifugal speeds and hence different centrifugal forces in order to separate subcellular elements grossly on the basis of their relative densities. The classical approach to the separation of the major organelles in liver from a crude homogenate is velocity sedimentation. Sample tubes are spun in a metal rotor at high speed in a vacuum chamber. The vacuum reduces friction and prevents the rotor from heating. A centrifugal force of 600 to 1000 g (g = the acceleration of one earth gravity) is used to sediment the heaviest particles, including unbroken cells and nuclei, within a few minutes. When the remaining supernatant is subjected to forces of 20 000 to 30 000 g, for 30 min to an hour, the resulting pellet at the bottom of the centrifuge tube contains mitochondria, peroxisomes, and lysosomes, which are all similar in size (about 0.5–2 μm). Recentrifugation of the supernatant at forces around 100 000 g for 1 to 3 h separates the membranous structures of the endoplasmic reticulum (the microsomal fraction), as well as the Golgi apparatus and plasma membranes. The term microsomes is routinely applied to the subcellular fraction enriched in membranes of the endoplasmic reticulum and derives from the fact that the homogenization procedure extensively disrupts this subcellular fraction, producing small, closed vesicles—the so-called microsomes. The microsomal fraction can be subdivided further into membranes of rough and smooth endoplasmic reticulum. Because of the high RNA and protein content, the rough microsomes can be readily separated from the smooth fraction. In the liver, most of the lighter microsomes correspond to the highly abundant smooth endoplasmic reticulum. In other cell types, this fraction is more difficult to separate from the Golgi or plasma-membrane components. These structures are about one logarithmic order of magnitude smaller than the prior sedimented fraction and can be further separated using more sophisticated centrifugation techniques described in detail below. Further ultracentrifugation of the remaining supernatant at maximally achievable rotor speeds (generating forces of 300 000–500 000 g) will pellet large macromolecules including viruses, different RNA species, and high molecular-weight proteins. The final supernatant is called the cytosol fraction. This represents the soluble fraction of the cell and comprises a complex mixture of proteins, enzymes, and metabolites including several that are released from various organelles during homogenization and centrifugation.

Equilibrium sedimentation also takes advantage of the different densities of the organelles, but is capable of much finer discrimination than simple velocity centrifugation, in which organelles with similar sizes usually cosediment. In equilibrium sedimentation, a density gradient is created using hypertonic solutions of one of several solutes ideally suited to this purpose. These include sucrose, caesium salts, isotonic Percoll, Nycodenz, Ficoll, and metrizamide. A crude mixture of subcellular fractions is layered on top of the density gradient. During centrifugation, each type of organelle will migrate, in a manner depending on its density and permeability to the surrounding solution, to an equilibrium point where the density of the surrounding gradient fluid equals that of the organelle (see Table 4). Of importance in a polarized cell such as the hepatocyte is the fact that regional domains of the cell membrane, notably the basolateral and canalicular membranes, can also be separated from one another through the application of equilibrium-sedimentation techniques. Plasma membranes can also be further processed by passing them through a fine needle to form vesicles. By this means, two forms of vesicles can be generated: vesicles with the normally exocellular surface on the outside ('rightside out') and those with a reversed orientation in which the intracellular surface now forms the exterior of the vesicle ('inside-out').

An ingenious variation on the theme of organelle preparation by equilibrium-density centrifugation has been to modify the density of the organelle itself either *in vivo* or *in vitro* before centrifugal separation.[10] For example, colloidal gold and other dense, nondegradable substances have been used to aid the isolation of lysosomal and endosomal fractions after their introduction by endocytosis either *in vivo* or *in vitro*. Also, the induction of swelling or causing the selective accumulation of a dense reaction product in an organelle has been used to create a shift in density of the subcellular structure in order to facilitate its subsequent isolation. The final purity of an isolated subcellular fraction—that is to say, the extent to which it is uncontaminated by other fractions—is assessed by several methods. These include morphological assessment by electron microscopy and by the measurement of the activity of specific marker enzymes or proteins that are well characterized in terms of their specific subcellular location (Table 5).

Table 4 Density of subcellular organelles

Organelle	Density (g/cm³)
Peroxisomes	1.23–1.32
Mitochondria	1.18
Lysosomes	1.12–1.21
Rough endoplasmic reticulum	1.2
Golgi vesicles	1.14
Plasma membranes	1.12–1.17
Endosomes	1.09–1.13
Plasma	1.027

Table 5 Marker enzymes for subcellular organelles	
Subcellular structure	**Marker enzyme**
Peroxisomes	Urate oxidase
	Catalase
	D-Amino acid oxidase
Mitochondria	Succinate cytochrome c reductase
	Cytochrome oxidase
	Glutamate dehydrogenase
Lysosomes	Acid phosphate
Smooth endoplasmic reticulum	Glucose 6-phosphate
Golgi apparatus	Galactosyltransferase
Endoplasmatic reticulum	NADPH-cytochrome c reductase
Basolateral plasma membrane	Na^+–K^+-ATPase
Canalicular plasma membrane	Alkaline phosphatase
	Mg^{2+}-ATPase
	5′-Nucleotidase
	Dipeptidylpeptidase IV

In the study of receptor-mediated endocytosis and the traffic of intracellular vesicles, radiolabelled tracers have proved particularly useful to track intercompartmental movements. Depending on the pathway being studied, specific tracers are used. For example, the degradation pathway of endocytosed glycoproteins is typically traced using asialofetuin, which is physiologically removed from the circulation by the galactose-specific receptor of the hepatocyte. IgA is taken up from the blood via a specific receptor and secreted into bile. Radio-iodinated IgA has been productively used to study this transcellular endosomal pathway (Kennedy, BiochemJ, 1988; 252: 739; Van Dyke, Hepatol, 1993; 18:604; Stieger, Hepatol, 1994; 20: 201).

Techniques other than, or in addition to, centrifugation have begun to prove their usefulness in the preparation of subcellular organelles. Theses techniques include the decidedly different approach of free-flow electrophoresis (Schmid, SubcellBioch, 1993; 19:1). This uses the property of net electrical surface-charge density to achieve separation of various subcellular elements. In this method, a thin layer of buffer containing the subcellular fractions is run in a particular direction through a chamber with an electric field applied perpendicularly to the direction of buffer flow. The subcellular elements migrate laterally in the electric field according to their surface-charge density. The buffer is collected at the outflow end of the chamber in defined spatial intervals, allowing recovery of the separated organelles in separate fractions. Finally, specific proteins expressed on the surface of the various organelles have allowed immunoprecipitation of specific subcellular structures as well as their separation following fluorescent labelling using FACS techniques.

Applications

The ability to isolate specific subcellular fractions has made a vast contribution to the advancement of knowledge in cell biology in general and hepatology in particular. Its detailed discussion is beyond the scope of this chapter, and only selected important or illustrative examples will be described. Subcellular fractionation has enabled the precise subcellular localization and characterization of many processes that had previously been only quantitatively determined in the liver. It has provided an extensive understanding of the subcellular anatomical realm that subserves and complements the study of cellular physiology, biochemistry, and molecular biology (Table 6). Important mechanistic and compartmental models of cell function have been formulated from studies at this level. Of great importance, the methods described in this section have permitted, in conjunction with the cloning of specific genes, a better understanding of the cell biology of many human genetic diseases.

Subfractions of plasma membrane and fractions of intracellular vesicles have been extensively used to elucidate the mechanisms of traffic at the intracellular membranes, including the sorting and targeting of intracellular vesicles derived from endocytosis or arising from the protein synthetic and exporting machinery collectively represented by the endoplasmic reticulum and Golgi apparatus. Vesicles formed from isolates of either basolateral or canalicular membranes, with their resident membrane-associated proteins, are a fundamental tool *in vitro* for the study of the uptake of organic anions and cations, including bile pigments and bile acids. Right-side-out vesicles have generally been used to characterize uptake processes while inside-out vesicles have lent themselves to the study of efflux processes.[11]

A significant amount of our knowledge about the physiological processes of cell replication, nutrient metabolism, energy metabolism and utilization, protein synthesis and degradation, and xenobiotic detoxification has been made possible through the use of subcellular fractionation techniques. The intracellular localization of all the major metabolic pathways, many of which are predominantly or even exclusively found in parenchymal liver cells, has been achieved largely through the use of these methods. Recently, isolated mitochondria have become an important tool for the study of mechanisms of hepatotoxicity. Indeed, these studies have helped to focus considerable attention on the role of mitochondrial damage and disruption of mitochondrial function in the pathogenesis of liver-cell dysfunction or death resulting from a variety of mechanisms (Fromenty, PharmTher, 1995; 67:101).

Table 6 Main metabolic pathways in cell organelles

Subcellular structure	Metabolic pathway
Mitochondria	Krebs' cycle
	Oxidative phosphorylation
	Fatty-acid β-oxidation
	Ketone-body synthesis
	Urea cycle (part)
	Haem synthesis
Peroxisomes	Alternative fatty-acid β-oxidation
	Oxidation of very long-chain fatty acids
	Plasmalogen biosynthesis
	Cholesterol biosynthesis (part)
	Side-chain oxidation of bile acids
	Oxidase and catalase activity
Lysosomes	Proteases
	Nucleases
	Acid phosphatases
	Glucosidases
	Glucuronidases
Smooth endoplasmic reticulum	Drug metabolism
	Glycerolipid biosynthesis
Rough endoplasmic reticulum	Protein synthesis
Golgi apparatus	Modification and targeting of proteins
Cytosol	Glycolysis
	Gluconeogenesis
	Glycogen synthesis
	Fatty-acid synthesis
	Pentose phosphate cycle

In recent years, there has been a considerable increase in understanding of the importance of the peroxisome in health and disease. The liver is particularly enriched in these spherical organelles, which are typically bounded by a single membrane and contain an abundance of the enzyme catalase. Peroxisomes may be remarkably increased in the livers of animals treated with certain xenobiotics or drugs, collectively referred to as peroxisome proliferators. Peroxisomes tend to be highly permeable and may lose substrates and even enzymes during isolation, making their study *in vitro* more challenging. Appreciation of their multiple metabolic functions in the hepatocyte has nevertheless grown. Defects in peroxisomal protein import and in the biogenesis of this organelle result in a variety of rare disorders including the cerebrohepatorenal syndrome (Zellweger disease), Refsum disease, and X-linked adrenoleucodystrophy.

Lysosomal lipid-storage diseases such as Niemann–Pick or Tay–Sachs result from specific defects in the enzymatic process of lipid degradation and have a significant impact on liver function.

Almost 50 per cent of the membrane structure of the hepatocyte is contributed by the smooth endoplasmic reticulum, a structure that is largely absent in other cell types. In contrast, in the liver, this subcellular compartment may proliferate extensively following exposure of the animal or isolated hepatocytes to certain xenobiotics. Most of the abundant and versatile drug-metabolizing enzyme machinery of the liver, including the phase I cytochromes P_{450} and phase II conjugation enzymes, reside in this fraction. The rough endoplasmic reticulum derives its name from the studding of this membrane with ribosomes. This component of the microsomal fraction is thus the main tool for the study, at the subcellular level, of protein synthesis and export. Recent work has opened up new areas of inquiry into the function of the endoplasmic reticulum and the derangement of this function in metabolic disease of liver. For example, disturbances in the degradation of misfolded mutant α_1-antitrypsin in the endoplasmic reticulum seem to have a significant impact on the clinical expression of α_1-antitrypsin deficiency (Wu, PNAS, 1994; 91:9014). Similarly, misassembly of the lipid core of very low-density lipoproteins in the endoplasmic reticulum resulting from a mutation in a cisternal protein of endoplasmic reticulum (microsomal triglyceride transfer protein) is the basis for the hepatic lipid accumulation and, rarely, more serious damage in abetalipoproteinaemia (Gregg, CurrOpinLipidol, 1994; 5:81).

Shortcomings

The study of subcellular fractions has the potential to characterize one homogeneous intracellular compartment with limited 'background' resulting from other compartments. The high resolution provided by this approach is hampered mainly by the imperfection of isolation methods. Due to the minuscule size of the particles of interest as well as the fact that they often overlap in size, density, electrochemical, and immunological properties, their perfect separation is not usually feasible. The separation process also may potentially alter the characteristics of the subcellular fraction of interest. For these reasons, the supplementation of conventional subcellular research methods with alternative protocols is often important in order to validate the data obtained.

The level of separation of subcellular components usually attained by current approaches also carries the disadvantage of removing both recognized and as yet unappreciated interactions between compartments. To address this issue, attempts at reconstituting organelles in a functional juxtaposition have been made, particularly in the study of protein synthesis, post-translational modification, and export (Verner K, EMBOJ, 1987; 6:2449; Miura, JBiochem (Tokyo), 1994; 115:1064).

References

1. Gores GJ, Kost LJ, and LaRusso NF. The isolated perfused rat liver: conceptual and practical considerations. *Hepatology*, 1986; **6**: 511–17.

2. Pang KS *et al.* Effects of perfusate flow rate on measured blood volume, Disse space, intracellular water space, and drug extraction in the perfused rat liver preparation: characterization by the multiple indicator dilution technique. *Journal of Pharmacokinetics and Biopharmaceutics*, 1988; **16**: 595–632.

3. Parrish AR, Gandolfi AJ, and Brendel K. Precision-cut tissue slices: applications in pharmacology and toxicology. *Life Sciences*, 1995; **57**: 1887–901.

4. Alpini G, Phillips JO, Vroman B, and LaRusso NF. Recent advances in the isolation of liver cells. *Hepatology*, 1994; **20**: 494–514.

5. Isom HC, Woodworth CD, Meng Y, Kreider J, Miller T, and Mengel L. Introduction of the ras oncogene transforms a simian virus 40-immortalized hepatocyte cell line without loss of expression of albumin and other liver-specific genes. *Cancer Research*, 1992; **52**: 940–8.

6. Darlington GJ. Liver cell lines. *Methods in Enzymology*, 1987; 151: 19–38.

7. Brill S, *et al.* Extracellular matrix regulation of growth and gene expression in liver cell lineages and hepatomas. In Arias IM, ed. *The liver: biology and pathobiology*. 3rd edn. New York: Raven Press, 1994: 869–98.

8. Rojkind M and Ponce-Noyola P. The extracellular matrix of the liver. *Collagen and Related Research*, 1982; **2**: 151–75.

9. Boyer JL and Soroka CJ. Vesicle targeting to the apical domain regulates bile excretory function in isolated rat hepatocyte couplets. *Gastroenterology*, 1995; **109**: 1600–11.

10. Courtoy PJ. Analytical subcellular fractionation of endosomal compartments in rat hepatocytes. *Subcellular Biochemistry*, 1993; **19**: 29–68.

3

Pathology

3.1 Histological features

Valeer J. Desmet and Tania Roskams

Hepatocellular changes

The ground-glass hepatocyte (Hadziyannis, ArchPathol, 1973; 96:327) displays a more homogeneous, paler eosinophilic staining than the normal hepatocyte in all or part of its cytoplasm (Plate 1 and see Plate 30). It is most typically observed in carriers of hepatitis B virus (**HBV**), in whom its appearance is due to hypertrophy of the endoplasmic reticulum, loaded with HBsAg.

A more or less similar appearance of hepatocytes may be observed in drug induction, in myoclonal epilepsy (Lafora's disease), in alcoholics treated with aversion drugs (disulfiram, cyanamide), in glycogenosis type IV (Andersen's disease), and in fibrinogen storage disease (Callea, Histopath, 1986; 10:65). In HBV-infected patients, HBsAg can be demonstrated in ground-glass hepatocytes by special stains (Shikata's orcein stain, Victoria blue), immunohistochemical techniques, and regular and immunoelectron microscopy.[1–3]

Acidophil condensation refers to a hepatocyte of reduced size, with increased density and eosinophilia of its cytoplasm, and usually pyknosis of the nucleus. The cell may assume a rhomboid outline.[1, 4]

Ballooning or hydropic swelling describes hepatocytes characterized by an increased volume with pale, 'empty' appearance of most of their cytoplasm; the remaining cytoplasm appears condensed in the perinuclear region (Plate 2 and see Plate 8). This lesion is thought to represent a precursor stage of lytic necrosis. It is observed in viral, toxic, and ischaemic liver damage, predominantly in acinar zone 3.[1,4]

Alcoholic clear cells ('hépatite alcoolique à cellules claires', Albot, SemHopParis, 1956; 45:1705) are enlarged and rounded hepatocytes with pale, rarefied cytoplasm; nuclei may be enlarged with prominent nucleoli. The cell borders are usually distinct, accentuated by pericellular fibrosis. Mallory bodies often occur in 'alcoholic clear cells'.[2]

Feathery degeneration of hepatocytes is seen in cholestasis, mostly of longer duration. This lesion resembles 'hydropic swelling' with, in addition, bilirubin impregnation of the visible threads of cytoplasm. Ultrastructurally, such cells display whorls of membranous material, thought to result from intracellular membrane damage due to the detergent action of retained bile acids.[5,6]

Alcoholic hyaline or Mallory body refers to an intracellular inclusion in hepatocytes, which are often pale and swollen (alcoholic clear cells). In its typical form, the Mallory body is an irregular, intensely eosinophilic mass (Plate 3). The lesion corresponds to clumps of aggregated cytokeratin filaments. Small Mallory bodies are better identified by immunostaining for cytokeratins.

The term alcoholic hyaline may be misleading because the lesion occurs in numerous other diseases besides alcoholic liver damage, especially in chronic cholestasis (Desmet, ActaMedScand, 1985; 703:111).

In alcoholic liver disease, Mallory body-containing hepatocytes may be encircled by polymorphonuclear and/or mononuclear inflammatory cells; this lesion is known as satellitosis. 2

Megamitochondria (giant mitochondria) appear as round or cigar-shaped, intensely eosinophilic inclusions of variable size, up to the size of a nucleus (Plate 3); they are negative on periodic acid–Schiff (**PAS**)–diastase stained sections, in contrast to α_1-antitrypsin inclusions and phagolysosomes, with which they might be confused.[2]

Mitochondriosis (oxyphil or oncocytic change) (Lefkowitch, AmJClinPath, 1980; 74:432) corresponds to an increase in number of mitochondria in hepatocytes, rendering the latter more granular and strongly eosinophilic than normal parenchymal cells. Oncocytic hepatocytes are often found in clusters.

Sanded nuclei (Bianchi, LabInvest, 1976; 35:1) are hepatocellular nuclei stuffed with hepatitis B core particles causing peripheral margination of the chromatin. In light microscopy, the central part of the nucleus appears occupied by faintly eosinophilic, finely granular ('sand') material. They may be found in small numbers during the viral replicative phase of chronic viral hepatitis B. Sanded nuclei should not be confused with nuclear vacuolation.[1,2]

Cytomegalovirus (CMV) inclusions may be found in all types of cells in the liver, most often in hepatocytes and bile duct cells. These are characterized by cytomegaly and the development of intranuclear basophilic inclusions, surrounded by a clear halo. The cytoplasm may be strongly basophilic. Appropriate immunostaining reveals CMV antigens (Vanstapel, ApplPathol, 1983; 1:41).

Herpes simplex viral inclusions occur as two types. The more common type renders the nucleus homogeneously basophilic, with effacement of the nucleolus and most of the chromatin granules. The second type corresponds to the classic Cowdry type A inclusion: an eosinophilic, rounded or irregular inclusion surrounded by a clear halo with margination of the chromatin. Viral antigens can be identified by appropriate immunostaining.[2,7]

Nuclear vacuolation corresponds to hepatocellular nuclei which appear empty on light microscopy. The vacuolation may be due to glycogen (e.g. in diabetics) or to invagination of cytoplasm or accumulation of lipid into the nucleus. This change is not very helpful in diagnosis.[2,4,7]

Atrophy of hepatocytes is reflected in reduced size and increased cytoplasmic density and lipofuscin content of hepatocytes (see Plate 19).

Hypoxic vacuoles are formed in anoxic conditions by invagination of the cell membrane of hepatocytes with engulfment of plasma proteins. They occur in acinar zone 3, and appear as pale-staining smaller or larger vacuoles. Appropriate immunostaining reveals the presence of albumin, fibrinogen, and other plasma proteins. Electron microscopy shows that the membrane surrounding the vacuoles is not part of the endoplasmic reticulum, which differentiates the lesion from 'endoplasmic reticulum storage disorders' such as α_1-antitrypsin or fibrinogen storage (Nakanuma, Liver, 1982; 2:212).

Necrosis and inflammation

Acidophil body (single cell acidophil necrosis; coagulation necrosis) refers to a rounded clump of intensely eosinophilic cytoplasm, with or without a pyknotic nucleus, corresponding to necrosis of a single hepatocyte. The acidophil body is disconnected from the liver cell plate and becomes phagocytosed by Kupffer cells. The lesion is often incorrectly referred to as Councilman (-like) body.[2,4,7]

Apoptosis represents a physiological, preprogrammed mode of cell death, characterized by budding and fragmentation of a liver cell into smaller and larger 'acidophil bodies' (Plates 2, 4). Apoptosis is an essential and vital component in liver development and growth, in physiology, and in the most diverse pathological conditions. It is the way in which senescent cells are eliminated in normal liver; it plays a role in embryonic development of intrahepatic bile ducts, in regression of ductular reaction, and in vanishing bile duct diseases. Apoptosis is part and parcel of focal necrosis and piecemeal necrosis in chronic hepatitis, it is a common feature in acute and fulminant hepatitis and in liver allograft rejection. Furthermore, apoptosis is a key phenomenon in several forms of toxic liver injury, in carcinogenesis, and in the cell kinetics of hepatocellular carcinoma (Patel, Hepatol, 1995; 21:1725).

Lytic necrosis represents a mode of liver cell death followed by rapid disappearance of the dead cells; it is histologically recognized by lack of cells.[8,9]

Confluent (lytic) necrosis refers to disappearance of groups of contiguous hepatocytes, resulting in denudation of the reticulin framework. According to the extent of confluent necrosis, it is graded as focal or zonal, the latter occupying an entire acinar zone, usually zone 3, occasionally zone 1 (for example in severe viral hepatitis A).

Bridging hepatic necrosis represents more extensive degrees of confluent necrosis, leading to necrotic 'bridges' between adjacent vascular structures.

Central–central bridging necrosis links adjacent central veins; it corresponds to confluent necrosis in the microcirculatory periphery of a complex acinus (Desmet, YaleJBiolMed, 1988; 61:61).

Portal–central bridging necrosis links portal tracts and central veins; it corresponds to confluent necrosis in the microcirculatory periphery of the simple acinus.

Still higher degrees of confluent necrosis are described as panlobular, multilobular, submassive, and massive necrosis.[8,9]

Surgical necrosis (Christoffersen, ActaHepatoSplenol, 1970; 17: 240) is observed in liver specimens taken during abdominal surgical interventions. It appears as acidophil necrosis of hepatocytes surrounded by neutrophil polymorphs (Plate 5). It is usually observed in acinar zone 3; the extent of the lesion increases with the duration of the operation and the degree of manipulation of the liver. This lesion is often observed after revascularization of the donor liver in liver transplantation.

Piecemeal necrosis occurs at the interphase between mesenchyme (portal tracts or septa) and parenchyma (interphase hepatitis). Mononuclear lymphoid cells infiltrate the mesenchyme and extend into the adjacent parenchyma, associated with progressive apoptotic cell death and disappearance of hepatocytes, thus leading to an unsharp mesenchymal–parenchymal border and gradual expansion of the mesenchymal area (Plate 6).[9]

Lymphocytic piecemeal necrosis represents the 'classic' lesion and is characterized by predominance of lymphocytes and plasma cells (Plate 6).[2,10]

Biliary piecemeal necrosis occurs in periportal (zone 1) locations in chronic biliary disease; it is characterized by cholate stasis of zone 1 hepatocytes, periportal ductular reaction, and infiltration by inflammatory cells, including neutrophils. This lesion also creates an unsharp mesenchymal–parenchymal interphase, and thus resembles classic piecemeal necrosis architecturally, but not cytologically.[2,4,10]

Fibrous piecemeal necrosis apparently represents a late stage of (biliary) piecemeal necrosis, in which connective tissue strands surround entrapped groups of hepatocytes with little cellular inflammation. Around portal tracts, it leads to formation of new limiting plates that border seemingly enlarged portal tracts. 10

Ductular piecemeal necrosis describes a lesion which is close to biliary piecemeal necrosis, with less emphasis on periportal or paraseptal cholate stasis.[10]

Liver cell rosettes 11 correspond to small groups of hepatocytes in lymphocytic or fibrous piecemeal necrosis; the cells appear hydropic, and are often arranged around a central lumen (Nagore, Liver, 1989; 9:43) (Plate 7).

Focal necrosis describes cell death (usually apoptotic in nature) of a small group of hepatocytes, associated with local accumulation of mononuclear cells (lymphocytes, histiocytes); apoptotic liver cell fragments are not always identifiable between the infiltrating cells.[4,12]

Spotty necrosis is virtually synonymous with focal necrosis, referring to involvement of single or very small groups of parenchymal cells (Plate 4).[4]

Emperipolesis refers to the intracellular location of a cell (usually a lymphocyte) inside a hepatocyte (Plate 8). The lymphocyte is often surrounded by a narrow clear halo. Peripolesis describes the close association between a lymphocyte and a hepatocyte; the former may be located in an indentation of the latter.[2]

Biliary and cholestatic lesions
Parenchymal changes

In its histological meaning, the term cholestasis used to refer to a microscopically visible deposition of bilirubin in the liver tissue. In a strict sense, it corresponds to bilirubinostasis. Since cholate stasis (see below) is another important parenchymal feature in chronic cholestatic conditions, it is more appropriate to replace the histological term cholestasis by the more precise term bilirubinostasis.[2,13]

Hepatocellular bilirubinostasis corresponds to intracellular accumulation of bilirubin-stained granules in the parenchymal cells, especially in toxic cholestasis (e.g. due to drugs and endotoxinaemia) (Plate 9 and see Plate 22).[6,11]

Canalicular bilirubinostasis is recognized as inspissated bile plugs in more or less dilated intercellular bile canaliculi. It first occurs in acinar zone 3, but may extend up to acinar zone 1 in cholestasis of long duration (Plate 9).[6]

Kupffer cell bilirubinostasis is represented by smaller and coarser bilirubin-stained inclusions in hypertrophic Kupffer cells. It is only observed in cholestasis of several days' duration (Plate 9).[6]

Ductular bilirubinostasis corresponds to inspissated, bilirubin-stained concrements in more or less dilated bile ductules. It is occasionally seen in long-standing extrahepatic bile duct obstruction, especially in extrahepatic bile duct atresia in the neonate. It also occurs in severely necrotizing hepatitis (Schmid, HumPath, 1972; 3:209). In septicaemia, large bile concrements are formed in unusually dilated periportal ductules (Lefkowitch, HumPath, 1982; 13:19) (Plate 10).

Cholate stasis is a lesion of zone 1 hepatocytes in long-lasting cholestasis.[2,4,13] The parenchymal cells are pale and swollen and coarsely granular. Some of the granules correspond to copper accumulation, and stain with rhodanine (copper) and orcein or Victoria blue (copper-binding protein or metallothionein). Later on, bilirubin granules may also accumulate, and Mallory bodies may develop. The term cholate stasis refers to the presumed intracellular accumulation of bile salts as the suspected mechanism for this lesion.

The appearance of *cholestatic liver cell rosettes* (Nagore, Liver, 1989; 9:43) is a sign of long-lasting cholestasis. It may be particularly pronounced in contraceptive steroid-induced cholestasis. Scattered through the parenchyma, groups of liver cells are arranged in tubular fashion around a smaller or larger lumen, which may appear empty or filled with eosinophilic or bilirubin-stained material (Plate 11). The composing hepatocytes express bile duct-type cytokeratins, indicating an intermediate differentiation of these hepatocytes.[13]

Xanthomatous cells (foam cells) occur as single cells or in clusters, in the parenchyma or portal tracts or both, in the case of long-lasting cholestasis. They correspond to lipid-laden histiocytes, related to hyperlipidaemia and hypercholesterolaemia.[14]

Bile infarct (Charcot–Gombault infarct) represents an area of paraportal necrosis of liver parenchyma; the central part of the necrotic zone in particular is impregnated with bilirubin (which has affinity for necrotic tissue) (Plate 12). With time, the necrotic mass becomes organized in a fibrous scar. This lesion is mainly (but not exclusively) observed in long-standing extrahepatic bile duct obstruction.[14]

Bile lake refers to a large mass (larger than the usual extracellular bile plug of canalicular bilirubinostasis) in the parenchyma of a cholestatic liver.[11,14]

Portal and periportal changes

Bile extravasates are mainly seen in late stages of large-duct obstruction; they represent inspissated bile concrements in ducts associated with erosion and necrosis of the epithelial lining of the duct. The bile mass in contact with portal connective tissue may incite a foreign-body giant cell reaction.

Lymphocytic cholangitis[10] describes a normal or damaged portal bile duct in a dense lymphocytic infiltrate, sometimes organized as a lymph follicle (e.g. early primary biliary cirrhosis).

Pleomorphic cholangitis[10] refers to a normal or altered portal bile duct surrounded (or even infiltrated) by a mixed inflammatory infiltrate (e.g. in liver allograft rejection and graft-versus-host disease).

Granulomatous cholangitis 10 indicates the presence of a noncaseating epithelioid cell granuloma close to or around a damaged portal bile duct (e.g. in primary biliary cirrhosis and sarcoidosis with chronic cholestasis) (Plate 13). This lesion is also referred to as florid bile duct lesion in primary biliary cirrhosis.

Fibro-obliterative cholangitis 10 corresponds to prominent layers of concentric dense connective tissue ('onion-skinning') around a portal bile duct, which may show features of atrophy and epithelial damage. The lesion indicates chronic irritation of the duct, but is not disease specific.

Purulent (suppurative) cholangitis[10] is characterized by accumulation of polymorphs in the lumen and in the wall of bile ducts; destruction of the epithelial lining may proceed to the formation of cholangitic abcesses.

Paucity of intrahepatic bile ducts (ductopenia) is morphometrically defined as a portal bile duct to portal tract ratio of less than 0.5 (normal value 0.9 to 1.8) (Alagille, JPediat, 1975; 86:63). The disappearance of the ducts seems to result from pleomorphic cholangitis. The entity is part of the 'vanishing bile duct' disorders.[15]

'Vanishing bile duct' disorders are recognized by the occurrence of portal tracts in which a portal bile duct of approximately the same size as the accompanying hepatic artery branch is missing (Nakanuma, Gastro, 1979; 76:1326). These disorders include extrahepatic bile duct atresia, paucity of intrahepatic bile ducts, idiopathic adulthood ductopenia, primary biliary cirrhosis, autoimmune cholangiopathy, sarcoidosis with chronic cholestasis, primary sclerosing cholangitis, hepatic graft-versus-host disease, liver allograft rejection, and some rare forms of prolonged drug-induced cholestasis.[10,15]

Hepatitic bile duct lesion (Poulsen–Christoffersen lesion) (Poulsen, HumPath, 1972; 3:217) represents a form of pleomorphic cholangitis, with stratification, vacuolation, and mononuclear cell infiltration of the affected bile duct segment (Plate 14). It appears to occur most frequently in viral hepatitis C.[1,2]

The ductal plate is the primitive shape of intrahepatic bile ducts during embryonic development.[15] It corresponds to a partly double layer of bile duct epithelium around the primitive portal tracts (Plate 15). Its normal fate is to become remodelled into the normal network of portal bile ducts (Van Eyken, Hepatol, 1988; 8:1586).

The ductal plate malformation represents a lack of remodelling of the embryonic ductal plate, with persistence of primitive bile duct structures (Jörgensen, ActaPMIScand, 1977; 257(Suppl):1). It is observed in infantile polycystic disease, congenital hepatic fibrosis, Caroli's disease, Meckel's syndrome, and Von Meyenburg complexes (Plate 16). Ductal plate malformation associated with features of duct destruction and inflammation (pleomorphic cholangitis) is also part of early, severe forms of so-called extrahepatic bile duct atresia.[15,16]

Ductular reaction ('cholangiolitis') refers to a periportal increase in the number of ductular profiles in histological sections. The ductules are accompanied by oedema and neutrophil polymorphs (inflammation of the ductules or cholangioles) (Plate 17). It is observed to a variable extent in all varieties of biliary disease.[11,13, 17]

In the case of acute, complete mechanical obstruction of larger bile ducts, the ductular reaction is mainly the result of ductular proliferation (so-called 'typical ductules', 'elongation type' of ductular proliferation, or 'marginal bile duct proliferation') (Christoffersen, ActaPMIScand, 1970; 212(Suppl):150) resulting from multiplication of pre-existing ductules at the margin of portal tracts.[17]

In the case of chronic, incomplete obstruction of larger bile ducts (e.g. in primary biliary cirrhosis, primary sclerosing cholangitis) the ductular reaction results from ductular metaplasia of zone 1 hepatocytes and from activation, proliferation, and differentiation of 'facultative stem cells' or progenitor cells (so-called 'atypical' or 'sprouting type' of ductular proliferation).[17]

Pericholangitis (Mistilis, AnnIntMed, 1965; 63:1), reported as a hepatic complication of ulcerative colitis, corresponds to the 'isolated small-duct sclerosing cholangitis' variant of primary sclerosing cholangitis.[10]

Fibrosis

The term fibrosis indicates an increase in connective tissue in the liver; it may occur in various patterns.

Portal fibrosis describes increased density and fibrous enlargement of portal tracts.

Concentric periductal fibrosis is a synonym of fibro-(obliterating) cholangitis.

Periportal fibrosis refers to fibrous extensions irradiating from portal tracts.

Centrolobular (acinar zone 3) fibrosis describes fibrous scarring around the terminal hepatic venules. When conspicuous, as in some forms of alcoholic liver disease, it has been described as 'sclerosing hyaline necrosis' (Edmondson, AnnIntMed, 1963; 59:646).

Perivenular fibrosis (Van Waes, Gastro, 1977; 73:646) indicates a fibrous thickening of the wall of the terminal hepatic venule. The lesion comprises a fibrotic rim more than 4 mm in thickness involving at least two-thirds of the perimeter of hepatic venules.

In pericellular or perisinusoidal fibrosis, collagen is laid down around single liver cells or small groups of hepatocytes. It occurs mostly in acinar zone 3. In alcoholic liver disease this pattern was described as 'chicken-wire fibrosis'.[2,11]

Septal fibrosis indicates fibrosis in the form of fibrous sheets. It occurs in various topographical patterns (portal–portal septa, portal–central septa, central–central septa; incomplete septa, etc.) according to the type of vascular canals linked by the connective tissue membranes.[9]

Active septa represent connective tissue sheets which are infiltrated by mononuclear inflammatory cells, with imprecise delineation from the adjacent parenchyma. They can be conceived as extensive degrees of piecemeal necrosis (Plate 6).[9]

Passive septa are fibrous membranes which are rich in fibres and poor in cells, with sharp delineation from the adjacent parenchyma (Plate 18). They derive from postnecrotic collapse and scarring after extensive confluent lytic necrosis.[2,9] Older (more than 6-month) passive septa contain elastic fibres, demonstrable by orcein or Victoria blue staining (Scheuer, Histopath, 1980; 4:487).

Primary collapse indicates postnecrotic collapse and scarring after confluent necrosis in a previously normal parenchyma; the topographical spacing of the approximated portal tracts and terminal hepatic veins is more or less preserved.[4]

Secondary collapse refers to postnecrotic scarring following necrosis in abnormal parenchymal territories (e.g. in cirrhosis), resulting in irregular spacing of afferent and efferent vessels.[4]

Hepatoportal sclerosis corresponds to phlebosclerosis of portal vein branches, as a result of organized mural thrombi or of portal hypertension, usually associated with some degree of portal and periportal fibrosis.[2,4,6,11]

Biliary fibrosis is often confused with true biliary cirrhosis. It represents an advanced but potentially reversible state of chronic bile duct disease, characterized by periportal or portal–portal septa, and garland-shaped parenchymal nodules; the basic lobular architecture and vascular relationships are preserved.[4,10,13]

Cirrhosis is a diffuse type of septal fibrosis of the liver, associated with regenerative parenchymal nodules and disturbed intrahepatic circulation (see Chapter 7.1).[18]

Vascular changes
Hepatic artery

Obliterative endarteritis is a feature of chronic vascular rejection of a liver allograft. It consists of the obstruction of arteries by subintimal fibrosis or the accumulation of foamy lipid-loaded cells.[6]

Afferent and efferent veins

Endothelialitis consists of lymphocytic infiltration of the portal or central vein endothelium, which appears damaged and lifted from its basement membrane. Endothelialitis is a helpful diagnostic feature in graft-versus-host disease and in acute liver allograft rejection (Snover, AmJSurgPath, 1987; 11:1).

Endophlebitis of the (terminal) hepatic veins consists of lymphocytic infiltration in the intima of the vessels. It is seen in acute (sub)massive necrosis in fulminant hepatitis. A lymphocytic phlebitis has been described in the (pre)cirrhotic stages of alcoholic liver disease.[7]

Veno-occlusive disease corresponds to narrowing of the lumen of terminal hepatic venules and larger draining hepatic veins, due to subintimal fibrosis. First observed in bush tea intoxication (senecio and crotalaria alkaloids), it may be due to several drugs, alcohol, graft-versus-host disease, and irradiation.[6,7,11]

Phlebosclerosis corresponds to fibrous thickening of the walls of veins, with or without an increase in elastic fibres. Phlebosclerosis of terminal hepatic venules occurs in several conditions, for example chronic passive congestion, alcoholic liver disease, and graft-versus-host disease. Phlebosclerosis of portal vein branches is part of the lesion of hepatoportal sclerosis.[6,7,11]

Prolapse of hepatocytes into terminal hepatic venules may result in partial occlusion and disruption of the wall of terminal hepatic venules. It has been reported in long-term anabolic–androgenic steroid therapy.[7]

Sinusoids and Disse space

Disse space lies between the sinusoidal wall and and the sinusoidal surface of the hepatocyte, from which abundant microvilli project into the space. The sinusoidal endothelium is discontinuous and extensively fenestrated and lacks a basement membrane. Therefore, the space of Disse is freely permeable to blood plasma and constitutes the immediate exchange area between blood and hepatocytes. The space of Disse contains collagen type I and III, constituting the 'reticulin' framework of the liver. However, several other extracellular matrix components are also present, for instance collagen type IV, laminin, and perlecan, in spite of the absence of a morphologically recognizable basement membrane.

Sinusoidal congestion occurs in acinar zone 3 as a result of venous outflow block; the sinusoids appear dilated and the parenchymal cells atrophic with pericellular fibrosis (Plate 19); all changes are variable according to the degree or duration, or both, of the venous congestion.

Sinusoidal dilatation in acinar zone 1[19] may occur in patients using contraceptive steroids. It is often accompanied by slight perisinusoidal fibrosis in that area (Winkler, ScaJGastr, 1975; 10: 699).

Peliosis indicates irregular blood-filled cavities corresponding to sinusoidal dilatation without constant zonal topography. The dilatation may be huge, creating blood pools in which liver cells are missing.[6,7,11]

Fibrin deposition in sinusoids is typically seen in acinar zone 1 in eclampsia (Plate 20), and in irregular topography in disseminated intravascular coagulopathy.

Capillarization of the sinusoids refers to important modifications of the space of Disse in fibrotic liver, as a morphologically distinct basement membrane-like structure appears, containing collagen type IV and laminin. In addition, increased amounts of collagen types I, III, V, and VI, fibronectin, tenascin, and undulin are deposited along the sinusoids. These changes are associated with loss of fenestrations of endothelial cells, further impairing exchange between blood and hepatocytes.[20] Hepatic stellate cells (Ito cells) increase in number and acquire an activated myofibroblast-like phenotype.

Hairy cell leukaemia may produce a characteristic 'angiomatous' picture, consisting of dilated sinusoids lined by leukaemic cells that have replaced the sinusoidal lining cells. Hairy cells display a clear rim of cytoplasm, and are positive for tartrate-resistant acid phosphatase and non-specific esterase.[7]

Extramedullary haematopoiesis is recognized by the occurrence in sinusoids of clusters of haematopoietic precursor cells, of the erythropoietic, granulopoietic, and thrombopoietic series. Normoblasts and megakaryocytes are the most easily identifiable precursor cells.[7]

Amyloidosis is characterized by the linear deposition of homogeneous eosinophilic material in vessel walls and in Disse spaces. Occasionally, globular deposition occurs. Advanced linear deposition of amyloid in parenchymal territories leads to atrophy of parenchymal cells. Amyloid is identified by the special stains Congo red and Sirius red, displaying characteristic green dichroism in polarized light.[7]

Light chain (deposit) disease resembles amyloidosis with granular and fibrillar material in Disse spaces; the deposited material is PAS-positive but does not stain as amyloid. Immunohistochemical stains for κ and λ light chains identify the deposits (Plate 21).[7]

Kupffer cell reaction and granuloma

Sinusoidal cell activation refers to excess sinusoidal cells, often of different type, including activated Kupffer cells and increased endothelial cells admixed with lymphocytes, monocytes, and plasma cells.[4]

Ceroid macrophages represent a phagocytic reaction to parenchymal necrosis, occurring as single cells or in clusters (also termed retothelial nodules).[7] These large mononuclear cells are filled with coarse PAS-positive, diastase-resistant inclusions, representing the phagocytosed debris of degenerated parenchymal cells. They are found near areas of necrosis in the early stage, and later on migrate to portal tracts; their long lifespan explains their interpretation as 'tombstones' of hepatic injury.[4,7]

Epithelioid granuloma. The term granuloma is not strictly defined; it refers to a focal accumulation of histiocytic cells, assuming epithelioid and multinucleated giant cell appearance in its most typical form (epithelioid granuloma). Histiocytic and epithelioid granulomas, with or without associated significant parenchymal inflammation (hepatitis), occur in numerous conditions.[21]

Lipogranuloma describes the accumulation of histiocytes and mononuclear cells around a parenchymal cell with large droplet steatosis.[19]

Mineral oil granulomas are a special form of foreign-body granuloma, consisting of histiocytes and vacuolated macrophages around clear spaces (mineral-oil deposits) in portal tracts and near terminal hepatic venules.[7]

Doughnut granuloma (fibrin ring granuloma) has a characteristic appearance with a central empty-appearing fat globule surrounded by a collar of histiocytes sprinkled with some lymphocytes, neutrophils, and sometimes eosinophils, and encircled by a ring of fibrin. Although highly characteristic of Q fever, this lesion is also observed in other conditions (for instance Hodgkin's disease, allopurinol hypersensitivity).[7]

Storage phenomena

Several metabolic diseases (storage diseases) are associated with deposition of metabolites in liver tissue.[22] Many of them require ultrastructural investigation for adequate identification. Their description is beyond the scope of this chapter.

Fat storage (steatosis, fatty metamorphosis) in hepatocytes is a feature common to numerous liver diseases. Neutral fat can be stained with oil red O or Sudan black in frozen sections; in paraffin-embedded tissue, fat appears as clear holes in parenchymal cells. The fat droplets may be small (microvesicular steatosis) with retained central position of the nucleus (Plate 22) or large (macrovesicular steatosis) in which case the nucleus is pushed to one side of the cell (Plate 23). The simultaneous presence of macro- and microvesicular steatosis indicates the presence of the inciting agent until the time of biopsy (e.g. alcohol abuse). Exclusive macrovesicular steatosis indicates a steady state of fat overload. Some special conditions with almost exclusive microvesicular steatosis have been emphasized (microvesicular fat diseases) (Sherlock, Gut, 1983; 24:265), including Reye syndrome, acute fatty liver of pregnancy, Jamaican vomiting sickness, and tetracycline and valproate intoxication.

Acute alcoholic foamy degeneration is a type of severe alcoholic liver damage with nearly exclusive microvesicular steatosis (Uchida, Gastro, 1983; 84:683).

Morula cells or spongiocytes correspond to hepatocytes with microvesicular steatosis, observed in Labrea fever in the Amazon river basin, which appears to represent delta hepatitis superinfection of hepatitis B virus carriers (Buitrago, Hepatol, 1986; 6:1285)[4] perhaps by a more pathogenic strain (Parana, JHepatol, 1995; 22:468).

Phospholipidosis is reflected in light microscopy in very small clear droplets and eosinophilic fine granules, often associated with Mallory bodies in some drug reactions (amiodarone, perhexiline maleate).[4,7]

Hepatic stellate cell hyperplasia (Ito cell hyperplasia) is recognized by an increased number of hepatic stellate cells (Ito cells, perisinusoidal cells); they appear as sinusoidal cells containing smaller or larger fat droplets indenting the nucleus (Plate 24). It is a diagnostic feature of vitamin A intoxication.[3]

Iron storage (siderosis) is reflected in the accumulation of Prussian blue-positive haemosiderin granules in hepatocytes (parenchymal siderosis) (Plate 25) and/or in Kupffer cells and macrophages (reticuloendothelial siderosis) (Plate 26).

Copper storage is recognized by the accumulation of intrahepatocellular granules which stain positively with rhodanin (copper) and orcein or Victoria blue (copper-binding protein or metallothionein).[6,11]

Glycogen storage is reflected by a clear appearance of enlarged hepatocytes with accentuated cell wall (plant cell-like appearance), often associated with glycogen vacuolation of the nucleus.[22]

α_1-*Antitrypsin storage* in the endoplasmic reticulum appears as eosinophilic inclusions of variable size in zone 1 hepatocytes. The inclusions are strongly PAS-positive and diastase resistant (Plate 27), and can be identified by immunohistochemical stains and electron microscopy.[22]

Fibrinogen storage may take the appearance of eosinophilic inclusions (resembling α_1-antitrypsin inclusions) or of ground-glass hepatocytes. The fibrinogen nature of the inclusions is ascertained by immunohistochemical staining.[23]

Lipofuscin (wear and tear pigment) appears as brownish pericanalicular granules in acinar zone 3 hepatocytes, which represent the ageing cells of the liver acinus. The amount of lipofuscin may increase (lipofuscinosis), for example in abuse of analgesics.

The pigment in Dubin–Johnson syndrome (Plate 28) resembles lipofuscinosis. The nature of this pigment (possibly melanin) is still debated (Kitamura, Hepatol, 1992; 15:1154).

Malaria pigment accumulates as dark granules in Kupffer cells in chronic malaria and schistosomiasis. The pigment is Prussian blue-negative and birefringent in polarized light.[7]

Ceroid pigment is an ill-defined material, appearing as granules and coarse clumps in hypertrophic Kupffer cells and macrophages ('ceroid macrophages') in all conditions associated with hepatocellular necrosis. The material represents phagocytosed debris from necrotizing liver cells. Ceroid macrophages thus attest to liver cell damage. They lay in the parenchyma in early stages, and later on migrate to portal tracts. Ceroid pigment is PAS-positive, diastase resistant, stains partly with fat stains, and is fluorescent under ultraviolet light.

Erythropoietic protoporphyria causes deposition of protoporphyrin as dark granules in hepatocytes and Kupffer cells and larger clumps of black material in dilated canaliculi and ductules. Under polarized light, the material is birefringent (appearing red in Maltese cross configuration in the larger deposits) and autofluorescent under ultraviolet light (Plate 29).[7]

Uroporphyrin crystals accumulate in hepatocytes in porphyria cutanea tarda. Difficult to recognize on haematoxylin–eosin stained sections, they are best visualized in unstained sections examined by polarizing microscopy (birefringence) or under ultraviolet light (red autofluorescence).[7]

Foreign material which may be stored in Kupffer cells includes talc, cellulose (in drug abusers), silica and anthracitic pigment (in coal workers), polyvinyl pyrrolidone (from plasma expanders), silicone (for instance from prosthetic heart valve devices), and thorotrast (a former contrast medium).[7]

Hepatitis (inflammation)

The term *liver cell pleomorphism* summarizes the complex set of histological changes of the liver parenchyma in several forms of acute viral- and drug-induced hepatitis (ballooning, acidophil condensation, apoptosis, regeneration). It is usually most marked in acinar zone 3 (Plates 2, 8).[1]

Lobular disarray refers to the disruption of the normal regular arrangement of liver cell plates caused by liver cell pleomorphism and focal necrosis in acute hepatitis (Plate 8).[4]

Acute hepatitis is characterized by mononuclear cell infiltration in portal tracts (portal hepatitis) and in the parenchyma, associated with signs of parenchymal damage (Plates 2, 8). The last depends on the severity of the hepatitis, corresponding to lobular disarray, liver cell pleomorphism, and spotty necrosis in milder forms, and various extents of confluent necrosis in severe cases.[1]

Portal hepatitis refers to mononuclear cell infiltration in portal tracts. Portal hepatitis without significant parenchymal damage is the hallmark of what was termed chronic persistent hepatitis, although of itself it is a non-specific lesion.[9]

Periportal hepatitis describes necroinflammatory changes in acinar zone 1 parenchyma around the portal tracts. It is a feature of viral hepatitis A. As a morphological descriptive term, it also refers to piecemeal necrosis (e.g. in active chronic hepatitis).[24]

Central (centrolobular) hepatitis refers to necroinflammatory lesions in acinar zone 3.

Non-specific reactive hepatitis indicates mild inflammatory changes, combining portal hepatitis and mild focal necrosis without demonstrable causative agent in the liver. It is observed in systemic and extrahepatic diseases, apparently due to circulating toxins and breakdown products.[4,25]

Chronic lobular hepatitis is not a morphological entity. Histologically, it corresponds to a picture of mild acute hepatitis. The notion of chronicity relies on the clinical history.[4,11]

Chronic active hepatitis is the older terminology (see initial classification of chronic hepatitis in ref. 26), combining periportal hepatitis (piecemeal necrosis) and parenchymal necroinflammatory lesions. With longer duration, increasing degrees of septal fibrosis supervene, eventually ending in liver cirrhosis.[9]

In the cirrhotic stage, the portal and parenchymal lesions of chronic active hepatitis may burn out (inactive cirrhosis) or persist (active cirrhosis).

Hepatitis B can be recognized in several cases by the presence of ground-glass hepatocytes. In acute episodes, liver cell pleomorphism is often marked and hepatocyte degeneration tends to be of a ballooning or lytic type and is localized in acinar zone 3.

Features suggestive for *hepatitis C* include: portal lymphoid aggregates or lymph follicles, bile duct damage, intra-acinar necroinflammatory changes with numerous apoptotic bodies, some steatosis, and a mild degree of piecemeal necrosis.[27]

Hepatitis D superinfection of chronic hepatitis B is usually characterized by severe lobular lesions with extensive piecemeal necrosis and rapid progression to cirrhosis. Marked panacinar inflammation with a morphology similar to hepatitis C is typical.[28, 29] 'Morula cells' (hepatocytes with microvesicular steatosis) have been described in some instances[30] and may be related to a more pathogenic strain (Parana, JHepatol, 1995; 22:468).

The histopathology of *hepatitis G* is not yet well established. Multilobular necrosis may be seen in fulminant cases, and chronic forms occur in varying degrees of severity.

Fibrosing cholestatic hepatitis, a peculiar morphological pattern of hepatitis B, was first observed after liver transplantation.[31] It is characterized by unusually high-level expression of intracytoplasmic HBsAg and HBcAg associated with only mild necrosis and inflammation. In addition, there is severe bilirubinostasis and a characteristic perisinusoidal fibrosis, encasing groups of liver cells or entire liver cell plates. It is apparently related to the immunosuppressed state of the patient, since it has also been reported in coinfection by HBV and HIV (Fang, Lancet, 1993; 342:1175) and in renal transplant recipients (Chen, Gastro, 1994; 107:1514; Booth, JHepatol, 1995; 22:500).

Drug-induced chronic hepatitis can be suspected in some cases on the presence of small granulomas, eosinophilic infiltration, and bile duct damage involving the finest biliary radicles.

Autoimmune hepatitis admittedly has no specific histopathology; however, a picture of severely active hepatitis including extensive piecemeal necrosis, bridging confluent necrosis, hepatitic liver cell rosettes, and abundance of plasma cells is quite suggestive.

Wilson's disease is the result of tissue injury due to copper overload in the liver and other organs. Clinically as well as histopathologically, it may manifest itself as acute hepatitis mimicking acute viral hepatitis, as fulminant hepatitis, as chronic active hepatitis indistiguishable from that due to viral and other aetiologies, or as cirrhosis. Helpful differential clues in the diagnosis of Wilson's disease include the presence of steatosis, glycogenated nuclei, the presence of Mallory bodies in periportal liver cells, and moderate to marked copper storage (best seen on rhodanine stain).

α_1-*Antitrypsin deficiency* can histologically resemble chronic hepatitis of viral and other aetiologies. Recently, a high prevalence of hepatotrophic viral infection (HCV and HBV) in predominantly heterozygote patients with chronic liver disease has been documented.[32] However, other studies suggest that α_1-antitrypsin deficiency *per se* may be the cause of chronic liver disease (Geller, Hepatol, 1994; 19:389).

Immunohistochemical stains (immunofluorescence and immunoperoxidase methods) are based on the binding of antibodies to specific antigens in tissue sections. Several procedures are available, the two most commonly used at present being the peroxidase–antiperoxidase immune complex method and the biotin–avidin immunoenzymatic technique. In the latter procedure, the high affinity of avidin for biotin is used to couple the peroxidase label to the primary antibody. Their use in demonstrating viral antigens has enormously increased the diagnostic impact of liver biopsy in confirming or establishing the viral aetiology of hepatitis. Some of the most frequently used are for hepatitis A, B (HBsAg, HBcAg, HBeAg, HBxAg), C, D, and E, herpes, and cytomegalovirus. Demonstration of HBsAg and HBcAg on paraffin sections of liver biopsies from patients with chronic hepatitis B is helpful in determining whether the patient is still in the viral replicative phase, and hence a potential candidate for interferon therapy, or whether the patient has already evolved into the so-called viral integration phase.[29]

In situ *hybridization* finds increasing application in diagnostic pathology in general.[33] It is applied to liver tissue for the assessment of viral replication in hepatitis A, B, C, and D, cytomegalovirus hepatitis, and Epstein–Barr viral hepatitis.[34] Combination of the *polymerase chain reaction* with *in situ* hybridization becomes possible, providing the pathologist with an extremely sensitive detection method.

Acute alcoholic hepatitis (acute hepatitis of the alcoholic type, fatty liver hepatitis, steatohepatitis) comprises several changes; there is no general agreement on minimum requirements. Usually the histological changes comprise steatosis, Mallory bodies, and satellitosis. In most cases, some degree of fibrosis (periportal, pericentral, pericellular) is also present. In the face of continuing alcohol abuse, the lesions may persist in the cirrhotic stage. It must be realized that in a minority of cases, this lesion is not due to alcohol (e.g. diabetes and obesity, amiodarone and perhexiline maleate toxicity, abetalipoproteinaemia).[2,7]

Regeneration

Parenchymal giant cells (multinucleated hepatocytes) correspond to huge, often pale parenchymal cells with multiple nuclei; they result from fusion rather than from incomplete division of hepatocytes. They occur most typically in neonatal cholestasis (so-called neonatal hepatitis and bile duct atresia), but are occasionally observed in adults, for example in viral hepatitis C and some forms of drug-induced hepatitis.[4]

Anisokaryosis refers to unequal size of the liver cell nuclei. It increases with advancing age, due to increasing ploidy of liver cell nuclei.

Liver cell dysplasia (dysplastic liver cells) (Anthony, JClinPath, 1973; 26:217) usually occurs in groups of hepatocytes. They are characterized by unequal size and shape and increased staining density (hyperchromatism) of their nuclei (Plate 30). Dysplasia seems to be related to HBV and HCV infection;[35] its presence heralds an increased risk for hepatocellular carcinoma.[36] Two types of liver cell dysplasia, small cell dysplasia and large cell dysplasia, are recognized.

Twin-cell plates. In the normal liver beyond the age of 5 years, hepatocytes are arranged in single-cell plates (muralium simplex). Plates of two or more cells in thickness (muralium duplex or multiplex) indicate regeneration (Plate 18).

Nodular regeneration refers to regenerative expansion of smaller or larger parenchymal territories.

Micronodules are conventionally defined as 3 mm or less in diameter. They comprise regenerative parenchymal masses which may correspond to different parts or combinations of architectural liver units, as follows:[6,7,11,18]

1. Segments of simple acini dissected by portal–central septa (pseudolobular nodules without vascular landmarks)
2. Segments of simple acini encircled by portal–portal septa, carrying a central draining venule (monolobular nodules in biliary fibrosis and cirrhosis)
3. Complex acini delineated by central–central septa and centred by a portal tract (in congestive or cardiac cirrhosis).

Macronodules (more than 3 mm in diameter) consist of large areas of parenchyma equivalent to several acini, presumably regenerating acinar agglomerates (multilobular nodules). A macronodule reveals a substructure, identified by draining veins, often in excess to portal tracts which may appear diminutive; these anatomical landmarks show a less regular distribution than in normal liver parenchyma.[6, 7,11,18]

Nodular regenerative hyperplasia is characterized by diffuse nodularity of the liver parenchyma, due to regeneration and hyperplasia of acinar zones 1 and 2, associated with parenchymal atrophy and compression in the intervening acinar zones 3, without obvious internodular septum formation.[6,7,11]

References

1. Bianchi L. Liver biopsy interpretation in hepatitis. Part II: histopathology and classification of acute and chronic viral hepatitis/differential diagnosis. *Pathological Research Practice*, 1983; 178: 180–213.
2. Bianchi L. Liver biopsy interpretation in hepatitis. Part I. Presentation of critical morphologic features used in diagnosis (Glossary). *Pathological Research Practice*, 1983; 178: 2–19.
3. Phillips MJ, Poucell S, Patterson J, and Valencia P. *The liver. An atlas and text of ultrastructural pathology.* New York: Raven Press, 1987: 524.
4. Popper H. General pathology of the liver: light microscopic aspects serving diagnosis and interpretation. *Seminars in Liver Disease*, 1986; 6: 175–84.
5. Desmet VJ. Current problems in diagnosis of biliary disease and cholestasis. *Seminars in Liver Disease*, 1986; 6: 233–45.
6. MacSween RNM, Anthony PP, Scheuer PJ, Portmann B, and Burt AD. *Pathology of the liver.* Edinburgh: Churchill Livingstone, 1994.
7. Ishak KG. New developments in diagnostic liver pathology. In Farber E, Phillips MJ, and Kaufman N, eds. *Pathogenesis of liver diseases.* Baltimore: Williams & Wilkins, 1987: 223–373.
8. Bianchi L. Necroinflammatory liver diseases. *Seminars in Liver Disease*, 1986; 6: 185–98.
9. International Group. Acute and chronic hepatitis revisited. *Lancet*, 1977; ii: 914–19.
10. Ludwig J. New concepts in biliary cirrhosis. *Seminars in Liver Disease*, 1987; 7: 293–301.
11. Scheuer PJ and Lefkowitch JH. *Liver biopsy interpretation*, 5th edn. London: WB Saunders, 1994.
12. Desmet VJ and De Vos R. Structural analysis of acute liver injury. In Keppler D, Bianchi L, and Reutter W, eds. *Mechanisms of hepatocyte injury and death.* Lancaster: MTP Press, 1984: 11–30.
13. Desmet VJ. Current problems in diagnosis of biliary disease and cholestasis. *Seminars in Liver Disease*, 1986; 6: 233–45.
14. International Group. Histopathology of the intrahepatic biliary tree. *Liver*, 1983; 3: 161–75.
15. Desmet VJ. Cholangiopathies: past, present and future. *Seminars in Liver Disease*, 1987; 7: 67–76.
16. Desmet VJ and Callea F. Cholestatic syndromes of infancy and childhood. In Zakim D and Boyer TD, eds. *Hepatology. A textbook of liver disease*, Vol. 2, 3rd edn. Philadelphia: WB Saunders, 1996: 1649–98.
17. Desmet V, Roskams T, and Van Eyken P. Ductular reaction in the liver. *Pathological Research Practice*, 1995; 191: 513–24.
18. Anthony PP, Ishak KG, Nayak NC, Poulsen HE, Scheuer P, and Sobin LH. The morphology of cirrhosis. *Journal of Clinical Pathology*, 1978; 31: 395–414.
19. Poulsen H and Christoffersen P. *Atlas of liver biopsies.* Copenhagen: Munksgaard, 1979.
20. Martinez-Hernandez A and Martinez J. The role of capillarization in hepatic failure: studies in carbon tetrachloride-induced cirrhosis. *Hepatology*, 1991; 14: 864–74.
21. Denk H, *et al.* Guidelines for the diagnosis and interpretation of hepatic granulomas. *Histopathology*, 1994; 25: 209–18.
22. Ishak KG. Hepatic morphology in the inherited metabolic diseases. *Seminars in Liver Disease*, 1986; 6: 246–58.
23. Callea F. In Lowe GDO *et al.*, eds. *Fibrinogen 2, Biochemistry, physiology and clinical relevance.* Amsterdam: Elsevier Science Publishers BV (Biomedical Division), 1987: 75.
24. Baptista A, *et al.* The diagnostic significance of periportal hepatic necrosis and inflammation. *Histopathology*, 1988; 12: 569–79.
25. Gerber MA and Thung SN. Histology of the liver. *American Journal of Surgical Pathology*, 1987; 11: 709–22.
26. De Groote J, *et al.* A classification of chronic hepatitis. *Lancet*, 1968; ii: 626–8.
27. Dhillon AP and Dusheiko GM. Pathology of hepatitis C virus infection. *Histopathology*, 1995; 26: 297–309.
28. Bianchi L and Gudat F. Chronic hepatitis. In MacSween RNM, Anthony PP, Scheuer PJ, Portmann B, and Burt AD, eds. *Pathology of the liver*, 3rd edn. Edinburgh: Churchill Livingstone, 1994: 349–95.
29. Desmet VJ. Immunopathology of chronic viral hepatitis. *Hepato-Gastroenterology*, 1991; 38: 14–21.
30. Buitrago B, *et al.* Specific histologic features of Santa Marta hepatitis. A severe form of hepatitis delta-virus infection in northern South America. *Hepatology*, 1986; 6: 1285.
31. Davies SE, *et al.* Hepatic histological findings after transplantation for chronic hepatitis B virus infection, including a unique pattern of fibrosing cholestatic hepatitis. *Hepatology*, 1991; 13: 150–7.
32. Propst T, Propst A, and Dietze O. High prevalence of viral infection in adults with homozygous and heterozygous a1-antitrypsin deficiency and chronic liver disease. *Annals of Internal Medicine*, 1992; 117: 641–5.
33. Crocker J. *Molecular biology in histopathology.* Chichester: John Wiley & Sons, 1994.
34. Desmet V and Fevery J. Liver biopsy. *Baillières Clinical Gastroenterology*, 1995; 9: 811–28.
35. Lefkowitch JH, *et al.* Pathological diagnosis of chronic hepatitis C: a multicenter comparative study with chronic hepatitis B. *Gastroenterology*, 1993; 104: 595–603.
36. Borzio M, *et al.* Liver cell dysplasia is a major risk factor for hepatocellular carcinoma in cirrhosis: a prospective study. *Gastroenterology*, 1995; 108: 812–17.

3.2 Histological classification of chronic liver disease

Valeer J. Desmet and Tania Roskams

Chronic hepatitis

Chronic hepatitis is not a single disease entity, but rather a clinical and pathological syndrome of multiple aetiology and characterized by varying degrees of hepatocellular necrosis, inflammation, and fibrosis.

The first classification of chronic hepatitis was proposed in 1968.[1] Distinction was made between non-cirrhotic and cirrhotic stages of the disease. At that time the causes of chronic hepatitis were largely unknown and most cases were assumed to be autoimmune in nature (so-called lupoid hepatitis) and, as such, treated with steroids and immunosuppressive drugs. The proposed classification was aimed at distinguishing subgroups according to the degree of disease activity in order to provide prognostic information and criteria for the use of immunosuppressive therapy. In the initial classification, distinction was made between a milder category of disease, termed chronic persistent hepatitis, and variants with more severe disease activity, termed chronic aggressive or chronic active hepatitis. The emphasis for identifying more severe variants of the disease was on periportal piecemeal necrosis. Later on, lobular parenchymal lesions, in particular bridging hepatic necrosis, were included as markers of severity.[2] Chronic persistent hepatitis and chronic active hepatitis were not considered as distinct disease entities, but as variations in the degree of disease activity.

Since 1968, impressive progress has been achieved in the understanding of chronic hepatitis, including recognition of various causes of the syndrome: viral hepatitis B,[3] C (Alter, Blood, 1995; 85: 1681), D,[4] and G; several forms of autoimmunity;[5] and adverse drug reactions.[6] Parallel progress has been made in the therapy of chronic hepatitis, which has evolved separately according to aetiology: corticosteroids for autoimmune and α-interferon for viral hepatitis. Several metabolic diseases (Wilson's disease and α_1-antitrypsin deficiency) have been shown to resemble chronic hepatitis clinically and histologically in some cases. Moreover, it was realized that piecemeal necrosis, considered an important diagnostic criterion in chronic active hepatitis, may also be present in biliary diseases like primary biliary cirrhosis and primary sclerosing cholangitis, and that some forms of periportal necrosis in acute hepatitis may easily be mistaken for piecemeal necrosis.[2,7] Finally, problems arose concerning possible overlap syndromes between autoimmune hepatitis and other chronic liver diseases such as primary biliary cirrhosis[8] and primary sclerosing cholangitis (Rabinovitz, DigDisSci, 1992; 37:1606), and overlap syndromes between chronic hepatitis C and other chronic liver diseases such as autoimmune hepatitis[9] and chronic alcoholic liver disease (Brillanti, JHepatol, 1991; 13:347).

Better insight into the aetiology and pathogenesis of chronic hepatitis also caused a shift in emphasis for the classification from purely histological features to a combination of histological, clinical, and serological factors. A comprehensive and clinically useful categorization of a patient with chronic hepatitis has to consider: (i) aetiology, (ii) disease activity, (iii) stage of the disease, and also additional items such as superinfection with other viruses, viral mutants, immunosuppression (congenital, drug-induced, or HIV-induced), and lifestyle of the patient.

In 1994, two proposals for a new classification of chronic hepatitis were published.[10,11] One proposal came from a panel of experts from the International Association for the Study of the Liver (IASL).[10] This proposal does not insist on terminology or specific scoring systems, but rather provides guidelines for classifying chronic hepatitis. It recognizes that chronic hepatitis is a multi-aetiological syndrome that is characterized by varying degrees of hepatocellular necrosis and inflammation. For lack of a better definition, chronicity is still defined as continuing disease without improvement for at least 6 months. It acknowledges that several other liver diseases may appear to have the clinical and histological features of chronic hepatitis and need to be considered in the differential diagnosis, but does not include them under the heading 'chronic hepatitis'. Diseases to be excluded are: biliary diseases (primary biliary cirrhosis and primary sclerosing cholangitis), since these diseases are primarily caused by bile duct lesions; metabolic diseases (α_1-antitrypsin deficiency and Wilson's disease), since they represent genetic defects including extrahepatic lesions; and alcoholic liver disease.

The classification should be primarily based on aetiology because of the substantial differences in course, prognosis, and therapy of the various aetiological categories. The aetiology may be viral (HBV, HBV + HDV, HCV, HGV), autoimmune, drug-induced, or unknown (cryptogenic chronic hepatitis). Combined aetiologies (e.g. viral B + C) may occur, and should be specified as such. Within these aetiological categories, histological details are important in grading and staging of the disease.

Table 1 Example of correlation between semiquantitative grading and verbal assessment of biopsies

Histological activity index[a]	Brief description	Possible diagnosis in old nomenclature
1–3	Minimal chronic hepatitis	Non-specific reactive hepatitis CLH CPH
4–8	Mild chronic hepatitis	Severe CLH, CPH Mild CAH
9–12	Moderate chronic hepatitis	Moderate CAH
13–18	Severe chronic hepatitis	Severe CAH with bridging necrosis

CAH, chronic active hepatitis; CLH, chronic lobular hepatitis; CPH, chronic persistent hepatitis.
[a] Components 1, 2, and 3 only.

The second proposal was prepared by an international working party for the 1994 World Congress of Gastroenterology.[11] This proposal is largely comparable with the guidelines of the IASL panel. There are some differences, however, in that it includes primary biliary cirrhosis, primary sclerosing cholangitis, α_1-antitrypsin deficiency, and Wilson's disease under the heading of chronic hepatitis; it insists on abandoning the older terminology (chronic persistent hepatitis, chronic active hepatitis); it emphasizes the compatibility of the proposed terminology with the SNOMED codes (codes from the Systematized Nomenclature of Human and Veterinary Medicine published by the College of American Pathologists);[11] and recommends particular scoring systems.

Grading

Grading of chronic hepatitis is a measure of the severity of the disease and is important for prognostic and therapeutic purposes. Disease activity can be evaluated by clinical symptoms, by aminotransferase levels, and by histopathology of the liver biopsy.[10]

In the complex histopathological picture of liver cell damage, necrosis, and inflammation, the main components that have to be considered to evaluate disease activity are: portal inflammation, periportal piecemeal necrosis, intralobular focal necrosis, and confluent lytic necrosis of variable extent, especially the portal–central bridging and multilobular type (Desmet, YaleJBiolMed, 1988; 61: 61). Several grading systems can be utilized. The old categories of chronic persistent hepatitis and chronic active hepatitis essentially represent a grading system. For those rejecting the old terminology, new terms for describing various degrees of severity can be used, such as minimal, mild, moderate, and severe chronic hepatitis[10] (Table 1).

Another method, semiquantitative grading, or the assignment of numerical scores to different grades, has become an important requirement of therapeutic trials and can also be used to supplement (but not replace) verbal descriptions in routine diagnostic practice. Several scoring systems have been described (Lok, JClinPath, 1985; 38:530; Ludwig, Gastro, 1993; 105:274; Bedossa, Hepatol, 1994; 20: 15; Reichard, Hepatol, 1995; 21:918) (Table 1).[12-15]

The most widely used is the histological activity index (**HAI**), also known as the Knodell score.[13] It has the advantage of widespread use and therefore comparability between different published series. Its wide range of possible scores for necroinflammation

(from 0 to 18) provides a useful level of fine tuning which is not possible with more restricted ranges.

However, the HAI causes several problems, which create a need for modification (Bedossa, Hepatol, 1994; 20:15).[12,15] The first three categories of the HAI (periportal and/or bridging necrosis, intralobular degeneration and focal necrosis, and portal inflammation) represent components of a grading system, whereas the fourth category (fibrosis) represents a lesion to be evaluated for staging. Therefore, the generated scores should not be added to make a total score.[10,12] The first category combines piecemeal necrosis with bridging necrosis. Since both lesions probably have different pathogenetic mechanisms,[16] it may be preferable to score these histological variables separately, in order to evaluate their respective response to therapy. To avoid these problems, several alternative semiquantitative grading systems have been proposed (Bedossa, 1994; Ishak, JHepatol, 1995; 22:696; Reichard, Hepatol, 1995; 21:918).[15]

An acceptable semiquantitative grading system should evaluate all histological lesions which are meaningful in the assessment of disease severity and of prognosis, should be as simple and practical as possible, should be shown to be reasonably reproducible with low intra- and interobserver variation, and should produce results which are clinically useful.[17] Scoring systems may be adapted for particular purposes, such as rating steatosis and noting the presence of portal lymph follicles or bile duct lesions in chronic viral hepatitis C (Bedossa, Hepatol, 1994; 20:15).

Staging

Staging is a measure of disease progression and has significant prognostic and therapeutic implications. Its histological evaluation is based on the severity of fibrosis and development of cirrhosis.

The original 1968 classification of chronic hepatitis distinguished between non-cirrhotic and cirrhotic stages.[1] Recent, more elaborate classifications distinguish intermediate stages of lobular architectural disturbance.[12] As is the case for histological grading, histological staging of fibrosis and cirrhosis can be adequately assessed by verbal descriptions (Table 2).

For statistical purposes, staging can be expressed in numerical scores, such as the fibrosis score in the HAI,[13] or the fibrosis score according to Scheuer[15] or Ishak et al.[17] (Table 2).

Table 2 Scoring system for staging of chronic hepatitis

Score	Description	Knodell et al.[13]	Scheuer[15]
0	No fibrosis	No fibrosis	None
1	Mild fibrosis	Fibrous portal expansion	Enlarged, fibrotic portal tracts
2	Moderate fibrosis		Periportal or portal–portal septa, but intact architecture
3	Severe fibrosis	Bridging fibrosis (portal–portal or portal–central linkage)	Fibrosis with architectural distortion, but no obvious cirrhosis
4	Cirrhosis	Cirrhosis	Probable or definite cirrhosis

Any scoring system should be carefully prepared, and a consensus among the participants in a study should be reached about the precise definition of histological variables to be included (Bedossa, AnnPath, 1993; 13:260).[18]

There is a general consensus that the old classification should be replaced by one that considers all clinical, aetiological, and histological information available. Consequently, the final diagnosis of chronic hepatitis should be based on (i) aetiology, (ii) grade, and (iii) stage of the disease.

Chronic biliary diseases

Chronic biliary diseases comprise diseases of the extrahepatic and intrahepatic biliary tree, usually associated with cholestasis. Extrahepatic biliary disease implies mechanical obstruction to large bile ducts outside the liver or within the porta hepatis. The most common aetiologies include lithiasis, tumours, atresia, choledochal cyst, and strictures.[19]

Intrahepatic biliary diseases are those conditions in which there is injury to the intrahepatic bile ducts. In some of these, especially primary biliary cirrhosis, liver allograft rejection, and graft–versus-host disease, the interlobular bile ducts up to a diameter of 100 μm are damaged and progressively disappear, resulting in ductopenia— the so-called vanishing or disappearing bile duct disorders. In others, like primary sclerosing cholangitis, interlobular ducts may be affected together with larger intrahepatic and extrahepatic bile ducts.

In contrast to extrahepatic biliary obstruction, chronic intrahepatic bile duct lesions may evolve over many years without obvious morphological bilirubinostasis. This period of evolution is characterized by profound changes at the interface between portal tracts and parenchyma—cholestasis, ductular reaction, and biliary piecemeal necrosis—which are attributable to the effects of prolonged impairment of bile excretion.

In children and in adults, progressive destruction and loss of bile ducts lead to portal–portal bridging fibrosis and eventually development of a biliary cirrhosis.

Just as for chronic hepatitis, the classification of chronic biliary diseases can be based on (i) aetiology, (ii) grade or severity of the disease, and (iii) stage of the disease.

Aetiology

Chronic biliary diseases should be classified primarily according to aetiology (e.g. extrahepatic bile duct obstruction). In several of these

conditions, however, the aetiology remains unclear. Such diseases can nevertheless be more or less precisely defined by a set of clinical, biochemical, histopathological, and other changes. Table 3 gives an overview of disorders which today are considered as separate (aetiological?) disease entities in the category of chronic cholestatic biliary diseases.

Grading

The liver lesions occurring in chronic cholestatic biliary diseases can be assessed semiquantitatively. Besides verbal descriptions, and mainly for the purpose of particular studies and for therapeutical trials, the various tissue changes due to cholestasis and inflammation can be subject to semiquantitative numerical scoring.

For instance, in a study on the efficacy of ursodeoxycholic acid in the treatment of primary biliary cirrhosis, Poupon et al.[21] scored nine lesions on a scale from 0 to 3: fibrosis, inflammation (portal, parenchymal, portal–parenchymal interface), parenchymal necrosis, and cholestatic features (bilirubinostasis, cholate stasis, cholestatic liver cell rosettes, and ductular reaction). Such semiquantitative numerical scoring of the severity of histopathological lesions in pre- and post-treatment biopsies allowed conclusions to be drawn about the efficacy of ursodiol treatment in primary biliary cirrhosis.

We suggest, however, that estimation of the amount and pattern of fibrosis should be used for staging of the disease rather than for grading the severity of the process. As was mentioned under grading in chronic hepatitis, appropriate scoring systems could be tailored to individual disease entities, such as granulomas in sarcoidosis and plugging of dilated ductules in mucoviscidosis.

Staging

Several histological staging systems have been proposed for primary biliary cirrhosis.[22-24] In contrast to the staging systems of Scheuer[22] and Popper and Schaffner[23] that are specific for primary biliary cirrhosis, the staging system of Ludwig[24] can be used for any chronic biliary disease. There are four stages, based on pathological features that reflect the progression of the disease:

Stage I, portal stage: characterized by portal inflammation and possibly bile duct lesions.
Stage II, periportal stage: characterized by periportal ductular reaction, inflammation, and fibrosis.
Stage III, septal stage: characterized mainly by fibrous septa linking adjacent portal tracts (portal–portal septal fibrosis).

Table 3 An overview of chronic cholestatic biliary diseases

I. Extrahepatic bile duct obstruction (complete or incomplete obstruction, due to several possible causes)[19]

II. Diseases of intrahepatic bile ducts[20]
    A. In neonates and children
        Extrahepatic bile duct atresia (which also involves intrahepatic bile ducts)
        Paucity of interlobular bile ducts:
            syndromic variety (Alagille's syndrome)
            non-syndromic variety
        Mucoviscidosis
    B. In adults
        Primary biliary cirrhosis
        Immune cholangitis or autoimmune cholangiopathy
        Sarcoidosis with chronic intrahepatic cholestasis
        Primary sclerosing cholangitis
        Idiopathic adulthood ductopenia
        Graft-versus-host disease
        Liver allograft rejection (ductopenic rejection)
        Drug-induced lesions of interlobular bile ducts
        Histiocytosis X and Hodgkin's disease

Stage IV, cirrhotic stage: characterized by true biliary cirrhosis—fibrous septa and nodular regeneration.

The presence of portal–portal bridging fibrosis has been shown to correlate inversely with survival (Roll, NEJM, 1983; 308:1), and the presence of cirrhosis seems to be more frequent in specimens taken within 2 years of death (Portmann, Gastro, 1985; 88:1777).

Other chronic liver diseases

Chronic liver diseases other than chronic hepatitis and cholestatic biliary disease should be classified according to the same basic principle of categorizing according to aetiology, with further characterization by grading and staging.

Two examples, partly documented in the literature, are haemochromatosis and alcoholic liver disease.

Haemochromatosis

An adequate histological grading system for semiquantitative numerical scoring of iron overload in the liver has been elaborated by Deugnier et al. (Hepatol, 1993; 17:30). Dividing the total histological iron score by the age of the patient (in years) yields a 'histological iron index', which compares favourably with the biochemical iron index, and even allows differentiation between homozygous and heterozygous patients with genetic haemochromatosis. However, the 'histological iron index' is not entirely specific for genetic haemochromatosis.[25]

Staging of the disease should be based on an estimation of the quantity and pattern of fibrosis. Several scoring systems can be considered for this purpose: the fibrosis score of the HAI;[13] or the fibrosis scores according to Scheuer,[15] Ishak et al.,[17] or Chevallier et al.[26]

Alcoholic liver disease

The severity of alcoholic liver lesions can be estimated and expressed in verbal descriptions, and also semiquantitatively assessed in numerical scoring systems. An example of semiquantitative scoring (grading) of disease severity can be found in the study of Trinchet (JHepatol, 1994; 21:235). As a general rule, it seems appropriate to reserve the item 'fibrosis' for determining the stage of progression of the disease rather than including it amongst the parameters for grading the severity. A possible exception might be the lesion 'pericellular or perisinusoidal fibrosis', in view of the apparent direct effect of ethanol on activating collagen gene expression (Walton, Hepatol, 1996; 23:310).

Staging of alcoholic liver disease should be based on the amount and the pattern of fibrosis. The scoring system which at present appears the most suitable for staging alcoholic liver disease is the semiquantitative scoring system of fibrosis according to Chevallier et al.[26]

References

1. De Groote J, et al. A classification of chronic hepatitis. *Lancet*, 1968; **ii**: 626–8.
2. Bianchi L, et al. Acute and chronic hepatitis revisited. *Lancet*, 1977; **ii**: 914–19.
3. Koff RS. Viral hepatitis. In Schiff L and Schiff ER, eds. *Diseases of the liver*, Vol. 1, 7th edn. Philadelphia: JB Lippincott, 1993: 492–577.
4. Negro F and Rizzetto M. Pathobiology of hepatitis delta virus. *Journal of Hepatology*, 1993; **17**: S149–S153.
5. Manns MP and Kruger M. Immunogenetics of chronic liver diseases. *Gastroenterology*, 1994; **106**: 1676–97.
6. Pessayre D and Larrey D. Acute and chronic drug-induced hepatitis. *Baillière's Clinical Gastroenterology*, 1988; **2**: 385–422.
7. Baptista A, et al. The diagnostic significance of periportal hepatic necrosis and inflammation. *Histopathology*, 1988; **12**: 569–79.
8. Ben Ari Z, Dhillon AP, and Sherlock S. Autoimmune cholangiopathy: part of the spectrum of autoimmune chronic active hepatitis. *Hepatology*, 1993; **18**: 10–15.
9. Strassburg CP and Manns M. Autoimmune hepatitis versus viral hepatitis C. *Liver*, 1995; **15**: 225–32.
10. Desmet VJ, Gerber M, Hoofnagle JH, Manns M, and Scheuer PJ. Classification of chronic hepatitis: diagnosis, grading and staging. *Hepatology*, 1994; **19**: 1513–20.
11. Working Party. Terminology of chronic hepatitis, hepatic allograft rejection, and nodular lesions of the liver: summary of recommendations developed by an international working party, supported by the World Congresses of Gastroenterology, Los Angeles, 1994. *American Journal of Gastroenterology*, 1994; **89**: S177–S181.

12. Bianchi L and Gudat F. Chronic hepatitis. In MacSween RNM, Anthony PP, Scheuer PJ, Portmann B, and Burt AD, eds. *Pathology of the liver*, 3rd edn. Edinburgh: Churchill Livingstone, 1994: 349–95.

13. Knodell RG, *et al.* Formulation and application of a numerical scoring system for assessing histological activity in asymptomatic chronic active hepatitis. *Hepatology*, 1981; **1**: 431–5.

14. Goodman ZD and Ishak KG. Histopathology of hepatitis C virus infection. *Seminars in Liver Disease*, 1995; **15**: 70–81.

15. Scheuer PJ. Classification of chronic viral hepatitis: a need for reassessment. *Journal of Hepatology*, 1991; **13**: 372–4.

16. Desmet VJ. Immunopathology of chronic viral hepatitis. *Hepato-gastroenterology*, 1991; **38**: 14–21.

17. Ishak K *et al.* Histological grading and staging of chronic hepatitis. *Journal of Hepatology*, 1995; **22**: 696–9.

18. Desmet V and Fevery J. Liver biopsy. *Baillière's Clinical Gastroenterology*, 1995; **9**: 811–28.

19. Desmet VJ. Cholestasis: extrahepatic obstruction and secondary biliary cirrhosis. In MacSween RNM, Anthony PP, Scheuer PJ, Burt AD, and Portmann BC, eds. *Pathology of the liver*, 3rd edn. Edinburgh: Churchill Livingstone, 1994: 425–76.

20. Desmet VJ. Vanishing bile duct disorders. In Boyer JL and Ockner RK, eds. *Progress in liver diseases*, Vol. 10. Philadelphia: WB Saunders, 1992: 89–121.

21. Poupon RE, Balkau B, Eschwège E, Poupon R, and DCA and PBC Study Group. A multicenter, controlled trial of ursodiol for the treatment of primary biliary cirrhosis. *New England Journal of Medicine*, 1991; **324**: 1548–54.

22. Scheuer PJ. Primary biliary cirrhosis. *Proceedings of the Royal Society of Medicine*, 1967; **60**: 1257–60.

23. Popper H and Schaffner F. Nonsuppurative destructive chronic cholangitis and chronic hepatitis. In Popper H and Schaffner F, eds. *Progress in liver diseases*, Vol. 3. New York: Grune & Stratton, 1970: 336–54.

24. Ludwig J, Dickson ER, and McDonald GSA. Staging of chronic non-suppurative destructive cholangitis (syndrome of primary biliary cirrhosis). *Virchows Archiv. A. Pathological Anatomy and Histopathology*, 1978; **379**: 103–12.

25. George P, Conaghan C, Angus H, Walmsley T, and Chapman B. Comparison of histological and biochemical hepatic iron indexes in the diagnosis of genetic haemochromatosis. *Journal of Clinical Pathology*, 1996; **49**: 159–63.

26. Chevallier M, Guerret S, Chossegros P, Gerard F, and Grimaud JA. A histological semiquantitative scoring system for evaluation of hepatic fibrosis in needle liver biopsy specimens: comparison with morphometric studies. *Hepatology*, 1994; **20**: 349–55.

4

Symptoms and signs of liver disease

4 Symptoms and signs of liver disease

Neil McIntyre

The collection of clinical information

The care of patients starts with collection of information by history taking, physical examination, and investigations. All three components are essential; their relative value varies from case to case. Some hepatologists argue that the history and physical examination are of limited value in managing liver disease, because investigations (e.g. ultrasound, CT scanning, cholangiography, liver biopsy and serological tests) often provide a precise diagnosis. Other specialists argue similarly; chest physicians and cardiologists may look at the chest radiograph or echocardiogram before examining the patient. This tends to bias both the detection and the interpretation of symptoms and physical signs, and so limits their value.[1,2]

Such an attitude stems from thinking about the history and physical examination just in terms of diagnosis of the presenting complaint, not as a search for problems needing explanation (and sometimes urgent management). We should try to identify all important problems, as disease may exist in more than one system.

Symptoms, signs, and routine laboratory tests are the basis on which further, more specialized, investigations are ordered. The better the initial assessment, the more likely it is that problems will be dealt with appropriately. This may involve a search for additional, and more specific, features of diagnostic, prognostic, or therapeutic value. Many special investigations are invasive, particularly in hepatology, and carry a small but significant risk of serious complications; not all clinicians have the facilities to carry them out. In developing countries, and in small, isolated hospitals in developed countries, physicians have to rely heavily on the clinical picture when making diagnostic and therapeutic decisions, or when deciding to refer the patient to another more specialized unit (often at great inconvenience and cost to the patient).

While we may be confident that liver disease is present, from details in referral letters, it is important to realize that referring physicians may have missed other problems, or omitted to mention them in referral letters, thinking them irrelevant to the liver problem. If, as a result, an important and treatable disease in another system is missed, excellent management of the liver disease may be nullified. Furthermore, there may be two hepatobiliary problems, not one, or problems in both the gut and liver; careful clinical evaluation may reveal additional problems and alter the management plan.

It is useful to be aware of the patient's clinical details when reviewing the results of special investigations. Sometimes a report is in error. One may look inadvertently at the wrong radiograph or CT scan (one having the wrong date, or belonging to another patient). Familiarity with the patient's story and physical signs enables us to spot inconsistencies. Confidence in the reliability of our own clinical findings justifies the repetition of invasive tests when the initial results are equivocal. Finally, the recognition of new symptoms and signs may allow early detection of complications in patients with liver disease, but for this, one must be fully aware of the details in the initial evaluation.

The history

The patient's story is as important in hepatology as in other areas of clinical medicine. A full history records:

(1) the history of the present illness (starting with a list of current complaints);
(2) systematic enquiry;
(3) past medical history;
(4) family history;
(5) drug history and allergies;
(6) psycho-social history;
(7) risk factors—including an occupational history and a history of foreign travel (see Appendices 1 and 2)

History of the present illness

A patient's 'illness' is essentially the set of symptoms from which he or she is suffering; the doctor's task is to decide whether they are due to a single disease, or to a combination of different diseases. Many doctors write a 'history of presenting symptoms or complaints', but this is poor clinical practice; presenting symptoms may be dramatic and important, but often, when the full story unfolds, they prove to be of little diagnostic relevance. Many liver diseases are a consequence of earlier problems, and underlying relationships may be missed by concentrating only on the story of the presenting complaints. For this reason one should take a 'history of the present illness' starting from the time when the patient last felt perfectly fit and well, even if this was many years before. New symptoms can then be seen as part of the natural history of a disease, as a complication of another condition or of previous treatments, or as manifestations of a new disease in someone with other problems.

Furthermore, in hepatology, details of current symptomatology are often unhelpful for differential diagnosis, as patients with liver disease tend to have similar symptoms regardless of cause, for example asthenia, anorexia, nausea, right upper quadrant discomfort, dark urine. Other, earlier features are usually of far greater diagnostic importance, for example previous episodes of upper abdominal pain, surgery, treatment with hepatotoxic drugs, and a history of blood transfusion or administration of blood products.

There are many possible causes of liver disease; few doctors remember to ask all the relevant questions. The initial collection of information can be improved by using a check list, or by giving the patient a self administered questionnaire; both save time in collecting routine information. It is particularly useful to take a 'secondary' history, which reviews the story and probes for points which may have been missed, particularly if the patient was clerked initially by an inexperienced clinician. Often patients cannot supply necessary details, for example about drugs or previous surgery; it is then crucial to contact clinicians who were involved earlier, or to look at their clinical notes.

Symptoms of liver disease
Weakness (asthenia), tiredness, and malaise

Weakness (asthenia), easy fatiguability, and tiredness are very common symptoms in patients with liver disease. They have little diagnostic value as they often occur in diseases of other systems, and in depression, but when they are present, liver disease should be considered as a cause. With chronic liver disease tiredness and easy fatiguability may be present for months, or even years, before the diagnosis is made. These symptoms usually get worse during the day; patients who feel worse in the morning, and improve during the day, are usually suffering from depression. The asthenia of liver disease may also be longstanding, but there is rarely objective evidence of weakness unless liver disease is advanced. The mechanisms underlying these symptoms are unknown and deserve further study. In a recent study no evidence of muscle weakness was found in patients with primary biliary cirrhosis (using supramaximal stimulation of the ulnar nerve to produce contraction of the adductor pollicis muscle); 'central' fatigue was identified using questionnaires, including the fatigue severity scale, a depression index, and a mental fatigue questionnaire (Jalan, Hepatol, 1996; 24:167A).

These symptoms contribute to the generalized 'malaise' which is a presenting feature in about a third of patients with acute hepatitis, chronic hepatitis, cirrhosis, or tumours, and in almost two-thirds of those with acute alcoholic liver disease. Although they may improve rapidly after an acute hepatitis, they may persist for many months. They constitute a major problem for patients with primary biliary cirrhosis ((Jalan, Hepatol, 1996; 24:167A). There is no effective symptomatic treatment for weakness and tiredness, but there may be rapid improvement when specific therapy is available for the liver disease (e.g. with steroids for autoimmune hepatitis, with long-term abstention from alcohol, or with successful liver transplantation).

Anorexia

Anorexia, or decrease in appetite, is a common symptom of liver disease, particularly in jaundiced patients with either hepatocellular failure or biliary obstruction. It is present in 89 per cent of patients with acute viral hepatitis (Henkin, Lancet, 1971; i:823), in which it is often a presenting feature; it is common in alcoholic hepatitis, the prevalence increasing with the severity of the liver disease (Mendenhall, AmJMed, 1984; 76:211). Anorexia may be profound; loss of adipose tissue and muscle, and other features of malnutrition,

are then an inevitable consequence, but this is not always reflected in the body weight if fluid retention is also present. In chronic liver disease the onset of severe anorexia is an ominous sign, unless it is caused by a drug or by another treatable condition.

Unfortunately, anorexia occurs in many other diseases. It is worth establishing whether there is another obvious cause, or whether anorexia is exacerbated by the thought of eating particular foods. It is also important to distinguish it from 'satiety', from food intolerance, and from 'sitophobia' (fear that eating will produce discomfort); these conditions often have specific causes. Satiety (in which the desire to eat is reduced during a meal, even though it may be normal before the meal) may result if the effective volume of the stomach is reduced; it is commonly associated with marked ascites.

Little is known about the cause(s) of anorexia (Russek, Appetite, 1981; 2:137; Kissileff, AnnRevNutr, 1982; 2:371; Baile, ProcNutrSoc, 1983; 42:113; Nicholl, AnnRevNutr, 1985; 5:213). Several factors have been proposed to account for anorexia, mainly from animal experiments. They include size of meals, periodicity and rate of eating, availability of food, changes in energy stores, and the nature of ingested food; these seem unlikely causes in liver disease. Changes in energy expenditure or in apparent palatabilty of food, or changes in the levels of circulating hormones (such as leptin, glucagon, somatostatin, cholecystokinin, gastrin and bombesin), or nutrients (glucose, free fatty aids, or amino acids) seem more likely causes in liver disease. In a recent study, rats with an obstructed bile duct seemed to have a complete absence of central responsiveness to neuropeptide Y induced food and water intake. This whole area deserves further study.

Disordered taste and smell

Patients with liver disease occasionally complain of disturbed taste and, less often, of problems with their sense of smell. This probably explains why smokers give up cigarettes when they become jaundiced (this is not, as often claimed, a specific pointer to acute hepatitis). In acute viral hepatitis decreased subjective taste acuity, and increased use of salt or sugar, was noted in 84 per cent of patients; an obnoxious taste or smell was attributed to fried foods (by 74 per cent) and to meat (by 90 per cent) (Henkin, Lancet, 1971; i:823). In a more objective study the thresholds for the detection and recognition of salt, sucrose, hydrochloric acid, and urea were elevated (Smith, Gastro, 1976; 70:568). Disordered taste and smell may contribute to anorexia in liver disease.

In alcoholic cirrhotics supplementation with both zinc (Weissmann, ActaMedScand, 1979;205:361) and vitamin E (Garrett-Laster, HumNutrCN, 1984; 38C:203) was reported to improve taste sensation.

Nausea and vomiting

Nausea and vomiting are common complaints in liver disease. Nausea often occurs without vomiting; much less commonly vomiting occurs without nausea. Many patients are familiar with the term 'nausea', using it to describe a sick feeling or a sensation that vomiting is imminent. Others use nausea erroneously to describe a sinking feeling in the stomach, or other sensations. Vomiting is a forceful expulsion of gastric contents, to be distinguished from 'regurgitation', 'retching', or 'dry heaves' (which may precede vomiting). 'Regurgitation', a very common symptom, is the reflux of gastric contents into the mouth, without the forceful efforts which accompany vomiting; it usually results from incompetence of the lower oesophageal sphincter and may respond to appropriate therapy. With 'retching' there is no expulsion of gastric contents; it is common in alcoholics, with or without liver disease, and usually occurs in the morning.

Even in acute viral hepatitis nausea and vomiting are uncommon initial symptoms (when compared with anorexia, malaise, or flu-like symptoms). Vomiting is often a striking feature in patients with acute biliary obstruction due to gallstones, but may be absent. Nausea and vomiting both occur commonly, at some stage of the disease, in jaundiced patients with either parenchymal liver disease (including tumours) or biliary obstruction; nausea appears before jaundice in most patients, particularly in those with alcoholic liver disease. Persistent nausea, which often leads to referral to a hepatologist, may occur without organic cause: of 77 such patients, 11 had undergone cholecystectomy, and it was suggested that surgery was performed because investigation of the nausea had revealed asymptomatic gallstones (Swanson, MayoClinProc, 1976; 51:257).

Detailed analysis of these symptoms in patients with liver disease is rarely of value, except to distinguish between them, but clearly it is important to ask about the nature and colour of vomitus. Patients nearly always mention the vomiting of black material or blood, which indicates bleeding from a site above the ligament of Treitz (the 'black' colour is actually dark brown, due to the presence of haematin). It is also important to check for obvious factors causing nausea, such as alcohol, and to assess whether prolonged nausea and/or vomiting might be related to the administration of a drug. Although nausea and vomiting are usually attributable to liver disease *per se*, particularly in acute hepatobiliary disorders, their appearance in patients with chronic disease should trigger the search for a remediable cause.

In a controlled trial in cirrhotic patients metoclopramide was shown to suppress nausea and heartburn (Uribe, Gastro, 1985; 88: 757), but it should be used cautiously in patients with fluid retention as it stimulates secretion of aldosterone; domperidone is to be preferred in such patients (D'Arienzo, Hepatol, 1985; 5:854).

Weight loss and gain

Weight loss is common in patients with acute and chronic liver disease, due mainly to anorexia and reduced food intake. It is an unusual presenting feature but may occur at some stage with all the major causes of liver disease, particularly acute hepatitis or malignancy. Weight loss regularly accompanies endstage liver disease, when loss of muscle mass, and of adipose tissue, is often a striking feature; it also occurs with superimposed hypercatabolic states, such as localized infections or bacteraemia.

In a series of 91 patients, investigated for loss of 5 per cent or more of the body weight, 35 per cent had no identifiable cause of weight loss; in the others the major causes were malignancy and gastrointestinal diseases. Abnormal biochemical results were found in 22 per cent of those with an organic cause but, although the most common abnormalities were of liver function tests, a primary disease of the liver was found in only one patient, who had alcoholic liver disease (Marton, AnnIntMed, 1981; 95:568).

The most common causes of weight gain in patients with chronic liver disease are simple obesity and fluid retention, but with the latter the patient usually complains of ankle or abdominal swelling rather than weight gain.

Abdominal discomfort and pain

Abdominal pain or discomfort is common in hepatobiliary diseases. Because the liver extends across the upper abdomen, pain or discomfort may be felt in the right hypochondrium or under the right lower ribs (front, side, or back), in the epigastrium, or in the left hypochondrium. However, although the liver is embryologically a midline organ, pain and discomfort originating in the liver are usually experienced under the right lower ribs. Pain results if an inflammatory or malignant lesion spreads to the surface of the liver or gallbladder; it may be exacerbated by breathing, and if the surface of the right diaphragm is involved, pain may also be felt in the right shoulder.

Pain or discomfort may occur if there is rapid or gross enlargement of the liver or spleen. Pain limited to the middle or lower abdomen is unlikely to be due to hepatic or biliary problems, but low retrosternal pain commonly results from acute biliary tract disease. Generalized discomfort may occur with abdominal distension due to ascites, and appears to be related to the rate of fluid accumulation and the tension in the abdominal wall.

The patient may complain of tenderness over the liver rather than pain or discomfort; this can occur with acute or chronic hepatitis, is found occasionally in cirrhosis, and is a common feature with an abscess. Some tumours (primary or secondary) are extremely tender on palpation.

Right upper quadrant pain

Chronic pain or discomfort in the right upper quadrant, or over the right lower ribs laterally or posteriorly, is a very common symptom in medical and surgical clinics', and patients (and many doctors) tend to assume that it originates in the liver or gallbladder. Hepatobiliary disease is an unlikely cause if the patient has no other features of liver or biliary disease (and if an ultrasound examination is normal); it is more likely then to be due to colonic distension with gas. Right upper quadrant pain is, however, very common in many different types of liver disease, and with chronic cholecystitis. Discomfort in this region often seems to appear after the patient has been told there is something wrong with the liver!

It may be difficult to get a clear description of the pain. If it has been present for weeks or months it is likely to be mild or moderate, as patients seek assistance early when a pain is truly severe. Persistent right upper quadrant pain or discomfort may occur in acute or chronic hepatitis, or with cirrhosis; the cause is unclear but it may be due to stretching of the hepatic capsule, or to inflammation near the surface of the liver.

Laurin *et al.* (AmJGastr, 1994; 89:1840) found that 31 of 178 patients with primary biliary cirrhosis (17 per cent) complained of abdominal pain at entry to the study, usually in the right upper quadrant. In a third of them the pain was still present after 12 months, and in 20 per cent it persisted after 24 months. Four had asymptomatic cholelithiasis, one oesophageal erosions, four gastric erosions, two duodenal erosions, and one a gastric ulcer. The authors concluded that upper gastrointestinal endoscopy was the best test to exclude treatable causes of the pain.

Although it is now assumed that there is no relationship between dyspeptic symptoms and the presence of gallstones, Kraag *et al.* (ScaJGastr, 1995; 30:411) found, on meta-analysis, that there was a relationship with upper abdominal pain, but with no preference for the right side. There was no association with classical dyspeptic symptoms such as flatulence, heartburn, acid regurgitation, bloating, and belching, and fat intolerance; there was a relationship with nausea and vomiting and with unspecified food intolerance.

Acute right upper quadrant pain is a common feature of cholecystitis, but in about half of patients with this condition the pain is felt across the upper half of the abdomen, is vague and generalized, or is felt diffusely across the right half of the abdomen. It is usually an intermittent pain, severe pain being interspersed with pain-free periods of an hour or two. The pain of acute cholecystitis is often aggravated by deep inspiration.[3] A previous history of jaundice, or of episodes of similar pain, is of diagnostic help in this condition.

Acute right upper quadrant pain may occur in pancreatitis, with hepatic neoplasm or abscess, and with acute biliary obstruction due to a common bile duct stone. When pain occurs with hepatic abscesses and tumours it tends to be more severe.

The pain of bile duct obstruction

This has been studied experimentally[4] (Schein, SGO, 1968; 126: 591; Schein, AmJSurg, 1970; 119:261). It results from distension and increased pressure within the bile duct and appears to have two phases. The first, due to lesser degrees of increased pressure, is usually described as a tolerable fullness and discomfort in the middle and upper abdomen, and is associated with nausea. The second, usually called 'biliary colic', is not a colic in the usual sense of the term, as it does not make the patient double up, nor does it wax and wane; it tends to persist as long as the elevated pressure is maintained. In experimental studies the severe pain is not produced until the pressure in the duct is above that required to produce maximal bile duct distension; it improves when the perfusion pressure is reduced (Doran, BrJSurg, 1967; 54:599). With cholangitis both the pain and the initial phase of fullness and discomfort are produced at lower intraluminal pressures. The severe pain is usually localized to the upper abdomen, is often central (being visceral in nature), and lasts for several hours.

In most patients with pancreatic tumours, and in many with complete obstruction due to gallstones, biliary pain is absent, even though the bile duct may be markedly dilated; presumably the pressure within the bile duct, and wall tension, is relatively low.

Jaundice and dark urine

Patients sometimes complain that they are, or have been, jaundiced, or 'looked yellow'; relatives or friends may have commented on their appearance. A history of jaundice, even in the past, is important; the simultaneous presence of dark urine establishes hepatobiliary disease as the most likely explanation for the jaundice.

Patients should be asked specifically whether their dark urine is a brown colour (like dark beer, Coca-cola, or tea without milk). 'Dark' orange or deep yellow urine does not suggest bilirubinuria, but should suggest the possibility of dehydration. Dark brown urine is usually due to the presence of bilirubin esters; it often occurs before the appearance of jaundice. Bilirubinuria should be confirmed with a dipstick as there are other causes of dark urine (see

Chapter 5.1). Conjugated bilirubin covalently bound to plasma proteins is not excreted in the urine in detectable amounts and may be present in plasma in the absence of dark urine. For reasons that are not understood, bilirubin esters may also be absent from the urine, despite high levels in the blood, in some patients with obstructive uropathy or parenchymal renal disease, and also when liver disease is associated with haemolysis.

Bowel function and stools

It is important to ask about the frequency, consistency, and colour of stools. A moderate increase in stool frequency, with passage of soft or loose stools, is common with all major causes of liver disease even in the absence of jaundice, and particularly in alcoholics and in acute viral hepatitis. If diarrhoea is severe, or if there is a marked alteration in bowel habit in patients with otherwise stable chronic liver disease, another cause should be sought. In some cases, diarrhoea may be due to increased faecal fat resulting from a lowered intraluminal concentration of bile salts. Obvious steatorrhoea is an uncommon presenting symptom except with malignant biliary obstruction, and higher levels of faecal fat result if the pancreatic duct is also blocked. Diarrhoea sometimes occurs with development of hepatocellular carcinoma; the reason is unknown. Liver disease may also be associated with conditions that cause diarrhoea, e.g. primary sclerosing cholangitis with ulcerative colitis, and hepatic secondaries with carcinoid syndrome (Chapters 24.2 and 22.3.2).

With bile duct obstruction, and in acute hepatitis with jaundice, the stools are usually pale, and the colour change is due to a reduction in the faecal excretion of pigments derived originally from the bile; the exact nature of the pigments is not known. Pale stools are also found in pancreatic steatorrhoea. It is particularly important to ask if the stools are black or very dark. If the patient is not taking oral iron or bismuth, or drinking Guinness, and if the stools tend to stick to the toilet pan, the most likely cause is upper intestinal bleeding; stool frequency, volume, and consistency may give a rough guide to the severity of the bleed.

Constipation is not usually a consequence of liver disease, although it may persist in those who habitually suffer from it. In patients with decompensated liver disease it may be a precipitating factor in the development of encephalopathy and should be treated. It may develop as a result of drug therapy.

Oedema and abdominal swelling (see Section 9)

In patients with liver disease, fluid retention causes swelling of the ankles and legs (or other types of dependent oedema), and/or abdominal distension (due to ascites). There are many causes of dependent oedema; when no other cause is obvious, liver disease should be considered as an explanation, even if there are no other obvious clinical features of liver involvement.

Abdominal distension, due to an increased volume of the abdominal cavity, may result from ascites (of which there are many causes), gaseous distension, or from enlargement of intra-abdominal organs (including the liver and spleen). Patients may complain of abdominal distension because their clothes become tight, or because of visible enlargement which may be gross. Ascites is the most common cause of abdominal distension in patients with established cirrhosis. Intermittent abdominal distension of short duration is a common complaint, usually due to intestinal gas and not to ascites or organomegaly.

With gross abdominal distension, patients often suffer abdominal discomfort, due presumably to increased intra-abdominal pressure, or to stretching of the visceral peritoneum in those with massive organomegaly. Patients with gross ascites may complain of the appearance or enlargement of hernias, of breathlessness due to elevation of the diaphragm, and occasionally of numbness on the lateral aspect of the thigh (due to pressure on the lateral cutaneous nerve, which emerges beneath the inguinal ligament). In some patients breathlessness may be unduly severe because of pleural effusion (usually right sided and sometimes gross), which is a well-recognized complication of ascites (see Chapters 8.1 and 25.1).

Ascites has also been described in acute viral hepatitis (Viola, Hepatol, 1983; 3:1013), but when it is a presenting feature in liver disease one should be suspicious of the development of the Budd–Chiari syndrome or of Wilson's disease (particularly in young patients).

Oliguria and nocturia

Patients with liver disease rarely complain of oliguria, but they may admit to reduced urine volume on direct questioning. It is a common feature in patients with overt fluid retention due to cirrhosis, and with hepatic venous outflow block. It may also occur in patients with severe acute liver disease, either as a secondary effect of the liver disease, or because the hepatitis is due to an agent which affects both the liver and kidneys; for example, poisoning due to paracetamol or carbon tetrachloride, or with leptospirosis (see Chapters 8.1, 13.1.2, 17, 18.1).

Nocturia may occur early in the course of fluid retention, presumably because recumbency causes a return of fluid to the central compartment, and also a change in the circulating levels of hormones such as renin, angiotensin, ADH, and atrial natriuretic peptide, thus promoting a transient diuresis (see Chapter 8.1).

Pruritus

Pruritus is an important symptom of liver disease. It is usually associated with cholestatic conditions, such as extrahepatic biliary obstruction, primary biliary cirrhosis (in which it is often the presenting symptom and may precede other features of the disease by months or years), sclerosing cholangitis, cholestasis of pregnancy, benign recurrent cholestasis, and biliary atresia in children. It is not always present in these conditions. It is also a feature in some patients with viral hepatitis (particularly hepatitis A) and occurs more commonly in adults than in children. It is rare in alcoholic liver disease, even when cholestatic features are present.

The pruritus of liver disease is of variable severity. It may be intermittent or mild, or generalized and severe. It tends to be most marked on the extremities, is present less often on the trunk, rarely on the neck and face, and hardly ever on the genitals (Sarkany, ProgrDerm, 1969; 4(i):1). It is often more troublesome after a hot bath, and at night, when the skin is warm, and when there is little else to divert the patient's attention.

The pruritus of liver disease has been attributed to the high plasma concentration of bile salts (or the retention of other biliary components), but there is still no convincing evidence to support this hypothesis (Ghent, YaleJBiolMed, 1979; 52:77; Freedman,

AmJMed, 1981; 70:1011). As opiate agonists, e.g. morphine, cause scratching in animals after injection into the brain, and opioid antagonists, e.g. naloxone, seem to relieve itching in patients with primary biliary cirrhosis, the suggestion has been made that itching due to liver disease is of central origin (Jones, Gut, 1996: 38:644).

The most effective therapy for the pruritus of liver disease is still oral cholestyramine, an anion-binding resin, which usually relieves itching within a few days. Colestipol, which has a similar action, is also effective and may be better tolerated. In patients resistant to these compounds other approaches can be tried, for example androgens such as methyltestosterone or stanozolol (Walt, BMJ, 1988; 296:607) which exacerbate the jaundice; rifampicin (Ghent, Gastro, 1988; 94:488); ursodeoxycholic acid; cortico-steroids; flumecinol (Turner, AlimPharmTher, 1994;8:337); pro-pofol (Borgeat, Gastro, 1993; 104:244); phototherapy (Rosenthal, ActaPaediat, 1994; 83:888); also phenobarbitone; methotrexate; evening primrose oil; S-adenosylmethionine (Gillespie, JGast-Hepatol, 1993; 8:168). The large number of agents tried is an eloquent testimony to the inadequacy of most of them! In some patients with primary biliary cirrhosis, pruritus may be unduly resistant to treatment, and so distressing that liver transplantation may be justified.

Bleeding and bruising (see Chapter 25.4)

Patients with either acute or chronic liver disease may complain of spontaneous (or easily induced) bleeding, from the nose or gums, or of easy bruising. The severity of the complaint is usually related to the degree of hepatic decompensation.

Fever and rigors (see also under Physical examination, below)

Fever is common in liver disease. It may be associated with the underlying cause of the liver disease, as in acute viral, alcoholic, or drug-induced hepatitis, or it may be due to a tumour or an infective complication (see Chapter 25.11). Rigors are uncommon in viral hepatitis; they are a classical feature of acute cholangitis, and in cirrhosis they should suggest a bacteraemic complication, although many bacteraemic cirrhotics have no obvious symptoms suggesting infection.

Encephalopathic symptoms, sleep[5] (see Section 9)

Patients in hospital with advanced liver disease often complain of somnolence during the daytime and may find it difficult to get off to sleep at night, but this is also true of patients with many other conditions. In cirrhotics this disturbance of the sleep-wake cycle may result from disruption of the diurnal rhythm of melatonin secretion, with markedly elevated levels of plasma melatonin during daylight hours (Steindl, AnnIntMed, 1995; 123:274).

Striking changes in mental function can occur with hepatic encephalopathy. In the early stages patients may sleep more during the day and suffer insomnia at night; sometimes there is clearly a reversed sleep pattern. At a more advanced stage there are changes in the conscious level. Patients tend to respond slowly to various stimuli, and may drift gradually into confusion, stupor, semi-coma, and eventually coma. Intellectual function deteriorates; initially the changes are subtle, but later there is a shortened attention span, an inability to solve mental problems or do simple calculations, memory loss, and finally an inability to communicate effectively at any level. Patients may develop personality disorders, showing undue euphoria or depression, become garrulous, irritable or angry, anxious or apathetic, and they may display inappropriate or bizarre behaviour. The patients themselves rarely complain of these disturbances, but they are a source of distress to relatives and friends. Methods of grading the degree of hepatic encephalopathy are presented at the end of this chapter.

Impotence and sexual dysfunction

Impotence is a symptom of cirrhosis (Cornley, Hepatol, 1984; 4: 1227); it was present in 14 of 20 patients with alcoholic cirrhosis, and in 10 out of 40 with non-alcoholic cirrhosis (the latter having been admitted for evaluation of liver transplant). In the alcoholics, impotence had been present for a longer time, and was more severe, than in the non-alcoholic cirrhotics, even though their liver disease appeared less advanced on biochemical grounds. In this study alcoholics had lower plasma testosterone levels and higher gonadotrophins than the non-alcoholic patients, but Kaymakoglu et al. (JGastroenterol, 1995; 30:745) found no significant differences between alcoholic and viral cirrhotics in with respect to clinical signs of hypogonadism, serum levels of sex steroids, and the results of seminal fluid analysis. They concluded that the degree of hypogonadism and feminization correlated well with the severity of liver failure.

Sexual behaviour was studied in women with a wide variety of liver diseases (Bach, Hepatol, 1989; 9:698). Liver disease was considered a significant factor interfering with sexual function in only 17 per cent, fatigue and depression being the usual reasons given. The frequency of intercourse decreased in 27 per cent following the onset of the disease. Reduced sexual desire was experienced in 33 per cent, difficulty in arousal in 18 per cent, lack of orgasm in 25 per cent, and dyspareunia in 21 per cent (usually attributed to poor vaginal lubrication). However, there appeared to be no statistical difference in sexual desire and function between these patients and women without liver disease who have participated in large-scale studies. Bach et al. stressed that women with liver disease could be reassured that they could maintain normal sexual relations.

Muscle cramps

Cirrhotic patients often complain of muscle cramps (Joekes, JRSM, 1982; 75:546). Konikoff and Theodor (JClinGastro, 1986; 8:669) found a much higher incidence of cramps in cirrhotics (88 per cent) than in age- and gender-matched controls (21 per cent). The cramps tended to be very painful, lasted for minutes, occurred mainly in the calves (but also in the fingers, toes, and thighs), were usually nocturnal and aggravated by rest. They occurred at varying intervals (more than once a week in another study) and seemed unrelated to diuretic therapy. Although the mean serum sodium, phosphate, and albumin levels were lower in cirrhotics with, than in those without, cramps the differences were not significant. The mean serum calcium level was significantly lower, but not the ionized calcium. Others reported similar findings (Chao, ChinJGastro, 1989; 6:169; Abrams, AmJGastr, 1996; 91:1363). Recently, Angeli et al. (Hepatol, 1996; 23:264) found that the prevalence of cramps was related to the duration of recognized cirrhosis and to the severity of liver functional impairment. In a multiple regression analysis, ascites, low mean arterial pressure, and high values of plasma renin activity were independent predictive factors for the occurrence of cramps in cirrhosis. Weekly intravenous infusion of albumin reduced cramp frequency.

The cramps may respond to quinine sulphate, which should probably be tried first. Konikoff et al. (IsrJMedSci, 1991; 27:221) investigated the role of vitamin E in the pathophysiology and treatment of muscle cramps. Patients suffering from cramps had a lower mean serum vitamin E level than those without cramps; after oral administration of tocopherol acetate (200 mg three times a day) there was a significant improvement in the frequency and duration of cramps and in their severity in terms of the associated pain.

Kobayashi et al. (ActaHepatolJpn, 1993; 34:960) treated patients with cramps occurring more than once a week with eperisone hydrochloride, an antispastic agent; cramps disappeared completely in 11 of 18 patients and they suggested that muscle cramps have a neural component, as eperisone hydrochloride is known to inhibit reflexes in the spinal cord. Yamamoto et al. (IntHepatolComm, 1994; 2:393) found that mean plasma taurine levels were lower in cirrhotics with cramps than in those without cramps; oral administration of taurine (3 g/day for 4 weeks) led to an improvement.

Systematic review

Systematic enquiry about symptoms relating to other body systems is important in patients with hepatobiliary disease. Patients often forget to mention symptoms, or they may feel that they are not relevant to their liver problem. A systematic enquiry allows detection of unsuspected diseases of other systems, and of complications of, or diseases associated with, the underlying liver disease. The links between the liver and other systems are fully discussed in Sections 24 and 25.

Past medical history

In many types of liver disease the past history is of great importance. In some cases relevant events may have occurred in the 'distant' past, in others more recently. Previous jaundice suggests the possibility of a previous acute hepatitis; if it was due to hepatitis B or hepatitis C infection, chronic liver disease may have resulted. Recurrence of jaundice suggests the possibility of reactivation, infection with another virus (including hepatitis D in HBsAg-positive patients), or the onset of hepatic decompensation. Previous jaundice may also have been due to gallstones, or drug-induced liver disease (often undiagnosed) which may have recurred with administration of the same drug. Jaundice soon after surgery suggests the possibility of halothane hepatitis, particularly with multiple exposures.

A history of blood transfusion or administration of various blood products, at any time in the past, is particularly important; it suggests the possibility of chronic hepatitis or cirrhosis due to hepatitis B, D, or C, or of HIV infection).

Previous surgery for tumours is important because liver involvement may be due to secondaries. A story of cholecystectomy, or other forms of upper abdominal surgery, suggests that subsequent liver disease may be due to retained gallstones, damage to the biliary tree causing stricture formation, or damage to the portal venous system.

A history of schistosomiasis, often in childhood, may be obtained in patients from countries in which it is endemic (see Chapters 13.4.1 and 32.1); this may explain clinical features suggesting portal hypertension. Schistomiasis now seems to be rather uncommon, and the high prevalence of hepatitis C in countries such as Egypt suggests that schistosomiasis may have been overdiagnosed as a cause of portal hypertension.

Family history

A family history of liver disease helps to establish the cause of genetically determined or infectious liver disease. This is particularly true for hereditary liver diseases such as Wilson's, galactosaemia, or hereditary fructose intolerance, which are often missed. Parental consanguinity should be noted, particularly in children.

When a genetically determined or infectious disease is found, it is crucial to check for family members who may be affected; the prognosis may be completely altered if certain diseases (e.g. Wilson's disease, galactosaemia, hereditary fructose intolerance) are detected early in siblings or other family members. With hepatitis B infection affected relatives require follow-up, and unaffected close relatives should be vaccinated.

Drug history

Drugs are an important cause of liver disease. A careful drug history often helps to establish the diagnosis. In puzzling cases of liver disease it is essential to check details of drug ingestion, not only with the patient or members of the family but also with other doctors who may have been involved in the patient's care. It may be necessary to obtain earlier clinical notes and to peruse them carefully, as details of the administration of the offending drug may be difficult to find. Sometimes the agent responsible; such as paracetamol, aspirin, oxyphenisatin, or anabolic steroids, may have been bought over the counter; many herbal medicines also cause liver damage and their importance is being increasingly recognized (see Section 17 and Chapter 29.1). A list of drugs causing various types of liver disease is presented in Section 17.

Psycho-social history and risk factors

Other risk factors for liver disease may emerge from a carefully taken psycho-social history. The most important of these, at least in Western countries, is alcohol abuse (see Section 15). While some patients give an accurate statement about their consumption, many do not; sometimes alcohol abuse is vehemently denied. Patients seem more willing to admit excessive alcohol consumption in a self-administered questionnaire, or in a computer-taken history, than to a doctor. If alcohol abuse is denied, if there is no other obvious explanation, and if the clinical picture would fit with alcohol-induced liver disease, it is essential to check the history with relatives, friends, or with other sources. Measurements of 'spot' blood alcohol levels are sometimes necessary to establish abuse.

A history of intravenous drug abuse, particularly involving the use of shared or dirty needles, suggests the possibility of acute or chronic viral hepatitis. The patient's sexual history and habits are also important. Homosexuality and heterosexual promiscuity are associated with increased risk of viral hepatitis, of perihepatitis due to gonococcus and chlamydia (in women and homosexuals), and of secondary syphilis, which occasionally presents with jaundice and/or abnormal liver function tests. Although many doctors are reluctant to probe into a patient's sex life it is important that this reluctance is overcome. Since the advent of AIDS the vast majority of patients no longer consider such questions to be inappropriate.

Previous treatment for psychiatric disorders is often hidden from physicians. As many of the drugs used may cause liver disease it is important to enquire specifically about such treatment and to check other possible sources of information.

There are many industrial causes of liver disease due to exposure to toxins; these are covered in Chapters 18.1 and 32.2.

Many hepatobiliary diseases are the consequence of residence in, or of travel to, countries in which these diseases are prevalent; they are considered in Chapter 32.1.

Physical examination

The physical examination is a cornerstone of clinical evaluation, one involving all the senses of the clinician (and particularly common sense!). Physicians, over centuries, have identified many physical signs of disease, and have argued over their value in diagnosis. Signs vary in importance. In liver disease some are relatively specific pointers to a particular condition (e.g. the Kayser–Fleischer ring of Wilson's, or a large gallbladder in jaundiced patients with carcinoma of the pancreas), or to certain complications of liver disease (e.g. asterixis in hepatic encephalopathy, abdominal collaterals with portal hypertension, and a fluid thrill with ascites, signs which may also give an indication of the severity of the disease).

However, other signs are relatively non-specific; they may be found in otherwise normal subjects (e.g. clubbing and Dupuytren's contracture), in diseases of other systems (clubbing, petechiae, and generalized skin pigmentation), or in so many different types of liver disease that they are of little value for differential diagnosis (e.g. spider naevi). Many of them are epiphenomena, of little practical value, but their recognition as features of liver disease is important as one does not then have to search for other causes of the signs. Sometimes several signs denote the same underlying abnormality; if the cause is obvious from one sign, there is little point in eliciting others (e.g. percussion for the lower edge of the liver is of little value if it is easily palpable, and percussion for ascites is superfluous if there is gross abdominal distension and a fluid thrill). Such 'complementary' signs are, however, valuable when initial findings are equivocal; for this reason beginners should use them regularly in order to gain experience in their use, both to learn the range of normal and to become familiar with the nature of the abnormal sign.

There is considerable inter- and intraobserver variation in the elucidation of physical signs in liver disease.[3,6-8] This stems partly from bad technique, partly from inattention during routine examination (observers tending to find what they expect to find), and partly because many signs are genuinely difficult to elicit. Even experienced hepatologists may miss a liver or spleen which they detect easily on the next visit to the bedside.

The general examination

Physical examination should start with a general examination of the patient, not only as part of a 'full' examination, but before a follow-up examination of any system.

The most important single question is whether the patient looks ill or well; many students (and some doctors) find it difficult to answer. If a patient with liver disease looks very ill on presentation, or if there is sudden deterioration in the appearance of a patient with chronic liver disease, it suggests the possibility of malignancy or a serious infection, such as bacteraemia or subacute bacterial peritonitis. Urgent admission for further investigation should be considered.

Body build is relevant. Loss of muscle bulk is a sign of advanced liver disease, and is particularly common in alcoholic cirrhotics. It is most easily recognized in the arms and legs. Unduly large muscles should suggest the possibility of anabolic steroid abuse. Loss of adipose tissue tends to occur with endstage liver disease from any cause. Obesity is now recognized as a common cause of abnormal liver function tests, often due to fatty liver or less commonly to non-alcoholic steatohepatitis.

Some diseases can be diagnosed at first sight; indeed, if they are not spotted straightaway it may be difficult to detect them on subsequent physical examination. Hyperthyroidism, hypothyroidism, and acromegaly may all be associated with abnormal liver function tests. Widely set eyes, a prominent forehead, flat nose, and small chin are characteristic of Alagille's syndrome (Alagille, JPediat, 1975; 86:63), although it has been suggested that this facies occurs with any form of persistent intrahepatic cholestasis in childhood (Sokol, JPediat, 1983; 103:203). Many alcoholics have a typical facial appearance.

Other facial signs may be seen. Marked subconjunctival haemorrhage occurs with leptospirosis icterohaemorrhagiae, but is also seen with severe acute hepatic failure from many causes, and occasionally in normal subjects for no obvious reason. Xanthelasma around the eyes suggests chronic cholestasis, while bruising of periorbital skin suggests the possibility of amyloid.

Parotid enlargement

Enlarged parotids are occasionally found as an epiphenomenon in cirrhotic patients and are thought to be related to alcohol abuse and/or malnutrition. The sign is often missed, but when marked there is a characteristic facial appearance. The glands are neither painful nor tender. The ducts are patent and secretion from the glands tends to be increased (Bonnin, PressMed, 1954; 62:1449; Wolfe, NEJM, 1956; 256:491; Brick, AnnIntMed, 1958; 49:438;).

Body temperature

Fever often accompanies infectious diseases involving the liver, such as acute viral hepatitis, Epstein–Barr virus and cytomegalovirus infections, Q fever, leptospirosis, amoebic and pyogenic liver abscesses, relapsing fever, typhoid, and many other infections (see Sections 12 and 13).

Secondary bacterial infection with fever is common in patients with chronic hepatitis and/or cirrhosis, who have a particular predisposition to bacteraemia (and to spontaneous bacterial peritonitis when ascites is present); patients with liver disease are also prone to other infections (see Chapter 25.11). Infection may cause a low temperature in patients with liver disease, as do haemorrhage or shock.

Patients with established liver disease may present with fever for which no cause can be found; and patients without known or obvious liver disease may suffer fever accompanied by abnormal liver function tests. The latter occurs in many systemic infections, and may result from malignancies, connective tissue disorders (see Chapter 24.7), sarcoidosis (see Chapter 14.2), and recurrent pulmonary thromboembolism. When fever is prolonged and unexplained it is referred to as 'pyrexia of unknown origin'.

Unexplained fever in established liver disease

Tisdale and Klatskin (YaleJBiolMed, 1960; 33:94) drew attention to fever in cirrhotics which was not explained by infection, gastrointestinal haemorrhage, or hepatocellular carcinoma. It occurred in about 40 per cent of alcoholics, but only 12 per cent of postnecrotic cirrhotics. In alcoholics there was a high incidence in women under the age of 50 years, many being in their late twenties or early thirties. Patients with fever had drunk more heavily and had poorer diets; they had more advanced clinical and biochemical signs of liver disease, hepatomegaly was more common, and the liver was often tender. Two-thirds had a white count above 10×10^9/litre, and in one-third it was greater than 15×10^9/litre. Liver biopsy showed more advanced hepatocellular damage, with polymorphonuclear infiltration of the parenchyma in about 50 per cent. The maximal temperature was usually between 38.3 and 39.4 °C (101–103 °F), but in a few it exceeded 39.4 °C. In more than half, the fever lasted more than 2 weeks, and in a quarter more than 4 weeks.

This picture is now recognized as common in alcoholic hepatitis. Unfortunately fever in this condition remains a diagnostic problem, as in non-alcoholics, because of the many intercurrent infections which also cause fever. The diagnosis of fever due to cirrhosis *per se* is essentially one of exclusion.

It was claimed that fever is an important sign in metastatic disease of liver (Fenster, AmJMed, 1961; 31:238), but in patients with primary cancers of colon, pancreas, stomach, and breast, the incidence of fever was no greater in those with metastatic liver disease than in those without; nor was fever more common with 'massive liver metastases' (Adeka, Cancer, 1985; 55:2830).

Pyrexia of unknown origin and the liver

Abnormal liver function tests are found in many infectious diseases in which the liver is not primarily involved. These infections are usually short lived; the diagnosis usually becomes obvious or the condition improves spontaneously. In some viral conditions fever resolves before the results of diagnostic tests become available.

Prolonged fever without obvious cause, and which resists vigorous investigation, is often associated with hepatomegaly and/or abnormal liver function tests. It is commonly due to an infection, to malignancy, or to a connective tissue disorder; there may not be any direct involvement of the liver in these cases. Occasionally the liver or biliary tree is the main site of the problem, as in chronic granulomatous hepatitis, with carcinoma of the liver or gallbladder, or with hepatic abscess or empyema of the gallbladder; in the last few examples diagnosis may be particularly difficult if hepatic imaging techniques fail to detect the lesions.

Pallor

Anaemia is common in liver disease (see Chapter 25.3), and may be detected clinically by inspecting the colour of the conjunctiva of the lower eyelids.

Cyanosis

'Cyanosis' denotes blue discoloration of the mucous membranes and/or skin, and is usually due to an excess of deoxygenated haemoglobin in the blood; it also occurs when chemical modification of haemoglobin, due to certain drugs or chemicals, results in sulphaemoglobinaemia or methaemoglobinaemia.

Cyanosis due to deoxygenated haemoglobin, or to an abnormal haemoglobin, may be observed in the tongue, lips, and peripheries. It is easier to detect cyanosis, indicating a low oxygen saturation, in patients with polycythaemia. It is much more difficult to detect in the presence of anaemia, and with marked anaemia cyanosis cannot be seen even with severe hypoxia. The intensity of cyanosis depends on the size of capillaries; when they are dilated the colour is rich, when constricted the colour is pale. The causes of cyanosis in liver disease are discussed in Chapter 25.1.

Dehydration

'Dehydration' implies a low total body water which may result from a low fluid intake or excessive loss of fluid (due to vomiting, diarrhoea, polyuria, diuretic therapy, or excessive sweating). When water is lost without equivalent amounts of sodium (as in sweating) both intracellular and extracellular spaces share the fluid deficit; such loss is tolerated relatively well. When isotonic fluids are lost (as with diarrhoea, vomiting, or gastrointestinal suction) fluid loss is predominantly from the extracellular space, including plasma, and important physiological consequences may result, including a fall in blood pressure and reduction of renal blood flow.

Similar effects may result from an internal loss of fluid if, for example, secretions accumulate in the gut due to intestinal obstruction or ileus; this removes fluid from the blood and interstitial space. Sometimes the effective intravascular volume, and the extracellular fluid space in the upper part of the body, is reduced in liver disease, even when there is lower limb oedema and/or ascites. Such maldistribution is common in cirrhotics, particularly after diuretic therapy.

Several physical signs have been proposed for detecting extracellular dehydration. The most useful is loss of skin turgor over the centre of the upper sternum. When a small fold of skin is pinched in young people it resumes its original position almost instantaneously. With ageing, however, there is increasing delay in the return to normal skin contour when the skin on the back of the hand is pinched. This is due to loss of skin elasticity. The response to pinching the skin over the upper sternum is unaffected by loss of elasticity, even in the very old; delayed return is thus a valuable sign of lower skin turgor due to a reduced extracellular space. When sternal skin turgor is reduced one should check the blood pressure (lying and standing) and jugular venous pressure, as low values (and/or an increased plasma urea) suggest the need for expansion of the intravascular volume.

Dyspnoea and tachypnoea

Patients with liver disease may suffer from the common causes of dyspnoea (difficult breathing) and tachypnoea (rapid breathing) which affect those with other conditions (e.g. cardiac or pulmonary diseases). Some conditions, such as cystic fibrosis (Chapter 20.4) and α1-antitrypsin deficiency (Chapter 20.3), may affect lungs and liver, and jaundice may occur with several types of pneumonia (Chapter 13.1.1). Tachypnoea is common with ascites, gross abdominal organomegaly, or large space-occupying lesions in the right lobe of the liver, presumably from elevation and restricted movement of the diaphragm. Dyspnoea may occur with large pleural effusions (often associated with ascites). Other causes of dyspnoea associated with liver disease are considered in Chapters 24.1 and 25.1.

Jaundice

The words 'jaundice' and 'icterus' are often used as if synonymous with the yellow or yellow-green discolouration of tissues seen with an increased plasma bilirubin. Hyperbilirubinaemia is by far the most common cause of jaundice, but other yellow pigments also cause jaundice. People with food fads may ingest excessive amounts of carrots, tomatoes, or papaya fruit, and develop yellow skin discoloration, particularly on the palms, caused by deposition of carotene or lycopenes. Mepacrine (once commonly used as an antimalarial), picric acid, fluorescein, and acriflavin also cause yellow staining of the skin (but neither these compounds nor the carotenoid pigments discolour the sclerae). Such compounds may be taken in order to feign liver disease; the absence of hyperbilirubinaemia can be established by measuring the serum bilirubin.

Jaundice due to increased bilirubin varies in severity. It is best detected by careful examination of the sclerae, because bilirubin binds selectively to fibrous tissue; the serum bilirubin must rise above 35 µmol/l (2 mg/dl) before a yellow tinge appears. Some clinicians advocate examination of the palate or the floor of the mouth to detect minor degrees of jaundice: while palatal jaundice may be pronounced it is not seen without scleral icterus; it is an epiphenomenon of little clinical value. Patients with an acute hepatic disturbance causing conjugated hyperbilirubinaemia, for example viral hepatitis, usually notice dark urine before jaundice. Bilirubinuria should be confirmed by testing. With unconjugated hyperbilirubinaemia, or with conjugated hyperbilirubinaemia due predominantly to the presence of a bili-protein (see Chapter 2.9), bilirubinuria does not occur and scleral icterus is then a crucial sign, which should raise suspicion of disorders such as haemolysis, cirrhosis, or biliary obstruction.

Pigmentation

The colour of human skin depends on the relative amounts of melanin, oxyhaemoglobin, deoxygenated haemoglobin, and carotene that are present. The content and nature of haemoglobin account for pallor, pinkness, and cyanosis; carotene gives skin its slight yellowish discoloration. The major pigmentary changes are caused by changes in the amount of melanin, which may be increased or decreased, either diffusely or patchily.

The common reasons for diffuse hyperpigmentation are racial origin and the degree of exposure to the sun. Increased skin pigmentation is less obvious in dark-skinned people, and reduced pigmentation less obvious in fair-skinned people. The patient (or a close relative) is the best opinion on such changes.

A diffuse increase in melanin pigmentation is seen with many chronic liver diseases, including primary biliary cirrhosis and other chronic cholestatic disorders, other forms of cirrhosis, haemochromatosis, and porphyria cutanea tarda. In these conditions there rnay be local areas of hyperpigmentation, particularly at sites of minor trauma or irritation (e.g. around the waist—due to pressure of elastic in the underwear).

Vitiligo

Vitiligo is a common autoimmune skin disease, due to patchy destruction of melanocytes with total depigmentation of affected skin. It affects about 1 per cent of the population, but it is usually a cause for complaint only in dark-skinned populations. There is a clear association with other autoimmune diseases; in primary biliary cirrhosis vitiligo is often seen against the generalized pigmentation, but it also occurs in autoimmune hepatitis.

Skin and body hair

The skin is the largest organ of the body; many dermatological abnormalities are found with liver disease (see Chapters 24.3 and 25.6). Sometimes the skin lesion suggests the diagnosis of the liver disease, e.g. striae in autoimmune hepatitis (Plate 1), skin lesions of cryoglobulinaemia in hepatitis C (Chapter 12.1.2.5), hereditary haemorrhagic telangiectasia (Chapter 24.1), CREST syndrome with primary biliary cirrhosis, and papular acrodermatitis with hepatitis B virus-related Giannotti Crosti syndrome (Chapter 25.6). Tattoos, and needle marks in intravenous drug abusers, suggest the mode of transmission of viral hepatitis (particularly B, C, and D). Erythemas and urticaria may be seen in the prodrome of acute viral hepatitis B and A (Scully, AmJGastr, 1993; 88:277). Xanthomas (Plates 2 and 3), and xanthelasma around the eyes, are found in patients with long-standing biliary obstruction and elevated plasma cholesterol levels (see Chapter 2.12). Scratch marks result from severe pruritus, and suggest its presence in those who cannot complain of this symptom, for example the very old or very young.

Spider naevi (Plates 4 and 5) are a clue to the presence of chronic liver disease, and may be large and numerous in alcoholic liver disease. Related signs include white spots, paper-money skin, and palmar (and plantar) erythema. The cause of these vascular abnormalities is not known. Excessive bruising is easily seen, but careful examination is needed to detect tiny petechial haemorrhages, which may be the first sign of thrombocytopenia. They tend to be most pronounced over the lower legs, but also appear on the arms or abdomen, particularly at points of trauma or pressure from tight clothing. They are relatively common in chronic liver disease with hypersplenism. It is important to detect an outbreak of new lesions; this may indicate a rapid fall in the platelet count, due to bacteraemia or disseminated intravascular coagulation (and therefore the need for urgent treatment). Haemorrhagic lesions are also seen in pseudomonas septicaemia, which may cause ecthyma gangrenosum, a relatively specific sign of this type of infection (Dorff, ArchIntMed, 1971; 128:591).

Lichen planus (Chapter 24.3) is associated with primary biliary cirrhosis (Powell, BrJDermatol, 1982; 107:616), and there is also a higher prevalence of other types of liver disease when compared

with control subjects (GISED, BMJ, 1990; 300:227). Seven of 30 patients with lichen planus were positive for anti-hepatitis C virus by second-generation ELISA, and five of these were positive for hepatitis C virus RNA by PCR (Bellman, Lancet, 1995; 346:1234). The reason for the association with liver disease is not known.

Lymphadenopathy

Palpable lymph glands are uncommon with liver disease. They are sometimes found early in the course of acute viral hepatitis, particularly with Epstein–Barr infection, and with leukaemia and lyphomas involving the liver.

Gynaecomastia

Gynaecomastia occurs in some males with liver disease, and with other causes of feminization. True gynaecomastia means that there is palpable enlargement of glandular tissue under the areola; it may be tender, with enlargement and pigmentation of the areola. Breast enlargement due to obesity should not be confused with true gynaecomastia which results from sex hormone imbalance in liver disease (Chapter 25.2), and is a troublesome side-effect of spironolactone. Potassium canrenoate, which like spironolactone is converted to the active metabolite canrenone, may be free of this side-effect (Dupont, Lancet, 1985; ii:731)

Mouth and throat

Examination of the mouth and throat is rarely of specific value in liver disease (Beitman, DigDisSci, 1981; 26:741). Telangiectasia may be seen in hereditary haemorrhagic telangiectasia associated with liver disease. Superficial glossitis is common, particularly in alcoholics and with carcinoid syndrome. The tongue may enlarge in AL amyloidosis, which can also cause superficial erosions, loose teeth, and purpura due to involvement of the vessels of the mouth and tongue. Measures of oral hygiene, dental care, and periodontal indices were worse in alcoholics with or without cirrhosis than in healthy subjects and non-alcoholic patients, and more teeth required treatment. Alcoholics had fewer teeth than patients without alcohol abuse. The severity and duration of liver disease had no influence on dental and periodontal disease (Novacek, JHepatol, 1995; 22:576).

The most important reason for examining the fauces in liver disease is the early detection of candidal infection, which occurs in patients with severe liver disease, particularly those on immunosuppressive therapy.

Green teeth have been reported in young children with hyperbilirubinaemia at birth or early in the neonatal period (Rosenthal, JPediat, 1986; 108;1030).

The breath of some patients with liver disease has an odour ('foetor hepaticus'). It occurs in fulminant hepatitis and with portal-systemic encephalopathy of any cause and has been noted in hepatitis, cirrhosis, and obstructive jaundice (Butt, Gastro, 1954; 26:829). It is of little value as a clinical sign because many clinicians are unable to detect it. Its biochemical basis is unclear: methanethiol and dimethylsulphide have been incriminated, but the causative substance may differ in different patients.[5] Recently, Tangerman et al. (Lancet, 1994; 343:483) concluded that foetor hepaticus is due to dimethylsulphide, but there was no relationship between breath levels and signs of encephalopathy. There was a relationship between dimethylsulphide levels and the presence of a surgical shunt in cirrhotics.

Hands and nails

Examination of the hands is rarely useful in liver disease. Palmar erythema, localized to the thenar and hypothenar eminences ('liver palms'), occurs in many patients with cirrhosis and less commonly in acute and chronic hepatitis. The skin of the hands is often warm, due to vasodilatation, even in the absence of palmar erythema (Chapter 25.1). Carrella *et al.* (Angiol, 1992; 42:969) concluded that capillary flow is not increased with the hyperdynamic circulatory changes of cirrhosis, and that the increased flow occurs through arteriovenous anastomoses. Plevris *et al.* (AmJGastr, 1991; 86:467) found that significantly more patients with alcoholic liver disease (particularly males) complained of cold hands than did normal individuals. The awareness of cold hands appeared to be more common in an intermediate group, between those with non-cirrhotic liver disease without varices and those with cirrhosis with varices. They confirmed these findings using a liquid crystal contact thermography system (Steele, JHepatol, 1994; 21:927): Child's A patients had warm hands of normal thermographic appearance; Child's B patients had cold hands and Child's C warm hands, and in these groups the thermographic appearance was abnormal. Autonomic dysfunction did not appear to be the main cause of these changes.

Patients with primary biliary cirrhosis may suffer from the CREST syndrome, with hands exhibiting sclerodactyly, Raynaud's phenomenon and calcinosis, and sometimes ulceration, pitting, and gangrene of the fingers. Digital vasospasm and infarction of the skin of the fingers may occur early in the course of acute hepatitis B (Cosgriff, JAMA, 1976; 235:1362).

Dupuytren's contracture

Dupuytren's contracture is a condition in which the palmar fascia becomes thickened and shortened, often causing fixed flexion deformities of the fingers. The prevalence in Caucasian populations is between 4 and 6 per cent, rising to 20 per cent in men aged over 65 years (Evans, BrJHospMed, 1986; 36:198). It is common in alcoholic cirrhotics and has been attributed to the liver damage. However, in one study the prevalence was similar in alcoholic cirrhotics (33 per cent), in patients with non-cirrhotic alcoholic liver disease (22 per cent), and in alcoholics without liver disease (28 per cent); in non-alcoholic chronic liver disease it was only 6 per cent and was 12 per cent in their controls (Attali, ArchIntMed, 1987; 147:1065). Six times as much hypoxanthine has been found in the palmar fascia of patients with Dupuytren's contracture compared to the amount found in control subjects; it was suggested that free radical formation, generated by the action of xanthine oxidase on hypoxanthine, may be important in the pathogenesis of Dupuytren's contracture (Murrell, BMJ, 1987; 295:1373).

Nails

A normal nail is smooth, evenly pink and has a proximal visible white lunula. The nail and finger meet at the lunula at an angle of less than 180°. In patients with severe pruritus, the nails may have a shiny appearance, due to repeated 'polishing'.

Terry (Lancet, 1954; i:757) described nails which were white to within 1 to 2 mm of the end where there was a strip of normal pink; the lunulas were often obscured. Although originally described in cirrhosis, similar findings occur in other conditions, for example congestive cardiac failure, rheumatoid arthritis, nephrotic syndrome, tuberculosis, diabetes mellitus, multiple sclerosis, and various carcinomas.

Muehrcke's lines also occur in cirrhosis (BMJ, 1956; 1:1327); they are transverse white lines, parallel to the lunula, which result from prolonged periods in which the serum albumin falls below 22 g/l; they are most common in the nephrotic syndrome.

Blue lunulas have been described in Wilson's disease (Bearn, JAMA, 1958; 166:904), and in argyria when they may be associated with corneal changes resembling Kayser–Fleischer rings (Whelton, ArchIntMed, 1968; 121:267).

Clubbing

Clubbing is an abnormal shape best seen from the side of the finger. The emergent angle is equal to or greater than 180° and the nail itself has an exaggerated convexity which, when severe, extends over the tip of the finger. In severe clubbing the end of the finger enlarges, giving a 'drumstick' appearance. The proximal end of the nail is easily depressed, giving a 'spongy' feeling. Clubbing is classically associated with chronic suppurative and interstitial lung disease, carcinoma of the bronchus, mesothelioma, cyanotic heart disease, infective endocarditis, malabsorption, and certain chronic gastrointestinal diseases. It can be familial. Mild clubbing is common in cirrhosis, and may be more marked in primary biliary cirrhosis, or when there is hypoxia or pulmonary hypertension. Hypertrophic osteoarthropathy may also be present with periostitis (subperiosteal new bone formation) at the distal diaphyses of the long bones (Epstein, AmJMed, 1979; 67:88).

Examination of the abdomen

Inspection

Abdominal inspection is often helpful in liver disease, and it should include a search for inconspicuous, but often important, skin lesions (such as petechiae or skin rashes), as well as for gross abnormalities. Skin lesions also found in other parts of the body are discussed above and in Chapter 25.6. Surgical scars indicate previous surgery, and possibly its nature. Lower abdominal striae result from rapid abdominal distension, due to pregnancy or ascites; purplish striae, a sign of Cushing's disease and corticosteroid administration, may be found in young women with autoimmune hepatitis.

Abdominal swelling may be localized, or generalized due to obesity or intra-abdominal distension. Ascites is the most common cause of distension in chronic liver disease. Small amounts of ascites cause little or no distension, but with increasing ascites there is bulging or convexity of the flanks, and then anteroposterior bulging of the abdomen. If the patient is also obese, ascites may be difficult to detect. With marked ascites the abdomen is grossly distended, there may be splaying of the lower ribs and, as Frehrichs noted over 100 years ago, the distance between the xiphisternum and the umbilicus is usually much greater than the distance between the umbilicus and the symphysis pubis (Plate 6).

Ascites is often associated with peripheral oedema which, when gross, may involve the abdominal wall and genitalia. Localized abdominal wall oedema, often unilateral, may also occur with ascites—after paracentesis (Conn, AnnIntMed, 1971; 74:943) or after abdominal surgery (Conn, AnnIntMed, 1972; 76:459), presumably because of leakage of peritoneal fluid. Localized chest wall oedema may occur after thoracocentesis for hepatic hydrothorax.

Localized bulgings of the abdominal wall may result from diffuse or focal enlargement of the liver, or from an enlarged spleen or gallbladder, and may be more evident when the organs move with respiration. With ascites, there may be localized bulging due to fluid-filled hernias (umbilical, femoral, inguinal, or incisional); umbilical hernias tend to be particularly prominent in the presence of ascites.

Abdominal wall veins

Small veins are sometimes visible on the abdominal wall in normal subjects; they are less apparent in obese subjects. Veins over the lower abdomen normally run downwards to the groin to join the ilio-femoral system; upper abdominal veins run upwards to drain into thoracic wall and axillary veins.

Portal hypertension results from obstruction to the flow of portal blood. When the obstruction is intrahepatic, due to cirrhosis (or other, less common, liver diseases), the high portal pressure may open up the obliterated umbilical vein (which in fetal life terminates in the left branch of the portal vein), although Lafortune *et al.* (AJR, 1985; 144:549) considered that the enlarged vessels carrying blood away from the left branch of the portal vein are para-umbilical veins and not the umbilical vein itself, which remains closed. Whichever veins are involved, they carry blood away from the liver in the ligamentum teres, which joins the falciform ligament and runs down to the umbilicus; they act as feeder veins, via the umbilicus, to the abdominal wall veins which radiate away from the umbilicus. These veins are usually prominent, but are only obvious at some distance from the umbilicus (Plate 7). Abdominal wall veins are seen more easily if the skin is stretched (either by hand, or as a result of intra-abdominal distension). (The 'caput medusae', described by many authors, with numerous dilated veins radiating out from the umbilicus itself, like the snakes on the head of the gorgon Medusa, appears to be a mythical sign. I have never seen this sign, or even a photograph of it, unless (1) the whole abdomen is meant to be the head, (2) Medusa was very bald on top, and (3) they were very thin snakes—the bottle of champagne offered in our first edition for the most convincing picture is still unclaimed!)

The para-umbilical veins may also supply small veins which penetrate the rectus sheath to reach the surface; the blood then runs upwards—often in large collaterals which are visible close to the midline above the umbilicus (Plate 8). If distended abdominal wall veins are seen which clearly have their origin in the umbilical venous system, portal hypertension is due to diffuse abnormality within liver parenchyma (cirrhosis in the vast majority), as the block must be distal to the left branch of the portal vein. In classical extrahepatic portal vein block there are no umbilical collaterals on the abdominal wall, and in cirrhotics with umbilical collaterals the abdominal wall veins tend to disappear if the main portal vein subsequently becomes thrombosed.

However, if abdominal surgery has been performed, adhesions can develop between the viscera and the abdominal wall. Then, with portal hypertension, collaterals may appear around the scar; they may be unilateral, depending on the position of the incision,

and are often prominent (Plate 9). Collaterals radiating out from a scar occur with intrahepatic portal hypertension and with portal vein block; unlike true umbilical collaterals, they indicate only a high portal pressure and not the site of the block.

Prominent abdominal wall veins also appear with inferior vena caval obstruction. They differ from portal collaterals in two ways. First, the distended veins found with inferior vena caval block appear to run up from the lower abdomen and legs, not from the umbilicus or a scar, and are usually most prominent at the sides of the abdomen (Plate 10). Secondly, the direction of venous flow is upwards, even over the lower abdomen; with umbilical collaterals the direction of venous flow is normal, that is upwards above the umbilicus and downwards over the lower abdomen. The direction of flow in collaterals coming from abdominal scars depends, of course, on the site of the scar. With an inferior vena caval block collaterals also tend to be visible over the skin of the lower back; this is rarely if ever seen as a result of portal hypertension. Both types of venous abnormality can be present in patients with the Budd–Chiari syndome (because hepatic venous thrombosis may be associated with an inferior vena caval block, or because the large caudate lobe seen in the Budd–Chiari syndrome may cause secondary obstruction of the cava). The sudden development of abdominal wall collaterals in a patient known to have cirrhosis suggests the possibility of an acute hepatic vein block.

Abnormal veins will also be visible on one side of the lower abdomen if there is a block to the ilio-femoral veins on that side. These are sometimes mistaken for collaterals due to portal hypertension, but their origin is obvious from their distribution, from the upward flow of blood, and because the patient often has more pronounced leg oedema on the affected side.

It is worth feeling a visible abdominal vessel just to make sure that it is not an arterial collateral due to a blocked aorta.

Palpation

Even if liver disease is suspected, the whole abdomen should be palpated to avoid missing other abnormalities, particularly in the lower abdomen. First use light palpation, to assess muscle tone and to detect obvious masses or tenderness. Then re-examine with deeper palpation, exerting greater pressure. The whole of the palmar surface of the fingers should be used, with large circular movements of the hand, in order to detect organs or masses; when something is felt, use small movements with the fingertips to delineate the organ or mass.

Tenderness may be superficial or deep. Press on the tender area while the patient tries to sit up (thus contracting the abdominal muscles). Deep tenderness, due to intra-abdominal disease, is abolished by this manoeuvre, while superficial tenderness (of muscle or subcutaneous tissues) persists. Occasionally with deep inflammatory lesions, e.g. cholecystitis, touching or scratching the skin gives an unpleasant sensation (hyperaesthesia) over the dermatomes corresponding to the nerve supply of the parietal peritoneum overlying the inflamed organ. Percussion over the right lower ribs can also produce pain, particularly with a hepatic abscess.

'Guarding' is due to voluntary contraction of abdominal muscles over a tender area, the patient expecting palpation to be painful. It can often be overcome by reassurance, by distracting the patient's attention, and by gentle palpation.[3] Guarding occurs without true tenderness if the patient is not lying comfortably with relaxed abdominal muscles, if your hands are cold, or if you are abrupt during palpation (particularly with children). Localized guarding in an otherwise soft abdomen is an important physical sign. Guarding may be mimicked if there is a large 'flat' mass or organ under the examining hand.

'Rigidity' is involuntary reflex spasm of the muscle of the whole abdominal wall. It cannot be overcome by reassurance, by distracting the patient's attention, or by warming the hands. If the abdomen is rigid (and silent, see below) the patient probably has peritonitis.

If tenderness is present, look for rebound tenderness.[3] Press the tender area with the flat of the hand, firmly but gently, for 30 to 60 s. There may be pain initially, which often improves during the period of pressure. Without warning, and preferably while the patient's attention is distracted, remove the hand suddenly to just above skin level. 'Rebound tenderness' is signified by an exacerbation of pain, usually accompanied by a facial grimace. Rebound tenderness, properly elicited, suggests inflammation of the underlying peritoneum.

Palpation of the right hypochondrium, liver, and gallbladder

Obvious enlargement of the liver, or a mass, may be felt on initial light or deep palpation of the upper abdomen. A large, hard liver in a soft abdomen is easy to feel, and technique is then relatively unimportant. Often, however, the liver is not obvious; good technique is necessary for 'difficult' livers.

Place your right hand with the index finger parallel to, but well below, the costal margin and lateral to the edge of the rectus sheath (Fig. 1). Press firmly but gently with the palmar surface of the fingers, angling the palm slightly so that maximum pressure is exerted by the radial border of the index finger—which should now be several centimetres closer to the posterior abdominal wall than the costal margin itself (because it needs to be below the edge of the descending liver). Ask the patient to take a very deep inspiration. If the liver is palpable you will feel its edge touch the side of your right index finger. Exert a little upward pressure in order to resist downward movement of the liver; otherwise your hand may move down with the liver and it is then more difficult to feel. Keep the right hand still while the patient is taking the deep inspiration; if you move it you may feel the 'bump' of a muscle bundle during inspiration and misinterpret it as the liver. It is important that the fingers should be parallel to the costal margin; this is usually the line of the liver edge; as the liver descends you should feel it 'flip' over your index finger (this is the best evidence that you are feeling the liver). If your hand is placed horizontally across the abdomen (Fig. 2), the right side of the liver edge may already be under your hand; as the liver descends it can slip easily under the rest of your hand without being 'flipped' or even felt.

It is much easier to feel a firm or hard liver than a soft one. Indeed, it is sometimes impossible to feel a very large, soft liver even when the edge is clearly demonstrable by ultrasound examination. One technique suggested for detecting the liver edge in difficult cases is to listen over the right side of the abdomen with the stethoscope diaphragm, while you 'scratch' the abdominal wall gently with a fingernail; the noise of the scratching changes pitch as you cross the edge of the liver.

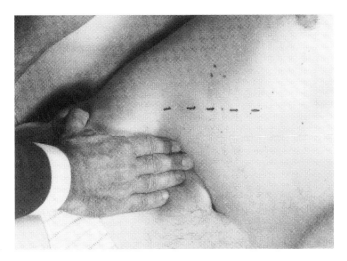

Fig. 1. Palpation of the liver. Note that the index finger is parallel to the costal margin, and the palm angled slightly to exert most pressure with the index finger, which is several centimetres closer to the posterior abdominal wall than the costal margin itself (because it needs to be below the edge of the descending liver).

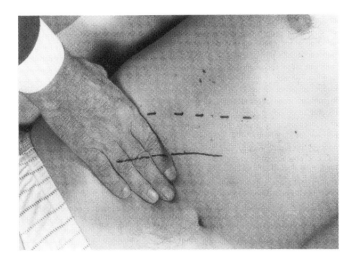

Fig. 2. The wrong way to palpate the liver! If the hand is placed horizontally across the abdomen the right side of the liver edge may already be under your hand, and when it descends the liver can slip under the hand without being felt.

Once the liver is felt, it is usually easy to map the line of its lower edge. Draw its position reasonably accurately in the notes (not just a straight line parallel to the costal margin!), recording the distance of the liver edge from the costal margin at a measured distance from the midline (and indicating whether the. measurement was made in quiet respiration or in deep inspiration). Although the surface projection of most livers is roughly triangular, with the base along the line of the right lower ribs laterally and the apex under the left nipple, there may be striking variations in shape, particularly in diseased livers. The consistency of the liver should be recorded, with a comment on the smoothness or nodularity of the surface. When the liver is easily palpable such a report is much more useful than a measurement of liver span by percussion (see below).

The fact that a liver is palpable does not mean that it is enlarged; it may be pushed down by emphysema and a normal-sized liver may be palpable in many healthy subjects on very deep inspiration. A normal right kidney is often palpable in slim women (but rarely in men), and may be mistaken for the liver if you do not perform bimanual palpation; this usually allows correct identification of the kidney, although a Riedel's lobe of liver may also be palpable bimanually.

Zoli *et al.* (AmJGastr, 1995; 90:1428) cast doubt on the value of physical examination (palpation and percussion) of the liver. They studied 100 healthy subjects and 100 cirrhotics, using ultrasound to establish the upper and lower borders of the liver (and also to calculate liver volume). With ultrasound the liver edge on deep inspiration was below the right costal margin in 92 of the 100 controls (somewhat surprisingly) and in 81 patients with cirrhosis. It was palpable in only 47 controls but in 78 of the cirrhotics. In the controls in whom the liver edge was below the costal margin on ultrasound but was not palpable, extension below the rib margin was as much as 10 cm. In the whole control population palpation underestimated the distance of the liver edge below the rib margin by an average of 2.9 cm, but only by 0.3 cm in the cirrhotics.

Difficulty in palpation of the liver edge in healthy subjects may have been related to the consistency of the liver; this was considered 'soft' in 39 of the 47 controls in whom the liver was actually palpable, and of grade 1 firmness in the other eight. No cirrhotics were thought to have a soft liver, 37 of the 78 were grade 1 firmness, 39 grade 2, and the other two were grade 3 ('firm' or 'ligneous'). The liver edge was thought to be 'sharp' in 37 of the 47 controls, but in only 38 of the 78 cirrhotics; the rest had a blunted liver edge. Zoli *et al.* considered that 'only the palpatory characteristics and consistency of the lower liver edge still have a diagnostic role, mainly when combined with US [ultrasound]'.

Results such as these have led some hepatologists to argue that physical examination of the liver is valueless and should be replaced by ultrasound examination. As they concede that the rest of the body should be examined properly, it seems bizarre to think that a liver doctor might refrain from examining the liver. Other physicians clearly have to feel the liver as it is clearly impractical to refer all their patients for ultrasonography, and patients with large livers and significant liver pathology may have no symptoms suggesting liver disease. Furthermore, ultrasonographers, like other doctors, are prone to error.

Pulsatile liver

Sometimes careful palpation of the liver reveals that the liver is pulsatile. This is common in tricuspid incompetence, when the right ventricular pressure is transmitted to the larger veins. 'Expansile' pulsation is felt during systole if two fingers are placed well apart on the surface of the enlarged liver. Hepatic pulsations are also found, less commonly, in other heart diseases, such as tricuspid stenosis, other conditions associated with systolic or diastolic overloading of the right atrium (George, ClinCard, 1988; 11:349), and constrictive pericarditis. In the presence of cardiac cirrhosis or significant centrilobular fibrosis these hepatic pulsations may be lost (Calleja, AmJMed, 1961; 30:302). Hepatic pulsations are considered in more detail in Chapter 24.1.

Gallbladder

The position of the gallbladder is quite variable (as evidenced by CT scanning). It usually lies in a shallow fossa on the underside of the right lobe of the liver; its tip, or fundus, tends to peep out from the inferior border of the liver at a point just below the ninth costal cartilage where the lateral border of the right rectus abdominis crosses the costal margin. A normal gallbladder is fairly soft, even when full, and is not palpable. If the gallbladder can be felt, it is probably both large and firm (due to increased pressure within). It may enlarge with obstruction to the biliary tree below the entry of the cystic duct, usually due to a carcinoma of the pancreas or ampulla. Enlargement is uncommon if the block is due to a gallstone, as the gallbladder is then usually thick walled and non-distensible due to coexisting chronic cholecystitis—this reasoning is known as 'Courvoisier's law'. The gallbladder also enlarges if the cystic duct itself is blocked, due to a gallstone or tumour; even a chronically diseased gallbladder may enlarge with cystic duct block.

If the liver is also palpable, as it is in most (but not all) patients with extrahepatic obstruction, the gallbladder is felt as a smooth, rounded mass projecting towards the umbilicus from below the liver edge. Because it tends to lie under the rectus, it may be difficult or impossible to feel in patients with firm abdominal musculature. In patients without a palpable liver a large gallbladder is often mistaken for a large liver. Because biliary obstruction causing gallbladder enlargement is usually relieved quickly, there is relatively little opportunity for practice at feeling large gallbladders, and the sign is often missed.

Right upper quadrant tenderness is the most common form of tenderness found in patients with hepatobiliary disorders. It may be due to liver tenderness, which can result from acute or chronic hepatitis, cirrhosis, abscesses or tumours, or it may be due to cholecystitis.

Epigastrium

If the recti are firm it may be extremely difficult to feel anything behind them, even when you know (from ultrasound or CT scan) that the liver or a mass is present in the epigastrium. Over 100 years ago the great German hepatologist Frehrichs pointed out the difficulty of interpreting signs when examining over the recti. If you move your right hand over the recti you will often feel the bumps of the recti and it is easy to confuse them with the presence of an abdominal mass. If, however, the abdominal musculature is lax, or if there is divarication of the recti or an incisional hernia, it is easy to feel a mass, or the edge of the liver if it crosses the epigastrium below the xiphisternum (as it does in many normal subjects). Even large pancreatic masses are difficult to feel.

If you press firmly, you will nearly always be able to feel aortic pulsation, and with practice will become familiar with the size of a normal aorta. An 'aortic aneurysm is a pulsatile swelling, and if fingers are placed on both sides of the swelling they move apart with each pulse beat.

Left hypochondrium and spleen

A mass may be felt in the left hypochondrium during initial palpation. If it is the spleen, it will move downwards and inwards during deep inspiration. If a mass is not palpable, ask the patient to take a deep breath; an enlarged spleen may become palpable during inspiration. If the spleen is massively enlarged, you may not detect it if you only examine the left hypochondrium, as its tip may be down as far as the right iliac fossa and its borders will be outside

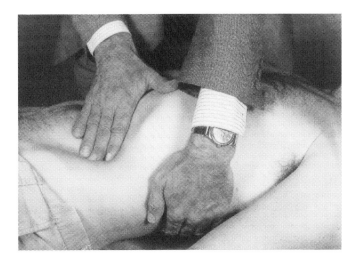

Fig. 3. Palpation of the spleen. If a mass is not obvious in the left hypochondrium, even on deep inspiration, a special technique should be used. Place the fingers of the left hand horizontally under the left lower ribs, and the palm vertically against the lateral chest wall. Press the fingers upwards and the palm inwards (as if you are trying to squeeze the spleen out from under the costal margin). Note that radial side of the index finger and the palm of the right hand are parallel to the costal margin, allowing contact with the descening spleen over a considerable length of the costal margin.

the domain of the left hypochondrium. However, a spleen of this size is almost always felt on initial light palpation of the whole abdomen. A very large spleen has easily defined borders and the splenic notch may be palpable on the medial border.

If a mass is not obvious in the left hypochondrium, even on deep inspiration, a special technique should be used for splenic palpation. With the patient lying flat, place the fingers of the left hand horizontally under the left lower ribs, and the palm vertically against the lateral chest wall (Fig. 3). Press the fingers of the left hand upwards and the palm inwards (as if you are trying to squeeze the spleen out from under the costal margin). Place the right hand so that its index finger is parallel to and below the costal margin. Press, firmly but gently, with the palmar surface of the fingers of the right hand, angling the palm slightly so that most pressure is exerted by the radial border of the index finger—which should be several centimetres below the costal margin (i.e. closer to the posterior abdominal wall). Now ask the patient to take a very deep breath. A palpable spleen will touch the right index finger. You should start a few centimetres away from the costal margin, and work up to the costal margin if you cannot feel the spleen initially.

You should exert a little pressure upwards and laterally, in order to resist the spleen as it descends, but it is important not to move the right hand during inspiration, as the 'bump' of a contracting muscle bundle is often misinterpreted as the splenic tip. As with the liver the best evidence of a spleen is when your finger 'flips' over the tip, but this occurs less commonly with splenic palpation. You may have to try several positions along the costal margin, as the position at which the spleen tip emerges is variable; sometimes it may be close to the epigastrium, sometimes closer to the mid-axillary line. For this reason the whole length of the index finger should be placed along the costal margin and not just a couple of

fingertips. The size and position of the spleen should be recorded as for the liver.

Instead of using the left hand to try to coax the spleen out, some clinicians prefer to roll the patient over on to the right side (right lateral decubitus position), so that the spleen shifts a little due to gravity. Another method is Middleton's method, in which patients place their left fist posteriorly and inferior to the left scapula; the examiner positions himself on the patient's left and hooks his fingers under the left costal margin. Barkun *et al.* (AmJMed, 1991; 91:512) used these two methods and palpation in the supine position; no one method was significantly superior to the others but the authors felt that the supine position was preferable to the right lateral decubitus position. Whichever method is used, a lot of practice is needed to become good at feeling spleens! In Barkun's study the three observers only felt 50 to 60 per cent of the spleens which were considered enlarged (13–23 cm) on ultrasound, but some of these might not have been palpable using any technique.

A number of clinical features, including the presence of a splenic notch, support the conclusion that a large mass felt in the left loin is a spleen rather than a kidney or another structure. The spleen moves towards the right iliac fossa on inspiration while a kidney moves vertically downwards; other masses tend not to move. It is sometimes possible, in deep inspiration, to get above the kidney and to insert the right hand between it and the left costal margin, but this is not possible with the spleen. As the kidney usually has bowel in front of it, the percussion note over it tends to be resonant.

The left lobe of a very large liver may be mistaken for the spleen, particularly if there is a deep fissure between it and the right side of the liver. The distinction can usually be made if the lower border of the liver is carefully mapped across the upper abdomen, although the true situation may only be revealed by ultrasound or CT scanning.

A palpable spleen usually indicates splenic pathology of some kind, but a spleen was felt in about 3 per cent of 2200 apparently healthy college students, and in a third of these it was still palpable 3 years later (McIntyre, AnnIntMed, 1967; 66:301).

Right and left loins and kidneys

The right kidney is palpable in the right loin in about 10 per cent of slim, healthy women when bimanual palpation is used during deep inspiration (Bearn, Lancet, 1959; ii:212). It is rarely palpable in men, and a normal left kidney, which lies higher than the right, is rarely palpable in either sex. Correct technique is very important for bimanual palpation of the kidneys. Place the left hand underneath the patient in the gap between the lower ribs and the iliac crest, with the tips of the fingers lateral to the sacrospinalis muscle mass. Place your right hand transversely across the abdomen, fingers pointing to the patient's left. Exert firm but gentle downwards pressure with the palmar surface of the distal phalanges, and without moving your right hand ask the patient to take a deep breath; with inspiration the kidney descends. As the patient breathes in, flip the fingers of your left hand upwards (at a rate of about 80 per min, i.e. several times faster than the respiratory rate); when the kidney is palpable it is felt to bump up against the fingers of the right hand, and you may be able to trap the kidney momentarily between your hands before it rises again on expiration.

A large right kidney is often mistaken for a palpable liver, especially in obese subjects. Percussion may help as there is usually a resonant note over the kidney. A Riedel's lobe of liver is also palpable on bimanual palpation, and is often mistaken for the right kidney, although it usually lies more laterally and has a relatively sharp edge. A very large liver may extend down into the right loin (and sometimes into the right iliac fossa), but masses other than kidney and liver are unusual findings in the right loin. Renal and hepatic enlargement may be found in patients with polycystic disease.

'Dipping'

In patients with tense ascites it is very difficult to feel enlarged organs or masses with the usual methods of palpation. They can often be palpated by 'dipping', a method which may also allow delineation of their outlines. Place the tips of the index, middle, and ring fingers on the abdominal wall and make a sudden, sharp inward movement. The inertia of an underlying organ or mass prevents rapid movement away from the examining hand and the surface or edge may be felt momentarily.

Testicular size

Testicular atrophy is common in cirrhotic males, particularly those with alcoholic liver disease or haemochromatosis, but is difficult to detect unless there is an obvious reduction in size. The size can be documented by comparison with a set of 'model' testicles, but this is rarely necessary in patients with liver disease (except for research purposes). Testicular atrophy is usually accompanied by thinning of body hair and other signs of feminization.

Percussion

Percussion of the abdomen is valuable for several purposes. It is useful for detecting the liver when it is enlarged but not palpable, and may help to detect a very small liver. Percussion over a mass indicates whether it is solid or fluid filled (when the note will be dull), or whether it contains gas (when the note is resonant). It is particularly valuable in the detection of ascites. When percussing it is customary to percuss from a resonant to a dull area.

To find the liver edge you should place your pleximeter finger on the abdominal wall and percuss at various points, working upwards from the right iliac fossa and from the umbilical region. With a normal liver the percussion note is usually resonant over the abdomen, even during deep inspiration, but it becomes dull on reaching the costal margin. This technique is useful for locating the liver edge (but when it is found below the costal margin it does not necessarily mean that the liver is enlarged; see above under palpation).

Percussion is unquestionably useful in detecting a liver edge below the costal margin when subjects are obese, when the abdominal musculature is firm, and when the liver is soft (in these situations even a very large liver may be impalpable). If the percussion note is resonant above the costal margin, it suggests either that the liver is small (due to cirrhosis, or due to shrinkage in severe hepatitis), or that bowel is present between the liver and the abdominal wall; in either case further investigation is needed.

Some clinicians advocate measurement of the percussion span, i.e. the distance between the lower edge of the liver and its upper border, both being assessed by percussion. It is usually measured in the 'mid–clavicular line' (bearing in mind that few observers bother

to check the correct position of this line), or in the midline. Not surprisingly, the percussion span varies with the patient's height, and to decide whether the span is normal (within a 95 per cent confidence interval of 3 cm) you must know the relationship between span and height, or use a formula taking height and body weight into account (Castell, AnnIntMed, 1969; 70:1183). In the 'mid-clavicular line' the span is about 3 cm greater with soft than with hard percussion. Although intra-observer error is relatively small, there is considerable inter-observer error (up to 2.5 cm). Using percussion, Zoli et al. (AmJGastr, 1995; 90:1428) found a higher liver span in cirrhotics than in controls, but in the same subjects the liver span by ultrasonography was higher in controls.

The current vogue for measurement of the percussion span seems absurd. Students often present this measurement before, and sometimes instead of, commenting on their findings on palpation. Although there is debate about its accuracy (Naftalis, AmJDigDis, 1963; 8:236; Rosenfield, AJR, 1974; 122:313; Espinoza, DigDisSci, 1987; 32:244), palpation of the liver allows you to decide whether it is obviously enlarged, permits delineation of the liver edge, allows assessment of its consistency (which gives a clue to the presence of cirrhosis or malignancy), and findings on palpation are more important and reproducible than those on percussion. The main use of percussion span is to detect a small liver. It is of little value for deciding whether a palpable liver is enlarged, or if it is a normal-sized liver pushed down by hyperinflated lungs, because other clinical signs are of more value for identifying emphysematous lungs.

Percussion of the spleen

Many teachers suggest percussion over the left lower ribs in order to detect an enlarged spleen which is not palpable. In my opinion this is rarely useful. In one study there was no correlation between spleen size on percussion and the size of the spleen on a radionuclide scan; many patients were thought to have large spleens when the scintigraphic image was normal.[8] Barkun et al. (AmJMed, 1991; 91:512) used two methods of percussion to assess splenic enlargement. They either percussed Traube's space (delineated by the sixth rib superiorly, the mid-axillary line laterally, and the left costal margin inferiorly), or used the splenic percussion sign (percussing at the point where the lowest intercostal space, eighth or ninth, crosses the left anterior axillary line). In their study on 118 patients (43 having an enlarged spleen on ultrasound, i.e. 13–23 cm) sensitivity and specificity for the splenic percussion sign were 79 and 46 per cent, while Traube's space percussion gave results of 62 and 72 per cent, respectively. Diagnostic accuracy was better with Traube's space percussion, and the authors believed that optimal clinical assessment of splenic enlargement should include this method. Curiously, they concluded that 'If Traube's space is dull, palpation of the spleen is warranted.'

Percussion for ascites

Gross ascites is usually obvious on inspection because there is distension of the whole abdomen, and a fluid thrill can be elicited (i.e. palpable vibrations are felt on one side of the abdomen when the opposite side is flicked with the fingers of the other hand). When there is only bulging of the flanks, or if there is doubt about the presence of ascites, percussion is useful. With ascites the percussion

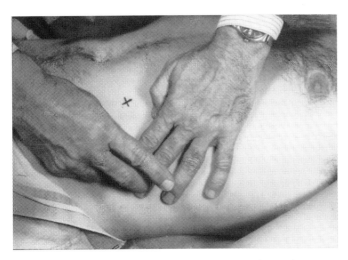

Fig. 4. Percussion for ascites. It is important to go well past the junction between resonance and dullness, and pick a spot on that side which is definitely dull.

note around the umbilicus is usually hyperresonant due to gas in the 'floating' bowel; as you percuss out towards the flanks you will find a dull percussion note on both sides. Go well past the junction between resonance and dullness, and pick a spot on that side which is definitely dull (Fig. 4). Now ask the patient to roll over on to the other side so that your chosen point is uppermost (Fig. 5). Allow about 20 s for the fluid to settle and percuss again. If the note is now clearly resonant, there is 'shifting dullness'—a cardinal sign of ascites—which should be present on both sides.

A number of other techniques have been proposed for detecting ascites. With the patient lying flat you can mark two points, one on each side, where resonance changes to dullness; if you now roll the patient to one side or the other and percuss again, you will find that the junction point on the dependent side will have moved closer to the umbilicus and you will not be able to detect a junction point on the uppermost side. (This appears to be the origin of a nonsensical technique, taught by some and which actually appears in print. It involves keeping the finger on the point at which resonance changes to dullness, rolling the patient over on the other side, and then

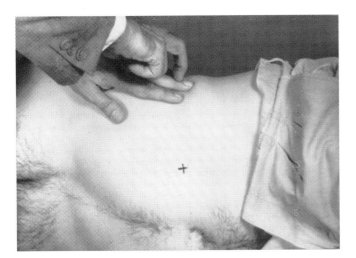

Fig. 5. Percussion for ascites. The patient has rolled over on to his side so that your chosen point is now uppermost.

percussing again at the same point. It is difficult to know what the sign is meant to be; without shifting dullness there may now be resonance if the pleximeter finger has accidentally shifted a centimetre or so towards the umbilicus, and dullness if it has moved in the other direction. If there is shifting dullness, the chances of detecting it are reduced because the original position was not one of maximal dullness. DO NOT USE THIS METHOD.)

If the patient lies face down for a few minutes, fluid accumulates around the umbilicus; if he then rises on to his hands and knees, dullness may be noted around the umbilicus; alternatively, a change in note may be heard at the edge of the fluid accumulation if a stethoscope diaphragm is moved laterally from the umbilicus while the flank is percussed lightly with the finger (this is known as the 'puddle' sign; Lawson, NEJM, 1959; 260:652). The 'puddle' sign is said to detect small amounts of ascites (in excess of 120 ml). Elicitation of these signs is clearly impracticable in sick patients (and is a bit of a performance in any patient).

Unfortunately, these signs are of limited value in doubtful cases, when they would be most useful; while ascites is unlikely to be present in the absence of flank dullness (<10 per cent of cases), the converse is not true (Cattau, JAMA, 1982; 247:1164). The presence of ascites can usually be detected or confirmed by ultrasound (or by CT scanning), and the best confirmation of the presence of ascites is aspiration of peritoneal fluid.

Ascites is not the only cause of gross abdominal swelling. Gross obesity, gaseous distension, abdominal masses, and large organs can usually be distinguished from ascites by careful physical examination. Massive ovarian or hydatid cysts, and occasionally pregnancy with hydramnios, can be more confusing as they may be associated with a fluid thrill; the finding of shifting dullness on percussion helps to distinguish ascites from these conditions.

Auscultation

Auscultation of the abdomen is performed in order to check for bowel sounds (and particularly their absence), and to detect vascular sounds and friction rubs.

Vascular sounds

There are two types of vascular noises—'arterial' bruits and 'venous' hums.

Arterial bruits

Bruits are intermittent noises, with the same rhythm as the radial pulse, which are assumed to occur when pulsatile arterial flow is greatest. They may be very quiet and the best way to detect bruits is to feel the pulse while listening for a bruit; knowing the rhythm makes it easier to hear them. It may also help if you ask the patient to stop breathing for a few seconds.

Epigastric bruits are common in normal subjects, the reported frequency varying from about 6 to 30 per cent. They tend to be more common in younger subjects. These benign bruits are highly localized (in the midline or just to the left, and in the mid or high epigastrium); they tend to be faint, but are louder and longer during expiration; they are systolic when compared to a phonocardiogram. Sometimes a benign bruit disappears when a patient changes position and may not return on resuming the original position; presumably such a bruit is due to transient pressure of an organ on the aorta.

Epigastric bruits occur with coeliac artery stenosis, when they are louder and longer than benign bruits and may extend into diastole (Watson, AnnIntMed, 1973; 79:211). Bruits also occur with disease of the abdominal aorta or its main branches; the site of maximum intensity then depends on the site of the lesion. A renal artery bruit may be heard over the corresponding side, either over the front of the abdomen or in the renal angle posteriorly. A splenic artery bruit (a sign of a tumour of the pancreatic body) may be heard high in the epigastrium anteriorly, in the left hypochondrium (Serebro, Lancet, 1965; i:85), or over the left side of the back at about the level of the twelfth rib. Bruits may also result from external pressure on vessels by tumours or large organs; these usually disappear when the patient changes position.

Bruits may be heard over the liver, when they suggest the presence of a vascular tumour, usually a hepatocellular carcinoma or, less commonly, an arteriovenous malformation. They occur rarely with a cholangiocarcinoma or a metastasis (Motoki, AmJ-Gastr, 1979; 71:582; Sherman, JAMA, 1979; 241:1495). They may also be audible in severe alcoholic hepatitis (Clain, Lancet, 1966; ii: 516), and may be heard for a day or two after a liver biopsy (due presumably to creation of a temporary arteriovenous fistula). Hepatic bruits have been described with large tortuous arteries in cirrhosis (very rare; Goldstein, JAMA, 1968; 206:2518), and in association with severe anaemia (<3 g/dl; Konar, BMJ, 1967; 4: 154).

Bruits in the left hypochondrium may occur with a tortuous, aneurysmal splenic artery, and with splenomegaly and splenic arteriovenous fistulae.

Venous hums

Venous hums are continuous noises and in subjects without liver disease are usually heard in the neck. They are occasionally audible in patients with portal hypertension as a result of rapid, turbulent flow in collateral veins, and can be heard over the xiphisternum or lower sternum, near the umbilicus, and less often over the liver, left hypochondrium, or back (Bloom, BrHeartJ, 1950; 12:343). Hums may originate in deep veins or in visible superficial collaterals, which may be large or very small, and there may be a thrill over the distended vein (the Cruveilhier–Baumgarten syndrome); there may be a hum, arising presumably from internal veins, even when there are no obvious surface collaterals. The source of the hum is obvious if it disappears when one or more visible veins (often surprisingly small) are occluded by finger pressure. Hums are usually louder when the patient breathes in, sits up, or stands.

A hum may be audible over the inferior vena cava (just above and to the right of the umbilicus), particularly with severe anaemia.

Friction rubs

When there is inflammation or infiltration of the capsule of the liver a friction rub may be heard over the liver when the patient breathes deeply. This is common when a tumour (primary or secondary) or abscess invades the visceral peritoneum, and with hepatic infarction. A transient rub is commonly heard for a day or two at the site of a liver biopsy, and after other percutaneous procedures. A rub heard in a young sexually active woman or homosexual male (usually associated with right upper quadrant pain, made worse by breathing

deeply) suggests the possibility of gonococcal or chlamydial perihepatitis (the Fitz-Hugh-Curtis syndrome). A hepatic friction rub has also been described in uraemic patients with a prior history of uraemic pericarditis (Kothari, ArchIntMed, 1979; 140:419).

A friction rub may also be heard over the spleen if splenic infarction has occurred, due to a splenic embolus or in association with massive splenomegaly, or if there is infection in or around the spleen.

Physical signs found in other systems with liver disease

Many physical signs are found in other systems in patients with liver disease. These are discussed in Section 25. There are, however, two signs (the Kayser–Fleischer ring, and the flapping tremor of hepatic encephalopathy) which are of particular interest in patients with liver disease.

Kayser–Fleischer rings

The Kayser–Fleischer ring (Plate 11) is a brown ring at the periphery of the cornea; it is present in virtually all cases of Wilson's disease with neurological signs, and in most cases of hepatic Wilson's disease. The ring is caused by copper deposition in Descemet's membrane; it extends from the limbus, fades gradually towards the centre, and is most marked at the upper and lower poles. When the iris is green or blue the ring may be visible to the unaided eye, but when the iris is brown, slit-lamp examination is required, preferably by an experienced ophthalmologist, and this should be requested in all patients with unexplained chronic liver disease, particularly in children and adolescents.

Kayser–Fleischer rings are also found occasionally in patients with primary biliary cirrhosis (Fleming, Gastro, 1975; 69:220), in other forms of chronic cholestasis (Kaplinsky, Pediat, 1980; 65:782), with chronic active hepatitis (Fleming, AnnIntMed, 1977; 86: 285; Frommer, Gastro, 1977; 72:1331), and cryptogenic cirrhosis (Rimola, ArchIntMed, 1978; 138:1857). They may also occur with an intraocular copper-containing foreign body.

Pigmented peripheral rings may be seen with an arcus stained with carotene, with bilirubin in prolonged jaundice, and in some patients with hypercupricaemia associated with myeloma (when the ring is densest at the centre and fades towards the limbus).

Hepatic encephalopathy
'Flapping tremor' (asterixis)

The most important physical sign of hepatic encephalopathy is the 'flapping tremor' or 'asterixis', first described by Adams and Foley (TrAmNeurolAss, 1949; 74:217). Ask the patient to raise both arms horizontally in front of him (palms downwards), to dorsiflex the wrists and spread the fingers wide apart, and to hold this posture for about 15 s (Fig. 6). The term 'asterixis', or flap, is used to describe the small, brief, intermittent movements of individual fingers, either of flexion or laterally in an ulnar direction, with rapid return of the fingers to the original position. With more severe asterixis the flap spreads proximally, movements involve the wrists and even the shoulders (the whole arm suddenly dropping), and in extreme cases you may see movements of the head if it is held erect. There may also be a background tremulousness of the hands.

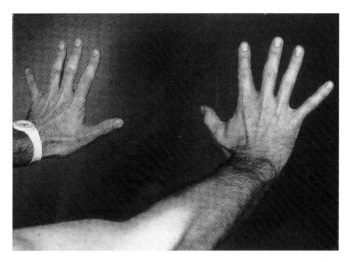

Fig. 6. Demonstrating a 'flap'. The patient has both arms raised horizontally in front of him (palms downwards), the wrists are dorsiflexed, and the fingers are spread wide apart. This posture should be held for about 15 s before concluding that a flap is absent.

Asterixis is not seen in resting limbs, or during voluntary movements.

Asterixis is random and asymmetrical. It is not due to contraction, but to sudden relaxation of muscles; electromyograms (EMG) from the contracted muscles holding the posture show frequent short periods of reduced electrical activity or 'silence', which may account for the tremulousness. Asterixis occurs when longer periods of absolute silence coincide in different muscles (Plate 12; Leavitt, ArchNeurol, 1964; 10:360).

Asterixis is not specific for hepatic encephalopathy, and occurs in uraemia, respiratory failure, hypokalaemia, hypomagnesaemia, and intoxication with certain drugs.[5]

Grading of encephalopathy

Most of the clinical features of hepatic encephalopathy were presented earlier. The clinical features of encephalopathy range from mild euphoria and slight confusion to deep coma with absent deep reflexes. For prognostic and therapeutic studies in liver disease it is usual to grade encephalopathy, and a number of systems have been used for this purpose. Two of these are presented in Tables 1 and 2.

Grading the overall severity of liver disease

A number of systems have been designed to assess the overall functional severity of liver disease, in order to quantify responses to therapy and, more importantly, to serve as a prognostic index. Two have been used widely: Child's grading, and Pugh's modification of Child's grading.

Child's grading[9,10]

Child and Turcotte, in 1964, introduced a system of grading (Table 3) to assess the risk of surgery in patients with liver disease. It was based on five variables: the levels of serum bilirubin and albumin, the absence or severity of ascites and encephalopathy, and the nutritional status. It is unquestionably a crude system, but it appears to have served surprisingly well for classifying patients into those who represent a good, moderate, or poor risk for surgery. The main problem in the use of Child's grading is that the findings in an individual patient may be a mixture of those in columns A, B, and C (Conn, Hepatol, 1987; 7:660). If patients are only categorized as A or C if they have a 'full house' of the appropriate findings, there will be an excessive number of grade B patients. For this reason some have given scores to each observation (e.g. 1 for those

Table 2 Grading of hepatic coma (Conn, Gastr, 1977; 72:573)	
Grade 0	No abnormality detected
Grade 1	Trivial lack of awareness, euphoria or anxiety. Shortened attention span. Impairment in performing addition or subtraction
Grade 2	Lethargy or apathy. Disorientation for time. Obvious personality changes, inappropriate behaviour
Grade 3	Somnolence to semi-stupor, but responsive to stimuli. Confused. Gross disorientation
Grade 4	Coma. Mental state not testable

Table 1 Stages in the onset and development of hepatic coma (Trey, NEJM, 1966; 274:473)			
Grade of stage	**Mental state**	**Tremor**	**EEG changes**
Stage Prodrome (often diagnosed in retrospect)	Euphoria, occasionally depression; fluctuant mild confusion; slowness of mentation and affect; untidy slurred speech; disorder in rhythm	Slight	Usually absent
Stage 2 Impending coma	Accentuation of stage 1; drowsiness; inappropriate behaviour; ability to maintain sphincter control	Present (easily elicited)	Abnormal; general slowing
Stage 3 Stupor	Sleeps most of time but rousable; speech incoherent; confusion marked	Usually present if patient co-operative	Always abnormal
Stage 4 Deep coma	May or may not respond to painful stimuli	Usually absent	Always abnormal

Table 3 Child's grading of the severity of liver disease

Clinical and biochemical measurements	Child's grade		
	A	B	C
Bilirubin (mg/100 ml)	<2.4	<2.3–2.9	>2.9
Albumin (g/l)	>35	30–35	<30
Ascites	Absent	Easily controlled	Poorly controlled
Encephalopathy	None	Minimal	Coma
Nutrition	Good	Moderate	Poor, wasting

Table 4 Pugh's grading of the severity of liver disease

Clinical and biochemical measurements	Points scored for increasing abnormality		
	1	2	3
Encephalopathy[a]	None	1 and 2	3 and 4
Ascites	Absent	Slight	Moderate
Bilirubin (mg/100 ml)	1–2	2–3	>3
Albumin (g/l)	>35	28–35	<28
Prothrombin (seconds prolonged)	1–4	4–6	>6
For primary biliary cirrhosis Bilirubin (mg/100 ml)	1–4	4–10	>10

[a] According to the grading of Trey *et al.* (NEJM, 1966; 274:473).

in column A, 2 for B, and 3 for C) and have then taken the sum of these scores in order to obtain an overall result (Campbell, AmJSurg, 1973; 126:748). This is the approach taken in Pugh's modification of Child's grading, which is now more widely used. Another problem with Child's grading is that there is sometimes disagreement between observers about the subjective components, i.e. ascites, neurological disorder, and particularly the nutritional state.

Pugh's modification of Child's grading

In 1973 Pugh and his colleagues (BrJSurg, 1973; 60:646) published a modification of Child's grading (Table 4), originally designed to assess operative risk in patients undergoing surgical transection of the oesophagus for variceal bleeding. Prolongation of the prothrombin time was added to, and nutritional assessment omitted from, the grading of Child. The individual measurements are allocated either 1, 2, or 3 points, depending on the result, and the points for the five variables are added to give a score (ranging from 5 to 15). Patients whose score totals 5 or 6 are considered to be grade A; those scoring 7, 8, or 9 are grade B, and those with a score of 10 to 15 are labelled grade C. Allowance is made in the scoring system for patients with primary biliary cirrhosis, as the level of bilirubin in these patients is usually out of proportion with other evidence of hepatic failure.

There are some problems in the use of the Child–Turcotte and Child–Pugh scoring systems.[10] Different clinical groups have used different total scores for allocation to grades A, B, and C. This affects prognosis; if fewer patients are allocated to group C because

a higher total score is needed for this purpose, the mortality for grade C patients will inevitably be higher than if a lower total score is needed. Another problem is that gradings are usually done at one point in time, usually just before a procedure is carried out. The grading may therefore be influenced by other factors; for example, the bilirubin may be higher because of recent transfusion, or encephalopathy may seem worse due to medication. No one has checked whether patients who have been persistently grade C do worse than those who have been tipped from grade A or B into grade C as a result of recent events. Another issue is whether one can legitimately claim to improve the grade, and thus the prognosis, by treating ascites or encephalopathy, or by increasing serum albumin by infusing large amounts of albumin.

Even so, the Pugh's score is a very useful method of assessing prognosis in cirrhosis (Infante-Rivard, Hepatol, 1987; 7:660). However, because of the great advances in hepatic surgery, it is increasingly important to be able to assess prognosis in patients with liver disease, and a large amount of work is currently in progress which is designed to improve our knowledge of prognostic factors.

References

1. Johnson Abercrombie ML. *The anatomy of judgment*. London: Hutchinson, 1960.
2. Feinstein AR. *Clinical judgment*. Baltimore: Williams and Wilkins, 1967.
3. De Dombal FT. *Diagnosis of acute abdominal pain*. Edinburgh: Churchill Livingstone, 1980.

4. Schein CJ. *Postcholecystectomy syndromes*. Hagerstown, MD: Harper and Row, 1978.

5. Conn HO and Lieberthal MM. *The hepatic coma syndromes and lactulose*. Baltimore: William and Wilkins, 1979.

6. Theodossi A, Knill-Jones RP, and Skene A. Inter-observer variation of symptoms and signs in jaundice. *Liver*, 1981; **1**: 21–32.

7. Espinoza P, *et al*. Interobserver agreement in the physical diagnosis of alcoholic liver disease. *Digestive Diseases and Sciences*, 1987; **32**: 244–7.

8. Chalmers TC, *et al*. Clinical examination of liver and spleen size. In Paumgartner G and Preisig R, eds. *The liver: quantitative aspects of structure and function*. Basel: Karger, 1973: 76–86.

9. Child CG and Turcotte JG. Surgery and portal hypertension. In Child CG, ed. *The liver and portal hypertension*. Philadelphia: WB Saunders, 1964.

10. McIntyre N. The Child–Turcotte and Child–Pugh classifications. In Poupon RE and Reichen J, eds. *Surrogate markers to assess efficacy of treatment in chronic liver diseases*. Dordrecht: Kluwer Academic Publishers, 1996.

5

Investigation of hepatobiliary disease

5.1 Biochemical investigations in the management of liver disease

S. B. Rosalki and Neil McIntyre

The chemical pathology laboratory plays a major role in the management of patients with liver disease. It provides various types of information, as set out in Table 1.

Liver function tests

All clinical laboratories employ a small battery of biochemical tests for the initial detection and subsequent management of liver disease. Although termed 'liver function tests' they are of little value for assessing liver function *per se*. A large number tests have been proposed (Table 2), but many provide similar information. In individual laboratories chemical pathologists tend to select tests with which they are familiar, and which they believe will satisfy the needs of their clinical colleagues.

Most laboratories routinely measure serum (or plasma) total bilirubin, aspartate and/or alanine aminotransferase, alkaline phosphatase, and serum albumin; some add serum γ-glutamyltransferase, bile acids, and/or other tests mentioned in Table 2. Tests for urinary bilirubin and urobilinogen are performed in the ward or clinic. Prothrombin and partial thromboplastin times, useful markers of the severity of liver disease, are usually measured in the haematology laboratory; they are valuable in managing liver disease but are not generally considered under the heading 'liver function tests'.

These tests, except possibly for bile acids (but see below), are not specific for liver disease; increased levels of plasma total bilirubin, aspartate and alanine aminotransferases, alkaline phosphatase and γ-glutamyltransferase, and low levels of albumin may all result from pathological processes outside the liver.

A few tests measure specific aspects of hepatic function. They include galactose elimination, bile acid clearance, aminopyrine breath tests, and measurement of the excretion of certain dyes. They are all inconvenient to perform, and tend to be costly in terms

---

Table 1 Role of the chemical pathology laboratory in liver disease

'Liver function tests'
Quantitative tests of liver function
'Specific' diagnostic tests
Other biochemical tests used in managing liver disease

Table 2 Tests used as 'liver function tests'

Tests used as indices of uptake, conjugation, and excretion of anionic compounds
   Serum total bilirubin (and direct and indirect)*
   Urinary bilirubin (and urobilinogen)*
   Bile acids*

Tests reflecting hepatocellular damage
   Aspartate and/or alanine aminotransferase*
   Glutathione-S-transferase*
   Lactate dehydrogenase and LD5 isoenzyme*
   Serum ferritin*
   Vitamin B_{12}*
   (Also the following enzymes presumed to be released from damaged hepatocytes)
   Isocitrate dehydrogenase
   Malate dehydrogenase
   Sorbitol dehydrogenase
   Ornithine carbamyltransferase
   Glutamate dehydrogenase
   Glutamine deaminase
   Guanase
   Fructose-1,6-aldolase
   Phosphohexoseisomerase
   Urocanase
   Alcohol dehydrogenase
   β-Glucuronidase
   Xanthine oxidase

Tests used to indicate obstruction to bile flow
   Alkaline phosphatase*
   γ-Glutamyltransferase*
   5'-Nucleotidase*
   Leucine aminopeptidase*
   Lp-X*
   Secretory component and IgA

Tests of synthetic function
   Serum albumin*
   Prealbumin*
   Cholinesterase*
   Lecithin cholesterol acyltransferase*
   Serum proteins – electrophoresis*
   Prothrombin and partial thromboplastin times

Test suggesting increased hepatic collagen formation
   Procollagen peptide*

* Tests discussed in the text.

of materials and laboratory time. They are, however, of great importance for our understanding of liver disease and for assessing the effects of therapy. Such tests are discussed in detail in Chapter 5.2.

If we are to use liver function tests properly we must know how to interpret them, appreciate when they are useful, and understand their limitations in clinical practice. In this chapter individual tests are discussed, and then the various ways in which they should be used.

Serum bilirubin (total and conjugated, bilialb and biliproteins)

The biochemistry and physiology of bilirubin is discussed in Chapter 2.9. A major early contribution to the clinical chemistry of jaundice was made by van den Bergh and Muller (BiochemZ, 1916; 77:90) who found two types of bilirubin in jaundiced sera; one reacting directly with Ehrlich's diazo reagent ('direct' bilirubin), the other requiring addition of alcohol for colour development ('indirect' bilirubin). Direct-reacting bilirubin was found with obstruction of the large bile duct and some other types of liver disease, but not with haemolytic jaundice.

The van den Bergh test was qualitative. In 1937 Malloy and Evelyn modified it and made quantitative measurements of 'direct' and 'indirect' bilirubin in plasma (JBC, 1937; 119:481). Cole *et al.* (BiochemJ, 1954; 57:514) identified bilirubin itself as the indirect reacting material, and Billing and Lathe (BiochemJ, 1956; 63:6p) and Schmid (Science, 1956; 124:76) showed that direct-reacting bilirubin was a mixture of bilirubin mono- and diglucuronides (i.e. bilirubin esters). It was soon found that bilirubin is conjugated in the liver and that its glucuronides are efficiently excreted in bile, little normally appearing in blood. Impaired excretion of conjugated bilirubin by hepatocytes explained the jaundice of hepatocellular disorders.

Bilirubin is insoluble in water, binds to albumin, and does not appear in urine. Bilirubin glucuronides are water soluble and are excreted in urine when their plasma level increases (see Urinary bilirubin, below). When serum bilirubin glucuronides are elevated, some bilirubin is found to be covalently bound to serum albumin and other proteins (Lauff, ClinChem, 1982; 28:629); this fraction (bilialb or biliprotein) may be a major component of serum total bilirubin, particularly during recovery from jaundice (Weiss, NEJM, 1983; 309:147). Its protein binding explains why bilirubinuria is absent in some patients with 'direct' hyperbilirubinaemia, supporting the early hypothesis of Nosslin (ScaJCLI, 1960; 12,Suppl. 49:1). For this reason a negative test for urinary bilirubin does not exclude the presence of conjugated hyperbilirubinaemia.

Methods

In most laboratories total serum bilirubin is measured by adding a diazo reagent (e.g. diazotized sulphanilic acid) to serum in the presence of ethanol or another accelerator. The depth of the violet colour produced is proportional to the total bilirubin concentration. Without ethanol colour development is less intense and the reading is taken as the amount of 'direct' bilirubin; 'indirect' bilirubin is the difference between total and 'direct' measurements. Bilirubin is altered by exposure to light so serum or plasma samples must be kept in the dark, preferably in a refrigerator, before measurements are made.

Some laboratories routinely provide results for direct and indirect bilirubin; but they are not accurate measurements of bilirubin and bilirubin esters as some free bilirubin appears to react directly with the reagent. Measurement of 'direct' bilirubin overestimates bilirubin esters at low bilirubin levels, and underestimates them at high concentrations. This is unfortunate; it is of little value to measure bilirubin and bilirubin esters at high bilirubin levels, but important to measure bilirubin esters when there is only a slight elevation of total bilirubin; this allows identification of 'unconjugated hyperbilirubinaemia', as in Gilbert's syndrome and haemolysis.

Several methods give accurate measurements of bilirubin and its conjugates (see Chapter 2.9), but are rarely used in routine laboratories. They show that conjugated bilirubins account for only 4 to 5 per cent (less than 1 μmol/l) of total bilirubin in normal subjects. However, the upper limit for 'direct-reacting' bilirubin is usually taken as about 3 μmol/l; levels above 5 μmol/l, with a normal total bilirubin, suggest hepatobiliary disease, but only if measured in a good laboratory (on a good day!). Accurate measurement of bilirubin conjugates (e.g. by alkaline methanolysis and high-performance liquid chromatography) is the most sensitive marker of hepatobiliary disease; it even allows the distinction to be made between the 'unconjugated hyperbilirubinaemia' of Gilbert's syndrome and that of haemolysis, as the proportion of bilirubin conjugates (as a percentage of total bilirubin) is normal in patients with haemolysis but low (less than 1.7 per cent) in Gilbert's syndrome.

Interpretation of bilirubin levels

The 'normal' range for total bilirubin concentration in serum or plasma is between 3 and 15 μmol/l, though many laboratories use an upper limit of 17 μmol/l. The mean total bilirubin level is about 3 to 4 μmol/l higher in men than in women; as Gilbert's syndrome (Chapter 20.6) is often 'diagnosed' when the plasma bilirubin is only just above the upper limit of 17 μmol/l, this explains, in part, why the condition appears more prevalent in men. In Gilbert's syndrome the total bilirubin increases with fasting or with a low fat intake; this is an important factor when interpreting bilirubin results.

Causes of an isolated elevation of serum bilirubin are listed in Table 3. In patients with benign unconjugated hyperbilirubinaemia (i.e. without an obvious increase in conjugated bilirubin) it is unusual to find bilirubin levels higher than 70 μmol/l, and other liver function tests are usually normal. The same is true with simple haemolysis. The clinical features of the benign hyperbilirubinaemias are presented in Chapter 20.6. Haemolysis is usually confirmed by haematological investigations which often suggest the cause. When haemolysis occurs in the presence of underlying liver damage, bilirubin levels tend to be much higher.

When other liver function tests are also abnormal, bilirubin levels above 17 μmol/l usually indicate liver disease of some kind and bilirubin esters are elevated. The major causes of a high serum bilirubin are presented in Table 4. The actual level of total bilirubin is rarely of diagnostic value. An elevated serum total bilirubin reflects increased production, reduced hepatic uptake and/or conjugation, or decreased biliary excretion of the pigment.

Table 3 Causes of isolated increase of serum bilirubin (hyperbilirubinaemia with normal or near-normal liver function tests)

Unconjugated
   Ineffective haemopoiesis, e.g. pernicious anaemia
   Haemolysis—transfusion, drugs, etc.
   Defective uptake or conjugation—newborn, Gilbert's syndrome,
                    Crigler–Najjar syndrome

Conjugated
   Dubin–Johnson syndrome
   Rotor syndrome
   Cholestasis of pregnancy or of oral contraceptive therapy

Table 4 Causes of hyperbilirubinaemia*

Unconjugated (premicrosomal)
   Excessive bilirubin production (haemolytic)
   Ineffective haemopoiesis
   Haemolytic disorders
   Abnormal bilirubin metabolism (congenital)
   Immaturity of enzyme systems:
      Physiological jaundice of new born
      Jaundice of prematurity
   Inherited defects:
      Gilbert's syndrome
      Crigler–Najjar syndrome
   Drug effects

Conjugated and unconjugated (postmicrosomal)
   Hepatocellular abnormality (hepatocellular)
   Primary hepatocyte disease (hepatitis, cirrhosis, neoplasm, drugs)
   Intrahepatic cholestasis (drugs, pregnancy)
   Benign postoperative jaundice
   Congenital conjugated hyperbilirubinaemia:
      Dubin–Johnson syndrome
      Rotor syndrome
   Mechanical obstruction of bile ducts (obstructive)
   Extrahepatic (calculus, neoplasm, stricture, atresia)
   Intrahepatic (infantile obstructive cholangiopathy, sclerosing cholangitis,
   primary biliary cirrhosis)

* After Rossoff L and Rossoff C, SurgClinNAm, 1977; 57:257.

In bile duct obstruction, even if complete, serum bilirubin tends to plateau between 170 and 500 µmol/l; the major pathway for the removal of bilirubin appears to be urinary excretion, but there is also breakdown of bilirubin to unidentified compounds. Extreme hyperbilirubinuria (up to 1500 µmol/l or greater) is more likely to occur in severe parenchymal liver disease, and usually in association with renal failure and/or with haemolysis (e.g. in sickle cell disease; Klion, AmJMed, 1964; 37:829; Sheehy, ArchIntMed, 1980; 140: 1364; Shao, AmJGastr, 1995; 90:2048), with glucose-6-phosphate dehydrogenase deficiency (Fulop, ArchIntMed, 1971; 127:254), or with blood tranfusion.

In acute liver diseases the serum bilirubin level is also of relatively little prognostic value; complete recovery usually occurs, even after deep jaundice, with resolution of underlying conditions such as acute viral hepatitis or biliary obstruction. With chronic liver diseases, however, a gradual and pronounced increase in serum bilirubin, without obvious cause (such as blood transfusion or administration of certain drugs), is an ominous prognostic sign; this has been well documented in the case of primary biliary cirrhosis (Shapiro, Gut, 1979; 20:137),

and in this condition a level of 100 µmol/l has been used to trigger consideration of liver transplantation.

Urinary bilirubin

When bilirubin esters are present the urine is usually a dark brown colour. As other compounds also cause dark urine (Table 5), the presence of bilirubin should be confirmed. Test strips impregnated with a diazo reagent are easy to use and can detect as little as 1 to 2 µmol of bilirubin per litre. This test is underused.

Bilirubinuria is important as it establishes the presence of liver damage; it occurs even with small increases in plasma conjugated bilirubin (if it is not protein bound) and usually precedes jaundice. When frank jaundice is present, bilirubinuria is less important; it simply confirms an increase in the plasma level of bilirubin esters (not bound to protein).

In patients with jaundice the absence of bilirubinuria is important, particularly if other liver function tests are normal, as it suggests an unconjugated hyperbilirubinaemia or haemolysis. However, with long-standing jaundice, absence of bilirubinuria may

Table 5 Causes of dark urine other than bilirubinuria

Colour	Cause
Orange	Concentrated urine, urobilin, drugs
Orange-reddish brown	Drugs, rhubarb ingestion
Dark brown	Altered blood, myoglobin, porphyrins*, phenolic drugs*
Red	Blood, beetroot, or blackberry ingestion (acid urine); food dyes, drugs, urates
Purple-red	Phenolphthalein laxatives (alkaline urine)
Port-wine	Porphyrin*, altered blood
Brown-black	Melanin*, homogentisic acid, altered blood, phenolic drug poisoning*

* Colour develops on standing.

simply indicate that conjugated pigment is present in plasma mainly as bilialb; this often occurs during recovery from an acute hepatitis, when bilirubin may be absent from the urine even at serum bilirubin levels as high as 170 μmol/l. At the onset of acute viral hepatitis, however, bilirubinuria may be found before jaundice appears.

Urinary urobilinogen

Bilirubin esters entering the gut undergo bacterial hydrolysis and degradation in the ileum and colon with the production of 'urobilinogen' (a term referring to a mixture of isomers). Some urobilinogen is excreted in the faeces; some is absorbed and travels via the portal vein to the liver, where most is removed and excreted in bile. A small amount escapes hepatic uptake and is excreted in the urine.

Urinary urobilinogens give a purple reaction with Ehrlich's aldehyde reagent. A dipstick containing this reagent allows rough and ready quantification, and can be used to monitor urinary urobilinogen on repeated occasions. Freshly voided urine should be used. Although much emphasis is placed on urobilinogen metabolism in undergraduate texts, the detection of urinary urobilinogen is of little clinical value. We do not test for urobilinogen at the Royal Free Hospital in London.

Increased amounts of urobilinogen are made when there is overproduction of bilirubin (for example with haemolysis) or with constipation or bacterial contamination of the small bowel. In the presence of liver damage more urobilinogen escapes hepatic uptake and biliary excretion, and is excreted in urine. When biliary obstruction is more or less complete, urinary levels fall, as less bilirubin enters the intestine for conversion to urobilinogen and less urobilinogen is absorbed. Urobilinogen production and urinary excretion are also reduced with diarrhoeal states and following treatment with antibiotics. Thus, increases and decreases in urinary urobilinogen may occur which are unrelated to changes in hepatic function.

The urinary excretion of urobilinogen is markedly dependent on urine pH; tubular reabsorption increases with increasing urinary acidity, which also renders urobilinogen unstable. Estimation of urinary urobilinogen in an acid urine is thus an unreliable index of plasma urinobilinogen levels. The peak urinary output of urobilinogen tends to occur between 12 noon and 1600 h, probably in association with the 'alkaline tide'.

Aspartate and alanine aminotransferases[1]

In 1955 De Ritis *et al.* (MinMed, 1955; 46:120) found marked elevations of serum aspartate aminotransferase (**AST**; glutamic oxaloacetic transaminase) in viral hepatitis; Wroblewski and LaDue (AnnIntMed, 1955; 43:345) reported high activity in many other hepatic disorders. It was considered an index of liver cell injury. Subsequently, a high serum alanine aminotransferase (**ALT**; glutamic pyruvate transaminase) was found in hepatic disorders in which AST was elevated. Increased activity of these enzymes in serum serves to identify or confirm liver disorder, but because such an increase is found in many liver diseases, an abnormal result is of limited value for differential diagnosis (see below).

Properties of the aminotransferase enzymes

The coenzyme for both enzymes is pyridoxal phosphate; it binds to a lysine residue in the enzyme, forms a transient Schiff base reaction with the amino acid, receives the amino group, and transfers it to the oxoacid.

Aspartate aminotransferase catalyses the reaction:

$$\text{aspartate} + \alpha\text{-ketoglutarate} = \text{oxaloacetate} + \text{glutamate.}$$

AST is found in high concentrations in liver, cardiac and skeletal muscle, kidney, pancreas, and red cells. When these tissues are damaged they release AST into the blood, and its serum level rises. There is no method of identifying the organ source of serum AST. However, we can identify two AST isoenzymes, one found in cytoplasm, the other in mitochondria, and they can be measured individually in serum.

Alanine aminotransferase catalyses the reaction:

$$\text{alanine} + \alpha\text{-ketoglutarate} = \text{pyruvate} + \text{glutamate.}$$

Because ALT was found in low concentration in tissues other than liver, where it is confined to the cytoplasm, a high serum ALT has been considered to be relatively specific for hepatic damage. However, this specificity has been overemphasized as serum ALT and AST levels may both rise when there is a significant myopathy (see below). ALT tends to rise and fall in parallel with AST, but a slight or moderate elevation of ALT is often found without an increase of AST, and this is a feature of chronic hepatitis (especially hepatitis C) and of fatty liver.

Both enzymes are released from damaged cells, due to increased permeability of the cell membrane or to cell necrosis. Release of mitochondrial AST from hepatocytes is thought to imply more severe cellular damage than release of the cytoplasmic isoenzyme or of ALT. The ratio of the mitochondrial to cytoplasmic or total AST has been proposed as a 'diagnostic' or differential diagnostic test, being especially increased in severe cell necrosis and in alcoholic liver disease, but few, if any, routine laboratories measure mitochondrial isoenzyme activity.

Measurement

Haemolysis causes only a small but definite increase in serum AST levels, but gross haemolysis may interfere with the measurement of the enzyme. Plasma or serum should be separated soon after blood collection to avoid release of erythrocyte AST, which occurs with storage even without obvious haemolysis. It has been claimed that

Table 6 Causes of high serum aminotransferases
Hepatobiliary disease
Myocardial disease
Pancreatic disease
Muscle disease
Alcohol
Non-hepatobiliary disease with liver involvement
Obesity/diabetes mellitus
Haemochromatosis
α_1-Antitrypsin deficiency
HIV infection
Hyperthyroidism
Coeliac disease
Immunoglobulin bound

aminotransferase levels are spuriously low in uraemia (Cohen, AnnIntMed, 1976; 84:275), possibly as a result of vitamin B_6 deficiency. Serum aminotransferase levels were found to be very low in patients undergoing long-term haemodialysis; this did not appear to result from vitamin B_6 deficiency (Yasuda, Gastro, 1995; 109:1295).

Some laboratories determine both of these enzymes, others measure only one, and there has been debate over their relative value. ALT has the advantage of somewhat greater specificity for liver disease, but this is of little practical value since it is rarely difficult on clinical grounds to decide whether an elevated AST is due to hepatic damage. Measurement of ALT activity is of little value except in relation to liver disease; furthermore, for the laboratory which wishes to perform only one test, AST can also be used to detect damage to cardiac and skeletal muscle. However, it is now appreciated that the measurement of both enzymes is required in hepatological practice. In patients with fatty liver or hepatitis C, for example, ALT may be elevated when AST does not exceed the normal range; in alcoholic hepatitis and cirrhosis, AST may rise without an increase in ALT. These conditions may therefore be missed if only one aminotransferase is measured.

The major value of aminotransferase measurements is in detecting hepatocellular damage, and in monitoring the patient's subsequent progress; return to normal suggests resolution of the factors causing hepatocellular damage. For this purpose ALT activity is generally more sensitive, and it is more often elevated than AST.

Because they increase in so many conditions (Table 6), even quite marked elevations of aminotransferase levels (up to 500 U/l) are of limited value in differential diagnosis. It is often stated that they help to differentiate jaundice which is 'hepatocellular' (when they are supposed to be high) from that which is 'obstructive' (when they are supposed to be low). There are, however, many exceptions to this 'rule' (see below), and the classification of jaundice into hepatocellular and obstructive causes is unhelpful (see Chapter 5.8). In particular, acute obstruction due to a gallstone is often associated with a marked elevation of aminotransferases.

Very high AST and ALT levels are of diagnostic value. An aminotransferase level which is more than 20 times the upper reference limit (about 1000 units/l) strongly suggests an acute hepatitis, due to a virus or drugs. However, blood must be taken near the onset of the illness because levels usually drop rapidly and aminotransferase levels are then of little diagnostic value. Normal levels or only modest elevations of serum aminotransferases early in an illness virtually exclude acute hepatitis as a cause.

A marked elevation is also seen with a profound fall in blood pressure, as in shock, with acute biliary obstruction due to gallstones (see below), and with acute heart failure, but these diagnoses are usually obvious on clinical grounds (although an erroneous diagnosis of acute hepatitis may be made). In a study of 56 patients with a serum AST over 3000 U/l, acute hypotension accounted for more than half of the cases; in this group there was a high mortality (Johnson, AmJGastr, 1995; 90:1244).

If baseline levels are available (e.g. for patients in hospital) it is easier to establish the cause of a very high aminotransferase level. In viral hepatitis, and with most drugs causing acute hepatitis, there is a gradual rise in aminotransferase levels for a week or two before the onset of jaundice. In shock and acute heart failure there is usually an abrupt rise, and a rapid fall if the underlying problem can be treated effectively.

Occasionally, striking elevations are seen in patients with extrahepatic obstruction (Ginsberg, DigDis, 1970; 15:803), with ascending cholangitis, and with autoimmune hepatitis; under these circumstances diagnostic problems may result and an erroneous diagnosis of acute hepatitis is often made. Rare cases have been described of an elevation of serum AST, often marked, due to the presence of 'macro-AST', formed by complexing of the enzyme with immunoglobulin of high molecular weight. This finding, analogous to macroamylasaemia, may cause diagnostic confusion. The immunoglobulin is usually IgG (Nagamine, ClinChem, 1983; 29:379; Weidner, ClinChem, 1983; 29:382; Fex, CCActa, 1987; 164: 11; Litin, MayoClinProc, 1987; 62:681; Connelly, Lancet, 1989; i: 847) but IgM was responsible in a patient with primary biliary cirrhosis (Matsuda, JGastro, 1994; 29:222).

In uncomplicated acute viral hepatitis (A and E, and many cases of B and B plus D hepatitis), the very high initial aminotransferase levels approach normal within 5 weeks of onset of illness; normal values are achieved in about 75 per cent of cases within 8 weeks. In acute hepatitis C the aminotransferase levels tend to be lower (usually less than 1000 IU/l). In hepatitis B, C, and D infections the elevations often persist and this suggests the development of chronic liver disease, but one cannot be certain about chronicity until about 6 months have elapsed. Even in hepatitis A infections, which have no long term sequelae, aminotransferase levels may take many months to return to normal, and during this time levels may rise again suggesting exacerbation of the disease (Sjogren, AnnIntMed, 1987; 106:221; see also Chapter 12.1.2.2).

More modest aminotransferase increases, up to about 10 times normal, are seen in many liver diseases, such as chronic hepatocellular disease, cirrhosis, hepatic infiltration or neoplasia, and cholestatic jaundice, and also after the initial stage of acute hepatitis. ALT is more frequently increased, except in alcoholic cirrhosis and infiltrative disease. In a study on 19 877 blood donors an elevated ALT (> 2.25 × SD, or > 55 U/l) was found in 99 (0.5 per cent). Four had acute hepatitis B, four were positive for anti-HCV, two had autoimmune disease, one had cholelithiasis, and one an acute appendicitis (Kundrotas, DigDisSci, 1993; 38:2145). In 87 the cause of the elevation in ALT could not be explained. It is now clear that fatty liver associated with obesity is the cause in many such patients in developed countries (Hulcrantz, JIntMed, 1993; 233:7; Chapter 5.8), while in other areas hepatitis C is the major cause (see Chapter

12.1.2.5). In both of these conditions the modest elevation of ALT is often accompanied by a similar elevation of γ-glutamyltransferase.

Minor aminotransferase increases, generally below twice the upper reference limit, are occasionally found when there is little evidence of significant liver disease on liver biopsy. This is particularly true for ALT, which rises in many conditions (e.g. with many drugs), and for AST after short periods of binge drinking in healthy subjects.

While aminotransferase levels usually rise in acute liver diseases, relatively small increases are sometimes encountered, even in fulminant hepatitis. For reasons which are not understood AST levels may appear disproportionately low in patients with Wilson's disease, even with severe illness presenting as fulminant hepatitis or subacute hepatic necrosis.

Liver disease does not always result in aminotransferase elevation; levels may be normal in patients with established but well compensated cirrhosis, and in patients with chronic and incomplete biliary obstruction. At least 50 per cent of patients with chronic hepatitis C have normal serum aminotransferase activity (Healey, Gut, 1995; 37:274). Patients on haemodialysis have low aminotransferase levels (Yasuda, Gastro, 1995; 109:1295), a factor of diagnostic importance particularly in terms of suspicion of chronic hepatitis C; this is common in such a group and markers for hepatitis C virus should be sought routinely.

Not surprisingly, many workers have tried to use the AST–ALT ratio to differentiate between various types of liver disease. In general, ALT activity exceeds that of AST in toxic and viral hepatitis, chronic active hepatitis, and cholestatic jaundice, but this can only serve as a guide in the individual case. AST is the higher of the two in alcoholic liver disease, neoplastic and infiltrative liver disease, and in non-biliary cirrhosis. It is claimed that an AST–ALT ratio greater than 2 is evidence of alcoholic hepatitis and/or cirrhosis, and that it distinguishes patients with these conditions from those with extrahepatic obstruction and viral hepatitis, in whom the ratio is normally less than 2 (Cohen, DigDisSci, 1979; 24:835). However, this distinction is rarely difficult on clinical grounds and the sensitivity and specificity of this ratio are only about 70 per cent; values more than 2 are seen in a significant proportion of patients with post-necrotic cirrhosis and chronic hepatitis, with Wilson's disease (Shaver, Hepatol, 1987; 6:615), and occasionally with viral hepatitis. Low hepatic ALT has been suggested as the reason for the high serum AST–ALT ratio seen in plasma in alcoholics. An increase in the AST–ALT ratio suggests development of cirrhosis in patients with chronic viral hepatitis (B, δ, and non-A, non-B) and 'primary biliary cirrhosis' (Williams, Gastro, 1988; 95:734), but there is considerable overlap in individual cases.

Attempts have been made to use the degree of abnormality, and change in AST relative to change in bilirubin, alkaline phosphatase, and other biochemical markers to identify different hepatobiliary diseases. They have proved disappointing (Clermont, Medicine, 1967; 46:197). The AST:bilirubin ratio is not of value, even in hepatitis. The AST:alkaline phosphatase ratio has been claimed to be useful in distinguishing between acute hepatitis and obstructive jaundice; although there is a characteristic relationship between these variables in the two conditions, about 5 to 10 per cent of patients still show inappropriate results.

Serum AST activity increases in many diseases other than in those affecting the liver. It rises with myocardial infarction and myocarditis, and with pulmonary embolism. AST and ALT are both increased with some myopathies (e.g. Duchenne dystrophy, active polymyositis, or hypothyroidism) and with trauma (even with intramuscular injections). Measurement of serum creatine kinase is usually of great value in identifying aminotransferase elevations due to muscle disease, but in patients of Afro-Caribbean origin quite marked elevations of creatine kinase may be found without an obvious cause (Johnston, JRSM, 1996; 89:462); the upper limit of the reference range for creatine kinase in this group is twice the normal upper limit found in white Caucasians. There may be confusion when diseases of skeletal muscle occur with liver disease. In chronic alcoholics, painless chronic myopathy is frequent, and acute myopathy can follow a drinking bout; these conditions may contribute to the serum aminotransferase elevations seen in such patients (Perkoff, AnnIntMed, 1967; 67:481).

Other tests indicating the presence of hepatocellular damage or necrosis (Table 2)

Glutathione-S-transferase (GST)[2]

Glutathione-S-transferases are widely distributed detoxification enzymes (Awasthi, IntJBiochem, 1994; 26:295; Takamatsu, Toxicology, 1994; 88:191). A cationic B form is found in liver as a bilirubin-binding protein (ligandin), whereas anionic forms are present in lungs, muscle, and erythrocytes. Serum GST-B has attracted interest as a highly sensitive index of hepatocellular integrity (Adachi, CCActa, 1980; 106:243) but its potential is somewhat offset by the limited availability and inconvenience of the radioimmunoassay used for its determination. The enzyme has a short plasma half-life, which facilitates early recognition of cessation of active cellular damage. It is especially high in acute hepatitis of viral or drug origin (increases 5- to 10-fold higher than those of aminotransferases), and massive increases have been observed with paracetamol toxicity and fulminant hepatitis. High values have also been observed with primary and secondary hepatic malignancies, and in untreated hyperthyroidism (presumably due to subclinical liver damage). In patients with chronic hepatitis C treated with interferon, GST correlated with biochemical relapse, and in some patients who responded to interferon and then relapsed, GST was elevated intermittently or continuously during therapy despite normal aminotransferase levels (Nelson, AmJClinPath, 1995; 104:193). Raised values have been noted in alcoholic liver disease, particularly in response to binge drinking.

Lactate dehydrogenase and the LD5 isoenzyme

Modest elevation of serum lactate dehydrogenase (LD) activity, generally averaging twice the upper reference limit, may be found early in acute viral hepatitis; LD activity appeared to be greater in hepatitis due to paracetamol and ischaemia than in viral hepatitis; in patients in whom the serum ALT and/or AST was at least five times the upper limit of normal, the mean ALT–LD ratio was 4.65 in viral hepatitis, 1.46 in paracetamol-induced hepatitis, and 0.87 in ischaemic hepatitis (Cassidy, JClinGastro, 1994; 19:118). The authors claimed that an ALT–LD ratio of 1.5 differentiated acute viral hepatitis from ischaemic hepatitis and paracetamol injury with a sensitivity of 94 per cent and a specificity of 84 per cent.

In most other types of liver disease normal (or near normal) values of LD are usual. With malignant involvement of the liver there are increased values in up to 80 per cent of patients, the frequency depending on the extent of metastatic disease, and high levels may be found.

Although there are many causes of a raised total serum LD, only liver disease, malignancy, and muscle disorders cause a preferential increase in the LD5 isoenzyme (Wieme, AnnNYAcadSci, 1961; 94: 898; Nathan, ClinChem, 1971; 19:1036). Thus determination of LD5 has greater specificity for liver disorders and greater sensitivity for their detection than measurement of total LD.

The plasma concentrations of other substances rise with hepatocellular damage (Table 2). Some are other enzymes, presumably released from damaged hepatocytes. The pattern of response does not necessarily mirror that of aminotransferases; for example, in acute viral hepatitis, lactate dehydrogenase and sorbitol dehydrogenase return to normal much more quickly. Serum glutamate dehydrogenase tends to rise in large duct obstruction. Glutamate dehydrogenase is principally located centrizonally and its activity in liver tissue, as well as in serum, may rise with biliary obstruction.

Not surprisingly, many of these have been advocated as useful liver function tests in their own right, or as contributors to patterns of abnormality that might help in differential diagnosis. They have not been widely employed and seem to have little advantage over aminotransferase estimations. Few have been widely used in hepatology and it is difficult to assess their merits relative to the aminotransferase tests which are commonly used.

Plasma vitamin B_{12} levels increase in patients with various kinds of liver disease and there is good evidence that it is released from damaged hepatocytes. More vitamin B_{12} is bound to transcobalamin I, the major B_{12} carrier in normal blood, and there is a more striking rise in the amount bound to transcobalamin II. Dialysable B_{12} levels are markedly increased and there is an accompanying rise in urinary B_{12} excretion. Serum B_{12}-binding proteins may be increased in hepatocellular carcinoma; there seems to be a particular association with the fibrolamellar form of the tumour (Paradinos, BMJ, 1982; 285:840).

Serum ferritin levels rise in patients with hepatocellular damage from almost any cause and are also elevated in patients with iron overload (see Chapters 2.16.1 and 20.2).

Alkaline phosphatases (liver, biliary, tumour, bone, intestinal, placental) [1,3]

Alkaline phosphatases are a family of zinc metalloenzymes, with a serine at the active centre; they release inorganic phosphate from various organic orthophosphates and are present in nearly all tissues. The natural substrates are thought to include pyrophosphate, phosphoserine, and phosphatidylethanolamine; intestinal alkaline phosphatase may act as a Ca^{2+}-dependent ATPase. In liver, alkaline phosphatase is found histochemically in the microvilli of bile canaliculi and on the sinusoidal surface of hepatocytes. The genes for various alkaline phosphatases have been sequenced. Alkaline phosphatases from liver, bone, and kidney are thought to be transcribed from the same gene, while the alkaline phosphatases from intestine and placenta are derived from different genes (Stein, FASEBJ, 1990; 4:3111).

Alkaline phosphatase activity in normal serum is due mainly to bone and liver isoenzymes; an intestinal phosphatase is present in about 20 per cent of normal subjects and may contribute up to 20 per cent of total activity (Langman, Nature, 1966; 212:41).

Measurement

In most laboratories measurement of total serum alkaline phosphatase activity is done as a standard 'liver function test', although an elevated alkaline phosphatase is often found in the absence of liver disease.

Several methods have been used for the measurement of its activity. The internationally recommended 'reference' method uses p-nitrophenol phosphate as substrate, in an alkaline transphosphorylating buffer such as 2-amino-2-methyl-1-propanol (IFCC, CCActa, 1983; 135;339F).

Fresh, unhaemolysed serum is the specimen of choice for the estimation. Heparinized plasma may also be used. The test should not be done on plasma if citrate, oxalate, or EDTA were used as anticoagulants; they form a complex with the zinc in the alkaline phosphatase, causing irreversible enzyme inactivation.

The reference range (and units) for total alkaline phosphatase activity varies with the method of determination, age and gender of the patient, and with other factors. Alkaline phosphatase activity is above the normal adult range until about 20 years of age; there is a peak in the neonatal period and another in adolescence (i.e. during periods of increased bone growth). Levels also tend to rise in older subjects, with more liver phosphatase in elderly males and more bone phosphatase in postmenopausal females (Table 7; reference limits: CCActa, 1988; 173:273). A post-prandial increase, due to the intestinal isoenzyme, occurs after a fatty meal in some normal subjects, usually those from blood groups A and O who also carry the ABH red cell antigen and are negative for Lewis antigen.

In normal pregnancy, alkaline phosphatase activity begins to increase during the third month, rises to twice the usual adult female level in late pregnancy, and may remain elevated for a few weeks after delivery (Fishman, AmJClinPath, 1972; 57:65; Romslo, ActaObGyn, 1975; 54:437). The main source of this increase during pregnancy is the placenta. Serum bone-specific alkaline phosphatase is higher in women who breast feed for at least 6 months than in those who bottle feed their babies; serum osteocalcin, another marker of bone formation, is also higher, as is the urinary collagen N-telopeptide, which is a marker of bone resorption (Sowers, JClinEndoc, 1995; 80:2210).

The various alkaline phosphatase isoenzymes in serum can be identified and measured by a number of methods; an elevation of one of them may be found even when the total alkaline phosphatase is normal.

For routine analysis of alkaline phosphatase isoenzymes, electrophoresis (on cellulose acetate, agarose, or polyacrylamide gels) is the method of choice, separation depending mainly on charge. The liver ('slow' liver band) and bone isoenzymes in normal sera are found in similar proportions, but may be difficult to distinguish from each other. The placental and intestinal isoenzymes are easily identified. The question usually asked by clinicians is whether an increased alkaline phosphatase level is due to liver or bone isoenzyme. These can be distinguished, and quantified, using wheatgerm lectin affinity electrophoresis (Rosalki, ClinChem, 1984; 30:

1182). Tumour isoenzymes, a 'biliary' (or fast liver) isoenzyme of high molecular weight, and one or more unusual hepatic isoenzymes can also be identified by electrophoresis.

Chemical, physical, and immunological methods

A number of other methods have been used to distinguish between alkaline phosphatase isoenzymes. Liver and bone alkaline phosphatases show different inhibition by urea or guanidine, but these inhibitors are not commonly used because the differences are small and determination errors large. In addition, inhibitors of intestinal alkaline phosphatase must be employed to compensate for a possible contribution from this fraction. Liver alkaline phosphatase is more heat stable than bone, but assays based on heat sensitivity are tedious and subject to considerable inaccuracy unless performed scrupulously. Monoclonal antibodies can distinguish between bone and liver isoenzymes, with some cross-reactions but without interference from alkaline phosphatase from other tissues. However, convenient clinical assays are not yet available. Measurement of bone and non-bone (mainly liver) enzyme using wheatgerm lectin precipitation provides a convenient and increasingly popular procedure for distinguishing the contribution of these fractions to plasma total alkaline phosphatase.

Alkaline phosphatase and liver disease

In 1933 Roberts found an elevated serum alkaline phosphatase activity with bile duct obstruction, and lower but still high levels in 'toxic, infective, and catarrhal' jaundice (BMJ, 1933; i:734); the increase was attributed to regurgitation of bile phosphatase. In 1934 King and Armstrong (CanMedAssJ, 1934; 31:376) introduced their classic method for measuring serum alkaline phosphatase. Levels more than 30 King-Armstrong (KA) units were common in large bile duct obstruction; unfortunately this was accepted as a diagnostic criterion for an extrahepatic block, even though early workers cast doubt on the value of phosphatase measurements in the differential diagnosis of jaundice (Morris, QJMed, 1937; 6:211) because values above 30 KA units were sometimes found in hepatitis and cirrhosis, and because the plasma phosphatase rose in subjects with a bile fistula.

The serum alkaline phosphatase activity goes up in many types of liver disease; the highest levels are seen with obstruction to the flow of bile, either intrahepatic or extrahepatic, or with intrahepatic space-occupying lesions such as primary or metastatic liver tumours. The high plasma alkaline phosphatase of liver disease is not a failure of the liver to excrete it. The phosphatase accumulating is produced in the liver, and animal studies show that hepatic synthesis of alkaline phosphatase increases after biliary ligation. There appear to be two hepatic isoenzymes, one from hepatocytes ('slow' liver) and a biliary (or 'fast' liver) alkaline phosphatase of high molecular mass which originates from the plasma membrane. With biliary obstruction, canalicular membrane alkaline phosphatase, solubilized by retained bile salts or shed as fragments, reaches the plasma by paracellular regurgitation or via transcellular endocytosis. 'Biliary' enzyme seems a better marker of biliary obstruction than total serum alkaline phosphatase activity.

In acute viral hepatitis, alkaline phosphatase is usually either normal or moderately raised,[1] but up to 40 per cent of patients have levels two and a half times the upper reference limit (Becker,

AmJMedSci, 1962; 243:222). Hepatitis A may present a cholestatic picture with marked and prolonged itching and elevation of alkaline phosphatase (Gordon, AnnIntMed, 1984; 101:635); cholestatic features may also be seen with chronic HDV infection. A very high alkaline phosphatase has been reported in Epstein-Barr virus infection ('glandular fever'), even with normal bilirubin levels (Futterweit, ArchIntMed, 1961; 108:143; Shuster, JAMA, 1969; 209:267).

Serum alkaline phosphatase is increased by drugs which cause cholestatic liver disease; an elevation has also been found with cimetidine (Payne, BMJ, 1982; 285:100), frusemide (furosemide) (Math, ClinChem, 1982; 28:1812; Nanji, ClinChem, 1982; 28: 240), phenobarbitone (phenobarbital) (Balazs, ArchToxicol, 1978; 1(Suppl):159), and phenytoin (Moss, Enzyme, 1975; 20:20).

An increase of a serum alkaline phosphatase having the properties of hepatic alkaline phosphatase has been described in Hodgkin's disease, congestive heart failure, and in infectious and inflammatory diseases not primarily involving the liver, such as polymyalgia rheumatica (Brensilver, Gastro, 1975; 68:118). The origin of this phosphatase is not clear; alkaline phosphatase may also act as an acute-phase reactant (Parker, ClinSci, 1989; 76(Suppl 20):19P).

Although a high alkaline phosphatase is usually found in 'cholestatic' liver disease, this is not always the case. Even with a confirmed extrahepatic block, due to tumour or stones, the alkaline phosphatase may be normal or only slightly raised in a small proportion of cases (Stern, BMJ, 1973; 1:533), even in the presence of bacterial cholangitis (George, AmJGastr, 1993; 88:771), particularly in the early stage. A normal alkaline phosphatase may also be seen in patients with primary biliary cirrhosis (Sherlock, NEJM, 1973; 289:674; Leslie, PostgradMedJ, 1978; 54:281; Mitchison, Hepatol, 1986; 6:1279), and in primary sclerosing cholangitis (Cooper, AmJGastr, 1988; 83:308). This may cause diagnostic confusion.

A low serum alkaline phosphatase has been found in Wilson's disease presenting with haemolytic anaemia and evidence of severe liver dysfunction (Shaver, Hepatol, 1986; 6:859).

In about 25 per cent of patients with cirrhosis an intestinal band is seen on electrophoresis and in some it may be the major alkaline phosphatase in serum (normally it does not exceed 20 per cent of total phosphatase activity). Increased serum intestinal alkaline phosphatase activity in cirrhosis is thought to result from diminished hepatic uptake, as a consequence of destruction of receptors for intestinal alkaline phosphatase on the liver cell surface; diminished hepatic excretion or catabolism might also be contributory. In some patients with jaundice an increase of bone isoenzyme can be detected (presumably as a result of secondary bone disease). This may result from osteoblastic activity in hepatic osteodystrophy, particularly when osteomalacia complicates liver disease (Long, BrJHospMed, 1978; 20:312; Chapter 25.10).

Tumours may secrete alkaline phosphatase into plasma, and there are tumour-specific isoenzymes, such as the Regan, Nagao, and Kasahara isoenzymes. Regan isoenzyme (a heat-stable placental-type isoenzyme) is found with bile duct carcinoma. Kasahara isoenzyme (a fetal intestinal-type phosphatase) is found in about 30 per cent of patients with hepatocellular carcinoma (Higashino, AnnIntMed, 1975; 83:74), and in this condition another alkaline phosphatase (heat labile) may be found which differs from the other tumour-produced enzymes. Unfortunately, such isoenzymes are of little diagnostic value; they are found in a small proportion of patients with tumours, and generally at a low level of activity so that sensitive immunological methods are needed for their identification. If detected they may be of value for monitoring antitumour therapy; successful treatment is associated with a fall or disappearance of the isoenzyme from plasma.

Identification of alkaline phosphatase isoenzymes is of limited value in distinguishing between various kinds of liver disease; 'biliary' enzyme is more frequently raised in cholestatic and neoplastic disorders, and intestinal alkaline phosphatase more often elevated in parenchymal disease, but there is considerable overlap. However, isoenzyme studies certainly help to decide whether an elevated alkaline phosphatase activity is due to liver disease or bone disease. When methods to identify alkaline phosphatase isoenzymes are not available, clinicians tend to look for raised levels of other markers of biliary obstruction (γ-glutamyltransferase or 5'-nucleotidase) in order to confirm a hepatic origin for raised alkaline phosphatase levels (Table 2). The measurement of γ-glutamyltransferase has 90 per cent sensitivity and specificity for this purpose, as it is normal in bone disease. When a marked alkaline phosphatase elevation is accompanied by a modest γ-glutamyltransferase elevation the possibility of concomitant bone and liver disease should be considered (but see below).

Occasionally, serum liver phosphatase is increased due to binding with serum immunoglobulins. This occurs in association with autoimmune hepatitis and ulcerative colitis. Binding interferes with normal clearance of the enzyme from plasma (Rosalki, AdvClinEnzym, 1986; 4:12). In rare families, serum liver phosphatase activity is increased without any evidence of a disease to account for this finding (Wilson, NEJM, 1979; 301:983; McEvoy, BMJ, 1981; 282:1272; Rosalki, Enzyme, 1988; 39:95). A liver-like enzyme was found to be transiently increased in plasma in association with a gastrointestinal infection in the condition of transient hyperphosphatasaemia of infancy (Stein, ClinChem, 1987; 33:313).

Alkaline phosphatase elevation occurs in many diseases other than those involving the liver. A list of causes of an isolated increase in serum alkaline phosphatase activity is given in Table 7 (and in ref.[3]).

5'-Nucleotidase[1]

5'-nucleotidase is an alkaline phosphatase which attacks nucleotides with a phosphate at the 5' position of the pentose. It is present in all human tissues but only liver disease appears to cause significant elevation of its activity in serum (the normal range is from 1 to 15 IU/l, measured at 37°C).

The highest levels are found with either intrahepatic or extrahepatic obstruction to bile flow, but increases are also found with chronic hepatitis, cirrhosis, and other hepatocellular disorders. In routine practice, measurement of 5'-nucleotidase activity has been used to confirm that liver disease is indeed the cause of an elevated alkaline phosphatase, but for this purpose it was superseded by measurement of γ-glutamyl transferase. It may still have a role in infancy and in pregnancy. In infancy, bone alkaline phosphatase and γ-glutamyl transferase levels are high for physiological reasons. In pregnancy the placental isoenzyme causes an elevated alkaline phosphatase in the third trimester, but γ-glutamyl transferase levels may fall or be unchanged in pregnancy cholestasis (Bertrand,

AnnMedIntern, 1973; 3:172). However, in both infancy and pregnancy, alkaline phosphatase isoenzyme studies are a better method of establishing that liver disease is the cause of an elevated alkaline phosphatase than 5'-nucleotidase activity.

Leucine aminopeptidase[1]

Leucine aminopeptidase is an enzyme which hydrolyses peptides in which an L-leucine residue contains the free amino group. It is widely distributed in the body, and is present in bile, bile ducts, and canaliculi. Blood levels are highest when there is intrahepatic or extrahepatic obstruction to bile flow. Levels also increase in acute hepatitis, cirrhosis, hepatic malignancy, and in the last three months of pregnancy. Like 5'-nucleotidase its major use has been to confirm that increased phosphatase activity is due to liver disease. This test is rarely used in routine practice.

γ-Glutamyl transferase[4,5]

γ-Glutamyl transferase is a membrane bound glycoprotein which catalyses the transfer of γ-glutamyl groups from γ-glutamyl peptides, particularly glutathione, to other peptides, to amino acids, and to water. It is found mainly in the membranes of cells with a high rate of secretory or absorptive activity. Large amounts are found in the kidneys, pancreas, liver, intestine, and prostate, and it is also found in many other tissues. The γ-glutamyl transferase of bile is is approximately 100 times greater than that of normal serum.

The gene for human γ-glutamyl transferase is on chromosome 22, and codes for a precursor protein of about 61 400 (RajpertDeMeyts, PNAS, 1988; 85:8840).

Several isoenzymes of γ-glutamyl transferase have been described, but there is no clear evidence of tissue specificity. The heterogeneity appears to be related to the number of sialic acid residues, to the degree of glycosylation, and to binding to lipoproteins (Nemezansky, ClinChem, 1985; 31:797).

Measurement

The reference interval for serum γ-glutamyl transferase is higher in men than in women. The γ-glutamyl transferase level is very high in neonates and infants up to 1 year, and appears to increase above the age of 60. Levels over the usually accepted upper limit of normal (50 U/l in men, 30 U/l in women) were found in about 15 per cent of those screened at the BUPA centre and as a result the upper limit of their normal range was readjusted to 80 in men and 50 in women. Even then, 6 per cent of men had an abnormal level and in 4 per cent the level was greater than 100 U/l. Reference levels are lower in lifelong abstainers from alcohol than in the general population.

Serum levels of γ-glutamyl transferase rise in almost all kinds of liver disease; its determination is therefore of little value in differentiating between them. Abnormal levels are found in about 90 per cent of patients suffering from hepatobiliary disease. It is undoubtedly a very sensitive indicator of the presence of liver disease (0.87 to 0.95), but specificity is limited by the many other conditions, not primarily hepatic, which increase γ-glutamyl transferase, possibly as a consequence of mild, clinically insignificant hepatic involvement. The highest levels of γ-glutamyl transferase (10 to 20 times the upper limit of normal) are found with intrahepatic biliary obstruction or with primary or secondary hepatic malignancies. However, a normal or low γ-glutamyl transferase is seen

Table 7 Causes of 'isolated' increases in serum alkaline phosphatase

Increased liver isoenzyme
    Hepatic metastases or infiltrative disease
    Primary biliary cirrhosis
    Cholelithiasis
    (NB all usually accompanied by γ-glutamyltransferase increase)
    Minor increase with age

Increased bone isoenzyme
    Physiological—childhood, puberty; postmenopausal (minor)
    Osteoblastic bone disease, e.g. Paget's disease, osteomalacia, metastases

Increased intestinal isoenzyme
    Liver disease (cirrhosis)
    Diabetes mellitus
    Chronic renal failure
    Intestinal disease (lymphoma, α-chain disease)
    Physiological (minor) increase after fat ingestion especially in H-substance
    secretors of blood group O and B

Placental isoenzyme
    Physiological pregnancy
    Malignant disease (minor activity increase)
    Indian childhood cirrhosis

Variant or unusual forms
    Immunoglobulin bound—autoimmune disease, inflammatory bowel disease
    Tumour-derived—ovarian, testicular, hepatocellular cancer (minor activity
    increase)
    Liver-like plus bone—benign transient hyperphosphatasaemia (massive increase)

Genetically determined increase
    Any or all isoenzyme form(s)

occasionally in patients with intrahepatic cholestasis, even with a very high bilirubin and alkaline phosphatase (Kajiwara, JapJGastr, 1983; 80:2224). In such patients there was no inhibitor in plasma, and the activity of the enzyme in liver was raised (Kajiwara, JapJGastr, 1984; 81:880). In infants with idiopathic cholestasis, a normal γ-glutamyl transferase was found to be of poor prognostic significance (Maggiore, JPediat, 1987; 111:251).

In acute viral hepatitis, serum levels of γ-glutamyl transferase rise to reach a peak in the second or third week of the illness, but in some patients the levels are still raised at 6 weeks. Levels remain high with the development of chronic hepatitis or cirrhosis, and the level is usually elevated in chronic hepatitis C.

γ-Glutamyl transferase levels are of definite, though limited, value in the management of alcoholic patients. In this group, levels may rise, presumably due to enzyme induction, even when there is no significant underlying liver disease; but there is a poor correlation between alcohol intake and the serum γ-glutamyl transferase activity. On cessation of drinking, γ-glutamyl transferase falls to normal over 2 to 5 weeks; if it does not return to normal, continued alcohol intake is likely, liver damage may have occurred, or there may be another reason for the high enzyme level. Unfortunately, about one-third to one-half of heavy drinkers show no elevation of γ-glutamyl transferase in the absence of liver disease, so it is not a sensitive screening test for alcoholism (Penn, BMJ, 1983; 286: 531; Moussavian, DigDisSci, 1985; 30:211). γ-Glutamyl transferase levels do not rise as the result of an alcoholic binge in healthy subjects, but may do so in alcoholics and patients with other liver disorders.

An increased γ-glutamyl transferase level is found in many patients who do not drink alcohol or drink only modest amounts. It is important that such patients are not labelled as alcoholics. The most common cause is fatty liver associated with obesity or hypertriglyceridaemia (see Chapter 5.8).

Elevated serum γ-glutamyl transferase activity is found in about 20 per cent of patients with uncomplicated diabetes mellitus; levels are rarely more than three times the upper limit of normal. The source of the enzyme is probably the liver but other clinical or biochemical evidence of liver disease is rarely found. Some authors have disputed the association with diabetes mellitus arguing that the raised γ-glutamyl transferase seen in these patients is due to associated conditions (Joubaud, SemHopPar, 1987; 63:1851). It seems likely that fatty liver is a cause in many patients with diabetes.

An increase in γ-glutamyl transferase activity is seen in several conditions other than liver disease and alcoholism. It increases in acute pancreatitis, and in 50 to 70 per cent of cases of acute myocardial infarction. The source of the enzyme in patients with myocardial infarction is not clear, as there is no measurable activity in cardiac or skeletal muscle; it may be due to secondary effects on the liver, as high levels are also found in congestive cardiac failure.

Serum γ-glutamyl transferase activity increases with the administration of enzyme-inducing drugs.[6,7] Moderate increases are seen with phenobarbitone, phenytoin (Keeffe, DigDisSci, 1986; 31:1056) and other anticonvulsant drugs, paracetamol (aminopyrine; Bartels, JPediat, 1975; 86:298), tricyclic antidepressants, and glutethimide. Smaller increases are seen with anticoagulants, oral contraceptives, and antihyperlipidaemic drugs.

Table 8 Causes of increased plasma levels of γ-glutamyl transferase

Hepatobiliary disease
Pancreatic disease
Alcohol
Drugs (especially enzyme-inducers)
Non-hepatobiliary disease with liver involvement (slight increase)
   Anorexia nervosa (Umeki, JNervMentDis, 1988; 176:513)
   Dystrophia myotonica (Ronnema, ActaMedScand, 1987; 222:267)
   Guillain–Barré syndrome (Kornhube, EurArchPsychNeurSci, 1988; 237:317)
   Hyperthyroidism
   Obesity—hyperlipidaemia/diabetes mellitus
   Porphyria cutanea tarda
   After myocardial infarction
Neurological disease (slight increase)
Malignant disease/radiotherapy (possibly from shedding of enzyme-containing plasma
  membrane fragments)

Causes of an isolated increase of γ-glutamyl transferase are presented in Table 8. Sometimes very high levels of serum γ-glutamyl transferase are found (approximately 1000 U/l) with no obvious cause.

Plasma proteins

The liver makes many circulating plasma proteins. Not surprisingly, liver disease affects the plasma concentration of many of them. However, the effects are complex and depend not only on changes in protein synthesis, but also on the effects of liver disease on the volume and distribution of extracellular fluids, on the half-life of the individual proteins, and on their catabolism by various tissues. There may also be changes in the metabolism of plasma proteins produced outside the liver. The estimation of 'total plasma protein' alone is of relatively little value. It is often normal even when there are gross disturbances of individual components. When the total level is either high or low its significance can only be interpreted by measurement of the major fractions. Measurement of total protein together with albumin is used to calculate globulin by difference.

Serum protein electrophoresis gives patterns which can be characteristic, but not diagnostic, of certain types of liver disease. Patients with non-biliary cirrhosis may show a low albumin and high gammaglobulin, those with autoimmune hepatitis a marked rise in gammaglobulin (Eliakim, ProgLivDis, 1972; 4:403). An excess of α_2- and β-globulins may be found with biliary obstruction due to accumulation of abnormal lipoproteins, and a low α_2-band with intravascular haemolysis (due to decreased haptoglobin concentration). A poor α-band suggests the possibility of α_1-antitrypsin deficiency.

Despite these characteristic patterns the electrophoretic strip is generally of little value. The various abnormalities are found in conditions other than liver disease and the changes found in patients with jaundice are of little help in diagnosis.

Serum or plasma albumin[8]

Albumin is the most abundant circulating protein. The total exchangeable pool of albumin is usually about 3.5 to 5.0 g/kg body weight, 38 to 45 per cent of it being present within the intravascular space. Serum levels of albumin are normally between 35 and 50 g/l. It accounts for most of the colloid osmotic pressure of plasma and has binding sites with great affinity for many naturally occurring compounds (including bilirubin) and for many drugs. Liver is the only site of synthesis (about 15 g/day in a 'normal' 70-kg person). About 1 g is lost each day into the gut; most of the rest is degraded by an unknown mechanism. When synthesis is reduced, the drop in plasma albumin is minimized by a reduction in its fractional catabolic rate.

The serum albumin level is widely regarded as a test of liver function, as it reflects hepatic protein synthesis. Unfortunately, other factors affect it; low values result from increased gastrointestinal or renal loss, increased catabolism, altered vascular permeability, or overhydration. Furthermore, it may take many days before reduced synthesis causes an obvious change in serum albumin because it has a long half-life (about 20 days). When patients without pre-existing liver disease suffer fever or trauma, the albumin halflife may fall to about 7 days; serum albumin levels drop rapidly, often to below 30 g/l (Rayner, QJMed, 1988; 69:907), which suggests a marked increase in albumin removal as well as inhibition of albumin synthesis.

The low serum albumin level often found with severe chronic liver disease is due mainly to reduced albumin synthesis; but low serum levels may also result from expansion of the plasma volume and extracellular space, which may contain more albumin than normal despite the low concentration. Although the fractional catabolic rate is low, the absolute rate of degradation and synthesis may be normal or even high. In patients with cirrhosis who have ascites, hepatic secretion of albumin is disturbed; while some enters the bloodstream directly via the sinusoids, much is released directly into the ascites.

Changes in serum albumin concentration should be interpreted with caution because many conditions other than liver disease are associated with low serum albumin levels (Table 9).

Specific protein measurements

The changes in the plasma protein electrophoretic pattern associated with liver disease are outlined above. They result from changes in one or more of the specific proteins which constitute the globulin fraction. α_1-Globulin is composed mainly of α_1-antitrypsin and α_1-acid glycoprotein (orosomucoid); both are acute-phase proteins which increase in many inflammatory disorders, orosomucoid being especially responsive in liver disease. Haptoglobin is found within

Table 9 Causes of low plasma albumin concentration

Impaired albumin synthesis
    Malnutrition
    Malabsorption
    Liver disease
    Malignant disease

Increased albumin loss
    Proteinuria, e.g. nephrotic syndrome
    Protein-losing enteropathy—inflammatory bowel disease
    Burns
    Exudative skin disease

Increased albumin catabolism
    Hypercatabolic states—injury, postoperation

Altered distribution between intra- and extravascular compartments from increased vascular permeability
    Inflammatory states—acute-phase reaction

Overhydration

Genetic variation
    Analbuminaemia

Interrupted synthesis
    Acute (and chronic) inflammatory conditions

the α_2-globulin complex; it is also an acute-phase protein. Increased clearance of haptoglobin–haemoglobin complexes causes the low level seen with intravascular or severe extravascular haemolysis. In non-biliary cirrhosis the β-globulin iron-binding protein, transferrin, may be reduced; it is sometimes considered as a negative acute-phase protein because it shows a non-specific reduction in many inflammatory disorders. The immunoglobulins (principally IgG, IgA, and IgM) are located within the gammaglobulin fraction and extend anodally from it. A diffuse (polyclonal) increase of staining in this region is common in chronic liver disease (especially autoimmune hepatitis) and in chronic inflammatory and other autoimmune disorders. IgA runs in the β–γ-region; it may increase in non-biliary cirrhosis (especially alcoholic), and this results in the appearance of β–γ-'fusion' or 'bridging' on an electrophoretic strip.

Although changes in the specific proteins considered above may be inferred from the electrophoretic appearances, they are better determined by quantitative immunological measurement. Specific proteins whose concentration is of particular interest in relation to liver disease include prealbumin, α_1-antitrypsin, α-fetoprotein, caeruloplasmin, procollagen-III peptide, and the immunoglobulins.

Prealbumin (transthyretin) [9]

Prealbumin consists of four identical subunits; it binds iodothyronines. It also binds one molecule of retinol-binding protein, which probably reduces urinary loss of the latter. The serum prealbumin concentration is 0.2 to 0.3 g/l; that of retinol-binding protein is 0.04 to 0.05 g/l. Measurement of prealbumin has been proposed as a liver function test (Rondana, Digestion, 1987; 37:72). It tends to fall in liver disease, presumably due to reduced synthesis. Because of its short half-life (1.9 days), changes may precede alterations in serum albumin. Determination of prealbumin has been considered particularly useful for identifying drug-induced hepatotoxicity (Hutchinson, Lancet, 1980; i:121). Reduction in the plasma level of retinol-binding protein in chronic liver disease may be associated with impaired dark adaptation.

Serum caeruloplasmin (see Chapter 20.1)

Caeruloplasmin is an intensely blue α_2-globulin, normally present in plasma at a concentration of 0.2 to 0.4 g/l. Its gene is on chromosome 3 (Yang, PNAS 1986; 83:3257). It is synthesized in liver and is an acute-phase protein. The plasma concentration (determined immunologically) rises in pregnancy, and with oestrogens, infections, rheumatoid arthritis, some malignancies, active non-Wilson's liver disease, and obstructive jaundice.

It is an oxidase for certain aromatic amines and phenols, for cysteine, ascorbic acid, and also for Fe^{2+} ions (Frieden, SemHemat, 1983; 20:114). Its physiological function is still not entirely clear; however, with hereditary absence of caeruloplasmin there is marked iron overload indicating that it plays a key role in iron metabolism (Yoshida, NatureGenet, 1995; 9:267).

Serum caeruloplasmin is an important diagnostic marker in Wilson's disease, in which the plasma level is usually low. A low caeruloplasmin is also found in neonates, Menkes' disease, kwashiorkor and marasmus, protein-losing enteropathy, nephrotic syndrome, severe hepatic insufficiency, copper deficiency, and in hereditary hypocaeruloplasminaemia (Edwards, ClinGenet, 1979; 15:311) and acaeruloplasminaemia.

Procollagen-III peptide (see Chapter 2.15)

Type III collagen is produced when a specific sequence of amino acids (procollagen-III peptide) is removed from the N-terminal end of its precursor molecule (procollagen III) during post-translational modification. The serum concentration of the peptide appears to increase not only with hepatic fibrosis but also with inflammation and necrosis. The value of serum procollagen-III peptide as a marker of fibrosis is uncertain, but serial measurement may be of value in the follow-up of chronic liver disease (Collazos, ClinBioch, 1994; 27:189). Although serum procollagen-III peptide increases in all liver diseases, serum levels of type IV collagen, 7S collagen, and laminin seem to increase mainly with chronic liver diseases associated with hepatic fibrogenesis (Hirayama, JGastro, 1996; 31: 242).

α_1-Antitrypsin (see Chapter 20.3)

α_1-Antitrypsin is a glycoprotein of M_r approximately 54 000, synthesized by the liver, and is an inhibitor of serine proteinases, especially elastase. Its normal serum concentration is 1 to 1.6 g/l. It is an acute-phase protein; serum levels increase with inflammatory disorders, pregnancy, and in women taking oral contraceptives. Liver disease occurs with α_1-antitrypsin deficiency, an inherited disorder sometimes identified by a reduced α_1-band on electrophoresis; deficiency should be confirmed by quantitative measurement. α_1-Antitrypsin shows genetic polymorphism. Approximately 90 per cent of Caucasian populations are homozygous for the M allele (i.e. MM phenotype); other alleles coded at the α_1-antitrypsin locus include F, S, Z, and null forms. The α_1-antitrypsin phenotype is best determined by isoelectric focusing; allelic variation may be associated with both low plasma concentration and deficient functional (inhibitory) capacity. Plasma levels of α_1-antitrypsin vary with phenotype; they are approximately 15 per cent of normal with *ZZ*, 38 per cent with *SZ*, and about 60 per cent with *MZ* and FZ.

The presence of the *Z* allele, particularly in homozygotes, is associated with defective processing of the protein in the liver. The precursor protein, deficient in sialic acid, is poorly secreted by hepatocytes; its intrahepatic accumulation may be a factor in the genesis of liver damage. Neonatal hepatitis is seen in *Pi ZZ* homozygotes, and less frequently with *MZ* and *SZ* phenotypes. Cirrhosis in adults has been found with *ZZ*, *MZ*, *SZ*, and *FZ* phenotypes.

α-Fetoprotein[10]

This protein, the principal one in fetal plasma in early gestation, is subsequently present at very low levels (reference limit 25 μg/l); it is generally measured by a radio- or enzyme immunoassay. It is increased in hepatocellular carcinoma, and more than 90 per cent of such patients have increased serum levels. Raised values are also found in other liver diseases, for instance in up to 15 per cent of patients with cirrhosis without hepatocellular carcinoma, in chronic hepatitis, in the regeneration phase of viral hepatitis, and with hepatic metastases. However, such elevations are generally minor compared with those observed in hepatocellular carcinoma, and they are often transient. To improve specificity for hepatocellular carcinoma (but with some loss of sensitivity), α-fetoprotein levels above 400 μg/l are generally regarded as a diagnostic prerequisite; at such levels 70 per cent or more of patients with hepatocellular carcinoma will show abnormality with less than 5 per cent false positives, many of the latter being transient; high α-fetoprotein levels are more often found in association with hepatocellular carcinoma in black and Chinese persons, and less often in white Europeans.

α-Fetoprotein elevation is less frequent when hepatocellular carcinoma arises in non-cirrhotic liver, and may not be detected in hepatocellular carcinoma associated with oral contraceptive therapy. Serial determination of α-fetoprotein is very valuable for monitoring patients with cirrhosis; if the level rises and continues to rise, one should search for hepatocellular carcinoma. It is also valuable in monitoring treatment of hepatocellular carcinoma, as levels fall with successful therapy.

Cholinesterase[11,12]

Cholinesterase is a plasma enzyme capable of hydrolysing a variety of choline esters. It is produced by the liver, and serum levels fall when liver disease causes decreased protein synthesis. The changes generally parallel those seen with serum albumin. Low values are occasionally encountered with genetic polymorphism, recognizable by the altered inhibition characteristics of the plasma enzyme.

In acute hepatitis, of infective or toxic origin, mildly reduced levels of plasma cholinesterase are found within a few days of onset, returning gradually to normal with recovery. Chronic hepatitis, cirrhosis, and neoplastic and other infiltrative diseases of the liver are also accompanied by low levels. In obstructive jaundice, normal values are the rule unless there is concomitant liver disease or if the obstruction is due to malignancy, when reduced values are found. Malignant disease, even if localized and not involving the liver, can give low enzyme levels due to impaired enzyme synthesis. With steatosis levels are normal or somewhat increased.

Cholinesterase has been used as an aid to the assessment of liver function before and after hepatic transplantation. Cholinesterase is best studied serially and is of greatest value as a prognostic tool. A sudden or marked fall to one-quarter of the usual activity indicates ominous deterioration. Many drugs have been reported to cause a reduction in cholinesterase activity.[12]

Serum bile acids (see Chapter 2.10)

Bile acids are derived from catabolism of cholesterol. The two main primary bile acids, cholic and chenodeoxycholic acids, are produced in the liver, conjugated with glycine or taurine, and excreted in bile. They play a key role in the digestion and absorption of fat and fat-soluble compounds. They are reabsorbed from the terminal ileum by an efficient active transport mechanism, but some reach the colon where bacteria cause deconjugation and/or dehydroxylation of the molecule at the 7α-position. The latter reaction converts cholic acid to deoxycholic acid, and chenodeoxycholic to lithocholic acid. These secondary bile acids are absorbed from the colon into the portal venous blood; the normal liver removes primary and secondary bile acids very efficiently from portal blood and excretes them rapidly into bile. This completes the enterohepatic circulation of bile acids (ie. liver–bile–intestine–portal vein–liver).

Liver disease affects bile salt metabolism in several ways. It may impair primary bile acid synthesis, change the relative proportions of cholic and deoxycholic acids (normally about twice as much cholic acid is produced), or lead to the production of unusual bile acids. There may be a change in the amount of bile acid which is conjugated or a change in the taurine–glycine ratio. As less primary bile acid enters the intestine there is sometimes less secondary bile acid synthesis and a reduction in plasma levels of deoxycholate. Impaired liver function, or diversion of portal blood, reduces hepatic bile acid removal from portal blood leading to an increase in the level of plasma bile acids, particularly after meals. Biliary obstruction causes a rise in plasma bile acids due to their regurgitation into the bloodstream. High plasma levels of bile acid increase urinary excretion of bile acids.

Few of these effects are of value in the clinical assessment of patients. The simplest bile acid measurement is the total bile acid concentration, either in the fasting state or after a meal, but even this test is rarely available in routine laboratories. The normal fasting level of serum bile acid is up to about 15 μmol/l (depending on the method used, which varies from laboratory to laboratory). The fasting level of serum bile acid is elevated in only about two-thirds of patients with a variety of types of liver disease. It is therefore of relatively limited value in screening for patients who might have liver disease.

Levels remain high in almost all patients with significant liver disease and the bile acid level measured 2 h after a meal is therefore a useful screening test for liver disease.

It has been suggested that serum bile acid measurements should be added to the conventional battery of 'liver function tests', or that they might replace measurement of direct-reacting bilirubin. The finding of a high level of serum bile acid has high specificity for the detection of liver disease (compared with other individual tests), but its sensitivity is limited. Adding a bile acid test would be unlikely to improve the specificity already obtained with the usual batteries of tests.

Ammonia

Arterial ammonia levels tend to be raised in chronic liver disease, particularly if there are features of hepatic encephalopathy or a significant degree of portal systemic shunting; they also increase in severe acute hepatitis and with fulminant hepatic failure. There is a poor correlation between ammonia levels and the degree of encephalopathy. The measurement of blood ammonia is of little clinical value in liver disease.

A high blood ammonia is also seen in hereditary deficiencies of urea cycle enzymes, in which the blood ammonia is usually higher than in acquired liver diseases; other liver function tests tend to be normal in these conditions (see Chapter 2.13.2).

Other tests which may be useful in managing patients with liver disease
Glucose

Blood glucose measurements are often valuable in patients with liver disease. Their frequent use is mandatory in patients with fulminant hepatic failure who may become hypoglycaemic despite intravenous administration of relatively large amounts of glucose (see Chapter 2.11). Hypoglycaemia is also common in acute fatty liver of pregnancy (Pockros, Medicine, 1984; 63:1).

High glucose levels and frank diabetes mellitus are also common in patients with cirrhosis, particularly when corticosteroids are used in the management of autoimmune chronic hepatitis. Glucose metabolism in liver disease is fully discussed in Chapter 2.11.

Cholesterol, triglyceride, and lipoproteins

The level of serum total cholesterol is often elevated in patients with biliary obstruction, and may reach very high levels in some patients with certain types of chronic intrahepatic cholestasis, such as primary biliary cirrhosis. It tends to fall in severe parenchymal liver disease, whether acute or chronic; in acute hepatitis there may be a rebound hypercholesterolaemia during the recovery phase. Serum triglyceride levels may be moderately increased in various types of liver disease, often showing reciprocal changes with the total serum cholesterol. In patients with either obstructive jaundice or severe parenchymal disease, lipoprotein electrophoresis may show an abnormal pattern, with loss of the α- (HDL) and pre-β-(VLDL) bands and a prominent β-band.

An abnormal lipoprotein, LP-X, was considered diagnostically useful, because it was said to be present in 99 per cent of patients with histological cholestasis, and absent in 97 per cent of those without cholestasis (Seidel, ClinChem, 1973; 19:86). However, it is of little practical value as 'cholestasis' is sometimes found in hepatitis and cirrhosis as well as in extrahepatic obstruction and intrahepatic cholestases. Furthermore, LP-X may be undetectable when there is clear evidence of surgical or other forms of obstruction to the biliary tree (Ross, Gut, 1970; 11:1035; Ritland, CCActa, 1973; 49:251; Vergani, CCActa, 1973; 48:243; Magnani, Gastro, 1976; 71:87). This limits the value of LP-X even for screening.

The abnormalities underlying the lipoprotein changes of liver disease are complex, and are fully discussed in Chapter 2.12.

Patients with primary or secondary hypertriglyceridaemias may have abnormal liver function tests as a result of an associated fatty liver. These are usually increases in alanine aminotransferase and γ-glutamyl transferase; increases in aspartate aminotransferase and alkaline phosphatase are less common, and jaundice is rare unless the fatty liver takes the form of a non-alcoholic steatohepatitis (see Chapter 5.8 and Section 16).

Lecithin cholesterol acyltransferase (**LCAT**)

LCAT is a glycoprotein produced in the liver; it is secreted into plasma, where it catalyses the formation of cholesteryl ester. Reduced plasma LCAT activity is an important determinant of the plasma lipid and lipoprotein changes found in liver disease (see Chapter 2.12). It has a short half-life in plasma and some workers believe that, as a single test, it is the most sensitive index of hepatocellular dysfunction (De Marties, JIntMedRes, 1983; 11:232; Simko, JIntMedRes, 1985; 13:249).

Blood alcohol

Measurement of blood ethanol is a valuable method of checking whether an alcoholic patient is telling the truth when he or she denies continuing alcohol consumption. Obviously it only detects recent consumption.

Urea and electrolytes

Blood or plasma urea is an important measurement in patients with liver disease. In severe liver disease, plasma urea may be low because of reduced hepatic urea synthesis; it then reflects hepatocellular function. A high level of urea may occur as a result of vascular or extravascular volume depletion (particularly due to diuretic therapy for oedema and/or ascites), renal failure secondary to liver disease and/or drugs, or gastrointestinal bleeding which increases urea production due to protein loading.

The plasma creatinine level is a better test for poor renal function than urea because it is unaffected by protein catabolism or liver function. However, high bilirubin levels may interfere with the laboratory detemination of creatinine and give rise to spuriously low values, particularly with kinetic methods using alkaline picrate, and enzyme methods using peroxidase detection systems (Spencer, AnnClinBioch, 1986; 23:1). Measurements of serum creatinine level and creatinine clearance fail to give an accurate assessment of the degree of renal failure in patients with cirrhosis with a low inulin clearance, because of increased tubular secretion of creatinine (Caregaro, ArchIntMed, 1994; 154:201). This has important implications with regard to dosage of potentially nephrotoxic drugs and failure to recognize renal impairment resulting from diuretics or paracentesis. Patients with well compensated alcoholic cirrhosis may have an elevated glomerular filtration rate (Wong, Gastro, 1993; 104:884).

Plasma electrolyte levels are often abnormal in severe liver disease and may change rapidly, either spontaneously (with complications such as bleeding, fluid retention, or infections), with diuretic therapy, or with inappropriate administration of fluid and electrolytes (either intravenously or orally). Careful monitoring is necessary for effective therapeutic control.

Hyponatraemia is much more common than hypernatraemia, although the latter may occur with gastrointestinal bleeding (as a result of a urea diuresis), following the use of lactulose, and from severe fluid restriction and increased insensible water loss; hypernatraemia may also occur in fulminant hepatic failure (Wilkinson, BMJ, 1974; i:186). Hyponatraemia usually results from excessive intake of water, either orally or intravenously (usually as 5 per cent glucose). In normal subjects, water loading (20 ml/kg in 45 min) causes excretion of 8 to 18 ml/min of hypotonic urine, of which 6 to 16 ml is 'free water', but the ability of many patients with liver disease to excrete a water load is reduced. If, as in many patients with cirrhosis with ascites, free water clearance falls below 1 ml/min or less, then dilutional hyponatraemia is a constant finding. A full discussion of the mechanisms underlying hyponatraemia is found in Chapter 8.1.

The handling of potassium in liver disease is complex.[13] Many reports suggest a low total body potassium in chronic liver disease (expressed per kilogram of body weight), possibly due to an excess extracellular volume; little difference is seen when results are expressed per kilogram of dry body weight. The intracellular potassium level appears normal in most studies, and it is difficult to increase total body potassium with potassium supplements (Birkenfeld, JCI, 1958; 37:687; Casey, Gastro, 1965; 48:198).

In compensated chronic liver disease (without ascites), serum potassium levels are usually normal. In patients with fluid retention, serum potassium levels vary. Low levels are common, usually associated with diuretic therapy, a poor diet, vomiting, or diarrhoea (which may also cause hypokalaemia in patients with compensated cirrhosis). A low serum potassium suggests a low total body potassium, but a low total body potassium may be found with normal serum levels (Soler, Gut, 1976; 17:152; Wheeler, Gut, 1977; 18:683). When serum levels are low, potassium-losing diuretics such as frusemide should be stopped and potassium chloride supplements should be given (preferably orally). If diuretic therapy needs to be continued, spironolactone should be used (but without potassium supplements).

In fulminant hepatic failure, hypokalaemia and hyponatraemia occur in about one-half of the cases (Wilkinson, BMJ, 1974; i:186; Gut, 1976; 17:501); hypokalaemia is often present on admission, while hyponatraemia tends to develop later in the illness.

Hyperkalaemia often occurs in patients with cirrhosis if they develop acute renal failure, or if they take spironolactone or a 'potassium-retaining' diuretic such as amiloride. Potassium supplements should not be given with such drugs, nor should these drugs be given together.

Both hypokalaemia[13] and hyperkalaemia are potentially dangerous; serum potassium levels therefore need close monitoring in severe liver disease, particularly during diuretic therapy. Urinary sodium and potassium are also useful measurements in patients with fluid retention—for monitoring the onset of the hepatorenal syndrome, and for assessing the efficacy of diuretic therapy; this is particularly true for spironolactone, the dose of which should be increased until the urinary sodium–potassium ratio is greater than 1.

Magnesium[14]

It is worth measuring serum magnesium levels occasionally in patients with cirrhosis, particularly alcoholics and decompensated patients. Chronic alcoholism is a common cause of hypomagnesaemia, attributed to urinary loss of magnesium, and to factors such as dietary deficiency, diarrhoea, and vomiting.

There have been few studies on magnesium metabolism in cirrhosis. Hypomagnesaemia has been reported, but not usually with clinical evidence of deficiency (Stutzman, JLabClinMed, 1953; 41:215). Magnesium deficiency may occur in cirrhosis (Cohen, Magnesium, 1985; 4:1). In patients with cirrhosis suffering from anorexia, muscle weakness, and cramps, muscle magnesium levels were low although plasma and bone magnesium concentrations were normal; symptoms resolved with magnesium supplementation for 6 weeks (Lim, QJMed, 1972; 41:291). In four patients with non-alcoholic cirrhosis, Cohen (Magnesium, 1986; 5:39) found that incomplete distal renal tubular acidosis was corrected by administration of magnesium.

Hypomagnesaemia may play a role in the genesis of severe hypokalaemia (Petersen, ActaMedScand, 1963; 174:595; Shils, Medicine, 1969; 48:61; Webb, JAMA, 1975; 233:23), which in patients with alcoholic cirrhosis may respond only to magnesium therapy (Bletry, SemHopPar, 1977; 53:1175; Fossaluzza, MinMed, 1979; 70:3503). In this group of patients, hypomagnesaemia may also be associated with hypophosphataemia due to inappropriate loss of phosphate in the urine (Adler, MinElecMetab, 1984; 10:63).

The mechanism for hypomagnesaemia (and magnesium depletion) is not clear, but increased urinary losses may result from secondary hyperaldosteronism and from loop diuretics such as frusemide. Aldosterone antagonists reduce urinary excretion of magnesium in patient with cirrhosis who have fluid retention (Lim, BMJ, 1978; i:755).

Calcium and phosphate

Serum calcium and phosphate levels are usually normal in patients with cirrhosis, although the mean serum phosphate tends to be lower in patients with liver disease than in normal controls (Long, CCActa, 1978; 87:353). Hypophosphataemia occurs in patients with alcoholic cirrhosis (Adler, MinElecMetab, 1984; 10:63).

Severe hypophosphataemia (less than 0.3 mmol/l) has been reported in several patients with acute hepatic failure due to paracetamol overdose. The levels in two patients were 0.01 and 0.06 mmol/l; they were treated with intravenous phosphate supplementation (Dawson, BMJ, 1987; 295:1312).

Patients with hepatocellular carcinoma may show hypercalcaemia which seems to be associated with an increase in plasma parathyroid-related protein (Yen, Liver, 1993; 13:311).

Acid–base disturbances and bicarbonate

Acid–base disturbances, particularly alkalosis, are common in chronic liver disease.[15] The alkalosis is usually respiratory (about 38 per cent), or mixed respiratory and metabolic (30 per cent); isolated metabolic alkalosis occurs in about 13 per cent. The alkalosis and hypocapnia can often be identified in mixed venous blood as well as in arterial specimens (Moreau, Liver, 1993; 13:20). The degree of hyperventilation leading to respiratory alkalosis is usually relatively mild; the cause of the hyperventilation remains obscure. Hypokalaemia, due to diuretics, vomiting, or diarrhoea, seems to be a major factor in the development of metabolic alkalosis.

Acidosis is less common, and is usually found in association with hypotension and/or renal failure (or with renal tubular acidosis, see Chapter 25.7). Lactic acidosis may be present in some cases, usually with sepsis, shock, or bleeding; it has been suggested that respiratory alkalosis may predispose to the development of lactic acidosis (Mulhausen, Medicine, 1967; 46:185). A hyperkalaemic hyperchloraemic metabolic acidosis has been described with use of spironolactone (Gabow, AnnIntMed, 1979; 90:338; Nierenberg, AnnIntMed, 1979; 91:321), and a hypokalaemic hyperchloraemic metabolic acidosis with lactulose (Kaupkc, AnnIntMed, 1977; 86: 745).

In fulminant hepatic failure, alkalosis (respiratory, meatabolic, or mixed) is very common; the mechanism is unknown. Mixed respiratory alkalosis–metabolic acidosis is also relatively common. Lactic acidosis occurs, particularly with overdose of paracetamol, and is inversely related to the oxygen extraction ratio (Bihari, JHepatol, 1985; 1:405; CritCareMed, 1985; 13:1034).

Clearly, serum bicarbonate concentrations must be interpreted with caution in patients with liver disease, because mixed disturbances are so common.

Urate

Patients with cirrhosis have been found to have a lower mean serum urate level than normal controls, and in some the serum urate was clearly subnormal. There was an inverse correlation between serum bilirubin and serum urate and, although urinary excretion of urate was the same in the two groups, urate clearance was greater in those with cirrhosis (Michelis, ArchIntMed, 1974; 134:681; Higuchi, IsrJMedSci, 1981; 17:1015). It has been suggested that the high urate clearance is related to a high 'effective vascular volume' (Decaux, AmJMed, 1982; 73:328); fractional urate excretion correlated positively with cardiac output, and negatively with peripheral resistance and urinary aldosterone (Decaux, Metabolism, 1984; 33:750; Nephron, 1986; 44:226). In one patient with alcoholic cirrhosis and cholestasis secondary to a gallbladder carcinoma, the serum urate became undetectable, in association with an increased renal urate clearance, mild glycosuria with a normal serum glucose, and a decreased tubular reabsorption of phosphate. These abnormalities returned to normal when the serum bilirubin fell following surgery (Arranzcaso, Nephron, 1995; 71:354).

Similar results were found in primary biliary cirrhosis, in which urinary copper is increased, and it was suggested that copper deposition in the renal tubules might play a part in the increased urate clearance (Izumi, Hepatol, 1983; 3:719). In this series the patients with hypouricaemia had the highest bilirubin levels, and also showed evidence of renal tubular acidosis on the basis of an acid loading test; in another study, patients with incomplete renal tubular acidosis were found to have lower mean serum urate levels than those without (Pares, Hepatol, 1984; 4:1265).

Hypouricaemia is a well recognized feature of Wilson's disease, and thought to result from impaired urate reabsorption due to renal tubular damage induced by copper (Leu, AmJMedSci, 1970; 260: 381; Wilson, KidneyInt, 1973; 4:331).

In acute fatty liver of pregnancy, and in toxaemia, a very high level uric acid is often seen, and is a useful pointer to the diagnosis (Burroughs, QJMed, 1982; 51:481). A high level of uric acid may also be seen with benign fatty liver and hyperlipidaemia.

The use of liver function tests

Most standard liver function tests are simple to perform, are relatively inexpensive and, as they are easily automated, they are included in the output of multichannel automatic analysers. For this reason, physicians may receive the results of liver function tests even if they did not request them, or they may ask for them without apparent reason. Often, of course, liver function tests are requested because the doctor suspects the presence of liver disease; he hopes that the tests will confirm his suspicions and give him a clue to the nature of the underlying hepatic pathology. If the results are normal, no further action will occur in the vast majority of cases, and little harm will result. If the results are abnormal, problems may arise. The doctor may not look at the test results (if he did not request them), he may ignore them (if they do not fit within his clinical preconceptions), or he may be stung into action!

Applications of liver function tests

Like all special investigations, liver function tests can be used for:

(1) screening (or profiling) to detect the presence of unsuspected liver disease;
(2) confirmation of the presence of liver disease in patients in whom it is suspected (with varying degrees of probability) on clinical grounds;
(3) differential diagnosis;
(4) prognosis;
(5) monitoring the progress of a patient with liver disease and assessing the response to therapy;
(6) clinical research.

One can define, in theoretical terms, the characteristics that are desirable in tests used for screening, monitoring, or diagnosis (and for the other purposes mentioned previously). Unfortunately, no investigation is equally useful for all of these purposes.

Screening and profiling

'Screening' may be defined as the routine performance of investigations on an apparently healthy population; 'profiling' the routine use of tests on patients, regardless of the clinical presentation. Screening and profiling are done mainly to detect unsuspected conditions for which treatment would be beneficial. Profiling has the added potential that it might shed light on the cause of the patient's symptoms and, if the results are negative, it may allow confident exclusion of many common and important conditions. Profiling is also useful for providing background data that may subsequently be helpful in assessing new clinical events, or for predicting or evaluating complications of therapy. For example, if jaundice occurs during treatment with a potentially hepatotoxic drug, it is clearly useful to know that liver function tests were normal at the start of therapy.

For screening or profiling, the main concern is to detect unsuspected disease and we want to be confident that a negative test excludes the disease. Usually, it does not matter if there are a relatively large number of false positive results, as the position can be clarified by further diagnostic tests; false positive results are a major problem only if further diagnostic tests are costly or if they are potentially hazardous to the patient. For screening or profiling, therefore, a test must have high sensitivity (see Appendix).

Screening and profiling tests are done on very large numbers of patients. Such tests must therefore be cheap to perform, and they must not cause patients discomfort or inconvenience.

'Batteries' of liver function tests

A single liver function test is of little value for screening for liver disease because several serious liver diseases may be associated with normal serum levels of either bilirubin, aspartate or alanine aminotransferase, alkaline phosphatase, albumin, or γ-glutamyl transferase. With any of these tests, employed individually, the number of false negatives would be unacceptably high. Furthermore, a positive result for only one of these tests has limited value in indicating the presence of liver disease, since many other diseases cause an increase in bilirubin, aspartate and/or alanine aminotransferase, alkaline phosphatase, and γ-glutamyl transferase, or a reduction in albumin (see Tables; and Chapter 5.8).

The use of a battery of liver function tests, however, constitutes a highly sensitive procedure; the number of false negatives must be minimized by this strategy. Few subjects with significant liver disease have a complete set of normal results with the commonly used batteries of liver function tests, although this does occur (e.g. in patients with well compensated cirrhosis), and if such patients are missed it is unlikely that there would be any untoward clinical consequences; they would tolerate drugs, surgical procedures, and other treatments far better than those in whom there was clear evidence of liver damage.

The use of a battery of liver function tests is also associated with high specificity; when more than one liver function test is abnormal, the probability of liver disease is very high. False positives are uncommon; they do however occur (e.g. a patient with chronic malabsorption may have a high serum alkaline phosphatase (from bone) and a low serum albumin; a patient with myocardial infarction may have a high aspartate aminotransferase (from cardiac muscle) and an elevated bilirubin, due perhaps to a functional and relatively trivial hepatic disturbance).

We believe that a battery of liver function tests should be performed routinely on hospital inpatients and outpatients. In a hospital population about 4 per cent have a raised aspartate aminotransferase, and a greater proportion an increased alanine aminotransferase. Alcoholic liver disease (often just a fatty liver) is a major cause, and mild elevations may fall with cessation of drinking; obesity is also an important factor (Chapter 5.8). About 4 to 5 per cent of patients show an increased alkaline phosphatase; bone disease, such as Paget's disease, is an important cause in the elderly. Only in a small number of patients does the finding of a high alkaline phosphatase lead to a new diagnosis of liver disease.

Similar results have been found in a 'healthy' outpatient population (Bates, JAMA, 1972; 222:74). Most of these abnormalities (approximately 90 per cent) had not been previously recognized. Confirmatory action was taken in only 20 to 25 per cent of cases, and a new diagnosis was established in only about 10 per cent of those with the abnormal results. Similar results were obtained by Whitehead and Wootton (Lancet, 1974; ii:1439). Although there did not appear to be a high diagnostic yield from profiling, other advantages were pointed out in both studies—reassurance for the patient, data that make other tests unnecessary, and baseline investigations against which to compare future test results. The last is a particularly valuable feature in the hospital setting.

Is it worth screening an apparently healthy population for evidence of liver disease? At the British United Provident Association (**BUPA**) centre, diabetes mellitus, hypercholesterolaemia, and liver

Table 10 Unexpected abnormalities of liver function tests
1. Value outside ± 2.5 SD or 95th percentile reference range: anticipated in 5 per cent of healthy individuals.
2. Inappropriate reference range: gender, age, body mass, ethnic origin.
3. Laboratory error.
4. State of the art analytical variation (frequently 10 per cent or more change on repeat).
5. Intraindividual biological variation (frequently up to 20 per cent).
6. See Table 9 (albumin), Table 4 (bilirubin), Table 7 (alkaline phosphatase), Table 8 (γ-glutamyl transferase), Table 6 (aminotransferases) for disorders affecting individual tests.

disease were the conditions found most frequently as a result of investigation of a 'normal' (but not necessarily unselected) population. Unsuspected liver disease, usually on the basis of excessive alcohol intake, was found in approximately 1 per cent of the subjects studied. Abnormal results of individual liver function tests were found in a larger proportion of subjects (Wilding, CCActa, 1972; 41:375).

A plasma total bilirubin above 17 μmol/l was found in about 5 per cent of those attending the BUPA centre; approximately 2 per cent of men had a level greater than 25 μmol/l, but only 0.5 per cent of women. Bilirubin was usually absent from the urine and other liver function tests were normal. This hyperbilirubinaemia is almost always benign and due to Gilbert's syndrome. The consequences of finding this high bilirubin may be deleterious, as the patients may then be subjected to unnecessary, expensive, and potentially hazardous medical or surgical intervention! However, knowledge of the presence of Gilbert's syndrome may explain the jaundice which is sometimes seen in patients with abdominal pain, who may reduce their food intake and thus put up their bilirubin level.

The value of γ-glutamyl transferase as a screening test is controversial (Penn, BMJ, 1983; i:531). It is undoubtedly a very sensitive indicator of the presence of liver disease (0.87 to 0.95) but lacks specificity, since many conditions with only minimal liver disturbance cause an increase of this enzyme. Levels exceeding the usually accepted upper limit of normal (50 mU/l in men, 30 mU/l in women) were found in about 15 per cent of those screened at the BUPA centre and as a result the upper limit of their normal range was readjusted to 80 in men, and 50 in women. Even then, 6 per cent of men had an abnormal level and in 4 per cent the level was greater than 100 mU/l.

Some causes of unexpected liver function test abnormalities and their frequencies in hospital medical admissions are shown in Tables 10 and 11.

Role in diagnosis

Standard liver function tests have a very limited role in the differential diagnosis of liver disease. Diagnostic considerations and strategy are considered in Chapter 5.8.

Monitoring

Much of the work of chemical pathology and haematology laboratories involves repetition of tests that are done to monitor progress. Greater attention needs to be paid to the use of tests for monitoring, but there is little theoretical basis for deciding on the most efficient and effective way of using them. Tests done to follow progress should be either quantititive (measures of a continuous variable) or semiquantitative (giving points on a scale with sufficient intervals to allow adequate documentation of change). The methods used should be reasonably precise in order to ensure that observed changes are real and not the result of experimental error. When repeated measurements are done on a single patient, it may be possible to detect clinically significant trends, even if all of the results remain within the conventional normal range. Clinicians should therefore be aware of the precision of the laboratory tests they use and of normal biological variations, so that the significance of a change between consecutive tests can be estimated. Tests for monitoring tend to be repeated on many occasions. They should, therefore, be cheap; expensive tests would be justified only if they were to be used to make important clinical decisions.

Conventional liver function tests are satisfactory for monitoring progress. They are quantitative, precise, and cheap. When results change with deterioration of liver disease, they tend to change only in one direction, that is, increasing in the case of bilirubin, aminotransferases, alkaline phosphatase, and γ-glutamyl transferase, and decreasing in the case of albumin. However, the results of individual tests sometimes change in opposite directions; for example, in acute hepatitis the aminotransferase levels may fall from a very high level while the bilirubin level continues to rise. The degree of change of aminotransferases and alkaline phosphatase may be of little prognostic significance, but increasing levels of bilirubin and falling levels of albumin (or clotting factors) suggest increasing severity of liver disease. Improvement in hepatic status is usually, but not invariably, accompanied by a return of all tests towards normal values.

Hepatology has made striking advances since the introduction of tests to measure serum bilirubin, alkaline phosphatase, and aminotransferases. Much of the effort that has been expended has gone into the search for improved diagnostic techniques and in many instances the results have been outstandingly successful. There are now excellent methods which allow us to delineate gross alterations in the biliary tree, to localize gross intrahepatic lesions, and to take biopsies of or aspirate these lesions. Advances in histopathology allow precise diagnosis of many types of hepatic disorder. New immunological techniques, some of which can be applied to biopsy samples, have revolutionized diagnosis, particularly in the field of viral disease of the liver. However, when the effort has been to search for tests to replace or supplement the long-established tests of liver function, or to look for aetiological clues in patterns of test responses, the results have been disappointing. The search will, we feel sure, continue; attempts are still being made to use mathematical and computer-aided procedures for this purpose. Such procedures may well prove valuable if they are based on analysis of clinical and laboratory data, but we suspect that analysis of laboratory data alone will prove fruitless. The major diagnostic advances are likely to come from the further development of tests with a high degree of specificity for individual hepatobiliary diseases.

The diagnostic limitations of conventional liver function tests, and their general limitations when employed individually, do not mean that these tests are without value. As we have indicated, the commonly used batteries of liver function tests are of considerable value for screening and profiling, are helpful in monitoring the progress of liver disease, and aid in predicting prognosis. For these purposes, they are tried and tested, although not perhaps well documented. They will continue to play an important role in the detection and management of liver disease.

Appendix
Sensitivity, specificity, and predictive accuracy

It can be assumed that in a large population some patients will have a particular disease.[16] If a test for that disease is applied to the whole population, then a certain number of those with the disease will have a positive result (true positives) and some will have a negative result (false negatives). Of those without the disease, some will have a positive result (false positives) and some a negative result (true negatives). Yerushalmy[17] defined the sensitivity of a diagnostic test as the number of true positive results divided by the total number of subjects who have the disease (that is, true positives plus false negatives). A test is therefore considered sensitive to the extent that it detects patients with the disease and minimizes false negatives.

Specificity is calculated by dividing the true negatives by the number of subjects without the disease (that is, true negatives plus false positives). A test is specific to the extent that it identifies those who do not have the disease, particularly in that it minimizes false positives.

These indices are of relatively little value to the practising clinician who does not need to know the sensitivity or the specificity of a test, but its predictive accuracy. In other words he needs to know the probability that a positive test indicates the presence of disease (that is, true positives divided by true positives plus false positives) or that a negative test indicates the absence of disease (that is, true negatives divided by true negatives plus false negatives). Unfortunately, the predictive accuracy of a test is markedly dependent on the type of population studied and the proportion of those who have the disease. When there are very few subjects with the disease, even a small percentage of false positives in the large healthy subgroup would mean that a positive result would have little predictive value; this would be true even if the test was highly sensitive and highly specific. The predictive accuracy of a negative result would be very high under these circumstances. By contrast, a positive result of a test with a specificity and sensitivity no better than tossing a coin might have a high predictive accuracy if there was a very high prevalence of the disease.

These principles have been ignored in many of the studies done to evaluate tests for hepatobiliary disease. Often they have been done on selected groups of patients in whom the prevalence of various diseases is high. This is particularly unsatisfactory if the tests are then used in another population in whom the prevalence is quite different (for example, if a test evaluated on inpatients is applied to a quite different outpatient population).

References

1. Rosalki SB. Enzyme tests in disease of the liver and biliary tract. In Wilkinson SH, ed. *Principles and practice of diagnostic enzymology*. London: Edward Arnold, 1976.

2. Beckett GJ and Hayes JD. Plasma glutathione-*S*-transferase measurements and liver disease in man. *Journal of Clinical Biochemistry and Nutrition*, 1987; **2**: 1–24.

3. Nemezansky E. Alkaline phosphatase. In Lott JA and Wolf PL, eds. *Clinical enzymology*. New York: Field Rich and Assoc, distributed by Year Book Publishers, 1986.

4. Rosalki SB. γ-Glutamyl transpeptidase. *Advances in Clinical Chemistry*, 1975; **17**: 53–107.

5. Nemezansky E. γ-Glutamyltransferase (GGT). In Lott JA and Wolf PL, eds. *Clinical enzymology*. New York: Field Rich and Assoc, distributed by Year Book Publishers, 1986.

6. Siest G, *et al*. References et variations biologique de la γ-glutamyltransferase. *Bulletin de la Societé Française D'Alcoologie*, 1983; **5**: 13–20.

7. Henny J, *et al*. Use of the reference state concept for interpretation of laboratory tests: drug effects on γ-glutamyltransferase. *Advances in Biochemical Pharmacology*, 1982; **3**: 209–13.

8. Rothschild MA, Oratz M, and Schreiber SS. Serum albumin. *Hepatology*, 1988; **8**: 385–401.

9. Hutchinson DR, Halliwell RP, Smith MG, and Parke DV. Serum 'prealbumin' as an index of liver function in human hepatobiliary disease. *Clinica Chimica Acta*, 1981; **114**: 69–74.

10. Kew MC. α-Fetoprotein. In Read A, ed. *Modern Trends in Gastroenterology*, Vol. 5. London: Butterworth, 1975.

11. Brown SS, *et al*. The plasma cholinesterases: a new perspective. *Advances in Clinical Chemistry*, 1981; **22**: 1–123.

12. Sawhney AK and Lott JA. Acetylcholinesterase and cholinesterase. In Lott JA and Wolf PL, eds. *Clinical enzymology*. New York: Field Rich and Assoc, distributed by Year Book Publishers, 1986.

13. Perez GO and Oster JR. Altered potassium metabolism in liver disease. In Epstein M, ed. *The kidney in liver disease*. 2nd edn. New York: Elsevier Biomedical, 1983: 183–201.

14. Knochel JP. Derangements of univalent and divalent cations in chronic alcoholism. In Epstein M, ed. *The kidney in liver disease*. 3rd edn. Baltimore: Williams & Wilkins, 1988: 132–53.

15. Oster JR. Acid–base homeostasis and liver disease. In Epstein M, ed. *The kidney in liver disease*. 2nd edn. New York: Elsevier Biomedical, 1983: 147–82.

16. Galen RS and Gambino SR. *Beyond normality—the predictive value and efficacy of medical diagnosis*. New York, John Wiley, 1975.

17. Yerushalmy J. Statistical problems in assessing methods of medical diagnosis with special reference to X-ray techniques. *Public Health Reports*, 1947; **62**: 1432–49.

5.2 Hepatic removal of circulating substances: importance for quantitative measurements of liver function

S. Keiding and Bernhard H. Lauterburg

The liver is ideally evolved for removal of substances from the circulation. The blood flows through a highly interconnected, sponge-like system of sinusoids, lined by hepatocytes in a single layer. The endothelial cells have fenestrae so that large molecules, but not the corpuscular elements of the blood, have direct access to the space of Disse (Wisse, Hepatol, 1985; 5:683). Numerous microvilli of the hepatocytes point, digit-like, into the space of Disse. These unique anatomical arrangements allow for direct access of blood-borne substances to a large area of the sinusoidal surface of hepatocytes. After transport across the liver-cell membrane, the ultimate intracellular conversion to metabolites or excretion to bile take place.

From a functional point of view the bloodstream is unidirectional from the inlet to the outlet of the sinusoids. This is in contrast to the *in vitro* experimental condition, where substrate and enzyme molecules move freely around each other, and all enzyme molecules are exposed to a uniform substrate concentration.

When attempting to describe quantitatively the dynamics of hepatic removal of substances from the circulation, the following problems must be considered.

1. Concepts developed experimentally *in vitro* must be adapted to the sinusoidal arrangement of hepatocellular anatomy and microcirculation.
2. Expressions used to describe liver function must be limited to terms that can be measured, such as liver blood-flow rate (Q), inlet substrate concentration (c_i), and outlet substrate concentration (c_o).
3. The model concepts should adequately express the complex physiological conditions in the intact organ. They should, however, be limited to few pertinent variables until the experimental results justify the inclusion of further terms.

This review starts from enzyme kinetics *in vitro* and then transposes those concepts to the liver structure in terms of a mathematical–physiological model. This model has proved to be comprehensive and applicable to many experimental and clinical conditions. Its limitations point to areas of further research.[1] Finally, the implications for the design and use of clinical tests to measure various liver functions are discussed.

In vitro Michaelis–Menten kinetics

In test-tube experiments, the enzymatic conversion of a substrate is characterized by Michaelis–Menten saturation kinetics with the relation between the conversion rate V and the substrate concentration c depending on the maximal conversion rate V_{max} and the half-saturation concentration K_m (Michaelis, BiochemZ, 1913; 49: 333)

$$V = V_{max} c / (K_m + c) \qquad (1)$$

At low concentrations, i.e., $c \ll K_m$, an increase in concentration causes a proportional increase in conversion rate; the kinetics is first-order. At high concentrations, i.e., $c \gg K_m$, an increase in concentration causes only a small increase in conversion rate; the enzymes are saturated with substrate and the kinetics is zero-order.

In vivo Michaelis–Menten kinetics

In the intact liver, the removal rate,

$$V = Q(c_i - c_o) \qquad (2)$$

where c_i is the substrate concentration in the inlet blood and c_o the concentration in the outlet blood; Q is the liver blood-flow rate. This relation is model-independent, being based on mass conservation only. It should be noted that throughout this chapter, the term 'liver removal rate' means 'splanchnic removal rate' in studies in the intact organism with no sampling from hepatic inlet blood.

During the passage of blood through the sinusoid, substrate removal by the hepatocytes gradually depletes the substrate. A concentration gradient develops along the direction of flow. We will first consider the simplest possible physiological approach, the removal of water-soluble substances by equivalent sinusoids. The sinusoids are perfused by blood containing red cells with about the same diameter as the sinusoid (Wisse, Hepatol, 1985; 5:683). This causes complete mixing of the substrate within each transection of the sinusoid. Diffusion is assumed to be much faster than the uptake rate, so the substrate concentration is similar throughout each transection from the sinusoidal bulk and throughout the space of Disse up to the liver-cell membrane. Removal of substrate by the

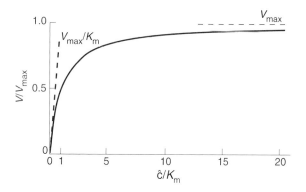

Fig. 1. *In vivo* hepatic removal kinetics. Michaelis–Menten relation between removal rate V and logarithmic average sinusoidal blood substrate concentration $\hat{c}$, normalized by division by $V_{\max}$ and K_m, respectively. K_m is the half-saturation concentration. $\hat{c} = (c_i - c_o)/\ln(c_i/c_o)$ where c_i and c_o are the sinusoidal inlet and outlet substrate concentrations, respectively. At high concentration, V approximates the maximal removal rate $V_{\max}$ (------). At low concentration, $V/\hat{c}$ approximates $V_{\max}/K_m$ (------).

hepatocytes is governed by irreversible Michaelis–Menten kinetics of the rate-limiting step, whether this is membrane transport, metabolic conversion within the cell or biliary excretion; it is a 'barrier removal' model (Winkler, in Preisig and Paumgartner, eds. *The liver: quantitative aspects of structure and function I*, Basel: Karger; 1973; 144–55).[1] The removal kinetics is described in relation to the local sinusoidal blood (or rather plasma water) substrate concentration. K_m is accordingly given in terms of blood (or plasma) concentration attributable to the rate-limiting process. In the first approach, all sinusoids are assumed to contain the same amount of enzymes (not necessarily evenly distributed along the sinusoid) being perfused by identical flow rates. It is a single equivalent sinusoidal perfusion model.[2]

This leads to a mathematical description of the sinusoidal substrate concentration gradient.[2,3] At low concentrations the gradient is exponential and flow-dependent (first-order kinetics). At high concentrations it is linear and flow-independent, with all enzymes along the sinusoid being saturated (zero-order kinetics). An example is given in Fig. A1 of ref.[3].

For the whole liver, integration of these relations for all sinusoids gives:[3]

$$V = V_{\max}\hat{c}/(K_m + \hat{c}), \quad \text{where } \hat{c} = (c_i - c_o)/\ln(c_i/c_o) \qquad (3)$$

This is an *in vivo* Michaelis–Menten relation where the concentration $\hat{c}$ is the logarithmic mean of the observable concentrations c_i and c_o (Fig. 1). The $\hat{c}$ concentration lies between c_i and c_o; it is smaller than $(c_i + c_o)/2$ and larger than the integrated mean concentration.[2] The $\hat{c}$ formulation should by no means be interpreted as if all hepatocytes were offered the uniform substrate concentration $\hat{c}$ throughout the liver. On the contrary it accounts for the decreasing sinusoidal concentration gradient.

It is seen that the flow rate Q does not appear in equation (3). This flow-independence of the relation of V and $\hat{c}$ is a salient feature of the model. It has been used in parameter-free, model-testing sets of experiments: on keeping a steady V from a constant galactose infusion into a recirculating rat-liver perfusion system, experimental changes in flow did not alter galactose $\hat{c}$ significantly (Keiding,

JPharmExpTher, 1976; 205:465). There are similar findings for the removal of indocyanine green in the intact cat (Krarup, ScaJCLI, 1976; 36:183), propranolol in perfused rat liver (Keiding, JPharmExpTher, 1984; 230:474), indocyanine green in human liver (Keiding, EurJClinInv, 1988; 18:507), as well as for estimated values of ethanol $V_{\max}$ and K_m in perfused rat liver (Keiding, BiochemPharm, 1984; 33:3209).

The model allows for determination of *in vivo* $V_{\max}$ and K_m of the rate-limiting removal process. $V_{\max}$ and K_m have been estimated from sets of steady-state values of c_i, c_o, and Q of galactose removal in perfused pig liver,[3] intact pig,[4] and intact cat,[5] for ethanol in perfused pig liver, intact pig and man,[6] for antipyrine in perfused pig liver,[7] and for parathyroid hormone in perfused rat liver (D'Amour, AmJPhysiol, 1989; 256:E87).

A direct estimate of $V_{\max}$ can be obtained from sets of c_i, c_o, and Q, as mentioned above. $V_{\max}$ is determined by the number of enzyme molecules, and as such it must be flow-independent at physiological variations in flow. An approximate estimate can be obtained from the removal rate at high concentrations [at $\hat{c} \gg K_m$ where equation (3) reduces to $V \approx V_{\max}$]. This can be obtained, in practice, from the arterial–hepatic venous concentration difference multiplied by the liver blood-flow rate (Jacobsen, ScaJCLI, 1969; 24:279). It can also be obtained from peripheral concentration measurements alone as utilized in the clinical estimate of hepatic galactose $V_{\max}$ (see later). The flow-independence of galactose $V_{\max}$ has been verified experimentally.[8]

Intrinsic hepatic clearance

An indirect measure of $V_{\max}$ may be obtained by the so-called intrinsic hepatic clearance, Cl_{intr}. From equation (3) we have, at low concentrations where $\hat{c} \ll K_m$ ensures first-order kinetics:[2,9]

$$Cl_{\text{intr}} = V/\hat{c} = V_{\max}/K_m \qquad (4a)$$

This is illustrated in Fig. 1. At $\hat{c} < 0.1K_m$, the approximation of $V/\hat{c}$ to $V_{\max}/K_m$ is 90 per cent or better. The lower the $\hat{c}$, the better the approximation. Intrinsic hepatic clearance is thus a flow-independent variable reflecting the total number of enzymes ($V_{\max}$) for the particular liver function studied.

Intrinsic hepatic clearance of indocyanine green is calculated from the same concentrations as used to estimate the liver blood-flow rate Q by the Fick's principle [compare equations 2,3, and 4(a)]. Its predicted flow-independence has been validated in man (Keiding, EurJClinInv, 1988; 18:507). The use of intrinsic clearance as a measurement of liver function in terms of an indirect measurement of $V_{\max}$ requires that K_m is not changed by the experimental or pathophysiological conditions studied.

Using the hepatic extraction fraction, $E = (c_i - c_o)/c_i$, and replacing V in equation (4a) by the term in equation (2) and $\hat{c}$ by the term in equation (3), we get:

$$Cl_{\text{intr}} = Q \ln (1E). \qquad (4b)$$

This expression is identical to that used in capillary physiology since its introduction in 1909 by Bohr (SkandinaviskArchivPhysiol, 1909; 22:240) and later by Crone (ActaPhysiolScand, 1963; 58:292).

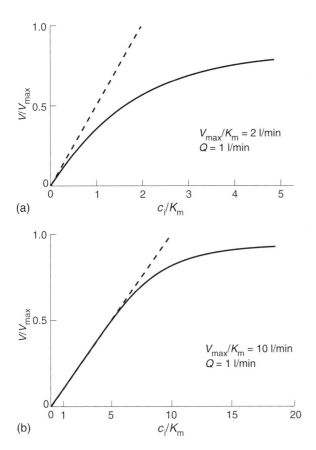

Fig. 2. *In vivo* hepatic removal kinetics in relation to sinusoidal inlet concentration c_i (i.e. peripheral substrate concentration). Flow-dependent saturation kinetics: $V = Qc_i(1 - \exp[-(V_{max} - V)/QK_m])$. The straight lines give the amount of substrate offered to the liver by the blood flow. (a) $V_{max}/K_m = 2$ litre/min, $Q = 1$ litre/min; (b) $V_{max}/K_m = 10$ litre/min, $Q = 1$ litre/min.

Removal kinetics in relation to peripheral blood concentration

The relation of the removal rate to the peripheral blood concentration is of interest in many experimental and clinical conditions, because it does not involve taking blood from a liver vein. This advantage is gained at the expense of introducing a number of theoretical and practical limitations. In the present context, peripheral blood concentration [as measured in a peripheral vein, or preferably in arterialized blood (Tygstrup, ScaJCLI, 1977; 37: 333)] is assumed identical with the sinusoidal inlet blood with concentration c_i.

The relation between the removal rate V (normalized with respect to V_{max}) and the peripheral substrate concentration c_i is illustrated in Fig. 2. The equation given in Fig. 2 is valid for values of c_i (and V) varying from first-order kinetics to saturation.[2,9] The relation is flow-dependent; the more, the larger the value of V_{max}/K_m.

Maximal removal rate

At high concentrations, $c_i \gg K_m$, the removal saturates and becomes approximately flow-independent. The degree of saturation, V/V_{max}, increases the higher the concentration relative to K_m.

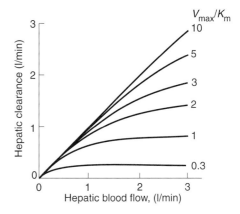

Fig. 3. Hepatic clearance (*Cl*) in relation to liver blood-flow rate (*Q*) at different values of V_{max}/K_m according to: $Cl = Q(1 - \exp[-V_{max}/QK_m])$. Flow-determined clearance for $V_{max}/K_m \gg Q$: $Cl = V/c_i \approx Q$. Enzyme-determined clearance for $V_{max}/K_m \ll Q$: $Cl = V/c_i \approx V_{max}/K_m$.

In quantitative evaluation of liver function the aim is to obtain estimates of V_{max} for various liver-cell functions (Tygstrup, JGast-Hepatol, 1990; 5:468). An example is the galactose elimination capacity test (Tygstrup, ScaJCLI, 1966; 18 (Suppl.): 118; Tygstrup, ScaJCLI, 1977; 37:333), where the galactose elimination rate at blood galactose higher than 2 mmol/l is assumed to reflect the enzyme activity of the rate-limiting galactokinase enzyme in the cytosol.[3] At these concentrations, V approximates V_{max} with 85 per cent or more, provided K_m and Q in man are about the same as in the pig[4] and cat.[5] Estimates of V_{max} can be interpreted clinically to give estimates of the 'functional liver-cell mass' (Tygstrup, in *Diagnostic procedures in the evaluation of hepatic diseases*. New York: Liss, 1983:17). These measurements are potentially prognostic, as found, for example, for the galactose elimination capacity test in fulminant liver failure (Tygstrup, SemLivDis, 1986; 6:129).

Clearance measurements

The principle of using clearance measurements to estimate liver blood-flow rate was suggested in 1945 by Bradley *et al.* (JCI, 1945; 24:890). In 1948, Lewis (AmJClinPath, 1948; 18:789) proposed the use of clearance to estimate liver-cell function. Application to clinical practice is, however, still a challenge to hepatologists. New procedures are currently being proposed, not always with sufficient acknowledgement of their limitations. Let us first define hepatic clearance *Cl* as

$$Cl = V/c_i \qquad (5a)$$

and steady-state systemic clearance Cl_{syst} as

$$Cl_{syst} = \text{infusion rate}/c_i. \qquad (5b)$$

When extrahepatic (extrasplanchnic) elimination is negligible, *Cl* equals Cl_{syst}. At low concentrations with first-order kinetics, the general equation in Fig. 2 for all concentrations reduces to the general clearance equation in Fig. 3 for all possible values of $V_{max}/(QK_m)$.

The first requirement, and common for both hepatic and systemic clearance, is that the clearance estimate must be approximately independent of the concentrations used. The removal must follow first order kinetics, with V and c_i being proportional. Before a substance is chosen for clearance measurements, its removal kinetics therefore has to be evaluated carefully to ensure that it is first-order. The consequences of using clearance measurements by a substance whose kinetics deviates from first-order is that the calculated clearance value depends on the dose given and, further, that the clearance varies with changes in liver function in a not easily comprehensible manner.[9] The decrease in the calculated caffeine clearance when the dose was increased (Bonati, ClinPharmTher, 1982; 32:98) may be an example of this.

Figure 3 shows the relation of Cl to Q at various values of V_{max}/K_m. At low V_{max}/K_m, clearance is practically independent of the liver blood-flow rate. At high V_{max}/K_m, clearance in practice depends only on flow. For substances between these limits, clearance depends on both V_{max}/K_m and on Q; the substance belongs to the mixed enzyme–flow-clearance regimen (see below).

Flow-determined clearance

Liver blood-flow rate can be measured directly by Fick's principle (Fick, PhysMedGesellschWurzb, 1872; 1870d: 16; Caesar, ClinSci, 1961; 21:43). The procedure is based on constant intravenous infusion of indocyanine green and measurements of concentrations in a peripheral artery and a liver vein. Indocyanine green has negligible extrahepatic elimination (Hunton, Gastro, 1960; 39: 713),[15] which implies that V equals the infusion rate (if necessary corrected for non-steady state).[14] The flow rate is calculated from equation (2).

For substances removed by a process with high capacity (and high affinity = low K_m) relative to Q, i.e., $V_{max}/(QK_m) \gg 1$, the liver will remove most of the substrate offered to it. Clearance will approach Q as $V_{max}/(QK_m)$ increases (see Fig. 3).

To obtain 90 per cent approximation of Cl to Q, $V_{max}/(QK_m)$ has to be larger than 2.3 (equation in Fig. 3). Clearance may then be used as an estimate of flow.[9,14] The approximation of Cl to Q equals the extraction fraction E, since $Cl/Q = E$.

For steady-state removal of sorbitol (corrected for urinary excretion), $V_{max}/(QK_m)$ ranges from 2.3 to 7.3 (see Table 1), with negligible extrahepatic extrarenal elimination in those with no liver disease.[10,11] Sorbitol clearance may thus prove useful as an estimate of liver blood flow in healthy individuals.

The suggestion by Tygstrup and Winkler (ClinSci, 1958; 17:1) to use galactose clearance as a measurement of liver blood flow has been examined under steady-state conditions (Henderson, Gastro, 1982; 83:1090). In individuals with no liver disease the extraction was high, but a significant extrahepatic elimination in man[13] as well as in cats (Burczynski, CanJPhysPharm, 1986; 64:1310) prevents its use as a flow measurement.

Indocyanine green clearance is sometimes used as a measure of liver blood-flow rate. This is not justified, since E is approximately 2/3 in controls and 1/3 in patients with liver disease, with large variations;[14] thus indocyanine green belongs to the mixed enzyme–flow-clearance regimen. These results support the doubts of Grozsman (Hepatol, 1983; 3:1039) and Keiding (JHepatol, 1987; 4:393), who both stressed the limitations of clearance measurements of liver blood-flow rate with no sampling from the liver vein.

Enzyme-determined clearance

For substances with low enzymatic capacity (as assessed by V_{max}/K_m) compared to the amount of substrate offered to the liver by the blood flow (Q), the removal rate is determined by the enzymatic capacity. Clearance will approach V_{max}/K_m as $V_{max}/(QK_m)$ reduces (see Fig. 3).

This clearance does not vary with flow and is proportional to V_{max}. To obtain 90 per cent approximation of Cl to V_{max}/K_m, $V_{max}/(QK_m)$ has to be less than 0.10. For smaller $V_{max}/(QK_m)$ the approximation improves. It can be used as a measurement of liver-cell function (Lewis, AmJClinPath, 1948; 18:789), provided that K_m is not changed under the experimental or pathophysiological conditions studied.

For such substances the sinusoidal substrate concentration gradient is small, and Cl and Cl_{intr} become nearly identical [cf. equation (4a) and equation in Fig. 3]. The extraction fraction E is small, even though the removal is first-order. Thus samples from the liver vein are not needed to obtain an approximate estimate of intrinsic hepatic clearance.

Antipyrine offers an example of a substance (Andreasen, EurJClinInv, 1974; 4:129) with negligible extrahepatic elimination, low $V_{max}/(QK_m)$ (around 0.05 in pigs,[7] not yet determined in man), and first-order kinetics at the doses used in clinical practice (Danhof, BrJClinPharm, 1979; 8:529).

Classification of clearance substances
Hepatic extraction fraction

In many studies, test substances are classified according to their hepatic extraction fraction E (Wilkinson, ClinPharmTher, 1975; 18: 377). It is true that a high E generally indicates a high degree of flow-dependence, and a low E a high degree of enzyme-dependence, as discussed above, but the influence of the enzyme capacity and of the flow on E cannot be separated. From the equation in Fig. 3, we obtain

$$E = 1 - \exp[-V_{max}/(QK_m)]. \qquad (6)$$

It is seen that E depends not only on V_{max}/K_m (being smaller with smaller values of V_{max}/K_m), but also on Q (being smaller with larger values of Q). Consequently, the extraction fraction neither gives an unambiguous measure of liver function nor is it suitable as a basis for classification of hepatic clearance substances.

$V_{max}/(QK_m)$

It appears from the above discussion that the comparative importance of enzyme activity and liver blood flow for the clearance measurements can be evaluated by means of the V_{max}/K_m for the substance studied relative to Q. Accordingly a classification based on $V_{max}/(QK_m)$ gives an unambiguous classification of liver clearance-test substances (Keiding, Pharmacol, 1979; 19:105).[9] Table 1 illustrates this for substances where V_{max} and K_m have been estimated directly or have been calculated approximately from clearance (and flow) values. The classification refers to hepatic clearance (excluding possible extrahepatic elimination). It is seen that in those with no liver disease, clearances of sorbitol and ethanol are flow-determined, while galactose clearance is on the border between the flow- and the

Table 1 Classification of substances removed by the liver according to the removal kinetics in individuals with no liver disease, based on their values of $V_{max}/(QK_m)$

Test substance	Experimental model*	$V_{max}/(QK_m)$ mean (range)	Reference
Enzyme-determined clearance: $V_{max}/(QK_m) < 0.1$			
Antipyrine	Pig (a)	0.05 (0.03–0.08)	7
Flow-determined clearance: $V_{max}/(QK_m) > 2.3$			
Sorbitol	Man (b)	3.6 (2.3–5.1)	10
Sorbitol	Man (b)	3.9 (2.3–7.3)	11
Ethanol	Man (a)	10 (5.6–13)	6
Ethanol	Pig (a)	5.2 (1.6–8)**	6
Ethanol	Cat (a)	5.5	12
Galactose	Man (b)	2.5 (1.9–4.2)	13
Galactose	Pig (a)	4.5 (2.3–6.9)	4
Galactose	Cat (a)	3.2 (2.0–6.3)**	5
Mixed enzyme–flow-determined clearance: $0.1 < V_{max}/(QK_m) < 2.3$			
ICG	Man (b)	0.7 (0.4–1.6)	14
ICG	Cat (a)	0.4	15
ICG	Monkey (b)	0.3	16
Ethanol	Isolated perfused pig liver (a)	1.6 (0.7–3.2)	6
Galactose	Isolated perfused pig liver (a)	2.2 (1.5–3.6)	3
Caffeine	Man (c)	0.20	17
Caffeine	Man, smokers (c)	0.15 (0.1–0.3)	18

* Experimental models: (a) Isolated perfused liver or liver-vein catheterization in man or intact animal. Measurements of sets of steady c_i, c_o, and Q. Calculation of V_{max} and K_m [equation (3)]. (b) Liver-vein catheterization in man or intact animal. Constant intravenous infusion at first-order kinetics. Measurements of steady c_i and c_o. Calculation of $E = (c_i - c_o)/c_i$ and of $V_{max}/(QK_m) = -\ln(1 - E)$ [from equations (4a, b)]. (c) Intravenous bolus injection in man: peripheral concentration measurements, assumed Q 0.02 ml/min per kg body weight for the present purpose. Calculation of $E = Cl/Q$ and of $V_{max}/(QK_m)$ as in (b). (d) Oral administration in man: peripheral concentration measurements, assumed Q 1.2 l/min for the present purpose. Calculation of $E = Cl/Q$ (assuming oral Cl and intravenous Cl identical, i.e., low E), and $V_{max}/(QK_m)$ as in (b).
** $Cl > 0.85 Q$ at $V_{max}/(QK_m) > 1.9$.
ICG, indocyanine green.

mixed enzyme–flow-determined regimens. Only antipyrine fulfils the criteria for enzyme-determined hepatic clearance. Indocyanine green clearance belongs to the mixed enzyme–flow-determined regimen.

In individuals with liver disease the situation is more complex. If the possible influence of intrahepatic vascular and functional shunting is ignored (see below), clearance of both galactose (Keiding, Gastro, 1983; 85:986) and sorbitol (Keiding, Gastro, 1989; 96:1227) provides examples of shift from flow-determined clearance in controls to mixed enzyme–flow-determined clearance in liver patients.

Physiological complexities
Sinusoidal heterogeneity

In the intact liver there is heterogeneity of the sinusoidal blood flow (Lautt, CanJPhysPharm, 1993; 71:128) and of the enzyme activity and flow rates in different sinusoids, yet common K_m values. The sinusoids are not identical, parallel tubes but form a highly interconnected, labyrinthine system. Thus a substrate concentration measured in the liver vein will be a flow- and enzyme-weighted mean of the sinusoidal distribution. This has been described in the distributed sinusoidal perfusion model (Bass, JTheorBiol, 1978; 72:161). The so-called dispersion model (Roberts, JPharmacokinBiopharm, 1986; 14:227; 261:289) aims at describing the axial flow distribution but disregards the effect of the unidirectional liver blood flow.

Heterogeneity of liver-cell functions along the direction of sinusoidal flow, 'metabolic zonation', with, for example, a glycogenetic zone at the inlet and a glycolytic zone at the outlet, has been demonstrated (Gumucio, Hepatol, 1989; 9:154). Removal kinetics is insensitive to a possibly uneven distribution of the enzymes along the sinusoid.[1] In contrast to this, the kinetics of the production of metabolites (Pang, JPharmExpTher, 1978; 207:178) may give information about heterogeneity along the sinusoid (Bass, JTheorBiol, 1980; 82:347).

Flow variations

Liver blood flow varies under different physiological or pharmacological conditions. In human studies, food intake increased the hepatic blood-flow rate (Buchardt Hansen, AnnSurg, 1977; 186: 216) and vasopressin decreased it (Jacobsen, ScaJCLI, 1969; 24: 279). As expected, neither of these flow changes was followed by changes in estimates of galactose V_{max}. As long as the perfusion rate was above 0.9 ml blood/min per g liver, flow changes in perfused rat livers were similarly not followed by changes in estimates of galactose V_{max}, whereas lower perfusion rates reduced the estimates (Keiding, ScaJCLI, 1980; 40:355). Similar results were found in the intact cat liver.[5] As the flow rate is gradually reduced, the effect of sinusoidal heterogeneity becomes significant, followed by derecruitment, and finally collapse of sinusoids (Bauer, PhysRev, 1963; 43:115; Lautt, EurJClinInv, 1989; 19:A89).

Deviations from Michaelis–Menten kinetics

Enzymatic reactions are sometimes better described by other kinds of non-linear kinetics than by the simple Michaelis–Menten kinetics. Mathematically this has been formulated by an extension of the simple sinusoidal perfusion model, for example for allosteric enzyme reactions (Johnansen, JTheorBiol, 1981; 89:549).

This discussion has so far been confined to hepatic removal processes. Important liver functions, however, include production of metabolites released to the blood. The production of urea from alanine in pigs and humans (Vilstrup, DanMedBull, 1989; 36:415) was described by a model similar to the sinusoidal perfusion model described above.

Systemic availability during saturation kinetics

The fraction of an orally administered substance passing through the liver is often called systemic availability A. If the intestinal absorbtion is complete,

$$A = 1 - E = c_o/c_i. \tag{7}$$

The hepatic removal of a substrate during its passage from the intestines to the systemic blood is sometimes called the hepatic first-pass effect. In clinical pharmacological studies of systemic availability, hepatic removal is often assumed to follow first-order kinetics. However, for several drugs hepatic removal follows saturation kinetics, as shown for acetylsalicylic acid (Levy, JPharmaceutSci, 1965; 54:959). The systemic availability during saturation kinetics can be calculated from the sinusoidal perfusion model by the equation given in Fig. 4. It is seen that the availability approximates 1.0 at doses (V) approximating (or exceeding) the maximal removal capacity (V_{max}). At lower doses, the systemic availability decreases. In general, the lower the $V_{max}/(QK_m)$, the higher the systemic availability.

Binding to circulating plasma proteins

Hydrophobic substances circulate in plasma bound to plasma proteins. Despite tight protein binding, they are efficiently extracted by the liver. Because of the binding to plasma proteins, more substrate can be transported in the circulating blood than if it were unbound only. On the other hand, a high plasma protein concentration reduces the fraction of unbound drug ultimately taken up by the hepatocytes. In cirrhosis, reduced plasma albumin correlates with a reduced fraction of bound drugs in plasma (Blaschkle, ClinPharmacokin, 1977; 2:32).

The effects of protein binding on the balance between hepatic and renal excretion can be illustrated by the removal of salicylic acid in patients with severe alcoholic cirrhosis (Roberts, EurJClinPharmacokin, 1983; 25:253). Hepatic removal was diminished, but total removal was roughly unaffected, owing to increased urinary excretion. This was probably because of low plasma albumin with an increased unbound fraction of salicylic acid in plasma.

Traditionally, it has been thought that for highly protein-bound drugs only the unbound fraction is available for removal by the liver (Rowland, JPharmokinBiopharm, 1973; 1:123). Instantaneous equilibrium between bound and unbound drug was believed to exist not only in the bulk of the sinusoid bloodstream, but also all the

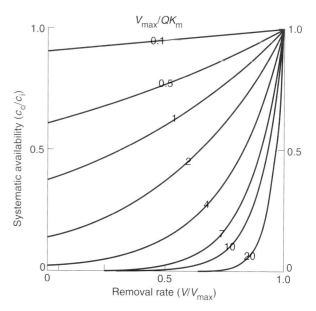

Fig. 4. Systemic availability $A = 1 - E = c_o/c_i$ in relation to dose (i.e., V/V_{max}) at saturation kinetics: $A = \exp[-(V_{max} - V)/QK_m]$. The different curves represent the relations for different $V_{max}/(QK_m)$ as given by the numbers.

way through the space of Disse to the plasma membrane of the hepatocytes. It has been shown for several substances, however, that more substrate is removed than can be explained by this traditional view: As the concentration of binding protein was increased, the hepatic removal of unbound substrate was enhanced (Weisiger, Gastro, 1980; 79:1065; Forker, JPharmExpTher, 1982; 223:342; Keiding, JHepatol, 1993; 19:327; Sorrentino, JHepatol, 1994; 21: 551).

These enhancement phenomena led Bass and co-workers[8,19] to examine the influence of diffusion barriers in the unstirred water layer adjacent to the hepatocyte plasma membrane, in the space of Disse. Their codiffusion model takes into account binding interactions between bound and unbound substrate, and diffusional transport from the sinusoidal lumen through the unstirred layer to the hepatocyte plasma membrane. The uptake of unbound drug by the hepatocytes creates disequilibrium between bound and unbound substrate in a thin layer near to the hepatocyte membrane. In this thin layer the rate of dissociation of the protein–substrate complex is higher than the rate of complex formation. Binding protein (albumin) is not taken up by the hepatocytes: after unloading the drug, it returns to the sinusoidal bulk. In the lumen of the sinusoid, bound and unbound substrate are assumed to be in equilibrium; or a small reduction of the unbound fraction could take place if the dissociation from the binding protein becomes rate-determining (Weisiger, AmJPhysiol, 1991; 261:G872; Ott, AmJPhysiol, 1997; 273:6227). The higher the concentration of the binding protein, the more protein–substrate complexes can be transported through the unstirred water layer to the disequilibrium layer where the unbound substrate is ultimately removed from the plasma.

Thus, following an increase in plasma protein concentration, more substrate can be transported in plasma. Clearance of total (bound plus unbound) substrate will decrease because of the reduced concentration of unbound substrate, but less so because of the codiffusion–disequilibrium processes. In the simplest version of the model, no additional membrane facilitation is assumed.

The codiffusion model is able to explain hitherto inexplicable observations on protein enhancement of hepatic removal of substrates.[1,19] Findings in studies of the hepatic removal of indocyanine green in intact pigs (Ott, EurJClinInvest, 1992; 22:347) and in humans (Keiding, JHepatol, 1993; 19:327) where the plasma protein concentration was experimentally changed, violated the traditional view and were in agreement with the codiffusion model. More recent data on the uptake of palmitate in isolated rat hepatocytes (Pond, AmJPhysiol, 1994; 267:G656), however, indicate that the albumin enhancement exceeds that predicted by the codiffusion model, suggesting the existence of some albumin-mediated facilitation of the uptake process.

It will be important to clarify the relative importance of changed protein binding and reduced liver-cell function during various liver diseases to the hepatic removal of plasma protein-bound substances.

Efflux

Efflux of substrate from the liver to the blood is known to occur with several compounds. The biexponential decay of the plasma concentration curve after bolus injection of bromosulphthalein (BSP) is usually assumed to reflect efflux from the liver cells. In rat livers first loaded with dibromosulphthalein (not metabolized, but otherwise similar to bromosulphthalein) and subsequently perfused with a dibromosulphthalein-free perfusate, the rate of efflux increased with increasing albumin concentration in the perfusate (Nijssen, EurJClinInvest, 1989; 19:A90). This suggests a possible role of plasma proteins for the efflux that 'mirrors' their role for the removal processes. For indocyanine green, Ott (AmJPhysiol, 1994; 266:G1108) demonstrated, in the pig, that a biexponential decay in concentration was due to transient extrahepatic, extravascular distribution and not to efflux from the liver cells.

Time dependence

Interpretation of experiments with time-dependent concentration changes requires major extensions of the modelling detailed above. A bolus of substrate, injected into the hepatic artery, will appear in the liver vein dispersed by the variation in sinusoidal transit times and substrate removal rates. This has been utilized in the multiple-indicator diffusion method introduced by Goresky (AmJPhysiol, 1963; 204:1101) to estimate transit times, intrahepatic volumes of distribution, and uptake rates of various substrates and indicators (not being removed). Unfortunately, since sampling inevitably must be at some distance from the sinusoidal inlet and outlet, with arterioles, venules, and other blood vessels as well as sampling tubes intervening, the concentration measurements will include the effect of dispersion in these non-removal pathways, which must be corrected for (Goresky, AmJPhysiol, 1963; 204:626).[8] Experiments on steady-state removal are not burdened with extrasinusoidal transit times, but do not allow evaluation of sinusoidal volumes of distribution.

In the intact organism, time-dependent studies must also account for (known or unknown) time-dependent changes of concentrations in the volume of distribution. An example of this is the clinical measurement of the galactose elimination capacity by a single injection method as proposed by Tygstrup. Hepatic removal depletes galactose in the blood. This again removes galactose from the extravascular volume of distribution, which has a higher galactose concentration than in the blood at a given point in time. This necessitates a correction for time delay in the calculations (Tygstrup, ScaJCLI, 1966; 18 (Suppl.):118). Another example is shown by indocyanine green, where a transient extrahepatic, extravascular volume of distribution was demonstrated in the pig (Ott, AmJPhysiol, 1994; 224:G118).

Extrahepatic elimination

Some examples can be used to illustrate the problems. At near-saturated concentration, galactose has a 10 per cent renal excretion, measured and corrected for in the galactose elimination capacity test (Tygstrup, ScaJCLI, 1966; 18 (Suppl.):118). At low galactose concentrations, a high hepatic extraction fraction led to the suggestion that systemic galactose clearance can be used as a measure of Q (cf. equation for flow-determined clearance in Fig. 3) (Henderson, Gastro, 1982; 83:1090). However, a small, but in this context significant, extrahepatic (i.e., extrasplanchnic) galactose elimination leads to about 30 per cent overestimation of liver blood flow by the systemic galactose clearance measurement both in normal man[13] and in cats (Burczynski, CanJPhysPharm, 1986; 64:1310).

The hepatic ethanol clearance (at concentrations below 0.5 mmol/l) is flow-determined (cf. Table 1 and ref.[6]). Unfortunately, there seems to be up to 50 per cent extrahepatic elimination in man (Keiding, JHepatol, 1986; 3 (Suppl.):S134). In cats, extrahepatic ethanol removal was negligible and ethanol clearance a valuable estimate of liver blood-flow rate (Greenway, CanJPhysPharm, 1988; 66:1192).

For indocyanine green, negligible extrahepatic elimination (Hunton, Gastro, 1960; 39:713)[15] makes it a suitable test substance for measurements of liver blood-flow rate by Fick's principle[14] and for measurements of intrinsic hepatic clearance (Keiding, EurJClinInvest, 1988; 18:507).

Liver disease
Impaired liver-cell function

Liver disease may reduce the number of liver cells as well as their function, resulting in a reduced 'functional liver cell mass' (Tygstrup, in *Diagnostic procedures in the evaluation of hepatic diseases*. New York: Liss, 1983; 17). This is reflected in diminished estimates of V_{max}, exemplified by measurements of the galactose elimination capacity (Tygstrup, ActaMedScand, 1964; 175:291) and antipyrine clearance in individuals with liver diseases. Also taurocholate V_{max} was reduced in isolated hepatocytes from cirrhotic rat livers (Reichen, Hepatol, 1987; 7:67).

When V_{max} is reduced during liver disease, the assumptions made by using V_{max} estimates and enzyme-determined clearance values (i.e., V_{max}/K_m) to evaluate liver-cell functions are still valid. However, caution should be used in transposing flow-determined clearance measurements to pathological conditions, since this principle is confined to conditions with high V_{max}. For example, as stated in Table 1, 90 per cent approximation of Cl to Q requires that $V_{max}/(QK_m)$ be larger than 2.3. For sorbitol, this seems to be fulfilled in controls (Molino, DigDisSci, 1987; 32:753).[10,11] However, in patients with liver disease, $V_{max}/(QK_m)$ can be estimated to be about 0.1 to 0.95,[10] shifting sorbitol clearance to the mixed enzyme–flow-clearance regimen (Keiding, Gastro, 1989; 96:1227). This implies that liver disease may shift the clearance regimen from being flow-determined in controls to the mixed enzyme–flow determined regimen during liver disease (see Table 1).

Capillarization of sinusoids

In cirrhosis there are often increased deposits of collagen in the space of Disse and a reduced number of endothelial cell fenestrae as demonstrated by scanning electron microscopy (Horn, in Wisse E, ed. *Sinusoidal cells.* Amsterdam: Elsevier, 1988; 189). The extravascular space accessible to albumin is reduced, as assessed by the multiple indicator method (Huet, JCI, 1982; 70:1234). The functional importance of this is not clear, but it is possible that it reduces the diffusional flux of protein-bound substrates towards the liver cell.

Intra- and extrahepatic vascular shunting

Portal–hepatic venous shunting often develops in long-lasting cirrhosis (Popper, AmJClinPath, 1952; 33:717). An intrahepatic shunt will carry the concentration c_i undiminished through the liver into the liver vein. The liver-vein blood with concentration $c_{o\,(mix)}$ will therefore consist of blood coming from functioning sinusoids with concentration c_o (possibly influenced by a reduced V_{max} of the sinusoids) and from the shunts (with concentration c_i). If the shunt takes some part pQ of the total flow Q ($0 < p < 1$), we have

$$c_{o(mix)} = (1-p)c_o + pc_i \qquad (8)$$

Attempts have been made to estimate the vascular shunting by comparison of measurements of total liver blood flow Q [as estimated by constant indocyanine green infusion and calculation according to Fick's principle (equation (2))] with clearance of sorbitol, assumed to give an estimate of the flow rate through functioning sinusoids. This proposal is based on the assumed flow-determined sinusoidal removal of sorbitol, i.e., functioning sinusoids with E close to 1.0, i.e., $V_{max}/(QK_m)$ higher than 2.3 (Table 1), which may not be fulfilled during liver disease with reduced V_{max} (Keiding, Gastro, 1989; 96:1227).

Since $c_{o\,(mix)} > c_o$, the calculated $\hat{c}$ concentration will be 'too high', and intrinsic clearance [equation (3)] 'too low'. Thus an observed low intrinsic clearance may be due to either reduced V_{max} or intrahepatic vascular shunting.

Intrahepatic shunting will result in increased systemic availability ($c_{o\,(mix)}/c_i$) during liver disease. Patients with cirrhosis often have extrahepatic vascular shunting, as reflected in the presence of oesophageal varices. This is of also of importance for the systemic availability.

Rationale for quantitative liver function tests

Conventional so-called liver function tests provide information on the integrity of hepatocytes (transaminases, etc.) and of bile formation (alkaline phosphatases, γ-glutamyl transferase, etc.). With the exception of serum albumin and prothrombin time these tests do not, however, reflect hepatic function. In a patient with inactive cirrhosis the activity of hepatic enzymes in serum may be normal in spite of decreased hepatic function. In contrast, hepatic function may be well preserved in the presence of markedly elevated transaminases.

Hepatic failure is ultimately the major cause of death in patients with severe liver disease. It is, therefore, reasonable to assume that single or serial quantitative assessments of different aspects of hepatic function might provide clinically valuable, complementary information on the severity, natural history, and prognosis of diseases of the liver and the effects of therapeutic interventions.

Tests to measure liver function quantitatively

The quantitative liver function tests in clinical use (Table 2) are based on the various functions of the liver and reflect hepatic blood perfusion, the functional, metabolic capacity of the liver, and blood–hepatocyte exchange to a variable extent.[1,20] Suitable test substances such as galactose, sorbitol and indocyanine green, with their limitations, have been mentioned above. Moreover, a number of compounds that are metabolized by cytochrome P_{450}-dependent processes are used to probe hepatic function, since the bulk of these enzymes is located in the liver. A drawback of tests based on the activity of cytochrome P_{450} enzymes is that environmental factors, diet, smoking, and concomitant drug therapy can either induce or inhibit the mono-oxygenases, independent of the presence or absence of liver disease. Suitable substrates are antipyrine (Poulsen, JHepatol, 1988; 6:374), caffeine (Renner, Hepatol, 1984; 4:38), erythromycin (Watkins, JCI, 1989; 83:688), and lidocaine (Oellerich, Lancet, 1989; i:640). In the case of aminopyrine, liver function can be probed with a breath test. Its metabolism generates labelled CO_2 that appears in breath when the methyl groups are labelled with either ^{14}C or ^{13}C (Bircher, ClinPharmTher, 1976; 20:484; Irving, JLabClinMed, 1982; 100:356).

Clinical utility of quantitative liver function tests

Even in healthy individuals there is considerable interindividual variability in the results of quantitative liver function tests such that normal ranges tend to be rather wide. The reproducibility of the test results in a given individual, however, is quite good. Thus, serial determinations in an individual patient are probably more informative than group comparisons. Liver function decreases with advancing age in parallel to the loss of liver volume (Schnegg, JHepatol, 1986; 3:164). These age-dependent changes in hepatic function should be taken into account when quantitative liver function tests are interpreted.

The result of liver injury from viruses, toxins, and chronic inflammation is ultimately a decrease in hepatic function. Clearly, quantitative liver function tests cannot be expected to provide an aetiological diagnosis, nor can they reflect specific morphological alterations or replace liver biopsy. However, once the diagnosis is known, quantitative liver function tests can provide more pertinent information on the severity of the liver disease. Hepatic perfusion and various liver functions may be well preserved in a patient

Table 2 Quantitative liver function tests in humans		
Test	**Provides an estimate of:**	**Reference**
Galactose elimination capacity	Metabolic capacity	Tygstrup, ActaPhysiolSca, 1963; 58:162
Aminopyrine demethylation	Microsomal function	Bircher, ChemPharmTher, 1976; 20:484
Caffeine clearance	Microsomal function	Renner, Hepatol, 1984; 4:38
Antipyrine clearance	Microsomal function	Poulsen, JHepatol, 1988; 6:374
Sorbitol clearance	Hepatic flow in normal individuals	Molino, DigDisSci, 1987; 32:753
Bromosulphthalein clearance	Biliary excretion	Haecki, JLabClinMed, 1976; 88:1019
Intrinsic clearance of indocyanine green	Biliary excretion	Keiding, EurJClinInvest, 1988; 18:507
Formation of monoethylglycine xylidide from lidocaine	Microsomal function	Oellerich, Lancet, 1989; i:640
Decarboxylation of ketoisocaproic acid	Mitochondrial function	Lauterburg, Hepatol, 1993; 17:418

with cirrhosis. Not surprisingly, many patients with documented cirrhosis have normal quantitative liver function tests. In general the results of quantitative liver function tests agree with subjective assessments of the severity of chronic liver disease such as the Child classification or the Pugh score. In a series of 187 patients with cirrhosis of mixed causation, 52 per cent of the patients with cirrhosis in Child class A, 11 per cent in class B, but none in class C had a normal aminopyrine breath test.[21] In chronic hepatitis, for example, the aminopyrine breath test was a better index of histological severity than conventional biochemical tests. A subnormal breath test predicted chronic active hepatitis with bridging necrosis or cirrhosis with a sensitivity of 86 per cent and a specificity of 84 per cent (Monroe, Hepatol, 1982; 2:317).

Prognostic value in acute liver disease

Now that liver transplantation is a treatment option in fulminant hepatic failure it will become more and more important to predict who will recover spontaneously and who will die unless a new organ is implanted. In fulminant hepatic failure, quantitative liver function tests may provide additional information on short-term survival. In fulminant failure due to viral hepatitis, patients with a galactose elimination capacity of less than 13 µmol/min per kg will most probably not recover (Ramsoe, ScaJGastr, 1980; 15:65). In addition, most of the patients in whom the galactose elimination capacity failed to increase during the first 10 days following admission died. Following an overdose of paracetamol, the aminopyrine breath test performed 24 to 36 h after admission predicted a fatal outcome when it was decreased to less than 5 per cent of the normal value (Saunders, BMJ, 1980; 280:279). Whether routine tests alone would also have predicted a fatal outcome is not known. In alcoholic hepatitis the aminopyrine breath test predicted survival with a sensitivity of 70 per cent and a specificity of 86 per cent (Schneider, Gastro, 1980; 79:1145). The test showed a better correlation with histological severity and clinical outcome than conventional biochemical tests when performed sequentially. The metabolism of lidocaine has shown some promise in assessing short-term survival of patients waiting for a liver transplant (Luketic, TranplProc, 1993; 25:1072).

Assessment of surgical risk

Surgical interventions in patients with chronic liver disease are associated with an increased risk (Aranha, AmJSurg, 1982; 143:55), particularly so when the operative procedure results in a further reduction of hepatic function as with hepatic resections and portosystemic shunts (Chandler, AnnSurg, 1985; 201:476; Yamanaka, AnnSurg, 1984; 200:658). A reliable, preoperative assessment of the risk of surgery and postoperative liver failure would be of clinical value. In a small group of patients with known or suspected liver disease the aminopyrine breath test was the best prognostic indicator of perioperative mortality following abdominal surgery (Gill, AnnSurg, 1983; 198:701). Likewise, in patients with extrahepatic obstruction the clearance of antipyrine provided an estimate of the outcome (McPherson, AmJSurg, 1985; 149:140). In contrast, the Pugh's score, but not the intrinsic clearance of indocyanine green, was the variable significantly related to survival in cirrhotic patients undergoing an end-to-side portocaval shunt (Pomier-Layrargues, Hepatol, 1988; 85:609). A frequently encountered question in patients with tumours or other focal lesions is whether the patient, who often suffers from cirrhosis, will tolerate a hepatic resection. The rate of removal of indocyanine green combined with a volumetric estimate of the residual liver after resection provides an estimate of surgical risk in these patients (Okamoto, Surgery, 1984; 95:586). No similar data are available for other quantitative liver function tests. The galactose elimination capacity may not be suitable in these conditions because some hepatocellular carcinomas can metabolize galactose, and a preoperative estimate of the residual functional capacity after resection is thus not possible.

Prognostic indices in chronic liver disease

With the advent of liver transplantation and effective drug treatments for various liver diseases, estimates of prognosis and of therapeutic efficacy have become increasingly important. A much used prognostic index is the classification of patients with chronic liver disease according to Child–Turcotte or a modification of their original scheme, such as that by Pugh et al. (BrJSurg, 1973; 60: 646).[22] These classifications are based on the combination of subjective and semiquantitative assessments of clinical and laboratory findings. The resulting scores are rather crude and reflect response to treatment or progression rather poorly in individual patients. Determination of hepatic function by one or a combination of the tests mentioned above at a single point in time does not generally provide more useful prognostic information than the classification according to Child (Villeneuve, Hepatol, 1986; 6:928; Henry, DigDisSci, 1985; 30:813; Albers, ScaJGastr, 1989; 24:269). This is not surprising considering the variable natural history of chronic liver diseases of different aetiology and the highly variable time course of the evolution of chronic liver disease in individual patients. Prognostication might improve if more homogeneous groups of patients were analysed. Thus, in a series of 94 patients with chronic hepatitis, a depressed aminopyrine breath test was one of the statistically significant predictors of death (Lashner, AmJMed, 1988; 85:609).

Since not only the natural history, but also individual rates of progression, are highly variable, sequential assessments of the patients' status might permit more accurate prognostication. In patients with primary biliary cirrhosis, serial determinations of the galactose elimination capacity may provide prognostic information in addition to a clinical risk score, which is based on clinical assessment and some routine laboratory tests (Reichen, Hepatol, 1991; 14:504).

In liver transplantation the formation of mono-ethyl-glycine-xylidine (MEGX) from lidocaine in potential organ donors has been proposed to predict short-term graft function, but the clinical utility of the test is controversial (Reichen, JHepatol, 1993; 19:4). An erythromycin breath test has been used to predict the dosage of cyclosporin after liver transplantation (Cakaloglu, Hepatol, 1994; 20:309) but it is doubtful that it provides clinically more useful information than measuring the blood cyclosporin concentration.

Assessment of therapeutic effects

Because of the prolonged course of chronic liver diseases, hard end-points of treatment, such as survival, are difficult to evaluate. Some studies have shown that the galactose elimination capacity and the aminopyrine breath test improve in patients with chronic hepatitis B who respond to interferon (Williams, Hepatol, 1989; 10:192; Reichen, JHepatol, 1994; 20:168) and that bromosulphthalein clearance improves in patients with cholestatic liver diseases treated with ursodeoxycholic acid (Poupon, Lancet, 1987; i:834). Thus, quantitative liver function tests may in some instances be used as markers of therapeutic efficacy.

References

1. Keiding S. Drug administration to liver patients: aspects of liver pathophysiology. *Seminars in Liver Disease*, 1995; **15**: 268–82.

2. Bass L, Keiding S, Winkler K, and Tygstrup N. Enzymatic elimination of substrates flowing through the intact liver. *Journal of Theoretical Biology*, 1976; **61**: 393–409.

3. Keiding S, Johansen S, Winkler K, Toennesen K, and Tygstrup N. Michaelis–Menten kinetics of galactose elimination by the isolated perfused pig liver. *American Journal of Physiology*, 1976; **230**: 1302–13.

4. Keiding S, Johansen S, and Winkler K. Hepatic galactose elimination kinetics in the intact pig liver. *Scandinavian Journal of Clinical and Laboratory Investigation*, 1982; **42**: 253–9.

5. Greenway CV and Burczynski FJ. Effects of liver blood flow on hepatic uptake kinetics of galactose in anaesthetized cats: parallel tube model. *Canadian Journal of Physiology and Pharmacology*, 1987; **65**: 1193–9.

6. Keiding S, Johansen S, Midtboel I, Raboel A, and Christiansen L. Ethanol elimination kinetics in human liver and pig liver *in vivo*. *American Journal of Physiology*, 1979; **237**: E316–24.

7. Andreasen PB, Raboel A, Toennesen K, and Keiding S. Michaelis–Menten kinetics of phenazone elimination by perfused pig liver. *Acta Pharmacologica et Toxicologica*, 1977; **40**: 1–13.

8. Bass L and Keiding S. Physiologically based models and strategic experiments in hepatic pharmacology. *Biochemical Pharmacology*, 1988; **37**: 1425–31.

9. Winkler K, Bass L, Keiding S, and Tygstrup N. The physiologic basis for clearance measurements in hepatology. *Scandinavian Journal of Gastroenterology*, 1979; **14**: 439–48.

10. Zeeh J, *et al.* Steady-state extra-renal sorbitol clearance as a measure of hepatic plasma flow. *Gastroenterology*, 1988; **95**: 749–59.

11. Avagnino P, *et al.* Assessment of liver circulation by *d*-sorbitol kinetics. *European Journal of Clinical Investigation*, 1989; **19**: A90.

12. Greenway CV and Lautt WW. Hepatic blood flow: Estimation from clearances of very low dose infusions of ethanol in cats. *Canadian Journal of Physiology and Pharmacology*, 1988; **66**: 1192–7.

13. Keiding S. Galactose clearance and liver blood flow. *Gastroenterology*, 1988; **94**: 477–81.

14. Skak C and Keiding S. Methodological problems in the use of indocyanine green to estimate hepatic blood flow and ICG clearance in man. *Liver*, 1987; **7**: 155–62.

15. Burczynski FJ, Greenway CV, and Sitar DS. Hepatic blood flow; accuracy of estimation from infusion of indocyanine green in anaesthetized cats. *British Journal of Pharmacology*, 1987; **91**: 651–59.

16. Branch RA, Shand DG, Wilkinson GR, and Nies AS. Increased clearance of antipyrine and *d*-propranolol after phenobarbital treatment in the monkey. *Journal of Clinical Investigation*, 1974; **53**: 1101–17.

17. Renner E, Weitholtz H, Huguenin P, Arnaud MJ, and Preisig R. Caffeine: a model compound for measuring liver function. *Hepatology*, 1984; **4**: 38–46.

18. Joeres R, Klinker H, Heusler H, Epping J, Zilly W, and Richter E. Influence of smoking on caffeine elimination in healthy volunteers and in patients with alcoholic liver cirrhosis. *Hepatology*, 1988; **8**: 575–9.

19. Bass L and Pond SM. The puzzle of rates of cellular uptake of protein-bound ligands. In Pecile A and Rescigno A, eds. *Pharmacokinetics: mathematical and statistical approaches to metabolism and distribution of chemicals and drugs.* London: Plenum, 1988: 245–69.

20. Reichen J. Assessment of hepatic function with xenobiotics. *Seminars of Liver Disease*, 1995; **15**: 189–201.

21. Villeneuve JP, *et al.* Prognostic value of the aminopyrine breath test in cirrhotic patients. *Hepatology*, 1986; **6**: 928–31.

22. Conn HO. A peak at the Child–Turcotte classification. *Hepatology*, 1981; **1**: 673–6.

5.3 Immunological investigations in liver diseases

Karl-Hermann Meyer zum Büschenfelde and Michael P. Manns

Introduction

The basic function of the immune system is to distinguish between 'self' and 'non-self'. Infectious agents like viruses are recognized by the immune system as 'non-self' and numerous cellular and humoral immune reactions are elicited to eliminate the infectious agent. The intact function of the immune system is necessary to guarantee the physical integrity of an individual. Development of specific antibodies and elimination of infectious agents without any clinical symptoms, or a self-limited acute disease with a following long-lasting immunity, may be the result. Alternatively, there may be an equilibrium between the infectious agent and the immune system of the infected organism (symbiosis). This is one of the major characteristics of chronic infectious diseases. The spectrum of results between the immune system of infected organisms and invading infectious agents is observed in clinical manifestations of virus-induced liver diseases such as hepatitis B.

A further pathogenetic mechanism of chronic inflammatory liver disease is a loss of tolerance against autologous liver tissue leading to autoimmune liver diseases. Autoimmune hepatitis and primary biliary cirrhosis are the two main groups of autoimmune liver disease. Specific rare forms of autoimmune liver disease are autoimmune cholangitis, and the overlap syndromes of primary biliary cirrhosis/autoimmune hepatitis and primary sclerosing cholangitis/ autoimmune hepatitis. Primary sclerosing cholangitis may also be regarded as an autoimmune liver disease.

The immune system consists of various cellular elements, among them lymphocytes and cells of the reticuloendothelial system. T and B lymphocytes are the main cellular components that contribute to the ability of the immune system to distinguish between 'self' and 'non-self'. The close collaboration between these various components of the immune system is mediated by lymphokines. After contact with foreign antigens, B lymphocytes differentiate into plasma cells and eventually secrete specific antibodies. The development from B lymphoblasts to antibody-secreting plasma cells is supported by T-helper cells, which are characterized by the CD4 membrane antigen. A further T-cell subpopulation expresses the CD8 membrane glycoprotein. CD8+ and CD4+ T lymphocytes are part of the T-cell compartment responsible for regulatory and cytotoxic functions. The physiological function of the immune system in distinguishing between 'self' and 'non-self' is maintained by a well-balanced network between the T-helper and T-suppressor

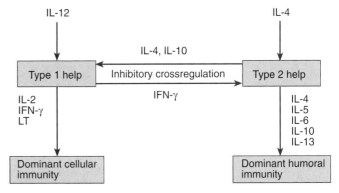

Fig. 1. Helper T-cell subsets: T_{H1} and T_{H2}.

lymphocytes. The CD4+ T-helper (T_H) population may be further divided into T_{H1}, T_{H2}, and T_{H0} cells (Fig. 1). T_{H1} cells secrete the cytokines interleukin 2 (**IL-2**) and interferon-γ (**IFN-γ**), while T_{H2} cells secrete IL-4, IL-5, IL-6, IL-10, and IL-13. T_{H1} cells stimulate the cytotoxic T-cell response, while T_{H2} cells stimulate B cells and antibody production. T_{H1} cells proliferate in response to IL-12, which is under clinical evaluation as a therapeutic cytokine for viral hepatitis.

In this chapter the value and application of immunological techniques in the diagnosis of liver disease will be presented. Where appropriate, the question of whether the detected abnormalities of the immune system contribute to our knowledge of the pathogenesis of liver disease will be discussed. Immunological techniques for the diagnosis of liver disease primarily detect antigen–antibody reactions. Several techniques have been introduced, starting with the complement fixation test and followed by immunofluorescence, immunodiffusion, counterimmunoelectrophoresis, radioimmunoassay, enzyme immunoassay, immunoblotting, and lately, recombinant DNA technology. Immunofluorescence is used as the screening method of choice for the detection of most autoantibodies in serum and for the detection of viral antigens in liver tissue. Radioimmunoassay and enzyme immunoassay techniques are used for the detection of autoantibodies and viral antigen–antibody systems in serum. The advent of immunoblotting techniques facilitated the definition of autoantigen–antibody systems on a molecular level, including the definition of the molecular masses of the antigens. Immunoblotting or enzyme-linked immunosorbent assay (**ELISA**)

Table 1 Major autoantibodies in liver disease

	Antigen	Disease association
Antinuclear antibodies (ANA)	Very heterogeneous	Autoimmune hepatitis Minor: PBC, PSC, viral hepatitis, drug-induced hepatitis
Liver–kidney microsomal antibodies (LKM)		
LKM-1	Cytochrome P-450 2D6	Autoimmune hepatitis type 2
LKM-2	Cytochrome P-450 2C9	Ticrynafen-induced hepatitis
LKM-3	UDP-glucuronosyl-transferases	Hepatitis D, autoimmune hepatitis
LM	Cytochrome P-450 1A2	Dihydralazine-induced hepatitis Hepatitis in APS-1
Anti-smooth muscle antibodies (SMA)	F-actin	Autoimmune hepatitis Chronic viral hepatitis C
Antibodies to cytosolic antigens		
Soluble liver antigen (SLA)	Cytokeratins	Autoimmune hepatitis type 3
Liver–pancreas (LP)	?	Autoimmune hepatitis type 3
Antiliver cytosol (anti-LC-1)	?	Autoimmune hepatitis type 2
(anti-LC-2)	?	Autoimmune hepatitis type 2
Autoantibodies to hepatocellular membrane antigens	ASGPR	Autoimmune liver diseases, namely autoimmune hepatitis
Antimitochondrial antibodies (AMA)	Acyltransferases	PBC
Antineutrophilic cytoplasmic antibodies (ANCA)	Actin?	PSC Minor: autoimmune hepatitis

APS-1, autoimmune polyendocrine syndrome type 1; PBC, primary biliary cirrhosis; PSC, primary sclerosing cholangitis.

techniques with recombinant autoantigens are nowadays used to further define and identify diagnostically relevant specific auto-antigen–antibody systems once a positive autoantibody result is obtained by screening tests such as immunofluorescence.

Autoantibodies

The diagnosis of autoimmune liver disease is based on the finding of characteristic autoantibody patterns in serum in the absence of overt viral, toxic, or metabolic factors that may themselves cause liver disease. It is important to realize that the diagnosis rests as much on positive autoantibody findings as on negative virological findings. Virus-induced liver disease (as well as toxic and metabolic liver disorders) may also be associated with autoantibody production. As a rule, however, the levels of autoantibodies detectable in viral hepatitis are much lower than the levels in autoimmune liver disease.

Whether and how autoantibodies are involved in the pathogenesis of inflammatory liver diseases remains unclear. In this chapter, emphasis will be placed on diagnostically relevant autoantibodies (Table 1).

Serologically, subgroups of autoimmune hepatitis can be distinguished. Autoimmune hepatitis type 1 is associated with antinuclear antibodies (ANA) with or without smooth muscle antibodies (SMA). A second subgroup is characterized by autoantibodies against a microsomal antigen of liver and kidney, the so-called LKM-1 antibodies. A third subgroup of autoimmune hepatitis is characterized by autoantibodies against cytosolic antigens such as soluble liver antigen (SLA) and liver–pancreas antigen (LP). It is still unknown whether the occurrence of high-titre smooth muscle antibodies, when directed against F-actin, *per se* characterizes a

fourth subgroup of autoimmune hepatitis. Primary biliary cirrhosis-specific subtypes of antimitochondrial antibodies (AMA) are well established diagnostic markers for this disease. Recently, anti-neutrophilic cytoplasmic antibodies (ANCA) have been found in primary sclerosing cholangitis and other liver diseases.

Antinuclear antibodies (ANA)

ANA are found in several liver diseases. They were first detected in patients with autoimmune hepatitis, which led to the term 'lupoid hepatitis'. This group of patients is now termed autoimmune hepatitis type 1. Other liver diseases with a significant prevalence of ANA are primary biliary cirrhosis, primary sclerosing cholangitis, drug-induced liver disease, and in some patients, viral hepatitis B and C. The most frequent method of detection of ANA is indirect immunofluorescence on Hep-2 cells. Dependent on the auto-antigens detected, different patterns of fluorescence are found: homogeneous perinuclear (58 per cent), speckled (21 per cent), homogeneous speckled (10 per cent), centromere (9 per cent), or homogeneous perinuclear (6 per cent).[1] Each pattern is associated with the recognition of several nuclear antigens with a wide range of molecular masses. The cut-off titre for a positive autoantibody result may vary depending on the laboratory. However, 1:40 for ANA and 1:80 for SMA are cut-off values in many laboratories. Among ANAs are autoantibodies directed against ssDNA, dsDNA, snRNPs, tRNA, and lamin A and C.[1] Recently, cyclin A was discovered as another species of antigens of antinuclear antibodies (Strassburg, JHepatol, 1996; 25:859).

ANA in primary biliary cirrhosis include anticentromeric auto-antibodies (Parveen, JGastHepatol, 1995; 10:438), antibodies directed against nuclear membrane proteins, and antibodies against nuclear regulatory proteins (Szostecki, JImmunol, 1990; 145:4338; Strassburg, JHepatol, 1996; 25:859). About 12 per cent of patients with primary biliary cirrhosis have anticentromeric antibodies which react with the scleroderma-specific antigen CENP. Although scleroderma is sometimes associated with primary biliary cirrhosis, not all patients with anticentromeric antibodies have evident scleroderma (Powell, QJMed, 1987; 237:75).

The second set of ANA in primary biliary cirrhosis is directed against nuclear membrane proteins; 25 per cent of sera from patients with this condition react with gp210, a nuclear pore membrane glycoprotein. This gp210 antibody has so far been described solely in sera from these patients (Nickowitz, Gastro, 1994; 106:193). Other nuclear membrane reactants include lamin B receptor (**LBR**) to which autoantibodies occur less frequently, and these also seem to be specific for primary biliary cirrhosis (Courvalin, JExpMed, 1990; 172:961). Immunoblotting of fusion proteins demonstrated an autoepitope within the nucleocytoplasmic domain for both gp210 and LBR autoantigens (Nickowitz, JExpMed, 1993; 178:2237; Lin, Hepatol, 1996; 23:57).

The third set of ANA in primary biliary cirrhosis reacts with nuclear regulatory proteins. About 8 per cent of patients with this disease have antibodies against cyclin A, a nuclear protein involved in cell cycle regulation and DNA synthesis (Strassburg, JHepatol, 1996; 25:859). Another autoantibody associated with this disease is anti-Sp100, which shows an intranuclear dot-like pattern (fine speckling) on the Hep-2 cell line by immunofluorescence. Anti-Sp100 is found in about 30 per cent of primary biliary cirrhosis sera, and the reactant is a 100-kDa protein as determined by immunoblotting (Szostecki, ClinExpImmun, 1987; 68:108). The biological function of this nuclear protein is still unknown. After cloning the cDNA for Sp100 and subsequent protein sequencing, sequence homologies with MHC class I molecules and several transcriptional regulatory proteins were discovered (Szostecki, Sca-JImmunol, 1990; 145:4338). Recently, Sternsdorf and coworkers (ScaJImmunol, 1995; 42:257) reported that PML, a transformation and cell growth-suppressing protein, causes the same dot-like pattern on immunofluorescence as does Sp100. It also seems to be as specific for primary biliary cirrhosis as the Sp100 autoantibody and often occurs concomitantly with it (Sternsdorf, 1995). So far, neither a liver-specific nuclear antigen nor a liver disease-specific ANA has been identified.

Smooth muscle antibodies (SMA)

SMA are directed against structures of the cytoskeleton. They are measured by indirect immunofluorescence on smooth muscle cells that have a well-developed cytoskeleton due to their contractile function. Antibodies to actin represent a subset of SMA antibodies which are particularly frequent in autoimmune hepatitis type 1. In autoimmune hepatitis, SMA are predominantly directed against F-actin.[2] This is a consituent of the cytoskeleton of the liver cell with a close association with the plasma cell membrane. F-actin antibodies seem to be diagnostically more relevant in children. Recently, antiactin antibodies in autoimmune hepatitis were further analysed. Actin antibody-positive patients with autoimmune hepatitis were younger, were more commonly HLA DR3 positive, and death and transplantation occurred more frequently in these patients than in actin antibody-negative patients with ANA-positive autoimmune hepatitis type 1.[3]

Antimicrosomal antibodies

LKM-1 autoantibodies

Autoimmune hepatitis type 2 is characterized by the presence of LKM-1 autoantibodies.[4] These autoantibodies were first described by Rizzetto et al.[5] using indirect immunofluorescence on rodent liver and kidney sections. Their characteristic feature is the exclusive staining of the P3 portion of the proximal renal tubules. Western blots with hepatic microsomes revealed a protein band at 50 kDa. In addition to the 50-kDa protein, a 55- and a 64-kDa protein were detected at a lower frequency (Codoner-French, ClinExpImmun, 1989; 54:232; Manns, JCI, 1989; 83:1066). In 67 per cent of patients with autoimmune hepatitis type 2, antibodies to liver cytosol type 1 (**anti-LC-1**) are detected (Martini, Hepatol, 1988; 8:1662; Abuaf, Hepatol, 1992; 16:892). The significance of anti-LC-1 autoantibodies in autoimmune hepatitis type 2, however, is not clear (Czaja, AmJGastr, 1995; 90:1206). Cytochrome P-450 2D6 is the major antigen for LKM-1 autoantibodies (Zanger, PNAS, 1988; 85:8256; Gueguen, BBResComm, 1989; 159:542; Manns, 1989) (Table 2). *In vitro* the enzymatic activity of cytochrome P-450 2D6 is inhibited by LKM-1 autoantibodies (Zanger, 1988; Manns, Hepatol, 1990; 12:127). However, this activity is not inhibited *in vivo*, and adequate expression of P-450 2D6 seems to be a prerequisite for the development of LKM-1 autoantibodies directed against P-450 2D6 (Manns, 1990). The epitopes recognized by LKM-1 autoantibodies have been characterized. A short minimal epitope of eight amino acids spanning amino acids 257 to 269 (DPAQPPRD) was identified first.[6] Further work on epitope mapping resulted in the identification of three other autoepitopes on P-450 2D6.[7] However, the autoantibodies of most patients with autoimmune hepatitis type 2 recognize the epitope of amino acids from 257 to 269, including the core sequence of DPAQPPRD. The autoantibodies of about 50 per cent of patients with this type of hepatitis recognize in addition an epitope from amino acids 321 to 351, and in some cases an epitope of amino acids from 373 to 389 or 410 to 429 (see Fig. 1 in Chapter 14.3).

LKM-2 autoantibodies

LKM-2 autoantibodies have so far only been observed in drug-induced hepatitis caused by tienilic acid and not in autoimmune hepatitis (Homberg, ClinExpImmun, 1984; 55:561). These autoantibodies are directed against cytochrome P-450 2C9 (Beaune, PNAS, 1987; 84:551) (Table 2). Since the antidiuretic drug tienilic acid has been withdrawn from the market, LKM-2 antibodies are no longer discovered.

LKM-3 autoantibodies

LKM-3 autoantibodies were first described in 10 to 20 per cent of patients with chronic hepatitis D.[8] These autoantibodies are also seen in 10 per cent of patients with autoimmune hepatitis type 2 (Manns, JCI, 1989; 83:1066; Durazzo, Gastro, 1995; 108:455; Obermayer-Straub, Gut, 1995; 37:A100). LKM-3 antibodies react with family 1 proteins of UDP-glucuronosyl transferases (**UGT-1**).[9] The main epitope is expressed on the constant regions of exons 2 to 5 of UGT-1. A minor autoepitope is expressed on UGT-2 proteins. This minor autoepitope has so far only been recognized by hepatitis D sera. In autoimmune hepatitis, LKM-3 antibodies

Table 2 Heterogeneity of cytochrome P-450s and UDP-glucuronosyl transferases (UGT) as human autoantigens

Antibody	kDa	Target antigen	Disease association
LKM-1	50	Cytochrome P-450 2D6	Autoimmune hepatitis, hepatitis C
LKM-2	50	Cytochrome P-450 2C9	Tienilic acid-induced hepatitis
LKM-3	55	UGT-1 UGT-2	Hepatitis D, autoimmune hepatitis
LM	52	Cytochrome P-450 1A2	Dihydralazine-induced hepatitis, autoimmune polyendocrine syndrome type 1
	54	Cytochrome P-450?	Halothane-induced hepatitis
	57	Disulphide isomerase	Halothane-induced hepatitis
	59	Carboxylesterase	Halothane-induced hepatitis
	59	?	Chronic hepatitis C
	64	?	Autoimmune hepatitis
	70	?	Chronic hepatitis C
	50	Cytochrome P-450 c21	Adrenal and ovarian failure
	50	Cytochrome P-450 scc	
	50	Cytochrome P-450 c17a	
	53	Cytochrome P-450 3A1	Anticonvulsant hypersensitivity: phenobarbital, phenytoin, carbamazepine
	53	Cytochrome P-450 2C11	

are usually associated with LKM-1; rarely are LKM-3 the only marker for this disease (Strassburg, Gastro, 1996; 111:1582). It is unknown whether LKM-3 antibodies characterize a subgroup of patients with hepatitis D that differs in disease progression or treatment response. Epitope mapping revealed a minimum epitope sequence of amino acids from 264 to 373, indicating that the LKM-3 autoepitope is conformation dependent (Straub, Hepatol, 1994; 20:427). LKM-3 autoantibodies against UGT-1 can be detected at a dilution of 1:1000 or above by Western blotting or with an ELISA based on baculovirus-expressed recombinant UGT protein (Table 2).

LM autoantibodies

Antimicrosomal antibodies that react only with liver tissue are called LM antibodies. These were found in drug-induced hepatitis caused by dihydralazine and react with cytochrome P-450 1A2 (Bourdi, JCI, 1990; 85:1967). At the same time, LM antibodies were found in one patient with autoimmune hepatitis (Manns, Arch-BiochemBiophys, 1990; 280:229) and these were also directed against cytochrome P-450 1A2. Recently, it became clear that antibodies against cytochrome P-450 1A2 in non-drug-induced liver disease are diagnostic markers for hepatitis as part of the autoimmune polyendocrine syndrome type 1.[10] There does not seem to be a serological overlap between LKM-1 antibodies in autoimmune hepatitis type 2 and LM antibodies in autoimmune polyendocrine syndrome type 1 (Table 2).

Autoantibodies against the asialoglycoprotein receptor

Autoantibodies against the asialoglycoprotein receptor (**ASGPR**), a liver-specific membrane receptor, have been demonstrated in patients with inflammatory liver disease. Worldwide studies on their prevalence clearly show that anti-ASGPR autoantibodies binding to human substrate are found preferentially in autoimmune hepatitis irrespective of serological subtype and genetic background.[11,12]

However, they may also be detected in primary biliary cirrhosis and viral liver disease, but very rarely in other forms of liver disease, non-hepatic autoimmune disorders, and healthy adults. Anti-ASGPR autoantibodies are polyclonal, bind to multiple epitopes, and correlate with the disease activity of autoimmune hepatitis.[12] Mapping of immunoreactivity on biochemical modifications of native ASGPR indicates that confirmational, protein-structural and glycoside antigens represent potential autoepitopes on the ASGPR (Treichel, ZGastr, 1997; 35:92). Among these autoepitopes, glycoside-directed anti-ASGPR seem to be highly disease specific for autoimmune hepatitis.

The ASGPR was the first liver-specific autoantigen which was found to stimulate proliferation of liver-infiltrating lymphocytes after autologous antigen presentation (Löhr, Hepatol, 1990; 12: 1314). This recognition was restricted to the MHC class II complex and not inhibitable by ASGPR ligand. The organ-specific T-cell reactivity was predominantly found in patients with autoimmune hepatitis and primary biliary cirrhosis. This reactivity suggests pathophysiological relevance considering the morphological finding that the ASGPR is preferentially expressed in the periportal area of the liver, the hallmark site of inflammation in chronic hepatitis (McFarlane, Hepatol, 1990; 11:408). Furthermore, it was shown that liver-infiltrating T-helper cells from patients with autoimmune hepatitis which specifically proliferate in the presence of ASGPR peptides stimulate the production and secretion of autoantibodies against the human ASGPR by autologous B cells *in vitro* (Löhr, ClinExpImmun, 1992; 88:45).

All studies on anti-ASGPR autoantibodies carried out worldwide have been performed using affinity-purified ASGPR as the target in two different assays: a liquid-phase radioimmunoassay using ASGPR from rabbit liver, the anti-ASGPR RIA (McFarlane, JHepatol, 1986; 3:196), and a solid-phase enzyme immunoassay with human ASGPR, the anti-ASGPR EIA (Treichel, Hepatol, 1990; 11:606). A further difference beyond the substrate specificity exists between the assays. The anti-ASGPR radioimmunoassay is based on the precipitation of complexes formed by radiolabelled

Table 3 Mitochondrial autoantigens: molecular identity, earlier designation, molecular mass function, and frequency of the corresponding autoantibody in patients with primary biliary cirrhosis

Subunits of the 2-oxo-acid dehydrogenase complex

Molecular identity	Earlier designation	Molecular mass (kDa)	Function	Autoantibody frequency (%)
PDH E1-α decarboxylase	M2d	41	Decarboxylates pyruvate with thiamine pyrophosphate (TPP) as a cofactor	66
E1-β decarboxylase	M2e	36	Decarboxylates pyruvate with TPP as a cofactor	1–7
E2 acetyltransferase	M2a	74	Transfers acetyl group from E1 to coenzyme A (CoA)	92
Protein X	M2c	56	Unknown	NA
BCOADC E2 acyltransferase	M2c	52	Transfers acyl group from E1 to CoA	54
OGDC E2 succinyl transferase	M2c	48	Transfers succinyl group from E1 to CoA	66

According to Galperin and Gershwin, ref. 18.
BCOADC, branched-chain 2-oxo-acid dehydrogenase; OGDC, 2-oxo-gluterate dehydrogenase; PDH, pyruvate dehydrogenase.

ASGPR and autoantibodies. Anti-ASGPR antibodies measured by enzyme immunoassay are detected indirectly using an enzyme-labelled antihuman immunoglobulin antiserum. Notably, both assays were demonstrated to give congruent results in a blind-conducted studies.[12] In addition to these two assays, both dot-blot and immunoblot analyses have been performed using human substrate.

Antimitochondrial antibodies (AMA)

A long-standing observation is that almost all patients with primary biliary cirrhosis have high levels of AMA. These autoantibodies were found to react with trypsin-sensitive antigens located on the inner mitochondrial membrane (Berg, JExpMed, 1967; 126:277). It was not until 1985 that several groups, using immunoblotting, showed up to five mitochondrial autoantigens with molecular masses ranging from 74 to 36 kDa (Frazer, JImmunol, 1985; 135:1739; Ishii, ImmunolLett, 1985; 9:325; Lindenborn-Fotinos, Hepatol, 1985; 5:763; Manns, JHepatol, 1985; 1(Suppl.1):S85). The cited molecular masses of the antigens varied slightly between the laboratories due to technical differences in estimating migration of the molecules in gels. Cloning of cDNA for the major mitochondrial autoantigen identified the proteins as enzyme subunits of the 2-oxo-acid dehydrogenase enzyme complexes (Surh, Hepatol, 1989; 9:63; Moteki, Hepatol, 1996; 23:436).[13,14] The enzymes catalyse the reductive transfer of an acetyl group from its substrate to coenzyme A for oxidation in the Krebs' cycle.

The AMA most frequently found in serum of patients with primary biliary cirrhosis are directed against the 74-kDa E2 subunit enzyme of the pyruvate dehydrogenase complex (PDC) (Table 3). These antibodies are found in high titre in about 95 per cent of patients with this disease. Anti-PDC-E2 antibodies cross-react with protein X (56 kDa) of the pyruvate dehydrogenase complex,

presumably due to a shared epitope. Some primary biliary cirrhosis sera react with PDC-E1-α or -β, although the frequency of such antibodies is only about 7 per cent. Other common autoantibodies specific for this disease are directed against the 52-kDa E2 subunit of the branched-chain 2-oxo-acid dehydrogenase complex (BCOADC) and the 48-kDa E2 subunit of the 2-oxo-gluterate dehydrogenase complex (OGDC). A summary of the different autoantigens including molecular mass, function, and frequency of autoantibodies is shown in Table 3. The AMA found in primary biliary cirrhosis are of the IgM and IgG classes with an isotype bias to IgG3 (Surh, Hepatol, 1988; 8:290). This isotype bias is also found in other autoimmune diseases. The AMA to the 2-OADC enzymes inhibit specifically the catalytic function of their corresponding autoantigen in vitro. Fregeau et al. (Hepatol, 1990; 11: 975) demonstrated this with sera that reacted exclusively with OGDC-E2; these inhibited only OGDC activity, whereas sera that reacted exclusively with PDC-E2 and/or BCOADC-E2 failed to inhibit OGDC activity. This was confirmed by experiments performed with primary biliary cirrhosis sera that was affinity purified on PDC. The purified antibodies reacted with and inhibited PDC-E2, but did not react with BCOADC-E2 or OGDC-E2, or inhibit the activity of the OGDC enzyme. These studies illustrate the lack of cross-reaction among the different 2-OADC antibodies, with exception of protein X which shares the 'lipoyl' epitope with PDC-E2.

The question arises of whether there is any direct role of the various autoantibodies in the pathogenesis of primary biliary cirrhosis. This has been disputed because the expression of disease does not correlate with the antibody titre. However, the titre of autoantibodies might not be the only consideration, since pathogenicity could relate to other properties of antibodies including affinity, isotype, subclass, or epitope specificity. For example, there is the interesting idea that AMA of the IgA isotype in transit through the biliary ductular epithelium undergo reactivity with a mitochondrial antigen (Van de Water, JCI, 1993; 96:723).

Antineutrophilic cytoplasmic antibodies (ANCA)

ANCA are autoantibodies directed against components in the cytoplasm of human granulocytes. They were first reported in 1982 in patients with systemic vasculitis and glomerulonephritis.[15] Later ANCA were described as a seromarker in Wegener's disease (van de Woude, Lancet, 1985; i: 425; Lüdemann, ClinExpImmun, 1987; 69:350). Two different ANCA patterns can be seen in ethanol-fixed human granulocytes, namely a cytoplasmic staining (cANCA), and an artefactual perinuclear staining (pANCA) caused by translocation of basic proteins to the negatively charged nucleus (Falk, NEJM, 1988; 318:1651; Venning, QJMed, 1990; 77:1287). In 1990 Saxon et al. (JAllClinImmunol, 1990; 86:202) demonstrated pANCA autoantibodies in patients with inflammatory bowel disease. Then several groups reported pANCA in sera of patients with autoimmune liver disease (Rump, Immunobiology, 1990; 181:406; Duerr, Gastro, 1991; 100:1385).

ANCA were demonstrated in 65 to 88 per cent of primary sclerosing cholangitis sera, in 49 to 92 per cent of autoimmune hepatitis sera, and in 0 to 5 per cent of primary biliary cirrhosis sera (Seibold, Gut, 1992; 33:657; Hardarson, AmJClinPath, 1993; 99: 277; Mulder, Hepatol, 1993; 17:411; Vidrich, JClinImmunol, 1995; 15:293; Targan, Gastro, 1995; 108:1159; Bansi, JHepatol, 1996; 24: 581). The reason for the differences in the percentage of ANCA-positive patients is not clear. Perhaps it results from the differences in the quality of granulocytes used as substrate or in the method used to stain the neutrophils. There is a predominance of the IgG1 subclass in autoimmune liver disease. Targan et al. (1995) found that 80 per cent of autoimmune hepatitis sera had only the IgG1 subtype, whereas primary sclerosing cholangitis sera had both IgG1 and IgG3. Bansi et al. (Gut, 1996; 38:384) compared the ANCA subclasses of ulcerative colitis and primary sclerosing cholangitis in combination with ulcerative colitis and found that IgG3 was increased in the latter group. Vidrich et al. (1995) were able to distinguish the pANCA found in ulcerative colitis from the ANCA found in primary sclerosing cholangitis and autoimmune hepatitis type 1 by subjecting the neutrophils to DNAase digestion. While there was a loss of the antigenic recognition in ulcerative colitis sera, the majority of primary sclerosing cholangitis and autoimmune hepatitis sera still recognized cytoplasmic constituents.

To distinguish the different diseases from one another and to learn more about autoimmune liver disease it would be helpful to know which autoantigen is recognized by these ANCA associated with liver disease. The autoantigen for cANCA in Wegener's granulomatosis was demonstrated to be serine proteinase 3 (Niles, Blood, 1989; 74:1888). The autoantigens for pANCA are much more heterogeneous. Several have been identified, namely myeloperoxidase (Falk, NEJM, 1988; 318:1651), lactoferrin (Peen, Gut, 1993; 34:56), elastase (Goldschmeding, KidneyInt, 1988; 34:558), BPI (Zhao, ClinExpImmun, 1995; 99:49), lysozyme (Savige, RheumInt, 1996; 16:1091), and cathepsin G (Halbwachs-Mecarelli, ClinExpImmun, 1992; 90:79), but there are many antigens, especially in inflammatory bowel disease and liver diseases, that have not been determined. Peen et al. (Gut, 1993; 34:56) found primary

sclerosing cholangitis sera to be positive for myeloperoxidase and lactoferrin. However, Haagsma et al. (JHepatol, 1993; 19:8) reported that their primary sclerosing cholangitis sera did not react with myeloperoxidase, proteinase 3, elastase, or lactoferrin. Gur et al. (Pathobio, 1995; 63:76) found that 35 per cent of their primary sclerosing cholangitis sera reacted with cathepsin G and Stoffel et al. (ClinExpImmun, 1996; 104:54) demonstrated a reaction with BPI in 44 per cent of their primary sclerosing cholangitis sera. Klein et al. (Hepatol, 1991; 6:1147) found five unknown primary sclerosing cholangitis autoantigens with molecular masses ranging from 30 to 95 kDa. In a study by Mulder et al. (Hepatol, 1993; 17:411), autoimmune hepatitis sera recognized a 66/67-kDa unknown protein and primary sclerosing cholangitis sera recognized lactoferrin and 66/67-kDa and 40-kDa unknown proteins. A disease-specific autoantigen for autoimmune liver diseases has yet to be found. However, recent data suggest that actin is an antigen for ANCA in liver diseases.[16]

Several methods are used to detect ANCA in patient sera: indirect immunofluorescence, radioimmunoassay, ELISA, Western blotting, dot blotting, and immunoprecipitation (Gross, ClinExpImmun, 1993; 91:1). The first and most widely employed method is indirect immunofluorescence on ethanol-fixed human granulocytes. Its reliability depends on the quality of the substrate, the incubation conditions, the washing steps, and the experience in interpreting the ANCA pattern. In conclusion, no specific ANCA antigens have been demonstrated in liver diseases, nor has it been demonstrated that the detection of ANCA is of clinical significance. Indirect immunofluorescence is still the method of choice until a specific autoantigen is found.

Cellular immune reactions

T-cell mediated immune reactions are relevant for the pathogenesis of virus-induced liver diseases as well as for autoimmune liver diseases.[17,18] It is possible that an autoantibody-mediated cytotoxicity is involved in the pathogenesis of autoimmune hepatitis. The role of liver cell damage mediated by antibodies and complement directed against viral antigens and autoantigens has not yet been extensively studied. Methods analysing the various functions of the cellular immune system are rather complicated and their diagnostic relevance is limited. T lymphocytes have been isolated from liver tissue showing antigen specificity for autoantigens recognized by disease-associated autoantibodies such as the asialoglycoprotein receptor, cytochrome P-450 2D6, and the mitochondrial acyltransferases, in particular the E2 subunit of pyruvate dehydrogenase. In recent years the T-cell epitopes for viral antigens have been identified in acute and chronic hepatitis B and C. A strong helper T-cell response is seen in self-limited acute hepatitis B. These helper and cytotoxic T-cell responses are directed against various epitopes expressed on the core as well as the S and the preS antigen and the HBV DNA polymerase. While the cytotoxic and helper T-cell responses are strong in self-limited acute hepatitis B, they are weak or absent in chronic hepatitis B. In contrast, strong cytotoxic and helper T-cell responses are seen in acute and chronic hepatitis C against numerous viral epitopes. A helper T-cell response against the non-structural region NS3 of the hepatitis C virus is associated with viral clearance. (For further details see Chapters 12.1.2.3 and 12.1.2.5 or recent review articles.)[19]

Immune complexes

Circulating immune complexes can be detected by various techniques, including the Raji cell test and the C1q binding assay. In primary biliary cirrhosis as well as in primary sclerosing cholangitis an increased prevalence of circulating immune complexes has been detected. Some antigens involved in these complexes have been identified, such as the SSB/Ro antigen in primary biliary cirrhosis (Penner, Gastro, 1986; 90:724). However, the detection of circulating immune complexes does not help in therapeutic management.

Immunoglobulins

The quantitative evaluation of immunoglobulin classes is of diagnostic value in primary biliary cirrhosis, in which IgM immunoglobulins are increased. This is due to an insufficient switch of synthesis from IgM to IgG antibody formation that usually occurs in natural infections. Furthermore, low IgA levels have been found in LKM antibody-positive autoimmune hepatitis type 2. IgA levels are increased in alcohol-induced liver disease. In autoimmune hepatitis, polyclonal hypergammaglobulinaemia is an established diagnostic criterion. Sometimes monoclonal gammopathy is associated with autoimmune hepatitis.

Clinical relevance of immunological investigations in liver diseases

Autoantibody testing is well established in everyday clinical practice. Once the diagnosis of chronic liver disease is made, antinuclear antibodies, smooth muscle antibodies, liver–kidney microsomal antibodies, and antimitochondrial antibodies should be tested. These are tested by indirect immunofluorescence on rodent liver, kidney, and stomach tissue in a routine laboratory. Immunofluorescence testing for ANA is sufficient for clinical diagnosis, although this method cannot distinguish different antigen–antibody systems. A further identification of the antigen specificity is not feasible for ANA. The costly determination of the various antigen specificities for ANA does not provide information that would influence the management of the patient. The same is true for the specificity of SMA. However, F-actin based assays may become useful in the future. If liver–kidney or liver microsomal antibody testing is positive by immunofluorescence, a further definition of the antigen specificity is diagnostically helpful (Table 2). Serum may be shipped to specialized laboratories capable of identifying the antigen specificity of such microsomal antibodies. In the case of microsomal autoantibodies, namely LKM-1 to -3 or LM, the distinction between autoimmune hepatitis and viral hepatitis C and D is of particular relevance concerning the choice of either antiviral or immunosuppressive treatment. On the other hand, the identification of drug-induced liver disease and autoimmune polyendocrine syndrome type 1 (**APS-1**) is particularly helpful for the individual patient, although immune-mediated drug-induced liver diseases as well as APS-1 are rare.

Antibodies to cytosolic antigens, such as anti-SLA and anti-LP, are only detectable by radioimmunoassay or enzyme immunoassay. Furthermore, these assays are not widely used or available. Clinically, these antibodies may be helpful in isolated cases where the diagnosis of autoimmune hepatitis is difficult and the usual autoantibody markers are negative. Antibodies to the asialoglycoprotein receptor may have a similar diagnostic relevance. Anti-LC1 and anti-LC2 are also cytosolic antibodies, but their antigen specificity has not been identified yet. Usually they occur together with LKM-1 antibodies in autoimmune hepatitis type 2.

Antimitochondrial antibodies are among the most specific autoantibodies in medicine and they are detected by immunofluorescence. If AMA are positive by immunofluorescence, at least assays with specificity for anti-PDC-E2 antibodies should be used to support the diagnosis of primary biliary cirrhosis. Anti-PDC-E2 antibodies are found in up to 95 per cent of patients with primary biliary cirrhosis, but it is still unclear whether they occur in other diseases. The determination of antibodies against the other mitochondrial acyltransferases (Table 3) may be helpful if anti-PDC-E2 assays are negative despite a positive AMA immunofluorescence test. Studies have suggested that certain subtypes of AMA specific for primary biliary cirrhosis are diagnostic markers for a more aggressive course of the disease. These data have not been confirmed. Therefore, at present, a determination of the various subtypes of AMA specific for this disease cannot be recommended for everyday clinical practice.

Antineutrophilic cytoplasmic antibodies may underline the diagnosis of primary sclerosing cholangitis. However, the diagnostic 'gold standard' for primary sclerosing cholangitis still is endoscopic retrograde cholangiopancreatography. Since the antigen specificity of ANCA in liver diseases is not well defined yet, and ANCA are not specific for a particular liver disease, it is premature to include them in the panel of diagnostically relevant autoantibodies for liver diseases.

Autoantibodies are useful as markers for the diagnosis of autoimmune hepatitis. They may be used to classify autoimmune hepatitis further into various subgroups. They are very helpful in the diagnosis of primary biliary cirrhosis. Anti-PDC-E2 antibodies are the most specific and sensitive diagnostic marker for primary biliary cirrhosis. Furthermore, hepatitis C and D may be associated with autoantibodies also seen in autoimmune hepatitis. Such autoimmune phenomena observed in viral hepatitis may identify patients whose condition is at risk of exacerbation by specific antiviral treatment, including an increase in aminotransferases under interferon therapy. Although autoantibodies in autoimmune and viral liver diseases may identify the same antigen, autoepitopes seem to differ between autoimmune liver disease and viral hepatitis C or D. In a rare group of drug-induced liver diseases the pathogenesis seems to be immune mediated. However, once LKM antibodies are detectable in serum, they should be further analysed regarding their antigen specificity. Antigens like cytochrome P-450 1A2, which is a target in dihydralazine-induced hepatitis, or P-450 2C9, which is associated with tienilic acid-induced hepatitis, may be helpful. Very recently, cytochrome P-450 2E1 was identified as an autoantigen for autoantibodies in alcoholic liver disease and halothane hepatitis (Table 2). Antibodies to the asialoglycoprotein receptor may help to diagnose autoimmune liver disease if the classic autoantibody markers are negative. The ASGPR antigen is of particular interest in studies on the pathogenesis of liver diseases as it is liver specific and membrane expressed.

The analysis of the antigen specificity for tissue-infiltrating T lymphocytes is an area of intensive research concerning the pathogenesis of all inflammatory liver diseases. However, the analysis of the T-cell response to either autoantigens or viral antigens is not useful yet for the management of the patient and should not be performed routinely. Determination of immune complexes and complement turnover studies are nowadays not necessary for the diagnosis nor for the follow-up of patients with liver diseases. In contrast, the determination of the immunoglobulins IgG, IgM, and IgA is useful in liver diseases. In the future, ELISA systems based on recombinant antigens will further improve the differential diagnosis of liver diseases.

References

1. Nishioka M. Nuclear antigens in autoimmune hepatitis. In Meyer zum Büschenfelde KH, Hoofnagle J, and Manns M, eds. *Immunology and liver*. Dordrecht: Kluwer Academic Publishers, 1993: 193–205.
2. Kurki P. Cytoskeleton antibodies in chronic active hepatitis. In Meyer zum Büschenfelde KH, Hoofnagle J, and Manns M, eds. *Immunology and liver*. Dordrecht: Kluwer Academic Publishers, 1993: 206–14.
3. Czaja AJ, Cassani F, Cataleta M, Valenti P, and Bianchi FB. Frequency and significance of antibodies to actin in type 1 autoimmune hepatitis. *Hepatology*, 1996; **24**: 1068–73.
4. Homberg JC, *et al.* Chronic active hepatitis associated with anti-liver/kidney microsome antibody type I: a second type of 'autoimmune hepatitis'. *Hepatology*, 1987; **7**: 1333–9.
5. Rizzetto M, Swana G, and Doniach D. Microsomal antibodies in active chronic hepatitis and other disorders. *Clinical and Experimental Immunology*, 1973; **15**: 331–44.
6. Manns MP, Griffin KJ, Sullivan KF, and Johnson EF. LKM-1 autoantibodies recognize a short linear sequence in P-450 2D6, a cytochrome P-450 monooxygenase. *Journal of Clinical Investigation*, 1991; **88**: 1370–8.
7. Yamamoto AM, Crestil D, Homberg JC, and Alvarez F. Characterization of anti-liver–kidney microsome antibody (anti-LKM-1) from hepatitis C virus positive and negative sera. *Gastroenterology*, 1993; **104**: 1762–7.
8. Crivelli O *et al.* Microsomal autoantibodies in chronic infection with HBsAg associated delta (δ) agent. *Clinical and Experimental Immunology*, 1983; **54**: 232–8.
9. Philipp T, *et al.* LKM-3 autoantibodies in chronic hepatitis D recognize the UDP-glucuronosyltransferases. *Lancet*, 1994; **344**: 578–81.
10. Clemente MG, *et al.* Cytochrome P-450 1A2 is a hepatic autoantigen in autoimmune polyglandular syndrome type 1. *Journal of Clinical Endocrinology and Metabolism*, 1997; **82**: 1853–61.
11. McFarlane IG, McFarlane B, Major GN, Tolley P, and Williams R. Identification of the hepatic receptor (hepatic lectin) as a component of liver specific membrane lipoprotein (LSP). *Clinical and Experimental Immunology*, 1984; **55**: 347–54.
12. Treichel U, *et al.* Demographics of anti-asialoglycoprotein receptor autoantibodies in autoimmune hepatitis. *Gastroenterology*, 1994; **107**: 799–804.
13. Gershwin ME, Mackay IR, Sturgess A, and Coppel RL. Identification and specificity of a cDNA encoding the 70 kDa mitochondrial autoantigen recognized in primary biliary cirrhosis. *Journal of Immunology*, 1987; **138**: 3525–31.
14. Yeaman SJ, Danner DJ, Mutimer DJ, Fussey SPM, James OFW, and Bassendine MF. Primary biliary cirrhosis: identification of two major M2 mitochondrial autoantigens. *Lancet*, 1988; **i**: 1067–70.
15. Davis P, *et al.* M4 and M9 antibodies in the overlap syndrome of primary biliary cirrhosis and chronic active hepatitis: epitopes or epiphenomena? *Hepatology*, 1992; **16**: 1128–36.
16. Orth T, Gerken G, Kellner R, Meyer zum Büschenfelde K-H, and Mayet W-J. Actin is a target antigen of anti-neutrophil cytoplasmic antibody (ANCA) in AIH type 1. *Journal of Hepatology*, 1997; **26**: 37.
17. Rehermann B. Immunopathogenesis of viral hepatitis. In Manns MP, ed. *Liver and gastrointestinal immunology. Baillière's Clinical Gastroenterology*, Vol. 10. London: Baillière Tindall, 1996.
18. Galperin C and Gershwin ME. Immunopathology of primary biliary cirrhosis. In Manns MP, ed. *Liver and gastrointestinal immunology. Baillière's Clinical Gastroenterology*, Vol. 10. London: Baillière Tindall, 1996: 461–81.
19. Manns MP. *Liver and gastrointestinal immunology. Baillière's Clinical Gastroenterology*, Vol. 10. London: Baillière Tindall, 1996.

5.4 Biopsy and laparoscopy

5.4.1 Liver biopsy

Françoise Degos and Jean-Pierre Benhamou

Despite advances in imaging procedures and laboratory investigations, histological examination of a liver specimen remains essential for the diagnosis of most diseases of the liver and intrahepatic bile ducts (Morisod, SchMedWoch, 1988; 118:125). In addition, special investigations (such as special stainings; measurement of enzyme activities; culture or inoculation for the demonstration of fungal, bacterial, rickettsial, or protozoal infections; chemical analysis for the measurement of iron or copper content) can be performed on liver specimens for the diagnosis of certain conditions. As liver biopsy is an invasive procedure, purely scientific investigations cannot, *per se*, be an indication for it, but it can be performed ethically on part of a liver specimen when another part is required for diagnostic purposes.

Liver biopsy must be performed by a trained, experienced physician for the procedure to be safe and for a large liver specimen to be obtained.[1,2] The main purpose of liver biopsy is a useful interpretation of lesions by a histopathologist familiar with the pathology of the liver.

The main problem is the choice of an adequate procedure for liver biopsy in a particular patient, in order that an accurate diagnosis be obtained (Fig. 1). The availability of ultrasound-guided biopsy and the transvenous approach make liver biopsy a feasible diagnostic procedure, without major risks in most cases.

Techniques

The choice of the technique of liver biopsy is dictated by coagulation disorders, the presence of ascites, and the results of the previous ultrasound examination. One must then consider the ability of the patient to co-operate; general anaesthesia can be used in children

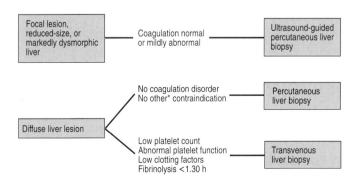

Fig. 1. Indications for the different techniques of liver biopsy. *Contraindications include dilatation of intrahepatic ducts, amyloidosis, myeloproliferative disorders, and emphysema.

and psychotic patients. In all other cases the procedure is carried out under local anaesthesia. Sedation with 10 mg of diazepam (sublingual or intramuscularly) and premedication with atropine to avoid vagal shock are often used. The patient's blood group should be known and facilities for blood transfusion must always be available.

Before making a decision for a liver biopsy, results of two important tests must be available—the coagulation tests (see Chapter 25.4) and the ultrasound examination of the liver. The exploration of haemostasis must include: (i) platelet count (Sharma, JClinGastro, 1982; 4:451), (ii) bleeding time by a sensitive method (Ivy), (iii) measurements of prothrombin time and, when possible, of factors II, VII + X, and V levels, (iv) measurement of activated partial thromboplastin time (**APTT**), and (v) fibrinolytic activity (euglobulin lysis time). One must be aware that in patients with uraemia or a high gammaglobulin level, a prolonged bleeding time is common, even in patients with a normal platelet count; this disorder is due to an acquired thrombopathy. Combined deficiencies of factors II, VII + X, and V are common in liver disease, and are responsible for a prolonged APTT. Percutaneous liver biopsy is not contraindicated if the levels of these factors are 50 per cent or more of normal values. APTT must not exceed 1.5 times the control value. Isolated prolonged APTT contraindicates liver biopsy and requires further investigation.

Fibrinolysis must also be checked, especially in patients with cirrhosis (Violi, Hepatol, 1993; 17:78). The euglobulin lysis time must be above 3 h. When the euglobulin lysis time is slightly shortened (ranging from 1.5 to 3 h), it can be corrected transiently before liver biopsy either by infusion of aprotinine (with special attention to the risk of allergic or anaphylactic reactions) or with lysin analogues (with special attention to contraindications of the product).

Ultrasound examination of the liver must be performed in every patient before liver biopsy. Information provided by ultrasound examination contributes to the choice of procedure for liver biopsy and is essential in recognizing two contraindications to blind liver biopsy, namely the dilatation of intrahepatic bile ducts (Conn, Gastro, 1975; 68:817) and presence of a hydatic cyst. Moreover, the size of the right lobe of the liver and the absence of vascular tumours (haemangiomas) must be assessed by ultrasound examination. Amyloidosis and myeloproliferative disorders (Nelson, AnnIntMed, 1960; 53:179) are relative contraindications to percutaneous biopsy: in such conditions the transvenous route is considered safer than the percutaneous route. Severe emphysema is also a relative contraindication since it does not allow a safe evaluation of the size and position of the liver by percussion; in such patients, ultrasound-guided biopsy is required. Moreover, the occurrence of pneumothorax in a patient with previous respiratory failure can be dangerous. When a biopsy is decided upon for the diagnosis of a space-occupying lesion, it must be guided by ultrasound.

With the disposable Menghini needle, a liver tissue specimen is obtained by aspiration; the diameter of the Menghini needle usually employed ranges from 1.4 to 1.8 mm.[1] With the Tru-cut needle (2G), the liver specimen is obtained without aspiration; the diameter of the needle is 2.05 mm. The former procedure is easier, quicker, and cheaper than the latter, although it more often yields a fragmented specimen (Bateson, JClinPath, 1980; 33:131); identification of cirrhosis is made more frequently on a specimen obtained with the Tru-cut needle than with a Menghini needle (Vargas-Tank, Liver, 1985; 5:178; Colombo, Gastro, 1988; 95:548).

The intercostal route is the most common approach. The size of the liver is assessed by light percussion or ultrasound examination. The 8th or 9th intercostal space on the midaxillary line is generally chosen for the puncture site. After adequate local anaesthesia, with careful infiltration of 5 to 10 ml of lignocaine into the different layers (subcutaneous tissue, intercostal space, diaphragm, and capsule of the liver), the patient is taught how to exhale fully. Then after checking the efficacy of local anaesthesia, the needle is inserted in the intercostal space (the direction is slightly cranial to avoid the gallbladder) and is advanced into the liver and rapidly withdrawn, while the patient maintains the expiration position. The specimen is discharged from the needle into the appropriate solution.

Percutaneous guided liver biopsy

If a focal lesion is recognized by ultrasound examination (or by computed tomography), or if the small size of the liver makes the blind transparietal biopsy uncertain, an ultrasound-guided biopsy is required. The recommended procedure has been controversial, but a consensus has now been reached (Menu, GastrClinBiol, 1988; 12:505). The needles used are similar to those used for the blind percutaneous liver biopsy (14 to 18G). Some workers use a thin needle, similar to the Chiba needle which provides small specimens for cytological, and sometimes histological, study (Sangalli, Gastro, 1989; 96:524).

Percutaneous liver biopsy can be CT guided (Martino, Radiol, 1984; 152:755), although from a practical point of view, ultrasound guiding is much easier.

In centres where laparoscopy is available, liver biopsy can be guided under the control of the operator's sight. Laparoscopically guided biopsy can be especially useful for sampling tumours located at the anterior surface of the liver (Fornari, GastrEnd, 1988; 34:231).

Percutaneous plugged liver biopsy

When coagulation disorders do not allow conventional percutaneous biopsy, and when the transvenous approach is not available or has been unsuccessful, the injection of 2 ml of gelatin sponge through the cannula of a Tru-cut needle has been used (Riley, Lancet, 1984; ii:436; Tobin, Lancet, 1984; ii:694; Tobin, DigDisSci, 1989; 34:13; Sawyer, Gut, 1989; 30:A746). Embolization of the biopsy track with steel coils has also been proposed (Allison, Radiol, 1988; 169:261). However, these procedures do not completely avoid the risk of significant bleeding in patients with severe coagulation disorders (Sawyerr, JHepatol; 17:81).

Transvenous transjugular approach[3,4]

The transvenous liver biopsy is performed after an overnight fast, when the patient is positioned supinely. The right internal jugular vein is punctured under local anaesthesia. When venous blood is aspirated, a vessel dilator with a polypropylene sheath is introduced percutaneously into the lumen of the jugular vein according to the Seldinger technique. The transvenous catheter is then introduced into the sheath and guided into the right hepatic vein under fluoroscopic control. The transvenous biopsy needle is slipped inside the catheter and advanced down to the tip of the catheter. When a correct position of the tip of the needle is confrmed by injection of contrast medium, the needle is rapidly advanced 1 to 2 cm beyond the tip of the catheter and withdrawn. The specimen of hepatic tissue is retained within the needle by a strong suction on a syringe connected to the needle.

Open-abdomen liver biopsy

A liver biopsy can be performed safely during intra-abdominal surgery (Michel, ArchSurg, 1977; 112:959). Haemostasis is easy to achieve. Wedge liver biopsy is usually performed. The reliability of open-abdomen liver biopsy is enhanced by performing a needle liver biopsy simultaneously (Menghini, AmJSurg, 1977; 133:383). A laparotomy for surgical biopsy should be considered in a small number of cases: (i) when a percutaneous or transvenous approach is contraindicated or has not been contributive, and (ii) when a large specimen is needed. It is important to take a sample of adequate size as the material may be unsuitable for histological examination if it is too close to the capsule.

Fine-needle aspiration of the liver

This technique, usually performed under ultrasound guidance by a radiologist, uses either 20- or 22-gauge needles. Numerous passes (as many as six) may be undertaken to achieve a satisfactory sample (Axe, AmJClinPath, 1986; 86:281). Tissue samples obtained by fine-needle aspiration allow cytological diagnosis; however, histological examination of small tissue specimens is sometimes possible and may contribute to the accuracy of the diagnosis (Farnum, JClinGastro, 1989; 11:101; Bolzio, JHepatol, 1994; 20:117).

The main advantage of fine-needle aspiration is that complications occur less frequently than with conventional liver biopsy. However, fine-needle aspiration has two limitations: (i) it cannot be used for the diagnosis of non-tumorous liver disease, and (ii) accuracy in the diagnosis of liver tumour is less than that of conventional liver biopsy (Seitz, GastrClinBiol, 1990; 14:529).

After-care of percutaneous and transvenous liver biopsy

The pulse rate and blood pressure should be recorded twice an hour for the first 6 h and every 3 h during the following 24 h; the physician should be called if a rise in pulse rate or a decrease in blood pressure is observed. Bed rest is essential for 24 h although some studies have reported safe liver biopsy without serious complications on a day-care basis (Knauer, Gastro, 1978; 74:101; Westaby, BMJ, 1980; 281:331; Jones, AnnIntMed, 1993; 118:96), with monitoring after biopsy for 3 h and discharge of the patient 6 h

Table 1 Contraindications to percutaneous liver biopsy
Amyloidosis Myeloproliferative blood diseases Extrahepatic cholestasis with intrahepatic bile duct dilatation Hydatic cyst Congestive liver Hypervascular tumours Rendu Osler disease

Table 2 Complications following liver biopsy

Complications after blind percutaneous liver biopsy
  Pain immediately or during the hours following the biopsy
  Vagal shock
  Bleeding: intraperitoneal, intrahepatic bleeding
  Intrahepatic arteriovenous fistula, haemobilia
  Pleural effusion: haemothorax, pneumothorax.
  Puncture of other organs: gallbladder, kidney, colon, and small
    intestine
  Sepsis: bacteraemia, septicaemia
  Reaction to anaesthetics
  Breaking the needle
  ? Cutaneous, muscular, intraperitoneous diffusion of malignant
    cells
 	
Complications of transvenous liver biopsy
  Haematoma at the site of puncture
  Transient Horner's syndrome, transient dysphonia
  Pneumothorax
  Supraventricular tachycardia
  Transient abdominal pain
  Perforation of the liver capsule: symptomatic (haemoperitoneum),
    or asymptomatic (aspiration of ascitic fluid during the
    procedure)

after the procedure. Recommendations have recently been made regarding liver biopsy in outpatient departments; this procedure is acceptable only: (i) when the patient can easily return within 30 min to the hospital where the biopsy was performed, (ii) if the patient has a reliable companion during the first postbiopsy night, and (iii) if the patient has no associated medical problem (Jacobs, DigDisSci, 1989; 34:322). The use of ultrasonography guided biopsy may lead to a lower rate of complications (Lindor, Hepatol, 1996; 23:1079).

Liver biopsy after liver transplantation

Liver biopsy is a frequently used diagnostic tool in transplantation centres. The experience of the Pittsburg centre, based on 12 750 liver biopsies, was reported (Van Thiel, Transpl, 1993; 55:1087) and showed that this procedure can be carried out safely; complications (arterioportal fistulas) occurred in 0.1 to 3.6 per cent of cases and required surgery or interventional radiological procedures that resulted in additional morbidity (Jabbour, DigDisSci, 1995; 40:1041). Patients with a choledochojejunostomy are no longer considered at particular risk of sepsis (Ben-Ari, JHepatol, 1996; 24:324).

Contraindications to blind percutaneous biopsy

Contraindications to blind percutaneous biopsy are well defined. Other techniques are now available to obtain a liver tissue specimen in patients in whom blind percutaneous biopsy is contraindicated.

Severe coagulation disorders, hydatid cyst, and intrahepatic bile dilation are regarded as contraindications. Liver biopsy of a superficial vascularized tumour is potentially dangerous. Transvenous liver biopsy should be preferred to percutaneous biopsy in amyloidosis, congestive liver disorders (heart failure, veno-occlusive disease, and peliosis), and in myeloproliferative disorders (Table 1).

Complications and risk[5–7]

The morbidity and mortality of liver biopsy are difficult to ascertain as large series of liver biopsies are no longer published. In two large series, the mortality was 0.015 per cent (Lindner, MedKlin, 1971; 66:924; Piccinino, JHepatol, 1986; 2:165). It is certain that ultrasound examination systematically performed before liver biopsy and in patients with complications induced by liver biopsy has improved the management and reduced the mortality (Henderström, JHepatol, 1989; 8:94). In a recent series, the rate of complications in liver biopsy was related mainly to the experience and training of the operator (Froehlich, DigDisSci, 1993; 38:1480). Table 2 summarizes the complications following liver biopsy.

Pain

Transient pain in the upper right quadrant and/or the tip of the right shoulder and epigastric discomfort are common after liver biopsy, and only require administration of paracetamol. More severe pain is likely to indicate a subcapsular accumulation of blood or bile. Very severe pain of sudden onset suggests biliary peritonitis due to puncture of the gallbladder.

Vagal shock

This common complication affects mainly young, neurotonic patients. It can be prevented partly by the administration of atropine before liver biopsy. When there are bradycardia and sweats, subcutaneous or intravenous administration of 0.25 mg atropine is again required.

Bleeding

Severe bleeding is usually intraperitoneal, but may be intrathoracic from an intercostal artery. Bleeding can result from the perforation of a distended portal vein, the direct puncture of the hepatic artery or its intrahepatic branches, or a tear of the liver following deep breathing during the procedure. Clinically significant haemorrhage has been reported in 0.2 per cent of over 7000 biopsies: four patients required laparotomy (Terry, BMJ, 1952; i:1102). Haemorrhage after liver biopsy should be managed initially with blood transfusion, and haemodynamic and haematocrit monitoring. However, persistent hypotension, increasing abdominal distension, or increasing volume of the intraperitoneal haemorrhage detected at ultrasound examination are indications for laparotomy by a surgeon trained in difficult hepatic surgery. Delayed haemorrhage has been observed up to 15 days (Reichert, JClinGastro, 1983; 5:263) or even 30 days (personal experience) after liver biopsy.

Intrahepatic haematoma

Intrahepatic haematoma (Forsell, DigDisSci, 1981; 26:631; Raines, Gastro, 1974; 67:284) is usually asymptomatic, but can induce fever, and/or a rise in serum aminotransaminases, and/or diminution of haematocrit. Intrahepatic haematoma can be detected easily by ultrasound examination. Occasionally, haematoma can be followed by delayed intraperitoneal haemorrhage.

Intrahepatic arteriovenous fistula

Intrahepatic arteriovenous fistula (shown by hepatic arteriography) follows 5.4 per cent of liver biopsies (Okuda, Gastro, 1978; 74:1204; Satava, Gastro, 1975; 69:492), but is usually asymptomatic. A bruit may be audible; spontaneous closure of small fistulas is frequent.

Haemobilia

Haemobilia results from rupture of an intrahepatic haematoma into a bile duct. It can develop at any time between 1 and 21 days after the liver biopsy (Attiyeh, Radiol, 1976; 118:559; Lee, Gastro, 1977; 72:941), and is indicated by biliary pain, jaundice, and melaena. The use of a fine needle for aspiration of the liver does not prevent the occurrence of the complication (Verhille, Gastro, 1991; 101: 1731). Ultrasound examination may raise suspicion of the diagnosis. The best evidence is provided by hepatic arteriography which demonstrates the pseudoaneurysm. The treatment is arterial embolization.

Pneumothorax

Pneumothorax, resulting from a lesion of the lower part of the right lung, can develop early after liver biopsy. When limited, pneumothorax requires no treatment.

Puncture of the gallbladder or intrahepatic dilated bile duct

This complication affects patients with an unusually positioned gallbladder or with a small cirrhotic liver. The patient complains of severe abdominal pain and hypotension during the minutes following the biopsy. Biliary peritonitis is usually self-limited, and should be managed conservatively with analgesics and antibiotics. Occasionally, surgical repair is required. Bile peritonitis may result from the puncture of a dilated intrahepatic bile duct. The risk of puncture of the gallbladder or a dilated intrahepatic bile duct should be markedly reduced if an ultrasound examination is performed before a liver biopsy. Moreover, a small meal before a liver biopsy would empty the gallbladder and avoid the risk of puncture.

Puncture of other organs

Other organs can be punctured, usually because of incorrect positioning of the needle. Most common is puncture of the colon, which can be detected when aspiration through the needle obtains intestinal fluid. Puncture of the kidney, pancreas, or adrenal glands is recognized at histological examination of the specimen.

Transient bacteraemia and septicaemia

The prevalence of bacteraemia in a prospective series of 69 liver biopsies was 5.8 per cent (McCloskey, ArchIntMed, 1973; 132: 213); in one-half of the patients, bacteraemia was asymptomatic. Septicaemia is uncommon after liver biopsy, but it has been reported in patients with cirrhosis or with cholangitis (Loludic, Gastro, 1977; 72:949); because of the risk of septicaemia, patients with valvular heart disease should receive prophylactic antibiotic cover before and after liver biopsy.

Tumorous dissemination

Well-documented subcutaneous implantation of hepatic tumour has been reported after liver biopsy (Davies, JAMA, 1968; 205:700; Evans, Lancet, 1987; i:620); this complication is uncommon and is not related to the size of the needle, as it has been reported after fine needle aspiration (Vergara, JHepatol, 1993; 18:276). Neoplastic seeding has also been reported following ethanol injection procedures, either for primary hepatocellular carcinomas or for liver metastases (Cedrone, Radiol, 1992; 183:787; Goletti, Radiol, 1992; 183:785). Intraperitoneal dissemination of tumorous tissue from the site of puncture of the liver is a possible, but not well-documented, complication; however, because of the risk of this complication, a few liver specialists are reluctant to perform liver biopsy when the diagnosis is otherwise obvious (John, HBPSurgery, 1993; 6:199).

Complications of transvenous liver biopsy

Transvenous liver biopsy can be regarded as a remarkably safe procedure. Large haematomas at the site of puncture of the jugular vein have been reported, especially if the puncture of the vein has been difficult. Transient Horner's syndrome and transient dysphonia have been described. Pneumothorax can be caused by puncturing the lung with the guide. Perforation of the liver capsule (from inside) may occur in patients with a small liver; in such cases, intraperitoneal haemorrhage may develop and massive intraperitoneal bleeding has resulted in the death of a patient with cirrhosis (Lebrec, Gastro, 1982; 83:338).

Reliability and representativeness of needle biopsy

Most liver lesions such as cholestasis, cirrhosis, chronic hepatitis, and acute hepatitis are diffuse, and a large enough specimen (i.e. containing at least four portal spaces) is representative of the whole liver. This is true for micronodular, but not necessarily for macronodular, cirrhosis. The distribution of granulomas within the liver is not regular and therefore serial sections are needed; granulomas may be present in one preparation and absent in another.

In some cases of diffuse hepatic lesion, the specimen, although of adequate size, may be considered normal erroneously. This situation occurs mainly in three conditions: (i) macronodular cirrhosis, (ii) regenerative nodular hyperplasia, and (iii) idiopathic portal hypertension (with perisinusoidal fibrosis recognized only on electron microscopic examination).

Preparation of the specimen

The specimen (about 1 to 3 cm in length) is usually fixed in 4 per cent neutral, buffered formaldehyde solution (10 per cent formalin) or in Bouin solution. The former is most commonly used but gives minor artefacts. The latter provides a very satisfactory light microscopic picture, but is not convenient for most histochemical investigations. Fixation should be maintained for at least 3 h at room temperature, or in case of emergency for 1 h at 37°C. With Bouin solution, fixation must be prolonged. The choice of routine stains varies according to the preferences of the pathologist. Haematoxylin and eosin staining, staining for collagen (Masson trichrome, or aniline blue chromotrope), and staining for reticulin (Gordon–Sweet method) are essential. Other staining may be requested, such as Perl's blue method for iron, rubanic acid for copper, or periodic acid–Schiff after diastase digestion for the demonstration of some intracytoplasmic globules in liver or Kupffer cells.

Characterization of fatty cells and especially microvesicular steatosis requires immediate deep-frozen samples for Oil Red-O staining; this technique must be decided upon before biopsy as the routine method of fixation must be avoided.

Specimens for electron microscopic studies are fixed briefly in glutaraldehyde solution, and preserved thereafter in solution at 4°C. Specimens for immunofluorescence techniques are usually deep-frozen immediately and placed in liquid nitrogen.

Interpretation and use of liver biopsy in clinical research

The quality of the interpretation of liver biopsy depends on the skill and experience of the pathologist (Theodossi, Gastro, 1980; 79: 232). However, the specimen should be at least 2 cm in length and a reliable evaluation of the liver structure can be given only if at least four portal zones can be examined. The reliability of the biopsy depends not only on the size of the liver specimen (Holund, ScaJGastr, 1980; 155:329), but also on the distribution of the lesions within the liver; in the case of diffuse disease, the lesions can be recognized by the examination of a small fragment; when the distribution is irregular, the interpretation is much more difficult. The recommendation that at least three preparations be examined certainly improves the diagnostic yield (Maharaj, Lancet, 1986; i: 523).

Transvenous liver biopsy has been found to be an efficient procedure, yielding a hepatic tissue specimen in most patients (in our experience more than 98 per cent). Hepatic tissue specimens obtained with transvenous liver biopsy are smaller than those obtained with percutaneous biopsy, because the diameter of the needle used is smaller than that of a Menghini needle or a Vim-Silverman needle. Moreover, the transvenous needle is advanced only 1 to 2 cm into the liver parenchyma. The hepatic tissue specimen, however, has been found to be large enough to allow correct evaluation of liver architecture in 99 per cent of patients without fibrotic lesions and in 75 per cent of patients with extensive fibrosis or cirrhosis. In 25 per cent of patients with extensive fibrosis or cirrhosis, the specimen of hepatic tissue was small or fragmented, and the liver architecture could not be assessed.

Liver samples are of great interest in clinical research as some immunofluorescence techniques can be used not only on frozen

Table 3 What can be studied with a liver specimen?

Immunohistology
Biochemical measurements (iron, copper)
Enzyme activity
Microbiological cultures
Virological cultures
DNA or RNA extraction for virological purposes (HBV DNA, HDV RNA, etc.)

sections (the most reliable technique) but also on paraffin-embedded sections: various antibodies can be used, such as mono- or polyclonal antibodies against HBV antigens, and various cellular infiltrates (e.g. antilymphocyte antibodies) can be sampled. Liver fragments can also be used in Southern blotting for the detection and analysis of HBV DNA or in polymerase chain reaction techniques for the detection and quantification of HCV RNA. Table 3 lists some studies performed on liver specimens.

References

1. Perrault J, McGill DB, Ott BJ, and Taylor WF. Liver biopsy: complications in 1000 inpatients and outpatients. *Gastroenterology*, 1978; **74**: 103–6.
2. Menghini G. One second biopsy of the liver; problems of its clinical application. *New England Journal of Medicine*, 1970; **283**: 582–5.
3. McAffe JH, Keeffe EB, Lee RG, and Rösch, J. Transjugular liver biopsy. *Hepatology*, 1992; **15**: 726–32.
4. Lebrec D, Goldfarb G, Degott C, Rueff B, and Benhamou JP. Transvenous liver biopsy; an experience based on 1000 hepatic tissue samplings with this procedure. *Gastroenterology*, 1982; **83**: 338–40.
5. Piccinino F, Sagnelli E, Pasquale G, and Guisti G. Complications following percutaneous liver biopsy; a multicentre retrospective study on 68 276 biopsies. *Journal of Hepatology*, 1986; **2**: 165–73.
6. Hegarty JE and Williams R. Liver biopsy: techniques, clinical applications and complications. *British Medical Journal*, 1984; **288**: 1254–6.
7. Sherlock S, Dick R, and Van Leeuwen DJ. Liver biopsy today. The Royal Free Hospital experience. *Journal of Hepatology*, 1984; **1**: 75–85.

5.4.2 Laparoscopy

Alberto Ferrari and Federico Manenti

Introduction

Laparoscopy is an old technique. It is employed widely throughout medicine in such differing fields as hepatology, gynaecology, and oncology. Its popularity as a diagnostic tool is more the result of tradition than the consequence of a rational evaluation of its usefulness. In hepatology, to the best of our knowledge, and with some oversimplification, it is largely used in Germany, Italy, and France; in the United States it has been the object of interest only recently, and in the United Kingdom it is used very little.

Instrumentation

Instrumentation has become standardized: two types of endoscope are used universally, having either a lateral or frontal view. The latter has an operative channel for endoscopic manoeuvres. The introduction of optical fibres and the wider practice of laparoscopic surgery have made the manoeuvres easier but there has been no real improvement in the diagnostic efficacy. Very high magnification lenses for close observation, although able to produce magnificent images, represent no true diagnostic advantage. Laparography is now an integral part of the examination. Cine photography during the procedure has no place except for didactic reasons.

Needles for biopsy, probes for liver palpation, cutters to improve the visual field in the presence of adhesions, and probes for electro-coagulation can be used through the operating laparascope as required.

The technique[1]

The standard procedure is well established. It differs from other gastrointestinal endoscopic techniques in requiring a pneumo-peritoneum and an artificial hole in the abdominal wall. The pneumoperitoneum is obtained with a Verres needle. This has a hollow internal cannula with a rounded end which stays retracted during penetration of the wall and protrudes immediately on entering the peritoneal cavity, thus avoiding lesions to the viscera.

The examination may be performed under light sedation; general anaesthesia is required only for very anxious or very young patients. Before insertion of the laparoscope, a pneumoperitoneum of the correct tension is created. The right paraumbilical approach is usually employed for the insertion of the laparoscope, as being the best compromise for the exploration of both liver lobes. However, when the usual entrance site is impeded due to the size of the liver or the presence of surgical scars, other insertion points can be used; the projection sites of the round ligament and the hypogastric vessels must be avoided because of the risk of vascular lesions. It is advisable to explore the whole thickness of the abdominal wall with a fine needle, in order to exclude the presence of enlarged veins, before inserting the laparoscope. The umbilical entrance, preferred by gynaecologists for aesthetic reasons, is not recommended in liver disease because it is possible that a patent umbilical vein will be perforated.

It is advisable to examine the different intraperitoneal organs in a standard sequence to guarantee thorough inspection. The pneumoperitoneum needle must be checked first for bleeding at the site of insertion or for lesions of the viscera; the peritoneum, omental and peritoneal vessels, liver, gallbladder, and spleen should then be examined. A search must be made for ascites in the lowest recesses of the peritoneal cavity. In females the exploration of ovaries and fallopian tubes should conclude the examination in the Trendelenburg posture, and is mandatory in the presence of peritoneal disease or ascites of unknown origin.

During the procedure, biopsy specimens of liver, spleen, or peritoneum can be taken, using needles or forceps, through the endoscopic operative channel or through the abdominal wall under visual guidance. Peritoneal adhesions may be a serious obstacle to examination of the viscera and/or execution of the biopsy.

Bleeding after liver biopsy can usually be stopped by moderate compression with a probe or with electrocoagulation. The so-called 'bioplug' device, which allows the insertion of a small fibrin sponge exactly at the biopsy site, can also help in effective control of bleeding.

Some refinements and extensions of 'simple' laparoscopy, such as cholangiography, portal pressure measurement and portography have never been widely used and have been outdated by newer imaging methods (see Chapter 5.5). Liver echography, with a very small probe inserted in the laparoscopic operative channel, increases the precision of liver examination, avoiding the interposition of the abdominal wall between the instrument and the liver parenchyma. This improvement with high resolution probes can aid the diagnosis, especially in cases of metastatic liver neoplasms, but technical problems and costs have hampered its use.

The risks

Laparoscopy is a safe procedure (Debray, AnnIntMed, 1976; 127: 689; Henning, ActaEndoscop, 1978; 8:329; Takemoto, GastrJap, 1980; 15:140): in published surveys the mortality is between 0.09 and 0.009 per cent in more than 100 000 procedures. Fatal events usually follow additional manoeuvres such as needle biopsy (Manenti, ActaEndoscop, 1983; 13:21), which has been shown to have a mortality of 0.26 per cent in 1147 biopsies performed during laparoscopy.

Pathological findings

Peritoneum

The surface should be bright and smooth. Loss of brightness is an indirect sign of pathological change. The most important findings are the regular grey-white nodules of tuberculous peritonitis and the jelly-like nodules which suggest peritoneal spreading of neoplastic tissue, usually arising from the pancreas, stomach, and, in the female, from the ovary (Plates 1 and 2).

Ascites

Fluid can be seen even when it is too scarce for clinical recognition. The gross appearance of ascites may give clues to its origin. In cirrhosis the fluid is transparent and pale yellow; a blood-stained fluid usually indicates peritoneal carcinosis or the spontaneous rupture of a carcinoma arising from cirrhosis, but it makes consideration of the possibility of a lesion due to the endoscopic procedure mandatory.

Portal hypertension[2]

Splenomegaly, large omental vessels, the vascular reopening of the round ligament, and the presence of many fine vessels on omentoperitoneal adhesions are all findings that indicate an augmented portal pressure and the development of significant porto-systemic shunting. The appearance of the collateral circulation may vary from a slight increase in peritoneal vascularity to huge tortuous vessels larger than 1 cm in diameter. Study of groups of patients shows that the different extension and evidence of collateral circulation are generally proportional to the levels of portal pressure (Zuin, ItalJGastr, 1982; 14:214). Important endoscopic signs of portosystemic collateral circulation appear to correlate with an increased proportion of patients with endotoxinaemia and a bad prognosis (Piai, ItalJGastr, 1982; 14:193).

In the presence of increased portal pressure engorged lymphatic vessels may be also seen, mainly on the falciform ligament and on the liver itself. 'Lymphatic microcysts', whitish spotty enlargements of lymphatic structures on the hepatic surface, also indicate increased portal pressure.

Findings in the assessment of liver diseases

Size

An enlargement of the liver, especially when limited to the left lobe, is an almost certain sign of liver disease.

Hardness

The normal liver is soft under the pressure of the endoscopic probe; the presence of more fibrous tissue than normal, as is seen in cirrhosis and many other types of liver disease, makes it firm to palpation. In occasional cases the firmness can be due to engorgement with blood resulting from venous outflow obstruction, as in the Budd–Chiari syndrome or congestive heart failure.

Margin

The liver margin usually follows the shape of the contiguous organs. A rigid, raised edge suggests fibrosis of the parenchyma. In cirrhosis, nodules can be found on the margin or can even, as in the macronodular form, fully obscure it.

Surface

In normal liver the surface is smooth and bright, reflecting the light of the scope (Plate 3). Depressions, undulations, or nodules can be seen, pointing to a progressive change of the structure of the liver. Frank nodularity suggests a complete structural change within the liver, and laparoscopy of a firm, diffusely nodular liver can frequently make a definite diagnosis of liver cirrhosis (Plate 4). The nodules can vary in diameter from a few millimetres to several centimetres. At laparoscopy the macronodular form (nodules of more than 3 mm in diameter) is most frequently seen. True micronodular cirrhosis is very rare and corresponds to the 'flat' (in endoscopic terms) fatty liver cirrhosis of alcoholic origin.

Isolated nodules are always suggestive of neoplastic lesions of epithelial or lymphatic origin. Shape, size, or colour can be diagnostic. The metastasis is a grey-white, volcano-like lesion surrounded by a hyperaemic halo (Plate 5); hepatocellulr carcinoma, usually associated with cirrhosis, is characterized by one or few nodules, without central depression, budding from the liver surface, with a yellow-reddish colour (Plate 6).

Colour

In a number of instances the laparoscopist can feel confident enough to make a precise diagnosis of the type of liver disease from the colour of the liver surface: yellow due to massive steatosis, usually from alcohol abuse; dark-brown in haemochromatosis; bright red in active chronic hepatitis; green in cholestatic jaundice (but it is impossible to distinguish biliary obstruction from parenchymal disease); bluish in the obstruction of the venous outflow as in the Budd–Chiari syndrome or constrictive pericarditis; with black spots in metastatic melanoma; brown-greenish and red, with a leopard-like aspect in chronic porphyria cutanea tarda.

White liver, the German 'Kandelzucker Lieber', sugar-candy liver, caused by a layer of fibrin on the liver surface, may suggest a past episode of bacterial (tuberculous) peritonitis.

Clinical use and indications of laparoscopy

We stated at the beginning of this chapter that laparoscopy is an old technique. Is it still a useful diagnostic tool? We feel that it can be in relation to well-defined diagnostic aims.

1. Ascites is probably the most fruitful area of application of laparoscopy which is very easy in this condition and is extremely

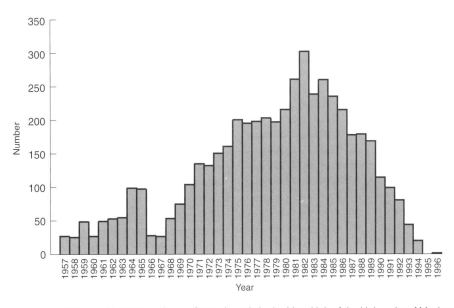

Fig. 1. Increase and decrease of the number of laparoscopies performed yearly in the Liver Unit of the University of Modena, Italy: the mirror of the evolution of the instrumental approach to liver disease in a setting of strong laparoscopic traditions.

well tolerated by the patient. Its main advantage is its ability to identify causes of ascites other than cirrhosis (Budd–Chiari syndrome, constrictive pericarditis, and peritonitis): in a single examination the problem can be resolved and the diagnosis confirmed by taking biopsies, thus saving time and money

2. Diagnosis of cirrhosis (compared with blind liver biopsy). The differing diagnostic yield of macroscopic and histological techniques in the presence of liver nodules is essentially due to the sampling error of biopsy in macronodular cirrhosis. Large nodules exceed the diameter of the biopsy needle and may not be recognized at histological examination (Pagliaro, DigDisSci, 1983; 28:39). Laparoscopic findings are more specific and almost equally sensitive. The interobserver agreement on liver nodularity is better at laparoscopy than at histology, because the concordance on the histological presence of cirrhosis is governed by the dimensions of the biopsy specimen (Orlandi, ItalJGastr, 1979; 11:5) and sometimes by its fragmentation. The diagnosis of cirrhosis has a strong impact on the prognostic judgement, but very little on the therapeutic decisions, where liver biopsy alone is more important and usually adequate. On the other hand, laparoscopy can allow a biopsy to be carried out even in patients with prolonged coagulation time.

3. Laparoscopy is an important diagnostic tool for focal lesions of the liver, yielding almost no false-positive results. Its sensitivity is limited in the presence of deep lesions without superficial involvement (Fornari, GastrEnd, 1988; 34:231). In spite of the diagnostic advantages offered by echography, CT, and echo-guided fine-needle biopsy, it has been found that requests for laparoscopy have recently increased. Laparoscopy may be useful to clarify or confirm the nature of a lesion found by other techniques (Lightdale, GastrEnd, 1985; 31:47). In the staging of neoplastic diseases the

difficulty of finding deep lesions is counterbalanced by the possibility of recognizing minute lesions of the liver and peritoneal surface, which are still out of reach of non-invasive techniques. As a consequence, laparoscopy can modify the diagnostic work-up, with avoidance of useless laparotomies for cancers of the stomach, pancreas, and oesophagus (Van den Velpen, Gut, 1994; 35:1617) and improvement in the diagnosis and staging of lymphoma.[3]

4. Laparoscopy is a sensitive tool in the evaluation of portal hypertension, but is only able to define its presence and is not predictive of its clinically relevant consequences, namely haemorrhage from ruptured oesophageal varices.

In conclusion, laparoscopy can still be a very important diagnostic tool and such expertise[4] should be maintained in the hands of gastroenterologists who continue to play a major role in the management of patients with chronic liver disease (Lightdale, GastrEnd, 1992; 38:392). However, its use must be limited to a small number of clinical situations when its results may be of substantial clinical usefulness. For this reason, even in areas where it was supported by local tradition, the number of purely diagnostic laparoscopies performed for liver disease has fallen dramatically and is bound to remain low (Fig. 1).

References

1. Beck K. *Color atlas of laparoscopy.* Philadelphia: WB Saunders, 1984.
2. Manenti F and Ferrari A. Assessment of liver cirrhosis. Laparoscopy. In Tygstrup N and Orlandi F, eds. *Cirrhosis of the liver. Methods and fields of research.* Amsterdam: Elsevier Science Publishers, 1987: 365–70.
3. Nord HJ and Boyd WP. Diagnostic laparoscopy. *Endoscopy*, 1996; **28**: 147–52.
4. Vargas C *et al.* Diagnostic laparoscopy: a 5-year experience in a hepatology training program. *American Journal of Gastroenterology*, 1995; **90**: 1258–62.

Imaging of the liver and biliary tract

*Jonathan M. Tibballs and Anthony F. Watkinson with a
contribution from Yves Menu*

Imaging methods such as ultrasonography and computed tomography (**CT**) have dramatically modified the investigation of liver and biliary-tract diseases over the past 20 years. Technical advances in ultrasonography, such as duplex, colour and power Doppler, endoscopic transducers, and intravascular contrast media, have extended its role, while the development of spiral CT has revolutionized hepatobiliary CT imaging. The development of fast-imaging and motion-suppression techniques, plus the development of intravascular, oral, and hepatic contrast agents has made magnetic resonance imaging (**MRI**) a clinically viable method. Other more invasive examinations, such as cholangiography and arteriography, are of value in selected cases, but increasingly there are non-invasive methods of obtaining the same information.

In this chapter, technical considerations and normal results of hepatobiliary imaging techniques will be discussed, followed by an overview of their relative roles in various pathological conditions.

Ultrasonography

Ultrasonography is the most commonly used hepatobiliary imaging method; it is easy to perform, is relatively cheap, and is well accepted by patients. It is generally agreed that patients who need imaging for suspected hepatobiliary disease should first be examined by ultrasonography.

Technical considerations

Ultrasonography should be performed after a 6-h fast, allowing the gallbladder to be distended with bile. Modern ultrasonographic devices are real-time, high-resolution machines. The probe frequency is generally 3.5 MHz; occasionally a 5-MHz probe is used in children or thin adults. Sector scanning is preferred to linear scanning, as it facilitates both sub- and intercostal approaches, both of which may be required to examine the entire liver. Mechanical or curved-array probes are available for sector scanning.

The procedure is done with the patient in the supine position. The left lateral decubitus position may be helpful in studying the right upper quadrant, because it displaces the air in the hepatic flexure of the colon, allowing better anatomical display of the liver and biliary tract.

Results

Table 1 summarizes the main points of interest of hepatobiliary sonography. Every examination should attempt to answer all these questions.

Liver size

Ultrasonography does not provide a reliable measurement of liver size. Early reports provided normal values for liver height in sagittal slices: it was suggested that the left lobe on the mid-sagittal slice should be under 12 cm, and that the height of the liver through the right mid-clavicular line should be less than 15 cm. These values proved of little use, because of large intra- and interobserver errors and the wide variation between normal individuals. No single measurement is reliable in detecting or excluding hepatomegaly. Finally, for technical reasons, the sector angle of an ultrasonographic image often does not allow the entire liver to be included in a single image, making accurate measurement impossible. However, ultrasonographic assessment of liver size is useful in some circumstances, for example when clinical findings are equivocal and when semiquantitative values are sufficient for diagnosis. Ultrasonography does allow the detection of pseudoenlargement of the liver, as with a Riedel's lobe or with flattening of the diaphragm. In patients with lung emphysema, ultrasonography may show that the liver volume is normal. When palpation of the liver is difficult, for example in obese patients or when there is ascites, ultrasonography allows assessment of liver size.

The most important role of ultrasonography in the evaluation of liver size is in the assessment of lobar or segmental atrophy/hypertrophy, which cannot be detected by clinical examination. It allows the recognition of anatomical landmarks, and therefore the precise evaluation of segmental anatomy of the liver.

Liver parenchyma

In normal individuals, the ultrasonographic image of the liver is made up of fine echoes with a homogeneous amplitude. When compared with the right kidney, which can be seen on the same image, the normal liver is of equal or slightly higher echogenicity than the renal cortex.

Hepatic vessels

The hepatic artery is usually visible at its origin from the coeliac trunk, and in the porta hepatis where it obliquely crosses the portal vein and common bile duct. Ultrasonography cannot depict the exact anatomy of hepatic arteries when there is an aberrant left or right hepatic artery. An aberrant artery may be suspected, but its exact distribution in the hepatic parenchyma cannot be assessed.

Table 1 Main points of interest in hepatobiliary sonography

Liver
What is the liver size (semiquantitative, see text)?
Are there any single modifications of liver anatomy (localized atrophy or hypertrophy)?
Is the intensity of parenchymal echoes normal (compared to kidney)?
Are there any focal liver lesions?

Gallbladder
Are the gallbladder localization and size normal?
What is the gallbladder-wall thickness?
Are there any endoluminal echoes?
If so, is there any shadowing?

Bile ducts
What is the transverse diameter of the common bile duct (at least two measurements)?
Is there any intrahepatic-duct dilatation?
In case of bile-duct dilatation, is there any internal or extrinsic obstructing process (stone or mass)?

Vessels
Is the inferior vena cava patent?
Are the hepatic veins visualized?
Are the portal vein and intrahepatic radicles patent?
What is the portal-trunk axial diameter?
Are there any collateral veins in cases of portal hypertension?
If duplex Doppler is available, are the flow recordings normal?

Other organs
Are the pancreas and the Wirsung duct normal?
What is the spleen size?
Is there any intra-abdominal lymph-node enlargement?
Is there any peritoneal fluid?

A normal portal vein is always visible in the porta hepatis, and its branches can be identified in the parenchyma, where they are surrounded by an echogenic tissue (containing arteries and bile ducts). The normal diameter of the main portal vein is 13 mm or less. Enlargement of the portal vein is strongly suggestive of portal hypertension, but is insensitive, occurring in only 75 per cent of cases (see below). Hepatic veins can be readily differentiated from portal radicles by their different orientation and lack of echogenic wall. The hepatic veins should be examined in all cases because they allow the delineation of liver segmental anatomy.

The most commonly used scheme for describing the segmental anatomy of the liver is that proposed by Couinaud, as adapted by Bismuth. The liver is considered to be divided by three oblique vertical scissura, corresponding to the vertical planes along which run the three main hepatic veins, and by an oblique horizontal scissura, corresponding to the plane of the left and right portal veins. Segment I ('caudate lobe') lies posteriorly, between the fissure for the ligamentum venosum and the inferior vena cava. Segments II and III lie to the left of the left hepatic scissura and are separated by the horizontal scissura, segment II lying superiorly. Segment IV ('quadrate lobe') lies between the left and middle hepatic scissura, and is subdivided into segments IVa and IVb by the horizontal scissura, IVa lying superiorly. Segments V and VIII lie between the middle and right hepatic scissura, with segments VI and VII lying lateral to the right hepatic scissura. Segments VII and VIII lie superiorly, separated from segments V and VI by the horizontal scissura (Fig. 1).

Identification of segmental anatomy is mandatory in patients with focal lesions who are being considered for surgery, as it aids planning of surgical liver resection.

Gallbladder and bile ducts

The gallbladder is easily identified, usually on the right mid-clavicular sagittal slice. It is generally pear-shaped, but its configuration varies, and internal septations, for example the 'Phrygian cap' appearance, are well-known normal variants. In rare instances the gallbladder is ectopic; it then usually appears 'intrahepatic', but actually lies in a deep fissure rather than within the liver parenchyma. The gallbladder may also be found in a retrohepatic or subdiaphragmatic location. It should be stressed that the end of the cystic duct remains in its normal position. Agenesis is very rare, and it should be considered as a possibility only if one is certain that the patient was fasting (because an empty gallbladder is sometimes difficult to identify); obviously previous surgery (including laparoscopic cholecystectomy) must be ruled out. The gallbladder wall is smooth and slightly hyperechoic in comparison to the liver. It should not be thicker than 3.5 mm in normal individuals. Many conditions are associated with thickening of the gallbladder wall.

Gallbladder size is difficult to assess. The upper limits of normal are usually about 10 cm in length and 5 cm in anteroposterior diameter, but it is not possible to assess the possibility of obstruction on the basis of measurements alone. In individual cases, distended gallbladders may be smaller than the usual upper limits, whereas hypotonic, non-distended gallbladders may be larger (as with cirrhosis, analgesia, parenteral feeding). A palpable gallbladder is a better sign of distension, and the ultrasonographer should palpate the upper abdomen when he or she thinks there is a possibility of cystic-duct obstruction.

The common bile duct is visible in the porta hepatis in most cases. When this area is not obscured, it is usually possible to

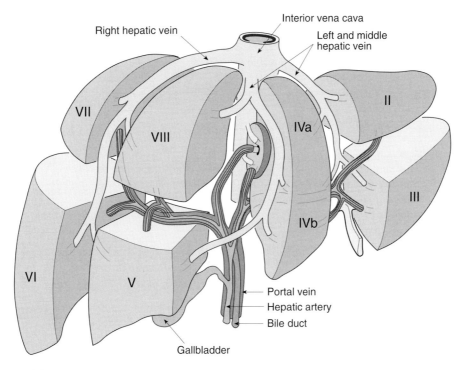

Fig. 1. Segmental anatomy of the liver.

follow the common bile duct down to the intrapancreatic portion. Ultrasonography cannot distinguish between the common duct and common hepatic duct because, in normal individuals, the confluence with the cystic duct is not visible.

The size of the common bile duct remains controversial. It is now accepted that the average diameter increases with age (roughly 1 mm per 10 years after the age of 50) (Wu, JClinUltrasound, 1984; 12:473). It appears that the common bile duct is not enlarged after cholecystectomy. When the common bile duct is enlarged before surgery, it may stay enlarged or it may diminish in size. When normal, it shows only the change in size associated with ageing (Graham, Radiol, 1980; 135:137; Mueller, AJR, 1981; 136:355; Feng, AJR, 1995; 165:859).

As a rough guide, a common bile duct of less than 7 mm internal transverse diameter should be considered of normal size; obstruction is a possibility when it is larger. It is important to realize that, in some individuals, a common bile duct under 7 mm is found in association with early obstruction, and that the duct may not be dilated if there is a diffuse, infiltrative tumour of the common bile duct, or with sclerosing cholangitis or common bile-duct stones.

Some workers have attempted to improve the sensitivity of ultrasonography for the diagnosis of obstruction by using a fatty meal test (Simeone, Radiol, 1982; 143:211; 1985; 154:763), because after a fatty meal a non-obstructed common bile duct gets smaller or its size does not change. If the common bile duct is obstructed its diameter increases. This test is most helpful in patients with suspected obstruction but a normal-sized duct, and in patients without clinical evidence of obstruction but with a large duct on ultrasonography; the reported sensitivity of this test is 84 per cent.

Normal intrahepatic bile ducts may be detected, using modern ultrasonographic equipment, as hypoechoic linear structures running parallel to the segmental portal radicle within the echogenic sheath. When dilated, intrahepatic ducts become obvious, and are sometimes larger than the adjacent portal-vein radicle. Doppler ultrasonography (see below) is a useful tool to differentiate vessels and bile ducts, as no signal is recordable from the latter. Intrahepatic dilatation is more obvious in the left lobe, even with a symmetrical obstruction, because this area is more readily evaluated. When intrahepatic ducts are dilated, biliary obstruction is almost certain.

Doppler examinations

Doppler examination can now be performed in association with conventional ultrasonography (i.e., duplex-Doppler ultrasonography), and may be included in many ultrasonographic devices dedicated to abdominal exploration. The same probe is used to record the image and the frequency-coded Doppler information. A comprehensive explanation of the duplex-Doppler technique can be found in other texts;[1] in simple terms it detects flows and their direction, and allows one to evaluate the velocity of blood flow in a vessel. Difficulties arise when attempts are made to quantify the flow rate, owing to errors in measurement of vessel size, and owing to the difference in blood velocity at different sites within the cross-sectional area of a vessel depending on the type of flow (i.e., laminar or not).

On duplex-Doppler ultrasonography the portal vein shows a steady flow directed towards the liver. Subtle modifications are seen with respect to the cardiac cycle and respiration. Hepatic arterial flow shows a low-resistance waveform with a systolic peak and continuous forward flow during diastole. Hepatic veins mirror the haemodynamics of the right atrium, with irregular hepatofugal flow and a short reversal during atrial systole. Recordings in the hepatic veins and inferior vena cava are similar.

Clinically, duplex–Doppler ultrasonography is useful in numerous circumstances, as follows.

1. It helps to assess vessel patency when this is questionable on conventional ultrasonographic images. However, failure to demonstrate flow should be interpreted with caution, as this can be due to technical factors.
2. It helps to identify collaterals in patients with portal hypertension; flow can be seen in collaterals, and bidirectional or even reversed portal flow may be detected.
3. It helps to evaluate the patency of surgical portosystemic shunts.
4. It may be used to assist in the creation of transjugular intrahepatic portosystemic stent (**TIPS**) shunts, and to assess subsequent patency. Alterations in hepatic and portal venous flow within the liver, and changes in flow velocity, may be used to detect stent stenosis, allowing revision of the stent before occlusion occurs, as this usually presents as recurrent and often life-threatening variceal bleeding (Dodd, AJR, 1995; 164:1119).

Colour Doppler techniques make duplex–Doppler ultrasonographic examinations easier, as they superimpose a colour-coded map of Doppler signals on the grey-scale image. This greatly facilitates the selection and localization of flow signal, but its sensitivity is lower than that of conventional duplex–Doppler ultrasonography.

Power Doppler, unlike duplex and colour Doppler, is not dependent upon the angle of insonation between the ultrasonographic probe and vessel of interest. This greatly increases its sensitivity for detecting flow, but gives no information about the direction of flow.

Contrast media and ultrasonography

Ultrasonographic contrast media increase the sensitivity of grey-scale and Doppler ultrasonography, and therefore increase detection of small lesions and of low-velocity flow within vessels [Balen, ClinRadiol, 1994; 49:77; Cosgrove, ClinRadiol, 1996; 51 (Suppl. 1.):1]. Several types of agent have been used for liver imaging [Leen, ClinRadiol, 1996; 51 (Suppl. 1): 35]. Carbon dioxide microbubbles can be injected directly into the hepatic artery via a selective catheter, producing short-lived enhancement of vascular structures. Ultrasonographic examination during the injection, so-called sonographic angiography, reportedly aids lesion detection and characterization (Kudo, Radiol, 1992; 182:155; AJR, 1992; 158:65). The most promising agents, however, are the saccharide microparticle suspensions, such as Levovist (Schering AG, Berlin, Germany). These microparticles stabilize the microbubbles, enabling them to survive passage through the pulmonary circulation. They can therefore be injected into a peripheral vein and produce systemic enhancement for up to 60 min. Reported uses include reliable exclusion of portal venous thrombosis, and detection and characterization of primary and secondary liver tumours.

Endoscopic ultrasonography

Recent work with ultrasonographic probes mounted on an endoscope has shown that it is possible to assess the common bile duct by positioning the tip of the endoscope in the vertical portion of the duodenum. The ampulla is clearly demonstrated as well as the lower portion of the duct. This appears to be the only method of imaging the ampulla. Initial work suggests that this method has a high

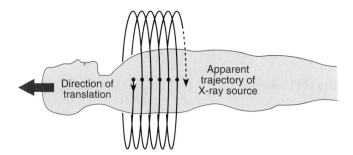

Fig. 2. The X-ray source describes an apparent spiral as the patient is moved through the gantry. Consequently a continuous volume of data is acquired.

sensitivity and specificity for the diagnosis of carcinoma of the ampulla and for stones in the common bile duct (Jaffe, DigDis, 1995; 13:39).

Computed tomography

CT of the hepatobiliary tract, as in other areas of the body, has been revolutionized by the introduction of spiral (or helical) CT. Previous generations of CT scanners acquired data one slice at a time, with incremental changes in table position ('conventional CT'). First- and second-generation scanners employed an X-ray source and detector(s) gantry that was rotated incrementally through 180° for each scan slice, with an exposure at each degree of rotation, producing scan times of many seconds to several minutes. Third- and fourth-generation scanners featured a dynamically rotating gantry, but were limited to a maximum of two to three revolutions at a time before having to reverse the direction of rotation due to constraints of the electrical cables. They reduced scan times to the order of 1 s, but at best could only acquire 8 to 12 scans/min, largely due to the 'dead' time taken to move the table between each scan. This necessitated multiple breath-holds by the patient to complete each examination, thereby introducing the problem of respiratory misregistration and the potential to miss small lesions.

Spiral CT (SCT)

In SCT the X-ray tube/detector gantry is able to rotate continually, thanks to the development of 'slip-rings' that allow electrical connection between the rotating and stationary parts of the scanner through brush contacts rather than the previously limiting electrical cables. By moving the patient constantly through the gantry the X-ray source describes a spiral or helix about the patient's long axis (Fig. 2). Consequently, data are acquired from an entire volume of tissue, rather than from individual slices, although the data are analysed by the computer and presented in slice format.

Resolution and pitch

Increasing the X-ray beam width (i.e., slice thickness) reduces image resolution. Increasing the speed of table movement increases the length of the spiral and therefore the volume imaged, but reduces resolution due to blurring.

Pitch may be defined as the speed of table feed (mm/s) divided by the slice thickness (mm), multiplied by the time taken for one complete revolution of the gantry (s), usually 1 s. A pitch of more than 1.7 generally produces too much blurring, and therefore is seldom exceeded. Reducing slice thickness is the best way of improving resolution, but this also limits the volume studied in a given breath-hold. As ever, a compromise is required to image the required volume of tissue whilst maintaining resolution.

Image reconstruction—overlapping slices

The spiral CT data are acquired at a given slice thickness (= X-ray beam width), e.g. 10 mm. As a continuous volume of data is acquired, the computer can reconstruct a 10 mm-thick slice at any point along the spiral. If slices are reconstructed at, say, 5-mm intervals, 'overlapping' slices are produced. This significantly reduces the problem of partial voluming, thereby improving lesion detection.

Advantages of SCT

The main practical advantages of spiral over conventional CT are as follows.

1. Reduced scan-acquisition times: typically the entire liver can be scanned in 20 to 30 s. This can be done during one breath-hold, thereby eliminating respiratory misregistration.
2. Targeted use of intravascular iodinated contrast: following an intravenous bolus of contrast there are three phases of hepatic enhancement (Baron, AJR, 1994; 163:323); exact timings depend upon the rate and volume of contrast injection, but the phases are essentially arterial (20–50 s), portal venous (50–90 s), and equilibrium (>120 s). Maximal parenchymal enhancement is achieved toward the end of the portal phase. The aim of contrast-enhanced CT is to maximize the contrast between focal lesions and liver parenchyma, and to image the liver during that time. Lesion:liver contrast diminishes as contrast equilibrates between the intravascular and extravascular spaces, the equilibrium phase, and therefore imaging should be completed before this phase begins, i.e., within 120 s of contrast injection. The majority (75–80 per cent) of the liver blood supply is from the portal vein. Some focal liver lesions, in particular tumours, derive their blood supply primarily from the hepatic artery, and can appear more conspicuous during the arterial phase of hepatic enhancement than during the later phases. Combining SCT scans during both the arterial and portal venous phases following a single intravenous injection of contrast can maximize lesion detection and aid characterization (Bonaldi, Radiol, 1995; 197:357). This principle of differential blood supply also underlies the techniques of hepatic CT angiography and CT arterioportography (see below).
3. Multiplanar and three-dimensional image reconstruction: acquisition of data from a volume of tissue rather than a series of slices allows image reconstruction in multiple planes, including curved planes, and dimensions, thanks to the dramatic increase in data-handling capacity of computer systems. The two main techniques are maximum-intensity projection (Fig. 3(a)) and surface-shaded display (Fig. 3(b)). These are computer-generated rather than 'real' images, and numerous technical pitfalls must be borne in mind when creating and interpreting them.[2]
   Three-dimensional images produced by these techniques may be rotated on a computer workstation console enabling them to be

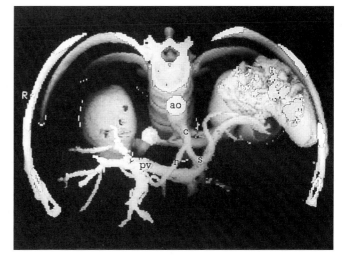

(a)

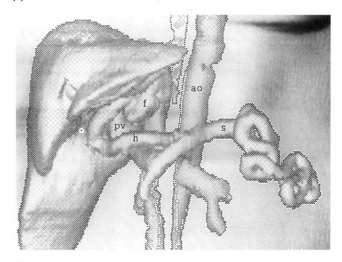

(b)

Fig. 3. (a) Maximum-intensity projection of a normal coeliac axis and portal venous system. (b) Surface-shaded display showing a markedly hypertrophied hepatic artery feeding a post-laparoscopic cholecystectomy arteriovenous fistula. The portal vein is clearly seen. ao, aorta; c, coeliac artery; h, hepatic artery; s, splenic artery; pv, portal vein; f, arteriovenous fistula.

viewed from any direction. This can be very useful for separating structures that overlie one another on a given projection, particularly blood vessels.

Practical considerations

Patients are typically fasted for 4 to 6 h, as intravenous iodinated contrast injection can cause nausea and occasionally vomiting. The procedure is routinely done in the supine position, although the left lateral decubitus position may be helpful in studying the left lobe of the liver, because it shifts the streak artefacts due to the air–fluid level in the stomach.

Oral contrast helps to differentiate intestinal loops from retroperitoneal structures, but it is not always necessary if the examination is focused on the liver. In particular, it should be omitted if common bile-duct stones are suspected, as the resulting high density may then be misinterpreted as contrast in the duodenum. Water is an alternative contrast agent for outlining the stomach and duodenum, and intravenous Buscopan or glucagon may be used to reduce duodenal peristalsis, particularly when imaging the periampullary region (Winter, Radiol, 1996; 201:365).

The liver is typically imaged with a slice thickness of 7 to 10 mm and a table feed of 10 mm/s (i.e., a pitch of 1–1.4), with image reconstruction at 5- to 10-mm intervals.

Plain studies, before intravenous contrast injection, are useful when planning dynamic contrast studies and also for the detection of calcification. With conventional CT, when scanning before the equilibrium phase could not be reliably accomplished, plain studies were advocated to aid detection of lesions that might subsequently appear isodense following contrast, such as angiomas and some primary and secondary malignant tumours. With SCT, imaging before the equilibrium phase is easily accomplished, and the value of plain studies has been questioned.

Contrast studies remain essential for the detection and characterization of many liver lesions, as outlined above. Studies acquired during the portal phase are routinely done. Arterial-phase studies may further obviate the need for plain studies by detecting hypervascular lesions that may subsequently become isodense with liver.

SCT angiography

Scanning during the arterial phase of intravenous contrast injection (e.g. 100–150 ml of 300 mg I/ml contrast at 2–3 ml/s) can be used to study the arteries themselves. By using thin slices (e.g. 3–5 mm, pitch $= 1$, reconstructed at 1.5- to 3-mm intervals) and timing the scan to the period of maximal hepatic arterial enhancement (typically 20–50 s after the start of injection), contrast between the arteries and liver parenchyma can be maximized. The subsequent data volume can be reconstructed by techniques such as maximum-intensity projection or surface-shaded display to demonstrate the arteries only, a technique known as SCT angiography. This technique is able to delineate the aorta and visceral arterial origins down to luminal diameters of 2 mm. It can detect anatomical variants such as an aberrant or replaced right hepatic artery, and may therefore be used to provide an arterial 'road map' before surgery.

If scanning is delayed until the portal phase of hepatic enhancement (typically 50–70 s after the start of contrast injection), the portal and hepatic veins are maximally enhanced and can be displayed using similar three-dimensional reconstruction techniques.

It should be noted, however, that specific preparation of the patient is required for SCT angiography, for example avoiding positive oral contrast, which interferes with subsequent image reconstruction. It is therefore a specific technique, and cannot be simply 'added on' to the end of a liver CT examination. Disadvantages include the need for a large volume of intravenous contrast and its limited resolution compared to conventional and digital-subtraction angiography. Also, current enhanced magnetic-resonance angiographic techniques can achieve similar resolution without the intravenous contrast load or use of ionizing radiation. Consequently, SCT angiography does not have widespread use in the abdomen.

SCT cholangiography

Intravenous cholangiographic contrast agents, such as iodipamide meglumine, undergo biliary excretion following intravenous infusion. SCT scanning during iodipamide infusion demonstrates the intra- and extrahepatic bile ducts. The SCT data can then be three-dimensionally reconstructed to display the biliary tree (Fig. 4). The resolution of this technique is inferior to that of conventional cholangiography, but it reliably shows the confluence of the intra- and extrahepatic ducts, and can identify major anatomical variations and ductal stones. It can only demonstrate unobstructed bile ducts, as a normal serum bilirubin is required for biliary excretion. It has been advocated as a non-invasive way of assessing the biliary tree before laparoscopic cholecystectomy (Van Beers, AJR, 1994; 162: 1331), but its cost-effectiveness has been questioned.

Obstructed, dilated bile ducts can be imaged without positive cholangiographic contrast. If SCT is performed during the period of maximal parenchymal enhancement following intravenous contrast injection, contrast between the liver parenchyma and unenhanced dilated bile ducts is maximized, the bile effectively acting as a negative contrast agent. Three-dimensional reconstruction techniques allow display of the unenhanced biliary tree, and can confirm the level of obstruction (Gillams, BrJRadiol, 1994; 67:445).

CT hepatic angiography

An angiographic catheter is placed selectively into the common hepatic artery and the liver scanned during contrast infusion. Lesions with mainly hepatic arterial supply, namely most tumours, enhance more than the surrounding liver parenchyma, which has a predominantly portal venous supply. Arterial injection allows the detection of more lesions than an intravenous bolus of contrast (Freeny, Radiol, 1983; 148:193). Contrast is injected (100 ml at 2–3 ml/s) with a mechanical injector. Pitfalls are misinterpretation of irregularities of the normal hepatic parenchymal pattern, and difficulties in differentiating between small hypervascular lesions and vessels. If the patient has diffuse disease of the liver, the parenchymal pattern may be heterogeneous and difficult to distinguish from tumour.

Three-dimensional reconstructions of spiral CT hepatic angiographic data reportedly show liver tumours and their associated arterial supply more clearly than conventional angiography (Kanematsu, AJR, 1996; 166:585).

CT arterioportography

With this technique, contrast is delivered via an angiographic catheter placed selectively in either the superior mesenteric or

---

Fig. 4. Hepatic artery aneurysm: SCT cholangiography was combined with SCT angiography to demonstrate the relation of the common bile duct to the aneurysm. (a) Late arterial phase-enhanced SCT scan showing a large hepatic artery aneurysm (arrowheads) with mural thrombus and a dilated lumen, and the enhanced common bile duct (arrow). (b) Coeliac angiogram showing the dilated hepatic artery. (c) Maximum-intensity projection reconstruction clearly showing the relation of the common bile duct to the hepatic artery (h) and portal vein (pv).

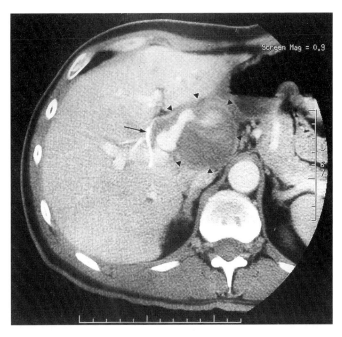

(a)

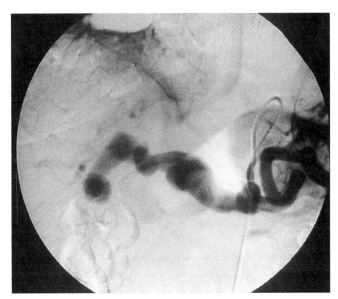

(b)

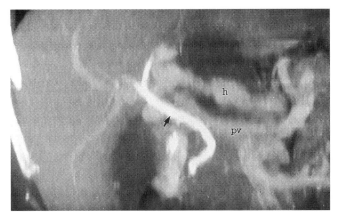

(c)

splenic artery. A single breath-hold spiral is acquired during pump injection of contrast (150 ml at 2 ml/s). A delay of 30 to 40 s from the beginning of contrast injection to the start of scanning allows contrast to reach the portal venous system. Tumours should appear hypodense because normal liver is greatly enhanced, whereas they are fed by unopacified blood from the hepatic artery (Lupetin, Radiographics, 1996; 16:723). Comparison with an intravenously enhanced SCT is advisable, as regional flow variations may simulate tumour infiltration (Peterson, Radiol, 1992; 185:149). According to various investigators, it is the most sensitive technique for detection of small liver lesions (0.5 cm and above).

Lipiodol intra-arterial injections

Lipiodol has been used for delineation of hepatocellular carcinoma. Staining of liver tumours with this oily suspension is seen after its injection into the hepatic artery. Hepatocellular carcinoma preferentially retains this suspension, but other tumours may also retain it. The reason for this uptake is not clearly explained. Lipiodol (10–15 ml) is injected slowly into the hepatic artery, under fluoroscopic control. CT is performed 10 to 14 days later (Yumoto, Radiol, 1985; 154:19).

The affinity of Lipiodol for hepatocellular carcinoma has been exploited as a possible therapeutic measure by labelling it with chemotherapeutic agents, such as epirubicin, or radioactive iodine (^{131}I).

Artefacts

The possibility of artefacts should be remembered when analysing images, as follows.

1. Partial-volume effect results from the inclusion within a single slice of structures with different densities. The measured density is an average of the single densities of each object. The resulting image usually has blurred contours. It is especially common for small structures that are only partially included in the slice plane. A small biliary cyst may exhibit a high measured density. This artefact is reduced by thin slices.
2. Respiratory artefacts occur because apnoea is necessary during slice acquisition to avoid motion blurring. Respiratory misregistration may occur if differing degrees of inspiration are taken between individually acquired slices. Both factors are greatly reduced by using SCT.
3. Air artefacts, seen as streaks across the liver, may be observed due to an air–fluid level in the stomach. Examination in the left lateral decubitus position can be used to eliminate these if they cause problems.

Normal anatomy

The liver occupies the entire right subdiaphragmatic area and extends to the left upper quadrant. The peritoneal attachments are not visible in normal cases.

Liver size

Evaluation of liver size and volume is possible, particularly if a single breath-hold SCT scan is performed, but this is time-consuming and of little clinical relevance, as discussed in the section on ultrasonography. CT, like ultrasonography, is much more useful in

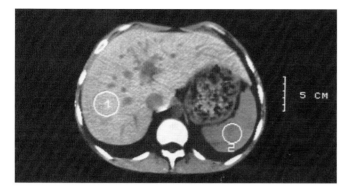

Fig. 5. Haemochromatosis: plain CT shows that the liver density is 88 HU and spleen density 53 HU.

delineating the regional anatomy, and in searching for localized hypertrophy or atrophy with respect to segmental anatomy.

Individual variations of normal liver morphology are commonly seen. 'Riedel's lobe' is a hypertrophy of the inferior part of the right lobe, usually seen in thin women; the inferior aspect of the liver may then be located in the right iliac fossa. The size of the left hepatic lobe varies considerably from one patient to another. Rare instances of complete absence of the left lobe have been described (Belton, Radiol, 1983; 147:184).

Hepatic vessels and segmentation

Before injection of contrast, the vessels appear hypodense. After injection into a peripheral vein, the hepatic arteries appear maximally enhanced from 15 to 30 s. The portal vessels appear maximally enhanced from 50 to 70 s.

The hepatic veins are the major landmarks of the segmental anatomy of the liver (see above under ultrasonography). Under normal conditions the parenchymal liver density is related mainly to portal enhancement and partly to arterial enhancement. It should be noted that the hepatic veins may enhance later than the inferior vena cava, which is opacified by the renal vessels; hepatic veins may then be seen as hypodense areas and misinterpreted as focal lesions.

Conventional CT will not usually detect variations of the hepatic artery, but arterial-phase SCT reportedly does so, although it cannot reliably define the intrahepatic distribution of aberrant arteries (this can be achieved with SCT angiography). An aberrant left hepatic artery can be seen within the fissure for the ligamentum venosum. An aberrant right hepatic artery is occasionally seen at its origin from the superior mesenteric artery.

Liver enhancement

The normal density of the liver on plain slices is usually between 50 and 75 Hounsfield Units (**HU**). The liver is homogeneous and slightly hyperdense to the renal cortex, pancreas, and spleen. The difference between the density of liver and spleen is 7.5 ± 4 HU (Piekarski, Radiol, 1980; 37:727). Fatty infiltration and ischaemia are the major cause of lower hepatic CT numbers; glycogen storage disease, haemochromatosis, and amiodarone intoxication are the main causes of higher CT numbers (Fig. 5).

Gallbladder and bile ducts

The gallbladder can always be seen on CT. It is located at the inferior aspect of the liver, except in the rare cases in which it is ectopic. The middle hepatic vein usually lies in close relation to the gallbladder bed. The density of the gallbladder bile varies according to viscosity (0–25 HU) and in a normal, fasting individual it is between 0 to 10 HU. The gallbladder wall is thin and enhances after injection; when contrast is injected via an arterial hepatic catheter, the enhancement is massive.

Intrahepatic bile ducts are not detected in normal examinations, unless a specific cholangiographic contrast agent is injected. If intrahepatic ducts are dilated, they appear as hypodense, tubular structures parallel to the portal radicles. They are more easily seen on postcontrast slices as the contrast between the enhanced liver parenchyma and blood vessels and non-enhanced bile ducts is then increased.

The common bile duct is usually visible in the porta hepatis. Measurements are similar to those with ultrasonography. When the common bile duct is measured, only the anteroposterior diameter is considered because the duct runs obliquely towards the pancreas, and a transverse measure would thus overestimate the real diameter. This is why the common bile duct appears on CT as an ovoid area, with a larger transverse diameter. Even when dilated, this ovoid shape is still evident as the superior portion of the common bile duct bows horizontally. By contrast the intrapancreatic duct remains vertical in most circumstances, and appears as a round, hypodense area in the dorsal aspect of the pancreas.

Magnetic resonance imaging

MRI is the most recent advance in cross-sectional imaging of the liver and bile ducts. Its clinical application is changing too rapidly for its final boundaries to be delineated. Recent advances in fast (including single breath-hold) imaging, motion-suppression techniques, and contrast agents have greatly increased its importance in liver and biliary-tract imaging.

Technical considerations

The physics of MRI is complex. An introduction is presented below, but for a detailed discussion the reader is referred to the review by Wehrli.[3]

Basic physical principles

Certain atomic nuclei demonstrate angular momentum, or spin. Those containing an odd number of protons induce a magnetic field, which can be expressed as a magnetic moment that has a definite magnitude and direction and is commonly likened to that of a microscopic bar magnet. When an external magnetic field is applied, two phenomena occur:

Firstly, the magnetic moments align with the external field, either parallel to it (i.e., in the same direction) or antiparallel to it (in the opposite direction). Those nuclei that are parallel to the external field are at a slightly lower energy state and therefore more stable. Slightly more nuclei align parallel than antiparallel, producing a small net magnetic vector within the sample, in the direction of the external field, known as longitudinal magnetization.

Secondly, the nuclei precess, a spinning and rotating motion analogous to that of a spinning top or gyroscope. The frequency of precession, or resonance frequency, is determined by the strength of the external magnetic field and the gyromagnetic constant, which is specific for each nucleus. This precessional frequency lies within the radiofrequency range of the electromagnetic spectrum. Although nuclei of the same element precess at the same frequency, they are not in phase (synchronous) with each other.

Resonance

Nuclei have their own natural frequency of oscillation. When exposed to this frequency of oscillation from another source, energy transfer occurs between the two. When a short radiofrequency pulse at or near the resonance frequency is applied, energy transfer to the nuclei occurs. The absorbed energy produces transitions between the parallel and antiparallel states. This deflects the net magnetic vector of the sample, typically through 90 or 180°, and the nuclei temporarily precess in phase, or synchronously. When deflected through 90° the net magnetic vector is directed in the transverse plane, and is known as transverse magnetization. This forms the basis of the MR signal.

Magnetic relaxation

After radiofrequency excitation the precessing nuclei dephase and the overall net magnetic vector returns to its original direction, aligned with the external magnetic field. This occurs by an exponential recovery of longitudinal magnetization (T_1 recovery) and decay of transverse magnetization (T_2 decay), processes known as magnetic relaxation.

Magnetic relaxation results in a return to a lower-energy state, and the energy difference is emitted as radiofrequency waves that induce electrical charge in a suitably positioned antenna or receiver coil. This constitutes the MR signal, which is mathematically analysed to produce the final MR image.

T_1 and T_2

Two time constants, T_1 and T_2, describe magnetic relaxation. The longitudinal relaxation time (T_1) describes T_1 recovery. It is the time taken for 63 per cent of the original longitudinal magnetization to recover, and is in the order of 300 ms to 3 s. The transverse relaxation time (T_2) describes T_2 decay. It is the time taken until 37 per cent of the transverse magnetization remains, and is of the order of 50 to 100 ms. These are time constants for a given nucleus in a given external field strength.

T_1 recovery occurs due to energy transfer from the excited nuclei to the surrounding molecular lattice ('spin-lattice relaxation'). T_2 decay occurs due to energy transfer to adjacent molecules as a result of local magnetic-field interactions and inhomogeneities ('spin-spin relaxation). These processes are less efficient if molecular mobility is high, as in water, and then T_1 and T_2 are long. Where molecular mobility is low, as in fat, T_1 and T_2 are short.

Some examples of T_1 and T_2 times are given in Table 2.

T_1 and T_2 weighting

The MR pulse sequence can be organized in such a way that either the T_1 or T_2 time of the tissues has the greatest influence on MR

Table 2 T_1/T_2 times in various tissues		
Tissue	**T_1 at 1.5 T (ms)**	**T_2 (ms)**
Fat	260	84
Liver	490	43
Kidney	650	58
Spleen	780	62
Water	>4000	>2000

signal and hence the final image. An image influenced mainly by T_1 times is known as T_1 weighted. Long T_1 produces low signal, short T_1 produces high signal; therefore water appears dark and fat bright. On T_2-weighted images, long T_2 produces high signal and short T_2 produces low signal; therefore water appears bright and fat appears dark.

Clinical MRI

In clinical MRI the hydrogen nucleus, a single proton, is used for imaging as it possesses nuclear spin and is abundant in biological tissue. Those hydrogen nuclei that are physically constrained, for example those in bone, are unable to change alignment in response to the external magnetic field, and therefore generate no MR signal. Hydrogen nuclei in body tissues and fluids have varying concentrations and degrees of mobility and hence have different T_1 and T_2 relaxation times, thereby producing different MR signals. MRI can therefore be thought of as a chart of the regional density of mobile hydrogen nuclei throughout the body.

Pulse sequences

The timing and strength of radiofrequency pulses applied to the sample can be varied to alter the MR signal generated. Each combination of radiofrequency pulses constitutes a pulse sequence, of which there are many, with new variations being described daily, spawning a host of bewildering acronyms (UTSE, GRASS, GRASE, FISP, STIR, FLASH, etc.). To make matters worse, many of these acronyms are manufacturer-specific, therefore one pulse sequence may be known by several names depending upon the equipment manufacturer.

Spin-echo sequences are the most commonly used. They provide good spatial resolution (particularly T_1-weighted images) and superior contrast resolution (particularly T_2-weighted images). They originally took several minutes (2–15 min) to acquire, but fast, or turbo, spin-echo imaging can acquire T_2-weighted images in a single breath-hold.

Gradient-echo sequences were developed to achieve single breath-hold image acquisition. Image contrast is more complex to analyse, and spatial resolution is poorer. They may give significant information about flowing blood and are used to acquire dynamic images following intravenous contrast enhancement. They are also more subject to artefacts.

Inversion-recovery sequences initially produced highly T_1-weighted images, but spatial resolution was poor. Short T_1 inversion-recovery (STIR) sequences suppress the signal from fat, eliminating respiratory-motion artefact from fat in the anterior abdominal wall. This technique is sensitive for fatty infiltration, periportal changes, and biliary dilatation.

Chemical-shift, or phase-contrast, sequences are sensitive for fatty infiltration and for liver neoplasms, which are frequently accompanied by some degree of fatty infiltration.

Echo-planar imaging is the fastest MR technique, acquiring data in milliseconds. This speed is currently at the expense of image resolution, but this will doubtless improve.

In addition to the basic pulse sequence, 'saturation bands' can be applied during image acquisition to cancel the signal from various structures, such as fat ('fat sat') and flowing blood in adjacent planes.

It is not possible to prescribe an exact protocol for liver MRI, as there are many variations in technique between imaging departments and equipment manufacturers. As a rule, most examinations include T_1- and T_2-weighted spin-echo sequences supplemented by gradient-echo and contrast-enhanced sequences as required (Saini, Radiol, 1995; 197:575).

Cautions and contraindications

An MRI examination involves exposure to high magnetic-field strengths and radiofrequency pulses. The latter result in energy deposition within the tissues in the form of heat. Guidelines exist to limit the power deposition during an MRI examination.

Non-aneurysmal surgical clips, metallic prostheses, and vascular stents are considered safe. Conventional cardiac pacemakers, ferromagnetic aneurysm clips, neurostimulators, some early prosthetic heart valves, metallic foreign bodies in the eye, and other implanted ferromagnetic devices are contraindications to MRI due to possible displacement in the external magnetic field, or current induction. Systematic screening for foreign bodies is routinely performed by questionnaire, supplemented with radiographs if required, before every MRI scan.

Although no harmful effects to pregnant women or fetuses have been shown, current guidelines are that MRI should only be used in pregnancy when there is a definite medical indication and potential benefit over other imaging techniques. Some patients are too claustrophobic to tolerate an MRI examination, despite sedation.

Normal results

Liver parenchyma

A few guidelines may help in image interpretation. When the sequence is T_1-weighted, the liver appears grey and homogeneous, with a higher intensity than the spleen. On T_2-weighted sequences, signal intensity from the liver is lower than that of the spleen. In this way, a quick glance at the images allows distinction between T_1- and T_2-weighting. Most liver tumours, including metastases, behave like the spleen, that is, they appear darker than the liver on T_1-weighting and brighter on T_2-weighting.

Some tissues are brighter than the liver on T_1-weighting; for example fat and cysts containing fluid of high protein content. Iron (haemochromatosis), air, calcification, and dense fibrosis are darker than the liver on both T_1- and T_2-weighting. Fluid-filled lesions (cysts, necrosis), or lesions with highly vascular components (angiomas, some metastases), appear extremely bright on T_2-weighting.

Non-flowing blood (haemorrhage, haematoma) has complex signal characteristics depending on the state of oxidation of the haemoglobin (**Hb**) molecule (oxyHb → deoxyHb → metHb → haemosiderin). Acute haemorrhage is high signal on both T_1- and T_2-weighted images, and the final product, haemosiderin, is low signal.

Blood vessels

Blood vessels have a different appearance according to the type of sequence. With the spin-echo technique, vessels appear black, as areas of low signal. This is due to the 'time-of-flight' effect: when a single slice is examined, a radiofrequency pulse gives energy to the slice and waits for the subsequent signal from the relaxing nuclei. Excited protons within flowing blood may have left the examination slice by the time the MR signal is emitted. They are replaced by non-excited protons flowing into the examination slice, which obviously generate no signal. In fact, there are many exceptions and sometimes blood vessels may appear bright, mixed, or grey depending on the blood velocity, type of spin-echo sequence, and orientation of the vessel (perpendicular or parallel to the slice axis). In summary, the interpretation of the blood-vessel signal from the spin-echo technique is difficult, and we can only say that the blood vessel is patent when no signal is observed in it.

On gradient-echo sequences, all the excitation and recording times are shorter, so that blood vessels may appear bright. In this way MRI is able to provide an 'angiographic contrast'. Three-dimensional reconstruction may lead to images of abdominal blood vessels, but this is not routinely done in everyday practice. In conclusion, one can say that the gradient-echo technique may assess the patency of blood vessels when they are filled with a bright signal.

MR contrast agents

As for CT, contrast agents are available for MRI. The role of these pharmaceutical compounds is to alter the T_1 and T_2 characteristics of the tissue, increasing the lesion:liver contrast ratio.

Intravascular contrast

Gadolinium (Gd) is a paramagnetic element. It is chelated with diethylenetriamine penta-acetic acid (**DTPA**) to counteract its toxicity. When injected intravenously its biodistribution is very similar to that of iodinated contrast agents. The main effect of this contrast agent is to shorten T_1, therefore increasing signal on T_1-weighted pulse sequences. T_2 is also shortened, producing a reduction in signal on T_2-weighted sequences, but this is not utilized clinically. The pattern of enhancement produced is in many ways similar to that of iodine-enhanced CT. However, Gd-DTPA does not enhance blood vessels on conventional spin-echo sequences, owing to the time-of-flight phenomenon discussed above, and it is expensive.

The development of fast gradient-echo sequences, however, has allowed dynamic-contrast imaging. Multiple acquisitions made after intravenous injection of gadolinium can be used to study the arterial and portal phases of liver enhancement, a technique directly analogous to the dual-spiral CT technique described above. Again, a volume of data can be acquired permitting image reconstruction, such as maximum-intensity projection and surface-shaded display, to display arterial and portal venous anatomy. Such techniques are being evaluated in the assessment for liver transplantation and may enable routine angiography to be omitted (Ward, ClinRadiol, 1996; 51:191).

Oral contrast

Oral Gd-DTPA and magnetic iron oxide particles may be used to delineate the bowel in much the same way as oral contrast in CT.

Hepatic contrast (Saini, Radiol, 1992; 182:12)

Intravenously injected superparamagnetic iron oxide (**SPIO**) particles are phagocytosed by the Kupffer cells of the hepatic reticuloendothelial system. As iron lengthens T_1 and shortens T_2, the liver appears dark on all sequences. Because tumours are devoid of phagocytic Kupffer cells they do not take up the particles and appear brighter on all sequences. Early studies reported a high rate of adverse reaction such as hypotension, nausea, and vomiting. More recent studies using slower injection rates have reported fewer side-effects, and definite superiority of SPIO-enhanced T_2-weighted images over non-enhanced T_2-weighted and contrast-enhanced CT images in terms of image quality and lesion detection (Winter, AJR, 1993; 161:1191). SPIO-enhanced, T_2-weighted images detected additional lesions in 27 per cent of patients when compared to non-enhanced, T_2-weighted images, and in 40 per cent when compared to contrast-enhanced CT scans (Ros, Radiol, 1995; 196:481).

Manganese is also paramagnetic, and is taken up by hepatocytes, increasing their signal on T_1-weighted images. Tissue devoid of hepatocytes, such as metastases, does not enhance and therefore becomes more conspicuous. In cases of hepatocellular carcinoma, the degree of enhancement correlates with histological differentiation (Murakami, Radiol, 1996; 200:69). Like gadolinium, manganese is toxic (particularly to cardiac tissue), and the toxicity is counteracted by chelation. Mangafodipir trisodium (Mn-DPDP) is the most extensively studied chelate.

Magnetic resonance angiography (MRA)

All forms of angiography are based on the principle of increasing the contrast between blood vessels and surrounding tissue. In conventional and CT angiography this is achieved by the injection of iodinated contrast material. MRA, however, utilizes blood flow itself to generate contrast between vessels and stationary tissue, and is therefore totally non-invasive.

The two common techniques used are time-of-flight and phase-contrast angiography. Each has its relative merits and disadvantages. Both can be performed as a two-dimensional slice or three-dimensional volume acquisition. As with SCT angiography, the data are postprocessed and reconstructed, typically using a maximum-intensity projection technique. The more recent technique of dynamic gadolinium-enhanced scanning has been described above.

Magnetic resonance cholangiopancreatography (MRCP)

As with all MRI techniques there are various strategies for performing MRCP. They all basically utilize heavily T_2-weighted sequences in which stationary fluids, such as bile and pancreatic secretions, have high signal intensity relative to surrounding liver and pancreas (Reinhold, AJR, 1996; 166:1285).

Normal intra- and extrahepatic bile ducts are visualized in over 90 per cent of cases. Anatomical variants are accurately depicted (Taourel, Radiol, 1996; 199:521). The presence and site of biliary

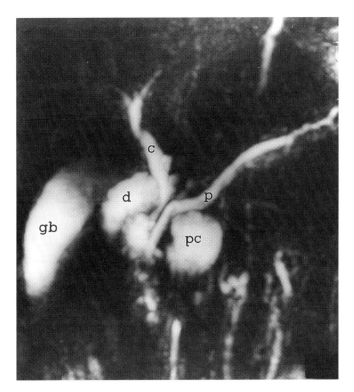

Fig. 6. Magnetic resonance cholangiopancreatography. The pancreatic duct (p) and common bile duct (c) are well seen and shown to enter the duodenum (d) separately. The confluence of the intrahepatic ducts is just seen. The gallbladder (gb) is shown. The high-signal focus seen medially is a small pseudocyst (pc).

obstruction are determined in 90 to 100 per cent and 85 to 100 per cent of cases, respectively. Benign and malignant lesions are distinguished in at least 80 per cent of cases.

Compared to endoscopic retrograde cholangiopancreatography, MRCP is safer, has a lower technical failure rate, and provides at least comparable diagnostic information (Fig. 6). A current, short-term disadvantage is restricted availability of MRI, but a longer-term disadvantage will remain its lack of therapeutic potential.

Angiography

Liver angiography has lost much of its diagnostic importance as newer techniques provide useful information about the vascularization of liver parenchyma and neoplasms. There are, however, still some indications for angiography: (i) portal hypertension, for assessment of portal venous patency and flow direction, and detection of varices and other spontaneous portosystemic shunts, e.g. splenorenal; (ii) presurgical evaluation for liver resection; (iii) chemoembolization of liver tumours; (iv) therapeutic embolization in cases of haemobilia, hepatic arterial aneurysm, and liver trauma; (v) characterization of focal hepatic lesions, e.g. cavernous haemangioma.

Technique

Selective catheterization is obtained using precurved catheters via the femoral route, or exceptionally through a brachial approach.

Injection into the coeliac trunk demonstrates the hepatic and splenic arteries, and subsequently the splenic and portal veins. Selective catheterization of the hepatic artery provides more detail of the intrahepatic arteries, facilitating assessment of cirrhotic and malignant change, arterioportal shunting, and reversal of portal venous flow. Injection into the superior mesenteric artery demonstrates an aberrant right hepatic artery if present, and in the subsequent portal venous phase outlines the superior mesenteric and portal veins ('indirect arterioportography'). Varices and spontaneous portosystemic shunts may be demonstrated during this phase.

Results
Anatomical considerations

There are important variations in the anatomical display of the hepatic artery. Every single artery may originate from the coeliac trunk (middle artery), the left gastric artery (usually an aberrant left hepatic artery), or the superior mesenteric artery (usually an aberrant right hepatic artery). In rare instances, the hepatic artery may originate from the aorta. Up to three hepatic arteries may coexist in the same individual.

As a rule, the description of a liver artery should refer to its origin and distribution. The most usual variants are a single middle hepatic artery feeding the whole liver (50 per cent), or an aberrant right hepatic artery (40 per cent), associated or not associated with another artery.

When there are multiple arteries, there are communications between them at the hilar level, so that the proximal obstruction or ligation of one branch has no lasting effect on arterial liver perfusion.

Liver arterial diseases

Angiography is the 'gold standard' for the exploration of vascular disease. Aneurysms, dissections, or dysplasias are promptly diagnosed. Arterioportal fistulas give early and massive opacification of the portal radicles, before the parenchymal phase, and should be differentiated from portal flow reversal. In the reversal the portal radicles are opacified more faintly, from the periphery of the liver towards the portal trunk, and appear only on late exposures, after the parenchymal phase of arteriography.

Liver and biliary-tract neoplasms

The only tumour with a specific arterial pattern is cavernous haemangioma (Freeny, Radiol, 1979; 132:143). Lakes of contrast, 1 to 15 mm in diameter, appear at the end of the arterial phase, and persist through the parenchymal and venous phase. There is no modification of the calibre of the hepatic artery.

Hepatic adenomas and focal nodular hyperplasia are highly vascular, and are seen as a very intense blush during the arterial phase. Details may differ from one tumour to another (central arteries in focal nodular hyperplasia, peripheral arteries in adenoma), but interpretation is difficult in most cases and angiography should not be considered as the principal tool for specific diagnosis.

Hepatocellular carcinoma may present in a similar way, but association with irregular intratumoral vessels is usual in this case. More importantly, hepatocellular carcinoma is associated in 40 per cent of cases with portal venous invasion. The precise, and still important, role of angiography in hepatocellular carcinoma will be discussed later.

For metastases, angiography has little value for diagnosis, except in cases of hypervascular tumours. In these cases (endocrine neoplasias, kidney adenocarcinoma, mesenchymal tumours), angiography may detect more tumours than other methods, because of the tumoral blush seen in the arterial phase.

A special application for angiography is its role in the evaluation of Klatskin tumours. These tumours are scirrhous and may invade the main branches of hepatic artery and portal vein. When there is obvious invasion of both left and right branches, either of arteries or veins, curative surgery is no longer possible. When unilateral invasion is seen, resection should usually be possible (Voyles, AnnSurg, 1983; 197:188).

Portal hypertension

Angiography is an anatomical tool for display of the portal vein when shunt surgery is planned. This technique has no special value for diagnosis and, in fact, it should be realized that it may be misleading in some cases. When partial thrombosis occurs, angiography may miss the clot if its margins are smooth; more often, if the clot is stuck to the posterior aspect of the portal trunk, an anteroposterior view of the portal vein may seem unremarkable. Axial techniques are better for detection of partial clots.

In cases of portal flow reversal, non-opacification of portal radicles, or even of the portal trunk, may be falsely interpreted as thrombosis. Comparison with arterial injection and Doppler studies should help in this situation.

Special techniques
Portography

Portal branches can be opacified by direct puncture of portal radicles with transhepatic insertion of the needle in the mid-axillary line, or by direct splenic puncture (direct splenoportography). These techniques are technically simple, but in view of the risk of haemorrhage have been almost totally superseded by the far less invasive indirect techniques.

Portal pressure may be estimated by hepatic venous-wedge pressures following puncture of the internal jugular or femoral vein. Direct access to the portal vein may now be achieved transhepatically from the hepatic vein [transjugular intrahepatic portosystemic stent (**TIPS**) shunt].

Hepatic venography and cavography

Catheterization of hepatic veins can be achieved through direct transhepatic puncture, but as in the case of the portal vein this has been superseded by the safer transfemoral or, more commonly, transjugular routes. Indications include evaluation of hepatic venous morphology, for example in suspected Budd–Chiari syndrome, pressure evaluation and liver biopsy in liver disease and portal hypertension, and the creation of TIPS shunts.

As the inferior vena cava has a close anatomical relation to the liver, cavography with pressure studies is often useful in cases of suspected obstruction to the hepatic outflow, or for precaval tumours. MRI can be used to assess the anatomy and patency of the inferior vena cava, but cannot assess caval pressure.

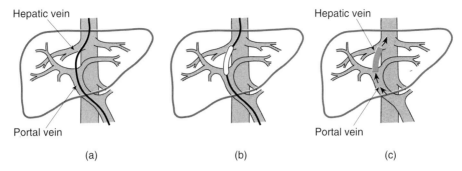

Fig. 7. TIPS shunt technique: (a) a needle/guidewire assembly is advanced from hepatic to portal vein; (b) the liver tract is dilated by balloon angioplasty; (c) stent deployed through liver tract.

Portocaval shunt opacification

When necessary, the opacification of surgical shunts may be achieved in two different ways. Opacification via the superior mesenteric artery allows a physiological approach to the shunts but requires arterial catheterization. Retrograde catheterization through the femoral route is useful for the direct opacification of shunts and allows the evaluation of the pressures on the two sides of the shunt.

TIPS shunt

This technique, developed in response to the persistently high mortality (35–50 per cent) associated with portal hypertensive variceal bleeding despite the use of established medical and surgical therapy, allows creation of a portosystemic shunt entirely within the liver. Following puncture of the right internal jugular vein a catheter/needle/guidewire assembly is advanced from a hepatic vein (usually the right) through liver parenchyma into a branch of the portal vein (usually the right). This track is then dilated with an angioplasty balloon and held open by a self-expanding metallic stent (Fig. 7).

The TIPS shunt reliably decreases the portal venous pressure and stops uncontrolled variceal bleeding in over 90 per cent of cases. This remains the main indication for the procedure. Other established indications are as a trial of shunt surgery and in selected patients with Budd–Chiari syndrome. Potential but unproven indications include treatment of refractory ascites and the hepatorenal syndrome. A TIPS allows unique access to the portal venous system for subsequent imaging, pressure studies, and intervention.

Complications include capsular perforation with potentially fatal intraperitoneal haemorrhage, hepatic encephalopathy, stent stenosis and occlusion, acceleration of liver failure, haemolysis, and right heart failure.[4]

Biliary-tract opacifications

Modern imaging, including sonography, leaves a smaller field of diagnostic interest in biliary-tract opacification.

Oral cholecystography

Since the development of ultrasonography, oral cholecystography is no longer a routine test for gallbladder stones, although there are still some indications for it that are related to therapeutic considerations.

On planning extracorporeal shock-wave lithotripsy or stone dissolution there is a need to assess gallbladder function because if the gallbladder is non-functional these methods are not indicated. Oral cholecystography provides a simple test for this; when the gallbladder opacifies after giving oral contrast it can be assumed that it is functioning and that the cystic duct is patent. Non-opacification may be observed in certain circumstances: for example, vomiting, diarrhoea, cholestasis, lack of contrast absorption, and competition with antibiotics for biliary excretion. These conditions should be excluded before concluding that there is a non-functioning gallbladder. Oral cholecystography is also better for showing stone size and number than ultrasonography, and thus allows better evaluation of the treatment.

Intravenous cholangiography

Opacification of the bile ducts is obtained after perfusion of hexa-iodinated contrast. The reported mortality (Nahum, JRadiol, 1975; 56:595) was 1 in 8000 examinations, which is much higher than that with other tests using intravenous contrast. Moreover, the detection rate for common bile-duct stones is low (Goodman, Gastro, 1980; 79:642). These factors explain why the use of this examination declined.

However, with the development of laparoscopic cholecystectomy, interest in intravenous cholangiography as a relatively non-invasive means of assessing the biliary tract preoperatively has been revived. The risk of reaction to modern contrast agents has not been clearly evaluated, but it does appear to be much lower than with the older agents.

Percutaneous transhepatic cholangiography (PTC) and endoscopic retrograde cholangiography (ERC)

PTC with a fine-needle technique is now a routine examination of the biliary tract (Okuda, AmJDigDis, 1974; 19(1):21). It is also an easy method for therapeutic approaches. Puncture is usually performed in the mid-axillary line under fluoroscopic control, but with guidance by ultrasound any dilated bile duct may be punctured (including those in the left lobe via an epigastric approach). Complications are few (under 5 per cent) (Mueller, AJR, 1981; 136:85). Infection may be prevented by antibiotic therapy and the injection of a only small quantity of contrast. Intraperitoneal haemorrhage and bile leaks are rare if the examination is done only in patients with normal coagulation, and provided that no more than five attempts at opacification are made using a fine needle. Ascites and impaired coagulation are contraindications. Opacification is obtained in 100 per cent of cases if the bile ducts are dilated, and in 70 to 90 per cent if they are not, depending on operator experience (Harbin, Radiol, 1980, 135:15). If biliary obstruction is demonstrated, external biliary drainage is indicated and can be done immediately. Access to the biliary tract is guaranteed and allows subsequent balloon dilatation and/or deployment of an endoprosthesis as necessary.

ERC can be used when an endoscopic approach to the papilla is possible; this excludes patients already subjected to duodenal resection, Roux-en-Y procedures, and most patients with enterogastric surgical anastomoses. Although dependent on operator skill, the success rate is generally over 90 per cent. The major complication is infection of the bile ducts, and the procedure is associated with a mortality quoted at 1 per cent.

These procedures are complementary rather than concurrent. Advantages of PTC include low cost, ease of use, fine delineation of intrahepatic ducts, and visualization of the upper pole of the obstruction. ERC requires an experienced operator, but is possible even in cases of abnormal coagulation or ascites. It shows the lower pole of the obstruction and allows a sphincterotomy when necessary, as well as visualization and biopsy of the papilla of Vater. If an obstructing lesion can be negotiated, an endoprosthesis may be deployed from below.

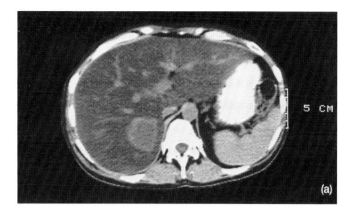

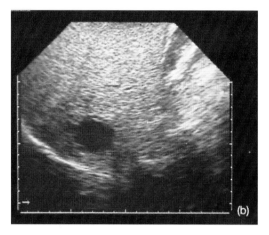

Fig. 8. Liver steatosis. (a) On plain CT, the entire liver appears hypodense (-15 HU) and non-enhanced blood vessels are more dense than parenchyma. In the posterior segment of the right lobe, a focal lesion appears spontaneously hyperdense. (b) Ultrasonography shows that the lesion is in fact a biliary cyst.

Imaging in the clinical setting

Parenchymal diseases of the liver

Fatty infiltration

Ultrasonographic features of fatty infiltration include increased parenchymal echogenicity with distal attenuation ('fade out') of the acoustic beam and loss of the echogenic walls of the portal veins. The degree of increased echogenicity is roughly proportional to the extent of fatty infiltration.

CT is the imaging technique of choice for assessing fatty infiltration as there is good correlation between the attenuation value of the hepatic parenchyma and the degree of fatty infiltration on biopsy. Fat deposition leads to a reduction in attenuation. Mild fatty infiltration may reduce the hepatic attenuation to that of the spleen. Moderate fat deposition reduces attenuation to below that of the spleen, whilst marked infiltration may produce negative HU numbers with blood vessels appearing hyperdense to liver parenchyma on plain scans (Fig. 8).

MRI is generally not helpful in assessing diffuse fatty infiltration, although it can be of use in characterizing focal fat deposition. Specialized techniques such as MR spectroscopy have been used to quantify fatty infiltration, but at present this is a research tool only.

Cirrhosis and portal hypertension

Imaging methods are not intended to provide the specific diagnosis of cirrhosis, which should be made by biopsy. They may, however, show a number of abnormalities that strongly suggest the diagnosis.

Ultrasonography, CT, and MRI may all demonstrate localized modifications of liver anatomy. The most frequent finding is hypertrophy of the caudate lobe and left lobe, and atrophy of the right lobe (see Fig. 22). This may be quantified (on CT) as the caudate lobe:right lobe ratio, which is reported to have high accuracy in diagnosing cirrhosis. A degree of fatty infiltration frequently coexists with cirrhosis.

In early cirrhosis the ultrasonographic appearances may be normal. Features of established cirrhosis include reduction in liver size, heterogeneous, coarse parenchymal echogenicity, irregular liver contour, and evidence of portal hypertension. The reported sensitivity for ultrasonographic diagnosis of cirrhosis varies from 65 to 95 per cent, but ultrasound is unable to assess aetiological factors.

Plain CT may show a nodular appearance, particularly in macronodular cirrhosis, with an irregular liver contour. The contrast-enhanced pattern is usually more homogeneous. CT arterio-portography may be of use in distinguishing between adenomatous hyperplastic nodules and hepatocellular carcinoma, as the nodules have a portal venous blood supply whereas only 6 per cent of hepatocellular carcinomas do. This distinction can now be made non-invasively with MRI, as adenomatous hyperplastic nodules are hyperintense on T_1-weighted images and hypointense on T_2-weighted, whereas hepatocellular carcinomas are hyperintense on T_2-weighted images. Regenerating nodules also show low signal on T_2-weighting. This may be striking and has been attributed to an increased haemosiderin content.

Angiography is used in the evaluation and planning of treatment in patients with cirrhosis rather than in initial diagnosis. Angiographic features of cirrhosis include a corkscrew appearance of the branches of the hepatic artery, a heterogeneous hepatogram, arterioportal shunting and, in endstage cirrhosis, reduction in liver size, hepatofugal portal venous flow, varices, and possibly tumour circulation.

Portal hypertension is inferred from the presence of varices, splenomegaly, and ascites, all of which can be readily demonstrated by ultrasonography, CT, and MRI.

Doppler ultrasonographic examination of the portal vein allows measurement of diameter, flow velocity, and respiratory variation. An increased diameter of the portal vein was considered a reliable sign in early reports. A diameter greater than 13 mm strongly suggests portal hypertension, but is seen in only 75 per cent of cases. In practice no single measurement is entirely reliable. Reversed (hepatofugal) portal venous flow is clearly shown. Doppler ultrasonography is also valuable in evaluating the patency of surgical and TIPS shunts.

The major venous collaterals are the coronary veins and associated oesophageal varices, the umbilical vein, the left gastric vein, and splenorenal shunts. Ultrasonography can demonstrate direction of flow in these channels. CT is better able to demonstrate retroperitoneal collaterals and other intra-abdominal collaterals such as mesentericogonadic veins or colonic varices.

MRI may show varices as tubular structures devoid of signal ('flow-void') on spin-echo sequences, but can show variable signal intensity in the presence of slow or turbulent flow. Dynamic Gd-enhanced MRI can demonstrate varices very elegantly.

One of the main roles of imaging is to assess the cause of portal hypertension. Prehepatic causes include thrombosis of the portal and splenic veins. A diagnosis of portal thrombosis (Fig. 9) is easily made by ultrasonography, CT or MRI (Parvey, AJR, 1994; 162:77). This may be at the early stage, when the intraportal clot is identified (Fig. 9(a,b)), or at the late stage of cavernous transformation of the portal vein (Fig. 9(c)). Whilst usually evident on angiography, it is often better appreciated on cross-sectional imaging (Fig. 9(a,b)). Portal venous thrombosis may be due to bland thrombus (Fig. 9) or tumour invasion (Fig. 10).

The imaging features of Budd–Chiari syndrome depend on the age and degree of venous obstruction. In the acute stage the liver is enlarged and there is usually splenomegaly and ascites. In the chronic stage the liver is nodular and irregular in shape, with caudate hypertrophy and peripheral atrophy.

Ultrasonography is the preferred method for the initial diagnosis of Budd–Chiari syndrome as it shows the modification of liver anatomy, and abnormalities of the hepatic veins (thrombosis, stenosis, intrahepatic collaterals), as well as the patency of the portal vein (Menu,

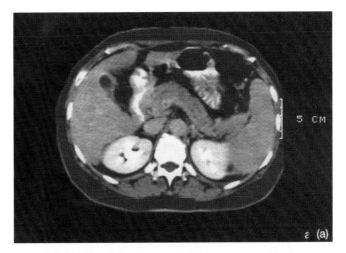

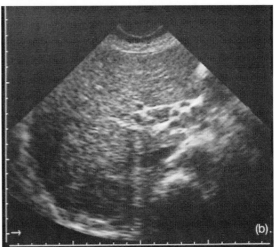

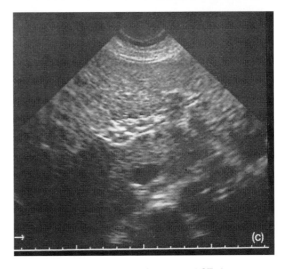

Fig. 9. Portal venous thrombosis: (a) enhanced CT shows a spot of low density in the portal vein; (b) ultrasonography on the same day shows echogenic material in the portal vein; (c) ultrasonography 20 days later shows multiple collaterals in the porta hepatis corresponding to cavernous transformation of the portal vein.

Radiol, 1985; 157:761). It should be noted that, in enlarged livers, the hepatic veins may be compressed and difficult to assess.

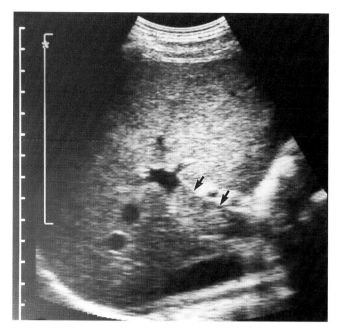

(a)

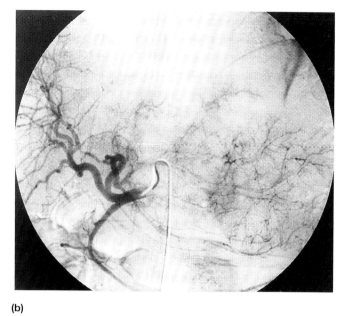

(b)

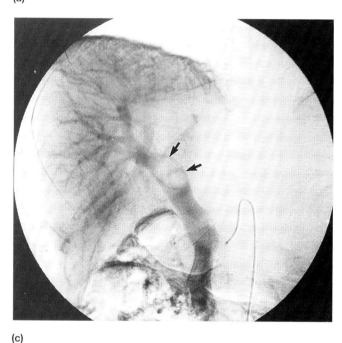

(c)

Fig. 10. Tumour thrombus in the portal vein. (a) Longitudinal ultrasonographic scan showing echogenic tissue in the main portal vein (arrows). (b) Coeliac angiogram showing neovascularization and expansion due to the large left-lobe tumour. (c) Portal-phase image of superior mesenteric arterial angiogram showing the portal venous filling defect *(arrows)* and occluded left portal vein. The patient had a large hepatocellular carcinoma of the left hepatic lobe, occluding the left portal vein and extending into the main portal vein.

CT shows 'patchy' contrast enhancement of liver parenchyma, often with more uniform enhancement of the caudate lobe. Like ultrasonography, it is still of limited value for evaluating the patency of the inferior vena cava (Mathieu, Radiol, 1987; 165:409).

The multiplanar capacity of MRI is useful in assessing the hepatic veins and inferior vena cava, although the potential for flow artefacts must be borne in mind. In cases secondary to tumour, Gd-DTPA enhanced T_1-weighted images may distinguish bland from tumour thrombus, as the latter enhances (Soyer, AbdomImag, 1994; 19:325).

Hepatic venography remains the definitive diagnostic examination, showing the pathognomonic 'spider's web' pattern of irregular, collateral intrahepatic veins. Cavography may show a membranous web and permits pressure studies.

Focal lesions of the liver

The main role of ultrasonography of the liver is the detection of focal lesions. As the technique is relatively cheap and easy to perform, it is the preferred method for tumour screening. The drawbacks of this method are its operator-dependence and the difficulty of comparing images between one examination and another.

The sensitivity for detection varies according to the size and structure of the focal lesion. When it is hypo- or hyperechoic, masses over 1 cm can be usually detected. In cases with an isoechoic pattern, much larger lesions may be missed.

Fluid-filled lesions

Ultrasonography is the only imaging method that allows a reliable diagnosis of fluid-filled lesions; such masses are completely anechoic and show posterior enhancement (Fig. 8). In most cases, fluid-filled lesions in the liver are simple biliary cysts, presenting as smoothly delineated, thin-walled, unilocular, fluid-filled masses. They should be distinguished from cystic secondary deposits, echinococcal cysts, biliary cystadenomas, and Caroli's disease. All these lesions present with a thicker wall, or with mural irregularities, internal septations or mural calcifications. In Caroli's disease, the relation between the cysts and the bile ducts is usually conspicuous.

CT is not generally performed in cases of simple biliary cyst as ultrasonography usually gives the diagnosis. When seen on CT the cysts are well defined with smooth, thin walls, devoid of internal architecture, and non-enhancing. Attenuation measurements are close to that of water (0 HU). In small cysts, partial-volume effect may lead to erroneous measurements of attenuation. However, CT is a useful tool in the evaluation of echinococcal cysts (Fig. 11), because it is more reliable than ultrasonography for the detection of mural calcification, analysis of the internal structure of heavily calcified cysts, and in searching for additional extrahepatic cysts (Kirshner, JComputAssistTomogr, 1978; 2:229).

On MR examinations, simple cysts appear as well-defined lesions that have very high signal on T_2-weighted and low signal on T_1-weighted images.

Solid lesions

The characterization of solid lesions on imaging has traditionally been poor. This remains true for grey-scale ultrasonography, where there is considerable overlap in appearances between different lesions. Duplex ultrasonography reportedly distinguishes between benign and malignant, primary and metastatic, focal liver lesions with high specificity but low sensitivity, based upon detection of Doppler frequency shifts (i.e., increased vascularity in malignant and primary lesions) (Reinhold, AJR, 1995; 164:1131). SCT and dynamic Gd-enhanced MRI allow imaging of the liver during two or more phases of vascular enhancement, resulting in improved characterization of lesions (Katsuyoshi, Radiographics, 1996; 1:273). A recent study of triphasic SCT (arterial-, portal-, and equilibrium-phase images) correctly characterized 87 per cent of lesions (van Leeuwen, Radiol, 1996; 201:327). Hepatic and hepatobiliary contrast agents also promise to improve characterization on MRI.

Focal fatty infiltration is a frequent finding. It presents either with focal areas of infiltration in a normal liver, or with localized areas of preserved normal liver in a diffusely fatty liver. In the former case, the lesion will appear as hyperechoic and homogeneous, with a sharp or lobulated pattern. In many cases, the outer limits of the hyperechoic area seem to run parallel to the segmental anatomy. In the latter cases, hypoechoic areas will appear in a hyperechoic liver. These lesions are most often localized in segment IV, in front of the left and right main branches of the portal trunk, and along the gallbladder bed. In some cases, focal fatty infiltration

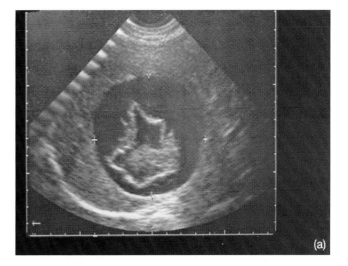

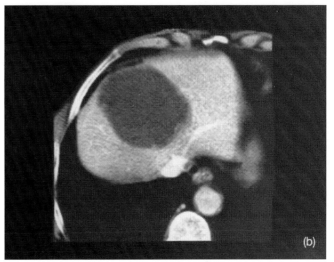

Fig. 11. Echinococcal cyst: (a) ultrasonography shows a floating membrane; (b) CT is not able to detect internal septations.

leads to diagnostic dilemmas, and fine-needle aspiration should be the next step (El-Hassan, BrJRadiol, 1992; 65:774).

Hepatic cavernous haemangioma (Fig. 12) is the single, most frequent, solid focal lesion detected by ultrasonography. As it is benign and requires no treatment in most cases, it should ideally be characterized with a single examination. In 60 per cent of cases it presents, usually incidentally, as a bright hyperechoic lesion, with sharp delineation and a homogeneous echo pattern. Posterior acoustic enhancement may be seen. It is generally agreed that such a lesion, when measuring less than 1.5 cm in diameter, should be considered as a haemangioma if detected in a patient with no relevant clinical or biological features (Jones, AJR, 1992; 158:535). It has been demonstrated (Bree, AJR, 1983; 140:41) that the sonographic appearance in itself is not specific, as it can be mimicked by various lesions such as metastases or lipoma (Fig. 13). If the lesion is over 3 cm in diameter, or if the echo pattern is atypical, further imaging is required.

Much has been written about CT in the exploration of cavernous haemangiomas. They classically show early peripheral globular

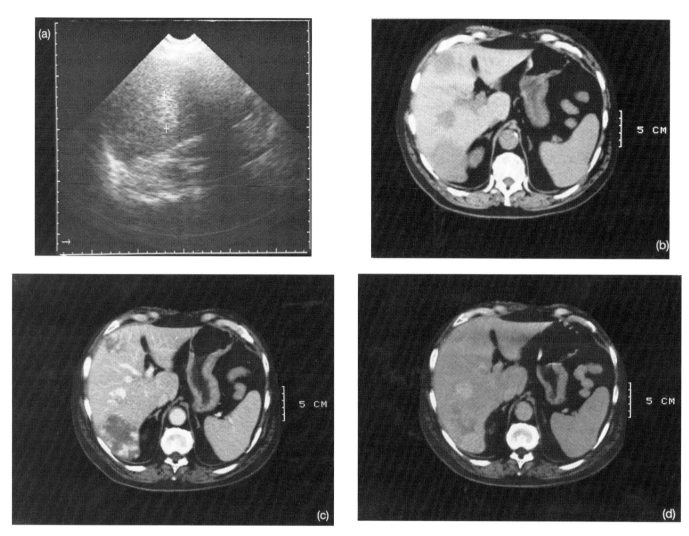

Fig. 12. Multiple cavernous haemangioma. (a) Ultrasonography shows a hyperechoic area, and the other lesions were similar. (b) On plain CT, three homogeneous lesions of blood density are seen. (c) Thirty seconds after injection, contrast enhancement is seen at the periphery of the lesion. (d) Five minutes later, the lesions are different. The smaller lesion is homogeneous and hyperdense. The posterior lesion is hyperdense but its centre remains hypodense. The anterior lesion is isodense but with a central hypodense area.

enhancement and subsequent partial or complete fill-in on delayed images (Quinn, Radiol, 1992; 182:545). Some haemangiomas may enhance slowly, necessitating repeat delayed scans after 10 to 15 min to assess fill-in. Central fibrosis, haemorrhage, or thrombosis may confuse the appearances.

On MRI, cavernous haemangiomas are best seen on heavily T_2-weighted sequences, when they demonstrate markedly high signal with a homogeneous pattern and sharp boundaries (Fig. 14). They show a similar enhancement pattern following intravenous contrast to that seen on CT, peripheral globular enhancement with delayed fill-in (Semelka, Radiol, 1994; 192: 401). When there are multiple lesions, all share the same pattern. MRI is more sensitive in lesion detection than either ultrasonography or CT. Cavernous haemangiomas need to be differentiated from simple cysts, which have a similar appearance, but ultimately this distinction is not clinically relevant. Hypervascular metastases (endocrine or kidney tumours) may also

have a similar pattern to haemangioma (Wittenberg, AJR, 1988; 151:79); therefore, as ever, clinical background remains a necessary basis for image interpretation.

If doubt persists despite the use of multiple methods of imaging, percutaneous biopsy may be performed relatively safely. Angiography is diagnostic but invasive (see above).

Focal nodular hyperplasia typically appears on ultrasonography as a well-defined, hypoechoic mass with homogeneous echogenicity except for a central scar, but the appearances are not specific. In particular a central scar may be seen in adenomas and larger haemangiomas.

The appearance on CT is sometimes characteristic enough to give a strong indication of the tumour type, as in the case of focal nodular hyperplasia (Fig. 15). The lesion is homogeneous on plain CT. After bolus injection, enhancement is massive, due to hypervascularization, but it disappears promptly. After a minute or even less, the lesion is isointense to the liver (Fig. 15(d)). This stresses

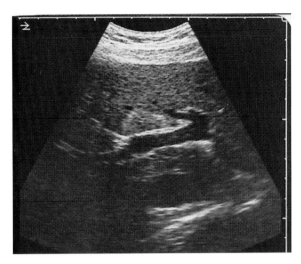

Fig. 13. Focal area of fatty infiltration mimicking haemangioma on ultrasonography.

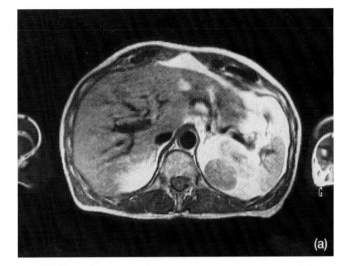

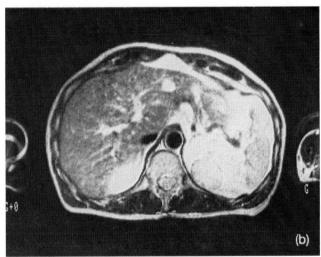

Fig. 14. MRI of cavernous haemangioma; T_2-weighted sequences (TR = 2000 ms) in a case of a small angioma of the left liver lobe. (a) Echo time (TE) 30 ms; (b) TE 80 ms. The latter is heavily T_2-weighted and the angioma appears brighter than in (a). This lesion had not been detected by CT, owing to its small size and location.

the importance of early slices after injection. A central fibrous scar, although not consistent, is usually seen during the bolus phase or later, and rarely on plain CT. Although indicative, these findings are still not specific as other tumours, including malignancies, may have a roughly similar appearance.

Focal nodular hyperplasia is usually isointense to liver on all pulse sequences. When a central scar is seen it is usually hyperintense on T_2-weighting. A capsule may be present, a feature that may also be seen in hepatocellular carcinoma. Angiography typically shows a hypervascular mass with arteries radiating from the periphery to the centre producing the classic 'spoke-wheel' appearance, but again this is not specific for focal nodular hyperplasia.

Hepatic adenomas are more difficult to characterize. They are highly variable in appearance depending upon the degree of central necrosis, haemorrhage and fibrosis, producing a mixed pattern on ultrasonography. On CT they are typically isodense on plain scans, show enhancement in the arterial phase, and subsequently become iso- or hypodense on delayed scans (Fig. 16). With MRI they often show increased signal on both T_1- and T_2-weighted images, the former being attributable to the presence of fat or haemorrhage. They are said to have a central arterial supply with radiating branches on angiography (Fig. 16), but this pattern is non-specific. In particular, differentiation from hepatocellular carcinoma may be difficult.

Metastases are the most common malignant lesions of the liver. Ultrasonography is the preferred method for detection, with a sensitivity of over 90 per cent. Five basic patterns are seen: hyperechoic (gastrointestinal tract, endocrine, renal primaries), 'bull's-eye' or 'target' lesions (bronchogenic primary) (Fig. 17), hypoechoic (lymphoma, pancreatic, cervical primaries), cystic (cystadeno-carcinoma of the pancreas and ovary, sarcoma, melanoma, carcinoid), and diffuse. Metastases from mucinous primary tumours, particularly of the colon, may calcify. Other features suggesting this diagnosis are a heterogeneous pattern from one lesion to another in the case of multiple lesions, or the appearance or growth of liver lesions on sequential sonograms. Ultimately, however, the diagnosis can only be unequivocally made histologically following biopsy, as

multifocal disease such as liver abscesses and heterogeneous fatty liver may mimic metastases.

Intraoperative ultrasonography is highly sensitive for detecting metastases. It may detect lesions additional to those shown on preoperative imaging, and clearly displays the relation of lesions to the hepatic and portal venous branches.

As on ultrasonography, a range of CT patterns may be seen. Most metastases are hypodense on plain CT, and enhance to a lesser degree than normal parenchyma, thereby improving their detectability. Hyperdense metastases are uncommon, but may be seen with endocrine, melanoma, thyroid, breast, and chorio-carcinoma primaries. They typically enhance greatly on arterial phase-enhanced scans. The hepatic arterial supply of metastases is exploited in the techniques of hepatic SCT angiography and SCT angiography, as explained previously. SCT angiography remains the 'gold standard' for evaluation of hepatic metastases. It has a

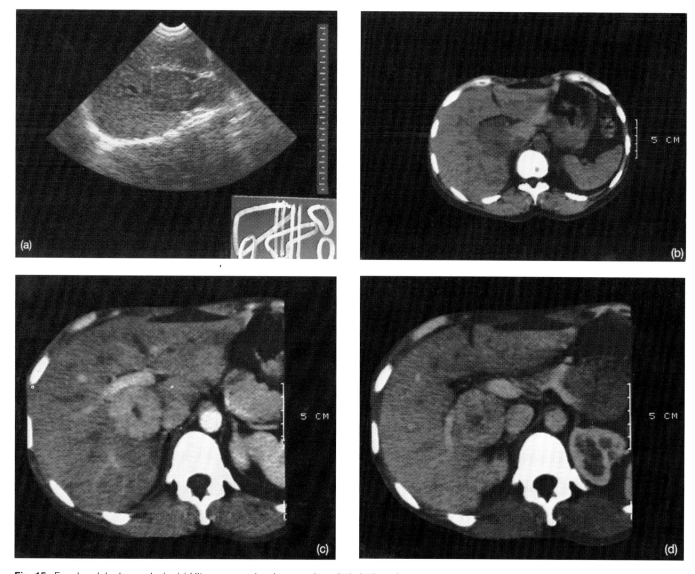

Fig. 15. Focal nodular hyperplasia. (a) Ultrasonography shows an isoechoic lesion of the caudate lobe. (b) On plain CT the lesion is hypodense, with a slight central hypodensity. On enhanced slices the lesion enhances soon after injection (c), and returns to isodensity after 60 s (d). A central hypodense area corresponds to the 'central scar' of focal nodular hyperplasia.

sensitivity of approximately 90 per cent, and is able to detect lesions as small as 5 mm in diameter (Fig. 18).

MRI with Gd enhancement is the most sensitive, non-invasive technique for detecting metastases, but is not widely practised owing to the present limited access to MRI and the availability of other methods to make the diagnosis in the majority of cases. Specific applications of MRI include differentiation between metastases and fatty infiltration, and the detection of diffuse, infiltrative disease. Its capacity for multiplanar imaging can be very useful in assessing lesions in the superior aspects of the liver, in particular in the context of possible invasion of the chest wall or diaphragm (Fig. 19).

Hepatocellular carcinoma (Fig. 20) is the most frequent primary malignant tumour of the liver. It may be focal, multifocal, or diffuse. In 85 per cent of cases it is associated with cirrhosis.

Every focal liver lesion in a patient with cirrhosis should be considered as hepatocellular carcinoma until another diagnosis is proven. Small hepatocellular carcinomas (under 3 cm in diameter) tend to be hypoechoic. Larger lesions are hyperechoic or of mixed pattern. A capsule may be present, seen as a thin, hypoechoic band. Doppler ultrasonographic examination may reveal high vascularity and helps in assessing portal and hepatic venous invasion. Tumour thrombus in the portal vein appears in 35 to 40 per cent of cases (Fig. 10), and is almost specific for the diagnosis of hepatocellular carcinoma. Invasion of the hepatic vein is less common, reported to occur in 6 per cent of cases. It is generally accepted that ultrasonography should be the method for detection, with a sensitivity of nearly 100 per cent for lesions over 2 cm, and 50 per cent for lesions between 1 and 2 cm. Sensitivity for lesions under 1 cm falls to 10 per

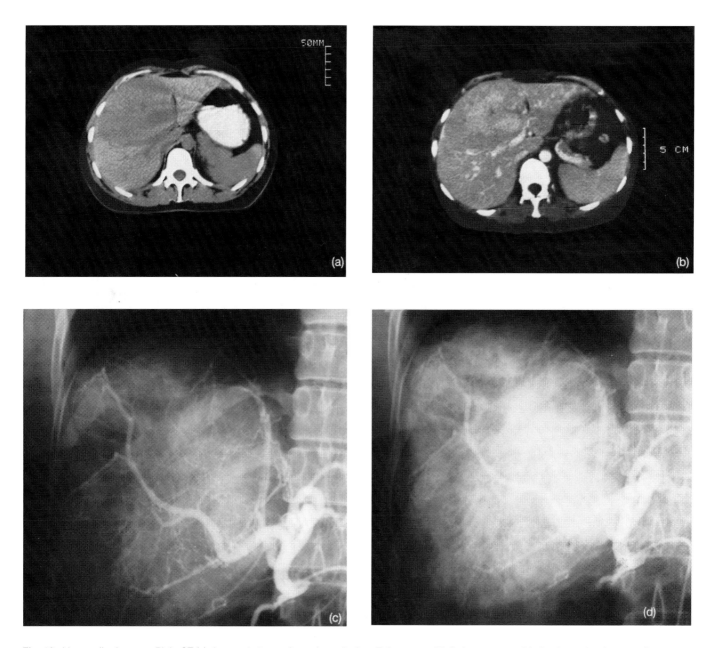

Fig. 16. Liver-cell adenoma. Plain CT (a) demonstrates an hypodense lesion. Enhancement is heterogeneous (b). Angiography shows radiate arteries feeding the lesion (c), and a heterogeneous parenchymal phase (d).

cent. The main differential diagnosis is the regeneration nodule, when the lesion diameter is about 1 cm. Usually regeneration nodules are multiple, all have a similar appearance, and they do not change size within months. Hepatocellular carcinoma, when disseminated, presents with heterogeneous nodules of various sizes and patterns. CT cannot reliably distinguish between regenerative nodules and hepatocellular carcinoma, but this can be achieved with MRI as regenerative nodules have low signal on T_2-weighted, whereas hepatocellular carcinoma has high signal.

On plain CT, the tumour is usually hypodense, often with central necrosis. CT evidence of cirrhosis is seen in 60 per cent of cases. Hyperdense areas may be related to haemorrhage (Fig. 21) or central

calcification, which may be found in 5 to 20 per cent of cases. Postcontrast dual-phase SCT scans maximize detection as 10 per cent of lesions are seen only in the arterial phase, becoming isodense to parenchyma on the portal-phase images (Fig. 22). The arterial-phase images may also demonstrate arterioportal shunting, or vascularity in a portal venous thrombus indicating tumour invasion (Baron, Radiol, 1996; 199:505). CT after intra-arterial injection of Lipiodol is of particular value; it is able to detect the oily contrast in the liver with a high sensitivity. This contrast is retained in hepatocellular carcinoma, while disappearing from normal liver within 7 to 14 days, improving lesion detection and characterization (Fig. 23).

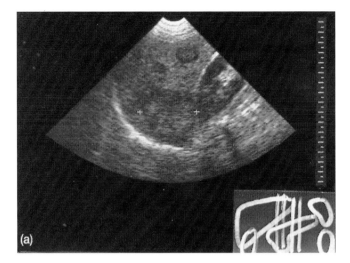

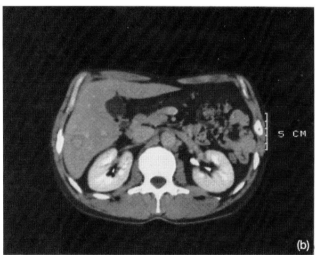

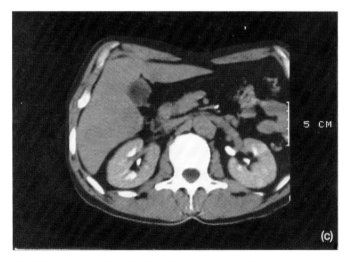

Fig. 17. Secondary deposits from lung cancer. A bull's eye pattern is seen on ultrasonography (a) and enhanced CT (b). On delayed slices (c) the lesion is less apparent.

When compared with CT, MRI is not able significantly to detect additional lesions. It has been reported (Ebara, Radiol, 1986; 159: 371) that 30 per cent of hepatocellular carcinomas were hyperintense on T_1-weighted sequences, in relation to the fatty components of the lesion. Other liver tumours, excepting hepatic-cell adenoma and lipoma, will appear hypointense on the same sequences. The same investigators suggested that a peritumoral capsule could be identified with MRI in 40 to 50 per cent of cases, a figure that seems to be superior to all other methods. It is also of interest that regeneration nodules appear different as they are hypointense on both T_1- and T_2-weighted sequences.

Hepatocellular carcinoma has a variable appearance on MRI, depending on the degree of necrosis, fibrosis, and fatty change. It may be used to demonstrate vascular invasion and to differentiate hepatocellular carcinoma from haemangioma or regeneration nodules.

The angiographic detection rate for hepatocellular carcinoma depends mainly on tumour size. About 45 per cent of nodules under 1 cm in diameter are detected, 64 per cent of those between 1 and 2 cm, and 93 per cent between 2 and 5 cm in diameter (Takayasu, Radiol, 1985; 154:25). Hepatocellular carcinoma is a hypervascular tumour with evidence of neovascularization and arterioportal shunting.

Angiography allows selective catheterization of the hepatic artery and injection of Lipiodol (Fig. 23). This may be used in a diagnostic screening role, as described above, or as a therapeutic tool by pharmaceutically linking Lipiodol to chemotherapeutic agents such as epirubicin. Preferential uptake of Lipiodol by tumour cells effectively targets the chemotherapy. Radioactive iodine (I^{131}) may also be linked with Lipiodol to achieve targeted radiotherapy.

Liver abscesses present with a heterogeneous pattern, mainly hypoechoic, depending on the amount of central fluid collection. Central gas bubbles, when present, are readily detected. Amoebic abscesses are usually more homogeneous and fluid-filled (Fig. 24), but differentiation is difficult on the basis of imaging methods alone. Diagnosis relies on the clinical and biological background. Abscess aspiration can be a diagnostic and therapeutic tool.

Gallbladder and bile ducts

Stones

The evaluation of gallbladder stones is one of the major roles of ultrasonography. The sensitivity and specificity are higher than 95 per cent, and the technique is considered the 'gold standard 'for detection of gallstones. The evolving therapeutic options (extracorporeal shock-wave lithotripsy, stone dissolution, coelioscopic surgery) have led to a new need for quantification of stones, in terms of number and diameter. It appears that ultrasonography might be less accurate than an oral cholecystogram for such quantification.

Evaluation of common bile-duct stones is much more difficult. The sensitivity of ultrasonography is low (50 per cent) and a normal sonogram does not rule out the diagnosis. CT seems to carry a higher sensitivity (Fig. 25).

Intrahepatic stones are rare. They can be accurately detected on sonograms as discrete foci of increased echoes, with distal acoustic shadowing, localized in dilated intrahepatic bile ducts. Ultrasonography is not sufficient for a complete evaluation of these stones

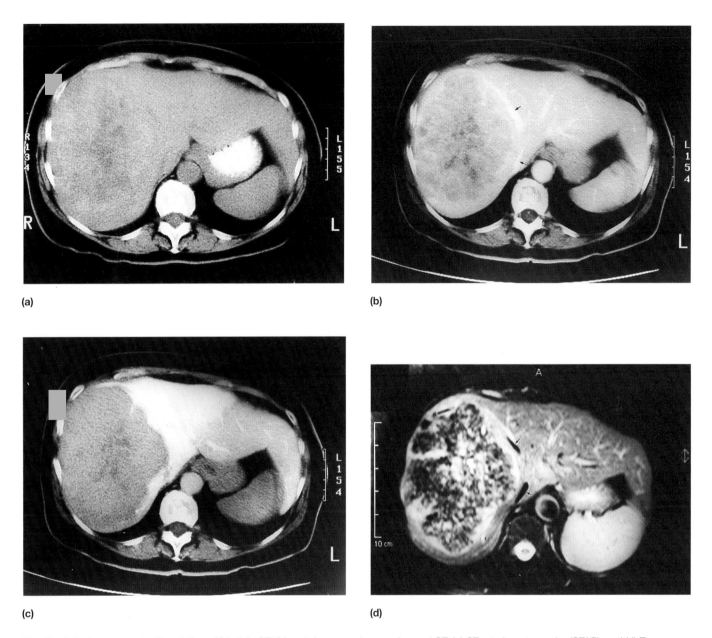

(a)

(b)

(c)

(d)

Fig. 18. Colonic metastasis. Correlation of (a) plain CT, (b) portal venous phase-enhanced CT, (c) CT arterioportography (CTAP), and (d) T_2-weighted, fat-saturated MR. The lesion is initially slightly hypodense on CT and heterogeneous to liver, becoming more conspicuous following intravenous contrast. It is hypodense on CTAP, and clearly seen on MR. Note the splaying of the right and middle hepatic veins in (b) and (d) (arrows).

as it may underestimate their number and topographical extent (Menu, AJR, 1985; 145:579).

Carcinoma

The most common appearance of gallbladder carcinoma is a large mass filling or replacing the gallbladder, and associated with gallstones. These findings may lead to the diagnosis. With CT contrast enhancement may be either diffuse or peripheral in the case of central necrosis. Infiltrating carcinoma is rare, presenting as a local thickening of the gallbladder wall. Scirrhous type with a contracted, fibrotic gallbladder may mimic a hilar carcinoma. Regional extension

involves the adjacent liver, bile ducts, and lymph nodes in the porta hepatis. This is best demonstrated by CT (Fig. 26).

Arteriography is performed as a preoperative procedure to depict invasion of hepatic vessels. Cholangiography provides the best preoperative determination of the site of obstruction and proximal extension.

In most cases, carcinoma of the common bile duct develops at the hilar level. Dilatation of intrahepatic bile ducts can be recognized with ultrasonography and CT, without any enlargement of the gallbladder or common bile duct. The tumour can be seen either as a focal thickening of the bile-duct wall or as a small intraductal

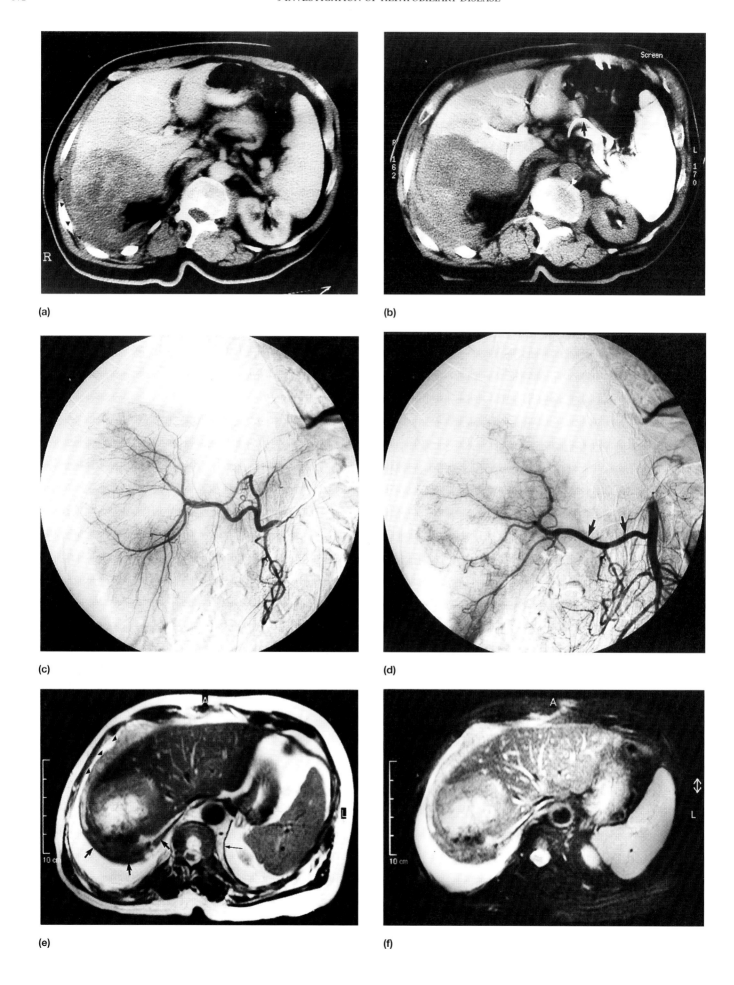

(a)

(b)

(c)

(d)

(e)

(f)

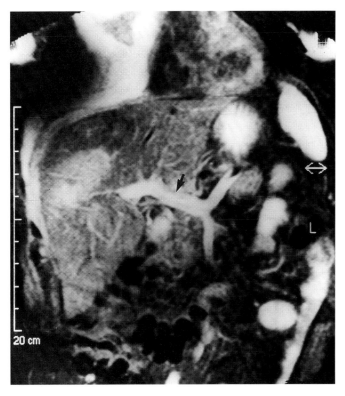

(g)

Fig. 19. Colonic metastasis with diaphragmatic invasion. (a) Portal venous phase-enhanced SCT shows a large segment VI/VII lesion distorting the liver contour. A pleural effusion is present (arrowheads). (b) SCT arterioportography shows non-enhancement of the lesion consistent with a metastasis. Note the catheter tip positioned in the splenic artery (arrow), because the patient had an accessory right hepatic artery arising from the superior mesenteric artery (SMA). (c) Common hepatic angiogram showing a hypovascular lesion. (d) SMA angiogram showing the accessory right hepatic artery (arrows) and the same hypovascular lesion. (e) T_2-weighted axial MR image showing mixed increased signal in the lesion. The crus of the right hemidiaphragm (thick arrows) is expanded and has increased signal when compared to that on the left (thin arrows). Abnormal soft tissue extends around the edge of the right hepatic lobe (arrowheads). (Findings confirmed on laparoscopy/thoracoscopy). (f) T_2-weighted image with fat suppression. Note the lack of signal from the mesenteric and abdominal-wall fat when compared to (e). The right pleural fluid remains high signal. (g) T_2-weighted coronal image with fat suppression. Note the demonstration of the patent portal vein (arrow).

mass. Occasionally, the tumour may not be detected. Unilobar atrophy is an ancillary finding related to long-standing obstruction. Local extension to the liver mostly involves segments I and IV (the 'caudate' and 'quadrate' lobes), and is clearly better demonstrated by CT than ultrasound. Cholangiography, either transhepatic or retrograde endoscopic, provides the best determination of tumour extension along the bile ducts. Transcatheter brushing and biopsy techniques are also available for cytological or histological examination. Infiltration of vessels in the liver hilum is seen frequently and requires angiographic examination, as the decision for curative or palliative methods will depend mainly on vascular extension.

References

1. Meire HB. Doppler. In Cosgrove DO, Meire HB, Dewbury KC, eds. *Clinical ultrasound—a comprehensive text: abdominal and general ultrasound.* Vol. 1. Edinburgh: Churchill Livingstone, 1993: 65–95.
2. Napel SA. Principles and techniques of 3D spiral CT angiography. In Fishman EK, Jeffrey RB, eds. *Spiral CT: principles, techniques and clinical applications.* New York: Raven Press, 1995: 167–82.
3. Wehrli FW. Principles of magnetic resonance. In Stark DD, Bradley WG, eds. *Magnetic resonance imaging.* St Louis: Mosby, 1992: 3–20.
4. Dick R, Patch D, Tibballs J. The transjugular intrahepatic portosystemic stent (TIPS) shunt. In Krasner N, ed. *Gastrointestinal bleeding.* London: BMJ Publishing Group, 1996: 175–86.

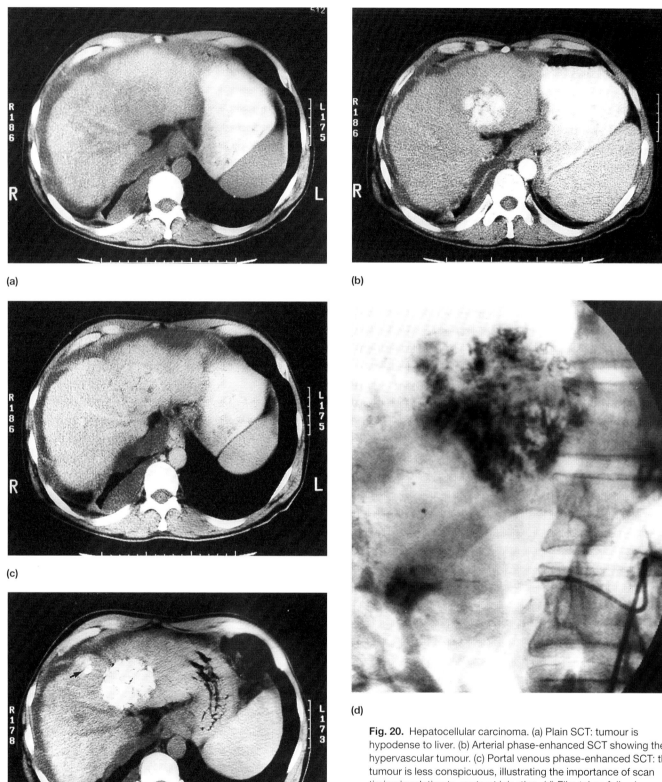

(a)

(b)

(c)

(d)

(e)

Fig. 20. Hepatocellular carcinoma. (a) Plain SCT: tumour is hypodense to liver. (b) Arterial phase-enhanced SCT showing the hypervascular tumour. (c) Portal venous phase-enhanced SCT: the tumour is less conspicuous, illustrating the importance of scan timing in relation to contrast injection. (d) Film taken following selective hepatic arterial Lipiodol injection; there is focal uptake by the tumour. (e) CT performed 9 days later shows retention of Lipiodol by the tumour. The second smaller focal uptake (arrow) is highly suspicious of a further small hepatocellular carcinoma not evident on the other scans.

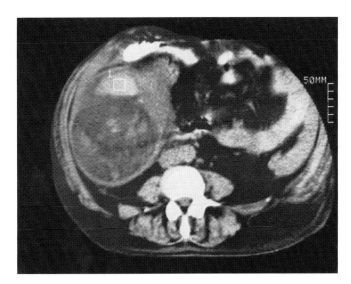

Fig. 21. Haemorrhagic hepatocellular carcinoma; haemorrhage present as an hyperdense area on plain CT (square).

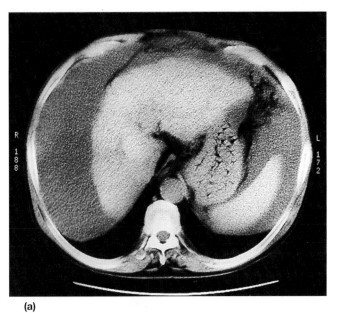

(a)

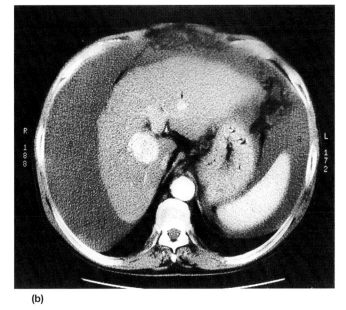

(b)

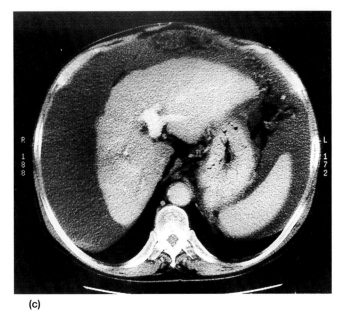

(c)

Fig. 22. Hepatocellular carcinoma. (a) Plain SCT, (b) arterial phase-enhanced SCT, and (c) portal venous phase-enhanced SCT. The large carcinoma can just be discerned in (a) and (c), but is most conspicuous in (b). The smaller-segment intravenous hepatocellular carcinoma (arrow) is only seen in (b). Note the irregular liver contour and right-lobe atrophy indicating cirrhosis. Ascites (a) indicates portal hypertension.

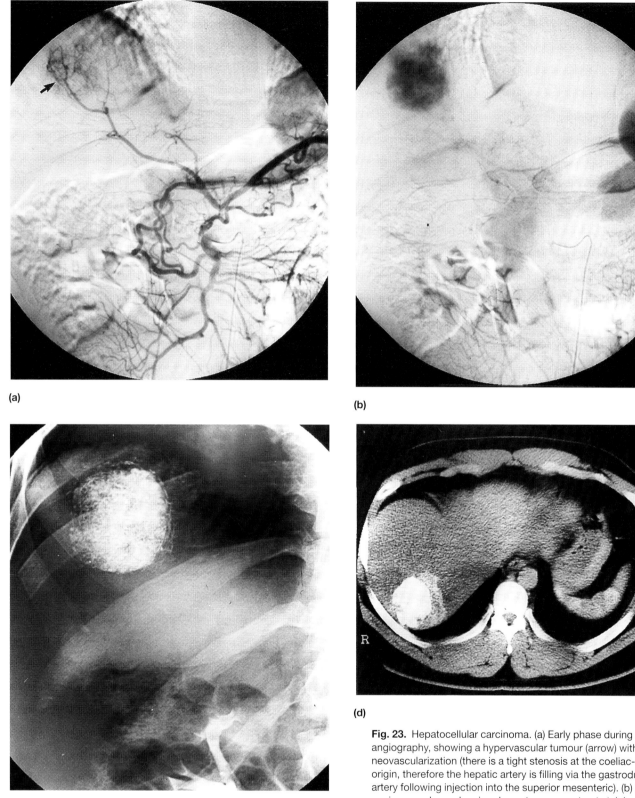

(a)

(b)

(c)

(d)

Fig. 23. Hepatocellular carcinoma. (a) Early phase during angiography, showing a hypervascular tumour (arrow) with neovascularization (there is a tight stenosis at the coeliac-axis origin, therefore the hepatic artery is filling via the gastroduodenal artery following injection into the superior mesenteric). (b) Late angiogram phase showing dense tumour contrast staining. (c) A film taken immediately after Lipiodol injection shows dense focal uptake. (d) CT scan 10 days later shows persistent focal uptake in the hepatocellular carcinoma and clearing from the remaining parenchyma.

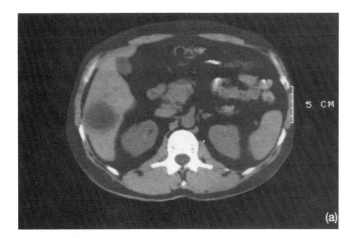

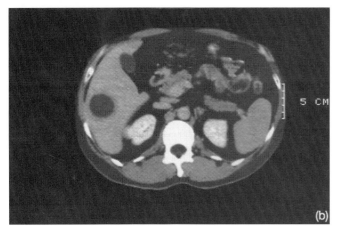

Fig. 24. Amoebic abscess: the lesion is homogeneous and fluid-filled; a peripheral area of intermediate density, seen on plain (a) and enhanced (b) CT corresponds to parenchymal oedema.

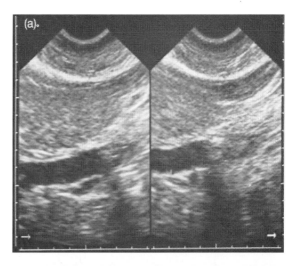

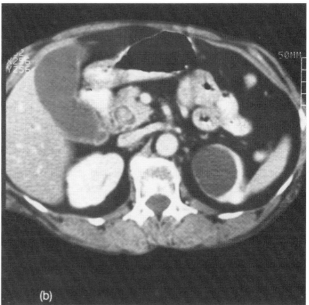

Fig. 25. Common bile-duct stone seen on ultrasonography (a) and CT (b).

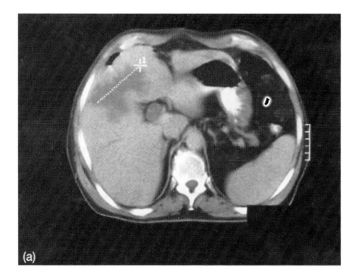

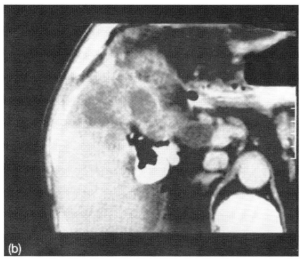

Fig. 26. Carcinoma of the gallbladder: CT demonstrates direct involvement of adjacent liver as well as bile-duct dilatation (a) and a heterogeneous mass in the gallbladder bed (b).

5.6 Radionuclide investigations of the liver

J. R. Buscombe and A. J. W. Hilson

Introduction

Radionuclide investigations of the liver are a powerful and often underused tool in the diagnosis of liver disease. Images obtained from radionuclide studies in disease reflect the difference in function between normal and pathological tissue. The resolution of the images is less than with ultrasound or CT; therefore it is often felt that the information is of poorer quality whereas, in fact, invaluable information on the underlying functional aspects of liver disease may be obtained. Indeed, many apparent discrepancies in liver imaging studies are explained by the difference between physiological/functional information from radionuclide studies and the anatomical/morphological information available from ultrasound or CT. These investigations are complementary; they should not be viewed as competitive.

This chapter will deal with the essentials of imaging liver function, perfusion, hepatocyte function, biliary excretion, and also with abnormal cell function arising from benign and malignant liver disease.

Non-invasive assessment of hepatic haemodynamics

Introduction

Radionuclide tracer techniques can be used in a variety of ways to provide information on hepatic haemodynamics. Several of these methods, such as the application of the Fick principle, indicator dilution techniques (Bradley, Surgery, 1974; 75:783), or the use of radioactive microspheres, are relatively invasive. While of value in providing accurate information for research, their use is limited in clinical practice. Some clinical applications of techniques involving direct injection are considered below. There are also techniques for measuring hepatic haemodynamics involving only intravenous injection and sampling; these are relatively non-invasive and can easily be incorporated into a general diagnostic strategy.

Techniques involving direct internal injection and sampling

Clinically useful data can be obtained from internal injection either of tracers that are distributed solely in the bloodstream (non-diffusible tracers) or of those that are extracted by the liver (extracted tracers).

Hepatic vascular catheter position checking

Direct injection of labelled microspheres into either the hepatic artery (Ziessman, JNuclMed, 1983; 24:871) or portal vein (Mooney, ClinRadiol, 1983; 34:657) enables the distribution of perfusion from these vessels, or catheters within them, to be imaged, and the degree of shunting assessed. It is most commonly used to confirm the position of catheters placed for intra-arterial chemotherapy.

Assessment of portal shunts by rectal tracers

The introduction of a radiopharmaceutical into the rectum has been used to a limited degree to study portacaval shunting. Both thallium-201 (Tonami, JNuclMed, 1982; 23:965), which is extracted by the liver, and [^{99}Tc^{m}]pertechnetate, which acts as a passive flow indicator during the first pass (Shiomi, JNuclMed, 1988; 29:460), have been used. The degree of shunting is increased in cirrhosis, and particularly so in patients with oesophageal varices. However, the pattern of flow changes with posture and patient movement (Tonami, NuclMedComm, 1995; 16:92).

Techniques using intravenous injection

Introduction

Following intravenous injection of a material that is removed from the circulation only by the liver, the blood clearance curve depends on the volume of distribution of the tracer, the liver blood flow, and the extraction efficiency of the tracer by the liver. If the extraction efficiency is very high, if there is a low concentration of tracer (so that no saturation of the extraction mechanism occurs), and if the volume of distribution is known or measured, then liver blood flow can be estimated.

The first successful estimation of total liver perfusion using the clearance rate of an extracted substance was by Dobson and Jones [ActaMedScand, 1952; 144 (Suppl. 273); Circul, 1953; 7:690]. They used ^{32}P-labelled chromic phosphate, which is a colloidal β-emitter.

Determination of the clearance rate required frequent blood sampling because of the short range of the β-particles. This technique was simplified by the use of γ-emitting pharmaceuticals, particularly colloidal ^{198}Au (Vetter, JCI, 1954; 33:1594), together with external probes to monitor blood clearance. It was shown that the clearance rate had a maximum of 94 per cent of directly

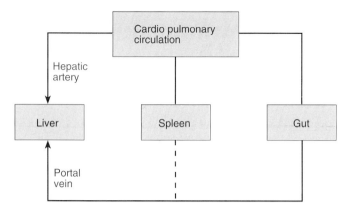

Fig. 1. Physiological model illustrating the firstpass dynamics of an intravenously injected tracer arriving at the liver. The splenic vein route is indicated by a broken line since, if colloid is used as the tracer, relatively little activity passes via this route.

measured hepatic blood flow. The remainder of the blood flow was felt to represent physiological portohepatic venous shunts at the level of sinusoids.

The advent of the gamma-camera and $^{99}\text{Tc}^{m}$-labelled colloid enabled the regional distribution of effective liver perfusion to be obtained as a static image. The development of computer acquisition of gamma-camera data enabled dynamic time series of images to be taken. Display of serial images covering the first pass of activity through the liver was used as a means of providing visual information on hepatic perfusion (Freeman, SemNuclMed, 1972; 2: 133). Later, quantification of images of colloid uptake was used to measure elements of total liver perfusion as an adjunct to static liver imaging. Information on the relative hepatic arterial and portal venous components of liver perfusion has been obtained by analysing the first-pass dynamics of both colloidal and non-diffusible tracers. More recently, the idea of combining the measurement of total liver perfusion and its relative components using either colloid (Walmsley, NuclMedComm, 1987; 8:613) or non-diffusible tracers (Dobson, Circul, 1953; 7:690) has been suggested as a means of further specifying hepatic haemodynamics. This combination is known as quantitative dynamic liver scintigraphy.

Relative components of liver perfusion

The relative magnitude of the hepatic arterial and portal venous components of hepatic perfusion can be assessed in first-pass scintigraphic studies with either extracted or non-diffusible tracers. The theory can be considered with reference to the physiological model shown in Fig.1.

Following intravenous injection, the tracer passes through the cardiopulmonary circulation and is then distributed to the various organs in amounts proportional to their perfusion. The arrival at the liver of tracer passing via the hepatic artery will be separated in time from that arriving via the portal vein, which is delayed by its passage through the gut and spleen.

If colloid is used, tracer that travels via the spleen is efficiently removed from the circulation, and thus the amount arriving via the portal vein will only reflect the mesenteric component of portal venous perfusion. By using the arrival times of activity in other organs as a reference, the times representing the two phases of

arrival in the liver can be estimated, and the corresponding amounts of colloid assessed.

Methods

Qualitative dynamic liver scintigraphy

Rapid sequential images of the liver following the first pass of an intravenously injected tracer can give qualitative information on hepatic haemodynamics (Waxman, JNuclMed, 1973; 13:522). The patient is imaged in a supine position from the anterior using a gamma-camera with a large field of view to cover the liver, spleen, and heart. Typically 20 images are recorded at 2-s intervals following intravenous injection of about 150 MBq of $[^{99}\text{Tc}^{m}]$colloid. The images are assessed visually by comparison with a normal pattern to see whether there is a biphasic arrival of tracer, and whether focal areas of hypo- or hypervascularity can be identified.

Measurement of total liver perfusion

Total liver perfusion can be measured by computer scintigraphy with radiolabelled colloid (Miller, EurJNuclMed, 1979; 4:1) by calculating the geometric mean of uptake into the liver and spleen (Fleming, PhysMedBiol, 1979; 24:176). Alternative methods using a simple index of clearance and principal components' analysis (Houston, BrJRadiol, 1980; 53:87) have also been applied.

Measurement of relative components of liver perfusion

This is carried out by dynamic computer scintigraphy on the first pass of tracer through the liver following a rapid bolus injection given intravenously. Images are acquired dynamically at 1-s intervals for approximately 40 s. Computer analysis of these studies involves careful choice of a region of interest over the liver, avoiding overlap with other organs in the field of view, and then production of the corresponding time–activity curve. Other regions, such as the left ventricle, left or right kidney or spleen, are used to produce reference curves for calculation of the times of the two phases of arrival at the liver. A typical set of curves is shown in Fig. 2. Several methods of analysis have been used to quantify the perfusion ratio. In colloid studies the actual amount of tracer arriving by the two routes can be assessed (Fleming, JNuclMed, 1983; 24:1108).

Findings in dynamic liver scintigraphy

In 20 per cent of the patients studied (David, ClinNuclMed, 1988; 13:402), analysis of the dynamic phase of the images by qualitative dynamic liver scintigraphy using radiocolloid gave additional information to that available from static images. The technique was useful for demonstrating the vascularity of individual large lesions in the liver. Most were shown to be hypovascular but some were hypervascular (Fig. 3). Early images were also useful in revealing delayed portal transit and unsuspected abnormalities in other abdominal vessels.

Normals

Relatively few workers have obtained absolute values of total liver effective perfusion rate from scintigraphy. The values obtained were shown to depend on the colloid used (Walmsley, NuclMedComm, 1987, 8:613). However, a hepatic arterial perfusion index can be

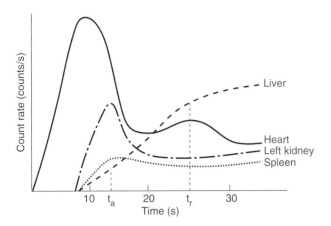

Fig. 2. A typical set of time–activity curves representing the first pass of colloid through the liver and some of the other organs used to produce time reference. Time t_a represent the end of the arterial phase assessed from the time of arterial arrival in other abdominal organs and t_r the end of the portal phase assessed by the onset of recirculation.

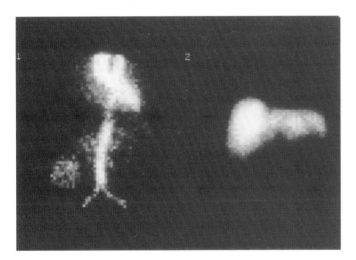

Fig. 3. Images showing the uptake of radiocolloid in a patient with a large carcinoid tumour at the base of the right lobe of the liver. (1) The arterial phase of the first pass; (2) the final colloid distribution. The hypervascularity of the tumour compared to the rest of the liver is demonstrated.

calculated, that is, arterial flow as a fraction of total hepatic perfusion, and mean values of 0.17 to 0.42 have been obtained (Sarper, JNuclMed, 1981; 22:318; Wraight, NuclMedComm, 1982; 3:273; Walmesley, NuclMedComm, 1987; 12:613). The results are in general agreement with previous estimates from using electromagnetic flow probes (Schenk, AnnSurg, 1962; 156:463) and constant-infusion indicator techniques (Strandell, JApplPhysiol, 1973; 35:755).

Cirrhosis

Total effective liver perfusion as measured by the colloid clearance rate is reduced in cirrhosis, but measured values overlap considerably with the normal range (Miller, EurJNuclMed, 1979; 4:1; McLaren, BrJSurg, 1985; 72:394). In contrast, the relative hepatic arterial perfusion index is markedly increased in cirrhosis irrespective of the technique (Wraight, NuclMedComm, 1982; 3:

273; McLaren, BrJSurg, 1985; 72:394). There is good correlation between the index and the degree of cirrhosis and the risk of bleeding in patients with oesophageal varices (Holbrook, BrJSurg, 1987; 74:527; Walmesley, NuclMedComm, 1987; 8:613).

Liver metastases

The relative arterial component of hepatic perfusion is increased in patients with metastases secondary to colorectal cancer. Two groups (Sarper, JNuclMed, 1981; 22:318; Leveson, BrJSurg, 1985; 75:128) found very high sensitivities (100 per cent and 94 per cent, respectively) for the detection of disease. One of these groups of patients has been followed for 3 years (Cooke, NuclMedComm, 1987; 8:970). The investigators have extended the definition of a true positive test to include patients (with a raised index at the time of the investigation) who went on to develop metastases within the 3-year period. The final sensitivity and specificity for detection of disease were 91 and 76 per cent, respectively, with a corresponding diagnostic accuracy of 82 per cent.

The hepatic arterial perfusion index increases in proportion to the percentage hepatic replacement by tumour (Hunt, BrJSurg, 1988; 75:611). By excluding patients with reduced portal perfusion, the index is useful when deciding about the treatment of liver metastases by hepatic arterial embolization. The index can also be used to monitor the effect of the embolization on haemodynamics (Flowerdew, BrJCanc, 1987; 55:269).

Role of dynamic liver scintigraphy

Both qualitative and quantitative dynamic studies using colloid can be regarded as adjuncts to the well-proven technique of static colloid imaging. The extra information provided is obtained with the same injection, but at the cost of some increase in the length and complexity of the procedure. Dynamic studies using non-diffusible tracers may have some minor theoretical advantages over colloid, but not enough to justify a separate radionuclide study.

Imaging studies
Hepatic
Kupffer cells

The conventional planar liver 'scan' or scintigram became a routine study with the introduction of ^{99}Tc^m-labelled sulphur colloid (Harper, Nucleonics, 1964; 22:50) (Table 1). The image obtained is of functioning Kupffer cells, not of morphological liver. This distinction is important when assessing images obtained, for instance, after radiotherapy; the Kupffer cells in the radiotherapy field lose their ability to take up colloid and so a defect is seen, but the morphology of the underlying liver remains unchanged.

Normal findings

The normal shape of the liver is highly variable (McAfee, ArchIntMed, 1965; 116:95) and changes with respiration. There are many methods of measuring the size of the liver, of varying degrees of complexity, but no good evidence that the information obtained justifies the effort involved; most centres rely on a simple subjective impression of size. The normal uptake of tracer is homogeneous throughout the liver and spleen (Fig. 4), and on the posterior view

Table 1 Standard protocol for [⁹⁹TCᵐ]sulphur colloid imaging

(1) Inject 100–150 MBq of [⁹⁹Tcᵐ]sulphur colloid intravenously
(2) Image 15–90 min after the injection
(3) If possible, image the patient standing against the gamma-camera
(4) Use a low-energy, high-resolution collimator, 256 × 256 matrix, minimum 600 000 counts per view
(5) Minimum four views, anterior, posterior and both laterals. In women, lift the right breast away from liver
(6) Additional right anterior and right posterior views may be obtained
(7) A costal margin marker view may be obtained; in addition, if there is a known liver mass this can be marked on a separate film using ⁵⁷Co markers

the density of uptake in the spleen and liver should be equal. There should only be minimal visualization of bone marrow.

Hepatocytes

Stadalnik and his co-workers in Sacramento, CA, have developed [⁹⁹Tcᵐ]neoglycalbumen (**NGA**), which is a tracer specifically taken up by the asialoglycoprotein receptor associated with hepatic binding protein (discussed more fully in Chapter 2.4). Using a complex mathematical analysis it is possible to derive the hepatic blood flow, receptor concentration, and a receptor binding constant (Stadalnik, JNuclMed, 1985; 26:1233). The ability of this test to quantify the volume of hepatic binding-protein receptors has been validated by comparing mathematical modelling with liver biopsy (Kudo, JNuclMed, 1991; 32:1177). Binding of hepatic binding protein and hence [⁹⁹Tcᵐ]NGA is reduced in patients with severe cirrhosis compared with normals (Virgolini, NuclMedComm, 1991; 12:507). Recovery of uptake of [⁹⁹Tcᵐ]NGA in fulminant liver failure may

precede both clinical and biochemical recovery (Moragas, Clin-NuclMed, 1995; 20:329).

Blood pool

It is possible to obtain an image of the hepatic blood pool by the use of ⁹⁹Tcᵐ-labelled red blood cells. This is of particular use in the identification of a haemangioma; initially such a lesion shows low blood-pool activity, but the activity increases with time and by 1 to 2 h after the injection the area of the liver showing the greatest activity is the one corresponding to the position of the haemangioma.

Clinical applications of radionuclide hepatic imaging

Diffuse parenchymal liver disease

With impairment of hepatocyte function, there is a reduction of colloid uptake in the liver, with a relative shift of uptake to spleen and to bone marrow. This is probably due to changes in blood flow rather than extraction efficiency. On a normal posterior planar image, the uptake in the spleen should be equal to or less than that in the liver. Increased splenic uptake should raise the suspicion of diffuse parenchymal liver disease. Splenomegaly due to infiltration shows reduced tracer uptake in the spleen. Visualization of bone marrow in the spine and ribs is a strong indicator of major liver damage. The technique is of value (McClees, JClinUltrasound, 1984; 12:75), but its accuracy is difficult to assess in the absence of any 'gold standard'.

Focal nodular hyperplasia

This is the only mass lesion of the liver that contains Kupffer cells. It follows that the demonstration of colloid uptake in a mass lesion allows accurate diagnosis of this condition.

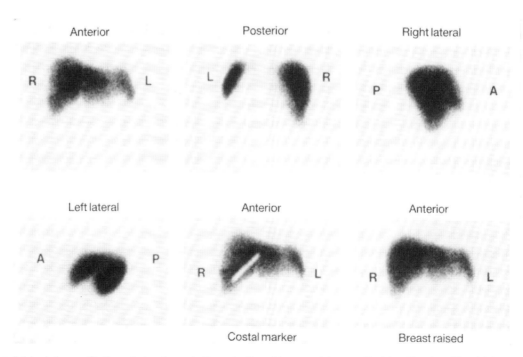

Fig. 4. Normal colloid scintigram. On the anterior view note the reduction of tracer uptake over the lateral border of the right upper pole due to absorption of photons by the breast, confirmed by the disappearance of this 'defect' on raising the breast.

Haemangioma

As described above, blood-pool imaging with $^{99}Tc^m$-labelled red blood cells is the method of choice in the identification of cavernous haemangioma. Additional colloid-subtraction and single-photon emission tomography (**SPECT**) imaging of the blood pool improves accuracy (Ziessman, JNuclMed, 1991; 32:2086).

Budd–Chiari syndrome

On the colloid image there is generalized reduction of tracer uptake, but with increased uptake in the caudate lobe, seen centrally in the anterior image, and posteriorly in the right lateral image (Tavill, Gastro, 1975; 68:509). This pattern is more clearly seen on a SPECT study.

Primary tumours

Hepatocellular cancer

Hepatocellular carcinoma is gallium-avid and can be imaged using gallium-67 citrate. Unfortunately, as the normal liver also takes up gallium it can be difficult to differentiate between physiological and pathological activity. A [$^{99}Tc^m$]colloid study will map normal liver tissue and subtraction of the two images should reveal the presence of the tumour (Loma, NEJM, 1972; 286:1323). This is a cumbersome method and the non-specific nature of gallium uptake, which also occurs in sites of infection and inflammation, reduces its usefulness in these patients.

It is possible to use [$^{99}Tc^m$]colloid imaging alone, with tumour having no uptake of tracer. Though sensitivity can be improved by tomography (Brenda, Radiol, 1984; 153:527), the method remains non-specific and similar appearances can be reported in liver cysts, infection, and metastases. However, in a patient with known disease it can provide a relatively cheap method of monitoring changes in the size of the tumour.

Other non-specific tracers that have been used include fluorine-18 fluorodeoxyglucose (**FDG**) positron-emission tomography (**PET**). In a series of 30 patients with hepatocellular cancer, some tumours appeared as areas of increased activity, others as decreased activity (Torizuka, JNuclMed, 1994; 35:1965). It was also suggested that PET might have a useful role in determining if active tumour remains after the therapeutic use of radio- or chemotherapy–iodinated poppy-seed oil (Lipiodol).

The portal blood supply of the hepatocellular cancer has been exploited in the use of thallium-201 chloride given per rectum (Tanami, NuclMedComm, 1985; 6:327): 7 out of 10 patients had accumulation of the thallium-201 chloride; interestingly, in all the patients other tissues such as the heart (which normally takes up thallium-201 chloride) were visible, suggesting a degree of portal–systemic shunting. In the three negative studies, no such shunt was found and it may be that in these patients the predominant blood supply to the tumour was via the hepatic artery and not the portal vein. Intravenous thallium-201 has a similar sensitivity though again there is normal liver uptake, which can obscure small tumours. The use of [$^{99}Tc^m$]phytate–thallium-201 subtraction imaging can help find small tumours within the liver (Mochizucki, JNuclMed, 1994; 35:1134).

More specific imaging of hepatocellular cancer has been possible with iodine-123 insulin. In 19 out of 20 patients, iodine-123 insulin was able to identify all known sites of tumour. In six patients with metastases from other cancers there was no accumulation of the radiolabelled insulin (Kurtaran, JNuclMed, 1995; 36:1875). At present it is not known if distant metastases can be identified by this method.

A different way to obtain specificity is to use a radiolabelled substance that is infused into the feeding artery of the tumour and has a very high first-pass extraction. Such a substance is iodinated poppy-seed oil (Lipiodol). This can be radiolabelled easily with iodine-123 or iodine-131. However, the use of this radio-pharmaceutical has been restricted to therapy (see below) rather than diagnosis.

Hepatocellular metastases

It may be possible to visualize metastases from hepatocellular carcinoma using non-specific tumour markers that have a reasonable sensitivity for identifying the primary tumour within the liver. These are limited at present to gallium-67 citrate and thallium-201 chloride, and fluorine-18 FDG used with PET. There is evidence that methods using these markers are generally more sensitive than CT or MRI for nodal disease; they also have the advantage of producing good-quality whole-body images that may help to find unexpected metastases. However, in the abdomen, the physiological bowel activity of both gallium-67 citrate and thallium-201 chloride may hinder identification of tumour in small lymph nodes (Kaneko, JpnJClinRadiol, 1983; 28:1067). Non-specific uptake, probably secondary to microcalcification, may be seen on standard [$^{99}Tc^m$]di-phosphonate bone scans (Fujimoto, ClinNuclMed, 1992; 17:99). The bone scan itself may give indirect evidence of bony metastases of hepatocellular cancer, and is often used to screen for extrahepatic disease if transplantation is being considered.

More specific uptake has been found using radiolabelled amphetamines, in particular iodine-123 N-isopropyl iodoamphetamine (IMP). The mechanism of uptake is unknown but this compound allowed identification of 92 per cent of hepatocellular metastases (Suto, ClinNuclMed, 1994; 19:302).

While hepatocellular cancer cells are relatively inactive within the liver, they still have some hepatocyte function, and hepatobiliary agents may therefore be used to identify the site of metastases, with particular success in the lungs (Wang, ClinNuclMed, 1991; 16:120).

The role of nuclear medicine in metastatic hepatocellular cancer beyond that of a standard, staging bone scan is not yet clear, but further work with either specific agents or PET may become of value in finding small amounts of residual disease.

Cholangiocarcinoma

Some cholangiocarcinoma cells express somatostatin receptors *in vitro*; subsequently, in one patient, uptake of indium-111 octreotide was observed within a confirmed cholangiocarcinoma (Tan, Gastro, 1995; 108:1908). This may provide a new method by which this tumour can be imaged.

Secondary tumours

Gallium

Gallium-67 citrate is a non-specific tracer that binds to plasma proteins involved with transport of iron, in particular transferrin

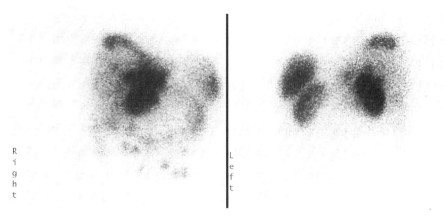

R
i
g
h
t

L
e
f
t

Fig. 5. Patient with disseminated carcinoid and multiple liver metastases showing uptake of indium-111 octreotide, a somatostatin analogue) in the liver imaged anteriorly (right-hand image) and posteriorly (left-hand image).

and lactoferrin. Though now used widely for imaging infection it was originally applied to tumour imaging. It has a high sensitivity in lymphoma (greater than 90 per cent in most high-grade tumours). However, in solid tumours the results are variable, with sensitivities as low as 50 per cent for metastases of breast and bronchial cancer. For this reason it is not recommended for use in identifying hepatic metastases in solid tumours, but may have a part to play in the assessment of patients with lymphoma.

Somatostatin

Many tumour cell types that have neural-crest origins express somatostatin receptors, which can be imaged with radiolabelled somatostatin analogues. The plasma half-life of somatostatin is too short to allow for reasonable imaging, and therefore the synthetic octapeptide analogue octreotide is used. This was initially labelled with iodine-123 (Krenning, Lancet, 1989; i:242), and was found to localize well in rare gastrointestinal tumours such as gastrinomas and insulinomas. There was a high hepatic uptake of the iodine-123 octreotide. An alternative indium-111 radiolabel was developed that is attached to the phenylalanine base in the octreotide via diethylenetriamino-pentaacetic acid (**DTPA**). The final labelled product, In-111-DTPA-Phe-octreotide, which is commercially available, has high specific binding for somatostatin-S_2 receptors, but lower hepatic uptake, and is cleared via the kidneys (Krenning, JNuclMed, 1992; 33:652)

Initially it was used to identify gastrointestinal endocrine tumours: sensitivity for localization of gastrinoma was 100 per cent, glucagonoma 100 per cent, and insulinoma 61 per cent (Krenning, SemOnc, 1994; 6:56). These tumours are rare, and though metastases to the liver are common, the number of patients imaged with this agent will remain small. However, there are other conditions in which liver metastases are more common; the sensitivity of indium-111-Phe-DTPA-octreotide in carcinoid is 96 per cent, phaeochromocytoma 86 per cent, and medullary thyroid cancer 71 per cent (Krenning, SemOnc, 1994; 21:56) (Fig. 5).

In a short series comparing the use of indium-111-DTPA-Phe-octreotide with CT and ultrasound in gut-related tumours with suspected liver metastases, 40 tumours were found with both methods, four were missed with indium-111-Phe-octreotide imaging, but 27 tumours were identified by somatostatin imaging alone. The investigators concluded that the sensitivity of indium-111-DTPA-Phe-octreotide imaging was 91 per cent, but that of CT and ultrasound only 68 per cent (Pauwels, SemOnc, 1994; 21:S21). Other tumours with neuroendocrine properties, such as small-cell lung cancer, breast cancer and Hodgkin's lymphoma, can be imaged with this method (Krenning, SemOnc, 1994; 21:56). In lymphoma, indium-111-DTPA-Phe-octreotide may be less useful in localizing tumour below the diaphragm, probably as result of normal physiological distribution of the tracer in the liver, kidneys, spleen, and colon (Sarda, EurJNucMed, 1995; 222:1105). Imaging quality does not appear to be affected by the administration of non-radiolabelled octreotide, and within the liver SPECT may also be of use.

Vasoactive intestinal peptide

Vasoactive intestinal peptide (**VIP**) labelled with iodine-123 has been used to image neuroendocrine tumours and metastases of carcinoma of the colon, both of which express VIP receptors *in vitro*. While only three patients with liver metastases have been studied, all had focal uptake of I-123-VIP (Virgolini, JNuclMed, 1995; 36:1732). There is little uptake in normal liver tissue and its possible utility in both diagnosis and therapy is being investigated.

Meta-iodobenzylguanadine

Radio-iodinated meta-iodobenzylguanadine (**MIBG**) is a guan-ethidine analogue that is actively taken up into presynaptic cells of the adrenaline/noradrenaline sympathetic medullary tissues. It is stored within the cells and can be imaged via its radiolabel. The MIBG can be labelled for imaging with either iodine-131 or iodine-123. Iodine-123 is preferred for imaging: it has a shorter half-life, emits only γ-irradiation, and the energy of that radiation is better imaged by modern gamma-cameras. It has been used to image phaeochromocytomas and also disseminated carcinoid (McEwan, SemNuclMed, 1985, 5:132; Jodrell, BrJCanc, 1988; 58:663). The sensitivity in phaeochromocytoma is between 79 and 95 per cent, and the specificity between 88 and 100 per cent. The main cause of a false-negative scan is that there is uptake within the normal adrenals, and it can be difficult to judge when the adrenal uptake is abnormal, particularly in bilateral disease. The high cost of the preparation, approximately twice the cost of a liver CT with contrast, has reduced its use, except when there is known disease and therapy with iodine-131 MIBG is being considered, or where there is biochemical evidence of a phaeochromocytoma but normal CT and ultrasonographic findings.

There is very little uptake of radio-iodinated MIBG within the liver and metastases from malignant phaeochromocytomas can be easily identified. The sensitivity of radio-iodinated MIBG for carcinoid in the liver is lower than for phaeochromocytoma, at about 50 to 60 per cent (Sinzinger, EurJNucMed, 1985; 11:A17; Feldman, JNuclMed, 1986; 27:1691).

Positron imaging

Positrons are produced by short-lived isotopes, normally generated within a cyclotron. After a very short distance (about 10^{-12} m) the positron will meet an electron. The resulting annihilation will result in two γ-rays of 511 keV being emitted at an angle of 180°. This can then be detected as two coincident events with detectors set at 180°. Using such a method, a PET image is formed.

The most useful of the positron-imaging isotopes is fluorine-18 (F-18), which has a half-life of 110 min and can be easily complexed to organic substances. For example, glucose uptake can be measured by use of F-18-FDG. As tumour cells tend to have a higher metabolic rate than surrounding tissue, focal accumulation of the F-18-FDG can be seen as an area of increasing activity within the tumour. Once phosphorylated the F-18-FDG is not metabolized further and remains within the cell.

Within the liver this agent has been used to image a range of metastatic tumours such as colorectal carcinoma, melanoma, breast carcinoma, and malignant melanoma (Hawkins, SemNuclMed, 1992; 22:268). The lack of uptake of F-18-FDG within normal liver makes recognition of liver metastases relatively easy. For example, in breast cancer the tumour activity of F-18-FDG is about six times that of normal liver tissue (Wahl, Radiol, 1991; 179:765). The sensitivity of F-18-FDG is high in many disseminated cancers: for example, in 33 patients with disseminated malignant melanoma the sensitivity was 92 per cent, with lesions of less than 3 mm only not detected (Steinert, Radiol, 1995; 195:705).

Its more general use in routine clinical work has been restrained by the high cost of the equipment and radiopharmaceuticals, and the need of a true understanding of the relation between data from PET and CT or MRI, and of which cases merit F-18-FDG.

As a research tool, PET remains very effective: for example, it is possible to predict the response of hepatic metastases from colonic carcinoma by the uptake of F-18-5-fluorouracil; if this is decreased while F-18-FDG activity remains unchanged it is a powerful predictor that the tumour will fail to respond to therapeutic 5-fluorouracil (Strauss, JNuclMed, 1991; 32:623). It is theoretically possible to follow any metabolic pathway using PET. In a few years time, it should enable us to improve our understanding of tumour growth and metabolism, and of the way tumours respond to chemotherapy.

Immunoscintigraphy

It is possible to image tumour metastases within the liver using radiolabelled antibodies directed against a tumour-specific antigen on the cell surface. A example of this is an antibody against carcinoembryonic antigen that is expressed by colon cancer cells (Abdel-Nabi, Radiol, 1987; 164:617). Initially, iodine-131 was used as a radiolabel, but it is less than ideal due to poor dosimetry and image quality. More recent studies have used monoclonal antibodies labelled with either indium-111 or technetium-99m. In both cases, good-quality imaging is possible up to 24 h with the $^{99}Tc^m$-labelled antibodies and up to 72 h with the indium-111.

The cancer that has been most closely studied is that of the colon. However, in the liver there is a significant problem in that the carcinoembryonic antigen is the same as, or resembles, the 95-kDa glycoprotein found on the surface of granulocytes and Kupffer cells. Consequently, most patients have significant physiological hepatic uptake of radiolabelled antibodies against carcinoembryonic antigen. In a series of 95 patients with suspected metastases from colonic cancer the sensitivity of immunoscintigraphy with the indium-111-labelled antibody (CYT103) for tumour was 69 per cent compared with 66 per cent for CT. The specificity for immunoscintigraphy was 89 per cent, the same as for CT. However, if the liver alone was considered the sensitivity of indium-111 CYT103 was 55 per cent and that of CT 87 per cent (Abdel-Nabi, Radiol, 1988; 166:747). These results have been repeated elsewhere. As a consequence, immunoscintigraphy of liver metastases has not proved as clinically useful as in lymph-node disease, for which immunoscintigraphy is clearly more sensitive than CT.

The use of antibody fragments or minichains may improve tumour targeting, with an increase in renal clearance of unbound activity, but as yet they have not been shown to improve localization within the liver. Immunoscintigraphy is expensive and is being directed towards therapy where uptake of antibody into normal liver tissue is not a major problem (Goldenberg, TumTarg, 1995; 1: 233).

Indirect imaging

Whilst it is possible to image metastases within the liver by positive uptake, it is also possible to use the fact that metastases result in a lack of normal hepatic tissue. Though hepatocyte imaging with [$^{99}Tc^m$]galactosyl–neoglycalbumin (Kutaran, JNuclMed, 1995; 36: 1875) can be used, this agent is not commercially available in Europe or North America, and therefore most commonly Kupffer-cell imaging with [$^{99}Tc^m$]sulphur colloid is used. There are no recent comparative studies with ultrasound and CT, but the sensitivities of all three methods are similar (Grossman, JNuclMed, 1977; 18: 327; Alderson, Radiol, 1983; 149:225). The advent of SPECT has allowed better localization of lesions within the liver; this method compares well with CT and is consistently more accurate than ultrasound (Strauss, JNuclMed, 1982; 23:1059; Dendy, AnnRadiol, 1983; 26:72; Kudo, Radiol, 1986; 159:697) (Fig. 6). The results of these tests are summarized in Tables 2 and 3. However, the anatomical methods have a better specificity, as direct visualization of the lesions often enables a definitive diagnosis to be made. Colloid scintigraphy may still have a part to play in monitoring the extent of disease in those patients with known hepatic metastases. Combination with indium-111 octreotide and iodine-123 MIBG imaging will also improve the detection of hepatic diseases by these methods (Buscombe, NuclMedComm, 1997; 18:289).

Different techniques have been used to determine the presence of metastatic disease within the liver. Greatest success has been achieved when the tumour cell expresses a unique biochemical property or contains specific surface receptor cells. This property

Table 2 Comparison of diagnostic accuracies of planar and SPECT scintigraphy, and CT

Technique	Number of patients	Overall diagnostic accuracy (%)	Range of diagnostic accuracies (%)
Planar scintigraphy	951	79	77–87
SPECT	1015	88	83–99
CT	743	92	78–94

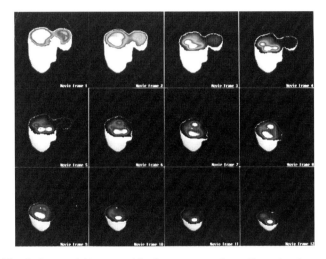

Fig. 6. Sequential tomographic slices across a three-dimensional rendered image obtained from a [⁹⁹Tcᵐ]sulphur colloid SPECT study. Multiple defects seen as dark areas in the liver are due to metastatic hepatocellular carcinoma.

Table 3 Detection sensitivities (%) for different lesion size

Technique	Diameter of lesion (cm)		
	0–2	2–4	4–6
Planar scintigraphy	5	48	91
SPECT	36	78	99
CT	35	79	100

tends to be limited to rarer tumour groups such as carcinoid and phaeochromocytoma. Tests for the more common tumours that metastasize to the liver (cancers of colon, breast, and ovary) rely on the different metabolic nature of the metastases compared to normal liver. While high sensitivities can be achieved, the cost of these tests compared to standard imaging such as CT may limit their use. Immunoscintigraphy within the liver has proved disappointing and has no clear clinical role.

Therapy

Treatment of hepatocellular cancer has been limited to palliation as only patients with advanced inoperable disease are offered for therapy using nuclear medical techniques. Early work used iodine-131-labelled antiferritin antibodies given intravenously, but results were disappointing (Order, JClinOncol, 1985; 3:1573). The same antibody given into the hepatic artery resulted in a small improvement in survival (Order, IntJRadiotOncolBiolPhys, 1991; 20: 953).

Non-immunological approaches have used iodine-131-labelled poppy-seed oil (Lipiodol) or yttrium-90-labelled theraspheres injected directly into the feeding artery of the tumour. Iodine-131 Lipiodol appears to give the better results (Novell, Lancet, 1991; 337:333; Bourguet, EurJNucMed, 1992; 19:608; Andrews, JNuclMed, 1994; 34:1637; Leung, JNuclMed, 1994; 34:1313). When compared with the combination of cytotoxic drugs attached to Lipiodol, iodine-131 Lipiodol proved to have similar efficacy but with significantly fewer side-effects (Battacharya, Cancer, 1995; 76: 2202).

Treatment of metastases within the liver has resulted in mixed results. In colon cancer, iodine-131-labelled antibodies against carcinoembryonic antigen have been used with some effect in a small group of patients (Lane, BrJCanc, 1994; 70:521), although others have reported a poor response (Begent, BrJCanc, 1991; 62:487). The treatment of liver metastases from metastatic phaeochromocytoma, carcinoids, and medullary-cell cancer of the thyroid using iodine-131-MIBG has been more successful, with response rates of 50 to 70 per cent (Clarke, JNuclMedBiol, 1991; 35:323; Hoefnagel, JNuclMedBiol, 1991; 35:408; Lewington, JNuclMedBiol, 1991; 35: 280). Therapy can be repeated at 6-monthly intervals and some patients have remained in remission or with static disease over many years. A single case report suggested that high-dose indium-111 octreotide may have a part to play in the treatment of carcinoid with liver metastases (Krenning, AnnNYAcadSci, 1994; 733:496).

Biliary imaging

Hepatobiliary scintigraphy enables information concerning the perfusion, uptake of tracer into the hepatocytes, and excretion through the biliary tree to be assessed. Initially I-131-Rose Bengal was used was used in association with a scintillation detector (a 'probe') to measure uptake and excretion of the tracer from the liver (Taplin, JLabClinMed, 1955; 45:665). A major advance came with the development of ⁹⁹Tcᵐ-labelled derivatives of iminodiacetic acid (**IDA**). The first of these compounds was H-IDA (Harvey, JNuclMed, 1975; 16:533), Newer halogenated compounds, such trimethylbromo IDA (Mebrofenin), with insignificant renal excretion, high uptake via the bilirubin pathway even at high concentrations of bilirubin, and rapid transit through the hepatocyte are recommended. Although, strictly speaking, only dimethyl IDA should be referred to as 'HIDA', the term has become generic and is used for the whole group of compounds (Table 4).

Normal findings

A normal liver (Fig. 7) shows good uniform uptake of tracer in both lobes, and by 5 min the cardiac blood pool should not be visible. The main biliary ducts should be visible by 7 min, and are often seen at 3 to 4 min. Activity is usually seen in the small bowel by 15 min, and is always seen by 30 min. The gallbladder is seen in 90 per cent of normal fasting patients by 30 min, and in 100 per cent by 60 min (Williams, JNuclMed, 1984; 25:160). Sometimes it is difficult to be sure whether activity is in the gallbladder or

Table 4 Standard protocol for hepatobiliary scintigraphy

(1) Fast the patient for 8 to 24 h before the study
(2) Position the patient supine under the gamma-camera
(3) Use a low-energy general-purpose collimator in a 256 × 256 matrix. Ensure the liver is fully within field of view
(4) Inject 150 MBq of [^{99}Tc^m]Mebrofenin (or another third-generation IDA) intravenously and start imaging
(5) Acquire dynamic images 1/sc for 60 s and 1/min for the subsequent 59 min
(6) Take anterior and right lateral static images at 60 min
(7) Further dynamic or static images can be acquired if needed

duodenal loop (or in the right kidney if a third-generation agent is not used). This is nearly always clarified on the right lateral view.

Findings in specific conditions

Acute cholecystitis

In acute cholecystitis there is obstruction of the cystic duct, and, by definition, HIDA cannot enter the gallbladder (Fig. 8). Therefore, if, on a HIDA study the gallbladder is seen, the patient cannot have acute cholecystitis. The converse is not true—failure of the gallbladder to fill occurs in many conditions, including chronic cholecystitis (when the gallbladder may fill by 4 h) and acalculous cholecystitis. However, if the imaging is performed for up to 4 h, visualization of the gallbladder has a sensitivity of 99 per cent for normality, and non-visualization has a sensitivity of 97 per cent for acute cholecystitis.[1]

Pharmacologically augmented studies

The diagnosis of acute cholecystitis may be improved by the use of either cholecystokinin or morphine. Cholecystokinin has the

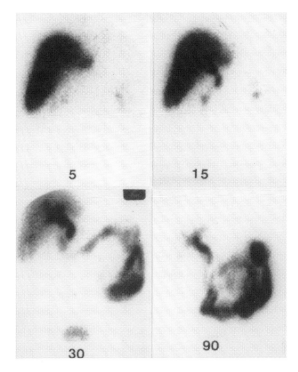

Fig. 8. Hepatobiliary scintigraphy in a patient with acute cholecystitis. Note that uptake and excretion are normal, but that the gallbladder is not seen, even at 90 min.

advantage of being more physiological but the disadvantage of causing more discomfort for the patient. Using either method, if the drug is administered 30 min before the hepatobiliary scintigraphy, non-visualization of the gallbladder at 30 min has a similar accuracy to the 4-h non-augmented study (Fink-Bennet, Sem-NuclMed, 1991; 21:133).

An additional use of cholecystokinin is in acalculous cholecystitis resulting in poor gallbladder emptying: 30 min after the start of a standard hepatobiliary study, when the gallbladder is full of activity, cholecystokinin is infused over 20 min; if less than 35 per cent of the activity has cleared the gallbladder 30 min after the cholecystokinin was started the patient has significant gallbladder dysfunction (Krishnamurthy, Gastro, 1981; 80:482).

Biliary obstruction

In acute biliary obstruction, hepatocyte function is well-maintained, and there is good uptake of HIDA, but with no excretion into the biliary system. This appearance is present immediately, and is a diagnostic pattern (Fig. 9). It is important to realize that this is true even before the ducts dilate. Ultrasonographic appearances will be unchanged at this stage. With partial obstruction, there will be delayed passage distal to the level of obstruction, and the dilated duct system will be visible on the HIDA study. If duct dilatation is marked, it appears as a defect radiating from the hilum on a colloid study.

Sclerosing cholangitis

Hepatobiliary scintigraphy has been used to assess patients with sclerosing cholangitis (Rodman, Gastro, 1987; 92:777). Classical features include an appearance of beading in the biliary tree,

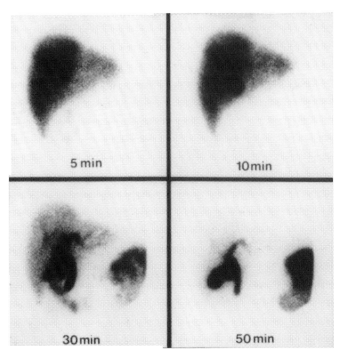

Fig. 7. Normal hepatobiliary study, showing lack of blood pool by 5 min, uniform uptake in parenchyma, clear activity in gut and gallbladder at 30 min, and excellent parenchymal clearance by 50 min.

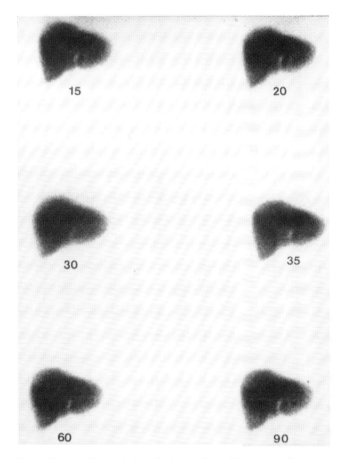

Fig. 9. Hepatobiliary scintigraphy in a patient with acute total obstruction. Note the well-maintained uptake of tracer with complete absence of excretion.

differential flow from right and left lobes of the liver, and delayed emptying into the small bowel.

The sensitivity in acquired immune deficiency syndrome-related sclerosing cholangitis appears to be the same as CT at 90 per cent and better than ultrasound at 67 per cent (Buscombe, NuclMed-Comm, 1992; 13:154).

It may provide an ideal screening test for those patients with suspected sclerosing cholangitis but in whom endoscopic retrograde pancreatography is not an ideal first-line test. The choice between CT and hepatobiliary scintigraphy will depend on the local costs and availability of each test.

Biliary leakage

Hepatobiliary scintigraphy is a very sensitive method for detecting biliary leakage, although it lacks the anatomical definition of the radiological methods. It is important to use a third-generation HIDA agent, and to review the study in dynamic mode on the computer to identify the site of leakage accurately.

Neonatal jaundice

In neonatal hepatitis, the biliary system is patent, and hepatobiliary agents will pass into the gut. Because of the immaturity of the fetal liver, tracer uptake may be poor, even in normals, but may be improved by enzyme induction with phenobarbitone, 5 mg/kg for

5 days preceding the study. By contrast, in biliary atresia, no activity passes into the gut. This is considered in more detail in Section 26.

Miscellaneous

LeVeen shunt studies

Radionuclide studies allow for simple assessment of the patency of LeVeen peritoneovenous shunts. Of several techniques, the simplest is that of Mededdu et al. (JNuclMed, 1983; 24:302). [99Tcm]albumen microspheres (200 MBq) are injected into the peritoneal cavity. If the shunt is patent, the microspheres are seen to have passed to the lungs. If this is not seen, a second injection directly into the tube allows localization of the level of block.

Hepatic and perihepatic infection

Pyogenic liver abscesses are probably best identified by ultrasound or CT, as aspiration can be performed, which will allow a microbiological diagnosis to be obtained (Pitt, WorldJSurg, 1990; 14:498). In those cases in which hepatic infection is suspected, but ultrasound or CT are unavailable or unhelpful, nuclear medical studies are indicated. Either gallium-67 citrate or labelled leucocytes can be used to identify hepatic infection. Leucocytes can be labelled either with indium-111 oxime (Thakur, JNuclMed, 1977; 18:1014) or [99Tcm]exametazime (Peters, SemNuclMed, 1994; 24:110). Imaging with indium-111 labelled leucocytes should be done at 4 and 24 h after reinjection of labelled white cells; with [99Tcm]exametazime-labelled cells, imaging is best done at 1 and 3 h after reinjection (Mountford, JNuclMed, 1990; 31:311). However, as all these imaging agents accumulate to some extent within the liver, it may be possible to miss either intrahepatic or associated perihepatic infection, for example in the subphrenic space. This explain why the sensitivity of labelled leucocyte imaging is the same as CT or ultrasound in the liver but greater elsewhere in the abdomen (Weldon, Gut, 1995; 37:557). Three simple strategies can be used to overcome this problem: (i) sequential imaging to see if initially photopenic liver accumulates gallium or labelled leucocytes over time; (ii) [99Tcm]colloid scans and subtraction imaging; (iii) SPECT, to increase contrast between the abscess and surrounding liver tissue.

In all patients with suspected infection, early use of gallium-67 citrate or labelled leucocytes will yield clinically useful results and will probably alter the management (Childs, JNuclMedTechnol, 1995; 23:262).

In patients with tuberculosis and those who are immunosuppressed, granulocyte involvement in the inflammatory response is often reduced, and leucocyte labelling (where over 90 per cent of labelled cells are granulocytes) will not be as useful as gallium-67 citrate. Furthermore, many of these infections are indolent and gallium allows imaging for up to 96 h.

Whilst [99Tcm]colloid imaging will show a defect at the site of infection, its use in diagnosis is limited in patients with either pyogenic or amoebic abscesses; however, it is cheap, allows one to monitor response to therapy, and as such is underused.

Reference

1. Goris ML. Sensitivity and specificity of common scintigraphic procedures. Chicago: Year Book Medical Publishers, 1985: 78–9.

5.7 Splanchnic haemodynamic investigations

Didier Lebrec

Introduction

Portal hypertension is characterized by an elevation of pressure in the portal vein and in its venous territory. This syndrome may be complicated by the development of portal systemic collaterals, which can be responsible for ruptured oesophageal or gastric varices. In general, the circulatory system is evaluated by blood flow, pressure, and volume. Vascular resistance is calculated from the ratio between pressure and blood flow. Portal pressure depends on two factors: portal intrahepatic vascular resistance (and vascular resistance of the portal systemic collaterals when portal hypertension is present) and portal tributary blood flow (the sum of gastro-intestinal, colic, splenic, mesenteric, and pancreatic blood flow). Splanchnic blood flow is the sum of portal tributary blood flow and hepatic arterial blood flow. In normal individuals it is essentially the same as hepatic blood flow. However, in portal hypertension, splanchnic blood flow is usually greater than hepatic since some portal blood bypasses the liver and enters the systemic circulation directly.

The haemodynamic investigation of the splanchnic circulation consists of the measurements of pressure and blood flow. In man, while pressures may be measured, there is no simple method for measuring either portal or hepatic arterial blood flows, or the flow through collateral vessels. Regional blood flow can, however, be measured in animals. Finally, since it is altered in portal hypertension, the systemic circulation must also be evaluated.

In this chapter, the main haemodynamic methods used in man are described. It must be emphasized, however, that results reported are those measured in fasted, conscious patients in a supine position. Results obtained under other conditions may differ widely from those reported below.

Measurement of portal pressure

The measurement of pressure in the portal venous system is the main method used to define and characterize portal hypertension. Normally, portal pressure ranges from 7 to 12 mmHg, and the pressure gradient between portal pressure and pressure in the vena caval territory ranges from 1 to 4 mmHg. Portal hypertension is present when portal pressure is higher than 12 mmHg or when the pressure gradient is higher than 4 mmHg. If the pressure in the vena caval territory increases, portal hypertension develops, but without a collateral circulation (unless another factor contributes to the portal hypertension). Portal pressure may be evaluated either directly or indirectly. Direct measurement of portal pressure is more invasive than the indirect method but is more valid, especially with cases of persinusoidal or extrahepatic portal hypertension.

Direct methods

During abdominal surgery, portal pressure may be measured directly by introducing a needle into the lumen of the portal vein or by inserting a catheter into a small ileal vein. These values for portal pressure differ from those measured without surgery, since anaesthetic agents modify the splanchnic and systemic circulation. Catheterization of the umbilical vein also allows direct measurement of portal pressure; but as this necessitates both general anaesthesia and surgery, it is not regularly used.

The most common direct technique is the percutaneous trans-hepatic puncture of the portal vein with a thin (Chiba) needle. The portal vein may be located by ultrasonography (Burchaarth, JGastroHepatol, 1987; 2:569). Larger needles may also be used, allowing a catheter to be inserted into the lumen of the portal vein in order to cannulate other smaller veins. If ascites or coagulation defects are present, these methods are contraindicated. The portal vein may be catheterized through a hepatic vein in the same manner as with a transvenous liver biopsy procedure. This method allows measurement of the pressure in the inferior vena cava, a hepatic vein, and the portal vein during one and the same procedure. It may cause abdominal pain.

Indirect methods

Intrasplenic pressure

Although splenic pressure, measured with a needle, has been widely used, this technique has a high risk of intraperitoneal haemorrhage. Splenic pulp pressure is similar to splenic vein pressure.

Intrahepatic pressure

It has been claimed that pressure in the hepatic tissue reflects sinusoidal pressure. This intrahepatic pressure measurement is performed blindly by introducing a needle percutaneously into the hepatic parenchyma (Fenyves, Hepatol, 1988; 8:211). While this pressure may be 'sinusoidal', it may also be intra-arterial, portal, or that of the hepatic vein or the biliary tract.

Hepatic venous pressures

Since it is simple and safe, measurement of wedged and free hepatic venous pressure is the most common procedure used to evaluate portal pressure indirectly. A radiopaque catheter is introduced into a hepatic vein (usually the right vein) with an approach through a jugular, femoral or brachial vein. This procedure is performed under radioscopic control.[1] The catheter is wedged to block the circulation in a small hepatic venule. The wedged position is verified by the absence of reflux of radio-opaque dye. Wedged hepatic venous pressure is similar to the occluded pressure obtained with a balloon catheter.

The hepatic venous pressure gradient (wedged minus hepatic venous pressure) ranges from 1 to 4 mmHg in normal individuals. The hepatic venous-pressure gradient remains normal in cases of extrahepatic portal hypertension and in certain cases of presinusoidal portal hypertension such as schistosomiasis (Lebrec, SemLivDis, 1986; 6:332). In presinusoidal portal hypertension, the pressure gradient may be elevated, in general to no more than 13 mmHg, thus indicating the presence of two blocks (presinusoidal and sinusoidal). In chronic liver disease with extensive fibrosis, as well as in non-cirrhotic portal hypertension, the hepatic venous-pressure gradient is increased from 5 to 20 mmHg but remains lower than the portal pressure. This increase in the pressure gradient is also observed in several acute liver diseases such as fulminant hepatitis (Valla, Hepatol, 1989; 10:482).

In alcoholic cirrhosis and in hepatitis-B-related cirrhosis, wedged hepatic venous pressure is generally similar to portal pressure.[1] The hepatic venous-pressure gradient exhibits a circadian variation with two peaks (9 a.m. and 11 p.m.) that may influence the moment of occurrence of variceal bleeding. Among these patients the hepatic venous-pressure gradient may differ widely from 10 to 30 mmHg. This value correlates with the severity of cirrhosis as estimated by the Child–Pugh classification (Braillon, Gut, 1986; 27:1204).

Liver lesions of acute alcoholic hepatitis increase the hepatic venous-pressure gradient (Poynard, DigDisSci, 1987; 32:337). The value correlates with the extent of fibrosis and the amount of liver-cell necrosis. In patients with cirrhosis, the presence of hepatocellular carcinoma may markedly increase the hepatic venous-pressure gradient to more than 30 mmHg, and this change may vary from one vein to another. In patients with alcoholic cirrhosis whose hepatic venous-pressure gradient is less than 12 mmHg, the gradient is not associated with the development of oesophageal varices or with the risk of gastrointestinal bleeding (Lebrec, Gastro, 1980; 79: 1139). When the hepatic venous-pressure gradient is less than 12 mmHg, ruptured oesophageal varices do not occur.

A hepatic venous-pressure gradient of more than 4 mmHg indicates sinusoidal portal hypertension but the mechanism causing this increase is not clear. It depends mainly on the reduction of hepatic vascular space, which increases intrahepatic vascular resistance (Lee, Gastro, 1987; 93:157). This pressure gradient also depends on several other factors such as portal pressure, portal tributary blood flow, and hepatic arterial blood flow.

Finally, in patients with alcoholic cirrhosis, a pharmacological decrease in the hepatic venous-pressure gradient indicates a reduction in portal pressure.[1] In this case, however, the reduction in the gradient may be more marked than the decrease in portal pressure.

Oesophageal variceal pressures

During oesophageal endoscopy, variceal pressures may be measured by different techniques. A first approach consists of puncturing the lumen of a varix with a needle (Staritz, Gut, 1985; 26:525). This should be done just before sclerotherapy because it may precipitate variceal bleeding. When measured by this technique, variceal pressure is elevated in cases with portal hypertension but no correlation with portal pressure or the hepatic venous-pressure gradient has been reported. Intravariceal pressure seems to correlate with the size of the varix and with a previous history of ruptured oesophageal varices.

A second approach uses an endoscopic gauge, allowing the measurement of variceal pressure without puncturing varices (Bosch, Hepatol, 1986; 6:667). This non-invasive method uses a hemispherical pressure gauge with a small chamber fed with a constant flow of gas. This chamber is covered by a latex membrane. When the gauge is placed over a varix, the pressure needed to fill the gauge, as measured by a pressure transducer, is equal to the variceal pressure. It is assumed that the pressure needed to compress a varix equals the pressure inside the varix. It has been recently demonstrated that this technique is reproducible, allowing repeated assessment of variceal pressure for evaluation of the effects of pharmacological therapy (Nevens, JHepatol, 1996; 24:66).

A third, recently described endoscopic method employs a transparent plastic balloon fixed to the tip of a gastroscope, with observation of the pressure equilibrium between varices and the balloon (Gerthsch, Gastro, 1993; 105:1159). The pressures obtained with this technique are correlated with those measured by needle puncture.

Measurement of splanchnic blood flow
Portal and hepatic arterial blood flows

During abdominal surgery, portal and hepatic arterial blood flow may be measured separately by means of an electromagnetic flow debitmeter. The results of this invasive method are difficult to evaluate because they are obtained under general anaesthesia. The ratio between portal and hepatic arterial blood flows can also be calculated by measuring hepatic radioactivity after the injection of a radioactive substance into a peripheral vein. A gamma-camera may evaluate both hepatic arterial and the portal radioactivity (Chapter 5.6). This method cannot be widely used because renal and pulmonary radioactivity interferes with hepatic and portal radioactivity measurements; moreover, it is difficult to dissociate arterial and portal curves.

Dilution indicator method

Hepatic blood flow can be estimated with the indicator dilution method (Cohn, AmJMed, 1972; 53:704). The indicator is injected either into the hepatic artery or the portal vein, and blood is drawn from a hepatic vein. Analysis of the curve for the hepatic vein gives the hepatic blood flow. This invasive technique is not widely used because there is inadequate mixing between the indicator and the blood. This method has been used to evaluate hepatic micro-circulation, transit time, and distribution volume (Huet, Sem-LivDis, 1986; 6:277).

Hepatic clearance method

The clearance method is at present the most widely used for estimating hepatic blood flow in man. It is based on the Fick principle (Caesar, ClinSci, 1961; 21:43). The hepatic clearance (Cl) depends on hepatic blood flow (HBF) and the extraction (E) of a substance by the liver

$$(Cl = HBF \times E)$$

Hence

$$HBF = \frac{Cl}{E}$$

Absolute hepatic clearance can be calculated by the continuous infusion method. When the peripheral concentration (C_p) of the substance has reached a plateau, the amount of substance removed by the liver is equal to the amount of perfused solution Q:

$$Cl = \frac{Q}{C_p}$$

Extraction depends on afferent (C_{aff}) and efferent (C_{eff}) concentrations of the substance. Thus,

$$E = \frac{C_{aff} - C_{eff}}{C_{aff}}$$

If this substance is captured only by the liver, the afferent concentration is equal to the peripheral venous or arterial concentration of this substance. The efferent concentration is obtained from blood drawn from a hepatic vein. Therefore, catheterization of an hepatic vein is necessary to measure hepatic blood flow by the clearance method. Hepatic clearance is hepatic blood flow only if extraction reaches 100 per cent. If extraction is lower than 10 per cent, hepatic blood flows are not calculated, as a slight error in the measurement of extraction will cause a large error in the calculation of flow. Thus, the clearance method cannot be used to measure hepatic blood flow in patients with severe liver disease. Moreover, a decrease in hepatic clearance does not indicate a decrease in hepatic blood flow since extraction may also decrease leaving hepatic blood flow constant.

The 'fractional clearance' (K) may also be used for the calculation of hepatic blood flow

$$K = \frac{Cl}{\text{blood volume}}$$

This method, using a bolus injection, is analogous to the continuous infusion method.

Substances used for these clearance methods must not be toxic, must diffuse only in the vascular space, and must only be removed by the liver. Two types of substance can be used, those cleared by hepatocytes (bromsulphthalein and indocyanine cardiogreen) and those cleared by Kupffer cells (colloid labelled with radiogold, denatured labelled albumin).

Galactose clearance has been proposed to estimate hepatic blood flow since hepatic extraction of this substance is more than 90 per cent in normal individuals (Keiding, Gastro, 1988; 94:477). In patients with liver disease, galactose extraction is markedly decreased and hence hepatic blood flow is not properly evaluated by the galactose clearance. Moreover, it has been demonstrated recently that extrahepatic uptake of galactose occurs in cirrhotic patients. These findings clearly indicate that galactose clearance cannot be used either for measurement of hepatic blood flow or for studying variations of hepatic blood flow in cirrhotics.

Values of hepatic blood flow

In normal, fasted, conscious individuals in the supine position, hepatic blood flow ranges from 1 to 2 l/min, that is, 1 ml/min per gram of liver tissue. In man it is accepted, although it has not been clearly demonstrated, that one-third of hepatic blood flow comes from the hepatic artery and two-thirds from the portal vein. In those with liver diseases, hepatic blood flow may differ widely from one patient to another. Whereas hepatic blood flow may be low, normal or elevated in patients with cirrhosis, acute alcoholic hepatitis increases hepatic blood flow (Cohn, AmJMed, 1972; 53: 704). In patients with acute hepatitis, hepatic blood flow may be increased; it is low in patients with extrahepatic portal hypertension. In cirrhotic patients, no correlation has been found between hepatic blood flow and either liver failure or portal pressure (Lebrec, ArchFrMalAppDig, 1973; 62:465). This observation is not surprising, because in portal hypertensive patients a certain percentage of the portal blood does not reach the liver but bypasses this organ through collateral circulation. Hence, portal pressure may decrease without a change in hepatic blood flow. In this case the reduction of portal pressure depends on a decrease in portal tributary blood flow.

Measurement of portal blood flow

Several invasive methods have been described for measuring portal blood flow. However, they necessitate the insertion of a catheter into the lumen of the portal vein. Portal blood flow can be measured by the continuous thermodilution method or by means of a catheter with an electromagnetic flowmeter.

The most common method for evaluating portal blood flow is based on the Doppler effect (Burns, Gastro, 1987; 92:824). This non-invasive procedure measures the velocity of red blood cells. At present, the pulsed-Doppler method is not accurate in man for the following reasons.

1. The mean angle between the Doppler beam and the axis of the portal vein may be too large, reaching up to 60°. In this case, a slight error of the angle results in a large variation in the cosine angle, which is related to flow velocity.
2. The ultrasound diffraction between the skin and the portal vein is not taken into consideration.
3. The measurement of maximal velocity in one area of the portal vein may differ from one position to another.

4. Since the measurement of blood flow depends on a cross-sectional area of the portal vein, a slight error in the estimated diameter of the portal vein results in a large variation in this section.

The pulsed-Doppler method has not yet been validated in man. The Doppler technique may, however, be used to assess the presence and direction of portal blood flow. In addition, in the same individual, physiological or pharmacological variations of blood velocity in the portal vein may be evaluated. Its accuracy and reproducibility are still in question for clinical application (Bolondi, JHepatol, 1991, 13:269).

Estimation of blood flow in the collateral circulation

Quantitation of portal–systemic circulation

The percentage of portal venous inflow shunted through portal–systemic collaterals may be estimated by comparing the area of an isotope dilution curve recorded from the hepatic vein after injecting an isotope into the superior mesenteric or splenic artery with the curve obtained after injecting an isotope into the hepatic artery (Groszmann, AmJMed, 1972; 53:715). In normal individuals, no shunting was detected but in patients with cirrhosis shunting of mesenteric or splenic flow ranged from zero to 100 per cent. A similar estimation may be obtained after intrasplenic injection of a radioactive indicator.

Comparing the bioavailability of drugs according to the method of their administration (intravenous or orally) allows the shunt fraction of the portal inflow to be measured (Nordlinger, Hepatol, 1982; 2:412). The liver must remove 100 per cent of the substance; the systemic availability of oral glyceryl trinitrate has been used. In this case, drug concentrations in plasma were replaced by assessments of pharmacological effects by using digital plethysmography (Porchet, Gastro, 1982; 82:629). None of these invasive and non-invasive methods, however, can be used to predict the complication of portal hypertension.

Azygos blood flow

The superior portal–systemic collateral circulation can be estimated by measuring blood flow in the azygos vein (Bosch, Hepatol, 1984; 4:424), which essentially drains the splenogastric collateral circulation. Azygos blood flow is measured by the local continuous thermodilution method. Under fluoroscopic control, a continuous thermodilution catheter with a curved tip is introduced into the azygos vein up to approx. 5 cm from its junction with the superior vena cava. Its position is verified by injection of a contrast medium into the catheter. During routine haemodynamic investigation, the azygos vein may be catheterized either from the femoral or from the right internal jugular vein. In normal individuals, azygos blood flow is approx. 100 ml/min. In patients with portal hypertension, azygos blood flow is higher than normal and ranges from 200 to 1500 ml/min.

An elevated azygos blood flow indirectly confirms the increased portal tributary blood flow observed in portal hypertensive animals. Azygos blood flow is correlated with portal pressure and depends on the severity of cirrhosis. Azygos blood flow is not correlated either with the presence and size of the oesophageal varices or with the risk of ruptured varices (Calès, JHepatol, 1984; 1:37). Finally, the measurement of azygos blood flow is more sensitive than the hepatic venous-pressure gradient for evaluating the change in splanchnic circulation after the administration of portal hypotensive drugs. Thus, the measurement of azygos blood flow seems to be the most viable method for the evaluation of portal hypertension.

Preliminary results showed that cine phase-contrast magnetic resonance angiography is a practical, non-invasive method for measuring absolute azygos blood flow and provides a non-invasive method of monitoring portal hypertension (Lommas, JHepatol, 1996; 22:399).

References

1. Valla D, Bercoff E, Menu Y, Bataille C, and Lebrec D. Discrepancy between wedged hepatic venous pressure and portal venous pressure after acute propranolol administration in patients with alcoholic cirrhosis. *Gastroenterology*, 1984; **86**: 1400–3.

5.8 Diagnostic approach to liver disease

Neil McIntyre

When liver disease is suspected the diagnostic approach must clearly depend on the initial clinical picture. Liver diseases present in many different ways. Sometimes it is easy to establish the cause; at other times it may be difficult to make a diagnosis, or even to decide whether significant liver disease is present. Diagnostic problems also arise in patients who are already known to have pre-existing liver disease.

The identification of liver disease

Liver disease is usually suspected when:

1. One or more 'liver function' tests are abnormal on routine testing, even if there are no clinical features of liver disease.
2. Vague symptoms or signs suggest the possibility of liver disease.
3. Abnormal liver function tests are found in patients at risk of liver disease (for example because of alcohol abuse, previous blood transfusion, gallstones).
4. Patients present with symptoms or signs which are strongly suggestive of liver disease (for example jaundice, bilirubinuria, florid spider naevi, a large liver and/or spleen, ascites, or umbilical collaterals).
5. Strong evidence of liver disease is found during the investigation of clinical disorders originally thought to be unrelated to the hepatobiliary system (particularly with imaging of the upper abdomen by conventional radiology, ultrasound, or CT scanning).
6. When a serious illness without obvious cause is associated with abnormal liver function tests (requested as part of a wide-ranging diagnostic search).
7. Patients have a relative or close contact suffering from liver disease, suggesting the possibility of a hereditary disorder or an infectious disease.

Patients falling into the first, second, third, sixth, and seventh categories pose problems for general practioners and general physicians; they must decide whether significant liver disease is present, and/or whether referral to a hepatologist is indicated. For patients in the fourth and fifth categories all that is usually required is a straightforward search for the cause of the underlying abnormality; if the diagnosis is not obvious, such patients should be referred to a specialist liver unit.

Abnormal liver function tests found during routine screening

The use of a battery of routine liver function tests is a highly sensitive procedure (see Chapter 5.1); relatively few patients with significant liver disease have a complete set of normal results with the commonly used tests (i.e. there are few false negatives). False negatives are found in some patients with well-compensated cirrhosis or space-occupying lesions, which would therefore remain unsuspected after routine biochemical screening. Fortunately, patients with cirrhosis who have normal test results tend to do well, and tolerate drugs, surgical procedures, and other treatments far better than those showing clear evidence of liver damage. However, the opportunity for early treatment of conditions such as haemochromatosis or tumours would clearly be lost. Furthermore, if liver disease is missed it is not possible to counsel patients about seeking help promptly when new symptoms arise, or about the need to reduce the dosage of, or to avoid, certain drugs which may be prescribed for unrelated conditions, but which are relatively contraindicated in patients with cirrhosis and other hepatic disorders (even if the disease is well compensated).

For this reason there are advantages in including other tests in the process of screening or profiling (see Chapter 5.1), such as haematological indices (including serum iron, total iron-binding capacity, and ferritin), thyroid function tests, autoantibodies, and markers of viral hepatitis. Not only do these additional tests have diagnostic value in the interpretation of abnormal liver function tests, they also have a high diagnostic 'pay-off' in their own right. Iron deficiency, thyroid disease, and autoimmune disorders are relatively common in patients without liver disease, while many carriers of hepatitis B and C have normal liver function tests.

Abnormalities of a single liver function test

The major hepatobiliary causes of abnormalities of a single liver function test are presented in Table 1. However, when only one liver function test is abnormal, consider causes other than liver disease, particularly if there are no other clinical features of liver disease.

Table 1 Hepatobiliary causes of an isolated abnormal liver function test (see also Chapter 5.1)

Increase in:	
Bilirubin	Gilbert's syndrome
	Crigler Najjar disease I and II
	Dubin–Johnson syndrome
	Rotor syndrome
	Drugs
	(? Cirrhosis/posthepatitis)
Alanine aminotransferase*	Fatty liver (see text)
	Hepatitis C
	Drugs
	Mild/treated autoimmune hepatitis
Aspartate aminotransferase*	Alcoholic cirrhosis/hepatitis
	Cirrhosis (other forms)
	(Macro AST—see Chapter 5.1)
Alkaline phosphatase	Primary biliary cirrhosis
	Sclerosing cholangitis/strictures
	Cholelithiasis
	Drugs (uncommon)
	Space-occupying lesions (including tumours)
	Cirrhosis (often intestinal enzyme)
γ-Glutamyl transferase	Fatty liver (see text)
	Alcohol
	Drugs (especially enzyme inducers)
	Space-occupying lesions
Decrease in:	
Albumin	Cirrhosis (especially with ascites)
	Analbuminaemia (genetic)

* An increase of both aminotransferases (without other abnormal results) occurs commonly in many other conditions, such as acute and chronic hepatitis and shock liver, as well as those listed above under the individual aminotransferases.

Strategy for these isolated findings

Serum bilirubin

A high total bilirubin may be due to an 'unconjugated hyperbilirubinaemia', or a hyperbilirubinaemia in which the conjugated bilirubin is also increased. The distinction is made by simultaneous measurement of serum bilirubin esters—conjugated or direct bilirubin—in order to assess the proportion of unconjugated bilirubin. However, it must be realized that our standard tests (Chapter 5.1) tend to overestimate conjugated bilirubin at relatively low levels of total bilirubin.

Conjugated hyperbilirubinaemia can also be identified by the finding of bilirubinuria, which may be present before overt jaundice appears. Bilirubinuria is absent in patients with 'unconjugated hyperbilirubinaemia', and also in some patients with a prolonged conjugated hyperbilirubinaemia because of the presence of 'bili-alb' (Chapter 5.1).

Gilbert's syndrome, an unconjugated hyperbilirubinaemia, is by far the most common cause of an isolated elevation of serum bilirubin, but haemolysis should be ruled out (see unconjugated hyperbilirubinaemia, below). The Dubin–Johnson and Rotor syndromes are rare causes of a mild conjugated hyperbilirubinaemia, which may also result from some drugs.

Alkaline phosphatase

When there is an isolated increase of alkaline phosphatase the best approach is to measure alkaline phosphatase isoenzymes (see Chapter 5.1). This may unearth a non-hepatic cause of a high alkaline phosphatase. Bone disease is most likely. A high intestinal phosphatase may be found in normal subjects, and is a relatively common finding in cirrhosis (see Chapter 5.1). Pregnant women have a high placental phosphatase.

If the liver isoenzymes are elevated one should search for a hepatobiliary disorder (see below). Other tests which usually rise with biliary obstruction (such as γ-glutamyl transferase, 5'-nucleotidase) have been used to try to confirm a hepatobiliary origin of an elevated alkaline phosphatase, but they lack specificity and are occasionally normal in patients with cholestasis.

γ-Glutamyl transferase

γ-Glutamyl transferase is a highly sensitive indicator of liver disease, but lacks specificity; many other conditions increase serum γ-glutamyl transferase (Chapter 5.1). Levels above the upper limit of normal (50 mU/l in men, 30 mU/l in women) are found in about 15 per cent of 'normal' subjects; even if the upper limit of the normal range is readjusted to 80 mU/l in men, about 6 per cent still have an abnormal level, and in 4 per cent the level is greater than 100 mU/l.

γ-Glutamyl transferase is mistakenly considered as a valuable marker of alcohol abuse, but about one-third of heavy drinkers show no increase in the serum activity of this enzyme. Because high levels are so common in other conditions, patients with a high γ-glutamyl transferase should not be labelled as alcoholics without confirmatory evidence.

Invasive investigations are probably unjustified in asymptomatic patients with an isolated elevation of γ-glutamyl transferase, as significant liver disease other than fatty liver is rare in such cases. They should be followed up, with clinical evaluation and measurement of γ-glutamyl transferase and other liver function tests, at intervals of a few months. If symptoms and/or signs appear, other tests become abnormal, or the γ-glutamyl transferase continues to rise over many months, an ultrasound and/or CT scan should be performed to exclude a space-occupying lesion (Chapter 5.5), and liver biopsy and/or cholangiography should be considered.

Albumin

The serum albumin may fall with many conditions which do not involve the liver (see Chapter 5.1). In the absence of other clinical features suggesting liver disease there should be a rigorous search for other causes of a low albumin.

Aminotransferases

An isolated elevation of aminotransferases (aspartate and/or alanine) is usually due to hepatic disease of some kind. Alanine aminotransferase is a highly sensitive test (except for serious alcoholic liver disease, when it is often normal in the presence of a raised aspartate aminotransferase) but lacks specificity. Aspartate aminotransferase is a less sensitive but more specific test. Conditions other than liver disease cause elevation of aminotransferases; the measurement of creatine kinase (Chapter 5.1) is particularly helpful as an obvious increase suggests that elevated aminotransferases may be due to unsuspected skeletal muscle damage (due to a myopathy or hypothyroidism), or excessive muscular work, as in bodybuilders even in the absence of androgen abuse. Both aspartate and alanine aminotransferases are released from muscle.

An isolated and modest increase of alanine aminotransferase alone is common in asymptomatic subjects, usually in association with hepatitis C, high alcohol intake, obesity or mild fatty liver from another cause, or drug-induced injury, but is often found in the absence of any significant liver disease. Appropriate 'routine' non-invasive diagnostic tests (Table 2) should be performed, but except for tests for hepatitis C are rarely found to be positive. A high fasting triglyceride, and ultrasonograpy or CT scanning, may support a diagnosis of fatty liver. Invasive investigations are rarely justified, except for liver biopsy to assess the stage of hepatitis C (see Chapter 12.1.2.5). Patients with an isolated increase of alanine aminotransferase should be followed-up with regular aspartate and alanine aminotransferase estimations.

If aspartate aminotransferase alone is raised, the likelihood of significant liver disease is much greater; this is particularly true for alcoholic cirrhosis (Chapter 5.1). A liver biopsy may be needed to establish the diagnosis. Because patients with alcoholic cirrhosis may have an isolated increase in aspartate aminotransferase, while

those with hepatitis C and fatty liver may show only an increased alanine aminotransferase, it is important that both tests are included in any routine battery of liver function tests.

When both aminotransferases are elevated the relative serum activities of these two enzymes may be of value. If alanine aminotransferase activity is clearly greater than that of aspartate aminotransferase, the most common causes are those which result in an

Table 2 Symptoms and signs suggesting hepatobiliary disease

Strong symptoms and signs of hepatobiliary disease
  Jaundice and dark urine
  Spider naevi, true palmar erythema
  Palpable liver, or spleen
  Small liver—percussion
  Palpable gallbladder
  Abdominal wall collaterals
  Bruit/friction rub over liver
  History of schistosomiasis
  Heavy alcohol abuse
  Kayser–Fleischer rings
  Pruritus, scratch marks
  Gynaecomastia
  Ascites
  'Flapping tremor'
  Venous hums
  Exposure to hepatotoxins
  Papular acrodermatitis
  Intravenous drug abuse

Intermediate symptoms and signs of hepatobiliary disease
  Haematemesis and/or melaena
  Bleeding and bruising
  Blood transfusion/blood products
  Family history of liver disease
  Hereditary haemorrhagic telangiectasia
  Homosexuality
  Tattoos
  Unexplained peripheral oedema
  Striae of autoimmune chronic hepatitis
  Unexplained loss of muscle bulk
  Pale stools
  Petechias
  Previous jaundice
  Previous malignancy
  Small testicles

Weak symptoms and signs of liver disease
  Asthenia, tiredness, and malaise
  Anorexia, disordered taste and smell
  Upper abdominal discomfort and pain
  Impotence/sexual dysfunction
  Heterosexual promiscuity
  Drugs for psychiatric disorders
  Erythemas/urticaria
  Residence/travel in certain countries
  Parotid enlargement
  Xanthomas and xanthelasma
  Cholecystectomy, or other forms of upper abdominal surgery
  CREST syndrome with primary biliary cirrhosis
  Weight loss and gain
  Nausea and vomiting
  Muscle cramps
  Oliguria and nocturia
  Pigmentation
  Dupuytren's contracture
  Lichen planus
  Vitiligo
  White nails
  Blue lunulas

isolated increase in alanine aminotransferase (see above), including patients with relatively trivial liver disease. This pattern is also seen commonly with other types of viral hepatitis, in mild cases of autoimmune hepatitis, and with drug-induced liver disease. Other diagnostic tests should help to identify viral or autoimmune hepatitis, and a careful drug history should be taken.

The most important (and common) cause for an aspartate aminotransferase increase which is clearly greater than that of alanine aminotransferase is alcoholic cirrhosis/hepatitis; but this relationship is also seen with neoplastic and infiltrative liver disease and in other non-biliary types of cirrhosis. These conditions are serious disorders and rigorous investigation, including liver biopsy, is usually justified in order to make a diagnosis.

If trivial liver disease is found on biopsy, and other relevant investigations (see below) are negative, the patient may need little in the way of follow-up, although it is prudent to perform liver function tests occasionally (at 6- or 12-month intervals) to check that there is no change in the clinical state.

Because aminotransferase levels may fluctuate, particularly with chronic hepatitis C (and sometimes with relapsing hepatitis A), it cannot be assumed that an acute liver disease has resolved when these tests have returned to normal; further tests should be performed at intervals in order to exclude chronic liver disease.

Abnormalities of more than one liver function test

When more than one liver function test is abnormal (aspartate/alanine aminotransferase being taken as one test), the probability of liver disease is very high, and in this situation the use of a battery of tests has high specificity and a high predictive value (in terms of the presence of some form of hepatobiliary disease). False positives are uncommon but do occur, for example a patient with malabsorption may have a high serum alkaline phosphatase (from bone) and a low serum albumin, or a patient with myocardial infarction may have a high aspartate aminotransferase of cardiac origin and an elevated bilirubin, due perhaps to a functional and relatively trivial hepatic disturbance.

The pattern of the test abnormalities is usually of little diagnostic value (see below) in apparently asymptomatic patients. However, some form of diffuse parenchymal disease is suggested when hyperbilirubinaemia (even without obvious jaundice) occurs with very high aminotransferases, although this pattern may be seen with acute biliary obstruction due to gallstones. Diseases of the bile ducts (large or small), or space-occupying lesions, are likely causes when an increase in bilirubin is seen with an increased alkaline phosphatase. The most common combination of findings is a modest increase in alanine aminotransferase (often with a smaller increase in aspartate aminotransferase) with a rise in γ-glutamyl transpeptidase. This occurs with fatty liver (the commonest cause in developed countries, see below), with hepatitis C (the commonest cause in many other countries), and as a result of ingestion of many drugs.

Because the predictive value for liver disease is so high when more than one liver function test is abnormal, the strategy for dealing with this situation is described below under 'Establishing the nature of liver disease'. It is important to persist with diagnostic efforts; if abnormal findings are ignored the chance of dealing with

problems such as alcoholism or haemochromatosis at a relatively early stage may be lost.

Abnormalities of liver function tests when liver disease is suspected

Although some symptoms and signs suggest the possibility of hepatobiliary disease (see Table 2 and Section 4), many of them may be present in diseases which do not involve the liver and bile ducts (for example tiredness, anorexia, abdominal discomfort). When clinical evidence is weak, and essentially indirect, the first step (from a hepatological point of view) is to establish that the patient does indeed have liver disease.

Abnormalities of a single liver function test

Although the finding of a single abnormal liver function test is of limited value for detecting liver disease (for the reasons given above), it is a more valuable pointer when liver disease is already suspected (when the prior probability of liver disease is high) than it is when found on routine testing (when the prior probability is low). For example, in the presence of hepatosplenomegaly, high levels of aminotransferases should suggest cirrhosis, and an increase of alkaline phosphatase the possibility of sclerosing cholangitis.

It is still sensible to check whether disease of another system is the cause of the abnormal result, particularly with isolated elevations of alkaline phosphatase or γ-glutamyl transferase, or with a low level of albumin. The general approach is similar to that employed when abnormal liver function tests are found in the absence of symptoms or signs.

Abnormalities of more than one liver function test

When the prior probability of liver disease is high (because there are clinical features which would fit with liver disease), the probability of liver disease is clearly very high when more than one liver function test is abnormal; the findings then demand explanation. False positives are uncommon in this situation (because specificity is high). The diagnostic approach should be determined both by the clinical story and by the nature of the abnormal test results, and is considered below under 'Establishing the nature of the liver disease'.

When aminotransferase levels are more than three times the upper limit of normal, significant, but not necessarily serious, liver disease is found in virtually all patients (Hay, Hepatol, 1989; 9:193); although high levels may also be found in patients with myopathies and hypothyroidism, there is usually no reason in these conditions to suspect liver disease on clinical grounds. Very high aminotransferases suggest acute hepatitis due to a virus or drugs, acute biliary obstruction, or an acute reduction in hepatic blood flow (see Sections 12 and 17 and Chapter 24.1). It is sensible to check whether more than one liver disease is present, as hepatitis B and C may coexist, and hepatitis C is commonly found in patients with alcoholic cirrhosis/hepatitis.

Clinical features strongly suggestive of hepatobiliary disease

Sometimes the clinical evidence of hepatic pathology is very strong (see Table 2), or there may be convincing radiological signs of

Table 3 Investigations which may be useful for precise diagnosis

'Routine' investigations giving 'specific' information

HBV markers (HBsAg, HBeAg; HBcAb, HBeAb, HBsAb; HBV DNA)	
HAV IgM Ab	
δ-Ab	
HVC Ab, HCV RNA	Acute/chronic viral hepatitis: (Section 12)
Antinuclear antibodies (to ds-DNA); smooth muscle antibodies (antiactin); liver-kidney-microsomal Ab; Ab to LSA	Autoimmune chronic hepatitis: (Chapter 14.3)
Antimitochondrial antibodies (M2, M4, M8)	Primary biliary cirrhosis: (Chapter 14.1)
α-Fetoprotein quantification; transcobalamin I	Primary liver cell carcinoma: (Chapter 22.2.1)
Serum copper and caeruloplasmin, urinary copper, Kayser–Fleischer rings	Wilson's disease: (Chapter 20.1)
Serum iron and iron-binding capacity, serum ferritin	Haemochromatosis: (Chapter 20.2)
VDRL, TPHA; hydatid serology; blood film; blood cultures	Infectious diseases: (Section 13)
(Detailed drug history)	Drug-induced liver disease: (Section 17)

'Other' investigations giving 'specific' information

Serum α₁-antitrypsin	α₁-Antitrypsin deficiency: (Chapter 20.3)
Fructose, galactose, tyrosine	Hereditary fructose intolerance, galactosaemia, tyrosinaemia: (Section 26)
Serum acid phosphatase	Gaucher's disease: (Chapter 20.7)
Creatine kinase and thyroid function tests	Myopathy, polymyositis, hypothyroidism
Markers for cytomegalovirus and herpesvirus	Acute viral hepatitis: (Section 12)

hepatobiliary disease. The diagnostic problem then is to establish the cause of the liver disease.

However, clinical features suggesting liver disease are sometimes found without disease of the liver or bile ducts. Ascites (Chapter 8.1), splenomegaly (Section 10), and distended abdominal wall veins (Section 4) may all, individually, be due to causes other than liver disease; these should be considered when assessing the patient, particularly when liver function tests are normal.

Establishing the nature of the liver disease

A major problem in hepatology is that many diagnostic investigations, although often definitive, are either expensive (for example CT scanning and MRI), or relatively invasive, and some carry a small but definite risk of serious complications (for example liver biopsy, various types of angiography, and percutaneous or endoscopic cholangiography). They also require expertise, for their performance or interpretation, that is not always available. It is not surprising that doctors try to make hepatological diagnoses using simpler and less hazardous methods.

Some investigations are very useful in providing a precise diagnosis (see Table 3). Some of these should probably be done routinely when the patient is first seen, in order to save time, for example viral markers, autoantibodies, α-fetoprotein, serum iron, total iron-binding capacity, and ferritin. Other tests need to be considered in puzzling cases. Often, however, these specific tests are not employed because they are forgotten, and it is sensible to use a checklist as an *aide-mémoire*.

Unfortunately many doctors rely too heavily on liver function tests for diagnostic purposes; they read more into the results of these tests than the confirmation of liver disease, even though common sense suggests that conventional liver function tests can have only a limited value in differential diagnosis. In most liver diseases there are usually abnormalities of one or more liver function

tests. Diagnostic discrimination would thus be possible only if it could be assumed that different diseases affect individual test results in a quantitatively different way, or that there are specific qualitative patterns of abnormality at some stage of the individual diseases.

Many authors have made claims about the diagnostic value of liver function tests on the basis of such assumptions. In most reports of this kind relatively small numbers of patients were studied, and results reported for only a limited number of hepatobiliary disorders. Successful discrimination has been claimed if the mean for one group of patients differed significantly from that of others, and little attention has been paid to the degree of overlap. Occasionally, only one type of liver disease was studied and the results found were then considered characteristic of that condition. Furthermore, tests are often performed on 'typical' cases, and it is assumed that the results would be the same even if the clinical presentation was different. Until recently, very few reports have considered the problems of the sensitivity, specificity, predictive accuracy, and efficiency of tests (or of combinations of tests), and little attention has been paid to the effect of the prevalence of different conditions on the diagnostic usefulness of the test (see Appendix to Chapter 5.1).

Undue reliance on liver function tests for diagnostic purposes led to an early classification of jaundice as haemolytic, hepatocellular, or obstructive (or cholestatic). The term 'haemolytic jaundice' was used when jaundice was acholuric (that is, urinary bilirubin was absent) and the serum bilirubin predominantly unconjugated; 'hepatocellular jaundice' when both unconjugated bilirubin and bilirubin esters were increased (although these were rarely measured), together with a normal or only slightly increased alkaline phosphatase and a moderate or marked increase in aminotransferases; and 'obstructive jaundice' (or 'cholestasis') when most of the serum bilirubin was conjugated, aminotransferase levels were only moderately elevated, and there was a more marked increase in alkaline phosphatase (more than two and a half times the upper reference limit). Unfortunately, the classification of jaundice on this

Table 4 Parenchymal liver diseases which may present with biochemical (and clinical) features suggesting extrahepatic biliary obstruction

Acute viral hepatitis
Alcoholic liver disease
Chronic active hepatitis and cirrhosis
Syphilitic hepatitis
Graft-versus-host disease
α_1-Antitrypsin deficiency
Intrahepatic cholestasis of pregnancy
Benign recurrent intrahepatic cholestasis
Drug-induced hepatitis
Primary biliary cirrhosis

Postoperative jaundice
Sarcoidosis
Lymphoma
Cystic fibrosis

Amyloidosis

Table 5 Diagnostic classification of hepatobiliary disease

A. Unconjugated hyperbilirubinaemia (see Chapter 20.6)
   Gilbert's syndrome
   Crigler Najjar disease (I and II)
   Haemolytic disorders

B. Large bile-duct disease (see Section 23)
   Tumours of pancreas, bile ducts, or gallbladder
   Gallstone obstruction of bile ducts
   Biliary strictures
   Sclerosing cholangitis
   Acute and chronic pancreatitis
   Caroli's syndrome
   Choledochal cysts
   Biliary atresia
   Parasites
   Biliary tract fistulas
   Mirizzi syndrome
   Duodenal diverticulum
   Trauma
   Acute cholangitis
   Biliary infections

C. Diffuse parenchymal liver disease (see relevant chapters)
   Alcoholic liver disease
   Viral or drug-induced acute hepatitis
   Chronic hepatitis
   Cirrhosis
   Fatty liver
   Graft-versus-host disease
   Granulomatous disorders
   Some storage disorders
   Cystic fibrosis
   Intrahepatic cholestases
   Schistosomiasis
   Other hepatic infections
   Nodular regenerative hyperplasia
   Congenital hepatic fibrosis
   Radiation injury

D. Space-occupying lesions (and infiltrations) (see relevant chapters)
   Primary and secondary hepatic malignancies
   Benign tumours
   Hepatic abscesses
   Inflammatory pseudotumour
   Haemangiomas
   Hydatid disease
   Simply cysts and polycystic disease
   Focal nodular hyperplasia
   Gaucher's disease
   Lymphomas and leukaemias
   Histiocytosis X
   Leishmaniasis
   Amyloidosis

E. Disorders of the hepatic circulation (see relevant chapters)
   Hepatic venous obstruction/thrombosis
   Veno-occlusive disease
   Constrictive pericarditis/heart failure/ischaemic hepatitis
   Portal venous obstruction/thrombosis
   Non-cirrhotic portal hypertension
   Hepatic arterial block/polyarteritis
   Arteriovenous fistula ·
   Pylephlebitis

basis was unsatisfactory for diagnostic purposes, although it is still advocated by some authors.

Diagnostic classification of liver disease

A sound diagnostic strategy must be based on a sound diagnostic classification. The classes should not only be collectively exhaustive, but should, ideally, be mutually exclusive (that is, all diagnostic possibilities should be included, but should not appear under more than one heading).

With the above classification into haemolytic, hepatocellular, and obstructive jaundice, many conditions called 'hepatocellular' also appear under the heading of obstructive or cholestatic jaundice: viral hepatitis, drug-induced hepatitis, alcoholic liver disease, chronic active hepatitis, and cirrhosis may all present with bio-chemical (and clinical) features considered 'typical' of extrahepatic biliary obstruction (Table 4). Furthermore, this classification does not extend into a general classification of liver disease, because it applies only to patients with jaundice, and because conditions which do not have a direct effect on hepatocytes or cause biliary obstruction are not easily included in this classification.

A more useful diagnostic classification, in which the groups are mutually exclusive (although more than one condition may be present in an individual patient), is the division of hepatobiliary diseases into:

(A) unconjugated hyperbilirubinaemia
(B) large bile-duct disease (identifiable on cholangiography)
(C) diffuse parenchymal liver disease
(D) space-occupying lesions (and infiltrations)
(E) disorders of the hepatic circulation.

This classification (Table 5) is applicable both for patients with jaundice and those with other types of presentation, and it takes into account the fact that diseases which cause jaundice may present without hyperbilirubinaemia; this is true even in patients with obstructive lesions of the main bile ducts (such as gallstones, tumours, or strictures), as the obstruction may be incomplete or intermittent.

With accurate methods patients can easily be categorized, on biochemical grounds, as having an unconjugated hyper-bilirubinaemia. It is clear that the other groups cannot be dis-tinguished on the basis of liver function tests, and that diagnosis must depend on other evidence.

Unconjugated hyperbilirubinaemia (see Chapters 2.9, 5.1 and 20.6)

A simple unconjugated hyperbilirubinaemia is present when there is a slight or moderate elevation of serum bilirubin without abnormality of other liver function tests. It is commonly found in men; about 5 per cent of 'normal' men have a total plasma bilirubin above 17 µmol/l, and about 2 per cent a level greater than 25 µmol/l. Almost all have the benign hyperbilirubinaemia known as Gilbert's syndrome, in which the total bilirubin is usually less than 50 µmol/l, although it may increase if food intake is reduced and then overt jaundice may develop. There are other rare familial causes of unconjugated hyperbilirubinaemia (see Chapter 20.6). It has been claimed that an isolated unconjugated hyperbilirubinaemia can occur with cirrhosis or after viral hepatitis, but many of these patients probably have coexisting Gilbert's syndrome. If bilirubinuria is present, the patient does not have an uncomplicated unconjugated hyperbilirubinaemia.

Haemolytic disorders must be excluded as a relatively rare cause of unconjugated hyperbilirubinaemia. The presence of haemolysis is suggested by a low haemoglobin and high reticulocyte count, and the underlying cause may be evident from the appearance of the red blood cells. In some rare red-cell disorders without obvious anaemia or haemolysis the diagnosis may be very difficult; special red-cell studies may be necessary.

The diagnosis of an unconjugated hyperbilirubinaemia can be confirmed by measurement of conjugated bilirubin. The diazo methods commonly used for this purpose are inaccurate, and tend to overestimate conjugated bilirubin. Modern methods, not yet widely available, allow differentiation between Gilbert's and haemolytic disorders (Chapters 2.9 and 20.6); with these techniques bilirubin esters are within the normal range in Gilbert's syndrome, but with haemolysis they rise in proportion to the total bilirubin.

Patients with a simple unconjugated hyperbilirubinaemia should not be subjected to unnecessary, expensive, and potentially hazardous investigations. Liver biopsy is not necessary for the diagnosis of Gilbert's syndrome.

Traditionally, the benign hyperbilirubinaemias have been classified under 'hepatocellular' jaundice (even though there is no increase in bilirubin esters), but they have few features in common with the other conditions in the group and it seems more logical for diagnostic purposes to group them, on the basis of the initial biochemical findings, under the heading 'unconjugated hyperbilirubinaemia' together with haemolytic disorders.

Large duct disease (B), parenchymal liver disease (C), space-occupying lesions and infiltrations (D), and disorders of the hepatic circulation (E)

Most patients being investigated for hepatobiliary disease fall into categories B and C (large duct or parenchymal liver disease). When conjugated hyperbilirubinaemia is present, several liver function tests are abnormal, and clinical features suggest the presence of liver disease, the most important clinical task is to decide between parenchymal disease and disease of the larger bile ducts (that is, those visible on cholangiography), but the possibility of a space-occupying lesion(s), or of disease of the hepatic vasculature, should

be borne in mind. If there is disease of the major ducts, surgery or therapeutic endoscopy may be needed, but surgery should be avoided in parenchymal liver disease; not only will it not relieve jaundice, but it may exacerbate the patient's condition.

The initial approach must clearly be dictated by the overall clinical picture. Sometimes clinical features may provide valuable clues, for example the age of the patient; the presence of risk factors such as alcohol, intravenous drug abuse, or homosexuality; an enlarged gallbladder; ascites; umbilical collaterals; or a hard and irregular liver. In these cases one can employ diagnostic methods which address the problem directly.

In many patients, however, the clinical picture is equivocal or even misleading. The classical features of obstructive jaundice (pale stools, dark urine, pruritus, and hepatomegaly) may be seen with some parenchymal liver diseases, and in patients with proven extrahepatic obstruction there may be no jaundice, dark urine, pale stools, pruritus, or hepatomegaly. In patients with 'cholestasis' due to parenchymal liver disease, the liver function tests may be just like those found in extrahepatic obstruction. With extrahepatic obstruction, on the other hand, serum bilirubin levels range widely and aminotransferase levels are often greater than 200 IU/l (and may exceed 1000 IU/l, particularly in acute gallstone obstruction). Alkaline phosphatase levels are less than two and a half times the upper reference limit (30 KA units/dl in the old notation) in approximately 20 per cent of cases of obvious bile duct obstruction; in a small proportion of cases with biliary obstruction, alkaline phosphatase levels remain normal despite the presence of jaundice (see Chapter 5.1).

The precise diagnosis of extrahepatic biliary obstruction can only be made on the basis of 'anatomical' evidence of biliary obstruction (by ultrasonography, CT scanning, MRI, or cholangiography; see Chapters 5.5 and 23.2); without it, there must always be doubt about the appropriateness of surgical intervention, even when extrahepatic obstruction seems highly likely on clinical grounds. Ultrasound should be used first because it is cheaper, more widely available, and can be performed at the bedside.

Ultrasonography, CT scanning, and MRI may all show clear evidence of dilatation of large bile ducts and so confirm large bile-duct obstruction. They may also give clues to the cause of the obstruction (such as gallstones, a large gallbladder, or enlargement of the pancreas), but often endoscopic or percutaneous cholangiography combined with bile cytology is necessary; even then the precise diagnosis may remain in doubt, particularly in patients with a bile duct carcinoma.

Bile duct obstruction may, however, be present without obvious duct dilatation, particularly with sclerosing cholangitis or with acute obstruction due to gallstones. If the clinical picture suggests large bile-duct disease (for example repeated attacks of upper abdominal pain, episodes of cholangitis, gallbladder stones, or the presence of ulcerative colitis), endoscopic cholangiography should be employed to delineate the biliary tree. This allows non-surgical management of gallstones within the ducts. If it fails to display the ducts, percutaneous cholangiography should be performed.

Even when the bile ducts are not involved, ultrasound, CT scanning (particularly with enhancement), and MRI are valuable diagnostic aids, because they also provide information about other hepatobiliary disorders (Chapter 5.5). Ultrasound examination and/or CT scanning are useful methods of confirming clinical findings such as ascites, a large and/or irregular liver, space-occupying lesions, and splenomegaly. Furthermore, some conditions (and often more than one) can be diagnosed with confidence on the basis of ultrasound, an enhanced CT scan, and/or MRI (for example fatty liver; cirrhosis, especially haemochromatosis; portal or hepatic venous block; and lesions such as polycystic disease, haemangioma, or hydatid disease). These tests, which are non-invasive, are therefore particularly valuable first-line procedures when there is no clue to the nature of the problem. Nuclear medicine studies may also be helpful in some patients (Chapter 5.6).

When ultrasound and/or CT scanning give no clues to the nature of the underlying disease, or when they simply provide evidence suggesting diffuse parenchymal liver disease, such as fatty liver, it is necessary to perform further diagnostic investigations. Before embarking on percutaneous liver biopsy it is sensible to perform other non-invasive tests which may be useful in differential diagnosis (Table 3). As pointed out above it is worth requesting some of these tests routinely, not only because they help in the diagnosis of liver disease, but because they may give information of general clinical importance and the results may prove useful in subsequent management. Furthermore, in hospital inpatients a diagnostic search should not be strictly sequential (considering one condition at a time), because the cost of delay in diagnosis, particularly in terms of the length of hospital stay, has to be set against the much smaller cost of the 'extra' tests.

If the bile ducts are not dilated and the specific tests are unhelpful, liver biopsy often suggests the nature of the underlying liver disease, such as acute or chronic hepatitis, cirrhosis, biliary tract disease, venous outflow block, or granulomatous disease. It may also give important clues to the aetiology in patients with diseases such as haemochromatosis, α_1-antitrypsin deficiency, amyloidosis, and infections with the hepatitis B and δ-viruses; special stains or electron microscopy may be needed. Full details of these various diseases are to be found in other chapters.

Patients with intrahepatic cholestasis often present a difficult diagnostic problem (Chapter 23.1); occasionally no precise classification of the disorder is possible even after a rigorous diagnostic evaluation.

Fatty liver

One of the commonest diagnostic problems in developed countries is that of fatty liver. Although it may present as palpable hepatomegaly, patients with fatty liver are usually detected when liver function tests (often done routinely) are found to be abnormal, or when fatty liver is suggested by ultrasonography or CT scanning done for the investigation of other clinical problems (especially pain or discomfort in the right upper quadrant).

Both forms of imaging have a relatively high specificity for fatty liver (a relatively low number of false positives) when there is diffuse involvement of the liver, but sensitivity is relatively poor, particularly when the fat content assessed histologically is less than 10 per cent (Hultcrantz, JIntMed, 1993; 233:7). Another major problem is that fatty liver may not be homogeneous, and focal areas of fat or fat sparing on CT scanning may cause confusion with other space-occupying lesions (see Chapter 5.5).

On biochemical testing, the usual abnormalities found are either an isolated increase of alanine aminotransferase or γ-glutamyl transferase, a combination of these results, or an increase of both alanine and aspartate aminotransferase activities (alanine aminotransferase having the higher value), usually with an increased γ-glutamyl transferase. The alanine aminotransferase is usually below 150 IU/l, but rarely both aminotransferases may be much higher (up to 500 IU/l) in patients who appear to have no cause for liver disease other than severe fatty liver. Hyperbilirubinaemia is rarely present; there is sometimes a modest increase in alkaline phosphatase (Golik, IntJObes, 1991; 15:797). There may also be an increased serum ferritin (Bacon, Gastro, 1994; 107:1103).

The finding of such biochemical changes is one of the major reasons for referral to a liver unit. The underlying liver disorder is usually fatty liver (Hulcrantz, ScaJGastr, 1986; 21:109), although hepatitis C and drug-induced damage may cause similar test results. In developed countries, obesity is the commonest cause of fatty liver (Van Ness, AnnIntMed, 1989; 111:473), which may also be associated with alcoholism, diabetes mellitus, and hypertriglyceridaemia. Obesity is also the commonest cause of these biochemical changes (Nomura, IntJObes, 1986; 10:349; Friedman, AnnIntMed, 1987; 107:137; Robinson, AnnClinBioch, 1989; 26:393), although when aspartate aminotransferase activity exceeds that of alanine aminotransferase, alcoholic liver disease is more likely (Van Ness, AnnIntMed, 1989; 111:473).

Unfortunately, as a result of the unwarranted emphasis which has been placed on γ-glutamyl transferase as a marker of alcohol abuse (Chapter 5.1), many doctors assume that an elevated γ-glutamyl transferase, often associated with high aminotransferases, indicates that a patient is drinking too much! This often causes unnecessary distress to patients. Although levels of this enzyme may be a little higher in patients drinking large amounts of alcohol (Robinson, AnnClinBioch, 1989; 26:393), it seems clear that this is of little diagnostic value in individual cases, given the effect of obesity on levels of this enzyme (Nilssen, AmJEpid, 1990; 132:318). A high MCV may be a better indicator of alcohol abuse in this situation.

Elevation of aminotransferases (alanine more than aspartate aminotransferase) and γ-glutamyl transferase, and fatty liver, are found in patients with diabetes mellitus (Stone, SemLivDis, 1988; 5:8) and with hyperlipidaemia, particularly hypertriglyceridaemia, occurring in about 50 per cent of patients seen in one large lipid clinic (Assy et al., personal communication). These abnormalities are more common in maturity-onset diabetes, and so the fatty liver may be related to the degree of obesity. The hypertriglyceridaemia is usually severe or a mixed hyperlipidaemia (Assy et al., personal communication).

The association of fatty liver with hypertriglyceridaemia may cause further diagnostic confusion with respect to alcohol, as alcohol abuse may also cause hypertriglyceridaemia with a type IV phenotype (i.e. a high level of very low density lipoprotein; see Chapter 2.12). In subjects with a predisposition to hyperlipidaemia, even a modest intake of alcohol may produce a striking increase in fasting triglycerides, and sometimes a secondary rise in cholesterol.

The prognosis for the vast majority of patients with non-alcoholic fatty liver appears excellent (Teil, Hepatol, 1995; 22:1714). The outlook is also good for those with alcoholic fatty liver, although some go on to develop more serious forms of alcoholic liver disease; it is not clear whether fatty liver plays a pathogenetic role in this process, or whether alcoholic hepatitis and cirrhosis develop independently.

Because patients who are obese, diabetic, or hyperlipidaemic with a modest increase of aminotransferase(s) and/or γ-glutamyl transferase are likely to have a fatty liver, invasive methods of investigation are probably unjustified, if chronic viral hepatitis or drug-induced liver damage can be ruled out. Patients who are obese should be advised to lose weight, diabetes should be strictly controlled, and hyperlipidaemia should be treated.

The diagnosis of fatty liver may be supported by ultrasound or CT scanning, but this does not exclude the simultaneous presence of cirrhosis, and fat is also found in patients with chronic hepatitis C. Liver biopsy should be considered in non-obese patients, and also if the level of aspartate aminotransferase is clearly higher than alanine aminotransferase (particularly in alcoholics), other liver function tests are clearly abnormal, or other clinical features (spleno-megaly, varices) suggest the possibility of cirrhosis—because fatty liver is sometimes associated with steatohepatitis and cirrhosis (Adler, AmJMed, 1979; 67:811; Ludwig, MayoClinProc, 1980; 55: 434; Powell, Hepatol, 1990; 11:74). Ursodeoxycholic acid therapy may be of benefit in the management of non-alcoholic steatohepatitis (Laurin, Hepatol, 1996; 23:1464).

Space-occupying lesions of the liver (and infiltrations)

The presence of one or more space-occupying lesions should ob-viously be suspected in patients with large, irregular livers. They should also be suspected, in the absence of hepatomegaly, if there are abnormal liver function tests such as a high alkaline phosphatase or γ-glutamyl transferase for which there is no other explanation. Space-occupying lesions can usually be detected by ultrasound (the best initial technique), CT scanning, MRI, or by nuclear medicine techniques, although some are undetectable by more than one of these methods (Chapters 5.5 and 5.6). If a space-occupying lesion is found, its nature should be established by the use of other investigations, such as liver biopsy, specialized CT scanning or MRI, angiography or cholangiography, or by aspiration of fluid for examination (including cytology).

Space-occupying lesions are sometimes present without hep-atomegaly or abnormal liver function tests. They may be found accidentally when imaging techniques are used to investigate con-ditions which are apparently unrelated to the liver or biliary tree, or during the investigation of unrelated hepatobiliary disorders. Early detection of some space-occupying lesions may be of therapeutic value (for example with small resectable tumours) but many benign lesions, such as haemangiomas, are also found, and when there is doubt about the diagnosis they require further work-up, preferably using relatively non-invasive techniques. The investigation of space-occupying lesions is best carried out in specialized centres, with experience in the performance and interpretation of the various diagnostic procedures that may be needed (Chapter 5.5).

Infiltration of the liver by abnormal cells (as in Gaucher's disease, lymphomas and leukaemias, histiocytosis X, and leishmaniasis), or by extracellular material (such as amyloid), may cause palpable hepatomegaly due to a 'space-occupying lesion' at a microscopic level. The diagnosis of the hepatic lesion is usually made by liver biopsy, but in many cases the correct answer comes only if the biopsy is examined by an experienced hepatic histopathologist and with the use of special stains. In some of these conditions the spleen may also be large, and a diagnosis may then be made by aspiration or biopsy of the spleen, but this is a more dangerous procedure than liver biopsy.

Vascular disease

Primary disorders of the hepatic vasculature are relatively rare (see Section 21). Hepatic and/or portal venous thrombosis may result when there is an underlying thrombotic tendency. Portal venous thrombosis may also be a complication of cirrhosis *per se*, and hepatocellular carcinoma is associated with thrombosis of portal and hepatic veins. Indeed, when features suggesting either hepatic or portal venous obstruction appear in a patient known to have cirrhosis (such as further enlargement of the liver or spleen, or the sudden onset of gastrointestinal bleeding or ascites), hepatocellar carcinoma should be suspected.

The diagnosis of these conditions is often missed because they are not considered; a high index of suspicion is required, and this justifies their separate inclusion in a diagnostic classification.

Extrahepatic portal venous obstruction usually presents with features of portal hypertension. Often the diagnosis is made after oesophageal varices are found at endoscopy for gastrointestinal bleeding. Splenomegaly may be the only sign. Because umbilical collaterals have their origin in the left branch of the portal vein, and appear only when the pressure at this site is elevated (see Section 4), abdominal wall collaterals are not visible in this condition, unless previous abdominal surgery has caused adhesions between viscera and the abdominal wall incisions; collateral vessels may then be seen emerging via the resulting scars. Liver function tests are usually normal in the absence of associated liver disease, although there is often a small and unexplained increase in the prothrombin time. Liver biopsy is usually unhelpful, although it may allow iden-tification of cirrhosis, hepatocellular carcinoma, or another disorder related to the extrahepatic block.

Confirmation of portal vein block requires specialized imaging techniques (see Chapter 5.5). It can be detected by Doppler ultra-sound, enhanced CT scanning, or MRI. However, for a definitive diagnosis, and for the diagnosis of other thromboses in the portal circulation such as splenic vein thrombosis, it may be necessary to display the block by splanchnic arteriography, or in some cases by splenic portography.

Hepatic vein block (Chapter 21.3) frequently presents with the sudden onset of ascites and hepatomegaly, although these are not always present. Often an initial diagnosis of cirrhosis is made, the correct diagnosis of hepatic outflow obstruction being made on a subsequent liver biopsy, although it should be made clinically if there are signs of inferior vena caval obstruction, for example marked ankle oedema, and typical abdominal wall collaterals (see Section 4) which may result either from an associated thrombosis of the inferior vena cava, or from external pressure on this vein from enlargement of the caudate lobe—a common finding when there is obstruction of the hepatic veins.

Strong support for the diagnosis may come from specialized imaging techniques, such as Doppler ultrasound, enhanced CT scanning, or MRI; the definitive diagnosis is usually made on the basis of hepatic venography (see Chapters 5.5 and 21.3).

Primary disorders of the hepatic arterial supply are rare (Chapter 21.1) except after liver transplantation. Polyarteritis nodosa affects the hepatic arteries, but clinical features suggesting hepatic involvement are rarely found, except when it is associated with hepatitis B; the liver is often found to be involved at autopsy. There may be aneurysms, which can rupture, and lesions of hepatic infarction. Patients may have features suggesting a connective tissue disorder (see Chapter 24.7), with fever and a polymorpholeucocytosis. The only abnormality of liver function tests may be an elevation of the alkaline phosphatase (Cowan, PostgradMedJ, 1977; 53:89), but polyarteritis may be suggested on a liver biopsy by the finding of an inflammatory angiitis in hepatic vessels.

Hepatobiliary involvement in serious illness without obvious cause

Patients sometimes have an illness in which the severity of the clinical features (such as prolonged fever, profound malaise, weakness, tachycardia, hypotension, weight loss, and/or mental confusion) causes great concern, and for which there is no obvious cause. It is then customary to perform a wide-ranging series of investigations in the hope that a diagnostic clue will be found. In these circumstances, abnormalities of liver function tests are often present.

The three major causes of such illnesses are infection, inflammation (as in the connective tissue disorders), and neoplasia. In all three there may be anaemia (of chronic disease), a high erythrocyte sedimentation rate, a high platelet count, and a high serum ferritin.

Infections

Some infectious diseases appear to cause abnormalities of liver function without direct involvement of the liver by the organism; the hepatic effects of these systemic infections are probably due to the effect of the toxins they produce, which may stimulate the release of cytokines. There is good evidence to suggest that other systemic infections invade the liver and produce their effects directly. The diagnosis of these conditions depends either on isolation of the organism or on the results of appropriate serological tests. If a common organism is not identified quickly from blood, urine, or other cultures, it is sensible to review a list of the infectious agents which are possible causes; these are presented in detail in Section 13.

The liver and/or biliary tract may also be the main site of an infection, for example a hepatic abscess, cholangitis, or infections of the gallbladder, which may present with fever, rigors, and other sytemic manifestations. If, as is often the case, the underlying cause is not apparent on clinical grounds (although organisms may sometimes be isolated from the blood), a diagnosis may be made with ultrasound, CT scanning, or MRI. Sometimes initial attempts at imaging prove fruitless or unconvincing, and repeated examinations may be necessary. When cholangitis is a likely cause of severe illness, cholangiography should be performed by the endoscopic route; this allows nasobiliary drainage of an obstructed biliary tree, and often an obstructing gallstone can be removed. Direct puncture of the liver in a patient with cholangitis, for percutaneous cholangiography and drainage (or for biopsy!), may cause shock.

Inflammation

The connective tissue disorders often cause difficulties in diagnosis, and in some of them abnormalities of liver function tests are found at some time during the course. In muscle diseases such as polymyositis both the aspartate and alanine aminotransferases may be strikingly elevated in the absence of liver disease; the finding of a marked increase in creatine kinase may suggest the correct diagnosis. The hepatological features of the connective tissue disorders are discussed in Chapter 24.9.

Malignancy

Malignancies of various organs are a frequent cause of puzzling clinical presentations. When there is a primary tumour of the liver or biliary tract, or when there are secondary deposits in the liver, liver function tests are often abnormal (particularly alkaline phosphatase and γ-glutamyl transferase), but abnormal liver function tests may also be found in association with tumours without direct involvement of the liver (for example Stauffer's syndrome with hypernephroma; Chapter 24.4).

Primary or secondary tumours of the liver are usually detectable by ultrasound examination or by the use of enhanced CT scanning or MRI. Each of these methods may fail to demonstrate a tumour mass(es); more than one method may be required, or it may be necessary to repeat them after an interval. Gallium scanning is a useful technique for detecting tumours and abscesses which may be undetectable by the other methods used.

It may also be difficult to demonstrate tumours outside the liver. CT scanning and MRI are of great value for this purpose. Bone tumours or metastases may show up on bone scans, and gallium scanning can often detect lesions in bone and other sites.

Patients in intensive care units often have abnormal liver function tests even in the absence of a primary hepatobiliary disorder. In 100 such patients severe infections, including bacteraemia, were the cause in about two-thirds of them; the postoperative or posttraumatic state, prolonged shock, severe gastrointestinal complications, and myocardial pump failure may either have been contributory factors or may have been causally related in some patients. Many also had renal and/or pulmonary failure and haematological complications (Kleinberger, LebMagDarm, 1985; 15:175). Blood transfusions for these conditions often cause a disproportionate elevation of the serum bilirubin.

In sick patients with abnormal liver function tests one should always consider the possibility of drug-induced liver damage. A careful review of the drugs administered over the previous few weeks often pays dividends.

Episodes of severe hypotension, of any cause and even of relatively short duration, may cause a marked increase in serum aminotransferases (Chapter 24.1). The cause is usually obvious if the hypotension is prolonged, as in shock, but the picture may be confusing if the hypotensive episode is brief and goes unnoticed, for instance with an inadvertent overdose of a hypotensive drug. The biochemical picture may be mistaken for an acute hepatitis, but if the patient recovers quickly from the hypotensive episode the aminotransferases fall rapidly to normal.

Sudden deterioration in patients with liver or biliary tract disease

Patients with pre-existing liver disease may, of course, suffer from other, unrelated diseases. Patients with cirrhosis are particularly prone to develop complications such as ascites, hepatic encephalopathy, and gastrointestinal bleeding from varices or from congestive gastropathy; these may occur individually or in combination. Patients with liver disease are also more susceptible to infections (see Chapter 25.11); bacteraemia is common, as is spontaneous bacterial peritonitis in those with ascites.

Acute deterioration, over a period of minutes or hours, and for no obvious cause, is usually due to bacteraemia or to gastrointestinal bleeding. Both conditions may cause tachycardia, hypotension, tachypnoea, mild fever and/or confusion, and impaired renal function with oliguria. Bleeding may become obvious with the appearance of haematemesis or melaena, but volume expansion may be necessary before it is evident in order to maintain the blood pressure. The white cell count may be lower than one would expect in a bacterial infection, due to hypersplenism. Cultures should be taken of blood, urine, ascites, and of intravenous drip lines and insertion sites, and the patient should be started on an appropriate antibiotic. The response to an antibiotic is the best 'diagnostic test' in many cases; although cultures may confirm the diagnosis, they are often negative. The appearance of new petechiae suggests bacteraemia as a cause, and there may be associated intravascular coagulation, which can be confirmed by the finding of fibrin degradation products.

More gradual deterioration, over days or weeks, may also result from infections such as spontaneous bacterial peritonitis or urinary infections; a chest radiograph may help in those who have recently vomited, have had surgery or an upper gastrointestinal endoscopy, or have been unconscious for some time. A gradual deterioration is also seen when the development of hepatocellular carcinoma results in a rapid worsening of hepatic function; the reason is rarely clear. Patients may deteriorate as a result of 'dehydration', often associated with vigorous diuretic therapy, or the failure to replace fluids lost in diarrhoea or drainage tubes. There may be a low intravascular volume, and loss of skin turgor in some parts of the body, even in the presence of ascites and dependent oedema.

The onset of confusion or coma may be due to hepatic encephalopathy, or to a fall in blood pressure due to haemorrhage or bacteraemia. However, in patients with liver disease, especially cirrhotics, impairment of cerebral function may also be due to drugs or alcohol, renal failure, hypoglycaemia (rarely), a subdural haemorrhage or a cerebral contusion (often due to only mild trauma, particularly in alcoholics), or an intracerebral haemorrhage (associated with a very low platelet count).

In patients with known biliary tract disease the most common cause of acute deterioration is bacteraemia associated with cholangitis, and a patient may become desperately ill within hours. Evidence of dilated ducts should be sought by ultrasound, CT scanning, or MRI, but their absence does not exclude bile duct infection due to stones or to sclerosing cholangitis.

A more prolonged deterioration in these patients may be seen due to the development of hepatic abscesses, which can usually be detected by imaging, or of a cholangiocarcinoma, which is often very difficult to identify by ultrasound, CT scanning, MRI, or even by cholangiography, especially if the ducts are already distorted by sclerosing cholangitis.

In some patients with liver disease there may be an exacerbation of jaundice without other features to suggest hepatic decompensation. This is common following blood transfusion, due to the increased bilirubin load, but it may also be due to the use of drugs which interfere with the excretion of bilirubin, and a detailed drug history should be taken.

6

Cirrhosis

6.1 Cellular and molecular pathobiology, pharmacological intervention, and biochemical assessment of liver fibrosis

A. M. Gressner and D. Schuppan

Introduction

According to a recommendation of a WHO expert group, 'cirrhosis of the liver is defined as a diffuse process characterized by fibrosis and the conversion of normal liver architecture into structurally abnormal nodules' (Anthony, JClinPath, 1978; 31: 395). Fibrosis, a hallmark of cirrhosis was defined 'as the presence of excess collagen due to new fibre formation' (Anthony, JClinPath, 1978; 31:395) but this description of fibrosis requires a redefinition on the basis of the detailed knowledge of the complex structure of the liver extracellular matrix under normal conditions and its perturbation under pathologic conditions (see Chapter 2.15).

Liver cirrhosis represents the terminal stage of a variety of chronic active liver diseases based on different aetiologies, among which nutritive-toxic (for example, alcoholic hepatitis and drug-induced hepatitis) (up to 50 per cent of all cirrhotic cases), viral-immunological (autoimmune hepatitis), and parasitic injuries (schistosomal cirrhosis and fibrosis) prevail (Fig. 1). Certain rare conditions are due to inborn errors of metabolism, for example haemochromatosis, hepatolenticular degeneration (Morbus Wilson), α1-proteinase inhibitor deficiency, Byler's disease (severe intrahepatic cholestasis with progressive liver cell damage), hereditary fructose intolerance, galactosaemia, and others. It should be noted that fibrosis might also exist in the absence of developing cirrhosis, for example in cases of congenital hepatic fibrosis, thrombocytopenic purpura, myeloid metaplasia, in diabetes, and after renal transplantation (Gressner, EurJClinChemClinBioch 1991; 29:293).

Cirrhosis is an important cause of long-lasting morbidity and death with a considerable social–economical impact.[1] In the USA it is the fourth leading cause of death in individuals under the age of 65 years and the annual costs of health care for cirrhosis are estimated to exceed $4 billion.[2] In other countries the death rates from cirrhosis might be even higher, as documented in a World Health Organization (**WHO**) report in 1985 which selected data from 20 reporting countries.[3]

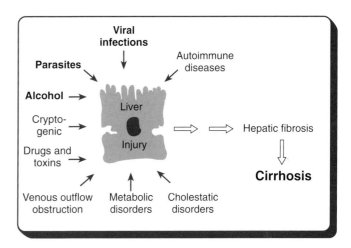

Fig. 1. Synopsis of various aetiologies of liver (cell) injury, fibrosis, and cirrhosis.

Principal pathobiochemical reactions in fibrogenesis

Fibrotic matrix changes in a chronically damaged liver are brought about by a loss of homeostatic mechanisms controlling matrix formation and deposition (fibrogenesis) and matrix degradation and removal (fibrolysis) leading to excessive connective tissue deposition (fibrosis). The data available indicate that stimulated matrix production in a chronically damaged liver is the main mechanism of exaggerated matrix accumulation. The inhibition of matrix degradation might support the accumulation of certain matrix molecules and contributes to changes in the distribution profile of the collagenous and non-collagenous components.

The pathogenesis of liver fibrosis has gained a model character for organ fibrosis in general, exemplifying the principal pathways and regulatory mechanisms along which tissue injury is converted to a strong accumulation and histologic redistribution of connective tissue.[4] The essential, extensively interrelated pathobiochemical

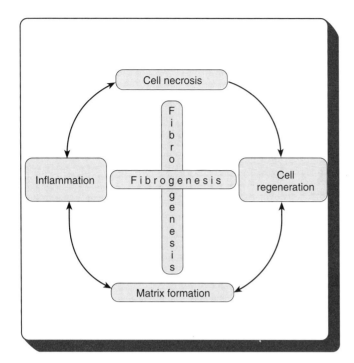

Fig. 2. The partial reactions of fibrogenesis and their interrelations ('fibrogenic circle').

reactions (Fig. 2) are considered to be (1) parenchymal cell injury, likely to be (with some exceptions) the initiating and perpetuating event followed by (2) inflammation, (3) hepatocellular regeneration, (4) extracellular matrix production, and (5) disorganization of the lobular architecture generating pseudolobules throughout the whole of the liver and a disturbed angioarchitecture (shunts). Fibrosis comprises all the complexity of the changes of the liver extracellular matrix including the following.

(1) A 3- to 10-fold increase of most of the extracellular matrix molecules.
(2) A disproportionate elevation of certain subspecies of individual extracellular matrix molecules (types of collagens, proteoglycans, hyaluronan, and structural glycoproteins).
(3) Subtle changes in the microcomposition of specific types of extracellular matrix molecules, for example concerning the degree of hydroxylation of collagen α-chains and the number, length, and degree of sulphation (charge density) of glycosaminoglycans occupying the core proteins of proteoglycans.
(4) The topographic redistribution of the extracellular matrix in injured liver leading to an early and preponderant subendothelial deposition of connective tissue in the space of Disse (perisinusoidal fibrosis) and to other forms of periportal, bridging, diffuse, or focal fibrosis.

It is likely that perisinusoidal fibrosis combined with the development of a subendothelial basement membrane (Hahn, Gut, 1980; 21:63) resulting in 'capillarization of the sinusoids' (Schaffner, Gastro, 1963; 44:239) contributes a major part to the clinical consequences of fibrosis since it hinders, by the development of diffusion barriers, the systemic functions of hepatocytes and non-parenchymal cells and/or interferes with the portal haemodynamics

due to stenosis of the intrasinusoidal blood flow and other disturbances of the hepatic microcirculation (Fig. 3). A vicious circle might develop from malnourished hepatocytes deprived of a sufficient supply with oxygen and nutrients leading to progredient hepatocellular damage (necrosis) and thereby to persistence of the initiating event. Unlike many other tissues, in the liver the excessive fibrogenic response is unnecessary for complete recovery of the damaged organ (Thompson, JPath, 1980; 130:65) since the high regenerative capacity of hepatocytes[5] can substitute in a complete and rapid way for the (necrotic) loss of parenchyma.

Cellular sources of extracellular matrix compounds
Non-parenchymal liver cells

The liver is composed of various epithelial and mesenchymal cell types having a quite different origin, lobular localization, and functions (Fig. 4). The principal question concerns the identification of the cellular sources of individual matrix components by means of *in situ* and *in vitro* techniques (metabolic tracer studies in cultured cells, immunocytochemistry, Northern blot analyses, and gene and mRNA amplification methods). The advantages and disadvantages of the various methods have been reviewed[6] and are in part responsible for some still existing controversies and discrepancies. Considerable progress has been made in recent years with the refinement of techniques for the isolation, culture, and assessment of the purity of the parenchymal and non-parenchymal liver cells from human and animal origin (Alpini, Hepatol, 1994; 20:494; Braet, LabInvest, 1994; 70:944), which contributes a major part to the validity of results obtained nowadays in cell culture studies. It is now well-established that perisinusoidal hepatic stellate cells (retinoid-storing cells, fat storing cells, hepatic lipocytes, parasinusoidal cells, and Ito cells), which are localized in the space of Disse (perisinusoidal space) and have the perikaryon embedded in recesses between adjacent hepatocytes with cellular extensions embracing the endothelial cell layer (Fig. 5), are the most important connective-tissue producing (precursor) cell type in the injured liver[6–11] (Geerts, JElectronMicroscTech, 1990; 14:247; Rockey, CellMotilCytoskel, 1992; 22:227). Normally, these cells have a low mitotic activity and are present in a ratio of 3.6:6 cells per 100 hepatocytes (Ito cell index). They are engaged in the storage and metabolism of retinoids[12] (Hendriks, Hepatol, 1987; 7:1368) and are related to pericytes, for example kidney mesangial cells (Pinzani, JCV, 1992; 90:642). Retinoid-storing cells contain, in large triacylglycerol-rich droplets, approximately 50 times more retinol (30 nmol total retinol per 10^6 cells) than parenchymal liver cells (0.5–0.8 nmol total retinol per 10^6 cells). Since endothelial cells (3 per cent) and Kupffer cells (1 per cent) contain only negligible amounts of retinol, it is calculated that in the whole liver 80 to 90 per cent of total retinol is present in this cell type.[12] There are indications of the intralobular heterogeneity of stellate cells as evidenced by a periportal/perivenous gradient of desmin expression, the vitamin A content, the size of the lipid droplets, and arborization of the dendritic processus (Wake, CellTissRes, 1993; 273:227; Ballardini, Hepatol, 1994; 19:440). In addition, the functional heterogeneity of stellate cells in culture has been documented

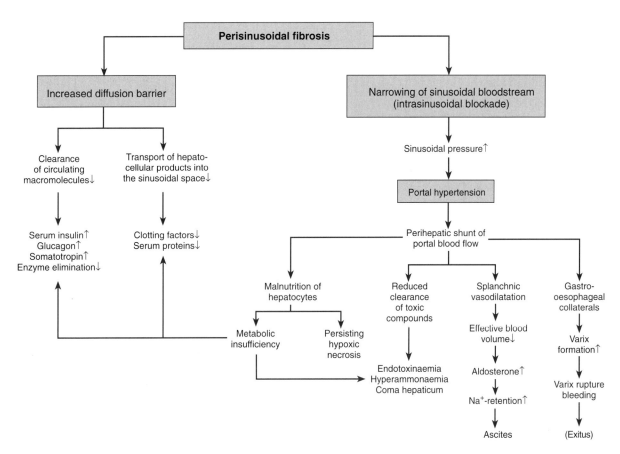

Fig. 3. Major functional consequences of connective tissue deposition in the perisinusoidal space of Disse (perisinusoidal fibrosis).

which might be important for their differential sensitivity to fibrogenic stimuli (Greenwel, LabInvest, 1991; 65:644; Ramm, AmJ-Physiolgastro, 1995; 32:G532; see below). Pathogenetically most relevant is the ability of hepatic stellate cells to be 'activated' *in situ* under necroinflammatory stimuli (Mak, Gastro, 1984; 87:188; Mak, Hepatol, 1988; 8:1027) and spontaneously during culture on plastic surfaces (Geerts, JHepatol, 1989; 9:59; Gressner, ProcSocExpBiolMed, 1991; 196:307). The process of activation, which is recognized as the key pathogenetic event in the initiation of fibrogenesis[11,13,14] (Bissell, Gastro, 1992; 102:180), includes the following.

(1) Stimulation of proliferation (Geerts, Hepatol, 1991; 13:1193).
(2) Phenotypic transformation (via so-called transitional cells) from the retinoid-'storing' to the 'synthetic' phenotype (myofibroblast) containing a reduced volume density of vitamin A-filled lipid droplets, a hypertrophied endoplasmic reticulum, and abundant desmin (only in rat but not in human liver), gelsolin, and smooth muscle α-actin filaments (Ballardini, VirchArchCP, 1988; 56:45; Ramadori, VirchArchCP, 1990; 59:349) but displaying reduced expression of glial fibrillary acidic protein (Fig. 6).
(3) Gene expression, synthesis, and secretion of a wide spectrum of matrix proteins, glycoconjugates, and glycosaminoglycans (hyaluronan) (Meyer, Hepatol, 1992; 16:204).
(4) Acquisition of contractility, for example in response to endothelin-1, angiotensin II, thrombin, and eicosanoids, suggesting vasoregulatory functions of activated hepatic stellate

cells in injured liver (Pinzani, JCI, 1992; 90:642; Housset, PNAS, 1993; 90:9266; Kawada, EurJBioch, 1993; 213:815; Pinzani, Gastro, 1996; 110:534).

Besides the expression of extracellular matrix components such as collagens (Friedman, PNAS, 1985; 82:8681), proteoglycans[15] (Schäfer, Hepatol, 1987; 7:680; Arenson, Gastro, 1988; 95:441, plasma and cellular fibronectin (Ramadori, Gastro, 1989; 97:163; Ramadori, Gastro, 1992; 103:1313), laminin (Maher, Hepatol, 1994; 19:764), nidogen/entactin (Schwoegler, LabInvest, 1994; 70:525), tenascin (van Eyken, Hepatol, 1992; 15:909), undulin (Casini, BBResComm, 1994; 199:1019), and hyaluronan (Gressner, BBRes-Comm, 1988; 151:222) (Table 1), transformed hepatic stellate cells (myofibroblasts) are able to synthesize a number of proinflammatory and fibrogenic cytokines, chemokines and growth factors, for example transforming growth factor (**TGF**)-α and -β, fibroblast growth factor (**FGF**), monocyte chemotactic peptide (**MCP**)-1, platelet activating factor (**PAF**), endothelin (**ET**)-1, insulin-like growth factor (**IGF**)-1, interleukin (**IL**)-6, and others (Fig. 7). In addition, activated hepatic stellate cells secrete the tissue inhibitor of metalloproteinases (**TIMP**)-1 providing the possibility of slowing down the degradation of certain types of newly formed collagens[16, 17] (Iredale, JCI, 1992; 90:282). During transformation to myofibroblasts, cultured hepatic stellate cells continuously increase the synthesis and secretion of various matrix proteins[15] (Friedman, PNAS, 1985; 82:8681; Geerts, JHepatol, 1989; 9:59; Gressner, ProcSocExpBiolMed, 1991; 196:307), change the expression of growth factors, chemokines, and cytokines (Pinzani, Endocrinol,

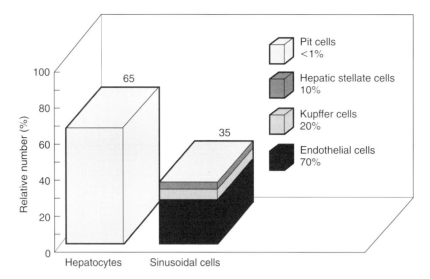

Fig. 4. Quantitative distribution of parenchymal (hepatocytes) and resident non-parenchymal (sinusoidal) cells in a normal liver.

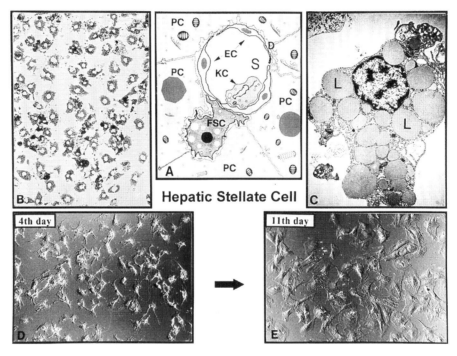

Fig. 5. (A) Schematic presentation of the localization of hepatic stellate cells (or fat-storing cells) in the tissue. The cell body is located in recesses between adjacent parenchymal cells in the perisinusoidal space of the liver. Two types of dendritic processes of stellate cells, that is perisinusoidal (subendothelial) and interhepatocellular extensions are distinguished. (B) Light microscopic appearance of lipid-laden retinoid-storing cells in early culture. (C) Electron micrograph of a retinoid-storing cell having numerous lipid droplets indenting the nucleus. The total retinol is stored in triacylglycerol-filled droplets of which two types can be discerned: type I has a limiting membrane between the cytosol and the vitamin A-containing triacylglycerol content, while type II is devoid of a limiting membrane. Differential interference contrast micrographs of (D) early (day 4) (mainly untransformed) and (E) late (day 11) (transformed) cultures of hepatic stellate cells. S, sinusoid; EC, endothelial cells; KC, Kupffer cell; FSC = HSC, hepatic stellate cells; PC, parenchymal liver cells; D, space of Disse; L, lipid droplets.

1990; 127:2343; Bachem, JCI, 1992; 89:19; Pinzani, AmJPhysiol, 1992; 262:C876; Marra, JCellPhysiol, 1996; 166:537; Pinzani, Gastro, 1996; 110:534), and modulate the expression of many cytokine receptors (Heldin, ExpCellRes, 1991; 193:364; Bachem, JHepatol, 1993; 18:40; Friedman, JBC, 1994; 269:10551; Pinzani, Gastro, 1996; 110:534). On the other hand, the expression of hepatocyte growth factor(**HGF**)/scatter factor in stellate cells is strongly downregulated during transformation to myofibroblasts (Ramadori, BBResComm, 1992; 183:739; Schirmacher, Hepatol, 1992; 15:5).

The participation of other types of non-parenchymal cells (Kupffer cells, endothelial cells, pit cells, bile duct cells, and fibroblasts) in liver extracellular matrix production has been reviewed; [6,7] the data suggest that relative to retinoid-storing cells their

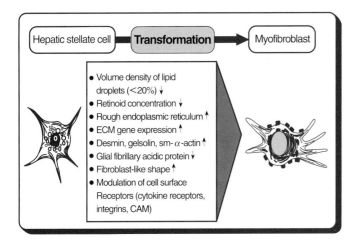

Fig. 6. Characteristic biochemical and morphological changes of activated hepatic stellate cells undergoing phenotypic transformation to myofibroblasts.

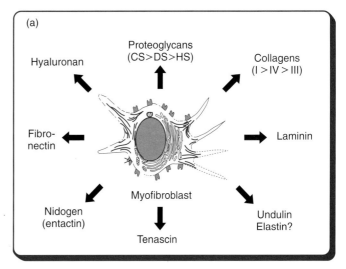

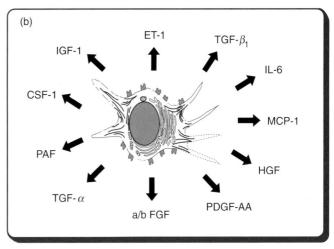

Fig. 7. Schematic presentation of (a) the extracellular matrix components and (b) the profibrogenic cytokines, chemokines, and growth factors expressed and secreted by myofibroblasts (transformed stellate cells) in culture. The data are compiled from the literature and are based on mRNA expression, immunological quantitation of the matrix components and cytokines, and the bioactivity of cytokines in the culture medium.

synthesis pattern is either restricted to certain types of extracellular matrix components, for example the synthesis of cellular fibronectin, type IV collagen, and thrombospondin by sinusoidal endothelial cells (Rieder, Hepatol, 1987; 7:856; Maher, JCI, 1990; 86:1641; Rieder, Hepatol, 1993; 18:937) and/or is only of minor magnitude[6] (Table 1). This conclusion, however, must be drawn with caution since it is based mainly on *in vitro* studies, which do not allow a simple extrapolation of quantitative data to the *in situ* function of the cells.

Parenchymal liver cells

A matter of controversy remains the potential of parenchymal liver cells (hepatocytes) to contribute to extracellular matrix production in health and disease. The experimental data obtained with a dual label method designed to measure hepatocyte-specific collagen synthesis in normal (Chojkier, JCI, 1986; 78:333) and fibrotic (Chojkier, Hepatol, 1988; 8:808) rat liver *in vivo*, Northern blotting of mRNAs from purified liver cells (Brenner, MolBiolMed, 1990; 7:105), *in situ* hybridization (Yamada, ActaPathJpn, 1989; 39:719; Brenner, MolBiolMed, 1990; 7:105) and earlier studies suggest a major role of hepatocytes in liver collagen formation but this conclusion is not supported by some other *in situ* hybridization studies which could not detect procollagen mRNAs in human

(Milani, AmJPathol, 1990; 137:59) and rat hepatocytes (Milani, Hepatol, 1989; 10:84; Milani, Gastro, 1990; 98:175; Nakatsukasa,

Table 1 Profile of matrix protein gene expression in liver cells

| Extracellular matrix protein | Hepatocytes | Hepatic stellate cells | | Endothelial cells | Kupffer cells | Bile duct epithelial cells |
		Fresh	Cultured			
Fibronectin	+	−	+ +	−	−	ND
Laminin B1	−	+	+	−	−	+
α_1(I)	(+)/ −	−	+	−	−	−
α_1(III)	(+)/ −	+	+ +	−	−	−
α_1(IV)	−	+	+	+	−	+
Decorin	−	+	+	ND	−	ND
Biglycan	−	+	+	ND	−	ND

+, present; −, absent; ND, not determined.

JCI, 1990; 85:1833) of normal and diseased livers. Another study also failed to measure significant collagen synthesis in the hepatocytes of fibrotic rat livers (Ogata, Hepatol, 1991; 14:361) using an approach similar to previous authors (Chojkier, JCI, 1986; 78:333; Chojkier, Hepatol, 1988; 8:808). The important question about the role of hepatocytes in collagen production needs further experimental clarification before a definite answer can be given. The hepatocytes appear to contribute only a minor (if any) fraction to extracellular matrix proteoglycan production since parenchymal cells, freshly isolated from normal and chronically injured livers, synthesize *in vitro* almost exclusively heparan sulphate proteoglycans (syndecan and glypican) which reside mainly intra- and pericellularly (Meyer, Liver, 1990; 10:94; Weiner, CellTissRes, 1996; 285:11). Their synthesis rate is reduced in cells from fibrotic livers (Meyer, Liver, 1990; 10:94). Matrix proteoglycans such as decorin and biglycan are not expressed in hepatocytes in culture or *in situ* (Meyer, Hepatol, 1992; 16:204; Krull, Hepatol, 1993; 18:581). Besides plasma fibronectin, cultured rat hepatocytes were identified to synthesize cellular fibronectin (Odenthal, ExpCellRes, 1992; 203:289). Together with the endothelial cells (Rieder, Hepatol, 1987; 7:856) and stellate cells (Ramadori, Gastro, 1989; 97:163; Ramadori, Gastro, 1992; 103:1313) parenchymal liver cells might be an important source of accumulating cellular fibronectin in fibrotic matrix (Odenthal, BBActa, 1993; 1181:266).

Cellular crosstalk mediating hepatic stellate cell activation via cytokines and growth factors

Extensive efforts have been made to clarify the mechanism of fibrogenesis by identifying the nature and origin of fibrogenic mediators which stimulate hepatic stellate cell activation and, hence, the amplification of extracellular matrix production in diseased livers.[9,13] (Rosenbaum, JHepatol, 1995; 22:65) Pathogenetically relevant cellular reactions contributing to stellate cell activation in damaged liver tissue include the following.

(1) Expansion of the pool of macrophages due to local proliferation of Kupffer cells and an influx of monocytes (Geerts, JHepatol, 1988; 6:50), cellular activation, and release of numerous fibrogenic mediators.
(2) Adhesion, influx, and disintegration of platelets (Ogawa, AmJPathol, 1985; 119:158) and release of growth factors at the site of injury (Bachem, JClinChemClinBioch, 1989; 27:555).
(3) Injury of the sinusoidal endothelial cells and release of fibrogenic mediators[18,19] (Rieder, KlinWschr, 1991; 69:387; Rosenbaum, BBResComm, 1989; 164:1099; McNeil, JCellBiol, 1989; 109:811; Feder, JLeukBiol, 1993; 53:126).
(4) Injury-dependent cessation of a hepatocyte-derived inhibitor of hepatic stellate cell proliferation (Chen, JHepatol, 1990; 11:330) and release of fibrogenic mediators by (damaged) hepatocytes (Gressner, Hepatol, 1992; 16:1250; Hoffmann, IntHepatolComm, 1994; 2:29; Gressner, Hepatol, 1995; 22:1507).

The changes in the microenvironment of the hepatic stellate cells by a greatly altered extracellular matrix and cellular composition imply that not only injured hepatocytes, but also endothelial cells, Kupffer cells, and aggregating platelets represent major effector cells, which release mediators, stimulating in a paracrine way, hepatic stellate cells and myofibroblasts. Thus, fibrogenesis is not only a cellular but a tissue phenomenon based on extensive cell–cell and cell–matrix interactions.

In addition, experimental data have been accumulated indicating autocrine stimulation of the myofibroblasts involving TGF-α, FGF, platelet-derived growth factor (**PDGF**), ET-1, and TGF-β (see below).

Paracrine stimulation of hepatic stellate cells by non-parenchymal cells

During injury the typical fenestration of the sinusoidal endothelial cells is reduced or even abolished and an incomplete subendothelial basement membrane-like structure is developed (Hahn, Gut, 1980; 21:63). In parallel with the 'capillarization of the sinusoids' (Schaffner, Gastro, 1963; 44:239), the volume of the endothelial cells increases (ballooning) and multiple intracellular vesicles suggest an enhanced phagocytosis. Endothelial cells have a function in the clearance of circulating matrix elements (Smedsrod, BiochemJ, 1990; 266:313) and, under certain conditions, synthesize and discharge several mediators including IL-1, FGF, PDGF, hydrogen peroxide, plasminogen activator inhibitor (**PAI**)-1, PAF, and MCP-1[18] (Rieder, Hepatol, 1993; 18:937; Nanji, AmJPathol, 1996; 148:739). The endothelial cells stimulate myofibroblast proliferation via PDGF and FGF, indirectly decrease matrix degradation by the synthesis of PAI-1, and, by producing PAF and MCP-1, attract inflammatory cells to the area of injury. A further important role of endothelial cells concerns their cooperation with other cell types in the activation of TGF-β (DeBleser, Hepatol, 1995; 21:1429). TGF-β is secreted by most cells in a latent form which requires cleavage of the latency-associated peptide (**LAP**) to yield active TGF-β. Only active TGF-β is able to bind to its receptors to induce a cellular response. During the incubation of myofibroblast- and Kupffer cell-conditioned media (containing latent TGF-β_1) with endothelial cells, latent TGF-β is efficiently activated. An even higher proportion of latent TGF-β is activated during the co-culture of myofibroblasts or Kupffer cells with endothelial cells. Since monocultures of myofibroblasts and Kupffer cells contain predominantly latent TGF-β, but co-cultures with endothelial cells have active TGF-β, cell–cell contact or close connection of the two different cell types is required to activate latent TGF-β. The addition of mannose-6-phosphate, whereby the IGF type II receptor is blocked, results in diminished TGF-β activation (Dennis, PNAS, 1991; 88:580). The data suggest that the binding of latent TGF-β via LAP to the mannose-6-phosphate receptor (IGF type II receptor) and plasmin or urokinase from endothelial cells are absolute requirements for TGF-β activation (DeBleser, Hepatol, 1995; 21:1429).

Media conditioned by Kupffer cells and monocytes (Gressner, JHepatol, 1987; 5:299; Zerbe, ExpMolPath, 1988; 49:87; Friedman, JCI, 1989; 84:1780; Meyer, BBResComm, 1990; 171:1122) and by myofibroblasts (Bachem, JCI, 1992; 89:19) but also platelet lysate (Bachem, JClinChemClinBioch, 1989; 27:555) can stimulate the proliferation (Zerbe, ExpMolPath, 1988; 49:87; Bachem, JClinChemClinBioch, 1989; 27:555; Friedman, JCI, 1989; 84:1780; Meyer, BBResComm, 1990; 171:1122; Bachem, JCI, 1992 89:19) and matrix synthesis (Friedman, JCI, 1989; 84:1780; Bachem, JCI,

1992; 89:19) of hepatic stellate cells and myofibroblasts. Kupffer cells and myofibroblasts promote the change of the hepatic stellate cell morphology from the 'storing' to the 'secreting' type (Friedman, JCI, 1989; 84:1780; Bachem, VirchArchCP, 1993; 63:123). Kupffer cells have broad stimulatory activity towards hepatic stellate cells, causing transformation into the activated phenotype (myofibroblast) characterized by (1) marked nuclear enlargement, cytoplasmic spreading, and apparent loss of retinoid vesicles, (2) a 3-fold enhanced protein synthesis, (3) a 2.5-fold stimulated collagen synthesis, (4) increased proliferation, and (5) responsiveness to PDGF (Friedman, JCI, 1989; 84:1780). The latter of these (resting, early cultured hepatic stellate cells are, in contrast to myofibroblasts, PDGF-receptor negative), is due to *de novo* expression of the β-type of the PDGF receptor during activation (Friedman, JCI, 1989; 84:1780). At present the factors and regulatory events underlying PDGF receptor induction are unknown but TGF-β might be responsible (Pinzani, Hepatol, 1995; 21:232). TGF-β induced a significant increase in the mitogenic effect of PDGF-BB but not of PDGF-AA and PDGF-AB, which suggests a selective action on the β-subunit of the PDGF receptor in human hepatic stellate cells (Pinzani, Hepatol, 1995; 21:232). It is proposed that this mechanism could indirectly perpetuate hepatic stellate cell proliferation by increasing the expression of PDGF-β receptors rendering the cells susceptible to this potent and ubiquitous mitogen.

TGF-β_1 is identified in Kupffer cell-conditioned media (Matsuoka, Hepatol, 1990; 11:599; Meyer, BBResComm, 1990; 171:1122). By transient acidification of the media collagen (Matsuoka, Hepatol, 1990; 11:599) and proteoglycan, the synthesis of hepatic stellate cells is enhanced but the proliferation is reduced (Meyer, BBResComm, 1990; 171:1122). These effects are neutralized completely by anti-TGF-β_1 antibodies which convert the proliferation inhibitory effect into a stimulatory action. The latter activity is suggested to be at least partially due to TGF-α (Meyer, BBResComm, 1990; 171:1122). The mRNAs of both TGFs are expressed preferentially in activated Kupffer cells (Meyer, BBResComm, 1990; 171:1122), but TGF-β_1 is secreted in an inactive, latent form and requires (proteolytic) activation before receptor binding as discussed.

In addition to TGF-β, Kupffer cells release a large number of cytokines[20,21] including TGF-α (Meyer, BBResComm, 1990; 171:1122), PDGF (Friedman, JCI, 1989; 84:1780), IL-1, IL-6 (Busam, JHepatol, 1990; 11:367), and tumour necrosis factor (**TNF**)-α (Estler, BiolChem, 1992; 373:271).

The main growth factors elaborated by and stored in the α-granules of platelets are TGF-β (Assoian, JBC, 1983; 258:7155), epidermal growth factor (**EGF**) (Oka, JCI, 1983; 72:249), PDGF, [22] and IGF-1. The following findings support the assumption that disintegrated platelets might be significantly involved in liver fibrogenesis by stimulating the growth, transformation, and extracellular matrix synthesis of hepatic stellate cells.

(1) An enhanced pool of platelets is found together with neutrophils and macrophages around necrotic areas (Ogawa, AmJPathol, 1985; 119:158).
(2) Platelets are the richest source of TGF-β and release this cytokine upon activation, adhesion, or aggregation at the site of injury into the surrounding tissue (Assoian, JBC, 1983; 258: 7155).

(3) PAF receptor antagonists attenuate hepatic injury and inflammation in rats after liver ischaemia/reperfusion (Zhou, Hepatol, 1992; 16:1236).
(4) Additional fibrogenic mediators such as PDGF, IGF-1, and EGF are discharged from α-granules following platelet activation (Oka, JCI, 1983; 72:249).

Experiments from this laboratory have shown that lysate from human platelets stimulates both the proliferation and proteoglycan synthesis of rat liver hepatic stellate cells kept in primary culture in a dose-dependent manner (Bachem, JClinChemClinBioch, 1989; 27:555).

The central role of TGF-β in liver fibrogenesis,[23] which affects matrix metabolism in a profibrogenic manner at different levels (Fig. 8), is documented by results showing that

(1) in acute CCl$_4$-induced liver injury the level of TGF-β mRNA rises strongly (Czaja, JCellBiol, 1989; 108:2477);
(2) hepatic stellate cells in culture express the TGF-β gene (Weiner, Hepatol, 1990; 11:111);
(3) TGF-β gene expression is significantly enhanced during experimental streptococcal cell wall-induced inflammation and fibrosis (Manthey, GrowthFact, 1990; 4:17) and during active fibrogenesis associated with human liver disease (Castilla, NEJM, 1991; 324:933; Annoni, JHepatol, 1992; 14:259; Llorente, JHepatol, 1996; 24:555);
(4) transgenic mice, which overexpress active TGF-β selectively in the liver, develop extensive hepatic fibrosis (Sanderson, PNAS, 1995; 92:2572).

TGF-β gene expression does not necessarily correlate with the amount of active TGF-β, because TGF-β undergoes extensive post-translational modification (activation) and the half-life of active TGF-β might be very short, since it binds efficiently to scavengers, that is α$_2$-macroglobulin[25] and the extracellular matrix components fibronectin, betaglycan (identical with type III TGF-β receptor) (Andres, JCellBiol, 1989; 109:3137), and decorin (Yamaguchi, Nature, 1990; 346:281) (Table 2). The efficiency of α$_2$-macroglobulin in binding TGF-β was demonstrated by experiments showing that the preincubation of transiently acidified media (containing active TGF-β) conditioned by myofibroblasts and Kupffer cells with α$_2$-macroglobulin results in a dose-dependent reduction of stimulated proteoglycan synthesis. This reduction is comparable to that obtained with neutralizing antibodies to TGF-β (Bachem, AnnNYAcadSci, 1994; 737:421). The reduction of active TGF-β at the site of injury, for example by the use of neutralizing antibodies, soluble TGF-β receptors, LAP, or elevation of TGF-β scavengers (α$_2$-macroglobulin or decorin), leads the way to potential future strategies for the inhibition of fibrogenesis (see below). In experimental glomerulosclerosis, fibrosis can be inhibited efficiently by anti-TGF-β, immunoglobulin (**Ig**) G (Border, Nature, 1990; 346:371) and by the TGF-β-binding proteoglycan decorin (Border, Nature, 1992; 360:361; Isaka, NatureMed, 1996; 2:418).

Paracrine stimulation of hepatic stellate cells by (damaged) parenchymal cells

Hepatocytes are closely connected with hepatic stellate cells in the tissue (Fig. 5) providing the opportunity for both soluble mediators

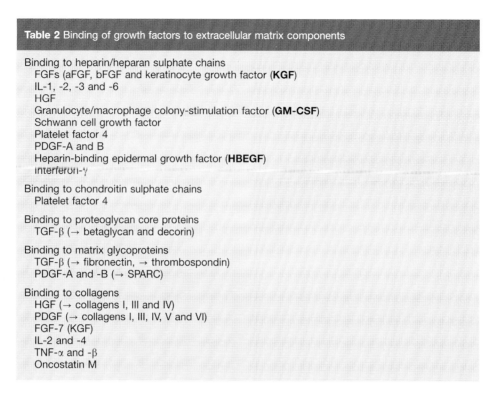

Table 2 Binding of growth factors to extracellular matrix components

Binding to heparin/heparan sulphate chains
  FGFs (aFGF, bFGF and keratinocyte growth factor (**KGF**)
  IL-1, -2, -3 and -6
  HGF
  Granulocyte/macrophage colony-stimulation factor (**GM-CSF**)
  Schwann cell growth factor
  Platelet factor 4
  PDGF-A and B
  Heparin-binding epidermal growth factor (**HBEGF**)
  Interferon-γ

Binding to chondroitin sulphate chains
  Platelet factor 4

Binding to proteoglycan core proteins
  TGF-β (→ betaglycan and decorin)

Binding to matrix glycoproteins
  TGF-β (→ fibronectin, → thrombospondin)
  PDGF-A and -B (→ SPARC)

Binding to collagens
  HGF (→ collagens I, III and IV)
  PDGF (→ collagens I, III, IV, V and VI)
  FGF-7 (KGF)
  IL-2 and -4
  TNF-α and -β
  Oncostatin M

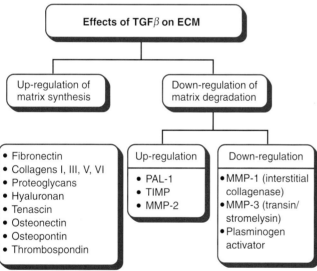

Fig. 8. Mechanisms by which active TGF-β affects extracellular matrix metabolism in a profibrogenic manner (modified from Massagué[24]).

and direct membrane contacts to be important in the mechanism of hepatic stellate cell activation. There are several observations which suggest that (injured) hepatocytes might be directly involved in the activation of stellate cells, thus forming a complementary pathway for their stimulation (Fig. 9). Since hepatocellular damage is frequently (if not necessarily) the primary event in the initiation of liver fibrogenesis, the deletion of membrane contact inhibition, the discharge of mitogenic factors from a (cytosolic) storage site ('wound hormone') (Gressner, Hepatol, 1992; 16:1250), and the loss of a putative hepatic stellate cell proliferation inhibitor normally produced by hepatocytes are potential ways in which damaged hepatocytes might contribute to hepatic stellate cell activation. Media

conditioned by primary cultures of normal rat hepatocytes are able to stimulate the proliferation of early cultured (untransformed) hepatic stellate cells (Gressner, Hepatol, 1992; 16:1250), an effect which is demonstrated in co-cultures of hepatocytes with stellate cells (Gressner, Hepatol, 1995; 22:1507; Rojkind, AmJPathol, 1995; 146:1508). An increasing number of cytokines, which are expressed and secreted by hepatocytes, is reported (Fig. 10), but their relation to the activation of stellate cells is not known. The mitogenic activity in the medium is not dependent on *de novo* synthesis; instead media of hepatocytes cultured under injurious conditions are highly active in promoting hepatic stellate cell proliferation. In fact, there is a significant positive correlation between LDH activity and the mitogenic potency of the conditioned media (Hoffmann, Int-HepatolComm, 1994; 2:29), which, however, does not promote transformation and matrix expression significantly (collagen types I and III, fibronectin, and laminin). The hepatocyte-derived mitogen(s), which is probably related to IGF-1 and IGF-binding proteins (Gressner, Hepatol, 1995; 22:1507), acts in concert (additive) with those growth factors provided by activated Kupffer cells (Gressner, JHepatol, 1993; 19:117). The injury-dependent loss of inhibitory signals normally secreted by hepatocytes (Choe, JBC, 1987; 262:5408), which curtail the proliferation of matrix-producing cells in normal tissue, might be an additional albeit not proven fibrogenic mechanism. Previously, arginase located at the external surface of liver cell membranes was identified as a potent inhibitor of hepatic stellate cell proliferation, protein synthesis, and matrix production in culture (Gressner, CellHepatSin, 1991; 3:237). The effect, which is due to a strong reduction of the arginine level in the medium, might also be potentially important *in situ* if the enzyme provides an arginine-depleted microenvironment for the hepatic stellate cells. In the case of hepatocyte damage, enzyme activity will be reduced, providing the opportunity for hepatic stellate cell proliferation.

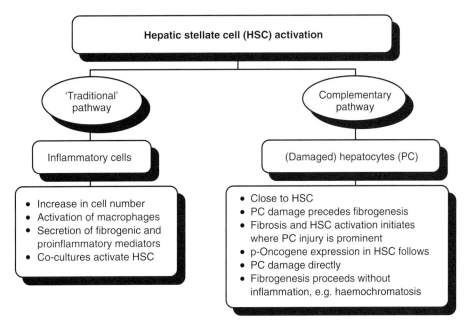

Fig. 9. Complementary pathways of hepatic stellate cell activation originating from inflammatory cells and (damaged) hepatocytes. PC, parenchymal cells.

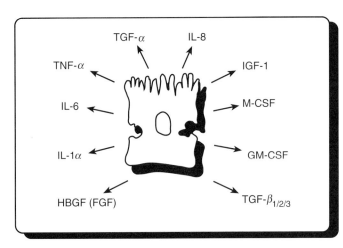

Fig. 10. Schematic presentation of cytokines produced by (murine) hepatocytes in culture. The data are compiled from the literature and are based on mRNA expression, immunological quantitation, and the bioactivity of cytokines in the culture medium.

Another mode of potentially important cell interactions is realized by hepatocytes metabolizing some profibrogenic xenobiotics to fibrogenic substances, which activate the transformation of hepatic stellate cells towards myofibroblasts and/or stimulate matrix gene expression (Table 3). An example of this pathway is given by the metabolism of ethanol, which by itself is not supposed to be fibrogenic (Holt, Hepatol, 1984; 4:843; Gressner, Gastro, 1988; 94: 797) although recently, ethanol-responsive regulatory elements in the rat α_1 (I) collagen gene have been identified (Walton, Hepatol, 1996; 23:310). Its oxidation product, acetaldehyde (and lactate), which is generated in hepatocytes or acetaldehyde–protein adducts, efficiently stimulates the expression of certain collagen types and fibronectin and the proliferation of (transformed) hepatic stellate cells (and fibroblasts) (Moshage, Hepatol, 1990; 12:511; Casini,

JHepatol, 1993; 19:385; Pares, Hepatol, 1993; 19:498). Proteoglycan metabolism, however, remains essentially unaffected (Gressner, Gastro, 1988; 94:797). The mRNA and protein expression of undulin are reduced by acetaldehyde (Casini, BBResComm, 1994; 199:1019) suggesting specific rather than uniform effects of this metabolite on matrix gene expression. Furthermore, ethanol- or chemically induced lipid peroxidation (in hepatocytes) stimulates collagen gene expression in fibroblasts (Parola, BBResComm, 1993; 194:1044) as well as in co-cultured human and rat hepatic stellate cells (Bedossa, Hepatol, 1994; 19:1262). Oxidative stress and malondialdehyde were shown to activate stellate cells through the induction of c-myb and NFκB (Lee, JCI, 1995; 96:2461). These alcohol-related non-peptide fibrogenic mediators (Table 3) suggest a specific fibrogenic role of ethanol (metabolites) in the pathogenesis of alcohol-related liver diseases (Friedman, Hepatol, 1990; 12:609). Comparative measurements of the serum levels of the N-terminal propeptide of type III procollagen and laminin in patients with alcoholic and matched non-alcoholic liver cirrhosis circumstantially support this hypothesis (Lotterer, JHepatol, 1992; 14:71).

Hepatic stellate cells and hepatocytes might also cooperate via direct cell–cell contacts. The pericellular matrix components and other cell surface-associated binding sites on the hepatic stellate cells and parenchymal liver cells such as fibronectin, laminin, and heparan sulphate proteoglycans (for example, syndecan and glypican) (Weiner, CellTissRes, 1996; 285:11), are potential candidates for the mediation of intercellular communications between both cell types. Extrapolated from findings in non-liver tissues (Ishihara, JCellPhysiol, 1989; 138:467), liver cell membrane-associated proteoheparan sulphate could be an important physiologic regulator of the mitotic activity of adjacent hepatic stellate cells in the normal liver. Injured hepatocytes, which have a strongly impaired synthesis of pericellular heparan sulphate (Gressner, JClinChemClinBioch, 1986; 24:821), will be unable to exert contact inhibition of hepatic stellate cells, which could then be rendered

Table 3 Non-peptide fibrogenic mediators

Mediator	Effect	Mechanism	Target/cell/tissue
Acetaldehyde	α_1(I) procollagen and fibronectin gene transcription ↑	Protein adduct formation?	Passaged hepatic stellate cells and skin fibroblasts
Lactate	Collagen synthesis ↑	?	Hepatic stellate cells, myofibroblasts, and 3T3 cells
Ethanol	Rat procollagen α_1(I) gene transcription ↑	Collagen enhancer-promoter ↑	Transgenic mice
Active oxygen species	Collagen gene transcription ↑ Prolyl hydroxylase ↑ Cell proliferation ↑	Lipid peroxidation ↑	Hepatic stellate cells and fibroblasts
Iron	Collagen synthesis ↑	Stability of type I procollagen mRNA ↑ Lipid peroxidation ↑	Fetal fibroblasts
Free proline	Collagen synthesis ↑	?	Liver slices

susceptible to growth factors secreted by resident and invaded inflammatory cells. Following this hypothesis, the interruption or abrogation of the membrane contact between the hepatocytes and hepatic stellate cells and the release of mitogens would be the initiating events of the activation of hepatic stellate cells (see below).

Autocrine stimulation of transformed hepatic stellate cells (myofibroblasts)

Besides endothelial cells, platelets, and Kupffer cells, myofibroblasts themselves have the capability to synthesize and secrete TGF-α, TGF-β (Bachem, JCI, 1992; 89:19), ET-1 (Pinzani, Gastro, 1996; 110:534), PDGF, and FGF-2 (Rosenbaum, Gastro, 1995; 109:1986; Hioki, JHepatol, 1996; 24:217). Since myofibroblasts express TGF-β receptors (Bachem, JHepatol, 1993; 18:40; Friedman, JBC, 1994; 269:10551), respond to TGF-β with enhanced proteoglycan (Bachem, FEBSLett, 1989; 257:134), fibronectin (Bachem, VirchArchCP, 1993; 63:123; Casini, Gastro, 1993; 105:245), and procollagen I, III synthesis (Casini, Gastro, 1993; 105:245), and synthesize TGF-β (Bachem, JCI, 1992 89:19) autocrine stimulatory loops have been suggested. TGF-β antisense oligonucleotides reduce the synthesis of fibronectin and proteoglycans in active myofibroblasts. The data provide evidence that TGF-β represents an autocrine-positive regulator of extracellular matrix synthesis in myofibroblasts. This autocrine loop might contribute to a self-perpetuation of fibrogenesis. Recently published experiments suggest that the autocrine production of FGF-2 and PDGF might mediate some of the effects of TGF-β (Win, Hepatol, 1993; 18: 137; Rosenbaum, Gastro, 1995; 109:1986), but TGF-β-induced production of reactive oxygen species has also been implicated. A further autocrine factor for activated stellate cells might be ET-1, which not only stimulates proliferation but also contraction. ET-1-induced contraction of the myofibroblasts might contribute to increased resistance of the portal blood flow in a fibrotic liver (Pinzani, Gastro, 1996; 110:534).

The extracellular matrix as a modulator of cell responsiveness

Adhesive cellular interactions and binding activities between cells and the insoluble meshwork of extracellular matrix proteins play a vital role in the regulation of gene expression and cell differentiation under normal and pathologic conditions. Principally, at least four types of cell adhesion molecules can be expressed on the cell surface (integrins, the immunoglobulin gene superfamily, cadherins, and selectins) (Stamatoglou, FASEBJ, 1994; 8:420). Integrins are a family of heterodimeric cell surface receptors consisting of at least 14 distinct α-subunits and eight or more β-subunits that can associate in various combinations.[26-29] Each integrin subunit has a large extracellular domain, a membrane-spanning region, and a short cytoplasmic domain (Fig. 11). The extracellular domain binds a great variety of matrix ligands expressing defined amino acid sequences (for example, RGD, DGEA, GPRP, and so on). After binding signal transfer into the cell occurs but the mechanism is not fully understood.[30] One concept suggests that integrins transmit signals by organizing the cytoskeleton to which the intracytoplasmic domain is linked via talin, vinculin, α-actinin to actin. Several reports have also indicated that tyrosine phosphorylation is associated with signal transduction of ligated integrins. These receptors are involved in the interactions of hepatocytes and stellate cells with the extracellular matrix, for example laminin and fibronectin (for further details see Chapter 2.15).

Matrix–hepatocyte interaction

In vivo, hepatocytes are surrounded by a framework of connective tissue to which the cells are anchored by specific receptors. The complex extracellular matrix and its individual components are used as culture substrata to improve the attachment, survival, and specific gene expression of cultured hepatocytes (Alpini, Hepatol, 1994; 20: 494). The maintenance of differentiated functions, which resemble those of cells *in situ* can be achieved in monolayers cultured on a defined matrix instead of pure plastic surfaces (Reid, Hepatol, 1984; 4:548). Sustained expression of liver-specific metabolic pathways by hepatocytes in culture is obtained when the cells are grown on a basement membrane-like matrix (Bissell, ScaJGastr, 1988; 23:1). Individual components of the matrix cannot substitute for the complex. The induction of albumin gene transcription (Bissell, MolBiolMed, 1990; 7:187; Caron, MolCellBiol, 1990; 10:1239), albumin secretion (Bissell, JCI, 1987; 79:801; Bissell, ScaJGastr, 1988; 23:1), and replicative DNA synthesis (Bissell, ScaJGastr, 1988; 23:1) are strongly affected by collagen culture substrata. The finding that the extracellular matrix affects the basal rate of DNA

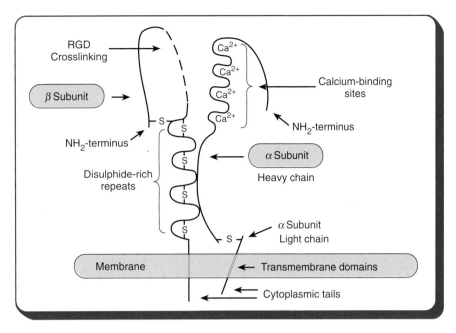

Fig. 11. Principal structure of a typical integrin; slightly modified from D'Souza (TrendsBiochemSci, 1991; 16:246).

synthesis in hepatocytes raises the possiblity that it may also modulate the response to various mitogens, for example EGF and TGF-α. The mitogenic reactivity of hepatocytes to EGF is strongly reduced if the cells are cultured on Matrigel®, an Engelbreth–Holm–Swarm (**EHS**) tumour matrix (Bissell, ScaJGastr, 1988; 23: 1). Proteoglycans have significant effects on maintaining a high albumin production of adult rat hepatocytes *in vitro* (Koide, BBRes-Comm, 1989; 161:385). A number of extracellular matrix receptors or binding sites have been defined (Bissell, EurJCellBiol, 1986; 40: 72; Clement, ExpCellRes, 1990; 187:320; Forsberg, JBC, 1990; 265: 6376), but the signal transduction pathways between the extracellular matrix components and gene activation are not clearly established. Hepatocyte–matrix interactions have potential pathogenetic implications not only for the development of liver fibrosis but also for the control of liver regeneration and the perturbation of hepatocellular functions in fibrosis, where the proximate matrix of the hepatocyte is greatly changed. Furthermore, epithelial–stromal interactions are also important in the pathobiology of primary hepatocellular carcinoma which is known to be associated with a qualitatively and quantitatively changed extracellular matrix (Donato, Cancer, 1989; 63:272).

Matrix–hepatic stellate cell interaction

Relatively little is known about the molecular interactions between hepatic stellate cells and matrices. So far, integrin receptors and cell adhesion molecules (**CAMs**) on hepatic stellate cells and myofibroblasts have only been partially characterized (Carloni, Gastro, 1996; 110:1127), but the phenotype and principal biochemical functions of these cells and their response to growth factors are greatly influenced by culturing them on a complete gel matrix consisting of basement membrane proteins (EHS matrix) (Friedman, JBC, 1989; 264:10756). Under these conditions, the spontaneous activation observed during culture on plastic surfaces is inhibited, the ultrastructure of hepatic stellate cells resembles that in a normal liver,

the cells do not exhibit proliferative activity, and the total collagen synthesis and proteoglycan production are strongly reduced (Friedman, JBC, 1989; 264:10756). The effects of the EHS gel are not reproduced by the individual components of the gel (laminin, type-IV collagen, and heparan sulphate proteoglycan) and are fully reversible. Other studies indicate that the culture of hepatic stellate cells on various types of collagens greatly influences the expression profile of collagens, the responsiveness to retinoids and the susceptibility to TGF-β. Only cells cultured on a type-I collagen matrix (but not those on type-IV collagen) respond to TGF-β with a significant increase of type-I and type-III collagen production (Davis, JBC, 1987; 262:10280; Davis, JCellPhysiol, 1988; 136:547). The stimulatory effect of hepatocyte-conditioned media on the proliferation of hepatic stellate cells described above (Gressner, Hepatol, 1992; 16:1250) is abolished if the cells are attached to matrigel. The mechanisms responsible for the effects of matrix on the phenotype of the cells are not clear, but one has to consider that matrigel and other matrices might include a complex mixture of growth factors and inhibitors bound to matrix molecules which could indirectly influence the cell behaviour.

Most cellular reactions are mediated via integrin receptors, but others might be due to the physical/mechanical environment provided by the gel and by the ability of the matrix molecules to bind and store a variety of cytokines. The core proteins of decorin and biglycan, both small chondroitin-dermatan sulphate proteoglyans, have been identified as binding sites for TGF-β, which suggests for these proteoglycans a role as components in a negative feedback system regulating cell growth and extracellular matrix production (Yamaguchi, Nature, 1988; 336:244; Ruoslahti, Cell, 1991; 64:867). Similarly, a number of cytokines are bound to defined domains of collagens, fibronectin, and laminin (Table 2; for further details see Chapter 2.15). Heparin/heparan sulphate is known to bind many growth factors (cytokines) and γ-interferon (Lortat-Jacob, JCI, 1991; 87:878; Lortat-Jacob, FEBSLett, 1991; 280:152).

Thus, the interplay of matrix, cytokines, and cells provides an almost indefinite number of regulatory mechanisms and actions, which are likely to be important in the pathogenesis of fibrotic organ transition. The sequestration of cytokines in the extra- and pericellular matrix, for which the term 'crinopexy' was recently proposed,[31] might be an efficient mechanism by which cells regulate the bioavailability of growth factors. A recently discovered, very special type of matrix–cell interaction is provided by the feedback inhibition of collagen synthesis in hepatic stellate cells involving the C-terminal propeptide of type-I procollagen (Ikeda, AmJPhysiol, 1993; 264:G157). This cleavage product reduces the expression of collagen in cells from normal but not from fibrotic rat livers (Ikeda, AmJPhysiol, 1993; 264:G157). It is speculated but not firmly proven that the loss of the feedback response of collagen synthesis in transformed hepatic stellate cells (myofibroblasts) could be an important mechanism of collagen overproduction in fibrosis.

A unifying concept of hepatic stellate cell activation: the cascade model

In an attempt to integrate conceptionally the present knowledge of the molecular and cellular interactions of hepatic stellate cells into a hypothetic model of cell stimulation, we propose a three-step cascade mechanism of hepatic stellate cell activation.[13] It implies sequential cross-talk between hepatic stellate cells, hepatocytes, Kupffer cells, platelets, endothelial cells, and myofibroblasts (transformed hepatic stellate cells) (Fig. 12). Accordingly, preinflammatory, inflammatory, and postinflammatory steps can be distinguished. In the preinflammatory phase (I), complete or only subtle hepatocellular damage leading to membrane leakage facilitates the release of paracrine-acting mitogens, which initiate like a 'wound hormone' proliferation of hepatic stellate cells (Fig. 12). In addition, ethanol-metabolizing hepatocytes produce acetaldehyde, reactive oxygen species, and lipid peroxides, which stimulate matrix gene expression in nearby hepatic stellate cells before the inflammatory mediators (second phase) become effective. The proliferation of hepatic stellate cells adjacent to hepatocytes might also be initiated by the decrease of membrane arginase as a consequence of hepatocellular damage, increasing the amount of arginine available for proliferation and matrix protein synthesis of hepatic stellate cells (Gressner, CellHepatSin, 1991; 3:237). In the subsequent inflammatory phase (II), cytokines of activated Kupffer cells/macrophages (for example, TGF-β, TGF-α, and TNF-α) and of disintegrated platelets (for example, TGF-β, EGF-like factors, and PDGF) stimulate hepatic stellate cells to proliferate and to transform to myofibroblasts (Fig. 12). The activation of the resident Kupffer cells and attracted monocytes is initiated immunologically and by phagocytosis of cell debris at the focus of necrosis. These activated cells might induce and perpetuate hepatocellular damage via the release of proteases, toxic cytokines (TNF-α), and reactive oxygen species. Toxic oxygen metabolites generated by polymorphonuclear leucocytes, which are attracted and activated by IL-8 producing ethanol-metabolizing hepatocytes (Shiratori, Hepatol, 1993; 18:1477), might further contribute to a pathogenetic vicious circle at least in alcoholic liver injury. In the inflammatory phase TGF-β, the prototype of a multifunctional fibrogenic cytokine[32] potently accelerates the transformation of hepatic stellate cells via intermediate stages (transitional cells) to myofibroblasts. The latter cell type is stimulated during the postinflammatory phase (III) via an autocrine loop generated by TGF-α, TGF-β, ET-1, PDGF, and FGF, which are expressed and secreted by myofibroblasts and for which these cells have the respective receptors (Fig. 12). In combination with further paracrine stimulation of still untransformed hepatic stellate cells by myofibroblasts, the postinflammatory phase potentially contributes to the self-perpetuation of fibrogenesis even after cessation of the initiating event. The matrix formed by the myofibroblasts might modulate the bioavailability of secreted cytokines and growth factors (for example, TGF-β) by forming a sink or sponge of cytokines providing the possibility of their storage, sustained release, protection against proteolytic attack, and site-directed liberation. In addition, α_2-macroglobulin, which is produced by hepatocytes as well as by myofibroblasts (Andus, EurJBioch, 1987; 168:641) might act as a pleiotropic scavenger of cytokines (for example, TGF-β, TNF-α, and PDGF).[25] The concept proposed ascribes (damaged) hepatocytes and myofibroblasts direct roles in the sequential activation of hepatic stellate cells. TGF-β, which is secreted by myofibroblasts, might also promote, after extracellular activation, hepatocyte death by induction of apoptosis in a paracrine way (Gressner, Hepatol, 1996; 23:571). The autocrine production of TGF-β in hepatocytes (Bissell, JCI, 1995; 96:447; Chunfang, JCellPhysiol, 1996; 167:394) and TGF-β generated by mesenchymal liver cells and bile duct epithelial cells (Milani, AmJPathol, 1991; 139:1221) could contribute to apoptotic cell damage by the release of mitogenic factors (Gressner, Hepatol, 1992; 16:1250) including reactive oxygen species to the stimulation of hepatic stellate cell proliferation (Gressner, IntHepatolComm, 1995; 4:94). These mechanisms could provide an explanation for the clinical finding

Fig. 12. The three-step cascade model of hepatic stellate cell (fat-storing cell and Ito cell) activation (Gressner, Gut, 1994; 35:1331). (A) The preinflammatory step is initiated by damage of the hepatocytes, which releases the stimulators of hepatic stellate cell proliferation and decreases membrane-associated inhibitors such as membrane arginase. In addition, the metabolism of ethanol (EtOH) to acetaldehyde (AcAld) and the generation of lipid peroxides initiate matrix gene expression in the stellate cells before the inflammatory stimuli (second step) become effective. (B) In the inflammatory step, mitogens from activated Kupffer cells, invaded macrophages, and disintegrated platelets are the most potent stimulators of hepatic stellate cell proliferation and transformation into myofibroblasts. Activated macrophages in turn can damage via the release of proteases, toxic cytokines (for example, TNF-α), and oxygen radical membrane damage of the hepatocytes. (C) In the postinflammatory step, fully transformed hepatic stellate cells (= myofibroblasts) release various cytokines, chemokines, and growth factors (TGF-α, TGF-β, ET-1, PDGF, and FGF-2), which stimulate non-transformed stellate cells in a paracrine way and, in an autocrine loop, the myofibroblast itself. The cytokines interact with and are sequestered by the extracellular matrix components and α_2-macroglobulin (α_2M) secreted by the myofibroblast. Abbreviations: CSF-1, colony-stimulating factor; PMN, polymorphonuclear leucocytes; all others as cited in the text.

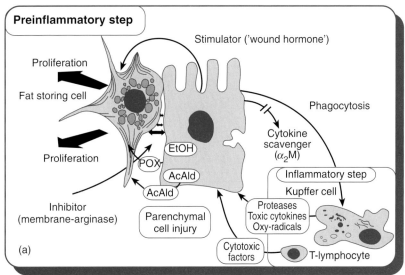

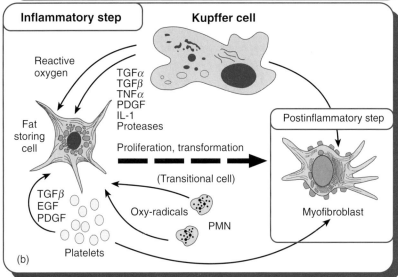

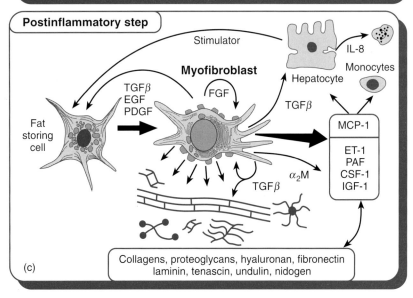

Table 4 Levels of pharmacological intervention with hepatic fibrogenesis

Fibroprevention
Reduction of liver cell damage by hepatocytoprotective agents

Fibrostasis
Inhibition of synthesis, secretion, processing, and deposition of extracellular matrix proteins

Fibrolysis
Dissolution and removal of extracellular matrix

that inflammation might not necessarily be required for developing fibrosis (Friedman, Hepatol, 1990; 12:609). Thus, therapeutic interventions should be focused both on anti-inflammatory and hepatocytoprotective effects.

Pharmacological therapy

The ultimate goal of the research on liver fibrogenesis is the development of a rational basis for an effective antifibrotic therapy. Pharmacological trials can take place at different levels (Table 4) using cytoprotective drugs (Table 5), inhibitors of extracellular matrix synthesis (Table 6), and accelerators of extracellular matrix breakdown (Table 7), respectively.[33] (Gressner, EurJClin-ChemClinBioch, 1991; 29:293). Most of the drugs listed in Tables 5,6 and 7 have been studied only in cell cultures and in various

Table 5 Drugs used in various experimental models for fibroprevention: reduction of cell damage by cytoprotection

Free radical scavengers/antioxidants
Glutathione
Superoxide dismutase (SOD)
α-Tocopherol
Desferrioxamine
(+) Cianidanol-3
Indole-3-carbinol
Tryptophan
Cysteine
Silymarin/silibinin

Dimethyl prostaglandin E_2
Prostacyclin (**PGI₂**)
Lipoxygenase inhibitors

Trifluoperazine
Diltiazem

Colchicine
Ursodeoxycholic acid
Proteinase inhibitors (**PMST** and **TLCK**)
Atrial natriuretic peptide (**ANP**)
$α_2$-Macrofetoprotein
Synthetic linear terpenoids (E-0712)
Cholestyramine
Malotilate

ε-Aminocaproic acid
Putrescine
HGFs/scatter factor
Phenylmethylsulphonyl fluoride
Glycyrrhizin
Fructose 1,6-bisphosphate

experimental models of liver fibrosis because severe side-effects (toxic reactions) prevent their systemic and continuous use. Therapeutic application in clinical situations is either very limited or of uncertain efficiency (Table 8). Among the cytoprotective agents (16,16-dimethyl)prostaglandin E_2 (Ruwart, Hepatol, 1984; 4:658; Abecassis, JCI, 1987; 80:881; Ruwart, Hepatol, 1988; 8:61) and other eicosanoids (Noda, JHepatol, 1986; 2:53; Bursch, Hepatol, 1989; 6:830) have found wide experimental and now also clinical interest. Through protection of the hepatocyte against noxious effects (and by additional mechanisms), prostaglandin E_2 significantly suppresses fibrogenesis and thereby the accumulation of collagen in a lipotrope-deficient diet-induced model of hepatic cirrhosis (Ruwart, Hepatol, 1988; 8:61; Peters, Prostagl, 1989; 37: 445). The precise mechanism of hepatocytoprotection by prostaglandin E_2, however, is presently not clearly defined. Potentially important for future antifibrotic trials could be the hepatocytoprotective effect of a continuous supply of HGF, which was shown to decrease the degree of acute CCl_4-induced liver injury significantly (Kaido, BBResComm, 1996; 218:1). Beneficial albeit contradictory effects have been reported for colchicine in human (Kershenobich, NEJM, 1988; 318:1709) and experimental (Poo, JHepatol, 1993; 19:90) antifibrotic trials, which need further clarification before its clinical usefulness can be firmly established.[33] (Palmerini, BiotechApplBiochem, 1995; 22:15). A concomitant acute phase reaction in rats renders the hepatocyte relatively insensitive to injuries (Gressner, JClinChemClinBioch, 1986; 24:821), suppresses inflammatory reactions (Van Gool, ExpMolPath, 1978; 29:228) and, therefore, might act antifibrogenically. Unexpectedly, the acute phase reaction was shown to aggravate fibrogenesis and fibrosis (Van Gool, ExpMolPath, 1986; 44:157). This effect might be partially due to the acute phase reaction-induced formation of $α_2$-macroglobulin, which is known to inactivate extracellular matrix-degrading enzymes (metalloproteinases and stromelysin) and to stimulate prolyl 4-hydroxylase activity in the liver (Van Gool, ExpMolPath, 1986; 45:160; Van Gool, ExpMolPath, 1988; 49:410). IL-6, the most important mediator of the acute phase reaction, stimulates the expression of $α_1$ (I) procollagen mRNA in cultured hepatic stellate cell lines and mediates stimulated hepatic collagen gene expression under acute phase conditions (Greenwel, LabInvest, 1995; 72:83). These observations might explain the overall profibrogenic effect of the acute phase reaction. The action of fibrostatic drugs, which are used predominantly (with some exceptions) in animal models and cell cultures but not in humans, is neither liver nor fibrosis specific (Table 6). Their clinical application is severely hampered by strong adverse side-effects if the drugs are applied systemically. Therefore, the development of site-directed (targeted) drug delivery systems that quite selectively affect the extracellular matrix-producing cells in the liver is required. Drug-loaded vesicle carrier systems such as liposomes and erythrocyte ghosts, that is transiently permeabilized haemoglobin-depleted and drug-filled erythrocytes, might be potentially useful. These particulate carriers are taken up and digested by liver macrophages and the liberated, pharmacologically active compound affects not only the Kupffer cells but by backflow also neighbouring cell types such as hepatic stellate cells. The selectivity for the liver is approximately 80 per cent, the remainder being taken up by macrophages in the spleen, lung, and bone marrow (Koch, JClinChemClinBioch, 1989; 27:749). This approach of targeting would offer the possibility

Table 6 Fibrostasis: pharmacological inhibition of collagen processing in cell cultures and various experimental models

Agent	Mechanism of action
Transcription and translation	
Glucocorticoids	Decrease of collagen mRNA by increased degradation and effect on collagen gene promoter (types I and IV)
Retinoids	Decrease of collagen mRNA
Interferon-γ	Decrease of collagen mRNA
N- and C-terminal procollagen propeptides	Decrease of collagen mRNA
Intracellular co- and post-translational modification	
Competitive inhibitors of prolyl 4-hydroxylase	Competitive inhibition with Fe^{2+}, oxygen; 2-oxoglutarate, and peptide substrate
Oxaproline peptides	Syncatalytic inactivation of prolyl 4-hydroxylase
Anthraquinone glycoside (*Streptococcus albogriseolus*)	Non-competitive inhibition of prolyl 4-hydroxylase
(+)-Catechin	Scavenging of activated oxygen
Proline analogues	Inhibition of triple helix formation by interference with *trans*-4-hydroxylation
Minoxidil	Inhibition of lysyl hydroxylase (not prolyl hydroxylase)
Doxorubicin	Inhibition of prolyl hydroxylase
Colchicine	Inhibition of collagen synthesis and secretion and anti-inflammatory and antimitotic suppression of cytokine release
Extracellular modifications	
β-Amino-propionitrile 2-Bromoethylamine 2-Chloroethylamine (lathyrogens)	Inhibition of lysyl oxidase, inhibition of cross-linking, and acceleration of degradation
D-Penicillamine	Interaction with lysine-derived aldehydes, inhibition of cross-linking, and acceleration of degradation

Table 7 Fibrolysis: acceleration of collagen breakdown

Agent	Mechanism of action
Cytochalasin B Colchicine Tumour-promoting phorbol esters TNF-α IL-1 Polyunsaturated lecithin Relaxin (?)	Stimulation of collagenase production and/or activation in mesenchymal cells
TNF-α	Suppression of production of tissue inhibitors of metalloproteinases

of influencing the fibrogenic effector activity of activated liver macrophages, of modulating the responsiveness of the target cell (hepatic stellate cell), and of a more liver-directed interference with the synthesis of collagen and other extracellular matrix components, depending on the drug of choice. Although the erythrocyte ghost delivery system has been used successfully in the past in enzyme replacement therapy (De Flora, PNAS, 1986; 83:7029; Zocchi, PNAS, 1989; 86:2040), its application in antifibrogenic trials has been not realized so far. An alternative approach of targeting an inhibitor of collagen synthesis is currently under investigation, utilizing proinhibitors (prodrugs) of prolyl 4-hydroxylase activity (pyridine-2,4-dicarboxylic-diethylamide and pyridine-2,4-dicarboxylic-di(2-methoxyethyl)-amide), which by themselves are ineffective but are metabolized to the active (competitive) inhibitor (pyridine-2,4-di-carboxylate) of the enzyme exclusively in the liver (Franklin, BiochemSocTrans, 1991; 19:812). Underhydroxylated collagen α-chains are not able to form stable helices and, therefore, are rapidly degraded. In experimental cirrhosis these drugs were reported to reduce the accumulation of collagen in the liver without producing major side-effects (Bickel, JHepatol, 1991; 13:S26; Böker, JHepatol, 1991; 13:S35), thus forming a basis for promising clinical trials. In addition, this drug might also inhibit the activation of

Table 8 *In vivo* data on potential antifibrotic drugs

| Drug | Antifibrotic effect | | Mechanism |
	Animal	Man	
Colchicin	no	(no)	Secretion of collagenase and cytokines ↓
d-Penicillamin	no	no	Collagen cross-links ↓ (lysylhydroxylase ↓)
Corticosteroids	no	(no)	Collagen synthesis ↓ and immunosuppressant
Ursodeoxycholic acid	?	?	Anticholestatic and anti-inflammatory
Silymarin	yes	(yes)	Membrane modulation? and anti-inflammatory
Polyunsaturated lecithin	yes	?	Collagenase activity ↑
Prostaglandins E_1/E_2	yes	?	Intracellular collagen degradation ↑ and collagen ↓
Prolylhydroxylase inhibitors	(no)	?	Intracellular collagen degradation ↑
Interferon-γ	yes	?	Collagenase ↑, collagen ↓ and proliferation ↓
Interferon-α/β	(yes)	(yes)	Collagen ↓(?)

The table lists experimental animal studies using suitable models of liver fibrosis, that is those lacking radical-induced damage or overt inflammation as major cause of fibrosis. Such studies are rat biliary fibrosis or alcoholic liver fibrosis in the baboon (see also Chapter 2.15); (yes)/(no), data suggest/do not indicate antifibrotic effect, but final proof is lacking; (?), major studies are still missing.

stellate cells in the diseased liver (Sakaida, Hepatol, 1996; 23:755). Polyunsaturated lecithin (**PUL**) was shown to prevent alcohol-induced fibrosis and cirrhosis in primates possibly due to stimulated collagenase activity in hepatic stellate cells and, thus, increased collagen breakdown (Lieber, Hepatol, 1990; 12:1390; Li, Hepatol, 1992; 15:373; Lieber, Gastro, 1994; 106:152; Ma, JHepatol, 1996; 24:604). Similarly, pentoxifylline, a methyl-xanthine derivative, prevents experimental fibrosis (Peterson, Hepatol, 1993; 17:486) and some important fibrogenic functions of cultured stellate cells (Windmeier, BiochemPharm, 1996; 51:577). Relaxin has been proven to decrease collagen accumulation in rodent models of non-hepatic fibrosis (Unemori, JInvDermatol, 1993; 101:280), which also suggests potential antifibrotic activity in liver fibrosis. Silymarin, a standardized hepatoprotective phytopharmacon with the polyphenole silibinin as the major active ingredient, was shown to reduce collagen accumulation in rat secondary biliary fibrosis (Boigk, JHepatol, 1995; 23:S142). The antifibrotic effects of both PUL and silymarin are currently being addressed by large multicentre clinical trials that include patients with alcoholic liver fibrosis and cirrhosis. Furthermore, it has been shown that ursodeoxycholic acid can decrease fibrogenesis and increase fibrolysis in rat secondary biliary fibrosis (Poo, Gastro, 1992; 102:1752) and in patients with primary biliary cirrhosis (Oesterling, Gut, 1995; 37:121A). Other and more sophisticated alternatives of future therapeutic strategies including molecular biological tools have been discussed.[34] One potentially successful approach is focused on the application of natural antagonists of growth factor receptors and cytokine-inactivating peptides or soluble receptors. Antifibrogenic and/or cytoprotective effects were obtained in experimental models with the administration of soluble TNF-α receptors (Czaja, Gastro, 1995; 108:1849), the IL-1 receptor antagonist (Mancini, VirchArchCP, 1994; 424:25), the ET-1 receptor antagonist bosentan (Rockey, Hepatol, 1995; 22:221A), and decorin proteoglycan (Border, Nature, 1992; 360:361; Harper, MethodsEnz, 1994; 245:241; Isaka, NatureMed, 1996; 2:418). The computational design and synthesis of growth factor analogues which inactivate the respective receptors might provide a novel clinical strategy in controlling abnormal cellular reactions in disease (Pietrzkowski, CancerRes, 1992; 52:6447). In future studies it might be feasible to use a liver-specific gene delivery

system[35,36] for the *in vivo* transfection of liver cells with genes encoding the respective antagonists or soluble cytokine receptors, thus, providing a sustained supply of cytokine scavengers at the site of action. The use of TGF-β antisense oligomers might also be of value for the treatment of fibrotic diseases in which TGF-β overexpression plays the most important pathogenetic role (Khanna, KidneyInt, 1996; 49:S2). Hepatic stellate cell activation (proliferation, transformation, and matrix gene expression) can be effectively inhibited by γ-interferon (Rockey, Hepatol, 1992; 16:776; Rockey, JInvMed, 1994; 42:660), α-interferon (Guido, JHepatol, 1996; 24:301), bosentan (Rockey, Hepatol, 1995; 22:221A), dexamethasone (Weiner, Hepatol, 1990; 11:111), and retinoic acid (Davis, JBC, 1987; 262:10280; Davis, JCI, 1990; 86:2062; Davis, BiochemJ, 1993; 294:785). The response of stellate cells to these and other inhibitors, however, may change during transformation, as shown recently for retinoids (Weiner, Hepatol, 1992; 15:336). The nuclear retinoic acid β-receptor decreases strongly during stellate cell transformation, which renders transformed cells less sensitive or even unresponsive to retinoids (Weiner, Hepatol, 1992; 15:336). Thus, the *in vivo* application of vitamin A has led to controversial effects (Geubel, Gastro, 1991; 100:1701; Schuppan, JLabClinMed 1992; 119:590; Seifert, Hepatol, 1994; 19:193; Seifert, Liver, 1995 15:1). Approaches directed at specific intervention with the activation of hepatic stellate cells may become promising areas of future antifibrotic research.

Clinical–chemical diagnosis, staging, and monitoring of fibrogenesis

The traditional way of confirming the presence of fibrosis and cirrhosis is based on the histological evaluation of a liver biopsy specimen, a procedure with several drawbacks.

(1) It is invasive and, therefore, cannot be repeated safely and with comfort in order to assess the progression of disease and the efficacy of treatment.

(2) Biopsy is associated with considerable sampling variability (error) in the detection of fibrosis/cirrhosis (Maharaj, Lancet,

1986; i:523), because of focal differences of inflammation and fibrosis.

(3) It allows a more or less static evaluation of fibrosis rather than an assessment of the dynamic process of ongoing fibrogenesis and fibrolysis, which is essential for the evaluation of the prognosis of the disease.

Accordingly, non-invasive, clinical–chemical procedures for identifying the existence of fibrosis and the progression of fibrogenesis and fibrolysis are needed.[37,38] The properties of an ideal clinical–chemical parameter for liver fibrosis should fulfil the following requirements.

(1) Specificity for the liver, with no major contribution by other organs.
(2) A sensitivity sufficient enough to detect minor changes of fibrogenesis and fibrolysis.
(3) A reflection of either fibrogenesis, fibrolysis, or the amount of connective tissue laid down in the liver and not merely an enhanced connective tissue turnover.
(4) A known biological half-life and known major routes of disposal and excretion, in order to allow a better interpretation of changing serum levels and the role of, for example, reduced kidney or liver function.
(5) Production by a defined cellular source in the diseased liver, preferably the activated hepatic stellate cells and not hepatocytes, in order to exclude, for example, interference by a functionally and synthetically compromised parenchyma.
(6) Measurement possible by sensitive, rapid, and easy to perform assay formats, such as the enzyme-linked immunosorbent assay (**ELISA**) technique that do not require expensive equipment or a nuclear medicine department.
(7) Standardization and validation by reference laboratories and external and internal quality control systems to ensure comparability of the results.

The available serum markers for liver fibrosis do not come up to the requirements of ideal parameters. However, biochemical, experimental, and clinical studies of the last few years have provided numerous data that permit a preliminary assessment of how validly certain markers mirror fibrogenesis and/or fibrolysis in the liver.

Several split products of the maturation and degradation pathways of extracellular matrix proteins and glycoproteins have been determined in the circulation,[37,39–41] using radioimmuno-, enzymeimmuno-, and radioligand assays. At present, the most frequently studied parameters are the cleavage products of different types of collagens (Schuppan, JCI, 1986; 78:241; Risteli, ClinChem, 1988; 34:715; Hartmann, ClinChem, 1990; 36:421; Hayasaka, JHepatol, 1990; 10:17; Melkko, ClinChem, 1990; 36:1328), basement membrane-related glycoproteins (Kropf, ClinChem, 1988; 34: 2026; Robert, AlcoholClinExpRes, 1989; 13:176; Misaki, ClinChem, 1990; 36:522; Niemelä, Gastro, 1990; 98:1621), and hyaluronan (Engström-Laurent, Hepatol, 1985; 5:638; Nyberg, Hepatol, 1988; 8:142). Table 9 lists the serum parameters that have been studied in man and/or rat and their preliminary assignment to either fibrogenesis, fibrolysis, or both.

The N-terminal propeptide of type III procollagen (**PIIINP**) arises from the extracellular processing of newly secreted or deposited, partially processed type III procollagen. Its serum level increases in fibrotic liver patients in correlation with the degree of histological inflammation and fibrogenic activity, but not in relation to the extent of fibrotic organ transformation (Surrenti, DigDisSci, 1987; 32:705; Annoni, Hepatol, 1989; 9:693). The determination of PIIINP concentration allows a powerful discrimination between chronic hepatitis with mild and moderate/severe activities and a prognostic assessment of patients with chronic alcoholic liver disease. A normal or slightly elevated level does not exclude pre-existing but slowly progressing fibrosis. The pathobiochemical mechanism of the changes in the PIIINP concentration in the serum (similar to other matrix components) of patients with chronic active liver diseases consists of stimulated synthesis and secretion, decreased hepatic (and renal) clearance, and alteration of the volume of distribution (Table 10) (Alcorn, Hepatol, 1987; 7:981). The liver and kidneys extract different types of N-terminal propeptide antigens of type III procollagen antigens; intact N-terminal propeptide is cleared in the liver by receptor-mediated endocytosis of sinusoidal endothelial cells, whereas smaller N-terminal propeptide antigens of type III procollagen are extracted by the kidneys (Bentsen, Hepatol, 1990; 11:957). The disappearance of radioactively labelled PIIINP from the serum, as determined in the normal pig, follows a two-order kinetics with half lives of approximately 45 min and 8 h (Thorbjorn Jensen, AmJPhysiol, 1993; 265:R139). These data are in accordance with previous findings that showed that PIIINP and **PIVCP** (synonymous with **NC1**, the C-terminal fragment of procollagen IV) have serum half-lives of approximately 25 min and 6 to 10 h in normal rats. Studies in man showed that enhanced PIIINP indicated an increase in bioactive liver prolyl hydroxylase, a key enzyme for the synthesis of stable collagen (Torres-Salinas, Gastro, 1986; 90:1241). In patients with chronic viral hepatitis subjected to treatment with interferon, the serum PIIINP correlated well with the mRNA encoding liver procollagen a1(I) and of the fibrogenic mediator TGF-β_1, but not with AST, a surrogate marker of inflammatory activity (Castilla, NEJM, 1991; 324:933). These more recent findings shed novel light on earlier studies performed in a follow-up design that demonstrated that PIIINP may be of great value in predicting the development of chronic hepatitis of different activities (gradings) when other serological parameters fail (Rohde, EurJClinInv, 1979; 9:451; Weigand, Hepatol, 1984; 4:835; Ballardini, Liver, 1984; 4:348; Annoni, JHepatol, 1986; 2:379; McCullough, Hepatol, 1987; 7:49), whereas the suggestion of PIIINP as a strong and independent predictor of the natural evolution of primary biliary cirrhosis (Eriksson, JHepatol, 1986; 2:370; Babbs, Lancet, 1988; 1021) has been challenged by others. PIIINP has been increasingly used in follow-up studies of patients with hepatitis C and to a minor degree hepatitis B who were treated with interferon-α. Most groups reported a normalization of PIIINP in complete responders (Camps, JHepatol, 1993; 17:390; Capra, JHepatol, 1993; 18:112; Gallorini, JHepatol, 1994; 14:257; Teran, Hepatol, 1994; 19:849; Suou, Hepatol, 1995; 22:426). Interestingly, two of these studies also reported a fall of PIIINP in interferon-treated patients who showed no or only a partial response (Camps, JHepatol, 1993; 17:390; Gallorini, JHepatol, 1994; 14:257; Teran, Hepatol, 1994; 19:849; Suou, Hepatol, 1995; 22:426). Since PIIINP remained suppressed in the latter patients, even 12 months after interferon was stopped, the agent might have a prolonged antifibrogenic effect that is independent of the serological response and a decrease of necroinflammation. This

Table 9 Serum assays for liver fibrosis

	Fibrogenesis	Fibrolysis	Liver specificity
PICP	+	−	(+), bone
PIIINP	+	(+), acute	+
PIVCP	− (?)	+	+ (fibrosis)
PIVNP	− (?)	+	+ (fibrosis)
Hyaluronan	+ (?)	+ (?)	(+), fibrosis
Laminin	+ (?)	+ (?)	(+) (fibrosis)
Collagen VI	−	+	(+)
Undulin	−	+ (portal)	+
Tenascin	+ (lobular)	−	+ (?)
TIMP-1	+	−	+ (?)
MMP-1/8	−	+	+ (?)
Integrin-β_1	+	(+)	(+)
Integrin-α chains	+	(+)	+ (?) (proliferation)
TGF-β_1	+	−	+ (?)

PICP, C-terminal propeptide of procollagen I; PIIINP, N-terminal propeptide of procollagen III; PIVCP, C-terminal propeptide of procollagen IV (NC1 fragment); PIVNP, N-terminal propeptide of procollagen IV (7-S collagen); TIMP-1, tissue inhibitor of metalloproteinases 1; MMP-1/8, interstitial collagenase as measured by enzyme activity; TGF-β_1, transforming growth factor β. The data on TGF-β_1 and integrin α-chains (own unpublished results) are preliminary. 'Liver specificity' denotes that most marked elevations are observed in liver diseases. PIIINP may reflect fibrolysis in acute bouts of hepatitis. For further details refer to the text.

Table 10 Determinants of the serum concentration of aminoterminal propeptide of type III procollagen PIIINP

Secretion	Liver
	Cellular secretion of type III procollagen
	Degradation of extracellularly deposited, partly
	processed procollagen
	Intracellular degradation of newly formed procollagen
	Extrahepatic
	Lung, skin, vessels, joints, and so on
Clearance	Renal (tubular reabsorption?)
	Extrarenal
	Biliary excretion
	Receptor-mediated uptake and degradation in sinusoidal
	endothelial cells
Distribution volume	Ascites

$$[PIIINP] = \frac{secretion - clearance}{distribution\ volume}$$

assumption is further supported by histological follow-up studies that suggested a decrease of the amount of hepatic collagen, irrespective of the clinical and serological response to interferon (Schvarcz, Liver, 1991; 11:30; Manabe, JHepatol, 1993; 18:1344).

Circulating collagen VI, a molecule that runs in filaments between large collagen fibrils, is a mixture of low molecular weight fragments, characterizing it as a marker of fibrolysis (Schuppan, AnalBioch, 1985; 148:238; Shahin, Hepatol, 1992; 15:637). Since both collagen VI and PIIINP derive from similar sites in the interstitial extracellular matrix, their simultaneous measurement in a patient could allow an assessment of the balance between fibrogenesis and fibrolysis. In this line, most but not all patients with primary biliary cirrhosis (**PBC**) stages I to IV who had been treated with ursodeoxycholic acid for 2 to 4 years showed a decrease of PIIINP and an increase in collagen VI, indicating a favourable

course in terms of the progression of fibrosis (Oesterling, Gut, 1995; 37:A121). In addition, serum collagen VI is not increased in young children, whereas other fibrosis markers, particularly PIIINP and, to a minor degree, basement membrane-related antigens, are not well suited for monitoring liver disease in this age group due to elevated levels that are related to body growth[42] (Trivedi, CCActa, 1986; 161:137). In small children serum collagen VI allowed the detection of chronic fibrotic liver disease with a sensitivity and specificity of almost 100 per cent (Gerling, Gut, 1995; 37:A122). However, generalized connective tissue diseases and renal fibrosis that can lead to elevated collagen VI levels have to be excluded (Schuppan, JHepatol, 1991; 13:S17; Marder, ClinNephrol, 1995; 44:178; Schuppan, JHepatol, 1995; 22:8288).

Undulin is a glycoprotein related to collagen XIV. It associates with the surface of mature fibrillar collagen (Schuppan, JBC, 264:

8823) in the dense interstitial extracellular matrix and appears to be removed rapidly when the normal collagen architecture is disturbed. Thus, it is not surprising that serum undulin increases 3- to 5-fold even in the early stages of alcoholic liver disease, schistosomiasis, and PBC when markers such as PIIINP are in the normal range (Shahin, Hepatogast, 1995; 42:22; Stickel, AlcAlc, 1995; 30:4). Since, as for collagen VI, the detected antigens derive from fibrolysis, serum undulin is now included in several clinical studies with potential antifibrotic drugs.

Tenascin, a non-collagenous glycoprotein, is absent from the portal tract stroma but found in the perisinusoidal space of a normal liver. It is highly expressed *de novo* in periportal zones, around vascular and bile ductular proliferations, and in the space of Disse during active fibrogenesis. In a cross-sectional study, serum tenascin has been found elevated in patients with acute and chronic liver diseases, but it was not judged superior to other fibrosis markers in the diagnosis of fibrosis and cirrhosis (Yamauchi, Liver, 1994; 14: 148). However, by using a different assay, tenascin was decreased by 50 per cent in all patients with chronic hepatitis B and C during and up to 6 months after interferon treatment, with comparable values for responders and non-responders, whereas it was in the normal range in 22 patients with PBC stages I to IV (Libuda, Hepatol, 1995; 22:369A). This led to the conclusion that tenascin could be a selective marker of sinusoidal fibrogenesis. The observation adds a novel dimension to the non-invasive assessment of local aspects of fibrogenesis in the liver.

Laminin, a large molecular mass glycoprotein constituent of basement membranes and some of its degradation products (fragment P1), are elevated in the circulation of patients with liver fibrosis (Kropf, ClinChem, 1988; 34:2026; Robert, Alcohol-ClinExpRes, 1989; 13:176; Misaki, ClinChem, 1990; 36:522; Niemelä, Gastro, 1990; 98:1621). Clinically sufficient diagnostic criteria for the assessment of hepatic fibrosis have been calculated for this assay (Kropf, ClinChem, 1988; 34:2026) and its potential usefulness has been stressed. Most importantly, a positive correlation between the serum level of laminin and the portal venous pressure has been established for fibrotic liver changes (Gressner, KlinWschr, 1986; 64:1240; Gressner, CCActa, 1986; 161:249; Gressner, Hepatogast, 1988; 35:95). Consequently, the criteria for the diagnostic effectiveness of serum laminin for portal hypertension were evaluated (Kropf, ClinChem, 1991, 37:30), which suggest serum laminin (but not PIIINP) as a clinically useful index of portal hypertension in ongoing fibrosis.

Hyaluronan (hyaluronic acid) is presently the only glycosaminoglycan which can be determined reliably by a radioligand assay, using specific binding proteins from bovine cartilage and brain tissue, respectively (Laurent, AnalBioch, 1980; 109:386; Delpech, AnalBioch, 1985; 149:555; Kongtawelert, AnalBiochem, 1989; 178: 367; Kongtawelert, AnalBioch, 1990; 185:313; Lindqvist, ClinChem, 1992; 38:127). Its concentration in the serum increases several fold in patients with fibrosing diseases (Engström-Laurent, Hepatol, 1985; 5:638; Frebourg, Hepatol, 1986; 6:392; Henriksen, JHepatol, 1988; 6:158; Nyberg, Hepatol, 1988; 8:142) but also in other pathological conditions affecting the extracellular matrix (for example rheumatoid arthritis, severe lung fibrosis, scleroderma, and advanced tumours). Elevated serum hyaluronan might be a sensitive parameter for the prediction of cirrhosis and for the progression of liver damage in biliary cirrhosis, but a firm correlation with the

Table 11 Mechanisms of increased circulating hyaluronan in cirrhotic liver disease

Decreased extraction	
Liver	Splanchnic extraction ratio ↓
	Endothelial cell clearance ↓
Kidney	Renal extraction ratio ↓
Increased supply	
Liver	Synthesis at inflammatory sites (hepatic stellate cells) ↑
Lymph	Portal hypertension → elevated lymph flow → decreased extraction by lymph nodes → spillover into circulation ↑

degree or severity of fibrotic organ changes has not been established so far.[43] It is suggested that the hyaluronan levels reflect both active fibrogenesis and hepatic failure, in particular damage of the sinusoidal endothelial cells (Deaciuc, Hepatol, 1993; 17:266; Shimizu, Hepatol, 1994; 20:1323; Nanji, JHepatol, 1996; 24:368). Hyaluronan has been proposed as the preferable marker for monitoring fibrosis in patients with chronic viral hepatitis C (Guechot, ClinChem, 1996; 42:558). The level of hyaluronan, like that of laminin, correlates positively with the portal venous pressure (Kropf, ClinChem, 1991; 37:30). Applying logistic regression analysis, formulas based on the serum concentrations of hyaluronan and laminin have been developed for the prediction of portal hypertension in alcoholic and non-alcoholic cirrhotic conditions (Kropf, ClinChem, 1991; 37:30). In this context, the serum hyaluronan levels were reported to reflect hepatic sinusoidal capillarization (Ueno, Gastro, 1993; 105:475). The concentration of hyaluronan in the circulation is strongly determined by the rates of hepatic and renal extraction, which are lowered in cirrhotic liver diseases (Table 11) (Fraser, JLabClinMed, 1986; 107:79; Henriksen, JHepatol, 1988; 6:158; Engström-Laurent, ConnTissRes, 1990; 24: 219). The half-life of serum hyaluronan, normally between 2.5 and 5.5 min, is prolonged under conditions of liver failure due to impairment of receptor-mediated endocytosis and catabolism by the sinusoidal endothelial cells and/or perihepatic haemodynamic shunting (Fraser, JLabClinMed, 1986; 107:79). It is hard to estimate the fraction of serum hyaluronan derived from the increased supply under conditions of active fibrosis, but it seems likely that this mechanism will be only of minor importance.

Circulating collagenases or their activities are of interest, since biochemical (Maruyama, LifeSci, 1982; 30:1379) as well as *in situ* hybridization studies (Milani, AmJPathol, 1994; 144:528) have demonstrated that the activity and expression of the enzyme that degrades fibrillar collagen I (interstitial collagenase and matrix metalloproteinase (**MMP**)-1) wanes with progression to advanced fibrosis. Recently, circulating collagen I degrading activity was determined enzymatically in patients with chronic liver diseases and found to be inversely correlated with the serum PIIINP (Murawaki, JHepatol, 1993; 18:328), suggesting that mechanisms that suppress collagenase activity and expression are operative during active fibrogenesis. In addition, *in situ* hybridization demonstrated a high level expression of tissue inhibitor of metalloproteinase (**TIMP**)-1, the most potent natural inhibitor of MMP-1, in hepatic stellate cells and occasional hepatocytes in areas of active fibrogenesis (Herbst, JHepatol, 1995; 23:140A). TIMP-1 can now been measured in the serum and a study showed it to be a sensitive marker of incipient alcoholic liver fibrosis (Li, Hepatol, 1994; 19:1418). Since only one other cross-sectional investigation of patients with chronic viral hepatitis was performed, in which TIMP-1 was correlated to histological scores of fibrosis and inflammation (Murawaki, JHepatol, 1995; 23:145) follow-up studies are needed for further evaluation.

A serum test for the β1 chain of integrins has been added to the spectrum of assayable fibrosis markers (Yamauchi, Hepatol, 1991; 14:244). Since essentially all cell types of the body bear a spectrum of β1 integrins on their surface, an increase of the serum β1 chain can be anticipated in multiple conditions of inflammation, fibrosis, and cell death. Accordingly, this parameter, which correlates with hepatic inflammation, necrosis, and fibrosis, shows little specificity (Yamauchi, Hepatol, 1991; 14:244).

Although significant progress has been made in defining and assaying the connective tissue-derived molecules in blood for the detection and monitoring of organ fibrosis, some major problems still remain:

(1) the molecules are not specific for tissue, organ, or disease;
(2) it is not clearly defined whether the elevated concentration is a sound indicator of stimulated synthesis or originates from perturbations of the catabolic rate of the marker protein in the tissue or circulation;
(3) the routes along which connective tissue-related components reach the blood are largely unknown.

To surmount some of these problems it will be necessary to analyse with more sophisticated methods those domains of the marker protein which clearly differentiate between the pro- or biosynthetic form and the mature (that is, the tissue-deposited) form, respectively. This would allow a clear-cut discrimination between the stimulated biosynthesis and tissue remodelling associated with an activated turnover of the extracellular matrix. Furthermore, it would be desirable to look for organ specificity of the various, almost ubiquitously distributed connective tissue components, but so far there are no indications that liver- or fibrosis-specific matrix molecules exist. It is doubtful whether the determination of those factors in the blood or in the supernatant of in vitro-cultured, blood-derived cells (monocytes), which are known to be potent stimulators of fibrogenesis, will be an alternative approach to a non-invasive monitoring of fibrogenesis. The determination of fibrogenic cytokines, for example of TGF-β (Hayasaka, CCActa, 1996; 244:117), either by immuno- or bioassays, has not proven useful so far in the diagnosis and monitoring of liver fibrogenesis.

There is a need for studies performing the quantitative reverse transcription polymerase chain reaction (**RT-PCR**) in liver biopsy material, quantifying mRNA levels for, for example procollagens I and III, MMP-1, and TGF-β1, that are expected to correlate with circulating fibrosis markers. However, the development of a quantitative RT-PCR from tiny biopsies is fraught with problems including those discussed above. Independent of the biochemical parameter under investigation, future follow-up studies have to be designed that apply improved scores of histological fibrosis.

References

1. Popper H, Davidson CS, Leevy CM, and Schaffner F. The social impact of liver disease. *New England Journal of Medicine*, 1969; 281: 1455–8.
2. Boyer JL and Bianchi L. *Proceedings of the 44th Falk Symposium. Liver cirrhosis.* Lancaster: MTP Press Ltd, 1986.
3. World Health Organization. *World Health Statistics Annual.* Geneva: WHO, 1989.
4. Gressner AM and Bachem MG. Cellular communications and cell–matrix interactions in the pathogenesis of fibroproliferative disease: liver fibrosis as a paradigm. *Annales de Biologie Clinique*, 1994; 52: 205–26.
5. Fausto N, Laird AD, and Webber EM. Liver regeneration 2—role of growth factors and cytokines in hepatic regeneration. *FASEB Journal*, 1995; 9: 1527–36.
6. Gressner AM and Bachem MG. Cellular sources of noncollagenous matrix proteins: role of fat storing cells in fibrogenesis. *Seminars in Liver Disease*, 1990; 10: 30–46.
7. Friedman SL. Cellular sources of collagen and regulation of collagen production in liver. *Seminars in Liver Disease*, 1990; 10: 20–9.
8. Ramadori G. The stellate cell (Ito-cell, fat storing cell, lipocyte, perisinusoidal cell) of the liver. *Virchows Archiv B Cell Pathology*, 1991; 61: 147–58.
9. Friedman SL. The cellular basis of hepatic fibrosis. *New England Journal of Medicine*, 1993; 328: 1828–35.
10. Pinzani M. Hepatic stellate (Ito) cells: expanding roles for a liver-specific pericyte. *Journal of Hepatology*, 1995; 22: 700–6.
11. Pinzani M. Novel insights into the biology and physiology of the Ito cell. *Pharmacology and Therapeutics*, 1995; 66: 387–412.
12. Blomhoff R and Wake K. Perisinusoidal stellate cells of the liver: important roles in retinol metabolism and fibrosis. *FASEB Journal*, 1991; 5: 271–7.
13. Gressner AM. Perisinusoidal lipocytes and fibrogenesis. *Gut*, 1994; 35: 1331–3.
14. Gressner AM and Bachem MG. Molecular mechanisms of liver fibrogenesis—a homage to the role of activated fat-storing cells. *Digestion*, 1995; 56: 335–46.
15. Gressner AM. Activation of proteoglycan synthesis in injured liver—a brief review of molecular and cellular aspects. *European Journal of Clinical Chemistry and Clinical Biochemistry*, 1994; 32: 225–37.
16. Arthur MJP. Matrix degradation in the liver. *Seminars in Liver Disease*, 1990; 10: 47–55.
17. Arthur MJP. Collagenases and liver fibrosis. *Journal of Hepatology*, 1995; 22: 43–8.
18. Rieder H, Meyer-zum-Büschenfelde KH, and Ramadori G. Functional spectrum of sinusoidal endothelial liver cells. Filtration, endocytosis, synthetic capacities and intercellular communication. *Journal of Hepatology*, 1992; 15: 237–50.
19. Smedsrod B, Debleser PJ, Braet F, Lovisetti P, Vanderkerken K, Wisse E, and Geerts A. Cell biology of liver endothelial and Kupffer cells. *Gut*, 1994; 35: 1509–16.
20. Decker K. Biologically active products of stimulated liver macrophages (Kupffer cells). *European Journal of Biochemistry*, 1990; 192: 245–61.
21. Nathan CF. Secretory products of macrophages. *Journal of Clinical Investigation*, 1987; 79: 319–26.
22. Meyeringold W and Eichner W. Platelet-derived growth factor. *Cell Biology International*, 1995; 19: 389–98.
23. Border WA and Noble NA. Mechanisms of disease: transforming growth factor-beta in tissue fibrosis. *New England Journal of Medicine*, 1994; 331: 1286–92.
24. Massagué J. The transforming growth factor-beta family. *Annual Review of Cell Biology*, 1990; 6: 597–641.
25. LaMarre J, Wollenberg GK, Gonias SL, and Hayes MA. Biology of disease: cytokine binding and clearance properties of proteinase-activated alpha2-macroglobulins. *Laboratory Investigations*, 1991; 65: 3–14.
26. Hynes RO. Integrins: versatility, modulation, and signaling in cell adhesion. *Cell*, 1992; 69: 11–25.

27. Juliano RL and Haskill S. Signal transduction from the extracellular matrix. *Journal of Cell Biology*, 1993; 120: 577–85.

28. Ruoslahti E. Integrins. *Journal of Clinical Investigation*, 1991; 87: 1–5.

29. Ruoslahti E. Fibronectin and its receptors. *Annual Review of Biochemistry*, 1988; 57: 375–413.

30. Yamada KM and Miyamoto S. Integrin transmembrane signaling and cytoskeletal control. *Current Opinion on Cell Biology*, 1995; 7: 681–9.

31. Feige JJ and Baird A. Crinopexy: extracellular regulation of growth factor action. *Kidney International*, 1995; 47: S15–18.

32. Border WA and Ruoslahti E. Transforming growth factor-beta in disease—the dark side of tissue repair. *Journal of Clinical Investigation*, 1992; 90: 1–7.

33. Wu J and Danielsson A. Inhibition of hepatic fibrogenesis: a review of pharmacologic candidates. *Scandinavian Journal of Gastroenterology*, 1994; 29: 385–91.

34. Chojkier M and Brenner DA. Therapeutic strategies for hepatic fibrosis. *Hepatology*, 1988; 8: 176–82.

35. Glaser V. Gene transfer to the liver. *Molecular Medicine Today*, 1996; 2: 47–51.

36. Alt M and Caselmann WH. Liver-directed gene therapy: molecular tools and current preclinical and clinical studies. *Journal of Hepatology*, 1995; 23: 746–58.

37. Schuppan D. Connective tissue polypeptides in serum as parameters to monitor antifibrotic treatment in hepatic fibrogenesis. *Journal of Hepatology*, 1991; 13: S17–25.

38. Risteli J. *Connective Tissue in Health and Disease*. Boca Raton: CRC Press, 1990: 61.

39. Plebani M and Burlina A. Biochemical markers of hepatic fibrosis. *Clinical Biochemistry*, 1991; 24: 219–39.

40. Wu JA and Danielsson A. Detection of hepatic fibrogenesis: a review of available techniques. *Scandinavian Journal of Gastroenterology*, 1995; 30: 817–25.

41. Horslev-Petersen K. Circulating extracellular matrix components as markers for connective tissue response to inflammations. *Danish Medical Bulletin*, 1990; 37: 308–29.

42. Danne. *Progress in Basement Membrane Research*. John Libbey, 1988: 315.

43. Guéchot J, Poupon RE, and Poupon R. Serum hyaluronan as a marker of liver fibrosis. *Journal of Hepatology*, 1995; 22: 103–6.

6.2 Cirrhosis: clinical aspects

Serge Erlinger and Jean-Pierre Benhamou

Definition

The word cirrhosis is derived from the Greek *scirrhus*, which means orange or tawny. It was proposed by Laennec in 1826. At the autopsy of a patient with cirrhosis, he observed a liver with a lightly mamellated and wrinkled surface with a greyish-yellow tint. He clearly described the nodules, whose colour was fawn or a 'yellowish russet', bordering on greenish.

Cirrhosis is best defined morphologically as a 'diffuse process characterized by fibrosis and the conversion of normal liver architecture into structurally abnormal nodules'.[1] The nodules lack normal lobular organization and contribute to the loss of the normal architecture. They are often referred to as 'regenerative' or 'hyperplastic': these terms imply concepts of pathogenesis and should not be included in the definition. The process is diffuse and should involve the whole organ: focal lesions, such as focal nodular hyperplasia, do not constitute cirrhosis, even if associated with fibrosis. Fibrosis without nodules, e.g. hepatoportal sclerosis, is not cirrhosis. Nodules without fibrosis, such as in regenerative nodular hyperplasia, are also not cirrhosis. Congenital hepatic fibrosis includes nodules surrounded by fibrosis: however, it is not considered to constitute cirrhosis because in the nodules the lobular architecture is maintained.[1] Hepatocellular necrosis, which is regarded as an important initial lesion in cirrhosis, may no longer be apparent at the time of diagnosis and is not included in most definitions.

Classification

One may classify cirrhosis according to morphological features, aetiology, stage of evolution and activity of the disease, and complications. Pathogenetic terms (for example, posthepatitic) are often difficult to apply because the pathogenesis may no longer be evident at the time of diagnosis, and because they may imply a cause. They should be avoided.

Micronodular cirrhosis

This is defined as a cirrhotic liver in which all or nearly all the nodules are less than 3 mm in diameter.[1] An important feature is the regularity of the nodule size. The nodules are uniformly surrounded by fibrosis septa. Micronodules may occasionally contain portal tracts or efferent veins, but, as a rule, they have lost their normal structures.

Often, a micronodular pattern is seen early in the development of the disease. With progression, larger nodules tend to appear.

Macronodular cirrhosis

This is characterized by septa and nodules that differ considerably in size, with many nodules more than 3 mm in diameter. Some nodules may be several centimetres in diameter. Some of the nodules may contain normal lobules. Some large nodules may contain portal tracts. While the macroscopic diagnosis is usually easy, the histological diagnosis may be difficult on a needle biopsy if the fragment is small and includes only a part of a nodule.

Mixed cirrhosis

This term applies to cirrhosis with micro- and macronodules in approximately equal proportions. In micronodular cirrhosis, the liver is often normal in size or enlarged, particularly when, in addition to cirrhosis, there is steatosis. In macronodular cirrhosis, the size of the liver may be normal, but is often reduced.

Aetiology

We will give here a list of the main causes of cirrhosis only. A more complete description will be found in the chapters dealing with a specific cause. Aetiological diagnosis is usually reached by a combination of epidemiological, clinical, biochemical, immunological, and histological features. In Table 1, the first category includes causes with an established relation to cirrhosis. The most frequent causes worldwide are alcohol and viral hepatitis, types B and C. The second category includes possible causes, with an unproven or debatable relation to cirrhosis. In the third category, the cause of cirrhosis is not known. Cryptogenic cirrhosis is cirrhosis without an identified cause: this should not be regarded as a disease entity, but most probably cirrhosis with several different potentially identifiable causes. At present, there is little evidence that 'cryptogenic' cirrhosis has an autoimmune or viral origin (Greeve, Hepatol, 1993; 17:593).

The role of autoimmunity as an initiating cause of chronic hepatitis and cirrhosis is highly probable. This diagnosis is usually made because there is no other cause, autoantibodies are found in the serum, and other autoimmune diseases may be present. Mycotoxins, of which aflatoxin has been the most studied, may induce cirrhosis in experimental animals. Their role in human cirrhosis is uncertain. Schistosomiasis may cause granulomas and extensive fibrosis. Whether it may also cause cirrhosis without other aetiological factors is not established. Malnutrition, as observed in

Table 1 Aetiology of cirrhosis

1. *Established causes*
Alcohol
Viral hepatitis, type B, B and D, and C
Autoimmune hepatitis
Metabolic disorders:
   Haemochromatosis
   Wilson's disease
   α_1-Antitrypsin deficiency
   Cystic fibrosis
   Glycogen storage diseases
   Galactosaemia
   Hereditary tyrosinaemia
   Hereditary fructose intolerance
   Hereditary haemorrhagic telangiectasia
   Byler's disease
   Abetalipoproteinaemia
   Porphyria
Biliary disease:*
   Extrahepatic biliary obstruction
   Intrahepatic biliary obstruction
   Primary biliary cirrhosis
   Primary sclerosing cholangitis
Venous outflow obstruction:
   Veno-occlusive disease
   Budd–Chiari syndrome
   Cardiac failure
Drugs and toxins
Intestinal bypass for obesity
Sarcoidosis
Syphilis

2. *Unproven causes*
Viral hepatitis, type G
Mycotoxins
Schistosomiasis
Malnutrition
Obesity
Diabetes mellitus

3. *Unknown cause*
Indian childhood cirrhosis
Cryptogenic cirrhosis

* Cirrhosis associated with extrahepatic biliary obstruction or with primary sclerosing cholangitis is usually designated as secondary biliary cirrhosis, as opposed to primary biliary cirrhosis.

Table 2 Estimated prevalence of cirrhosis

Condition	Number of cases per 10^6
Alcoholic (France)	3000[4]
Cryptogenic (Saunders, BMJ 1981; 282:263)	700
Haemochromatosis* (Lindmark, ActaMedScand, 1985; 218)	1000
α_1-Antitrypsin deficiency**	120[24]
Primary biliary cirrhosis (Eriksson, ScaJGastro, 1984; 19:971)	90
Wilson's disease (Sternlieb, NEJM, 1968; 278:352)	5

* Prevalence of homozygotes in the population.
** Prevalence in Scandinavia, assuming that cirrhosis occurs in approx. 20 per cent of homozygotes.
The prevalence of cirrhosis complicating viral hepatitis has not been indicated, because no reliable estimate is available.

kwashiorkor, induces steatosis. It is not proven that it may also cause cirrhosis.

Activity and evolution

Activity is assessed by the degree of liver-cell destruction and inflammatory infiltration. Piecemeal necrosis at the margin of septa, acidophilic bodies, focal necrosis, as well as alcoholic cirrhosis, should be taken into account. It is usual to grade activity as absent, slight, moderate, and severe, but it is important to remember that activity may have been modified by treatment, and that the sample may not be representative. The evolution is assessed by follow-up and serial clinical, biochemical and, whenever possible, histological observations. The complete characterization, in a given patient, should take into account the morphological features, aetiology, activity, complications of the disease, and its evolution.

Epidemiology

The prevalence of cirrhosis in the population is not exactly known. This is, in part, due to the fact that many cases are clinically silent. Up to 30 or even 40 per cent of cases may be discovered at autopsy, [2,3] and an unknown proportion remains undetected.

The prevalence of alcoholic cirrhosis in France has been estimated as approximately $3000/10^6$ population.[4] It is three times higher in men ($4500/10^6$) than in women ($1500/10^6$). In men over 30 years who drink more than 80 g of alcohol per day, and in women who drink more than 40 g of alcohol per day, it is about $25\,000/10^6$. According to a British study, the annual incidence of alcoholic cirrhosis in west Birmingham increased from $56/10^6$ in 1960, to $153/10^6$ in 1974 (Saunders, BMJ, 1981; 282:263). In the same period, the annual incidence of cryptogenic cirrhosis remained stable at approximately $30–40/10^6$ and that of cirrhosis of all other causes at about $10/10^6$. From 1981 to 1985, the annual incidence of alcoholic cirrhosis in Denmark was $190/10^6$ in men and $85/10^6$ in women, and that of non-alcoholic, non-biliary cirrhosis (i.e., viral and cryptogenic) was $110/10^6$ in men and $82/10^6$ in women (Almdal, Hepatol, 1991; 13:650). There may be marked geographical differences in incidence from one country to the other, or even between different regions in the same country (Marubini, in Tygstrup N, Orlandi F, eds. *Cirrhosis of the liver.* Amsterdam: Elsevier, 1987; 275). Moreover, the proportion of alcoholic and non-alcoholic cirrhosis differs from one country to the other, the prevalence of alcoholic cirrhosis being generally highest in wine-producing countries.

The age-standardized mortality rates due to cirrhosis in France increased between 1945 and 1967 from $100/10^6$ to $400/10^6$ per year in men (corresponding figures in women were $40/10^6$ per year in 1945, and $150/10^6$ per year in 1967). These rates have been decreasing since 1967 by approximately 2 per cent per year (Copperé, GastrClinBiol, 1986; 10:468).

For comparison, the estimated prevalence for alcoholic cirrhosis and several other causes of cirrhosis are indicated in Table 2. Detailed epidemiological data for specific causes will be discussed in the corresponding chapters.

Clinical features

Compensated cirrhosis

Clinically, cirrhosis may develop without giving rise to any symptom. As the lesion progresses, it has two major consequences, hepatic failure and portal hypertension, which are responsible for the main complications of cirrhosis, jaundice, encephalopathy, ascites, and digestive haemorrhage. Cirrhosis without any of these complications may be designated as compensated cirrhosis. Cirrhosis with one or several of these complications is usually referred to as decompensated cirrhosis.

Compensated cirrhosis is clinically latent and may be discovered at a routine clinical examination or biochemical screening, or during an abdominal operation for another condition, or at autopsy; 30 to 40 per cent of cases of cirrhosis may be asymptomatic.[2] In other cases, cirrhosis may be suspected because of low-grade fever or general deterioration with asthenia, anorexia or weight loss, or because of anaemia, thrombocytopenia or leucopenia due to hypersplenism.

Decompensated cirrhosis

The most frequent manifestations of decompensated cirrhosis are ascites, jaundice, hepatic encephalopathy, and gastrointestinal haemorrhage. These and other manifestations are discussed next.

Ascites

The pathophysiology, clinical manifestations, complications, and therapy of ascites are discussed in detail in Section 8. Ascites develops progressively and attracts attention when it becomes voluminous. It is frequently associated with oedema of the legs. It is painless, except when the abdomen is highly distended, or when there is bacterial peritonitis. Occasionally, ascites may be discovered because of a inguinal or umbilical hernia. Ascites may appear after abdominal surgery. When ascites is voluminous it contributes to anorexia, probably because of compression of abdominal viscera.

In about 5 to 10 per cent of cases, ascites is associated with pleural effusions.[5] Most effusions (approximately 70 per cent) are located on the right, but they may occur on both sides, or even only on the left. They are due to direct passage of ascitic fluid from the abdomen into the pleural cavity through defects in the diaphragm.[6] Sometimes a pleural effusion is present without any detectable ascites (Rubinstein, Gastro, 1985; 88:188), probably because the negative intrathoracic pressure favours the net transport of fluid from the peritoneal cavity into the pleural cavity at a rate equal to its rate of production. The diagnosis of ascites is easy when it is abundant. A small amount of fluid is best recognized by ultrasonography (or CT). Paracentesis should always be performed for protein determination, a red and white cell count, and aerobic and anaerobic cultures.

Jaundice

Jaundice in cirrhosis is due primarily to failure of the liver cell to excrete bilirubin. It is usually the result of mixed, conjugated and unconjugated, hyperbilirubinaemia, with a predominance of conjugated bilirubin. It is associated with dark urine and bilirubinuria. Jaundice is always a manifestation of severe liver dysfunction. However, several factors not directly related to hepatocellular damage may contribute to hyperbilirubinaemia and jaundice in a cirrhotic patient: the most frequent are (a) hyperhaemolysis, which increases the bilirubin load to the liver and contributes to unconjugated hyperbilirubinaemia; (b) functional renal failure in patients with ascites (the so-called hepatorenal syndrome), which decreases bilirubin excretion by the kidney and contributes to conjugated hyperbilirubinaemia; (c) bacterial infections (for example, bacterial peritonitis, or urinary infection), which may induce cholestasis and also contribute to conjugated hyperbilirubinaemia. Correction of these factors, whenever possible, will decrease the intensity of jaundice. In a patient with deep jaundice, alcoholic cirrhosis, and none of these contributing factors, the first diagnosis to be considered is alcoholic hepatitis. Finally, a patient with cirrhosis may have a coincidental cause of jaundice—acute viral hepatitis—or biliary obstruction due to a stone in the common bile duct, a tumour, or chronic pancreatitis.

Hepatic encephalopathy

The pathophysiology, symptoms, diagnosis, and therapy of hepatic encephalopathy are discussed in Section 9. Encephalopathy occurs either spontaneously or as a consequence of a precipitating factor. The most common precipitating factors are a gastrointestinal haemorrhage, a bacterial infection or the administration of some drugs, such as diuretics in patients with ascites, electrolyte disturbances, and hyperazotaemia, or neurosedatives, especially of the benzodiazepine family. Neurosedatives should always be given with extreme caution to a cirrhotic patient. Valproic acid (Zimmerman, Hepatol, 1982; 2:591) and propranolol (Tarver, BMJ, 1983; 287: 585; Wiesner, JClinGastro, 1986; 8:74) have also been incriminated, but the evidence is mostly circumstantial.

Several clinical classifications of encephalopathy are used. A convenient one distinguishes: stage 1, characterized by asterixis; stage 2, characterized by disorientation (confusion); stage 3, characterized by stupor or arousable coma; and stage 4, characterized by deep coma.[7] Neither these clinical manifestations nor the associated electroencephalographic changes have any specificity: they all may be observed in metabolic encephalopathy (or coma) of other causes.

Digestive haemorrhage

Digestive haemorrhage is a severe complication of cirrhosis and may be life-threatening. It is usually the consequence of the rupture of oesophageal or gastric varices. The pathogenesis, medical, and surgical management are discussed in Section 7. A digestive haemorrhage may also be due to acute erosions (ulcerations) of the gastric mucosa, or as a consequence of a gastropathy secondary to portal hypertension.[8] It may also be due to a gastric or duodenal ulcer. Emergency endoscopy is mandatory as soon as possible after the beginning of the bleeding episode to determine the most likely cause of the haemorrhage.

General deterioration

This is the most common clinical feature of cirrhosis. Anorexia, weight loss, weakness, and fatiguability are the chief complaints. Anorexia may be exaggerated by ascites. Weight loss may be masked by accumulation of ascitic fluid or oedema. Muscle wasting may be evident at clinical examination, in spite of a normal, or even increased, weight.

Fever: bacterial infections

Fever is frequent.[9] It is usually low-grade and continuous, in the range of 38 to 38.5°C. In alcoholic cirrhosis, fever is often due to alcoholic hepatitis (see Section 14). The most important problem when fever is present is to determine whether it is due to cirrhosis itself, or to an associated infection. Bacterial infections are frequent in cirrhosis, because of multiple defects in immune defence (Runyon JHepatol, 1993; 18:271) and macrophage function (Gomez, NEJM, 1994; 331:1122). The prevalence of infection in patients admitted to hospital with cirrhosis is 30 to 40 per cent. Community-acquired infections seem more frequent than nosocomial. The most frequent infections are bacterial peritonitis when ascites is present, urinary infection, upper respiratory or bronchopulmonary infection, and cutaneous infection (Caly, JHepatol, 1993; 18:353). The mouth should also be carefully examined for dental infection. Ascitic fluid (and/or pleural fluid if any) and urine cultures should be obtained in all cases.

Infection is an important cause of deterioration of the patient, and of death during a hospital admission: the mortality of an infected cirrhotic patient may be as high as 30 per cent (Caly, JHepatol, 1993; 18:353). When infection is suspected (i.e., ascitic-fluid neutrophil count > 250/mm^3, fever, pyuria), non-nephrotoxic antibiotics should be given empirically. Prophylactic oral quinolones should be used for prevention of infection (a) after a first episode of bacterial peritonitis, (b) when protein concentration in ascitic fluid is lower than 10 g/l, suggesting a high risk of infection, and (c) after a variceal haemorrhage (Runyon, JHepatol, 1993; 18:271).

Haematological complications

Anaemia

Anaemia is extremely frequent in decompensated cirrhosis. Its pathogenesis is often complex and includes decreased bone-marrow production and increased peripheral destruction. Anaemia is usually macrocytic, but may be microcytic and hypochromic after gastro-intestinal blood loss. Factors other than blood loss and iron deficiency that may contribute to anaemia are: (a) folate deficiency; (b) haemolysis, especially in advanced cirrhosis [haemolysis is a consequence of alterations of the erythrocyte membrane and increased red-cell fragility; in severe cases this causes deformities of red cells visible by optical microscopy, and the occurrence of echinocytes or acanthocytes (see Section 24)]; (c) hypersplenism, or sequestration of red cells in the spleen when there is splenomegaly. Anaemia may be associated with thrombocytopenia and leucopenia.

Impaired coagulation

Impaired coagulation is due to a decreased activity of coagulation factors synthesized by the liver, to fibrinolysis, to disseminated intravascular coagulation, and to thrombocytopenia (see Section 24). When moderate, impaired coagulation may have no clinical consequence. When severe, it may be responsible for spontaneous ecchymoses, gingival haemorrhage, nasal haemorrhage, or purpura. A thorough coagulation study must be carried out before a potentially haemorrhagic procedure, such as a liver biopsy.

Endocrine complications

Endocrine abnormalities occur, presumably as a consequence of the failure of the liver to conjugate or metabolize hormones, because of liver-cell failure or portal–systemic shunts, or both. Alcohol may also induce endocrine changes, and, in an alcoholic cirrhotic, it may be difficult to determine whether alcohol or cirrhosis is the cause.

Feminization

Feminization is manifested by gynaecomastia, spider angioma, palmar erythema, and changes in the pattern of body hair. It is thought to be due to increased conversion of androgenic steroids into oestrogens in peripheral tissues (skin, adipose tissue, muscle, bone). Thus, plasma oestradiol and oestrone may be normal or only moderately elevated.[10] Spironolactone may induce gynaecomastia by decreasing serum testosterone and reducing hepatic androgen-receptor activity (Francavilla, Gastro, 1987; 92:203).

Hypogonadism

Hypogonadism is manifested in men by testicular atrophy, loss of libido, impotence, and a high prevalence of infertility. Impotence is very common. It will not be commonly volunteered by the patient. There is no satisfactory therapy. It may improve with improvement of liver function. Hypogonadism is thought to be due to a direct effect of alcohol, rather than a consequence of liver disease itself.[11] In alcoholics, there is frequently a decrease in plasma testosterone, an increase in sex hormone-binding globulin, with, as a result, a decrease in the unbound testosterone in plasma.[10] There is also evidence for hypothalamic and pituitary defects.

In women, oligomenorrhoea, amenorrhoea, and sterility are frequent. Plasma oestradiol and progesterone are reduced.[10] Successful pregnancies have been achieved in cirrhotic patients.[12]

Diabetes

The prevalence of diabetes is increased in patients with cirrhosis.[13] It is manifested by hyperglycaemia, glucose intolerance, mild glycosuria, hyperinsulinaemia, and peripheral insulin resistance. It is often discovered incidentally during the evaluation of decompensated cirrhosis. In most cases, it can be treated by diet; occasionally, it requires oral agents and very occasionally insulin.

The diabetes in cirrhosis is characterized by hyperinsulinaemia and hyperglucagonaemia.[14] Hyperinsulinaemia is thought to result from decreased catabolism of insulin by the liver. Increased insulin secretion may also contribute (see Section 24).

Hypoglycaemia

Hypoglycaemia may be observed in advanced cirrhosis with severe hepatocellular failure. It may also be due to bacterial infection, to excessive alcohol consumption (Arky, NEJM, 1966; 274:426), or to hepatocellular carcinoma, because of increased glucose consumption by the tumour (McFazdean, AmJMed, 1969; 47:220).

Pulmonary complications (see Chapter 24.1)

Dyspnoea and lung abnormalities: hepatopulmonary syndrome

Dyspnoea is rare in cirrhosis, except when ascites or pleural effusion are present. It may also suggest pulmonary hypertension (see below). Frank cyanosis is rare. Clubbing of the fingers is frequent. These symptoms are the consequence of oxygen desaturation (Rodman, NEJM, 1960; 260:73).

Decreased arterial oxygen partial pressure is observed in about 50 per cent of decompensated cirrhotic patients, with Po_2 in the range 60 to 70 mmHg. Contributing factors are multiple and include: (a) pulmonary arteriovenous anastomoses, either microscopic (Berthelot, NEJM, 1966; 274:291), or involving larger vessels; (b) an altered ventilation–perfusion relation, especially in patients with ascites or pleural effusions; (c) a reduced pulmonary diffusing capacity, sometimes due to interstitial oedema or to dilatation of precapillary pulmonary vessels (Agusti, JHepatol, 1990; 10:251); (d) decreased oxygen affinity of red cells.[7]

The pulmonary circulation is usually markedly dilated in cirrhosis. This vasodilatation seems to be due to a loss of vascular tone, with poor reactivity to hypoxia. These functional abnormalities have been designated as the 'hepatopulmonary' syndrome (Agusti, JHepatol, 1990; 10:251; Cadranel, GastrClinBiol, 1994; 18:224). They seem to be best diagnosed by contrast echocardiography (Abrams, Gastro, 1995; 109:1283). Their precise pathophysiology is not known. Since most of the abnormalities are functional rather than organic, they should not be considered as a contraindication to liver transplantation (Krowka, Hepatol, 1990; 11:138; Krowka, Gastro, 1995; 109:1009). Transjugular intrahepatic portosystemic shunts may also improve hypoxaemia (Riegler, Gastro, 1995; 109:978).

Pulmonary hypertension

Pulmonary hypertension occurs in about 1 per cent of cirrhotic patients.[15] It is probably more prevalent after surgical portacaval shunts.[15,16] It is manifested by dyspnoea, syncope, precordial pain, and, rarely, haemoptysis. Accentuation of the pulmonic second sound, a murmur along the left lower sternal border, cardiac enlargement on radiographic examination, with right ventricular hypertrophy, are highly suggestive of the diagnosis. This should be confirmed by cardiac catheterization.

The pathogenesis is not established: the passing of emboli or humoral vasoconstrictors from the portal to the systemic and then to the pulmonary circulation has been suggested.[16] This could explain why pulmonary hypertension appears more prevalent after portacaval anastomosis.

Cardiac complications (see Chapter 24.1)

About 30 to 60 per cent of cirrhotic patients develop a circulatory hyperdynamic state that is characterized by an increase in cardiac output and a decrease in peripheral resistance.[17] These changes increase with exercise. Exercise capacity is decreased (Grose, JHepatol, 1995; 22:326) and there is a left ventricular dysfunction induced by exercise. Clinically, bounding pulses, warm hands, and capillary pulsations may be observed. Tachycardia and a moderate decrease in diastolic pressure are usual. The pathogenesis is not

fully elucidated. The decreased vascular resistance could be due to decreased arteriolar sensitivity to catecholamines. In cirrhosis, there is an increased catecholamine concentration in peripheral blood.[18] The mechanism of these abnormalities is not known. In spite of increased cardiac output, systemic blood pressure is often slightly decreased, because of the low systemic resistance. However, hypertension may occur (Heikal, EurJGastroHepatol, 1993; 5:463).

Gallstones (see Chapter 22.4)

The prevalence of gallstones is increased in cirrhosis.[19,21] This is due to an increase in pigment stones, not cholesterol stones. Gallbladder bile in cirrhotics is not saturated with cholesterol and cholesterol gallstones are rare. The increased prevalence of pigment stones may be related to hyperhaemolysis and increased excretion of bile pigments. It is often stated that gallstones in cirrhotic patients cause fewer complications than cholesterol gallstones in non-cirrhotic people; in particular, biliary obstruction appears less frequent (Dunnington, AnnSurg, 1987; 205:226). This has not been adequately documented.

Peptic ulcer (see Chapter 24.5)

The prevalence of peptic ulcer is reportedly higher in cirrhotics than in the general population.[2,22] Ulcer is observed in 10 to 15 per cent of cirrhotic patients. The life-time prevalence may be as high as 24 per cent (Siringo, JHepatol, 1995; 22:633). The annual incidence rate of ulcer is 4.3 per cent when studied prospectively by endoscopy (Siringo, JHepatol, 1995; 22:633). Ulcers are usually asymptomatic. However, the complication rate is 20 to 40 per cent. In contrast to an earlier belief, the prevalence is not greater after surgical portacaval shunt.[23] The exact mechanism of this increased prevalence of peptic ulcer is not known. In particular, any association with *Helicobacter pylori* infection has not been adequately studied.

Hepatocellular carcinoma

Hepatocellular carcinoma occurs in 10 to 25 per cent of cirrhotic patients, particularly in cirrhosis due to hepatitis B and hepatitis C virus infections, haemochromatosis, cirrhosis due to α_1-antitrypsin deficiency,[24] and alcoholic cirrhosis. It is rare in primary biliary cirrhosis and in cirrhosis due to autoimmune hepatitis. In cirrhosis due to hepatitis B virus infection, the annual incidence of hepatocellular carcinoma ranges from 1 to 1.5 per cent to approximately 5 per cent in Western patients (Colombo, NEJM, 1991; 325:675; Pateron, JHepatol, 1994; 20:65; Fattovich, Hepatol, 1995; 21:77) and 2 to 3 per cent in patients in the Far East (Liaw, Liver, 1989; 9:235). In Western patients, the incidence of hepatocellular carcinoma complicating alcoholic cirrhosis is similar to that observed in viral cirrhosis (Colombo, NEJM, 1991; 325:675).

Most authorities recommend a detection programme in patients with compensated cirrhosis who could benefit from a surgical resection of the tumour. This programme includes ultrasonographic examination of the liver and measurement of serum α_1-fetoprotein at least every 6 months. However, screening every 6 months may not be sufficient (Pateron, JHepatol, 1994; 20:65). In Japan, some authorities favour detection every 3 months, because of a short doubling time of cancer foci in some patients (Oka, Hepatol, 1990; 12:680; Okuda, Cancer, 1985; 56:918). It has not been demonstrated that such screening programmes significantly prolong survival (Collier, Hepatol, 1998; 27:273).

The pathogenesis, clinical features, diagnosis, and treatment of hepatocellular carcinoma are discussed in Section 21.

Diagnosis
Clinical

The diagnosis of cirrhosis may often be suspected clinically. At physical examination, the liver is enlarged, with firm edges, sometimes tender, although it may sometimes be normal or decreased in size. A palpable splenomegaly is found in 20 to 60 per cent of cases. Liver and spleen palpation are essential, but may be difficult because of thickness of abdominal wall, or ascites. Many clinical symptoms of cirrhosis are found on the skin.

Spider angioma (see Section 4)

Spider angioma[25] are most frequently observed on the vascular territory of the superior vena cava (face, upper limbs, hands and fingers, thorax), rarely on the upper part of the abdomen. They consist of a central arteriole surrounded by numerous small vessels resembling a spider's legs (see Plate 4, Section 4). Their diameter ranges from 1 to 10 mm. When large enough, they may be seen to pulsate. Pressure on the central arteriole causes disappearance of the lesion. They may decrease in size or disappear with improvement of hepatic function. They are probably the result of hormonal changes, especially in oestrogen metabolism, due to liver-cell failure.

Spider angiomas may also be observed transiently in acute viral hepatitis, in normal individuals (usually less than five in number), occasionally in rheumatoid arthritis, during oestrogen treatment, and during pregnancy (they appear during the second trimester, and disappear about 2 months after delivery). They should not be confused with telangiectasia (such as seen in hereditary haemorrhagic telangiectasia), Campbell de Morgan spots (bright red spots appearing in normal persons after the age of 30), or venous stars.

Palmar erythema (see Section 4)

Palmar erythema is an exaggeration of the normal speckled mottling of the palm. It mostly occurs on the thenar and hypothenar eminencies, pulps of fingers, and circumungueal areas in the dorsum of the fingers. It usually spares the central part of the palm. The soles of the feet may be similarly affected. It may be associated with spider angioma. It is also believed to be due to impaired oestrogen metabolism. It may be observed in rheumatoid arthritis, pregnancy, chronic febrile diseases, leukaemia, and thyrotoxicosis.

White nails (see Section 4)

White nails are due to a white opacity of the nailbed that replaces the normal pink colour of the nail. A small, pink zone is left at the top of the nail and the lunula may disappear.

Finger clubbing (see Section 4)

Finger clubbing is frequent and related to oxygen desaturation (see above). It may be associated with hypertrophic osteoarthropathy.

Dupuytren's contracture (see Section 4)

Dupuytren's contracture in cirrhosis is not a consequence of liver-cell failure, but is associated with alcoholism.

Muscle cramps

Muscle cramps (painful involuntary contractions of skeletal muscle) are more frequent in cirrhosis than in the general population. They occur frequently at rest, at night, are asymmetrical, and affect the muscles of legs and feet. They are related to the duration of the disease and the severity of liver function impairment (Hepatol, 1996; 23:264). They seem to be associated with the decrease in 'effective' plasma volume and may be corrected by weekly intravenous albumin infusions (Hepatol, 1996; 23:264).

Foetor hepaticus (see Section 4)

Foetor hepaticus is a sweetish smell of the breath, best perceived when entering the patient's room. It occurs in patients with severe liver-cell failure, or in those with extensive collateral circulation. It is presumably of intestinal origin and becomes less intense after treatment with broad-spectrum antibiotics. It is frequently associated with hepatic encephalopathy.

Collateral circulation (see Section 4)

Collateral circulation on the abdominal wall develops because of portal hypertension. Portal blood is deviated via paraumbilical veins to the umbilicus, where it reaches collaterals of the caval system. Collateral circulation develops predominantly above the umbilicus. Blood flows away from the umbilicus. In rare cases, prominent collateral veins radiate from and around the umbilicus. A murmur may be heard and a thrill may be felt. A prominent periumbilical circulation suggests the development of a large paraumbilical or umbilical vein from the left portal branch: this is designated as the Cruveilhier–Baumgarten syndrome. It is best diagnosed at ultrasonography. In some patients, collateral circulation may develop elsewhere in the body, for example in the flanks or in the back, because of a congenital venous anomaly or a previous surgical intervention.

Biochemical investigation

Biochemical tests considered to be useful in cirrhosis are serum bilirubin (conjugated and unconjugated), alanine and aspartate aminotransferases, alkaline phosphatase, γ-glutamyl transferase, serum proteins and protein fractionation, immunoglobulin concentration, and prothrombin time. A detailed discussion of these tests in liver diseases is found in Section 5. In the anicteric cirrhotic patient, serum bilirubin is normal or below 30 μmol/l.

Aminotransferases

Aminotransferases are moderately elevated, usually less than five times the upper normal limit. Aspartate aminotransferase (**AST**) is more elevated than alanine aminotransferase (**ALT**). AST is elevated in approximately 90 per cent of cases, and ALT in 65 per cent of cases.[26] Thus, a normal value does not exclude the diagnosis. In a patient with non-alcoholic chronic liver disease, a AST–ALT ratio above 1 strongly suggests the presence of cirrhosis, rather than chronic hepatitis.[27] In alcoholic liver disease, the AST–ALT ratio is usually above 1, irrespective of the presence of cirrhosis.

γ-Glutamyl transferase

γ-Glutamyl transferase is thought to be a more sensitive test than aminotransferases or alkaline phosphatase in patients suspected to have chronic liver disease. However, the specificity is poor when used alone. It is particularly useful in alcoholic cirrhosis: a γ-glutamyl transferase disproportionately elevated compared with AST, ALT, or alkaline phosphatase is suggestive of alcohol abuse, even in a patient without histological advanced liver disease.[28] A γ-glutamyl transferase:alkaline phosphatase ratio greater than 2.5 is highly suspicious of alcohol abuse.[29] Its usefulness in the diagnosis of hepatocellular carcinoma in patients with cirrhosis has not been adequately evaluated.

Alkaline phosphatase

Alkaline phosphatase is elevated in nearly 70 per cent of cases of cirrhosis. It is usually less than three times the upper limit of normal. A markedly elevated alkaline phosphatase may indicate hepatocellular carcinoma, or suggest a diagnosis of primary biliary cirrhosis or primary sclerosing cholangitis.

Serum albumin concentration

Serum albumin concentration is usually decreased. The origin of hypoalbuminaemia is multifactorial and includes decreased synthesis, haemodilution, and possibly decreased secretion. When marked, hypoalbuminaemia contributes to the formation of ascites and oedema.

Serum globulin

Serum globulins are increased. This is related to a polyclonal increase in immunoglobulins. IgA is preferentially increased in alcoholic cirrhosis: this results in a bridging of the gap between β- and γ-globulins in conventional electrophoresis. IgG is preferentially increased in cryptogenic cirrhosis and cirrhosis due to autoimmune or (to a lesser extent) viral hepatitis. IgM is preferentially increased in primary biliary cirrhosis.

Prothrombin time

Determination of the prothrombin time is useful before a liver biopsy, which should not be performed when prothrombin concentration is below 50 per cent of normal. Albumin and prothrombin time are useful diagnostic indices and are used to estimate liver function quantitatively (see below).

In addition to conventional biochemical tests, the aetiological investigation of a cirrhotic patient should include tests for hepatitis B, C, and D (delta) virus markers, a search for autoantibodies (mitochondrial, nuclear, smooth muscle, liver–kidney microsomes types 1 and 2) (see Chapter 5.3), serum iron and transferrin concentrations and saturation, serum copper and caeruloplasmin concentrations and urinary copper excretion, and α_1-antitrypsin determination. Detailed investigations aimed at determining the cause will be found in the chapters dealing with the specific causes. Finally, α-fetoprotein should be measured for screening of hepatocellular carcinoma.

Imaging techniques

Ultrasonography

Ultrasonography is used routinely in the evaluation of a cirrhotic patient. Its major indication is the early detection of hepatocellular carcinoma. Tumours of more than 2 cm in diameter are detected with a good sensitivity. Tumours appear usually as nodules of decreased, subnormal, or rarely increased echogenicity. Some 'hyperplastic' or 'regenerative' benign nodules may give a similar appearance.[30] Nodules smaller than 2 cm, or those located at the superior part of the liver (an area particularly difficult to examine by ultrasonography), may escape detection, as may diffuse, infiltrative tumours. The presence of thrombosis of the portal vein or of one of its main branches is a strong argument in support of the diagnosis.

A typical nodule at ultrasonography associated with an α-fetoprotein concentration above 300 ng/ml is practically diagnostic of hepatocellular carcinoma. In such cases, liver biopsy should not be performed, because of the risk of spread of the tumour, particularly at the puncture site (Hamazaki, Hepatogast, 1995; 42:601). In doubtful cases, whenever possible, a liver biopsy guided by ultrasonography should be performed to obtain a histological confirmation.

Apart from detection of hepatocellular carcinoma, ultrasonography is useful in assessing liver size and shape, in the diagnosis of steatosis associated with cirrhosis, in detecting ascites, and in evaluating portal hypertension. In cirrhosis, the shape of the liver is usually modified, with hypertrophy of the left lobe (segments II and III) and atrophy of the right lobe (mainly the posterior sector, or segments VI and VII). Hypertrophy of the Spigel lobe (or segment I) is also common. The margins of the liver may appear finely nodular, especially when ascites is present and enhances the contrast. The echogenicity of the liver parenchyma is increased and slightly irregular. This is probably related to fat and/or fibrosis, and simply indicates the presence of a diffuse liver disease: it is not specific for cirrhosis.[31] Echographic signs of portal hypertension are as follows.

1. An increased diameter of the portal vein: a diameter of more than 15 mm is diagnostic of portal hypertension with a specificity of 100 per cent and a sensitivity of about 50 per cent.
2. The presence of collateral veins: these are detectable in about 90 per cent of patients with portal hypertension; they are located mostly in the coronary vein, an umbilical or, more frequently, a paraumbilical vein, and in the splenic area territory, where they form splenorenal anastomoses.
3. Splenomegaly, which is not specific (see Section 4).

The gallbladder is often large (Finet, GastroenterolClinBiol, 1991; 15:678) and hypotonic; its wall is thickened because of ascites, dilatation of gallbladder veins, or portal hypertension; gallstones are observed in 20 to 30 per cent of cirrhotic patients (see above).

Computed tomography (CT)

CT is usually *not* useful in the evaluation of a cirrhotic patient, except when hepatocellular carcinoma is suspected. Abnormalities in size and shape are similar to those observed at ultrasonography (see Section 4). Density is homo- or heterogeneous. Steatosis produces areas of hypodensity. The sensitivity of CT for the diagnosis of hepatocellular carcinoma is similar to that of ultrasonography. Usually, a carcinoma appears as nodular zones of hypodensity. The nodules may be heterogeneous, probably because of necrotic areas. Haemorrhage in the tumours may produce areas of hyperdensity. Calcifications are found in 5 to 25 per cent of cases. After infusion of contrast agent, the tumour remains usually hypodense.

A rapid injection technique (angioscan) shows prominent arterial vascularization. Portal vein thrombosis can be detected by direct visualization of the thrombus, and hypodense areas in the liver with a lobar distribution, due to abnormal liver perfusion. CT after intra-arterial injection of lipiodol is probably more accurate than ultrasonography in determining the extension of the tumour before surgical resection (see below). If ultrasonography has established that the tumour cannot be removed surgically, CT is unnecessary.

CT is less sensitive and less specific than ultrasonography in the evaluation of portal hypertension.

Arteriography

Arteriography is usually *not* useful in the diagnosis of cirrhosis. It has two main indications: (i) the study of the anatomy of hepatic vessels before a surgical procedure, especially a liver transplantation; (ii) the evaluation of the extension of a hepatocellular carcinoma detected by ultrasonography. In this case, an intra-arterial injection of ultrafluid lipiodol is given during the arteriography and a CT scan obtained 2 to 3 weeks later. Foci of hepatocellular carcinoma retain lipiodol and appear as hyperdense areas.[32]

When arteries are visualized, their branches have a tortuous, 'corkscrew' appearance. Arteriography may help to differentiate hepatocellular carcinoma from a cirrhotic nodule. The venous phase allows visualization of the portal system and of the portacaval collateral circulation. Demonstration of a large, spontaneous, splenorenal shunt may explain the occurrence of hepatic encephalopathy in some patients (Takashi, JHepatol, 1985; 1:467).

Endoscopy

The diagnosis of oesophageal varices is routinely made by endoscopy. Endoscopic examination can best determine the existence of the varices, their size and extent, and their appearance. Grading of the varices is important since the risk of bleeding increases with their size,[33,34] and is high when mucosal abnormalities are present.[35] Examination of the stomach and duodenum is also important to detect the gastropathy of portal hypertension (Triger, JHepatol, 1989; 8:267)[8,36] or an associated ulcer. Upper gastrointestinal endoscopy should always be performed when the diagnosis of cirrhosis has been established because: (a) when medium-sized or large varices are present, prophylaxis of haemorrhage with β-blocking agents should be recommended whenever possible;[37] (b) gastric or duodenal ulcers are often asymptomatic.

Peritoneoscopy

Peritoneoscopy is used in some centres (see Section 5). However, many do not consider it necessary for the evaluation of a cirrhotic patient. It may help, in some cases, to establish the diagnosis when liver biopsy is not contributive, either because the fragment is too small for correct interpretation, or when the histological evidence of cirrhosis is not conclusive. This is sometimes the case in macronodular cirrhosis, which is easily diagnosed by direct visualization.

Other techniques

Radioisotopic scans

Radioisotopic scans can be obtained with a [^{99}Te^m]sulphur colloid, which is taken up by macrophages. It shows the size and shape of the liver, and the size of the spleen. In cirrhosis, uptake of the colloid by the liver is heterogeneous, the spleen is enlarged, and splenic uptake is increased (see Section 5). Most of the information, however, can be obtained by ultrasonography, which is less expensive and does not require administration of radioactivity. The technique has been abandoned for this purpose in most centres.

Magnetic resonance imaging (MRI)

MRI is currently being evaluated and has not yet been applied to large numbers of patients in order to determine its exact usefulness in cirrhosis. The main indications being evaluated, at present, are: (a) the quantification and follow-up of iron overload in haemochromatosis (Radiology, 1994; 193:533); (b) the differential diagnosis between a benign nodule and a small hepatocellular carcinoma (less than 3 cm in diameter). Hypervascularity of the nodule is a strong argument for malignancy (Radiology, 1991; 178:493); MRI after injection of a contrast agent, such as gadolinium, is useful to detect hypervascularity of the nodules.

Liver biopsy

Liver biopsy is necessary to prove the diagnosis of cirrhosis. It is simple, inexpensive, generally easily accepted by the patient, and safe. Most biopsy specimens are taken by the lateral percutaneous approach. When a localized lesion is suspected, an approach through the epigastrium may be preferred. Ultrasonography and CT are increasingly used to guide the biopsy needle. The transvenous route by jugular and hepatic vein catheterization is used when poor coagulation precludes the percutaneous route.[38] The tissue sample is usually adequate for diagnosis. A biopsy may also be obtained at laparoscopy or laparotomy. Details of these techniques and their indications, particularly as a function of coagulation problems, as well as their complications, are discussed in Section 5. The patient should always be properly informed of the possibility of complications, mostly intraperitoneal haemorrhage.

In cirrhosis, biopsy is useful in establishing the type and severity, and the degree of activity. It may be helpful in determining the cause. The presence of fat is suggestive of alcoholism, diabetes, and obesity; it is also observed with drugs such as perhexiline maleate. Ground-glass hepatocytes are observed in chronic infection with the hepatitis B virus. Bile-duct damage is observed in primary biliary cirrhosis and periductal fibrosis suggests primary sclerosing cholangitis. In both conditions, a prominent ductular proliferation may be observed. Accumulation of iron, when marked, suggests haemochromatosis. α_1-Antitrypsin globules should always be looked for in cirrhosis of uncertain aetiology, and, when suspected, confirmed by specific immunocytochemical staining. Dilatation of sinusoids and congestion is observed in the Budd–Chiari syndrome and cardiac failure or constrictive pericarditis. Biopsy is often essential in the diagnosis of hepatocellular carcinoma complicating cirrhosis.

The major problem in interpretation of biopsy in cirrhosis is that of sampling error. Biopsy is more reliable in micronodular cirrhosis, where nodules less than 3 mm in diameter are easily recognized. It may be much more difficult to recognize macronodular cirrhosis, where a sample of a large nodule may appear normal. Special stains, such as for reticulin, are necessary to detect subtle changes in lobular architecture. It should be stressed again that not all samples are easily classified as micronodular or macronodular cirrhosis, and that mixed forms are frequent.

Finally, in cirrhosis, the sample is often fragmented: fragmentation, by itself, may be an indication that cirrhosis is present.

Differential diagnosis

In compensated cirrhosis, the main problem is to distinguish cirrhosis from other chronic liver diseases producing abnormalities of liver function or portal hypertension.

Chronic hepatitis of all causes (including virus B or C infections, autoimmune hepatitis, Wilson's disease, α_1-antitrypsin deficiency, or drug-induced chronic hepatitis) may induce abnormalities in liver function tests similar to those of cirrhosis. In a chronic carrier of hepatitis B surface antigen (HBsAg), it is sometimes impossible to predict whether or not cirrhosis is present on the basis of clinical examination and liver function tests alone. Conditions associated with extrahepatic portal vein thrombosis or presinusoidal intrahepatic portal hypertension may also mimic cirrhosis. These include congenital hepatic fibrosis, hepatoportal sclerosis, hepatic schistosomiasis, and regenerative nodular hyperplasia.[39] Ultrasonography will usually detect obstruction of the portal vein with a good sensitivity. If the portal vein is patent, the intrahepatic causes should be considered. A liver biopsy is necessary.

In decompensated cirrhosis, depending on the patient's presentation, the causes of jaundice (Section 2), hepatic encephalopathy (Section 9), gastrointestinal bleeding (Section 7), and ascites (Section 8) should be considered. Conditions that may closely mimic decompensated cirrhosis are the Budd–Chiari syndrome, venoocclusive disease, and constrictive pericarditis. Ultrasonography is essential to examine the hepatic veins and vena cava. In the Budd–Chiari syndrome (Section 20), ultrasonography allows an accurate diagnosis in the majority of cases. The Spigel lobe (segment I) is markedly enlarged in about 70 per cent of cases. The echogenicity of the liver is heterogeneous. Abnormalities of the wall and distribution of hepatic veins are seen. Sometimes the hepatic veins are not visible and an hepatic venous collateral circulation is seen. It should be remembered that hepatic veins may not be detectable in cirrhosis. In such cases, CT may be helpful. MRI allows a better visualization of the inferior vena cava. It is also useful in examining the patency of hepatic veins when Budd–Chiari syndrome is suspected (Radiology, 1995; 195:117). Finally, hepatic venography should be performed in difficult cases to visualize the abnormal hepatic veins and collateral circulation directly.

Chronic veno-occlusive disease (Section 20) has been observed after the consumption of bush tea containing pyrrolizidine alkaloids, after hepatic irradiation, azathioprine administration, chemotherapy for leukaemia, or as part of a graft-versus-host reaction. It can only be proven by liver biopsy.

Constrictive pericarditis may also mimic cirrhosis. Characteristically, gross ascites and hepatomegaly are present, and jaundice is absent. The diagnosis will be made on clinical signs, pericardic calcifications at radiographic examination, echocardiography, electrocardiography, and cardiac catheterization.

Prognosis

The prognosis of cirrhosis depends on its aetiology, epidemiological setting, clinical and laboratory manifestations, severity of histological lesions, and possibilities of treatment. Few studies on prognosis provide all this information and it is probably appropriate to try to determine prognosis in separate aetiological groups.

As an example, reported series suggest that the 5-year survival may be as high as 90 per cent in alcoholic cirrhosis in the absence of ascites, jaundice, digestive haemorrhage, or continued alcohol drinking.[40] At the other extreme, it may be as low as zero in patients with alcoholic cirrhosis with encephalopathy (Saunders, BMJ, 1981; 282:263). Intermediate 5-year survivals of 7 to 19 per cent have been observed for patients with cirrhosis and ascites, jaundice, and haematemesis.[41] In a very large series of cirrhotic patients from southern Italy (many of them having viral cirrhosis), those originally compensated became decompensated (i.e., developed a complication) at a rate of 10 per cent per year. Ascites was the most frequent first sign. The 6-year survival was 54 per cent in compensated and 21 per cent in decompensated cirrhotics. Indicators of risk of death were advanced age, male sex, encephalopathy, haemorrhage, varices, prothrombin time, HBsAg positivity, and hepatocellular carcinoma.[42] In another large series of western European patients (Fattovich, Hepatol, 1995; 21:77) with compensated cirrhosis due to hepatitis B virus infection, the probability of decompensation was 23 per cent in 5 years, and the probability of survival after the first decompensation was 35 per cent in 5 years.

With the increasing use of liver transplantation in patients with life-threatening liver disease, it has become extremely important to use criteria that allow determination of prognosis in an individual patient with the best possible accuracy. This ideal goal has not yet been reached, but several attempts have been made. Historically, the first of these attempts was made by Child and Turcotte[43] to help select cirrhotic patients for portacaval shunt surgery. They graded patients on the basis of (i) serum albumin concentration, (ii) serum bilirubin concentration, (iii) presence and severity of ascites, (iv) presence and severity of encephalopathy, and (v) the state of nutrition. Their criteria, presented in Table 3, allowed separation of the patients into three classes (A, B, and C) of increasingly poor prognosis. In its initial form, the classification is easily made, but the patients who satisfy the criteria of groups A and C will be extremely rare (each 5 per cent of all cirrhotics), while 90 per cent of patients will be graded B (Conn, Hepatol, 1981; 1:673). Nevertheless, it appears very useful not only as a predictor of survival, but also as a reliable index of the occurrence of the complications.[2]

Several modifications of the original Child and Turcotte classification have been proposed. The most widely used is that of Pugh et al.[44] They have omitted the assessment of body nutrition, included prolongation of the prothrombin time, and made use of a weighting system whereby 1, 2, or 3 points are scored for increasing

Table 3 Criteria for Child–Turcotte classification

	Class designation		
	A	B	C
Serum bilirubin (mg/100 ml)	<2.0	2.0–3.0	>3.0
Serum albumin (g/100 ml)	>3.5	3.0–3.5	<3.0
Ascites	None	Easily controlled	Poorly controlled
Neurological disorders	None	Minimal	Severe, coma
Nutrition	Excellent	Good	Poor, 'wasting'

abnormality of each of the five variables 'measured' (Table 4). They have also acknowledged that in patients with primary biliary cirrhosis, serum bilirubin was usually 'out of proportion' to other evidence of hepatic failure. The qualities of simplicity, availability, low cost, and good predictive power with regard to short-term (1-year) survival makes the 'Pugh' score very useful: sensitivity and specificity (for this criterion) reach approximately 80 per cent.[45] More complex, computer-derived formulas have been proposed, using multiple variables and Cox regression models of proportional hazards.[34,46-48] Poor prognosis is generally associated with a low prothrombin index, marked ascites, gastrointestinal bleeding, high age, high daily alcoholic consumption, high serum bilirubin and alkaline phosphatase activity, low serum albumin, little connective tissue inflammation, poor nutrition, and presence of encephalopathy, and, in viral B cirrhosis, persistent viral replication (Realdi, JHepatol, 1994; 21:656). With a still more complex model, large varices at endoscopy, high hepatic-vein pressure gradient, and low indocyanine green clearance were independently associated with a high risk of bleeding[34] and a poor prognosis. This approach certainly holds promise for the future, but, at present, there is no evidence that it has a proven superiority over the Child–Pugh score and it is not used in most hepatology centres.

Other prognostic indices or functions have been used in particular clinical situations and will be discussed in the relevant sections of this book. This is the case of the discriminant function

Table 4 Criteria for the scoring system of Pugh *et al.*

	Points		
	1	2	3
Serum bilirubin (mg/100 ml)	<2.0	2.0–3.0	>3
Serum albumin (g/100 ml)	>3.5	2.8–3.5	<2.8
Prothrombin time (seconds prolonged)	1–4*	4–6*	>6***
Encephalopathy (grade)	None	1 and 2	3 and 4
Ascites	Absent	Slight	Moderate
For primary biliary cirrhosis:			
Bilirubin (mg/100 ml)	1–4	4–10	>10
Bilirubin (μmol/l)	17–68	68–170	>170

* >50% of normal; ** 40–50% of normal; *** <40% of normal.

Table 5 Discriminant function in alcoholic liver disease

Score indicating discriminant function (poor prognosis)

1. Initial[50]
[4.6 × prothrombin time (s)] + serum bilirubin (mg/dl): >93
2. Modified[51]
4.6 (prothrombin time − control) + serum bilirubin (mg/dl): >32

of Maddrey *et al.* (Table 5),[49,50] the combined clinical laboratory index of the University of Toronto[51] for alcoholic liver disease (Table 6), and the 'Mayo Clinic' risk factors for primary biliary cirrhosis[52] and primary sclerosing cholangitis.[53]

Treatment

General measures

The treatment of well-compensated cirrhosis (i.e., cirrhosis without complications) has nothing specific: adequate mixed diet and avoidance of alcohol are probably most useful. A daily intake of 1 g protein/kg body weight is generally adequate. In malnourished patients, more protein may be needed. Additional choline, methionine, or various hepatoprotective agents, as well as avoidance of butter, eggs, fats, coffee, or chocolate, are of no proven therapeutic value and should not be advised.

Treatment of complications

The treatment of complications, especially ascites and oedema (Section 8), encephalopathy (Section 9), or gastrointestinal bleeding (Section 7) will be discussed in the appropriate chapters.

Prophylaxis of variceal haemorrhage

In patients with cirrhosis, the most important indicator of bleeding is variceal size. Endoscopic screening every other year in patients without varices, and every year in patients with varices is recommended. For the prevention of the first bleeding, several controlled trials have shown that treatment with β-blocking agents significantly decreases the risk. Both propranolol (40–160 mg/day) and nadolol (80–160 mg/day) are effective. Meta-analyses of the published trials have shown a significant benefit on prevention of bleeding,[37,54] and on survival (Pagliaro, AnnIntMed, 1992; 117: 59). Prophylactic sclerotherapy is not recommended because of its potentially severe complications. For the prevention of rebleeding after a first haemorrhage, both β-blocking agents and sclerotherapy have been shown to reduce the risk of bleeding recurrence and of death.[54] Combining sclerotherapy with β-blocking agents is recommended after these drugs have failed to prevent the first haemorrhage.[54] Endoscopic banding ligation appears as effective and more convenient than sclerotherapy (Stiegmann, NEJM, 1992; 326:1527; Laine, AnnIntMed, 1993; 119:1; Gimson, Lancet, 1993; 342:391). Shunt surgery virtually abolishes rebleeding, but does not prolong survival and causes more encephalopathy. It should be considered only in patients in whom the combination of β-blocking

Table 6 Combined clinical and laboratory index (CCLI)[51]

Clinical abnormalities			Laboratory abnormalities		
Type	Grade	Score	Type	Grade	Score
Encephalopathy	1–3	2	Prothrombin (s prolonged)	4–5	1
				>5	2
Collateral circulation	1–2	1	Haematocrit (% normal)	75–89.9	1
				<75	3
Oedema	1	1	Albumin (g/dl)	2.5–2.9	2
	2–3	2			
				<2.5	3
Ascites	1–3	2	Bilirubin (mg/dl)	2.1–8	2
				>8	3
Spider naevi	>10	1	Alkaline phosphatase (IU/dl)	>330	2
Weakness	—	1			
Anorexia	—	1			

The sum of the scores is the CCLI. The range of the CCLI is 0–25.

agents and sclerotherapy or ligation has failed or is not easily available. In these patients, hepatic transplantation, when available, should also be considered. Transcutaneous intrahepatic porto-systemic shunts are still being evaluated (LaBerge, JVascSurg, 1992; 16:258) and must be assessed in randomized controlled trials.[54]

Antifibrotic drugs

The use of antifibrotic drugs is logical in cirrhosis.[55] Penicillamine has been used in primary biliary cirrhosis in several controlled trials, with a total of 767 patients (see Section 14): it has no proven benefit on symptoms and survival, and has numerous toxic effects. Colchicine is a drug that, experimentally, disrupts microtubules and inhibits procollagen secretion (as well as the secretion of other proteins). One long-term, double-blind, placebo-controlled, clinical trial of this drug (1 mg/day, 5 days per week) on 100 patients in good condition followed for up to 14 years has been published.[56] The overall median survival was significantly longer in the colchicine-treated group (11 years) than in the placebo group (3.5 years). There was also some evidence of histological improvement. Although these results appear impressive, 19 patients were lost to follow-up, and 22 did not take their medication, transiently or permanently. This study requires confirmation. At present, the evidence does not seem sufficiently strong to recommend long-term use of colchicine in all patients with cirrhosis.

Future approaches for the treatment of fibrosis include interferon-γ, 2-oxo-glutarate analogues, prostaglandins, agents increasing the activity of extracellular proteases, and somatic gene therapy.[55] None of these approaches has so far been subjected to clinical trials.

Other treatments

The use of immunosuppressive agents and of ursodeoxycholic acid in cholestatic liver diseases (primary biliary cirrhosis, primary sclerosing cholangitis), D-penicillamine in Wilson's disease, iron removal in haemochromatosis, antiviral agents in cirrhosis due to hepatitis B or C, and corticosteroids in cirrhosis due to autoimmune hepatitis will be discussed in the relevant chapters.

Surgical operations in cirrhosis

All surgical operations in cirrhotic patients potentially have a higher risk and mortality than in non-cirrhotic patients. Surgery in cirrhotic patients without gastrointestinal bleeding has an overall mortality of 30 per cent and an additional morbidity rate of 30 per cent.[57] Mortality and morbidity are related to the severity of the disease: mortality is 10 per cent in Child's grade A patients, 31 per cent in grade B, and 76 per cent in grade C patients. Operations on the biliary tract, including cholecystectomy[58,59] for peptic ulcer disease or for colon resection, have a particularly poor prognosis in Child's B or C patients. These risk criteria probably apply to hepatic resection for small hepatocellular carcinomas arising in a cirrhotic liver.[60]

Surgical operations should be carried out in patients with cirrhosis only when there is a clear indication for a potentially life-threatening condition.

Follow-up and general management

Once the diagnosis of compensated cirrhosis is established, an upper gastrointestinal endoscopy should be performed to detect oesophageal varices. If grade 2 or 3 varices are present, primary prevention of variceal bleeding with a β-blocking agent should be started (unless there is a contraindication to these drugs). The patient should be clearly informed that this will be a lifelong treatment and that interrupting the drug may lead to a 'rebound' of portal hypertension and to variceal bleeding. General dietary advice should be given.

Follow-up is aimed at helping patients comply with dietary advice and drug therapy, at detecting early signs of hepatocellular failure, and early detection of hepatocellular carcinoma. Compliance with dietary advice is especially important in those with alcoholic cirrhosis: recurrence of alcohol abuse should be promptly diagnosed and treated. Diagnosis of recurrence is by careful history, variation of biochemical tests (aminotransferases, γ-glutamyl transferase) or unexplained occurrence of a complication. Detecting early signs of hepatocellular failure should be by clinical examination, ultrasonography to detect ascites, and routine liver function tests (serum bilirubin and albumin concentration, prothrombin time). Development of hepatic failure (serum albumin less than 30 g/l, prothrombin activity less than 30 per cent of normal), as well as complications (recurrent variceal haemorrhage, ascites resistant to medical therapy, episodes of spontaneous bacterial peritonitis, hepatic encephalopathy) should prompt consideration of hepatic transplantation. This should be the case both in non-alcoholic cirrhosis, and in alcoholic cirrhosis if an abstinence from alcohol of at least 6 months has been convincingly established.[61]

Early detection of hepatocellular carcinoma (see Section 21) should be advised in patients with an acceptable operative risk (who might benefit from a resection). The risk of development of hepatocellular carcinoma is especially high in men over 50 years with an elevated α-fetoprotein concentration. Detection should be by ultrasonography, liver function tests (especially alkaline phosphatase), and α-fetoprotein determination. Desgamma-carboxyprothrombin may also be helpful. In suitable patients, this should be tested at least every 6 months. Some authorities, especially in Japan, recommend screening for hepatocellular carcinoma every 3 months (see above: Hepatocellular carcinoma). Confirmation and evaluation of extension is best made by arteriography and CT scanning after injection of ultrafluid lipiodol in the hepatic artery. Unfortunately, the number of patients who might benefit from such a detection programme has not been determined accurately and the cost-effectiveness has not been established.

Treatment and follow-up of the patient with decompensated cirrhosis will be considered in the relevant chapters and the indications for transplantation in these patients are discussed in Chapter 29.5.

References

1. Anthony PP, Ishak KG, Nayak NC, Poulsen HE, Scheuer PJ, and Sobin LH. The morphology of cirrhosis: definition, nomenclature, and classification. *Bulletin of the World Health Organization*, 1977; **55**: 521–40.

2. Conn HO and Atterbury CE. Cirrhosis. In Schiff L and Schiff ER, eds. *Diseases of the liver*, 6th edn. Philadelphia: Lippincott, 1987: 725–864.

3. Hällen J and Norden J. Liver cirrhosis unsuspected during life: a series of 79 cases. *Journal of Chronic Disease*, 1965; **17**: 951–8.

4. Rueff B. *Alcoologie clinique*. Paris: Flammarion Médecine-Sciences, 1989: 83–4.

5. Johnston RF and Loo RV. Hepatic hydrothorax: studies to determine the source of the fluid and report of thirteen cases. *Annals of Internal Medicine*, 1964; **61**: 385–401.

6. LeVeen HH, Piccone VA, and Hutto RB. Management of ascites with hydrothorax. *American Journal of Surgery*, 1985; **148**: 210–13.

7. International Hepatology Informatics Group. *Diseases of the liver and biliary tract. Standardization of nomenclature, diagnostic criteria and prognosis.* Leevy CM, Sherlock S, Tygstrup N, and Zetterman R, eds. New York: Raven Press, 1994.

8. McCormack TT, *et al*. Gastric lesions in portal hypertension: inflammatory gastritis or congestive gastropathy? *Gut*, 1985; **26**: 1226–32.

9. Tisdale WA and Klatskin G. The fever of Laennec's cirrhosis. *Yale Journal of Biology and Medicine*, 1960; **33**: 94–106.

10. Van Thiel DH, Gavaler JS, and Schade RR. Liver disease and the hypothalamic pituitary gonadal axis. *Seminars in Liver Disease*, 1985; **5**: 35–45.

11. Van Thiel DH, *et al*. Patterns of hypothalamic pituitary gonadal dysfunction in men with liver disease due to differing etiologies. *Hepatology*, 1981; **1**: 39–46.

12. Warma RR. Course and prognosis of pregnancy in women with liver disease. *Seminars in Liver Disease*, 1987; **7**: 59–66.

13. Felig P and Sherwin R. Carbohydrate homeostasis, liver and diabetes. *Progress in Liver Disease*, 1976; **5**: 149–71.

14. Sherwin R, Joshi P, Hendler R, Felig P, and Conn HO. Hyperglucagonemia in Laennec's cirrhosis. The role of portal–systemic shunting. *New England Journal of Medicine*, 1974; **290**: 239–42.

15. McDonnell PJ, Toye PA, and Hutchins GM. Pulmonary hypertension and cirrhosis: are they related? *American Reviews of Respiratory Disease*, 1983; **127**: 437–41.

16. Lebrec D, Capron JP, Dhumeaux D, and Benhamou JP. Pulmonary hypertension complicating portal hypertension. *American Reviews of Respiratory Disease*, 1979; **120**: 849–56.

17. Murray JF, Dawson AM, and Sherlock S. Circulatory changes in chronic liver disease. *American Journal of Medicine*, 1958; **24**: 358–67.

18. Henriksen JH, Christensen NJ, and Ring-Larsen H. Noradrenaline and adrenaline concentrations in various vascular beds in patients with cirrhosis. *Clinical Physiology*, 1981; **1**: 293–304.

19. Bouchier IAD. Postmortem study of the frequency of gallstones in patients with cirrhosis of the liver. *Gut*, 1969; **10**: 705–10.

20. Nicholas P, Rinaudo PO, and Conn HO. Increased incidence of cholelithiasis in Laennec's cirrhosis: a postmortem evaluation of pathogenesis. *Gastroenterology*, 1972; **63**: 112–21.

21. Samuel D, Sattouf E, Degott C, and Benhamou JP. Cirrhose et lithiase biliaire en France: une étude nécropsique. *Gastroentérologie Clinique et Biologique*, 1988; **12**: 39–42.

22. Kirk AP, Dooley JS, and Hunt RH. Peptic ulceration in patients with chronic liver disease. *Digestive Diseases and Sciences*, 1980; **25**: 756–60.

23. Phillips MM, Ramsby GR, and Conn HO. Portacaval anastomosis and peptic ulcer: a non-association. *Gastroenterology*, 1975; **68**: 121–31.

24. Eriksson S, Carlson J, and Velez R. Risk of cirrhosis and primary liver cancer in alpha-1-antitrypsin deficiency. *New England Journal of Medicine*, 1986; **314**: 736–9.

25. Bean WB. *Vascular spiders and related lesions of the skin*. Oxford: Blackwell Scientific, 1959.

26. Ellis G, Goldberg DM, Spooner RJ, and Ward AM. Serum enzyme tests in diseases of the liver and biliary tree. *American Journal of Clinical Pathology*, 1978; **70**: 248–58.

27. Williams ALB and Hoofnagle JH. Ratio of serum aspartate to alanine aminotransferase in chronic hepatitis. Relationship to cirrhosis. *Gastroenterology*, 1988; **95**: 734–9.

28. Rosalski S and Rau D. Serum gamma-glutamyl-transpeptidase activity in alcoholism. *Clinica Chimica Acta*, 1972; **39**: 41–7.

29. Reichling JJ and Kaplan MM. Clinical use of enzymes in liver disease. *Digestive Diseases and Sciences*, 1988; **33**: 1601–14.

30. Kondo F, *et al*. Histological features and clinical course of large regenerative nodules: evaluation of their precancerous potentiality. *Hepatology*, 1990; **12**: 592–8.

31. Sandford NL, Walsh P, Matis C, Baddeley H, and Powell LW. Is ultrasonography useful in the assessment of diffuse parenchymal liver disease? *Gastroenterology*, 1985; **89**: 186–91.

32. Merine D, Takayasu K, and Wakao F. Detection of hepatocellular carcinoma: comparison of CT during arterial portography with CT after intraarterial injection of iodized oil. *Radiology*, 1990; **175**: 707–10.

33. Lebrec D, *et al*. Portal hypertension, size of esophageal varices, and risk of gastrointestinal bleeding in alcoholic cirrhosis. *Gastroenterology*, 1980; **79**: 1139–44.

34. Gluud C, Henriksen JH, Nielsen G, and the Copenhagen Study Group for Liver Diseases. Prognostic indicators in alcoholic cirrhotic men. *Hepatology*, 1988; **8**: 222–7.

35. North Italian Endoscopic Club for the Study and Treatment of Esophageal Varices. Prediction of the first variceal haemorrhage in patients with cirrhosis of the liver and esophageal varices. A prospective multicenter study. *New England Journal of Medicine*, 1988; **319**: 983–9.

36. Papazian A, Braillon A, Dupas JL, Sevenet F, and Capron JP. Portal hypertensive gastric mucosa: an endoscopic study. *Gut*, 1986; **27**: 1199–203.

37. Hayes PC, Davis JM, Lewis JA, and Bouchier IAD. Meta-analysis of value of propranolol in prevention of variceal haemorrhage. *Lancet*, 1990; **336**: 153–6.

38. Lebrec, D, Goldfarb G, Degott C, Rueff B, and Benhamou JP. Transvenous liver biopsy: an experience based on 1000 hepatic tissue samplings with this procedure. *Gastroenterology*, 1982; **83**: 338–40.

39. Lebrec D and Benhamou JP. Non-cirrhotic intrahepatic portal hypertension. *Seminars in Liver Disease*, 1986; **6**: 332–40.

40. Powell WJ and Klatskin G. Duration of survival in patients with Laennec's cirrhosis. *American Journal of Medicine*, 1968; **44**: 406–20.

41. Ratnoff OD and Patek AJ Jr. The natural history of Laennec's cirrhosis of the liver: analysis of 386 cases. *Medicine*, 1942; **21**: 207–68.

42. D'Amico G, Morabito A, Pagliaro L, Marubini E, and the Liver Study Group of 'V. Cervello' hospital. Survival and prognostic indicators in compensated and decompensated cirrhosis. *Digestive Diseases and Sciences*, 1986; **31**: 468–75.

43. Child III CG and Turcotte JG. Surgery and portal hypertension. In Child III CG, ed. *The liver and portal hypertension*. Philadelphia: Saunders, 1964: 50.

44. Pugh RNH, Murray-Lyon IM, Dawson JL, Pietroni MC, and Williams R. Transection of the oesophagus for bleeding oesophageal varices. *British Journal of Surgery*, 1973; **60**: 646–9.

45. Infante-Rivard C, Esnaola S, and Villeneuve JP. Clinical and statistical validity of conventional prognostic factors in predicting short-term survival among cirrhotics. *Hepatology*, 1987; **7**: 660–4.

46. Schlichting P, *et al.* Prognostic factors in cirrhosis identified by Cox's regression model. *Hepatology*, 1983; **3**: 889–95.

47. Christensen E, *et al.* Updating prognosis and therapeutic effect evaluation in cirrhosis with Cox's multiple regression model for time-dependent variables. *Scandinavian Journal of Gastroenterology*, 1986; **21**: 163–74.

48. Pignon JP, *et al.* Analyse multidimensionnelle selon le critère de Cox de la survie de patients atteints de cirrhose alcoolique. *Gastroentérologie Clinique et Biologique*, 1986; **10**: 461–7.

49. Maddrey WC, Bointnott K, Bedine MS, Weber FL, Mezey E, and White RI Jr. Corticosteroid therapy of alcoholic hepatitis. *Gastroenterology*, 1978; **75**: 193–9.

50. Carithers RL Jr, *et al.* Methylprednisolone therapy in patients with severe alcoholic hepatitis. *Annals of Internal Medicine*, 1989; **110**: 685–90.

51. Orrego H, Israel Y, Blake JE, and Medline A. Assessment of prognostic factors in alcoholic liver disease: toward a global quantitative expression of severity. *Hepatology*, 1983; **3**: 896–905.

52. Dickson ER, Grambsch PM, Fleming TR, Fisher LD, and Langworthy A. Prognosis in primary biliary cirrhosis: model for decision making. *Hepatology*, 1989; **10**: 1–7.

53. Wiesner RH, *et al.* Primary sclerosing cholangitis: natural history, prognostic factors and survival analysis. *Hepatology*, 1989; **10**: 430–6.

54. D'Amico G, Pagliaro L, and Bosch J. The treatment of portal hypertension: a meta-analytic review. *Hepatology*, 1995; **22**: 332–54.

55. Chojkier M and Brenner DA. Therapeutic strategies for hepatic fibrosis. *Hepatology*, 1988; **8**: 176–82.

56. Kershenobich D, *et al.* Colchicine in the treatment of cirrhosis of the liver. *New England Journal of Medicine*, 1988; **318**: 1709–13.

57. Garrison RN, Cryer HM, Howard DA, and Polk HC. Clarification of risk factors for abdominal operations in patients with hepatic cirrhosis. *Annals of Surgery*, 1984; **199**: 648–55.

58. Schwartz SI. Biliary tract surgery and cirrhosis. A critical combination. *Surgery*, 1981; **90**: 577–83.

59. Aranha GB, Sontag SJ, and Greenlee HB. Cholecystectomy in cirrhotic patients: a formidable operation. *American Journal of Surgery*, 1982; **143**: 55–60.

60. Franco D, *et al.* Resection of hepatocellular carcinoma. Results in 72 European patients with cirrhosis. *Gastroenterology*, 1990; **98**: 733–8.

61. Kumar S, *et al.* Orthotopic liver transplantation for alcoholic liver disease. *Hepatology*, 1990; **11**: 159–64.

7

Portal hypertension and gastrointestinal bleeding

7.1 Anatomy of the portal venous system in portal hypertension

J. Michael Henderson

Normal anatomy of the portal system

Embryology[1]

The development of the portal circulation builds around the two vitelline veins bringing blood from the yolk sac and the two umbilical veins returning the blood from the placenta. The vitelline veins intercommunicate in the septum transversum which is the site of development of the liver sinusoids. The extrahepatic portal venous system develops primarily from the left vitelline vein, which is later joined by the splenic vein to establish to the portal vein. Portions of both the right and left vitelline veins disappear and the remnant of the right vitelline vein continues as the right branch of the intrahepatic portal vein, while the left branch of the intrahepatic portal vein is formed from the left vitelline vein. The right umbilical vein atrophies; the left maintains its patency and communicates with the liver sinusoids but is directly connected to the sinus venosus. The duct venosus communicates directly to a large common hepatic vein, bypassing much of the hepatic sinusoids in the fetal circulation, allowing most of the placental blood to bypass the developing liver. Despite this complex development, there are surprisingly few congenital anomalies of the portal venous system.

Gross anatomy[2]

The adult portal venous system includes all the veins that collect blood from the abdominal portion of the alimentary tract, the spleen, and the pancreas. The portal vein itself is formed behind the neck of the pancreas by the confluence of the superior mesenteric and splenic veins. It is approximately 6 to 8 cm long, 1 to 1.2 cm in diameter, and passes superiorly from the upper margin of the pancreas, behind the duodenum, in the free edge of the lesser omentum, to terminate at the right end of the portahepatis.

The superior mesenteric vein is primarily formed by all the veins draining the small bowel, with significant further contributions of the ileocolic, right colic, and middle colic veins. It runs in the root of the mesentery, in front of the third portion of the duodenum to unite with the splenic vein behind the neck of the pancreas. The splenic vein originates at the splenic hilus and runs on the posterior surface of the pancreas transversely to join the superior mesenteric vein behind the neck of the pancreas. The splenic vein receives numerous small feeding branches from the body and tail of the pancreas. The short gastric veins enter the spleen pulp superior to

the origin of the splenic vein as does the left end of the gastroepiploic arcade. The third vein to contribute to portal venous inflow is the inferior mesenteric vein which drains blood from the rectum and the left colon. It enters the splenic vein in approximately two-thirds of patients within 1 to 2 cm of the splenic veins union with the superior mesenteric vein. In one-third of subjects, the inferior mesenteric vein enters directly into the superior mesenteric vein or at its confluence with the splenic vein. Finally, the left gastric, or coronary vein, has a variable entry into the portal venous system usually within 1 to 2 cm of the confluence, entering the splenic vein approximately 50 per cent of the time and the portal vein in the other 50 per cent.

The portal system carries all the blood from the alimentary tract to the liver and thus in the normal subject all of the above named veins have blood flow directed towards the liver. This is of particular pertinence in portal hypertension, because in these patients some of these vessels show reversal of blood flow with blood going away from the liver to collateral veins which shunt directly to the systemic circulation.[3]

The gastro-oesophageal junction

The normal venous anatomy of the gastro-oesophageal junction and lower oesophagus is particularly relevant to this chapter on portal hypertension.[4–7] This has been extensively studied by Vianna and colleagues.[4] Their work used the three techniques of radiological study, corrosion casting, and morphometry. These studies were performed in specimens of a block of tissue that comprised the lower two-thirds of the oesophagus and the entire intra-abdominal portal circulation. Injections for corrosion casting and for radiographic studies were made by cannulating the splenic vein, ligating obviously leaking sites in the tissue block, and proceeding to injection with the test substance. The morphometric studies examined 1 cm slices in the region of interest to document luminal areas of the main venous channels.

These studies documented four distinct zones of venous drainage:

1. The gastric zone, which extends for 2 to 3 cm just below the gastro-oesophageal junction, is the junctional zone between the stomach and lower oesophagus; the veins are longitudinal rather than the irregular network seen in the rest of the stomach. These veins are in the submucosa and lamina propria and come together

at the lower (gastric) end to drain into the short gastric and left gastric veins. This configuration can be seen in Figs 1 and 2—marked as GZ.

2. The palisade zone extends 2 to 3 cm superiorly from the gastric zone into the lower oesophagus. The veins are uniformly distributed, parallel, and run longitudinal in four groups which correspond to the oesophageal mucosal folds. The corrosion casting and radiological imaging of this zone (PZ) are illustrated in Figs 1 and 2. There are multiple anastomoses between these veins which occupy the lamina propria as illustrated in Fig. 3. There are no perforating veins in the palisade zone linking the intrinsic and extrinsic veins of the distal oesophagus. Morphometric study shows that the cross sectional area of the veins at this level is increased compared to other levels. These observations strongly support the palisade zone as being the watershed between the portal and systemic circulation. This is the anatomic location of the lower oesophageal sphincter—a region of the oesophagus of major physiological importance in swallowing and in control of gastro-oesophageal reflux.

3. The perforating zone extends approximately 2 cm further up the oesophagus above the palisade zone. The organized longitudinal structure is lost, with veins looping and forming a network. The main feature of this zone is perforating veins through the muscle wall of the oesophagus linking the internal and external veins. These perforating veins occur circumferentially around the oesophageal wall and are best illustrated in Fig. 2.

4. The truncal zone is 8 to 10 cm long and is characterized by four or five longitudinal veins in the lamina propria, as illustrated in Fig. 2. Perforating veins penetrate from the submucosa at irregular intervals to the external oesophageal venous plexus.

The summary of these zones is schematically illustrated in Fig. 4, as conceptualized by Vianni and colleagues.[4] This diagram represents the blood flow directions in the four zones described above.

Changes with portal hypertension

Obstruction of portal venous flow, whatever the aetiology, results in a rise in portal venous pressure. The first response to increased venous pressure is the development of a collateral circulation diverting the obstructed portal flow to the systemic veins.[8] The sites and extent of these collaterals' paths vary and are illustrated in some of the following figures. While some of these collaterals are relatively 'benign', clinically the most important and dangerous are gastro-oesophageal varices. The patterns of development and anatomic variations of these will be described in more detail.

Collateral pathways

Figure 5 illustrates a large inferior mesenteric vein shown at angiography in a patient with cirrhosis and portal hypertension. The flow in this vein is away from the liver towards the rectum and anal canal, which is one of the natural portal systemic collateral sites. Retrograde flow in the inferior mesenteric vein is a consistent finding in portal hypertension, but only occasionally does the vein enlarge to the size illustrated in this figure.

Figure 6 illustrates a large umbilical vein in a patient with cirrhosis and portal hypertension. The umbilical vein can enlarge

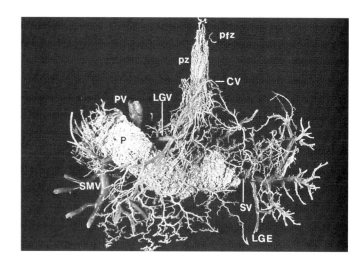

Fig. 1. A corrosion cast of the portal venous system, with emphasis of the upper stomach and lower oesophagus. P = pancreas, SMV = superior mesenteric vein; PV = portal vein; LGV = left gastric vein; LGE = left gastric epiploeic vein; SV = splenic vein; pz = palisade zone; pfz = perforating zone. This corrosion cast of normal blood vessels illustrates how the portal venous system condenses at the gastric fundus to form a tight longitudinal plexus of veins through the lower oesophagus in the palisade zone. (Used with the permission of Vianna and colleagues, Gastroenterology.[4])

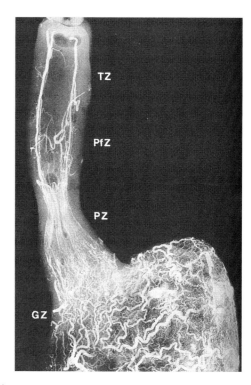

Fig. 2. A postmortem radiograph study of the venous anatomy at the gastro-oesophageal junction in a normal subject. The vessels have been injected with a barium gelatine solution to demonstrate the venous anatomy. GZ = gastric zone; PZ = palisade zone; PfZ = perforating zone; TZ = truncal zone. The network of veins in the gastric fundus condense just below the gastro-oesophageal junction and come together with longitudinal channels in the palisade zone. The perforating veins in the perforating zone can be identified. (Used with the permission of Vianna and colleagues, Gastroenterology.[4])

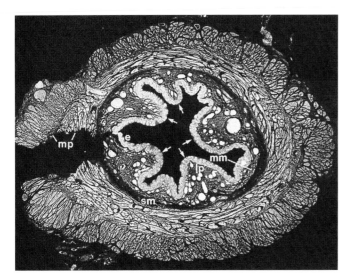

Fig. 3. A morphometric study of a transverse section of the distal oesophagus in a normal subject. This specimen has been injected with barium gelatine and transected 3 cm above the gastro-oesophageal junction. lp = lamina propria; sm = submucosa; mm = muscularis mucosa; e = epithelium; mp = muscularis propria. The white channels in the lamina propria represent the venous channels of the palisade zone which can clearly be seen to congregate in the longitudinal folds of the oesophagus. (Used with the permission of Vianna and colleagues, Gastroenterology.[4])

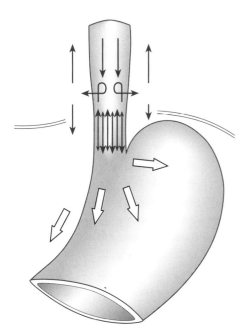

Fig. 4. Diagrammatic representation of the postulated pattern of normal venous drainage of the lower oesophagus. Venous drainage from the gastric fundus and lesser curvature is inferiorly to the portal vein. In the palisade zone, there is to/fro flow that is probably respiration dependent. The perforating veins connect the intrinsic and extrinsic oesophageal plexuses. Flow in the truncal zone is inferior to the perforating zone. (Used with the permission of Vianna and colleagues, Gastroenterology.[4])

from its vestigial size up to 2 cm in diameter and this always communicates with the left portal vein. It runs in the falciform

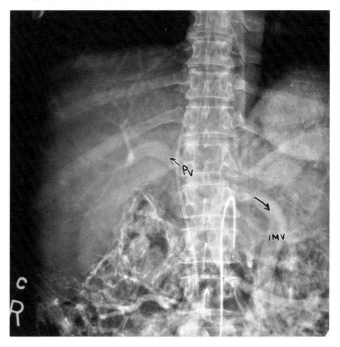

Fig. 5. Venous phase of a superior mesenteric artery injection in a patient with cirrhosis. PV = portal vein; IMV = inferior mesenteric vein. The inferior mesenteric vein fills in a retrograde pattern indicating blood flow away from the liver in this patient with portal hypertension. This large inferior mesenteric vein fills pararectal varices and anastomosis to the haemorrhoidal veins.

ligament and may give rise to the clinical finding of a caput medusae at the umbilicus. Although the umbilical vein may not always be visualized at angiography, a prominent dye pattern in the left portal vein is usually due to the origin of an umbilical vein. Flow in this is again away from the liver depriving the liver sinusoids of portal flow.

Figure 7 illustrates retroperitoneal collaterals with spontaneous shunting to the gonadal vessels. This is more common in female patients where the retroperitoneal collaterals will often communicate with larger ovarian vessels and spontaneously shunt into the iliac veins.

Figure 8 illustrates a patient with portal vein thrombosis and cavernous transformation of the portal vein. Rather than a single portal vein going to this liver, there are three or four very large channels, which demonstrate the preferred collateralization route when there is portal vein thrombosis. It is easier for the obstructed, high pressure superior mesenteric vein to collateralize to the low pressure sinusoids in the liver than to seek the more complex routes illustrated above. A clinical correlation with this abnormality is that an ultrasound exam may demonstrate an apparently good portal flow to the liver, when in reality one is only visualizing one of the large collateral vessels.

Gastro-oesophageal varices

This collateral pathway is of particular clinical importance because of the propensity of these abnormal veins to bleed. Thirty per cent of patients identified with compensated cirrhosis and 60 per cent of patients with decompensated cirrhosis have gastro-oesophageal

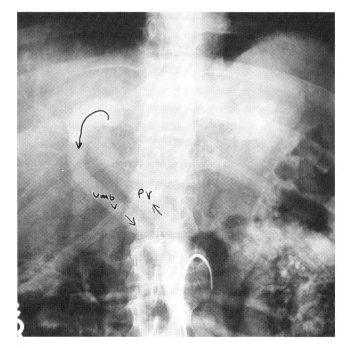

Fig. 6. This venous phase superior mesenteric artery injection demonstrates prograde flow in the portal vein (PV) and hepatofugal flow in the umbilical vein (UMB V) carrying blood away from the liver towards the umbilicus. This patient had a caput medusae fed by this large umbilical vein.

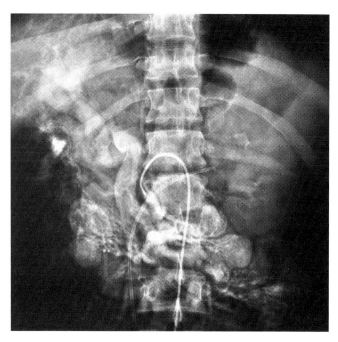

Fig. 8. Venous phase superior mesenteric artery study of cavernous transformation of the portal vein in a patient with portal vein thrombosis. Three large collateral venous channels can be seen in the region of the portal vein and have developed from the obstructed superior mesenteric vein to the low pressure sinusoids in this normal liver.

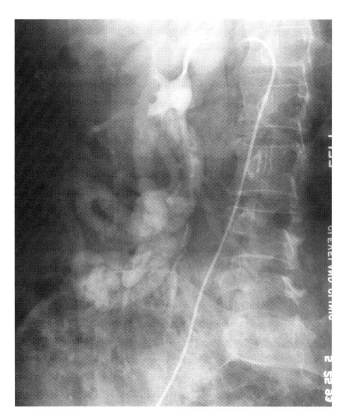

Fig. 7. Venous phase of a superior mesenteric artery injection showing large retroperitoneal collaterals around the terminal ileum, cecum, and the right pelvis.

varices at the time of presentation. The risk of bleeding from gastro-oesophageal varices is 30 per cent in the first year after their identification.[9] An understanding of the pathophysiology leading to the development of varices and of the anatomic changes around the gastro-oesophageal junction provide some basis for therapies used to reduce the risk of bleeding.

There are two main inflows to gastro-oesophageal varices. The first of these is the left gastric or coronary vein. This may be a major contributor to variceal inflow as illustrated in Fig. 9 where virtually all the portal venous flow is diverted into the left gastric vein to gastric fundal and oesophageal varices. In contrast, the patient illustrated in Fig. 10 also had a major bleed from gastro-oesophageal varices, yet the left gastric vein is of a very small calibre.

The other major route of inflow for gastro-oesophageal varices is from the splenic hilus through the short gastric veins. This is illustrated in Fig. 11, where the dominant venous outflow from the spleen is into gastric varices. The splenic vein is open in this patient with cirrhosis. However, the finding of isolated gastric fundus varices raises the question of isolated splenic vein thrombosis, where all the splenic outflow traverses the short gastric veins to the gastric fundus. The importance of identifying these patients is that they have a normal liver and are cured by splenectomy. The impact of these inflow changes on the venous anatomy at the gastro-oesophageal junction has been studied with the same techniques to those described previously for normal anatomy. The gastric, palisade, perforating, and truncal zones can again be identified, but undergo significant change in portal hypertension. The two main features of adaptation are dilatation and tortuosity, which are highly variable and do not occur in any constant or regular manner. Dilatation of the veins in the palisade zone are the most clinically problematic as

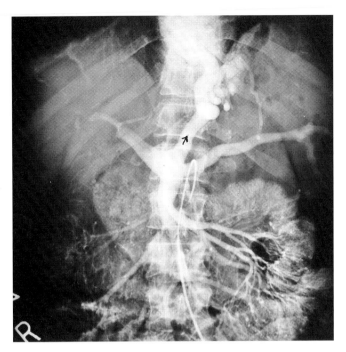

Fig. 9. Superior mesenteric artery injection in a patient with cirrhosis in whom there is no prograde portal flow into the liver although the portal vein is patent. Virtually all of the superior mesenteric venous flow is diverted into a large left gastric vein (↑) filling varices at the gastric fundus (gastric zone) and large paraoesophageal varices around the oesophagus. Note that there is also retrograde filling of the splenic vein.

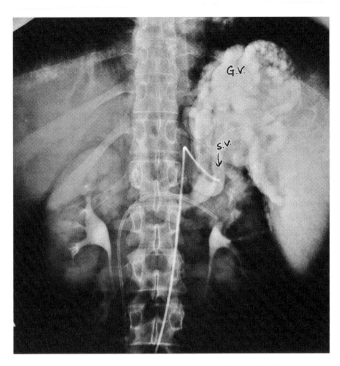

Fig. 11. The venous phase of a splenic artery injection in this patient with cirrhosis demonstrates a tortuous splenic vein (SV), and large gastric fundal varices (GV). It should be noted that these gastric varices drain through the retroperitoneum into a spontaneous splenorenal shunt with faint visualization of the inferior vena cava. The lower catheter is in the left renal vein which can be seen to drain some of the contrast on this venous phase study.

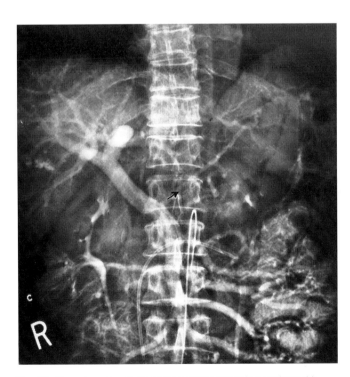

Fig. 10. Superior mesenteric venous phase study in a patient with cirrhosis who still has good prograde portal flow to the liver. The increased density in the left branch of the portal vein is probably the origin of a large umbilical vein. The arrow indicates a small left gastric vein filling small gastric fundal varices. It should be noted that this patient had significant variceal bleeding.

this is the commonest site of rupture and bleeding. In contrast, enlargement of the paraoesophageal varices has less clinical consequence in terms of bleeding risk, but has physiological significance in terms of diverting portal flow.

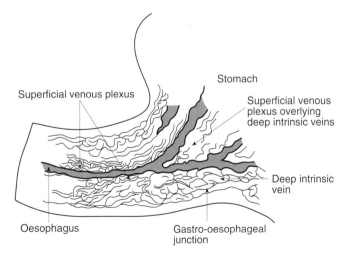

Fig. 12. Schematic representation of a resin cast of the lower oesophagus and upper stomach in a patient with portal hypertension. This cast has been partially dissected with the anterior wall removed to demonstrate the enlarged superficial venous plexus of veins as well as large deep intrinsic veins. These intercommunicate in the gastric zone. (Reprinted with permission from Kitano *et al.*, *British Journal of Surgery*.[10])

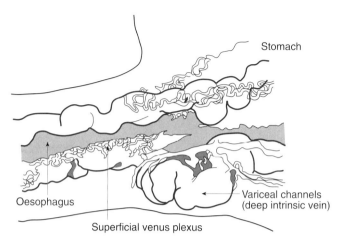

Fig. 13. A resin cast of the lower oesophagus and upper stomach at a later stage of dissection. Two very large, tortuous deep intrinsic variceal channels are demonstrated with overlying superficial venous plexus. For this dissection some of the superficial venous plexus illustrated in the prior figure have been removed. (Reprinted with permission from Kitano *et al.*, *British Journal of Surgery*.[10])

Resin cast studies by Kitano and coworkers[10] demonstrate the dilation and tortuosity of both the deep and superficial venous plexuses and are illustrated in Figs 12 and 13. When the deep veins become very large, they can displace the superficial veins and be lie immediately beneath the mucosa as illustrated in Fig. 13.

Further interesting data were generated by Spence *et al.*[11] who showed blood-filled channels in the oesophageal squamous epithelium as illustrated in Fig. 14. These are apparently fed by communicating channels which erode into the epithelium. The precise relationship of each of these anatomic abnormalities to the event of variceal bleeding has not been fully clarified.

The main vascular patterns that develop in portal hypertension, demonstrated by these various studies can be summarized as:

1. Varices in the fundus of the stomach are predominantly fed by the short gastric veins but may also be fed by the left gastric vein. From a clinical perspective, gastric varices may either occur 'in continuity' with oesophageal varices or be 'isolated' in the fundus. The latter group have a higher propensity to bleed and are particularly problematic in management.

2. Varices in the gastric and palisade zones form most of the varices seen in clinical practice, are markedly tortuous, numerous, and dilated. They run longitudinally in these two zones and are usually in continuity. Because there are no perforating veins in the palisade zone, the submucosal veins are particularly prone to rupture and bleeding. This is the main anatomical site for the clinical problem of bleeding gastro-oesophageal varices.

3. Varices at the perforating and truncal zones—the perforating vessels above the palisade zone provide a communication between the paraoesophageal varices and the submucosal varices. These perforating pathways can increase the pressure in the submucosal varices and in some patients flow to submucosal vessels will increase the risk of bleeding. Doppler ultrasound studies of perforating veins in patients with portal hypertension have suggested that these may be incompetent and there may be bidirectional flow through the perforators.[12] It has been

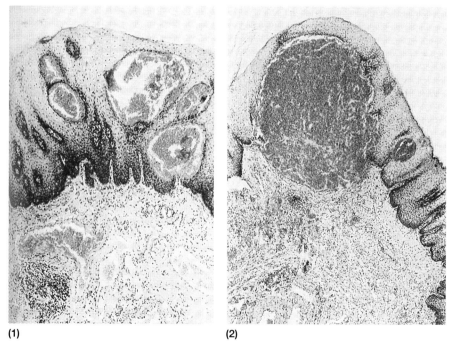

Fig. 14. (1) Blood-filled channels in the oesophageal epithelium in a patient with portal hypertension. In addition, there are dilated vessels in the lamina propria. Magnification × 40. (2) A large subepithelial blood-filled channel in a patient with portal hypertension. The smaller intraepithelial channel appears to be arising from papillary capillary present to the right of the larger lesions. Magnification × 26. (Reproduced with permission from Spence *et al.*, Surgery, Gynecology and Obstetrics.[11])

speculated that turbulence of flow through these incompetent perforators are risk factor in further bleeding.

4. Paraoesophageal varices are not at risk of bleeding but may develop as very large veins with significant flow. This flow can be measured clinically as azygos blood flow. These channels become important when there are incompetent perforators allowing this high flow to increase submucosal venous pressure and flow.

Anatomic studies of the portal circulation, and particularly the detailed studies of the gastro-oesophageal junction, have increased knowledge as to why and how gastro-oesophageal varices form. This information also provides pointers as to the therapeutic options.

References

1. Davies DV and Davies F. *Gray's anatomy—descriptive and applied.* Longmans, Green and Co., 1962.
2. Douglas BE, Baggenstoss AH, and Hollinshead WH. The anatomy of the portal vein and its tributaries. *Surgery, Gynecology and Obstetrics*, 1979; **91**: 562–76.
3. Salam AA and Warren WD. Anatomic basis of the surgical treatment of portal hypertension. *Surgical Clinics of North America*, 1974; **54**(6): 1247–57.
4. Vianna A, Hayes PC, Moscoso G, *et al.* Normal venous circulation of the gastroesophageal junction. A route to understanding varices. *Gastroenterology*, 1987; **93**(4): 876–89.
5. Butler H. The veins of oesophagus. *Thorax*, 1951; **6**: 276–96.
6. Kegaries D. The venous plexus of the oesophagus. *Surgery, Gynecology and Obstetrics*, 1934; **58**: 46–51.
7. Noda T. Angioarchitectural study of esophageal varices. With special reference to variceal rupture. *Virchows Archiv. A Pathological Anatomy and Histopathology*, 1984; **404**(4): 381–92.
8. Sikuler E, Kravetz D, and Groszmann RJ. Evolution of portal hypertension and mechanisms involved in its maintenance in a rat model. *American Journal of Physiology*, 1985; **248**: G618–25.
9. The North Italian Endoscopic Club for the Study and Treatment of Esophageal Varices. Prediction of the first variceal hemorrhage in patients with cirrhosis of the liver and esophageal varices. A prospective multicenter study. *New England Journal of Medicine*, 1988; **319**(15): 983–9.
10. Kitano S, Terblanche J, Kahn D, and Bornman PC. Venous anatomy of the lower oesophagus in portal hypertension: practical implications. *British Journal of Surgery*, 1986; **73**(7): 525–31.
11. Spence RA, Sloan JM, and Johnston GW. Histologic factors of the esophageal transection ring as clues to the pathogenesis of bleeding varices. *Surgery, Gynecology and Obstetrics*, 1984; **159**(3): 253–9.
12. McCormack TT, Rose JD, Smith PM, and Johnson AG. Perforating veins and blood flow in oesophageal varices. *Lancet*, 1983; **ii**: 1442–4.

7.2 Pathophysiology of portal hypertension and its complications

Jaime Bosch and Juan Carlos García-Pagán

Definition

Portal hypertension is a common syndrome characterized by a chronic increase of the portal venous pressure. Portal hypertension promotes the formation of collateral vessels through which portal blood is diverted to the systemic circulation bypassing the liver. These portal–systemic collaterals form by the opening and dilatation of pre-existing vascular channels connecting the portal venous system and the superior and inferior vena cava that are closed in normal conditions and that dilate because of the high portal pressure. It is not known whether other factors, such as active angiogenesis, are also involved in the development of the collateral circulation. The most important anastomotic system, by far, is the gastro-oesophageal collateral system draining into the azygos vein, as this includes the oesophageal varices, which are responsible of the main complication of portal hypertension—massive upper gastrointestinal bleeding. Other manifestations of the portal hypertension syndrome include ascites, hepatic encephalopathy, disturbances in the metabolism of drugs and endogenous compounds, bacteraemia, splenomegaly, anaemia, thrombopenia, and leucopenia.[1]

Aetiology

Any disease interfering with portal blood flow can result in portal hypertension. Causes of portal hypertension are usually classified according to their location as prehepatic, intrahepatic, or posthepatic (Table 1). All categories can cause the formation of varices and bleeding. However, there are some differences in other clinical manifestations. Thus, ascites is a prominent finding in posthepatic portal hypertension, but very rare when this is prehepatic. This latter group is characterized by the formation of 'bridging' collaterals carrying portal blood to the liver ('hepatopetal' collaterals), which often give rise to large gastric (fundal) varices. Intrahepatic portal hypertension can be caused by many liver diseases (Table 1). Cirrhosis accounts for over 90 per cent of the cases in developed countries, to the point that all other intrahepatic causes have been often grouped as 'non-cirrhotic portal hypertension'. This is clearly inadequate, since schistosomiasis is a very common cause of portal hypertension in South America and North Africa.

Table 1 Causes of portal hypertension

Prehepatic
  Splenic vein thrombosis
  Portal vein thrombosis
  Cavernomatosis of the portal vein
  Hypoplasy and congenital stenosis of the portal vein
  Extrinsic compression of the portal vein
Intrahepatic
  Partial nodular transformation
  Nodular regenerative hyperplasy
  Congenital hepatic fibrosis
  Hepatic peliosis
  Polycystic disease of the liver
  Idiopathic portal hypertension
  Hypervitaminosis A
  Arsenic, copper sulphate, and vinyl chloride toxicity
  Chronic bile duct obstruction and sclerosing cholangitis
  Sarcoidosis
  Tuberculosis
  Amyloidosis
  Mastocytosis
  Liver infiltration in haematological diseases
  Rendu–Osler disease
  Schistosomiasis
  Primary biliary cirrhosis
  Acute fatty liver of pregnancy
  Severe acute viral hepatitis with multilobular necrosis
  Fulminant hepatic failure of any aetiology
  Chronic active hepatitis
  Hepatocellular carcinoma
  Hepatic metastasis
  Haemocromatosis
  Wilson's disease
  Hepatic porphyria
  α_1-Antitrypsin deficiency
  Cyanamid hepatotoxicity
  Alcoholic hepatitis
  Alcoholic cirrhosis
  Hepatitis virus B and C related cirrhosis
  Veno-occlusive disease of the liver
Posthepatic
  Budd–Chiari syndrome
  Thrombosis and congenital malformations of the thoracic segment of the inferior vena cava
  Constrictive pericarditis
  Tricuspid valve disease
  Severe congestive myocardiopathy
Other
  Arteriovenous fistulas (intrasplenic, aortomesenteric, aortoportal, hepatic artery–portal vein)

Factors influencing portal pressure

As in any vascular system, the pressure gradient along the portal venous system is the product of portal blood flow and the vascular resistance that opposes this flow. According to Ohm's law, this relationship is defined by the equation:

$$\Delta P = Q \times R$$

in which ΔP is the portal pressure gradient, Q is blood flow within the entire portal venous system (which in portal hypertension includes also the portal–systemic collaterals), and R is the vascular resistance of the portal venous system, which in turn represents the sum of the serial resistance of the portal vein and the hepatic vascular bed, and of the parallel resistance of the collaterals. This relationship clearly indicates that portal pressure may increase because of an increase in portal blood flow, in vascular resistance, or by a combination of both. An important implication of this relationship is that an increased portal pressure may be reduced by decreasing portal blood flow, vascular resistance, or both. This provides the rational basis for the treatment of portal hypertension.

Factors influencing vascular resistance are interrelated by Poiseuille's law in the equation:

$$R = 8\mu L / \pi r^4$$

in which μ is the coefficient of blood viscosity, L is the length of the vessel, and r its radius. It follows that changes in the radius of the vessels is the main factor influencing vascular resistance and this is, therefore, of major influence in the pathophysiology of portal hypertension.[1] The relationship between the above mentioned parameters is completely applicable to flow through rigid tubes. In the vascular system other factors may also be considered. Thus, contrary to what happens in rigid tubes, as pressure increases elastic blood vessels will distend offering less resistance to flow. This relationship between changes in the volume of a blood vessel for a given change in transmural pressure is known as compliance.

Increased vascular resistance

In normal conditions, the portohepatic circulation is highly compliant and can accommodate large variations in blood flow with only minor changes in portal pressure. This is the reason why increased resistance to portal blood flow is the primary factor in the pathophysiology of portal hypertension, and may occur at any site within the portal venous system. As stated before, resistance to portal blood flow is exerted both at the intrahepatic vascular bed and at the portal and portal–collateral vessels.

Intrahepatic resistance

In cirrhosis, increased intrahepatic vascular resistance is thought to be located mainly at the hepatic sinusoid and is the consequence of the distortion of the liver vascular architecture caused by fibrosis, scarring, and nodule formation.[2] In addition, recent, elegant pathological studies have suggested that thrombotic events occurring in small hepatic or portal veins, usually involving lymphocytic phlebitis, are important—not only causing progression of the architectural distortion present in liver cirrhosis, but also increasing intrahepatic vascular resistance and therefore worsening portal hypertension (Wanless, Hepatol, 1995; 21:1238).

Although morphological changes occurring in chronic liver diseases probably are the most important factors involved in the increased intrahepatic resistance, there is now increasing evidence that the hepatic circulation is also modulated by an active component that can be modified by several endogenous and pharmacological stimuli.

It has been suggested that such a modifiable component can be due, in part, to the active contraction or relaxation of activated hepatic stellate cells. These cells, which are located around the sinusoids, have perisinusoidal and interhepatocellular branching processes that contain actin-like filaments and have been shown to acquire contractile properties (Pinzani, Gastro, 1996; 110:534; Housset, PNAS, 1993; 90: 9266). Activated stellate cells evolve into myofibroblasts, which are very abundant in the cirrhotic scar tissue and allow the contraction of the fibrous septas surrounding the cirrhotic nodules, thereby further contributing to active changes in the hepatic vascular resistance.[3] Therefore, some vasoactive mediators, either vasoconstrictors or vasodilators, may modulate intrahepatic vascular resistance through the contraction–relaxation of these cells.

There is some evidence suggesting that endothelin may play a role in modulating intrahepatic vascular resistance. Circulating plasma levels of endothelin are increased in patients with cirrhosis (Asbert, Gastro, 1993; 104:1485). The exact mechanism promoting such increases is not well known but it seems conceivable that an increase in its production may be the main factor, although a decreased clearance cannot be excluded. Recent experimental studies have shown that endothelin promotes the contraction of activated stellate cells (Rockey, Hepatol, 1996; 24:233; Pinzani, Gastro, 1996; 110:534; Housset, PNAS, 1993; 90:9266) and its infusion in the isolated perfused liver preparation may increase the portal perfusion pressure, that may be decreased by endothelin antagonists (Rockey, Hepatol, 1996; 24:233). However, the latter has not been observed in some *in vivo* studies (Leivas, Gastro, 1995; 108:1842).

Studies in perfused cirrhotic livers have suggest that adrenergic receptors may be involved in the regulation of intrahepatic resistance in cirrhosis. Thus, noradenaline is able to increase intrahepatic vascular resistance and this increased resistance is completely blunted by the administration of α-adrenergic antagonists such as prazosin. On the other hand, administration of β-adrenergic agonists, such as isoproterenol, reduces intrahepatic vascular resistance in the perfused cirrhotic liver. Angiotensin II and vasopressin have also been shown to increase intrahepatic vascular resistance in the perfused cirrhotic liver.[7] However, the mechanisms of this increase have not been well characterized. The high plasma concentrations of these three circulating vasoactive factors (noradrenaline, angiotensin II, and vasopressin), usually found in cirrhosis, could contribute to the increased intrahepatic vascular resistance observed in this situation. In that regard, it is known that both angiotensin II blockade with saralasin and α-adrenergic blockade with prazosin markedly decrease the hepatic venous pressure gradient in patients with cirrhosis (Albillos, Gastro, 1995; 109:1257).

Nitric oxide may also play a role in the regulation of the intrahepatic portal circulation in portal hypertension. Thus, the hepatic resistance is markedly increased *in vivo* in cirrhotic rats after the administration of nitric oxide antagonists (Pizcueta, Gastro, 1992; 103:1909). In addition, preliminary data in an experimental model of cirrhosis suggested that nitric oxide may contribute to the basal vascular tone of the intrahepatic portal bed (Mittal, Gastro, 1993; 104:A956). Moreover, it has also been suggested that the synthesis of nitric oxide may be limited in the cirrhotic liver in comparison with normal livers (Mittal, Hepatol, 1992; 16:123A). Thus, a relative deficit of the release of nitric oxide in the intrahepatic circulation, which has been ascribed to endothelial sinusoidal dysfunction, may contribute to the increased intrahepatic vascular resistance observed in cirrhosis. Other vasoactive substances, such as prostaglandins, the hyperpolarizing factor, and carbon monoxide (Suematsu, JCI, 1995; 96: 2431), may also play a role in the modulation of intrahepatic vascular resistance.

Portal–collateral resistance

In advanced portal hypertension the collateral circulation may carry over 90 per cent of the blood entering the portal system (Chojkier, AmJPhysiol, 1981; 240:G371). In these circumstances, it is obvious that the vascular resistance of these vessels may markedly influence the overall resistance to portal blood flow and, therefore, portal pressure.[1] These vessels have a substantial amount of smooth muscle and may thus exhibit active changes in diameter promoted by vasoactive substances.

Although lower than that of the cirrhotic liver, the resistance of this collateral bed is higher than that of a normal liver. The elements that modulate collateral resistance are not well known. Studies performed with isolated perfused portosystemic collateral bed suggest that nitric oxide may play a role in the control of portocollateral vascular resistance (Mosca, AmJPhysiol, 1992; 263: G544). This has also been substantiated by *in vivo* studies in rats with prehepatic portal hypertension (Pizcueta, BrJPharmacol, 1992; 105:184). The collateral vessels are probably also hypersensitive to serotonin (Cummings, BrJPharmacol, 1986; 89:501), which markedly increases their vascular resistance, while this can be decreased by β-adrenergic stimulation (Mosca, AmJPhysiol, 1992; 263:G544). Further evidence on the active modulation of resistance in portal–collateral vessels has been reported in studies in intact portal hypertensive animals, in which the administration of selective 5-hydroxytryptamine receptor blockers causes a significant decrease in portal pressure without modifying the systemic haemodynamics and portal inflow, suggesting that portal–collateral resistance is responsible for part of the increase in portal pressure (Kaumann, Gastro, 1988; 95:1601; Fernández, Hepatol, 1993; 18:389). The mesenteric vein and collateral vessels from portal hypertensive rats also show an enhanced response to vasopressin (Cummings, BrJPharmacol, 1986; 89:501) and electric field stimulation, while they show impaired responses to norepinephrine and β₂-adrenergic stimulation (Martínez-Cuesta, Gastro, 1996;111: 727). The latter has been related to impaired neural release of nitric oxide (Martínez-Cuesta, Gastro, 1996; 111:727).

Increased blood flow

An increased portal venous inflow is characteristically observed in advanced stages of portal hypertension.[8] Such an increased blood flow plays a contributory role in maintaining and aggravating the portal hypertensive syndrome.

Increased portal venous inflow is the result of a marked arteriolar vasodilation in splanchnic organs draining into the portal vein. Thus, in portal hypertension a vascular territory—the portal venous system—simultaneously exhibits increased blood inflow and increased outflow resistance.[9] An important concept is that vasodilatation is not limited to the splanchnic arterial bed, but rather it is almost generalized. Thus, the systemic circulation is also hyperkinetic in portal hypertension, where there is an increased cardiac index and reduced arterial blood pressure and peripheral (systemic) vascular resistance.[8] The increase in the cardiac index is preceded by peripheral vasodilatation and expansion of the plasma volume (Albillos, Gastro, 1992; 102:931). The increased blood volume also contributes to increase further portal pressure[1] and is required to promote and maintain the increased cardiac index characteristic of portal hypertension.

These disturbances of the systemic haemodynamics promoted by portal hypertension (systemic arteriolar vasodilatation, reduced peripheral resistance, hypervolaemia, and increased cardiac output) are extremely important since they play a central role in the pathophysiology of sodium retention and ascites formation, as well as in other complications of portal hypertension, such as the hepatopulmonary syndrome. The mechanism and implications of these circulatory disturbances are extensively discussed in Chapter 8.1.

Role of increased release of endogenous vasodilators

Several studies have focused on the potential role of circulating vasodilators in promoting the splanchnic hyperaemia observed in portal hypertension. Cross-circulation studies between portal hypertensive and normal animals have demonstrated the development of splanchnic vasodilation in the recipient, indicating that transferable humoral factors are implicated in its pathogenesis.[10] Many candidate substances have been proposed—mainly vasodilators of splanchnic origin that undergo hepatic metabolism and may accumulate in the systemic circulation because of reduced hepatic uptake due to liver disease and/or portal–systemic shunting.[1] Those for whom evidence has been reported are discussed above.

Glucagon, a 29-amino acid peptide secreted by pancreatic α-cells and the oxyntic mucosa of the stomach, is probably the humoral vasodilator for which there is most evidence for a significant role promoting splanchnic hyperaemia in portal hypertension (Benoit, AmJPhysiol, 1986; 251:G674; Kravetz, AmJPhysiol, 1988; 254: G322).[10] Plasma glucagon levels are elevated in patients with cirrhosis and in experimental models of portal hypertension. This hyperglucagonism results, in part, from decreased hepatic clearance of glucagon, but more importantly from increased secretion of glucagon by pancreatic α-cells (Gomis, Hepatol, 1994;19:1257). Studies increasing the circulating glucagon of normal rats to levels similar to those observed in portal hypertension have shown a significant increase in splanchnic blood flow. Conversely, in an experimental model of portal hypertension, the normalization of circulating glucagon by means of glucagon antibodies (Benoit, AmJPhysiol, 1986; 251:G674) or by somatostatin infusion partially reverses the increased splanchnic blood flow (Kravetz, AmJPhysiol, 1988; 254:G322), a response that can be specifically blocked by preventing the fall in circulating glucagon by a concomitant glucagon infusion (Pizcueta, Gastro, 1991; 101:1710). On the basis of these studies, it has been suggested that hyperglucagonism may account for approximately 30 to 40 per cent of the splanchnic vasodilation of chronic portal hypertension.[10] Therefore, other factors must also be involved. Moreover, some studies have yielded divergent results by suggesting that in experimental portal hypertension, splanchnic vasodilation is not necessarily associated with hyperglucagonism (Sikuler, Hepatol, 1986; 6:414).

Recently, much interest has been paid to the physiological role of vasoactive factors produced by the vascular endothelium. There is increasing evidence indicating that some of these agents, such as nitric oxide and prostacyclin, may play a major role in the pathogenesis of the circulatory abnormalities associated with chronic portal hypertension.

Nitric oxide is a powerful endogenous vasodilator generated in several tissues by constitutive and inducible nitric oxide synthases from the amino acid L-arginine and has been identified as the endothelial derived relaxing factor. Nitric oxide is the natural ligand for soluble guanylate cyclase with a subsequent increase in cGMP, the final agent responsible for the relaxation of the vascular wall.[11] It has recently been suggested that excessive nitric oxide biosynthesis may be involved in the pathogenesis of the hyperdynamic circulation associated with portal hypertension (Pizcueta, Gastro, 1992; 103:1909; Pizcueta, BrJPharmacol, 1992; 105:184; Clària, Hepatol, 1992; 15:343). This evidence has been described in experimental studies using specific nitric oxide inhibitors that have shown this factor to be implicated in the regulation of splanchnic and systemic haemodynamics in portal hypertensive animals. Thus, the acute administration of specific nitric oxide antagonists to experimental models of portal hypertension provoked splanchnic and systemic vasoconstriction, attenuating the hyperdynamic circulation of these animals (Pizcueta, Gastro, 1992; 103:1909; Pizcueta, BrJPharmacol, 1992; 105:184; Clària, Hepatol, 1992; 15:343). The vasoconstrictor effect of nitric oxide inhibition was significantly higher in portal hypertensive animals in comparison with controls animals, suggesting that an excessive amount of nitric oxide may be responsible for the vasodilatation observed in portal hypertension. The recent finding that patients with cirrhosis have increased serum and urinary concentrations of nitrites and nitrates, which are products indicative of nitric oxide oxidation, also supports a role for nitric oxide in the genesis of the circulatory disturbances of portal hypertension (Guarner, Hepatol, 1993; 18:1139). However, it has been shown that nitric oxide inhibition attenuates but does not 'normalize' the hyperkinetic syndrome in portal hypertension, suggesting that other factors may also contribute to the vasodilatation of portal hypertension. Moreover, a recent study indicated that chronic nitric oxide inhibition by specific antagonists, although precluding the development of systemic vasodilatation (Lee, Hepatol, 1993; 17:84; Lee, Gastro, 1993; 105:1464; García-Pagán, AmJPhysiol, 1994; 30:G984), delayed, but did not prevent, the development of splanchnic vasodilatation. These data suggest that factors other

than nitric oxide may also be involved in the pathogenesis of the hyperdynamic circulation.

The production of nitric oxide is catalysed by the enzyme nitric oxide synthase of which there are at least three different types. One is constitutive and is Ca^{2+} dependent. Another nitric oxide synthase is inducible by cytokines and endotoxin and is partially or totally Ca^{2+} independent.[11] Whether the increased nitric oxide activity observed in portal hypertension is due to a stimulation of the constitutive nitric oxide synthase, which is normally present in the endothelium or, as it has been suggested, to the *de novo* formation of the inducible nitric oxide synthase still remains controversial (Vallance, Lancet, 1991; 337:776; Fernández, Gastro, 1995; 108:1487; Kanwar, JHepatol, 1996; 23:85). Recent studies suggest that tumour necrosis factor α, a mononuclear-derived cytokine that has been found to be elevated in portal hypertension, may play a role in the hyperkinetic circulation observed in portal hypertensive rats, probably by increasing nitric oxide synthesis (López-Talavera, Gastro, 1995; 108:761; López-Talavera, Hepatol, 1996; 23:1616).

Several studies have supported a role for prostaglandins in the hyperdynamic circulation of portal hypertension (Sitzmann, AnnSurg, 1989; 209:322; Hamilton, Hepatol, 1982; 2:36). It has been shown that patients with cirrhosis may have increased systemic levels of prostacyclin (Guarner, Gastro, 1992; 102:303). Prostacyclin has also been found to be increased in the portal vein of portal hypertensive rats (Hamilton, Hepatol, 1982; 2:236). In addition, the inhibition of prostaglandin biosynthesis by indomethacin reduced the hyperdynamic circulation and portal pressure in patients with cirrhosis and portal hypertension (Bruix, Gastro, 1985; 88:430). There could be an interaction between prostacyclin and nitric oxide contributing both to the hyperkinetic splanchnic circulation (Fernández, Gastro, 1996; 110:1529).

Other vasodilators have also been involved in the pathogenesis of the splanchnic vasodilatation. Bile acids are increased in portal hypertension and have vasodilatory properties. However, data in the literature are controversial (Genecin, AmJPhysiol, 1990; 259:G21; Thomas, DigDisSci, 1991; 36:1243) and their role in mediating hyperdynamic circulation is not well defined. Other candidates include calcitonin gene-related peptide, neuropeptides, adenosine, endotoxin, and a variety of vasodilatory gastrointestinal hormones. However, available evidence is scarce for most of them.

All together, these data suggest that none of these vasoactive factors should be regarded as 'the' factor responsible for the splanchnic vasodilation present in portal hypertension, which is likely to be multifactorial in origin. In addition, experimental studies suggest that when one of these vasoactive mediators, such as nitric oxide biosynthesis (García-Pagán, AmJPhysiol, 1994; 30:G984) or prostaglandins (Fernández, Gastro, 1996; 110:1529), are chronically inhibited, other vasoactive systems may be enhanced, maintaining the splanchnic vasodilation. Thus, it is possible that splanchnic vasodilatation represents an adaptive response to the presence of portal hypertension that stimulates all the physiological mechanisms regulating the splanchnic blood flow.

Reduced vascular sensitivity

Increased levels of endogenous vasodilators may contribute to splanchnic hyperaemia by a dual mechanism: relaxing the vascular smooth muscle and decreasing the sensitivity to endogenous vaso-constrictors, such as noradrenaline, angiotensin II, and vasopressin (Pizcueta, AmJPhysiol, 1990; 258:G191).

Initial studies showed that increasing the circulating glucagon levels in normal rats to values similar to those observed in portal hypertensive rats allowed the reproduction, in the normal animals, of the impairment in vascular sensitivity to noradrenaline observed in rats with portal hypertension. A similar observation was made when assessing the response to vasopressin and to angiotensin II (Pizcueta, AmJPhysiol, 1990; 258:G191). More recently it has been shown that the impaired vascular sensitivity to vasoconstrictors observed in portal hypertensive rats can be reversed by pre-treatment with somatostatin analogues (Sieber, Hepatol, 1996; 23: 1218), further supporting the concept that an increased release of endogenous vasodilatory peptides can be responsible for the reduced vascular sensitivity to vasoconstrictors. The non-specific nature of this abnormality is emphasized by the observation that the vascular sensitivity can be restored by infusing small amounts of terlipressin (Heinemann, JHepatol, 1996; 24:739). In addition, nitric oxide inhibition has been shown to correct the vascular hyporesponsiveness to vasoconstrictors present in portal hypertension (Castro, Hepatol, 1993; 18:367; Lee, Hepatol, 1992; 16: 1043; Sieber, Gastro, 1992; 103:235). Although it has been proposed that such an attenuated response to endogenous vaso-constrictors may contribute to arterial vasodilatation in portal hypertension, the fact that this is non-specific and that it can be reversed by infusing small doses of exogenous constrictors suggests that, rather than the cause, this abnormality may represent another consequence of the excessive release of endogenous vasodilators.

Pathophysiology of the complications of portal hypertension

Formation of oesophageal varices

As stated before, portal hypertension is the main factor leading to the formation of portosystemic collaterals that divert portal blood to the systemic circulation, bypassing the liver, in an attempt to decompress the portal venous system.[1] The most common and clinically more important part of this collateral circulation are the gastro-oesophageal collaterals connecting the portal system with the thoracic vessels (i.e. the azygos and hemiazygos veins) via the coronary vein and the short gastric veins, as these collaterals include the gastro-oesophageal varices, which often rupture and cause massive gastrointestinal bleeding.

Portal hypertension is defined by the finding of an increased portal pressure gradient (the difference between portal venous pressure and free hepatic venous pressure, or its equivalent, the hepatic venous pressure gradient) above the normal value (up to 5 mmHg). However, collateralization of the portal venous system requires that the portal pressure gradient increases above a critical threshold value, which is 10 to 12 mmHg for the formation of gastro-oesophageal varices and 12 mmHg for the rupture of the varices (Groszmann, Gastro, 1990; 99:1401).[12] This threshold value is also required for bleeding from portal hypertensive gastropathy and for the appearance of ascites. These observations suggest that it could be possible to prevent the development of the complications of portal hypertension (formation of varices,

bleeding, and ascites) if early pharmacological intervention could prevent the portal pressure increasing above this threshold. In practice, there is experimental evidence indicating that development of portal–systemic collaterals can be prevented by portal pressure reducing agents (Sarin, JCI, 1991; 87:1032; Lin, Hepatol, 1991; 14:325). Furthermore, it has been shown that reduction of the portal pressure gradient below this threshold value in patients with varices caused a significant reduction in the size of the varices (Groszmann, Gastro, 1990; 99:1401).

Therefore, the 12 mmHg threshold gradient defines what should be considered as a clinically significant increase in portal pressure. However, this does not mean that above these values all patients will develop complications. In a recent survey at our institution, over 40 per cent of cirrhotic patients without oeso-phageal varices were found to have a portal pressure gradient above the threshold. It is likely that these patients are at a much higher risk of developing varices than those with a portal pressure gradient below these values.

Approximately 50 per cent of the compensated cirrhotic patients already have oesophageal varices at the time of the diagnosis of their liver disease. In patients with liver cirrhosis and no oesophageal varices, the incidence of new varices varies between 8 and 23 per cent after 1 year of follow-up (Calès, Gut, 1990; 31: 1298).[13] Multivariate analysis did not identify any clinical variable that predicted which patients will develop oesophageal varices and which will not. As already discussed, it is likely that the severity of portal hypertension and the period of time that patients maintain an increased portal pressure gradient may be important in determining the rate of formation of varices. Finally, formation of varices may be influenced by angiogenic factors. This is suggested by the fact that the collaterals are not only dilated vessels, on the contrary they show a marked hyperplasy of the muscular wall layer.

Pathophysiology of variceal haemorrhage

In patients with cirrhosis and oesophageal varices the incidence of first variceal bleeding ranges from 19 to 40 per cent after 2 years of follow-up.[14] This means that there are some patients with oesophageal varices that are never going to bleed. Obviously, being able to predict the patients at higher risk of bleeding is of great interest to provide effective therapy for those who are more likely to benefit from it. Up to now, such prediction has been based on the observation that some clinical and endoscopic parameters are statistically related to an increased bleeding risk.[16] A better approach, however, would be first to identify the factors involved in the pathophysiology of variceal haemorrhage and then to assess its prognostic value in prospective investigations.

Two theories have been proposed to explain variceal bleeding (Bosch, MedicinaClin, 1984; 82:401; Conn, Gastro, 1980; 79: 1333).[15] The erosion theory suggested that varices bleed because of external trauma to the thin, fragile walls of the varices caused by swallowing of solid food and by gastro-oesophageal reflux. This theory was abandoned because of the lack of objective evidence supporting it: there is no proven relationship between eating and bleeding, neither the incidence of gastro-oesophageal reflux nor of oesophagitis is greater in patients with bleeding varices than in those without. At present, the most widely accepted hypothesis of the pathophysiology of variceal haemorrhage is the so-called explosion theory, that suggests that the main event leading to bleeding is an excessive hydrostatic pressure inside the varices due to portal hypertension. In this hypothesis, more important than intravariceal pressure is the strength exerted on the wall of the varices: bleeding probably occurs when the expanding force inside the varices can no longer be counterbalanced by increasing wall tension; at this moment the varix bulges and bursts.[15] The factors regulating the tension exerted by the wall of the varices are interrelated by Laplace's law in the equation:

$$\text{Tension} = (P\text{i} - P\text{e}) \times r/w$$

in which $P\text{i}$ is the intravariceal pressure, $P\text{e}$ the pressure in the oesophageal lumen, r is the radius of the varix, and w the thickness of its wall. It follows that an increased variceal size and decreased wall thickness will multiply the deleterious effects of a high intravariceal pressure increasing variceal wall tension to values close to the rupture point; a big varix with thin walls (indicated by the presence of 'red signs' on endoscopy) will reach a high wall tension (and risk of bleeding) at much lower variceal pressures than a small varix with thick walls.[16]

These concepts fit well with the results of clinical studies showing that variceal size, the presence of red colour signs in the wall of the varices at endoscopy, and the degree of liver failure, estimated by the Child–Pugh classification, are the main variables correlating with the risk of variceal bleeding.[16] Haemodynamic variables were also shown to be useful. A prophylactic propranolol placebo trial clearly showed that the risk of experiencing the first episode of bleeding was abolished when the portal pressure gradient (or its equivalent, the hepatic venous pressure gradient) was decreased to 12 mmHg or below (Groszmann, Gastro, 1990; 99:1401) and that after surviving from an episode of bleeding, the risk of further bleeding episodes is much reduced if the hepatic venous pressure gradient is decreased by over 20 per cent of baseline values (Feu, Lancet, 1995; 346:1056). In addition, it has been shown that variceal pressure is significantly higher in variceal bleeders than in non-bleeders (Rigau, Gastro, 1989; 96:873) and that, when variceal pressure is measured repeatedly during the follow-up, patients that will experience variceal bleeding maintain higher variceal pressures than in those who will not (Feu, JHepatol, 1990; 11:S22). Therefore, available data fit perfectly with the predictions of the explosion theory. It is likely that prognostication could be improved if the variceal wall tension itself could be measured, which has not been possible because of lack of adequate methods for an accurate quantitation of the radius and thickness of the wall of the varices. Studies combining measurements of variceal pressure with semiquantitative assessment of variceal size allowed rough estimation of a variceal wall tension 'index' (as the product of variceal pressure and estimated diameter). These studies showed that variceal wall tension was much higher in variceal bleeders than in non-bleeders (Rigau, Gastro, 1989; 96:873). Endoluminal sonography is a new, promising technique that by improving assessment of variceal size (Escorsell, JHepatol, 1995; 23:70) and of variceal wall thickness (Miller, Gastro, 1995; 108:A1223) may allow a more precise calculation of variceal wall tension. Clinical studies will have to show whether the use of these techniques proves useful in the

investigation of the pathophysiology of variceal haemorrhage and in the assessment of the risk of bleeding in individual patients.

Probably the most important factor in the chain of events that leads to variceal haemorrhage is the increased portal pressure that promotes the formation and dilatation of the varices and that is responsible for the increased intravariceal pressure. As the varices dilate their walls will become thinner, bringing variceal wall tension to a 'high risk' level. At this moment, any further increase in variceal pressure or size, or any defect in the variceal wall, will determine leakage of the varices and clinical haemorrhage. In that regard, it is worth noting that in patients with cirrhosis, portal pressure should not be considered a static but as a dynamic parameter. In these patients it has been shown that the portal pressure gradient exhibits circadian variations (García-Pagán, Hepatol, 1994; 19:595). The periods of the day in which there is a spontaneous decrease and increase in portal pressure have been shown to be coincidental in time with the lower and higher prevalence of acute variceal bleeding in epidemiological surveys (García-Pagán, Hepatol, 1994; 19:595; Siringo, Gastro, 1992; 102: A890; Merican, JHepatol, 1993; 19:15). Other physiological stimuli such as meals (Lee, Hepatol, 1988; 8:647) or physical exercise (García-Pagán, Gastro, 1996; 111:1300-6) have also been shown to modify portal pressure in patients with cirrhosis. Why such relatively small changes in portal pressure may influence the moment of onset of bleeding is unknown. However, it is likely that in patients that already are at a high risk of haemorrhage, even moderate changes in portal pressure may be clinically significant.

Pathophysiology of ascites and of other complications of portal hypertension

The pathophysiology of sodium retention, ascites, and of the hepatorenal syndrome are discussed in Chapters 8.1 and 8.2. The pathophysiology of hypersplenism is reviewed in Section 10. Regarding the mechanism of bleeding from portal hypertensive gastropathy, see Chapter 8.3.

References

1. Bosch J, Pizcueta P, Feu F, Fernández M, and García-Pagán JC. Pathophysiology of portal hypertension. *Gastroenterology Clinics of North America*, 1992; **21**: 1–14.
2. Shibayama Y and Nakata K. Localization of increased hepatic vascular resistance in liver cirrhosis. *Hepatology*, 1985; **5**: 643–7.
3. Bathal PS and Grossmann HJ. Reduction of the increased portal vascular resistance of the isolated perfused cirrhotic rat liver by vasodilators. *Journal of Hepatology*, 1985; **1**: 325–9.
4. García-Pagán JC, Bosch J, and Rodés J. The role of vasoactive mediators in portal hypertension. *Seminars in Gastrointestinal Diseases*, 1995; **6**: 1–9.
5. Lautt WW, Greenway CV, and Legare DJ. Effects of hepatic nerves, norepinephrine, angiotensin, elevated central venous pressure on post-sinusoidal resistance sites and intrahepatic pressures. *Microcirculation*, 1987; **33**: 50–61.
6. Marteau P, Ballet F, Chazouillères O, *et al.* Effects of vasodilators on hepatic microcirculation in cirrhosis: a study in the isolated perfused rat liver. *Hepatology*, 1989; **9**: 820–3.
7. Ballet F, Chretien Y, Rey C, *et al.* Differential response of normal and cirrhotic liver to vasoactive agents. A study in the isolated perfused rat liver. *Journal of Pharmacology and Experimental Therapeutics*, 1988; **244**: 233–5.

8. Vorobioff J, Bredfeldt J, and Groszmann RJ. Hyperdynamic circulation in a portal hypertensive rat model: A primary factor for maintenance of chronic portal hypertension. *American Journal of Physiology*, 1983; **244**: G52–6.

9. Sikuler E and Groszmann RJ. Interaction of flow and resistance in maintenance of portal hypertension in a rat model. *American Journal of Physiology*, 1986; **250**: G205–12.

10. Benoit JN, Barrowman JA, Harper SL, *et al*. Role of humoral factors in the intestinal hyperemia associated with chronic portal hypertension. *American Journal of Physiology*, 1984; **247**: 486–93.

11. Moncada S, Palmer RMJ, and Higgs EA. Nitric oxide: Physiology, pathophysiology and pharmacology. *Pharmacology Review*, 1991; **43**: 109–42.

12. Garcia-Tsao G, Groszmann RJ, Fisher RL, Conn HO, Atterbury CE, and Glickman M. Portal pressure presence of gastrovarices and variceal bleeding. *Hepatology*, 1985; **5**: 419–24.

13. Pagliaro L, D'Amico G, Pasta L, Politi F, Vizzini G, Traina M, Madonia S, Luca A, Guerrera D, Puleo A, and D'Antoni A. Portal hypertension in cirrhosis: Natural history. In Bosch J and Groszmann RJ, ed. *Portal hypertension. Pathophysiology and treatment*. Oxford: Blackwell Scientific Publications, 1994: 72–92.

14. D'Amico G, Pagliaro L, and Bosch J. The treatment of portal hypertension: a meta-analytic review. *Hepatology*, 1995; **22**: 332–54.

15. Polio J and Groszmann RJ. Hemodynamic factors involved in the development and rupture of esophageal varices: a pathophysiologic approach to treatment. *Seminars in Liver Disease*, 1986; **6**: 318–31.

16. The North Italian Endoscopic Club for the study and the treatment of esophageal varices. Prediction of the first variceal hemorrhage in patients with cirrhosis of the liver and esophageal varices. *New England Journal of Medicine*, 1988; **319**: 983–9.

7.3 Intrahepatic portal hypertension

Jean-Pierre Benhamou and Dominique Valla

Introduction

Portal hypertension can be defined as an increase in the gradient between portal venous pressure and inferior vena caval pressure.[1,2] An increased resistance to portal blood flow plays a major part in the mechanism of portal hypertension. A secondary increase in splanchnic blood flow contributes to the maintenance of high portal pressure in spite of the development of portosystemic collaterals.[3] The causes of portal hypertension can be classified according to the site of the increased vascular resistance. Suprahepatic blocks refer to obstruction of the hepatic veins or suprahepatic inferior vena cava; infrahepatic blocks refer to obstruction of the portal vein; only intrahepatic blocks will be considered in this chapter.

Haemodynamic studies based on the measurement of portal venous pressure, wedged hepatic venous pressure, and free hepatic venous pressure or inferior vena caval pressure allow a precise analysis of the site of increased intrahepatic vascular resistance.[1,2] These studies allow further classification of intrahepatic blocks as follows. (a) Presinusoidal block is characterized by an elevated portal venous pressure but a normal hepatic venous-pressure gradient (wedged minus free hepatic venous pressure (**HVPG**)); this type of block is determined by lesions of portal venules. (b) Sinusoidal block is characterized by an increased HVPG with wedged hepatic venous pressure being equal to portal venous pressure. It is generally admitted that this type of intrahepatic block is related to sinusoidal lesions leading to a loss of the normal communications between contiguous hepatic lobules.[1] Compression of central or intercalated venules may also explain the haemodynamic characteristics of sinusoidal block but this point remains controversial (Laut, Hepatol, 1987; 7:952). (c) Mixed presinusoidal and sinusoidal blocks are characterized by an increased HVPG and an increased portal venous pressure that is higher than wedged hepatic venous pressure.

Most causes of portal hypertension are associated with various types of intrahepatic blocks either sequentially during the course of the disease or in various forms of the disease. Therefore, the classification of intrahepatic blocks according to the results of haemodynamic studies is of great interest for understanding the pathogenesis of portal hypertension but not for determining its aetiology.

Conditions usually complicated by portal hypertension

Cirrhosis

HVPG is constantly increased in cirrhosis (Reynolds, JCI, 1955; 34: 213; Viallet, Gastro, 1970; 59:372; Boyer, Gastro, 1977; 72:584;

Valla, Gastro, 1984; 86:1400).[4] Values for HVPG range from 8 to 30 mmHg. Ruptured oesophageal varices almost exclusively affect patients with HVPG greater than 12 mmHg (Garcia-Tsao, Hepatol, 1985; 5:419). Within 10 days after variceal haemorrhage, there is a spontaneous decrease in portal pressure, approximately 20 per cent in magnitude (Pomier-Layrargue, Gastro, 1987; 93:1218). The prevalence of portal hypertension in cirrhosis would be underestimated if its recognition were based on the only presence of oesophageal varices. The prevalence of oesophageal varices is about 40 per cent at the time of diagnosis of cirrhosis and 90 per cent after 10 years of follow-up (Christensen, Gastro, 1981; 81:944).

The influence of the cause of cirrhosis on the natural history of portal hypertension has not been clearly evaluated. A decrease in portal pressure has been documented in patients with alcoholic cirrhosis in whom liver lesions have improved after abstinence (Gluud, JHepatol,, 1987; 4:168; Poynard, DigDisSci, 1987; 32:337) and in patients with non-alcoholic cirrhosis in whom spontaneous portosystemic shunts have enlarged (Onishi, JClinGastro, 1984; 6: 447).

In patients with alcoholic cirrhosis, portal venous pressure equals wedged hepatic venous pressure (Reynolds, JCI, 1955; 34:213; Viallet, Gastro, 1970; 59:372; Boyer, Gastro, 1977; 72:584; Valla, Gastro, 1984; 86:1400).[4] In a few patients wedged hepatic venous pressure is higher than portal venous pressure and reversal of portal vein flow occurs (Valla, Gastro, 1984; 86:1400, Rector, Hepatol, 1988; 8: 16–20; Bauret, GastrClinBiol, 1989; 13:132). Studies of hepatic microcirculation have identified several mechanisms that may explain the increased intrahepatic vascular resistance:[5] a reduction of sinusoidal calibre due to hepatocyte enlargement (Vidins, Hepatol, 1985; 5:408) or to compression by regenerative nodules (Popper, AmJPathol, 1977; 87:228; Krosgaard, ScaJGastr, 1987; 22:82); an alteration in the elastic properties of the sinusoidal wall due to collagen deposition in the Disse space (Schaffner, Gastro, 1963; 44:239; Orrego, Gastro, 1981; 80:546); compression of hepatic venules by regenerative nodules (Sherlock, AmJSurg, 1974; 127:121); central vein lesions such as perivenous fibrosis (Lieber, ClinRes, 1976; 24:478A, Nakano, Gastro, 1982; 83:777), phlebitis, veno-occlusive changes, or phlebosclerosis (Goodman, Gastro, 1982; 83:786). Whatever the lesion, it should be pointed out that the organization of the sinusoidal bed results in a maximal increase in resistance at the termination of sinusoids (Henriksen, Liver, 1988; 8:88). Haemorrheological changes probably contribute to the increased intrahepatic vascular resistance (Matos, Hepatol, 1988; 8:1424). In 20 per cent of patients with non-alcoholic cirrhosis, portal venous pressure exceeds wedged hepatic venous pressure, which indicates some degree of presinusoidal block.[4] Portal fibrosis, piecemeal necrosis, and portal inflammation may account for this additional presinusoidal block.

Non-cirrhotic alcoholic and alcoholic-like liver disease

Alcoholic liver injury can be complicated by portal hypertension in the absence of cirrhosis. Increased HVPG is very uncommon in steatosis, although oesophageal varices have been described in patients who died of massive alcoholic steatosis. Alcoholic hepatitis and especially the so-called acute sclerosing hyaline necrosis is associated with an increased HVPG; however, wedged hepatic venous pressure in these patients is less markedly increased than in patients with alcoholic cirrhosis (Reynolds, AnnIntMed, 1969; 70: 497). In patients with alcoholic fibrosis, even in the absence of cirrhosis, HVPG is constantly increased and oesophageal varices are present in half the cases.[4] The sinusoidal and perivenular lesions implicated in the pathogenesis of portal hypertension of alcoholic cirrhosis are also implicated in non-cirrhotic alcoholic liver injury.

Similar findings have been reported in patients with alcoholic-like hepatic injury associated with morbid obesity or jejunoileal bypass (Capron, DigDisSci, 1982; 27:265).

Chronic hepatitis

Chronic active hepatitis is associated with portal hypertension in the absence of cirrhosis. The prevalence of oesophageal varices, gastrointestinal bleeding, and ascites is about 20, 5, and 30 per cent, respectively (Czaja, Gastro, 1976; 71:901).[4] There is a significant relation between the severity of the liver lesions and the magnitude of the increase of HVPG[4] (Ampelas, GastrClinBiol, 1989; 13:136). In patients with mild chronic hepatitis, HVPG is not increased. In patients with moderate to severe chronic hepatitis without cirrhosis, the increase in HVPG is mild to moderate; the highest values for HVPG are recorded in patients with severe chronic hepatitis and cirrhosis. Portal venous pressure is higher than wedge hepatic venous pressure, which indicates the presence of both sinusoidal and presinusoidal blocks (Boyer, Gastro, 1977; 72:584). Portal and periportal fibrosis might be the mechanism for portal hypertension (Ampelas, GastrClinBiol, 1989; 13:136).

Primary biliary cirrhosis

In patients with primary biliary cirrhosis, portal hypertension is present before true cirrhosis has developed (Kew, Gut, 1971; 12: 830).[6,7] The prevalence of oesophageal varices is 20 per cent within a year after the onset of symptoms and 90 per cent 9 years later.[6] At the early stage of primary biliary cirrhosis, portal hypertension results from a presinusoidal block; at the late stage of the disease, sinusoidal block is superimposed. HVPG is poorly related to the presence of regenerative nodules,[6] portal or sinusoidal fibrosis,[7] or granulomas.[7] Portal and periportal inflammation[7] and periportal nodular hyperplasia (Nakanuma, AmJGastr, 1987; 82:8; Chazouillères, GastrClinBiol, 1986; 10:764) might play a part in the mechanism of the presinusoidal increase in vascular resistance. Portosystemic shunting may be better tolerated in patients with primary biliary cirrhosis than in those with alcoholic or posthepatitic cirrhosis (Bauer, AnnSurg, 1976; 183:324); however, this point has been questioned (Sepersky, DigDisSci, 1982; 27:507). End-to-side portacaval shunting may make a subsequent liver transplant difficult and therefore should be avoided in patients in whom liver transplantation might be considered. For this reason, propranolol or sclerotherapy of oesophageal varices are recommended for prevention of recurrent gastrointestinal bleeding in patients with primary biliary cirrhosis.

Chronic biliary obstruction

Oesophageal varices are present in 20 per cent of patients with chronic biliary obstruction.[8,9] Signs of portal hypertension usually appear within 2 to 5 years after the onset of obstruction.[10] This explains why the cause of biliary stricture complicated by portal hypertension is, in most of the cases, a non-malignant lesion, with a long silent course, such as biliary strictures following surgical bile-duct injury.[8–10] However, in a few cases, portal hypertension develops within a year or less and may then be caused by a malignant biliary stricture (Gulsrud, DigDisSci, 1979; 24:166). Portal pressure is elevated in patients with chronic biliary obstruction, well before the development of true cirrhosis. In such patients, portal hypertension mainly results from portal fibrosis. Hyperplasia of periportal hepatocytes has been suggested to play as a great part as fibrosis.[10] Portal vein thrombosis is associated with bile-duct injury in 10 per cent of cases.[9]

The relief of biliary obstruction may not be followed by the disappearance of portal hypertension.[8] The construction of portosystemic shunts using the portal vein may be difficult or dangerous due to scarring and inflammation induced by prior surgery or cholangitis.[8,9] Furthermore, the relief of portal hypertension facilitates surgical repair of bile-duct injury; therefore, portosystemic shunting, such as with splenorenal or mesocaval shunts, is recommended before the surgical repair of bile-duct strictures.[8,9] Multiple operations on the biliary tract may make liver transplantation difficult and should be avoided in patients in whom transplantation might be envisaged.

Haemochromatosis

Portal hypertension may be present in idiopathic (genetic) or secondary haemochromatosis before the development of true cirrhosis; [11] it is then related to fibrosis. In patients with true cirrhosis, portal hypertension is more marked than in patients with non-cirrhotic fibrosis. Gastrointestinal bleeding due to portal hypertension is rare but may occur when HVPG is lower than 10 mmHg. This observation indirectly suggests that both sinusoidal and presinusoidal intrahepatic blocks are present. The development of *de novo* varices is prevented and the regression of previous varices is favourably influenced by phlebotomy (Fracanzani, Hepatol, 1995; 22:1127).

Hepatosplenic schistosomiasis

It has been estimated that 100 million individuals worldwide suffer from schistosomiasis mansoni or japonicum.[12–14] Haemodynamic studies have showed that portal pressure is increased in 80 per cent or more infected patients,[15] but these studies are probably biased by being based only on symptomatic patients admitted to hospital. In endemic areas, such as Nairobi, hepato-splenic schistosomiasis is the cause of portal hypertension in one-third of unselected patients with documented oesophageal varices.[13]

The natural history of portal hypertension is closely related to the number of eggs deposited in the liver, which is roughly parallel to the number of eggs excreted in stools in untreated patients (Sheever, AmJTropMedHyg, 1968; 17:38). Gastrointestinal bleeding from ruptured oesophageal varices is the major complication and the main cause of death in these patients.[13] Multiple episodes of gastrointestinal bleeding extending over many years are characteristic. The risk of gastrointestinal bleeding is positively correlated with splenic pulp pressure.[15] Splenomegaly is very common: it is not only related to portal hypertension, but also to reticuloendothelial hyperplasia following continued antigenic stimulation (Kloetzel, AmJTropMedHyg, 1962; 11:472). Ascites is uncommon but may occur following gastrointestinal bleeding.[13] There is no manifestation of liver failure. Spontaneous hepatic encephalopathy does not occur. When the manifestations of liver failure are present, superimposed chronic viral hepatitis and post-hepatitic cirrhosis should be suspected. The association of schistosomiasis and chronic viral hepatitis is common for two reasons: (i) in the areas where hepatosplenic schistosomiasis is endemic, the prevalence of hepatitis B or C viral infections is also very high, and (ii) bleeding patients with hepatosplenic schistosomiasis are at high risk of acquiring chronic viral hepatitis through blood transfusion (Dunn, Hepatol, 1981; 1:653).

Haemodynamic studies have showed that there are two stages in the development of portal hypertension. In the early stage, wedged hepatic venous pressure is normal whereas portal venous pressure is increased:[15] the presinusoidal block results from the obstruction of portal venules by the eggs and the granulomatous reaction. Intrahepatic cavernomas connecting the segments of portal venules unobstructed by the eggs and granulomas develop.[15] The portal vein and its major branches are dilated. Portal vein thrombosis may be present.[15] The entire hepatic arterial bed is dilated. Total hepatic blood flow is maintained at normal values (Ramos, Gastro, 1964; 47:241).[15] At a late stage, wedged hepatic venous pressure is increased in the absence of cirrhosis (Ramos, Gastro, 1964: 47: 241).[15] This superimposed sinusoidal block might result from several factors: the development of perisinusoidal fibrosis (Grimaud, LabInvest, 1977; 36:268), the increased arterial supply to the liver sinusoids (Alves, Gastro, 1977; 72:126), or focal nodulation of hepatic parenchyma (Alves, Gastro, 1977; 72:126).

Various forms of surgical therapy have been attempted to prevent recurrent bleeding. Splenectomy may be complicated by portal vein thrombosis (Cheever, TrRevSocTropMedHyg, 1967; 61:626). Hepatic encephalopathy following portosystemic shunting is as frequent in schistosomiasis as in cirrhosis (Warren, NEJM, 1964; 271:921; Da Silva, AnnSurg, 1986; 204:148; Raia, Hepatol, 1994; 20:398). Oesophagogastric devascularization with splenectomy was found to be superior to proximal and distal splenorenal shunt in a prospective randomized trial (Raia, Hepatol, 1994; 20:398). Sclerotherapy of oesophageal varices (Bessa, Surgery, 1985; 97:164), or propranolol administration (Küre, ZGastr, 1986; 24 (Suppl. 1):39) have been reported to reduce the risk of recurrent bleeding in patients with hepatosplenic schistosomiasis.

Congenital hepatic fibrosis

Congenital hepatic fibrosis is a genetically transmitted condition characterized by enlarged portal spaces containing abundant connective tissue and numerous ectatic bile ducts. This lesion is frequently associated with various cystic lesions of the kidneys (Kerr, QJMed, 1961; 30:91). The main consequence of congenital hepatic fibrosis is portal hypertension and gastrointestinal bleeding from oesophageal varices.[16] Two-thirds of the patients present with haematemesis or melaena, most of them between 5 and 20 years of age, but, in a few, after 40 years. Splenomegaly and hypersplenism are common; ascites is uncommon.

Portosystemic shunting appears to be better tolerated in patients with congenital hepatic fibrosis than in patients with cirrhosis.[17] Macronodular transformation occurring 18 years after surgical portosystemic shunting raises the possibility that deprivation of portal venous inflow in this disease may precipitate the development of nodular transformation (Bertheau, JHepatol, 1994; 20:213). Recurrent ascending cholangitis is a major cause of death (de Vos, JHepatol, 1988; 6:222).[17]

Hepatoportal sclerosis. Idiopathic portal hypertension. Incomplete septal cirrhosis

Various denominations have been given to a clinicopathological entity characterized by portal hypertension and moderate to minimal portal fibrosis without cirrhosis: hepatoportal sclerosis,[18] non-cirrhotic portal fibrosis,[19] idiopathic portal hypertension,[20–24] non-cirrhotic intrahepatic portal hypertension,[25] benign intrahepatic portal hypertension,[26] idiopathic presinusoidal portal hypertension,[27] sinusoidal portal hypertension.[28] The so-called Banti syndrome might well be a variant of this entity.[27,29] Some confusion has arisen from the restriction of the term 'idiopathic portal hypertension' to those cases in which no lesion was found by light microscopy, but in which perisinusoidal fibrosis was demonstrated by electron microscopy.[24] Recently, incomplete septal cirrhosis, characterized by slender and often incomplete septa that demarcate large, rather inconspicuous nodules, has been related to hepatoportal sclerosis (Nevens, Gastro, 1994; 106:459; Bernard, JHepatol, 1995; 22:495)

A cause for hepatoportal sclerosis can be found only in a minority of cases: chronic arsenical intoxication (Morris, Gastro, 1974; 64: 86; Huet, Gastro, 1975; 68:1270; Datta, Gut, 1979; 20:378); chronic exposition to vinyl chloride monomers (Thomas, NEJM, 1975; 292: 17; Smith, Lancet, 1976; ii:602; Blendis, Gastro, 1978; 75:206); chronic exposure to copper sulphate in vineyard sprayers (Cortez-Pimentel, Gastro, 1977; 72:275); protracted treatment with methotrexate (Podurgiel, MayoClinProc, 1973; 48:787); treatment with 6-mercaptopurine, azathioprine, and prednisone in renal transplant recipients[24] (Bordfeldt, JClinGastro, 1982; 4:157); irradiation and chemotherapy following resection of Wilms' tumour (Barnard, Gastro, 1986; 90:1054); hypervitaminosis A (Jacques, Gastro, 1979; 76:599; Verneau, GastrClinBiol, 1984; 8:121; Geubel, Gastro, 1991; 100:1701). Hepatoportal sclerosis without apparent cause is rare in Western countries, but common in India and Japan.

Clinical features include bleeding from ruptured oesophageal varices and splenomegaly with hypersplenism. Ascites is uncommon. Liver function is normal. The main histological features are: (a) irregular thickening of the liver capsule; (b) thickening of some portal tracts with fine fibrous septa radiating out from some of them; and (c) distortion of lobular architecture with hyperplastic expansion of some areas and atrophy of other areas, and irregularly distributed central veins (Okuda, Liver, 1982; 2:176).[26] Fibrosis and nodule formation, when present, affect the subcapsular areas, but not deeper parts of the liver. At electron microscopy, perisinusoidal fibrosis has been found in most cases (Tandon, Gut, 1970; 11:905).[24]

HVPG may be normal or mildly increased; portal venous pressure is much higher than wedged hepatic venous pressure in all cases; thus the presinusoidal component of the intrahepatic block is predominant or exclusive (Boyer, Gastro, 1977; 72:584).[24,27,29] The presinusoidal block may be the consequence of obliteration of large- and medium-sized (Nayak, ArchPathLabMed, 1969; 87:359; Bernard, JHepatol, 1995; 22:495). Portal scarring and replacement of terminal portal venules with tiny, multiple vascular channels may also participate in the presinusoidal block (Nayak, Arch-PathLabMed, 1969; 87:359; Bernard, JHepatol, 1995; 22:495). Thrombosis of the portal vein is present in a number of cases (Kameda, JGastrHepatol, 1986; 1:139).[18–20] Portal venography shows a paucity of medium-sized branches with occasional abrupt interruptions and avascular areas beneath the liver surface.[21,22] There is approximation of portal and hepatic vein branches, which suggests atrophy of the liver parenchyma resulting from obliterative portal venopathy (Okuda, Liver, 1981; 1:255). Perisinusoidal fibrosis, which may be the only significant lesion and may be missed at light-microscopic examination, would be a likely explanation for the increased HVPG.[24]

Prognosis is much better in patients with hepatoportal sclerosis than in those with cirrhosis.[20,21,25] However, the prognosis of incomplete septal cirrhosis, which might represent a late stage of hepatoportal sclerosis, is similar to that of classical viral macronodular cirrhosis and may progress to endstage liver disease (Nevens, Gastro, 1994; 106:459; Bernard, JHepatol, 1995; 22:495). Portosystemic shunting is reported to be well tolerated in these patients;[20] however, postshunt chronic portal systemic encephalopathy has been reported.[21,25]

Nodular regenerative hyperplasia

Nodular regenerative hyperplasia is an uncommon disorder of the liver characterized by multiple regenerative nodules of a diameter smaller than that of the lobule without fibrosis.[30–36] The extracellular liver-cell plates are normally orientated, but may be atrophic. In a few cases, nodular regenerative hyperplasia is associated with peliosis hepatis [37] (Ihara, MedJOsakaUniv, 1982; 33:13) or perisinusoidal fibrosis (Degott, Liver, 1985; 5:276). The pathogenesis of nodular regenerative hyperplasia is incompletely understood. According to a widely accepted hypothesis, the regenerative nodules would result from heterogeneous perfusion of liver tissue with atrophy of the poorly perfused areas and hyperplasia of the normally perfused areas.[32,33,36] In support of this hypothesis is the frequent finding of obliterative lesions in portal venules[32,36] or hepatic arterioles (Reynolds, JRheum, 1984; 11:838). The association with peliosis hepatis and perisinusoidal fibrosis suggests that uneven perfusion may also result from irregularly distributed sinusoidal lesions.[36] This view is supported by an

experimental model in rodents given selenium orally in whom capillarization of sinusoids seems to precede nodule formation. Nodular regenerative hyperplasia is associated with systemic disorders (listed in Table 1) in 80 per cent of cases. These associated conditions are commonly characterized by hypergammaglobulinaemia and/or the presence of circulating immune complexes. An attractive hypothesis would be the that the obliterative vascular lesions would be the consequence of an immune-complex disease.[36]

The main manifestations of nodular regenerative hyperplasia are hepatomegaly, splenomegaly, increased serum alkaline phosphatases, and increased γ-glutamyl transpeptidase. Other liver tests are minimally altered and, occasionally all liver tests can be completely normal (Colina, Liver, 1989; 9:253). Portal hypertension is the main complication. The prevalence of oesophageal varices, and of gastrointestinal bleeding and ascites, are approximately 60, 30, and 30, respectively.[31,33-35] Liver failure rarely develops.

Increased portal venous pressure is a constant finding (Miyai, AmJClinPathol, 1980; 73:267).[31,35] Wedged hepatic venous pressure is increased to a much smaller degree.[31,35] This observation is compatible with obliterative portal venopathy resulting in a presinusoidal block. Superimposed increased sinusoidal resistance may be the consequence of a decreased sinusoidal diameter due to compression by hyperplastic nodules.

Prevention of recurrent gastrointestinal bleeding has been achieved with portosystemic shunting (Naber, JHepatol, 1991;12: 94).[31,35] Although liver function is usually preserved, chronic portosystemic encephalopathy may occur after portosystemic shunting (Samuel, GastrClinBiol, 1985; 9:162). Prognosis is mainly dependent on the associated extrahepatic disorder (Naber, JHepatol, 1991;12:94).

Partial nodular transformation

Partial nodular transformation is a very uncommon lesion characterized by large nodules of hepatocytes, 3 to 80 mm in diameter, which predominate in the perihilar region of the liver.[38,39] The periphery of the liver may be normal, atrophic, or affected by nodular regenerative hyperplasia.[40] This last finding suggests that partial nodular transformation and nodular regenerative hyperplasia may be two different aspects of a unique entity.[39,40]

Peliosis hepatis

Peliosis hepatis is characterized by blood-filled cavities of various sizes, bordered by hepatocytic plates, and randomly distributed throughout the hepatic lobule.[41–44] The hepatocytes bordering the peliotic cavities are often atrophic or compressed.[44] Peliosis hepatis, sinusoidal dilatation, perisinusoidal fibrosis, and nodular regenerative hyperplasia may coexist.[37,44–46] The peliotic cavities consist of dilated sinusoids and Disse spaces.[44,45] The pathogenesis is unknown. Indirect evidence suggests two mechanisms: (i) obstruction at the junctions of sinusoids and central veins (Paradinas, Histopath, 1977; 1:225);[44,46] (ii) a primary lesion of the sinusoidal (mainly endothelial) cells.[44,45] Peliosis hepatis is frequently associated with extrahepatic diseases (listed in Table 2). Most of these associated diseases share the following features: (a) a chronic, debilitating condition, (b) frequently associated with severe infections, and (c) leading commonly to the

Table 1 Reported conditions associated with nodular regenerative hyperplasia of the liver*

Conditions	References
Drugs and chemicals	
Androgenic-anabolic steroids	Sweeney, JClinPath, 1976; 29:626
Contraceptive steroids	[34]
Immunosuppressive drugs	[32,34]; Ihara, MedJOsakaUniv, 1982; 33:13; Key, Lancet, 1987; 2:1050
Corticosteroids	[34]
Arsenic	Popper, AmJPathol, 1978; 92:349
Vinyl chloride	Popper, AmJPathol, 1978; 92:349
Toxic oil syndrome	Sollis-Herruzo, Hepatol, 1986; 6:687
Bacterial infections	
Endocarditis	[30,32]
Tuberculosis	[31,32]
Monoclonal gammapathies	
Multiple myeloma	[32]
Waldenström's macroglobulinaemia	[36,37]
Chronic lymphocytic leukaemia with plasmocytoma	[36]
Monoclonal gammapathy immunoglobulin Gκ	[31]
Malignancies	
Malignant tumours	[33,34]
Lymphoma	[34]
Hodgkin's disease	[34]
Myeloproliferative disorders	
Polycythaemia vera	[32]
Myeloid metaplasia	[32]; Degott, Liver, 1985; 5:276
Primary thrombocythaemia	[32]
Immune-complex diseases	
Rheumatoid arthritis with or without Felty syndrome	[32,34]; Blendis, OJMed, 1974; 43:35; Thorne, AmJMed, 1982; 73:35
Scleroderma	[32]; Russel, JRheum, 1983; 10:748
Mixed cryoglobulinaemia	[36]
Polyarteritis nodosa	Nakanuma, ArchPathLabMed, 1984; 108:133
Disseminated lupus erythematosus	[34,36]
Other conditions	
Renal transplantation	[32,34]; Ihara, MedJOsakaUniv, 1982; 33:13
Crohn's disease	[34]
Diabetes	[34]; Thung, Cancer, 1982; 49:543

* Modified from Voinchet et al. (37).

administration of androgenic–anabolic steroids (Bragheri, Ann-IntMed, 1974; 81:610; Nadell, ArchPathLabMed, 1977; 101:405).[41–46] Several drugs and chemicals have been incriminated; however, rather than a direct toxic effect, these substances may only potentiate the action of as yet unidentified endogenous factors.[47] Comparison of Tables 1 and 2 indicates that nodular regenerative hyperplasia and peliosis hepatis have a number of associated conditions in common.[37] In patients with acquired immune deficiency syndrome, an infectious form of peliosis hepatis has been characterized under the name of bacillary peliosis hepatis (Perkocha, NEJM, 1990; 323:1581). It is related to infection by a newly identified pathogen: *Rochmalinea henselae*.

Manifestations of peliosis hepatis are related to the severity of the lesions:[46] mild lesions induce no signs or symptoms, whereas in severe lesions, hepatomegaly, ascites, oesophageal varices or liver failure are present.[41–46] Death results from intraperitoneal bleeding, liver failure or a complication of the associated conditions, but not from portal hypertension.

HVPG is increased.[46] The mechanism for increased intrahepatic resistance is unknown. Perisinusoidal fibrosis is a late sequel after resolution of the peliotic cavities (Gerlag, JHepatol, 1985; 1:339), but can be demonstrated by electron microscopy in the early stages.[44,45] Perisinusoidal fibrosis could thus explain the intrahepatic block observed in peliosis hepatis.

Sinusoidal dilatation

The lesion of sinusoidal dilatation differs from peliosis hepatis in the following characteristics: (a) the ectatic sinusoids do not take the cystic appearance that is typical of peliosis hepatis; (b) the dilatation is not randomly distributed, but affects a distinct part (pericentral, and mid-zonal or periportal) of the lobule. However, the separation between the two entities may be difficult to draw, morphologically and aetiologically. Like peliosis hepatis, sinusoidal dilatation has been reported in association with nodular regenerative hyperplasia and perisinusoidal fibrosis.[37] Table 3 lists the conditions that have been reported to be associated with sinusoidal dilatation; these conditions are almost identical to those associated with peliosis hepatis (Table 2) and nodular regenerative hyperplasia (Table 1). A distinction should be made between sinusoidal dilatation induced by oral contraceptives (Winkler, ScaJGastr, 1975; 10:699) and pregnancy (Fisher, CardiovascIntRadiol, 1984; 7:299), which predominates in the periportal region (zones I and II), and sinusoidal dilatation associated with the other conditions, which

Table 2 Reported conditions associated with peliosis hepatis*

Conditions	References
Drugs and chemicals	
Androgenic-anabolic steroids	[41–44]; Bragheri, AnnIntMed, 1974; 81:610; Nadell, ArchPathLabMed, 1977; 101:405
Contraceptive steroids	Serrano-Martinez, GastroHepato, 1986; 9:344
Antineoplastic drugs	[41]; Heberling, InnMed, 1976; 3:414; Nadell, ArchPathLabMed, 1977; 101:405
Azathioprine-6 thiocyanine	[46]; Gerlag, JHepatol, 1985; 1:339; Larrey, Gut, 1988; 29:1265
Corticosteroids	[42]
Arsenic	Popper, AmJPathol, 1978; 92:349
Thorium dioxyde	Okuda, Liver, 1981; 1:110
Vinyl chloride	Popper, AmJPathol, 1978; 92:349
Copper sulphate	Pimentel, Gastro, 1977; 72:275
Toxic oil syndrome	Solis-Herruzo, Hepatol, 1986; 6:687
Bacterial infections	
Endocarditis	Nadell, ArchPathLabMed, 1977; 101:405; Molle, NouvPresseMed, 1979; 8:2481
Pneumonia, bronchopneumonia	[41,43]; Bragheri, AnnIntMed, 1974; 81:610; Nadell, ArchPathLabMed, 1977; 101:405
Cellulitis	[41,43]
Tuberculosis	[44]; Zak, AmJPathol, 1950; 26:1; Kent, ArchPathol, 1961; 72:658
Monoclonal gammapathies	
Multiple myeloma	[42]; Bragheri, AnnIntMed, 1974; 81:610
Waldenström's macroglobulinaemia	[37]
Systemic light-chain deposition	[37,44]
Myeloproliferative disorders	
Myelofibrosis	Nadell, ArchPathLabMed, 1977; 101:405
Polycythaemia vera	Nadell, ArchPathLabMed, 1977; 101:405
Malignancies	
Solid tumours	[41,43]; Heberling, InnMed, 1976; 3:414
Hodgkin's disease	[42,44]
Anaemias	
Fanconi anaemia	Bragheri, AnnIntMed, 1974; 81:610; Nadell, ArchPathLabMed, 1977; 101:405
Sideroblastic anaemia	Nadell, ArchPathLabMed, 1977; 101:405
Other conditions	
Renal transplantation	[46]; Gerlag, JHepatol, 1985; 1:339; Hankey, MedJAust, 1987; 146:102
Chronic haemodialysis	Hankey, MedJAust, 1987; 146:102; Hillion, Nephron, 1983; 35:205
Diabetes	Hamilton, ArchPathol, 1952; 54:5
Acquired immunodeficiency syndrome	[45]; Devars du Mayne, PresseMed, 1985; 14:1177; Czapar, ArchPathLabMed, 1986; 110:611
Marasmus	Simon, Gastro, 1988; 95:805

* Modified from Voinchet *et al*. (37).

Table 3 Reported conditions associated with sinusoidal dilatation

Conditions	References
Drugs and chemicals	
Contraceptive steroids	[47]; Winkler, ScaJGastr, 1975; 10:699; Bretagne, SemHopParis, 1984; 60:3331; Weinberger, ArchIntMed, 1985; 145:927
Azathioprine	Gerlag, JHepatol, 1985; 1:339
Thorium dioxide	[48]
Bacterial infections	
Brucellosis	[49]
Tuberculosis	[49]
Malignancies	
Solid tumours	[48,49]; Winkler, ScaJGastr, 1975; 10:699
Hodgkin's disease	[49]
Lymphoma	[49]
Other conditions	
Renal transplantation	Gerlag, JHepatol, 1985; 1:339
Diabetes	Fisher, Radiol, 1984; 7:299
Pregnancy	Winkler, ScaJGastr, 1975; 10:699; Fisher, Radiol, 1984; 7:299
Cirrhosis	[48]
Amyloidosis	[49]
Infectious mononucleosis	Weinberger, ArchIntMed, 1985; 145:927
Histiocytosis X	Fiorello, JPediatGastrNutr, 1983; 2:332

predominates in the centrilobular region (zones II and III).[48,49] The pathogenesis is unknown.

Manifestations of sinusoidal dilatation may be absent, or include pain in the right upper quadrant, fever, and hepatomegaly. Ascites and oesophageal varices have been reported (Gerlag, JHepatol, 1985; 1:339).[48] The erythrocyte sedimentation rate and serum gammaglobulin are almost constantly raised (Weinberger, ArchIntMed, 1985; 145:927). Liver function tests are moderately abnormal. Perisinusoidal fibrosis may persist as a late sequel (Bretagne, SemHopPar, 1984; 60:3331). In few cases, the disease progresses to fibrosis and cirrhosis with oesophageal varices, splenomegaly, and hypersplenism (Bragheri, AnnIntMed, 1974; 81:610).

Haemodynamic findings may further distinguish periportal from centrilobular sinusoidal dilatation. In the former, HVPG was normal (Fisher, Radiol, 1984; 7:299), whereas, in the latter, it was increased (Gerlag, JHepatol, 1985; 1:339).[48]

Veno-occlusive disease

This cause of portal hypertension is described elsewhere.

Acute hepatitis

A slight increase in HVPG or intrasplenic pulpal pressure is common in acute symptomatic, benign hepatitis (Reichman, Gastro, 1957; 33:609; Preisig, Circul, 1966; 34:188; Lundbergh, ActaMedScand, 1974; 196:315). Oesophageal varices do not develop (Reichman, Gastro, 1957; 33:609). Ascites is absent or, when present, can be ascribed to an exudative mechanism (Viola, Hepatol, 1983; 3:1013).

In severe or fulminant hepatitis, however, portal hypertension is common.[50,51] Rupture of oesophageal varices has been reported (Nouel, GastrClinBiol, 1981; 5:91). Ascites is frequently present,[50, 51] especially in the patients with HVPG higher than 10 mmHg.[51] The increase in HVPG is related to the severity of hepatitis.[51] The magnitude of centrilobular sinusoidal collapse, a hallmark of the severity of acute hepatitis,[52] seems to be a major determinant of increase in HVPG.[51] The cause of hepatitis, viral, drug-induced, or unknown, has no influence on the degree of portal hypertension.[50, 51]

Acute fatty liver of pregnancy

In acute fatty liver of pregnancy, moderate portal hypertension seems to be frequent and might be due to compression of the sinusoids by the hepatocytes affected by microvesicular steatosis.[53]

Conditions uncommonly complicated by portal hypertension

Sarcoidosis

About 50 cases of portal hypertension due to hepatic sarcoidosis have been reported.[54] In two series of patients with hepatic sarcoidosis, the prevalence of increased HVPG was 30 and 45 per cent.[54,55] This prevalence is probably overestimated since it was based only on symptomatic patients. Portal hypertension occurs in two forms of hepatic sarcoidosis. Sarcoidosis with chronic intrahepatic cholestasis is clinically and histologically very similar to

primary biliary cirrhosis (Rudzki, AmJMed, 1975; 59:373); in this form of sarcoidosis, portal hypertension has many features in common with that complicating primary biliary cirrhosis or chronic biliary obstruction.[54] In sarcoidosis without major cholestasis, portal hypertension may be the presenting manifestation of hepatic involvement. In this form of hepatic sarcoidosis, two types of intrahepatic block have been documented. Presinusoidal block might be due to compression of the portal venules by granulomas.[54] A sinusoidal or postsinusoidal block can be superimposed and might be due to extensive fibrosis or cirrhosis.[54]

Corticosteroids have no influence on portal hypertension and do not prevent its development. Surgical portacaval shunts for the prevention of recurrent bleeding are complicated by hepatic encephalopathy in 16 per cent of cases.[54,55] No evaluation of other surgical or medical treatments is available because of the small number of treated patients.

Polycystic disease of the liver

In patients with polycystic disease, even those with numerous large cysts, portal hypertension and hepatic dysfunction are usually absent. However, these complications have been described in a few patients (Bernard, ArchMalAppDigNutr, 1961; 50:513; Ratcliffe, BMJ, 1984; 288:1330; Van Erpecum, JHepatol, 1987; 5:109). Portal hypertension can be due to direct compression of the portal vein (Bernard, ArchMalAppDigNutr, 1961; 50:513) or the hepatic veins (Uddin, Gut, 1995; 36:142) by large cysts. Oesophageal varices can disappear after fenestration of the cysts (Van Erpecum, JHepatol, 1987; 5:109).

Amyloidosis

Massive hepatic amyloidosis can cause portal hypertension; however, this complication is uncommon (Melkebeke, Digestion, 1980; 20:351; Case Records of the Massachusetts General Hospital, NEJM, 1987; 317:1320; Horsman, Liver, 1995; 15:332). Involvement of the heart or the digestive tract is certainly a more common cause of ascites or gastrointestinal bleeding than portal hypertension.

Infiltration of the liver by malignant cells

Portal hypertension is an uncommon complication of the infiltration of the liver by malignant cells. When it occurs, it is usually associated with rapidly developing neoplasia. Ascites and severe hepatic failure are frequently present.

This presentation has been reported in patients with metastatic carcinoma,[56,57] chronic lymphoid or myeloid leukaemia,[58,59] and Waldenström's macroglublinaemia.[60] The type of intrahepatic block may be related to the type of infiltration: in patients in whom malignant cells are present only in portal tracts, a presinusoidal type of block is usually present;[59,60] in patients in whom the malignant cells infiltrate the sinusoids, the intrahepatic block is of the sinusoidal type and ischaemic necrosis of hepatocytes causing liver failure is common.[56,58] Obstruction of hepatic vein radicles and portal vein branches by intraluminal neoplastic invasion may contribute to the disorganization of intrahepatic circulation.[57]

Systemic mastocytosis

Although hepatic involvement is common in systemic mastocytosis (Mican, Hepatol, 1995; 22:1163),[61] few cases of symptomatic portal hypertension have been reported (Silvain, GastrClinBiol, 1989; 13:834).[62–66] Ascites can be due to peritoneal involvement by mast cells.[62] Gastrointestinal bleeding can be related to duodenal ulcers, which are common in patients with systemic mastocytosis (Cherner, Gastro, 1988; 95:657). HVPG is increased.[62, 63,65] Sinusoidal block may be related to massive infiltration of sinusoids by mast cells,[62–65] and to extensive portal and periportal fibrosis.[61,66] In addition, increased splenic blood flow may contribute to portal hypertension through an increased portal inflow.[63,66]

Primary myeloproliferative disorders

Occasionally, portal hypertension may be the presenting manifestation of primary myeloproliferative disorders. In patients with polycythaemia vera or essential thrombocythaemia, portal hypertension usually results from thrombosis of the portal vein or the hepatic veins. In patients with myeloid leukaemia, massive infiltration of the sinusoids with malignant cells is the usual mechanism for portal hypertension.[58] In patients with myeloid metaplasia, infiltration of sinusoids by foci of extramedullary haemopoiesis, perisinusoidal fibrosis, and nodular regenerative hyperplasia may cause a sinusoidal block (Shaldon, AmJMed, 1962; 32:758; Degott, Liver, 1985; 5:276; Roux, JClinGastro, 1987; 9:483; Roux, Gastro, 1987; 92:1067).[59] The increased splenic blood flow related to splenomegaly, and elevated presinusoidal resistance, may also play a part in the mechanism of portal hypertension (Blendis, ClinSci, 1970; 38:73).

Hereditary haemorrhagic telangiectasia

In patients with hereditary haemorrhagic telangiectasia (or Rendu–Osler–Weber disease), portal hypertension may develop (Feizi, Gastro, 1972; 63:660; Capron, AmJGastr, 1981; 76:47; Bernard, Gastro, 1993; 105:482).[67] Large bands of fibrosis dissecting the liver parenchyma or cirrhosis are present in cases with portal hypertension. These lesions may be due to transfusion-transmitted chronic viral hepatitis or to the vascular malformation itself.[67] HVPG is elevated in these patients. Increased hepatic blood flow due to arteriovenous shunting in the liver may contribute to portal hypertension.

References

1. Reynolds T, Ito S, and Iwatsuki S. Measurement of portal pressure and its clinical application. *American Journal of* Medicine, 1970; **49**: 649.
2. Bosch J, Mastai R, Kravetz D, Navasa M, and Rodes J. Hemodynamic evaluation of the patient with portal hypertension. *Seminars in Liver Disease*, 1986; **6**: 309–17.
3. Benoit JN and Granger DN. Splanchnic hemodynamics in chronic portal hypertension. *Seminars in Liver Disease*, 1986; **6**: 287–98.
4. Pomier-Layrargues G, *et al*. Presinusoidal portal hypertension in non-alcoholic cirrhosis. *Hepatology* 1985; **5**: 415–18.
5. Huet PM, Pomier-Layrargues G, Villeneuve JP, Varin F, and Viallet A. Intrahepatic circulation in liver disease. *Seminars in Liver Disease*, 1986; **6**: 277–86.
6. Lebrec D, Sicot C, Degott C, and Benhamou JP. Portal hypertension and primary biliary cirrhosis. *Digestion*, 1976; **14**: 220–6.
7. Navasa M, Pares A, Bruguera M, Caballeria J, Bosch J, and Rodes J. Portal hypertension in primary biliary cirrhosis. Relationship with histological features. *Journal of Hepatology*, 1987; **5**: 292–8.
8. Sedgwick CE, Povlantzas JK, and Kune GA. Management of portal hypertension secondary to bile duct strictures: review of 18 cases with splenorenal shunt. *Annals of Surgery*, 1966; **163**: 949–53.
9. Adson MA and Wyuchulis AR. Portal hypertension in secondary biliary cirrhosis. *Archives of Surgery*, 1968; **96**: 604–12.
10. Hadjis NS and Blumgart LH. Role of liver atrophy, hepatic resection and hepatocyte hyperplasia in the development of portal hypertension in biliary disease. *Gut*, 1987; **28**: 1022–8.
11. Möhrl M, Schwalback G, and Wannagat L. Portale hypertension bei idiopathischer Hämochromatose. *Zeitschrift fur Gastroenterologie (München)*, 1979; **6**: 381–6.
12. Warren KS. The relevance of schistosomiasis. *New England Journal of Medicine*, 1980; **303**: 203–6.
13. Nash TE, Cheever AW, Ottesen EA, and Cook JA. Schistosome infections in humans: perspectives and recent findings. *Annals of Internal Medicine*, 1982; **97**: 740–54.
14. De Cock KM. Hepatosplenic schistosomiasis: a clinical review. *Gut*, 1986; **27**: 734–5.
15. Coutinho A. Hemodynamic studies of portal hypertension in schistosomiasis. *American Journal of* Medicine, 1968; **44**: 547–56.
16. Fauvert R and Benhamou JP. Congenital hepatic fibrosis. In: Schaffner F, Sherlock S, and Leevy CM, eds. *The liver and its diseases*. New York: Stratton Intercontinental Medical Books, 1974; 283–8.
17. Kerr DNS, Okonkwo S, and Choa RE. Congenital hepatic fibrosis: the long term prognosis. *Gut*, 1978; **19**: 514–20.
18. Mikkelsen WP, Edmondson HA, Peters RL, Redeker AG, and Reynolds TB. Extra- and intra-hepatic portal hypertension without cirrhosis (hepatoportal sclerosis). *Annals of Surgery*, 1965; **162**: 602–20.
19. Sama SK, *et al*. Non cirrhotic portal fibrosis. *American Journal of* Medicine, 1971; **51**: 160–9.
20. Boyer JL, *et al*. Idiopathic portal hypertension. Comparison with the portal hypertension of cirrhosis and extrahepatic vein obstruction. *Annals of Internal Medicine*, 1967; **66**: 41–68.
21. Okuda K, *et al*. Clinical study of eighty-six cases of idiopathic portal hypertension and comparison with cirrhosis with splenomegaly. *Gastroenterology*, 1984; **86**: 600–10.
22. Villeneuve JP, *et al*. Idiopathic portal hypertension. *American Journal of* Medicine, 1976; **61**: 459–63.
23. Feneyrou B, *et al*. Hypertension portale idiopathique. Intérêt diagnostique du cathétérisme direct de la veine porte (à propos de 6 observations). *Gastroentérologie Clinique et Biologique*, 1982; **6**: 472–6.
24. Nataf C, *et al*. Idiopathic portal hypertension (perisinusoidal fibrosis) after renal transplantation. *Gut*, 1979; **20**: 531–7.
25. Kigham JGC, Levison DA, Stansfeld AG, and Dawson AM. Non-cirrhotic intrahepatic portal hypertension: a longterm follow-up study. *Quarterly Journal of Medicine*, 1981; **50**: 259–68.
26. Levison DA, Kingham JGC, Dawson AM, and Stansfeld AG. Slow cirrhosis—or no cirrhosis? A lesion causing benign intrahepatic portal hypertension. *Journal of Hepatology*, 1982; **137**: 253–72.
27. Polish E, Christie J, Cohen A, and Sullivan BS. Idiopathic presinusoidal portal hypertension (Banti's syndrome). *Annals of Internal Medicine*, 1962; **56**: 624–7.
28. Kluge T, Sommerschild H, and Flatmark A. Sinusoidal portal hypertension. *Surgery*, 1970; **68**: 294–300.
29. Ohnishi K, *et al*. Portal hemodynamics in idiopathic portal hypertension (Banti's syndrome). Comparison with chronic persistent hepatitis and normal subjects. *Gastroenterology*, 1987; **92**: 751–8.
30. Knowles DM, Kaye GI, and Godman GE. Nodular regenerative hyperplasia of the liver. *Gastroenterology*, 1975; **69**: 746–51.
31. Rougier P, Degott C, Rueff B, and Benhamou JP. Nodular regenerative hyperplasia of the liver. Report of six cases and review of the literature. *Gastroenterology*, 1978; **75**: 169–72.

32. Wanless IR, Godwin TA, Allen F, and Feder A. Nodular regenerative hyperplasia of the liver in hematologic disorders: a possible response to obliterative venopathy. A morphometric study of nine cases with an hypothesis on the pathogenesis. *Medicine*, 1980; **59**: 367–79.

33. Wanless IR. Micronodular transformation (nodular regenerative hyperplasia) of the liver: a report of 64 cases among 2500 autopsies and a new classification of benign hepatocellular nodules. *Hepatology*, 1990; **11**: 787–97.

34. Stromeyer FW and Ishak KG. Nodular transformation (nodular 're-generative' hyperplasia) of the liver. A clinicopathologic study of 30 cases. *Human Pathology*, 1981; **12**: 60–70.

35. Capron JP, *et al*. L'hyperplasie nodulaire régénérative du foie. Etude de 15 cas et revue de la littérature. *Gastroentérologie Clinique et Biologique*, 1983; **7**: 761–9.

36. Wanless IR, Solt LC, Kortan P, Dec JHN, Gariner GW, and Prokipchuk EJ. Nodular regenerative hyperplasia of the liver associated with macroglobulinemia. *American Journal of Medicine*, 1981; **70**: 1203–7.

37. Voinchet O, Degott C, Scoazec JY, Feldmann G, and Benhamou JP. Peliosis hepatis, nodular regenerative hyperplasia of the liver and light chains deposition in a patient with Waldenström's macroglobulinemia. *Gastroenterology*, 1988; **95**: 482–6.

38. Sherlock S, Feldman CA, Moran B, and Scheuer PJ. Partial nodular transformation of the liver with portal hypertension. *American Journal of Medicine*, 1966; **40**: 195–203.

39. Wanless IR, Lentz JS, and Roberts EA. Partial nodular transformation of liver in an adult with persistent ductus venosus. Review with hypothesis on pathogenesis. *Archives of Pathology and Laboratory Medicine*, 1985; **109**: 427–32.

40. Shedlofsky S, Koehler RE, Deschermver-Kecskemeti K, and Alpers DH. Non cirrhotic nodular transformation of the liver with portal hypertension: clinical, angiographic, and pathological correlation. *Gastroenterology*, 1980; **79**: 938–43.

41. Yanoff M and Rawson AJ. Peliosis hepatis. Anatomic study with demonstration of two varieties. *Archives of Pathology*, 1964; **77**: 73–9.

42. Taxy JB. Peliosis hepatis: a morphologic curiosity becomes an iatrogenic problem. *Human Pathology*, 1978; **9**: 331–40.

43. Karasawa T, Shikata T, and Smith RS. Peliosis hepatis. Report of nine cases. *Acta Pathologica Japonica*, 1979; **29**: 457–9.

44. Zafrani ES, Cazier A, Baudelot AM, and Feldmann G. Ultrastructural lesions of the liver in human peliosis. A report of 12 cases. *American Journal of Pathology*, 1984; **114**: 349–59.

45. Scoazec JY, *et al*. Peliosis hepatis and sinusoidal dilatation during infection by the human immunodeficiency virus (HIV). An ultrastructural study. *American Journal of Pathology*, 1988; **131**: 38–47.

46. Degott C, Rueff B, Kreis H, Duboust A, Potet F, and Benhamou JP. Peliosis hepatis in recipients of renal transplants. *Gut*, 1978; **19**: 748–53.

47. Valla D and Benhamou JP. Drug-induced vascular and sinusoidal lesions of the liver. In Bircher J, ed. *Adverse drug reactions in the differential diagnosis of GI and liver diseases*, vol. 2, *Baillière's Clinical Gastroenterology*, 1988: 481–500.

48. Poulsen H, Winckler K, and Christoffersen P. The significance of centrilobular sinusoidal changes in liver biopsies. *Scandinavian Journal of Gastroenterology*, 1970; Suppl. 7: 103–9.

49. Bruguera M, Aranguibel F, Ros E, and Rodes J. Incidence and clinical significance of sinusoidal dilatation in liver biopsies. *Gastroenterology*, 1978; **75**: 474–8.

50. Lebrec D, Nouel O, Bernuau J, Rueff B, and Benhamou JP. Portal hypertension in fulminant viral hepatitis. *Gut*, 1980; **21**: 962–4.

51. Valla D, Fléjou JF, Lebrec D, Bernuau J, Rueff B, and Benhamou JP. Portal hypertension and ascites in acute hepatitis. Clinical, hemodynamic and histological correlations. *Hepatology*, 1989; **10**: 482–7.

52. Bianchi L, Zimmerli-Ning M, and Gudat F. Viral hepatitis. In MacSween RNM, Anthony PP, and Scheuer PJ, eds. *Pathology of the liver*. New York: Churchill Livingstone, 1979: 164–91.

53. Bernuau J, Degott C, Nouel O, Rueff B, and Benhamou JP. Non-fatal acute fatty liver of pregnancy. *Gut*, 1983; **24**: 340–4.

54. Valla D, Pessegueiro-Miranda H, Degott C, Lebrec D, Rueff B, and Benhamou JP. Hepatic sarcoidosis with portal hypertension. A report of seven cases with review of the literature. *Quarterly Journal of Medicine*, 1987; **63**: 531–44.

55. Maddrey WC, Johns CJ, Boitnott JK, and Iber FL. Sarcoidosis and chronic hepatic disease: a clinical and pathological study of 20 patients. *Medicine*, 1970; **49**: 375–95.

56. Hyun BH, Singer EP, and Sharret RH. Esophageal varices and metastatic carcinoma of liver. *Archives of Pathology*, 1964; **77**: 292–8.

57. Nouel O, Bernuau J, Lebrec D, Laraki R, Rueff B, and Benhamou JP. Insuffisance hépatocellulaire grave et hypertension portale due à un cancer secondaire du foie. *Gastroentérologie Clinique et Biologique*, 1979; **3**: 135–7.

58. Datta DV, Grover SL, Saini VK, Datta BN, Aikat BK, and Chhuttani PN. Portal hypertension in chronic leukaemia. *British Journal of Haematology*, 1975; **31**: 279–85.

59. Dubois A, *et al*. Portal hypertension in lymphoproliferative and myeloproliferative disorders: hemodynamic and histological correlations. *Hepatology*, 1993; **17**: 246–250.

60. Brooks AP. Portal hypertension in Waldenström's macroglobulinemia. *British Medical Journal*, 1976; **1**: 689–90.

61. Yam LT, Chan CH, and Li CY. Hepatic involvement in systemic mast cell disease. *American Journal of Medicine*, 1986; **80**: 819–26.

62. Capron JP, Lebrec D, Degott C, Chivrac D, Coevoet B, and Delobel J. Portal hypertension in systemic mastocytosis. *Gastroenterology*, 1978; **74**: 595–7.

63. Grundfest S, Cooperman AM, Ferguson R, and Benjamin S. Portal hypertension associated with systemic mastocytosis and splenomegaly. *Gastroenterology*, 1980; **78**: 370–3.

64. Sawers AH, Dawson J, Biaganza J, and Geary CG. Systemic mastocytosis, myelofibrosis and portal hypertension. *Journal of Clinical Pathology*, 1982; **35**: 617–19.

65. Le Jeune C, Hugues FC, Rolle G, Jaubert F, and Dufat R. Hepatomegalie avec hypertension portale révélatrice d'une mastocytose systémique. *Revue de Médecine Interne*, 1986; **7**: 253–7.

66. Sumpio BE, O'Learn G, and Gusberg RJ. Variceal bleeding, hypersplenism and systemic mastocytosis. Pathophysiology and management. *Archives of Surgery*, 1988; **123**: 767–9.

67. Martini GA. The liver in hereditary haemorrhagic telangiectasia: an inborn error of vascular structure with multiple manifestations: a reappraisal. *Gut*, 1978; **19**: 531–7.

7.4 Clinical manifestations and management of bleeding episodes in cirrhotics

Jaime Bosch and A. K. Burroughs

Gastrointestinal bleeding in patients with chronic liver disease is a serious complication which often induces a deterioration in liver function as well as having a high mortality. It is usually related to portal hypertension, the most common cause being ruptured oesophageal or gastric varices and less commonly gastric mucosal lesions. Bleeding from varices in other sites, for example the rectum, is far less common.

Its management can be considered in three distinct clinical situations: the acute bleeding episode, the prevention of variceal and gastric mucosal rebleeding, and the primary prevention of the first bleeding episode.

Randomized clinical trials (**RCTs**) of the available treatments are best summarized using a meta-analysis. A meta-analysis provides a more stable and reliable estimate of the treatment effects, overcoming the problems of low power in small trials. Pooled estimates of the treatment effects are presented as pooled odds ratios (**PORs**) according to the Mantel–Haenszel–Peto method (Collins, BMJ, 1985; 290:17). Values of PORs less than 1.00 indicate a favourable effect of the experimental treatment as compared to the control treatment. This effect is statistically significant when the 95 per cent confidence interval (**CI**) of the POR does not include values greater than or equal to 1.00.

The acute bleeding episode
Natural history of the variceal bleeding episode
Early rebleeding

Patients with variceal bleeding frequently have early rebleeding occurring within the first few days of hospital admission (Fleischer, Gastro, 1983; 84:538; De Dombal, Endoscopy, 1986; 18(Suppl.2): 6).[1,2] In the survey by De Dombal 54 per cent of 544 patients with bleeding varices had early rebleeding by the tenth day of admission, compared to 20 per cent of 1426 patients with bleeding peptic ulcers.

There is a relationship between the severity of liver disease and an increased risk of early rebleeding. In a prospective study of 311 consecutive admissions for bleeding oesophageal varices in cirrhotics, early rebleeding (within 5 days of admission) occurred in 21 per cent of patients classified as Pugh's grade A, 40 per cent of grade B patients, and 63 per cent of grade C patients. The severity of portal hypertension is another risk factor for early rebleeding, as this is more frequent in patients with higher portal and/or variceal pressures (Vinel, Hepatol, 1986; 6:116; Ready, Gastro, 1991; 100: 1403; Ruiz del Arbol, JHepatol, 1992; 16:S36).

Thus, the clinical problems of acute variceal bleeding span several days during which there is a high risk of continued bleeding or rebleeding. Treatment regimens to stop bleeding should be evaluated in terms of the immediate cessation of bleeding and in terms of providing a bleed-free interval and preventing early rebleeding. However, it is important to realize that approximately 40 to 50 per cent of patients with variceal bleeding (depending on the spectrum of severity of the chronic liver disease) will settle rapidly with simple measures and will not rebleed within the first few days.

Survival

It is well established that the degree of liver cell failure is an important prognostic indicator for both the short- and long-term survival of cirrhotics who have bled from varices (Pagliaro, AnnIntMed, 1992; 117:59).[3] Although the deterioration in liver function can be minimized in patients with variceal bleeding, there are no measures in the short-term to improve liver cell function. This means that there will always be a small proportion of patients who will inevitably die despite early and effective control of variceal bleeding. However, the optimal control of bleeding and the prevention of very early variceal rebleeding is the major factor which can be changed by therapy, thus improving the prognosis.

Smith and Graham[2] have shown that short-term survival following acute variceal bleeding is the major determinant of long-term survival. Using a hazard model for death, they estimated that if a cirrhotic who had bled from varices survived 3 months, then the risk of death returned to that which was present before the bleed. In their series, most patients were in Child's C class with a very high 2-day mortality of 36 per cent. A similar hazard model has been shown in a series where the 2-day mortality was 3 per cent.[4]

General management

Variceal bleeding is a medical emergency and its management should be undertaken in an intensive care setting by a team of experienced medical staff, including a clinical hepatologist, endoscopist, and surgeon.[5] It is essential to have well-trained nurses. A specific plan of management should always be used, following a protocol adapted to the particular resources available. This is greatly facilitated by the establishment of gastrointestinal bleeding units. Early referral is warranted if there is a lack of either medical or surgical expertise in techniques to control bleeding. Clinical and laboratory evidence of the severity of haemorrhage and of liver disease should be included in the initial assessment, as these have prognostic significance. The following should be evaluated: haemoglobin/haematocrit, white cell count, platelet count, plasma urea and electrolytes, creatinine, prothrombin and partial thromboplastin times, baseline liver function tests, routine blood cultures, urine culture, ascitic fluid culture, chest radiograph, and electrocardiograph. Blood gases (in decompensated cirrhosis or those with chest problems) should also be considered.

The initial therapy is aimed at correcting hypovolaemic shock, preventing complications associated with gastrointestinal bleeding, and achieving haemostasis at the bleeding site. The first two goals, which are independent of the cause of the haemorrhage, demand immediate management. Specific therapy to stop bleeding is usually given when the patient has had initial resuscitation and following diagnostic endoscopy, with the important exception of pharmacological therapy, that can be started earlier in the course of the bleeding episode, on arrival to hospital or even during transfer to hospital.

Replacement of blood volume

Variceal bleeding in cirrhosis is often massive; it is therefore essential to introduce at least one large-bore intravenous cannula to allow rapid transfusion if required. In addition, a central venous line should be inserted for the monitoring of central venous pressure. A minimum of four units of blood should be kept cross-matched and ready for transfusion. Blood volume replacement should be initiated as soon as possible to avoid complications from hypovolaemic shock and a decreased perfusion of vital organs. It is important to emphasize that the replacement of the blood volume should not be considered solely in terms of blood transfusion. If plasma proteins and other colloid expanders are used, only a few units of blood may be needed. After the systolic blood pressure is restored to between 80 and 90 mmHg in this way, the transfusion policy using packed red cells should be to maintain the haematocrit at approximately 25 to 30 per cent (not above) or the haemoglobin at 9 g/dl and the urine output at 40 ml/h or more.[5] Frequent measurements of the blood pressure, heart rate, and central venous pressure during therapy are mandatory. The haematocrit or haemoglobin should be measured every 6 to 8 h.

Overtransfusion should be avoided, not only because of the risks inherent with blood transfusion, but also because there may be a rebound increase in the portal pressure with a consequent risk of continued bleeding or rebleeding.[6] Experimental studies in rats with portal hypertension, due to portal vein constriction or carbon tetrachloride-induced cirrhosis, have shown an increase in portal pressure beyond the basal values when restoring lost blood volume (Kravetz, Gastro, 1986; 90:1232; Kravetz, Hepatol, 1989; 9:808). Furthermore, hypovolaemia and low blood pressure are very powerful stimuli for the activation of vasoactive neurohumoral systems aimed at maintaining the arterial pressure within normal limits. This is achieved by a marked systemic vasoconstriction, which is particularly accentuated in the splanchnic area, resulting in a reduction in the portocollateral blood flow with a concomitant fall in portal pressure (Kravetz, Gastro, 1986; 90:1232). Thus, variceal bleeding tends to stop spontaneously during hypovolaemia, but may continue or start up again with overtransfusion of any fluids. However, it is important to correct anaemia progressively on the following days, since persistent anaemia is associated with a worsening of the hyperkinetic syndrome and of portal hypertension and may be a risk factor for rebleeding (Panés, Gastro, 1992; 103:407).

Prevention of complications

The main complications associated with gastrointestinal bleeding in patients with chronic liver disease are airway aspiration causing pneumonia, hepatic encephalopathy, infections by enteric organisms, hypoxaemia, and renal/electrolyte imbalance, with an increase of ascites and renal failure. These frequently lead to the deterioration of liver function and may be the ultimate cause of death.

The aspiration of blood or gastric secretions is particularly frequent in patients with impaired consciousness due to shock or hepatic encephalopathy.[7] Although aspiration may occur at any time during the bleeding episode, the highest risks are during haematemesis and during emergency endoscopy and the placement of balloon tamponade tubes. Suspected or proven aspiration should be treated immediately with antibiotics; monitoring with pulse oximetry is useful. Its prevention is based on the following measures: close supervision by a well-trained nurse, positioning the patient in a semireclined position, preferably the left lateral decubitus, orotracheal intubation in comatose patients, and aspiration of the gastric contents through an indwelling nasogastric tube.[7]

Nasogastric aspiration through an indwelling large bore tube is not universally used; however, it allows the enteral administration of drugs in comatose patients and is a useful method of monitoring the activity of bleeding.[5] In addition, the removal of blood from the upper gastrointestinal tract may help to prevent and correct hepatic encephalopathy, which is a frequent complication of variceal haemorrhage. Encephalopathy also requires the administration of lactulose (15 to 30 ml/6 h) via the nasogastric tube and cleansing enemas. In the presence of renal failure, electrolytes in the enemas cannot be excreted—magnesium-containing enemas should be avoided in these situations (Collinson, BMJ, 1986; 293:1013).

Severe infections are common complications of gastrointestinal bleeding in cirrhosis and may be present on admission. In addition to aspiration pneumonia, these patients are prone to develop systemic infections and spontaneous bacterial peritonitis due to enteric organisms. Thus, blood and urine cultures and ascitic taps should be performed routinely. The administration of oral nonabsorbable antibiotics has been shown to reduce the incidence of these serious complications and this should reduce the mortality due to bleeding (Rimola, Hepatol, 1985; 5:463). Norfloxacin (400 mg twice a day via the nasogastric tube) has been shown to be safe and effective (Soriano, Gastro, 1992; 103:1267), as well as systemic antibiotics (Blaise, Hepatol, 1994; 20:34). The presence of sepsis was independently associated with early rebleeding in a prospective study (Bernard, Gastro, 1995; 108:1828). Suspected sepsis should be treated immediately with broad-spectrum antibiotics (avoiding aminoglycosides which may cause renal damage).

The support of vital organ functions relies on the maintenance of adequate tissue perfusion and oxygenation. Aspiration of the blood, prolonged shock, and multiple blood transfusions may markedly impair pulmonary gas exchange and result in significant hypoxaemia and acute respiratory failure. Arterial hypoxaemia is frequent in cirrhotics with advanced liver failure (Rodriguez-Roisin, AmRevRespDis, 1987; 135:1085). This results from functional abnormalities such as pulmonary vasodilation, impaired hypoxic vasoconstriction, ventilation/perfusion mismatching, and shunts (Agusti, JHepatol, 1990; 10:25). Therefore, it is essential to perform close haemodynamic monitoring, measurements of blood gases or pulse oximetry, and serial chest radiographs. Chest physiotherapy and the provision of an adequate oxygen supply are integral parts of therapy (Krowka, Chest, 1994; 105:1528). There is experimental evidence that portal hypertensive gastric mucosa is more susceptible to injury following haemorrhage shock than normal mucosa (Stremmer, JSurgRes, 1990; 48:313).

Renal function should be supported by adequate fluid and electrolyte replacement (saline infusions should be avoided) and should be monitored with strict attention to fluid balance. Close haemodynamic monitoring should prevent hypotension and allow rapid correction of any hypovolaemia. It is crucial to avoid the administration of nephrotoxic drugs, particularly aminoglycosides and non-steroidal anti-inflammatory agents. Daily measurements of serum creatinine, urea and electrolyte concentrations, and the rate of urinary output are used as markers of renal perfusion. The urine output should be maintained at over 40 ml/h; an output below 20 ml/h indicates poor renal perfusion and impending renal failure.[5] Massive or tense ascites should be treated by paracentesis, preferably with albumin replacement (Ginès, JHepatol, 1993; 17(Suppl.2):14). This has been shown to improve the haemodynamic conditions and to decrease the portal pressure and portal–collateral blood flow transiently (Luca, Hepatol, 1994; 20:30; Luca, Hepatol, 1995; 22:753).

Patients with advanced cirrhosis frequently show wasting of muscle and adipose tissue. Malnutrition may contribute to an increased susceptibility to infections and to impaired renal function. The suppression of oral intake during the acute bleeding episode significantly worsens the nutritional state; feeding should be resumed as soon as a 24-h interval free of bleeding has been achieved. There are difficulties in providing balanced nutrition in patients with cirrhosis. Enteral nutrition is always preferable, as parenteral nutrition further complicates the fluid balance, and leads to an added risk of sepsis.

Alcoholic patients may exhibit withdrawal symptoms when admitted because of bleeding. These often require sedation. Intravenous heminevrin or propofol has a shorter half-life than other sedatives and can be easily titrated; close supervision of the fluid and electrolyte balance is mandatory.

Diagnostic endoscopy

Diagnostic endoscopy does not improve survival (Koff, DigDisSci, 1981; 26:12s), but an early diagnosis improves and rationalizes its management, including the use of therapeutic endoscopic procedures, such as sclerotherapy or banding ligation for varices. Endoscopy should be performed as soon as resuscitation is adequate and always before the use of balloon tamponade or surgery is considered. Usually it can be performed within 6 h of admission. In difficult or comatose patients endotracheal intubation and light anaesthesia should be used. This may also be necessary during alcohol withdrawal, if an immediate diagnosis is required.

At endoscopy a diagnosis of bleeding varices is made if there is a venous (non-pulsatile) spurt or a venous ooze, an adherent clot, or if a platelet aggregate or fibrin clot (white in colour) is seen on a varix. In the absence of these signs, variceal bleeding can only be diagnosed in the absence of other lesions in the stomach or duodenum. If active bleeding is seen it is usually located just above the oesophagogastric junction. If more than one non-bleeding lesion is seen immediate re-endoscopy is mandatory if rebleeding occurs (Mitchell ScaJGastr, 1982; 17:695). Gastric variceal bleeding accounts for no more than 10 per cent of patients in most series, but it is more difficult to establish whether gastric varices are the source of bleeding rather than oesophageal varices (Sarin, Hepatol, 1992; 16:1343). Non-variceal lesions have been considered to be a frequent cause of bleeding in cirrhotics with varices. However, recent series in which early endoscopy was used have shown that variceal bleeding was the source of bleeding in 80 per cent of cases (Mitchell, ScaJGastr, 1982; 17:965; Sutton, AmJMed, 1987; 83:273; Taibibian, JClinGastro, 1989; 9:279). Erosions and portal hypertensive gastropathy (gastric mucosal lesions without inflammation, due to dilatation of mucosal vessels) are frequently found, but are an uncommon cause of acute bleeding.

Specific therapy

Different techniques have been used to control variceal haemorrhage, including drugs, oesophageal tamponade, endoscopic sclerotherapy or banding ligation, and surgery. The optimal therapy should stop bleeding and prevent early rebleeding. This will usually require the combination of several of these procedures in a therapeutic regimen which ideally should be available in any hospital. The interpretation of the results of clinical trials of these therapies does have some important problems.

Firstly, the time of starting treatment (randomization), relative to the time of admission to the first hospital to which the patient is taken, is an important variable in evaluating the efficacy of therapy. Clearly, the longer the time interval from admission, the less the residual risk of early rebleeding (Burroughs, Hepatol, 1989; 9:801). Patients may be sent to referral centres having spent several hours or days in the referring hospital free of early rebleeding or they may be referred only when an early rebleed has occurred. Secondly, as many patients with bleeding varices, particularly those with better liver function, respond rapidly to simple measures, invasive measures such as sclerotherapy or surgery will be required more often in those patients with poorer rather than better liver function. Thirdly, if the pattern of bleeding can be predicted soon after admission, on clinical, haemodynamic, or endoscopic criteria (such as the visible vessel in a bleeding peptic ulcer), this will provide a better chance of altering the course of variceal bleeding following admission. For example, it could be used as a basis for 'immediate' invasive therapy (sclerotherapy or surgery). Early rebleeding is associated with a high mortality within 30 days, independently from indices of liver dysfunction (Burroughs, Hepatol, 1986; 6:115(Abstr.); Garcia-Pagan, SeronoSymposiaRev, 1989; 22:287).

Pharmacological therapy

From a theoretical point of view, pharmacological therapy is the optimal treatment for variceal bleeding, because it can be given virtually immediately, which is not the case with endoscopic sclerotherapy or surgical procedures. Moreover, it does not require sophisticated equipment or specialized training. Thus, if a safe and effective drug were available, therapy could not only be given at arrival to the emergency room before diagnostic endoscopy but also while the patient is being transferred to hospital. It is useful to keep in mind these unique advantages of pharmacological therapy when considering the different alternatives for the treatment of acute variceal haemorrhage.

Pharmacological treatment is aimed at arresting variceal haemorrhage by decreasing the pressure and blood flow in the oesophageal varices, thus allowing haemostasis at the bleeding site. Splanchnic vasoconstrictors, such as vasopressin and somatostatin and their synthetic derivatives, are the principal agents. Constrictors of the physiological lower oesophageal sphincter have also been used.

Vasopressin

This drug has been widely used in the treatment of variceal haemorrhage, but its use is still controversial.[8] Vasopressin (ADH) is a very powerful vasoconstrictor. At pharmacological doses, it reduces blood flow in all splanchnic organs and thereby decreases the portal blood flow and portal pressure. Vasopressin is also effective in reducing the collateral (azygos) blood flow (Bosch, JHepatol, 1985; 1:125) and variceal pressure (Bosch, Hepatol, 1988; 8:861). This is important because it is thought that both the risk of bleeding and the severity of variceal haemorrhage are directly proportional to the transmural pressure gradient at the varices.[9] The adverse haemodynamic effects of vasopressin derive from systemic vasoconstriction with increased peripheral vascular resistance and reduced cardiac output, heart rate, and coronary blood flow (Bosch, Gastro, 1981; 80:518; Groszmann, Hepatol, 1982; 2:756). Moreover, vasopressin infusion may lead to water retention and dilutional hyponatraemia. These effects may result in serious complications such as myocardial ischaemia or infarction, arrythmias, mesenteric ischaemia, limb ischaemia, heart failure, pulmonary oedema and cerebrovascular accidents. In 25 per cent of cases vasopressin has to be withdrawn because of these complications (Conn, Gastro, 1975; 68:211, Kravetz, Hepatol, 1984; 4:442). Superior mesenteric artery infusions of smaller doses of vasopressin have been used in an attempt to decrease the systemic toxicity of the drug; however, three trials failed to show any advantage of the intra-arterial administration (Table 1) (Johnson, AnnSurg, 1977; 186:369; Clanet, ActaGastroBelg, 1978; 41:539; Chojkier, Gastro, 1979; 77:540). Because of these limitations vasopressin is rarely used at present. When used, vasopressin is administered as a continuous intravenous infusion, starting at 0.4 U/min, which is increased if necessary to 0.6 U/min. Therapy is usually maintained until bleeding has been controlled for 24 h. If more than 0.4 U/min are required, the rate of infusion is decreased stepwise before discontinuation of therapy.

Vasopressin was compared with non-active treatment in four RCTs, including a total of only 157 patients (Merigan, NEJM, 1962; 266:134; Conn, Gastro, 1975; 68:211; Mallory, ArchSurg, 1980; 115:30; Fogel, AnnIntMed, 1982; 96:565) (Table 1). The first of these studies (Merigan, NEJM, 1962; 266:134) assessed the treatment outcome just 1 h after starting a 20-min vasopressin infusion (and did not report on the side-effects). The pooled results from these trials show a significant beneficial effect of vasopressin in reducing the failure to control bleeding although the mortality rate was unaffected. From 32 to 64 per cent of vasopressin-treated patients experienced one or more complications requiring the withdrawal of therapy in approximately 25 per cent of cases. Three out of 85 vasopressin-treated patients died because of complications from therapy.[3]

Combined vasopressin and nitroglycerine administration

This drug combination allows an enhancement in the reduction in portal pressure while decreasing the systemic side-effects of vasopressin therapy (Groszmann, Hepatol, 1982; 2:757).

Vasopressin associated with nitroglycerine has been compared with vasopressin alone in three trials (Gimson, Hepatol, 1986; 6:410; Tsai, Hepatol, 1986; 6:406; Bosch, Hepatol, 1989; 10:962) (Table 1), only one of which was double blind. Nitroglycerine was given sublingually (Tsai, Hepatol, 1986; 6:406), intravenously (Gimson, Hepatol, 1986; 6:410), or transdermally (Bosch, Hepatol, 1989; 10:962). The pooled estimate of the treatment effect shows a significant reduction in the failure to control bleeding with the combination therapy, as well as a significant reduction in the complications associated with vasopressin treatment, but the decrease in mortality was not significant.[3] A significant reduction in blood transfusions was reported in the double-blind trial (Bosch, Hepatol, 1989; 10:962). These results suggest that if a decision to use vasopressin is made, it should be used in association with nitroglycerine. Transdermal preparations are the easier way of administration.

Terlipressin (Glypressin)

Terlipressin (glypressin) is a synthetic triglycyl analogue of lisine-vasopressin with dual effects. Its intrinsic activity causes immediate vasoconstrictor effects, which are followed by those due to its slow transformation *in vivo* into vasopressin by enzymatic cleavage of the triglycyl residues (Blei, Hepatol, 1986; 6:146). Glypressin, unlike vasopressin, does not enhance fibrinolysis (Douglas, Gut, 1979; 20: 565; Prowse, EurJClinInv, 1980; 10:49) and has a longer biological activity that allows its administration by intravenous injection every 4 h (Blei, Hepatol, 1986; 6:146).

The clinical efficacy of glypressin was assessed in three placebo-controlled trials (Walker, Hepatol, 1986; 6:112; Freeman, JClinGastro, 1989; 11:58; Soderlund, ScaJGastr, 1990; 25:622). The pooled estimates showed a highly significant reduction in the failure to control bleeding and also in mortality (Table 1).[3] Glypressin controlled the bleeding in 79 per cent of the cases. It is important to note that this is the only pharmacological treatment that has been shown to reduce mortality from variceal bleeding. A recent double-blind ambulance study that evaluated its use at a prehospital stage (at the patient's home and during transferral) had a decreased

Table 1 RCTs of drug therapy and balloon tamponade for acute variceal bleeding

Trial	Number of patients	Failure to control bleeding (%)			Death rate		
		Control	Treated	Odds ratio (95% CI)	Control	Treated	Odds ratio (95% CI)
Vasopressin compared with non-active treatment							
Merigan et al.	53	100	45	0.07 (0.02–0.24)	80	93	3.05 (0.38–24.1)
Conn et al.	33	75	29	0.17 (0.04–0.65)	62	53	0.68 (0.18–2.67)
Mallory et al.	38	85	55	0.25 (0.06–0.99)	45	44	0.98 (0.28–3.46)
Fogel et al.	33	63	71	1.43 (0.34–6.07)	42	50	1.36 (0.34–5.33)
POR (95% CI)				0.22 (0.12–0.43)			1.11 (0.54–2.28)
Intra-arterial compared with intravenous vasopressin							
Johnson et al.	25	36	50	1.70 (0.36–8.08)	45	28	0.49 (0.09–2.48)
Clanet et al.	26	7	45	8.17 (1.34–49.9)	60	18	0.19 (0.04–0.90)
Chojkier et al.	22	50	50	1.00 (0.19–5.15)	70	75	1.27 (0.27–8.02)
POR (95% CI)				2.20 (0.84–5.74)			0.44 (0.17–1.15)
Vasopressin plus nitroglycerine compared with vasopressin							
Tsai et al.	39	79	55	0.35 (0.94–1.30)	58	55	0.89 (0.25–3.11)
Gimson et al.	72	56	32	0.38 (0.15–0.95)	26	24	0.86 (0.29–2.49)
Bosch et al.	65	46	27	0.45 (0.16–1.22)	29	30	1.07 (0.37–3.10)
POR (95% CI)				0.39 (0.22–0.72)			0.94 (0.50–1.79)
Glypressin compared with placebo							
Walker et al.	50	48	20	0.29 (0.09–0.93)	32	12	0.32 (0.08–1.20)
Freeman et al.	31	62	40	0.42 (0.10–1.67)	25	20	0.76 (0.14–3.97)
Soderlund et al.	60	45	16	0.26 (0.09–0.78)	38	10	0.21 (0.06–0.69)
POR (95% CI)				0.31 (0.15–0.61)			0.32 (0.15–0.70)
Glypressin compared with vasopressin							
Freeman et al.	21	91	30	0.08 (0.01–0.47)	27	20	0.68 (0.09–4.86)
De Saint et al.	16	17	20	1.23 (0.10–15.1)	33	30	0.86 (0.10–7.16)
Lee et al.	45	67	81	2.04 (0.55–7.56)	33	48	1.79 (0.55–5.83)
Chiu et al.	54	46	50	1.15 (0.39–3.31)	36	46	0.52 (1.52–4.48)
D'Amico et al.	111	24	9	0.34 (0.12–0.93)	16	25	1.68 (0.67–4.19)
POR (95% CI)				0.64 (0.36–1.14)			1.48 (0.85–2.57)
Glypressin compared with balloon tamponade							
Colin et al.	54	12	12	1.00 (0.18–5.41)	22	15	0.62 (0.16–2.41)
Fort et al.	47	21	22	1.05 (2.65–4.20)	8	13	1.62 (0.26–10.2)
POR (95% CI)				1.03 (0.35–3.00)			0.87 (0.29–2.59)
Glypressin compared with somatostatin							
Silvain et al.	87	43	54	1.50 (0.65–3.46)	22	27	1.31 (0.49–3.50)
Walker et al.	50	32	20	0.54 (0.15–1.89)	24	16	0.61 (0.15–2.41)
VBSG	161	16	20	1.30 (0.58–2.91)	17	20	1.19 (0.54–2.63)
POR (95% CI)				1.18 (0.70–1.99)			1.10 (0.63–1.93)
Somatostatin compared with placebo							
Valenzuela et al.	84	25	44	2.24 (0.91–5.18)	28	31	1.18 (0.46–3.01)
Burroughs et al.	120	59	36	0.39 (0.18–0.81)	11	15	1.28 (0.45–3.65)
Somatostatin compared with vasopressin							
Kravetz et al.	61	42	47	1.21 (0.44–3.29)	45	47	1.06 (0.39–2.88)
Jenkins et al.	22	67	30	0.24 (0.05–1.27)	33	20	0.53 (0.08–3.32)
Bagarani et al.	49	68	33	0.26 (0.09–0.78)	40	25	0.51 (0.16–1.67)
Cardona et al.	38	44	60	1.83 (0.52–6.46)	17	30	2.05 (0.47–8.99)
Hsia et al.	46	63	45	0.51 (0.16–1.61)	62	63	1.05 (0.32–3.43)
Saari et al.	54	48	35	0.53 (0.18–1.58)	36	34	0.92 (0.23–2.83)
Rodriguez-Moreno et al.	31	37	60	0.42 (0.10–1.67)	19	20	1.08 (0.19–6.24)
Hwang et al.[a]	48	54	37	0.52 (0.17–1.59)	50	46	0.85 (0.28–2.60)
POR (95% CI)				0.68 (0.45–1.04)			0.92 (0.59–1.43)
Somatostatin compared with balloon tamponade							
McKee[b]	40	30	50	2.25 (0.64–7.86)	25	0	0.11 (0.02–0.69)
Jaramillo et al.	39	50	42	0.73 (0.21–2.54)	25	26	1.07 (0.26–4.42)
Avgerinos et al.	61	33	32	0.95 (0.33–2.75)	33	23	0.59 (0.19–1.79)
POR (95% CI)				1.13 (0.57–2.24)			0.52 (0.23–1.15)
Balloon tamponade compared with vasopressin							
Pinto Correia et al.	37	35	30	0.79 (0.20–3.09)	12	20	1.02 (0.45–2.30)
Terés et al.	108	34	13	0.33 (0.14–0.79)	30	31	1.80 (0.32–10.2)

[a] Octreotide compared with vasopressin.
[b] Octreotide compared with balloon tamponade.

mortality in the glypressin group, but did not have any effect on the haemodynamic or transfusion parameters during the period of administration. Thus, the cause–effect on mortality needs cautious interpretation (Levacher, Lancet, 1995; 346:865).

Glypressin was compared with vasopressin in five RCTs[10] (Freeman, Lancet, 1982; ii:66; Lee, ChinJGastro, 1988; 5:131; Chiu, JGastroHepatol, 1990; 5:549; D'Amico, JHepatol, 1994; 20:206) in two of which vasopressin was associated with nitroglycerine (Lee, ChinJGastro, 1988; 5:131; D'Amico, JHepatol, 1994; 20:206). A total of 247 patients were included. These studies found a significantly lower complication rate with glypressin, even when vasopressin was associated with nitroglycerine.[3] The failure to control bleeding was almost significantly reduced with glypressin. Glypressin was found to be safe when used for longer periods, to prevent early rebleeding (Variceal Bleeding Study Group, Hepatol, 1993; 18:140A). Finally, glypressin was found to be as effective as balloon tamponade in two trials[11] (Fort, Hepatol, 1990; 11:678) and as somatostatin in three trials (Silvain, Hepatol, 1993; 18:61; Walker, Hepatol, 1992; 15:1023; Variceal Bleeding Study Group, Hepatol, 1993; 18:140A), in terms of both the control of bleeding and mortality. Therefore, there is evidence indicating that in variceal haemorrhage glypressin is effective in controlling bleeding and in reducing mortality, that it is simpler, more effective, and safer than vasopressin (even when this is associated with nitroglycerine), and as effective as balloon tamponade or somatostatin.

Somatostatin

This was introduced for the treatment of variceal haemorrhage because of its capacity to decrease the portal pressure without the adverse effects of vasopressin on the systemic circulation (Bosch, Gastro, 1981; 80:518). Somatostatin causes splanchnic vaso-constriction and thereby decreases the portal and collateral blood flow and portal pressure. This is due in part to the inhibition of the release of vasodilatory peptides by somatostatin (Kravetz, AmJPhysiol, 1988; 254:G322). Its effects are much more pronounced following bolus injections than during continuous infusions (Cirera, Hepatol, 1995; 22:106); because of this, it has been recommended to give bolus injections at the start of therapy, that can be repeated until the bleeding is controlled and when there is any rebleeding during treatment. A direct vasoactive effect may contribute to the marked, immediate falls in portal pressure and azygos blood flow caused by bolus injections of somatostatin (Bosch, Gastro, 1981; 80:518; Mastai, JHepatol, 1986; 3:S1). The usual dose for a bolus injection is 250 μg and 250 to 500 μg/h are given as continuous infusions. When successful, therapy is maintained for 2 to 5 days.

The effectiveness of somatostatin in controlling variceal bleeding was assessed in two placebo controlled trials (Valenzuela, Hepatol, 1989; 10:958; Burroughs, Gastro, 1990; 99:1388) (Table 1). Two placebo-controlled trials have come to opposite conclusions; one showed no effect (Valenzuela, Hepatol, 1989; 10:958) and the other a significant benefit of somatostatin (Burroughs, Gastro, 1990; 11:1388). However, in the study where somatostatin was not effective (Valenzuela, Hepatol, 1989; 10:958) there was an 83 per cent response rate in the placebo group, which is the highest response rate to any drug in any trial of variceal bleeding. Some inadvertent selection must have occurred. The two trials also differed in the

duration of treatment which was of 30 h in one study (Valenzuela, Hepatol, 1989; 10:958) and 5 days in the other (Burroughs, Gastro, 1990; 11:1388) as well as in the definition of treatment success, including a 4-h bleeding-free interval in the former and 5 days in the second. These differences make it difficult to compare the two studies and meaningless to pool their results. Two unblinded trials compared somatostatin with 'non-active treatments', ranitidine (Loperfido, RecProgMed, 1987; 78:82) and cimetidine (Testoni, CurrTherRes, 1986; 39:759), but the differences did not reach statistical significance. Other placebo-controlled trials on the use of somatostatin in acute variceal bleeding are in progress.

Seven trials compared somatostatin with vasopressin (Kravetz, Hepatol, 1984; 4:442; Jenkins, BMJ, 1985; 290:275; Bagarani, Ital-JSurgSci, 1987; 17:21; Cardona, GastroHepato, 1989; 12:30; Hsia, ChinJGastro, 1990; 7:71; Saari, AmJGastr, 1990; 85:804; Rguez-Moreno, JHepatol, 1991; 13:S162). Octreotide, a synthetic peptide still under investigation, has part of the amino acid sequence of somatostatin and shares many of its properties and was used in another study (Hwang, JHepatol, 1992; 16:320) (Table 1). These studies showed an important reduction of the failure to control bleeding with somatostatin, approaching statistical significance, without any difference in mortality. In all the trials complications were virtually absent with somatostatin (median 6.5 per cent and range 0 to 18 per cent), whereas the median complication rate was 49 per cent (range 17 to 74 per cent) with vasopressin. Three trials compared somatostatin or octreotide with glypressin, failing to show differences either in the control of bleeding or in mortality (Silvain, Hepatol, 1993; 18:61; Walker, Hepatol, 1992; 15:1023) (Table 1). Somatostatin was also shown to be equivalent to balloon tamponade in three trials (McKee, Digestion, 1990; 45:60; Jaramillo, JHepatol, 1991; 12:100; Avgerinos, JHepatol, 1991; 13:78) (Table 1) and to endoscopic sclerotherapy in five further studies (Di Febo, Gastro, 1990; 98:A583; Jenkins, Gut, 1990; 31:A627; Shields, JHepatol, 1992; 16:128; Planas, Hepatol, 1994; 20:370; Sung, Lancet, 1993; 342:637) (Table 2).

Therefore RCTs comparing somatostatin with other active treatments support the fact that somatostatin is effective in the treatment of variceal bleeding. Moreover, somatostatin is certainly the safest therapy available, which makes it possible to start therapy earlier (prior to diagnostic endoscopy) and to maintain treatment for several days to prevent early rebleeding. While there is a large experience with somatostatin, there is not yet enough data regarding the use of octreotide in the treatment of acute variceal bleeding, although this drug has been reported to be useful as an adjunct to emergency sclerotherapy (**EST**) (Besson, NEJM, 1995; 333:555) in one study, but not in another (Burroughs and International Octreotide Varices Study Group, Hepatol, 1996).

Metoclopramide and domperidone

These drugs increase the lower oesophageal sphincter pressure and have been suggested for the management of variceal bleeding since on acute administration these have been shown to reduce the inflow of blood into the varices in portographic studies, and to reduce azygos blood flow significantly. However, their value for arresting or preventing variceal bleeding is uncertain (Hosking, Gut, 1988; 6:523; Feu, JHepatol, 1989; 9:S149).

Table 2 RCTs of emergency sclerotherapy (EST) for acute variceal bleeding

Trial	Number of patients	Failure to control bleeding (%)			Death rate		
		Control	Treated	Odds ratio (95% CI)	Control	Treated	Odds ratio (95% CI)
EST compared with sham procedure							
Gregory	87	39	5	0.13 (0.05–0.36)	49	25	0.39 (0.17–0.95)
EST compared with vasopressin							
Soderlund and Ihre	107	16	5	0.32 (0.09–1.09)	36	28	0.69 (0.31–1.58)
Larson et al.	82	NR	NR	–	13	5	0.33 (0.07–1.56)
El-Zayadi et al.	118	NR	NR	–	20	11	0.51 (0.19–1.38)
Westaby et al.	64	35	12	0.28 (0.09–0.87)	39	27	0.60 (0.21–1.69)
Alexandrino et al.	83	29	29	1.03 (0.40–2.65)	41	39	0.94 (0.39–2.26)
POR (95% CI)				0.51 (0.27–0.97)			0.65 (0.42–1.01)
EST compared with somatostatin							
Di Febo et al.	47	22	8	0.35 (0.07–1.74)	26	21	0.75 (0.20–2.86)
Jenkins et al.	40	10	10	1.00 (0.13–7.69)	–	–	–
Shields et al.	80	23	17	0.69 (0.23–2.05)	31	19	0.55 (0.20–1.55)
Planas et al.	70	20	17	0.83 (0.25–2.74)	28	23	0.74 (0.26–2.14)
Sung	98	31	26	0.82 (0.34–1.96)	29	41	1.71 (0.75–3.91)
POR (95% CI)				0.70 (0.40–1.22)			0.97 (0.56–1.65)
EST compared with balloon tamponade							
Barsoum et al.	100	NR	NR	–	42	26	0.49 (0.22–1.12)
EVASP	187	NR	NR	–	48	47	0.98 (0.55–1.73)
Paquet and Feusener	43	27	5	0.20 (0.04–0.99)	27	9	0.32 (0.07–1.45)
Moreto	43	20	0	0.09 (0.1–0.76)	30	30	1.02 (0.28–3.70)
POR (95% CI)				0.15 (0.04–0.53)			0.75 (0.49–1.15)
EST compared with surgery							
Cello et al.	13	NR	NR	–	71	66	1.28 (0.48–3.39)
Huizinga et al.	76	NR	NR	–	33	24	0.65 (0.24–1.74)
Terés et al.	32	29	27	0.88 (0.18–4.01)	53	47	0.78 (0.20–3.08)
Burroughs et al.	101	4	18	4.20 (1.21–14.6)	37	44	1.32 (0.59–2.91)
Cello et al.	64	NR	NR	–	56	50	0.78 (0.29–2.07)
POR (95% CI)				2.24 (0.85–5.87)			0.91 (0.56–1.46)

Balloon tamponade

Balloon tamponade is aimed at obtaining a temporary haemostasis by direct compression of bleeding varices. Balloon tamponade is effective in controlling the bleeding temporarily, but is a dangerous treatment. Fatal complications occur in 6 (Haddock, DigDisSci, 1989; 34:913) to 20 per cent (Chojkier, DigDisSci, 1980; 25:267) of cases. Aspiration pneumonia occurs in 10 per cent of patients, even in experienced hands. Many patients experience thoracic pain, which often requires analgesia or withdrawal of the tube. However, the most life-threatening complication is airway obstruction by the oesophageal balloon, caused by its migration due to external traction or because the patient pulls out the tube. A pair of scissors should be kept ready at the bedside to cut through the tube should this emergency arise. This emphasizes that tamponade should only be used by skilled and experienced staff in intensive care facilities.[7]

The double-balloon Sengstaken–Blakemore tube is recommended in patients bleeding from oesophageal varices, while the single-balloon Linton–Nachlas tube is used in gastric varices (Teres, Gastro, 1978; 75:566). The following recommendations are important for the safe and effective use of balloon tamponade: the procedure should be performed by an experienced doctor assisted by well-trained nurses, the patient should be in a left lateral decubitus position, encephalopathic patients require endotracheal intubation before passage of the tamponade tube, the channels of the tube should be checked for patency and the balloons should be

tested for leaks, and the tube is lubricated and passed through the mouth or nose into the stomach. When using the Sengstaken–Blakemore tube, the gastric balloon is then inflated with a minimum of 250 ml of air and the tube is slowly withdrawn until firm resistance is encountered at the oesophagogastric junction; at this point, while an assistant nurse is keeping a gentle traction to the tube, the oesophageal balloon is inflated to a pressure of between 50 and 60 mmHg measured using a sphygmomanometer linked to the system. The pressures in the oesophageal balloon should be checked hourly. Continuous aspiration of the oesophagus should be undertaken for the duration of tamponade and gastric aspiration should be performed hly. If the tube does not have an oesophageal aspiration channel then a nasogastric tube should be tied alongside the main tube to perform this. When using the Linton–Nachlas tube, the single, large gastric balloon is inflated with 600 ml of air; the tube is kept under an external traction of 1 kg to compress the gastric varices at the fundus and to stop bleeding from the oesophageal varices by interrupting the blood flow through the submucous venous plexus at the cardia, thereby decreasing the inflow of blood into the oesophageal varices. The possibility of aspiration is much greater than with the Sengstaken-Blakemore tube and therefore extreme caution must be used.

In experienced hands and provided the balloon is in the correct position, balloon tamponade is highly effective in controlling variceal bleeding,[7] with bleeding control rates of 40 to 90 per cent (Chojkier, DigDisSci, 1980; 25:267; Hunt, DigDisSci, 1982; 27:

413).[7] However, a recurrence of bleeding is observed in almost 50 per cent of the patients within 24 h of balloon deflation.[7] Balloon tamponade was compared to vasopressin ($\pm$ nitroglycerine) in two RCTs (Pinto Correia, Hepatol, 1984; 4:885; Terés, Hepatol, 1990; 11:964), to glypressin ($\pm$ nitroglycerine) in two[11] (Fort, Hepatol, 1990; 11:678), to somatostatin in two (Jaramillo, JHepatol, 1991; 12:100; Avgerinos, JHepatol, 1991; 13:78), and to octreotide in one (McKee, Digestion, 1990; 45:60) (Table 1). There were no differences between tamponade and either glypressin or somatostatin, but tamponade is slightly more effective than vasopressin ($\pm$ nitroglycerine) (Table 1). Pooling the results of these seven RCTs shows a trend in favour of balloon tamponade for arresting bleeding, without differences in mortality.[3]

Ballon tamponade is therefore effective for temporarily controlling variceal bleeding, but because of its brief effects and complications, it should be restricted to patients with massive bleeding, not controlled by initial therapy, while waiting for definitive treatment.[12]

Endoscopic therapy
Sclerotherapy

Endoscopic sclerotherapy (EST) has become widely used because of the high success rate reported. It has also been shown that EST reduces the rate of early rebleeding.[13] It is either performed at the diagnostic endoscopy or after the use of drugs or balloon tamponade. Intravariceal, paravariceal, and combined injections of sclerosants have been used, the most common sclerosants being 5 per cent ethanolamine, 5 per cent sodium morrhuate, and 1 per cent polidocanol. The immediate effect is mostly due to sealing off of the bleeding point by local oedema; thrombosis of varices is probably a secondary effect. No more than two injection sessions should be used to arrest variceal bleeding following admission (Burroughs, NEJM, 1989; 321:857; Borman, SAfrMedJ, 1986; 70:34). Following the first emergency injection, the usual approach is to continue to inject electively at days 3 to 7.

Sclerotherapy has the potential of starting specific therapy at the time of diagnosis. However, it is often difficult to have experienced endoscopists available on a 24-h basis. Moreover, EST is associated with a considerable risk of causing significant complications, which is greater than with elective injections (Sanowski, JClinGastro, 1987; 9:504; Schuman, AmJGastr, 1987; 82:823; Kahn, Surgery, 1989; 105:160). The more common complications of sclerotherapy are oesophageal ulceration (70 to 80 per cent of patients) (Westaby, Gut, 1984; 25:129), bleeding from oesophageal ulcers (5 to 20 per cent), oesophageal stenosis (5 to 10 per cent), and, less frequently, perforation of the oesophagus and sepsis. The overall rate of serious complications is in the range of 10 to 20 per cent with an overall mortality of 2 to 5 per cent (Westaby, Bailliere'sClinGastro, 1992; 3:465). Less severe but frequent adverse effects are transient dysphagia (60 to 80 per cent), chest pain (40 to 60 per cent), and pleural effusions (20 to 30 per cent).

EST has been assessed in 20 RCTs (Gregory, Gastro, 1990; 98:A53; Soderlund, ActaChirScand, 1986; 151:449; Larson, JAMA, 1986; 255:497; El-Zayadi, GastrEnd, 1988; 34:314; Westaby, Hepatol, 1989; 9:274; Alexandrino, JHepatol, 1990; 11(Suppl):S1; Di Febo, Gastro, 1990; 98:A583; Jenkins, Gut, 1990; 31:A627; Shields, JHepatol, 1992; 16:128; Planas, Hepatol, 1994; 20:370; Sung,

Lancet, 1993; 342:637; Barsoum, BrJSurg, 1982; 69:76; Copenhagen Esophageal Varices Sclerotherapy Project, NEJM, 1984; 311:1594; Paquet, Hepatol, 1985; 5:580; Moretó, SGO, 1988; 167:331; Cello, Surgery, 1982; 91:333; Huizinga, SGO, 1985; 160:539; Terés, JHepatol, 1987; 4:159; Burroughs, NEJM, 1989; 321:857; Cello, NEJM, 1987; 316:11) (Table 2). One RCT compared EST with a sham procedure (Gregory, Gastro, 1990; 98:A53) and showed a significant reduction in mortality but not in early rebleeding. It was not specified whether the controls were given any active treatment. EST was compared with drug therapy in 10 RCTs: vasopressin in five (Soderlund, ActaChirScand, 1986; 151:449; Larson, JAMA, 1986; 255:497; El-Zayadi, GastrEnd, 1988; 34:314; Westaby, Hepatol, 1989; 9:274; Alexandrino, JHepatol, 1990; 11(Suppl):S1) and somatostatin or octreotide in five (Di Febo, Gastro, 1990; 98:A583; Jenkins, Gut, 1990; 31:A627; Shields, JHepatol, 1992; 16:128; Planas, Hepatol, 1994; 20:370; Sung, Lancet, 1993; 342:637). When these are combined, a significant beneficial effect of EST is found both reducing the failure to control bleeding and reducing early rebleeding, mainly because of better results with EST than with vasopressin. The impact of EST reducing early rebleeding is difficult to assess because of the use of additional sclerotherapy sessions. Three trials compared EST with somatostatin (Di Febo, Gastro, 1990; 98:A583; Jenkins, Gut, 1990; 31:A627; Planas, Hepatol, 1994; 20:370) and two with octreotide (Shields, JHepatol, 1992; 16:128; Sung, Lancet, 1993; 342:637); no significant differences were found in terms of bleeding control and rebleeding. The inhospital mortality rate was similar with each treatment. EST was compared with balloon tamponade in four trials (Barsoum, BrJSurg, 1982; 69:76; Copenhagen Esophageal Varices Sclerotherapy Project, NEJM, 1984; 311:1594; Paquet, Hepatol, 1985; 5:580; Moretó, SGO, 1988; 167:331), but only two (Paquet, Hepatol, 1985; 5:580; Moretó, SGO, 1988; 167:331) reported the effect on control of bleeding. However, the reported bleeding control rates with EST of 100 per cent (Moretó, SGO, 1988; 167:331) and 95 per cent (Paquet, Hepatol, 1985; 5:580) are not easy to reproduce in clinical practice. Four trials compared EST with esophageal transection (Cello, Surgery, 1982; 91:333; Huizinga, SGO, 1985; 160:539; Terés, JHepatol, 1987; 4:159; Burroughs, NEJM, 1989; 321:857) and one with portacaval shunt (**PCS**) (Cello, NEJM, 1987; 316:11), in failures of medical treatment. The failure to control bleeding was significantly higher with EST in one study (Burroughs, NEJM, 1989; 321:857). Rebleeding was significantly higher with EST (Cello, Surgery, 1982; 91:333; Huizinga, SGO, 1985; 160:539; Cello, NEJM, 1987; 316:11). No significant differences in mortality were found.

Severe complications, including bleeding from postsclerosis ulcers, stenosis and perforation of the oesophagus were observed in 18 per cent of the patients who underwent EST; 15 per cent of the complications were fatal.[3]

The available data therefore suggest that EST is better than balloon tamponade and vasopressin, but not better than somatostatin, although it is too early to draw definite conclusions. There are no comparisons with glypressin. Emergency surgery is better than EST in controlling bleeding and reducing rebleeding, particularly in severe patients not responding to medical treatment or balloon tamponade, but the mortality is equal. Injection of cyanoacrylate has also been used for active bleeding oesophageal varices and found to be superior to sclerotherapy alone in a single trial (Feretis, Endoscopy, 1995; 27:355).

Endoscopic banding ligation of varices

This technique has been recently developed for the treatment of oesophageal varices and has also been used in acute variceal bleeding. It is based on the same concept as for banding ligation of internal haemorrhoids. The technique is not difficult for skilled endoscopists; multiple banding devices have been developed that do not require an outer sheath which was used for repeated intubation and responsible for perforation. The procedure takes more time and may require deeper sedation than sclerotherapy, increasing the risk of airway aspiration during acute bleeding. A comparison of the effects of banding and EST in comparative RCTs have not shown marked differences in efficacy in patients treated early during the bleeding episode. It has been claimed that band ligation may control bleeding in more than 80 per cent of patients with a low rate of complications (Stiegmann, NEJM, 1992; 326:1527). In a recent study (Lo, Hepatol, 1995; 22:466), banding ligation was effective in arresting acute variceal bleeding in 94 per cent of cases (18 out of 19) as compared with 80 per cent (12 out of 15) of patients treated with sclerotherapy (statistically non-significant) but a review of all trials shows no difference (Hou, Hepatol, 1995; 21:1517; Gimson, Lancet, 1993; 342:391; Laine, AnnIntMed, 1993; 119:1; Lo, JHepatol, 1994; 21:1048; Jensen, GastroEnd,. 1993; 39:279). Ulceration at the site of banding is considered normal (Westaby, BailClinGastro, 1992; 3:465) and recurrent bleeding from banding-related ulcers has been observed in approximately 10 per cent of cases (Stiegmann, NEJM, 1992; 326:1527).

Emergency surgery

Portacaval shunt and staple transection

In many centres surgery is used as second-line treatment following EST. Emergency surgery should only be used when medical and endoscopic therapy has failed to control variceal haemorrhage or when there is recurrent, massive bleeding. Surgery carries least risk in patients in Child's classes A and B. In patients with advanced liver failure, who have a poor prognosis, transjugular intrahepatic portal -systemic shunt (**TIPS**) is likely to be a better option. When surgery is decided upon the operation should not be delayed. Both portacaval shunt surgery and staple transection of the oesophagus, using an automatic transection and suturing device (or a more extensive disconnection and devascularization procedure) are highly effective emergency measures to stop bleeding. Staple transection can be highly effective in arresting variceal bleeding (Hoffman, ScaJGastr, 1983; 18:707) and has a lower risk of encephalopathy than shunts.

Four RCTs have compared staple transection to endoscopic sclerotherapy (Table 2) (Cello, Surgery, 1982; 91:333; Huizinga, SGO, 1985;160:539; Terés, JHepatol, 1987; 4:159; Burroughs, NEJM, 1989; 321:857). Huizinga (SGO, 1985; 160:539) reported similar major complications, but rebleeding was significantly less in transected patients (3 versus 49 per cent). The mortality within 30 days was also less, but not significantly so (24 versus 33 per cent). Terés (JHepatol, 1987; 4:159) selected high-risk patients who were randomized after rebleeding or if conservative measures had failed. Cessation of bleeding was achieved in 83 per cent of injected patients

versus 71 per cent of transected patients. Rebleeding during follow-up was 50 per cent in the injected group (with further elective injections) and 43 per cent in the transected group (with no elective treatment of varices). The long-term survival was similar. In the largest study patients were randomized only when conservative therapy failed within the first 5 days following. A 5-day bleed-free interval was achieved in 62 per cent using one injection session and in 80 per cent of transected patients, using an intention-to-treat analysis. There were no differences in complications or in mortality. These trials show that oesophageal staple transection does not increase the mortality as compared to sclerosis and is associated with a lower rate of rebleeding.[3] Transection may be followed by injection/banding ligation when varices regrow across the transection line. Bleeding from the transection line is common, but it is rarely severe. Omeprazole may reduce the frequency of rebleeding from this lesion (Kaye, Hepatol, 1992; 15:1031). Transection is not recommended when transplantation is considered. These patients are better managed using emergency shunt surgery or TIPS.

Calibrated portacaval-H-graft shunt

Small diameter interposition portacaval or mesocaval graft (**PCHG**) shunts have been proposed by Sarfeh *et al.* (Surgery, 1986; 100:52) to maintain the hepatic blood flow partially and reduce the risk of encephalopathy and liver failure of portacaval anastomosis. This might decrease the mortality from liver failure while affording effective protection against the bleeding risk. Eight or 10 mm PCHGs usually cause a reduction of portal pressure of more than 40 per cent. The liver blood flow was significantly higher than after the total shunts and postoperative encephalopathy lower (Sarfeh, AnnSurg, 1986; 204:356). A late patency of more than 90 per cent has been reported (Rypins, AnnSurg, 1984; 200:706). In addition, a PCHG is easy to manage in the case of subsequent liver transplantation. From a haemodynamic point of view, PCHG is quite similar to TIPS. Even though preliminary results from uncontrolled series are promising, the clinical advantages of small diameter interposition PCHG over distal splenorenal shunt (**DSRS**) or TIPS have not been proven.

Liver transplantation

Liver transplantation should always be considered in patients with advanced cirrhosis who have bled from varices. Survival data after shunt surgery for variceal bleeding is not comparable with survival after liver transplantation following variceal haemorrhage, because of the usually good liver function of patients submitted to shunt surgery in contrast to endstage disease patients submitted to liver transplantation, resulting in a worse survival after transplantation (Henderson, AnnSurg, 1992; 216:248). However, as could be anticipated, when only Child's C patients are considered, the survival is better after liver transplantation (Iwatsuki, BailClinGastro, 1992; 6:517).

The possibility that a patient with relatively good liver function may later require liver transplantation should be kept in mind when indicating surgical treatments for portal hypertension to avoid therapies that may interfere with transplantation. In that regard, it has been suggested that staple transection may complicate dissection for transplantation. In a similar way, when TIPS is used, care should be taken to avoid placing stents too far into the portal vein or hepatic veins.

Transjugular intrahepatic portal-systemic shunt (TIPS)

TIPS is an intrahepatic shunt performed percutaneously using interventional radiological techniques to communicate a hepatic vein and an intrahepatic branch of the portal vein. This communication is dilated by means of forced balloon angioplasty and the parenchymal tract is stabilized by placing an expandable metallic stent. The final diameter of the shunt is set at 8 to 12 mm. Several types of stents are available, with similar efficacy (Palmaz, AJR, 1985; 145:821; Gillams, Radiol, 1990; 174:137).

TIPS markedly decreases portal pressure, the average initial reduction being approximately 50 per cent (Ring, AnnIntMed, 1992; 116:304; Zemel, JAMA, 1991; 266:390; Ganger, Hepatol, 1992; 16(Suppl):240A; LaBerge, JVascSurg, 1992; 16:258; Sanyal, AmJGastr, 1992; 87:1305). This is followed by a reduced bleeding risk, a progressive reduction of variceal size (Rössle, Hepatol, 1991; 14:96A; Sanyal, AmJGastr, 1992; 87:1305), and ammelioration of ascites (Rössle, Hepatol, 1991; 14:96A; LaBerge, JVascSurg, 1992; 16:258) and renal function. The main problem with the use of TIPS is the marked tendency of the stents to become progressively stenosed over time. This is due to proliferation of the neointima which covers the stents and to fibrosis around the vascular intersections, which makes that portal pressure returns to pre-TIPS values. TIPS dysfunction may be managed by balloon dilatation and/or restenting. Other frequent problems are the development of liver failure (5 to 10 per cent) and of hepatic encephalopathy (20 to 40 per cent). Nevertheless, encouraging results are reported with TIPS for the treatment of acute bleeding and for the prevention of rebleeding (Rössle, Hepatol, 1991; 14:96A; LaBerge, JVascSurg, 1992; 16:258; Sanyal, AmJGastr, 1992; 87:1305). However, this needs confirmation in RCTs. At present its main indication is the treatment of variceal bleeding episodes uncontrolled by medical and endoscopic therapy in patients with poor liver function (Sanyal, Gastro, 1996; 11:138).

The main advantage of TIPS over surgical shunts is that the mortality associated with the procedure is probably lower, particularly in patients with advanced liver failure. Criteria to select the best candidates are still not available.

Other procedures

Percutaneous embolization of varices via transhepatic catheterization of the portal vein is useful in arresting bleeding, but carries a high rate of complications, including intra-abdominal bleeding and portal vein thrombosis and has been practically abandoned. However, percutaneous occlusion of the coronary vein is easy to perform at the time of TIPS and is used sometimes as complementary treatment in patients undergoing TIPS for acute variceal bleeding, especially from fundal varices (Terabayashi, Gastro, 1987; 93:1205; Bernman, Surgery, 1988; 104:500; L'Hermine, AJR, 1989; 152:755).

Treatment of gastric varices

Prominent gastric varices are more common with portal vein thrombosis than with intrahepatic portal hypertension. Therefore, the

patency of the portal vein should be investigated in all such patients. Isolated gastric varices are a feature of isolated splenic vein thrombosis. The treatment of choice in the latter case is splenectomy.

Bleeding from subcardial varices is treated and responds like bleeding from oesophageal varices. Bleeding from fundal varices requires a different clinical approach, since their tendency to rebleed is higher than that of oesophageal varices (Hosking, BrJSurg, 1988; 75:195; Sarin, AmJGastr, 1989; 84:1244). These varices may bleed at relatively low portal pressures, which may be due to its usually large size, which causes the variceal wall tension to be be quite high even at low intravariceal pressures. In addition, the fact that unlike the oesophageal varices, these are intra-abdominal vessels can determine different haemodynamic correlations. The main differences in management are the following.

1. Balloon tamponade. The single large gastric balloon (Linton–Nachlas tube) should be used rather than the Sengstaken–Blakemore tube.
2. Sclerotherapy. Fundal varices are not usually responsive to sclerotherapy. They can be injected with bucrylate (Soehendra, Endoscopy, 1986; 18:15; Raymond, Hepatol, 1989; 10:488) or 1 per cent thrombin (Williams, Gut, 1994; 35:1287). Neither the precise treatment schedule, the complications, nor the applicability of these techniques are well established due to the lack of controlled trials (Binmoeeler, Endoscopy, 1995; 27:392).
3. Banding—early results are mixed. It does not appear to be better than sclerotherapy.
4. Surgery. Some authors believe that bleeding from fundal varices is still the province of the surgeon (Trudeau, GastrEnd, 1986; 32:264). Most groups prefer derivative shunt surgery if this is possible.
5. TIPS: for effective control of the bleeding, large shunt diameters (greater than 10 mm) may be necessary.

Ectopic varices

While in most instances portal hypertension leads to the formation of oesophageal and gastric varices, some patients develop varices at unusual locations—'ectopic varices'. These are rarely the sole manifestation of portal hypertension. Usually they are associated with oesophageal varices (Lebrec, ClinGastroent, 1985; 14:105). Anorectal varices are more frequently detected as they are easily accessible (Hosking, Lancet, 1989; ii:349).

Ectopic varices can develop and rupture in many different places. There are anecdotal reports of bronchial, vaginal, vesical, gallbladder, and common bile duct varices. Bleeding from ectopic varices may thus result in unusual manifestations (that is, haemobilia, haemoperitoneum, and haematuria). However, the more frequent locations of ectopic varices are at the stoma of an enterostomy (27 per cent), the duodenum (18 per cent), jejunum and ileum (18 per cent), colon (15 per cent), rectum (9 per cent), and peritoneum (10 per cent). It has been suggested that the overall incidence of ectopic varices ranges between 1 and 3 per cent in patients with cirrhosis, whereas the incidence is higher in extrahepatic portal hypertension (20 to 30 per cent). It is likely that previous operations favour the development of ectopic varices, since these are much more common in patients with portal hypertension and previous abdominal surgery.

Ectopic varices have frequently been treated by surgery, using local resection, ligation of the varices, or portacaval shunts. Local resection for anorectal varices is contraindicated as major bleeding complications may ensue (Hosking, Lancet, 1989; ii:349). There have been reports of good results using endoscopic sclerotherapy with 1 per cent thrombin injection for bleeding duodenal varices (Sans, Endoscopy, 1996), and more recently with TIPS.

Non-variceal bleeding

Patients with portal hypertension frequently bleed from non-variceal sources. This makes necessary the use of emergency endoscopy to diagnose the specific cause of bleeding, since the treatment for non-variceal haemorrhage may differ substantially from treatment for variceal haemorrhage.

Portal hypertensive gastropathy

Portal hypertensive gastropathy (**PHG**), which is also known as 'congestive' gastropathy, is a very frequent complication of portal hypertension, although in most cases it is asymptomatic. It is characterized by a marked dilatation of the gastric mucosal vessels, which is responsible for its endoscopic appearance. Mild PHG is characterized by the finding of a 'mosaic' pattern (pale lines drawing a snake-like pattern over a hyperaemic mucosa). Severe PHG is characterized by multiple small red spots or its equivalent, the brown or black spots, that occasionally may ooze some blood. The PHG lesions may be located anywhere in the stomach. Experimental studies have shown that the gastric mucosal blood flow is not reduced but markedly increased in portal hypertension (Piqué, Gastro, 1988; 95:727) indicating that the gastric mucosa is hyperaemic rather than congestive in portal hypertension. The hyperaemia is due in part to an excessive release of nitric oxide (Casadevall, Hepatol, 1993; 18:628) and can be reduced by nitric oxide inhibitors as well as by several vasoconstrictors, such as terlipressin (Panés, Hepatol, 1994; 19:55), somatostatin (Panés, Hepatol, 1994; 20:336), and propranolol (Panés, Hepatol, 1993; 17: 213) and by oestrogen-progestagen administration (Panés, Hepatol, 1994; 20:1261). There is no association with *Helicobacter pylori* (D'Amico, Gastro, 1990; 9:1558; McCormick, Gut, 1991; 32:351).

Clinically, the disease may cause episodes of overt gastrointestinal bleeding (often only manifested by melaena), but these are usually less severe than variceal bleeds or it may cause chronic occult blood loss and microcytic anaemia, requiring repeated blood transfusion and oral iron therapy (Quintero, Gastro, 1987; 93: 1054). PHG occurs more frequently after repeated endoscopic sclerotherapy for oesophageal varices (Sarin, Gastro, 1992; 102: 994). The observation that this lesion rarely occurs after portacaval shunts has justified the use of shunting procedures for the treatment of refractory bleeding from PHG (Sarfeh, SGO, 1982; 155:167). Propranolol (Hosking, Hepatol, 1987; 7:437), somatostatin (Panés, Hepatol, 1994; 20:336), and terlipressin (Panés, Hepatol, 1994; 19: 55) have been suggested for the treatment of acute bleeding from PHG. Antacids, H_2 blockers and sucralphate are not helpful. Rebleeding from severe PHG is very frequent, with an actuarial incidence of 70 per cent at 1 year. Propranolol therapy significantly reduces the incidence of recurrent bleeding and the transfusion requirements in patients who have bled from PHG (Perez-Ayuso, Lancet, 1991; 337:1431). There is no need to treat PHG if the endoscopic lesions are not associated with clinical manifestations (acute or chronic blood loss).

Peptic ulcer

Haemorrhage from gastric or duodenal ulcers is common in patients with portal hypertension, who are reported to have an increased incidence of peptic ulcer disease (Terés, Gut, 1976; 17:37; Siringo, JHepatol, 1995; 22:633; Tabinowitz, DigDisSci, 1990; 35:705). The diagnosis of bleeding from peptic ulceration should be based on endoscopic findings. It is important to emphasize that a visible vessel on a peptic ulcer at endoscopy has the same significance as it does in non-cirrhotic patients and indicates a high potential for recurrent haemorrhage.

The treatment of a bleeding ulcer in cirrhosis should be conservative, if possible. Antisecretory drugs are useful in accelerating healing of the ulcer but are less useful in arresting bleeding. More aggressive therapeutic procedures should be used in patients with a visible vessel, if it shows active bleeding or stigmata of recent haemorrhage. A variety of endoscopic techniques has been used in these cases, including Nd:YAG lasers, electrocoagulation, heater probes, clips, and sclerotherapy. Injection sclerotherapy is performed using a variety of substances (thrombin, polidocanol, ethanol, and adrenaline 1:10:000), either alone or in combination. These are highly effective treatments for arresting bleeding and may reduce the need for emergency operations (Panés, Lancet, 1987; ii:1292), which are poorly tolerated by patients with advanced liver failure. However, the rare patient with massive haemorrhage not responding to therapeutic endoscopic procedures should undergo surgery. After the acute episode therapeutic eradication of *H. pylori* should be instituted.

Acute gastric erosions

Decompensated cirrhotics, particularly those with renal failure, spontaneous bacterial peritonitis, and acute respiratory failure, frequently bleed from acute gastric erosions. Haemorrhagic shock and reperfusion injury predispose the portal hypertensive mucosa to injury in an experimental model (Stremmer, JSurgRes, 1990; 48: 313). The administration of H_2 blockers or omeprazole may prevent the development of acute erosions in these high-risk situations. Haemorrhage from gastric erosions is rarely massive and should be treated conservatively. H_2 blockers accelerate the healing of acute gastric erosions, but do not stop bleeding (Terés, DigDiscSci, 1980; 2:92). The more important aspect of therapy is the correct management of the underlying disease.

Prevention of rebleeding from varices

Cirrhotics who survive the first variceal haemorrhage have a 70 per cent risk of rebleeding from varices (Schalm, ClinGastroent, 1985; 14:209). Although most cirrhotics who have bled from varices will usually rebleed from varices, they may rebleed from gastric mucosal lesions particularly following long-term sclerotherapy (McCormack, Gut, 1985; 26:1226). The calculation of a rebleeding index depends on the interval from the last bleed at which the analysis of rebleeding is started, given that rebleeding is more frequent close to the initial bleed than later on.[4] Thus, different rebleeding frequencies may only reflect different definitions due to different starting points for analysis used by different authors.

The proportion of deaths following the first variceal haemorrhage which are due to rebleeding from varices is between 20 and 35 per cent. There will be considerable variability in different populations due to the underlying differences in the severity of liver disease and the rate of its deterioration in the interval between episodes of bleeding. Graham and Smith[1] showed that in a population of decompensated alcoholic cirrhotics the major risk of death (which includes that due to rebleeding) is in the first 6 weeks following variceal bleeding. They estimated that 3 months afterwards, the risk of death is probably very similar to that before the bleed, that is similar to that of patients who had never bled. A similar pattern was found in a cirrhotic population with much better liver function.[4] Thus, therapy to prevent rebleeding starting a long time after the last bleed might not be expected to influence the survival significantly.

Because of the frequency and severity of recurrent variceal bleeding, effective preventive treatment is mandatory in patients surviving an episode of acute variceal bleeding. Preventive therapy should be started as soon as possible after controlling the acute bleeding episode. It is strongly recommended that treatment protocols for variceal bleeding leave no gaps between treatment of acute bleeding and prevention of rebleeding.

Different treatment options can be used to prevent variceal rebleeding, including surgical, endoscopic, and pharmacological therapy. These are summarized in the following sections using meta-analysis whenever available.

Shunt surgery
Elective portacaval shunt versus no shunt

In four randomized trials (Jackson, AnnSurg, 1971; 174:672; Resnick, Gastro, 1974; 67:843; Rueff, Lancet, 1976; i:655; Reynolds, Gastro, 1981; 80:1005), portacaval shunts did not increase survival compared to no treatment, despite a markedly significant reduction in rebleeding (Table 3). The overall rebleeding rate in shunted patients was 12 to 22 per cent, whereas in the control groups it was 65 to 98 per cent. With meta-analysis an increase in survival is approached but it does not reach statistical significance (POR 0.7 and CI 0.5 to 1.03).[3] This was due to operative deaths and an increase in deaths due to liver failure because of the diversion of the portal vein blood flow. Variceal rebleeding following elective portacaval shunts is usually related to shunt thrombosis, which is estimated to occur in approximately 10 per cent of patients. However, the different sources of rebleeding were not identified.

The results of survival analysis in the therapeutic shunt trials are confusing for the following reasons.

1. Shunts were not performed in 9 to 23 per cent of patients randomized to surgery and these patients were excluded from analysis, except in the study of Resnick (Gastro, 1974; 67: 843), that is there was no analysis using the 'intention-to-treat' principle.
2. Shunt surgery was performed several weeks after the bleeding episode (mean values between 1 and 8 weeks), so most of the patients had already survived the early period following bleeding when the risk of death is highest.

3. The interval between the bleeding episode and randomization differed considerably between the treatment groups, for example in the study of Reynolds (Gastro, 1981; 80:1005) the shunt group was randomized at 57 ± 4.4 days and the control group at 41 ± 4.5 days; Rueff (Lancet, 1976; i:655) randomized and performed shunts at a mean of 7 days following bleeding (range 4 to 14 days), while the control group patients were randomized 14 days or more following bleeding. These differences in time of entry mean that the trial groups had different risks of death at randomization.
4. The selection of patients may have been important in all the trials; most were Pugh's grade A. Resnick (Gastro, 1974; 67:843) took 7 years to recruit 89 patients, Jackson (AnnSurg, 1971; 174: 672) recruited only 30 per cent (89 out of 300), and Rueff (Lancet, 1976; i:655) only 9 per cent (79 out of 832) implying a strict selection.

All the trials, except that of Jackson (AnnSurg, 1971; 174:672), showed that chronic (spontaneous) encephalopathy was increased in the shunted patients (POR 4.9 and CI 2.11 to 11.3).[3] This difference disappears if mild transient encephalopathy following rebleeding in control patients is included (POR 1.0 and CI 0.6 to 1.6).[3] Moreover, the proportion of shunted patients with severe incapacitating encephalopathy (13 to 20 per cent) was smaller than the proportion of control patients with recurrent bleeding who died (3 to 53 per cent). As 16 to 37 per cent of control patients eventually had shunt surgery, the difference in the incidence of chronic and severe encephalopathy may not be as dramatic as is commonly believed.

On the basis of these results one should probably reassess the value of therapeutic portacaval shunts, were it not for the advent of liver transplantation. If possible, elective surgery which involves the hilar structures or involves dissection in the right upper abdomen should not be used. However, several other types of shunt, for example mesocaval shunts (**MCS**s) (including H-grafts) (Lillemoe, SurgClinNAm, 1990; 70:379) or distal splenorenal shunts, do not interfere with liver transplantation. PCHGs are less of a technical problem than end-to-side portacaval shunts (Rypins, SurgClinNAm, 1990; 70:395).

Distal splenorenal shunts versus non-selective shunts

The incidence of liver failure and severe encephalopathy following total shunting of portal blood led Warren and Zeppa to devise a selective shunt—the distal splenorenal shunt. There are six randomized studies (Table 3) comparing shunts in which alcoholic cirrhotics comprised at least 75 per cent of the patients; three compared portacaval shunts with distal splenorenal shunts (Conn, Hepatol, 1981; 1:151; Langer, Gastro, 1985; 88:424; Harley, Gastro, 1986; 91:802), one a mixture of shunts (Reichle, AmJSurg, 1979; 137:13), one with proximal splenorenal shunts (**PSRS**s) (Fischer, AnnSurg, 1981; 194:531), and one with mesocaval shunts (Millikan, AnnSurg, 1985; 201:712). All trials excluded the most decompensated patients and most included a high proportion of Child's grade A cirrhotics. The recruitment period lasted 10 years for 80 patients in the study by Langer (Gastro, 1985; 88:424)—this suggests marked selection. The survival analysis in three trials

Table 3 Therapeutic shunt-surgery trials

Trial	Number of patients	Rebleeding rate (%)			PSE rate (%)			Death rate		
		Control	Treated	Odds ratio (95% CI)	Control	Treated	Odds ratio (95% CI)	Control	Treated	Odds ratio (95% CI)
Portacaval shunt compared with non-active treatment										
Jackson et al.	155	65	9	0.09 (0.05–0.17)	NR	NR	–	64	44	0.45 (0.24–0.84)
Resnick et al.	79	72	18	0.10 (0.04–0.27)	4	11	2.38 (0.45–12.5)	48	44	0.87 (0.34–2.23)
Rueff et al.	89	71	15	0.11 (0.05–0.24)	4	20	4.85 (1.30–18.1)	47	52	1.25 (0.54–2.86)
Reynolds et al.	89	98	20	0.44 (0.18–0.98)	0	18	8.57 (2.02–36.3)	66	58	0.71 (0.30–1.66)
POR (95% CI)				0.08 (0.05–0.12)			4.9 (2.11–11.3)			0.7 (0.47–1.03)
Portacaval compared with distal splenorenal shunt										
Reichle et al.	27	NR	NR	–	NR	NR	–	31	29	0.90 (0.18–4.58)
Fischer et al.	42	17	16	0.89 (0.18–4.47)	4	5	1.22 (0.07–20.4)	22	0	0.13 (0.02–0.84)
Langer et al.	78	24	12	0.47 (0.15–1.49)	21	40	2.40 (0.92–6.25)	53	48	0.82 (0.34–1.97)
Millikan et al.	55	31	45	1.79 (0.61–5.28)	4	17	3.87 (0.72–20.8)	58	72	1.89 (0.63–5.71)
Harley et al.	53	42	33	0.69 (0.23–2.06)	35	30	0.80 (0.26–2.50)	54	66	1.69 (0.57–5.03)
Grace et al.	81	32	32	0.96 (0.38–2.42)	46	39	0.75 (0.31–1.81)	46	68	2.41 (1.01–5.80)
POR (95% CI)				0.88 (0.54–1.45)			1.29 (0.76–2.17)			1.28 (0.82–2.01)
Shunt surgery compared with sclerotherapy										
Rikkers et al.	57	57	18	0.20 (0.07–0.59)	7	15	2.25 (0.42–12.0)	40	37	0.88 (0.30–2.54)
Terés et al.	112	51	23	0.30 (0.14–0.64)	6	19	3.25 (0.92–11.4)	24	23	0.95 (0.39–2.28)
Henderson et al.	72	59	3	0.07 (0.02–0.20)	12	16	1.45 (0.32–6.43)	32	57	2.68 (1.06–6.75)
Spina et al.	66	31	6	0.18 (0.05–0.64)	7	7	0.96 (0.12–7.22)	25	12	0.41 (0.12–1.44)
Cello et al.[a]	65	–	–	–	12	12	1.00 (0.23–4.34)	75	84	1.76 (0.52–5.92)
Korula et al.[a,b]	53	51	12	0.16 (0.06–0.45)	–	–	–	31	8	0.52 (0.15–1.80)
Planas et al.[b]	69	51	12	0.18 (0.12–0.28)	11	29	8.09 (0.81–80.5)	23	15	0.59 (0.17–1.96)
POR (95% CI)				0.18 (0.12–0.28)			2.00 (1.10–3.60)			1.00 (0.67–1.51)

[a] Portacaval shunt.
[b] Trial published only as abstract.

(Langer, Gastro, 1985; 88:424; Harley, Gastro, 1986; 91:802; Millikan, AnnSurg, 1985; 201:712), is complicated by the failure to use an intention-to-treat principle. The interval between randomization and the last episode of bleeding and that between randomization and operation was of the order of several weeks in most trials. Only Conn (Hepatol, 1981; 1:151) specified these intervals for the whole trial population; randomization was carried out at a mean of 41 days (range 1 to 243 days) following bleeding and shunt surgery was performed at a mean of 4 days (range 0 to 51 days) following randomization. As in the therapeutic portacaval shunt trials, most of the patients had already survived the period following variceal bleeding in which the risk of death was highest. Rebleeding was similar in both trial groups but several types of non-selective shunts were used. Compared to portacaval shunts, distal splenorenal shunts resulted in slightly more rebleeding from all sources (13 to 42 versus 9 to 33 per cent). Compared to mesocaval and proximal splenorenal shunts there was less rebleeding with distal splenorenal shunts (35 versus 41 per cent (mesocaval shunts) and 13 versus 21 per cent (distal splenorenal shunts), respectively).

There is less encephalopathy in the short-term following distal splenorenal shunts (Henderson, Gastro, 1986; 91:1021). Although the overall encephalopathy rates are not significantly different, they are somewhat reduced in distal splenorenal shunt groups (4 to 39 versus 11 to 76 per cent in the non-selective groups). Two studies showed a reduction in severe or incapacitating encephalopathy (Langer, Gastro, 1985; 88:424; Millikan, AnnSurg, 1985; 201:712) but three others showed similar frequencies and one study (Reichle, AmJSurg, 1979; 137:13) did not give rebleeding and encephalopathy rates. The mortality was reduced in three trials (significantly in one; Fisher, AnnSurg, 1981; 194:531), and non-significantly increased in three others (Millikan, AnnSurg, 1985; 201:712; Harley, Gastro, 1986; 91:802; Grace, Hepatol, 1988; 8:1475).

Thus, distal splenorenal shunt appears to be as effective as portacaval shunt in terms of rebleeding. There is slightly less encephalopathy and long-term mortality, although this is not statistically significant. However, distal splenorenal shunt is a much more demanding operation and requires skilled surgeons. Moreover, variceal rebleeding is more common after distal splenorenal than portacaval shunt, and it is not suitable in decompensated cirrhotics with ascites nor in the emergency situation. Following distal splenorenal shunt, alcoholic cirrhotics have a worse survival than non-alcoholic cirrhotics (Henderson, WorldJSurg, 1984; 8:722; Zeppa, AnnSurg, 1978; 187:510).

However, in today's era of liver transplantation, portacaval shunts should be avoided in potential transplant candidates. distal splenorenal shunt does not hinder a future liver transplant (Esquivel, Surgery, 1987; 101:430). The calibrated small diameter portacaval H-graft shunt designed by Sarfeh (AnnSurg, 1986; 204: 356) could also result in reduced portosystemic encephalopathy in comparison with portacaval shunt, and has the advantage of being easier to handle in the case of transplantation. As yet, there are no fully published RCTs comparing this procedure with portacaval shunt for the risk of encephalopathy.

Devascularization procedures

Many devascularization procedures have been used. All have a significant risk of recurrent bleeding (Wexler, SurgClinNAm, 1990;

70:425), except for the Sugiura procedure in Japanese patients. This two-stage operation consists of a transthoracic oesophageal devascularization, oesophageal transection, and transabdominal paraoesophageal devascularization with splenectomy. The mortality was less than 5 per cent and rebleeding less than 2 per cent (Sugiura, WorldJSurg, 1984; 8:673). However, results in non-Japanese patients have shown a high mortality in the emergency situation and in the elective situation (Orozco, AmJSurg, 1986; 152:539) with a high rebleeding rate of 37 per cent in survivors (Gouge, AmJSurg, 1986; 151:47). The long-term results of simpler operations, such as oesophageal transection using mechanical stapling, also have rebleeding rates of up to 50 per cent (Wexler, SurgClinNAm, 1990; 70:425). Rebleeding is not always from varices; the transection line is frequently the site of rebleeding and this can be prevented with omeprazole (Kaye, Hepatol, 1992; 15:1031; Johlin, DigDisSci, 1992; 37:1373). Using an oesophageal button Prioton (SGO, 1986; 163: 121) achieved a remarkable 21 per cent variceal rebleeding rate at 5 years. Devascularization has been submitted to a controlled comparison with long-term sclerotherapy; there was a similar survival but the rebleeding rate was lower than with sclerotherapy (Table 2) (Triger, Gut, 1992; 33:1553). In general, devascularization procedures are not the surgical procedures of choice and should be reserved for those patients who are not suitable for shunt surgery or TIPS, and in whom sclerotherapy or drugs are not an option or have failed.

Long-term sclerotherapy

Trials of sclerotherapy versus controls

There are eight controlled trials in cirrhotic patients comparing acute and elective sclerotherapy versus solely conservative measures for bleeding (Rossi, J Hepatol, 1991; 12:283; Terblanche, Lancet, 1983; ii:1328; Copenhagen Esophageal Varices Sclerotherapy Project, NEJM, 1984; 311:1594; Westaby, Hepatol, 1985; 5:827; Soderlund, ActaChirScand, 1985; 151:449; Korula, Hepatol, 1985; 5: 584; Burroughs, JHepatol, 1989; 9(Suppl.):S12; Gregory, Hepatol, 1994; 20:618) (Table 4) including a total of 1111 patients. In half of the trials (Copenhagen Esophageal Varices Sclerotherapy Project, NEJM, 1984; 311:1594; Westaby, Hepatol, 1985; 5:827; Soderlund, ActaChirScand, 1985; 151:449; Korula, Hepatol, 1985; 5:584) EST was avoided, if possible, in the control group, that is when rebleeding occurred the management of the acute bleed was different in the two treatment groups. The same treatment protocol for rebleeding was used in three studies (Rossi, JHepatol, 1991; 12:283; Terblanche, Lancet, 1983; ii:1328; Burroughs, JHepatol, 1989; 9(Suppl.):S12). The patients were randomized within 10 days of admission in seven trials (Rossi, JHepatol, 1991; 12:283; Terblanche, Lancet, 1983; ii:1328; Copenhagen Esophageal Varices Sclerotherapy Project, NEJM, 1984; 311:1594; Westaby, Hepatol, 1985; 5:827; Soderlund, ActaChirScand, 1985; 151:449; Korula, Hepatol, 1985; 5:584; Burroughs, JHepatol, 1989; 9(Suppl.):S12). A recent meta-analysis shows that acute and chronic sclerotherapy, compared with no sclerotherapy, significantly reduces rebleeding (POR 0.63 and CI 0.49 to 0.79).[3] The mortality was reduced by sclerotherapy (POR 0.78 and CI 0.61 to 0.94).[3]

Rebleeding from varices was uncommon after achieving eradication of varices (surprisingly 'eradication' was not defined in any of the studies). Eradication was not achieved in 17 to 56 per cent of

Table 4 Non-surgical treatments for the prevention of rebleeding

Trial	Number of patients	Rebleeding rate (%)			Death rate		
		Control	Treated	Odds ratio (95% CI)	Control	Treated	Odds ratio (95% CI)
β-Blockers compared with non-active treatment							
Burroughs et al.	48	59	54	0.81 (0.26–2.51)	23	5	0.62 (0.14–2.63)
Lebrec et al.	74	64	21	0.17 (0.07–0.44)	22	8	0.32 (0.09–1.16)
Villeneuve et al.	79	81	76	0.75 (0.25–2.18)	38	45	1.35 (0.55–3.29)
Queniet et al.	99	64	57	0.72 (0.32–1.62)	21	23	1.16 (0.45–2.99)
Gatta et al.	24	67	25	0.20 (0.04–0.96)	25	8	0.31 (0.03–2.59)
Colombo et al.[a]	62	47	25	0.39 (0.14–1.10)	23	12	0.48 (0.13–1.75)
Colombo et al.[b]	62	47	31	0.52 (0.19–1.45)	23	9	0.36 (0.09–1.38)
Sheen et al.	36	55	28	0.32 (0.08–1.21)	11	0	0.12 (0.01–2.12)
Garden et al.	81	84	53	0.23 (0.09–0.60)	44	37	0.74 (0.30–1.79)
Rossi et al.	54	63	48	0.55 (0.19–1.60)	33	26	0.70 (0.22–2.24)
Cerbelaud et al.	84	78	40	0.21 (0.08–0.49)	NR	NR	–
Colman et al.	52	50	35	0.54 (0.18–1.60)	4	4	1.00 (0.06–16.4)
POR (95% CI)				0.40 (0.30–0.54)			0.70 (0.48–1.02)
Sclerotherapy compared with non-active treatment							
Terblanche et al.	75	55	57	1.06 (0.42–2.62)	63	62	0.95 (0.37–2.42)
EVASP	187	54	48	0.79 (0.44–1.40)	78	64	0.52 (0.28–0.99)
Westaby et al.	116	82	55	0.29 (0.13–0.64)	53	32	0.42 (0.20–0.88)
Soderlund et al.	107	66	56	0.66 (0.30–1.44)	70	56	0.55 (0.25–1.20)
Korula et al.	120	84	49	0.21 (0.10–0.45)	33	33	1.00 (0.46–2.13)
Rossi et al.	53	63	50	0.60 (0.20–1.75)	33	23	0.61 (0.19–1.99)
Burroughs et al.	204	60	56	0.85 (0.48–1.48)	54	47	0.76 (0.44–1.31)
Gregory	153	63	55	0.70 (0.43–1.65)	56	63	1.32 (0.80–2.17)
POR (95% CI)				0.62 (0.49–0.79)			0.77 (0.61–0.98)
Sclerotherapy compared with β-blockers							
Alexandrino et al.	65	73	55	0.44 (0.16–1.22)	32	29	0.85 (0.30–2.44)
Dollet et al.	55	41	64	2.52 (0.88–7.21)	41	53	1.65 (0.58–4.73)
Westaby et al.	108	56	50	0.79 (0.37–1.68)	42	37	0.82 (0.38–1.76)
Rossi et al.	53	48	50	1.07 (0.37–3.12)	26	23	0.86 (0.24–2.97)
Martin et al.	76	53	55	0.36 (0.16–0.83)	23	31	1.44 (0.52–3.93)
Dasarathy et al.	91	67	42	0.36 (0.16–0.83)	41	22	1.04 (0.45–2.38)
Fleig et al.	105	52	47	0.82 (0.38–1.77)	32	36	1.21 (0.54–2.70)
Liu et al.	118	57	33	0.38 (0.18–0.80)	39	28	0.60 (0.28–1.29)
Terés et al.	116	64	45	0.47 (0.23–0.97)	40	36	0.86 (0.41–1.82)
POR (95% CI)				0.66 (0.50–0.88)			0.96 (0.71–1.28)
Sclerotherapy plus β-blockers compared with sclerotherapy							
Westaby et al.	53	30	27	0.87 (0.26–2.86)	26	35	1.49 (0.46–4.79)
Jensen and Karup	31	75	20	0.11 (0.03–0.47)	6	7	1.06 (0.06–17.9)
Lundell et al.	39	50	63	1.68 (0.49–5.71)	NR	NR	–
Vicker et al.	73	41	44	1.10 (0.44–2.78)	26	23	0.83 (0.29–2.41)
Vinel et al.	74	40	18	0.34 (0.12–0.94)	14	13	0.79 (0.21–3.02)
Bertoni et al.[c,d]	28	28	7	0.24 (0.04–1.63)	21	7	0.32 (0.04–2.60)
Gerunda et al.[c,d]	60	23	20	0.82 (0.24–2.78)	10	3	0.34 (0.04–2.60)
Avgerinos et al.	85	52	31	0.41 (0.18–0.99)	23	18	0.75 (0.26–2.15)
Villanueva et al.[c]	40	39	55	1.84 (0.54–6.32)	0	9	6.46 (0.38–108)
Acharya et al.	114	21	17	0.76 (0.30–1.93)	12	9	0.66 (0.20–2.19)
POR (95% CI)				0.66 (0.46–0.93)[e]			0.83 (0.52–1.33)
Sclerotherapy plus β-blockers compared with β-blockers							
O'Connor et al.	62	87	68	0.33 (0.10–1.96)	81	55	0.31 (0.11–0.90)
Ink et al.	125	53	38	0.55 (0.28–1.11)	35	26	0.66 (0.32–1.39)
POR (95% CI)				0.49 (0.27–0.89)			0.52 (0.28–0.95)
Endoscopic ligation compared with sclerotherapy							
Stiegmann et al.	129	48	36	0.62 (0.31–1.24)	45	28	0.49 (0.24–1.00)
Laine et al.	77	44	26	0.47 (0.19–1.19)	15	10	0.65 (0.17–2.45)
Gimson et al.	103	53	30	0.38 (0.17–0.84)	NR	NR	–
POR (95% CI)				0.49 (0.31–0.78)			0.53 (0.28–0.99)

[a] Propranolol.
[b] Atenolol.
[c] Trial published only as an abstract.
[d] Sclerotherapy plus nadolol compared with sclerotherapy.
[e] Statistically significant heterogeneity. By excluding Jensen's trial, POR = 0.74 (CI 0.52 to 1.06) without heterogeneity.

patients, mainly due to early death. However, even after eradication was achieved, 10 to 23 per cent of patients still rebled. Complications were frequent and contributed to death in 2 to 11 per cent of patients (Soehendra, ActaEndoscop, 1986; 16:39; Sanowski, JClin-Gastro, 1987; 9:504; Schuman, AmJGastr, 1987; 82:823; Kahn, Surgery, 1989; 105:160). Bleeding due to ulceration was only reported separately in one study (9 per cent of sclerosed patients of Soderlund and Ihre (ActaChirScand, 1985; 151:449) and it is not clear if this was included in the calculation of rebleeding in all studies. Long-term studies (Westaby, ScaJGastr, 1984; 19(Suppl. 102):71; Sauerbruch, Endoscopy, 1987; 19:181; Sakai, Endoscopy, 1988; 20:134) show that in one-third of patients varices never recur following eradication, while new varices rebleed in approximately 30 per cent of the remainder.

Trials of sclerotherapy versus shunt surgery

Sclerotherapy was compared to distal splenorenal shunt in four RCTs (Rikkers, AnnSurg, 1987; 206:261; Terés, Hepatol, 1987; 7:430; Henderson, AnnIntMed, 1990; 112:262; Spina, AnnSurg, 1990; 211:178; Spina, JHepatol, 1992; 16:338) and to portacaval shunt in three (Cello, NEJM, 1987; 316:11; Korula, Hepatol, 1988; 8:1242; Planas, Gastro, 1991; 100:1078) (Table 3). A total of 493 patients were included, of whom 307 were in distal splenorenal shunt trials. Patients were randomized soon after bleeding in only one trial (Cello, NEJM, 1987; 316:11). In the other trials the patients were randomized at least 10 days after the index bleed. Rebleeding was more markedly and significantly reduced by shunt surgery in five trials (Rikkers, AnnSurg, 1987; 206:261; Terés, Hepatol, 1987; 7:430; Henderson, AnnIntMed, 1990; 112:262; Spina, AnnSurg, 1990; 211:178; Spina, JHepatol, 1992; 16:338; Planas, Gastro, 1991; 100:1078). The POR was significantly reduced with shunt surgery as compared with sclerotherapy (0.18 and CI 0.12 to 0.28).[3] Chronic or recurrent PSE was greater after shunt surgery in four RCTs (Rikkers, AnnSurg, 1987; 206:261; Terés, Hepatol, 1987; 7:430; Henderson, AnnIntMed, 1990; 112:262; Planas, Gastro, 1991; 100:1078) and was unchanged in two (Cello, NEJM, 1987; 316:11; Spina, AnnSurg, 1990; 211:178). No information was available in one (Korula, Hepatol, 1988; 8:1242). The POR was significantly increased with shunt surgery (2.00 and CI 1.1 to 3.6). The risk of death was lower in shunted patients (but non-significantly) in five RCTs (Rikkers, AnnSurg, 1987; 206:261; Terés, Hepatol, 1987; 7:430; Spina, AnnSurg, 1990; 211:178; Spina, JHepatol, 1992; 16:338; Korula, Hepatol, 1988; 8:1242; Planas, Gastro, 1991; 100:1078) and higher in two (Cello, NEJM, 1987; 316:11; Henderson, AnnIntMed, 1990; 112:262). The suggestion in the study by Henderson (Henderson, AnnIntMed, 1990; 112:262) that the sclerotherapy group had less mortality because of rescue shunt surgery is not supported by the other studies. The pooled estimates of the seven studies disclosed no differences in mortality between the two treatments (POR 1.00 and CI 0.67 to 1.51).[3]

Similar results are obtained when only the four studies comparing elective sclerotherapy vs distal splenorenal shunt are considered, except that the increase in PSE after distal splenorenal shunt does not reach statistical significance (POR 2.03, CI 0.94 to 4.38). Prior identification of patients who continue to rebleed despite sclerotherapy would avoid a trial by sclerotherapy before performing shunt surgery but this is not possible. Seen in this light, elective sclerotherapy needs to be improved.

Trials of sclerotherapy versus TIPS

The preliminary results of randomized controlled trials comparing TIPS with endoscopic sclerotherapy in the prevention of variceal rebleeding are available (Table 5). These studies suggest that the risk of rebleeding is significantly reduced by TIPS, although there is an increased risk of hepatic encephalopathy and a trend towards a higher mortality. The fact that most of these studies are available only in abstract form precludes a more detailed analysis, but makes it unlikely that TIPS will become the first-line therapy for prevention of rebleeding in all patients.

Endoscopic variceal banding ligation compared with sclerotherapy

Following the promising results of initial reports in terms of the control of variceal bleeding and of the prevention of recurrent bleeding (Van Stiegmann, AmJSurg, 1990; 159:21), endoscopic banding ligation was compared with sclerotherapy in three RCTs (Stiegmann, NEJM, 1992; 326:1527; Laine, AnnIntMed, 1993; 119:1; Gimson, Lancet, 1993; 342:391) (Table 4). A total of 309 patients were included. The rate of recurrent variceal bleeding was significantly reduced in one study (Gimson, Lancet, 1993; 342:391). The pooled results show a significant benefit from banding ligation (POR 0.49 and CI 0.31 to 0.78). The mortality was almost significantly reduced by ligation in one study (Stiegmann, NEJM, 1992; 326:1527) and unchanged in the others (Laine, AnnIntMed, 1993; 119:1; Gimson, Lancet, 1993; 342:391); the POR was non-significantly reduced (0.72 and CI 0.44 to 1.18). In all three studies, the number of sessions to eradicate varices was significantly less with endoscopic ligation. Complications were less with ligation in two studies (Stiegmann, NEJM, 1992; 326:1527; Laine, AnnIntMed, 1993; 119:1), but not in the other (Gimson, Lancet, 1993; 342:391). Recently, endoscopic banding ligation has been compared with the combined use of banding ligation and sclerotherapy with equivalent results (Laine, Gastro, 1996; 110:529).

The results of these studies therefore indicate that there is a significant advantage of using endoscopic banding ligation, which is at present the recommended long-term endoscopic treatment.[14] Future trials should compare endoscopic banding against other active treatments (drug combinations, surgery and TIPS).

Randomized trials of β-blocker versus placebo for the prevention of recurrent variceal bleeding

Haemodynamic basis

In patients with cirrhosis, the administration of propranolol and other non-selective β-blockers, such as nadolol or timolol, reduces the portal pressure by decreasing the portal–collateral blood flow (Lebrec, Lancet, 1980; ii:180; Bosch, Hepatol, 1984; 4:1200; García-Tsao, Hepatol, 1986; 6:101). This is due to splanchnic vasoconstriction, promoted by the blockade of vasodilating β_2-adrenoceptors in the splanchnic circulation and by the decrease in the heart rate and cardiac output caused by the blockade of cardiac β_1-adrenoceptors. β_2-Blockade is an important determinant of the

Table 5 Preliminary results of RCTs comparing TIPS versus endoscopic sclerotherapy in the prevention of recurrent variceal bleeding

	Number of patients		Rebleeding (%)		Mortality (%)		Encephalopathy (%)		Follow up
	TIPS	EST	TIPS	EST	TIPS	EST	TIPS	EST	
Sanyal (1994)	40	39	25	20	28	10*	23*	15**	
Cabrera (1996)	31	32	23	52**	20	16	33	13*	15 months
Merli (1996)	39	42	18	50**	27	16	50*	17*	15 months
Rössle (1994)	26	27[a]	8	26*	8	4	19	0	
Cello (1995)	21	19	0	37**	19	16	52	42	
Sauer (1996)	42	41[a]	9 (1 y)	44*	23 (1 y)	15	29	9*	18 months
			23 (2 y)	71*	31 (2 y)	33			
Jalan (1995)	18	21[b]	11	52*	28	24	22	10	
Vinel (1995)[c]	32	33[a]	41	61	50	42	?	?	

[a] EST + propranolol.
[b] Endoscopic banding ligation of varices instead of EST.
[c] Child–Pugh's class C.
* $p < 0.05$, ** $p < 0.01$.

haemodynamic effects of these drugs on portal hypertension; because of this, atenolol and other cardioselective β_1-blockers have less potential in the treatment of portal hypertension.

The decrease in portal pressure and blood flow caused by propranolol is accompanied by a marked reduction in azygous blood flow (reflecting blood flow through gastroesophageal collaterals and varices) (Bosch, Hepatol, 1984; 4:1200) as well as in variceal pressure (Feu, Hepatol, 1993; 18:1082). A reduction in variceal pressure and collateral blood flow is likely to represent the mechanism by which non-selective β-blockers reduce the risk of variceal bleeding, since these parameters are the major determinants of variceal wall tension (Rigau, Gastro, 1989; 96:873).[15]

The total hepatic blood flow decreases moderately following propranolol administration, because the hepatic artery blood flow does not increase enough to match the fall in portal blood flow (Mastai, Hepatol, 1989; 10:269). The reduction in liver perfusion is accompanied by impairment in some quantitative liver function tests, such as the hepatic clearance of indocyanine green (**ICG**) and the hepatic intrinsic clearance. However, the galactose elimination capacity is not altered (Vinel, JHepatol, 1988; 7:186). Similarly, there is no evidence of adverse effects of propranolol on renal or cerebral perfusion.

Variability in response to propranolol

The portal pressure response to propranolol is not homogeneous and varies markedly from patient to patient. While some patients exhibit a pronounced reduction in portal pressure, others do not. An absence of response is defined as a less than 20 per cent decrease in the portal pressure (estimated from the hepatic venous pressure gradient, **HVPG**) or a failure to reduce the HVPG to 12 mmHg or below (Feu, Lancet, 1995; 346:1056; Groszmann, Gastro, 1990; 99: 1401). These values represent the decrease in portal pressure which is associated with protection from the risk of variceal bleeding; therefore, propranolol non-responders probably do not benefit from continued β-blocker therapy. The prevalence of propranolol non-responders ranges between 50 and 70 per cent in different series (Bosch, Hepatol, 1984; 4:1200; Garcia-Tsao, Hepatol, 1986; 6:101; Feu, Lancet, 1995; 346:1056). The mechanism of non-response is

not related to an inadequate dose, insufficient blockade of β_1-adrenoceptors (Bosch, Hepatology, 1984; 4:1200), the aetiology or severity of portal hypertension (Garcia-Tsao, Hepatol, 1986; 6:101), circulating levels of adrenaline and noradrenaline, or down-regulation of β_2-adrenoceptors (García-Pagán, Gastro, 1992; 102: 2015). The more important factor determining non-response is an increase in the portal–collateral vascular resistance, which attenuates the reduction in portal pressure achieved as a consequence of the fall in portal venous inflow caused by β-blockade. Such an increase in the portal–collateral resistance has been well documented in experimental models (Kroeger, Hepatol, 1985; 5:97) and may depend on the extent of the collateral circulation (Pizcueta, Hepatol, 1989; 10:953; Escorsell, Hepatol, 1995; 22:156A).

There is no accurate way of predicting the portal pressure response to propranolol therapy in a given patient, except by invasive haemodynamic studies. Patients with a marked reduction in portal pressure after propranolol administration (a decrease in the HVPG to 12 mmHg or less) have been shown to be completely protected from their first variceal haemorrhage (Groszmann, Gastro, 1990; 99:1401) or patients treated after the first variceal haemorrhage, from the risk of recurrent bleeding. A decrease in HVPG greater than 20 per cent of the baseline value is also associated with a dramatic decrease in the risk of recurrent variceal haemorrhage (Feu, Lancet, 1995; 346:1056), which is supported by the results of another recent study comparing pharmacological treatment to sclerotherapy (Villanueva, NEJM, 1996; 335:1624); this however was not observed in another study (McCormick, Hepatol, 1995; 22:255A(Abstr.)). Therefore, an assessment of the effects of therapy on the portal pressure may provide useful prognostic information. The measurement of the propranolol plasma levels and heart rate may be used to monitor compliance to therapy, but do not correlate with the changes in portal pressure.

The dose of propranolol or nadolol required by each patient varies markedly. Since these agents have a marked first-pass effect, the bioavailability is markedly influenced by the extent of portal-systemic shunting and by the degree of liver failure. Most patients require 40 to 80 mg twice a day (once a day if using nadolol), but some require much more. The dosage is usually matched against the heart rate; this is not an index of the effect on portal pressure, but allows one to assess if therapy achieves an adequate blockade of β_1-adrenoceptors. It is customary to increase the dose stepwise until the resting heart rate is reduced by 25 per cent of baseline values (to a limit of 55 beats/min). Frequently, the dose has to be adjusted again during the course of therapy. Cimetidine impairs propranolol metabolism; it is therefore preferable to use other H_2 antagonists if they are needed. Nadolol is less lipid soluble than propranolol, which results in less first-pass uptake and longer biological activity. The usual dose is 40 to 80 mg once a day. The haemodynamic effects of nadolol and propranolol are superimposable.

Propranolol and nadolol are well tolerated, the proportion of patients discontinuing treatment because or poor tolerance or side-effects being approximately 15 per cent. Contraindications to propranolol/nadolol are present in approximately 15 per cent of the patients.

Results of trials

Eleven randomized controlled trials have been published (two in abstract form), including a total of 755 patients (Burroughs, NEJM, 1983; 309:1539; Lebrec, Hepatol, 1984; 4:355; Villeneuve, Hepatol, 1986; 6:1239; Queuniet, GastrClinBiol, 1987; 11:41; Gatta, Digestion, 1987; 37:22; Colombo, Hepatol, 1989; 9:433; Sheen, Liver, 1989; 9:1; Garden, Gastro, 1990; 98:185; Rossi, JHepatol, 1991; 12:283; Cerbelaud, GastrClinBiol, 1986; 18:A10; Colman, Hepatol, 1990; 12:851). One trial comparing propranolol with atenolol and with placebo (Colombo, Hepatol, 1989; 9:433) was analysed as two separate trials. Comparative data are shown in Table 4. No fatal complications of propranolol have been reported. Propranolol was assessed in 10 studies and nadolol in one (Gatta, Digestion, 1987; 37:22). None was double blind. The patients were randomized more than 3 weeks after bleeding in five trials (Lebrec, Hepatol, 1984; 4:355; Gatta, Digestion, 1987; 37:22; Colombo, Hepatol, 1989; 9:433; Sheen, Liver, 1989; 9:1; Colman, Hepatol, 1990; 12:851).

Rebleeding was reduced by β-blockers in all trials, significantly in four (Lebrec, Hepatol, 1984; 4:355; Gatta, Digestion, 1987; 37:22; Garden, Gastro, 1990; 98:185; Cerbelaud, GastrClinBiol, 1986; 18:A10). A meta-analysis of these trials shows a highly significant reduction of rebleeding (POR 0.40 and CI 0.30 to 0.53).[3] The death risk was reduced with β-blockers in eight trials and unchanged or non-significantly increased in three (Villeneuve, Hepatol, 1986; 6:1239; Queuniet, GastrClinBiol, 1987; 11:41; Colman, Hepatol, 1990; 12:851). One study (Cerbelaud, GastrClinBiol, 1986; 18:A10) did not report on the mortality. The POR was 0.7 (CI 0.48 to 1.02), approaching statistical significance. The side-effects of the β-blockers were not frequent and mild.

Only one trial (Kiire, BMJ, 1989; 298:1363) has been published evaluating non-cirrhotic portal hypertensive patients (mainly with schistosomiasis); in these patients propranolol reduced rebleeding compared to no treatment.

New pharmacological perspectives
Vasodilators

Many vasoactive agents have been found to decrease portal pressure after oral administration. These include the vasodilating nitrates, nitroglycerine (García-Tsao, Hepatol, 1987; 7:805), isosorbide dinitrate (Blei, Gastro, 1987; 93:576), and isosorbide 5-mononitrate

(Navasa, Gastro, 1989; 96:1110; García-Pagán, JHepatol, 1990; 11:189; Escorsell, JHepatol, 1996; 24:423), which are predominantly venous dilators that reduce portal pressure by decreasing the portal–collateral resistance, the serotonin S_2 antagonists, ketanserin (Vorobioff, Hepatol, 1989; 8:88) and ritanserin (Fernández, Hepatol, 1993; 18:389), the central α-agonist, clonidine (Albillos, Gastro, 1992; 102:248), and the α_1-adrenergic blocker, prazosin (Albillos, Gastro, 1995; 109:1257). These drugs reduce portal pressure without a further decrease in liver perfusion. Molsidomine has many similarities to isosorbide dinitrate (Vinel, Hepatol, 1990; 11:239). It is not known if these agents will prove good alternatives to propranolol. The decrease in portal pressure achieved is of the same order of magnitude as that caused by propranolol (Garcia-Pagan, JHepatol, 1996; 24:430). However, many of them cause a significant fall in the arterial blood pressure, which may be detrimental, and may cause symptoms in patients with advanced liver failure. Calcium channel blockers appear to be of no benefit.

Combination therapy

It has been shown that the association of a nitrovasodilator enhances the reduction in portal pressure achieved with vasopressin (Groszmann, Hepatol, 1982; 2:757) and, more importantly, with propranolol (García-Pagán, AnnIntMed, 1991; 114:869). The rationale for such combination therapy comes from the finding that propranolol increases the portal–collateral resistance, which suggests that the association of a venous dilator may cause a further fall in the portal pressure. Both isosorbide 5-mononitrate and isosorbide dinitrate have been shown to achieve this goal, although the former is safer in terms of not causing hypotension and impaired renal function (Morillas, Hepatol, 1994; 20:1502). The association of molsidomine with propranolol was not found to be useful in a recent study (García-Pagán, JHepatol, 1996; 24:430). The combination of propranolol and prazosin may have greater effects on the HVPG than that of propranolol and isosorbide 5-mononitrate, but the latter is safer and better tolerated and is the only one that has been used in large-scale clinical trials.

The combination of propranolol and isosorbide-5-mononitrate results in a greater reduction in portal pressure than with either drug alone, while maintaining the decrease in the azygos blood flow and improving hepatic perfusion (García-Pagán, Hepatol, 1990; 11:230). This beneficial effect was particularly evident in patients who do not respond to propranolol. Combination therapy achieved a marked decrease in the HVPG (greater than 20 per cent of baseline values or below 12 mmHg) in a significantly greater proportion of patients than propranolol alone (García-Pagán, AnnIntMed, 1991; 114:869). Since the intensity of the decrease of portal pressure correlates with the clinical benefit from propranolol therapy (Feu, Lancet, 1995; 346:1056), it is likely that the association of propranolol and isosorbide 5-mononitrate can improve the results of long-term drug therapy for portal hypertension.

The clinical efficacy of this drug combination is still under investigation, but three large studies have yielded very promising results. The first of these trials (McCormick, Hepatol, 1994; 20:106A) showed similar results using the combination of propranolol and isosorbide 5-mononitrate than with aggressive therapy (shunt surgery in Child's A and B patients and sclerotherapy in Child's C patients). The second trial (Villanueva, NEJM, 1996; 335:1624) demonstrated significantly better results with the association of nadolol and isosorbide 5-mononitrate than with endoscopic sclerotherapy. The mortality however was not reduced. The third study is a prophylactic trial of nadolol plus isosorbide 5-mononitrate against nadolol alone (Merkel, JHepatol, 1995; 23(Suppl.1):69), showing a significantly lower incidence of variceal bleeding in the group of patients that were treated with combination therapy. Therefore, the combination of β-blockers and isosorbide 5-mononitrate is preferable to β-blockers alone in the prevention of variceal haemorrhage.

Randomized trials of β-blockers compared with sclerotherapy

Nine randomized controlled trials have been reported, including a total of 787 patients (Rossi, JHepatol, 1991; 12:283; Alexandrino, J Hepatol, 1988; 7:175; Dollet, GastrClinBiol, 1988; 12:234; Westaby, Hepatol, 1990; 11:353; Martin, GastrClinBiol, 1991; 15:833; Dasarathy, Hepatol, 1992; 16:89; Fleig, Hepatol, 1987; 7:355; Fleig, JHepatol, 1988; 7(Suppl):S32; Liu, GastrWorldCongr, 1990; FP1181; Terés, Gastro, 1993; 105:1508) (Table 4). EST was used for rebleeding in both groups in two studies (Westaby, Hepatol, 1990; 11:353; Fleig, Hepatol, 1987; 7:355), was systematically used in the sclerotherapy group but only occasionally in the medical group in two trials (Alexandrino, JHepatol, 1988; 7:175; Dollet, GastrClinBiol, 1988; 12:234), and not used in either groups in two further studies (Rossi, JHepatol, 1991; 12:283; Dasarathy, Hepatol, 1992; 16:89). Treatment for acute rebleeding was not reported in three trials (Martin, GastrClinBiol, 1991; 15:833; Liu, GastrWorldCongr, 1990; FP1181; Terés, Gastro, 1993; 105:1508). Therefore, it is possible that differences in management of acute bleeding episodes in the two treatment arms may have influenced the results of some of these studies.

The rebleeding rate was lower with sclerotherapy in six studies (Alexandrino, JHepatol, 1988; 7:175; Westaby, Hepatol, 1990; 11:353; Dasarathy, Hepatol, 1992; 16:89; Fleig, Hepatol, 1987; 7:355; Liu, GastrWorldCong, 1990; FP1181; Terés, Gastro, 1993; 105:1508) and increased in three (Rossi, JHepatol, 1991; 12:283; Dollet, GastrClinBiol, 1988; 12:234; Martin, GastrClinBiol, 1991; 15:833). This qualitative heterogeneity approached statistical significance ($p = 0.07$). Because of such heterogeneity, the significant reduction of rebleeding observed with sclerotherapy in the metaanalysis (POR 0.68 and CI 0.50 to 0.88) should not be considered as definite evidence of the superiority of sclerotherapy over propranolol. Moreover, despite the slight reduction in rebleeding, no trial showed differences in survival; the POR was 0.96 (CI 0.71 to 1.28). Not surprisingly, complications were more common and severe with sclerotherapy. Therefore, these studies suggest that sclerotherapy is slightly more effective than β-blockers in the prevention of recurrent variceal bleeding, but this does not result in improved survival and is associated with more frequent and severe complications.

As already mentioned, a recent study (Villanueva, NEJM, 1996; 335:1624) comparing sclerotherapy with the combination of nadolol and isosorbide 5-mononitrate showed drug therapy to be significantly better and safer than sclerotherapy in the prevention of variceal rebleeding, supporting the concept that combination therapy may offer greater protection from the risk of variceal bleeding than β-blockers alone. If these results are confirmed, drug therapy would represent the first treatment option in the prevention of variceal rebleeding. It is clear that further trials are required to compare combined drug therapy with improved endoscopic treatments such as endoscopic banding ligation of the varices.

Randomized trials of β-blockers combined with sclerotherapy for the prevention of variceal rebleeding

From a theoretical point of view, since β-blockers and sclerotherapy prevent variceal rebleeding through different mechanisms, its combination should improve the results obtained separately with either therapy. Moreover, since when using drug therapy the benefit of reduced portal pressure is achieved very rapidly, the association of β-blockers and sclerotherapy may have the potential for decreasing the risk of variceal rebleeding before 'eradication' of the varices by sclerotherapy. However, β-blockers should not be expected to prevent the rebleeding episodes due to sclerotherapy-related oesophageal ulceration.

There are 10 randomized trials of propranolol plus repeated injection versus repeated sclerotherapy alone (Table 4). A total of 573 patients were included (Westaby, Hepatol, 1986; 6:673; Jensen, ScaJGastr, 1989; 24:339; Lundell, ActaChirScand, 1990; 156:711; Vickers, JHepatol, 1994; 21:81; Vinel, Gastro, 1992; 102:1760; Bertoni, JClinGastro, 1990; 12:364; Gerunda, Hepatol, 1990; 12: 988; Avgerinos, JHepatol, 1993; 19:301; Villanueva, RevEspEnfermAparDig, 1994; 86:499; Acharya, JHepatol, 1993; 19: 291). Propranolol was associated with sclerotherapy in seven trials and nadolol in three (Bertoni, JClinGastro, 1990; 12:364; Gerunda, Hepatol, 1990; 12:988; Villanueva, RevEspEnfermAparDig, 1994; 86:499). Rebleeding was reduced with the combination therapy in six trials (Westaby, Hepatol, 1986; 6:673; Jensen, ScaJGastr, 1989; 24:339; Vinel, Gastro, 1992; 102:1760; Bertoni, JClinGastro, 1990; 12:364; Gerunda, Hepatol, 1990; 12:988; Villanueva, RevEspEnfermAparDig, 1994; 86:499), significantly in two (Jensen, ScaJGastr, 1989; 24:339; Vinel, Gastro, 1992; 102:1760). One of the two trials with significant bleeding risk reduction (Jensen, ScaJGastr, 1989; 24:339) should probably be considered an outlier because of the particularly high rebleeding rate with sclerotherapy (75 per cent), which is the highest ever reported. This may be related to the long interval (30 days) between sclerotherapy sessions, as suggested by the fact that eight out of 12 patients who rebled, did so within the first 50 days. The pooled estimates show no significant differences (POR 0.79 and CI 0.51 to 1.20) and with significant heterogeneity ($p = 0.009$). No significant difference in the mortality was observed in any trial. Therefore, these studies do not support the use of β-blockers together with sclerotherapy, but it should be noted that β-blockers were not continued after eradication in most of these studies. A recent large study, which included patients with schistosomiasis has shown a 14 versus 39 per cent rebleeding rate in favour of the combination group (Elsayed, Gut, 1996; 38:770).

The association of propranolol and sclerotherapy has been compared with propranolol alone in two trials (O'Connor, Gastro, 1989; 96:899; Ink, Hepatol, 1992; 16:912), including 193 patients (Table 4). The minimum follow-up was 2 years. Both trials showed a reduction in the risk of rebleeding and death with the combined therapy.

Bories *et al.* (JHepatol, 1987; 5:S13) compared propranolol with oesophageal transection using a clip. The rebleeding rates were 73 per cent with propranolol and 17 per cent with surgery.

Transplantation

As the prognosis of cirrhotic patients with variceal bleeding is related to the severity of the underlying liver disease, successful transplantation of the liver will dramatically improve their survival (Garrett, Surgery, 1988; 104:819). However, because the risk of death falls dramatically once the patient has survived a few weeks from the bleeding episode, that is returns to that pertaining to the underlying liver disease,[1,4] liver transplantation will only improve the prognosis related to the bleeding episode if it is performed in the acute period. It may be difficult to justify a higher priority for transplantation, in order to find a donor quickly for the patient who has bled (but has already survived the first few days) than for those with terminal liver disease who have not bled recently. At present, immediate transplantation for bleeding will probably be reserved for patients already accepted into a programme. In any case the bleeding must still be stopped and the techniques used should take into account the fact that transplantation may be performed in the near future (Wood, SurgClinNAm, 1990; 70:449). Sclerotherapy ulcers may cause bleeding, perforation and death following transplantation (Vickers, GastrEnd, 1989; 35:45). Only skilled endoscopists should perform sclerotherapy in transplant candidates and omeprazole may be useful for rapid healing of ulcers (Gimson, Gut, 1988; 29:A728; Johlin, DigDisSci, 1992; 37:1373; Shephard, GastrEnd, 1993; 39:474; Garg, DigDisSci, 1995; 40:1569). Sclerotherapy can also cause portal vein thrombosis (Schuman, AmJGastr, 1987; 82:823; Ashida, AmJGastr, 1989; 84:306; Korula, DigDisSci, 1991; 36:1164). TIPS probably represents the best shunting procedure in this situation, but should not be used prophylactically to prevent bleeding. If surgery is considered, a mesocaval interposition Goretex or autologous vein graft shunt or a high H–graft portacaval shunt or a distal splenorenal shunt should be preferred, as a standard portacaval shunt may complicate the transplant procedure.

Prevention of the first variceal bleeding episode

The natural history of cirrhotics with varices who have never bled and potential pitfalls in study design have recently been reviewed.[16] Approximately one-third of cirrhotics with oesophageal varices bleed and the average mortality due to the first variceal bleed is approximately 50 per cent. Thus, prophylactic treatment to prevent variceal haemorrhage may offer the best opportunity to improve prognosis. Much of what we know about the natural history is based on the control groups of prophylactic shunt studies, in which 30 per cent of patients bled and half of these died because of the bleeding. Although it is commonly assumed that these cirrhotic patients were unselected, they were, in most cases, patients who were already in hospital because of their liver disease. The risk of bleeding cannot be considered to be the same as in those with an abnormal biochemistry without complications of cirrhosis in whom varices are found at endoscopy during a diagnostic work up. This type of selection accounts for part of the high variability found in trials of prophylactic therapy. Recently the use

of indices of the severity of liver disease and of endoscopic markers shown to indicate a high risk of bleeding (large varices and red signs) have been the basis for prophylactic trials (NIEC, NEJM, 1988; 319:983). In Japan, in a trial evaluating devascularization (Inokuchi, AnnSurg, 1984; 200:61), only cirrhotic patients with a high endoscopic risk score, based on the presence of red signs (Beppu, GastrEnd, 1981; 27:213), were randomized. Despite the selection, bleeding occurred in only 19 per cent of patients in the control group. This is important when designing prophylactic trials; yet, most studies have insufficient power (that is, too few patients were included) to identify favourable treatment effects. In such a situation, meta-analysis is very helpful in assessing the efficacy of the different treatments that have been proposed.

Shunt surgery compared with non-active treatment

The prophylactic shunt trials were among the first randomized controlled studied in hepatology. Four trials are reported including a total of 412 patients with varices of any size (Jackson, AmJSurg, 1968; 115:22; Resnick, AnnIntMed, 1969; 70:675; Rueff, Lancet, 1976; ii:655; Reynolds, Gastro, 1981; 80:1005). These trials showed that shunt surgery was very effective in preventing variceal bleeding (4 to 16 versus 19 to 39 per cent in untreated control patients), but significantly increased the risk of chronic or recurrent encephalopathy (21 to 37 control versus 38 to 52 per cent shunted patients) and most importantly, resulted in a significant reduction of survival (POR 0.31 and CI: 0.17–0.56) (Table 3). Prophylactic shunt surgery was abandoned on the basis of these results.

In a recent trial comparing a variety of devascularization procedures or selective shunts with conservative treatment, Inokuchi *et al.* (Hepatol, 1990; 12:1) reported a significant bleeding risk reduction with prophylactic surgery: 8 versus 32 per cent after a median follow up of 49 months. The mortality was also significantly reduced in the surgical group (22 versus 49 per cent). However, there are important problems in interpreting these results. Different operations were used in 22 centres, based on the surgeon's choice (each team operated on a mean of two to three patients with different operations). The mortality rate was unusually high in the control group of well-compensated patients (none was Child C). Furthermore, nine patients in the surgical group but none in the control group were withdrawn from the analysis. Because of these pitfalls the conclusions of this study are difficult to accept.

Prophylactic sclerotherapy compared with non-active treatment

There are 19 trials (Andreani, Hepatol, 1990; 12:1413; The PROVA Study Group, Hepatol, 1991; 14:1016; Strauss, Hepatol, 1988; 8:1395; Paquet, Endoscopy, 1982; 14:4; Witzel, Lancet, 1985; i:773; Koch, Endoscopy, 1986; 18:40; Kobe, Endoscopy, 1990; 22:245; Wordehoff, DeutschMedWoch, 1987; 112:947; Santangelo, NEJM, 1988; 318:814; Sauerbruch, NEJM, 1988; 319:8; Piai, Hepatol, 1988; 8:1495; Potzi, Gut, 1989; 30:873; Russo, WorldJSurg, 1989; 13:149; Triger, Hepatol, 1991; 13:117; VA Cooperative Variceal Sclerotherapy Group, NEJM, 1991; 324:1779; De Franchis, Gastro, 1991; 101:1087; Saggioro, DigDisSci, 1986; 31:504S; Fleig, Hepatol, 1988; 7(Suppl.):S128; Quer, MedClin(Barc), 1991; 96:352)

Table 6 Non-surgical treatments for prevention of first bleeding

Trial	Number of patients	Bleeding rate (%) Control	Treated	Odds ratio (95% CI)	Death rate Control	Treated	Odds ratio (95% CI)
Sclerotherapy compared with non-active treatment							
Paquet	71	61	9	0.10 (0.04–0.27)	39	6	0.15 (0.05–0.46)
Witzel et al.	109	57	9	0.12 (0.05–0.26)	55	21	0.25 (0.11–0.53)
Koch et al.	60	33	30	0.86 (0.29–2.53)	33	37	1.16 (0.40–3.31)
Kobe et al.	63	73	30	0.19 (0.07–0.50)	58	47	0.65 (0.24–1.73)
Wordehoff and Spech	49	63	20	0.18 (0.06–0.55)	67	56	0.64 (0.21–2.00)
Santangelo et al.	95	15	35	2.77 (1.10–6.97)	24	24	1.03 (0.40–2.63)
Sauerbruch et al.	113	43	32	0.63 (0.29–1.33)	45	28	0.49 (0.23–1.05)
Piai et al.	140	42	14	0.25 (0.12–0.52)	38	23	0.49 (0.24–1.00)
Potzi et al.	82	34	29	0.80 (0.32–2.02)	46	24	0.39 (0.16–0.95)
Russo et al.	41	15	0	0.12 (0.01–1.18)	10	0	0.12 (0.00–2.03)
Adreani et al.	83	32	21	0.59 (0.23–1.57)	44	43	0.96 (0.40–2.27)
Triger et al.	68	40	39	0.97 (0.37–2.56)	60	61	1.02 (0.39–2.69)
Gregory et al.	281	17	22	1.36 (0.76–2.45)	17	32	2.19 (1.28–3.77)
NIEC	106	37	36	0.96 (0.44–2.11)	47	35	0.60 (0.28–1.29)
PROVA	145	18	18	1.00 (0.43–2.33)	19	25	1.38 (0.63–3.01)
Saggioro et al.	29	75	23	0.13 (0.03–0.57)	25	15	0.57 (0.10–3.35)
Fleig et al.	49	18	14	0.77 (0.17–3.52)	29	29	1.00 (0.29–3.45)
Strauss et al.	37	0	22	9.42 (1.21–72.9)	32	39	1.36 (0.36–5.18)
Planas et al.	46	8	27	3.63 (0.80–16.4)	21	23	1.11 (0.28–4.46)
POR (95% CI)				0.58 (0.47–0.72)[a]			0.76 (0.62–0.94)[a]
β-Blockers compared with non-active treatment							
Pascal et al.	227	27	17	0.57 (0.30–1.06)	36	22	0.49 (0.29–0.88)
Ildeo et al.	79	22	3	0.23 (0.07–0.81)	18	10	0.53 (0.15–1.85)
Lebrec et al.	106	19	13	0.66 (0.23–1.85)	19	19	1.00 (0.38–2.63)
IMPP	174	35	21	0.51 (0.26–0.99)	31	43	1.67 (0.91–3.08)
Adreani et al.	84	32	5	0.16 (0.05–0.49)	44	30	0.56 (0.23–1.35)
Conn et al.	102	22	4	0.21 (0.06–0.66)	22	16	0.68 (0.25–1.84)
PROVA	140	18	18	0.99 (0.42–2.35)	19	10	0.49 (0.20–1.26)
Strauss et al.	36	25	20	0.76 (0.16–3.59)	44	35	0.67 (0.19–2.64)
Colman et al.	48	8	35	4.90 (1.23–19.5)	28	26	0.91 (0.26–3.21)
POR (95% CI)				0.54 (0.39–0.74)			0.75 (0.57–1.06)

[a] Clinically meaningless because of statistically significant heterogeneity.

(Table 6), of which three are in abstract form (Strauss, Hepatol, 1988; 8:1395; Saggioro, DigDisSci, 1986; 31:504S; Fleig, Hepatol, 1988; 7(Suppl.):S128). A total of 1630 patients were included with quite heterogeneous criteria. Ten trials required the presence of large varices as an inclusion criterion; nine included patients with varices of any size. Only in one was a HVPG greater than or equal to 12 mmHg required (Triger, Hepatol, 1991; 13:117). The sclerotherapy technique varied across trials: various sclerosants in different doses were injected intra- or perivariceally or both.

There was a striking heterogeneity of results for the effect of sclerotherapy on both the risk of bleeding and death, with three trials reporting a beneficial and the others no effect or even a harmful effect (Table 6). This heterogeneity is not only qualitative, but refers also to the magnitude of the treatment effect and is statistically significant (Pagliaro, AnnIntMed, 1992; 117:59).

The first study selected patients with large varices with cherry-red spots and/or smaller varices with poor coagulation (Paquet, Endoscopy, 1982; 14:4): 66 per cent of the control group bled versus 6 per cent of the sclerosis group, which showed a significantly increased survival. However, to date, these results have not been reproduced. In unselected cirrhotic populations prophylactic sclerotherapy was of benefit in one study (Witzel, Lancet, 1985; i:773),

but 60 per cent of the control group bled—selection must have occurred but it is not clear how. These studies have been criticized because of the unusually high bleeding rates in the control groups and defects in the randomization process.[17] Another trial showed a significantly favourable effect on mortality, but no reduction in bleeding risk (Potzi, Gut, 1989; 30:873). Two of these three studies did not use EST for acute bleeding episodes in the patients randomized to medical treatment as opposed to those in the sclerotherapy groups (Paquet, Endoscopy, 1982; 14:4; Witzel, Lancet, 1985; i:773). In contrast to these results, the remaining trials failed to support the use of prophylactic sclerotherapy. The largest trial was interrupted because of a significant excess mortality in the sclerotherapy arm that ceased after the termination of treatment (VA Cooperative Variceal Sclerotherapy Group, NEJM, 1991; 324:1779).

Although a meta-analysis of these trials shows a beneficial pooled effect of sclerotherapy both on bleeding and death (Table 6), these pooled estimates are of questionable value because of such an important intertrial heterogeneity. The results of sclerotherapy tended to be favourable in trials with a high bleeding rate in untreated controls and unfavourable in those with low baseline bleeding risk. A positive effect in high-risk patients would be consistent with the efficacy of sclerotherapy for the prevention of rebleeding while the harmful effect in low-risk patients probably results from the fact that the side-effects and complications (which include bleeding and deaths) may exceed the potential advantage. Recently a further study, which also used a HVPG of greater than 16 mmHg as a stratification variable, together with large varices demonstrated a lower bleeding rate (25 versus 76 per cent) and a lower mortality in the group which received sclerotherapy (Paquet, Endoscopy, 1994; 26:734). This trial needs to be repeated using banding.

Thus, the clinical role of prophylactic sclerotherapy remains unsettled. However, *a priori*, sclerotherapy is too invasive to use in asymptomatic patients, considering that bleeding will occur before eradication in a small minority and that iatrogenic bleeding is potentially a problem. Furthermore, compliance in this asymptomatic group is particularly important. Most of these limitations also apply to banding ligation. If bleeding occurs from new varices that have not been injected (or ligated) all prior treatment will have been to no purpose. To assess whether sclerotherapy (or banding ligation) may be beneficial in patients at very high risk of bleeding, a further investigation in comparison with β-blockers (alone or associated with isosorbide 5-mononitrate) would be required.

Randomized controlled trials of β-blockers for prevention of the first upper gastrointestinal haemorrhage

The optimal prophylactic treatment should be easy to administer, have relatively few side-effects and be reasonably effective. Drug therapy best fulfils these criteria.

Nine prophylactic trials of β-blockers in cirrhotics with large varices have now been published, seven studies as full reports (Ideo, Hepatol, 1988; 8:6; Lebrec, JHepatol, 1988, 7:118; Italian Multicenter Project for Propranolol, JHepatol, 1989; 9:75; Pascal, NEJM, 1987; 317:856; Andreani, Hepatol, 1990; 12:1413; Conn, Hepatol, 1991; 14:1016; The PROVA Study Group, Hepatol, 1991; 14:1016) and two in abstract form (Strauss, Hepatol, 1988; 8:1395; Colman, Hepatol, 1990; 12:851). Only two trials were double blind (Conn, Hepatol, 1991; 14:1016; Colman, Hepatol, 1990; 12:851). A total of 996 patients were included mainly on the basis of the presence of large oesophageal varices or any size varices with a portal pressure gradient greater than 10 mmHg (Colman, Hepatol, 1990; 12:851) or greater than or equal to 12 mmHg (Conn, Hepatol, 1991; 14:1016). Propranolol was assessed in seven studies and nadolol in two (Ideo, Hepatol, 1988; 8:6; Lebrec, JHepatol, 1988, 7:118).

The main results of these trials are shown in Table 6. The bleeding risk was reduced by β-blockers in seven studies (Ideo, Hepatol, 1988; 8:6; Lebrec, JHepatol, 1988, 7:118; Italian Multicenter Project for Propranolol, JHepatol, 1989; 9:75; Pascal, NEJM, 1987; 317:856; Andreani, Hepatol, 1990; 12:1413; Conn, Hepatol, 1991; 14:1016; Strauss, Hepatol, 1988; 8:1395), significantly in four (Ideo, Hepatol, 1988; 8:6; Italian Multicenter Project for Propranolol, JHepatol, 1989; 9:75; Andreani, Hepatol, 1990; 12:1413; Conn, Hepatol, 1991; 14:1016) and was unchanged in one (The PROVA Study Group, Hepatol, 1991; 14:1016); only one trial, available as an abstract, reported an increase in risk with propranolol

(Colman, Hepatol, 1990; 12:851). The results of this trial are clearly not comparable with the others and it should be considered an outlier. This study had a small sample size (48 patients) which may have resulted in unbalanced randomization, as suggested by the unusually low bleeding rate among the controls (8 per cent) as opposed to the unusually high rate in treated patients (34 per cent). A recent meta-analysis showed a far more homogeneous and significant therapeutic effect of β-blockers than in the secondary prevention studies and suggested a consistent treatment effect in reducing bleeding.[3] The bleeding risk reduction in β-blocker-treated patients was highly significant either including (POR 0.54 and CI 0.39 to 0.74) or excluding (POR 0.48 and CI 0.35 to 0.66) the outlier trial.

The mortality rate was reduced with β-blockers in seven trials (Ideo, Hepatol, 1988; 8:6; Pascal, NEJM, 1987; 317:856; Andreani, Hepatol, 1990; 12:1413; Conn, Hepatol, 1991; 14:1016; The PROVA Study Group, Hepatol, 1991; 14:1016; Strauss, Hepatol, 1988; 8:1395; Colman, Hepatol, 1990; 12:851), significantly in one (Pascal, NEJM, 1987; 317:856). The pooled estimate showed an important risk reduction approaching statistical significance (POR 0.75 and CI 0.57 to 1.06). The failure to achieve a statistically significant effect on mortality probably reflects a type II error; more patients should have been included to show a treatment effect on mortality. A recent meta-analysis based on individual data from 586 patients included in four RCTs showed that patients given β-blockers had significantly lower rates of bleeding, fatal bleeding, and death from bleeding with a trend towards a reduction in the total mortality (Poynard, NEJM, 1991; 324:1532).

Side-effects of β-blockers were reported in less than 15 per cent of patients and were usually minor (mainly weakness), requiring withdrawal of therapy in less than half of them. No mortality from treatment has been reported. The efficacy of therapy was limited to the time of drug administration; after stopping propranolol therapy bleeding occurred in one trial (Conn, Hepatol, 1991; 14:1016), suggesting that therapy should be maintained for life. An exciting finding of a double-blind study (Conn, Hepatol, 1991; 14:1016) is that in patients whose HVPG dropped to 12 mmHg or below, whether on propranolol or placebo, no bleeding was observed, the size of the varices was significantly reduced, and the survival probability significantly prolonged (Groszmann, Gastro, 1990; 99:1401). This was the first time a haemodynamic index was shown to predict the absence of bleeding and other clinical events in patients with varices. This finding strongly suggests that if the reduction of portal pressure achieved with drug therapy could be potentiated (for instance, by combination therapy associating isosorbide 5-mononitrate to the β-blocker), this will result in a significant improvement of the efficacy of preventive treatment. This is supported by the findings of a recent study showing that the association of nadolol and isosorbide 5-mononitrate was significantly better in preventing the first variceal bleeding than nadolol alone (Merkel, JHepatol, 1995; 23(Suppl.1):69).

Therefore, these trials show that treatment with β-blockers is safe and that it is beneficial in cirrhotic patients with varices who have not previously bled. Since most studies were conducted in patients with moderate or large varices and given the fact that the risk of bleeding is low in patients with small varices, this treatment is not yet recommended for all patients with varices, but just for those with moderate to large varices. However, it is conceivable that β-blockers are also useful in the earlier stages of portal hypertension syndrome. Indeed, there is evidence in experimental studies, that the early treatment with β-blockers significantly reduces the formation of portal–systemic collaterals (Sarin, JCI, 1991; 87:1032; Lin, JHepatol, 1991; 13:213), suggesting that early treatment with β-blockers in compensated cirrhotics without varices may be useful in preventing the formation of varices and decompensation of the disease. This is probably one of the more stimulating areas requiring further investigation.

References

1. Graham DY and Smith JL. The course of patients after variceal haemorrhage. *Gastroenterology*, 1981; 80: 800–9.
2. Smith JL and Graham DY. Variceal haemorrhage, a critical evaluation of survival analysis. *Gastroenterology*, 1982; 82: 968–72.
3. D'Amico G, Pagliaro L, and Bosch J. The treatment of portal hypertension: a meta-analytic review. *Hepatology*, 1995; 22: 332–54.
4. Burroughs AK, Mezzanotte G, Phillips A, McCormick PA, and McIntyre N. Cirrhotics with variceal haemorrhage: the importance of the time interval between admission and the start of analysis for survival and rebleeding rates. *Hepatology*, 1989; 9: 801–7.
5. Bosch J, Navasa M, García-Pagán JC, De Lacy AM, and Rodés J. Portal hypertension. *Medical Clinics of North America*, 1989; 73: 931–53.
6. McCormick PA, Jenkins SA, McIntyre N, and Burroughs AK. Why portal hypertensive varices bleed and bleed: a hypothesis. *Gut*, 1995; 36: 100–3.
7. Panés J, Terés J, Bosch J, and Rodés J. Efficacy of balloon tamponade in treatment of bleeding gastric and esophageal varices. Results in 151 consecutive episodes. *Digestive Diseases and Sciences*, 1988; 33: 454–9.
8. Hussey KP. Vasopressin therapy for upper gastrointestinal tract haemorrhage. Has its efficacy been proven? *Archives of Internal Medicine*, 1985; 145: 1263–7.
9. Rigau J, Bosch J, Bordas JM, *et al.* Endoscopic measurement of variceal pressure in cirrhosis: correlation with portal pressure and variceal haemorrhage. *Gastroenterology*, 1989; 96: 873–80.
10. Desaint. In Lebrec D and Blei AT, eds. *Vasopressin analogs in portal hypertension*. 1987: 157.
11. Colin. In Lebrec D and Blei AT, eds. *Vasopressin analogs in portal hypertension*. 1987: 149.
12. Bosch J, D'Amico G, Luca A, García-Pagán JC, Feu F, and Escorsell A. *Drug therapy for variceal haemorrhage. Portal hypertension: pathophysiology and treatment*. Oxford: Blackwell Scientific Publications, 1994: 108–23.
13. Burroughs AK. Sclerotherapy of varices. In Rodés J and Arroyo V, eds. *Therapy in liver diseases*. Barcelona: Ediciones Doyma, 1992: 114–27.
14. Laine L and Cook D. Endoscopic ligation compared with sclerotherapy for treatment of esophageal variceal bleeding. A meta-analysis. *Annals of Internal Medicine*, 1995; 123: 280–7.
15. Polio J and Groszmann RJ. Haemodynamic factors involved in the development and rupture of esophageal varices: a pathophysiological approach to treatment. *Seminars in Liver Disease*, 1986; 6: 318–31.
16. Burroughs AK, D'Heygere F, and McIntyre N. Pitfalls in studies of prophylactic therapy for variceal bleeding in cirrhosis. *Hepatology*, 1986; 6: 1407–13.
17. Fleig. In Burroughs AK, ed. *Methodology and reviews of clinical trials in portal hypertension*, 1987: 291.

8

Ascites and renal dysfunction in hepatic cirrhosis

8.1 Pathogenesis, diagnosis, and treatment of ascites in cirrhosis

Vicente Arroyo, Pere Ginès, Ramón Planas, and Juan Rodés

Introduction

The aim of this chapter is to review the pathogenesis, diagnosis, and treatment of ascites in cirrhosis. The reader should see Chapter 8.2 dealing with renal dysfunction in cirrhosis for a better understanding of the current chapter. Since the publication of the first edition of the *Oxford textbook of clinical hepatology,* there have been few advances concerning the pathogenesis and diagnosis of ascites in cirrhosis. However, major changes have occurred in the management of ascites. Therapeutic paracentesis has been a topic of major interest during recent years and numerous trials have assessed different aspects of this procedure. Additionally, several studies have shown that the transjugular intrahepatic portacaval shunt may be useful in the management of patients with ascites refractory to diuretics. The introduction of aquaretic agents, which are extremely effective in normalizing renal water metabolism in experimental cirrhosis, may be important for the management of patients with spontaneous or diuretic-induced dilutional hyponatraemia. Finally, there have also been important studies on the treatment of hepatorenal syndrome.

Ascites: historical hallmarks

The accumulation of fluid within the peritoneal cavity is such an outstanding phenomenon that it has interested physicians throughout history. The link between ascites and liver disease had already been recognized by Erasitratus of Cappadocia around 300 BC (Daunson, Gastro, 1980: 39:790). However, it was not until 1671 that ascites was first related experimentally to portal hypertension; Richard Lower (1631–1691) produced ascites in a dog by ligating the inferior vena cava just below the diaphragm.[1,2] Heidenhain and Starling were the first investigators to assess the effect of portal hypertension on thoracic-duct lymph flow.[3-5] They demonstrated that obstruction of the suprahepatic inferior vena cava or of the portal vein were followed by increased lymph flow through the thoracic duct. The characteristics of the thoracic lymph depended on the site of obstruction, being more concentrated when the inferior vena cava was obliterated. In 1931, Bolton and Barnard (JPatholBacteriol, 1931; 34:701) first produced evidence implicating increased lymph production by the liver in the formation of ascites. They suggested that with a blocked hepatic outflow, ascites occurs if the efferent liver lymphatics cannot remove the increased amount of lymph produced by the liver.

As early as the first century AD, Celsus, discussing dropsy in his book *De medicina*, recognized the importance of renal function in the pathogenesis of ascites.[6] He recommended that the amount of liquid taken and of urine excreted should be measured in patients with dropsy 'for if more fluid is excreted than is taken, so at length there is hope of good health'. The relation between the formation of ascites and the reduction of urine volume, however, was not clearly established until the middle of the nineteenth century. Fr Th. von Frerichs reported the development of oliguria in his patients with ascites and proposed a hypothesis that is similar to our current theories on the pathogenesis of renal dysfunction in cirrhosis: 'the more blood that is accumulated in the portal vein, the less blood is felt within the arterial system, the latter significantly influencing urinary secretion'. In 1863, Austin Flint (AmJMedSci, 1863; 45:306) first showed that renal histology is normal in patients with cirrhosis, ascites and oliguria, thus demonstrating the functional nature of this abnormality. The first renal functional abnormality identified in cirrhosis with ascites was the reduced ability to excrete free water (Aldersberg, AnnIntMed, 1943; 19:642). The role of sodium retention in the pathogenesis of ascites was not known until the middle of the twentieth century (Farnsworth, JLabClinMed; 1948; 33:1545; Eisenmenger, JLabClinMed, 1949; 34:1029). Finally, hepatorenal syndrome was first recognized by Hecker and Sherlock in 1956 (Hecker, Lancet, 1956; ii:1221).

Circulatory abnormalities in patients with cirrhosis and ascites were identified at the same time as the impairment in renal function. Parera *et al.* reported in 1946 that plasma volume is increased in these patients (AnnIntMed, 1946; 24:643). On the other hand, in 1953 Kowalsky and Abelmann (JCI, 1953; 32:550; 1025) described that cardiac output was increased and systemic vascular resistance reduced in patients with decompensated cirrhosis. In the middle of the 1960s, several studies reported increased plasma renin and noradrenaline in patients with cirrhosis and ascites (Genost, Hypertension, 1965; 13:97; Joly, Lancet, 1967; ii: 121), thus demonstrating an increase in the activity of endogenous vasoconstrictor systems. Finally, in the 1970s, Cohn *et al.* and Groszmann *et al.* presented indirect evidence for the existence of splanchnic arteriolar vasodilation in patients with cirrhosis.[7,8]

Therapeutic paracentesis was the leading treatment of ascites from the time of Hippocrates until the middle of the twentieth century. The first detailed description of this procedure was made by Aulus Cornelius Celso (30 BC–AD 50) in his work 'The Eight

Books of Medicine', a compendium of the teachings of Hippocrates, other Hellenistic physicians, and the School of Alexandria.[9] In the seventeenth century, Sanctorius Sanctorio from the University of Padova designed the first trochar for paracentesis.[10] Finally, in the 1950s, Nelson *et al.* were the first to show that therapeutic paracentesis may induce abnormalities in the systemic circulation (JCI, 1951; 30:738). The decline of therapeutic paracentesis started at the beginning of the 1960s with the introduction of spironolactone and the loop diuretics.[11,12] In 1972, LeVeen *et al.* introduced peritoneovenous shunting for the management of refractory ascites (AnnSurg, 1974; 180:580). Finally, in 1985, Quintero *et al.* published a randomized controlled study on cirrhotic patients admitted to various hospitals in the area of Barcelona with tense ascites, demonstrating that paracentesis together with intravenous albumin is more effective than the standard diuretic therapy, is associated with a lower incidence of complications (renal impairment and hepatic encephalopathy), and considerably reduces the duration of the hospital stay and, therefore, the cost of treatment.[13] Subsequent investigations confirming their findings have led to the reintroduction of therapeutic paracentesis as one of the treatments of choice of tense ascites in cirrhosis.

Aetiology and diagnosis of ascites
Causes

Many diseases are known to lead to the formation of free fluid within the peritoneal cavity (Table 1). Basically, the causes of ascites may be grouped into those conditions in which the pathological process does not directly affect the peritoneum and those in which the peritoneum itself is involved. The first group includes diseases associated with sinusoidal portal hypertension (cirrhosis, acute alcoholic hepatitis, fulminant or subacute viral or toxic hepatitis, congestive heart failure, constrictive pericarditis, inferior vena caval obstruction, Budd–Chiari syndrome, and hepatic veno-occlusive disease), hypoalbuminaemia (nephrotic syndrome, protein-losing enteropathy, and malnutrition), and a variety of disorders that may cause ascites through different mechanisms, such as myxoedema, ovarian diseases (carcinoma, benign tumours, ovarian hyperstimulation syndrome), chronic pancreatitis, biliary-tract leakage (secondary to liver trauma, biliary-tract surgery, or transhepatic cholangiography), diseases affecting the lymphatic system of the splanchnic area, and chronic renal failure. In the second group, ascites is formed as a consequence of primary peritoneal disease or as a result of peritoneal involvement in systemic processes; tuberculous, fungal (*Candida albicans, Coccidioides immitis*), parasitic and granulomatous peritonitis (sarcoidosis, Crohn's disease, peritoneal granulomatous reaction to talc, cotton and wood fibres, starch, and barium), primary or metastatic peritoneal tumours, vasculitis (systemic lupus erythematosus, Henoch–Shönlein purpura), eosinophilic gastroenteritis, and Whipple's disease are the most characteristic causes of ascites in this group. By far the most frequent cause of ascites in Europe and in North America is hepatic cirrhosis, followed by neoplasms, and to a lesser extent, congestive heart failure and tuberculous peritonitis. These four conditions account for more than 90 per cent of the ascites in these areas (Tavel, JAMA, 1959; 237:727; Berner, ArchIntMed, 1964; 113:687).

Detection

The diagnosis of ascites is simple when large amounts of fluid accumulate in the peritoneal cavity. On physical examination the abdomen is distended, the flanks bulge, and a fluid wave may be demonstrable. Other characteristic signs of ascites, such as flank and shifting dullness, are also obvious. The diagnosis is much more difficult by physical examination when there is a small volume of ascitic fluid. It has been suggested that minimal amounts of ascites (less than 500 ml) can be detected by an exploratory manoeuvre that combines percussion and auscultation of the abdomen (Lawson, NEJM, 1959; 260:652). After 5 min in the prone position, the patient is asked to assume a position on hands and knees so that the middle portion of the abdomen is dependent. One flank is percussed by repeated, light flicking at a constant intensity, with the stethoscope being over the most dependent portion of the abdomen (the area of the ascitic 'puddle'). The stethoscope is then gradually moved toward the flank opposite the percussion site. A positive sign indicating the presence of ascites consists of a marked change in the intensity and character of the percussion note as the stethoscope is moved from the ascitic puddle to the flank opposite the point of percussion, where ascites is not present. A point of demarcation between the ascitic puddle and the area without intraperitoneal fluid can be obtained, correlating with the amount of ascitic fluid present. Nevertheless, in a recent prospective study in which five physical signs (bulging flanks, flank dullness, shifting dullness, fluid wave, and puddle sign) were compared with the ultrasonographic demonstration of ascites (which can detect as little as 100 to 200 ml of intraperitoneal fluid) in patients in whom the bedside diagnosis of ascites was in question, the puddle sign did not show greater specificity and sensitivity for the detection of intra-abdominal fluid than the other signs of ascites (Cattau, JAMA, 1982; 247:1164).

Peripheral oedema (oedema in the lower extremities) is common in patients with cirrhosis. In many cases it precedes the development of ascites by weeks or months, but it may also appear simultaneously with, or following, the accumulation of fluid within the abdomen. Massive peripheral oedema without ascites is occasionally seen in cirrhotic patients with severe hepatic insufficiency and a surgical portacaval shunt. Peripheral oedema in cirrhosis decreases or disappears with nocturnal rest and increases with ambulation. It is postulated that hypoalbuminaemia and increased venous pressure in the lower extremities due to constriction of the intrahepatic segment of the inferior vena cava or to the high intra-abdominal pressure caused by the presence of ascites are the main factors for peripheral oedema in cirrhosis.

Ultrasonography, computed tomography, and magnetic resonance imaging are very useful in the assessment of patients with ascites (Golberg, Radiol, 1970; 96:15; Golberg, ArchIntMed, 1973; 131:217; Huning, BrJRadiol, 1973; 46:325; Proto, AmJRoent, 1976; 126:974; Yeh, Radiol, 1977; 124:783; Jolles, AmJRoent, 1980; 135: 315; Cohen, Radiol, 1985; 155:705; Wall, JComputAssistTomogr, 1986; 10:746; Malde, JPostgradMed, 1993; 39:132; Branney, JTrauma, 1995; 39:375). In addition to their sensitivity in detecting minimal amounts of ascites they may suggest its cause, based on the characteristics of the intra-abdominal organs and vessels and the appearance of the intra-abdominal fluid. Ultrasonography is the best of these methods since it is not expensive, is as reliable as

Table 1 Causes of ascites

Ascites not associated with peritoneal disease
Intrahepatic sinusoidal portal hypertension:
    Cirrhosis
    Acute alcoholic hepatitis
    Fulminant hepatitis (toxic or viral)
    Subacute hepatitis (toxic or viral)
    Hepatic veno-occlusive disease
    Massive liver metastasis
Extrahepatic sinusoidal portal hypertension:
    Congestive heart failure
    Constrictive pericarditis
    Inferior vena cava obstruction
    Hepatic vein obstruction (Budd–Chiari syndrome)
Hypoalbuminaemia:
    Nephrotic syndrome
    Protein-losing enteropathy
    Malnutrition
Miscellaneous disorders:
    Myxoedema
    Ovarian disease:
      carcinoma
      benign tumours
      ovarian hyperstimulation syndrome
    Pancreatic ascites
    Bile ascites
    Chylous ascites
    Nephrogenic ascites
    Acquired immune deficiency syndrome

Ascites due to primary peritoneal disease
Malignant ascites:
    Primary peritoneal mesothelioma
    Secondary peritoneal carcinomatosis
Granulomatous peritonitis:
    Tuberculous peritonitis
    Chlamydia trachomatis peritonitis
    Fungal and parasitic peritonitis (*Candida albicans, Histoplasma capsulatum, Coccidioides immitis, Cryptococcus neoformans,*
      Schistosoma mansoni, Strongyloides stercoralis, Entamoeba histolytica)
    Sarcoidosis
    Starch granulomatous peritonitis
    Barium peritonitis
    Vasculitis (systemic lupus erythematosus, Henoch–Schönlein purpura)
Miscellaneous peritoneal disease:
    Eosinophilic gastroenteritis
    Whipple's disease
    Endometriosis

computed tomography, and is free of radiation hazards. Intraperitoneal fluid due to portal hypertension appears as homogeneous, echo-free areas surrounding and interposed between the loops of bowel and viscera in a relatively uniform manner. When the amount of ascites is small, the fluid tends to collect in the flanks and the superior right paracolic gutter, around the liver, and in the lowest peritoneal reflection in the pelvis. Rectal and transvaginal echography are particularly sensitive in the detection of small volumes of intra-abdominal fluid, the transvaginal approach being able to detect less than 50 ml of ascitic fluid (Steinkampf, JReprodMed 1991; 36:729; Gerdes, Chirurgie, 1994; 65:709). Atypical sonographic characteristics, such as the presence of multiple fine echoes (indicating the presence of debris) or septations and fibrous strands within the ascitic fluid, may be seen in exudative ascites. Matted loops of bowel, plastering of the liver to surrounding structures, and loculation of fluid, when present, are very suggestive of malignant ascites (Edell, AmJRoent, 1979; 133:111). Peritoneal

thickening, lymphadenopathy, and bowel thickening in the ileo-caecal junction are suggestive of a tuberculous aetiology (Kedar, ClinRadiol, 1994; 49:24).

Characteristics of cirrhotic ascites

The biochemical and cytological analysis of ascitic fluid provides important information for the differential diagnosis. The ascitic fluid in cirrhotics is transparent and yellow/amber in colour. Traditionally, ascites in these patients is considered to have the characteristics of a transudate, with a total protein concentration of less than 2.5 g/dl and with relatively few cells. However, recent studies show that cirrhotics with ascites do not constitute a homogeneous population with respect to the characteristics of the ascitic fluid. Total ascitic protein concentration ranges between 0.5 and more than 6 g/dl (Runyon, AnnIntMed, 1992; 117:215) and is greater than 3 g/dl ('exudative ascites') in up to 30 per cent of patients with otherwise uncomplicated cirrhosis.[14-18] The proportions of albumin and globulins in the total protein concentration are approximately 45 and 55 per cent, respectively.[14,16] There is a close, direct correlation between ascitic albumin and globulin concentrations, indicating that proteins of ascitic fluid in cirrhosis come from capillaries with relatively large pores, probably the hepatic sinusoids (García-Diaz, EurJGastroHepatol, 1995; 7: 963).[16,19] This contention is also supported by the observation of a similar ascites:plasma ratio for albumin and globulins (approximately 0.3 for both types of proteins).[14,16,19] However, although ascitic proteins may come mainly from the extremely permeable hepatic sinusoids, the relative contribution of the hepatic microvasculature and the splanchnic capillaries to the formation of ascites may vary markedly from patient to patient, since the ascitic fluid:plasma ratios for total proteins, albumin, and globulins range between 0.04 and 1.03 in patients with cirrhosis and ascites (Tarao, Gut, 1979; 20:205; Henriksen, ScaJCLI, 1980; 40:493).[14,16,19, 20] The total protein, albumin, and globulin concentrations in ascitic fluid in cirrhosis correlate directly with the corresponding plasma concentrations and inversely with portal pressure.[16] The mobilization of ascites with diuretics increases the concentration of proteins in the ascitic fluid (Hoefs, AmJGastr, 1981; 76:423; Runyon, Hepatol, 1986; 6:396; JHepatol 1992; 14:249). The total protein concentration in ascitic fluid in cirrhosis is an important predictive factor for spontaneous bacterial peritonitis. This syndrome, which consists of the spontaneous infection of ascitic fluid with no apparent intra-abdominal source, is thought to be due to the passage of Gram-negative bacilli from the intestinal lumen to the general circulation and to the ascitic fluid.[16] Spontaneous bacterial peritonitis usually occurs in cirrhotics with a low total protein concentration in ascitic fluid (<1 g/dl), whereas it is infrequent in cirrhotics with higher protein concentrations in ascitic fluid and in patients with cardiac or malignant ascites, who generally have a protein concentration over this limit (Kurtz, AmJGastr, 1982; 77:146; Runyon, AmJGastr, 1984; 79:796; Gastro, 1986; 91: 1343; Tító, Hepatol, 1988; 8:27; Llach, Hepatol, 1992; 16:724; Andreu, Gastro, 1993; 104:1133).[21] The ascitic fluid has opsonic and bactericidal activity, which seems to be mediated by complement and fibronectin (Fromkes, Gastro, 1977; 73:668; Simberkoff, JLabClinMed, 1978; 91:831; Michel, SGO, 1980; 151:55; Akalin, JInfDis, 1983; 147:1011).The total protein concentration in ascitic fluid correlates with the concentration of these proteins with antibacterial activity; the predictive value of the total protein concentration in ascitic fluid for the development of spontaneous bacterial peritonitis is probably a consequence of this relation (Runyon, Hepatol, 1985; 5:634; Such, JHepatol, 1988; 6:80). The ascitic fluid of cirrhotics contains immune complexes that consume complement and may contribute to reducing its antibacterial activity (Quismorio, IntArchAllApplImmunol, 1981; 64:190).

The ascitic fluid in the cirrhotic without spontaneous bacterial peritonitis usually has fewer than 300 to 500 white blood cells per mm^3; nevertheless 10 to 15 per cent may have more than 500 cells and 5 per cent more than 1000 cells (Paddok, NEJM, 1940; 223: 1010; Kline, Gastro, 1976; 70:408).[14,15,17,22] More than 70 per cent of these white cells are mononuclear leucocytes. In contrast, in cirrhotic patients with spontaneous bacterial peritonitis the ascitic fluid usually contains more than 500 white blood cells per mm^3 (frequently more than 2000), with more than 70 per cent of

them being polymorphonuclear leucocytes.[21,22] Nevertheless, there is an overlap between the two groups, particularly in cirrhotic patients with superimposed hepatocellular carcinoma (Colli, Cancer, 1993; 72:677; Wang, JHepatol, 1994; 20:79). The pH and the concentration of lactate in ascitic fluid in otherwise uncomplicated cirrhosis is similar to that in plasma (Brook, DigDisSci, 1981; 26: 1089; Gitlin, Hepatol, 1982; 2:408). Patients with spontaneous bacterial peritonitis have a significantly lower pH and higher lactate concentration in ascitic fluid than in plasma. Based on these findings, the ascitic-fluid pH, lactate concentration, and plasma–ascitic-fluid pH and lactate gradients have been proposed as rapid, sensitive markers of spontaneous bacterial peritonitis. However, they do not improve the results obtained with the absolute white-cell count and the polymorphonuclear count in ascitic fluid (García-Tsao, Hepatol, 1985; 5:91; Scemama-Clergue, Gut, 1985; 26:332; Yang, Hepatol, 1985; 5:85; Attali, Gastro, 1986; 90:1255; Pinzello, Hepatol, 1986; 6:244; Stassen, Gastro, 1986; 90:1247). The pH of the ascitic fluid had a high prognostic value in cirrhotics with spontaneous bacterial peritonitis (Navasa, GastroHepato, 1985; 8: 455). As with the total protein concentration, the absolute concentration of white cells in ascitic fluid increases during diuretic treatment while the concentration of polymorphs remains unchanged (Hoefs, Hepatol, 1981; 1:249). Therefore the percentage of polymorphs over the total leucocyte content of the ascitic fluid actually decreases during the mobilization of ascites with diuretics. The concentration of red blood cells in cirrhotic ascites is usually lower than 1000 cells per mm^3, although higher concentrations may occasionally be detected. In fact, bloody ascitic fluid, which indicates more than 50 000 red cells per mm^3 (haematocrit of about 0.5 per cent), occurs in approximately 2 per cent of cirrhotics (Mandel, Gastro, 1954; 27:231; Natelson, AmJGastr, 1969; 52: 523).[17] In one-third of these patients, bloody ascites is secondary to a superimposed hepatocellular carcinoma bleeding into the peritoneal cavity (Desitter, AmJGastr, 1984; 79:136). However, in as many as 50 per cent of patients no apparent cause for bloody ascites can be detected. The hepatic and the thoracic lymph of cirrhotics is often bloody also (Dumont, NEJM, 1960; 263:471; Denny, ArchSurg, 1966; 92:657). The mechanism of bloody ascites in cirrhotics without hepatocellular carcinoma could, therefore, be related to the leakage of bloody lymph from the liver lymphatics.

Alterations in the coagulation-related proteins in ascites have recently been reported in cirrhotic patients. The concentration of fibrinogen and plasminogen in ascitic fluid is lower than that expected from their molecular weights (Henderson, AnnSurg, 1980; 192:738), whereas the concentrations of plasminogen activators and fibrin/fibrinogen degradation products are higher than in plasma (Baele, AmJGastr, 1986; 81:440; Scott-Coombes, Gut, 1993; 34: 1120; Toschi, BiomedPharmacoth, 1993; 47:345; Buo; ScaJGastr, 1995; 30:1101). This suggests that fibrinolysis is occurring within the peritoneal cavity. In addition, there is apparently intraperitoneal coagulation in cirrhotic patients since the concentration of fibrin monomers in ascitic fluid is almost 10 times higher than in plasma (Hoefs, DigDisSci, 1981; 26:518). Therefore the alterations in the coagulation-related proteins in cirrhotic ascites are probably the consequence of a complex coagulation disturbance within the ascitic fluid resulting in intraperitoneal coagulation and primary and secondary fibrinolysis. The infusion of ascitic fluid into the general circulation, either directly or by the insertion of a peritoneovenous shunt, is often associated with disseminated intravascular coagulation, as manifested by a marked reduction in platelet count, prothrombin time, and fibrinogen concentration, and an increase in the plasma concentrations of fibrin degradation products, thus confirming the procoagulant activity of ascitic fluid (Wilkinson, PostgradMedJ, 1975; 51:583; Salem, AmJHemat, 1981; 11:153; Gut, 1983; 24:412; Stein, ArchIntMed, 1981; 141:1149; Tawes, AmJSurg 1981; 142:51; Ragni, AnnSurg, 1983; 198:91; LeVeen, AnnSurg, 1987; 205:305). This coagulopathy is clinically significant in 20 to 50 per cent of patients treated with a peritoneovenous shunt and sometimes requires ligation of the prosthesis (Ansley, Surgery, 1978; 83:181; Harmon, AnnIntMed, 1979; 90:774; Gibson, AustNZJMed, 1981; 11:8). Several substances present in the ascites, such as tissue thromboplastin, endotoxin, collagen, activated clotting factors, and fibrin degradation products, have been implicated in the procoagulant activity of the ascitic fluid.

Cirrhotic patients with ascites have a very high concentration of interleukin 6 in ascitic fluid. The ascitic fluid:plasma concentration ratio of interleukin 6 is approximately 100 in these patients, indicating intra-abdominal production of this cytokine (Andus, JHepatol, 1992; 15:378; Zeni, ClinInfDis, 1993; 17:218; Bac, Liver, 1995; 15:265). The concentration of tumour necrosis factor is also higher in ascitic fluid than in plasma in cirrhotic patients, although the differences are much less impressive than with interleukin 6 (Zeni, ClinInfDis, 1993; 17:218). Significant concentrations of soluble tumour necrosis-factor receptors have also been detected in the ascitic fluid of cirrhotic patients with and without spontaneous bacterial peritonitis, the significance of which is still unknown (Andus, Hepatol, 1992; 16:749). Activated peritoneal macrophages could be the origin of the intra-abdominal production of cytokines. Spontaneous bacterial peritonitis is associated with a marked increase of cytokines in the ascitic fluid (Propst, EurJClinInv, 1993; 23:832; Le Moine, JHepatol, 1994; 20:819). Intra-abdominal cytokines escape into the systemic circulation and may explain some of the complications observed in patients with spontaneous bacterial peritonitis, particularly the impairment in circulatory and renal function (Navasa, JHepatol, 1994; 21:S48).

The biochemical and cytological characteristics of ascitic fluid in other diseases causing intrahepatic sinusoidal portal hypertension, such as acute alcoholic hepatitis, fulminant or subacute viral or toxic hepatitis, and massive metastatic infiltration of the liver, are similar to those found in cirrhotic ascites.

Differential diagnosis of cirrhotic ascites

Malignant ascites

The macroscopic appearance of malignant ascites is generally similar to that of cirrhotic ascites (less than 10 per cent of malignant ascites are macroscopically bloody).[23] Thus the differential diagnosis must be based on exploratory findings and laboratory tests. Measurement of the total protein concentration of the ascitic fluid (generally over 3.0 g/dl in malignant ascites) and its cytological examination for malignant cells, which were the laboratory tests first used to differentiate malignant ascites from that secondary to portal hypertension, are still the most common methods used (Foot, AmJPathol, 1956; 32:961; Rovelstad, Gastro, 1958; 34:436; Gastro,

1959; 37:339; Ceelen, ActaCytol, 1964; 8:175; Cardozo, ActaCytol, 1966; 10:455; Johnson, ActaCytol, 1966; 10:161; Foot, AnnNY-AcadSci, 1967; 63:1324; Benedict, ActaCytol, 1972; 16:304; Krivinkova, ActaPMIScand, 1976; 84:455; Malden, QJMed, 1986; 58:221).[18,23]

Standard cytological examination is 60 to 90 per cent accurate in the diagnosis of malignant ascites, especially when adequate volumes of fluid (at least several hundred millilitres) and concentration techniques are used (García, ModPathol, 1994; 7:665). False-positive results are rare in skilled hands. The greatest source of confusion is the differentiation of malignant cells from atypical mesothelial cells. The use of immunocytochemical techniques with monoclonal or polyclonal antibodies against numerous tumour markers (oestrogen and progesterone receptors, cancer antigen 125, carbohydrate antigen 19–9, carcinoembryonic antigen, epithelial membrane antigen, human erythrocyte antigen, CD15, CD45, CD11c, epithelial glycoprotein 34, BW-495; tumour-associated antigen 72, epithelium-specific tumour-associated monoclonal antibody (Moab), cytokeratin, vimentin, lysozyme, and 83D4 antigen) are useful in differentiating malignant from non-malignant ascites in these cases (Lacassagne, ActaCytol, 1991; 35:315; Shinozuka, Nippon-SankaFujinkaGakkaiZass, 1991; 43:1355; Skov, VirchArchA 1991; 419:59; Daste, ArchAnatCytolPath, 1992; 40:183; Kocjan, JClin-Path, 1992; 45:358; Masood, DiagCytopathol, 1992; 8:161; Mezger, ActaCytol, 1992; 36:75; Mottolese, DiagCytopathol, 1992; 8:153; Berena, JClinLabAnal, 1993; 7:19; Athanassiadou, ActaCytol, 1994; 38:718; Shield, DiagCytopathol, 1994; 11:237; Ascoli, Diag-Cytopathol, 1995; 12:303; Beuzelin-Yvraut, JClinPath, 1995; 48:433; Nomoto, JSurgOncol, 1995; 60:30). These techniques may also help to differentiate primary (mesothelioma) from metastatic peritoneal malignancy (Betta, Pathologica, 1991; 83:99; Delahaye, JPath, 1991; 165:137; Donna, DiagCytopathol, 1992; 8:361; Maguire, DiagCytopathol, 1994; 10:130). False-negative results on standard cytological examinations are the rule when ascites is due to portal hypertension secondary to massive liver metastases with little peritoneal involvement.[23] In this type of ascites the total ascitic protein concentration is usually lower than 2.5 g/dl. The differential diagnosis between cirrhotic ascites and the ascites secondary to massive liver metastases, however, can easily be achieved by ultrasonography, computed tomography or liver scan. DNA analysis by flow cytometry or image analysis, and the detection of oncogene (c-Ha-*ras*) expression, are sophisticated techniques that have been explored in the differential diagnosis of effusion samples, but they do not improve the results obtained with conventional cytological examination (Rijken, AmJClinPath, 1991; 95:2; Pinto, AnalQuantCytolHistol, 1992; 14:222; Athanassiades, CancerDetectPrev, 1993; 17:585; Granados, ActaCytol, 1994; 38:711; Kehoe, BrJObsGyn, 1995; 102:656).

The serum–ascitic-fluid gradient for albumin improves the diagnostic accuracy of the total protein concentration in ascitic fluid (Pare, Gastro, 1983; 85:240; Lee, Cancer, 1992; 70:2057; Runyon, AnnIntMed, 1992; 117:215) (Fig. 1).[18,23,24] The concentration of lactic dehydrogenase in malignant ascites is higher than the corresponding values in plasma due to leakage of the enzyme from the malignant cells lining the peritoneum, whereas the reverse is the rule for cirrhotic ascites (Wroblensky, AnnIntMed, 1958; 48:813; Fleisher, Gastro, 1959; 37:325; Kirkeby, ScaJCLI, 1959; 11:

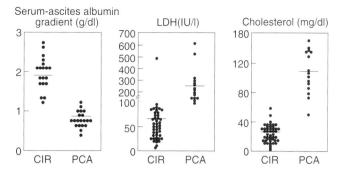

Fig. 1. Serum–ascites albumin gradient and ascitic-fluid concentration of lactic dehydrogenase and cholesterol in patients with cirrhosis (CIR) and peritoneal carcinomatosis (PCA).

185; De-Torregrosa, AmJMedSci, 1959; 238:552; Asada, AmJDig-Dis, 1962; 7:1001; Boyer, ArchIntMed, 1978; 138:1103).[25-28] The concentration of lactic dehydrogenase in ascitic fluid and its ascitic fluid–plasma ratio are, therefore, useful for differentiating malignant from cirrhotic ascites, although they do not improve the results obtained with the ascitic fluid–plasma albumin gradient (Greene, AmJGastr, 1978; 70:448) (Fig. 1).[23,25] Other measurements in ascitic fluid that have proved to be of value in differentiating malignant from cirrhotic ascites include total lipids (Rovelstad, Gastro, 1958; 34:436; Siddiqui, JGastHepatol, 1992; 7:161), free fatty acids (Greco, CCActa, 1995; 239:13), cholesterol (Jungst, JHepatol, 1992; 14:224; Guptal, JGastHepatol, 1995; 10:295),[23,24,26-28] fibronectin (Runyon, JHepatol, 1986; 3:219; Mortensen, ScaJGastr, 1988; 23:1085; Adamsen, EurJSurg, 1991; 157:325),[23,24,26-28] carcinoembryonic antigen and other tumour-associated antigens (CA-125, 83D4 soluble antigen, carbohydrate antigen 19–9, tissue polypeptide antigen) (Nystrom, ArchIntMed, 1977; 137:875; Lowenstein, AnnIntMed, 1978; 88:635; Couch, Cancer, 1981; 48:2475; Martinez-Vea, Cancer, 1982; 50:1783; Bergmann, Cancer, 1987; 59:213; Coenen, FortschrMed, 1991; 109:280; Daoud, ClinChem, 1991; 37:1968; Osinaga, Cancer, 1992; 69:1745; Chen, JGastHepatol, 1994; 9:396),[28] urokinase, tissue plasminogen activator, plasminogen activator inhibitor and fibrin/fibrinogen degradation products (Scholmerich, Gastro, 1984; 87:1160; Scoot-Coombes, Gut, 1993; 34:1120; Buo, ScaJGastr, 1995; 30:1101), and human chorionic gonadotropin-β (Gerbes, Digestion, 1996; 57:113). Of these last, the cholesterol concentration of ascitic fluid, which is higher in most malignant ascites than in cirrhotic ascites owing to higher permeability to lipoproteins (Jungst, JHepatol, 1992; 1992; 14:244) (Fig. 1), seems to be the most interesting because of its simplicity and cost-effectiveness.[24, 27] Laparoscopy and direct biopsy of the peritoneal metastases is a useful approach to confirm the diagnosis of malignant ascites in those cases with negative cytology (Chu, GastrEnd, 1994; 40:285).

Chylous ascites

Chylous ascites is an infrequent feature in patients with cirrhosis (Nix, AmJGastr, 1957; 28:40; Kelly, Gastro, 1960; 39:161; Vasko, ArchSurg, 1967; 95:355; Tsuchiya, Angiol, 1973; 24:576). In some cases it develops in the postoperative period after splenorenal shunt,

but in most instances it appears spontaneously (Rector, Gastro, 1984; 6:369). Chylous ascites is macroscopically turbid and white ('milky' ascites), and separates into layers on standing. These characteristics are due to a high concentration of chylomicrons very rich in triglycerides. The diagnosis of chylous ascites is based on triglyceride concentration in ascitic fluid, which is usually over 110 mg/dl and always higher than the corresponding value in plasma (Lesser, ArchIntMed, 1970; 125:1073).[29] The concentration of cholesterol and phospholipids in ascitic fluid is, however, similar to that of non-chylous ascites. Gross milkiness of chylous ascites correlates poorly with absolute triglyceride concentrations because turbidity also reflects the size of the chylomicrons.[29] In fact, a study on pleural effusions indicates that the macroscopic characteristics (chylous, bloody, turbid, or serous) may fail to detect chylous effusions (triglyceride concentration over 110 mg/dl) in almost one-third of the cases (Staats, MayoClinProc, 1980; 55:700). The proportion of lipids in chylous ascites is very similar to that of intestinal and human thoracic-duct lymph after the ingestion of a fat meal.[30] As patients with cirrhosis usually have elevated pressure within the splanchnic lymph vessels, it has been suggested that spontaneous chylous ascites in these patients may be a consequence of the rupture of these lymph vessels leading to the leakage of whole intestinal lymph into the peritoneal cavity.[30] Chylous ascites after splenorenal shunt is probably secondary to injury to retroperitoneal lymphatics (Maywood, AmJSurg, 1978; 135:700; Warren, AmJSurg, 1978; 135:607). In fact, chylous ascites is a well-recognized postoperative complication in patients submitted to renal transplantation, aortic aneurysmectomy, retroperitoneal lymph adenectomy, and pancreatoduodenectomy (Nixt, AmJGastr, 1957; 28:40; Vasko, ArchSurg, 1967; 95:355).[29] Hepatic cirrhosis is a relatively infrequent cause of chylous ascites. Primary abnormalities of the lymphatics (lymphangiectasia) and the obstruction of the lymphatic system due to malignancies, especially lymphomas, are by far the most common causes in adults (Kelly, Gastro, 1960; 39:161; Vasko, ArchSurg, 1967; 95:355; Browse, BrJSurg, 1992; 79:1145).[29] Other diseases associated with chylous ascites in adults include portal-vein thrombosis, sarcoidosis, nephrotic syndrome, tuberculosis, pancreatitis, abdominal trauma, constrictive pericarditis, encapsulating peritonitis, and pulmonary fibrosis with thoracic-duct obstruction. Congenital malformations of the lymphatic system, including stenosis or atresia of the lymphatics and lymphatic mesenteric cysts, are the main causes of chylous ascites in children. Chylous ascites should be differentiated from pseudochylous ascites in which, although the macroscopic appearance may be identical, the triglyceride concentration is lower than 110 mg/dl.

Clinically, chylous ascites is usually silent except for the distension of the abdomen. However, exceptionally it may simulate an acute peritonitis (Hardy, EurJSurg, 1992; 158:511; Currier, ANNA J, 1995; 22:157).

Tuberculous peritonitis

The differential diagnosis between cirrhotic ascites and ascites due to tuberculous peritonitis is particularly important since alcoholic cirrhosis may predispose to peritoneal tuberculosis (Burack, AmJMed, 1960; 28:510). Clinically, tuberculous peritonitis is characterized by fever, abdominal pain, anorexia, weight loss, abdominal tenderness, and ascites (Hyman, Gastro, 1962; 42:1; Battersby,

BrJSurg, 1967; 54:398; Sochocky, AmRevRespDis, 1967; 95:398; Singh, NEJM, 1969; 281:1091; Dineen, AnnSurg, 1976; 184:717; Karney, Chest, 1977; 72:310; Vyravanathan, PostgradMedJ, 1980; 56:649; Alvarez, Medicine, 1984; 63:25; Weir, AmJMed, 1985; 79: 467; Jakibowski, JInfDis, 1988; 158:687; Nafeh, AmJTropMedHyg, 1992; 47:470; Sandikci, JGastHepatol, 1992; 7:298; Marshall, AmJGastr, 1993; 88:989). However, none of these symptoms is invariably present. The proportion of patients with pleural or pulmonary tuberculosis or with a reactive tuberculin skin test ranges between 21 and 78 per cent and between 30 and 89, respectively, in the different series (Huges, DisChest, 1960; 38:42; Johnston, AnnIntMed, 1961; 54:1125; Gonella, ArchIntMed, 1966; 117:164; Snerman, ArchIntMed, 1980; 140:506; Linggenfelser, AmJGastr, 1993; 88:744; Lundstedt, ActaRadiol, 1996; 37:489). In females without active pulmonary tuberculosis, peritoneal tuberculosis may represent the local extension of a tuberculous salpingitis. However, in many cases no active focus of tuberculosis, apart from the peritoneal disease, can be detected. Ultrasonography and computed tomography may suggest the diagnosis of tuberculous peritonitis. Findings frequently seen in tuberculous peritonitis include diffuse, regular peritoneal thickening, infiltration of the greater omentum, ascites with fine, mobile septation or floating debris on ultrasonography, loculation of ascites, bowel thickening, particularly in the ileocaecal area, retroperitoneal lymph-node enlargement, lesions in solid organs (pelvic, adrenal, hepatic, splenic), cold abscesses, and adhesions (Rodriguez, JComputAssistTomogr, 1966; 20:269; Lee, ClinRadiol, 1991; 44:306; Ramaiya, AbdomImaging, 1993; 18: 23; Kedar, ClinRadiol, 1994; 49:24; Bankier, ClinRadiol, 1995; 50: 223; Sheikh, JClinUltrasound, 1995; 23:413; Demirkazik, ActaRadiol, 1996; 37:517; Lundstedt, ActaRadiol, 1996; 37:489). Results of examination of the peritoneal fluid are also suggestive of tuberculous infection if there is an increased concentration of proteins (over 3 g/dl) and lymphocytes. However, it has been shown that the ascitic fluid may be a transudate, particularly in cirrhotics with ascites and tuberculous peritonitis (Burak, AmJMed 1960; 28:510; Marshall, AmJGastr, 1988; 11:1259).[31] Ziehl–Nielsen-stained smears usually fail to show acid-fast bacilli. The proportion of cultures of ascitic fluid positive for *Mycobacterium tuberculosis* varies markedly from series to series (from 8 to 69 per cent), probably reflecting technical differences. It has been suggested that the proportion of positive cultures may be increased up to 80 per cent by concentrating 1 litre of the fluid by centrifugation. Nevertheless, the diagnosis of tuberculous peritonitis cannot be based on cultures of ascitic fluid since the usual techniques of culturing acid-fast bacilli may require several weeks to obtain a definite result. The activity of lactic dehydrogenase in ascitic fluid is greater in tuberculous peritonitis than cirrhosis. As in malignant ascites, the concentration of this enzyme in tuberculous ascites is higher than in plasma (De-Torregrosa, AmJMedSci, 1959; 238:552).[31] There are reports that the concentration of the tumour antigen CA125 in ascitic fluid may be very high in tuberculous peritonitis (Imai, ArchGynecolObstet, 1991; 248:157; Okazaki, JMed, 1992; 23:353). The activity of adenosine deaminase in the peritoneal fluid is a provenly sensitive and specific test for tuberculous peritonitis (Martinez-Vazquez, Gut, 1986; 27:1049; Lingenfelser, AmJGastr, 1993; 88:744) (Fig. 2). This is an enzyme in the catabolism of purine bases (catalysing the deamination of adenosine with the formation of inosine). It participates in the proliferation and differentiation of lymphocytes, and increases in tuberculous effusions probably as a consequence of the stimulation of cell-mediated immunity and T lymphocytes. The isozyme adenosine deaminase 2 is the dominant component of tuberculous pleural effusions (Shibagaki, JLabClinMed, 1996; 127:348). The concentration of interferon-γ in ascitic fluid is also greater in tuberculous peritonitis than cirrhotic ascites, although this does not improve on the results obtained with adenosine deaminase in the diagnosis of this condition (Ribera, Tubercle, 1991; 72:193; Sathar, Gut, 1995; 36:419). The concentration of adenosine deaminase in ascitic fluid in tuberculous peritonitis correlates directly with the total protein concentration in ascites (Soliman, JEgyptSocParasitol, 1994; 24:93). It is therefore not surprising that the number of false-negative results for adenosine deaminase in tuberculous peritonitis is higher in cirrhotic patients than in patients without chronic liver diseases.[32]

Open peritoneal biopsy during a laparotomy or minilaparotomy, blind needle biopsy of the peritoneum, and laparoscopy with direct biopsy of the affected areas have been used to confirm the diagnosis of tuberculous peritonitis (Wolfe, Lancet, 1979; i:852; Geake, GastrEnd, 1981; 27:66; Rodriguez-Lopez, Endoscopy, 1982; 14:178). Laparoscopy with direct peritoneal biopsy is the best of these methods (Bhargava, AmJGastr, 1992; 87:109; Mimica, Endoscopy, 1992; 24:588; Nafeh, AmJTropMedHyg, 1992; 47:470; Sandikci, JGastHepatol, 1992; 7:298). The peritoneum characteristically shows scattered or confluent miliary nodules of uniform size, with adhesions between bowel loops, liver capsule, and abdominal walls. The histological appearance is characterized by the presence of caseating granulomas. In some instances, tubercle bacilli may be seen by staining with auramine–rhodamine and microscopy under ultraviolet light. *Mycobacterium tuberculosis* can be cultured from the biopsy specimen of the peritoneum. The macroscopic and microscopic appearances of tuberculous peritonitis are similar to those of other conditions causing granulomatous peritonitis, such as sarcoidosis, Crohn's disease, and iatrogenic granulomatous peritonitis. The last condition occurs after 0.15 per cent of abdominal operations and is usually caused by a cell-mediated immune response to starch, talc, cotton fibres, and wood fibres originating from disposable surgical gowns and drapes (Holmes, Surgery, 1972; 71:85; Sternlieb, ArchSurg, 1977; 112:458). Iatrogenic granulomatous peritonitis appears 2 to 9 weeks postoperatively and is characterized by abdominal pain, tenderness and fever, and frequently by the accumulation of ascites. The observation of starch granules in the ascitic fluid obtained by paracentesis can be diagnostic.

Ascites due to hepatic venous-outflow block

Ascites secondary to postsinusoidal portal hypertension (congestive heart failure, constrictive pericarditis, obstruction of the inferior vena cava, Budd–Chiari syndrome) generally shows a total protein concentration and ascitic fluid–plasma albumin gradient similar to that reported in malignant ascites and tuberculous peritonitis (Runyon, JClinGastro, 1988; 10:410). The diagnosis can, however, be established by considering the clinical condition of the patient and the concentrations of leucocytes, lactic dehydrogenase, cholesterol, and adenosine deaminase in the ascitic fluid, which are lower in ascites secondary to hepatic outflow block. Patients with ascites due to constrictive pericarditis often lack symptoms of

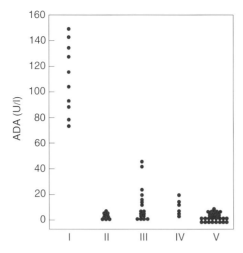

Fig. 2. Ascitic-fluid concentration of adenosine deaminase (ADA) in different groups of patients with ascites: group I, tuberculous peritonitis; group II, non-tuberculous septic peritonitis; group III, malignant ascites; group IV, miscellaneous; group V, cirrhosis (reproduced by permission from Martinez Vazquez, Gut, 1986; 27: 1049).

congestive heart failure. It is therefore important to seek physical findings characteristic of this entity (jugular venous distension with early diastolic collapse and inspiratory swelling, a diastolic knock that may be confused with a third heart sound, and pulsus paradoxus) in any patient with exudative ascites and no evidence of liver disease. Clear lung fields on radiographic examination and low voltage of the electrocardiogram suggest constrictive pericarditis. The diagnosis is confirmed by cardiac echography or catheterization. In patients with ascites due to a congenital web in the inferior vena cava, a cava-to-cava collateral circulation can be observed on the abdomen or back. The final diagnosis is based on inferior vena cavography. The differential diagnosis between chronic Budd–Chiari syndrome and cirrhosis is often difficult on clinical grounds. The protein concentration in ascitic fluid may be low in some of these patients as a result of the capillarization of the hepatic sinusoids (Roberts, AmJDigDis, 1978; 23:844). On the other hand, they may have hepatic stigmata, abnormal liver function tests, splenomegaly, and oesophageal varices (Powell-Jackson, QJMed, 1982; 51:79; Dilawari, Medicine, 1994; 73:21; Okuda, JHepatol, 1995; 22:1). If major hepatic veins are not visualized by computed tomography and ultrasonography this may suggest Budd–Chiari syndrome. The liver scintiscan sometimes shows a marked increase in isotope uptake centrally, possibly because of hypertrophy of the caudate lobule related to its autonomous venous drainage directly into the vena cava. However, in most cases the diagnosis is made by liver biopsy. Ascites with a high protein concentration is frequently found in the postoperative period of liver transplantation (Gane, Gastro, 1995; 109:1631). It is usually due to postsinusoidal portal hypertension secondary to deficient venous drainage from the implanted liver. Ascites due to obstructed hepatic venous outflow has also been reported in patients with polycystic liver disease (Torres, JAmSocNephrol, 1994; 5:1186; Uddim, Gut, 1995; 36:142).

Bile ascites

The leakage of bile into the peritoneal cavity may lead to two different clinical pictures.[33] Some patients develop signs and symptoms of peritonitis, including severe epigastric, right upper quadrant or diffuse abdominal pain, rigidity of the abdomen, rebound tenderness, hypotension, tachycardia, oliguria, and marked leucocytosis. Others have essentially no symptoms other than those caused by the accumulation of large quantities of bile ascites in the abdominal cavity (Santschi, ArchSurg, 1963; 87:851; Rosato, SGO, 1970; 130:494; Stein, Gastro, 1973; 64:1013; Auner, ArchIntMed, 1979; 139:245). In both circumstances, paracentesis yields a green ascitic fluid with a bilirubin concentration considerably higher than in plasma. Between these two extremes there is a wide spectrum of symptoms. Some patients may initially have a very brief period of apparent peritoneal signs followed by rapid, spontaneous resolution of symptoms and the accumulation of bile ascites, while others initially develop ascites with the signs of peritoneal irritation appearing posteriorly. Why intraperitoneal leakage of bile induces these two clinical pictures is unknown. Bile ascites usually occurs after biliary-tract surgery (mainly cholecystectomy), percutaneous diagnostic procedures (liver biopsy and percutaneous transhepatic cholangiography), and trauma with injuries to the gallbladder, common bile duct, hepatic duct or liver.[33] In contrast, the most common cause of bile peritonitis is spontaneous perforation of the gallbladder or bile ducts due to erosion by stones or cholecystitis.[33] It has been suggested that, in these last conditions, bacterial contamination of bile or a higher concentration of bile salts (which are capable of inducing chemical irritation of the peritoneum) are important factors in the development of bile peritonitis (Cain, Gastro, 1967; 53:600). The rate of leakage may also play a part. Bile ascites secondary to the spontaneous rupture of the common bile duct can also be observed in neonates as a consequence of congenital malformations of the biliary tract (stenosis, choledocal cyst) or stones.[33] Bile ascites should be considered as a possible diagnosis in any cirrhotic patient accumulating intra-abdominal fluid after a liver biopsy. The incidence of bile ascites and/or peritonitis has increased with the introduction of laparoscopic cholecystectomy (Morgenstern, SurgEndosc, 1993; 7:432)

Pancreatic ascites

Pancreatic ascites occurs in approximately 3 per cent of patients with chronic pancreatitis as a result of the leakage of fluid from a ruptured pancreatic duct, or from a pancreatic pseudocyst, into the peritoneal cavity (Sankaran, ArchSurg, 1976; 111:430; Cameron, Gastro, 1978; 74:134; Mann, AmJGastr, 1979; 71:186; Cabrera, MedicinaClin, 1986; 86:369; Fernández-Cruz, Hepatogast, 1993; 40:150). Other, less frequent causes include acute haemorrhagic pancreatitis (Maringhini, DigDisSci, 1996; 41:848), abdominal trauma, and pancreatic cancer. Since most patients with chronic pancreatitis are alcoholics and may develop massive ascites with little or no abdominal tenderness, the differential diagnosis of pancreatic from cirrhotic ascites may be difficult on clinical grounds. Laboratory analyses are therefore essential to establish a correct diagnosis. In virtually all cases, serum and especially ascitic-fluid amylase and lipase are dramatically increased (Polak, Digestion, 1968; 1:296; Schindler, Gastro, 1970; 59:453; Sileo, DigDisSci,

1975; 20:1110). The concentration of pancreatic enzymes in ascitic fluid is between 5 and 20 times greater than the plasma concentrations obtained simultaneously. The protein concentration in ascitic fluid is generally over 3 g/dl and the fluid is usually serous, but can be serosanguineous, turbid, or chylous. The concentration of methaemalbumin in ascites is markedly increased in patients with haemorrhagic pancreatitis and has prognostic significance (Sankaran, DigDisSci, 1978; 23:182). The concentration of leucocytes in ascitic fluid ranges between 70 and 2200 per mm^3, 80 per cent being lymphocytes (Boyer, ArchIntMed, 1978; 138:1103).[12] Ultrasonography or computed tomography are important diagnostic procedures for pancreatic ascites since they may detect the presence of a pseudocyst. Pseudocysts in patients with pancreatic ascites are usually small, due to continuous leakage of the cystic fluid into the peritoneal space.

Other types of ascites

Other causes of ascites easily differentiated from cirrhotic ascites include nephrogenic ascites, myxoedema, and Meig's syndrome. Nephrogenic ascites may become a severe problem in approx 5 per cent of patients maintained on chronic haemodialysis (Arismendi, AmJMed, 1976; 60:46; Hammond, JAmSocNephrol, 1994; 5:1173). The pathogenesis of ascites in these patients is unknown. The protein concentration in ascitic fluid is usually over 3 g/dl and the white blood-cell count ranges between 30 and 1500/mm^3 (Craig, ArchIntMed, 1974; 134:276). The amylase and lactic dehydrogenase activities in ascitic fluid are lower than the plasma concentrations obtained simultaneously. Peritoneal biopsies show only minor inflammation or fibrosis. The diagnosis of nephrogenic ascites is one of exclusion, so that it is important to rule out other causes.

Myxoedema is an infrequent cause of gross ascites (about 3 to 4 per cent of cases of myxoedema develop significant ascites). As the systemic changes of myxoedema may be mild, it may not be identified as the cause of the ascites, thus leading to unnecessary diagnostic procedures (Haley, ArchSurg, 1962; 85:328; Clancey, MedJAust, 1970; 2:415; deCastro, JClinGastr, 1991; 13:411). The ascitic fluid in myxoedema may be serous or gelatinous and characteristically has a high protein concentration. The pathogenesis of myxoedematous ascites is unknown.

Meig's syndrome consists of the association of ascites and hydrothorax with various types of benign ovarian tumours (fibroma, cystadenoma, struma ovarii). A 'modern' type of Meig's syndrome is the ovarian hyperstimulation syndrome occurring in patients treated with clomiphene and human menopausal gonadotrophins to induce ovulation (Schenker, FertSter, 1978; 30:255; Thaler, FertSter, 1981; 36:110). This syndrome is characterized by massive ascites, pleural effusions, signs of hypovolaemia (tachycardia, haemoconcentration, oliguria), and enlarged ovaries (more than 10 cm in diameter). A recent study has demonstrated that this syndrome is associated with a marked arterial vasodilation and activation of the renin–aldosterone and sympathetic nervous systems and antidiuretic hormone (**ADH**) (Balasch, AnnIntMed, 1994; 121:27). The formation of ascites and pleural effusions is due to increased capillary permeability in the ovarian vessels.

High-protein ascites may develop in patients with the acquired immune deficiency syndrome in the absence of portal hypertension or any other potential cause of ascites. Chronic non-specific peritonitis is found on laparoscopic peritoneal biopsy in these cases (Wilcox, Gastro, 1991; 100:745).

Cirrhotic hydrothorax

Pleural effusions, in the absence of primary pulmonary, pleural or cardiac disease, occur in approximately 5 per cent of patients with hepatic cirrhosis (Johnston, AnnIntMed, 1964; 61:385; Lieberman, AnnIntMed, 1966; 64:341). Clinical ascites is almost always evident and the pleural effusion is usually right-sided. Occasionally, however, effusion develops in the left pleura, on both sides, or in the absence of detectable ascites (Mirouze, DigDisSci, 1981; 26:984; Rubinstein, Gastro, 1985; 88:188; Giacobbe, JClinGastr, 1993; 17:271). The pathogenesis of cirrhotic hydrothorax involves, in most cases, the direct passage of ascitic fluid from the abdomen through acquired defects in the diaphragm into the pleural space (Fig. 3) (Okuda, JpnMedJ, 1967; 22:15; Lieberman, ArchIntMed, 1970; 125:114; Singer, Gastro, 1977; 73:575; Alberts, ArchIntMed 1991; 151:2383). The driving force leading to the peritoneal–pleural transfer of fluid is the hydrostatic gradient between the positive intra-abdominal pressure and the negative intrathoracic pressure. In cases of cirrhotic hydrothorax without detectable ascites the transport of fluid into the pleural space probably equals the rate of production of ascites. The presence of direct communications between the peritoneal and pleural cavities can be demonstrated by radioisotopic studies. The intraperitoneal injection of tracer amounts of [^{99m}Tc^m] sulphur colloid is followed by the rapid appearance of the isotope in the pleural cavity (Verreault, JNuclMed, 1986; 27:1706; Recoskie, ClinNuclMed, 1990; 15:97). The communications can be visualized by ultrafast echo-magnetic resonance imaging (MagnResImag, 1993; 11:1067). The biochemical and cytological characteristics of the pleural fluid are similar to those of the ascitic fluid obtained simultaneously. It is not unusual, however, to find slightly higher concentrations of total protein, albumin, cholesterol, and total lipids in pleural than ascitic fluid, probably related to a higher rate of water reabsorption from the pleural compartment. However, if there are marked differences in the biochemical or cytological characteristics between the pleural and the ascitic fluids one should search for another cause of the pleural effusion. Spontaneous bacterial empyema due to Gram-negative bacilli is a frequent complication in patients with cirrhotic hydrothorax. The pathogenesis of this complication is similar to that of spontaneous bacterial peritonitis.[34] Videothoracoscopy has been used effectively to localize and close the diaphragmatic defects causing cirrhotic hydrothorax.[35]

Factors involved in ascites formation in cirrhosis
Portal hypertension

In patients with liver disease, portal hypertension is essential to the formation of ascites. The accumulation of fluid within the peritoneal cavity is a common complication in diseases causing sinusoidal portal hypertension, for example Budd–Chiari syndrome (due to thrombosis of the hepatic veins or to compression of these veins by

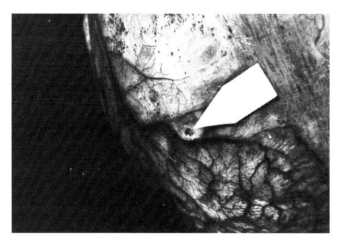

Fig. 3. Hole of 1 mm diameter in the right hemidiaphragm in a cirrhotic patient with right pleural effusion (reproduced by permission from Singer, Gastro, 1977; 73:575).

hepatic tumours, abscesses, or cysts), hepatic veno-occlusive disease, cirrhosis, and severe acute hepatitis of toxic, viral or alcoholic origin. By contrast, it is extraordinarily infrequent in liver diseases in which the block to portal flow occurs before the sinusoids (schistosomiasis, congenital hepatic fibrosis, idiopathic portal hypertension, hepatic sarcoidosis). Similarly, when portal hypertension develops as a consequence of an extrahepatic blockage of the hepatic or portal blood flow, ascites only occurs in those circumstances in which the vascular blockade increases sinusoidal pressure (right heart failure, constrictive pericarditis, obstruction of the inferior vena cava by congenital membranous webs) but not when the portal or the splenic veins are occluded. The relation between sinusoidal portal hypertension and the formation of ascites is also evident from experimental studies. Obstruction of the thoracic inferior vena cava or the hepatic veins is followed by rapid accumulation of fluid within the abdominal cavity. Ascites also occurs in several experimental models of cirrhosis (induced by carbon tetrachloride, dimethylnitrosamine, or chronic ligation of the bile duct). In contrast, partial or even complete obstruction of the portal vein is not followed by the formation of ascites.

Effect of sinusoidal portal hypertension on trans-sinusoidal fluid exchange

Differences in anatomical and functional characteristics between the hepatic and splanchnic microvasculature have been proposed to explain why ascites only develops in circumstances of sinusoidal portal hypertension. The hepatic sinusoids are structurally unique among microvessels since they do not have a basement membrane. They are lined by three main types of cells (see Chapter 1.4): endothelial, Kupffer, and fat-storing (Ito). The endothelial cells are by far the main component of the sinusoidal wall. Kupffer cells also contribute to the wall, although they are most often found within the lumen, attached by processes to the endothelial cells. Ito cells are found in the space of Disse, between the endothelial and liver cells. The endothelial cells form a very porous sinusoidal wall with large apertures, ranging from 100 to 500 nm in radius (Fig. 4).

Occasionally, microvilli from the hepatocytes cross the space of Disse and pass through these gaps in the endothelial membrane, thus reaching the sinusoidal lumen. This extremely porous membrane is almost completely permeable to macromolecules, including plasma proteins. These special characteristics of the sinusoidal wall are not surprising considering that the main function of the hepatic sinusoids is to promote intimate contact between the blood entering the liver and the hepatocytes. The space of Disse is relatively inconspicuous in normal conditions. It includes sparse bundles of collagen, glycosaminoglycans, occasional particles of very-low-density lipoprotein, Ito cells, and hepatocyte microvilli. Since no lymph vessels can be identified within the hepatic lobule, it has been suggested that the fluid in the space of Disse, in free communication with the interstitial spaces at the portal and central venous ends of the sinusoid, enters the lymphatics present in the portal tracts and in the central venous area as liver lymph. The highly porous nature of the sinusoidal wall explains why, in the normal liver, the protein concentration of hepatic lymph is approximately 95 per cent that of plasma measured simultaneously (Witte, AnnSurg, 1968; 168:567; Dumont, Lymphology, 1975; 8: 111).[36] A consequence of this high permeability is that the trans-sinusoidal oncotic gradient is virtually zero. Liver lymph is principally drained by vessels leaving at the liver hilus, although a small proportion passes through vessels accompanying the hepatic veins into the chest.[37] Lymph from the hilus, as well as that from other organs including the pancreas, spleen, kidney, adrenals, stomach, large and small intestines, gallbladder, and mesentery, all drains via the para-aortic plexus and cisterna chyli into the thoracic duct.[37] This duct is a lymphatic channel 36 to 45 cm long that begins at the upper end of the cisterna chyli near the lower border of the 12th thoracic vertebra, passes through the diaphragm, and ascends in the posterior mediastinum in close relation to the aorta and azygos vein. It passes into the neck behind the aortic arch, and then curves laterally, joining the left subclavian or internal jugular vein. The anatomical arrangement of the terminal thoracic duct is extremely variable. Only occasionally does it drain into the right jugular or subclavian vein alone. Usually there are many anastomotic sites between it and the venous system in the left side of the neck. In normal humans the thoracic lymph flow may reach 800 to 1000 ml/ day (Kessler, Gastro, 1969; 56:538).[38]

Constriction of the suprahepatic inferior vena cava or the hepatic veins in experimental animals has been the model most frequently used to investigate the effect of sinusoidal portal hypertension on fluid exchange through the sinusoidal wall. The increased pressure in the hepatic veins is almost completely transmitted back to the hepatic sinusoids, indicating that capillary pressure is not autoregulated in the liver.[39] In addition, because of the high permeability to plasma proteins of the sinusoidal wall, no oncotic force opposes the increase in hydrostatic sinusoidal pressure. Consequently, elevation of hepatic venous pressure is followed by a dramatic increase in the passage of fluid with a protein concentration similar to that of plasma, from the sinusoidal lumen to the space of Disse (Mitzner, AmJPhysiol, 1974; 227:513; Lautt, AmJPhysiol, 1976; 231:292; Orloff, AnnSurg, 1978; 188:494).[39-43] The relation between sinusoidal pressure and the hepatic production of lymph is such that an increase of 60 per cent in lymph production occurs for every millimetre rise in sinusoidal pressure.[39] The macroscopic consequence of this phenomenon is a marked enlargement of the

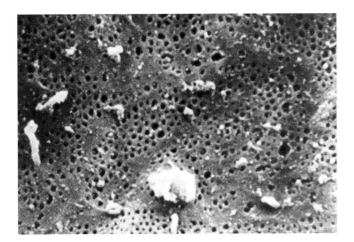

Fig. 4. Surface view of the endothelial lining of a liver sinusoid, as seen by scanning electron microscopy. Numerous fenestrae, with a pore size of 100 to 500 nm radius, are observed.

liver. However, the compliance of the liver, that is, the relation between interstitial pressure and interstitial volume, is very low.[44] This means that little interstitial fluid can accumulate without altering interstitial pressure. It has been estimated that for venous pressures between zero and 30 mmHg, approximately 65 per cent of the rise in hepatic venous pressure is transmitted to the hepatic interstitium.[51] The remaining 35 per cent is absorbed by the increase in intravascular and interstitial volume. This high interstitial pressure explains the two major consequences of experimental sinusoidal portal hypertension: a striking increase in lymph flow through the liver lymphatics and thoracic duct, and the direct passage of hepatic lymph with very high protein concentrations from the liver surface into the peritoneal cavity, forming ascites (Hyatt, JLabClinMed, 1955; 45:274; Van der Heyde, Surgery, 1964; 56:1121; Orloff, ArchSurg, 1966; 93:119; Orloff, AmJSurg, 1967; 114:213).[39,41-43]

Results of studies in cats with experimental constriction of the thoracic inferior vena cava strongly support the hypothesis that the ascitic fluid produced during acute experimental blockage of the hepatic outflow is mainly derived from the hepatic microvascular compartment. Greenway and Lautt investigated the effect of increasing hepatic venous pressure on the formation of hepatic lymph in anaesthetized cats.[40] The livers of these animals, with venous and arterial inflow intact, were inserted into a plethysmograph. The sequence of events occurring after the elevation in hepatic venous pressure consisted of a transient increase in hepatic volume, followed by a rapid accumulation of fluid with a protein concentration of approximately 80 per cent of the plasma concentrations within the plethysmograph. With obstruction of the hepatic lymphatics, the rate of fluid filtration through the liver surface was directly proportional to the sinusoidal pressure. Freeman (MedClinNAm, 1953; 37:109) and Mallet-Guy (LyonChirurg, 1954; 49:153) repositioned the liver supradiaphragmatically and subsequently constricted the thoracic inferior vena cava. Ascites only developed in the thoracic cavity. When a cellophane bag was placed around the liver, ascitic fluid only accumulated in the bag.

Effects of portal hypertension on splanchnic transmicrovascular fluid exchange

The structural and functional characteristics of the microvasculature of the stomach and small and large intestines are very different from those of the liver.[44] First, the splanchnic capillaries are much less porous than the hepatic sinusoids and have a well-defined basement membrane. Although most splanchnic capillaries are fenestrated, the estimated pore size, 3.7 to 12 nm in radius, is between 50 to 100 times less than that of the hepatic sinusoids. The oncotic reflection coefficient (**ORC**), which describes the fraction of the total protein oncotic pressure generated across a capillary membrane (impermeable proteins generate 100 per cent of their maximum oncotic pressure, ORC = 1; whereas freely permeable proteins generate no oncotic pressure, ORC = 0) has been estimated as 0 in the normal liver and 0.78, 0.92, and 0.85 in the stomach, small intestine, and colon, respectively (Granger, CircRes, 1979; 44:335; Gastro, 1981; 81:22).[42,45] Consequently, any increase in filtration in the splanchnic capillaries is quickly counterbalanced by an increase in the oncotic pressure difference between capillary lumen and interstitial space. This may explain the infrequency of ascites in presinusoidal portal hypertension.

Three other factors may contribute to the infrequency of ascites when the blockage to portal flow occurs before the sinusoids. First, the gastric and intestinal interstitium is much more compliant than the hepatic interstitium and considerable interstitial fluid can accumulate in these organs without causing any major changes in interstitial pressure.[44,46] Secondly, the intestines have a very efficient lymphatic system for removing interstitial oedema. In this respect, it is interesting that in normal conditions approximately 20 per cent of the fluid absorbed by the small intestine is carried out into the general circulation by the lymphatics (Granger, AmJPhysiol, 1978; 233:E429). The abrupt elevation of portal venous pressure increases lymph flow from the stomach, small intestine, and colon (Granger, AmJPhysiol, 1978; 232:E13; Perry, AmJPhysiol, 1981; 241:G478).[45,47] Because of the low permeability of intestinal capillaries to plasma proteins, the ratio between protein concentrations in the intestinal lymph and in plasma in conditions of portal hypertension is characteristically low (20 per cent).[36,48, 48] Finally, since most splanchnic capillaries are located within the submucosa[44] and the hydraulic conductance (permeability to submucosal interstitial fluid) of the muscular and serosal layers of the stomach, small bowel, and colon is probably low, it is not surprising that partial occlusion of the portal vein produces marked accumulation of fluid in the submucosa with no major changes in the serosal and muscular layers.[50] This also explains why transudation of fluid out of the gut in this condition occurs mainly into the lumen and not into the intraperitoneal space. In fact, net fluid and electrolyte secretion into the lumen of the small bowel occurs in animal models following acute elevation of portal pressure.[51]

Source of ascites in cirrhosis

All the findings discussed above offer a rational explanation for the absence of ascites in patients and experimental animals with presinusoidal portal hypertension. They also suggest that an imbalance between hepatic lymph production and the capacity of the lymphatic system of the liver and thoracic duct to return the hepatic lymph to the general circulation may be the predominant mechanism of ascites in experimental blockade of the hepatic venous outflow and in patients with constrictive pericarditis, Budd–Chiari syndrome, and hepatic veno-occlusive disease, who have increased lymph flow in the thoracic duct and ascites with a high protein content.[44,48,49,52] However, since hepatic cirrhosis differs in many respects from experimental blockade of the hepatic venous outflow, the pathogenesis of ascites in patients with chronic liver disease may vary from that in experimental sinusoidal portal hypertension.

First, it is well established that there are marked structural changes in the hepatic microvasculature in cirrhosis, the most characteristic being capillarization of the hepatic sinusoids (Fig. 5). This abnormality, which was originally described by Schaffner and Popper (Gastro, 1963; 44:239), has been extensively investigated by Huet *et al.* (JCI, 1982; 70:1234). These workers showed that the marginal areas of the regenerative nodules were perfused with capillaries rather than sinusoids, whereas sinusoids were present in the central areas of the micronodules. The sinusoids were fenestrated in a normal fashion and lacked a basement membrane. In contrast, capillaries exhibited a continuous endothelial lining lacking fenestrae, supported by a basement membrane and collagenous tissue. The structure was such that, along a single vascular pathway, capillary and sinusoidal structures were encountered in sequence. Variations in the degree of capillary change were found from patient to patient. Huet *et al.* also investigated the functional consequences in cirrhotic patients of this alteration in liver microcirculation by using a multiple-indicator dilution technique. Labelled red-blood cells and albumin were injected simultaneously into the portal vein or hepatic artery and the outflow dilution pattern was obtained from hepatic venous blood. In the normal liver, labelled red cells occupy the intravascular compartment, whereas the volume of distribution of albumin, which gains access to the space of Disse, includes both the intravascular and the interstitial compartments. This explains why in normal livers the volume of distribution of albumin exceeds that of red cells by 60 per cent. By contrast, in organs with less permeable capillaries in which no significant albumin exchange occurs during the time of a single passage, the difference between the volume of distribution of these two markers is only 7 per cent. In cirrhotic patients the calculated volume of distribution of albumin within the liver exceeded that of red cells by 7 to 60 per cent. Some patients showed a pattern similar to that expected in the normal liver, while in others the hepatic sinusoids were almost impermeable to albumin.

Second, there is evidence that, contrary to what occurs in other vascular territories, the intestinal microvasculature does not autoregulate its capillary pressure or the capillary filtration co-efficient in cirrhosis. Portal hypertension in cirrhotic patients and in animals with experimental cirrhosis is not associated with an increased splanchnic arteriolar resistance but rather with a generalized splanchnic arteriolar vasodilation.[53] As discussed later, the simultaneous occurrence of increased portal venous pressure and arterial blood inflow to the splanchnic microcirculation leads to a marked increase in splanchnic microvascular hydrostatic pressure and permeability, explaining why interstitial oedema in the mucosal, muscular, and serosal layers is prominent in human cirrhosis (Astaldi, AmJDigDis, 1960; 5:603; Norman, Gastro, 1980;

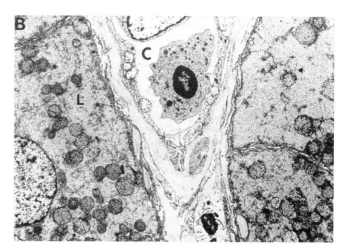

Fig. 5. Electron micrograph showing microvascular changes associated with cirrhosis: the sinusoidal lumen (C) is separated from the liver cells (L) by a non-fenestrated endothelial cell membrane, a basement membrane, and a layer of fibrillary collagen (reproduced by permission from Huet, JCI, 1982; 70:1234).

79:707).[54] The serosal oedema is manifested by a five-fold increase in the thickness of the jejunal peritoneum in cirrhotic patients compared with controls.[54]

Third, the total protein content in hepatic and thoracic-duct lymph and in ascitic fluid is remarkably lower in cirrhosis than in experimental blockage of the hepatic outflow. Increased flow of thoracic-duct lymph (usually 8–9 l/day) is a characteristic finding in cirrhosis, whether or not ascites is present (Fig. 6).[48] This is associated with a marked enlargement of the thoracic duct and an elevation in duct pressure,[38,55] which has been attributed to the presence of valves and endothelial folds at the duct–venous junction making the flow of lymph into the venous system of the neck difficult. The number, size, and thickness of lymphatics in the hilum of the liver, and in the mucosal and serosal layers of the intestine and mesentery, are markedly increased in cirrhosis (Johnson, AmJPhysiol, 1963; 204:31; CircRes, 1965; 16:294). The hepatic lymph:plasma ratio for total proteins in cirrhosis with ascites ranges between 20 and 80 per cent.[57] This low protein concentration of hepatic lymph is probably a consequence of the capillarization of hepatic sinusoids. The total protein content of intestinal lymph in cirrhotics with ascites is generally under 20 per cent of that in plasma.[57] Finally, the thoracic-duct lymph and the total protein concentration of ascitic fluid in these patients are between those of the hepatic and intestinal lymph (Boyer, AmJMedSci, 1969; 257: 32).[36,55,57] It is therefore very likely that ascites in cirrhosis derives from both the hepatic and splanchnic vascular compartments.

Studies evaluating the escape of radiolabelled albumin from the intravascular to the extravascular compartment and to the intraperitoneal space (which estimates the fluid dynamics through the capillary wall and peritoneum and liver surface, respectively) indicate that the lymphatic system is extremely efficient in returning most of the excessive hepatic and splanchnic lymph to the general circulation in cirrhotic patients with ascites (Henriksen, Clin-Physiol, 1983; 3:423; ScaJCLI, 1981; 41:289; 589; 601; 1984; 44: 143).[20] The transvascular escape rate of radiolabelled albumin in

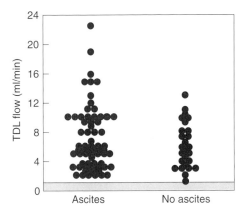

Fig. 6. Thoracic duct lymph (TDL) flow in patients with hepatic cirrhosis both with and without ascites: lymph flow was ascertained after cannulation of the thoracic duct in the left neck.; the horizontal line represents the upper limit of TDL flow in normal individuals (reproduced by permission from Witte, Gastro, 1971; 61:742).

these patients is remarkably high (8.5 per cent of the total intravascular mass of albumin per hour). The fraction of the transvascular escape of albumin passing into the peritoneal cavity is, however, very low (0.21 per cent). Ascites formation is therefore the consequence of a small spill-over of the increased rate of formation of hepatic and splanchnic lymph, most of which is returned directly to the circulation through the lymphatic system.

Studies on the effect of surgical (side-to-side and end-to-side) portacaval shunts in the formation of ascites have been performed in experimental animals to assess the site of origin of ascitic fluid. In conditions of sinusoidal portal hypertension, a side-to-side portacaval shunt decompresses both the splanchnic capillaries and the hepatic sinusoids. Side-to-side shunting reduces the sinusoidal pressure by shunting splanchnic blood away from the liver, thus decreasing the inflow of blood to the sinusoids, and also by allowing retrograde egress of sinusoidal blood through the portal vein into the inferior vena cava (Redeker, JCI, 1964; 43:1464; Mulder, Surgery, 1966; 59:923; Burchell, SGO, 1974; 138:359). An end-to-side portacaval shunt is as effective as a side-to-side shunt in decompressing the splanchnic vascular compartment. However, it is much less effective in decompressing the sinusoidal compartment since it does not allow the sinusoidal blood to be shunted to the inferior vena cava. In fact, haemodynamic studies in cirrhotic patients have shown a significantly greater reduction in wedged hepatic venous pressure (which estimates sinusoidal pressure) after a side-to-side shunt than after end-to-side portacaval anastomosis. Side-to-side, but not end-to-side, portacaval anastomosis prevented the formation of ascites in animals with blocked hepatic venous outflow and with experimental cirrhosis induced by the ligation of the common bile duct (Orloff, Surgery, 1964; 56:784).[58,59] These results have been interpreted as indicating that ascites in both conditions derives mainly from the intrahepatic sinusoidal vascular bed. However, these experimental data should be regarded cautiously, since in human cirrhosis both types of shunts have been proved equally effective in preventing the formation of ascites (Orloff, AnnNYAcadSci, 1970; 170:213; Franco, GastrClinBiol, 1983; 7:533).

Effects of portal hypertension on splanchnic arteriolar circulation

In addition to increasing hepatic and splanchnic lymph production, portal hypertension induces a profound alteration of the splanchnic circulation. Classically, portal hypertension was considered to be due solely to an increased resistance to portal venous flow. However, it is now clear that the pathogenesis of portal hypertension is much more complex and that increased portal venous inflow secondary to a generalized splanchnic arteriolar vasodilation also plays an important part in the increased portal pressure.[53,60–66] This high portal venous inflow may explain why, in experimental animals, portal pressure remains increased despite the development of a marked collateral circulation. The mechanism by which portal hypertension induces splanchnic arteriolar vasodilation and increased portal venous inflow is not entirely understood. There is evidence that some degree of portosystemic shunting is almost obligatory for its development.[67] Portosystemic shunts allow the systemic delivery, and perhaps enhance production and release, of vasodilating substances of splanchnic origin. In this regard, there is evidence that glucagon might be the most important of these substances, accounting for approximately 30 to 40 per cent of the splanchnic vasodilatation in rats with chronic portal hypertension.[66,68–70] Decreased sensitivity of the gastric and intestinal microvasculature to endogenous vasoconstrictor systems may also contribute to the splanchnic hyperaemia associated with portal hypertension.[71] Finally, as discussed in other chapters, increased activity of the vascular NO synthetic pathway seems to be an important mechanism of splanchnic hyperaemia in portal hypertension (Sieber, Gastro, 1993; 104:1750; Ros, Hepatol, 1995; 21: 554; Morales-Ruiz, Hepatol 1996; 24:1481).

There is indirect evidence that splanchnic arteriolar vasodilation also occurs in patients with cirrhosis and portal hypertension. Under normal conditions almost all the flow circulating in the splanchnic bed reaches the liver, so the hepatic equals the splanchnic blood flow. In patients with cirrhosis and portal hypertension, because there is important shunting of blood through the portosystemic collateral circulation, the hepatic blood flow represents only a part of the splanchnic blood flow. Between 60 and 80 per cent of the mesenteric and splenic blood flow is shunted through the collateral circulation in cirrhotic patients.[72,73] Since several investigations have shown that the hepatic blood flow is normal or even increased in most such patients,[74–76] it follows that in these there must be a marked increase in splanchnic blood flow secondary to arteriolar vasodilatation. The observation that the mean transit time in the splanchnic vascular bed is substantially reduced in alcoholic cirrhotics further indicates the occurrence of splanchnic arteriolar vasodilation in these patients.[77]

Renal sodium and water retention

In addition to portal hypertension, the renal retention of sodium and water is of major importance in the pathogenesis of ascites. The strongest arguments for this contention derive from daily clinical practice. Oliguria and low urinary sodium excretion are constant features in cirrhotic patients accumulating ascites. Ascites disappears in most cirrhotic cases when sodium intake is restricted and the urinary sodium excretion is increased by diuretics. Finally, in patients leaving a sodium-restricted diet and/or diuretic treatment, reaccumulation of ascites is the rule. Several experimental studies have shown that sodium retention precedes the formation of ascites (Levy, AmJPhysiol 1977; 233:F572; JLabClinMed, 1978; 92:560; López-Novoa, AmJPhysiol, 1980; 238:F353; Jimenez, Hepatol, 1985; 5:245). The mechanisms responsible for renal sodium and water retention in cirrhosis are discussed in detail in Chapter 8.2. The most important factors are increased activity of the renin–angiotensin–aldosterone and sympathetic nervous systems, and hypersecretion of ADH. The stimulation of these endogenous vasoconstrictor systems in cirrhosis, which is a compensatory mechanism to maintain arterial pressure within normal limits, is secondary to a reduction in effective arterial blood volume due to the splanchnic arteriolar vasodilation. Renal sodium and water retention would therefore be the final step of a sequence of events, initiated by portal hypertension, that would lead to splanchnic arteriolar vasodilation, arterial hypotension, and homeostatic activation of endogenous systems with vasoconstrictor and sodium- and water-retaining properties.[78]

Pathogenesis of ascites: the forward theory

The evolution of our concepts on the formation of ascites in cirrhosis is imitating that on congestive heart failure 25 years ago. The formation of oedema in heart failure was initially considered as secondary to the increase in venous pressure due to the impaired cardiac function. The disruption of the Starling equilibrium in the microcirculation due to the backward increase in capillary hydrostatic pressure would lead to the accumulation of fluid in the interstitial space and the formation of pulmonary and peripheral oedema (backward theory). With the demonstration of the importance of the renin–aldosterone and sympathetic nervous systems, ADH, and renal sodium and water retention in the pathogenesis of congestive heart failure, however, the described mechanism of cardiac oedema moved from the venous to the arterial vascular compartment (Schrier, NEJM, 1988; 319:1065; 1127; AnnIntMed, 1990; 113:155). According to this new concept, the predominant mechanism of oedema in congestive heart failure would be an impairment in effective arterial blood volume secondary to the decrease in cardiac output (forward theory). The high-pressure baroreceptors located in the aortic, carotid sinus, and juxta-glomerular apparatus would sense the underfilling of the arterial vascular compartment, stimulating the renin–aldosterone and sympathetic nervous systems and ADH, and inducing an increased renal tubular reabsorption of sodium and water. The retained fluid would extravasate in those areas with increased venous pressure. Additionally, the increased activity of these endogenous vasoconstrictor systems would produce systemic vasoconstriction and further decrease the cardiac output, thus closing a vicious circle. This 'forward theory' of oedema formation in congestive heart failure has been extremely important in improving the management of this condition. The administration of vasodilators decreases cardiac afterload, increases cardiac output, deactivates the endogenous vasoconstrictors systems, improves renal function, and increases the response to diuretics.

The traditional concept of ascites formation in cirrhosis also considers hepatic oedema to be a direct consequence of the 'backward' increase in hydrostatic pressure in the hepatic sinusoids and splanchnic capillaries due to the sinusoidal portal hypertension.[48, 49,55,57] This feature, together with the hypoalbuminaemia, would alter the Starling equilibrium within the hepatic and splanchnic microcirculation, leading to the accumulation of fluid in the intertitial space of these vascular territories. Leakage of fluid from the interstitial space to the peritoneal cavity would occur when the formation of interstitial oedema overcomes the capacity of the abdominal lymphatic system to return the hepatic and splanchnic lymph to the systemic circulation. Renal dysfunction in cirrhosis would be a consequence of a reduction in the circulating blood volume secondary to the formation of ascites. The fact that the blood volume is constantly increased in patients with cirrhosis would not invalidate this hypothesis, since the effective blood volume would be reduced, due to an enlargement of the intravascular venous compartment promoted by the increased portal pressure. The demonstration that cardiac output is markedly increased in cirrhosis, indicating an increased amount of blood reaching the arterial vascular system, and that peripheral vascular resistance is reduced, are strong arguments against this hypothesis.

During the last decade, data have been presented indicating that ascites formation in cirrhosis could be better explained on a 'forward' basis, as follows.

1. As indicated above, arteriolar vasodilation is a constant finding in cirrhosis with ascites. It is the primary event in the hyperdynamic circulation (hypervolaemia, high cardiac output, low peripheral vascular resistance, arterial hypotension) that characterizes patients with compensated and decompensated cirrhosis. Arteriolar vasodilation is also the primary event in the stimulation of the renin–aldosterone and sympathetic nervous systems and ADH, and renal dysfunction (sodium and water retention and hepatorenal syndrome) in patients with ascites.[78]

2. Arteriolar vasodilation in cirrhosis occurs predominantly if not exclusively in the splanchnic circulation, is due to the increase in portal pressure, and contributes significantly to the maintenance of portal hypertension. In fact, blood flow to the remaining major vascular territories (muscular and cutaneous, renal, and cerebral) is reduced in patients with cirrhosis and ascites (Bru, GastroHepato, 1997; 20:86).[79,80] In contrast, the splenic and mesenteric blood flows are increased in these patients.[81]

3. Investigations on portal vein-ligated rats have demonstrated that the increased hydrostatic pressure in the splanchnic microcirculation in portal hypertension is predominantly due to the increased inflow of blood to this vascular territory, secondary to the splanchnic arteriolar vasodilation.[65,68,82] The acute increase in portal pressure is not followed by splanchnic arteriolar vasodilation. In contrast, this feature is constantly observed during chronic portal hypertension. This is due to the existence of a delay of 24 to 48 h between the ligation of the portal vein and the onset of splanchnic arteriolar vasodilation. In experimental animals with chronic portal hypertension and, therefore, with splanchnic arteriolar vasodilation, splanchnic capillary pressure is approximately 70 per cent higher than in control animals. In contrast, when portal venous pressure is

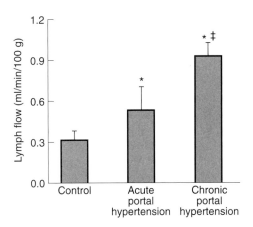

Fig. 7. Intestinal lymph flow in control rats at normal portal pressure, during acute elevations of portal pressure in control rats, and in rats with chronic portal hypertension. *Indicates values that are statistically different from controls. ‡ Indicates values that are statistically different from those obtained during acute elevations in portal venous pressure in control rats. (Reproduced by permission from Korthuis, AmJPhysiol, 1988; 254:G339.)

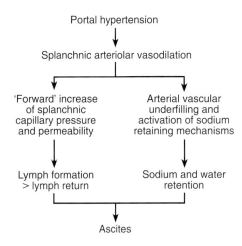

Fig. 8. The forward theory of ascites formation.

acutely elevated to achieve an equivalent degree of portal hypertension, capillary pressure is increased by only 10 to 20 per cent. Chronic portal hypertension is also associated with a greater increase in the capillary filtration coefficient in the splanchnic circulation than acute portal hypertension.[65] This is probably related to an increase in microvascular surface area secondary to splanchnic arterial vasodilation. The combination of the increased capillary hydrostatic pressure and filtration coefficient in the splanchnic microcirculation during chronic portal hypertension leads to a marked increase in intestinal lymph flow, a feature not observed during acute portal hypertension (Fig. 7).[65] Splanchnic arteriolar vasodilation is therefore the predominant mechanism of increased lymph formation during chronic portal hypertension.

4. Portal hypertension is higher in cirrhosis than in prehepatic portal hypertension. In experimental animals with chronic ligation of the portal vein, portal pressure averages 15 mmHg whereas it approaches 25 to 30 mmHg in experimental cirrhosis.[65] Among cirrhotic patients with ascites, the degree of portal hypertension is also higher in those with rather than without ascites.[76] Splachnic arteriolar vasodilation is also higher in patients with decompensated than compensated cirrhosis since they have a similar decrease in peripheral vascular resistance in the setting of marked overactivity of endogenous vasoconstrictor systems.[76] In fact, blocking the vascular effect of these systems is associated with a marked fall in systemic vascular resistance in patients and experimental animals with cirrhosis and ascites, indicating that the degree of 'baseline' arterial vasodilation (the one that would be present in the absence of the homeostatic stimulation of these systems) is greater in decompensated than compensated cirrhosis.[83–85]

These data suggest that the pathogenesis of ascites could be satisfactorily explained on the basis of the changes in the arterial circulation induced by portal hypertension (Fig. 8).[86] The hypothesis (forward theory of ascites formation) considers that the accumulation of fluid within the abdomen is a consequence of

the splanchnic arteriolar vasodilation, which would simultaneously produce arteriolar vascular underfilling and a 'forward' increase in the splanchnic capillary pressure and filtration coefficient. In patients with compensated cirrhosis or with prehepatic portal hypertension, the degree of portal hypertension and of splanchnic arteriolar vasodilation is moderate. Their arterial vascular underfilling can be compensated for by transient and undetectable episodes of sodium and water retention that increase the plasma volume and cardiac index, and refill the dilated arterial vascular bed.[78] On the other hand, the lymphatic system is able to return the moderate increase in lymph produced to the systemic circulation, thus preventing leakage of fluid into the abdominal cavity. As cirrhosis progresses, however, portal hypertension and the secondary fall in splanchnic vascular resistance are progressively more intense and a critical point is reached at which the consequences of splanchnic arteriolar vasodilation can no longer be compensated for by increasing the lymph return, plasma volume, and cardiac index. The maintenance of arterial pressure then requires persistent activation of the renin–aldosterone system, the sympathetic nervous system and ADH, which produces continuous water and sodium retention. The retained fluid is, however, ineffective in refilling the dilated arterial vascular bed because it escapes from the intravascular compartment, due to an imbalance between the excessive lymph production and the ability of the lymphatic system to return it to the systemic circulation. The final consequence of both disorders is continuous leakage of fluid into the abdominal cavity and the formation of ascites.

Reabsorption of ascites

Although the above discussion has exclusively emphasized factors involved in the formation of ascites, the amount of ascites present at any given time reflects the balance between the rates of formation and reabsorption. Information on reabsorption is limited. It appears that the lymphatics on the undersurface of the diaphragm are specially important in removing ascitic fluid from the peritoneal cavity. Electron-microscopic studies of diaphragmatic peritoneum have demonstrated an anatomical arrangement that facilitates absorption from the peritoneal cavity. The peritoneal surface of the diaphragm is covered by a single layer of two different populations of mesothelial cells (cuboidal and extremely flattened).[87,88] These cells rest on a connective tissue matrix within which lies a rich plexus of terminal lymphatic vessels (lymphatic lacunae). Cuboidal mesothelial cells are usually over the lymphatic lacunae and the submesothelial connective tissue between them is scant or even absent. The remaining areas of the diaphragm, which lack submesothelial lymphatic lacunae, are mainly covered by flattened cells. Areas with cuboidal and flattened cells differ markedly in the structure of their intercellular (lateral) surfaces. Flattened cells form a layer with no discontinuity between adjacent cells. In contrast, numerous gaps are present between the cuboidal mesothelial cells, large enough to allow the passage of particles of Indian ink, colloidal carbon, and of erythrocytes. Basically, two types of structurally different intercellular gaps may be found between the cuboidal cells (Fig. 9). One type, which is formed by interlacing filamentous processes from adjacent mesothelial cells, represents a 'true intercellular gap' and overlies a thin layer of connective tissue. The other type, which represents a 'stoma', consists of a circular pore formed among several mesothelial cells whose cell membranes form adhesions with the underlying lymphatic endothelium. This results in a well-defined channel leading directly from the peritoneal cavity to the lumen of the lymphatic lacunae. The submesothelial plexus of lymphatic vessels intercommunicates at regular intervals by way of transverse anastomoses that drain into a deeper plexus of valved collecting vessels, which penetrate connective tissue septa of the muscular fibres of the diaphragm. Drainage from the deeper lymphatics of the diaphragm is mainly via parasternal trunks on the ventral thoracic wall, right lymphatic duct, and right subclavian or internal jugular veins (Courtice, AustJExpBiolMedSci, 1950; 28:1161; JPhysiol, 1951; 114:336).[89,90] The lymphatic drainage of the diaphragm is therefore independent of the thoracic duct. The periodic respiratory movements of the diaphragm may be important in the passage of ascites into the lymphatic system and general circulation.[89] During inspiration, intercellular gaps and stomata close, intraperitoneal pressure is increased, and the lacunae are emptied through the combined effects of local compression, and increased intra-abdominal and reduced intrathoracic pressures (Morris, AustJExpBiolMedSci, 1953; 31:239). During expiration, the gaps and stomas are opened and free communication is re-established. The importance of diaphragmatic lymphatics in the reabsorption of intraperitoneal fluid has been demonstrated in animal studies showing that particles and cells of various sizes are rapidly removed from the peritoneal cavity by the lymphatics of the diaphragm; the obliteration of these diaphragmatic lymphatics by abrasion significantly delays the absorption of serum from the peritoneal cavity and increases the propensity of portal hypertension to produce ascites (Raybuck, AmJPhysiol, 1960; 198:1207; Raunbuck, AmJPhysiol, 1960; 199:1021; Lill, Gastro, 1979; 76:997).[87, 90]

Reabsorption of ascites from the peritoneal cavity into the general circulation is a rate-limited phenomenon. The average fractional reabsorption rate of radiolabelled albumin from the peritoneal cavity into the general circulation in cirrhotics with ascites has been estimated as 1.27 per cent of the intraperitoneal protein mass per hour, corresponding to a rate of ascitic fluid reabsorption of 1.4 l/24 h.[20] The rate of reabsorption of ascitic fluid, as estimated by the transport of radiolabelled proteins from the abdominal cavity into the circulating plasma, varies markedly from patient to patient

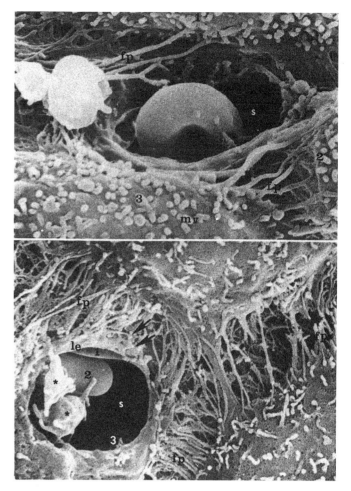

Fig. 9. Scanning electron micrographs of the peritoneal surface of the diaphragm. The upper figure shows a stoma (s) located at the junction of several cells (numbered 1–3). A red blood cell was caught in the process of entering the stoma. Numerous filamentous processes (fp) and intercellular gaps are also shown. In the lower figure, three red blood cells (numbered 1–3) and two platelets are in the process of entering the stoma. Margins of the lymphatic endothelial cells (le) extend on to the peritoneal surface and make contact with the margins and filamentous processes (fp) of cuboidal mesothelial cells (arrows). (Reproduced by permission from Leak, AmJAnat, 1978; 151:557.)

(Dykes, ClinSci, 1968; 34:85).[20,91] Henriksen *et al.* report a range of reabsorption rates of 0.57 to 4.42 l/24 h in six cirrhotics with a mean ascitic fluid volume of 6.2 l.[20] The values obtained by Buhac *et al.* in 12 patients with an average volume of ascitic fluid of 9.95 l ranged from 1.0 to 5.3 l/24 h (mean 2.25 l/24 h).[91] The time of appearance of radioactivity in plasma after the injection of radiolabelled albumin into the ascitic fluid in these patients was, on average, 0.5 h (range 0.1–1.2 h). This time lag between the intraperitoneal injection of tracer and the appearance of tracer in plasma suggests that the transport of ascitic fluid into the general circulation is slow and through tubes (lymphatic vessels) and not a transperitoneal absorption.[20] There are very few data on the factors influencing the reabsorption rate of ascitic fluid. Animal studies have demonstrated a positive relation between intra-abdominal pressure and reabsorption of intraperitoneal fluid (Zink,

Gastro, 1977; 73:1119; AmJPhysiol, 1977; 233:H185). However, this relation was not observed in cirrhotic patients, in whom a decrease in intra-abdominal pressure did not lead to significant changes in the reabsorption of ascitic fluid from the peritoneal cavity.[91] The low rates of ascites formation and reabsorption of ascitic fluid in cirrhotics with ascites should not be taken as an indication that in these patients the intraperitoneal cavity is a segregated compartment isolated from the rest of the body. In fact, the transperitoneal exchange of water and water-soluble substances (for example, antibiotics not bound to proteins) by diffusion is very rapid in cirrhotics with ascites. It has been demonstrated that the water content of ascitic fluid enters and leaves the peritoneal cavity very rapidly, approximating 40 to 80 per cent per hour (Prentice, AmJMed, 1952; 13:668).

Prognosis of patients with cirrhosis and ascites

The appearance of ascites in patients with cirrhosis carries a poor prognosis. The probability of survival 1 and 5 years after the first episode of ascites has been estimated as 50 and 20 per cent, respectively (Arroyo, SemLivDis, 1986; 6:353). Among cirrhotics with ascites, those with hepatorenal syndrome have the shortest survival. They usually die within weeks or months after the onset of renal failure, independent of the degree of hepatic insufficiency (Ginès, Gastro, 1993; 105:229). Studies in non-azotaemic cirrhotics with ascites have shown that sodium excretion and plasma renin activity have prognostic significance (Arroyo, AnnIntMed, 1981; 94:198; Genoud, SchMedWoch, 1986; 116:463). Non-azotaemic cirrhotics with elevated plasma renin activity or with marked sodium retention (urinary sodium excretion lower than 10 mEq/day) have a significantly lower survival than those with normal plasma renin concentrations or relatively high urinary sodium excretion. Two investigations have evaluated the prognostic value in cirrhotics with ascites of numerous variables based on history, physical examination, hepatic biochemical tests (including galactose elimination capacity), renal function tests, systemic and splanchnic haemodynamics, and endogenous vasoactive systems. Among 38 variables considered in the series by Llach et al. (Gastro, 1988; 94:482), composed of 139 patients in hospital for the treatment of an episode of ascites, only seven had independent prognostic value, including mean arterial pressure, plasma noradrenaline, glomerular filtration rate, urinary sodium excretion, nutritional status, hepatomegaly, and serum albumin (Fig. 10). In the multivariate analysis by Tage-Jensen et al. (JHepatol, 1988; 6:350) in 81 alcoholic cirrhotics with and without ascites, among the 25 variables considered only the presence of ascites, the plasma noradrenaline concentration, portal pressure, and serum bilirubin were independent predictors of survival. Thus both studies indicate that measures estimating systemic and portal haemodynamics and renal function are better predictors of survival than those used to estimate hepatic function in patients with cirrhosis and ascites. Other variables with prognostic significance in cirrhotic patients with ascites include the Child–Pugh score, the ascitic protein concentration, a history of spontaneous bacterial peritonitis, and the resistant of ascites to the diuretic therapy (Salerno, AmJGastr, 1993; 88:514; Guardiola, AmJGastr, 1995; 90:2086).

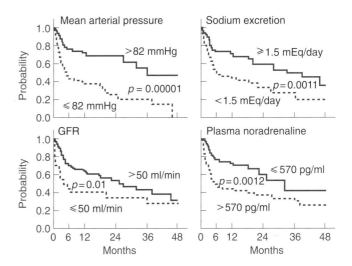

Fig. 10. Probability of survival in 136 cirrhotic patients with ascites classified according to mean arterial pressure, plasma noradrenaline concentration, urinary sodium excretion, and glomerular filtration rate (GFR) (reproduced by permission from Llach, Gastro, 1988; 94:482).

Treatment of ascites
Bed rest and low-sodium diet

The assumption of an upright posture by patients with cirrhosis and ascites is associated with a striking activation of the renin–angiotensin–aldosterone and sympathetic nervous systems, a reduction of glomerular filtration rate and sodium excretion, and a decreased response to loop diuretics (Bernardi, Gut, 1985; 26:629; Ring-Larsen, BMJ, 1986; 292:1351; Gerbes, ClinInvest, 1993; 71:894). These effects are even more striking when upright posture is associated with moderate physical exercise.[93,94] Therefore, from a theoretical point of view, bed rest could be useful for the treatment of ascites in cirrhosis, particularly in patients who respond poorly to diuretics.

The aim of the medical treatment of ascites is to mobilize the intra-abdominal fluid by creating a net negative balance of sodium. In approximately 10 to 20 per cent of cirrhotics with ascites, those who spontaneously excrete relatively high amounts of sodium in the urine, this can be obtained simply by reducing the sodium content in the diet to 40 to 60 mEq/day (Gerbes, JHepatol, 1993; 17 (Suppl. 2):S4).[95,96] A more intense dietary sodium restriction is not practical, since it is difficult to accomplish and may worsen the anorexia and malnutrition commonly present in these patients. In the remaining cases with marked sodium retention, a negative sodium balance cannot be obtained without the aid of diuretics to increase urinary sodium excretion over intake. However, even in these patients, dietary sodium restriction is very important since it reduces the diuretic requirements (Reynolds, Gut, 1978; 19:549; Descos, Hepatogast, 1983; 30:15; Gauthier, Gut, 1986; 27:705). In cirrhotics responding poorly to diuretic treatment, a negative sodium balance cannot be obtained unless sodium intake is limited. A frequent cause of diuretic-resistant ascites is inadequate sodium restriction. This 'apparently intractable' ascites should be suspected in any patient whose ascites does not decrease despite a good natriuretic response to diuretics. In this respect, it is important to note that many drugs, particularly the antibiotics, may contain relatively high amounts of sodium. Once ascites has disappeared, many cirrhotics continue to require a strict sodium diet and diuretics to avoid its reaccumulation. Other cases can, however, be maintained without ascites by moderate sodium restriction and low doses of diuretics. Finally, some patients may even recover their ability to excrete sodium normally and may be free of ascites despite normal sodium intake and no diuretics. Therefore, the long-term management of cirrhotics with ascites varies markedly from patient to patient, and every effort should be made to adjust sodium intake and diuretic dosage to individual requirements during the course of the disease.

Diuretics

Loop diuretics, in particular frusemide, and distal diuretics, especially spironolactone, are the drugs most commonly used in the treatment of ascites in cirrhosis (Arroyo, JHepatol, 1994; 21:667). Loop diuretics inhibit chloride and sodium reabsorption in the ascending limb of the loop of Henle but have no effect on the distal nephron (distal and collecting tubules).[97,98] They must reach the tubular lumen to be effective. Loop diuretics are all organic acids and are highly bound to plasma proteins. As a consequence, they can only reach the lumen by being actively secreted from the blood into the urine via the organic-acid transport pathway of the straight segment of the proximal tubule. Once in the luminal compartment, frusemide is carried with the luminal fluid to the ascending limb of the loop of Henle, where it inhibits a specific cotransport system, the Na^+-$2Cl^-$-K^+ carrier, located in the luminal membrane of the ascending-limb cells. This effect probably involves the interaction of the anionic site of frusemide with the Cl-binding sites of the carrier, thus resulting in inhibition of active chloride reabsorption. It is therefore not surprising that the urinary concentration of frusemide correlates best with the response. Loop diuretics also increase the renal synthesis of prostaglandins, and anti-inflammatory drugs reduce their natriuretic effect. Renal prostaglandins therefore appear to be involved in the natriuretic response to loop diuretics.

Loop diuretics such as frusemide are the most powerful diuretics presently available. High dosage of frusemide can increase sodium excretion up to 30 per cent of the filtered sodium in normal individuals. This high natriuretic potency can be attributed to two features. First, between 20 and 50 per cent of the filtered sodium is reabsorbed in the loop of Henle. Secondly, in the absence of hyperaldosteronism, the distal and collecting tubules, which are downstream from the loop of Henle, have a limited capacity for sodium reabsorption and are not capable of mitigating the diuresis induced by loop diuretics. Frusemide is rapidly absorbed from the gut. Onset of action is extremely rapid (within 30 min of oral administration), with peak effects occurring within 1 to 2 h; most of the natriuretic activity has finished in 3 to 4 h.

Spironolactone and other distal diuretics (triamterene, amiloride) have a much lower intrinsic natriuretic potency than loop diuretics. They are able to increase sodium excretion up to 2 per cent of the filtered sodium.[97,98] Spironolactone undergoes extensive metabolism in man, leading to numerous biologically active compounds, including canrenone, 6-β-hydroxy-7-α-thiomethyl-spironolactone, and 7-α-thiomethylspironolactone.[99] The anti-mineralocorticoid effect of spironolactone has traditionally been

attributed to its major metabolite, canrenone. However, recent studies show that canrenone only accounts for 10 to 25 per cent of the antimineralocorticoid activity. Other metabolites are therefore important in its diuretic effect. Spironolactone metabolites are tightly bound to plasma proteins from which they are released slowly to the kidney and other target organs; the half-life of these metabolites in healthy individuals has been estimated to range between 10 and 35 h after single or multiple doses of spironolactone. This explains the 24 to 48 h delay between drug withdrawal and the end of the natriuretic effect. Spironolactone metabolism is impaired in cirrhosis, so that the terminal half-lives of spironolactone and its metabolites are increased when compared to values in normal individuals (Sungaila, Gastro, 1992; 102:1680).

Spironolactone metabolites act by competitively inhibiting the tubular effect of aldosterone on the distal nephron. This hormone enters the collecting tubular cell through the basolateral membrane, interacts with a cytosolic receptor bound to heat-shock proteins, dissociates the receptor from these proteins, and exposes a region with high affinity for DNA. The aldosterone–receptor complex is then translocated to the nuclei and interacts with specific DNA sequences, stimulating the release of mRNA and the synthesis of specific proteins that participate in the tubular reabsorption of sodium, namely sodium channels inserted into the luminal membrane, favouring sodium transport from the tubular lumen to the intracellular space, and Na-K-ATPase, molecules of which are inserted into the basolateral membrane, favouring the extrusion of intracellular sodium into the perivascular space (Garty, JMembr-Biol, 1986; 90:193; Bodine, Receptor, 1990; 1:83; Funder, Trends-EndocrinolMetab, 1990; 1:145; Verrey, SemNephrol, 1990; 10:410; Bastl, KidneyInt, 1992; 42:250). The increased number of Na-K-ATPase molecules in the basolateral membranes and the activation of potassium channels in the luminal membrane are the predominant mechanisms for the kaliuretic effect of aldosterone.

The activity of spironolactone and spironolactone metabolites does not depend on their filtration or tubular secretion but rather on their plasma concentrations because they act on the capillary side of the collecting tubular cells. They enter the basolateral membrane and interact with the mineralocorticoid cytosolic receptor. However, contrary to what occurs with aldosterone, the interaction of spironolactone with the receptor does not result in the exposure of the high-affinity DNA region. Therefore, spironolactone acts as a specific antagonist of aldosterone (Marver, PNAS, 1974; 71:1431; Cheng, Endocrinol, 1976; 99:1097; Claire, Endocrinol, 1979; 104:1194; Corvol, KidneyInt, 1981; 20:1). This explains why spironolactone is effective in increasing sodium excretion in patients with primary or secondary hyperaldosteronism and in healthy people on a low-sodium diet; however, it has no effect on patients with adrenalectomy or healthy people on a high-sodium diet. The half-life of the aldosterone-induced proteins (sodium channels and Na-K-ATPase molecules) is relatively prolonged, explaining the lag of 2 days between the beginning of spironolactone treatment and the onset of the natriuretic effect. The effective dosage of spironolactone depends on the plasma aldosterone concentration. Patients with moderately increased plasma aldosterone require low doses (100–150 mg/day), but as much as 500 mg/day may be required to antagonize the tubular effect of aldosterone in cases with marked hyperaldosteronism.[100]

The administration of standard doses of loop diuretics to non-azotaemic cirrhotics with ascites gives rise to a good natriuretic response in only 50 per cent of patients (Moult, Gut, 1974; 15: 988).[100,101] The mechanism of this poor diuretic effect is not well established. The bioavailability of frusemide is reportedly normal in cirrhotics with ascites, indicating that the renal resistance to the drug cannot be explained by impaired intestinal absorption (Sawhney, Gastro, 1981; 81:1012). On the other hand, although there is one study that shows impaired tubular secretion of fru-semide in cirrhotics with ascites (Pinzani, Gastro, 1987; 922:294), others suggest that the pharmacokinetics and renal handling of frusemide in such patients are similar to those in healthy individuals (Allgulander, ClinPharmacokin, 1980; 5:570; Keller, EurJClin-Pharm, 1981; 20:27; Sawhney, Gastro, 1981; 81:1012; Gonzalez, EurJClinPharm, 1982; 22:315; Verbeeck, ClinPharmTher, 1982; 31: 719; Traeger, IntJClinPharmacol, 1985; 23:129; Villeneuve, Clin-PharmTher, 1986; 40:14). Therefore, the most likely mechanism for diuretic resistance to frusemide in cirrhosis with ascites is pharmacodynamic in nature; that is, frusemide does not increase sodium excretion either because the delivery of fluid to the loop of Henle is reduced, owing to enhanced proximal sodium reabsorption (Gatta, Hepatol, 1991; 14:231), or because most sodium not re-absorbed in the loop of Henle by the action of frusemide is sub-sequently taken up in the convoluted distal and collecting tubules, owing to secondary hyperaldosteronism. The latter proposal is supported by several studies showing that non-azotaemic cirrhotics with ascites who have renal resistance to frusemide or other loop diuretics are those with higher plasma aldosterone concentrations (Sawhney, Gastro, 1981; 81:1012).[100,101]

Treatment of non-azotaemic cirrhotics with ascites with spiro-nolactone is followed by a good natriuretic response in most patients (Eggert, BMJ, 1970; 4:401; Campra, DigDisSci, 1978; 23:1025). Therefore, contrary to what would be expected on the basis of their intrinsic natriuretic potencies, spironolactone is more effective than frusemide in non-azotaemic cirrhotics with ascites, which was also concluded in the only published, randomized study comparing frusemide with spironolactone in these patients.[100] The most rational treatment of cirrhotics with ascites is spironolactone alone or with frusemide. The simultaneous administration of frusemide and spironolactone increases the natriuretic effect of both drugs and reduces the incidence of the hypo- or hyperkalaemia frequently observed when these agents are given alone.

Two different approaches are commonly employed in the treat-ment of cirrhotic ascites with diuretics. The 'step care' medical treatment consists of progressive implementation of the therapeutic measures currently available.[102–105] Treatment is begun with a low-sodium diet; if there is no response, spironolactone is given at increasing dosage (starting with 100 mg/day) until a satisfactory diuresis is achieved. Where there is no response to the highest dosage of spironolactone (400 mg/day), frusemide is added, also at increasing dosage (40–160 mg/day). A more rapid therapeutic schedule, which may be particularly indicated in patients with tense ascites and avid sodium retention, is the 'combined treat-ment'.[106] It begins with the simultaneous administration of 40 mg/day frusemide and 100 mg/day spironolactone. If there is no response after 4 to 5 days, the dosage is increased stepwise up to 160 mg/day frusemide and 400 mg/day spironolactone. Cases not responding to this programme should be considered to have di-uretic-resistant ascites (see below). The best way to assess the effectiveness of diuretic therapy is by monitoring body weight. The goal of diuretic treatment should be to achieve a weight loss of 300 to 500 mg/day. Once ascites has been mobilized, diuretic treatment should be adjusted to maintain the patient free of ascites. In most non-azotaemic cirrhotics, this can be achieved with low doses of spironolactone (100–200 mg/day). The most important predictor of diuretic response in cirrhotic patients with ascites is the degree of impairment of circulatory and renal function. Patients with a low glomerular filtration rate and/or high plasma concentrations of renin, aldosterone, and noradrenaline require a high diuretic dosage or do not respond to medical treatment.[100,102,104,105]

Several studies have assessed the effect of a new loop diuretic, torasemide, in patients with non-azotaemic cirrhosis and ascites; they suggest that it may be more effective in increasing urine volume and sodium excretion than frusemide, with less kaliuretic effect (Ficcadori, ClinInvest, 1993; 71:579; Cardiol, 1994; 82 (Suppl. 2): 80; Gerbes, JHepatol, 1993; 17:353; Gentilini, CardiovascDrugsRes, 1993; 7 (Suppl. 1):81; Applefeld, AlimPharmTher, 1994; 8:397; Knauf, Cardiol, 1994; 82 (Suppl. 2):87). Amiloride is less effective than potassium canrenone in these patients (Angeli, Hepatol, 1994; 19:72).

A low-sodium diet and 100 mg/day spironolactone in patients with compensated cirrhosis and portal hypertension are associated with a significant decrease of portal pressure, azygos blood flow, and variceal pressure (Okamura, AmJGastr, 1991; 86:46; Katsuta, JHepatol, 1993; 17 (Suppl. 2):S19; García-Pagán, Hepatol, 1994; 19:1095; Nevens, Hepatol, 1996; 23:1047). The percentage decrease in portal pressure is similar to that obtained with propranolol. Since this effect is associated with a decrease in blood volume, an increase in plasma renin activity, aldosterone and noradrenaline, and a fall in atrial natriuretic peptide concentration it is considered secondary to a reduction in effective circulating blood volume. These findings open the question of whether sodium restriction and spironolactone can be given prophylactically in patients with compensated cirrhosis and portal hypertension to prevent or delay the development of gastrointestinal haemorrhage and ascites.

Complications of diuretic treatment in cirrhosis

The use of diuretics in cirrhotics with ascites may be associated with complications related to the effect of these drugs on the kidney and on extrarenal organs. Approximately 20 per cent of these patients develop azotaemia due to depletion of intravascular volume (Rodés, PostgradMedJ, 1975; 55:492). This diuretic-induced renal failure is usually moderate and always reversible after diuretic withdrawal; it is the consequence of an imbalance between the intravascular fluid loss caused by the diuretics and the net passage of fluid (ascites reabsorption minus ascites formation) from the peritoneal cavity into the general circulation (Shear, NEJM, 1970; 282:1391). If diuretic therapy produces a loss of fluid above the net passage of ascitic fluid into the intravascular compartment, a contraction of circulating blood volume and a concomitant decrease of glomerular filtration rate will occur. Interstitial fluid accumulated as oedema is more easily reabsorbed than ascites. This explains why diuretic-induced renal failure occurs less frequently in patients with both ascites and oedema than in those having only ascites.

Hyponatraemia, occasionally severe, is another common complication of diuretic therapy in cirrhotics with ascites (Sherlock, ScaJGastr, 1970; 7 (Suppl.): 9).[107,108] Although the pathogenesis of this abnormality is multifactorial, impairment of the renal ability to excrete free water induced by these drugs is probably the most important mechanism. Free-water formation in the kidney occurs in the ascending limb of the loop of Henle, where sodium chloride is reabsorbed without a concomitant reabsorption of water, leading to hypotonic urine. The second factor in water excretion is ADH, which regulates water reabsorption in the collecting tubules. Loop diuretics inhibit chloride and sodium reabsorption in the ascending limb of the loop of Henle. Moreover, the intravascular volume depletion produced by diuretic therapy increases fluid reabsorption in the proximal tubule, thus diminishing the delivery of sodium chloride to the loop of Henle. Both mechanisms impair the formation of free water in the diluting segment of the nephron. Finally, diuretic-induced hypovolaemia stimulates the release of ADH.

The distal nephron (distal and collecting tubules) plays a critical part in regulating acid balance. Sodium reabsorption in this segment generates a lumen-negative voltage that promotes passive potassium and H^+ excretion into the lumen (Arruda, AmJPhysiol, 1980; 239:F515). In cirrhotics with ascites, the inhibition of sodium reabsorption by spironolactone or other distally acting diuretics, such as triamterene or amiloride, may therefore produce metabolic acidosis (Gabow, AnnIntMed, 1979; 90:338; Batlle, KidneyInt, 1981; 20:389; Hulter, AmJPhysiol, 1981; 240:F381). The administration of loop diuretics alone markedly increases potassium excretion and may produce serious hypokalaemia. This is not due to a specific direct effect on potassium transport but to increased potassium secretion by the distal nephron promoted by a high delivery of fluid to this segment (Good, AmJPhysiol, 1979; 236: F192). Spironolactone, triamterene, and amiloride increase the serum potassium and may produce severe hyperkalaemia when used at high doses. This complication is particularly common in cirrhotics with hepatorenal syndrome. Spironolactone-induced hyperkalaemia is generally considered to be due to a reduction of urinary potassium excretion secondary to the inhibition of distal sodium reabsorption (Gussin, JClinPharm, 1977; 17:651). However, studies on cirrhotics with ascites have shown that spironolactone produces a small but significant increase in potassium excretion (Campra, DigDisSci, 1978; 23:1025; Stergiou; MinElecMetab, 1993; 19:86).[100] An alternative mechanism may be a shift of potassium from the intracellular to extracellular space due to inhibition of the aldosterone effect on internal potassium balance or to metabolic acidosis (Alexander, JCI, 1968; 47:740).

The most important complication of diuretic therapy is hepatic encephalopathy, which has been estimated to occur in approximately 25 per cent of cirrhotic patients admitted to hospital with tense ascites and treated with diuretics.[107,108] Diuretic-induced hepatic encephalopathy was traditionally considered to be secondary to hyperammonaemia because of increased renal ammonia production following diuretic-induced hypokalaemia and alkalosis (Baertl, JCI, 1963; 42:696). However, more recent studies show that some diuretics may also impair the urea cycle, leading to reduced hepatic transformation of ammonia to urea (Häussinger, KlinWschr, 1990; 68:1096). Finally, other more recent studies suggest that in cirrhotic patients with ascites there is an increase in arteriolar vascular resistance in the cerebral circulation that may result in a reduction

in cerebral blood flow (Almdal, ScaJGastr, 1989; 24:299; Dillon, EurJGastroHepatol, 1995; 7:1087). Since cerebral arterial vascular resistance correlates closely with renal vascular resistance in these patients (Guevara, GastroHepato, 1987; 20:86), the hypothetical mechanism of cerebral vasoconstriction in decompensated cirrhosis is arterial vascular underfilling. Since diuretic therapy may impair effective arterial blood volume, a further deterioration of cerebral blood flow could contribute to diuretic-induced hepatic encephalopathy.

Perhaps the most frequent side-effects of spironolactone in cirrhotics with ascites are those related to its antiandrogenic activity. Chronic spironolactone treatment is often associated with decreased libido, impotence, and gynaecomastia in men, and menstrual irregularities in women. The origin of these abnormalities is probably related to alterations in sexual steroid metabolism. At high dosage, spironolactone reduces testosterone biosynthesis and increases the peripheral conversion of testosterone to oestradiol (Loriaux, AnnIntMed, 1976; 85:630). In addition, *in vitro* experiments have shown that spironolactone inhibits the binding of testosterone to the cytosolic and nuclear receptors in the target organs (Carvol, Endocrinol, 1975; 97:52; Rose, AnnIntMed, 1977; 87:398).

Finally, cirrhotic patients treated with diuretics over a long period frequently complain of intense muscle cramps (Konikoff, JClinGastro, 1986; 8:669; Kobayashi, DigDisSci, 1992; 37:1145). They usually appear during the night, affect both the lower extremities and the hands, and disappear rapidly either following assumption of the upright position or spontaneously. The mechanism of diuretic-induced muscle cramps is unknown. They are clearly related to the reduced effective arterial blood volume present in these patients since muscle cramps particularly occur in cases with low mean arterial pressure and high plasma renin activity, and their frequency can be drastically reduced if diuretic treatment is combined with plasma volume expansion with albumin.[109] The oral administration of quinine reduces the frequency of muscle cramps.[110]

Refractory ascites

Although the term of refractory ascites (or intractable ascites, resistant ascites or problematic ascites) was introduced in the 1950s to define ascites not responding to sodium restriction and diuretics, there has been major confusion concerning the use of this term during the last few decades. For this reason the International Ascites Club recently organized a consensus conference to elaborate a new definition and the diagnostic criteria for refractory ascites in cirrhosis.[111] This conference extended the concepts proposed by a consensus conference held in Rome during the 13th International Congress of Gastroenterology in 1988.[112]

According to this organization, 'refractory ascites' is that which cannot be mobilized or the early recurrence of which (i.e., after therapeutic paracentesis) cannot be satisfactorily prevented by medical therapy. Two different subtypes of refractory ascites can be identified:

(1) 'diuretic-resistant ascites' is that which cannot be mobilized or the early recurrence of which cannot be prevented because of a lack of response to dietary sodium restriction and intensive diuretic treatment;

(2) 'diuretic-intractable ascites' is that which cannot be mobilized or the early recurrence of which cannot be prevented because of the development of diuretic-induced complications that preclude the use of an effective diuretic dosage.

The following criteria were considered important for the diagnosis of refractory ascites.

1. Ascites: the term ascites in these definitions refers to grade 2 or 3, clinically detectable ascites (grade 1, mild; grade 2, moderate; grade 3, massive or tense).
2. Mobilization of ascites: decrease of ascites to at least grade 1.
3. Treatment period to define refractory ascites: patients must have been on intensive diuretic treatment for at least 1 week.
4. Lack of response: mean loss of body weight of less than 200 g/day during the past 4 days on intensive diuretic therapy and urinary sodium excretion of less than 50 mEq/day.
5. Dietary sodium restriction: a 50-mEq sodium diet.
6. Intensive diuretic treatment: spironolactone, 400 mg/day, plus frusemide, 160 mg/day (bumetanide, 4 mg/day, or equivalent doses of other loop diuretics).
7. Early ascites recurrence: reappearance of grade 2 to 3 ascites within 4 weeks of initial mobilization; reaccumulation of ascites within 2 to 3 days of paracentesis must not be considered as early recurrence because it represents a shift of interstitial fluid into the intraperitoneal space.
8. Diuretic-induced complications: diuretic-induced hepatic encephalopathy is the development of hepatic encephalopathy in the absence of other precipitating factors. Diuretic-induced renal failure is an increase in serum creatinine by greater than 100 per cent to a value above 2 mg/dl in patients with ascites responding to diuretic treatment. Diuretic-induced hyponatraemia is a decrease in serum sodium by greater than 10 mEq/l to a concentration lower than 125 mEq/l. Diuretic-induced hypo- or hyperkalaemia are, respectively, a decrease of serum potassium to less than 3 mEq/l or an increase to more than 6 mEq/l despite appropriate measures to normalize potassium concentrations.

'Recidivant ascites' is defined as ascites that recurs frequently (on three or more occasions within a 12-month period) despite dietary sodium restriction and adequate diuretic dosage, and is not to be considered as a true refractory ascites.[111]

Most cirrhotics with diuretic-resistant ascites have type II hepatorenal syndrome,[111] or lesser, although significant, degrees of impairment in renal perfusion and glomerular filtration rate (increased serum creatinine to between 1.2 and 1.5 mg/dl) (Arroyo, PostgradMedJ, 1975; 51:558).[95,96,98] It is important to stress that the inverse relation between glomerular filtration rate and serum creatinine concentration is hyperbolic. This means that a small increase in creatinine over normal represents a marked impairment of renal haemodynamics and glomerular filtration rate. The mechanism whereby ascites is resistant to diuretic therapy in cirrhotics with renal failure is probably related to alterations in both the pharmacokinetics and pharmacodynamics. The access of loop diuretics to the organic-acid secretory site, and of spironolactone to the aldosterone receptors, which is mainly determined by the amount of blood flowing to the proximal tubule and distal nephron, respectively (Bratter, Drugs, 1985; 30:427), may be impaired in cirrhotics with functional renal failure due to the low renal perfusion. Moreover, the delivery of sodium chloride to the loop of Henle and distal nephron, the sites where frusemide and spironolactone inhibit sodium reabsorption, may be markedly reduced in cirrhotics with functional renal failure secondary to a low glomerular filtration rate and enhanced sodium reabsorption in the proximal tubule.[102] Therefore, both impaired access of diuretics to the effective sites on the tubular cells, and a reduced substrate for the diuretic action, are presumably the most important mechanisms of refractory ascites in cirrhosis. Additional factors that may contribute to the renal resistance to diuretics in cirrhotics with functional renal failure are hypoalbuminaemia, which reduces the delivery of diuretics to the kidney, and the increased activity of endogenous systems with sodium-retaining effects (renin–angiotensin–aldosterone and sympathetic nervous systems), which may inhibit the natriuretic effect of diuretics.

Non-steroidal anti-inflammatory drugs depress the diuretic response to frusemide and spironolactone in cirrhotics with ascites by a mechanism unrelated to the impairment in renal haemodynamics (Daskalopoulos, AmJKidneyDis, 1985; 6:217).[113,114] Evidence for the possible use of these agents should therefore be carefully sought in any cirrhotic patient not responding to sodium restriction and an adequate diuretic regimen.

Peritoneovenous shunting

In 1974, LeVeen and associates (AnnSurg, 1974; 180:580) introduced the peritoneovenous shunt for the treatment of cirrhotics with diuretic-resistant ascites. This device consists of a perforated intra-abdominal tube connected through a one-way, pressure-sensitive valve to a silicone tube that traverses the subcutaneous tissue up to the neck, where it enters one of the jugular veins (usually the internal jugular) (Fig. 11). The tip of the intravenous tube is located in the superior vena cava near the right atrium or in the right atrium itself. The aim of the shunt is to produce sustained expansion of the circulating blood volume by the continuous passage of ascites from the peritoneal cavity to the general circulation. Whenever a pressure gradient of 3 cmH$_2$O or more exists between the abdominal cavity and the superior vena cava, the valve remains open and ascitic fluid flows into the central venous system. If this gradient diminishes, the valve closes, thus preventing blood from reflushing into the venous limb of the shunt. The insertion of a LeVeen shunt is technically simple and can be performed under local anaesthesia (LeVeen, CurrProbSurg, 1979; 16:5). It is advisable to assess the correct placement of the venous tip by chest radiography in the operating room. Although the LeVeen is the most widely used peritoneovenous shunt, other types are available. The Denver shunt has a valvular system with a pumping mechanism (Lund, ContempSurg, 1979; 14:31).[115] The valvular system opens at low pressure gradients (1 cmH$_2$O) or when the pump chamber, placed in an intercostal space, is externally pressed. The Denver shunt was designed to reduce the high incidence of shunt obstruction observed with the LeVeen. It was thought that the compression of the pump chamber would avoid the formation of thrombi at, and within, the tip of the intravenous segment and the deposition of fibrin within the valve. However, a randomized study comparing LeVeen and Denver shunts in cirrhotics with medically intractable ascites showed a higher probability of shunt obstruction in patients treated

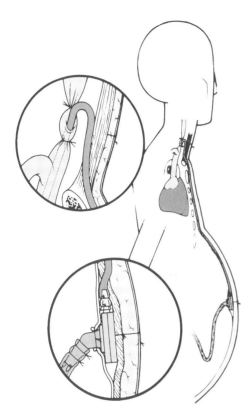

Fig. 11. Schematic drawing of the LeVeen shunt. The valve lies outside the peritoneum and deep to the abdominal muscles. The venous collecting tube traverses the subcutaneous tissue of the chest wall into the neck where it enters the internal jugular vein. The tip of the tubing is pushed into the superior vena cava. The two detailed views illustrate the valve lying subcutaneously and the tip of the venous tube entering the internal jugular vein. (Reproduced by permission from LeVeen, AnnSurg, 1976; 184:574.)

with the Denver, probably as a consequence of the reflux of blood into the valve during the release phase of the pumping cycle (Fulenwider, ArchSurg, 1986; 121:351). To avoid this problem a double-valve Denver shunt was later developed. Whether this new valvular system is effective in preventing shunt obstruction is unknown.

Numerous studies show that the peritoneovenous shunt is capable of correcting most abnormalities thought to be involved in the pathogenesis of ascites. It produces a striking increase of circulating blood volume and cardiac output (Darse, AnnSurg, 1981; 194:189). Since arterial pressure does not rise, there is a concomitant reduction in peripheral vascular resistance. These haemodynamic changes are associated with an increase in the plasma concentration of atrial natriuretic factor and a suppression of the plasma concentrations of renin, aldosterone, noradrenaline, and ADH (Berkowitz, Surgery, 1978; 84:120; Blendis, Gastro, 1979; 77:250; Reznick, Gastro, 1983; 84:713; Blendis, Hepatol, 1987; 7:143; Klepetko, Gastro, 1988; 95:764). Urine volume and free-water clearance increase in most patients, as is seen with the serum sodium in cases with dilutional hyponatraemia (Campbell, JClinNutrGastro, 1986; 1:59).[116] However, there is significant natriuresis in less than half of the patients (Greig, Gastro 1981;80:119). In cirrhotics with moderate functional renal failure, the peritoneovenous shunt may improve renal blood flow and glomerular filtration rate (Walpnick, JAMA,

1977; 237:131; Schroeder, KidneyInt, 1979; 15:54; Schwartz, AmJSurg, 1980; 139:370). Finally, a marked reduction in portal pressure and intrahepatic vascular resistance, as estimated by the wedged-to-free hepatic venous-pressure gradient, has been reported after the insertion of a peritoneovenous shunt (Greig, Gastro, 1981; 80:119; Henriksen, ScaJGastr, 1983; 18:529). The mechanism of this last effect is unknown. Follow-up studies show that these haemodynamic and hormonal changes persist in most cases and that a significant proportion of patients remain with minimal or no ascites despite a moderate sodium restriction and low diuretic dosage. Additionally, the nutritional status, as estimated by the arm-muscle circumference, improved significantly in patients successfully treated with a peritoneovenous shunt (Franco, AmJSurg, 1983; 146:652).

Unfortunately, the procedure is associated with a high rate of complications, which may occur early in the postoperative period or at any time during follow-up (Greig, AmJSurg, 1980; 139:125; Epstein, Gastro, 1982; 82:790; Rubinstein, Gut, 1985; 26:1070; Fulenwider, ArchSurg, 1986; 121:351).[116-118] Acute bacterial infection, generally caused by *Staphylococcus* spp., is the most serious early complication.[116] The prosthesis is usually colonized and in most cases the infection cannot be eradicated unless the shunt is removed. The prophylactic administration of antistaphylococcal antibiotics 24 h before and for 48 h after surgery reduces the incidence of early postoperative infections.[116] Postoperative fever, probably related to the passage of endotoxin contained in the ascitic fluid into the general circulation, is almost inevitable and disappears spontaneously within the second postoperative week.[118] Practically every cirrhotic patient treated with a peritoneovenous shunt develops biochemical signs of intravascular coagulation within the early postoperative period, including a decrease in plasma fibrinogen and platelets, prolongation of prothrombin, thrombin, and partial thromboplastin times, and a rise in the plasma concentrations of fibrin and fibrinogen-degradation products (Harmon, AnnIntMed, 1979; 90:774; Stein, ArchIntMed, 1981; 141:1149; Tawes, AmJSurg, 1981; 142:51; Ragni, AnnSurg, 1983; 198:91; Salem, AmJHematol, 1981; 11:153; Gut, 1983; 24:412). The mechanism of this complication is unknown, but it possibly be secondary to the massive passage of tissue thromboplastin and clotting factors, plasminogen activators, endotoxin, fibrin-split products, and collagen, which are present in the ascitic fluid, into the general circulation. The incidence of symptomatic intravascular coagulation was relatively high (25 per cent) within the years immediately following the introduction of the shunt when the shunt was inserted without prior removal of ascitic fluid. At that time the mortality rate attributed to intravascular coagulation was 5 per cent. However, at present, with the widespread acceptance of the need to evacuate ascitic fluid preoperatively, or during surgery before inserting the shunt, the rate of symptomatic intravascular coagulation after peritoneovenous shunting has decreased dramatically. Some investigators have suggested the removal of all ascitic fluid and its replacement with normal saline before insertion of the prosthesis (Biagini, SGO, 1986; 163:315). Antiplatelet therapy with aspirin (300 mg/day) and dipyridamole (400 mg/day) in the immediate pre- and postoperative periods prevented intravascular coagulation after peritoneovenous shunting (Salem, Gut, 1983; 24:412; Tang, Gastro, 1992; 102:1334). Other postoperative complications, such as bleeding from oesophagogastric varices (Markey, Gastro, 1979; 77:341) and congestive heart failure (Darsee, AnnSurg, 1981; 194:189), which are related to the acute expansion of the circulating blood volume, can also be prevented by reducing the volume of ascitic fluid before inserting the shunt. Postoperative mortality (within the first month after surgery) ranges between 0 and 26 per cent.[116]

Obstruction of the shunt is the most common complication during follow-up (Fulenwider, ArchSurg, 1986; 121:351).[116] It occurs in more than 30 per cent of patients and is usually due to deposition of fibrin within the valve or around the intravenous catheter, thrombotic obstruction of the venous limb of the prosthesis, or thrombosis of the superior vena cava or right atrium initiated at the venous end of the shunt or in damaged endothelium.[116,119] Although the thrombosis of the superior vena cava is usually incomplete, total occlusion may occur, resulting in the development of a superior vena cava syndrome.[119] Vascular thrombosis may result in pulmonary embolism. Obstruction of the shunt is frequently, but not necessarily, followed by reaccumulation of ascites. In these cases, Doppler ultrasonography or $^{99}Tc^m$ scintigraphy after intraperitoneal injection of radioisotope will show the absence of flow through the shunt (Kirchmer, AnnSurg, 1977; 185:145; Metzler, Surgery, 1980; 87:106; JUltrasoundMed, 1994; 13:959). When obstruction is confirmed by these techniques, a shuntogram after the injection of contrast medium into the proximal subcutaneous limb of the shunt should be performed in order to identify its exact site (LeVeen, AnnSurg, 1984; 200:212). Patients with obstruction at the venous limb of the shunt require venography or digital angiography to rule out vascular thrombosis.[119] It has been suggested that the insertion of a titanium tip 3 cm long into the venous end of the LeVeen shunt prevents thrombotic obstruction of its venous limb and the development of thrombosis in the superior vena cava (Hillaire, GastrClinBiol, 1988; 12:681; Surgery, 1993; 113:373). Titanium is highly thromboresistant, a characteristic that has been exploited extensively in intravascular devices such as prosthetic heart valves. The titanium tip was also designed to provide gradual, streamlined, flow convergence of ascites and blood. Finally, the weight and design of the tip may limit endothelial damage and mural thrombus formation in the superior vena cava. Unfortunately, in a study on a large series of patients, Ginès et al. were not able to confirm that the titanium tip reduces the incidence of obstruction in peritoneovenous shunts.[120]

Bacterial infections, particularly bacteraemia and spontaneous peritonitis, are also common complications during follow-up.[116] Bacteraemia can be successfully treated with antibiotics. Early recurrence indicates colonization of the shunt or bacterial endocarditis. Removal of the shunt has been recommended in patients with peritonitis (Wormser, AmJMed, 1981; 70:358), although some have successfully treated patients with bacterial peritonitis without this.[116] To prevent bacterial infections in patients with peritoneovenous shunts, prophylactic antibiotics should be administered whenever an invasive manoeuvre is to be performed.

Finally, another long-term complication of peritoneovenous shunting is small-bowel obstruction, which occurs in approximately 10 per cent of patients (Greenlee, ArchSurg, 1981; 116:518; Kravetz, GastroHepato, 1982; 5:347; Stanley, DigDisSci, 1996; 41:571). The small bowel is compressed and kinked inside multiple 'cocoons' and cysts consequent to marked peritoneal fibrosis. The shunt is usually not ensnared in the fibrosed areas but remains free. The cause is unknown.

Because of the high incidence of shunt-related complications, peritoneovenous shunting should be restricted to patients with refractory ascites. These patients, however, often have endstage liver disease and an extremely poor prognosis, which cannot be modified by successful treatment of ascites. In fact, an overall analysis of the four prospective, randomized trials comparing peritoneovenous shunting with conventional medical treatment in patients with refractory ascites does not disclose any benefit in terms of survival (Wapnick, BrJSurg, 1979; 66:667; Bories, JHepatol, (Suppl.), 1985; 1:23; Ring-Larsen; Hepatol, 1988; 8:S86; Stanley, NEJM, 1989; 321:1632). The role of peritoneovenous shunting in the management of patients with hepatorenal syndrome is also unclear: a beneficial effect has been observed in single cases, but the results obtained in the only two randomized trials published so far seem to indicate that peritoneovenous shunting, although preventing the progression of functional renal failure, does not improve the chances of survival (Daskalopoulos, Gastro, 1985; 88:1655; Linas, KidneyInt, 1986; 30:736). The reintroduction of therapeutic paracentesis has lead to a decline in the use of peritoneovenous shunting (Arroyo, JHepatol, 1994; 21:667). In the two randomized, controlled trials comparing paracentesis with the LeVeen shunt in patients with refractory ascites, shunting was superior in the long-term control of ascites, as estimated by the time to first readmission for ascites, the number of readmissions for ascites, and diuretic requirements.[120,121] However, these advantages had little impact on the natural course of the disease since patients treated in both groups did not differ significantly in their time to first readmission for any reason, total time in hospital during follow-up, and probability of survival. Furthermore, frequent reoperations were required in the surgical group due to shunt obstruction. At present, many groups consider paracentesis to be the treatment of choice in patients with refractory ascites, peritoneous shunting being indicated only in those intolerant of frequent paracentesis. The morbidity and survival of cirrhotics treated with the LeVeen shunt correlate with the degree of impairment of liver and renal function, patients with severe hepatic and renal failure having a higher incidence of complications and lower survival (Turner, AmJSurg, 1982; 144:619; Gleysteen, AmJGastr, 1984; 79:654; Smith, AmJGast, 1984; 79:659). Therefore, the best results with this procedure should be expected in those very few patients with diuretic-resistant ascites and preserved hepatic function.

Therapeutic paracentesis

For many centuries, paracentesis was the only effective way to relieve ascites. However, it was abandoned at the end of the 1950s. Several circumstances led to the decline of paracentesis as a treatment for cirrhotic ascites. The considerable width and length of the trocars used and the insufficiency of the aseptic measures taken during the procedure were the probable cause of the high incidence of local complications (Liebowitz, NYStateJMed, 1962; 62:1822; 1997; 2223). On the other hand, the rapid mobilization of ascites through the wide cannula was associated with disturbances in systemic haemodynamics and renal function (Nelson, JCI, 1951; 30:738). The classic study of Hecker and Sherlock (Lancet, 1956; ii:1221) describing the appearance of renal failure in close chronological relation to therapeutic paracentesis in six patients with cirrhosis was another important factor leading to the abandonment of paracentesis. Finally, with the introduction of frusemide and spironolactone at the beginning of the 1960s, an effective medical treatment for ascites was available. A critical analysis of the literature, however, indicates that the traditional concept that therapeutic paracentesis adversely influences systemic haemodynamics and renal function in cirrhosis was never substantiated by carefully controlled, prospective investigations, but rather by individual observations or studies of only a very few patients. In fact, various studies performed after the 1950s failed to find any major adverse effect in cirrhotic patients treated with large-volume paracentesis (Kowalski, JCI, 1954; 33:768; Gordon, AmJGastr, 1960; 33:15; Knauer, NEJM, 1967; 276:491; Shear, NEJM, 1970; 282:1391; Iwatsuki, Gastro, 1973; 65:294; Guazzi, AmJMed, 1975; 59:165; Carey, CleveClinQ, 1983; 50:397).

Numerous prospective investigations, including 14 randomized, controlled trials, have been published re-evaluating the usefulness of therapeutic paracentesis in the treatment of cirrhotics with ascites. The first study consisted of a controlled trial comparing repeated, large-volume paracentesis (4–6 l/day until the disappearance of ascites) plus intravenous albumin infusion (40 g after each tap) with standard diuretic therapy (frusemide plus spironolactone at increasing doses) in 117 patients with tense ascites and avid sodium retention who were admitted to several hospitals in the Barcelona area.[122] Patients with severe liver impairment (hepatic encephalopathy, serum bilirubin over 10 mg/dl, and prothrombin activity less than 40 per cent) or renal failure (serum creatinine over 3 mg/dl) were excluded. The results (confirmed later by three similar trials in Milan, Barcelona, and Paris)[123-125] showed the following.

1. Paracentesis was more effective than diuretics in eliminating ascites (96.5 compared to 72.8 per cent).
2. Paracentesis plus intravascular-volume expansion did not induce significant changes in hepatic and renal function, serum electrolyte concentrations, cardiac output, plasma volume, plasma renin activity, and plasma concentrations of noradrenaline and ADH in the whole group of 58 patients treated with this procedure nor in the subgroups of patients with functional renal failure (13 cases) or without peripheral oedema (22 cases).
3. The incidence of hyponatraemia, renal impairment, and hepatic encephalopathy was much lower in patients treated with paracentesis (5.1, 3.4, and 10.2 per cent, respectively) than in those receiving diuretics (30, 27, and 29 per cent). Other complications occurred with similar frequency in both groups. The high incidence of hyponatraemia, renal impairment, and encephalopathy in the diuretic group was similar to that reported by Sherlock et al. (41, 34, and 29 per cent), and by Strauss et al. (22, 24, and 27 per cent) in two series of 112 and 100 patients, respectively, with non-azotaemic normonatraemic cirrhosis and ascites treated with a variety of diuretic combinations.[107,108]
4. The duration of the hospital stay and therefore the cost of treatment were lower in patients treated with paracentesis.
5. There were no significant differences in the probability of readmission to the hospital during follow-up, the causes of readmission, the probability of survival, and the causes of death between the two groups of patients.

Another randomized controlled trial, also from the Barcelona group, which was aimed at establishing whether intravenous albumin infusion is necessary in cirrhotic patients treated with large-volume paracentesis, confirmed the efficacy and safety of repeated, large-volume paracentesis combined with intravenous albumin.[126] The inclusion criteria were identical to those of the previous trial. The incidence of hyponatraemia, renal impairment, and hepatic encephalopathy in the group of 52 patients treated with repeated, large-volume paracentesis plus intravenous albumin infusion (3.8, 0, and 11 per cent, respectively) was lower than that reported in patients treated with diuretics. In this group of patients the mobilization of ascites by paracentesis/intravenous albumin was also not associated with significant changes in renal and hepatic function, and in the plasma concentrations of renin and aldosterone. In contrast, the incidence of hyponatraemia (17 per cent) and renal impairment (11 per cent) was significantly higher in the group of 53 patients treated with repeated, large-volume paracentesis without intravenous albumin. In all these patients the mobilization of ascites was associated with a marked increase in the plasma concentrations of renin, indicating an impairment in systemic haemodynamics. This change was also found in a second randomized, controlled trial comparing paracentesis with and without albumin in 35 cirrhotic patients with tense ascites. Following an early decrease in plasma renin immediately after paracentesis, a significant post-treatment increase was observed only in patients not receiving albumin (García-Compean, Liver, 1993; 13:233). A pilot investigation (Simon, Hepatol, 1987; 7:423) in 13 patients with cirrhosis and ascites has confirmed that complete mobilization of ascites by large-volume paracentesis without intravenous albumin infusion increases the activity of the renin–angiotensin system and impairs renal and systemic haemodynamics. These adverse effects have not been observed in patients in whom the ascites was only partially mobilized by paracentesis without colloid replacement (Kao, Hepatol, 1985; 5:403; Pinto, Hepatol, 1988; 8:207).

Whether ascites can be safely mobilized by total paracentesis (complete removal in a single paracentesis session) plus intravenous albumin infusion (6–8 g/l of ascites removed) was investigated in 38 cirrhotics with tense ascites (6 with renal failure and 16 without peripheral oedema).[127] The aim was to assess if cirrhotic patients with tense ascites could be treated in a regimen involving admission to hospital for 1 day only. With the aid of a suction pump, a mean of 10.7 litres of ascites fluid was removed in approximately 1 h and no significant changes were observed in renal and hepatic function or in the plasma concentrations of noradrenaline, renin, and aldosterone over a 6-day period during which patients were kept in hospital but without diuretics. The incidence of hyponatraemia, renal impairment, and hepatic encephalopathy in this series of patients (3, 0 and 10 per cent, respectively) and the clinical course of the disease as estimated by the probability of readmission to hospital, causes of readmission, probability of survival, and causes of death, were similar to those reported by the same group of investigators in patients treated with repeated, large-volume paracentesis.

Five randomized, controlled trials have aimed at investigating whether albumin can be substituted by less expensive plasma expanders (dextran 70, dextran 40, and polygeline) (Planas, Gastro, 1990; 99:1736; Salerno, Hepatol, 1991; 13:707; Fassio, JHepatol, 1992; 14:310; Solá, JHepatol, 1994; 20:282).[128] These five studies have shown that total or repeated, large-volume paracentesis with

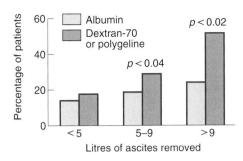

Fig. 12. Incidence of paracentesis-induced circulatory dysfunction in cirrhotic patients with ascites divided according to the volume of ascitic fluid removed and the type of plasma expander used (reproduced by permission from Ginès, Gastro, 1996; 111:1002).

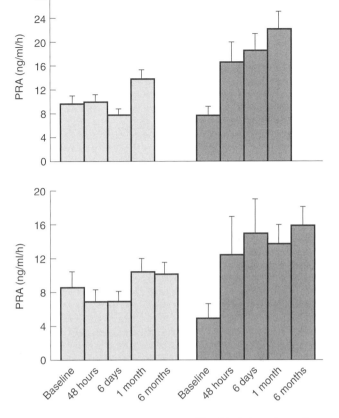

Fig. 13. Plasma renin activity at baseline (B), 48 h, 6 days, 1 month and 6 months (shown only in the lower figure) after discharge from hospital in four series of patients, two including patients who did (shadowed bars) and two who not develop paracentesis-induced circulatory dysfunction (empty bars); data are presented as mean + SEM; *$p<0.02$; **$p<0.001$; ***$p<0.0001$ vs baseline (reproduced by permission from Ginès, Gastro, 1996; 111:1002).

intravenous administration of dextran or polygeline (6–8 g or 125 ml, respectively, per litre of ascitic fluid removed) are not associated with significant changes in renal and hepatic function. The incidence of hyponatraemia, renal impairment, and hepatic encephalopathy after treatment in patients receiving dextran or polygeline (Haemaccel) was similar to that in patients receiving albumin. However, whereas in patients receiving albumin there is no significant change in plasma renin, a significant increase in the degree of activity of the renin–aldosterone system is constantly observed in patients receiving the synthetic plasma expanders, indicating an impairment in circulatory function. The clinical significance of this paracentesis-induced circulatory dysfunction has recently been assessed.[128] Two-hundred and eighty-nine cirrhotic patients admitted to hospital with tense ascites and treated by total paracentesis were randomly treated with intravenous albumin (97 patients), dextran 70 (93 patients), or polygeline (99 patients) at a dose of 8 g/l of ascitic fluid removed. Plasma renin was measured before and 2 and 6 days after treatment in all patients and 1 and 6 months after discharge in most patients. Paracentesis-induced circulatory dysfunction was defined as a 50 per cent increase in plasma renin activity over baseline at the sixth day after treatment up to a value greater than 4 ng/ml per h (upper normal limit). The incidence of the dysfunction was significantly lower in patients treated with albumin (18 per cent) than in those receiving dextran 70 (34 per cent) or polygeline (38 per cent). The only independent predictors of paracentesis-induced circulatory dysfunction were the type of the plasma expander used and the volume of ascitic fluid removed (Fig. 12). When that volume was less than 5 l, the incidence of circulatory dysfunction was similar in patients treated with albumin or with the synthetic plasma expanders. However, when it was greater than 5 l the incidence of circulatory dysfunction was higher in patients receiving dextran 70 or polygeline. Differences were particularly noteworthy when the volume of paracentesis was greater than 9 l. The induced circulatory dysfunction was not spontaneously reversible (Fig. 13) but persisted during the entire follow-up. More importantly, it was associated with more rapid reaccumulation of fluid and readmission for the treatment of tense ascites, and significantly shorter survival (Fig. 14).

The pathogenesis of paracentesis-induced circulatory dysfunction has been investigated by several groups in studies in which ascites was mobilized without plasma-volume expansion (Knauer,

NEJM, 1967; 276:491; Guazzi, AmJMed, 1975; 59:165; Simon, Hepatol, 1987; 7:423; Savino, AnnSurg, 1988; 208:504; Panos, Hepatol, 1990; 11:662; Lucca, Hepatol, 1994; 20:30; 1995; 22:753; Pozzi, Gastro, 1994; 106:709; Wang, JGastHepatol, 1994; 9:592). It is well established that circulatory function improves within the first 12 h after paracentesis, as indicated by a marked increase in cardiac output and stroke volume, a reduction in cardiopulmonary pressures, and suppression of plasma renin activity and aldosterone concentration, and of sympathetic nervous activity. This improvement in circulatory function is probably due to mechanical factors (reduction in intrathoracic pressure and increase in venous return) that improve cardiac function. This early phase is, however, followed by opposing haemodynamic changes, with a reduction in cardiac output and marked activation of the renin–angiotensin and sympathetic nervous systems. Renal function also improves during the first hours after paracentesis and worsens 24 to 48 h after the procedure. Plasma volume does not decrease and the transvascular escape of albumin (an estimate of the passage of fluid from the intra- to extravascular compartments) does not increase after paracentesis in patients developing circulatory dysfunction.[129] In contrast, the increase in plasma renin activity in these patients is closely related

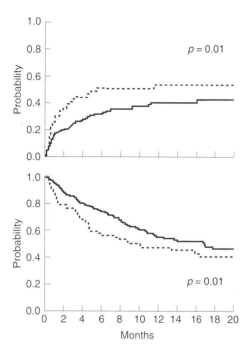

Fig. 14. Probability of readmission to hospital during follow-up for ascites (top) and probability of survival (bottom) in patients who did and did not develop paracentesis-induced circulatory dysfunction (reproduced by permission from Ginès, Gastro, 1996; 111:1002).

to a decrease in systemic vascular resistance.[130] Paracentesis-induced circulatory dysfunction is, therefore, not due to a decrease in circulating blood volume secondary to the rapid reformation of ascites, as it was traditionally considered, but rather to an accentuation of the peripheral arteriolar vasodilation in these patients. The mechanism by which the mobilization of ascites induces a reduction in systemic vascular resistance and why this circulatory dysfunction is prevented by albumin are unknown.

The aim of paracentesis associated with intravenous albumin infusion is the rapid mobilization of ascitic fluid without adverse circulatory effects. However, it does not improve circulatory and renal function. Therefore, patients with tense ascites treated by paracentesis require sodium restriction and diuretics after treatment to prevent the reaccumulation of ascites. The required diuretic dosage depends on the degree of impairment of renal function and diuretic requirements before paracentesis. Patients with normal blood urea nitrogen and serum creatinine require a standard diuretic dosage (150–200 mg/day spironolactone or 100 mg/day spironolactone plus 40 mg/day frusemide).[131] Higher diuretic dosages, however, are required in patients with abnormal blood urea nitrogen or serum creatinine, or in patients with refractory ascites before treatment.

As indicated above, two multicentre, randomized studies comparing repeated, large-volume paracentesis/intravenous albumin with the LeVeen shunt have been reported.[120,121] In these two investigations, 171 patients with refractory ascites (no response to 400 mg/day spironolactone and 160 mg/day frusemide) or recidivant ascites (more than three episodes of ascites within a period of 9 months despite adequate diuretic treatment) were included. Seventy-one patients had renal failure. Eighty-four patients were treated with paracentesis and 87 with the LeVeen shunt (39 with a

titanium tip). The patients were subsequently discharged from hospital with diuretics to avoid reaccumulation of ascites. Cases developing tense ascites during follow-up were treated according to their initial schedule. Both types of treatment were equally effective in mobilizing the ascites. The duration of the first hospital stay was significantly shorter in the paracentesis group than in the shunt group, there being no significant differences between the groups with respect to the proportion of patients developing complications during their stay in hospital or in the number who died. During follow-up a similar number of patients from both groups had to be readmitted to hospital for tense ascites. However, the number of readmissions for ascites (296 compared to 70) was significantly higher in the paracentesis group. In 37 of the 70 readmissions for ascites in the group of patients treated with the LeVeen shunt an obstruction of the prosthesis was recorded, and a new shunt had to be inserted in most cases. Obstruction of the valve was the most common cause of shunt blockage. The probability of shunt obstruction 1 year after the insertion of the prosthesis was 40 per cent. The number of patients readmitted to hospital for other reasons, the total time in hospital during follow-up, and the probability of survival were similar in both groups.

Mobilization of ascites by paracentesis is associated with a marked reduction in portal and variceal pressures, and it has been suggested that it could be of value in the initial management of cirrhotic patients with tense ascites admitted to hospital for the treatment of an episode of variceal bleeding (Lucca, Hepatol, 1994; 20:30; Kravetz, Hepatol, 1997; 25:59). Therapeutic paracentesis is also associated with an improvement of respiratory function (Angueira, Hepatol, 1994; 20:825; Chao, JHepatol, 1994; 20:101). Finally, and contrary to previous suggestions (Runyon, Gastro, 1989; 97:158; Ljubicic, Hepatol, 1994; 19:346), a recent randomized, controlled trial has shown that the treatment of ascites by paracentesis is not associated with an increased incidence of spontaneous bacterial peritonitis during follow-up (Sola, Hepatol, 1995; 21:340).

The following conclusions can be drawn from these investigations.

1. Therapeutic paracentesis, either repeated large-volume or total, combined with intravenous infusion of albumin is a rapid, effective, and safe treatment for ascites in patients with cirrhosis. Since therapeutic paracentesis is associated with a lower incidence of complications than standard diuretic therapy and considerably shortens the time in hospital, it is the first choice for patients with marked sodium retention and tense ascites.

2. The mobilization of ascites by paracentesis without intravenous colloid is almost constantly associated with an impairment in the effective circulating blood volume, as estimated by the plasma concentrations of renin and aldosterone, and induces renal impairment and/or dilutional hyponatraemia in approximately 20 per cent.

3. The incidence of this paracentesis-induced circulatory dysfunction is significantly lower in patients treated with albumin than in those receiving the less expensive synthetic plasma expanders dextran 40, dextran 70, and polygeline. Paracentesis-induced circulatory dysfunction is a clinically relevant disorder since it is not spontaneously reversible and is associated with an increased probability of ascites recurrence and shorter survival.

Albumin is therefore the best plasma expander for cirrhotic patients with tense ascites treated by paracentesis.

4. Therapeutic paracentesis does not improve systemic and renal haemodynamics or sodium retention. Therefore, cirrhotic patients treated with paracentesis require diuretics to avoid reaccumulation of ascites.

5. Although the LeVeen shunt is more effective than therapeutic paracentesis in preventing the reaccumulation of ascites in cirrhotics with refractory ascites, a high proportion of patients treated with the shunt need reoperation due to its obstruction. The total time in hospital during follow-up and the probability of survival are identical with both therapeutic procedures. Therefore, therapeutic paracentesis is an alternative treatment to peritoneovenous shunting in cirrhotics with refractory ascites.

6. All studies on therapeutic paracentesis have excluded cirrhotics with severe liver and renal failure. The safety of paracentesis in this subset of patients is therefore still unknown.

Although paracentesis is a very simple procedure, several precautions should be taken to avoid local complications. It is advisable to perform paracentesis under strict sterile conditions. The abdomen should be cleaned, disinfected, and draped in a sterile fashion, and the physician should wear a sterile gown, gloves, mask, and cap during the entire procedure. We use a modified Küss needle, which is a sharp-pointed, blind, metal needle within a 7-cm long, 17G, metal, blunt-edged cannula with side holes (Fig. 15). Similar needles are now available commercially. Under local anaesthesia, the Küss needle is inserted into the left lower abdominal quadrant. Once the needle has entered the peritoneal cavity, the inner part is removed and the cannula is connected to a large-volume suction pump. The physician remains at the bed side throughout the treatment. With this technique, the duration of treatment ranges from 20 to 90 min depending on the amount of ascitic fluid removed. In cases submitted to total paracentesis, the procedure is finished when the flow from the cannula becomes intermittent despite gentle mobilization of the cannula within the abdominal cavity and turning the patient on to the left side. After paracentesis, patients should recline for 2 h on the side opposite to the paracentesis site to prevent leakage of ascitic fluid. Samples of ascitic fluid should be routinely taken for cell counts, biochemical examination, and culture. The intravenous administration of albumin is begun at the end of the procedure. Peripheral oedema rapidly reabsorbs after the mobilization of ascites in most patients and usually disappears within the first 2 days after treatment.[122, 123,126,127] Most of this fluid goes to the intraperitoneal cavity in the form of ascites. It is, therefore, not uncommon for patients with massive peripheral oedema to require a second paracentesis to remove the fluid shifted from the interstitial space to the intraperitoneal compartment.

Surgical portacaval anastomosis and transjugular intrahepatic portacaval shunt

Ascites and its complications (hepatorenal syndrome and spontaneous bacterial peritonitis) are rare in cirrhotic patients submitted to end-to-side portacaval anastomosis for the treatment of variceal bleeding (Castells, Hepatol, 1994; 20:584), and the surgical relief of portal hypertension, either by end-to-side or side-to-side portacaval

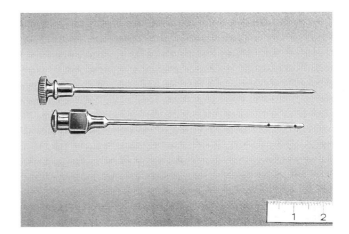

Fig. 15. Modified Küss needle used for paracentesis.

anastomosis, is an apparently effective treatment for ascites. It is therefore not surprising that portacaval anastomosis has been proposed as a treatment for refractory ascites. In 1970, Orloff (AnnNYAcadSci, 1970; 170:213), reviewing the literature on the surgical treatment of ascites, was able to collect data for 71 cirrhotics with ascites treated with end-to-side portacaval anastomoses and for 131 patients treated with side-to-side portacaval shunts. In most of these cases, ascites was refractory to diuretic treatment. Twenty-three patients treated with end-to-side shunts (32 per cent) and 24 treated with side-to-side anastomoses (18 per cent) died in the postoperative period. Of the surviving patients, 39 (81 per cent) in the end-to-side group and 100 (90 per cent) in the side-to-side group remained free of ascites during a follow-up period ranging from months to more than 10 years, despite a normal sodium diet and no diuretics. Subsequently, it was shown that, in cirrhotics treated with end-to-side portacaval shunts, the development of ascites during follow-up usually occurs in those cases who maintain a relatively high sinusoidal pressure and hepatic arterial blood flow (Nagoya, JMedSci, 1973; 35:133). More recently, Franco *et al.* (GastrClinBiol, 1983; 7:533) reported their experience with 41 patients submitted to side-to-side or end-to-side portacaval anastomoses for the treatment of refractory ascites. Almost all these patients had previously been treated with a LeVeen shunt that had to be removed because of complications such as thrombosis of the superior vena cava, infections, or gastrointestinal haemorrhage. The operative mortality (within 2 months of surgery) was exceptionally low (2 patients, 4.8 per cent), probably in relation to the relatively well-preserved hepatic function presented by most cases. Every patient reaccumulated ascites in the immediate postoperative period and 12 developed renal failure. However, ascites and renal impairment disappeared a few days after the operation in all but two cases. Only one of the survivors developed ascites during follow-up. The probability of survival 1 and 3 years after surgery was 73 and 39 per cent, respectively. The incidence of severe chronic hepatic encephalopathy (36 per cent), however, was very high. Other studies have shown that side-to-side portacaval shunting may be followed by a return to normal renal function in patients with hepatorenal syndrome (Schroeder, AnnIntMed, 1970; 72:923; KidneyInt, 1979; 15:54). The disappearance of ascites and renal failure in patients treated with portocaval shunts is associated with a return to normal plasma concentrations of renin and aldosterone. These data suggest that, although portacaval anastomosis is an effective treatment for refractory ascites in patients with cirrhosis and preserved hepatic function, it is associated with a high postoperative mortality and a high incidence of incapacitating chronic hepatic encephalopathy. Since no controlled trials have compared the portacaval shunt with other treatments such as the LeVeen shunt or therapeutic paracentesis, its role in the management of refractory ascites is unconfirmed. Nevertheless, it is important to point out that only a few patients with refractory ascites are suitable candidates for surgical portacaval shunts since they usually present with a severe hepatic insufficiency that precludes any major surgical procedure.

The development of the transjugular intrahepatic portacaval shunt (**TIPS**) for the treatment of gastrointestinal haemorrhage in cirrhosis has reintroduced the idea of treating ascites and its complications (hepatorenal syndrome and refractory ascites) by reducing portal pressure. TIPS can be performed in an angiography room within less than 2 h under conscious sedation. The complications associated with the surgical procedure, which were of great importance in cirrhotic patients with ascites treated by end-to-side or side-to-side portacaval anastomosis, can now be avoided by using this percutaneous technique. Numerous uncontrolled studies have been published assessing the effectiveness of TIPS in patients with refractory ascites (Ferral, Radiol, 1993; 189:795; Ochs, NEJM, 1995; 332:1192; Quiroga, Hepatol, 1995; 21:986; Somberg, Hepatol, 1995; 21:709; Wong, AnnIntMed, 1995; 122:816). TIPS functions as a side-to-side portacaval anastomosis. It reduces portal pressure and hepatic blood flow. In cirrhotic patients with ascites, TIPS reduces plasma renin activity and plasma aldosterone and norepinephrine concentrations, increases sodium excretion, and reduces the diuretic requirements. In fact, many patients can be maintained without ascites despite a normal sodium intake and no diuretic dosage. Some studies show that it may also improve renal function in patients with hepatorenal syndrome (Alam, Gastro, 1995; 108:1024A; Ochs, NEJM, 1995; 332:1192; Bresing, Gastro, 1996; 110:A1158). As expected, the main problem is hepatic encephalopathy after treatment, which may range from 15 to 75 per cent (Sanyal, Hepatol, 1994; 20:46). Although in many cases the encephalopathy can be controlled by medical therapy, in some it is associated with marked impairment in hepatic function and does not respond to treatment. TIPS has the additional problem of a high rate of shunt malfunction due to stenosis of the stent lumen or the segment of hepatic vein connecting with the prosthesis (Freedman, SemInterventRadiol, 1994; 11:161; Shiffman, Hepatol, 1995; 22:1591; Rössle; JHepatol, 1996; 25:224).

In the only randomized, controlled trial so far published comparing paracentesis/intravenous albumin with TIPS in patients with refractory ascites, TIPS was associated with a significant reduction in survival.[132] A second trial published in abstract form showed no difference in survival between patients with refractory ascites treated by paracentesis/albumin or TIPS (Ochs, Hepatol, 1995; 22:297A). Clearly more studies are needed before advocating the widespread use of TIPS for the treatment of refractory ascites or hepatorenal syndrome in cirrhosis (Arroyo, JHepatol, 1996; 25:221).

Other therapeutic approaches for ascites

Although some studies showed that expansion of the circulating blood volume with a salt-poor albumin infusion improves renal

haemodynamics, sodium retention, and the renal response to diuretics in patients with cirrhosis (McCoy, Gastro, 1967; 53:229; Reynolds, Medicine, 1967; 46:191), this procedure is of little value in the management of ascites. The cost of albumin for intravenous infusion is very high and its benefits are only short-lived. The half-life of radiolabelled human serum albumin in cirrhosis is approximately 4 weeks (Wilkinson, ClinSci, 1963; 25:281; Boyer, AmJMedSci, 1969; 257:32).

Paracentesis with reinfusion of unmodified or concentrated ascitic fluid into a peripheral vein has been used for the treatment of refractory ascites for more than 30 years (Kaiser, ArchSurg, 1962; 85:763; Pearlman, Surgery, 1967; 62:248; Eknoyan, NEJM, 1970; 282:713). In the 1970s, Levy et al. (PostgradMedJ, 1975; 51:564) designed a machine (Rhodioascit) that aspirates the ascitic fluid through a catheter located in the peritoneal cavity, concentrates this fluid by pressure ultrafiltration, and then reinfuses it into the central venous system, discharging the ultrafiltrate containing low molecular-weight substances (no proteins) (Smart, JClinNutrGastro, 1988; 3:10). Monitoring of the central venous pressure is necessary to avoid cardiovascular complications, and the procedure ranges from 4 h to more than 12 h depending on the volume of ascites and the patient's tolerance. The Rhodioascit machine was rather popular in Europe for the treatment of refractory ascites during the 1970s. However, it is now rarely used because it offers no advantages over therapeutic paracentesis associated with plasma-volume expansion and can induce serious complications, particularly pulmonary oedema, peritonitis, intravascular coagulation, and gastrointestinal haemorrhage (Arroyo, PostgrMedJ, 1975; 51:571; Davidson, PostgrMedJ, 1975; 51:583). Nevertheless, during the last few years, there have been several investigations published on treating patients with cirrhosis and refractory ascites by paracentesis and reinfusion of concentrated ascitic fluid using different methods of concentration (Tang, Gastro, 1992; 102:1344; Rossaro, DigDisSci, 1993; 38:903; Bernardi, JHepatol, 1994; 20:289). Moreover, two randomized, controlled trials have shown that paracentesis plus intravenous reinfusion of concentrated ascitic fluid is as effective and safe as paracentesis plus intravenous albumin infusion in patients with refractory ascites (Smart, JHepatol, 1990; 10:191; Bruno, BMJ, 1992; 304:1655). Nevertheless, it is easier and less expensive to infuse albumin than to concentrate and reinfuse the ascitic fluid.

An alternative approach to the patient with refractory ascites has been ultrafiltration of ascitic fluid with reinfusion of the concentrate into the peritoneal cavity (Raju, AmJGastr, 1984; 79:308; Landini, IntJArtifOrg, 1985; 8:277; Cadranel, IntJArtifOrg, 1992; 15:432). This procedure was designed to remove salt and water from the peritoneal cavity with no loss of proteins and with no risk of overloading the circulating volume. It involves the insertion of two catheters or a single double-lumen catheter into the peritoneal cavity, the removal of the ascitic fluid through one of the catheters by means of a roller pump, the circulation of this fluid through an ultrafilter, and the reinfusion of the concentrated, protein-rich, ascitic fluid into the abdominal cavity. Heparin has to be given intraperitoneally to prevent the formation of fibrin clots within the ultrafilter. Other methods proposed for the removal of fluid in patients with refractory ascites are intermittent haemodialysis, slow continuous ultrafiltration, continuous arteriovenous ultrafiltration, and continuous arteriovenous haemodialysis.[133] The aggressiveness of these procedures, their high cost, and their potential complications, make them inadvisable.

Treatment of hyponatraemia in cirrhosis with ascites: aquaretic drugs

Dilutional hyponatraemia is the most common abnormality of serum electrolytes in patients with cirrhosis and ascites. It is usually asymptomatic, even in patients with a markedly reduced serum sodium. On the other hand, the presence of hyponatraemia does not contraindicate diuretic treatment in patients with cirrhosis and ascites (Arroyo, AmJDigDis, 1976; 21:249). In fact, most cirrhotics with ascites and hyponatraemia respond satisfactorily to diuretics without a further reduction in serum sodium. Therefore, the use of aggressive procedures for the treatment of hyponatraemia in cirrhosis, such as the insertion of a LeVeen shunt, is not justified. Studies using isotopic techniques have shown that total body sodium is markedly increased in cirrhotic patients with ascites and hyponatraemia, indicating that the reduced serum sodium is the result of a dilution of body fluids secondary to the impairment of free-water excretion (Talso, Metabolism, 1956; 5:58; Leaf, NEJM, 1962; 267:77). Consequently, the treatment of hyponatraemia should be directed toward reducing total body water. The administration of sodium may produce a transient increase in serum sodium but at the expense of increasing the rate of ascites formation. Classically, the treatment of dilutional hyponatraemia consisted of water restriction. However, this therapy is difficult to carry out and is rarely effective. Demeclocycline, a tetracycline that inhibits the tubular effect of ADH, has been shown to correct water retention and hyponatraemia in cirrhotics with ascites, but its usefulness in these patients is limited by the high incidence of renal failure it produces (Carrilho, AnnIntMed, 1977; 87:195; Perez-Ayuso, Nephron, 1984; 36:30). It is interesting that demeclocycline does not produce renal failure in other conditions associated with non-osmotic hypersecretion of ADH. Decaux *et al.* (Nephron, 1986; 44:337) reported that the administration of urea (30–90 g/day) to five patients with refractory ascites and dilutional hyponatraemia was associated with an improvement in the renal response to diuretics and an increase in serum sodium. Further studies are necessary to confirm these findings.

During the last two decades a great effort has been made to develop specific antagonists of the tubular effect of ADH that could act as aquaretic agents and be used for the treatment of dilutional hyponatraemia in cirrhosis with ascites, and in congestive heart failure. The initial approach was to develop analogues of the ADH molecule with affinity for the V_2 receptors but lacking hydro-osmotic activity (Sawyer, ISIAtlasSci:Pharmacol, 1988; 2:252). Unfortunately, although several peptides with aquaretic activity in experimental animals were developed, they disclosed ADH agonistic activity when given to humans (Dubb, KidneyInt, 1987; 31:267; Thibonnier, HormRes, 1990; 34:124). It is interesting that the administration of one of these analogues to rats with carbon tetrachloride-induced cirrhosis, ascites, and dilutional hyponatraemia was associated with a normalization of renal water metabolism with polyuria and an increase in free-water excretion (Clària, Gastro, 1989; 97:1294). The investigation of non-peptidic substances with

aquaretic effects has had very promising results and several types of aquaretic agents have been developed that are effective in experimental animals as well as in man.

The first renal ADH antagonist identified was a benzazepine derivative named OPC-31260 (Yamamura, BrJPharmacol, 1992; 105:787), which is 100 times more selective for V_2 receptors than for V_1 receptors. It is active after oral and intravenous administration, has no agonistic effect, and increases the urine volume in normal rats and in rats treated with ADH without increasing urinary solute excretion, but not in Brattleboro rats with congenital diabetes insipidus. In normal man (Onishi, JCI, 1993; 92:2653; JPharmExpTher, 1995; 272:546), OPC-31260 also induces a marked increase in urine volume (it may be as high as that obtained with frusemide) with a decrease in urine osmolality towards very low values (it may reach concentrations below 100 mosmol/kg), resulting in a remarkable increase in free water, with minor effects in electrolyte excretion. The peak effects on urine volume and osmolality are observed between 1 and 2 h and last for 4 h. With the highest single dose used in normal individuals the aquaretic effect is so marked that it is associated with a significant increase in serum osmolality and sodium. The plasma ADH also increases in these individuals. OPC-31260 was aquaretic and increased serum sodium and osmolality in acute studies on rats with carbon tetrachloride-induced cirrhosis with ascites (Tsuboi, KidneyInt, 1994; 46:237) and in human cirrhosis with ascites.[134] However, long-term therapeutic studies are still not available. Other non-peptide V_2 antagonists have been developed and are currently being investigated.

A second type of aquaretic agents that may be relevant for the treatment of dilutional hyponatraemia in oedematous conditions are the κ-opioid agonists (ketazocine, ethylketazocine, bremazocine, R-84760, E-2078, U-62,066E, CI-997, and RU-51599), which increase urine volume in man and experimental animals with a reduction in urine osmolality and without changes in electrolyte excretion (Leander, JPharmExpTher, 1983; 224:89; 1983; 227:35; Rathbun, PharmBiochBehav, 1983; 19:863; Salas, JPharmExpTher, 1989; 250:992; 1992; 262:979; Fujibayashi, EurJPharm, 1994; 261:133). The mechanism of this aquaretic effect is complex but clearly mediated through κ-receptors since it is blocked by κ-opioid receptor antagonists (Yamada, EurJPharm, 1989; 160:229). The κ-opioid agonists act on the central nervous system, inhibiting the release of ADH from the neurohypophysis (Slizgi, JPharmExpTher, 1982; 220:585; Leander, JPharmExpTher, 1983; 224:89; 1983; 227:35; Bicknell, JPhysiol, 1987; 388:9P; Salas, JPharmExpTher, 1989; 250:992; Yamada, EurJPharm, 1989; 160:229). The observation that these substances increase urine flow in the isolated perfused kidney suggests the existence of a local, intrarenal mechanism of action. The efficacy of κ-opioid agonists in the treatment of water retention in human and experimental cirrhosis was recently evaluated by Bosch-Marcé (Gastro, 1995; 109:217) and by Gadano (Hepatol, 1996; 24:448A). The acute subcutaneous administration of RU-51599 (niravoline) to rats with cirrhosis, ascites, and impaired free-water excretion was associated with normalization of renal water metabolism. The plasma concentrations of ADH decreased after the administration of the drug but did not reach normal values The acute intravenous administration of RU-51599 to patients with cirrhosis and ascites induced a marked (five to seven times) increase in urine volume during the first 2 to 3 h, associated with a reduction of urine osmolality to values lower than plasma osmolality and a significant increase in serum sodium. Personality disorders and mild confusion were detected in only two of the eight patients treated and disappeared within 8 h.

There is only one study assessing the effect of these aquaretic drugs given long term (10 days). This is a comparative study of OPC-31260 and RU-51599 in rats with experimental cirrhosis (Bosch-Marcé; GastroHepato, 1997; 20 (Suppl. 1):11). The aquaretic effect of OPC-31260 was transitory, occurring only during the first 2 days. In contrast, RU-51599 showed an aquaretic effect throughout the whole study period. There are no such studies recorded in humans.

Treatment of hepatorenal syndrome

Since the mechanism of hepatorenal syndrome in cirrhosis is intense vasoconstriction of the renal arteries mediated by endogenous vaso-active systems, several attempts have been made to reverse this syndrome pharmacologically. The intrarenal infusion of non-spe-cific vasodilators such as acetylcholine and papaverine improved renal blood flow but not the glomerular filtration rate in cirrhotic patients with hepatorenal syndrome (Conn, MedAnnualDC, 1970; 39:1). Similar results have been obtained after the stimulation of renal dopaminergic receptors by the infusion of non-pressor doses of dopamine (Barnardo, Gastro, 1970; 58:524; Bennett, ArchIntMed, 1975; 135:964; Wilson, JAMA, 1977; 25:2719). The pharmacological blockade of vasoconstrictor α-adrenergic nerves by the intrarenal infusion of phentolamine or phenoxybenzamine, or the stimulation of vasodilator, β-adrenergic nerves with isoproterenol, also have no significant effect on the glomerular filtration rate in these patients (Epstein, AmJMed, 1970; 49:175). In the only study on cirrhotic patients with hepatorenal syndrome using the angiotensin II-block-ing agent saralasin, the renal plasma flow and glomerular filtration rate failed to increase.[135] In this study, however, the hypotensive effect of saralasin infusion could have masked a possible vasodilating effect of angiotensin II blockade on the renal circulation. Neither did the blockade of the renin–angiotensin system with the angiotensin-converting enzyme inhibitor captopril produce any improvement of renal blood flow and glomerular filtration rate in cirrhotics with ascites and impaired renal perfusion (Bataille, Gastro, 1984; 86:129; Lobden, JClinGastro, 1985; 7:354). Finally, no beneficial effects on renal function have been observed after the intrarenal infusion of prostaglandins E₁, E₂, and A₁ in cirrhotics with functional renal failure (Arieff, AmJMed, 1974; 56:695; Zusman, Prostagl, 1977; 13:819; Ginès, JHepatol, 1993; 220:1993). The pathogenesis of functional renal failure in cirrhosis is very complex, and many factors operate simultaneously to cause renal vasoconstriction in these patients. It is therefore not surprising that the pharmacological manipulation of only one of these factors fails to reverse this syndrome. Solis-Herruzo et al. (JHepatol, 1987; 5:167) have shown that lumbar sympathetic blockade by local anaesthesia produces a transitory improvement in creatinine clearance in cirrhotics with functional renal failure. This manoeuvre theoretically suppresses the renal sympathetic nervous activity and the adrenergically me-diated, intrarenal generation of angiotensin II.

A more rational approach to the treatment of functional renal failure is by improving the haemodynamic disturbance responsible for the activation of the endogenous vasoconstrictor systems in cirrhosis. This has been attempted by the intravenous ad-ministration of vasopressin analogues, which have a potent vaso-constrictor activity upon the splanchnic circulation, with little vasoconstrictor effect in the renal circulation. The first of these studies was performed some 30 years ago by Cohn et al. (Circul, 1968; 38:151), who infused the synthetic analogue of vasopressin, octapressin, in patients with decompensated cirrhosis without hep-atorenal syndrome. Low doses (0.004–0.02 U/min) increased renal blood flow, reduced renal vascular resistance, and produced a slight increase in arterial pressure and systemic vascular resistance in these patients. The fraction of the cardiac output delivered to the kidney was increased at all dose concentrations. These observations were later confirmed by Kew et al. (Gut, 1972; 13:293). More recently, Lenz et al. (Gut, 1989; 30:90; Gastro, 1991; 101:1060) investigated the effect of another vasopressin analogue, 8-ornithine vasopressin (ornipressin), on renal function in patients with cirrhosis and ascites and a creatinine clearance of less than 45 ml/min. The intravenous administration of ornipressin, at a dose of 6 IU/h over a period of 4 h, was associated with a reduction in cardiac output and heart rate, and an increase in arterial pressure and peripheral vascular resistance to almost normal. This was associated with a marked suppression of the plasma concentrations of renin and noradrenaline (which did not reach normal values), and a significant increase in urine volume and sodium excretion. Although creatinine clearance increased significantly, the magnitude of the change was clinically irrelevant. The achievement of normal arterial pressure following the acute administration of other vasoconstrictor drugs, such as angiotensin II and noradrenaline, in this type of patient is also associated with an increase in urine volume and sodium excretion (Lianos, KidneyInt, 1982; 21:70; Laragh, JCI, 1963; 42:1179). However, these agents do not increase either renal plasma flow or the glomerular filtration rate. The combined administration of vasoconstrictors (ornipressin or noradrenaline) and renal vaso-dilators (dopamine, prostacyclin) also fails to improve renal function in patients with hepatorenal syndrome (Saló, JHepatol, 1996; 25: 916). These data therefore suggest that the acute administration of systemic vasoconstrictors alone or associated with renal vasodilators, although it markedly improves systemic haemodynamics and sup-presses the endogenous vasoconstrictor systems, does not reverse hepatorenal syndrome.

One of the major problems in a critical analysis of the role of pharmacological treatment in hepatorenal syndrome is that most studies consist of acute investigations in which renal function is measured before and during a few hours of drug infusion whereas it may be that the syndrome requires longer periods of treatment to be reversed. This possibility is suggested by recent investigations assessing the effect of plasma-volume expansion plus vasoactive drugs over longer periods of time. Fevery et al. (JHepatol, 1990; 11: 153) have shown that suppression of the renal vasoconstrictor systems by expanding the plasma volume with albumin together with the oral administration of the prostaglandin E₁ analogue misoprostol for 5 to 12 days reversed hepatorenal syndrome in four cirrhotic patients with ascites. This beneficial effect was largely due to the volume expansion since the long-term administration of misoprostol alone does not affect renal function in patients with hepatorenal syndrome (Ginès, JHepatol, 1993; 17:220). A very recent study (Guevara, GastroHepato, 1997; 20 (Suppl. 1):12) shows complete normalization of plasma renin activity, plasma aldosterone and noradrenaline, and serum creatinine in 12 patients with severe hepatorenal syndrome after 2 weeks of treatment with ornipressin and albumin infusion. Renin and noradrenaline were normalized within the first 3 days of treatment, but at this time no significant changes in creatinine clearance were observed. It is possible that some intrarenal mechanisms, which could be activated by renal ischaemia, (i.e., increased intrarenal release of adenosine and endothelin and decreased intrarenal synthesis of prostaglandins and nitric oxide synthase), and which might be critical in the maintenance of renal vasoconstriction and in the pathogenesis of hepatorenal syndrome, require longer periods of treatment to be deactivated.

Several published studies have evaluated peritoneal dialysis and haemodialysis in the treatment of patients with functional renal failure and their results have been uniformly disappointing (Jacobson, MedClinNAm, 1973; 57:1569; Ring-Larsen, ScaJGastr, 1973; 8:33; Wilkinson, ClinNephrol, 1977; 8:287). In these a total of 35 cirrhotic patients with severe functional renal failure were treated with peritoneal dialysis and only one survived. Of 32 patients treated with haemodialysis by five different groups of investigators, only four survived.[136] Haemodialysis was frequently associated with serious complications, such as gastrointestinal haemorrhage and severe arterial hypotension.

Drug-induced renal impairment in cirrhosis

Antibiotics

Patients with cirrhosis and ascites are predisposed to aminoglycoside nephrotoxicity, the reported incidence of which (32 per cent) (Cabrera, Gastro, 1982; 82:97) is much higher than that found by other investigators in the general population (3–11 per cent). In that study, aminoglycoside nephrotoxicity was associated with a marked deterioration of renal function. A study of the risk factors in aminoglycoside toxicity found that the presence of liver disease was an independent predictor of nephrotoxicity (Moore, Lancet, 1978; ii:604). The mechanism of this high incidence of aminoglycoside nephrotoxicity in cirrhosis is not known. In the study by Cabrera et al., gentamicin or tobramycin were administered in association with cephalothin, which is known to increase the nephrotoxicity of aminoglycosides (Wade, Lancet, 1978; ii:604). However, this was not the case in the study of Moore et al. Another possibility is that patients with decompensated cirrhosis are prone to develop this complication; they frequently have impaired renal blood flow and glomerular filtration rates, and renal accumulation of aminoglycosides is greater with renal impairment (Chiu, AntimicrobAgentsChemother, 1978; 14:214). Cabrera et al. found that aminoglycoside nephrotoxicity was five times more frequent in patients with renal failure before treatment than in those with a normal baseline serum creatinine.

The diagnosis of aminoglycoside nephrotoxicity in cirrhotics with serious infection is difficult because these patients may also develop functional renal failure. The determination of urinary sodium concentration, fractional sodium excretion, and urine: plasma osmolality and creatinine ratios is not useful in differentiating functional renal failure from acute tubular necrosis in cirrhotic patients with ascites (Cabrera, Gastro, 1982; 82:97;

Diamong, AnnIntMed, 1982; 96:597; Dudley, Hepatol, 1986; 6: 248). The differential diagnosis, however, is of clinical importance. Aminoglycosides must be interrupted when nephrotoxicity develops, whereas careful dosage adjustment is necessary in the presence of functional renal failure. Furthermore, dialysis is indicated in cirrhotics with acute tubular necrosis but not in patients with functional renal failure. The measurement of other urinary markers of tubular damage, such as β_2-microglobulin and tubular enzymes, may help in differentiating these disorders (Gatta, EurJClinInv, 1981; 11:239; Cabrera, Gastro, 1982; 81:97; Solis-Herruzo, JHepatol, 1986; 3:123). The urinary concentration of β_2-microglobulin in alcoholic cirrhotics with superimposed acute alcoholic hepatitis, severe renal failure, and deep jaundice (serum bilirubin greater than 20 mg/dl) may be similar to that commonly observed in acute tubular necrosis, suggesting a spontaneous development of tubular damage in these patients (Rector, Hepatol, 1985; 5:321). Therefore, urinary β_2-microglobulin and tubular enzymes may not be useful in the diagnosis of aminoglycoside nephrotoxicity in patients with terminal hepatic and renal failure.

Non-steroidal anti-inflammatory drugs

The initial studies showing that patients with cirrhosis and ascites develop renal failure after cyclo-oxygenase inhibition with nonsteroidal anti-inflammatory drugs (NSAIDs) were made almost 20 years ago (Boyer, Gastro, 1979; 77:215; Zipser, JClinEndoc, 1979; 48:895; Arroyo, EurJClinInv, 1983; 13:271). The first group of investigators observed that the oral administration of indomethacin (50 mg every 6 h for a total of four doses) produced a significant reduction of renal plasma flow and glomerular filtration rate in a large series of cirrhotics with ascites, but not in patients without ascites. Zipser et al. gave indomethacin (200 mg for 1 day) or ibuprofen (2 mg for 1 day) to 12 cirrhotics with ascites and 8 normal individuals; both drugs induced a marked decrease of urinary prostaglandin E_2 excretion and of creatinine clearance in all patients, but in normal individuals they caused no change in creatinine clearance. Finally, Arroyo et al. gave an intravenous bolus of 450 mg lysine acetylsalicylate (equivalent to 250 mg acetylsalicylic acid) to 5 normal individuals, 9 cirrhotics who had never had ascites, and 19 cirrhotics with ascites; it did not alter renal function in normal individuals and cirrhotics without ascites, but it reduced the glomerular filtration rate in 11 of the 19 patients with ascites. Urinary prostaglandin E_2 was decreased in all individuals after lysine acetylsalicylate. In these three studies the degree of impairment of renal function after NSAIDs correlated with baseline values of urine sodium excretion and plasma renin and noradrenaline; patients with lower sodium excretion and higher plasma renin activity and noradrenaline concentrations developed greater reductions of renal plasma flow and glomerular filtration rate. These studies therefore indicate that cirrhotics with increased activity of the renin–angiotensin and sympathetic nervous systems and marked sodium retention are especially predisposed to develop renal failure after cyclo-oxygenase inhibition. The results of these three studies have been confirmed by subsequent investigations in cirrhotic patients with ascites receiving indomethacin, naproxen, lysine acetylsalicylate, and sulindac (Lianos, KidneyInt, 1982; 21:70; Mirouze, Hepatol, 1983; 3:50; Planas, Gastro, 1983; 84:247; Daskalopoulos, AmJKidneyDis, 1985; 6:217; Laffi, Gastro, 1986; 90:182; Quintero,

Nephron, 1986; 42:298), and in dogs with cirrhosis secondary to common bile-duct ligation (Zambraski, JLabClinMed, 1984; 103: 549). The decline in glomerular filtration rate and renal blood flow in the dogs with ligated common bile ducts and cirrhosis was preventable by prior administration of saralasin or captopril (Levy, AmJPhysiol, 1983; 245:F521), confirming that overactivity of endogenous vasoconstrictor systems as well as inhibition of renal prostaglandin synthesis is a major determinant of renal failure after NSAID administration.

Three studies have suggested that non-acetylated salicylates are less effective in inhibiting renal synthesis of prostaglandins than other NSAIDs, and do not impair renal function or the renal response to frusemide in patients and experimental animals with cirrhosis and ascites (Zambraski, JPharmExpTher, 1988; 247:983; Antillon, AmJGastr, 1989; 84:153; Salerno, JHepatol, 1993; 19:279). Further studies are needed to confirm these findings.

The most important practical conclusion of these investigations is that NSAIDs should be used with great caution, if ever, in patients with cirrhosis and ascites because they may induce renal failure, water retention and dilutional hyponatraemia, and diuretic-resistant ascites. Although these adverse renal effects have always been rapidly reversible after drug withdrawal, it is important to note that in these studies NSAIDs were given as an investigative tool, at low dosage, and for 1 or 2 days only. Whether renal impairment would be also quickly reversible after long-term treatment with therapeutic dosages of these drugs is unknown.

Drugs used in the treatment of portal hypertension

Reports on the renal effects of somatostatin, a drug used for the treatment of acute variceal bleeding, are conflicting. One study (Ginès, Gastro, 1992; 103:1868) shows a significant decrease in glomerular filtration rate, sodium excretion, and free-water clearance during the acute infusion of somatostatin. Conversely, another (Mountakalakis, NephrolDialTransp, 1988; 3:604) shows an increase in urine volume and creatinine clearance in patients with ascites who received otreotide, a synthetic analogue of somatostatin.

Propranolol, the drug most extensively used in the prophylaxis of variceal bleeding and rebleeding, has significant effects on systemic and splanchnic haemodynamics and on the endogenous vasoactive systems. It reduces cardiac output, increases systemic vascular resistance and circulating noradrenaline, and reduces plasma renin activity and aldosterone in patients with cirrhosis with and without ascites (Henriksen, Hepatol, 1993; 18:688). However, it has no significant effects on renal function in these patients (Bataillee, Gastro, 1984; 86:129; Rector, ArchIntMed, 1984; 144:1761; Bernardi, JHepatol, 1989; 8:279).

Nitrates have recently been introduced for the prophylaxis of variceal rebleeding, given alone or in combination with propranolol. They reduce portal pressure mainly by decreasing hepatic vascular resistance whereas propranolol is effective by reducing portal venous inflow and acting on the portocollateral circulation. This difference might explain the additive effects of the combined treatment in reducing portal pressure. The acute oral administration of isosorbide-5-mononitrate in cirrhotic patients with and without ascites is associated with a significant reduction in cardiac output, systemic vascular resistance and arterial pressure, an increase in plasma renin

activity and aldosterone concentration, a suppression of the plasma concentrations of atrial natriuretic peptide, and a reduction in renal blood flow, glomerular filtration rate, free-water clearance and sodium excretion (Salmerón, Hepatol, 1993; 17:800). These effects were particularly marked in the patients with ascites. These findings were later confirmed (Salerno, Hepatol, 1996; 23:1135) in a study which observed the same changes after the acute administration of isosorbide-5-mononitrate in 21 patients with and without ascites. Interestingly enough, Salerno et al. also found a significant reduction of arterial pressure, urine volume, and sodium excretion during long-term administration of the drug in the patients with ascites. Therefore, acute and chronic administration of nitrates alone impairs renal function in decompensated cirrhosis. The effect of the combined treatment (propranolol plus nitrates) on renal function is more controversial. Vorovioff et al. (Hepatol, 1993; 18:477) compared patients chronically treated with propranolol alone with those treated with propranolol plus isosorbide dinitrate. Eight of the 14 patients with ascites or a history of ascites receiving propranolol plus isosorbide dinitrate showed impairment in renal function and sodium metabolism, as reflected by the clinical development or worsening of ascites and a need for higher diuretic dosage. This high frequency of renal impairment did not occur in patients receiving propranolol alone, In contrast, others (Morillas, Hepatol, 1994; 20:1502; Merckel, Hepatol, 1995; 22:808) did not observe any detrimental effects on renal function after 3 or 6 months of therapy with a combination of isosorbide-5-mononitrate and β-blockers.

Prazosin is another drug investigated as a possible treatment for portal hypertension. It is an α-adrenergic blocker that reduces portal pressure by decreasing intrahepatic vascular resistance. Long-term administration of prazosin to compensated cirrhotic patients with portal hypertension caused vasodilation of the systemic circulation, which led to ascites or oedema formation in a significant number of patients (Albillos, Gastro, 1995; 109:1995).

References

1. Besnier E. Ascite. In Dechambre A and Hann L, eds. *Dictionnaire encyclopédique des sciences médicales*. Paris: Asselin et Masson, 1884: 475–506.
2. Lain-Entralgo P. *Historia de la medicina*. Barcelona: Salvat Editores, 1982: 260–2.
3. Heidenhain R. Veruche und fragen zur lehre von der lymphbildung. *Archiv fur die Gesamte Physiologie des Menschen und der Tiere*, 1891; **49**: 290–301.
4. Starling EH. The influence of mechanical factors on lymph production. *Journal of Physiology (London)*, 1884; **16**: 224–67.
5. Starling EH. Production and absorption of lymph. In Schaefer EA, ed. *Textbook of physiology*. London: Caxton, 1898: 285–311.
6. Celsus AC. *Los ocho libros de la medicina*. Barcelona: Editorial Iberia SA, 1966: 185–6.
7. Cohn JN, Khatri JM, Groszmann RJ, and Kotelanski B. Hepatic blood flow in alcoholic liver disease measured by an indicator dilution technique. *American Journal of Medicine*, 1972; **53**: 704–14.
8. Groszmann RJ, Kotelanski B, Cohn JN, and Khatri IM. Quantitation ofportosystemic shunting from the splenic and mesenteric beds in alcoholic liver disease. *American Journal of Medicine*, 1972; **53**: 715–22.
9. Chinchilla A. *Análes históricos de la medicina en general. Volumen II. Historia particular de las operaciones quirúrgicas. paracentesis*. Valencia: Imprenta López y Cia, 1841: 200–31.
10. Widal V. Paracentese. In Dachambre A and Hann L, eds. *Dictionnaire encyclopédique des sciences médicales*. Paris, 1884: 509–16.
11. Goldberg M. The renal physiology of diuretics. In Orloff J, Berliner RW, and Geiger SR, eds. *Handbook of physiology*. Section 8. *Renal physiology*. Washington DC, American Physiological Society, 1973: 1003–33.

12. Liddle GW. Sodium diuresis induced by steroidal antagonists of aldosterone. *Science*, 1957; **126**: 1016–18.

13. Quintero E, *et al.* Paracentesis versus diuretics in the treatment of cirrhotics with tense ascites. *Lancet*, 1985; **i**: 611–12.

14. Wilson JAP, Suguitan EA, Cassidy WA, Parker RH, and Chan CH. Characteristics of ascitic fluid in the alcoholic cirrhotic. *Digestive Diseases and Sciences*, 1979; **24**: 645–8.

15. Sampliner RF and Iber FL. High protein ascites in patients with uncomplicated hepatic cirrhosis. *American Journal of the Medical Sciences*, 1974; **267**: 275–9.

16. Hoefs JC. Serum protein concentration and portal pressure determine the ascitic fluid protein concentration in patients with chronic liver disease. *Journal of Laboratory and Clinical Medicine*, 1983; **102**: 260–73.

17. Bar-Meir S, Lerner E, and Conn HO. Analysis of ascitic fluid in cirrhosis. *Digestive Diseases and Sciences*, 1979; **24**: 136–44.

18. Rector WG Jr and Reynolds TB. Superiority of the serum–ascites albumin difference over the ascites total protein concentration in separation of 'transudative' and 'exudative' ascites. *American Journal of Medicine*, 1984; **77**: 83–5.

19. Henriksen JH. Permselectivity of the liver blood-lymph (ascitic fluid) barrier to macromolecules in decompensated cirrhosis: relation to calculated pore-size. *Clinical Physiology*, 1983; **3**: 163–71.

20. Henriksen JH, Lassen NA, Parving HH, and Winkler K. Filtration as the main transport mechanism of protein exchange between plasma and the peritoneal cavity in hepatic cirrhosis. *Scandinavian Journal of Clinical and Laboratory Investigation*, 1980; **40**: 503–13.

21. Hoefs JC and Runyon BA. Spontaneous bacterial peritonitis. *Disease-a-Month*, 1985; **31**: 1–48.

22. Conn HO and Fessel JM. Spontaneous bacterial peritonitis in cirrhosis. Variations on a theme. *Medicine*, 1971; **50**: 161–97.

23. Runyon BA, Hoefs JC, and Morgan TR. Ascitic fluid analysis in malignant-related ascites. *Hepatology*, 1988; **8**: 1104–9.

24. Prieto, M, Gomez-Lechón MJ, Hoyos M, Castell JV, Carrasco D, and Berenguer J. Diagnosis of malignant ascites. Comparison of ascitic fibronectin, cholesterol, and serum–ascites albumin difference. *Digestive Diseases and Sciences*, 1988; **33**: 833–8.

25. Castaldo G, *et al.* Total discrimination of peritoneal malignant ascites from cirrhosis and hepatocarcinoma-associated ascites by assays of ascitic cholesterol and lactate dehydrogenase. *Clinical Chemistry*, 1994; **40**: 478–82.

26. Hafter R, Klaubert W, Gollritzer R, Von Hugo R, and Graeff H. Crosslinked fibrin derivatives and fibronectin in ascitic fluid from patients with ovarian cancer compared to ascitic fluid in liver cirrhosis. *Thrombosis Research*, 1984; **35**: 53–64.

27. Gerbes AL, Jungst D, Xie YN, Permanetter W, and Paumgartner G. Ascitic fluid analysis for the differentiation of malignant-related and non-malignant ascites. Proposal of a diagnostic sequence. *Cancer*, 1991; **68**: 1808–14.

28. Lee CM, Changchien CS, Shyu WC, and Liaw YF. Serum–ascites albumin concentration and fibronectin in the diagnosis of malignant ascites. *Cancer*, 1992; **70**: 2057–60.

29. Press ON, Pres NO, and Kaufman SD. Evaluation and management of chylous ascites. *Annals of Internal Medicine*, 1982; **96**: 358–64.

30. Malagalada JR, Iber FL, and Linscheer WG. Origin of fat in chylous ascites of patients with liver cirrhosis. *Gastroenterology*, 1974; **67**: 878–86.

31. Shakil AO, Korula J, Kanel GC, Murray NG, and Reynolds TB. Diagnostic features of tuberculous peritonitis in the absence and presence of chronic liver disease: a case-control study. *American Journal of Medicine*, 1996; **100**: 179–85.

32. Hillebrand DJ, Runyon B, Yasmineh WG, and Rynders GP. Ascitic fluid adenosine deaminase insensitivity in detecting tuberculous peritonitis in the United States. *Hepatology*, 1996; **24**: 1408–12.

33. Ackerman N, Sillin LF, and Suresh K. Consequences of intraperitoneal bile: bile ascites versus bile peritonitis. *American Journal of Surgery*, 1985; **149**: 244–6.

34. Xiol X, *et al.* Spontaneous bacterial empyema in cirrhotic patients: a prospective study. *Hepatology*, 1996; **23**: 719–23.

35. Mouroux J, Perrin C, Venissac N, Blaive B, and Richelme H. Management of pleural effusion of cirrhotic origin. *Chest*, 1996; **109**: 1093–6.

36. Witte MH, Witte CL, and Dumont AE. Estimated net transcapillary water and protein flux in the liver and intestine of patients with portal hypertension from hepatic cirrhosis. *Gastroenterology*, 1981; **80**: 265–72.

37. Gnepp DR. Lymphatics. In Staub NC and Taylor AE, eds. *Edema*. New York: Raven Press, 1984: 263–98.

38. Dumont AE and Mulholland JH. Alterations in thoracic duct lymph flow in hepatic cirrhosis. Significance in portal hypertension. *Annals of Surgery*, 1962; **156**: 668–77.

39. Laine GA, Hall JT, Laine SH, and Granger HJ. Transsinusoidal fluid dynamics in canine liver during venous hypertension. *Circulation Research*, 1979; **45**: 317–23.

40. Greenway CV and Lautt WW. Effects of hepatic venous pressure on transsinusoidal fluid transfer in the liver of the anaesthetized cat. *Circulation Research*, 1970; **26**: 697–703.

41. Brauer R, Holloway RJ, and Leong GF. Changes in liver function and structure due to experimental passive congestion under controlled hepatic vein pressures. *American Journal of Physiology*, 1957; **197**: 681–95.

42. Granger DN, Miller T, Allen R, Parker RE, Parker JC, and Taylor AE. Permselectivity of cat liver blood–lymph barrier to endogenous macromolecules. *Gastroenterology*, 1979; **77**: 103–9.

43. Granger HJ and Laine GA. Consecutive barriers to movement of water and solutes across the liver sinusoids. *Physiologist*, 1980; **23**: 83–5.

44. Granger DN and Barrowman JA. Gastrointestinal and liver edema. In Staub NC and Taylor AE, eds. *Edema*. New York: Raven Press, 1984: 615–56.

45. Richardson PDI, Granger DN, Mailman D, and Kvietys PR. Permeability characteristics of colonic capillaries. *American Journal of Physiology*, 1980; **239**: 6300–5.

46. Granger DN, Mortillaro NA, Kvietys PR, and Taylor AE. Regulation of interstitial fluid volume in the small bowel. In Hargens AR, ed. *Tissue fluid pressure and composition*. Baltimore: Williams and Wilkins, 1981: 173–83.

47. Mortillaro NA and Taylor AE. Interaction of capillary and tissue forces in the cat intestine. *Circulation Research*, 1976; **39**: 348–58.

48. Witte MH, Witte CL, and Dumont AE. Progress in liver disease: physiological factors involved in the causation of cirrhotic ascites. *Gastroenterology*, 1971; **61**: 742–50.

49. Witte CL, Witte MH, and Dumont AE. Lymph imbalance in the genesis and perpetuation of the ascites syndrome in hepatic cirrhosis. *Gastroenterology*, 1980; **78**: 1059–68.

50. Yoffey IM and Courtice FC. *Lymphatics, lymph and the lymphomyeloid complex*. New York: Academic Press, 1970.

51. Iber FL. Normal and pathologic physiology of the liver. In Sodeman WA and Sodeman WA Jr, eds. *Pathologic physiology*. Philadelphia: Saunders, 1974: 790–817.

52. Levy M. Pathophysiology of ascites formation. In Epstein M., ed. *The kidney in liver disease*. 3rd edn. Baltimore: Williams and Wilkins, 1983: 209–43.

53. Vorobioff J, Bredfeldt JE, and Groszmann RJ. Increased blood flow through the portal system in cirrhotic rats. *Gastroenterology*, 1984; **87**: 1120–6.

54. Duhac J and Jarmolych J. Histology of the intestinal peritoneum in patients with cirrhosis of the liver and ascites. *Digestive Diseases and Sciences*, 1968; **23**: 417–22.

55. Dumont AE and Witte MH. Contrasting patterns of thoracic duct lymph formation in hepatic cirrhosis. *Surgery, Gynecology and Obstetrics*, 1986; **122**: 524–8.

56. Witte CL and Witte MH. The circulation in portal hypertension. *Yale Journal of Biology and Medicine*, 1975; **48**: 141–55.

57. Witte CL, Witte MH, Cole WC, Chung YC, Bleisch VR, and Dumont AE. Dual origin of ascites in hepatic cirrhosis. *Surgery, Gynecology and Obstetrics*, 1969; **129**: 1027–33.

58. Levy M and Wexler MJ. Renal sodium retention and ascites formation in dogs with experimental cirrhosis but without portal hypertension or increased splanchnic vascular capacity. *Journal of Laboratory and Clinical Medicine*, 1978; **91**: 521–36.

59. Unikowsky B, Wexler MJ, and Levy M. Dogs with experimental cirrhosis of the liver but without intrahepatic hypertension do not retain sodium or form ascites. *Journal of Clinical Investigation*, 1983; **72**: 1594–604.

60. Vorobioff J, Bredfeldt JE, and Groszmann RJ. Hyperdynamic circulation in portal-hypertensive rat model: a primary factor for maintenance of chronic portal hypertension. *American Journal of Physiology*, 1983; **244**: G52–7.

61. Blanchet L and Lebrec D. Changes in splanchnic blood flow in portal hypertensive rats. *European Journal of Clinical Investigation*, 1982; **12**: 327–30.

62. Bosch J, Enriquez R, Groszmann RJ, and Storer EH. Chronic bile duct ligation in the dog: hemodynamic characterization of a portal hypertension model. *Hepatology*, 1983; **3**: 1002–7.

63. Sugita S, Ohnishi K, Saito M, and Okuda K. Splanchnic hemodynamics in portal hypertensive dogs with portal fibrosis. *American Journal of Physiology*, 1987; **252**: G748–54.

64. Crissinger KD, Kvietys PR, and Granger DN. Developmental intestinal vascular responses to venous pressure elevation. *American Journal of Physiology*, 1988; **254**: G658–63.

65. Korthuis RJ, Kinden DA, Brimer GE, Slattery KA, Stogsdill P, and Granger DN. Intestinal capillary filtration in acute and chronic portal hypertension. *American Journal of Physiology*, 1988; **254**: G339–45.

66. Benoit JN and Granger DN. Splanchnic hemodynamics in chronic portal hypertension. *Seminars in Liver Disease*, 1986; **6**: 287–98.

67. Sikuler E, Kravetz D, and Groszmann RJ. Evolution of portal hypertension and mechanisms involved in its maintenance in a rat model. *American Journal of Physiology*, 1985; **248**: G618–25.

68. Benoit JN, Barrowman JA, Harper SL, Kvietys KR, and Granger ND. Role of humoral factors in the intestinal hyperemia associated with chronic portal hypertension. *American Journal of Physiology*, 1984; **247**: G486–93.

69. Korthuis RJ, Benoit JN, Kvietys PR, Townsley MI, Taylor AE, and Granger ND. Humoral factors may mediate increased hindquarter blood flow in portal hypertension. *American Journal of Physiology*, 1985; **249**: H827–33.

70. Kravetz D, *et al.* Hyperglucagonemia and hyperkinetic circulation after portocaval shunt in the rat. *American Journal of Physiology*, 1987; **252**: G257–61.

71. Kiel JW, Pitts V, Benoit JN, Granger ND, and Shepherd AP. Reduced vascular sensitivity to norepinephrine in portal hypertensive rats. *American Journal of Physiology*, 1985; **248**: G192–5.

72. Benoit JN, Korthuis RJ, Granger DN, and Battarbee HD. Splanchnic hemodynamics in acute and chronic portal hypertension. In Bomzom A and Blendis L, eds. *Cardiovascular complications of liver disease*. Boca Raton: CRC Press, 1990: 179–206.

73. Groszman RJ. Mechanism of portal hypertension. In Arroyo V, Bosch J, and Rodés J, eds. *Treatments in hepatology*. Barcelona: Masson SA, 1995: 3–8.

74. Huet PM, Pomier-Layrargues G, Villeneuve JP, Varin F, and Viallet A. Intrahepatic circulation in liver disease. *Seminars in Liver Disease*, 1986; **6**: 277–86.

75. Bosch J, Mastai R, Kravetz D, Bruix J, Rigau J, and Rodés J. Measurement of azygos venous blood flow in the evaluation of portal hypertension in patients with cirrhosis. Clinical and haemodynamic correlations in 100 patients. *Journal of Hepatology*, 1985; **1**: 125–39.

76. Bosch J, *et al.* Hepatic hemodynamics and the renin–angiotensin–aldosterone system in cirrhosis. *Gastroenterology*, 1980; **78**: 92–9.

77. Kotelanski B, Groszmann RJ, and Cohn JN. Circulation times in the splanchnic and hepatic beds in alcoholic liver disease. *Gastroenterology*, 1972; **63**: 102–11.

78. Schrier RW, Arroyo V, Bernardi M, Epstein M, Henriksen JH, and Rodés J. Peripheral arterial vasodilation hypothesis: a proposal for the initiation of renal sodium and water retention in cirrhosis. *Hepatology* 1988; **8**: 1151–7.

79. Fernández-Seara J, *et al.* Systemic and regional hemodynamics in patients with liver cirrhosis and ascites with and without functional renal failure. *Gastroenterology*, 1989; **97**: 1304–12.

80. Maroto A, *et al.* Brachial and femoral blood flow in cirrhosis. Relationship with renal dysfunction. *Hepatology*, 1993; **17**: 788–93.

81. Sato S, Ohnishi K, and Sugita K. Splenic artery and superior mesenteric artery blood flow: nonsurgical Doppler US measurement in healthy subjects and patients with chronic liver disease. *Radiology*, 1987; **164**: 347–52.

82. Benoit JN and Granger DN. Intestinal microvascular adaptation to chronic portal hypertension in the rat. *Gastroenterology*, 1988; **94**: 471–6.

83. Schroeder ET, Anderson GH, Goldman SH, and Streeten DHP. Effect of blockade of angiotensin II on blood pressure, renin and aldosterone in cirrhosis. *Kidney International*, 1976; **9**: 511–19.

84. Arroyo V, Bosch J, Mauri M, Rivera F, Navarro F, and Rodés J. Effect of angiotensin II blockade on systemic and hepatic hemodynamics and on the renin–angiotensin–aldosterone system in cirrhosis with ascites. *European Journal of Clinical Investigation*, 1981; **11**: 221–9.

85. Clària J, *et al.* Effect of V_1-vasopressin and angiotensin-II blockade on arterial pressure and endogenous vasoconstrictor systems in conscious rats with cirrhosis and ascites. *Gastroenterology*, 1991; **100**: 494–501.

86. Arroyo V and Ginès P. Arteriolar vasodilation and the pathogenesis of the hyperdynamic circulation and renal sodium and water retention in cirrhosis. *Gastroenterology*, 1992; **102**: 1077–9.

87. Leak LV and Rahil K. Permeability of the diaphragmatic mesothelium: the ultrastructural basis for 'stomata'. *American Journal of Anatomy*, 1978; **151**: 557–94.

88. Tsilibary AC and Wissing SL. Absorption from the peritoneal cavity: SEM study of the mesothelium covering the peritoneal surface of the muscular portion of the diaphragm. *American Journal of Anatomy*, 1977; **149**: 127–41.

89. Yoffey JM and Courtice FC. Lymph flow and regional lymphatics. In Arnold E, ed. *Lymphatics, lymph and the lymphomyeloid complex*. New York: Academia, 1970: 356–443.

90. French JE, Florey HW, and Morris B. The absorption of particles by the lymphatics of the diaphragm. *Quarterly Journal of Experimental Physiology*, 1960; **45**: 88–98.

91. Buhac I, Flesh L, and Kishore R. Intraabdominal pressure and resorption of ascites in decompensated liver cirrhosis. *Journal of Laboratory and Clinical Medicine*, 1984; **104**: 264–70.

92. Llach J, *et al.* Prognostic value of arterial pressure, endogenous vasoactive systems and renal function in cirrhosis with ascites. *Gastroenterology*, 1988; **94**: 482–7.

93. Saló J, *et al.* Effect of upright posture and physical exercise on endogenous neurohormonal systems in cirrhotic patients with sodium retention and normal plasma renin, aldosterone and norepinephrine levels. *Hepatology*, 1995; **22**: 479–87.

94. Saló J, *et al.* Impairment of renal function during moderate physical exercise in cirrhotic patients with ascites. Relationship with the activity of neurohormonal systems. *Hepatology* (in press).

95. Arroyo V and Rodés J. A rational approach to the treatment of ascites. *Postgraduate Medical Journal*, 1975; **51**: 558–62.

96. Ginès P, Arroyo V, and Rodés J. Pharmacotherapy of ascites associated with cirrhosis. *Drug*, 1992; **43**: 316–32.

97. Suki WN and Eknoyan G. Physiology of diuretic action. In Seldin DW and Giebisch G, eds. *The kidney: physiology and pathophysiology*. 2nd edn. New York: Raven, 1992: 3629–70.

98. Puschett JB and Winaver J. Effects of diuretics on renal function. In Ewindhager E, ed. *Handbook of physiology*. Section 8. *Renal physiology*. Oxford University Press, 1992: 2335–407.

99. Karim A. Spironolactone metabolism in man revisited. In Brumer HR, ed. *Contemporary trends in diuretic therapy*. Amsterdam: Excerpta Medica, 1986: 23–7.

100. Perez Ayuso RM, *et al.* Randomized comparative study of efficacy of furosemide versus spironolactone in non-azotemic cirrhosis with ascites. Relationship between the diuretic response and the activity of the renin–angiotensin–aldosterone system. *Gastroenterology*, 1983; **84**: 961–8.

101. Arroyo V, Bosch J, Casamitjana R, Cabrera J, Rivera F, and Rodés J. Use of piretanide, a new loop diuretic, in cirrhosis with ascites. *Gut*, 1980; **21**: 855–9.

102. Gatta A, Angeli P, Caregaro L, Menon F, Sacerdoti D, and Merckel C. A

pathophysiological interpretation of unresponsiveness to spironolactone in a stepped-care approach to the diuretic treatment of ascites in non-azotemic cirrhotic patients. *Hepatology*, 1991; **14**: 231–6.

103. Gerbes AL. Medical treatment of ascites in cirrhosis. *Journal of Hepatology*, 1993; **17** (Suppl. 2): S4–9.

104. Bernardi M, *et al.* Efficacy and safety of the stepped care medical treatment of ascites in liver cirrhosis: a randomized controlled clinical trial comparing two diets with different sodium content. *Liver*, 1993; **13**: 156–62.

105. Takaya A, *et al.* Stepped care medical treatment for cirrhotic ascites: analysis of factors influencing the response to treatment. *Journal of Gastroenterology and Hepatology*, 1995; **10**: 30–5.

106. Forns X, Ginès A, Ginès P, and Arroyo V. Management of ascites and renal failure in cirrhosis. *Seminars in Liver Disease*, 1994; **14**: 82–96.

107. Sherlock S, Senewiratne B, Scott A, and Walker JG. Complications of diuretic therapy in hepatic cirrhosis. *Lancet*, 1966; **i**: 1049–53.

108. Strauss E, De Sa MF, and Laut CM. Standardization of a therapeutic approach for ascites due to chronic liver disease. A prospective study of 100 cases. *Gastroenterologia Endoscopia Digestiva*, 1985; **4**: 79–86.

109. Angeli P, *et al.* Cirrhosis and muscle cramps: evidence of a causal relationship. *Hepatology*, 1966; **23**: 264–73.

110. Lee FY, *et al.* A randomized controlled clinical trial of kinidine in the treatment of cirrhotic patients with muscle cramps. *Journal of Hepatology*, 1991; **12**: 236–40.

111. Arroyo V, *et al.* Definition and diagnostic criteria of refractory ascites and hepatorenal syndrome in cirrhosis. *Hepatology*, 1966; **23**: 164–76.

112. Arroyo V, Epstein M, Gallus G, Gentilini P, Ring-Larsen H, and Salerno F. Refractory ascites in cirrhosis. Mechanism and management. *Gastroenterology International*, 1989; **2**: 195–207.

113. Planas R, Arroyo V, Rimola A, Perez Ayuso RM, and Rodés J. Acetylsalicylic acid suppresses the renal hemodynamic effect and reduces the diuretic action of furosemide in cirrhosis with ascites. *Gastroenterology*, 1983; **84**: 247–52.

114. Mirouze D, Zipser RD, and Reynolds TB. Effects of inhibitors of prostaglandin synthesis on induced diuresis in cirrhosis. *Hepatology*, 1983; **3**: 50–5.

115. Epstein M. Peritoneovenous shunt in the management of ascites and the hepatorenal syndrome. In Epstein M (ed). *The kidney in liver disease*. 4th edn. Philadelphia: Hanley and Belfus, 1996: 491–506.

116. Smajda C and Franco D. The LeVeen shunt in the elective treatment of intractable ascites in cirrhosis. A prospective study on 140 patients. *Annals of Surgery*, 1985; **201**: 488–93.

117. Bernhoft RA, Pellegrini CA, and Way LW. Peritoneovenous shunt for refractory ascites. Operative complications and long-term results. *Archives of Surgery*, 1982; **117**: 631–5.

118. Lund RH and Moritz WM. Complications of Denver peritoneovenous shunt. *Archives of Surgery*, 1982; **117**: 924–8.

119. Smajda C, Tridart D, and Franco D. Recurrent ascites due to central venous thrombosis after peritoneojugular (LeVeen) shunt. *Surgery*, 1986; **100**: 535–40.

120. Ginès A, *et al.* Treatment of patients with cirrhosis and refractory ascites by Leveen shunt with titanium tip: comparison with therapeutic paracentesis. *Hepatology*, 1995; **22**: 124–31.

121. Ginès P, *et al.* Paracentesis with intravenous infusion of albumin as compared with peritoneovenous shunting in cirrhosis with refractory ascites. *New England Journal of Medicine*, 1991; **325**: 829–35.

122. Ginès P, *et al.* Comparison of paracentesis and diuretics in the treatment of cirrhotics with tense ascites. Results of a randomized study. *Gastroenterology*, 1987; **93**: 234–41.

123. Salerno F, *et al.* Repeated paracentesis and i.v. albumin infusion to treat 'tense' ascites in cirrhotic patients: a safe alternative therapy. *Journal of Hepatology*, 1987; **5**: 102–8.

124. Hagege H, Ink O, Ducreux M, Pelletier G, Buffet C, and Etienne JP. Treatment de l'ascite chez les malades atteints de cirrhose sans hyponatrémie ni insiffisance rénale. Résultats d'une etude randomisée comparant les diurétiques et les ponctions compensées par l'albumin. *Gastroenterologie Clinique et Biologie*, 1992; **16**: 751–5.

125. Solà R, *et al.* Total paracentesis with dextran-40 vs diuretics in the treatment of ascites in cirrhosis: a randomized controlled study. *Journal of Hepatology*, 1994; **20**: 282–8.

126. Ginès P, *et al.* Randomized comparative study of therapeutic paracentesis with and without intravenous albumin in cirrhosis. *Gastroenterology*, 1988; **94**: 1493–502.

127. Tító L, *et al.* Total paracentesis associated with intravenous albumin in the management of patients with cirrhosis and ascites. *Gastroenterology*, 1990; **98**: 146–151.

128. Ginès A, *et al.* Randomized trial comparing albumin, dextran-70 and polygeline in cirrhotic patients with ascites treated by paracentesis. *Gastroenterology*, 1996; **111**: 1002–10.

129. Saló J, *et al.* Effect of therapeutic paracentesis on plasma volume and transvascular escape of albumin in patients with cirrhosis. Relationship with postparacentesis circulatory dysfunction. *Journal of Hepatology* (in press).

130. Ruiz del Arbol L, Monescillo A, Jiménez W, García-Plaza A, Arroyo V, and Rodés J. Paracentesis-induced circulatory dysfunction: mechanism and effect on hepatic hemodynamics in cirrhosis. *Gastroenterology* (in press).

131. Fernandez-Esparrach G, *et al.* Diuretic requirements after therapeutic paracentesis in non-azotemic patients with cirrhosis. A randomized doubleblind trial of spironolactone versus placebo. *Journal of Hepatology*, 1997; **26**: 614–20.

132. Lebrec D, *et al.* Transjugular intrahepatic portosystemic shunt: comparison with paracentesis in patients with cirrhosis and refractory ascites: a randomized trial. *Journal of Hepatology*, 1966; **25**: 135–44.

133. Perez GO, Epstein M, and Oster JR. Role of dialysis and ultrafiltration in the treatment of the renal complications of liver disease. In Epstein M, ed. *The kidney in liver disease*. 3rd edn. Baltimore: Williams and Wilkins, 1988: 613–24.

134. Inoue T, *et al.* Aquaretic effect of a potent orally active nonpeptide V_2 antagonist in cirrhosis. *Proceedings of the Biannual Meeting of the International Association for the Study of the Liver.* Cape Town, 1966; 26T.

135. Arroyo V, Bosch J, Rivera F, and Rodés J. The renin–angiotensin system in cirrhosis. Its relation to functional renal failure. In Bartoli E and Chianusi L, eds. *Hepato-renal syndrome*. Padova: Piccin Medical Books, 1979: 202–27.

136. Perez GO and Oster JR. A critical review of the role of dialysis in the treatment of liver disease. In Epstein M, ed. *The kidney in liver disease*. New York: Elsevier, 1978: 325–36.

8.2 Renal dysfunction in cirrhosis

Vicente Arroyo, Pere Ginès, Wladimiro Jiménez, and Juan Rodés

Renal dysfunction is an important event in cirrhosis. In addition to playing a critical role in the pathogenesis of ascites, it is one of the most sensitive prognostic markers in these patients and, therefore, an important selection criterion for liver transplantation. Although most of the controversies concerning renal dysfunction in cirrhosis described in the previous edition of the *Oxford Textbook of Clinical Hepatology* are still unsolved, new mechanisms have been recognized. The role of vascular endothelium and nitric oxide is specially relevant. This chapter describes the clinical features and mechanisms of renal dysfunction in cirrhosis. Renal dysfunction associated with other diseases (fulminant hepatitis, acute alcoholic hepatitis, or obstructive jaundice) and the treatment of the different abnormalities of renal function in cirrhosis are discussed in other chapters of this book.

Renal functional abnormalities

Sodium retention

Sodium retention is the most common abnormality of renal function in cirrhosis. It is constantly present in patients with ascites and plays a major role in the pathogenesis of this complication. Ascites disappears in most patients when sodium retention is inhibited by diuretics. Conversely, diuretic withdrawal or a high sodium diet leads to the reaccumulation of ascites. The degree of sodium retention in cirrhosis with ascites varies considerably from one patient to another, being practically non-existent in some patients, whereas it is relatively high in others (Arroyo, PostgradMedJ, 1975; 51:558). The observation that ascites may be made to disappear in the latter patients only by reducing sodium intake below sodium excretion is a further argument for the importance of sodium retention in the pathogenesis of ascites (Pecikyan, AmJMed, 1967; 42:359). Experimental studies have shown that sodium retention precedes ascites formation in cirrhosis (Levy, AmJPhysiol, 1977; 233:F572; Levy, JLabClinMed, 1978; 92:560; López-Novoa, AmJPhysiol, 1980; 238:F353; Jiménez, Hepatol, 1985; 5:245). The impairment of sodium excretion in most cirrhotics occurs in the setting of a normal glomerular filtration rate. Therefore, the predominant mechanism for sodium retention in these patients is an increased tubular sodium reabsorption.

Patients with compensated cirrhosis do not have sodium retention. However, they present subtle abnormalities of sodium metabolism. For example, these patients are unable to excrete an acute intravenous salt load normally (Nacarato, Gastro, 1981; 81:205; Caregaro, EurJClinInv, 1985; 15:360; Wood, Hepatol, 1988; 8:831; Wong, Hepatol, 1994; 20:873). On the other hand, compensated cirrhotics with severe portal hypertension may not 'escape' from an exogenously administered mineralocorticoid hormone. If a normal individual ingesting a diet containing a constant amount of sodium is given a salt-retaining mineralocorticoid daily, a transient period of sodium retention is experienced, and limited weight gain occurs, reflecting the expansion of the extracellular fluid volume. After 3 to 5 days, however, sodium excretion increases and equals dietary intake, so that no further weight gain or extracellular volume expansion occurs. In contrast, compensated cirrhotics with high portal pressure may not escape from the sodium retaining effect of mineralocorticoids, and they develop continuous renal fluid and sodium retention, leading to the formation of ascites and oedema (Wilkinson, ClinSci, 1979; 56:401; LaVilla, Gastro, 1992; 102:2114).[1] Finally, it has been shown that compensated cirrhotics retain sodium while they are in an upright posture whereas they show an exaggerated natriuresis during bed rest (Trevisani, JHepatol, 1992; 16:190; Bernardi, Gastro, 1993; 105:188).

Impaired free-water excretion

The oral or the intravenous (as 5 per cent glucose solution) administration of a water overload of 20 ml/kg body weight over 45 min to a normal individual is followed after a period of between 30 and 60 min by the excretion of hypotonic urine (60–110 mosm/kg), at a rate of 8 to 14 ml/min. The volume of water excreted per min by this individual can ideally be divided into two parts. The first consists of water which dissolves urinary solutes iso-osmotically with respect to plasma (osmolar clearance). The second part consists of water free of solutes (free-water clearance, C_{H_2O}). Since osmolar clearance in normal individuals is 1.5 to 2.5 ml/min, free-water clearance after a water overload in these subjects ranges between 6 and 12 ml/min. This means that a healthy person is able to maintain total body water within normal limits even if water ingestion is 10 litres or more per day.

C_{H_2O} after a water overload is normal in compensated cirrhotics and reduced in most patients with cirrhosis and ascites (Papper, JLabClinMed, 1952; 40:523; Papper, ArchIntMed, 1959; 103:750; Rivera, Metabolism, 1961; 10:1; Baldus, AnnIntMed, 1964; 60:326; Epstein, Gastro, 1985; 89:1415).[2,3] The degree of impairment of water excretion in cirrhosis with ascites also varies markedly from

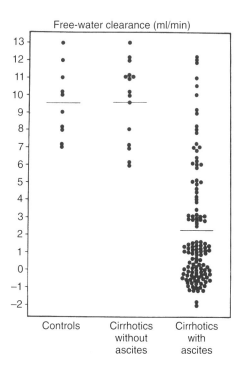

Free-water clearance (ml/min)

Fig. 1. Free-water clearance after an oral water overload of 20 ml/kg body weight in normal subjects and in patients with hepatic cirrhosis with and without ascites.

| Table 1 Diagnostic criteria for the hepatorenal syndrome* |

Major criteria

1. Low glomerular filtration rate, as indicated by serum creatinine greater than 1.5 mg/dl or 24-h creatinine clearance lower than 40 ml/min
2. Absence of shock, ongoing bacterial infection, fluid losses, and current treatment with nephrotoxic drugs
3. No sustained improvement in renal function (decrease in serum creatinine to 1.5 mg/dl or less or increase in creatinine clearance to 40 ml/min or more) following diuretic withdrawal and expansion of plasma volume with 1.5 litres of a plasma expander
4. Proteinuria lower than 500 mg/day and no ultrasonographic evidence of obstructive uropathy or parenchymal renal disease

Additional criteria

1. Urine volume lower than 500 ml/day
2. Urine sodium lower than 10 mEq/l
3. Urine osmolality greater than plasma osmolality
4. Urine red blood cells less than 50 per high power field
5. Serum sodium concentration lower than 130 mEq/l

* All major criteria must be present for the diagnosis of hepatorenal syndrome. Additional criteria are not necessary for the diagnosis, but provide supportive evidence. Reproduced from reference 5, with permission.

patient to patient (Fig. 1). Thus, whereas in some cirrhotics with ascites C_{H_2O} after a water overload is only slightly reduced, others present very low C_{H_2O} or may be unable to dilute the urine after the water load (negative C_{H_2O}). These patients with very low (<1 ml/min) or negative C_{H_2O} retain most water taken in with the diet, causing a dilution of the interieur milieu, hyponatraemia, and hypoosmolality.[4] Hyponatraemia in cirrhosis with ascites is, therefore, almost always a consequence of an excess of water and not of sodium deficiency. This concept is important from a therapeutic point of view. The incidence of hyponatraemia in cirrhotic patients with ascites is approximately 35 per cent.[4]

Hepatorenal syndrome (also called functional renal failure of cirrhosis)

Hepatorenal syndrome is a peculiar type of functional renal failure that occurs in patients with acute liver failure and cirrhosis with ascites. It is due to reduced renal perfusion and, in most cases, renal histology is normal or presents minor abnormalities. Recently, the International Ascites Club has proposed new definitions and diagnostic criteria for hepatorenal syndrome.[5] It is defined as 'a syndrome that occurs in patients with chronic liver disease and advanced hepatic failure and portal hypertension characterized by impaired renal function and marked abnormalities in the arterial circulation and activity of the endogenous vasoactive systems. In the kidney, there is marked renal vasoconstriction that results in low glomerular filtration rate. In the extrarenal circulation there is a predominance of arteriolar vasodilation, that results in reduction of systemic vascular resistance and arterial hypotension. A similar syndrome may also occur in the setting of acute liver failure.' The proposed criteria for the diagnosis of hepatorenal syndrome are

listed in Table 1. There are major criteria, which must be present for the diagnosis of hepatorenal syndrome, and additional criteria, which are not necessary for the diagnosis but provide supportive evidence.

Hepatorenal syndrome has interested hepatologists, nephrologists, and clinical physiologists. Several reasons explain this multidisciplinary interest. First, hepatorenal syndrome is a common complication of patients with cirrhosis and ascites. Retrospective studies indicate that it is present in approximately 17 per cent of patients admitted to hospital with ascites and in more than 50 per cent of the cirrhotics who die (Rodés, RevClínEsp, 1970; 117: 475). A recent study estimated that the probability of developing hepatorenal syndrome 2 and 5 years after the onset of ascites in patients with cirrhosis is 32 and 41 per cent, respectively (Fig. 2).[6] Secondly, hepatorenal syndrome represents the most accurate prognostic index in patients with cirrhosis and ascites: most of these patients die within weeks or months after the onset of the syndrome, independently of the degree of hepatic insufficiency (Fig. 2).[7,8] Thirdly, most cirrhotics with refractory ascites, i.e. the ascites that cannot be mobilized by maximal medical treatment, have renal failure, as manifested by abnormally high plasma levels of blood urea nitrogen (**BUN**) and serum creatinine concentration (Arroyo, GastrInternat 1989; 2:195) Finally, cirrhosis with ascites and hepatorenal syndrome represents a unique condition for the investigation of the relationship between systemic haemodynamics, endogenous vasoactive systems, and renal function in man.

There are two distinct types of hepatorenal syndrome in cirrhosis.[5,8] Type-1 hepatorenal syndrome is characterized by a rapid increase in BUN and serum creatinine, which reach extremely high levels within days after the onset of renal failure (over 100 mg/dl and 5 mg/dl, respectively) (Fig. 3). Most of these patients also present progressive oliguria, dilutional hyponatraemia (often below 120 mEq/l), and hyperkalaemia. This rapidly progressive renal

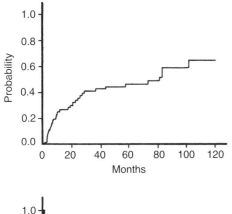

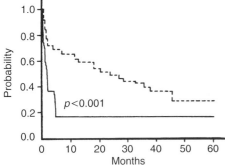

Fig. 2. (a) Cumulative probability of developing hepatorenal syndrome from the onset of ascites in a series of 136 patients. (b) Probability of survival in this series of patients classified according to the presence (continuous line, 24 patients) or absence (discontinuous line, 112 patients) of hepatorenal syndrome. (Reproduced by permission from Ginés P *et al.*, *Ballière's Clinical Gastroenterology*, 1989; 3:165–86).

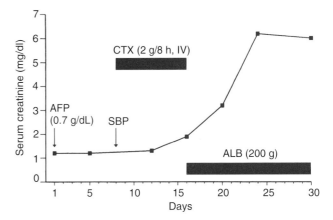

Fig. 3. Course of renal function in a cirrhotic patient admitted to hospital for the treatment of an episode of tense ascites. The ascitic fluid protein concentration (AFP) at admission was very low. The patient developed signs of spontaneous bacterial peritonitis (SBP) 8 days after admission and was treated with cefotaxime (CTX). Despite resolution of SBP a rapid deterioration of renal function developed that did not respond to plasma volume expansion with albumin (ALB).

impairment always occurs in patients with extremely poor hepatic function who, in addition to ascites, often present other complications of the underlying cirrhosis, such as jaundice or hepatic encephalopathy. Type-1 hepatorenal syndrome is commonly observed in alcoholic cirrhotics with superimposed severe alcoholic hepatitis or in any aetiological type of cirrhosis with ascites in which hepatic function deteriorates rapidly as a consequence of a serious bacterial infection, gastrointestinal haemorrhage, or a major surgical procedure. There is limited information on the incidence and predictive factors of type-1 hepatorenal syndrome after these events. A recent study has shown that this type of hepatorenal syndrome may develop in 15 per cent of cirrhotic patients during or after an episode of spontaneous bacterial peritonitis.[9] In this study, increased BUN or serum creatinine or reduced serum sodium concentration before the infection were identified as predictive factors of subsequent development of type-1 hepatorenal syndrome, thus confirming an early study showing that patients with pre-existing renal failure are especially predisposed to develop type-1 hepatorenal syndrome.[8] Type-1 hepatorenal syndrome occurs in 10 per cent of cirrhotic patients treated with large-volume paracentesis without plasma volume expansion, whereas it is extremely infrequent in patients treated with albumin as a plasma expander.[10] The development of type-1 hepatorenal syndrome carries an ominous prognosis since most of these patients die within days or weeks after the onset of the syndrome, independently of the

therapy used (haemodialysis, plasma volume expansion, peritoneovenous shunt, vasoactive agents); death results from a combination of hepatic and renal failure and the precipitating cause of the syndrome.[7]

The differential diagnosis between type-1 hepatorenal syndrome and acute tubular necrosis may be extremely difficult, and sometimes impossible.[11–13] First, patients with type-1 hepatorenal syndrome often present complications that may lead to acute tubular necrosis, i.e. arterial hypotension or serious infections requiring potentially nephrotoxic antibiotics. Secondly, the traditional markers of tubular integrity (urinary sodium concentration lower than 10 mEq/l; urine : plasma creatinine ratio lower than 30; urine : plasma osmolality ratio higher than 1; and fractional sodium excretion lower than 1 per cent) may be present in cirrhotics with well-documented acute tubular necrosis; conversely, type-1 hepatorenal syndrome may develop in the setting of a preserved urine volume and sodium excretion. Finally, type-1 hepatorenal syndrome may progress to acute tubular necrosis (Wilkinson, JClinPath, 1978; 31: 101; Mandal, AmJKidneyDis, 1982; 2:363).[22,23] According to the International Ascites Club, type-1 hepatorenal syndrome is defined by a doubling of the initial serum creatinine to a level greater than 2.5 mg/dl or a 50 per cent reduction of the initial 24-h creatinine clearance to a level lower than 20 ml/min in less than 2 weeks.[5]

Type-2 hepatorenal syndrome is characterized by a moderate increase in BUN and serum creatinine (usually lower than 60 mg/dl and 2 mg/dl, respectively) which remains steady for months.[5, 8] It is important to realize, however, that in cirrhosis a small increase in BUN or serum creatinine represents a marked fall in glomerular filtration rate (**GFR**). In fact, GFR in patients with type-2 hepatorenal syndrome is reduced by more than 50 per cent. Type-2 hepatorenal syndrome usually occurs in cirrhotics with a relatively preserved hepatic function, whose main clinical problem is an ascites refractory to diuretic treatment.[5] Survival of these patients, however, is considerably less than that of non-azotaemic cirrhotics with ascites.

The renal impairment that characterizes hepatorenal syndrome is functional in nature and related to disturbances in splanchnic and systemic haemodynamics and renal perfusion. GFR in patients with cirrhosis and ascites correlates closely with renal blood flow, patients with hepatorenal syndrome being those with lower renal perfusion.[3] Renal arteriographic studies and, more recently, studies with duplex Doppler ultrasonography have shown that impaired renal perfusion in patients with hepatorenal syndrome is secondary to an active vasoconstriction of the renal arteries, which takes place not only in the small arterioles but also in the large intrarenal arteries, including the primary branches of the main renal artery and the interlobar and proximal arcuate arteries (Epstein, AmJMed 1970; 49:175).[14,15] Hepatorenal syndrome in cirrhotics occurs in the setting of a circulatory dysfunction characterized by high cardiac output and marked overactivity of the renin–angiotensin and sympathetic nervous systems and high plasma levels of antidiuretic hormone and endothelin, which are powerful arterial vasoconstrictors.[6,16] However, arterial pressure is decreased, indicating the existence of an intense arteriolar vasodilation.[6,17–19] Hepatorenal syndrome may disappear after the expansion of the circulating blood volume that follows the insertion of a peritoneovenous shunt, following the correction of portal hypertension by a surgical side-to-side or a percutaneous transjugular intrahepatic portacaval shunt (TIPS), or after a successful liver transplantation (Schroeder, AnnIntMed, 1970; 72:923; Iwatsuki, NEJM, 1973; 289: 1155; Walpnick, JAMA, 1977; 237:131; Schroeder, KidneyInt, 1979; 15:54; Wood, AnnSurg, 1987; 205:415; Spahr, AmJGastr, 1995; 90: 1169; Sturgis, JClinGastr, 1995; 20:241). Finally, the kidneys of cirrhotics with hepatorenal syndrome are able to work normally when transplanted to patients with chronic renal failure (Koppel, NEJM, 1969; 280:1367).

Mechanisms of renal function abnormalities in cirrhosis

Several neurohumoral systems and endogenous substances with sodium- or water-retaining activities, or vasoactive properties, have been implicated in the pathogenesis of renal dysfunction in cirrhosis, including the renin–angiotensin–aldosterone and the sympathetic nervous systems[20,21] antidiuretic hormone,[22] prostaglandins[20] (Zipser, AmJMed, 1986; 81:95(Suppl. 2B); Epstein, Hepatol, 1987; 7:1359), leukotrienes,[23] natriuretic peptides,[24–27] endothelin,[16] nitric oxide,[28] natriuretic hormone,[29] renal-kallikrein–kinin system,[30] glomerulopressin (Alvestrand, Lancet, 1984; i:195), endotoxin (Wilkinson, AdvNephrol, 1978; 7:15; Coratelli, KidneyInt, 1985; 28:S143), false neurotransmitters (Fisher, Lancet, 1971; ii:75), platelet activating factor (Caramelo, EurJClinInv, 1987; 17:7), oestrogens (Preedy, JCI, 1956; 35:430), and vasoactive intestinal peptide (Calam, Peptides, 1984; 5:441). It is important to point out, however, that more than 100 different compounds with significant effects on renal function have been isolated in human urine. Therefore, the systems and substances cited above probably represent only a small fraction of the neurohumoral factors that may affect renal function in cirrhotics with ascites. In addition, alterations in intrarenal haemodynamics may also participate in the pathogenesis of sodium and water retention in these patients. Here we summarize the extensive data presently available implicating the renin–angiotensin–aldosterone system, sympathetic nervous system, antidiuretic hormone, natriuretic peptides, natriuretic hormone, nitric oxide, endothelin and arachidonic acid metabolites in the pathogenesis of renal dysfunction in cirrhosis.

The renin–angiotensin–aldosterone system

Through the secretion of renin, the kidney exerts powerful control over arterial pressure, extracellular fluid volume (including blood volume), sodium and potassium excretion, and the electrolyte composition of the body.[31,32] Renin is produced in the kidney by specialized cells of the juxtaglomerular apparatus, the granular cells of the wall of the afferent arteriola, which are in intimate contact with the macula densa in the ascending limb of the loop of Henle. The vascular and tubular components of the juxtaglomerular apparatus are richly innervated by sympathetic nerves. Renin is an enzyme with no biological activity and acts on an α-globulin (renin substrate or angiotensinogen), synthesized by the liver, releasing the inactive decapeptide angiotensin I (A-I). The plasma renin activity is the most common measurement used to estimate the activity of the renin–angiotensin–aldosterone system. It is calculated by measuring (using a radio-immunoassay) the amount of A-I generated by a plasma sample incubated for 3 h under conditions that inhibit further conversion of A-I to angiotensin II (A-II). Plasma renin activity, therefore, depends on the plasma concentration of renin and renin substrate. In healthy subjects the plasma is very rich in renin substrate and it does not affect the measurement of plasma renin activity. However, in patients with decompensated cirrhosis and hyper-reninism the plasma concentration of renin substrate may be extremely low and the measurement of plasma renin activity after an incubation period of 3 h may underestimate the degree of activity of the renin–angiotensin–aldosterone system (Asbert, JHepatol, 1992; 15:179). The incubation time for the measurement of plasma renin activity in these patients should be shorter (1 h or less) than in normal subjects to avoid this problem. An alternative approach is to measure total renin directly by radio-immunoassay.

Three major mechanisms control renin release from the kidney (Davis, PhysiolRev, 1976; 56:1; Peach, PhysiolRev, 1977; 57:313; Reid, AnnRevPhysiol, 1978; 40:377):

(1) the renal baroreceptor mechanism sensitive to changes in renal perfusion pressure;
(2) the macula densa mechanism, which responds to changes in sodium delivery or transport within the ascending limb of the loop of Henle;
(3) the renal sympathetic nervous activity which directly stimulates renin release by operating upon β_1-receptors present in the juxtaglomerular apparatus.

These three mechanisms operate in concert, since they are influenced in the same direction when there are changes in effective circulating blood volume or arterial pressure. In addition to these mechanisms, other factors are known to modify renin release.[31] A-II, vasopressin, and atrial natriuretic peptide inhibit renin secretion. In contrast, kallikrein–kinin and certain prostaglandins, most particularly prostacyclin, stimulate renin release. Available evidence suggests that all factors that affect renin release do so by changing the intracellular concentration of either calcium or cAMP (Churchill, AmJPhysiol, 1985; 249:F175). An increase in free cytosolic calcium suppresses renin release; a fall increases it. Conversely, a rise in cAMP stimulates renin secretion and a fall results in decreased secretion.

A-I is subsequently transformed to the octapeptide A-II by the action of the specific converting enzyme dipeptil carboxypeptidase. Since the largest concentration of this converting enzyme is found in the lung, it was believed that conversion of A-I to A-II was primarily systemic rather than intrarenal. However, subsequent investigations have demonstrated that the converting enzyme is also present in the juxtaglomerular apparatus, and that significant amounts of A-II are generated locally within the kidney (DiSalvo, CircRes, 1971; 29:398; Bailie, JCI, 1971; 50:119); this suggests that A-II is released immediately adjacent to the afferent and efferent glomerular arterioles. It is therefore likely that renal function could be influenced not only by the A-II reaching the kidney via the renal artery but also by that locally generated within or near the juxtaglomerular apparatus.

A-II is one of the active components of the renin–angiotensin–aldosterone system. It is among the most active endogenous vasoconstrictors so far identified. The arteriolar vasoconstrictor effect of A-II is mediated:

(1) by an interaction with specific receptors (AT1 receptors) located on the vascular smooth muscle cells, which results in a sequence of events characterized by activation of a G protein, stimulation of phospholipase C, release of inositol-3-phosphate and diacylglycerol from a membrane phospholipid, inositol-3-phosphate-induced calcium release from non-mitochondrial intracellular sites, phosphorylation of myosin light chain kinase, and contraction of the cells;

(2) by a stimulation of specific receptors in the area postrema of the central nervous system, resulting in an increase in the sympathetic nervous activity; and

(3) by an enhancement of neurotransmission at the peripheral noradrenergic neuroeffector junction.[31–34]

The renal vasculature is especially sensitive to the vasoconstrictor effect of A-II since a striking reduction of renal blood flow occurs with doses of A-II well below those required to induce a pressor response (Debon, ClinSciMolMed, 1963; 25:123; Hollenberg, JCI, 1974; 54:34). A-II also reduces the glomerular filtration rate. The latter effect is related to both a decrease in renal perfusion and to a direct contractile effect on glomerular mesangial cells (Blantz, JCI, 1976; 57:419). Finally, the increase in diacylglycerol induced by the interaction of A-II with AT_1 receptors in the adrenal glomerulosa cells stimulates the aldosterone biosynthetic pathway and increases the release of this hormone to the circulation.[31–34] Atrial natriuretic factor inhibits the aldosterone-stimulating effect of A-II. Activation of G proteins following the interaction of A-II with AT_1 receptors also activates phospholipase A_2, which releases arachidonic acid from membrane phospholipids and increases the synthesis of prostaglandins.

The second active component of the renin–angiotensin–aldosterone system is aldosterone, an important regulator of sodium, potassium, and acid–base balance.[31,34,35] The collecting tubule is the nephron segment responsive to aldosterone. The principal cells, located predominantly in the cortical segments, probably mediate the aldosterone-regulated sodium reabsorption and potassium secretion, whereas the intercalated cells, which predominate in the inner stripe of the outer medulla, participate in the aldosterone-regulated hydrogen ion transport. Aldosterone diffuses freely across the basolateral membrane of the principal cells and binds to a cytoplasmic receptor. The steroid–receptor complex is transported into the nuclear compartment and binds to specific promoters of a number of genes which are under aldosterone regulation. The interaction of the steroid–receptor complex with the promoter leads to the transcription of mRNAs which are, in turn, translated into their respective proteins, mediators of the sodium transport process. Among these proteins, the amiloride-sensitive sodium channel and the Na^+,K^+-ATPase are of particular importance in the antinatriuretic effect of aldosterone. The sodium channels are inserted into the luminal membrane and favour the passive transport of sodium from the tubular lumen to the intracellular space. The Na^+,K^+-ATPase (or sodium pump) molecules are located in the basolateral membrane and promote the active transport of intracellular sodium to the extracellular compartment and the entry of potassium from the extracellular to the intracellular space. The kaliuretic effect of aldosterone is related to its stimulatory effect on Na^+,K^+-ATPase and probably also to the activation of luminal-membrane potassium channels. The synthesis of the proteins activated by aldosterone takes time, and the half-life of these proteins is relatively prolonged. This explains the delay between the administration or withdrawal of spironolactone, a drug that competitively inhibits the binding of aldosterone to the cytosolic receptor, and the onset or finalization of the diuretic action.

The renin–angiotensin–aldosterone system is activated in most cirrhotics with ascites with marked sodium retention (urinary sodium excretion lower than 5 mEq/l) and in all patients with hepatorenal syndrome (Fig. 4) (Rosoff, Gastro, 1975; 69:698; Epstein, CircRes, 1977; 41:818; Arroyo, EurJClinInv, 1979; 9:69; Wilkinson, Hypertension, 1979; 1:125; Sellars, QJMed, 1985; 56: 485; Bernardi, Gastro, 1986; 91:683). In many of these patients the plasma levels of renin and aldosterone reach extraordinarily high values. In cirrhotic patients with ascites and moderate sodium retention, the plasma levels of renin and aldosterone may be normal or only slightly elevated (Fig. 4). Plasma renin activity and aldosterone are normal or reduced in compensated cirrhotics (Wernze, KlinWschr, 1978; 56:389; Bernardi, Gut, 1983; 24:761; Trevisani, JHepatol, 1992; 16:190).[36,37] Several lines of evidence indicate that aldosterone plays a major role in the pathogenesis of sodium retention in cirrhosis. Urinary sodium excretion in cirrhotics with ascites correlates closely with the degree of hyperaldosteronism, plasma aldosterone levels being higher in cirrhotics with marked sodium retention (Wilkinson, ClinSci, 1979; 56:169). On the other hand, sodium retention can be reversed in most of these patients following the blockade of the renal tubular effect of aldosterone with spironolactone (Eggert, BMJ, 1970; 4:401; Campra, DigDisSci, 1978; 23:1025; Pérez-Ayuso, Gastro, 1983; 84:961). Finally, longitudinal studies in rats with experimental cirrhosis have shown a close chronological relationship between the stimulation of the renin–angiotensin–aldosterone system and the onset of sodium retention (Jiménez, Hepatol, 1985; 5:245). Both features preceded the formation of ascites in these experimental animals. The observation that cirrhotics with ascites may present sodium retention in the absence of hyperaldosteronism is generally considered as an

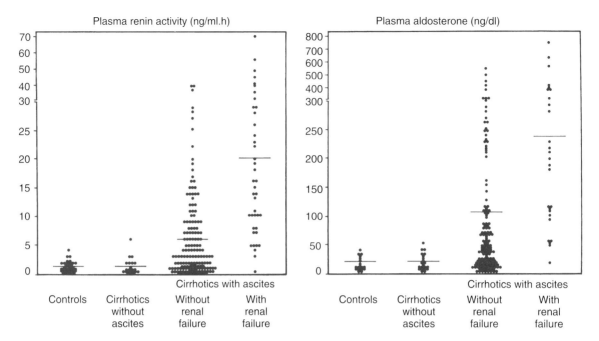

Fig. 4. Plasma renin activity and plasma aldosterone concentration in healthy subjects, cirrhotic patients without ascites, and cirrhotic patients with ascites with and without hepatorenal syndrome. Measurements were made after 5 days on a 50 mEq sodium diet and without diuretics. Plasma renin activity was measured after incubating for 1 h.

indication that factors other than aldosterone are involved in the excessive tubular sodium reabsorption.[37] However, cirrhotics with moderate sodium retention and normal plasma aldosterone concentration are extremely sensitive to spironolactone (Pérez-Ayuso, Gastro, 1983; 84:961; Bernardi, Digestion, 1985; 31:189); these patients may have an increased tubular sensitivity to aldosterone.

Although renin and aldosterone are catabolized by the liver, it is clear that both hyper-reninism and hyperaldosteronism in cirrhosis with ascites are due to an increased secretion and not to an impaired hepatic metabolism (Wernze, KlinWschr, 1972; 50:302; Mitch, AmJMed, 1979; 66:804).[38] Plasma aldosterone concentration in these patients correlates closely with plasma renin, indicating that the main stimulus for aldosterone secretion is A-II (Arroyo, EurJClinInv, 1979; 9:69). Plasma renin activity in cirrhotics with ascites correlates inversely with renal plasma flow and glomerular filtration rate.[24,39] This observation was interpreted initially as evidence that increased renin release in these patients was due to activation of the renal baroreceptor mechanism by impaired renal haemodynamics. However, studies in non-azotaemic cirrhotics with ascites have clearly demonstrated that the activity of the renin–angiotensin–aldosterone system, as estimated by the plasma renin activity and plasma renin concentration and by the renal renin release, may be highly increased in patients with normal renal blood flow and glomerular filtration rate (Arroyo, EurJClinInv, 1979; 9: 69). Therefore, alterations in renal perfusion are not major determinants of renin secretion in cirrhotics with ascites.

Studies using pharmacological agents that interrupt the renin–angiotensin–aldosterone system (inhibitors of the converting enzyme, and structural analogues that competitively antagonize A-II at the vascular AT1 receptor) have been important our understanding of the activation of the renin–angiotensin–aldosterone system in patients

with cirrhosis and ascites. These patients present a systemic circulatory dysfunction characterized by low arterial pressure, hypervolaemia, high cardiac output, and low peripheral resistance, findings consistent with marked arteriolar vasodilation.[19,40–48] Inhibition of the endogenous renin–angiotensin–aldosterone system in cirrhotic patients with increased plasma levels of renin by the intravenous injection of saralasin, a specific antagonist of A-II, or by converting enzyme inhibitors, is associated with a further decrease of arterial pressure and peripheral resistance (Schroeder, KidneyInt 1976; 9:511; Pariente, Gastro, 1985; 88:1255); this may be striking in patients with marked overactivity of the renin–angiotensin–aldosterone system.[49] The systemic circulatory disturbance of these patients would, therefore, be much more intense if endogenous A-II was not acting at the peripheral vasculature to maintain arterial pressure at normal or near-normal levels. Renin release in cirrhotics with ascites is, therefore, a homeostatic mechanism to maintain systemic haemodynamics, with arterial hypotension being the most likely mechanism of hyper-reninism in these patients.

Inhibition of renal prostaglandin synthesis in patients with cirrhosis and ascites using non-steroidal anti-inflammatory drugs is associated with a suppression of plasma renin activity. On the contrary, administration of prostaglandins increases the plasma levels of renin (Ginès, JHepatol, 1993; 17:220). These features indicate that renal prostaglandins contribute to the hyper-reninism in these patients. Natriuretic peptide receptor blockade in experimental cirrhosis is associated with a marked stimulation of the renin–angiotensin–aldosterone system in the absence of changes in systemic arterial blood pressure.[26] Natriuretic peptide receptor blockade also induces a marked increase in renal vascular resistance and fall in renal perfusion and glomerular filtration rate. Although the increase in renin could be related to stimulation of the intrarenal baroreceptor and macula densa mechanism, the most likely mechanism is that natriuretic peptides inhibit renin release in cirrhosis.

Plasma renin activity is particularly elevated in patients with hepatorenal syndrome (Fig. 4).[30,39] On the other hand, plasma renin activity in non-azotaemic cirrhotic patients with ascites is an independent predictor of hepatorenal syndrome development.[6] Therefore, it is reasonable to presume that endogenous A-II is involved in the pathogenesis of the active vasoconstriction, causing hepatorenal syndrome in cirrhosis. At present there is no direct evidence for this. The inhibition of the renin–angiotensin–aldosterone system with saralasin or converting enzyme inhibitors in patients with cirrhosis, ascites, and impaired renal perfusion is not followed by an improvement in renal blood flow and glomerular filtration rate.[50,51] The arterial hypotension that invariably follows the administration of these agents in cirrhotics with functional renal failure, however, could mask the renal vascular effect of inhibition of A-II.

The sympathetic nervous system

The sympathetic nervous system is another important endogenous mechanism controlling systemic haemodynamics and renal function in man (Börge-Person, PhysiolRev, 1996; 76:193). This system is influenced by high-pressure baroreceptors located in the carotid sinus and aortic arch and low-pressure baroreceptors (volume receptors) present in the cardiac atria and pulmonary veins. High-pressure baroreceptors are quiescent below an arterial pressure of 80 mmHg and show a progressive excitation with increasing arterial pressure up to approximately 180 mmHg. The activity from these receptors elicits a reflex inhibition of the sympathetic outflow and thus provides the afferent limb of the buffer reflexes that stabilize arterial pressure. When compared with the sympathetic activity directed to other visceral structures, efferent renal nerve activity appears to be particularly sensitive to inhibition by arterial baroreceptors (Tobey, AmJPhysiol, 1987;252:R26; Weaver, MinElecMetab, 1989; 15:24). Low-pressure baroreceptors are activated by distension of the cardiac atria and pulmonary veins and, therefore, function as intravascular volume receptors. Afferent impulses arising from high- and low-pressure baroreceptors travel via the glossopharyngeal and vagus nerves to an integrative site in the medulla, which alters the sympathetic nervous outflow according to the information received. Afferent impulses from high- and low-pressure baroreceptors are also sent to the supraoptic and paraventricular nuclei of the hypothalamus, thus modifying antidiuretic hormone secretion.[52] Therefore, three neurohormonal vasoactive systems, the sympathetic nervous system, the renin–angiotensin–aldosterone system, and antidiuretic hormone, are closely interrelated and operate simultaneously to regulate arterial pressure and intravascular volume. In this respect it is interesting to note that atrial distension not only stimulates low-pressure baroreceptors that inhibit the sympathetic nervous activity but also increases the synthesis and release of atrial natriuretic peptide from the cardiac myocytes, and it has been shown that there are close interactions between both systems. Atrial natriuretic peptide exaggerates the inhibitory effects of atrial receptors on sympathetic outflow (Thoren, AmJPhysiol, 1986; 251:H1252) and inhibits renin release, and both mechanisms influence tubular fluid reabsorption in the same direction to decrease intravascular volume.

Several studies suggests that baroreceptors may also exist within the liver, which may affect renal function by altering the renal sympathetic nervous activity. The existence of these receptors was first proposed by Ohm and Haberich (PfleugersArchPhysiol, 1969; 306:227) and Liang (JPhysiol, 1971; 214:571), who showed an antidiuretic response following a large increase in portal venous pressure. This response was abolished by application of local anaesthetics to the renal nervous plexus, suggesting a neurogenic effect whose efferent branch is provided by the renal sympathetic nervous system. Previous investigations showing that crush stimulation of the hepatic nervous plexus induced a reduction in glomerular filtration rate and renal sodium clearance were in keeping with this suggestion (Sawchenko, AmJPhysiol, 1979; 236:R5). However, in these studies arterial blood pressure also fell, so it was not possible to exclude a possible influence of high pressure and volume baroreceptors. The first strong data suggesting the existence of hepatic baroreceptors were provided by Kostreva et al. who showed that constriction of the inferior vena cava above the diaphragm resulted in a marked increase in hepatic afferent activity and a reflex increase in renal sympathetic nerve activity, which were eliminated by section of the hepatic nerves but not by carotid sinus denervation, bilateral cervical vagotomy and phrenectomy.[53] The increased renal sympathetic nervous activity was not observed after occlusion of the portal vein or the inferior vena cava below the liver. Constriction of the inferior vena cava in rats with biliary cirrhosis also increased afferent hepatic and efferent renal sympathetic nervous activity, an effect that is blocked by hepatic denervation (DiBona, AmJPhysiol, 1995; 269:G29). Finally, recent studies by Lang et al., showing that liver cell swelling, and presumably intrahepatic pressure increase, following the infusion of glutamine into the superior mesenteric artery of anaesthetized rats, leads to marked decreases in renal plasma flow, glomerular filtration rate, and urinary flow rate, also supports the existence of hepatorenal reflexes (Hepatol, 1991;14:590; PfleugersArchPhysiol, 1993; 425:268). This effect was abolished by spinal transection, renal denervation, or section of the vagal hepatic nerves, and was not observed following the injection of glutamine into the jugular vein.

The renin–angiotensin–aldosterone system is physiologically active only in circumstances in which the effective intravascular volume or the arterial pressure are compromised; in healthy subjects with normal sodium intake A-II blockade is not associated with significant changes in arterial pressure. However, in normal subjects the sympathetic nervous system is continuously operating to maintain arterial pressure and heart rate at normal levels. The haemodynamic effects of activation of the sympathetic nervous system result from the direct action of catecholamines, mainly noradrenaline, released from the terminal ends of the postsynaptic sympathetic neurones, upon the α- and β-receptors in the effector organs. Noradrenaline release stimulates β_1-receptors in the heart, causing increased cardiac rate and contractility. It also causes vasoconstriction in the peripheral arterioles via stimulation of α-receptors. The sympathetic nervous system also influences systemic haemodynamics indirectly by modifying renin release and antidiuretic hormone secretion (Reid, AnnRevPhysiol, 1978; 40: 377).[54]

The kidney is richly innervated by sympathetic noradrenergic fibres which reach the afferent and efferent arterioles, juxtaglomerular apparatus, proximal and distal convoluted tubules, thick ascending limb of the loop of Henle, and distal and collecting tubules (Barajas, JUltrastructRes, 1973; 43:107; Mueller, JUltrastructRes, 1973; 41:533). In contrast, there is neither physiological nor anatomical evidence supporting the existence of sympathetic cholinergic vasodilator fibres in the kidney. Direct electrical stimulation of the renal nerves produces a decrease in renal blood flow and GFR, and stimulates sodium reabsorption in the proximal tubule, loop of Henle, and distal nephron (Di Bona, AmJPhysiol, 1977; 233:F73; Di Bona, RevPhysiolBiochemPharmacol, 1982; 94:75).[55] These effects, which can also be demonstrated when the renal sympathetic nervous system is reflexly activated through high- and low-pressure baroreceptors, are mediated by α_1-adrenoreceptors.[55,56] The effect of the sympathetic nervous system on renal sodium metabolism is independent of its haemodynamic effect, since it can be observed with subpressor nerve stimulation in the absence of changes in renal perfusion and GFR. The cellular mechanism involved following α_1-adrenoreceptor stimulation is similar to that of A-II and includes a G protein that activates multiple phospholipases, including phospholipase C and phospholipase A_2. Phospholipase C generates inositol-3-phosphate that releases calcium from endoplasmic reticulum and diacylglycerol. Phospholipase A_2 generates arachidonic acid and prostaglandins.

The most commonly used method to assess the sympathetic nervous activity in man is by measuring the plasma levels of noradrenaline, since most noradrenaline circulating in plasma is derived from that released as a transmitter at postsynaptic sympathetic nerve terminals. Many studies have been performed using this method in patients with cirrhosis with and without ascites or hepatorenal syndrome; they demonstrate that the plasma noradrenaline concentration in peripheral venous samples is normal in compensated cirrhosis, and usually increased in patients showing sodium retention and ascites (Bernardi, Gut, 1985; 26:629; Epstein, MinElecMetab, 1985; 11:25; Burghardt, KlinWschr, 1986; 64:103) (see Fig. 10).[30,39,42,57–59] The arterial plasma concentration of noradrenaline is also increased in the latter group of patients and correlates with the corresponding values obtained in venous samples (Henriksen, ScaJCLI, 1986; 46:39).[60] To investigate whether the elevated plasma noradrenaline in cirrhotics with ascites is due to an increased rate of release or to a decreased rate of degradation, several studies have examined the rate of secretion versus clearance in these patients. These investigations have shown conclusively that the elevation of plasma noradrenaline is due to increased release and not impaired degradation.[59–62] In normal subjects, the plasma concentration of noradrenaline in renal vein samples is similar to, or lower than, that in arterial samples, the renal venous–arterial difference, therefore, being zero or slightly negative. In contrast, in cirrhotics with ascites this difference is usually positive, indicating an increased activity of the renal sympathetic nervous system.[57,59–61] Some workers have suggested that increased plasma concentrations of noradrenaline in peripheral venous samples in cirrhotics with ascites may not reflect general activation of the sympathetic nervous system, but that they are a consequence of the release of large amounts of noradrenaline into the general circulation by the kidneys due to a selective activation of the renal sympathetic nervous activity (Henriksen, JHepatol, 1984; 1:55). However, by using radiotracer techniques, it has been shown that both total body and renal release of noradrenaline were elevated in parallel in these patients.[93] Direct evidence of a generalized

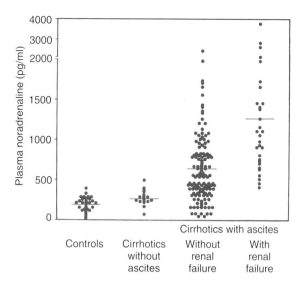

Fig. 5. Plasma noradrenaline concentration in healthy subjects, cirrhotic patients without ascites, and cirrhotic patients with ascites with and without hepatorenal syndrome. Measurements were made after 5 days on a 50 mEq sodium diet without diuretics.

overactivity of the sympathetic nervous system in cirrhosis has been provided by measuring the sympathetic nerve discharge rates from a peripheral muscular nerve. Muscular sympathetic nerve activity is markedly increased in patients with ascites and normal in patients without ascites and correlates directly with plasma noradrenaline (Floras, AnnIntMed, 1992; 116:446).

Since the sympathetic nervous activity stimulates sodium reabsorption and is vasoconstrictor in the renal circulation, it has been implicated in the pathogenesis of sodium retention and hepatorenal syndrome in cirrhosis. There is evidence supporting this contention. Plasma noradrenaline and total noradrenaline spillover are normal in compensated cirrhotics, and usually increased in patients with ascites and sodium retention. In the latter group, sodium excretion correlates inversely with these measurements.[58, 61] Experimental studies have provided direct evidence on the role of the sympathetic nervous system in sodium retention in cirrhosis. Acute bilateral renal surgical denervation is followed by increased urine volume and sodium excretion in bile duct-ligated miniature swine with cirrhosis and ascites; in conscious cirrhotic rats with ascites it improves renal excretion of both an intravenous and an oral sodium load (Zambraski, Physiologist, 1985; 28:268; Koepke, AmJPhysiol, 1987; 252:R1019). Such direct evidence has also been presented in patients with cirrhosis, in whom anaesthetic blockade of the lumbar sympathetic nervous system, a manoeuvre that reduces the renal sympathetic nervous activity, improves sodium excretion (Solis-Herruzo, JHepatol 1987;5:167). Among cirrhotics with ascites, patients with hepatorenal syndrome have the highest plasma concentration of noradrenaline (Fig. 5).[43,64] Moreover, the acute inhibition of the renal sympathetic outflow with clonidine in patients with cirrhosis is associated with a reduction in renal vascular resistance and an increase in GFR, indicating that the activation of the sympathetic nervous system participates in the pathogenesis of the renal vasoconstriction of cirrhosis (MacGilchrist, EurJClinInv, 1991; 114:373).

Factors other than the sympathetic nervous activity and aldosterone are involved in sodium retention in cirrhosis.[37] A series of non-azotaemic patients with ascites, moderate to intense sodium retention, and normal recumbent levels of plasma renin activity, aldosterone, and noradrenaline were studied in upright position and during moderate physical exercise and compared with a group of normal subjects and of patients with compensated cirrhosis. There were no significant differences in plasma renin activity, aldosterone, and noradrenaline between the three groups in any of the study conditions. Interestingly enough, the cirrhotic patients with ascites showed high circulating levels of atrial natriuretic peptide, indicating that sodium retention may occur in cirrhosis in the absence of detectable activation of the renin–angiotensin–aldosterone system and sympathetic nervous system and despite increased circulating levels of natriuretic peptides.

Antidiuretic hormone

Antidiuretic hormone (**ADH**) is produced by magnocellular neurones arising bilaterally in the supraoptic nuclei of the hypothalamus.[52] These neurones project medially to merge in the pituitary stalk and continue to form the posterior lobe of the pituitary gland. The neurones terminate as bulbous enlargements on capillary networks scattered through the stalk and body of the neurohypophysis. Biosynthesis of ADH occurs from the peptide precursor propressophysin, which is composed of ADH and the vasopressin-binding protein neurophysin. The precursor is synthesized in cell bodies in the supraoptic nuclei, packed in secretory granules, and cleaved progressively as it moves down to the axon to yield neurophysin and ADH. In the nerve terminals, ADH and neurophysin are stored in secretory granules and secreted by a calcium-dependent exocytotic process. Secretion is triggered by propagation of an electrical impulse that causes depolarization of the cell membrane, an influx of calcium, fusion of the secretory granules with the cell membrane, and extrusion of their contents.

The most important physiological stimulus for ADH secretion is the osmotic pressure of body water, which induces changes in the water content of a group neurones (osmoreceptor) concentrated in the anterior hypothalamus near the supraoptic nuclei.[52] The functional properties of these neurones resemble those of a set-point receptor. Plasma osmolality below a threshold level suppresses ADH to low or undetectable levels. Above that point, plasma ADH rises steeply in direct proportion to plasma osmolality. Secretion of ADH is also affected by changes in systemic haemodynamics.[52] Small decreases (<10 per cent) in blood volume or arterial pressure have little effect on plasma ADH. However, beyond that point, plasma ADH rises at a rapidly increasing rate. The ADH responses to haemodynamic changes are mediated by neurogenic stimuli that arises from high- and low-pressure baroreceptors. Changes in blood volume or pressure large enough to affect ADH secretion do not interfere with osmoreceptor regulation of the hormone but rather raise or lower the threshold level of hormone secretion. For example, in the presence of hypovolaemia, plasma ADH secretion can be suppressed if plasma osmolality falls, but the set point at which ADH decreases in response to hypo-osmolality is lower than under normal conditions. This concept is of importance in explaining the relationship between ADH and plasma osmolality in circumstances, such as cirrhosis, with simultaneous changes in systemic haemodynamics and extracellular osmolality.

The two major biological effects of ADH are to increase water permeability in the cortical and medullary collecting tubules (hydro-osmotic effect), thus allowing water to be reabsorbed passively from the tubular lumen to the isotonic cortical and hypertonic medullary interstitium, and to produce contraction of the vascular smooth muscle cells (vasoconstrictor effect).[52,63] The hydro-osmotic effect of ADH is mediated by the insertion of water channels (aquaporin-2), which are stored in cytoplasmic vesicles near the tubular lumen, in the luminal membrane of the collecting tubule epithelial cells (King, AnnRevPhysiol, 1966; 58:619). In the unstimulated state, this membrane is almost impermeable to water due to a lack of water channels. In contrast, the basocellular membrane, which is very rich in aquaporin-3 (a different water channel that also transports non-ionic solutes such as urea), is highly permeable to water. The hydro-osmotic effect of ADH is initiated by the binding of the hormone to a V2 receptor on the basolateral membrane of the collecting duct epithelial cells (Morel, KidneyInt, 1987; 31:512; Jard, KidneyInt, 1988; 32:S38; Thibonier, KidneyInt, 1988; 34:S52).[63] This receptor is coupled to adenylate cyclase by a guanine nucleotide-binding protein (**Gs**), which stimulates the enzyme. Adenylate cyclase stimulation results in the breakdown of ATP to cyclic AMP (**cAMP**), which in turn activates a cytosolic protein kinase that promotes the insertion of aquaporin-2 molecules into the luminal membrane. There is a second guanine nucleotide-binding protein (**Gi**) coupled to adenylate cyclase, which inhibits the enzyme.

The vasoconstrictor effect of ADH is initiated by the interaction of the hormone with V1 receptors placed in the plasma membrane of the vascular smooth muscle cells. The intracellular mechanism is similar to that of A-II and noradrenaline and involves phospholipase C, inositol-3-phosphate, and diacylglycerol. The final effect is an increase in cytosolic calcium and cell contraction. The vascular effect of ADH is particularly striking in the splanchnic, muscular, and cutaneous vasculature, with renal circulation being much less sensitive to its vasoconstrictor action (Hofbauer, JCardiolPharmacol, 1984; 6:S429). As with A-II and noradrenaline, the interaction of ADH with V1 receptors also activates phospholipase A_2, which increases the release of arachidonic acid and prostaglandin synthesis in the vascular smooth muscle cells.

There is evidence that V1 receptors are present on V2-responsive renal epithelia and that interaction of ADH with these receptors modulates the effect of the hormone on the water transport process.[63] The increase in the activity in intracellular calcium concentration promoted by the interaction of ADH with the V1 receptors inhibits vasopressin-sensitive adenylate cyclase activation. On the other hand, the activation of phospholipase A_2 increases the synthesis of prostaglandin E_2. This prostaglandin is released into the lumen and interacts in the luminal membrane of the same or nearby cells with specific receptors coupled to adenylate cyclase by a Gi protein. The result of this process is also an inhibition of the vasopressin-mediated activation of adenylate cyclase. Both mechanisms antagonize the hydro-osmotic effect of ADH.

The production of free water within the kidney occurs in the ascending limb of the loop of Henle by a process involving the reabsorption of sodium chloride without a concomitant reabsorption of water (this segment of the nephron is almost impermeable to water).[64] Free-water formation is, therefore, the result of a reabsorption of electrolytes from the tubular fluid rather than of an addition of water. In normal conditions, the kidney is continuously producing a hypotonic tubular fluid in the ascending limb of the loop of Henle. The final osmolality of the urine, therefore, depends on the degree of water reabsorption in the cortical and medullary collecting tubules, which is influenced by ADH.[64]

Impairment of free-water excretion in cirrhosis was initially considered the result of reduced delivery of sodium chloride to the ascending limb of the loop of Henle, a mechanism initially proposed by Schedl and Barter (JCI, 1960; 39:2258); they showed that free-water clearance in cirrhotics with ascites could be markedly increased by the intravenous administration of mannitol. Since the renal effect of mannitol was at that time considered to be due to inhibition of sodium reabsorption in the proximal tubule, the improved free-water excretion following mannitol was interpreted as the result of increased delivery of sodium chloride to the diluting segment of the nephron. Subsequent studies showed that C_{H_2O} in cirrhosis correlated closely with GFR, patients with negative C_{H_2O} after a water load being those with hepatorenal syndrome (Lancestremere, JLabClinMed, 1962; 60:967).[3] Accordingly, impaired free-water excretion in cirrhotics with ascites was considered a consequence of decreased filtered sodium and excessive proximal sodium reabsorption. It is now well established that the diuretic effect of mannitol takes place in the loop of Henle, but several studies performed during recent years support the original hypothesis of Schedl and Barter. Micropuncture studies provide evidence that proximal tubular sodium reabsorption is markedly increased in rats with experimental cirrhosis (Lopez Novoa, AmJPhysiol, 1977; 232: F315). Lithium clearance, thought to estimate distal delivery of filtrate, is reduced in cirrhosis with ascites (Angeli, EurJClinInv, 1990; 20:111; Gatta, Hepatol, 1991; 14:231; Angeli, Hepatol, 1992; 15:651). The expansion of the circulating blood volume, either by head-out water immersion or after the insertion of a LeVeen shunt, improves free-water excretion in ascitic cirrhotics (Reznic, Gastro, 1983; 84:713; Epstein, MinElecMetab, 1984; 10:155). Blood volume expansion depresses proximal sodium reabsorption. Finally, C_{H_2O} in cirrhosis correlates closely with sympathetic nervous activity.[58] Although the effect of the renal sympathetic nervous system is complex, it seems to cause marked stimulation of sodium reabsorption in the proximal tubule.

ADH also plays a major role in the impairment of free-water excretion in cirrhosis. Plasma levels of ADH are increased in most cirrhotics with ascites and correlate closely with the reduction in free-water excretion (Fig. 6).[58,65] Longitudinal studies in rats with experimental cirrhosis and ascites have shown that impairment of water excretion appears in close chronological relationship with the onset of ADH hypersecretion (Camps, Gastro, 1987; 93:498). Brattleboro rats (rats with a congenital deficiency of ADH) with cirrhosis do not develop an impairment in water excretion (Linas, KidneyInt, 1981; 20:173). Kidneys from cirrhotic rats with ascites show increased gene expression of aquaporin-2, the ADH-regulated water channel (Aschina, Hepatol, 1995; 21:169). The blockade of V2 receptors with specific peptide and non-peptide ADH antagonists returns the impaired renal water excretion to normal in rats with carbon tetrachloride-induced cirrhosis and ascites.[66,67] This effect has also been observed following the administration of niravoline (RU-51599), a kappa opioid agonist that inhibits the release and the tubular effect of ADH, to rats with cirrhosis and patients with ascites[68] (Gadano, Hepatol, 1996; 24:448A). Plasma levels of

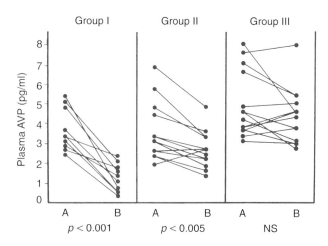

Fig. 6. Plasma antidiuretic hormone (AVP) concentration after 16 h of water restriction (A) and following a water overload of 20 ml/kg of body weight (B). Group I includes normal subjects (free-water clearance 9.6 ± 0.8 ml/min). Group II includes cirrhotics with ascites who were able to generate free water after the water load (free-water clearance 3.6 ± 0.6 ml/min). Group III includes cirrhotics with ascites who were unable to generate free water after the water load (free-water clearance 0.37 ± 0.07 ml/min). (Reproduced with permission from Perez-Ayuso et al., *Kidney International,* 1983; **26**: 72–80.)

ADH in patients with cirrhosis and ascites also correlate with renal perfusion and GFR, patients with hepatorenal syndrome having higher levels of ADH.[65] Therefore, ADH might contribute to the active renal vasoconstriction in hepatorenal syndrome.

The increased plasma ADH concentration in cirrhosis is due to an increased hypothalamic synthesis and not to a reduced systemic clearance of the peptide (Ardillou, AdvNephrol, 1984; 13:35; Solís-Herruzo, Hepatol, 1992; 16:974; Kim, Hepatol, 1993; 17:143). Evidence indicates that this increased synthesis of ADH is related to a non-osmotic haemodynamic stimuli. Most patients with high plasma levels of ADH have a degree of hyponatraemia that would suppress the release of this hormone in normal subjects.[65,69] Moreover, ADH in cirrhotic patients with ascites correlates with plasma renin activity and noradrenaline and is suppressed by manoeuvres that increase effective arterial blood volume, such as head-out water immersion or peritoneovenous shunting.[45,58,65] Finally, the blockade of V1 receptors with specific ADH antagonists in rats with experimental cirrhosis, ascites, and ADH hypersecretion is followed by a significant decrease in arterial pressure, an effect not observed in control animals.[66] This indicates that ADH hypersecretion contributes to the maintenance of arterial pressure in cirrhotics and suggests that the most likely mechanism of ADH hypersecretion in decompensated cirrhosis is arterial hypotension.

Arachidonic acid metabolites

The kidneys are able to synthesize substances that act locally to regulate renal function. Among these substances, the most extensively studied are prostaglandins (**PGs**), which are derived from arachidonic acid metabolism. The initial step in the formation of these compounds is the interaction of a stimulus, commonly a hormone, with a receptor on the cell surface, leading to an activation of phospholipase A_2 (Smith, MinElecMetab, 1981; 6:10) (Fig. 7). The net effect of this process is an increase in free arachidonic acid

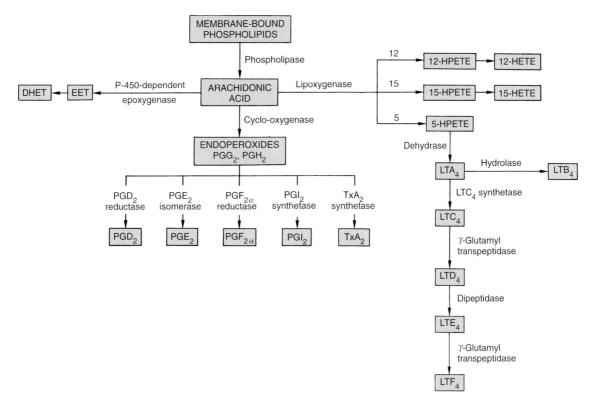

Fig. 7. General scheme of arachidonic acid metabolism. PG, prostaglandin; HPETE, hydroepoxyeicosatetranoic acid; HETE, hydroxyeicosatetranoic acid; LT, leukotriene; EET, epoxyeicosatrienoic acid; DHET, dihydroeicosatrienoic acid; Tx, thromboxane.

concentration, normally quite low, within the cell. The second step is the synthesis of the endoperoxides PGG_2 and PGH_2 from arachidonic acid. This is a complex process catalysed by a cyclo-oxygenase. Non-steroidal anti-inflammatory drugs (**NSAIDs**) are powerful inhibitors of this enzyme (Flower, PharmRev, 1974; 26: 33; Dunn, KidneyInt, 1980; 18:609). PGG_2 and PGH_2 are extremely unstable intermediates that are rapidly converted through various enzymes to the active compounds $PGF_{2\alpha}$, PGE_2, PGI_2 (or prostacyclin), PGD_2, and thromboxane A_2 by the action of specific enzymes. These enzymes have been poorly studied and they are difficult to inhibit.

For many years it was thought that cyclo-oxygenase was a single enzyme constitutively present in most tissues and that inhibition of this enzyme by NSAIDs leads to decreased production of pro-inflammatory PGs as well as beneficial PGs produced in the stomach and kidney. However, it has recently been disclosed that cyclo-oxygenase exists in at least two isoforms (Fletcher, JBC, 1992; 267: 4338; Hla, PNAS, 1992; 89:7384). Cyclo-oxygenase-1 is constitutively expressed in most of the tissues and is involved in the physiological production of PGs. Activation of cyclo-oxygenase-1 leads, for instance, to the production of PGI_2 which, when released by the renal vasculature, contributes to the maintenance of renal perfusion and GFR, and when released by the gastric mucosa is cytoprotective (Smith, AmJPhysiol, 1992; 263:F181). The inducible form, cyclo-oxygenase-2, is present in cells exposed to pro-inflammatory agents, including cytokines, and is expressed during certain inflammatory process (Kuujubu, JBC, 1993; 268:5425). It has been hypothesized that inhibition of inducible cyclo-oxygenase-2 by NSAIDs may well explain the therapeutic utility of these drugs

as anti-inflammatory agents, whereas inhibition of constitutive cyclo-oxygenase-1 may explain their unwanted side-effects on the stomach and the kidneys (Smith, AnnNYAcadSci, 1994; 134:50). The recent development of new NSAIDs with selective action on cyclo-oxygenase-2 (Seibert, PNAS, 1994; 91:12013) opens a new field in the pharmacology of the inflammatory process, particularly in patients who require PGs to maintain vital functions.

The kidney contains several structures capable of synthesizing PGs: epithelial cells of the cortical and medullary collecting ducts, epithelial cells of the descending limb of the loop of Henle, arterial vascular endothelial and smooth muscle cells, medullary interstitial cells, epithelial cells of the parietal layer of Bowman's capsule, and mesangial cells (Smith, AmJPhysiol, 1978; 235:F451). Glomeruli predominantly produce PGI_2 with lesser amounts of PGE_2, thromboxane A_2 and $PGF_{2\alpha}$; afferent and efferent arterioles produce PGI_2 and PGE_2, and medullary interstitial cells and collecting duct epithelial cells produce PGE_2 (Hassid, PNAS, 1979; 76:1155; Sun, KidneyInt, 1981; 19:760; Schlondorff, AmJMed, 1986; 81:1 (Suppl. 2B)). The descending limb of the loop of Henle also synthesizes PGE_2, whereas proximal and distal convoluted tubules and the ascending limb of the loop of Henle have very little PG production. PGs are rapidly metabolized to products with no biological activity (Anggard, KidneyInt, 1981; 19:771). Because of their rapid degradation, their biological actions are exerted at the site of synthesis. Therefore, PGI_2 and PGE_2 synthesized by the arterioles and glomeruli are thought to regulate renal perfusion and GFR; PGE_2 synthesized by the collecting duct epithelial cells are involved in the tubular handling of sodium and water in the distal nephron (Dunn, AmJPhysiol, 1977; 233:F169; McGiff, AnnRevPharmTox, 1981;

21:479; Schnermann, KidneyInt, 1981; 19:802); the dominant action of PGE_2 synthesized in the thin descending limb of the loop of Henle may be to regulate sodium and chloride reabsorption in the ascending limb of Henle's loop (Currie, AnnRevPhysiol, 1984; 46: 327). Renal medullary interstitial cells are capable of forming very high quantities of PGE_2 which are thought to regulate vasa recta blood flow and salt and water reabsorption in contiguous portions of the nephron, such as the medullary thick ascending limb of the loop of Henle and medullary collecting tubule.[70]

There is much evidence that PGs are involved in the control of renal haemodynamics. PGE_2 and PGI_2 have powerful vasorelaxant effects on the renal arterioles and the glomerular mesangium (Stevenson, AmJMed, 1982; 72:354).[70] This effect is mediated by a stimulation of adenylate cyclase and increased intracellular cyclic AMP (Mené, CircRes, 1988; 62:916). On the contrary, thromboxane A_2 and leukotrienes C_4 and D_4 stimulate phospholipase C, increase intracellular inositol-3-phosphate, diacylglycerol and calcium , and produce contraction of the mesangial cells and possibly also the renal arterioles.[70] A–II and ADH, by interacting with AT_1 and V1 receptors, respectively, in vascular smooth muscle and mesangial cells, stimulate phospholipase A_2 which releases arachidonic acid from membrane phospholipids and enhances the renal synthesis of PGI_2 and PGE_2 (Hassid, AmJPhysiol, 1982; 243:C205). Noradrenaline and efferent renal nerve activity also stimulate the renal synthesis of PGs, an effect that is mediated by α-receptors (Cooper, JPharmExpTher, 1985; 233:24). PGE_2 and PGI_2 antagonize the renal vasoconstrictor effect of these endogenous vasoactive compounds. Finally, cyclo-oxygenase inhibition by NSAIDs potentiates the renal vasoconstrictor effect of A–II, noradrenaline, ADH, and renal nerve stimulation, and impairs renal blood flow and GFR in circumstances of low sodium diet, haemorrhagic hypovolaemia, congestive heart failure, nephrotic syndrome, surgical stress, and renal failure (Lifschitz, KidneyInt, 1981; 19:781; Lifschitz, JLabClinMed, 1983; 102:313; Cooper, JPharmExpTher, 1984; 229:139; Dunn, AnnRevMed, 1984; 35:411; Olive, NEJM, 1984; 310:563; Seino, Hypertension, 1985; 7:53). These conditions have two features in common. First, the activity of the renin–angiotensin–aldosterone system, sympathetic nervous system, and ADH is elevated; secondly, the renal production of PGs is increased, probably as a homeostatic response to antagonize the renal vascular effects of these systems. Renal PGE_2 and PGI_2 therefore regulate renal haemodynamics by modulating the renal vascular effects of endogenous vasoconstrictors.

PGE_2 also modulates the renal tubular action of ADH.[70] ADH stimulates the production of PGE_2 by cortical and medullary collecting duct epithelial cells. This effect appears to be secondary to the interaction of ADH with V1 receptors present in these cells, leading to stimulation of phospholipase A_2. On the other hand, PGE_2 inhibits the hydro-osmotic effect of ADH. Several mechanisms are involved in this effect, including: decreased osmotic hypertonicity of the renal interstitial medulla due to inhibition of solute reabsorption in the ascending limb of the loop of Henle and of ADH-induced urea absorption in the inner medullary collecting duct and solute reabsorption in the ascending limb; increased renal medullary renal plasma flow which dissipates the osmotic interstitial gradient (Düsing, CircRes, 1977; 41:287; Roman, AmJPhysiol, 1981; 241: F53); and direct inhibition of ADH-stimulated water flow secondary to an inhibitory effect on the adenylate cyclase/cyclic AMP system

(Handler, KidneyInt, 1981; 19:831; Schuster, AmJPhysiol, 1985; 249:F645). Finally, inhibition of PGs with NSAIDs enhances the tubular effect of ADH. A negative feedback, therefore, exists in which ADH itself stimulates the synthesis of its antagonist PGE_2 in the collecting duct epithelial cells.

The following points support the suggestion that PGs play an important role in the homeostasis of renal blood flow and GFR in cirrhotic patients with ascites:

1. The urinary excretion of PGE_2 and 6-keto-$PGF_{1\alpha}$ (a stable metabolite of PGI_2), which is thought to estimate the renal production PGE_2 and PGI_2, respectively, is increased in non-azotaemic cirrhotics with ascites, while it is reduced in patients with hepatorenal syndrome (Zipser, JClinEndoc, 1979; 48:895; Guarner, ClinSci, 1986; 3:111; Laffi, Gastro, 1986; 90:274).[30, 39,71,72] Although it is difficult to ascertain whether the reduced PG excretion in patients with hepatorenal syndrome is a cause or a consequence of the renal impairment, the increased urinary excretion in cirrhotics with ascites without hepatorenal syndrome suggests that renal synthesis of PGs is increased in this group of patients. The content of PGH_2 synthetase in medullary collecting tubules, as estimated by immunofluorescence techniques, was found to be markedly reduced in kidney samples from cirrhotic patients with hepatorenal syndrome, compared with that found in cirrhotics with ascites and preserved renal haemodynamics and in non-cirrhotic patients with acute tubular necrosis and acute tubulointerstitial nephritis (Govindarajan, Hepatol, 1987; 7:654). This suggests that loss of renal PG synthetase activity might be the cause of the diminished urinary excretion of PGs in cirrhotics with hepatorenal syndrome. This syndrome could therefore be the result of an imbalance between the degree of activation of endogenous vasoconstrictor systems and the renal production of vasodilator PGs.

2. Non-azotaemic cirrhotics with ascites also show high urinary excretion of thromboxane B_2 (a stable metabolite of thromboxane A_2) and PGF_{2a},[71,72] which suggests that the stimulus promoting synthesis of PGs in these patients acts at the initial step of the arachidonic acid cascade, thus increasing the synthesis of all prostaglandins. Longitudinal studies in rats and dogs with experimental cirrhosis have shown a close chronological relationship between the increase in urinary excretion of PGs and the onset of hyperaldosteronism and sodium retention (Zambranski, JLabClinMed, 1984; 103:549; Sola, ClinSci, 1988; 75: 263), suggesting that the high renal PG synthesis in non-azotaemic cirrhosis with ascites is related to the stimulation of the renin–angiotensin–aldosterone system, sympathetic nervous system, and ADH.

3. The administration of NSAIDs induces a profound decrease in renal blood flow and GFR in non-azotaemic cirrhotics with increased activity of the renin–angiotensin–aldosterone system and sympathetic nervous system and marked sodium retention. In contrast, PG inhibition with these drugs in patients with ascites and normal plasma renin activity and plasma noradrenaline is not associated with significant changes in renal perfusion and GFR (Fig. 8) (Mirouze, Hepatol, 1983; 3:50; Planas, Gastro 1983; 84:247; Quintero, Nephron, 1986; 42: 298).[39,73,74]. These findings are the most persuasive arguments indicating that renal PGs are important factors in the

maintenance of renal blood flow and GFR in non-azotaemic cirrhotics with ascites, and that an equilibrium between the degree of activity of endogenous vasoconstrictors and the renal synthesis of vasodilator PGs is of crucial importance in the homeostasis of renal haemodynamics in these patients. The observation that the decline in renal perfusion and GFR induced by indomethacin in cirrhosis with ascites could be prevented by prior administration of saralasin or converting enzyme inhibitors is consistent with this hypothesis (Levy, AmJPhysiol, 1983; 245: F521).

4. The initial observation of an increased urinary excretion of thromboxane B_2 in patients with hepatorenal syndrome (Zipser, Gastro, 1982; 84:698) has not been confirmed. In fact, several studies have shown that its urinary excretion is increased in non-azotaemic cirrhotics with ascites and reduced in patients with hepatorenal syndrome.[71] The administration of thromboxane A_2 inhibitors to patients with alcoholic cirrhosis and hepatorenal syndrome is not associated with an improvement in renal function (Zipser, Gastro, 1984; 87:1128). Therefore, present evidence is not consistent with the hypothesis that hepatorenal syndrome in cirrhosis is related to a decrease in the ratio of the vasodilator PGE_2 and PGI_2 to the vasoconstrictor thromboxane A_2.

5. In patients with compensated cirrhosis the urinary excretion of PGs is similar to that in normal subjects.[39,72,75] On the other hand, there have been several studies showing that renal perfusion and GFR are normal in these patients and that PG inhibition with NSAIDs is not associated with significant changes in renal function.[39,73,74] These studies therefore indicate that PGs are not involved in the regulation of renal perfusion during the initial phases of cirrhosis, prior to the appearance of ascites. This feature is not surprising since it is well known that PGs are important in the maintenance of renal perfusion only in conditions of activated endogenous renal vasoconstrictors. However, it has recently been shown that renal perfusion and GFR may be increased in patients with compensated cirrhosis and that PG inhibition returns renal function to normal in these patients (Wong, AmJGastr, 1995;90:1465; Wong, JHepatol, 1995; 23:1).[75] Further studies are needed to confirm these observations which suggest a primary increase in PG synthesis and renal vasodilation in compensated cirrhosis.

The increased renal production of PGE_2 in non-azotaemic cirrhotics with ascites, by antagonizing the hydro-osmotic effect of ADH, also contributes to the maintenance of free-water excretion in these patients. Most cirrhotic patients with ascites can dilute the urine after a water load despite inadequate suppression of ADH, indicating a relative resistance to the tubular effect of this hormone.[65] This renal resistance to ADH is related to increased renal production of PGE_2, since PG inhibition in these patients is associated with marked impairment in free-water excretion, occurring in the absence of changes in plasma ADH and independent of changes in renal blood flow and GFR.[65]

In addition to the synthesis of the classical PGs, two other major pathways of arachidonic acid metabolism have been described, which lead to additional compounds of potential biological activity (Ardaillou, AmJMed, 1986; 81:12) (Fig. 7).[70] The first pathway involves the lypo-oxygenase enzymes and leads to mono- and di-hydroxyeicosatetranoic acids and the leukotrienes. The second uses

cytochrome P-450-dependent enzymes and generates a series of epoxygenase products. Whereas the renal effects of PGs are well known, there is very limited information regarding the renal effects of these compounds.

Leukotrienes are synthesized predominantly by macrophages in response to several chemotactic stimuli (bacterial endotoxins, platelet-activating factor, complement component C5a). Circulating leukotrienes are taken up rapidly and partially metabolized by the liver and the kidney which release active and inactive compounds into the bile and urine.[36] Lypo-oxygenase products may also be produced within the kidney since 12-hydroperoxyeicosatetranoic acid and 15-hydroperoxyeicosatetranoic acid have been found in rabbit renal medulla and in rat and human glomeruli incubated with arachidonic acid; the isolated perfused rat kidney produces leukotrienes C_4, D_4, and B_4 (Ardaillou, AmJMed, 1986; 81:12). Leukotrienes (C_4, D_2, and E_4) are potent vasoconstrictors. Infusions of these compounds via the renal artery increase renal vascular resistance (Rosenthal, CanJPhysPharm, 1983; 61:325; Piper, Prostagl, 1985; 29:61). In vitro these leukotrienes also cause glomerular contraction (Barnett, AmJPhysiol, 1986; 250:F838). The observation of markedly increased urinary excretion of leukotriene E_4 and N-acetyl-leukotriene E_4 in cirrhotics with hepatorenal syndrome, compared with normal controls and patients with compensated cirrhosis, suggest that leukotrienes may participate in the pathogenesis of this syndrome (Huber, EurJClinInv, 1989; 19:53; Moore, JHepatol, 1990;11:262). Whether the increased urinary excretion of leukotrienes in cirrhotics with hepatorenal syndrome is a consequence of an increased renal production, representing a shift of the arachidonic acid metabolic pathway from the synthesis of vasodilator PGs to that of vasoconstrictor leukotrienes, or is secondary to increased plasma levels and renal excretion due to an impaired hepatic clearance, is unknown (Uemura, Hepatol, 1994; 20:804).[23]

Eicosanoids arising from cytochrome P-450 mono-oxygenases are also probably involved in renal function since they have been shown to be produced by the kidneys, particularly in the thick ascending limb of the loop of Henle, to inhibit the hydro-osmotic effect of ADH, and to relax the vascular smooth muscle cells (Carrol, EurJPharm, 1987; 138:281; Schlondorff, AmJPhysiol, 1987; 253: F464). In the only study currently available on cirrhosis, Sacerdoti et al. (JHepatol, 1991; 12:230) found that cirrhotic rats with ascites show a reduced renal synthesis of these P-450-dependent arachidonic acid metabolites.

Natriuretic peptides

The natriuretic peptide family consists of four closely related peptides, atrial natriuretic peptide (**ANP**), brain natriuretic peptide (**BNP**), C-type natriuretic peptide (**CNP**), and urodilatin (**URO**, or renal natriuretic peptide) which have similar amino acid compositions and natriuretic and/or vasoactive properties (Goetz, AmJPhysiol, 1991; 261:F921; Mukoyama, JCI, 1991; 87:1402; Zeeuw, KidneyInt, 1992; 41:1115; Ana, PharmRev, 1993; 15:457; Davidson, AmJHypertension, 1994; 12:329; Totsune, Hypertension, 1994; 24:758; Forssmann, Nephron, 1995; 69:211).[76–79] They play an important role in the homeostasis of extracellular fluid volume and renal function. These peptides interact with specific receptors (A and B receptors) on the cell surface and activate

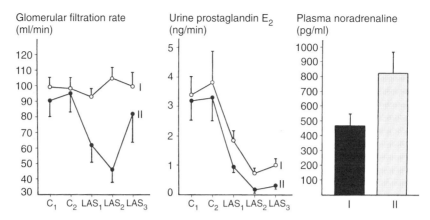

Fig. 8. Glomerular filtration rate and urinary excretion of prostaglandin E_2 (mean $\pm$ SEM) before and after the intravenous injection of 450 mg of lysine acetylsalicylate in 19 patients with cirrhosis and ascites. Patients are divided in two groups according to whether they developed renal insufficiency (II; 11 patients) or not (I; 8 patients) after the administration of the drug. C1 and C2 represent two 30-min periods before the administration of lysine acetylsalicylate. LAS1, LAS2, and LAS3 represent three 30-min periods after the administration of lysine acetylsalicylate. Values of plasma noradrenaline correspond to those of samples obtained before lysine acetylsalicylate injection. (Reproduced with permission from Arroyo V., *et al.*, *European Journal of Clinical Investigation*, 1983; **13**: 271–8.)

particulate guanylate cyclase, which catalyses the production of the second messenger, cGMP. ANP and BNP have high affinity for A-receptors *in vitro* and have potent *in vivo* vasodilatory and natriuretic effects. URO is synthesized within the kidney and thought to act locally, also by interacting with A-receptors. On the other hand, CNP has high affinity for B-receptors and low affinity for A-receptors, which presumably accounts for its failure to produce natriuresis *in vivo*. In addition, there is a third type of receptor, C-receptors, which are not coupled to guanylate cyclase, and therefore lack biological activity, functioning as clearance receptors. There are other major differences within this group of peptides regarding their physiological actions and site of production. ANP, BNP, and URO have a potent natriuretic effect, while CNP has only a modest effect on sodium handling in the kidney. On the other hand, CNP but not ANP has venodilatory action. Since the signal mechanisms are similar, differences in biological activity depend on the site of production of the peptide and distribution of their respective receptors (Gardner, JCI, 1993; 92:1606). The kidney is relatively deficient in type-B receptors. ANP and BNP are produced primarily by the myocardial cells and secreted into the circulation, where they are carried to distant target tissues to act in true hormonal fashion. CNP is mainly synthesized by the vascular endothelium and probably functions as a local autocrine or paracrine regulator, with its effects being confined to a specific vascular bed (Stingo, AmJPhysiol, 1992; 262:H308; Stingo, AmJPhysiol, 1992; 263:H1318; Wei, AmJPhysiol, 1993; 264:H71). Finally, URO appears to be synthesized by the distal nephron (connecting and cortical collecting tubules). It is considered that URO is released from these segments into the tubular lumen and induces natriuresis by interacting with A-receptors located downstream of the nephron, in the inner medullary collecting duct.

Among the different natriuretic peptides, the most extensively studied is ANP. It is a 28-amino-acid peptide synthesized by atrial myocytes; it exhibits potent vasodilator and natriuretic effects (Laragh, NEJM, 1985; 331:1330; Ackerman, ClinChem, 1986; 32: 241; DeBold, FedProc, 1986; 45:2081; Needleman, NEJM, 1986; 314:828; Goetz, AmJPhysiol, 1988; 254:E1; Lang, ISIAtlasSci:

Pharmacology, 1988; 2:295; Sonnenberg, ISIAtlasSci: Pharmacol, 1988; 2:171). This cardiac hormone is cleaved from an atrial peptide precursor of high molecular weight, stored in specific granules, and released into the circulation, mainly via the coronary sinus (Crozier, Hypertension, 1986; 8:III11), in response to atrial distension. The plasma levels of ANP are therefore an index of the fullness of the intrathoracic vascular compartment. In this respect, any manoeuvre 'or disease that produces central volume expansion (intravenous saline administration, high sodium intake, head-out water immersion, adoption of a supine position from standing, primary hyperaldosteronism, inappropriate ADH secretion, congestive heart failure, chronic renal failure) is associated with an increased synthesis and release of ANP, and with high plasma levels of this hormone. Conversely, the decrease in central blood volume and in atrial distension produced by water or sodium restriction, diuretic administration, mechanical ventilation with positive end-expiratory pressure, haemodialysis in patients with chronic renal failure, or by adequate treatment in patients with congestive heart failure, is accompanied by reductions in the plasma concentration of ANP. The intracellular mechanism involved in the release of ANP is mediated by a rise in intracellular calcium and activation of the phosphoinositide pathway. ANP release may be inhibited by the sympathetic nervous activity and stimulated by A-II, ADH and endothelin. The significance of these influences in physiological and pathophysiological conditions is unknown.

ANP is cleared rapidly from plasma, with a half-life of 1–4 min. The predominant clearance pathway is mediated by C-receptors, which are the major high-affinity cell surface receptors for ANP in many tissues, including vascular endothelium, vascular smooth muscle cells, and glomeruli (Maak, Science, 1987; 238:675; Nussenzveig, JBC, 1990; 265:20952).[80] This receptor, which is not coupled to any known effector system for biological activity, serves for uptake and internalization of circulating ANP, leading to hydrolysis of the peptide in the lysosomal compartment. Circulating ANP is filtered by the glomeruli and almost totally inactivated by a neutral endopeptidase present in the brush border of the proximal tubule epithelial cells (Wilkins, AmJPhysiol, 1992; 262:F161). Analogues of ANP have been constructed that are devoid of intrinsic ANP biological activity and that bind with high affinity to the C-receptor subtype.[80] These analogues have been shown to reduce the metabolic clearance, to raise the circulating plasma levels of ANP and to elicit natriuretic and arterial hypotensive effects (Almeida, AmJPhysiol, 1989; 256:R469). On the other hand, there are inhibitors of neutral endopeptidases (thiorphan and phophoramidon) that increase urinary excretion of ANP and of its second messenger cGMP, produce natriuresis, and potentiate the renal responses to infused ANP (Brand, JAmCollCard, 1993; 22:86A; Seymour, ClinExpPharmPhys, 1995; 22:63). The potential therapeutic usefulness of these compounds is currently being assessed.

ANP has complex effects within the kidney.[76,77] In the isolated kidney, which lacks innervation and circulating vasoconstrictive substances, ANP is known to produce a vasoconstrictor effect on the efferent arteriole, increasing total vascular resistance. In contrast, when isolated kidneys are preconstricted with A-II, noradrenaline, or ADH, ANP markedly decreases total renal vascular resistance toward normal values. On the other hand, experiments in isolated arcuate arteries have shown that ANP antagonizes the vasoconstrictor effect of all vasoconstrictor manoeuvres, and studies using videometric techniques in hydronephrotic rats have shown that ANP leads to a vasorelaxation of the renal arcuate, intralobular, and afferent arterioles, but significantly constricts the efferent arterioles. These studies indicate that ANP does not behave as a classic renal vasodilator, but rather as a powerful antagonistic of preglomerular vasoconstriction and that it consistently constricts the efferent vasculature, an effect that contributes to one of the major renal actions of the hormone, namely, the increase in GFR.

In addition to these effects on the renal vasculature, ANP causes a marked increase in natriuresis.[76,77] The natriuretic effect of ANP is so marked that it can increase urinary sodium concentration to levels above the plasma sodium concentration. The increased amount of the filtered sodium and other still poorly defined intrarenal haemodynamic changes are of major importance in this effect since natriuresis induced by ANP, but not that induced by furosemide, can be nearly totally abolished by manoeuvres such as aortic or renal artery clamping, which reduce renal perfusion pressure and prevent the rise in GFR. Although recent evidence suggests that ANP directly inhibits sodium reabsorption in the inner medullary collecting duct, the renal clamp experiments demonstrate that the intrarenal haemodynamic effects of ANP are the most important cause of its natriuretic effect.

ANP has striking inhibitory effects on the renin–angiotensin–aldosterone system.[76,77] It inhibits renin release at doses that increase the plasma levels of the hormone within the physiological range. This effect is mediated by increasing hydrostatic pressure at the juxtaglomerular cells through afferent arteriolar vasodilation and by increasing the amount of filtered sodium and the sodium delivery to the macula densa. ANP is also a powerful inhibitor of the vascular effect of A-II and of other endogenous vasoconstrictors. Finally, it also inhibits the stimulatory effect of A-II on aldosterone production by the adrenal glands. This effect is unspecific since ANP also inhibits the stimulation of aldosterone production by other factors, such as potassium and ACTH.

Pharmacological doses of ANP in normal subjects are associated with a decrease in arterial pressure.[76,77] This is generally associated with a decreased cardiac output and central venous pressure and an increase in systemic vascular resistance, suggesting that, in normal states, the primary haemodynamic response to exogenous ANP is a reduction in cardiac preload. Since ANP increases capillary permeability and does not affect venous compliance or capacitance, the reduction in cardiac output is likely to be due to a decrease of the intravascular fluid compartment. However, there is evidence that in pathological states characterized by increased vascular tone, as in patients with decompensated cardiac failure, which is characterized by activation of the renin–angiotensin–aldosterone system and sympathetic nervous system, ANP may induce a significant net reduction in systemic vascular resistance. These findings are consistent with *in vitro* studies showing that ANP functions as an antagonist of vasoconstrictor mechanism rather than as a true vasodilator. In fact, the vasodilatory effect of ANP is detected only in precontracted vessels. ANP antagonizes contractions induced by all vascular vasoconstrictors. For unknown reasons this effect is particularly pronounced toward the vasoconstrictor effect of A-II. There is also considerable variability in the sensitivity of vascular territories to ANP, the kidneys being one of the most sensitive territories.

The plasma level of ANP is increased in non-azotaemic cirrhotics with ascites, as well as in patients with hepatorenal syndrome (Campbell, AmJMed, 1988; 84:112; Klepetko, Gastro, 1988; 95:764; Morgan, Gastro, 1988; 95:1641; Skorecki, AmJMed, 1988; 85:375; Epstein, AmJNephrol, 1989; 9:133; Salerno, Gastro, 1990; 98:1063; Angeli, Hepatol, 1992; 16:1389). In patients without ascites ANP levels may be either normal or increased.[81,82] In one study, plasma levels of ANP were measured simultaneously in samples obtained from the coronary sinus, right atrium, pulmonary artery, hepatic vein, and femoral vein in cirrhotics with ascites with and without hepatorenal syndrome.[81] The coronary sinus blood flow was also measured in these individuals by thermodilution; therefore, the cardiac release and the splanchnic and peripheral extraction of ANP could be determined. The plasma concentration of ANP was significantly higher in cirrhotics than in controls in the venous blood of every vascular territory studied. The high plasma ANP in these patients was clearly related to increased production and release, and not to impaired splanchnic and peripheral extraction of the peptide (Fig. 9). A recent article showing that elevation of ANP in experimental cirrhosis was associated with increased ANP gene expression in the heart are in keeping with this study (Poulos, Gastro, 1995; 108:1496). The possibility that altered synthesis of ANP led to abnormal molecular forms without biological activity, was proposed to explain the paradoxical observation of sodium retention and increased plasma levels of ANP in cirrhosis with ascites. This was not supported by studies comparing the chromatographic pattern and the biological activity of ANP obtained from cirrhotic patients with ascites and from healthy subjects (Jiménez, Hepatol, 1991; 14:601).

Pharmacological doses of synthetic human ANP to patients or animals with cirrhosis and ascites result in a significantly lower increase in GFR, urine volume, and sodium excretion than in controls (Koepke, AmJPhysiol, 1987; 252:1210; Petrillo, JCardiol-Pharmacol, 1988; 12:279; Salerno, Hepatol, 1988; 8:21; Ferrier, AmJNephrol, 1989; 9:291; Laffi, Gastro, 1989; 96:167; López,

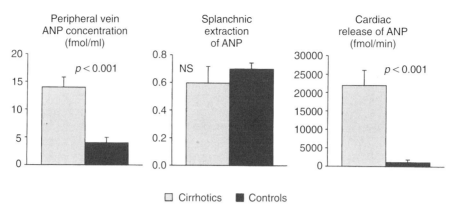

Fig. 9. Plasma levels, splanchnic extraction, and cardiac release of atrial natriuretic peptide (ANP) in patients with cirrhosis and individuals with atypical chest pain and normal coronary arteriograms (controls). (Reproduced with permission from Ginés, P. *et al. Hepatology*, 1988; **8**: 636–42.)

JHepatol, 1989; 9:217; Morali, AmJMed, 1991; 91:383; Ginès, Gastro, 1992; 102:280; Warner, Hepatol, 1993; 17:500; Moreau, GastrClinBiol, 1994; 18:568). In most patients with marked sodium retention and elevated levels of plasma renin activity, aldosterone, and noradrenaline, the renal response to high doses of ANP may be completely blunted. This renal resistance to the effects of ANP is probably unrelated to alterations at the receptor level, since the increase in the plasma levels of ANP after head-out water immersion in cirrhotics with ascites is associated with an appropriate increase in the urinary excretion of cGMP, the second messenger for ANP in the kidney. As renal denervation reverses the blunted diuretic and natriuretic responses to ANP in cirrhotic rats with ascites, the renal resistance to ANP in cirrhosis may be related to the increased activity of endogenous antinatriuretic and vasoconstrictor factors (renin–angiotensin–aldosterone system, noradrenaline, ADH) which overcomes the effects on ANP in intrarenal haemodynamics and excretory function.

The circulating plasma levels of BNP are also increased in cirrhotic patients with ascites with and without hepatorenal syndrome.[25] These patients also present a blunted natriuretic response to pharmacological doses of this peptide (LaVilla, Hepatol, 1995; 22:1745). BNP is preferentially produced by the ventricles from a prohormone different to that of ANP.[83] The mechanism regulating BNP release is probably the same as that for ANP, i.e. the degree of expansion of the central blood volume, and its pharmacological spectrum, including diuretic, natriuretic, hypotensive, and smooth muscle relaxant activity and suppressive effect on the renin–angiotensin–aldosterone system, is also similar to that of ANP.[83]

The mechanism responsible for the increased cardiac secretion of ANP and BNP is unknown. Plasma volume is increased in cirrhotics with ascites. Therefore ANP and BNP hypersecretion in these patients could be due to an expansion of the intrathoracic blood volume secondary to this hypervolaemia. However, recent studies have shown that although cirrhotic patients present an increased cardiac output, indicating an elevated amount of blood circulating through the intrathoracic vascular compartment per unit of time, the transit time in this compartment is extremely short, so that the amount of blood existing in a particular moment, which is that influencing the release of natriuretic peptides, is in fact decreased.[84] On the other hand, atrial pressure is usually normal in these patients.[81] Therefore, the increased release of ANP and BNP in cirrhosis occurs in the setting of a central hypovolaemia and normal atrial pressure.

The urinary excretion of URO, which probably reflects the renal production of this peptide, is normal in cirrhotic patients with and without ascites.[27] The circulating natriuretic peptides (ANP and BNP) and URO are, therefore, independently regulated in patients with cirrhosis and ascites. The circulating plasma levels of CNP are increased in cirrhotic patients with ascites as compared with compensated cirrhotics and normal subjects (Gerbes, Hepatol, 1996; 24:447A). However, the significance of this is unknown.

With the introduction of specific antagonists of natriuretic peptide receptors, their role in circulatory and renal function in physiological and pathological conditions will probably became more clear. In the only study so far published on cirrhosis, the natriuretic peptide receptor blocking agent HS-142–1 was given to conscious control rats and rats with carbon tetrachloride-induced cirrhosis with ascites.[26] No significant changes in arterial pressure were observed in either group of animals. In control rats HS-142–1 induced a significant decrease in GFR, urine volume, and sodium excretion. However, no significant changes were observed in these animals in renal plasma flow and renal vascular resistance. In contrast, in cirrhotic rats with ascites, HS-142–1 administration was associated with a dramatic decrease in renal blood flow and increased renal vascular resistance (Fig. 10). Cirrhotic rats also experienced a decrease in GFR, urine volume, and sodium excretion, which was significantly more marked than in control rats. HS-142–1 suppressed plasma renin activity and aldosterone in cirrhotic rats but not in control animals. These findings indicate that endogenous natriuretic peptides play a critical role in the maintenance of renal perfusion and GFR and in the regulation of the renin–angiotensin–aldosterone system in cirrhosis with ascites.

Natriuretic hormone (sodium pump inhibitor)

Natriuretic hormone is a still uncharacterized hormone of probable hypothalamic origin. Although its chemical nature is presently

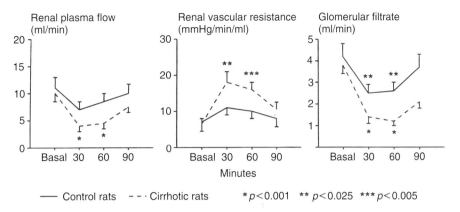

Fig. 10. Renal plasma flow, renal vascular resistance, and glomerular filtration rate in control (solid line) and cirrhotic rats with ascites (dotted line) under baseline conditions and at 30, 60, and 90 min after the administration of a specific antagonist of endogenous natriuretic peptide receptors. Significances denoted in the figure are versus baseline values. (Reproduced with permission from Angeli *et al. Hepatology*, 1994; **20**: 948–54.)

unknown, many of its biological effects are well established (De Wardener, PhysiolRev, 1985; 65:678; Haddy, NEJM, 1987; 316: 621; Hanlyn, ISIAtlasSci:Pharmacol, 1988; 2:339; Goto, PharmRev, 1992; 44:377; Woofson, KidneyInt, 1994; 46:299). It is a digitalis-like substance that crossreacts with antidigoxin antibodies and binds to ouabain receptors. It inhibits Na^+, K^+-ATPase (the sodium pump) *in vitro* and *in vivo*. Finally, in animals, it increases sodium excretion and arterial pressure. Natriuresis occurs without change in renal blood flow and glomerular filtration rate, indicating that it is due to inhibition of tubular sodium reabsorption. The hypertensive effect is due to increased arterial vascular resistance. Both effects may be due to inhibition of the Na^+, K^+-ATPase activity in renal tubular and vascular smooth muscle cells, respectively. Na^+, K^+-ATPase is located in the basolateral membrane of the tubular cells and promotes sodium transport from the intracellular to the extracellular compartment, and the entry of potassium into the cells. The resulting decrease in intracellular sodium favours reabsorption of sodium from the tubular lumen. Inhibition of Na^+, K^+-ATPase in smooth muscle cells promotes entry of calcium ions, thus increasing their contractility. The biological activities of natriuretic hormone are detected in specific fractions of plasma and urine obtained by gel chromatography. Its activity in plasma and urine increases in circumstances of extracellular volume expansion (high sodium diet, intravenous saline infusion, head-out water immersion, administration of mineralocorticoids, chronic renal failure). On the other hand, rats with lesions of the anteroventral third ventricle (in the central nervous system) fail to increase natriuretic hormone and are unable to increase sodium excretion in response to acute intravenous sodium loading. Natriuretic hormone is therefore considered an important factor in the regulation of extracellular fluid volume and sodium excretion. The fact that its activity in plasma and urine is elevated in patients and experimental animals with arterial hypertension suggests that it also may be involved in the pathogenesis of this disorder (Buckalew, AnnRevPhysiol, 1984; 46:343).[85]

The initial studies on natriuretic hormone in cirrhosis showed conflicting results. Naccarato *et al.* observed that the natriuretic effect of urinary extracts obtained by gel chromatography was significantly lower in eight compensated cirrhotics than in eight healthy subjects, both groups being submitted to extracellular volume expansion with saline; suggesting a deficient release of natriuretic hormone in response to volume expansion in the early phases of hepatic cirrhosis (Gastro 1981; 81:205). Favre (Adv-Nephrol, 1981; 11:3) and Kramer (PostgradMedJ, 1975; 51:532) also found decreased urinary excretion of natriuretic hormone in eight cirrhotics with ascites. However, others found that plasma activity of natriuretic hormone (estimated by ouabain displacement assay and digoxin-like immunoreactivity), was normal or increased in these patients (Yang, Hepatol, 1986; 9:363; Cunningham, KidneyInt, 1988; 34:570). Recently, LaVilla *et al.* evaluated activity of natriuretic hormone in urinary extracts obtained by gel chromatography in a large series of cirrhotics with ascites, with and without hepatorenal syndrome, compensated cirrhotics, and healthy volunteers (Hepatol, 1990; 12:464). Activity (assessed by inhibition of Na^+, K^+-ATPase, crossreaction with antidigoxin antibodies, and effect on sodium excretion in rats) was consistently increased in all subgroups of cirrhotic patients compared with healthy subjects. Plasma ANP was also increased in the subsets of patients with ascites. Interestingly, in a second study, this group of investigators found that human urinary extracts containing a material that inhibits the enzyme Na^+,K^+-ATPase and produces natriuresis in the bioassay control rat failed to increase sodium excretion in cirrhotic rats with ascites, suggesting a renal resistance to the effect of natriuretic hormone in cirrhosis (Asbert, JHepatol, 1994; 20:660). It is evident, therefore, that sodium retention in cirrhosis is not due to deficient production of natriuretic hormones (natriuretic peptides and natriuretic hormone) but rather to an increased activity of endogenous antinatriuretic systems.

Nitric oxide

The history of nitric oxide (NO) as a endogenous vasoactive factor synthesized by the vascular endothelium was initiated in 1980 by Furchgott and Zawadsky (Nature, 1980; 288:373), who showed that the vasodilator effect of acetylcholine in isolated aortic strips is dependent on the integrity of the endothelial lining of the vessels. They suggested the existence of an endothelium-derived relaxing factor that mediated the effect of acetylcholine. In 1987 Palmer *et al.* demonstrated that this factor was nitric oxide (Nature, 1987;

327:524), a highly diffusible and reactive, short-lived gas. Nitric oxide is also produced by vascular and non-vascular smooth muscle cells, macrophages, fibroblasts, central and peripheral neurones, renal tubular epithelial cells and mesangial cells, hepatocytes, Ito cells and neutrophils (Moncada, PharmRev 1991; 43:109; Moncada, NEJM, 1993; 329:2002). In addition to participating in the homeostasis of arterial blood pressure and regional haemodynamics (Navar, PhysiolRev, 1966; 76:425; Persson, PhysiolRev, 1966; 76:193), nitric oxide is known to be involved in the host immune response and to be a major neurotransmitter of the non-adrenergic–non-cholinergic nervous system and a cytotoxic and bactericidal agent (Ignarro, AnnRevPharmTox, 1990; 30:535; Moncada, PharmRev, 1991; 43: 109; Lowenstein, Cell, 1992; 70:705; Vane, JPhysiolPharmacol, 1992; 43:195; Lowenstein, AnnIntMed, 1994; 120:227).

Nitric oxide is formed from molecular oxygen and the guanidino nitrogen of L-arginine by the action of the nitric oxide synthases (Moncada, PharmRev, 1991; 43:109; Schmidt, CellCalcium, 1992; 13:427; Schmidt, BBActa, 1993; 1178:153; Marín, JAuton-Pharmacol, 1995; 15:279). Nitric oxide formation occurs in two steps. The first step consists of an N-oxygenation of L-arginine to Nw-hydroxy-L-arginine. The second step consists of an oxidative cleavage of the $C=N$ bond of Nw-hydroxy-L-arginine leading to citrulline and nitric oxide. There are three nitric oxide synthases (Forsterman, BiochemPharm, 1991; 42:1849). Neuronal and endothelial nitric oxide synthase, which are also termed nitric oxide synthase I and nitric oxide synthase III, respectively, are constitutively present in the cells. A third nitric oxide synthase, inducible or nitric oxide synthase II, is expressed primarily after transcriptional induction (Nathan, FASEBJ, 1992; 6:3051). Constitutive nitric oxide synthases I and III are Ca^{2+}/calmodulin dependent enzymes, while inducible isoform II is a Ca^{2+}-independent enzyme. Nitric oxide synthase II produces greater and longer-lasting nitric oxide release than do constitutive I and III nitric oxide synthases. Because nitric oxide synthase reacts directly with L-arginine, it is possible to interfere with this mechanism by providing excess quantities of various non-metabolizable L-arginine analogues such as NG-nitro-L-arginine (L-**NNA**), NG-nitro-L-arginine methyl ester (L-**NAME**), and NG-monomethyl-L-arginine (L-**NMMA**), which competitively inhibit the formation of nitric oxide (Moncada, PharmRev, 1991; 43:109; Nathan, FASEBJ, 1992; 6:3051). Other agents such as haemoglobin, methylene blue, and gossypol can interfere with the action of nitric oxide to increase cGMP formation. These agents inhibit the three isoforms of nitric oxide synthase. The recent development of specific inhibitors of nitric oxide synthase II will be of great value in the further understanding of the physiology and pathophysiology of nitric oxide.

In vascular tissue, the nitric oxide synthase III (constitutive nitric oxide synthase isoform) has been cloned in endothelial cells (Lamas, PNAS, 1992; 89:6348). The amount of nitric oxide generated by nitric oxide synthase III is small (nmolar quantities). Once synthesized within the endothelial cells, nitric oxide diffuses to adjacent vascular smooth muscle cells, where it binds to the haem moiety of the soluble guanylyl cyclase and catalyses increased formation of cGMP which produces relaxation, presumably by reduction of the intracellular free Ca^{2+} concentration (Schmidt, BBActa, 1993; 1178:153). The effect of nitric oxide is transient since it is rapidly inactivated. However, since endothelial nitric oxide synthase III is tonically active *in vivo*, there is a continuous basal

production of nitric oxide which leads to a nitric oxide-dependent vasodilator tone (Lowenstein, AnnIntMed, 1994; 120:227). This continuous effect of nitric oxide on vascular smooth muscle cells is essential for the regulation of arterial pressure and regional blood flow. In fact, the inhibition of nitric oxide synthesis with L-arginine analogues in normal animals is associated with a marked increase in arterial pressure and reduction in regional blood flow. The basal production of nitric oxide regulates blood flow in the brain, heart, lungs, gastrointestinal tract, and kidney. It appears that the kidney vasculature is more dependent than other vascular tissues on endogenous nitric oxide to maintain a low vascular resistance (Naver, PhysiolRev, 1996; 76:425). The nitric oxide-dependent vasodilator tone seems to be related to the continuous activation of nitric oxide synthase III by physical stimuli such as pulsatile flow and shear stress. Other stimuli that increase the activity of endothelial nitric oxide synthase III and the release of nitric oxide include several endogenous substances with vasodilator properties (endothelium-dependent vasodilators: substance P, acetylcholine, bradykinin, platelet activating factor, and ATP). The stimuli that increase nitric oxide synthase III activity generally cause an increase in endothelial cell cytosolic Ca^{2+} via activation of phospholipase C or activation of calcium channels that allow the influx of calcium. Calcium binds to calmodulin, and the calcium–calmodulin complex activates the nitric oxide synthase III constitutively present in the endothelial cells. Nitrovasodilators are nitric oxide donors and exert their pharmacological effect by releasing nitric oxide directly to the vascular smooth muscle cells without the co-operation of the endothelial cells.

Nitric oxide synthase II is not constitutively expressed in vascular tissue. However, it can be induced in endothelial and especially in the smooth muscle cells by endotoxin and cytokines (tumour necrosis factors and interleukin) (Lowenstein, PNAS, 1992; 89: 6711). Since nitric oxide synthase II is regulated at the transcriptional level, the initiation of nitric oxide synthesis and release is delayed after the stimulus (by several hours) but once initiated the synthesis of nitric oxide is long-lasting (Marín, JAuton-Pharmacol 1995; 15:279). Another differential characteristic of nitric oxide synthase II is that it induces the synthesis of large amounts of nitric oxide (mmolar quantities).

Nitric oxide synthase inhibition in experimental animals is associated with a 25 to 30 per cent reduction in renal blood flow without significant changes in GFR, suggesting a preferential vasodilatory effect of nitric oxide on the efferent arterioles (Navar, PhysiolRev, 1996; 76:425). There are closed interactions between nitric oxide and other renal vasoactive systems. Infusions of A-II at doses that have little effect on renal vascular resistance when given alone, cause massive renal vasoconstriction when the nitric oxide system is acutely inhibited (Alberola, AmJPhysiol, 1994; 267:R1472; Raij, KidneyInt, 1995; 48:20). Inhibition of nitric oxide also potentiates the renal vasoconstrictor effects of endothelin (Ito, Hypertension, 1991; 17:1052). These data suggest that, as occurs with prostaglandins, nitric oxide is an important mechanism in maintaining renal perfusion in circumstances of increased activity of the endogenous vasoconstrictor systems. There are also close correlations between nitric oxide and PGI_2 (Doni, EurJPharm, 1988; 151:19; Lahera, Hypertension, 1990; 15:659; Lahera, AmJHypertension, 1991; 4:260; Salom, AmJPhysiol, 1991; 260:F145; Salazar, AmJPhysiol, 1995; 268:R1442). PGI_2 inhibits endothelial nitric oxide release. On the other hand, the renal vasodilatory potential of nitric oxide is particularly evident in the presence of prostaglandin inhibition. These data suggest that the renal vasodilatory tone mediated by nitric oxide is especially important for the maintenance of renal perfusion in circumstances of impaired prostaglandin synthesis and that both systems probably operate simultaneously in the homeostasis of renal blood flow.

Valance and Moncada were the first to propose that nitric oxide could play a pathogenic role in the arterial vasodilation and hyperdynamic circulation in cirrhosis (Lancet, 1991; 337:776). Many studies using different approaches in animals with experimental cirrhosis and prehepatic portal hypertension, and in patients with compensated and decompensated cirrhosis, have subsequently given support to this hypothesis.

The first approach used to assess the role of nitric oxide in circulatory dysfunction in cirrhosis was to inhibit nitric oxide synthesis with L-arginine analogues in experimental animals. Clària et al. (Hepatol, 1992; 15:343) using increasing doses of L-NNA showed that the pressor effect of nitric oxide inhibition in the systemic arterial circulation was significantly greater in cirrhotics rats with ascites than in control animals, suggesting increased activity of endogenous vascular nitric oxide (Fig. 11). During the same year, Pizcueta et al. (Gastro, 1992; 103:1909) found that the administration of L-NAME to rats with prehepatic portal hypertension was associated with a significant increase in arterial pressure and systemic and splanchnic arterial vascular resistance and a reduction in cardiac output. However, since the dose of L-NAME used in this study was very high, the observed haemodynamic changes could be unspecific and related to the vasoconstrictor effect of nitric oxide inhibition. This problem was subsequently addressed by Niedberger et al. (Gastro, 1995; 109: 1624). Aortic tissue concentration of cGMP, the second messenger of nitric oxide, was used as an estimation of the vascular production of nitric oxide in rats with experimental cirrhosis and ascites and in control rats. The baseline aortic tissue concentration of cGMP was markedly increased in cirrhotic rats. L-NAME, at a dose that returned aortic cGMP to normal in cirrhotic rats, corrected the arteriolar vasodilation and the hyperdynamic circulation in these animals. These studies suggest that in cirrhosis there is increased activity of vascular nitric oxide which participates in the pathogenesis of the arteriolar vasodilation and hyperdynamic circulation.

A reduced pressor effect of vasoconstrictors is an important contributory factor to the systemic arteriolar vasodilation in cirrhosis (Laragh, JCI, 1963; 42:1179; Ames, JCI, 1965; 44:1171; Jiménez, Gastro, 1994; 107:1201). The arterial system in cirrhosis is not only relaxed but also responds poorly to the vasoconstrictor effect of A-II, endothelin, ADH, and catecholamines. Nitric oxide is involved in this feature. Studies in normal rats and rats with prehepatic portal hypertension (partial portal vein ligation) and cirrhosis have shown that the reduced pressor response to endothelin or methoxamine in the systemic arterial circulation returned to normal following nitric oxide inhibition with L-NNA or L-NAME (Lee, Hepatol, 1992; 16:1043; Hartleb, Gastro, 1994; 107: 1085). Studies in aortic rings from cirrhotic rats with ascites and control animals have shown that the reduced contractility of cirrhotic rings to A-II, noradrenaline, or phenylephrine was reversed after incubation with inhibitors of nitric oxide or endothelial denudation, but was not influenced by cyclo-oxygenase inhibition

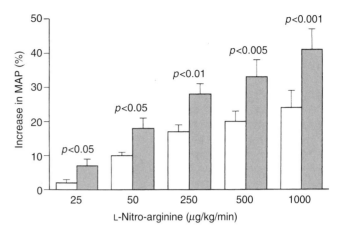

Fig. 11. Percentage increase in mean arterial pressure following nitric oxide inhibition with increasing doses of l-nitro-arginine in control (empty bars) and cirrhotic rats with ascites (shadowed bars). P values given in the figures represent differences between control and cirrhotic rats. (Reproduced with permission from Clària et al. *Hepatology*, 1992; **15**: 343–9.)

with indomethacin (Castro, Hepatol, 1993; 18:367; Karatapanis, Hepatol, 1994; 20:1516; Michielsen, JHepatol, 1995; 23:341). On the other hand, the effect of nitric oxide inhibition in returning the contractility of aortic rings to normal disappeared following endothelial denudation. Contrary to what occurs with vasoconstrictors, the responsiveness to endothelial nitric oxide-dependent vasodilators (acetylcholine and ADP) is increased in aortic rings from cirrhotic rats with ascites (Claria, Hepatol, 1994; 20: 1615), adding further support to the suggestion that the endothelial nitric oxide synthetic pathway is increased in cirrhosis. Finally, since arterial vasodilation in cirrhosis occurs predominantly in the splanchnic circulation, a similar set of experiments has been performed in perfused superior mesenteric arterial beds of normal rats and rats with prehepatic portal hypertension and with cirrhosis and ascites (Sieber, Gastro, 1992; 103:235; Sieber, Gastro, 1993; 104:1750). In both groups of portal hypertensive animals there was a significant hyporeactivity to the vasoconstrictor effect of noradrenaline, ADH and potassium chloride, and this hyporesponsiveness was overcome by preincubating vessel preparations with L-NNA. These data, therefore, suggest that the increased vascular nitric oxide activity may be located predominantly in the vascular endothelium and plays a major role in the hyporesponsiveness to vasoconstrictors in cirrhosis.

More direct evidence of increased vascular nitric oxide activity has been presented by other studies. Ros et al. (Hepatol, 1995; 21: 554), using a co-incubation assay, demonstrated that endothelial nitric oxide production is higher in arterial vessels of cirrhotic rats with ascites than in vessels of control rats. On the other hand, nitric oxide synthase III mRNA and protein expression have been shown to be increased in thoracic aorta of cirrhotic rats (Martin, AmJPhysiol, 1996; 270:F494; Morales-Ruiz, Hepatol, 1996; 24:1481). Finally nitric oxide synthase II has been reported to be expressed in arterial vessels of cirrhotic rats with ascites but not of control animals (Morales-Ruiz, Hepatol, 1996; 24:1481). Therefore, both the constitutive (nitric oxide synthase III) and the inducible (nitric oxide synthase II) nitric oxide synthase pathway appear to be activated in cirrhosis. Recent studies have suggested that tumour necrosis factor, a cytokine that has been found to be increased in cirrhosis, may participate in the stimulation of nitric oxide synthase II (López-Talavera, Gastro, 1995; 108:761; López-Talavera, Hepatol, 1996; 23:1696).

Preliminary data indicate that the expression of nitric oxide synthase III is decreased in the intrahepatic vasculature and that gene transfer of nitric oxide synthase III reduces portal pressure in rats with experimental cirrhosis (Van de Casteele, Hepatol, 1996; 24;313A; Roskams, Hepatol, 1996; 24:314A). A reduced intrahepatic nitric oxide synthase III could, therefore, contribute to the pathogenesis of sinusoidal portal hypertension in cirrhosis.

There have been very few investigations on nitric oxide in human cirrhosis, but they are all in agreement with the experimental studies reported above. The serum concentration of nitrite and nitrate, which are indicative products of nitric oxide oxidation, are significantly elevated in patients with cirrhosis and ascites compared to control subjects (Guarner, Hepatol, 1993; 18:1139), suggesting an increased production of nitric oxide. Also, the endogenous pulmonary nitric oxide production measured in exhaled air is increased in patients with cirrhosis (Sogni, JHepatol, 1995; 23:471). The pressor responsiveness to nitric oxide inhibition is higher in cirrhotic patients than in control subjects (Campillo, Hepatol, 1995; 22:1423). An increased response to nitric oxide-dependent vasodilators has also been reported in cirrhotic patients (Albillos, AmJPhysiol, 1995; 268:G459). Finally, the impaired pressor responsiveness to vasoconstrictors in hepatic arteries from patients with liver failure returns to normal following nitric oxide synthesis inhibition (Smith, Endothelium, 1993; 1:S90 (Abstr.)).

There is experimental evidence that nitric oxide plays a major role in the homeostasis of renal haemodynamics in cirrhosis (Clària, Hepatol, 1992; 15:343; Ros, Hepatol, 1995; 22:915). The inhibition of prostaglandin synthesis by lysine acetylsalicylate in rats with experimental cirrhosis and ascites is associated with a modest but significant decrease in renal perfusion and GFR, an effect not observed in control animals. Nitric oxide inhibition with L-NNA, at a dose that increases arterial pressure significantly and reduces renal perfusion by more than 50 per cent in control animals, does not significantly affect renal perfusion in cirrhotic rats with ascites. Since the urinary excretion of 6-keto-PGF$_{1\alpha}$ increased markedly in cirrhotic rats during nitric oxide inhibition, it may be possible that the renal vasoconstrictor effect of nitric oxide inhibition was overcome by a compensatory increase in the renal vascular synthesis of the PGI$_2$. In fact, when both prostaglandin and nitric oxide synthesis are inhibited simultaneously, there is a dramatic decrease of renal blood flow and GFR in cirrhotic rats with ascites. These data indicate that in experimental cirrhosis both nitric oxide and PGI$_2$ play an important role in the maintenance of renal blood flow and GFR within normal limits, and suggest that both systems operate synergistically in the sense that one takes control when the other is inhibited. The renal circulation in rats with prehepatic portal hypertension and experimental cirrhosis behaves in a similar way as the systemic circulation regarding the response to vasoconstrictors and to endothelium-dependent vasodilators. The renal vasoconstrictor response to methoxamine is blunted in rats with prehepatic portal hypertension, and this hyporesponsiveness is abolished by nitric oxide inhibition (García-Estañ, JHepatol, 1996; 25:206). On the other hand, the renal vasodilator response to

acetylcholine is increased in cirrhotic rats (García-Estañ, AmJPhysiol, 1994; 267:R549).

Nitric oxide may also participate in renal tubular sodium and water handling in cirrhosis (Clària, Hepatol, 1992; 15:343; Ros, Hepatol, 1995; 22:915; Tajiri, Hepatol, 1995; 22:1430). Inhibition of nitric oxide synthesis in rats with cirrhosis and ascites is associated with a significant increase in urine volume and sodium excretion, an effect not observed in control rats. However, since arterial pressure and GFR also increase after nitric oxide inhibition in cirrhotic rats, the diuretic and natriuretic effects could be non-specific and related to intrarenal haemodynamic changes, namely the increased filtered load and a pressure natriuresis. The administration of L-arginine, the natural substrate for nitric oxide synthase, to humans and experimental animals is associated with an increased synthesis of nitric oxide, as indicated by an elevation in the urinary excretion of cGMP and nitrates/nitrites. So far only one study has been published assessing the role of L-arginine administration in cirrhosis, and it was performed in patients with moderate ascites (Tajiri, Hepatol, 1995; 22:1430). L-Arginine administration produced a significant reduction in arterial pressure without significant changes in creatinine clearance in normal subjects and cirrhotic patients. The most relevant finding was that, despite the reduction in arterial pressure and the lack of changes in GFR, there was a marked increase in urine volume and sodium excretion in both groups, indicating an inhibition of tubular sodium reabsorption. The increase in the urinary excretion of cGMP was greater and the diuretic and natriuretic effect of L-arginine smaller in cirrhotics than in controls. Therefore these findings suggest that although nitric oxide is natriuretic in cirrhosis with ascites, there is a renal resistance to the tubular effect of this compound.

One of the most relevant functions of nitric oxide is its powerful microbicidal activity. The recent demonstration that nitric oxide synthase II is induced in peritoneal macrophages of rats with carbon tetrachloride-induced cirrhosis and that spontaneous bacterial peritonitis constantly develops in this experimental model following the administration of the specific nitric oxide synthase II inhibitor, L-NIL, suggests that nitric oxide may be extremely important in preventing acute bacterial infections in decompensated cirrhosis (Morales-Ruiz, Gastro, 1997; 112:2056). The studies of Laffi et al. (Hepatol, 1995; 22:1666) and Criado-Jiménez et al. (JMolMed, 1995; 73:31), showing an increased activity of the nitric oxide synthetic pathway in neutrophils and monocytes from cirrhotic patients with ascites, are in keeping with this suggestion.

Endothelins

Endothelins (ETs) are a family of three endogenous peptides, each of 21 amino acids, which have a variety of biological functions (Vane, JCardiolPharmacol, 1989; 13:S1; Yanagisawa, Biochem-Pharm, 1989; 38:1877; Rubanyi, FASEBJ, 1991; 5:2713; Macrae, TrendsEndocrinMetab, 1992; 3:153). ET-1 was identified from the medium of cultured endothelial cells (Yanagisawa, Nature, 1988; 332:411), it is the most potent vasoconstrictor peptide yet characterized. The vasoconstrictor activity of ET-1 is exceptionally long lasting. When a low intravenous bolus dose of ET-1 is given, a pressor response is detected for up to several hours. ET-1 is processed from a large prepropeptide precursor of approximately 200 amino acids (preproET-1) through the formation of a 38 to 39 amino acid intermediate form called big ET-1, which is probably secreted by endothelial cells (Yanagisawa, TrendsPharmacolSci, 1989; 10:374). Big ET-1 is then converted rapidly to ET-1 by the action of an ET converting enzyme (Opgenorth, FASEBJ, 1992; 6: 2653). In addition to being produced by endothelial cells, ET-1 is also produced by non-vascular cells from the brain, kidney, and lungs, and has a variety of actions in addition to its vasoactive effect. ET-2 and ET-3, the two other members of the family, are expressed in brain, kidney, adrenal glands, and gut but not in the endothelium. Detectable levels of ET-1 and ET-3 are found in plasma (Battistini, LabInvest, 1993; 68:601). ET-3 is relatively abundant in neural tissues and is thought to be a neural form of endothelin.

At least two endothelin receptor subtypes (**ETA** and **ETB**) have been identified (Sakurai, TrendsPharmacolSci, 1992; 13:103; Bax, TrendsPharmacolSci, 1994; 15:379). Interaction of endothelins with ETA and ETB receptors leads to activation of phospholipase C, which, in turn, increases the intracellular production of inositol-1, 4,5-triphosphate and the release of calcium from intracellular stores (Simonson, FASEBJ, 1990; 4:2989). Gating of receptor-operated calcium channels and indirect modulation of voltage-gated channels are also increased by endothelin. Endothelin-induced activation of phospholipase C also results in protein kinase C stimulation, which participates in various effects of endothelin, including its mitogenic effect (Simonson, PhysiolRev, 1993; 73:375). The binding of ET-1 to ETA receptor is about 100 times greater than that of ET-3 (Sakurai, Drugs, 1993; 46:795). The affinity of ET-2 to ETA receptor is between that of ET-1 and ET-3. ETB receptor shows similar affinity for the three endothelins. Endothelin receptor mRNA has been detected in several tissues, including brain, lung, heart, kidney, and liver (Hori, Endocrinol, 1992; 130:1885; Housset, PNAS, 1993; 90:9266). There is an important difference in the cellular distribution pattern of endothelin receptors in the vascular wall (Suraki, TrendsPharmacolSci, 1992;13:103). ETA receptor is found on the vascular smooth muscle cells. In contrast, ETB receptor predominates in the endothelial cells. Interaction of endothelins with ETA receptors in vascular smooth muscle cells results in intracellular release of calcium and vasoconstriction. The intracellular release of calcium induced by the activation of ETB receptors in the endothelial cells results in the stimulation of the constitutive nitric oxide synthase III and the release of nitric oxide (Rubanyi, PharmRev, 1994; 46:325). It is now clear that the initial vasodilator and hypotensive response to endothelin administration is mediated by this mechanism. However, this effect is very transient and is rapidly followed by a vasoconstrictor effect mediated by the irreversible interaction of endothelin with ETA receptors in the vascular smooth muscle cells. Interaction of endothelins with ETA and ETB receptors also stimulates phospholipase A_2 and the synthesis of PGI_2 and PGE_2 (Simonson, PhysiolRev, 1993;73:375). These vasodilator prostaglandins, together with nitric oxide, probably constitute negative-feedback signals attenuating endothelin-induced vasoconstriction in some vascular beds. Recent studies suggest the existence of two subtypes of ETB receptors (ETB1 and ETB2). ETB1 is related to nitric oxide production whereas ETB2 has similar effects to those of ETA (Sokolovsky, JBC, 1992; 267: 20551).

ET-1 is released in response to various stimuli, including shear stress, hypoxia, several vasoactive substances (thrombin, A-II, ADH, epinephrine, thromboxane A_2, and bradykinin), endotoxin, and some cytokines (interleukin-1 and tumour necrosis factor) (Simonson, PhysiolRev, 1993; 73:375; Rubanyi, PharmRev, 1994; 46:325). Once released, it acts as a local paracrine/autocrine peptide in the endothelial cells and in the underlying smooth muscle cells. The biological significance of the circulating plasma levels of endothelin is unknown (Battistini, LabInv, 1993; 68:600). It probably simply reflects spillover from local endothelin release. However, it has been suggested that in some conditions, the plasma concentration of endothelin may be sufficiently high to have biological activity. There are specific antagonists of ETA and ETB receptors for use in experimental animals and in man (Bax, TrendsPharmacolSci, 1994; 15:379).

In the kidney, ET-1 is produced by endothelial and non-endothelial cells, including mesangial cells and collecting tubule epithelial cells (Kohan, AmJKidneyDis, 1993;2 2:493; Nord, KidneyInt, 1993; 44:451; Simonson, AnnRevPhysiol, 1993; 55:249; Simonson, PhysiolRev, 1993; 73:375; Navar, PhysiolRev, 1996; 76: 425). ET-1 is a powerful renal vasoconstrictor and reduces GFR. In addition, endothelin is a powerful inhibitor of the hydro-osmotic effect of ADH.

The circulating plasma level of immunoreactive endothelin is increased in patients with cirrhosis, particularly in patients with ascites (Fig. 12) (Uchiara, Hepatol, 1992; 16:95; Moller, JHepatol, 1993; 19:285; Hartleb, GastroClinBiol, 1994; 18:407; Matsumoto, DigDisSci, 1994; 39:2665; Bernardi, JHepatol, 1996; 24:161).[16, 86] There is one study showing that among patients with ascites, endothelin is higher in those with hepatorenal syndrome.[16] Both ET-1 and ET-3 are increased. Based on these data it has been speculated that in cirrhosis endothelin would be a further endogenous vasoconstrictor system, activated to correct the arteriolar vasodilation. It would act in concert with the renin–angiotensin–aldosterone system, sympathetic nervous system, and ADH to maintain arterial pressure within normal limits. In cases with severely impaired circulatory function, a great increase in endothelin release could contribute to the renal vasoconstriction that characterizes hepatorenal syndrome. In fact, there is evidence that endothelin is involved in other types of acute renal failure, such as those secondary to the administration of cyclosporin or radiocontrast media (Kon, KidneyInt, 1991; 40:1; Cantley, KidneyInt, 1993; 44:12179; Nord, KidneyInt, 1993; 44:451).

Several lines of evidence, however, do not support this contention. First, whereas the activity of the renin–angiotensin–aldosterone system, sympathetic nervous system, and ADH in cirrhotic patients changes in parallel with alterations in effective extracellular volume, this is not the case with respect to the plasma levels of endothelin. For example, plasma renin activity and noradrenaline, but not endothelin, increase with the assumption of an upright posture in cirrhotic patients with and without ascites (Saló, JHepatol, 1995; 22:389). Conversely, plasma renin activity and noradrenaline, but not endothelin, decrease when the effective plasma volume is expanded. Secondly, other investigations have failed to confirm a relationship between plasma endothelin and the degree of impairment in renal function in cirrhotic patients with ascites.[86] Finally, the administration of BQ-123, a specific antagonist of ETA receptors, did not induce significant changes in arterial pressure in rats with carbon tetrachloride-induced cirrhosis

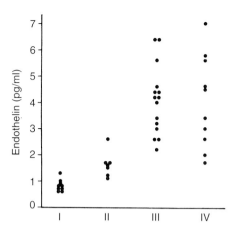

Fig. 12. Plasma concentration of immunoreactive endothelin in normal subjects (I), patients with compensated cirrhosis (II) and patients with cirrhosis and ascites without and with hepatorenal syndrome (III and IV). (Reproduced by permission of Asbert *et al. Gastroenterology,* 1993; **104**: 1485–91.)

with ascites.[87] A decrease in arterial pressure, however, is constantly observed in this model following the blockade of the A-II or V1-ADH receptors (Clària, Gastro, 1991; 100:494).

The tissue concentration of immunoreactive endothelin and ET-1 mRNA content in the lung, kidney, and aorta is similar in rats with carbon tetrachloride-induced cirrhosis and ascites and control rats.[87] Since these areas are highly vascular, this argues strongly against a generalized stimulation of vascular endothelin. In contrast, the hepatic tissue concentration of endothelin is ten times higher in the cirrhotic animals. ET-1 mRNA production is also very high in cirrhotic, and almost undetectable in normal, livers. These data strongly suggest that the increased circulating plasma level of endothelin in cirrhosis derives from the liver.

In rats with carbon tetrachloride-induced cirrhosis, hepatic ET-1 mRNA overexpression only occurs in Ito cells (Housset, PNAS, 1993; 90:9276). In hepatocytes, ET-1 mRNA is undetectable. On the other hand, although ETA and ETB receptors are present in hepatocytes, Ito cells express ETA/ETB receptors in far greater abundance than any other resident liver cell. These features suggest that the increased hepatic production of endothelin in cirrhosis originates from Ito cells and that endothelin, which acts principally as a local paracrine/autocrine agent, may be involved in Ito cell function in cirrhosis. During liver injury, Ito cells undergo proliferation and a process of activation characterized by loss of vitamin A droplets, enhanced collagen production, and expression of smooth muscle α-actin (Tanaka, JPath, 1991; 164:273; Friedman, NEJM, 1993; 328:1828). The mytogenic effect of endothelin could participate in this process. Moreover endothelin, which induces contractility of activated Ito cells and increases portal pressure in experimental animals, may contribute to the increased intrahepatic resistance and portal pressure in cirrhosis (Bauer, AmJPhysiol, 1994; 267:G143; Zhang, AmJPhysiol, 1995; 266:G269; Rockey, Hepatol, 1996; 24:233). The acute blockade of ETA receptor with BQ-123 in rats with experimental cirrhosis is not associated with significant changes in the increased portal pressure.[87] However, when both ETA and ETB receptors are simultaneously blocked with mixed ETA/ETB receptor antagonists, a marked reduction in

intrahepatic vascular resistance and portal pressure occurs (Gandhi, Hepatol, 1996; 24:316A; Lebrec, Hepatol, 1996; 24:316A), suggesting that endothelin participates in the pathogenesis of portal hypertension.

Other vasoactive substances

Very few studies have been performed assessing the kallikrein–bradykinin system in cirrhosis. However, this system is involved in the homeostasis of renal perfusion and in tubular function (Carretero, AmJPhysiol, 1980: 238:F247; Regoli, PharmRev, 1980; 32:1; Mayfield, AmJNephrol, 1983; 3:145; Margolius, AnnRevPhysiol, 1984; 46:309; Taylor, DrugDevRes, 1988; 16:1; Bhoola, PharmRev, 1992; 44:1; Burch, LifeSci, 1992; 50:829). Kinins are potent vasoactive peptides, formed by the action of specific peptidases, the kallikreins, on kininogen substrates. There are two types of kallikreins, the glandular kallikrein synthesized in salivary and sweat glands, pancreas, and kidney (distal and collecting tubules), and the plasma kallikrein. Both types of enzyme are synthesized as inactive precursors (prekallikreins) and differ in molecular weight, substrate specificity, and sensitivity to inhibitors. Kininogens are α_2-globulins, existing in multiple isoforms with different molecular weights. Plasma kininogen is the form of largest molecular weight. It is synthesized by the liver and leads to the formation of bradykinin. The distal nephron synthesizes a low molecular weight kininogen which is converted to lysine-bradykinin by the action of renal kallikrein and then to bradykinin. Kinins are degraded by the action of kininases I and II, the latter being the same enzyme that converts A-I to A-II (angiotensin-converting enzyme). The brush border in the proximal tubule is very rich in kininases which destroy most of the filtered kinins. The large amounts of kinins present in the urine are, therefore, of renal origin. Kinins have many functions, including a potent vasodilator effect, inhibition of the tubular effect of ADH and increase in renin release. The vasodilator and inhibitory effect on the tubular action of ADH may be partially mediated by prostaglandins, since kinins are known to stimulate the endothelial and renal tubular synthesis of these compounds. Bradykinin also stimulates the constitutive nitric oxide synthase III and increases the endothelial release of nitric oxide (Lahera, AmJHypertension, 1991; 4:260). There is evidence that this effect is the predominant mechanism of the vasodilatory activity of kinins (Navar, PhysiolRev, 1996; 76:425).

The urinary excretion of kallikrein, which is thought to estimate its renal synthesis, is increased in non-azotaemic cirrhotic patients with ascites and reduced in patients with hepatorenal syndrome. Since renal kallikrein production is stimulated by A-II, aldosterone, ADH, and prostaglandins (Bohola, PharmRev, 1992; 44:1), there are many potential candidates for the increased urinary kallikrein in non-azotaemic cirrhosis. However, the mechanism and significance of the reduced urinary excretion of kallikrein in patients with hepatorenal syndrome is unknown. It may be a consequence of impaired renal function. However, an alternative hypothesis is that, as proposed for prostaglandins, a reduced intrarenal synthesis of kallikrein and bradykinin may participate in the pathogenesis of hepatorenal syndrome. A recent study suggests that the plasma kallikrein–kinin system may also play a pathophysiological role in cirrhosis (McGilchrist, ClinSci, 1994; 87:329). The administration of aprotinin, a kallikrein inhibitor, to patients with cirrhosis and ascites, was associated with a significant increase in systemic vascular resistance and arterial pressure, suppression of plasma renin activity and A-II and aldosterone concentration, and increase in renal perfusion, GFR, and absolute sodium excretion. These data support the existence of an association between the plasma kallikrein–kinin system, systemic vasodilation, activation of the renin–angiotensin–aldosterone system, and renal dysfunction in this condition.

Adenosine is another substance that participates in the regulation of regional haemodynamics (Fredholm, ClinPhysiol, 1986; 6:1; Collis, PharmTher, 1989; 6:1; Naver, PhysiolRev, 1996; 76:425). It is a nucleoside derived from the intracellular catabolism of ATP. Under normoxic conditions, the intracellular concentration of adenosine is extremely low because of the efficacy of several enzymes in converting adenosine to other compounds. However, when oxygen consumption increases or oxygen supply decreases, conversion of ATP to adenosine increases markedly. Once formed in the cell, adenosine diffuses to the extracellular space and causes its biological effects by acting on specific receptors. Extracellular adenosine is then taken up rapidly by the cells, particularly red blood cells, and catabolized to inosine and uric acid. Dypiridamole blocks this process and increases the extracellular level of adenosine. Because the main biological activity of adenosine in most organs is production of arteriolar vasodilation, and because tissue levels of adenosine increase whenever ischaemia or increased oxygen consumption is present, this nucleoside is considered an important mediator in the regulation of regional blood flow. However, in the kidney adenosine does not produce arteriolar vasodilation but rather arterial vasoconstriction, particularly if the renin–angiotensin–aldosterone system is stimulated.

The renal vasculature of cirrhotic patients with ascites and increased activity of the renin–angiotensin–aldosterone system is extremely sensitive to the vasoconstrictor effect of adenosine. A syndrome indistinguishable from hepatorenal syndrome may develop in these patients following the intravenous administration of dypiridamole at a dose that induces a twofold increase in plasma adenosine levels in healthy subjects. This renal vasoconstrictor effect is not observed in normal subjects, patients with compensated cirrhosis, or patients with ascites and normal plasma renin activity or aldosterone.[88] It has been speculated that renal vasoconstriction in cirrhotic patients may be initiated by the systemic vasoconstrictor systems (renin–angiotensin–aldosterone system, sympathetic nervous system, and ADH) activated in response to effective arterial hypovolaemia. However, once a critical threshold of renal hypoperfusion is achieved, there would be an increased renal release of adenosine and other renal vasoconstrictors (i.e. endothelin, which is also stimulated by ischaemia), which would accentuate the renal vasoconstriction.[88]

Alterations in intrarenal haemodynamics

Under conditions of constant extracellular fluid volume or renal perfusion pressure, changes in GFR are accompanied by parallel changes in proximal tubular sodium reabsorption (glomerulotubular balance), thus preventing dramatic modifications in urinary sodium excretion. Altered physical factors in the capillary network surrounding the proximal tubule, which is anatomically connected with the glomerular capillary bed through the efferent arteriole, are of major importance in this homeostatic mechanism.[89] The increase in GFR leads to a reduction in hydrostatic pressure and increase in oncotic pressure in the peritubular capillaries, which enhances sodium reabsorption in the proximal tubule. The opposite occurs when GFR is reduced. However, alterations in extracellular fluid volume disrupt the glomerulotubular balance. Extracellular fluid volume expansion depresses proximal sodium reabsorption even when the GFR is held constant or reduced. The contrary occurs when there is contraction of extracellular fluid volume. Since it is well established that changes in sodium excretion caused by these manoeuvres are associated with parallel changes of peritubular hydrostatic pressure, intrarenal physical factors probably contribute to this feature. Cirrhotic patients with ascites behave as if they have a low effective extracellular fluid volume. Changes in intrarenal physical factors could, therefore, play a contributory role in the pathogenesis of sodium retention in these patients.

Pressure natriuresis is another important intrarenal homeostatic mechanism regulating sodium excretion (Mizelle, Hypertension, 1993; 22:102). It refers to the mechanism that mediates the changes in sodium excretion observed in response to changes in arterial pressure. Pressure natriuresis is independent of GFR, which remains unmodified during changes in arterial pressure owing to a potent autoregulatory mechanism of the cortical blood flow. Thus, it is secondary to changes in tubular sodium reabsorption. It has been proposed that pressure natriuresis occurs in the proximal tubule through changes in hydrostatic and colloid osmotic pressures in the peritubular capillary network. However, recent studies have presented evidence suggesting that the collecting tubule is the predominant site of pressure natriuresis, and that nitric oxide may mediate this process (Navar, CurrOpinNephrolHypert, 1996; 5:64). In contrast to the cortical circulation, the medullary circulation does not have a high efficiency of autoregulation. Therefore, any increase in renal perfusion pressure (which is mainly dependent of arterial pressure) would increase medullary blood flow and shear stress, leading to increased endothelial release of nitric oxide. Nitric oxide could reduce sodium reabsorption in the distal nephron either directly or indirectly through changes in medullary haemodynamics or interstitial hydrostatic pressure. There are conflicting data concerning the function of the pressure–natriuresis mechanism in cirrhosis. A recent experimental study in rats with carbon tetrachloride-induced cirrhosis with and without ascites suggests that the cirrhotic kidney is not normally able to increase sodium and water excretion in response to changes in arterial pressure (Atucha, AmJPhysiol, 1993; 265:G1045). In contrast, other studies have observed that the production of a moderate increase in mean arterial pressure by the intravenous infusion of A-II or noradrenaline is followed by a paradoxical increase in sodium excretion in most patients and experimental animals with cirrhosis and ascites, a phenomenon not observed under normal conditions (Laragh, JCI, 1963; 42:1179; Gutman, ClinSciMolMed, 1973; 45:19).[74] Noradrenaline administration also returns the natriuretic response to extracellular fluid volume expansion to normal in patients with cirrhosis and ascites.[44]

Pathogenesis of renal dysfunction in cirrhosis

An outstanding observation in cirrhotic patients with ascites is that sinusoidal portal hypertension correlates with the degree of stimulation of the endogenous vasoactive systems. In a large series of cirrhotic patients, with and without ascites, Bosch *et al.* reported that sinusoidal portal hypertension, as estimated by the free-to-wedged hepatic venous pressure gradient, correlated closely with urinary sodium excretion, plasma renin activity, and plasma renin and aldosterone concentrations.[68] Patients with more severe portal hypertension had a higher plasma renin and aldosterone and lower urinary sodium excretion. In cirrhotic patients there is also a positive correlation between portal pressure and sympathetic nervous activity.[60] Finally, since the plasma concentration of ADH parallels plasma renin activity and noradrenaline concentration in cirrhotic patients with ascites, it is likely that ADH release and the degree of impairment of water excretion also correlate with sinusoidal portal pressure in these patients.[58,65] Therefore, any theory concerning the pathogenesis of renal dysfunction must explain satisfactorily why sinusoidal portal hypertension activates these endogenous systems which, in turn, promote renal sodium and water retention.

At present three hypotheses have been proposed to explain renal dysfunction in cirrhosis—the classical 'underfilling hypothesis', the 'overflow hypothesis', and the 'peripheral arterial vasodilation hypothesis'. In all three, renal dysfunction is considered to be a consequence of a disruption of the mechanisms involved in homeostasis of circulatory function. However, they differ with respect to the nature of this disturbance.

Traditional underfilling hypothesis

This considers that the initial event is the disruption of the Starling equilibrium within the hepatic and splanchnic circulation (Witte, Gastro, 1971; 61:742; Witte, Gastro, 1980; 78:1059) (Fig. 13). The capillary hyperfiltration occurring in the hepatic sinusoids and splanchnic capillaries is initially buffered by lymphatic mechanisms, so that fluid is returned to the circulation via the thoracic duct. However, as the liver disease progresses, filtration exceeds the capacity for lymphatic return and fluid then accumulates in the peritoneal cavity as ascites. Loss of fluid from the intravascular compartment to the intraperitoneal space leads to contraction of the circulating plasma volume. This activates intrathoracic and arterial mechanoreceptors which signal to the kidney to retain sodium and water. The retained fluid cannot adequately fill the intravascular compartment and suppress the sodium and water retaining signals to the kidney because fluid is continuously leaking in the peritoneal cavity, thus creating a vicious circle. Hepatorenal syndrome is the extreme expression of circulating hypovolaemia.

There is much evidence against this hypothesis. First, if this theory was correct, plasma volume and cardiac index would be reduced and systemic vascular resistance increased. However, the plasma volume and cardiac index in cirrhotics with portal hypertension with or without ascites are invariably increased (Fig. 14) and systemic vascular resistance markedly reduced, thus reflecting peripheral vasodilation (Lancestremere, JCI, 1962; 41:1922; McCloy, AnnIntMed, 1967; 66:307).[19,40–47] Secondly, plasma

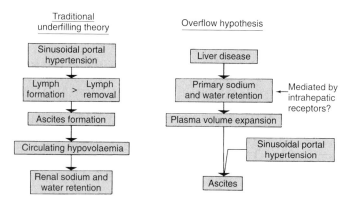

Fig. 13. Traditional underfilling theory and overflow hypothesis of ascites formation in cirrhosis.

volume does not change in cirrhotics during formation, or spontaneous loss, of ascites (Lieberman, JCI, 1969; 48:975). Finally, longitudinal studies in experimental animals with cirrhosis have shown that sodium retention precedes the formation of ascites, suggesting that sodium retention is a cause and not a consequence of ascites formation (Jiménez, Hepatol, 1985; 5:245).

Overflow theory

The overflow hypothesis was proposed in an attempt to relate the three most relevant features occurring in decompensated cirrhotic patients with portal hypertension: a hyperdynamic circulation (hypervolaemia, high cardiac index, increased heart rate, and low peripheral vascular resistance), sodium retention, and the formation of ascites. The hypothesis was proposed after demonstrating that oral administration of 9-α-fluorocortisone to compensated cirrhotics with portal hypertension caused ascites in many patients.[1] According to this hypothesis (Lieberman, AnnNYAcadSci, 1970; 170: 202), the initial event is 'primary' renal sodium and water retention (primary in the sense that it is not due to a decrease in intravascular volume) (Fig. 13). The cause of the primary sodium retention was not delineated in the initial proposal. Subsequently, several mechanisms have been suggested, including a hepatorenal reflex mediated by intrahepatic mechanoreceptors which predominate over normal volume regulatory mechanisms, a decreased hepatic clearance of a sodium-retaining hormone, or a reduced hepatic synthesis of a natriuretic substance (Levy, JLabClinMed, 1978; 91: 521; Unikowski, JCI, 1983; 72:1594; Levy, AmJPhysiol, 1987; 253:

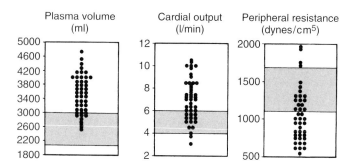

Fig. 14. Plasma volume, cardiac output, and calculated peripheral vascular resistance in a series of patients with cirrhosis and ascites. The shaded area represents the normal range.

F664; Wood, Hepatol, 1988; 8:831; Wensing, Hepatol, 1990; 11: 779; Wensing, Hepatol, 1990; 13:13; Levy, GastrInternat, 1992; 5: 186; Wong, Hepatol, 1994; 20:873). As sodium and water are retained, plasma volume expands, leading to adaptive circulatory changes (high cardiac index and low systemic vascular resistance) to accommodate the excess intravascular fluid. The encounter between abnormal Starling forces in the hepatic and splanchnic vascular beds and an expanded plasma volume leads to 'overflow' ascites formation. Support for this hypothesis derives from studies of experimental models of cirrhosis in the rat and dog in which renal sodium and water retention and blood volume expansion clearly preceded ascites formation.

However, the overflow theory of ascites cannot satisfactorily explain the systemic circulatory disturbance present in patients with cirrhosis. It proposes that in cirrhotics with ascites the systemic circulation is overfilled due to primary sodium retention. However, most evidence from clinical and experimental studies indicates that the systemic circulation is underfilled in cirrhosis, and that this underfilling occurs not because the circulating blood volume is reduced, but because the arterial vascular compartment is enlarged. Cirrhotic patients with ascites are usually hypotensive, yet the plasma volume and cardiac index may be considerably increased (Fig. 14).[19,40,42–48] Thus, the low arterial blood pressure is a consequence of a reduced peripheral arterial vascular resistance. This peripheral arterial vasodilation, and the concomitant arterial hypotension, occurs in a significant number of patients despite marked overactivity of the renin–angiotensin–aldosterone system and sympathetic nervous system, and ADH hypersecretion, suggesting that the systemic haemodynamic derangement would be much more intense in these cases if these endogenous vasoconstrictors were not acting on the peripheral vasculature. In fact, the acute blockade of A-II and ADH with specific vascular antagonists in patients and experimental animals with cirrhosis and ascites may be associated with a dramatic fall of arterial pressure secondary to arteriolar vasodilation (Clària, Gastro, 1991; 100: 494). Similar observations have been made after returning plasma noradrenaline spillover to normal with clonidine in cirrhotics with ascites and increased sympathetic nervous activity (Willett, Lancet, 1982; 2:939). This haemodynamic pattern of cirrhotics with ascites, characterized by a high circulating blood volume (high plasma volume and cardiac index) and signs of arterial underfilling (arterial hypotension and compensatory stimulation of the renin–angiotensin–aldosterone system and sympathetic nervous system, and ADH release), which is very similar to hyperdynamic circulation present in patients with traumatic arteriovenous fistula (Epstein, JCI, 1953; 32:233), is radically distinct and much more complex than that proposed by the overflow theory.

Much evidence suggests that the reduction in peripheral vascular resistance in cirrhosis takes place mainly in the splanchnic circulation. Studies in rats with ligated portal vein and in rats and dogs with experimental cirrhosis have shown that portal hypertension is associated with a generalized splanchnic arteriolar vasodilation, accounting for the hyperdynamic circulation in these models (Blanchet, EurJClinInv, 1982; 12:327; Bosch, Hepatol, 1983; 3: 1002; Vorobioff, AmJPhysiol, 1983; 244:652; Benoit, AmJPhysiol, 1984; 247:G486; Vorobioff, Gastro, 1984; 87:1120; Khiel, AmJPhysiol, 1985; 248:G192; Korthuis, AmJPhysiol, 1985; 249:H827; Sikuler, AmJPhysiol, 1985; 248:G618; Benoit, SemLivDis, 1986; 6:

287; Kravetz, AmJPhysiol, 1987; 252:G257; Sugita, AmJPhysiol, 1987; 252:G748; Crissiger, AmJPhysiol, 1988; 254:G658; Korthuis, AmJPhysiol, 1988; 254:G339). There is indirect evidence of marked splanchnic arteriolar vasodilation in patients with cirrhosis and portal hypertension, as hepatic blood flow is usually normal or even increased in these patients even though 60 to 80 per cent of the portal blood flow is shunted through the collateral circulation.[40, 90–92] It has also been shown that the mean transit time in the splanchnic vascular bed is substantially reduced in alcoholic cirrhotics, suggesting a hyperkinetic splanchnic circulation in these patients.[41] Recent studies using echo-Doppler techniques have documented increased splenic and mesenteric blood flow in patients with cirrhosis (Nakamura, NipponShokGakkaiZass, 1987; 84:210; Sato, Radiol, 1987; 164:347). Finally, the vascular resistance in other major vascular territories (kidney, skin, and muscle) is normal or increased in cirrhotics with ascites, and always increased in patients with hepatorenal syndrome.[19,93] Splanchnic arterial vasodilation in cirrhosis and prehepatic portal hypertension is related to the increased in portal pressure and results in a high portal venous inflow that maintains or aggravates the portal hypertensive syndrome.

The mechanism by which portal hypertension leads to reduced splanchnic arterial vascular resistance is unknown. Many endogenous vasodilators, including glucagon (Benoit, AmJPhysiol, 1984; 247:E486; Benoit, AmJPhysiol, 1986; 251:G674; Kravetz, AmJPhysiol, 1988; 254:G322), nitric oxide, calcitonin gene-related peptide, adenosine, vasoactive intestinal peptide, substance P, and platelet activating factor (Hortnagl, Lancet, 1984; iii:480; Henriksen, EurJClinInv, 1986; 16:211; Villamediana, LifeSci 1986; 39:201; Caramelo, EurJClinInv, 1987; 17:7; Bendtsen, JHepatol, 1991; 12: 118; Lee, Hepatol, 1992; 15:1107) have been proposed. Nitric oxide, calcitonin gene-related peptide, and substance P are neurotransmitters of the non-adrenergic non-cholinergic nervous system. This is a sensory component of the autonomic nervous system, widely distributed within the body and the splanchnic area, that responds to various stimuli (including chemical or mechanical stimuli) releasing these potent vasodilators locally (Sanders, AmJPhysiol, 1992; 262:G379). It is therefore possible that this system may participate in the decreased vascular resistance in the splanchnic circulation associated with portal hypertension.

Peripheral arteriolar vasodilation hypothesis

This hypothesis proposes that portal hypertension is the initial event of renal dysfunction in cirrhosis, with splanchnic arteriolar vasodilatation causing underfilling of the arterial vascular compartment and high-pressure baroreceptor-mediated stimulation of endogenous vasoconstrictor systems (renin–angiotensin–aldosterone system, sympathetic nervous system, and ADH) being the intermediate step, and renal sodium and water retention the final consequence (Fig. 15).[94] When sinusoidal portal hypertension is moderately increased, the systemic haemodynamic disturbance is corrected by transient sodium and water retention induced by these endogenous vasoconstrictor systems. The fluid retained by the kidneys remains in the intravascular compartment, increases the intravascular volume and cardiac output, refills the dilated arterial vascular bed, suppresses the signals stimulating the endogenous vasoactive systems, and returns sodium and water excretion to

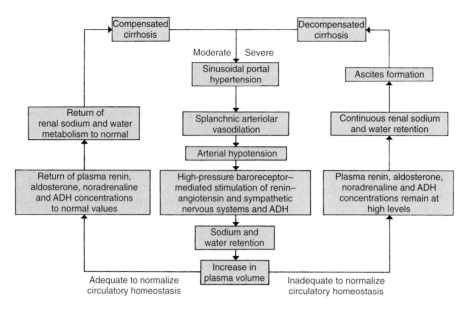

Fig. 15. Peripheral arteriolar vasodilation hypothesis.

normal. This sequence of events explains what occurs in patients with compensated cirrhosis, who show moderate portal hypertension, increased plasma volume and cardiac index, reduced peripheral vascular resistance, preserved renal ability to excrete sodium and free water, and normal renal blood flow and GFR.

Non-azotaemic cirrhotic patients with ascites represent a more advanced stage of the continuum in the process of portal hypertension-induced underfilling of arterial vessels. At this stage of cirrhosis, the increase in cardiac output and blood volume secondary to the transient sodium and water retention is no longer sufficient to maintain circulatory homeostasis. This could be due to the progression of sinusoidal portal hypertension causing greater splanchnic arteriolar vasodilation, as well as the extravasation of fluid from the sinusoidal and splanchnic capillaries to the peritoneal cavity caused by the higher portal pressure and portal venous inflow. The arterial baroreceptors sense the vascular underfilling, activate the endogenous vasoconstrictor systems, and promote sodium and water retention. However, the fluid retained by the kidneys is not effective in correcting the arterial underfilling, since it leaks in the peritoneal cavity as ascites. The activity of the renin–angiotensin–aldosterone system, sympathetic nervous system, and ADH release remains increased to maintain arterial pressure, thus perpetuating sodium and water retention and ascites formation. Renal blood flow and GFR are normal or only moderately decreased in these patients, despite the overactivity of these vasoconstrictor systems, since they are antagonized by increased production of the vasodilating substances such as natriuretic peptides, renal PGE_2 and PGI_2, and nitric oxide.

Hepatorenal syndrome represents the most extreme manifestation in the underfilling of arterial circulation. Arterial pressure in patients with hepatorenal syndrome is lower than in non-azotaemic cirrhotics with ascites.[19] On the other hand, the plasma concentrations of the three major vasoconstrictors in patients with hepatorenal syndrome are among the highest observed in patients with cirrhosis and ascites. Since the urinary excretion of prostaglandins is markedly reduced in these patients, it is attractive to

consider that hepatorenal syndrome in these patients with extreme arterial vascular underfilling occurs as a consequence of an imbalance between the activity of endogenous vasoconstrictor systems, which is very much increased, and the synthesis of renal vasodilators, which may be reduced. Nevertheless, the diminution in the urinary excretion of prostaglandins or the low renal PGH_2 synthetase activity, which are the main arguments supporting this hypothesis, may be a result of the decline in renal function rather than a contributor to the impaired renal haemodynamics.

Several lines of evidence support this sequence of events. First, as indicated above, the blockade of endogenous vasoconstrictor systems in patients with cirrhosis and ascites causes a marked arterial hypotension, which indicates that these systems contribute to the maintenance of arterial pressure. Secondly, central blood volume (i.e. the blood contained in the low-pressure intrathoracic vessels, heart, and thoracic aorta) is reduced in patients with cirrhosis with ascites. Since cardiac output is increased, this indicates a very rapid circulation through this vascular system due to the low systemic vascular resistance and increased heart rate (hyperdynamic circulation). In fact, central blood volume and systemic vascular resistance correlate directly in patients with cirrhosis.[95,96] Consistent with these features are the observations that the activity of the renin–angiotensin–aldosterone system and sympathetic nervous system in cirrhosis with ascites can be suppressed by the administration of vasoconstrictors or vasoconstrictors associated with plasma volume expansion, and that vasodilators may trigger sodium retention and ascites and/or oedema formation in compensated cirrhosis (Nichols, CircRes, 1985; 56:457; Shapiro, KidneyInt, 1985; 28:206; Lenz, Gastro, 1991; 101:1060; Salmerón, Hepatol, 1993; 17:800; Vorobioff, Hepatol, 1993; 18:477; Albillos, Gastro, 1995; 109:1257; Guevara, JHepatol, 1996; 25:710 (Suppl. 1)). Finally, longitudinal studies in rats with prehepatic portal hypertension and cirrhosis have been able to reproduced the sequence of events proposed by the peripheral arteriolar vasodilation hypothesis. In prehepatic portal hypertensive animals, peripheral arteriolar vasodilation precedes sodium retention and the hyper-dynamic circulation. Sodium retention in this model is only a transient phenomenon that leads to an increased plasma volume. Sodium restriction prior to portal vein ligation blunts the expansion of plasma volume (Genecin, AmJPhysiol, 1990; 259:G498; Colombato, Hepatol, 1991; 15:323; Albillos, Gastro, 1992; 102:931). In rats with experimental cirrhosis there is a close temporal relationship between the decrease in arterial pressure, the activation of the renin–angiotensin–aldosterone system and the onset of sodium retention (López, Hepatol, 1991; 13:585).

A weak point of the peripheral vasodilation hypothesis is that sodium retention occurs in a significant proportion of patients with cirrhosis and ascites in the setting of normal plasma levels of renin and aldosterone.[37] Nevertheless, it is well known that the activity of the renin–angiotensin–aldosterone system does not increase until there is a significant reduction in effective blood volume (greater than 10 per cent) (Hesse, PSEBM, 1974; 145:227; Hesse, Clin-SciMolMed, 1975; 49:515; Hesse, ScaJCLI, 1978; 38:155; Mark, AmJPhysiol, 1978; 235:H29). It is, therefore, possible that more sensitive mechanisms (i.e. intrarenal mechanisms such as pressure natriuresis) could be responsible for this apparently paradoxical feature.

References

1. Denison EK, Lieberman FL, and Reynolds TB. 9-α-fluorohydro-cortisone induced ascites in alcoholic liver disease. *Gastroenterology*, 1971; **61**: 497–503.
2. Vaamonde CA. Renal water handling in liver disease. In Epstein M, ed. *The kidney in liver disease*, 2nd edn. New York: Elsevier Biomedical, 1983: 55–86.
3. Shear L, Hall PW, and Gabuzda GJ. Renal failure in patients with cirrhosis of the liver. II. Factors influencing maximal urinary flow rate. *American Journal of Medicine*, 1966; **39**: 199–209.
4. Arroyo V, Rodés J, Gutierrez-Lizarraga MA, and Revert L. Prognostic value of spontaneous hyponatremia in cirrhosis with ascites. *American Journal of Digestive Disease*, 1976; **21**: 249–56.
5. Arroyo V, *et al*. Definition and diagnostic criteria of refractory ascites and hepatorenal syndrome in cirrhosis. *Hepatology*, 1996; **23**: 164–76.
6. Ginès A, *et al*. Incidence, predictive factors and prognosis of hepatorenal syndrome in cirrhosis with ascites. *Gastroenterology*, 1993; **105**: 229–36.
7. Llach J, *et al*. Prognostic value of arterial pressure, endogenous vasoactive systems and renal function in cirrhosis with ascites. *Gastroenterology*, 1988; **94**: 482–7.
8. Rodés J, Bosch J, and Arroyo V. Clinical types and drug therapy of renal impairment in cirrhosis. *Postgraduate Medical Journal*, 1975; **55**: 492–7.
9. Follo A *et al*. Renal impairment following spontaneous bacterial peritonitis in cirrhosis. Incidence, clinical course, predictive factors and prognosis. *Hepatology*, 1994; **20**: 1495–1501.
10. Ginès P, *et al*. Randomized comparative study of therapeutic paracentesis with and without intravenous albumin in cirrhosis. *Gastroenterology*, 1988; **94**: 1493–502.
11. Cabrera J, Arroyo V, Ballesta AM, Rimola A, Gual J, and Rodés J. Aminoglycoside nephrotoxicity in cirrhosis. Value of urinary beta-2 microglobulin to discriminate functional renal failure from acute tubular damage. *Gastroenterology*, 1982; **82**: 97–105.
12. Dudley FJ, Kanel GC, Wood LJ, and Reynolds TB. Hepatorenal syndrome without sodium retention. *Hepatology*, 1986; **6**: 248–51.
13. Diamong JR and Yoburn DC. Nonoliguric acute renal failure associated with low fractional sodium excretion. *Annals of Internal Medicine*, 1982; **96**: 597–600.
14. Sacerdoti D, Bolognesi M, Merkel C, Angeli P, and Gatta A. Renal vasoconstriction in cirrhosis evaluated by duplex Doppler ultrasonography. *Hepatology*, 1993; **17**: 219–24.
15. Maroto A, *et al*. Diagnosis of functional renal failure in cirrhosis by Doppler sonography. Prognostic value of resistive index. *Hepatology*, 1994; **20**: 839–44.
16. Moore K, Wendon J, Frazer M, Karani J, Williams R, and Badr K. Plasma endothelin immunoreactivity in liver disease and the hepatorenal syndrome. *New England Journal of Medicine*, 1992, **327**: 1774–8.
17. Levy M. Hepatorenal syndrome. *Kidney International*, 1993; **43**: 737–53.
18. Laffi G, LaVilla G, and Gentilini P. Pathogenesis and management of the hepatorenal syndrome. *Seminars in Liver Disease*, 1994; **14**: 71–81.
19. Fernandez-Seara J, *et al*. Systemic and regional hemodynamics in patients with liver cirrhosis and ascites with and without functional renal failure. *Gastroenterology*, 1989; **97**: 1304–12.
20. Arroyo V, Ginès P, Rimola A, and Gaya J. Renal function abnormalities, prostaglandins and effects of non-steroidal antiinflammatory drugs in cirrhosis with ascites. An overview with emphasis on pathogenesis. *American Journal of Medicine*, 1986; **81** (Suppl. 2B): 104–22.
21. Di Bona GF. Renal neural activity in hepatorenal syndrome. *Kidney International*, 1984; **25**: 841–53.
22. Arroyo V, Clària J, Saló J, and Jiménez W. Antidiuretic hormone and the pathogenesis of water retention in cirrhosis with ascites. *Seminars in Liver Disease*, 1994; **14**: 44–58.
23. Keppler D, Hagmann W, Rapps S, Denzlinger C, and Koch HK. The relation of leukotrienes to liver injury. *Hepatology*, 1985; **5**: 883–91.
24. Ginès P, *et al*. Atrial natriuretic factor in cirrhosis with ascites: plasma levels, cardiac release and splanchnic extraction. *Hepatology*, 1988; **8**: 636–42.
25. LaVilla G, *et al*. Plasma levels of brain natriuretic peptide in patients with cirrhosis. *Hepatology*, 1992; **16**: 156–61.
26. Angeli P, *et al*. Renal effects of endogenous natriuretic peptides receptors blockade in cirrhotic rats with ascites. *Hepatology*, 1994; **20**: 948–54.
27. Saló J, *et al*. Urinary excretion of urodilatin in patients with cirrhosis. *Hepatology*, 1996; 24:1428–32.
28. Ros J, *et al*. Role of nitric oxide and prostacyclin in the control of renal perfusion in experimental cirrhosis. *Hepatology*, 1995; **22**: 915–20.
29. LaVilla G, *et al*. Natriuretic hormone activity in the urine of patients with cirrhosis of the liver. *Hepatology*, 1990; **12**: 467–75.
30. Perez-Ayuso RM, *et al*. Renal kallikrein excretion in cirrhotics with ascites: relationship to renal hemodynamics. *Hepatology*, 1984; **4**: 247–52.
31. Laragh J and Sealey JE. Renin–angiotensin–aldosterone system and the regulation of sodium, potassium and blood pressure homeostasis. In Windhager EE, ed. *Handbook of physiology: renal physiology*, (Section 8) (1st edn). New York: Oxford University Press, 1992: 1409–542.
32. Knox FG and Granger JP. Control of sodium excretion: An integrative approach. In Windhager EE, ed. *Handbook of physiology: renal physiology*, (Section 8) (1st edn). New York: Oxford University Press, 1992: 927–67.
33. Ausiello DA, Holzman EJ, Gronich JH, and Ercolani L. Cell signaling. In Seldin DW and Giebisch G, eds. *The kidney: physiology and pathophysiology*, (2nd edn). New York: Raven Press, 1992: 645–706.
34. Hall JE and Brans MW. The renin–angiotensin–aldosterone system. Renal mechanism and circulatory homeostasis. In Seldin DW and Giebisch G, eds. *The kidney: physiology and pathophysiology*, (2nd edn). New York: Raven Press, 1992: 1455–502.
35. Rossier BC and Palmer LG. Mechanism of aldosterone action on sodium and potassium transport. In Seldin DW and Giebisch G, eds. *The kidney: physiology and pathophysiology*, (2nd edn). New York: Raven Press, 1992: 1373–409.
36. Simon MA, Diez J, and Prieto J. Abnormal sympathetic and renal response to sodium restriction in compensated cirrhosis. *Gastroenterology*, 1991; **101**: 1354–60.
37. Saló J, *et al*. Effect of upright posture and physical exercise on endogenous neurohumoral systems in cirrhotic patients with sodium retention and normal supine plasma renin, aldosterone and norepinephrine levels. *Hepatology*, 1995; **22**: 479–87.
38. Bosch J, Ginès P, Arroyo V, Navasa M, and Rodés J. Hepatic and systemic hemodynamics and the neurohumoral systems in cirrhosis. In Epstein M, ed. *The kidney in liver disease*, (3rd edn). Baltimore: Williams and Wilkins, 1988: 286–305.

39. Arroyo V, *et al.* Sympathetic nervous activity, renin–angiotensin system and renal excretion of prostaglandin E2 in cirrhosis. Relationship to functional renal failure and sodium and water excretion. *European Journal of Clinical Investigation*, 1983; **13**: 271–8.

40. Bosch J, *et al.* Hepatic hemodynamics and the renin–angiotensin–aldosterone system in cirrhosis. *Gastroenterology*, 1980; **78**: 92–9.

41. Kotelanski B, Groszmann RJ, and Cohn JN. Circulation times in the splanchnic and hepatic beds· in alcoholic liver disease. *Gastroenterology*, 1972; **63**: 102–11.

42. Nicholls KM, *et al.* Elevated plasma norepinephrine concentrations in decompensated cirrhosis. Association with increased secretion rate, normal clearance rate and suppressibility by central blood volume expansion. *Circulation Research*, 1985; **56**: 457–61.

43. Henriksen J, Ring-Larsen H, and Christensen N. Circulating noradrenaline and central hemodynamics in patients with cirrhosis. *Scandinavian Journal of Gastroenterology*, 1985; **20**: 1185–90.

44. Nichols KM, Shapiro MD, Kludge R, Chung HM, Bichet P, and Schrier RM. Interrelationship between cardiac output and vascular resistance as determinants of effective arterial blood volume in cirrhotic patients. *Kidney International*, 1985; **28**: 206–11.

45. Bichet DG, Groves B, and Schrier RW. Mechanism of improvement of water and sodium excretion by immersion in decompensated cirrhotic patients. *Kidney International*, 1983; **24**: 788–94.

46. Kontos HH, Shapiro W, Mauck HP, and Patterson JL. General and regional circulatory alterations in cirrhosis of the liver. *American Journal of Medicine*, 1964; **37**: 526–35.

47. Lieberman FL and Reynolds TB. Plasma volume in cirrhosis of the liver: its relation to portal hypertension, ascites and renal failure. *Journal of Clinical Investigation*, 1967; **46**: 1297–310.

48. Tristani FE and Cohn JN. Systemic and renal hemodynamics inoliguric hepatic failure: effect of volume expansion. *Journal of Clinical Investigation*, 1967; **46**: 1894–906.

49. Arroyo V, Bosch J, Mauri M, Rivera F, Navarro F, and Rodés J. Effect of angiotensin II blockade on systemic and hepatic hemodynamics and on the renin–angiotensin–aldosterone system in cirrhosis with ascites. *European Journal of Clinical Investigation*, 1981; **11**: 221–9.

50. Arroyo V, Bosch J, Rivera F, and Rodés J. The renin–angiotensin system in cirrhosis. Its relation to functional renal failure. In Bartoli E and Chiandusi L, eds. *Hepato-renal syndrome*. Padova: Piccin Medical Books, 1979: 202–27.

51. Lobden I, Shore A, Wilkinson R, and Record CO. Captopril in the hepatorenal syndrome. *Journal of Clinical Gastroenterology*, 1985; **7**: 354–60.

52. Robertson GL. Regulation of vasopressin secretion. In Seldin DW and Giebisch G, eds. *The kidney: physiology and pathophysiology*, (2nd edn). New York: Raven Press, 1992: 1595–614.

53. Kostreva D, Castañer A, and Kampine J. Reflex effects of hepatic baroreceptors on renal and cardiac sympathetic nerve activity. *American Journal of Physiology*, 1980; **238**: R390–R394.

54. Mancia G, Saino A, and Grassi G. Interactions between the sympathetic nervous system and the renin–angiotensin system. In Laragh JH and Brenner BM, eds. *Hypertension: pathophysiology, diagnosis and management*, (2nd edn). New York: Raven Press, 1995: 399–408.

55. Kopp UC and DiBona GF. Neural control of renal function. In Seldin DW and Giebisch G, eds. *The kidney: physiology and pathophysiology*, (2nd edition). New York: Raven Press, 1992: 1157–204.

56. González-Campo JM and Knox FG. Integrated responses of the kidney to alterations in extracellular fluid volume. In Seldin DW and Giebisch G, eds. *The kidney: physiology and pathophysiology*, (2nd edn). New York: Raven Press, 1992: 2041–88.

57. Ring-Larsen H, Hesse B, Henriksen JH, and Christensen NJ. Sympathetic nervous activity and renal and systemic hemodynamics in cirrhosis: plasma norepinephrine concentration, hepatic extraction and renal release. *Hepatology*, 1982; **2**: 304–10.

58. Bichet DG, Van Putten VJ, and Schrier RW. Potential role of increased sympathetic activity in impaired sodium and water excretion in cirrhosis. *New England Journal of Medicine*, 1982; **307**: 1552–7.

59. Henriksen J, Christensen N, and Ring-Larsen H. Noradrenaline and adrenaline concentrations in various vascular beds in patients with cirrhosis. Relation to haemodynamics. *Clinical Physiology*, 1981; **1**: 293–304.

60. Henriksen J, Ring-Larsen H, Kanstrup IL, and Christensen NJ. Splanchnic and renal elimination and release of catecholamines in cirrhosis. Evidence of enhanced sympathetic nervous activity in patients with decompensated cirrhosis. *Gut*, 1984; **25**: 1034–43.

61. Willet I, Esler M, Burke F, Leonard P, and Dudley F. Total and renal sympathetic nervous system activity in alcoholic cirrhosis. *Journal of Hepatology*, 1985; **1**: 639–48.

62. Esler M *et al.* Increased sympathetic nervous activity and the effects of its inhibition with clonidine in alcoholic cirrhosis. *Annals of Internal Medicine*, 1992; **116**: 446–55.

63. Skirecki KL, Brown D, Ercolani L, and Ausiello A. Molecular mechanism of vasopressin action in the kidney. In Windhager EE, ed. *Handbook of physiology. Section 8, renal physiology*. New York: Oxford University Press, 1992: 1185–218.

64. Jamison RL and Gehrig JJ Jr. Urinary concentration and dilution. In Windhager EE, ed. *Handbook of physiology. Section 8, renal physiology*. New York: Oxford University Press, 1992: 1219–80.

65. Perez Ayuso RM, *et al.* Evidence that renal prostaglandins are involved in renal water metabolism in cirrhosis. *Kidney International*, 1984; **26**: 72–80.

66. Clària J, *et al.* Blockade of the hydroosmotic effect of vasopressin normalizes water excretion in cirrhotic rats. *Gastroenterology*, 1989; **97**: 1294–9.

67. Tsuboi Y, Ishikawa SE, Fujisawa G, Okada K, and Saito T. Therapeutic efficacy of the non-peptide AVP antagonist OPC-31260 in cirrhotic rats. *Kidney International*, 1994; **46**: 237–44.

68. Bosch M, *et al.* Aquaretic effect of the kappa opioid agonist RV 51599 in cirrhotic rats with ascites and water retention. *Gastroenterology*, 1995; **109**: 217–23.

69. Bichet D, Szatalowicz V, Chaimovitz C, and Schrier W. Role of vasopressin in abnormal water excretion in cirrhotic patients. *Annals of Internal Medicine*, 1982; **96**: 413–17.

70. Conrad KP and Dunn MJ. Renal prostaglandins and other eicosanoids. In Windhager EE, ed. *Handbook of physiology, Section 8, renal physiology*. New York: Oxford University Press, 1992: 1708–57.

71. Rimola A, *et al.* Urinary excretion of 6-keto-prostaglandin-F1-alpha, thromboxane A2 and prostaglandin E2 in cirrhosis with ascites. Relationship to functional renal failure (hepatorenal syndrome). *Journal of Hepatology*, 1986; **3**: 111–17.

72. Moore K, Ward PS, Taylor GW and Williams R. Systemic and renal production of thromboxane A2 and prostacyclin in decompensated liver disease and hepatorenal syndrome. *Gastroenterology*, 1991; **100**: 1069–77.

73. Boyer TD, Zia P, and Reynolds TB. Effects of indomethacin and prostaglandin A1 in renal function and plasma renin activity in alcoholic liver disease. *Gastroenterology*, 1979; **77**: 215–22.

74. Lianos EA, Alavi N, Tobin M, Venuto R, and Bentzel CJ. Angiotensin induced sodium excretion patterns in cirrhosis: role of renal prostaglandins. *Kidney International*, 1982; **21**: 70–7.

75. Wong F, Massie D, Hsu P, and Dudley F. Indomethacin-induced renal dysfunction in patients with well compensated cirrhosis. *Gastroenterology*, 1993; **104**: 869–76.

76. Aras SA and Maak TH. Atrial natriuretic factor. In Windhager EE, ed. *Handbook of physiology, Section 8, renal physiology*. New York: Oxford University Press, 1992: 1577–673.

77. Lewicki JA and Protter AA. Physiological studies of the natriuretic peptide family. In Laragh J and Brenner BM, eds. *Hypertension: pathophysiology, diagnosis, and management*. New York: Raven Press, 1995: 1029–53.

78. Gunning M and Brenner BM. Urodilatin. In Laragh JH and Brenner BM, eds. *Hypertension: pathophysiology, diagnosis, and management*. New York: Raven Press, 1995: 1021–7.

79. Clavell AL, Stingo AJ, Wei CM, Heublein DM and Burnett JC Jr. C-type natriuretic peptide: a selective cardiovascular peptide. *American Journal of Physiology*, 1993; **264**: R290–5.

80. Maak T. Receptors of natriuretic peptides: Structure, function and regulation. In Laragh JH and Brenner BM, eds. *Hypertension: pathophysiology, diagnosis, and management*. New York: Raven Press, 1995: 1001–20.

81. Ginès P, *et al.* Atrial natriuretic factor in cirrhosis with ascites: plasma levels, cardiac release and splanchnic extraction. *Hepatology*, 1988; **8**: 636–42.

82. Fernádez-Rodriguez C, Prieto J, Quiroga J, Zozaya JM, Andrade A, and Rodriguez-Martinez D. Atrial natriuretic factor in cirrhosis: relationship to renal function and hemodynamic changes. *Journal of Hepatology*, 1994; **21**: 211–16.

83. Ogawa Y and Nakao K. Brain natriuretic peptide as a cardiac hormone in cardiovascular disorders. In Laragh JH and Brenner BM, eds. *Hypertension: pathophysiology, diagnosis, and management*. New York: Raven Press, 1995: 833–40.

84. Henriksen JH, Bendtsen F, Sorensen TI, Stadager C, and Ring-Larsen H. Reduced central blood volume in cirrhosis. *Gastroenterology*, 1989; **97**: 1506–13.

85. Haddy FJ and Buckalew VM Jr. Endogenous digitalis-like factors in hypertension. In Laragh JH and Brenner BM, eds. *Hypertension, pathophysiology, diagnosis, and Management*, (2nd edn). New York: Raven Press, 1995: 1055–67.

86. Asbert M, *et al.* Circulating levels of endothelin in cirrhosis. *Gastroenterology*, 1993; **104**: 1485–91.

87. Leivas A, *et al.* Endothelin-1 does not play a major role in the homeostasis of arterial pressure in cirrhotic rats with ascites. *Gastroenterology*, 1995; **108**: 1842–8.

88. Llach J, *et al.* Effect of dipyridamole on kidney function in cirrhosis. *Hepatology*, 1993; **17**: 59–64.

89. Wilcox CS and Baylis C. Glomerular-tubular balance and proximal regulation. In Seldin DW and Giebisch G, eds. *The kidney: physiology and pathophysiology*. New York: Raven Press, 1985: 985–1012.

90. Cohn JN, Khatri JM, Groszmann RJ, and Kotelanski B. Hepatic blood flow in alcoholic liver disease measured by an indicator dilution technique. *American Journal of Medicine*, 1972; **53**: 704–14.

91. Groszmann RJ, Kotelanski B, Cohn JN, and Khatri IM. Quantitation of portasystemic shunting from the splenic and mesenteric beds in alcoholic liver disease. *American Journal of Medicine*, 1972; **53**: 715–22.

92. Huet PM, Pomier-Layrargues G, Villeneuve JP, Varin F, and Viallet A. Intrahepatic circulation in liver disease. *Seminars in Liver Disease*, 1986; **6**: 277–86.

93. Maroto A, *et al.* Brachial and femoral artery blood flow in cirrhosis: relationship with kidney dysfunction. *Hepatology*, 1993; **17**: 788–93.

94. Schrier RW, Arroyo V, Bernardi M, Epstein M, Henriksen JH, and Rodés J. Peripheral arterial vasodilation hypothesis: a proposal for the initiation of renal sodium and water retention in cirrhosis. *Hepatology*, 1988; **8**: 1151–7.

95. Henriksen JH, Bendtsen F, Gerbes AL, Christensen NJ, Ring-Larsen H, and Sorensen TIA. Estimated central blood volume in cirrhosis: relationship to sympathetic nervous activity, beta adrenergic blockade and atrial natriuretic factor. *Hepatology*, 1992; **16**: 1163–70.

96. Henriksen JH and Moller S. Hemodynamics, distribution of blood volume, and kinetics of vasoactive substances in cirrhosis. In Epstein M, ed. *The kidney in liver disease*, (4th edn). Philadelphia: Hanley and Belfus, 1966: 241–58.

9

Hepatic encephalopathy

9 Hepatic encephalopathy

Andres T. Blei

Definition and classification

Hepatic encephalopathy, defined in broad terms as changes in neurological function that result from liver disease, encompasses a wide range of neuropsychiatric signs and symptoms that are associated with both acute and chronic liver failure.[1-3] The term is not used when specific liver diseases exhibit discrete neurological findings (e.g. Wilson's disease, Zellwegger syndrome, or bilirubin encephalopathy in Crigler–Najjar syndrome). Rather, it focuses on the changes in mental state seen in cirrhosis and fulminant hepatic failure. The development of encephalopathy carries important prognostic implications in such patients: In acute liver failure, individuals with deep encephalopathy can succumb from neurological complications such as brain oedema and intracranial hypertension.[4] In cirrhosis, the grade of encephalopathy is one of the five elements included in the Child–Pugh classification, a prognostic tool.[5]

Two major alterations underlie the development of encephalopathy in acute and chronic liver disease: on the one hand, hepatic insufficiency and, on the other, portal–systemic shunting, where the opening of collateral vessels as a result of portal hypertension allows elements in the portal blood to gain access to the systemic circulation. In fulminant hepatic failure, liver function is lost while extrahepatic portal–systemic shunting is not present. In cirrhotic patients with hepatic encephalopathy, the degree of hepatic failure and the extent of portal–systemic shunts are variable. In addition, even with similar degrees of shunting, flow through larger and wider collaterals increases the rate of delivery of substances from the portal blood to the systemic circulation (Coy, AmJPhysiol, 1991; 261:G1072). Still, the separation between liver function and portal–systemic shunting should not be a rigid one as there is an interplay between both elements: extensive and long-standing portal–systemic shunting (seen after a non-selective portacaval anastomosis) can result in liver insufficiency, while the ability of the cirrhotic liver to extract substances from the portal vein decreases with worsening liver function.[6] In fulminant hepatic failure, portal blood flowing through a necrotic liver can also be viewed as a total portal–systemic shunt.

These considerations lead to a classification of hepatic encephalopathy that is based on the clinical setting in which symptoms occur (Table 1). The encephalopathy of acute liver failure shares clinical characteristics with that of cirrhosis, but also exhibits unique features (see below). In cirrhosis, three major syndromes can be present:

(1) Precipitant-induced (or acute) encephalopathy, commonly seen in the hospital setting, where a superimposed event is a key factor.
(2) Chronic encephalopathy, seen with extensive portal–systemic shunts and after portacaval shunt surgery, can be recurrent (discrete episodes) or persistent (constant changes of mental state). The recent use of **TIPS** (transjugular intrahepatic portal–systemic stent shunt) to treat portal hypertension has seen the reappearance of patients with this condition. A more striking (but rare) type of chronic encephalopathy has been termed hepatocerebral degeneration, as it reflects discrete anatomical changes and neurological signs (see Chapter 25.8).
(3) Subclinical encephalopathy reflects alterations in cognitive function in patients who clinically exhibit a normal mental state. Its diagnosis requires the use of neuropsychological testing; many cirrhotic subjects (up to 70 per cent) appear to exhibit such deficits.

With the advent of surgical techniques to decompress the portal hypertensive territory, the term 'portal–systemic encephalopathy' has been coined to highlight the importance of the anatomical rearrangement. The term can also be applied to patients who exhibit clinical and structural changes in the brain with extensive portal–systemic shunts in the absence of parenchymal liver damage (McDermott, JCI, 1954; 33:1; Demirci, Neurology, 1992; 42:983). By now, the reader may be bewildered by the different nomenclature, as some terms are interchangeably used by many authors in the literature. In fact, a consensus on terminology in this area is sorely needed. What any classification does highlight is the wide spectrum of alterations in neurological status. Their pathogenesis and therapy share some elements but differ in several other aspects.

Pathogenesis

Seldom has an area of hepatology been so full of controversy as the study of the pathogenesis of hepatic encephalopathy. Several hypotheses have been postulated over several decades and their tenets argued vehemently.[7-10] The difficulties in obtaining information on human neurochemistry have led to the use of animal models, that reproduce some features of the human counterpart but do not replicate the picture in its entirety.[11] As in many other neurological conditions, the response to specific therapeutic measures has been one arbiter of the validity of a postulated hypothesis.

Table 1 Classification of hepatic encephalopathy

	Hepatic failure	Extrahepatic PSS	Special features
Acute liver failure	Maximal	Absent	Development of brain oedema and ↑ ICP
Cirrhosis			
Acute encephalopathy	Variable	Variable	Precipitant-induced
Chronic encephalopathy	Variable	Generally large	Most often seen after portacaval surgery
Subclinical encephalopathy	Variable	Variable	Requires neuropsychological testing

PSS, Portal–systemic shunting; ICP, intracranial pressure.

More recently, advances in human non-invasive imaging and quantification, such as **MR** (magnetic resonance) and MR spectroscopy, together with new tools to assess brain function, such as **PET** scanning (positron emission tomography), carry the promise of new insight into mechanisms of disease.

Interrelated concepts that facilitate the understanding of the pathogenesis of hepatic encephalopathy (Table 2) will be reviewed here:

(1) circulating neurotoxin(s) that arises from the splanchnic bed;
(2) the astrocyte and other neuroanatomical modifications; and
(3) alteration of neurotransmission as a major pathophysiological change.

Neurotoxin(s) derived from the splanchnic bed

In the 1950s, it was postulated that the liver synthesizes compounds that are critical for brain function, such as cytidine and uridine (Geiger, AmJPhysiol, 1954; 177:138). From this perspective, hepatic encephalopathy could be viewed as arising from the the lack of production of such compounds by a diseased liver. However, experimental and clinical evidence do not support this concept. Cross-perfusion experiments in a rat model of acute liver failure showed that depuration of its blood through a normal liver is far more critical for an adequate mental state than the provision of liver-derived blood from a normal animal (Roche-Sicot, ClinSciMolMed, 1974; 47:609). Clinical practice has taught that a cirrhotic patient can plunge into coma as a result of a precipitating factor and wake up after 48 h without any further deterioration of liver function. More recently, a diametrically opposite view of the role of a diseased liver has been raised: claims of a favourable response to total hepatectomy in some patients with an acutely failing liver have raised the possibility that products of a necrotic liver induce deleterious neurological effects (Ringe, AnnSurg. 1993; 218:3). This concept will be further reviewed, but could be termed as a 'liver-derived toxin' hypothesis. The nature of such deleterious activity is unknown.

In fact, for many years the controversy has centred around the nature of gut-derived toxin(s). The clinical evidence that supports the existence of such toxin(s) can be surmised from the response to therapy in cirrhosis: it is of nitrogenous origin, as witnessed by the

Table 2 Pathogenesis of hepatic encephalopathy; candidate toxins and possible mechanisms of altered neurotransmission

	Peripheral alterations	Related alterations in neurotransmission

Ammonia	Portal–systemic shunting
	Reduced intrahepatic elimination
	
	  • intrahepatic shunts
	  • decreased urea synthesis
	  • decreased glutamine synthesis
	Renal ammoniagenesis
	Decreased muscle metabolism
		Glutamatergic
		  Elevation of glutamine (Gln)
		  ↑ Extracellular
		  glutamate
		? GABAergic
		  Via neurosteroid synthesis after activation of
		  peripheral Bz receptors
		Dopaminergic
		  Plasma tyrosine (precursor) exchanges for Gln
		Serotoninergic
		  Plasma tryptophan (precursor) exchanges for Gln

'Endogenous' Bz	? Intestinal source ? Intracerebral generation	GABAergic Binding to GABA$_A$ receptors

False neurotransmitters	? Generated from intestinal bacteria
	? As a result of increased entry of
	  aromatic amino acids into brain,
	  • due to plasma imbalance
	  • in exchange for glutamine
		Dopaminergic/catecholaminergic
		  Synthesis shifted to octopamine and
		  other neurotransmitters

Manganese	Decreased biliary excretion Portal–systemic shunting	? Dopaminergic D$_2$ receptor alteration

Bz, Benzodiazepines. See text for further details.

precipitation of encephalopathy with different nitrogenous substances (Phillips, NEJM, 1952; 247:239) and the favourable response to protein restriction as a therapeutic measure. While constipation can precipitate encephalopathy, increased catharsis is a cornerstone of treatment. The main source of this activity appears to be the colon, as drugs that act at that level (non-absorbable disaccharides) improve mental state. Intestinal bacteria appear to be involved in the generation of the toxin(s), as non-absorbable antibiotics (e.g. neomycin) can improve an abnormal mental state. The toxin(s) must be at a high concentration in portal blood, as the construction of a portacaval anastomosis can precipitate encephalopathy. Four gut-derived toxins have been implicated:

(1) ammonia;
(2) synergistic compounds with ammonia;
(3) octopamine and other false neurotransmitters; and
(4) GABA/endogenous benzodiazepines.

Ammonia

In the early 1930s, it had already been noted that ammonia salts would induce neurological changes in cirrhotic patients (Van Coulaert, CRSocBio, 1932; 111:739). A role for ammonia in the pathogenesis of encephalopathy has been evaluated extensively over many years and much is known about its metabolism and mode of action.

Ammonia is generated in the intestine via two major mechanisms: as a result of the breakdown of urea by bacteria in the colonic lumen and from the metabolism of glutamine by small bowel mucosa.[13] It is absorbed via non-ionic diffusion and exhibits a high concentration in the portal vein, almost tenfold higher than arterial levels.[6] In the liver, both portal-derived ammonia and that derived from amino acid metabolism are taken up by periportal hepatocytes and used as a substrate for urea synthesis, in a reaction that exhibits a low affinity but a high capacity for ammonia metabolism. In periportal hepatocytes, ammonia combines with glutamate to form glutamine, a reaction catalysed by glutamine synthetase and exhibiting a high affinity but a low capacity for ammonia metabolism.[14] The net effect of the two metabolic systems in series is a tight control of the levels of ammonia in the hepatic vein (see Chapter 2.13.2)

In patients with cirrhosis, multiple mechanisms contribute to the development of hyperammonaemia, a frequent finding in these patients. The absorption rate from the intestine may be higher in view of the increased splanchnic inflow seen in the portal hypertensive state.[15] In view of the high hepatic extraction of ammonia (c. 0.9), portal–systemic shunts, both extra- and intrahepatic, will result in an increased systemic bioavailability. A reduction of hepatic mass will decrease the capacity to synthesize urea (Rudman, JCI, 1973; 52:2241) as well as glutamine. Furthermore, extrahepatic sites also contribute to the development of hyperammonaemia. The synthesis of glutamine in muscle, an important alternative site for ammonia metabolism,[16] may be decreased in patients who lose muscle mass, a common finding in advanced cirrhosis with ascites. Generation of ammonia by the kidney may be increased in the face of respiratory alkalosis, an alteration that arises from primary hyperventilation seen in cirrhosis (Wichsner, RespirPhysiol, 1974; 20:393), and as a result of potassium deficiency (Gabuzda, Medicine,

1966; 45:481), a frequent finding in cirrhosis irrespective of the use of diuretic therapy.

Recent studies using PET scanning have shown an increased passage of circulating ammonia into the brain in patients with cirrhosis.[17] Ammonia moves across membranes in its gaseous form (NH_3) and, with a pK of approximately 9, it circulates almost exclusively in its ionized form (NH_4^+). In the presence of systemic alkalosis, an increased proportion of diffusible ammonia may be present, favouring its entry into brain. On the other hand, the increased permeability–surface product seen on PET scanning[17] suggests that either that the blood–brain barrier is more permeable to ammonia or that an increased capillary surface is present, a finding that could be explained by cerebral vasodilatation.

In liver disease, the status of the blood–brain barrier, localized to the capillary endothelial cell of the brain, is a contentious issue (Horowitz, Gastro, 1983; 84:1003; Seda, Hepatol, 1984; 4:359; Lo, Hepatol, 1987; 7:452). Movement of hydrophilic solutes across the blood–brain barrier is mainly accomplished using carrier-mediated transport systems. A gross disruption of the barrier, with injury to the tight junctions that normally maintain the impermeability of the vascular endothelium, is not a feature in animals (Sarna, BrainRes, 1977; 138:550; Traber, Hepatol, 1987; 7:1272) or humans (Kato, Hepatol, 1992; 15:1060). Rather, activation of specific mechanisms may be present, such as the transport of neutral amino acids across the barrier (Mans, AmJPhysiol, 1983; 245:C74); the evidence for such an alteration is controversial.[18,19] In the case of ammonia, its rapid diffusion across membranes under normal circumstances argues against an alteration of the barrier as an explanation for the increased passage of ammonia into brain;[17] it would rather suggest an increased extraction, that could be explained if cerebral vasodilatation was present; this area is in need of more work.

Once inside neural tissue, ammonia may exert deleterious effects at many levels.[20] Brain glucose metabolism may be affected (Hindfeldt, JCI, 1977; 59:386; Lockwood, JCI, 1986; 78:86; Hawkins, AdvExpBiolMed, 1993; 341:13). Specific alterations may be present on neurones, astrocytes, and the interactions between both cell types.[21,22] Direct effects on cortical neurones include inhibition of chloride extrusion, affecting postsynaptic inhibitory potentials (Szerb, ProgNeurobiol, 1992; 39:135). In addition, ammonia may decrease the activity of the tricarboxylic acid cycle via inhibition of α-ketoglutarate dehydrogenase (Lai, JNeuroch, 1986; 47:1376). In astrocytes, detoxification of ammonia to glutamine may be a critical initial step in a cascade of events that alters astrocyte morphology and affects several neurotransmitter systems. Measurements of glutamine in the cerebrospinal fluid (CSF) of patients with hepatic encephalopathy correlate reasonably well with the degree of alteration in mental state (Hourani, ArchIntMed, 1971; 127:1033).

A wide range of medical disorders that affect mental state are also associated with hyperammonaemia. These include urea cycle enzyme deficiencies, Reye's syndrome and toxicity from drugs such as sodium valproate. Furthermore, medications that reduce ammonia levels (e.g. lactulose or sodium benzoate) or increase the activity of the urea cycle (zinc, ornithine–aspartate) have been reported to improve the altered mental state in all these conditions, including hepatic encephalopathy. Criticisms of the 'ammonia hypothesis' have also been expressed. Not all ammonium salts induce encephalopathy. Seizures, common in congenital hyper-ammonaemias,[23] are seldom observed in subjects with hepatic encephalopathy. The lack of correlation between circulating ammonia levels and the degree of encephalopathy has been a classic criticism; however, in the presence of an increased passage of ammonia into the brain, as seen in humans with hyperammonaemia, [17] a direct relationship between blood and brain levels need not necessarily be present.

Synergistic toxins

Other products of colonic bacterial metabolism may act synergistically with ammonia to aggravate encephalopathy. In experimental animals receiving intravenous doses of ammonia, administration of mercaptans, such as methanethiol and dimethyldisulphide, reduced the dose of ammonia that resulted in coma.[24] Mercaptans are sulphur-containing products of methionine metabolism and have been implicated in the genesis of fetor hepaticus, a unique odour detected in the breath of encephalopathic patients. However, they are difficult to measure in humans (Al-Mardini, Gut, 1984; 25:284). In one study, there was no relationship between the levels of methanethiol and the presence of encephalopathy (Blom, Hepatol, 1990; 11:682). However, administration of methionine to cirrhotic patients can result in an altered mental state (Phear, ClinSci, 1955; 15:93). The mechanisms by which mercaptans may affect brain function have not been studied extensively.

Short-chain and medium-chain fatty acids may also potentiate the effects of ammonia on the brain. Administration of octanoic acid to experimental animals can result in coma and, again, comagenic doses of ammonia can be reduced by the co-administration of this medium-chain fatty acid (Zieve, MetabolBrainDis, 1987; 2:147). Fatty acids can uncouple oxidative phosphorylation and block electron transport in mitochondria. Production of octanoic acid and C_3–C_5 short-chain fatty acids (such as propionate, butyrate, and valerate) is reduced with therapy of hepatic encephalopathy using non-absorbable disaccharides (Mortensen, Gastro, 1990; 98:353). Phenols, derived from the catabolism of phenylalanine and tyrosine, are another category of compounds that may affect mental state (Windus Podehl, JLabClinMed, 1983; 130:103); their role is uncertain.

Circulating false neurotransmitters

Intestinal bacteria can act on luminal protein to generate compounds derived from tyrosine that possess weak neurotransmitter activity, such as octopamine. Such compounds would be absorbed in the portal vein, escape hepatic uptake in chronic liver disease, and reach the brain where they would act as a 'false' neurotransmitter.[25]

It is possible that these compounds may be generated within the brain tissue itself. An increased transfer of neutral amino acids, such as phenylalanine and tryptophan, across the blood–brain barrier has been observed in experimental models (Mans, JNeuroch, 1982; 38: 705), a transport that occurs in exchange for glutamine, generated in astrocytes as a result of the detoxification of ammonia (Cangiano, JBC, 1983; 258:8949). In addition, the plasma levels of aromatic amino acids (phenylalanine, tyrosine) in chronic liver disease is increased, as a result of decreased hepatic uptake, favouring their

entry into brain (Fischer, Surgery, 1975; 78:276). The concomitant decrease in the plasma levels of branched-chain amino acids such as leucine, valine, and isoleucine (Morgan, Gut, 1978; 19:1068) reduces the competition for transport via the neutral amino acid carrier. Once in brain tissue, synthesis from tyrosine to noradrenaline and dopamine is diverted away to the genesis of octopamine, tyramine, and β-phenylethanolamine. The rationale for this shift is not totally clear, but could arise from phenylalanine-induced inhibition of tyrosine hydroxylase, the rate-limiting step in tyrosine metabolism.

In spite of the initial enthusiasm with which this hypothesis was received, clinical attempts at re-establishing the normal plasma aromatic/branched chain amino acid ratio have given inconclusive results. In fact, an abnormal amino acid ratio is also seen in patients without encephalopathy, as its values reflect poor hepatic function. To shed further doubt on this hypothesis, measurements of brain catecholamines in postmortem samples of cirrhotic patients have shown a decrease of brain octopamine with normal noradrenaline/adrenaline values.[26] An increased entry of aromatic amino acids into brain was not confirmed in a group of patients with cirrhosis.[19]

GABA/'endogenous' benzodiazepines

In the early 1980s, a new hypothesis was postulated (Baraldi, Science, 1982; 216:427; Schaefer, Lancet, 1982; ii:18). According to this view, GABA, a potent inhibitory neurotransmitter, which can also be generated within the intestine from the decarboxylation of glutamate, would gain access to the systemic circulation in the presence of liver failure and/or portal–systemic shunting. As a result, GABA would enter the brain via an abnormally permeable blood–brain barrier and induce neuroinhibition after binding to an increased number of GABA receptors.

This hypothesis, generated from data in animal models of acute liver failure (rats and rabbits with galactosamine-induced hepatitis) received intense scrutiny during the 1980s. Many of its tenets have been refuted. The increased GABA levels in plasma may reflect cross-reactivity with other amino acids (Ferenci, Hepatol, 1988; 8:69). The increased permeability of the normally impermeable blood–brain barrier to GABA was not observed in other animal models (Knudsen, JHepatol, 1988; 7:187). Furthermore, no alterations in GABA levels (Lavoie, JNeuroch, 1987; 49:692) or binding (Butterworth, Hepatol, 1988; 8:1084) were seen in human postmortem brain tissue; the original description of increased receptor numbers had methodological problems (Rössle, MetabolBrainDis, 1989; 4:203).

None the less, an alteration of GABAergic neurotransmission may still be present in hepatic encephalopathy. It has been proposed that endogenous benzodiazepines, ligands for the GABA receptor, may be of gut origin. Their nature will be discussed below.

Neuroanatomical changes

With the exception of brain oedema, the brain of patients dying in hepatic coma is surprisingly void of gross abnormalities. The only consistent change is the diffuse hyperplasia of astrocytes of the cerebral cortex, subcortical nuclei (such as the dentate and lenticular nucleus), and other brainstem nuclei.[27] Other parenchymal structures are minimally involved.

Astrocytes are the most abundant cellular element in the brain.[28] Their name reflects their stellar-like anatomy, with a small cellular body and extensive foot processes that surround capillary endothelial cells, neurones as well as axons. Functionally, this anatomical arrangement results in several key roles: neuronal function is optimized by controlling the extracellular environment (via mechanisms for the uptake of critical compounds such as CO_2, potassium, and glutamate (Walz, ProgNeurobiol, 1989; 33:309; Ransom, JClinNeurophys, 1992; 9:224)). The function of the endothelial cell is also affected; in isolated preparations, co-culturing with astrocytes allows endothelial cells to express blood–brain barrier properties, such as impermeable tight junctions (Janzer, Nature, 1987; 325:253). Astrocytes are the only cellular elements containing glutamine synthetase, the sole mechanism that the brain possesses to detoxify ammonia (Norenberg, BrainRes, 1979; 161: 303).

In animal models of fulminant hepatic failure, astrocyte swelling (Fig. 1(a)) is a prominent pathological feature in practically all preparations (Livingstone, Gastro, 1977; 73:697; Traber, Hepatol, 1987; 7:1272). Morphometric studies in cirrhotic patients dying in hepatic coma indicate an increase in size of astrocyte nuclei (Martin, ExpPath, 1987; 32:241). A characteristic appearance, the so-called Alzheimer type II astrocyte,[29] is commonly observed in brains examined after immersion-fixation (Fig. 1(b)). Human retinal glial cells undergo similar changes (Reichenbach, ActaNeuropath, 1995; 90:273). This can be reproduced in the experimental setting after administration of ammonia (Cavanagh, JNeurolSci, 1971; 12:63) and appears related to ammonia itself, as it can still be detected after inhibition of ammonia detoxification with methionine–sulphoximine, an inhibitor of glutamine synthetase (Gutierrez, ArchNeurol, 1975; 32:123). It is also seen in congenital hyperammonaemic conditions (Solitaire, JMentDefRes, 1969; 13:153; Bruton, Brain, 1970; 93:423). Coupled with other evidence of astrocyte pathology, such as loss of glial fibrillary acidic protein, an intermediate filament (Sobel, JNeuropathExpNeurol, 1981, 40:625; Kretzchmer, JNeuropathExpNeurol, 1985, 44:459), these changes highlight the need to consider a dysfunction of this cell in any theory of the pathogenesis of encephalopathy.[30]

Cortical atrophy can be seen on neuroradiological imaging (Tarter, Lancet, 1986, ii:892; Zeneroli, JHepatol, 1987, 4:283), but may also reflect the additive effects of alcohol, ageing, or other non-liver related processes. It plays a minor, if any, role in the symptomatology of hepatic encephalopathy. Discrete macroscopic changes can be detected in the so-called hepatocerebral degeneration.[31] This entity is characterized by a patchy, but diffuse, spongy degeneration of the cortex, where histologically neuronal degeneration of the deep cortical layer can be observed. Microcavitation can be seen in the striatum (Finlayson, Brain, 1981; 104: 79), a lesion that is also observed in Wilson's disease and hence the term 'acquired hepatolenticular degeneration' also used to define this condition. This is a feature of long-standing portal–systemic shunting, and can be seen many years after portacaval shunt surgery. Very rarely, spinal demyelination can occur after shunt surgery, with a symmetrical and variable loss of axons beginning in the spinal cord and becoming more conspicuous at lower levels. It predominates in the lateral pyramidal tracts and can give rise to a syndrome of spastic paraparesis.[32]

More recently, magnetic resonance imaging has raised the possibility that abnormalities of the basal ganglia may be more widespread than previously thought. A symmetrical hyperintense globus pallidus (Fig. 2) on T_1-weighted MR spin echo sequences can be observed in more than 70 per cent of stable cirrhotic subjects, even without evidence of encephalopathy.[33,34] It has been related to plasma ammonia levels in one series (Kulisevsky, Hepatol, 1992; 16: 1382) and to liver function in others (Pujol, Neurology, 1993; 43: 65). It persists (at least) over a 2-year period (Kulisevsky, Neurology, 1995; 45:995) and is reversible after hepatic transplantation. Direct measurements of human brain at autopsy indicate that the accumulation of manganese could explain the hyperintensity seen on MR.[35,36] Manganese intoxication is a discrete neurological entity characterized by the development of similar changes in basal ganglia (Shinotoh, Neurology, 1995; 45:1119). Manganese is neurotoxic, and possible pathogenic mechanisms include oxidative stress and excitotoxicity (Brouillet, ExpNeurol, 1993; 120:89). In liver disease, portal–systemic shunting and biliary excretory failure could contribute to hypermanganesaemia (Spahr, Hepatol, 1996, 24:1116). The reasons for selective brain deposition of manganese are unclear, although a recent study suggests that hyperintensity seen at MR may be more widespread than a sole change in basal ganglia (Norton, JHepatol, 1994; 21:764).

Alterations of neurotransmission

Metabolic diseases can alter the level of consciousness as a result of two major mechanisms: a brain energy failure or an alteration of neurotransmission. The first is exemplified by the encephalopathy that accompanies hypoglycaemia, where the lack of substrate results in a loss of the energy required to maintain transmembrane ionic gradients. Alterations in brain energy metabolism have been detected in patients with severe hepatic encephalopathy (Fazekas, AmJMed, 1956; 21:843). Recent studies measuring glucose utilization in rats after portacaval anastomosis using autoradiographic techniques have yielded conflicting results as both an increase and a reduction of this parameter in several brain regions have been noted (Lockwood, JCI, 1986; 78:86; Hawkins, AdvExpBiolMed, 1993; 341:13). Measurements of human glucose consumption with PET scanning have also yielded conflicting results (reviewed in ref.[12]). In one study with special attention to statistical analysis, only a selective loss of glucose consumption was noted, specifically in the area of the cyngulate gyrus.[37] Using ^{31}P-MR spectroscopy, a reduction in the ratio of phosphomonoesters to ATP was noted in human brain, a decrease that could reflect less breakdown of ATP to AMP;[38] however, changes in other chemical compounds (such as choline) may explain these findings. Studies in animal models, where a reduction of brain ATP was demonstrated,[39] were performed at a late stage of the neurological picture. While newer technology may shed further light on this issue, a consensus has emerged that energy failure, though possibly present at the end of the clinical course, is not a primary pathogenic mechanism in hepatic encephalopathy.[9]

Multiple neurotransmitter systems are altered in animal models of hepatic encephalopathy. This multiplicity is shared with other metabolic disorders of the brain and raises the question as to which change is primarily responsible for symptoms and which are secondary to earlier modifications. In order to study this complex

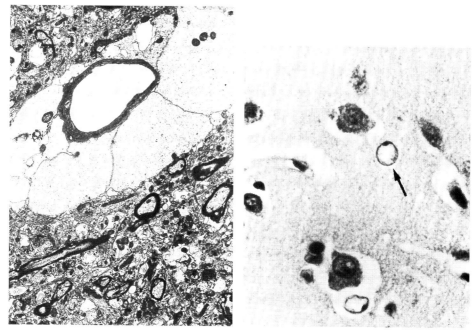

Fig. 1. Alterations of astrocytic morphology in liver failure. (a) Hydropic foot-processes of astrocytes surround a cerebral capillary from the cerebral cortex in a rabbit with galactosamine-induced fulminant hepatic failure (courtesy of Dr Mauro dal Canto, Northwestern University). (b) An Alzheimer type II astrocyte, with a large nucleus and its chromatin displaced to the side (by courtesy of Dr Roger Butterworth, Université de Montreal).

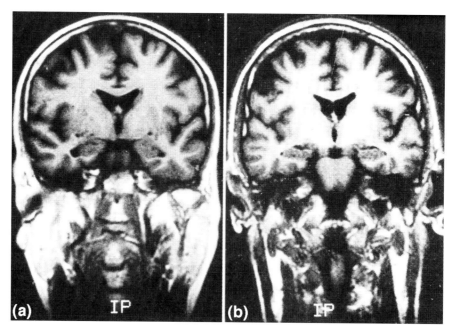

Fig. 2. Radiological alterations in cirrhosis. MR exam of a normal control (left) is compared to that of a cirrhotic individual, with conspicuous changes in the area of the basal ganglia. A hyper-resonant globus pallidus is seen. (Reproduced from Kulisevsky, Hepatol, 1992; 16:1382, with permission).

rearrangement, neurochemical measurements and behavioural testing are tools to probe such systems in the experimental animal. Recent technological advances, such as brain microdialysis, for example, have allowed measurements of transmitters in the extracellular space (deKnegt, JHepatol, 1994, 20:19; Rao, JNeuroch, 1995; 65:1221). Improved methods for monitoring behaviour in small rodents are also becoming available (Steindl, AmJPhysiol, 1996; 34:G555).

GABAergic neurotransmission

Under normal conditions, the GABAA receptor complex includes the presence of binding sites to benzodiazepines and barbiturates,

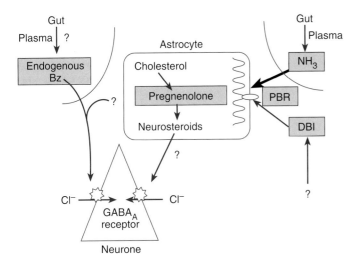

Fig. 3. Schematic diagram of possible mechanisms to explain opening of the chloride channel in neuronal GABA_A receptors in hepatic encephalopathy (HE). Shaded areas include reported abnormalities. Circulating 'endogenous' or 'natural' benzodiazepines may be receptor ligands (see Mullen, SemLivDis, 1996; 16:255), though their nature and origin (including a possible intracerebral source) have not been elucidated. An alternative pathway is via the production of neurosteroids in astrocytes. Activation of the mitochondrial peripheral benzodiazepine receptor (PBR), the density of which is increased in human brain (Lavoie, Hepatol, 1990; 11:874), can occur as a result of hyperammonaemia (Ducis, BrainRes, 1989; 499:362) or from the effects of diazepam-binding inhibitor (PBI), a peptide whose levels are increased in HE (Rothstein, AnnNeurol, 1989; 26:57). As a result, neurosteroids are synthesized from cholesterol; synthesis of the intermediate, pregnenolone, has been shown to be increased in two mouse models (Itzhak, BrainRes, 1995; 705:345).

drugs that exert their neurological efects by facilitating the action of GABA on the chloride channel. In hepatic encephalopathy, an increased concentration of compounds that bind to the GABA receptor (but not GABA) have been described in the plasma, cerebrospinal fluid, and brain of patients with acute and chronic liver failure (Fig. 3).[40] These compounds have been termed 'endogenous' or 'natural' benzodiazepines, as they cross-react in a benzodiazepine radioreceptor assay but do not appear to exhibit the structure of this group of pharmacological agents. Animals without any lifetime exposure to exogenous benzodiazepines also have measurable levels of this activity (Basile, JNeuroch, 1989, 53:1057; Olasmaa, JNeuroch, 1990; 55:2015). A small fraction corresponds to known benzodiazepine compounds[41] but the source and nature of the greater fraction is unclear. It has been proposed that precursors of these compounds are produced by specific intestinal micro-organisms (Yurdaydin, BrainRes, 1995; 679:42). To highlight these difficulties, there is also evidence of the presence in hepatic encephalopathy of endogenous ligands, such as diazepam-binding inhibitor (Rothstein, AnnNeurol, 1989; 26:57) that bind to the GABA receptor and exert opposite pharmacological effects (proanxiety and agitation).

Several observations suggest that alterations in GABAergic neurotransmission may be present. Cirrhotic patients exhibit an excessive sedative response to benzodiazepines (Bakti, Hepatol, 1987; 7:629) (although it should be noted that they are also susceptible to the sedative effects of many other agents). To single-cell recordings of Purkinje cerebellar neurones from rabbits with galactosamine-induced acute liver failure, addition of flumazenil, a benzodiazepine receptor antagonist, resulted in neuronal firing (Basile, JNeurosci, 1988; 8:244), a phenomenon not seen in such cells from normal rabbits. This suggested that flumazenil was displacing a ligand from its receptor, allowing neuronal function to proceed. Although a beneficial effect of flumazenil has not been observed in all experimental models, clinical experience with this drug indicates a subset of patients with hepatic encephalopathy in whom the mental state improves.[42] In the latter study, the lack of correlation between plasma levels of benzodiazepine receptor-ligands with the clinical response to flumazenil suggested that the drug may be working through other mechanisms.

Recent observations implicate the peripheral benzodiazepine receptor in the pathogenesis of hepatic encephalopathy.[8,9] In contrast to the central receptor, part of the GABA complex, the peripheral one is located on the outer mitochondrial membrane, mainly of astrocytes. It has been implicated in many cellular functions.[43] One of the best characterized is the regulation of the synthesis of neurosteroids, such as allopregnanolone and allotetrahydrodeoxycorticosterone, derived from cholesterol. The peripheral benzodiazepine receptor is involved in the process of transfer of cholesterol from the outer to the inner mitochondrial membrane. When neurosteroids are released, they bind to the GABA receptor, where they exert rapid non-genomic agonistic effects.

Ammonia may increase the affinity of ligands to the astrocytic peripheral benzodiazepine receptor (Ducis, BrainRes, 1989; 499: 362). Increased numbers of such receptors have been reported in rats after portacaval anastomosis[44] and, postmortem, in brains of patients with cirrhosis;[45] such changes are also observed in a rat model of acute liver failure (Itzhak, BrainRes, 1995; 705:345) and in hyperammonaemic mice with congenital ornithine transcarbamylase deficiency (Rao, PediatrRes, 1993; 34:377). Another agonist of the peripheral receptor is the neuropeptide, diazepam-binding inhibitor (Korneyer, JNeuroch, 1993; 61:1515), the levels of which are elevated in hepatic encephalopathy, and which exhibits antagonist activity at the level of the GABA receptor, as noted above,. The possibility that neurosteroids may intervene in the pathogenesis of hepatic encephalopathy is currently being explored.

Glutamatergic neurotransmission

Glutamate is a major excitatory neurotransmitter in the brain. Profound alterations have been observed at many sites involved in glutamatergic neurotransmisson. Total levels of brain glutamate are decreased in several animal models and in tissue of patients with cirrhosis;[46,47] this reduction reflects its consumption in the formation of glutamine. However, increased levels in the cerebrospinal fluid (Swain, Hepatol, 1992; 16:1028) and extracellular space (De-Knegt, JHepatol, 1994, 20:19; Michalak, Hepatol, 1996; 24:908) have been observed in animal models. Such an increase could be explained by an increased release, suggested from experimental preparations (Moroni, JNeuroch, 1983, 40:850; Tossman, Neuro-chemRes, 1987, 21:440), and/or a defect in glial reuptake. The

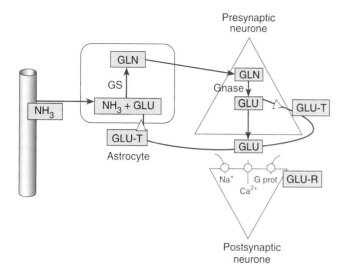

Fig. 4. Schematic diagram of possible mechanisms to explain alterations of glutamatergic neurotransmission in hepatic encephalopathy (HE). Shaded areas include reported abnormalities. Ammonia is detoxified in astrocytes to glutamine via the amidation of glutamate (GLU), whose total levels are decreased in HE (Record, EurJClinInv, 1976; 6:387). The activity of glutamine synthetase (GS) may actually be decreased (Girard, MetabolBrainDis, 1993; 8:207) but glutamine (GLN) levels markedly increase and are substrates for glutamate synthesis (via the action of glutaminase, Gnase) in presynaptic neurones, where they are released from vesicles into the cleft. Elevated extracellular glutamate has been found consistently (de Knegt, JHepatol, 1994; 20:19). Secondary alterations in glutamate receptors (Glu-R) may be present (Peterson, JNeuroch, 1990; 55:386; Michalak, Hepatol, 1996; 24:908), with involvement of ionotropic receptors (that mediate sodium and calcium entry) rather than metabotropic receptors (that activate G-protein). Preliminary reports indicate a decreased activity of glutamate transporters (Glu-T) (Huo, SocNeurosciAbstr, 1995; 21:108; Butterworth, Hepatol, 1996; 24:696, abstract) involved in glutamate reuptake.

latter was suggested in brain-slice preparations (Schmidt, MetabolBrainDis, 1990; 5:19) and can be reproduced by adding ammonia to isolated astrocytes.[48] This defect in glial reuptake may reflect effects on glutamate transporters, of glial and/or neuronal origin.

This increased extracellular glutamate may explain the alterations of receptor binding reported in several models. Glutamate binds to ionotropic [*N*-methyl-*d*-aspartate, **AMPA** (α-amino-3-hydroxy-5-methyl-4-isoxazolepropionic acid), and kainate subtypes] and metabotropic receptors in postsynaptic membranes,[49] while glial cells appear not to exhibit the *N*-methyl-*d*-aspartate type. A reduction in *N*-methyl-*d*-aspartate receptor number (Peterson, JNeuroch, 1990; 55:386) and in the affinity of non-*N*-methyl-*d*-aspartate receptors (Maddison, JNeuroch, 1991; 56:1881) has been reported in animal models.

Alterations in extracellular glutamate levels and in receptor function have the potential of affecting many cellular functions as well as the interactions between astrocytes and neurones (Fig. 4). The recent development of agonists/antagonists to the different receptor subtypes indicates new avenues for pharmacological testing.

Dopaminergic neurotransmission

As a result of the 'false neurotransmitter' hypothesis, the possibility was raised that a depletion of dopamine could be related pathogenically to hepatic encephalopathy. As in Parkinson's disease, the presence of extrapyramidal symptoms in patients with cirrhosis suggests that a dopamine deficiency may play a functional role. However, when dopamine levels in cirrhotic patients were increased by the administration of L-dopa, no clear improvement in clinical encephalopathy was noted (Michel, Gastro, 1980; 79:207).

Recent observations have rekindled the interest in possible alterations of the dopaminergic system. Autopsied brain tissue has shown increased levels of homovanillic acid, a dopamine metabolite (Bergeron, NeurochemRes, 1989; 14:853). Levels of monoamine oxidase-A, the enzyme responsible for dopamine degradation, were increased in the brains of cirrhotic individuals (Rao, BrainRes, 1993; 621:349). The number of the D_2 dopamine receptors was specifically decreased in human tissue.[50] Of even greater interest is the observation that manganese toxicity is exerted via its accumulation in the pallidum and neurodegenerative changes that result in a reduction of D_2 receptors.[51] At this time, we lack a chelating agent that could remove manganese specifically from brain tissue. If available, such a drug would allow the full assessment of the role of managanese in altered dopaminergic neurotransmission.

Serotoninergic neurotransmission

We have reviewed the evidence that indicates an increased entry of tryptophan, the serotonin precursor, into brain. In hepatic encephalopathy, cerebral levels of the stable metabolite of serotonin, 5-hydroxyindolacetic acid, are consistently elevated in animals (Bengtsson, JNeuroch, 1991; 56:1069) and human tissue (Bergeron, NeurochemRes, 1989; 14:853). This could reflect an increased turnover of serotonin metabolism (Bugge, WorldJSurg, 1987; 11: 810). More recent data have shown an increase in the activity of monoamine oxidase-A, the enzyme that is involved in the degradation of serotonin (Rao, BrainRes, 1993; 621:349), which would explain the increased levels of 5-hydroxyindolacetic acid (Fig. 5). An increased number of S_2 receptors has been noted in human postmortem tissue (Rao, NeurosciLett, 1994; 182:69), a factor that could account for the precipitation of overt hepatic encephalopathy by ketanserin, an S_2 receptor antagonist (Vorobioff, Hepatol, 1989; 9:88).

Serotonin exerts multiple effects in the brain and, at the time of writing, 13 receptor subtypes have been identified.[49] Methysergide, a non-specific receptor antagonist, had some beneficial effects on behavioural parameters of an animal model (reviewed in ref.[52]). More work is needed to assess the pathogenic implications of an altered serotoninergic system.

Other neurotransmitter systems

At the present time, up to 80 neurotransmitter systems have been identified in the brain. So far, I have covered four. Alterations in opioidergic neurotransmission may be involved in the alcohol preference of rats after portacaval anastomosis (Martin, AmJPhysiol, 1985; 248:G287), an alteration that is accompanied by region-selective alterations of μ and δ receptors and responds to treatment with the opioid antagonist, naloxone (de Waele, Hepatol. 1996; 24: 895). Its role in hepatic encephalopathy, proposed as a result of

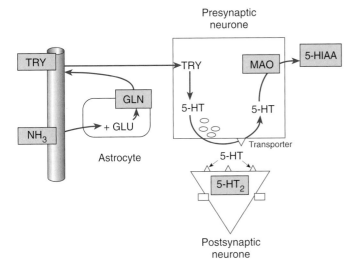

Fig. 5. Schematic diagram of possible mechanisms to explain activation of the serotoninergic system in hepatic encephalopathy (HE). Shaded areas include reported abnormalities. An increased entry of tryptophan (the precursor of serotonin, 5-HT) into brain, in exchange for glutamine generated in astrocytes, has been proposed (James, Lancet, 1979; 2:772). Cerebral levels of 5-hydroxyindolacetic acid (5-HIAA), a metabolic product, are elevated (Bengtsson, JNeuroch, 1991; 56:1059), indicating an increased degradation of serotonin (5-HT) via the activation of monoamine oxidase, MAO (Rao, BrainRes, 1993; 621: 349). The nature of synaptic 5-HT has not been fully ellucidated; an increase in the number of human S2 receptors has been shown (Rao, NeurosciLett, 1994; 182:69).

altered levels of enkephalins and endorphins, is uncertain (Panerau, BrainRes, 1982, 247:188; Yurdaydin, JPharmExpTher, 1995; 273: 185).

Clinical manifestations

A wide range of symptoms and signs can be elicited in patients with hepatic encephalopathy. Some of them are seen throughout the spectrum of clinical syndromes, some are noted only in specific entities.

Encephalopathy of acute liver failure

The development of encephalopathy in a subject with an acutely failing liver is a serious prognostic sign. It can occur within 1 or 2 weeks after the onset of jaundice (hyperacute liver failure or fulminant hepatic failure) or occur on a more protracted time interval (subacute or subfulminant hepatic failure). The stages of encephalopathy have been well delineated but some clinical manifestations are seldom seen in chronic liver disease (Table 3). Periods of excitation and mania can be present in the stage 1, prodromic phase of acute liver failure; this can be a difficult management problem, as pharmacological sedation obscures any spontaneous change in mental state. In stage 2, coma is impending, with drowsiness and inability to maintain sphincter control; a flapping tremor can be easily elicited. Seizure activity, myoclonic or focal, is a feature of late stages of acute hepatic failure and is rarely seen in chronic liver disease. The progression of changes in mental state can be very rapid, counted in hours, and in stages III (stupor) and IV (coma), brain oedema and intracranial hypertension can complicate the clinical course.

Brain oedema

The development of brain swelling is seldom observed in cirrhotic patients. The mechanisms that result in brain oedema in acute liver failure are the subject of controversy.[53] Two major pathogenic mechanisms have been proposed: in the first, cytotoxic (or cellular) oedema would arise from circulating toxins that, once in brain tissue, result in an increase of intracellular osmolarity. Sodium and glutamine have been proposed as possible osmolytes. In the case of sodium, circulating inhibitors of Na^+,K^+-ATPase activity (Seda, Hepatol, 1984; 4:74), whose presence can be determined indirectly, would enter brain tissue and prevent the exit of intracellular sodium. However, the existence of such inhibitors is controversial, and inhibition of brain Na^+,K^+-ATPase has not been demonstrated convincingly in animal models.

A role for glutamine has been the subject of recent investigations. Accumulation of this osmogenic amino acid in the brain has been demonstrated in human postmortem tissue (Record, EurJClinInv, 1976; 6:387) and *in vivo* with MR spectroscopy (McConnell, Hepatol, 1995; 22:69). Its generation within astrocytes occurs from the amidation of glutamate (Fig. 4). Inhibition of glutamine synthesis in animals infused with ammonia prevents the development of brain oedema (Takahashi, AmJPhysiol, 1991; 261:H825; Blei, Hepatol, 1994; 19:1431). There is clinical evidence that other acute conditions, such as chemotherapy-associated hyperammonaemia, are associated with brain swelling (Watson, Lancet, 1985; ii:1271). Thus, the question can be re-phrased. Why is brain oedema so exceptional in cirrhosis, where brain glutamine is also increased? Recent insight into mechanisms of brain water homeostasis provide a possible explanation. The accumulation of glutamine triggers mechanisms to restore osmotic compensation; they include the loss of other organic osmolytes (McManus, NEJM, 1995; 333:1260), of which myo-inositol is abundant in glial cells. Unchanged values of myo-inositol were seen in patients with acute liver failure (McConnell, Hepatol, 1995; 22:64), while an increase in glutamine and a reduction in myo-inositol is a characteristic feature of MR spectroscopy in cirrhosis (Ross, Radiol, 1994; 193:457). Such time-dependent changes in osmolytes have been seen in rats after a portacaval anastomosis (Cordoba, Hepatol, 1996; 24:919) and after placement of a TIPS in cirrhotic individuals (Haussinger, Gastro, 1994; 107:1475). A protective role against brain swelling of this osmotic adaptation remains uncertain.

A second major mechanism would imply a disrupted blood–brain barrier, also termed 'vasogenic' oedema. Indirect evidence suggests that a gross disruption, as in cerebral tumours or trauma, is not seen in acute liver failure. Computed tomography shows minimal changes (Muñoz, Hepatol, 1991; 13:209) or, when present, subtle but diffuse changes in the cerebral cortex (Wijdicks, MayoClinProc, 1995; 70:195); patchy involvement of both grey and white matter is noted in areas where the blood–brain barrier is broken. Brain biopsies of patients who had died with brain oedema showed intact tight junctions in the capillary endothelial cells (Kato, Hepatol, 1992; 15:1060). On the other hand, there is evidence in experimental models of alterations of blood–brain barrier permeability toward the end of their clinical course (reviewed in ref. [53]). It is unclear

Table 3 Grading of encephalopathy

Grade	Level of consciousness	Intellectual function	Neurological abnormalities	EEG abnormalities
0	Normal	Normal	None	None
1	Lack of awareness Change in personality Day/night reversal	Short attention span Easy forgetfulness	Slight tremor Uncoordination Asterixis	Symmetric slowing
2	Lethargy Unsuitable behaviour	Loss of orientation	Asterixis Abnormal reflexes	Symmetric slowing Triphasic waves
3	Asleep but rousable Confused when awake	Loss of interpersonal communication	Abnormal reflexes	Triphasic waves
4	Unarousable	Absent	Babinski/clonus Decerebrate	Delta (very slow) activity

Reproduced from Schafer DF, Jones EA. In Zakim D, Boyer T, eds. *Hepatology*, 2nd edn. 450. Philadelphia: Saunders, 1990: with permission.

whether these arise from specific alterations of endothelial cell function or from changes in the cerebral circulation.

Intracranial hypertension

Brain oedema is clinically silent, but once a critical point is reached, the normal intracranial pressure (0–10 mmHg) begins to rise within the limits of the rigid skull. Once brain compliance has been critically reduced, intracranial pressure can swiftly increase and reduce the cerebral perfusion pressure (mean arterial pressure – intracranial pressure) to the point where brain ischaemia develops. The clinical course culminates with the development of 'pressure waves' that elevate the pressure to critical levels and result in displacement of brain structures (Fig. 6). Herniation of the temporal or uncal lobe can be life-threatening. Brain oedema and intracranial hypertension are a major cause of death in acute liver failure.

An increased intracranial pressure can be clinically silent until high pressure values are reached. Patients are deeply encephalopathic and a sudden respiratory arrest can be a clinical presentation. Frequent monitoring of signs that indicate a high pressure, such as loss of the caloric or pupillary reflexes, is not an effective screening tool. Papilloedema is not detected. With this diagnostic difficulty, alternative methods for clinical monitoring have been examined (see below).

Acute encephalopathy in cirrhosis

This is the most common presentation in the hospital setting: a patient with known chronic liver disease develops an alteration in

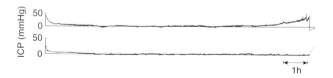

Fig. 6. Elevation of intracranial pressure in a rat model of acute liver failure (ALF). Pressure is recorded continuously from the onset of ALF, and initial higher values stabilize 1 hour after surgery in both ALF (top) and control (bottom). Within the last 2 hours of the course, intracranial pressure progressively rises in ALF and, in the last 30 min, episodic elevations occur with values above 50 mmHg. These culminate in brain herniation and demise of the animal. (Reproduced from Webster, Hepatol, 1991; 14:715, with permission.)

Table 4 Classification of coma

Glasgow coma scale

Eyes open	
Spontaneously	4
To command	3
To pain	2
No response	1
Best motor response	
Obeys verbal order	6
Painful stimulus, localizes pain	5
Painful stimulus, flexion response	3
Painful stimulus, extension	2
No response	1
Best verbal response	
Oriented and conversant	5
Disoriented and conversant	4
Inappropriate words	3
Incomprehensible sounds	2
No response	1

Total score from 3 (best) to 15 (worst)

mental state as a result of a precipitating factor. Gastrointestinal haemorrhage, uraemia, and the use of sedatives are incriminated most commonly. Less frequent, but clinically relevant, precipitants include constipation, infection, hypokalaemia, and excessive protein consumption. Removal or antagonism of the precipitant factor will result in neurological improvement.

Exploration of mental status (Table 3)

Difficulties can arise in the diagnosis of early encephalopathy. Subtle alterations of behaviour are first detected by family members. Abnormalities of sleep, including insomnia, hypersomnia, or inversion of sleep can be an initial complaint. A shortened attention span, irritability, or depression can be detected. In individuals with defined activities, abnormalities in handwriting or subtly impaired computations can become apparent. As encephalopathy progresses, intellectual function may show a loss of orientation to time, while an overt change in personality can occur in some individuals. A lethargic state of consciousness can evolve into confusion, stupor, and coma; a detailed classification of coma is available (Table 4).

Physical signs

Several physical signs can be detected in such patients. Asterixis, the most conspicuous, was first described in 1953.[27] It represents an intermittency of sustained muscle contraction with arrythmic lapses of sustained posture. Under normal circumstances a very short myoelectric silence can be detected when maintaining a constant contraction of a muscle group; asterixis represents the prolongation of this myoelectrical silence, such that the contraction cannot be sustained. Its pathogenesis is unclear, although it originates from derangements in central pathways rather than peripheral alterations.

The intermittency of the 'liver flap' distinguishes it from a tremor. It is most commonly elicited by asking the patient to extend his or her arm while retroflexing the wrist with separated digits. It is a feature of stages 1 and 2 encephalopathy; as the depth of encephalopathy progresses, the patient cannot co-operate with the request. In debilitated individuals, asterixis can also be elicited by asking the patient to extend the tongue or by having the examiner's fingers squeezed by the subject's hand; in both circumstances, the position cannot be maintained. Asterixis is not a pathognomonic finding in hepatic encephalopathy; it can also be observed in other metabolic encephalopathies, such as uraemia, carbon dioxide narcosis, in hypomagnesaemia, and with diphenylhydantoin intoxication. It can also be seen in focal neurological disease (Rio, ActaNeurolScand, 1995; 91:377).

Fetor hepaticus is a peculiar odour detected in the exhaled breath of patients with encephalopathy. It is difficult to define, but if sampled, it is easier to recognize in subsequent individuals. It is a pungent, somewhat sour odour noted at all stages of encephalopathy. Volatile sulphur-containing compounds, such as mercaptans, may account for this finding (Chen, JLabClinMed, 1970; 75:628).

A wide range of other neurological signs can be detected. Extrapyramidal abnormalities, including bradykinesia, dysarthria, rigidity, and tremor, have been described in cirrhotic patients.[34] Focal neurological findings can also be observed during the course of overt encephalopathy. Long-tract signs, such as Babinski and ankle clonus, can be unilateral or bilateral; they may be confusing in the individual that is stuporous or comatose, but in contrast to established neurological lesions, these focal signs characteristically wax and wane. Transient cortical blindness (Miyata, AmJGastr, 1988; 83:780) and alternating gaze deviation (Averbuch-Heller, Neurology, 1995; 45:191) have been reported. It should be remembered that metabolic encephalopathies, such as hepatic encephalopathy, can result in the clinical expression of previously silent small, focal lesions.

Diagnosis (Table 5)

Detection of a precipitating event is a critical initial step, which may require examinations to exclude gastrointestinal bleeding or infection; encephalopathy can be a presenting symptom of spontaneous bacterial peritonitis. The detection of the precipitant factor provides further evidence that the encephalopathy is of hepatic origin.

There are two clinical circumstances that pose difficulties in diagnosis. The first is the rare circumstance where encephalopathy is the presenting symptom of liver disease. As in other cases of a new abnormal mental state, a thorough physical examination and laboratory examination should provide diagnostic clues. In this setting measurement of plasma ammonia is useful; except for sedative-induced encephalopathy, most precipitating causes of encephalopathy are associated with an elevated ammonia level. Arterial blood provides a more accurate determination, as venous ammonia samples are influenced by the variable degree of peripheral metabolism. More recently, 'arterialized' samples (where the hand is warmed and the venous sample is drawn in a distal direction) or from the ear-lobe capillary (Huizenga, CCActa, 1995, 239.65) have been proposed. Immediate analysis and good laboratory practice are critical, as contamination should be rigorously avoided. Once the patient has been diagnosed as having hepatic encephalopathy, serial measurements of ammonia are unnecessary, as clinical examination is adequate to assess the evolution. In fact, as already discussed, blood ammonia levels have only a weak correlation with mental state abnormalities.

The second diagnostic challenge is the exclusion of other causes of encephalopathy in patients with known liver disease. Alcoholic subjects may develop Wernicke's encephalopathy, where a confusional state is associated with dysconjugate gaze. Fever and/or leucocytosis are not features of hepatic encephalopathy and a lumbar puncture may be necessary to exclude meningitis; such patients may already exhibit a coagulopathy, and the procedure should be done by an experienced individual. If available, determination of glutamine in the CSF can assist in the diagnosis of hepatic encephalopathy. The presence of focal neurological signs may prompt neuroimaging with CT or MR. Brain atrophy may be seen, especially in alcoholic subjects (Barthauer, AlcoholClinExpRes, 1992; 16:982), but its clinical relevance is questionable. A hyperresonant globus pallidus is not diagnostic of hepatic encephalopathy (Thuluvath, Hepatol, 1995; 21:440). Agitation and tremulousness, features of alcohol withdrawal, are seldom signs of hepatic encephalopathy. In other patients, extrapyramidal symptoms can be prominent; resistance to passive movements may increase with the velocity of limb displacement (*gegenhalten*). Parkinsonian features can be detected in up to 89 per cent of subjects (Spahr, Hepatol, 1996; 24:1116).

Chronic encephalopathy

This category includes patients with recurrent episodes of encephalopathy as well as those in whom a persistent alteration in mental state can be detected clinically. In those with recurrent episodes, dietary indiscretion and constipation are more conspicuous precipitants than gastrointestinal haemorrhage and uraemia. In cirrhotic patients with persistent abnormalities of mental state or in whom spontaneous episodes of encephalopathy recur, extensive spontaneous large-diameter portal–systemic shunts (e.g. splenorenal) can be detected (Takashi, JHepatol, 1985; 1:467; Ohnishi, AmJGastr, 1986; 81:450). Such cases may explain how, occasionally, patients can be discovered in psychiatric or neurological wards.

Individuals subjected to surgical portal–systemic anastomosis are especially prone to chronic encephalopathy, that can vary according to the type of anastomosis and the nature of liver function (Mutchnik, Gastro, 1974; 66:1005; Langer, Gastro, 1985; 88:424). Patients may develop an acute hypomanic or paranoid–schizophrenic reaction in the first months after the operation (Read,

Table 5 Diagnostic approach to overt encephalopathy in cirrhosis

1. Exclude other causes of encephalopathy

With fever and ↑ WBC	Consider lumbar puncture
In active alcoholism	Consider subarachnoid haemorrhage
Alcoholism and confusion	Consider Wernicke encephalopathy
	Obtain drug screen
Encephalopathy with asterixis	Rule out uraemia, CO_2 narcosis, ↓ Mg
Decerebrate posturing	Consider brainstem lesions, but neuro-ophthalmological examination is normal in liver cases
Exclude dementia	Normal consciousness + global cognitive defect
	Long duration; insidious onset
Exclude psychosis	Normal consciousness + selective cognitive defect
	Short duration; acute onset

2. Search for precipitating factor of hepatic encephalopathy

Most common	Gastrointestinal haemorrhage, uraemia, use of sedatives, diuretics
Other causes	Dietary indiscretion, infection, constipation, hypokalaemia
Also consider	Hypoxia, anaemia, hyponatraemia, and hypophosphataemia
When none found	Large spontaneous portal–systemic collaterals
	Acute deterioration of liver function

3. Obtain diagnostic tests

Arterial ammonia	For diagnostic uncertainty, not needed for follow-up
EEG	For diagnostic uncertainty
Search for precipitant	Blood count and chemistry, blood/urine/ascites culture
	Rectal/nasogastric examination for occult blood
	Drug screen
Imaging	Brain CT for exclusion of other pathology

QJMed, 1967; 36:135), but persistent changes tend to develop 1 year after surgery. Approximately 30 per cent of patients, in whom endoscopic and/or pharmacological techniques have failed to control portal hypertension-related bleeding that receive an emergency surgical anastomosis, or in whom a TIPS is placed,[54] develop episodes of encephalopathy. In non-alcoholic cirrhosis, persistent encephalopathy is more often seen with non-selective central shunts (end-to-side and side-to-side portacaval anastomoses, mesocaval shunt) than with selective derivations (distal splenorenal shunts).[55] No single hepatic or neurological test has emerged as a clear predictor of encephalopathy after shunt surgery (Huet, CanJSurg, 1979; 22:545; Pomier-Layrargues, Hepatol, 1988; 8: 1506; Planas, AmJGastr, 1992; 87:1792). In the case of TIPS, the procedure is employed in older subjects, and this may have emerged as a risk factor[54] (Somberg, AmJGastr, 1995; 90:549). The role of a previous episode of encephalopathy in predicting post-TIPS encephalopathy may depend on whether it occurred spontaneously or as a result of a precipitant factor (Blei, Hepatol, 1994; 20:249).

Hepatocerebral degeneration will develop many years after the surgical anastomosis[31] or in patients with large portal–systemic shunts (Summerskill, QJMed, 1956; 25:245). Patients develop a variety of extrapyramidal symptoms, including disturbances of gait, tremor, chorea, and ataxia (Mendoza, EurNeurol, 1994; 34:209). Muscle rigidity can be conspicuous. The patients can appear as somewhat jovial in spite of their severe limitations. If spastic paraparesis develops, movement may be severely limited;[32] loss of bladder control can be prominent.

Subclinical encephalopathy

A variable number of patients with cirrhosis, who appear to be clinically normal and whose neurological exam at the bedside appears unremarkable, exhibit cognitive deficits on neuropsychological examination.[56,57] The prevalence of these abnormalities is variable, and in the absence of a 'gold standard,' a true prevalence may be difficult to define; up to 70 per cent of patients have been reported to exhibit such changes.

Recent functional data point at subcortical alterations as a possible anatomical site responsible for subclinical changes (Kono, JNeurolSci, 1994; 126:162). In one series, the previously discussed alterations in the basal ganglia were associated with neuropsychological abnormalities (Kulisevsky, Neurology, 1995; 45:995). When neuropsychological testing is performed across different domains, results indicate a selective alteration in processes, such as attention and fine motor speed, that suggest involvment of basal ganglia (McCrea, ArchNeurol, 1996; 53:758). The selective reduction in glucose consumption in the area of the cyngulate gyrus, a nucleus involved in the attention process (Lockwood, Hepatol, 1993; 18:1061), coupled with focal alterations of cerebral perfusion (O'Carroll, Lancet, 1991; 337:1250) supports this notion of selective injury.

On the other hand, the relation of subclinical changes to protein metabolism[56] and plasma amino acid imbalance,[57] the reports of global reduction in cerebral blood flow noted in these patients (Rodriguez, JCerebrBloodFlowMetab, 1987; 7:768), coupled with the response of neuropsychological tests to therapeutic manipulations which are applied in overt encephalopathy, suggest a global impact of the liver disease on brain function, as seen in cases of clinical encephalopathy. As is the rule in controversial aspects of hepatic encephalopathy, there may be truth in both points of view.

The impact of subclinical encephalopathy on the daily life of patients is a matter of debate. Proscription of automobile driving was recommended to patients that exhibit abnormal visual reaction times (Schomerus, DigDisSci, 1981; 26:622). A recent pilot study, where the quality of automobile driving was assessed blindly in patients without prior episodes of overt encephalopathy, did not reveal differences between patients with and without abnormal neuropsychological tests nor in their comparison with carefully matched controls (Srivastava, JHepatol, 1994; 21:1023). In the absence of clear guidelines, it would appear prudent to evaluate fully patients who depend on driving or operating heavy machinery for their livelihood, and to examine the effects of therapy on their performance. If patients have already exhibited overt episodes of encephalopathy, limitation of driving may be necessary.

Sleep abnormalities are frequent in unselected cirrhotic patients.[58] They may be related to alterations of circadian function (Steindl, AnnIntMed, 1995; 123:274) but could also reflect elements of anxiety and depression that may arise as a result of living with chronic disease. They are not necessarily related to abnormal neuropsychological test results (Cabrera, Hepatol, 1996; 24:1103).

Quantitating hepatic encephalopathy

With the variability that characterizes the clinical expression of hepatic encephalopathy, it is not surprising that many tools are available for patient follow-up. In subjects with overt changes in mental state, no test supercedes a clinical assessment. It is in the diagnosis of the more subtle forms, such as subclinical encephalopathy, that a large number of tests have been developed.

Encephalopathy of acute liver failure

The development of brain oedema and intracranial hypertension poses diagnostic difficulties and influence the timing of liver transplantation. Brain swelling is not amenable to bedside clinical measurement as radiological techniques are imprecise and are not conducive to repeated measurements in these critically ill patients. Most of the effort is directed at measuring intracranial pressure. However, in the past few years, alternative non-invasive methods have been proposed.

Intracranial pressure monitoring

Patients with acute liver failure exhibit a severe coagulopathy, and placement of an intracranial pressure monitor may be associated with complications. A survey of clinical practice in the United States revealed a much lower incidence of haemorrhagic complications with the use of epidural transducers, while those monitors where the dura mater was pierced (such as subdural bolts or intraventricular catheters) were associated with considerably more bleeding and even death.[59] Epidural monitors are less precise and calibration can be problematic. The use of very thin transducers applied to the brain's surface has been suggested as an alternative, although complications do occur. Familiarity with the equipment and experience with such patients are important in reducing the complications. The procedure is reserved for patients in whom liver transplantation is being considered, as evidence of increased survival by measurement of intracranial pressure has not been demonstrated (Keays, JHepatol, 1993; 18:205).

Measurement of cerebral blood flow

Cerebral perfusion is decreased in the majority of patients with acute liver failure.[60] However, measurements of blood flow using radioactive xenon have shown that a subset of patients with acute liver failure may actually exhibit higher flows than would be expected for their cerebral metabolic rate, calculated as the product of cerebral blood flow and arteriovenous oxygen difference (the latter is estimated from measurements in a peripheral artery and in

the jugular bulb). The term 'luxury perfusion' can describe this phenomenon (Aggarwal, Hepatol, 1994; 19:80), a change that can increase cerebral blood volume and facilitate the development of intracranial hypertension. In addition, these patients lose the capacity to autoregulate their cerebral blood flow in the face of variations of arterial pressure (Larsen, JHepatol, 1995; 23:212). In this setting, an increase in arterial pressure may result in cerebral hyperaemia. These abnormalities in autoregulation appear to regress after liver transplantation and are not seen in the majority of patients with cirrhosis (Larsen, Hepatol, 1995; 22:730).

Tools are being developed to monitor cerebral perfusion. Repeated measurements using radioactive xenon are not a practical alternative. Use of Doppler insonation of the middle cerebral artery may provide a non-invasive measurement[60] but it requires further validation. The sole measurement of the arteriovenous oxygen difference across the brain (arterial and jugular vein samples) is theoretically insufficient, as changes in perfusion and in cerebral metabolism can independently affect its value. Elevated jugular venous lactate has been demonstrated in some patients, raising the possibility that these individuals may be suffering from brain ischaemia (Wendon, Hepatol, 1994; 19:1407). Whether any of these measurements could replace intracranial pressure monitoring remains to be proven, and they may be more likely to provide complementary information.

Auditory evoked potentials

In one study, serial recording of sensory evoked potentials in patients with fulminant hepatic failure provided prognostic information. Disappearance of the N70 wave was associated with the patient's demise or the lack of spontaneous recovery (Madl, Hepatol, 1994; 20:1487). This experience awaits confirmation from other centres.

Encephalopathy in cirrhosis
The PSE index

Many studies examining both precipitant-induced and chronic encephalopathy have utilized the portal–systemic encephalopathy (**PSE**) index (reviewed in ref.[3]). This method combines clinical features with objective data, scored in a semiquantitative fashion. For scoring, greater weight is given to mental state (factor of 3) than to arterial ammonia, asterixis, EEG findings, and score of the trailmaking test (factor of 1), each with scores of $1+$ to $4+$. Adding the contribution of these five parameters results in a PSE index value. The index has shortcomings, as separation in grades for some of its parameters (asterixis, trailmaking, ammonia) may be somewhat artificial; furthermore, repeated EEGs may not be readily available.

EEG

The electroencephalogram is part of the PSE index as it shows characteristic changes in hepatic encephalopathy.[61] These include the replacement of the normal background waves of 9 to 12 cycles/second by progressively slower waves, including φ waves, triphasic, and δ waves (the latter exhibit 2–3 cycles/second). These changes are not specific, as other metabolic encephalopathies and psychotropic agents can induce similar alterations. Quantitative and automated electroencephalographic analysis integrates the tracing and delineates the dominant signals (Van der Rijt,

ElectroencephaloClin Neurophys, 1984; 57:423 and 61:502). However, the use of the EEG has fallen behind that of other neurophysiological tools, mainly due to its low sensitivity. It still plays a role in patients where the diagnosis of the cause of encephalopathy is unclear.

Other neurophysiological testing

The integrated electrical response to visual, auditory, or somatosensory stimuli is the rationale for the use of evoked potentials.[62] Several parameters can be determined, including peaks and latencies; as a result, the function of afferent pathways and of the cerebral cortex can be evaluated. Results are expressed as time (in milliseconds) to positive (P) or negative (N) deflections. They have been used to detect subclinical encephalopathy as well as follow subjects with overt changes in mental state. For the latter, their sensitivity and specificity are questionable (Sandford, Hepatol, 1988; 8:1094; Van der Rijt, JHepatol, 1992; 14:141). Assessment of visual evoked potentials has been the tool most often evaluated, but differences in the type of light stimulus as well as in the liberal use of other waves than the P100 latency (100 ms between stimulation and peak) makes comparison between studies difficult.

For patients in whom subclinical encephalopathy is suspected, endogenous event-related potentials may exhibit a greater sensitivity. In this test, two aspects are combined: visual or acoustic signals are presented but, in addition, the patient is asked to identify a predefined stimulus (such as a high-frequency sound). A prolongation of the P300 latency to acoustic stimuli was observed in patients with early encephalopathy (Davies, Hepatol, 1990, 12: 688; Weissenborn, ElectroencephaloClinNeurophys, 1990; 75:829). Visual event related potentials appeared to be superior to neuropsychological testing in detecting abnormalities in such individuals ([63]; Kugler, ElectroencephaloClinNeurophys, 1994; 91:337).

Neuropsychological testing

A large number of tests have been utilized in the diagnosis of subclinical encephalopathy. The test most often utilized has been the number connection test, part of the PSE index. It can be administered as part A (number connection) and part B (Fig. 7). Though initially thought to reflect abnormalities corresponding to visuospatial perception, other neuropsychological areas appear to be involved in an abnormal result, including that of attention. The test is influenced by age and educational background, as well as subject to the effects of repeated learning (Zeneroli, JHepatol, 1992; 15:263). A battery of three tests (the trail test, the digit symbol substitution, and the block design test) was reported to be an accurate tool to diagnose subclinical encephalopathy.[57] More recent developments focus on the comparison between different neuropsychological domains as a useful diagnostic approach (McCrea, ArchNeurol, 1996; 53:758). However, in the absence of a 'gold standard', all these batteries require validation in the same patient over a period of time.

An important question is whether patients with alcoholic cirrhosis exhibit abnormalities due to the long-term neurological effects of alcohol. On a variety of neuropsychological tests, abstinent subjects with alcoholic cirrhosis perform comparably to their non-alcoholic counterparts (Tarter, AlcoholClinExpRes, 1988; 12:619).

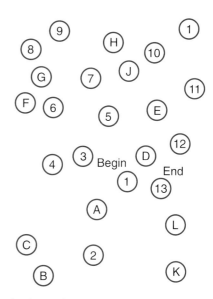

Fig. 7. Example of a number connection test (Reitan trail), part B. The patient is instructed to connect letters to numbers in a consecutive order (A,1,B,2,C,3....) and the time taken to perform the task is monitored.

After transplantation, the abnormalities in the alcohol group also improve (Arria, AlcoholClinExpRes, 1991; 15:956).

Treatment of hepatic encephalopathy—general aspects

Several reviews on therapy have been published recently.[3,52,64] A rational therapeutic scheme for hepatic encephalopathy targets four possible non-mutually exclusive sites (Fig. 8):

(1) the gut, decreasing the access of toxins to the systemic circulation;
(2) the liver, increasing the elimination of such toxins;
(3) the blood–brain barrier, by interfering with their entry into brain;
(4) the brain itself, by attempting to restore the abnormalities of neurotransmission.

The gut

The therapeutic goal at this site is interference with the formation and/or absorption of nitrogenous compounds arising from bacterial metabolism in the colon, and especially ammonia. Restriction of protein intake is one common approach to fulfilling this goal. However, malnutrition may arise from excessive protein restriction. A positive nitrogen balance may actually benefit subjects with encephalopathy by increasing the ability of liver and muscle to carry out detoxification functions (Morgan, JAmCollNutr, 1995; 14:152). In the catabolic state of cirrhosis, a high protein intake, *c.* 1.2 g/kg, may be necessary to accomplish this objective (Swart, ClinNutr, 1989; 8:329). In addition, the type of ingested protein is important. Vegetable (Uribe, DigDisSci, 1982; 27:1109) and dairy-based protein (Fenton, Lancet, 1966; i:164) are better tolerated than animal-derived protein, as a high calorie to nitrogen ratio seen in the former reduces gluconeogenesis and has anabolic effects on the utilization

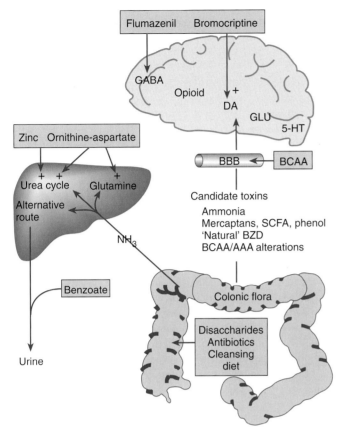

Fig. 8. Schematic diagram of therapeutic strategies in hepatic encephalopathy. Treatments reported to be successful are shaded. However, most effective therapy has been directed to the gut, where several options are available, The ability to increase urea and glutamine synthesis in a cirrhotic liver, as well as the activation of alternative pathways of nitrogen excretion (via the administration of benzoate), has not been fully evaluated. Branched-chain amino acids (BCAA) may work at the level of the blood–brain barrier (BBB) but their effectiveness is still matter of conjecture. Two neurotransmitter systems have been manipulated pharmacologically, with limited results. It is anticipated that new drugs will become available for testing based on agonism/antagonism of different neurotransmitter systems.

of dietary proteins (Zieve, Hepatol, 1987; 7:196). Vegetable-based diets have a high content of fibre, which increases the elimination of nitrogen products in the stool (Weber, Gastro, 1985; 89:538). For those intolerant of vegetable-based diets, administration of soluble forms of fibre can be added to a therapeutic regimen.[65] Standard amino acid formulations can satisfy nitrogen requirements, 70 g/day, in patients who need prolonged protein restriction. The enteral route is always preferred.

Bowel cleansing is another mainstay of therapy. Colonic cleansing reduces the luminal content of ammonia, decreases bacterial counts, and lowers blood ammonia in cirrhotic patients. Although different laxatives could accomplish this effect, non-absorbable disaccharides have additional benefits and are widely used for this effect. The use of mannitol as an oral cleansing solution has been proposed for patients with gastrointestinal haemorrhage in order to prevent the development of encephalopathy (Rolachon, GastrClinBiol, 1994; 18:1057).

Non-absorbable disaccharides have been widely used since their original description (Bircher, Lancet, 1966; 1:890). They include lactulose (β-galactosido-fructose) and lactitol (β-galactosido-sorbitol). When administered orally, they are not broken down by intestinal disaccharidases and thus reach the caecum, where enteric bacteria cleave the molecules and metabolize them, mainly to acetate; as a result, caecal pH drops (Florent, JCI, 1985; 75:608; Mortensen, Hepatol, 1992; 16:1350). In fact, acidification of the stool (pH < 6) can be used to monitor therapy. The acidification results in a cathartic effect and favours non-ionic diffusion of ammonia into the lumen, where it is assimilated for bacterial metabolism. As a result, faecal nitrogen excretion is increased while plasma levels of ammonia and the total body pool of urea decrease (Weber, Gastro, 1982; 82:213).

Oral dosing (15–30 ml four times a day) is titrated to result in two to three soft bowel movements/day. In comatose patients, a more rapid onset of action may occur by administration via enema (Uribe, Hepatol, 1987; 7:639), with the patient in the Trendelenburg position to favour passage of the enema into the right colon. Complaints with oral administration include an excessively sweet taste, abdominal cramping, and flatulence; these improve with continued administration. Excessive stool depositions as a result of overdosing can lead to loss of hypotonic colonic fluid with a resultant hypertonic dehydration with hypernatraemia, a factor that can by itself alter mental state.

Comparisons of lactitol to lactulose indicate similar effects but better palatability of the former agent (Blanc, Hepatol, 1992; 15: 222). The use of crystalline lactulose has been proposed to reduce potential contamination with other saccharides. In patients with known intestinal lactase deficiency, oral lactose will have similar effects (Uribe, DigDisSci, 1980; 25:924).

Antibiotics affect the intestinal flora that generates the putative toxins. In the case of neomycin, the most widely used antibiotic (Fisher, NEJM, 1957; 256:1030), non-bacterial effects may also be present at the level of the intestinal mucosa (van Berlo, JHepatol, 1988; 7:250). Although poorly absorbed, oto- and nephrotoxicity can develop (as with the use of other aminoglycosides), especially after chronic use. Thus, it is less commonly used as a first line of therapy. The starting dose is 3 to 6 g/day, in divided doses, and reduced to 1 to 2 g/day for maintenance. Other antibiotics have also been evaluated. Metronidazole, 800 mg/day in divided doses, has been shown to have similar effects to neomycin, although its bacterial spectrum of action is dissimilar (Morgan, Gut, 1982; 23:1). Metronidazole is metabolized in the liver, and adjustment of the dose may be necessary with liver failure (Loft, ScaJGastr, 1987; 22: 117). Limited experience with other poorly absorbable antibiotics, such as vancomycin (Tarao, Gut, 1990; 31:702) and rifaximin, also suggests beneficial effects.

The liver

The potential of the diseased liver to increase its metabolic capacity is limited, as a reduction of hepatic mass, intrahepatic shunting, and alterations of the sinusoidal architecture impose fixed restrictions. None the less, improvement of the capacity of the liver to clear ammonia has been sought. Zinc is a cofactor for many enzymes in the urea cycle and a deficiency may exist in cirrhosis as a result of malnutrition and increased urinary excretion. An improvement in the capacity to synthesize urea and in clinical status has been reported after administration of zinc acetate or sulphate, 600 mg/day in divided doses (Reding, Lancet, 1984; ii:493; Marchesini, Hepatol, 1996; 23:1084). This has not been confirmed in other studies (Riggio, DigDisSci, 1991; 36:1024; Bresci, EurJMed, 1993; 2:414). However, overt hepatic encephalopathy can be precipitated by overt zinc deficiency (Vander Rijt, Gastro, 1991; 100:114).

Ornithine–aspartate provides substrates for both urea and glutamine synthesis. It is undergoing clinical evaluation. It appears to prevent the rise of blood ammonia after a nitrogenous load (Staedt, JHepatol, 1993; 19:424).

Children with urea cycle enzyme deficiencies are treated with drugs that allow an alternative pathway for nitrogen excretion. In the case of sodium benzoate, conjugation of one molecule of benzoyl-CoA with glycine results in one atom of nitrogen excreted in the urine as hippurate. In one clinical trial, the drug was equally effective as lactulose in the treatment of acute encephalopathy in cirrhosis (Sushma, Hepatol, 1992; 16:138). A second drug is phenylbutyrate; it is a precursor for the malodorous phenylacetate, which is conjugated in the liver with glutamine, and the product, phenylacetylglutamine, is excreted in the urine, resulting in the loss of two nitrogen atoms per molecule. Preliminary results are difficult to evaluate as patients were being treated with other medications (Mendenhall, AmJGastr, 1986; 81:540). The effectiveness of the conjugation process for both drugs in patients with advanced cirrhosis remains to be established.

The blood–brain barrier

We have reviewed the false neurotransmitter hypothesis, where one of its basic tenets is the increased passage of precursor aromatic amino acids into brain. This led to the testing of the effects of branched-chain amino acid solutions, both in oral and intravenous forms, in order to restore the altered aromatic/branched-chain amino acid ratio and thus prevent the entry of phenylalanine, tyrosine, and tryptophan into brain. Numerous trials have been published in both acute precipitant-induced encephalopathy as well as in chronic encephalopathy.[66] Meta-analyses have yielded conflicting results (Eriksson, Gastro, 1989; 98:228; Naylor, Gastro, 1989; 97:1033). Critical review of these studies does not indicate a major beneficial effect but, given on a long-term basis, it may improve encephalopathy by increasing protein body stores (Marchesini, JHepatol, 1990; 12:92). It may provide a source of protein in patients with dietary protein intolerance. Even if beneficial for subclinical encephalopathy, as recently suggested (Plauth, JHepatol, 1993; 17:308), in most patients its use is not justified due to its relatively high cost.

The brain

We have reviewed how, once toxins enter into brain tissue, several neurotransmitter systems appear to be affected. Ammonia has been implicated in potential glutamatergic and serotoninergic alterations, false neurotransmitters have been proposed to account for abnormalities in dopaminergic neurotransmission, and endogenous or 'natural' benzodiazepines (and now neurosteroids) in an elevated GABAergic tone. Central effects of agonists/antagonists of these different systems provide new therapeutic options as well as clues

to the pathogenesis of encephalopathy. However, only two have received extensive evaluation.

Flumazenil is a selective antagonist of the benzodiazepine receptor. In several controlled studies in patients with variable degrees of encephalopathy, the mental state of a subset of individuals, c. 40 per cent, was improved with a bolus of intravenous flumazenil, albeit transiently. A source of controversy is whether such patients had received exogenous benzodiazepines (a common occurrence in hospitalized patients) but in some, no detectable benzodiazepines could be found in their serum. A favourable response occurs typically within a few minutes of administration and a repeat injection is possible. An oral preparation is as yet unavailable. The drug undergoes hepatic clearance and its elimination half-life is doubled in cirrhotics (Pomier-Layrargues, Hepatol, 1989; 10:969).

Enhancement of dopaminergic neurotransmission by increasing dopamine levels has been sought with the use of L-dopa and bromocriptine. With the latter and when used to improve consciousness, no major benefits were seen (Uribe, Gastro, 1979; 76:1347). However, bromocriptine, in association with non-absorbable disaccharides, at a dose of 10 mg twice a day, resulted in an improvement of extrapyramidal symptoms (Morgan, Gastro, 1980; 78:663). Manipulation of glutamatergic and serotoninergic neurotransmission has been tried in experimental models of hepatic encephalopathy but, as yet, has not reached the stage of clinical testing.

Treatment of hepatic encephalopathy—specific strategies (Table 6)

Encephalopathy of acute liver failure

Many of the measures that are used in the acute encephalopathy of cirrhosis are also applied in this setting, such as protein restriction and bowel cleansing with non-absorbable disaccharides. Their effectiveness, never tested in a controlled trial, may be at best marginal. Correction of other factors that may affect mental state, such as hypoglycaemia, pharmacological sedation, or infection, is mandatory.

Tracheal intubation is recommended at the onset of grade 3 coma to minimize the risk of sudden respiratory arrest. Intracranial hypertension, defined as a persistent elevation of intracranial pressure above 25 mmHg for more than 5 min or the appearance of sudden elevations of pressure (the so-called 'pressure waves') are treated with mannitol, 0.5 to 1 mg/kg intravenously.[67,68] The drug should not be re-administered at fixed doses, but bolused again when needed. In patients with renal failure, hyperosmolarity is a risk, and the patients may require dialysis. Emergency liver transplantation should be considered in the appropriate candidate. As a last resort, the patient can be treated with a barbiturate infusion, such as thiopental 180 to 500 mg administered intravenously over 15 min (Williams, Hepatol, 1989; 10:306).

Acute encephalopathy in cirrhosis

Establishing the nature of the precipitating factor is critical, as removal or correction of the inciting cause is the most important

Table 6 Therapeutic strategy in hepatic encephalopathy

Acute encephalopathy in cirrhosis
Identify, remove, and treat precipitating event
  Removal of blood from the gastrointestinal tract
  Reversal of azotaemia
  Specific antagonists for sedative-induced encephalopathy
  Antibiotics for spontaneous bacterial peritonitis or other infections
  Correct electrolyte disturbances
Bowel cleansing
  Disaccharide enemas may be better than tap-water enemas
Start oral non-absorbable disaccharides
  Lactulose or lactitol 30 ml every 1–2 h until bowel evacuation
  Then 15–45 ml every 6 h titrated to 2–3 soft bowel movements/day
Dietary management
  Provide calories as intravenous glucose in the first day
  Advance protein from 20 g/day to maximal tolerated
Chronic encephalopathy in cirrhosis
Search for precipitants
  Dietary indiscretion and constipation more prominent than in acute encephalopathy
Oral medications
  If intolerance or ineffectiveness of non-absorbable disaccharides:
  Replace with neomycin (3–6 g/day); monitor for toxicity
  Replace with metronidazole (up to 800 mg/day); monitor for toxicity
  Consider addition of zinc sulphate, or zinc acetate, 600 mg/day
  Consider addition of neomycin to non-absorbable disaccharides
Dietary manipulation
  Increase consumption of vegetable and dairy sources of protein
  Feeding at bedtime (to decrease nocturnal gluconeogenesis)
  For those intolerant to protein, consider branched-chain amino acid supplements
For problematic encephalopathy
  Consider occlusion of large spontaneous portal–systemic shunt
  Reduction of lumen of TIPS or portal–systemic shunt
  Consider colonic exclusion in patient with reasonable liver function who is not a transplant candidate

therapeutic aspect. Dietary protein is withheld for a few days and carbohydrates are administered intravenously. Protein is reintroduced once the mental state is improved and enteral feeding provided for those patients in whom encephalopathy persists; branched-chain amino acids are seldom necessary.

There are few controlled studies comparing therapeutic agents to placebo for this type of acute encephalopathy. The ones that are available do not indicate a striking drug effect. In a small group of 21 patients, oral lactulose was superior to placebo (Simmons, Gastro, 1970; 59:827); however, 10 days elapsed between randomization and evaluation, a period when other variables could be affecting results. When compared to placebo, neomycin was not more efficacious than standard therapeutic measures (bowel cleansing, removal of precipitating factor), although precipitating factors were not randomly distributed between groups (Strauss, Hepatogast, 1992; 39:342). In yet another controlled evaluation, a combined treatment with lactulose and neomycin was not superior to placebo in the management of such episodes, with removal of the precipitating factor common to both groups (Blanc, GastrClinBiol, 1994; 18:1063).

It is difficult to interpret results in such patients, as allocation of precipitating factors during randomization cannot be fully controlled. Still, they highlight the importance of control of the precipitating factor as a key therapeutic step. Lactitol or lactose enemas appear to improve encephalopathy at a faster rate when compared to cleansing enemas, as seen in a small group of 20 patients (Uribe, Hepatol, 1987; 7:1278). Oral lactulose can be given as 30 to 60 ml

of syrup every 1 to 2 h until stooling occurs, at which time the dose is adjusted to 15 to 30 ml three to four times a day.

Flumazenil, 1 mg intravenous bolus, is certainly indicated for patients in whom benzodiazepines are identified or suspected as a precipitating factor. In a recent study, 6 of 13 patients in deep encephalopathy transiently improved their mental state, in contrast to none with placebo. Similar results have been reported by other groups (Cadranel, EurJGastroHepatol, 1995; 7:325; Van der Rijt, GastrClinBiol, 1995; 19:572). The effect is prompt but transient, and at 24 h, the two groups were indistinguishable. The impact of multiple dosing has not been evaluated. More information is needed on this type of agent.

Chronic encephalopathy

Protein restriction may be necessary to manage this type of patient, although high protein requirements may be needed for these catabolic patients. Consultation with a dietitian should be considered in order to provide alternative sources to animal protein, such as vegetable or casein-based protein. Oral branched-chain amino acids are seldom needed.

Non-absorbable disaccharides are also indicated. Two small studies showed improvement of chronic encephalopathy when oral lactulose was compared to placebo (Germanin, ArchFrMalAppDig, 1973; 62:293; Elkington, NEJM, 1969; 281:408). Comparison against neomycin has shown improvement in mental status in over 70 per cent of treated patients (Conn, Gastro, 1977; 72:573).

Furthermore, in crossover studies, reinstitution or switch to lactulose/lactitol is associated with an improvement in mental status. Results in this group are more easily interpretable as the role of a precipitating factor is not as marked as in the acute precipitant-induced episode.

Oral, poorly absorbable antibiotics are seldom used as a first line of therapy, as concerns with long-term toxicity and bacterial resistance arise. If chronic neomycin is used, periodic auditory examinations and renal function testing are mandatory. For patients with difficulties in symptom control, zinc supplementation can be entertained. For those with prominent extrapyramidal symptoms, a trial of bromocriptine may be considered. Embolization of large spontaneous collaterals can be performed as a measure of last resort (Uflacker, Radiol, 1987; 165:721; Vavasseur, CardvascIntRadiol, 1994; 17:293).

Encephalopathy after portacaval anastomosis can be crippling, and requires tight dietary control as well as the use of many drugs (preferably acting at different sites). Revision of the shunt (Dagenais, WorldJSurg, 1991; 15:109) or occlusion of the TIPS (Hauerstein, Radiol, 1995; 194:175) is recommended for intractable cases. In suitable candidates, chronic encephalopathy is a clear indication for hepatic transplantation, although the procedure carries a greater mortality in patients with altered mental status at the time of the transplant. There are a few reports of improvement of the picture of hepatocerebral degeneration after the transplant procedure (Powell, Gastro, 1989; 98:1079). In non-transplant candidates with acceptable liver function, a surgical exclusion of the colon, preferably a colonic bypass, can provide relief from intractable encephalopathy (Resnick, Gastro, 1968; 74:1057).

Subclinical hepatic encephalopathy

The indications to treat subclinical encephalopathy would be clearer if the natural history of this condition was better defined. In the meantime, it may be prudent to separate patients according to a past history of an overt episode of encephalopathy. Consideration of the risk of driving an automobile may be more important if encephalopathy had been previously diagnosed. Sleep abnormalities, which cause considerable distress to patients, seldom respond, in the author's experience, to usual measures employed to treat hepatic encephalopathy; general hygienic measures can be considered (van Someren, BehavBrainRes, 1993; 57:235).

Neuropsychological tests do improve with many of the treatments that have been reviewed. These include protein restriction (De Bruijn, Gut, 1983; 24:53), non-absorbable disaccharides (McClain, JClinGastro, 1984; 6:325; Morgan, JHepatol, 1989; 8:208; Salerno, JHepatol, 1994; 21:1092) and branched-chain amino acids (Egberts, Gastro, 1985; 88:887; Plauth, JHepatol, 1993; 17:308). The case of flumazenil is controversial, as one study showed benefit (Gooday, Psychopharm, 1995; 119:295) while the other did not (Kapczinski, Psychopharm, 1995; 120:220); in the latter, patients with alcoholic cirrhosis developed more anxiety.

Concluding remarks

The World Health Organization has designated the 1990s as the 'decade of the brain'. As a result, the explosion of knowledge in the neurosciences should result in a better understanding of the mechanisms that underlie the pathogenesis of encephalopathy. One can anticipate that the next edition of this textbook will require further expansion of these sections. Better therapy for individuals with hepatic encephalopathy will focus on the altered neurochemistry as well as improving the ability to prevent the exposure of the brain to the diverse neurotoxins responsible for the multiple manifestations of this syndrome.

References

1. Conn HO and Lieberthal MM. *The hepatic coma syndromes and lactulose*. Baltimore: Williams and Wilkins, 1978.
2. Conn HO and Bircher J, eds. *Hepatic encephalopathy, syndromes and therapies*. Bloomington: Medi-Ed Press, 1994.
3. Capocaccia L, Merli M, and Riggio O, eds. *Advances in hepatic encephalopathy and metabolic nitrogen exchange*. Boca Raton: CRC Press, 1995.
4. Blei AT. Cerebral edema and intracranial hypertension in acute liver failure: Distinct aspects of the same problem. *Hepatology*, 1991; **13**: 376–9.
5. Pugh RNH, Murray-Lyon IM, Petroni MC, and Williams R. Transection of the esophagus for bleeding esophageal varices. *British Journal of Surgery*, 1973; **60**: 646–9.
6. Nomura F, *et al.* Effect of intrahepatic portal-systemic shunting on hepatic ammonia extraction in patients with cirrhosis. *Hepatology*, 1994; **20**: 1478–81.
7. Ferenci P, Puspok A, and Steindl P. Current concepts in the pathophysiology of hepatic encephalopathy. *European Journal of Clinical Investigation*, 1992; **22**: 573–81.
8. Mousseau DD and Butterworth RF. Current theories on the pathogenesis of hepatic encephalopathy. *Proceedings of the Society for Experimental Biology and Medicine*, 1994; **206**: 329–44.
9. Butterworth RF. The neurobiology of hepatic encephalopathy. *Seminars in Liver Disease*, 1996; **16**: 235.
10. Norenberg MD. Astrocytic-ammonia interactions in hepatic encephalopathy. *Seminars in Liver Disease*, 1996; **16**: 245.
11. Blei AT, Omary R, and Butterworth RF. Animal models of hepatic encephalopathies. In Boulton AA, Baker GB, and Butterworth RF, eds. *Animal models of neurological disease, Neuromethods 22*. Clifton: Humana, 1992: 183–222.
12. Morgan MY. Non-invasive neuroinvestigation in liver disease. *Seminars in Liver Disease*, 1996; **16**: 293.
13. Powers-Lee SG and Meister A. Urea synthesis and ammonia metabolism. In Arias IM, Jakoby WB, Popper H, Schachter D, and Shafritz D, eds. *The Liver: biology and pathobiology*. New York: Raven Press, 1988: 317–29.
14. Haussinger D. Nitrogen metabolism in liver: structural and functional organization and physiological relevance. *Biochemical Journal*, 1990; **267**: 281–90.
15. Rikkers LF. Portal hemodynamics, intestinal absorption and postshunt encephalopathy. *Surgery*, 1983; **94**: 126–33.
16. Lockwood AH, *et al.* The dynamics of ammonia metabolism in man. Effects of liver disease and hyperammonemia. *Journal of Clinical Investigation*, 1979; **63**: 449–60.
17. Lockwood AH, Yap EWH, and Wong WH. Cerebral ammonia metabolism in patients with severe liver disease and minimal encephalopathy. *Journal of Cerebral Blood Flow and Metabolism*, 1991; **11**: 337–41.
18. James JH, Escorrou J, and Fischer JE. Blood brain neutral amino acid transport activity is increased after portacaval anastomosis. *Science*, 1978; **200**: 1395–7.
19. Knudsen GM, Schmidt J, Paulson OB, and Vilstrup H. Passage of amino acids and glucose across the blood–brain barrier in hepatic encephalopathy. *Hepatology*, 1993; **17**: 987–92.
20. Cooper AJL and Plum F. Biochemistry and physiology of brain ammonia. *Physiological Reviews*, 1987; **2**: 440–519.
21. Norenberg MD, Neary JT, Bender AS, and Dombro RS. Hepatic encephalopathy: a disorder in glial-neuronal communication. *Progress in Brain Research*, 1992; **94**: 261–9.

22. Butterworth RF. Portal–systemic encephalopathy: a disorder of neuron-astrocytic metabolic trafficking. *Developmental Neuroscience*, 1993; **15**: 313–19.

23. Ampola MG. The urea cycle: enzymes and defects. In Arias IM, Boyer J, Fausto N, Jakoby WB, Schachter D, and Schafritz D, eds. *The liver*. New York: Raven Press, 1994: 365–78.

24. Zieve L, Doizaki WM, and Zieve J. Synergism between mercaptans and ammonia on fatty acids in the production of coma: a possible role for mercaptans in the pathogenesis of hepatic coma. *Journal of Laboratory and Clinical Medicine*, 1974; **83**: 16–28.

25. Fischer JE and Baldessarini RJ. False neurotransmitters and hepatic failure. *Lancet*, 1971; **ii**: 75–80.

26. Cuilleret G, Pomier-Layrargues G, Pons F, Cadilhac J, and Michel H. Changes in brain catecholamine levels in human cirrhotic hepatic encephalopathy. *Gut*, 1980; **21**: 565–9.

27. Adams RD and Foley JM. The neurological disorder associated with liver disease. *Association for Research into Nervous and Mental Disease Proceedings*, 1953; **32**: 198–237.

28. Murphy S, ed. *Astrocytes: pharmacology and function*. San Diego: Academic Press, 1995.

29. Hösslin CV, Alzheimer A. Ein betrag zur klinik und patologischen anatomie der Westphal-Strumpellachen pseudosklerose. *Zeitschrift fur die Gesamte Neurologie und Psychiatrie*, 1912; **8**: 183–209.

30. Norenberg MD. Hepatic encephalopathy. In Ketterman H and Ransom BR, eds. *Neuroglia*. New York: Oxford; 1995: 950–63.

31. Victor M, Adams RD, and Cole M. The acquired (non-Wilsonian) type of chronic hepatocerebral degeneration. *Medicine*, 1965; **44**: 345–96.

32. Zieve L, Mendelson DF, and Goopfert M. Shunt encephalopathy: II. Occurrence of permanent myelopathy. *Annals of Internal Medicine*, 1960; **53**: 53–63.

33. Pujol A, Graus F, Peri J, Mercader JM, and Rimola A. Hyperintensity in the globus pallidus on T1-weighted and inversion-recovery MRI: a possible marker of advanced liver disease. *Neurology*, 1991; **41**: 1526–7.

34. Krieger S, Jaub M, Jansen O, Theilmann L, Geibler M, and Krieger D. Neuropsychiatric profile and hyperintense globus pallidus on T1-weighted magnetic resonance images in liver cirrhosis. *Gastroenterology*, 1996; **111**: 147–56.

35. Pomier-Layrargues G, Spahr L, and Butterworth RF. Increased manganese concentration in pallidum of cirrhotic patients. *Lancet*, 1995; **345**: 735.

36. Krieger D, Krieger G, Jansen O, Gass P, Theilmann L, and Lichtnecker H. Manganese and chronic hepatic encephalopathy. *Lancet*, 1995; **346**: 270–4.

37. Lockwood AH, Yap EWH, Rhoades HM, and Wong W. Altered cerebral blood flow and glucose metabolism in patients with liver disease and minimal encephalopathy. *Journal of Cerebral Blood Flow and Metabolism*, 1991; **11**: 331–6.

38. Taylor-Robinson SD, *et al*. Cerebral phosphorus-31 magnetic resonance spectroscopy in patients with chronic hepatic encephalopathy. *Hepatology*, 1994; **20**: 1173–8.

39. Hindfelt B, Plum E, and Duffy TE. Effect of acute ammonia intoxication on cerebral metabolism in rats with portacaval shunts. *Journal of Clinical Investigation*, 1977; **59**: 386–96.

40. Basile AS, Jones EA, and Skolnick P. The pathogenesis and treatment of hepatic encephalopathy: evidence for the involvement of benzodiazepine receptor ligands. *Pharmacological Reviews*, 1991; **43**: 27–71.

41. Basile AS, *et al*. Elevated brain concentrations of 1,4 benzodiazepines in fulminant hepatic failure. *New England Journal of Medicine*, 1991; **325**: 473–8.

42. Pomier-Layrargues G, *et al*. Flumazenil in cirrhotic patients in hepatic coma: a randomized double-blind placebo-controlled crossover trial. *Hepatology*, 1994; **19**: 32–7.

43. Parola AL, Yamamura HI, and Laird II HE. Peripheral-type benzodiazepine receptors. *Life Science*, 1993; **52**: 1329–42.

44. Giguere JF, Hamel E, and Butterworth RF. Increased densities of binding sites for the 'peripheral-type' benzodiazepine receptor ligand [³H]PK 11195 in rat brain following portacaval anastomosis. *Brain Research*, 1992; **585**: 295–8.

45. Lavoie J, Pomier-Layrargues G, and Butterworth RF. Increased densities of peripheral-type benzodiazepine receptors in brain autopsy samples from cirrhotic patients with hepatic encephalopathy. *Hepatology*, 1990; **11**: 874–80.

46. Record CO, Buxton B, Chase RA, Curzon G, Murray-Lyon IM, and Williams R. Plasma and brain aminoacids in fulminant hepatic failure and their relationship to hepatic encephalopathy. *European Journal of Clinical Investigation*, 1976; **6**: 387–94.

47. Lavoie J, Giguere JF, Pomier-Layrargues G, and Butterworth RF. Amino acid changes in autopsied brain tissue from cirrhotic patients with hepatic encephalopathy. *Journal of Neurochemistry*, 1987; **49**: 692–7.

48. Bender AS and Norenberg MD. Effects of ammonia on l-glutamate uptake in cultured astrocytes. *Neurochemical Research*, 1996; **21**: 567–73.

49. Cooper J, Bloom F, and Roth RH. *The biochemical basis of neuropharmacology*. New York: Oxford University Press, 1996.

50. Mousseau DD, Perney P, Pomier-Layrargues G, and Butterworth RF. Selective loss of pallidal dopamine D2 receptor density in hepatic encephalopathy. *Neuroscience Letters*, 1993; **162**: 192–6.

51. Butterworth RF, Spahr L, Fontaine S, and Pomier-Layrargues G. Manganese toxicity, dopaminergic dysfunction and hepatic encephalopathy. *Metabolic Brain Disease*, 1995; **4**: 259–67.

52. Ferenci P, Herneth A, and Steindl P. Newer approaches to therapy of hepatic encephalopathy. *Seminars in Liver Disease*, 1996; **16**:329.

53. Córdoba J and Blei AT. Brain edema and hepatic encephalopathy. *Seminars in Liver Disease*, 1996; **16**: 271.

54. Sanyal AJ, *et al*. Portosystemic encephalopathy after transjugular intrahepatic portosystemic shunt: Results of a prospective controlled study. *Hepatology*, 1994; **20**: 46–55.

55. Langer B, Taylor BR, and Greig PD. Selective or total shunts for variceal bleeding. *American Journal of Surgery*, 1990; **160**: 75–9.

56. Rikkers L, Jenko P, Rudman D, and Freides D. Subclinical hepatic encephalopathy: Detection, prevalence and relationship to nitrogen metabolism. *Gastroenterology*, 1978; **75**: 462–9.

57. Gitlin N, Lewis DC, and Hinkley L. The diagnosis and prevalence of subclinical hepatic encephalopathy in apparent healthy, ambulant, nonshunted patients with cirrhosis. *Journal of Hepatology*, 1986; **3**: 75–82.

58. Tarter RE, Hegedus AM, Van Thiel DH, Schade RR, Gavaler JS, and Starzl TE. Nonalcoholic cirrhosis associated with neuropsychological dysfunction in the absence of overt evidence of hepatic encephalopathy. *Gastroenterology*, 1984; **86**: 1421–7.

59. Blei AT, Olafsson S, Webster S, and Levy R. Complications of intracranial pressure monitoring in fulminant hepatic failure. *Lancet*, 1993; **341**: 157–8.

60. Larsen FS. Cerebral circulation in liver failure: Ohm's law in force. *Seminars in Liver Disease*, 1996; **16**: 281.

61. Parsons-Smith B, Sumerskill W, Dawson AM, and Sherlock S. The electroencephalograph in liver disease. *Lancet*, 1957; **ii**: 866–71.

62. Kullmann F, Hollerbach S, Holstege A, and Schölmerich J. Subclinical hepatic encephalopathy: the diagnostic value of evoked potentials. *Journal of Hepatology*, 1995; **22**: 101–10.

63. Kugler C, *et al*. Visual event related P300 potentials in early portosystemic encephalopathy. *Gastroenterology*, 1992; **103**: 302–10.

64. Córdoba J and Blei AT. Treatment of hepatic encephalopathy. *American Journal of Gastroenterology*, 1997; **92**: 1429–39.

65. Mullen KD and Weber FL Jr. Role of nutrition in hepatic encephalopathy. *Seminars in Liver Disease*, 1991; **11**: 292–304.

66. Morgan MY. Branched chain amino acids in the management of chronic liver disease. Facts and fantasies. *Journal of Hepatology*, 1990; **11**: 133–41.

67. Córdoba J and Blei AT. Cerebral edema and intracranial pressure monitoring. *Liver Transplant Surgery*, 1995; **1**: 187–94.

68. Muñoz SJ. Difficult management problems in fulminant hepatic failure. *Seminars in Liver Disease*, 1993; **13**: 395–413.

10

The spleen, hypersplenism, and other relationships between the liver and spleen

10 The spleen, hypersplenism, and other relationships between the liver and spleen

P. Aiden McCormick

Structure and function of the spleen

The spleen is the largest lymphoid organ in the body and has important immunological, filtering, and reservoir functions.[1] It is largest in relation to body size in infants but, in common with other lymphoid tissue, reaches its maximum size in late adolescence. Thus the finding of an enlarged spleen may be more significant clinically in older patients. The normal adult spleen weighs about 150 g and becomes smaller in old age.[2] The spleen lies parallel to the long axis of the left tenth rib, the surface markings of the upper border being 4 to 5 cm lateral to the tenth thoracic spine and those of the lower border being where the tenth rib meets the midaxillary line.[3] If the spleen enlarges, its lower border moves downwards and forwards in contact with the diaphragm and anterior abdominal wall. As it must at least double in size before it becomes palpable below the costal margin,[4] it is not usually palpable. However, it may be felt in up to 3 per cent of apparently healthy young adults,[5] but is rarely associated with long-term morbidity in these subjects as 10-year follow-up revealed only a slight increase in minor infections (Ebaugh, AnnIntMed, 1979; 90:130).

The spleen receives its arterial supply from the splenic artery, a branch of the coeliac axis, and drains via the splenic vein into the portal venous system. Both splenic artery and vein lie close to the pancreas for much of their length and are prone to damage in patients with pancreatic disease, for example acute or chronic pancreatitis, pancreatic pseudocyst, and pancreatic tumours. Damage to the splenic artery may cause splenic infarction or torrential haemorrhage, whereas damage to the vein may cause splenic vein thrombosis with the development of left-sided (sinistral) portal hypertension and gastric varices.[6]

The spleen is surrounded by a tough capsule from which trabeculas of fibrous tissue extend into the splenic substance, which contains red pulp and white pulp (Fig. 1). These are so named because of the macroscopic appearance of the cut surface of the spleen. White pulp is visible as tiny white or grey spots (Malpighian corpuscles) seen against the dark red background of the red pulp. The white pulp is lymphatic tissue, which surrounds the splenic arterioles to form the periarterial lymphatic sheath. It contains lymphocytes, monocytes, and lymphoid follicles. The red pulp consists of a reticular meshwork, containing phagocytic reticular

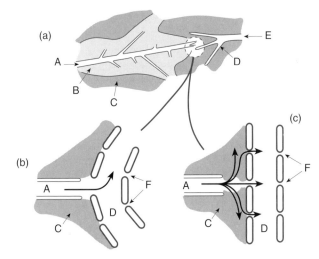

Fig. 1. Microcirculation of the spleen. (a) The splenic arteriole surrounded by the periarterial lymphatic sheath. The splenic arterioles terminate in the red pulp which then drains into the venous sinuses. Most of the blood enters the venous sinuses through fenestrations in its wall called interendothelial slits. If the interendothelial slits are wide open, blood flow from the splenic arteriole into the venous sinus is rapid (b). If, however, the interendothelial slits are narrow, blood flow is impeded. This results in slower flow and diversion of more blood into the red pulp (c). A, splenic arteriole; B, periarterial lymphatic sheath (white pulp); C, reticular meshwork (red pulp); D, venous sinus; E, splenic venule; F, interendothelial slit.

cells and endothelial macrophages, which lies between the splenic arterioles and the venous sinuses (Fig. 1). This reticular meshwork also contains contractile cells which are involved in the regulation of the microcirculation.[7]

Microcirculation of the spleen

The microcirculation of the spleen has, of necessity, been studied mainly in experimental animals and the results have been extrapolated to man.[7] The splenic microcirculation has two functional components, one having a short and the other a long transit time. Transit time in this context refers to red cell transit. The anatomical pathways corresponding to the short and long transit circulations have been a matter of controversy. Controversy has centred on how red cells travel from the arteriole to the venous sinuses. From corrosion-casting experiments in animals and man it appears that there may be three routes:[7]

(1) direct arteriovenous connections;
(2) via large terminal openings in venous sinuses which cause little resistance to flow from the red pulp;
(3) via narrow gaps in the walls of the venous sinuses called interendothelial slits (Fig. 1).

Red cells passing through the arteriovenous connections or through the large terminal openings in venous sinuses would have a rapid transit time whereas red cells traversing the interendothelial slits would have a longer transit time. The speed by which red cells enter the venous sinuses through the interendothelial slits is variable and depends on the size of these slits and the distance between the termination of the splenic arteriole and the wall of the venous sinus. Both of these factors can be altered by surrounding contractile cells.

Thus, if the termination of the arteriole is close to a wide-open interendothelial slit, then blood flow is rapid (Fig. 1(b)). However, if the arteriolar termination is not closely apposed to the venous sinus and the interendothelial slits are narrow, blood flow is slow and blood is diverted into the red pulp (Fig. 1(c)). It is estimated that in normal subjects 90 per cent of blood flow passes rapidly through the spleen while 10 per cent passes slowly through the red pulp.[7] The rapid component passes through the region bordering the white pulp, bypassing the filtration regions of red pulp. This suggests that under normal circumstances the immunological functions of the spleen take precedence over the filtration functions (Schmidt, ScanMicrosc, 1993; 7:613). The fast component of blood flow is usually referred to as the closed circulation, because it has the characteristics of a circulation without a break in the endothelial continuity; the slow circulation is referred to as the open circulation.[8]

In the splenic sinuses of the red pulp abnormal cells are exposed to phagocytic cells for long periods and may be destroyed. The precise mechanisms by which the red cells are destroyed are not well understood. It has been suggested that the red pulp has a microenvironment characterized by relative hypoxia, hypoglycaemia, and acidosis and that this metabolic strain may be responsible for red cell death. Recent work has not confirmed this hypothesis.[7] Another suggested mechanism is that the distortion of red cells necessary to allow them to pass through the narrow interendothelial slits means that abnormal red cells with diminished deformability are held up and can be removed from the circulation. Erythrocytes with intracellular inclusions such as Heinz bodies, Howell Jolly bodies, and intracellular parasites are also held up (Fig. 2). In this situation the part of the cell membrane including the inclusion may be pinched off and phagocytosed, thus allowing the erythrocyte to squeeze through the interendothelial slit and re-enter the circulation. Alternatively if the cell contains many inclusions, such as malaria parasites, it may be destroyed.

Immunological functions

As the spleen contains 25 per cent of the body's lymphoid tissue and receives 5 per cent of cardiac output it is well placed to respond

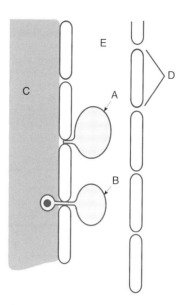

Fig. 2. Microcirculation of the spleen. Red blood cells traversing narrow interendothelial slits in the venous sinus. The normal red cell squeezes through but the red cell with an intracellular inclusion is held up. A, normal red cell; B, red cell with intracellular inclusion; C, red pulp; D, interendothelial slits; E, venous sinus.

to bloodborne antigens.[1] Small arterial branches feeding the white pulp leave the splenic arterioles at right angles, thus preferentially skimming off plasma, containing soluble antigens, into the surrounding lymphoid tissue. The spleen is a major site of antibody production in man and evidence of antibody production can be found there as soon as 16 h after initial exposure to bloodborne antigens.[9] Splenectomized patients appear to have diminished circulating levels of IgM (Lockwood, ClinHaem, 1983; 12:449). The ability of a splenectomized patient to mount an antibody response to new polysaccharide antigens appears to be significantly impaired (Amlot, Lancet, 1985; i:1008). This may explain the clinical observation that postsplenectomy sepsis is more common in children than in adults. Adults may be protected by the fact that they have been previously exposed to many common bacterial antigens and thus already have had a primary immunization process.[10]

The main splenic arterioles end in the red pulp where particulate antigens are exposed to phagocytic cells. The spleen and liver are the body's principal filters of bloodborne particles, including bacteria. Because of its much larger size the liver is quantitatively more important. However, the Kupffer cells of the liver require the presence of type-specific antibody, and opsonization of particles, to produce rapid and efficient uptake of bacteria.[11] Splenic macrophages are more efficient than Kupffer cells at dealing with bacteria in the non-immune host, and are particularly important in dealing with malarial parasites.[12] The difference in phagocytic efficiency may be explained by sluggish blood flow through the splenic sinuses, in comparison to the very rapid flow through the hepatic sinusoids, which ensures that splenic macrophages have adequate time to phagocytose bacteria. The increased incidence of overwhelming sepsis with encapsulated bacteria, such as pneumococci in patients who have had a splenectomy, attests to the importance of the spleen in dealing with bloodborne bacteria.[11] A number of roles concerning immune regulation and control have recently been ascribed to the spleen in experimental animals but their relevance to man, and more particularly splenectomized man, have yet to be determined.[13]

Reservoir function

In addition to its filtering and immunological functions, the spleen acts as a reservoir for blood cells.[14],[15] In normal subjects it contains approximately 30 per cent of the circulating pool of platelets; these can be released under conditions of stress or following an infusion of adrenaline. There is some evidence suggesting that granulocytes may be stored in a similar fashion.[16] In man the spleen contains about 3 to 5 per cent of red cell volume and there is no significant storage of erythrocytes.

Imaging of the spleen

The spleen may be imaged using various techniques including nuclear medicine scanning, ultrasonography, computed tomography (**CT**), angiography, and magnetic resonance imaging.[17] Ultrasound and radionuclide measures of spleen volume give comparable results (Shah, AmJGast, 1996; 91:2580). Ultrasound and CT are useful for defining the size of the spleen and the presence or absence of focal lesions. The splenic vein is usually seen on ultrasound, and splenic venous blood flow may be estimated using Doppler ultrasound (Sato, Radiol, 1987; 164:347). Splenic vein thrombosis may frequently be diagnosed using ultrasound imaging but occasionally splenic arteriography or splenoportography is necessary to confirm the diagnosis. Splenoportography produces excellent images of the splenic and portal veins but has fallen out of favour because of the risks of intraperitoneal bleeding. The risk is minimized by gelfoam plugging of the needle track (Brazzini, Radiol, 1987; 162:607). Three-dimensional vascular reconstruction using spiral CT can now produce very elegant studies of the splanchnic vasculature (Fig. 3) (Stehling, AJR, 1994;163:947). This may reduce the need for splenoportography. Magnetic resonance imaging may also be useful in the assessment of portal vein patency (Torres, AJR, 1987; 148:1109).

Splenomegaly

Many liver diseases are associated with splenomegaly (Table 1) which may occur even in patients with uncomplicated biliary tract disease (Gregory, Gastro, 1972; 62:436). The hepatologist most frequently encounters splenomegaly in patients with portal hypertension due to cirrhosis, schistosomiasis, or extrahepatic portal vein obstruction. The incidence of splenomegaly in cirrhotics varies between 36 and 92 per cent in different series.[18] The spleen may be very enlarged in patients with idiopathic portal hypertension. In a series of 350 patients with this condition from Japan the mean spleen weight at time of splenectomy was 723 g with 20 per cent weighing more than 1.5 kg.[19] Minor degrees of splenomegaly may be encountered in patients with viral infections such as viral hepatitis, infectious mononucleosis, and cytomegalovirus infection. Massive splenomegaly may be seen in amyloidosis, sarcoidosis, Gaucher's disease, kala-azar, lymphomas, myelofibrosis, and other conditions characterized by infiltration of the liver and spleen.

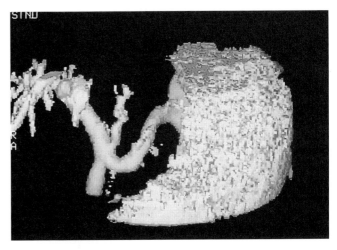

Fig. 3. Three-dimensional vascular reconstruction of the splanchnic veins using images obtained using spiral CT. A section of the spleen with splenic vein, part of the portal vein, and part of the superior mesenteric vein are shown. A number of intrahepatic portal vein branches may be seen. The coronary vein arises from the junction of the splenic and portal veins. (Reproduced by courtesy of F. Flanagan and Dr D. E. Malone.)

Patients with the last conditions may complain of abdominal pain and discomfort due to the very enlarged spleen. While most storage diseases present in childhood, adult Niemann-Pick disease may manifest in middle age with isolated splenomegaly (Dawson, HumPath, 1982; 13:1115).

In congestive splenomegaly there is thickening of the splenic capsule, and considerable white pulp hyperplasia and fibrosis superimposed on congestion of the red pulp.[20] Although the term congestive 'splenomegaly' implies that enlargement of the spleen is due primarily to portal hypertension or splenic vein block, the poor correlation between splenic size and level of portal pressure suggests that passive congestion is not the sole mechanism involved (Westaby, Digestion, 1978; 17:63; Merkel, ClinPhysiol, 1985; 5:531).[21] The cause of the liver disease appears to be important as non-alcoholic cirrhotics frequently have larger spleens than alcoholic cirrhotics.[22] In many patients with alcoholic cirrhosis the spleen may be impalpable. It has been reported that splenic size decreases in alcoholic patients after abstinence from alcohol (Sato, JHepatol, 1989; 8:150). In contrast, patients with primary biliary cirrhosis appear to have significantly heavier spleens than other forms of cirrhosis (Terayama, PathInt, 1994; 44:753). Splenomegaly may occur before cirrhosis is established and may be due to an element of presinusoidal portal hypertension in primary biliary cirrhosis.

Another factor which may be important in the causation of splenomegaly in patients with portal hypertension is increased stimulation by intestinal antigens which bypass the hepatic Kupffer cells leading to lymphoid hyperplasia of the spleen (Rozga, ActaChirScand, 1985; 151:125). It has also been suggested that there is a relationship between the splenic and intestinal circulations with reciprocal changes in flow occurring in the two circulations to maintain portal venous pressure and flow (Nishida, Gastro, 1990; 98:721). This would imply that the splenic circulation may have an important role in the maintenance of portal hypertension. A number of studies have shown that splenic blood flow is increased in portal hypertensive patients with splenomegaly (Williams, ClinSci, 1968;

Table 1 Causes of splenomegaly

Congestive splenomegaly
    Cirrhosis of any aetiology, e.g. alcoholic, posthepatitic, cryptogenic, autoimmune chronic hepatitis, primary biliary cirrhosis, primary sclerosing cholangitis, haemochromatosis, Wilson's disease, cystic fibrosis, α_1-antitrypsin deficiency, type IV glycogen storage disease
    Schistosomiasis
    Portal vein or splenic vein thrombosis
    Hepatic vein outflow obstruction, e.g. Budd–Chiari syndrome, veno-occlusive disease or cardiac causes of increased hepatic vein pressure, particularly constrictive pericarditis
    Idiopathic portal hypertension
    Nodular regenerative hyperplasia
Infectious disorders involving the liver and spleen
    Viral infections, e.g. hepatitis A, B, C, D, non-A, non-B, infectious mononucleosis, cytomegalovirus
    Bacterial infections, e.g. typhoid, brucellosis, tuberculosis, syphilis, leprosy
    Fungal infections, e.g. systemic candidiasis, histoplasmosis and other disseminated fungal infections
    Protozoal diseases, e.g. malaria and visceral leishmaniasis
Infiltrative disorders involving the liver and spleen
    Storage disorders, e.g. Gaucher's disease, Hurler syndrome, Niemann–Pick disease
    Cellular infiltration, e.g. lymphoma, sarcoidosis, extramedullary haematopoiesis
    Others, e.g. amyloidosis
Causes of splenomegaly more frequently seen in children
    Biliary atresia
    Sickle-cell anaemia (hyposplenism is common in adults because of splenic infarction)
    Cystic fibrosis
    Giant cell hepatitis
    α_1-Antitrypsin deficiency
    Storage diseases, e.g. Gaucher's disease, Niemann–Pick disease, Hurler syndrome and the mucopolysaccharidoses, neurovisceral storage disease with ophthalmoplegia, Wolman's disease, galactosaemia

34:441) but there is a poor relationship between splenic blood flow and the level of portal hypertension (Merkel, ClinPhysiol, 1985; 5: 531). The increased splenic blood flow is associated with dilatation of the splenic artery and may result in aneurysm formation (Blendis, Gut, 1969; 10:85). There is a further increase in splenic blood flow following portacaval shunting (Gitlin, Gastro, 1970; 59:208). The increased flow is probably temporary and returns to baseline values 1 year after distal splenorenal shunt and splenopancreatic connection (Takagi, Hepatol, 1994; 20:342). Spleen size has been reported to fall by about 50 per cent 1 year following distal splenorenal shunt (Takagi, Hepatol, 1994; 20:342). Thus, splenomegaly in portal hypertension may be due to a combination of passive venous congestion, increased splenic blood flow, and immune stimulation.

Hypersplenism

The term hypersplenism was first introduced by Chauffard in 1907 and is not precisely defined.[23] The cardinal features are splenomegaly, a reduction in one or more cellular elements of the blood in the presence of a normal or hypercellular bone marrow, and correction of the blood cytopenia by splenectomy,[24] although this is not usually recommended as treatment (see below). Other causes of peripheral cytopenias, such as folate deficiency, drug toxicity, and gastrointestinal blood loss, must be considered and, if necessary, corrected before the diagnosis of hypersplenism is accepted. Hypersplenism has been reported in 11 to 55 per cent of patients with portal hypertension in different series.[24] Hypersplenism may occur in any condition which causes splenomegaly and it is not unique to patients with liver disease and portal

hypertension. A number of mechanisms have been proposed to explain the presence of cytopenias in patients with splenomegaly. These include excessive pooling of blood elements in the spleen, increased destruction of blood elements, and haemodilution due to increased plasma volume.

Anaemia in hypersplenism

The anaemia of cirrhotic patients with hypersplenism is usually mild and does not require specific treatment. It is thought to be due to sequestration of red blood cells in the enlarged spleen. In the normal spleen there is no significant pooling of red cells.[15] However, in experimental animals, it has been demonstrated that an acute increase in splenic venous pressure, to levels seen in patients with portal hypertension, causes marked splenic pooling of erythrocytes and the development of peripheral anaemia. This is due to a marked reduction in the fast component of splenic blood flow with diversion of a major part of blood flow into the splenic cords (Levesque, JLabClinMed, 1980; 96:606). The exposure of larger numbers of red blood cells to phagocytic cells in the splenic cords probably contributes to the marginally reduced red cell survival times noted in these patients. Another factor which may contribute to the anaemia is the increased plasma volume noted in patients with splenomegaly of any aetiology. Although increased plasma volume appears to be a significant contributory factor to the anaemia in many haematological conditions complicated by splenomegaly, it appears to be less important in cirrhotics with hypersplenism as splenectomy seldom returns the plasma volume to normal in these patients (Blendis, EurJClinInv, 1970; 1:54).

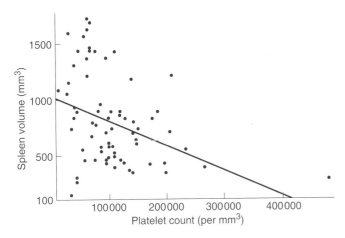

Fig. 4. Platelet count compared with spleen size. The platelet count is inversely related to spleen size although the relationship is very variable between different patients. (Reproduced from El-Khishen *et al.*, with permission.[25])

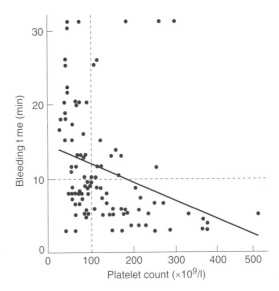

Fig. 5. Bleeding time compared with platelet count in cirrhotic patients. Overall there is a weak but significant correlation between platelet count and bleeding time (rs = −0.0483; p < 0.001). (Reprinted from Blake, BMJ, 1990; 301:12, with permission.)

Thrombocytopenia in hypersplenism

The normal spleen stores between 30 and 45 per cent of the circulating platelet pool and this figure may rise to over 90 per cent in patients with splenomegaly. Splenic pooling of platelets causes marked thrombocytopenia in the peripheral blood in many patients.[24] There is a significant inverse correlation between the size of the spleen and the platelet count, although the relationship is very variable between individual patients (Fig. 4).[25] It has also been suggested that the presence of platelet-associated immunoglobulin in many cirrhotic patients may contribute to thrombocytopenia (Pereira, AmJHematol, 1995; 50:173). Anticardiolipin antibodies in patients with hepatitis C virus infection may also be associated with thrombocytopenia and this should be distinguished from hypersplenism. Platelets are not irreversibly confined to the enlarged spleen and may be released under conditions of stress or during an intravenous infusion of adrenaline.[26] In splenomegalic patients the platelet count may double during an infusion of adrenaline but rarely reaches normal levels. As the spleen preferentially stores large, young platelets (megathrombocytes), it has been suggested that the released platelets may be particularly effective for haemostasis.[25] However, there is also evidence of defective platelet function in patients with liver disease (Desai, Lancet, 1989; 333:693; Ordinas, Hepatol, 1996; 24:1137) (see Chapter 25.3). Thrombocytopenia may be associated with an increased risk of cerebrovascular accidents in cirrhotic patients (Guanabens, GastroHepato, 1983; 6:119), but this is not a common problem.

In cirrhotics with thrombocytopenia the bleeding time is prolonged and is significantly correlated with platelet count (Fig. 5) (Blake, BMJ, 1990; 301:12). The importance of thrombocytopenia in variceal haemorrhage is unclear. Studies from our unit suggest that thrombocytopenia may predict early failure to control acute variceal bleeding (Burroughs, JHepatol, 1985; 1:s203) but that it is not predictive of early mortality. In patients with acute variceal bleeding and thrombocytopenia, platelet transfusions are rarely used, because of cost and because the majority of infused platelets are rapidly sequestered in the spleen. Furthermore most patients stop bleeding, either spontaneously or after treatment, and do not require platelets. The difficulty lies in patients with poor liver function and severe thrombocytopenia, who continue to bleed despite emergency sclerotherapy and balloon tamponade. There is no information as to whether these patients benefit from platelet transfusions. Our policy is to reserve platelet transfusions for use preoperatively in patients with severe thrombocytopenia (platelet count <25000), who continue to bleed following emergency sclerotherapy and require emergency surgery. This policy is purely empirical and is recorded merely to illustrate the difficulties in dealing with this problem. Other less expensive methods of improving haemostasis in these patients, for example fresh frozen plasma, desmopressin, and tranexamic acid,[27] are always used first.

Granulocytopenia in hypersplenism

Granulocyte kinetics in man are difficult to study because of methodological problems. The size of the splenic granulocyte pool in normal and enlarged spleens is somewhat controversial.[15] It has been suggested that about 30 to 50 per cent of the circulating granulocyte pool is stored in the normal spleen.[16] This proportion is increased in patients with splenomegaly. Many cirrhotic patients with splenomegaly have mild to moderate granulocytopenia and there is a significant inverse relationship between the size of the spleen and the total white cell count (Fig. 6).[25] Granulocytopenia is rarely a significant clinical problem in these patients, as they are able to mount a significant granulocytosis in the face of infection. Plasma myeloperoxidase levels are elevated in patients with cirrhosis and it has been suggested as a possible marker of hypersplenism (Nakamuta, Hepatol, 1993; 18:1377). Myeloperoxidase is contained in the primary granules of neutrophils. It is believed that increased neutrophil destruction in the spleen along with portal systemic

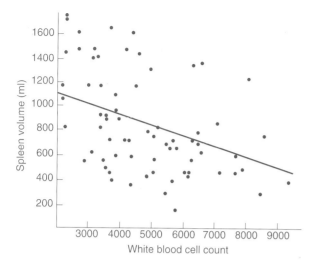

Fig. 6. Peripheral blood white cell count compared with spleen size. The white cell count is inversely related to spleen size although the relationship is very variable between different patients. (Reproduced from El-Khishen *et al.*, with permission.[25])

shunting may explain the increased plasma levels of myeloperoxidase in cirrhosis.

Treatment of hypersplenism

Hypersplenism rarely requires specific treatment. The anaemia is seldom troublesome and despite low granulocyte or platelet counts in the peripheral blood, cirrhotics with splenomegaly can usually mobilize granulocytes in the face of infection and platelets in the face of bleeding. Treatment for hypersplenism may be considered when a cirrhotic with splenomegaly and severe thrombocytopenia presents with life-threatening, recurrent variceal haemorrhage, particularly if the patient is from a remote area[11] or there is difficulty in finding compatible blood for transfusion. In this situation treatment aimed at stopping the recurrent bleeding, for example shunt surgery or endoscopic sclerotherapy, may be more beneficial than any attack on the spleen. Reversal of hypersplenism is unlikely to affect long-term survival as prognosis is related, in most cases, to the severity of the underlying liver disease. Nevertheless, in occasional patients, treatment aimed primarily at reversing the effects of hypersplenism may be considered and some of the treatments which have been used are described below.

Liver transplantation

Orthotopic liver transplantation is now frequently performed in patients with end-stage liver disease. Following transplantation portal pressure returns to normal although splanchnic haemodynamics may still be deranged for a considerable time (Henderson, Hepatol, 1989; 10:288). This is accompanied by a fall in spleen size and a rise in peripheral blood platelet count (Yanaga, AnnSurg, 1989; 210:180). Auxiliary heterotopic liver transplantation has also been reported to cause reduction in splenic size and normalization of platelet and leucocyte counts (Rinkes, Gastro, 1991;100:1126). Thus, although hypersplenism is not perceived as an indication for

liver transplantation, liver transplantation is probably the most effective treatment for the hypersplenism of chronic liver disease.

Splenectomy

Splenectomy by definition cures hypersplenism. However in patients with portal hypertension the operation is technically difficult and associated with considerable morbidity and mortality. It is now rarely performed in Western countries for cirrhotic patients except·as part of portal decompressive surgery. Splenectomy is still widely performed in countries where schistosomiasis is endemic, for the treatment of abdominal pain associated with marked splenomegaly or for hypersplenism. Splenectomy is rarely performed in patients with portal vein thrombosis as it appears to be the least effective surgical intervention in this group of patients (Webb, QJMed, 1979; 48:627). An exception is the rare syndrome of left-sided, or sinistral, portal hypertension, where isolated splenic vein thrombosis causes splenomegaly and the development of gastric varices. In this instance splenectomy may cure the portal hypertension and any associated hypersplenism.[6] Splenectomy has been performed after liver transplantation in children with recurrent rejection who could not tolerate azathioprine because of leucopenia (Megison, JPediatSurg, 1990; 25:881).

Overwhelming sepsis with organisms such as *Pneumococcus* and *Haemophilus influenzae* is a well-described complication following splenectomy, particularly in young patients (Selby, QJMed, 1987; 63:523). This is less common since the introduction of pneumococcal vaccination and long-term oral penicillin therapy, although recommendations for adults postsplenectomy vary (Reid, Lancet, 1994; 344:970). Recently, some surgeons have advocated partial splenectomy in order to preserve the immunological functions of the spleen while reducing its mass. A number of reports have appeared suggesting that this is a useful treatment for Gaucher's disease (Guzzetta, SGO, 1987; 164:359; Rodgers, AnnSurg, 1987; 205:693) and hypersplenism complicating cystic fibrosis (Louis, EurJPaediatSurg, 1993; 3:22). Patients with Gaucher's disease develop hepatosplenomegaly due to infiltration with glucocerebroside and often present with massive splenomegaly and hypersplenism. Most patients with the disease are young and do not have portal hypertension; thus partial preservation of the spleen may be technically feasible and may reduce the risk of postsplenectomy sepsis. However, clinical experience with this procedure is limited and long-term results are awaited. The success of treatment with glucocerebrosidase in reducing liver and spleen volumes in Gaucher's disease may make partial splenectomy unnecessary in this disease (Hollak, Lancet, 1995; 345:1474).

Shunt surgery

There is controversy about the effects of shunt surgery on hypersplenism. Splenorenal shunting significantly reduces splenic size (Takagi, Hepatol, 1994; 20:336). Most authors report an increase in white cell and platelet counts after various types of shunts. Serial platelet counts have even been recommended as a test of shunt patency (Koyanagi, AmJSurg, 1988; 156:29). However two controlled studies have given discrepant results.[18,28] Both included patients randomized to prophylactic or therapeutic portocaval shunt surgery compared with non-shunted patients. While in both studies splenomegaly disappeared more frequently in the shunt patients, only one study showed an improvement in white cell and platelet counts.[28] The effects of transjugular shunting on shunting has also been disappointing. In one study a transjugular shunt was inserted in 60 patients for bleeding or ascites (Sanyal, Hepatol, 1996; 23:32). Mean platelet count prior to transjugular shunting was 58 000 and did not significantly increase over 1-year follow-up. However five of the 40 had a sustained increase in platelet count of greater than 25 per cent but this was not predictable from changes in portal venous pressure. If the portal venous system is adequately decompressed following shunt surgery or transjugular shunting and the risk of variceal bleeding eliminated, the residual platelet count may not be of great importance.

Splenic embolization

Partial embolization of the spleen using autologous blood clot was first reported by Maddison in 1973.[29] Since then numerous authors have reported marked increases in peripheral white cell and platelet counts following this procedure (Alwmark, AnnSurg, 1982; 196:518; Shah, AmJSurg, 1990; 56:774; Brandt, JPediatSurg, 1989; 24:642). Partial splenic embolization has also been used to treat painful splenomegaly (Grassi, CardiovascIntRadiol, 1987; 10:291). Most workers now use gelfoam or steel coils rather than autologous blood clot. Radio-embolization with yttrium-90 has also been described (Becker, Radiol, 1995; 195:183). Initial enthusiasm for splenic embolization was tempered by reports of a high incidence of serious side-effects including splenic abscess, splenic rupture, acute pancreatitis, and septicaemia. However, complication rates can be substantially reduced by the use of strict aseptic technique, prophylactic antibiotics, and the avoidance of total splenic embolization. To avoid complete splenic embolization, it is recommended that only 70 to 80 per cent of the splenic parenchyma is embolized at any one time. If necessary repeated procedures can be performed to achieve a satisfactory result. Even with these precautions local pain, small pleural effusions, and prolonged fever are frequently encountered, particularly in children. In a series of 40 adult patients with cirrhosis and hypersplenism, partial splenic embolization resulted in significant increases in white cell and platelet counts in all.[30] Twenty five patients received treatment to allow interferon therapy for chronic viral hepatitis. A dose reduction because of thrombocytopenia or leucopenia was required in only two out of 20 who subsequently received interferon. In another series splenic embolization in 17 patients resulted in significant improvement in the endoscopic grade of portal hypertensive gastropathy (Ohmagari, AmJGastr, 1993; 88:1837). Successful partial splenic embolization has also been described in a patient with severe hypersplenism who continued to require platelet transfusions following liver transplantation (Herrero, Transpl, 1997; 63:482).

Colony stimulating factors (cytokines)

Both granulocyte colony-stimulating factor (**G-CSF**) and granulocyte-macrophage colony-stimulating factor (**GM-CSF**) have been used in the treatment of hypersplenism. Nine patients with cirrhosis and hypersplenism were treated for 7 days with GM-CSF (Gurakar, JHepatol, 1994; 21:582). There was an increase in absolute neutrophil count (2600 ± 1100 versus 1300 ± 200) but no significant change in platelet numbers. G-CSF was given to three children with severe hypersplenism after living related liver transplantation

with improvement in circulating granulocyte counts (Ishizone, JPediatSurg, 1994; 29:510). Unfortunately these agents have relatively little effect on platelet counts. Recently the cytokine thrombopoietin has been identified and cloned. It stimulates the proliferation and differentiation of megakaryocytic precursors and enhances platelet production in animal models (Kaushansky, Blood, 1995; 86:419). In addition it also appears to augment erythropoeisis after myelosuppressive therapy (Kaushansky , JCI, 1995; 96:1683). Thrombopoietin levels appear to be inappropriately low in patients with liver disease and thrombocytopenia and increase following liver transplantation suggesting improved hepatic synthesis (Fried, Hepatol, 1996; 24:178A). Thrombopoietin levels were not affected by TIPS shunting, which appears to have little effect on platelet numbers (Peck-Radosavljevic, Hepatol, 1996; 24:178A). Exogenous thrombopoietin may prove useful in the treatment of thrombocytopenia due to hypersplenism.

Other relations between the spleen and liver

Hyposplenism

Although hypersplenism is very common, functional hyposplenism has also been reported in patients with liver disease. In a study of 82 patients with alcoholic liver disease, splenic function was assessed by counting pitted erythrocytes (Muller, Gut, 1994; 35:679). Five patients (6 per cent) had pitted erythrocyte counts comparable to splenectomized patients. Abstinence from alcohol significantly reduced the pitted erythrocyte counts suggesting that this functional hyposplenism may be a direct toxic effect of alcohol. The authors suggest that this defect in splenic function may contribute to the susceptibility to infection in these patients. Susceptibility to infection may also be related to impaired function of splenic and other tissue macrophage Fcγ receptors (Gomez, NEJM, 1994; 331: 1122). Defective clearance of IgG-sensitized autologous red cells was demonstrated in 37 out of 49 alcoholic cirrhotics but not in alcoholics without liver disease or control subjects. This defect was related to the severity of the liver disease but not to the presence or absence of splenomegaly. Functional hyposplenism has not been confirmed in non-alcoholic liver disease (Markus, JHepatol, 1993; 18:106). Hyposplenism may occasionally occur in patients with hepatic amyloidosis (Gertz, Hepatol, 1997; 25:118).

Splenomegaly causing portal hypertension

The development of portal hypertension and oesophageal varices have been reported in a number of conditions associated with gross splenomegaly (Aufses, ArchSurg, 1960; 80:655; Blendis, ClinSci, 1970; 38:73). The presumed mechanism is increased splenic blood flow but many of these patients also have infiltration of the liver which may increase intrahepatic resistance, and some may have had portal vein or splenic vein thrombosis. Some investigators believe that abnormalities of the intrahepatic portal venous system rather than splenomegaly and secondary increases in portal venous flow are responsible for the pathogenesis of most types of non-cirrhotic portal hypertension (Ohbu, Hepatol, 1994; 20:302). However Japanese workers described increased splenic blood flow in idiopathic portal hypertension compared to a control group of cirrhotic patients with similar sized spleens (Aoki, Hepatogast, 1995; 42: 1030).[19] Thus, the relative contributions of increased splenic blood flow and increased portal venous resistance in this condition are still controversial.

Left-sided (sinistral) portal hypertension

This rare form of portal hypertension is characterized by portal pressure in the territory of the splenic vein. It is usually caused by isolated splenic vein thrombosis due to inflammatory diseases of the pancreas.[6] Patients usually have gastric varices without obvious oesophageal varices. Splenectomy may be curative. A variant is the rare splenic arteriovenous fistula. This is usually caused by the rupture of a splenic artery aneurysm into the splenic vein. The onset is generally sudden with abdominal pain followed by diarrhoea, ascites, and gastrointestinal bleeding. Ultrasound or dynamic CT scanning is often diagnostic and splenectomy is usually curative (McClary, AmJGastr, 1986; 7:572).

Peliosis of the spleen

Peliosis hepatitis is a rare condition characterized by the presence of multiple, small blood-filled cavities in the liver substance. Splenic peliosis also occurs, usually associated with hepatic peliosis. Cases of fatal and non-fatal haemoperitoneum have been described following rupture of peliotic cysts in the spleen (Parsons, PostgradMedJ, 1980; 56:796). In patients with immunodeficiency or cancer hepatosplenic peliosis may be due to infection with *Bartonella henselae* or *Bartonella quintana* (Liston, ClinInfDis, 1996; 22:951). *Bartonella quintana* is linked to contact with cats and is presumed to cause visceral cat-scratch disease. The organisms may be identified in liver biopsy specimens using Warthin-Starry staining or electron microscopy (Perkocha, NEJM, 1990; 323:1581). Various antibiotics including erythromycin, doxycycline and rifampicin may be effective. In immunosuppressed patients 3 months of treatment may be required. Hepatosplenic peliosis has also been associated with the use of drugs such as androgenic steroids (Warfel, ArchPathLabMed, 1982; 106: 99).

Spontaneous rupture of the spleen

Spontaneous rupture of the spleen in patients with liver disease is very rare but has been described in patients with portal hypertension, infectious mononucleosis (Peters, AmJMed, 1986; 80:123), Gaucher's disease, amyloidosis, angiosarcoma of the liver and spleen (Mahony, AJR, 1982; 138:965), and viral hepatitis (Van Landingham, ArchSurg, 1984; 119:224). It usually presents as an acute intra-abdominal catastrophe and is often fatal. Spontaneous rupture of the splenic vein may also occur rarely in patients with portal hypertension (Almgren, ActaChirScand, 1983; 149:109).

Splenic infarction

Liver disease is a rare cause of splenic infarction (Jaroch, Surgery, 1986; 100:743) but one case of spontaneous infarction of the entire spleen with resolution of hypersplenism has been described in a patient with cirrhosis and portal hypertension (Capron, Gastro, 1976; 71:308). Liver–spleen scintigraphy may be superior to ultrasound or CT scan in the diagnosis of splenic infarct in patients with congestive splenomegaly (Chin, PostgradMedJ, 1993; 69:715).

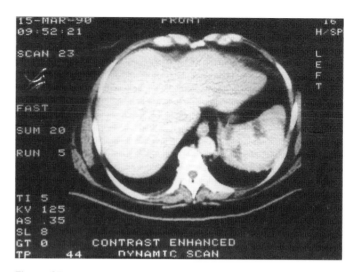

Fig. 7. CT scan in a patient with visceral leishmaniasis involving the liver and spleen. The patient presented with left upper quadrant pain and three low density splenic infarcts are visible in the spleen substance. (Reproduced by courtesy of Dr R. E. Pounder.)

Splenic infarction may occur in patients with marked splenomegaly due to any cause (Fig. 7).

Biliary atresia and polysplenia

An association has been noted between extrahepatic biliary atresia and the presence of multiple spleens in neonates. The polysplenia syndrome is characterized by other abnormalities including cardiovascular anomalies and intestinal malrotation (Sullivan, ClinNuclMed, 1987; 12:55). The presence of polysplenia is most easily diagnosed using scintigraphy.

Infections of the spleen

Pyogenic abscess of the spleen is not a common problem in patients with cirrhosis (Gleich, SGO, 1988; 167:211). However it may occur in situations where the arterial supply to the enlarged spleen is compromised, for example following splenic artery embolization or when the splenic artery is used to arterialize a liver graft in patients in whom the hepatic artery is damaged or unsuitable.

The spleen and the liver may both be affected by systemic *Candida* infection in immunocompromised patients (Bondestam, BMJ, 1981; 282:1514). Occasionally the spleen may contain an amoebic abscess (Wagner, ObsGyn, 1975; 45:562) or a hydatid cyst (Jain, JPostgradMed, 1988; 34:117). Brucellosis is a rare cause of hepatosplenic abcesses (Vallejo, ClinInfDis, 1996; 22:485).

Thrombocytopenia and hepatitis C

Thrombocytopenia has recently been described as a complication of hepatitis C virus infection and should be distinguished from hypersplenism in hepatitis C virus-related cirrhosis. It appears to be associated with the presence of antiphospholipid antibodies (Prieto, Hepatol, 1996; 23:199). In addition to thrombocytopenia, these patients may also have arterial or venous thrombotic complications such as deep venous or portal vein thrombosis. Portal hypertension may coexist in approximately 40 per cent of patients with anticardiolipin antibodies. Platelet associated antibodies and associated thrombocytopenia have also been described in patients with hepatitis C virus infection (Dine, PressMed, 1993; 22:269).

The spleen and hepatitis B

It has been demonstrated that splenic mononuclear cells contain replicative forms of hepadnaviruses in animal models of hepatitis B (Hosoda, Hepatol, 1990; 11:44). The importance of the spleen as a reservoir of hepatitis B in patients transplanted for hepatitis B-related liver disease remains to be determined.

The spleen and liver transplantation

In experimental xenograft transplantation the production of anti-graft antibodies by B lymphocytes may be important in rejection. In a rat model of liver transplantation low-dose tacrolimus and splenectomy were found to be additive in suppressing rejection and graft failure (Kashu, Transpl, 1996; 61:1522). Thus, splenectomy may represent a possible immunosuppressive strategy in liver transplantation.

The spleen and endotoxin-induced liver injury

The spleen is believed to contain approximately 15 per cent of the fixed tissue macrophages in the body. A recent study in rats suggested that both activated Kupffer cells and splenic macrophages may be responsible for endotoxin-induced liver injury following partial hepatectomy. Splenectomy attenuated liver injury in these animals and improved survival (Suzuki, Hepatol, 1996; 24:219). The relevance of this finding to human surgery remains to be established.

References

1. Sills RH. Splenic function: physiology and splenic hypofunction. *CRC Critical Reviews in Oncology and Haematology*, 1987; **7**: 1–36.
2. Krumbhaar EB and Lippincott SW. The postmortem weight of the 'normal' human spleen at different ages. *American Journal of Medical Sciences*, 1939; **197**: 344–58.
3. Robinson JO (ed). *Rawling's landmarks and surface markings of the human body*, (9th edn). London: HK Lewis, 1973: 65–6.
4. Last RJ. *Anatomy: regional and applied*, (5th edn). Edinburgh: Churchill Livingstone, 1973: 469–71.
5. McIntyre OR and Ebaugh FG. Palpable spleens in college freshmen. *Annals of Internal Medicine*, 1967; **66**: 301–6.
6. Lankisch PG. The spleen in inflammatory pancreatic disease. *Gastroenterology*, 1990; **98**: 509–16.
7. Groom AC and Schmidt EE. Microcirculatory flow through the spleen. In Bowdler AJ, ed. *The spleen, structure, function and clinical significance*. London: Chapman and Hall, 1990: 45–102.
8. Chen LT. Microcirculation of the spleen. An open or closed circulation? *Science*, 1978; **201**: 157–9.
9. Koren A, Haasz R, Tiatler A, and Katzuni E. Serum immunological levels in children after splenectomy. *American Journal of Diseases of Childhood*, 1984; **138**: 53–5.
10. Kopp WC. The immune functions of the spleen. In Bowdler AJ, ed. *The spleen, structure, function and clinical significance*. London: Chapman and Hall, 1990: 103–26.
11. Hosea SW, Brown EJ, Hamburger MI, and Frank MM. Opsonic requirements for intravascular clearance after splenectomy. *New England Journal of Medicine*, 1981; **304**: 245–50.
12. Looareesuwan S, *et al*. Dynamic alteration in splenic function during acute falciparum malaria. *New England Journal of Medicine*, 1987; **317**: 675–9.
13. Borek F. Previously unrecognised functions of the spleen; development and maintenance of immune competence and regulation. *CRC Critical Reviews of Immunology*, 1986; **6**: 287–93.
14. Peters AM. Splenic blood flow and blood cell kinetics. *Clinical Haematology*, 1983; **12**: 421–47.
15. Wadenvik H and Kutti J. The spleen and pooling of blood cells. *European Journal of Haematology*, 1988; **41**: 1–5.
16. Peters AM, Saverymuttu SH, Keshavarzian A, Bell RN, and Lavender JP. Splenic pooling of granulocytes. *Clinical Science*, 1985; **68**: 283–9.
17. Friedman AC. Magnetic resonance imaging of the spleen. In Friedman AC, ed. *Radiology of the liver, biliary tract, pancreas and spleen*. Baltimore: Williams and Wilkins, 1987: 1031–8.
18. Mutchnick MG, Lerner E, and Conn HO. Effect of portocaval anastomosis on hypersplenism. *Digestive Diseases and Sciences*, 1980; **25**: 929–38.
19. Okuda K. Idiopathic portal hypertension (hepatoportal sclerosis). In Okuda K and Benhamou JP, eds. *Portal hypertension*. Tokyo: Springer Verlag, 1991: 271–87.
20. McMichael J. The pathology of hepatorenal fibrosis. *Journal of Pathology and Bacteriology*, 1934; **39**: 481–582.
21. Witte CI, Witte MH, and Dumont AE. The portal triad in hepatic cirrhosis. *Surgery, Gynecology Obstetrics*, 1978; **146**: 965–74.
22. Soper NJ and Rikkers LF. Effect of operations for variceal haemorrhage on hypersplenism. *American Journal of Surgery*, 1982; **144**: 700–3.
23. Chauffaud M. Apropos de la communication de M Vaquez. *Bulletins et Memoires de la Societé Medicale des Hopitaux de Paris*, 1907; **24**: 1201–3.
24. Toghill PJ. The syndromes of splenic dysfunction. In Bowdler AJ, ed. *The spleen, structure, function and clinical significance*. London: Chapman and Hall, 1990: 209–32.
25. El-Khishen MA, Henderson JM, Millikan WJ, Kutner MH, and Warren WD. Splenectomy is contraindicated for thrombocytopenia secondary to portal hypertension. *Surgery, Gynecology Obstetrics*, 1985; **160**: 233–8.
26. Aster RH. Pooling of platelets in the spleen: role in the pathogenesis of 'hypersplenic' thrombocytopenia. *Journal of Clinical Investigation*, 1966; **45**: 645.
27. Burroughs AK, *et al*. Desmopression and bleeding time in patients with cirrhosis. *British Medical Journal*, 1985; **291**: 1377–81.
28. Felix WR Jr, Myerson RM, Sigel B, Perrin EB, and Jackson FC. The effect of portocaval shunt on hypersplenism. *Surgery Gynecology Obstetrics*, 1974; **139**: 899–904.
29. Maddison F. Embolic therapy of hypersplenism. *Investigative Radiology*, 1973; **8**: 280–1.
30. Sangro B, Bilbao I, Herrero I, *et al*. Partial splenic embolization for the treatment of hypersplenism in cirrhosis. *Hepatology*, 1993; **18**: 309–14.

11

Non-parasitic cystic diseases

11.1 Non-cystic malformations of the biliary tract

Valeer J. Desmet, Tania Roskams, and Peter Van Eyken

Atresia of extrahepatic bile ducts

Introduction (historical overview)

Atresia of the extrahepatic bile ducts is defined as absence of a lumen in part or all of the extrahepatic biliary tract, causing complete obstruction to bile flow. The earliest observations on extrahepatic bile duct atresia date from the middle of the nineteenth century (Heschl, WienMedWoch, 1865; 15:493). Surgical treatment of this condition was first discussed by Holmes in 1916 (AmJDisChild, 1916; 11:405); he predicted that a conventional biliary–enteric anastomosis might be feasible in patients (16 per cent of the total) with dilated, bile-containing proximal segments of extrahepatic ducts (the 'correctable' variant of extrahepatic bile duct atresia). Successful surgery was first reported by Ladd in 1928 (JAMA, 1928; 91:1082). One of his early patients was reported as doing well 37 years later (Lou, ArchSurg, 1972; 105:771), although few reports of survival were published in the next four decades (Bill, ArchSurg, 1974; 109:367).

A new era in the study and therapy of extrahepatic bile duct atresia was inaugurated by a new surgical management of this disease, which was developed in Japan by Dr Morio Kasai in 1957. This new approach, hepatic portoenterostomy or the 'Kasai operation', was published in the English literature in 1968 (Kasai, JPediatSurg, 1968; 3:665). Kasai and his colleagues introduced two important concepts into the pathology of biliary atresia (Howard, BrJSurg, 1983; 70:193). First, they showed that intrahepatic bile ducts are patent from the interlobular ducts of the liver to the porta hepatis in nearly all patients during the first 2 or 3 months after birth. Interlobular bile ducts appeared to be destroyed rapidly and to decrease progressively in number after 2 months of age. This explained why surgery was most effective for patients under 10 weeks of age and made early and rapid investigation mandatory. Second, the radical approach of portoenterostomy with resection of the obliterated extrahepatic ducts provided unique specimens not hitherto available. Histopathological study of these fibrous remnants confirmed the concept that extrahepatic bile duct atresia represents a necroinflammatory process leading to progressive destruction of the extrahepatic bile ducts (Witzleben, p.339 in reference 1; Witzleblen, p.53 in reference 2). It soon became clear that the intrahepatic bile ducts participate in the dynamic inflammatory process, and are subject to progressive destruction (Haas, World-JSurg, 1978; 2:561).

Increased experience with hepatic portoenterostomy worldwide has revealed that the intrahepatic component of ductal inflammation and destruction is of great importance in determining prognosis, even in patients with good postoperative bile flow soon after surgery. Hepatic portoenterostomy, including all subsequent variants and technical improvements of the operation, is not tantamount to cure (Alagille, p.233 in reference 3).[4] A considerable proportion of patients retain abnormalities of liver function tests and develop signs of portal hypertension (Alagille, p.233 in reference 3).[5]

Although the results today are encouraging, the situation is not ideal; the cause(s) of extrahepatic bile duct atresia are unknown, diagnosis is difficult, and only a minority of infants are truly cured by radical surgery (Jenner, AnnRCSurg, 1978; 60:367). It appears as if a completely satisfactory solution will not be reached without an understanding of the fundamental aetiology(ies) and/or pathogenesis involved (Jenner, 1978; Witzleben, LabInvest, 1978; 38:525; Witzleben, p.28 in reference 6).

Incidence of extrahepatic bile duct atresia

The incidence of biliary atresia is about 1 per 10 000 to 13 000 live births (Jenner, AnnRCSurg, 1978; 60:367). The incidence is similar in studies from Japan, North America, and the United Kingdom. It occurs more frequently in females than in males (Balistreri, JPediat, 1985; 106:171), and only a few familial cases have been reported. Coincidence of extrahepatic bile duct atresia with other disorders is reported occasionally, for example with the heterozygous state of galactosaemia, α_1-antitrypsin deficiency, and small bowel atresia. Such patients apparently represent fortuitous and unusual associations of different pathogenic processes.[7]

Extrahepatic bile duct atresia may be associated with a number of malformations, some of them constituting the 'polysplenia syndrome' (Chandra, JPediat, 1974; 85:649; Karrer, JPediatSurg, 1991; 26:524; Davenport, p.11 in reference 8). This comprises multiple spleens, venous anomalies (partial absence of inferior vena cava with azygos drainage; preduodenal portal vein, bilateral superior vena cava), dextro- or laevocardia, cardiac anomalies, tendency to laevoisomerism, and inversion of abdominal viscera. Associated malformations of this type are reported in about 11 per cent of patients with extrahepatic bile duct atresia (Rickham, ZKinderchir, 1979; 26:114; Karrer, 1991; Silveira, ActaPaedScand, 1991; 80:1192; Davenport, p.11 in reference 8). Besides their importance with respect to surgical techniques, these associated malformations suggest that the causal agent responsible for extrahepatic bile duct atresia may be operative relatively early during intrauterine development.

Pathology of extrahepatic bile duct atresia
Pathology of the extrahepatic bile ducts
Macroscopic lesions

It is useful to distinguish between correctable and non-correctable types. Correctable variants of extrahepatic bile duct atresia occur in patients in whom only limited segments of the extrahepatic bile ducts have interrupted permeability; the obliterated segment can be resected and the preserved proximal parts of the extrahepatic system can be reimplanted in the duodenum.[4] Kasai proposed a classification of the observed anatomical variants.[9] The main groups (types I, II, and III according to Kasai) are represented in Fig. 1. Type I corresponds to atresia of the common bile duct, where the more proximal extrahepatic bile duct segments are intact. Type IIa represents obliteration in the common hepatic duct with or without atresia of its main branches; the common bile duct, the cystic duct, and gallbladder are normal. Reanastomosis in this type is performed through cystically dilated ducts near the porta hepatis. Type IIb also belongs to the correctable category, although all main branches of the extrahepatic system of bile ducts (common duct, hepatic ducts, and cystic duct) are obliterated or missing. Reanastomosis with the duodenum is possible through cystically dilated ducts in the hilum. Unfortunately, the 'correctable' types I, IIa, and IIb represent less than 10 per cent of all patients with extrahepatic bile duct atresia; 90 per cent or more of patients cannot be corrected by these reanastomoses (Lilly, JPediatSurg, 1987; 22: 522). They belong to Kasai's type III, which represents non-correctable biliary atresia—absence or atresia of common, hepatic, and cystic ducts. There are no cystically dilated hilar ducts that can be used for anastomosis in these patients. The presence of a peculiar prehilar fibrous cone can often be seen. The gallbladder is involved in the atretic process in about 80 per cent of patients.[10]

Microscopic lesions

Numerous studies have been published on the histopathology of fibrous remnants of the resected extrahepatic biliary tree (Gautier, JPediat, 1976; 89:704; Chandra, JPediat, 1978; 93:196; Gautier, ArchPathLabMed, 1981; 105:397; Kasai, p.351 in reference 1; Ohi, p. 157 in reference 11). These have focused on (i) the topography and the nature of the lesions observed in the extrahepatic ductal remnants and (ii) the correlation between the numbers and sizes of identifiable ductal structures at the porta hepatis and the success of postoperative bile flow after hepatic portoenterostomy.

Topography and types of lesions

A constant finding is complete fibrous obliteration of at least a segment of the extrahepatic biliary tree, confirming the diagnosis of extrahepatic bile duct atresia at the microscopic level. Usually, however, one segment only is reduced to a fibrous cord, and the remaining parts contain remnants of lumina and inflammatory changes in variable amounts. The histological appearances can be divided into three types (Gautier, JPediat, 1976; 89:704; Chandra,

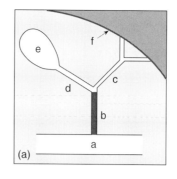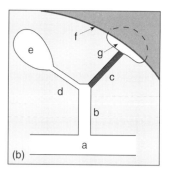
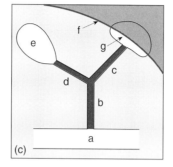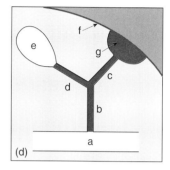

Fig. 1. Anatomical types of extrahepatic bile duct atresia according to Kasai (redrawn after Fig.1 in Witzleben, p.339 in reference 1, with permission). (a) Type I. Correctable form of atresia. The common bile duct is partially or completely occluded or reduced to a fibrous cord. (b) Type IIa. Correctable form of atresia. Obliteration of common hepatic duct; the common bile duct and cystic duct are patent, and the gallbladder is intact. There are cystically dilated bile ducts at the porta hepatis. (c) Type IIb. Correctable form of atresia. Obliteration of common, hepatic, and cystic ducts. The gallbladder is not involved. There are cystically dilated bile ducts at the porta hepatis. (d) Type III. Non-correctable form of atresia. There is obliteration of common, hepatic, and cystic ducts, and no anastomosable ducts at the porta hepatis. A prehilar fibrous cone is present. Explanation of symbols: a, duodenum; b, ductus choledochus; c, ductus hepaticus communis; d, ductus cysticus; e, gallbladder; f, liver; g, dilated ducts.

JPediat, 1978; 93:196). One histological picture (type 1 according to Gautier et al., 1976) corresponds to absence of any lumen lined by biliary epithelium (Plate 1). The bile duct segment is reduced to a fibrous cord, often with a concentric arrangement of collagen bundles and without inflammatory infiltration. A second type of appearance (type 2 according to Gautier et al., 1976) corresponds to lumina lined by epithelium. The lumina may be distributed randomly or grouped in clusters. Periluminal inflammatory cells are usually found, and signs of necrosis and sloughing of epithelial cells are often observed. Bile plugs may be present in the lumina. A third pattern (type 3 according to Gautier et al., 1976) is characterized by a central structure which unquestionably corresponds to an altered bile duct (Plate 2). In some specimens, the structure contains a loose network of connective tissue without visible epithelium. In a larger proportion of specimens, the lumen is filled either with cellular debris and macrophages containing bile, or with a biliary concrement. In other instances, the lumen appears free but narrowed by surrounding inflammatory tissue; in 75 per cent of such specimens the epithelial lining is columnar in type but lines the perimeter of the lumen only incompletely. Smaller epithelial structures may be seen at the peripheral part of the section, similar to those of type 2.

All investigators agree that the variable histological appearance reflects a dynamic process of progressive inflammatory destruction of the extrahepatic bile ducts. The early stage corresponds to periductal inflammation with necrosis and sloughing of the epithelial lining, followed by progressive periductal fibrosis and narrowing of the lumen. The endstage is a complete fibrous scar of a destroyed epithelium-lined tube which remains identifiable as a fibrous cord (Witzleben, p.28 in reference 6).

An important observation is that fibrous obliteration of the extrahepatic ducts increases with the age of the patient, in parallel with increasing fibrosis in the liver (Miyano, JPediatSurg, 1977; 12: 19). Equally interesting is the finding that epithelial necrobiosis and inflammatory infiltration may be observed distal to regions of complete obstruction, indicating that these changes are not secondary to occlusion of bile ducts (Haas, WorldJSurg, 1978; 2:561).

Correlation between number and size of bile ducts near the porta hepatis and postoperative drainage of bile

The rationale of hepatic portoenterostomy lies in establishing continuity between the bile ducts near the porta hepatis and the intestinal lumen. Theoretically, successful restoration of bile flow is expected in those patients with patent biliary structures near the porta hepatis and greatest flow in patients with the largest diameter and/or greatest numbers of such structures. Kasai et al.[9] indicated that a satisfactory postoperative flow of bile is obtained only when the diameter of the patent ducts near the porta hepatis is at least 200 μm. Suruga et al. (JPediatSurg, 1982; 17:1) concluded that duct lumens of 100 mm in diameter were sufficient for assuring adequate flow of bile. Some authors recommend intraoperative confirmation by frozen section of the presence of microscopically patent ducts at the level of anastomosis in portoenterostomy (Ohya, JPediatSurg, 1990; 25:801; Altman, p.391 in reference 1). However, in the studies mentioned above, the correlation between presence of patent ducts and postoperative flow of bile was not 100 per cent. Furthermore, other workers reported no correlation between postoperative drainage of bile and numbers or sizes of bile ducts at the porta hepatis (Gautier, JPediat, 1976; 89:704). Gautier et al. (1976) found, for example, that 6 of 13 patients with no demonstrable bile ducts at the porta hepatis developed an adequate bile flow postoperatively. In later studies, workers have applied a sophisticated computer analysis of the sizes of bile ducts to the problem (Matsuo, ZKinderchir, 1984; 39:46).

Matsukawa (ArchJpnChir, 1984; 53:47) concluded from three-dimensional histometry of bile ducts in the porta hepatis that the sites of obstruction may be located very close to the liver tissue, and that interruptions of bile duct continuity are found at any level of the fibrous, scarred tissue cone, This finding suggests a preponderant importance of the bile duct configuration high up in the porta hepatis. Finally, it was concluded (Suruga, JPediatSurg, 1985; 20: 252) that the size of the bile ducts at the porta hepatis has little influence on operative results. A recent study found that bile canalicular membrane filament accumulation has a prognostic value (Segawa, JPediatSurg, 1993; 28:851).

While refinement in recognition and measurement of bile ducts draining at the porta hepatis may be helpful for better prediction of surgical results, the occurrence of adequate bile flow in some patients without recognizable epithelial structures remains unexplained. These puzzling cases raise the question of how bile is drained in the absence of ductal continuity, and point to alternative pathways such as lymphatic drainage of bile constituents. The concept of lymphatic drainage forms the basis for some modifications of the Kasai procedure (omentopexie).[4]

Pathology of the liver and intrahepatic bile ducts in extrahepatic bile duct atresia

Classic extrahepatic bile duct atresia

Introductory remarks

There has been much discussion about the value of liver biopsy in the diagnosis of extrahepatic bile duct atresia. In more recent years the diagnostic accuracy of liver biopsy is reported to be 90 per cent, or even 95 per cent (Brough, p.381 in reference 1; Witzleben, p.28 in reference 6).[4] The improved accuracy of histopathological interpretation of liver biopsies in the diagnosis of extrahepatic bile duct atresia is due to attributing less importance to parenchymal giant cells, paying more attention to changes in the portal tracts, including interlobular bile duct damage, and above all to awareness that the histopathological changes are influenced profoundly by the age of the patient (Witzleben, p.28 in reference 6). The most important message for the histopathologist is that he is studying a snapshot of a dynamic process.

Optimal time for diagnostic liver biopsy

'Ductular reaction' is accepted as the most reliable, although not pathognomonic, criterion in diagnosing extrahepatic obstruction in liver tissue specimens (Brough, p.381 in reference 1). It should be realized that this alteration takes some time to develop. This explains why some authors recommend postponing liver biopsy until the end of the 6th postnatal week in order to assure an optimal chance for confident diagnosis of extrahepatic bile duct atresia (Vazquez-Estevez, JPediatSurg, 1989; 24:48).[4] However, our own experience and that of others[12] indicates that there is a broad variability in the extent of liver alteration and 'ductular reaction' in patients of the same age, that diagnostic histological features may be observed in some infants at a younger age than 6 weeks (e.g. 4 weeks), and that in some 'early severe' cases the lesions may be far advanced and close to biliary cirrhosis at the age of 4 to 6 weeks. Hence it appears that the optimal time for diagnostic liver biopsy depends to a large extent on clinical judgement and the experience of the paediatrician or paediatric surgeon. A liver biopsy, obtained too early in the course of the disease, may not be diagnostic, necessitating a second, later biopsy (Ferry, ClinPediat, 1985; 24:305).

Histopathological features

The 'classic' features of extrahepatic bile duct atresia comprise alterations that change in the course of the disease, allowing some chronological staging of the lesions in successive periods.[4] As emphasized before, the timing of the stages is only approximate. The earliest stage (from about 1 to 4 weeks)[4] is characterized by non-specific features of bilirubinostasis, consisting of granules of bile pigment in hepatocytes and intercellular bile plugs. A few hepatocytes may show degeneration and necrosis. Parenchymal giant cells may be seen, but usually in small numbers and without striking hydropic change. There is no inflammatory infiltration, either in the parenchyma or the portal tracts. The amount of bilirubin in Kupffer cells increases with the duration of cholestasis. Foci of extramedullary haematopoiesis may persist to a variable extent. The histopathology in this early period does not allow a firm diagnosis.

In the second stage of the disease, from about 4 to 7 weeks, [4] the portal tracts show changes characteristic of extrahepatic obstruction of the bile duct. These consist of rounding of the portal tract, oedema, dilatation of lymph vessels, and 'ductular proliferation'. Some authors also insist on the proliferation of interlobular portal ducts, recognizable by positive immunostaining for epithelial membrane antigen (Witzleben, p.28 in reference 6). The increase in ductules occurs typically at the periphery of the portal tracts—so-called marginal bile duct proliferation. The 'ductular reaction' becomes associated with an inflammatory infiltration, including lymphocytes and polymorphonuclear leucocytes. The density of the inflammatory infiltrate is variable. The ductular reaction in the periphery of the portal tracts creates an indistinct borderline between portal connective tissue and periportal parenchyma (acinar zone 1). This stage is considered diagnostic of extrahepatic bile duct atresia and explains the recommendation by some workers to postpone diagnostic liver biopsy until the 6th week of life.[4]

Equally important from a diagnostic point of view are the lesions of the portal bile ducts, which can be grouped under the heading inflammatory destruction, although this is evaluated by some as an inconsistent finding (Witzleben, p.28 in reference 6). The ducts show permeation by inflammatory cells, disruption of their basement membrane, and epithelial abnormalities including increased acidophilia, vacuolization, flattening, and shedding or necrosis of the epithelium (Plate 3). The ductal inflammatory lesions bear striking resemblance to those observed in the extrahepatic bile duct remnants, and are responsible for progressive disappearance of intrahepatic bile duct segments.

During a subsequent third stage (from 7 to 8 weeks), portal and periportal fibrosis develops associated with periportal extension of the 'ductular reaction.[4] The density of the inflammatory infiltrate may decrease and portal oedema and lymphangiectasis become less prominent. Bile concrements appear in the lumen of some of the ductular segments, which show signs of biliary reabsorption as vacuolization, lipofuscin, and bilirubin pigment and reduplication of the basement membranes on electron microscopic examination. The parenchymal changes by themselves remain non-diagnostic. The extent and topography of bilirubinostasis is variable; coarse bile plugs are scattered throughout the parenchyma and some hepatocytes show feathery degeneration: damage to liver cells and necrosis of single cells seem to depend on the degree of bile stasis. There is no appreciable intralobular inflammation. Pigmented macrophages tend to cluster in periportal regions.

In the fourth stage, after about the 10th week, the periportal fibrosis gradually extends into the surrounding parenchyma, while the density of the inflammatory infiltration tends to decrease.[4] Also, the number of ductular structures seems to decrease, and the remaining ductules often show dilatation of the lumen and bile concrements. The interlobular bile ducts display 'fibrous cholangitis', with irregular narrowing of their lumen, thickening of their basement membrane, and development of concentric periductal

fibrosis. The strangulated ducts show progressive atrophy of their epithelial lining. The progressing periportal fibrosis causes linkage of adjacent portal tracts, reaching the stage of biliary fibrosis, but not yet fully developed biliary cirrhosis.[13] The liver lesions at this time are advanced beyond the optimal stage for successful hepatic portoenterostomy, and indicate a high-risk patient with regard to successful postoperative drainage of bile. One study, however, found better prognostic indicators in parenchymal giant cell transformation and degeneration (Vazquez-Estevez, JPediatSurg, 1989; 24:48). The final (or fifth) stage (beyond 12 weeks) corresponds to further progression to secondary biliary cirrhosis, characterized by nodular regeneration of the parenchyma and perinodular septal fibrosis.[4] The diagnosis of biliary cirrhosis on diagnostic liver biopsy (the fifth stage of disease) is a contraindication for corrective surgery (Schweizer, p.88 in reference 2).[4]

Several authors have emphasized specifically the alterations that can be observed at the level of the interlobular bile ducts in the central part of the portal tracts (Bill, JPediatSurg; 1977; 12:977; Haas, WorldJSurg, 1978; 2:561; Suruga, JPediatSurg, 1992; 27:707; Ito, p.62 in 14). These changes consist of a spectrum of lesions of the lining cells of bile ducts, including intracellular vacuoles, flattening and condensation of cells with pyknotic nuclei, and necrosis of bile duct cells, as well as mitoses of these cells. Similar lesions of the lining epithelium of bile ducts were observed in larger intrahepatic ducts at the porta hepatis (Haas, 1978; Witzleben, Lab-Invest, 1978; 38:525). Consideration of the distribution of these changes in the original specimens, and their persistence after corrective surgery, indicated that they are not secondary to distal obstruction alone and that they apparently represent an intrahepatic component of the basic disease process affecting the extrahepatic ducts (Haas, 1978; Fabbretti, p.70 in reference 8). However, there is still some controversy as to the extent to which these lesions might be secondary to obstruction (Nietgen, Gastro, 1992; 102:2126; Witzleben, p.28 in reference 6; Perez-Atayde, p.60 in reference 8).

Ongoing damage to the bile ducts leads to a progressive disappearance of the interlobular bile ducts (Kasai, p.351 in reference 1; Alagille, p.233 in reference 3), also confirmed on hepatectomy specimens at the time of liver transplantation (Fabbretti, p.70 in reference 8). Extrahepatic bile duct atresia thus represents a 'disappearing bile duct disease' (Sherlock, Lancet, 1987; ii:493).[15] Absence of the interlobular bile ducts in late stages of extrahepatic bile duct atresia probably results from various causes: damage from distal extrahepatic obstruction; strangulation by progressive fibrosis; ischaemia due to compression of the peribiliary capillary plexus by portal fibrosis (International Group, Liver, 1983; 3:161); and, perhaps most importantly, from a relentless progression of the primary process of 'sclerosing cholangitis' which affects the bile ducts (Bill, ArchSurg, 1974; 109:367; Altman, JPediatSurg, 1975; 10:685; Haas, WorldJSurg, 1978; 2:561; Howard, p.167 in reference 3; Ohi, p.1 in 3; Fabbretti, p.70 in reference 8).

Lesions of the intrahepatic bile ducts can be recognized by radiographic investigation which demonstrates hypoplasia of the intrahepatic biliary tree (Lilly, PediatClinNAm, 1985; 32:1233).[12] Rare lesions which are mentioned in exceptional instances include islands of cartilage near the porta hepatis (Witzleben, p.28 in reference 6) and palisading granulomas around damaged interlobular ducts (Calder, Histopath, 1993; 23:585).

Progression of extrahepatic bile duct atresia is not only associated with disappearance of intrahepatic bile ducts; the branches of the portal vein also often appear strikingly hypoplastic in the sclerosing portal tracts (Ohuchi, JPediatSurg, 1986; 21:10). In later biopsies from patients with extrahepatic bile duct atresia, fusion between large preterminal portal tracts may be observed, resulting in enlarged fibrous areas. There is an apparent lack of the finer ramifications of portal tracts. This picture suggests a lack of continued outgrowth of terminal ramifications of the portal tracts and the vessels they contain. Such apparently stunted growth of portal tracts may be part of a retardation in growth and differentiation of intrahepatic bile ducts, and may also be responsible for the hypoplastic pattern of the portal vein (Ohuchi, 1986).

The intrahepatic lesions in untreated or unsuccessfully treated extrahepatic bile duct atresia were shown to follow a particular time course (Landing, PediatPath, 1985; 4:309). An early phase of rapid proliferation of bile ductules, peaking at 205 days, is followed by rapid regression to approximately 400 days. There is a slower progressive loss of intrahepatic ducts thereafter. The connective tissue in the portal tracts increases on a slower course and continues to increase after maximum regression of ducts is reached, indicating a dissociation between the ductular reaction and fibrosis in extrahepatic bile duct atresia. It was also found (Wells, PediatPath, 1985; 4:321) that males with extrahepatic bile duct atresia show statistically significant longer survival than females. Females show a more stormy progression with a greater degree of proliferation of ductules in the early phase (less than 200 days), and greater regression of ducts and more rapid development of fibrosis compared with males between 200 and 400 days.

Extrahepatic bile duct atresia with 'hyperplasia of intrahepatic bile ducts'

In about 20 per cent of patients with extrahepatic bile duct atresia, the damaged intrahepatic bile ducts in the liver biopsy appear as unusually shaped duct structures in excessive numbers, suggesting a congenital 'hyperplasia' of the bile ducts. Congenital hyperplasia of the intrahepatic bile ducts is described in the English literature as 'congenital hepatic fibrosis' (Kerr, QJMed, 1961; 30:91), in the German literature as 'cholangiodysplastische Pseudo-Zirrhose' (Fink, ZblAllgPath, 1955; 93:497) and 'cholangiodysplasia of the hyperplastic type',[4] and in the French literature as 'fibroangioadénomatose' (Kerneis, PressMed, 1961; 69:1406). The basic lesion of the intrahepatic bile ducts in this entity corresponds to a lack of resorption and remodelling of the excess of epithelial structure which is formed in the first embryonic stage of intrahepatic development of bile ducts, namely the so-called 'ductal plate' (Hammar, ZMikroskAnatForsch, 1926; 5:59). Lack of remodelling into mature bile ducts with persistence of the original embryonic ductal plate structure is termed the 'ductal plate malformation' (Jørgensen, ActaPMIScand, 1977; 257(Suppl):1). The bile ducts appear hyperplastic in this condition.

The ductal plate malformation constitutes a basic lesion of congenital hepatic fibrosis, infantile polycystic disease, von Meyenburg complexes, Ivemark syndrome, Meckel syndrome, and Caroli's disease (Desmet, SemLivDis, 1987; 7:67; Desmet, Hepatol, 1992; 16:1069).

However, ductal plate malformation of the intrahepatic bile ducts may also be associated with extrahepatic bile duct atresia

(Plate 4) (Raweily, Histopath, 1990; 17:521; Desmet, Hepatol, 1992; 16:1069; Woolf, SemLivDis, 1993; 13:261; Terracciano, VerDschGesPath, 1995; 79:297; Desmet, p.27 in reference 8). In the German literature this was described as 'association between extrahepatic bile duct atresia and cholangiodysplasia of the hyperplastic type' (so-called 'cholangiodysplastische Pseudozirrhose') in 7 of 69 patients with extrahepatic bile duct atresia.[4] The histological picture of preoperative liver biopsies showed a combination of 'intrahepatic bile duct hyperplasia' (ductal plate malformation) together with the typical features of extrahepatic bile duct atresia: oedema, inflammatory infiltrate, and marginal ductular proliferation. Similar patterns were observed at the time of Kasai operation in 10 patients out of a series of 41 patients (Desmet, p.27 in reference 8).[7] The age of these 10 patients at the time of surgical intervention ranged from 30 to 70 days. In all cases, even in the youngest at 4 weeks of age, histology revealed already advanced biliary fibrosis, with serpiginous fibrous bands connecting portal tracts. These patients thus can be considered 'early severe' cases. The original portal tracts are enlarged and characterized by excess numbers of branches of the hepatic artery and a relatively small size of the portal vein(s). The portal bile ducts display a peculiar pattern, of curved segments of variable length surrounding the portal vessels, assuming the basic configuration of an embryonic ductal plate (Plate 4). In several instances, the portal vessels are surrounded by two and even three concentric structures, corresponding to interrupted and partially remodelled ductal plates. This observation suggests that repetitive formation of ductal plates may occur in successive waves during the first few weeks of life in patients with early severe extrahepatic bile duct atresia. Concentric ductal plates may represent an embryonic type of 'ductular reaction', recognized as ductal 'hyperplasia'. Several enlarged portal areas apparently correspond to fused clusters of smaller portal tracts since multiple aggregates of complex ductal plates surrounding arterial sprouts may be observed in the same large mesenchymal area. Apparently, such histological features result from sectioning through abnormally branching portal tracts: instead of growing by regular tree-like branching, resulting in individualized portal tracts separated by intervening parenchyma, the portal tracts give rise to multiple sprouts of smaller portal twigs which remain in close proximity. Such features may indicate a stunted growth of portal tracts, presumably due to inadequate development (hypoplasia) of the branches of the portal vein (Desmet, Hepatol, 1992; 16:1069). This finding would correlate with the observation that portal pressure is often increased at the time of corrective surgery.[16] The immature ducts with ductal plate configuration appear to be subjected to the same fate as their normal or mature counterparts in untreated or progressive extrahepatic bile duct atresia. They show variable degrees of necrobiosis of their lining cells, and become subject to progressive atrophy and fibrous obliteration.

To summarize, the 'natural course' of extrahepatic bile duct atresia is comparable in both 'classic' and 'early severe' cases. In both instances progress of the disease is accompanied by variably progressive destruction of intrahepatic segments of bile ducts, either normally-shaped, mature ducts in classic cases, or immature types of ducts with ductal plate configuration in the early severe cases. Reduplication of ductal plates, followed by variable destruction of ducts, results in a varying degree of 'ductal hyperplasia' and resemblance to the pattern of congenital hepatic fibrosis. It is possible that the ductal patterns peculiar to early severe cases are responsible for the later development of a congenital hepatic fibrosis-like pattern (Desmet, Histopath, 1992; 20:465). The histological features and clinical course of early severe forms of extrahepatic bile duct atresia strongly support the concept of an antenatal start to the basic disease process of this condition, which apparently interferes with the normal maturation and remodelling of the embryonic ductal plates and with the normal development of portal vein branches.

Aetiology and pathogenesis of extrahepatic bile duct atresia

Pathogenesis

Extrahepatic bile duct atresia has been considered to be a congenital anomaly due to failure of recanalization of the bile duct, which was thought to be occluded by proliferated epithelial cells early in fetal life (Ylppö, ZKinderheilk, 1913; 9:319). The other prevailing concept has been that this condition represents a progressive destruction of developed extrahepatic and even intrahepatic bile ducts by an inflammatory process of unspecified nature. Landing (ProgPediatSurg, 1974; 6:113) proposed the concept of 'infantile obstructive cholangiopathy', based on the histopathological similarity of the liver lesions in patients with neonatal hepatitis, extrahepatic bile duct atresia, and choledochal cyst. According to this concept, extrahepatic bile duct atresia is the result of a cholangiopathic process which starts in postnatal life in most cases. The cholangiopathy is due to an inflammatory process, which affects and destroys the liver parenchymal cells as well as the bile duct epithelium, the latter resulting in obliteration of the bile duct lumina. According to the predominance of parenchymal or ductal lesions, the disease corresponds to either neonatal hepatitis or extrahepatic bile duct atresia.

Schweizer and Müller[4] presented a new theory on the pathogenesis of extrahepatic bile duct atresia, which takes into account most of the observed facts and available information. They propose to distinguish between two types of extrahepatic bile duct atresia, a fetal/embryonic form and a prenatal-, perinatal-, or postnatal-acquired form of the disease.

The fetal/embryonic form is characterized clinically by an early onset of jaundice. Without a jaundice-free interval, the physiological jaundice of the newborn child turns into a pathological, conjugated hyperbilirubinaemia in the 2nd or 3rd week of life. An analysis of the clinical records of 342 children with extrahepatic bile duct atresia from 10 hospitals indicates that this type of clinical course is observed in 34 per cent of patients.[4] This type of the disease is characterized morphologically by complete absence of epithelial bile duct remnants in the hepatoduodenal ligament. In their own patients of this type, Schweizer and Müller[4] found associated malformations of malrotation in all four patients and ectopic pancreas in the hepatoduodenal ligament in one. This group of findings was taken as evidence that the atresia of bile ducts started in the embryonic or fetal period. The bile duct was missing at the time of birth either because it had not been formed or because it became obliterated completely in the embryonic or fetal period. These patients have a bad prognosis. Postoperative bile flow was not achieved after hepatoportoenterostomy in any of them.

The prenatal, perinatal, or postnatal form of extrahepatic bile duct atresia is characterized clinically by a shorter or longer jaundice-free period following the physiological jaundice of the newborn child. As a rule, the pathological jaundice develops after a latent period in the 3rd to 5th week of life. From a study of 342 children with extrahepatic bile duct atresia observed in 10 different hospitals it appeared that 66 per cent had had a jaundice-free period with a mean duration of 6 days.[4] Bile duct remnants were demonstrated regularly in the hepatoduodenal ligament of these patients, in the form of segments with epithelium-lined lumina or epithelial clusters. In none of the patients with this form of extrahepatic bile duct atresia could associated malformations be demonstrated. The range of findings in this group suggests that the bile duct was present at birth, but that subsequently it became obliterated, as an acquired disease. The prognosis in these children is better than for the former type. Adequate postoperative flow of bile was achieved in 12 of 16 of these patients.

Aetiology

The aetiology of extrahepatic bile duct atresia remains unknown. Two main possibilities are usually considered: (i) a congenital structural anomaly, or (ii) an inflammatory sclerosing acquired lesion.[4]

Observations in favour of a congenital structural anomaly or malformation are: the association of extrahepatic bile duct atresia with other congenital anomalies in about 20 per cent of cases (Silveira, ActaPaedScand, 1991; 80:1192), including the biliary atresia–splenic malformation syndrome in about half of these patients (Karrer, JPediatSurg, 1991; 26:524; Davenport, p.11 in reference 8); the rare, but occasional, occurrence of extrahepatic bile duct atresia in fetuses and stillborns;[17] and the occurrence of ductal plate malformation of intrahepatic bile ducts in a variable percentage (Raweily, Histopath, 1990; 17:521; Terracciano, VerDschGesPath, 1995; 79:297; Callea, p.304 in reference 14) of patients.

The biliary atresia–splenic malformation syndrome is thought to be caused by a prenatal insult to the embryo at approximately the 5th week of gestation (Karrer, JPediatSurg, 1991; 26:524; Davenport, p.11 in reference 8). Concordance between ductal plate malformation of interlobular bile ducts and other associated congenital abnormalities could not be established until recently (Witzleben, p.28 in reference 6). In any case, extrahepatic bile duct atresia as a congenital malformation does not correspond to a static abnormality, in view of the progressive and sclerosing nature of the lesions. A novel type of analysis of segregation patterns of the anomalies in individual patients suggested the existence of two major groups: one with various combinations of anomalies within the laterality sequence, and another in which the anomalies did not follow any recognizable pattern (Carmi, AmJMedGen, 1993; 45:683). Such congenital forms could conceivably arise through a malformation, a disruption, or a chromosome abnormality (Silveira, ActaPaedScand, 1991; 80:1192).

Such observations support the hypothesis that extrahepatic bile duct atresia is an aetiopathogenetically heterogeneous entity. The majority of cases have no associated congenital anomalies and presumably are caused by factors acting after organogenesis is complete. Whether these act late in gestation, at birth, or postnatally is unknown (Silveira, ActaPaedScand, 1991; 80:1192; Balistreri, p.293 in reference 8).

The influence of genetic factors in this condition is likely to be indirect, possibly in the form of increased susceptibility of the biliary epithelium to infectious or toxic agents (Silveira, BrazJMedBiolRes, 1991; 24:67). The inflammatory destruction of the bile ducts could be of infectious, ischaemic, or toxic origin.

Infectious aetiology

From the beginning of this century (Rolleston, BMJ, 1901; i:758), it has been suggested that extrahepatic bile duct atresia is the result of an infectious hepàtitis resulting in destructive cholangitis. Infectious agents, which are considered possible aetiological agents in extrahepatic bile duct atresia include cytomegalovirus, herpes simplex, hepatitis viruses A, B, and C, group A and C rotaviruses, and reovirus type 3.[7] Although an infectious aetiology remains unproven, the debate has been reopened as the result of several case reports (Guerra Aguirre, AnnEspPaediat, 1989; 30:91; Le Luyer, ArchFrancPediat, 1990; 47:361; Hart, AmJDisChild, 1991; 145:302; Parashar, JPediatSurg, 1992; 27:843; Riepenhoff-Talty, PediatRes, 1992; 31:115A; Riepenhoff-Talty, PediatRes, 1993; 33:394; Tanaka, ActaPathJpn, 1993; 43:360; Iwami, p.7 in reference 8; Sasaki, p.3 in reference 8).

Ischaemic aetiology

It has been proposed (Gautier, ArchFrancPediat, 1979; 36:3) that extrahepatic bile duct atresia could be related to insufficient vascularization of the biliary tree (Ho, JPediatGastrNutr, 1993; 16:53). Fibrous obliteration of the common duct could be produced experimentally by inducing ischaemia of bile ducts (Schweizer, ZKinderchir, 1974; 15:90). Definite proof for an ischaemic origin in human extrahepatic bile duct atresia, however, is lacking.

Exogeneous toxic origin

No aetiological link could be demonstrated with teratogenic drugs or ionizing radiation (Howard, BrJSurg, 1983; 70:193). Some epidemiological studies on extrahepatic bile duct atresia have revealed a time–space clustering compatible with an exogeneous toxic origin of the disease (Strickland, JPediat, 1985; 100:749). Epidemiological studies in lambs and calves in South Wales, Australia, further support the environmental theory of the aetiology of extrahepatic bile duct atresia (Harper, AustVetJ, 1990; 67:18).

Endogeneous toxic origin

An irritation of the bile passages by pathological bile salts has been proposed (Harris, AmJDisChild, 1960; 100:783). A remarkable case report mentions a neonate with an ectopic liver in the umbilicus in conjunction with extrahepatic bile duct atresia in the liver proper and an ectopic pancreas in the jejunum; the pathological features of the ectopic liver and the liver were quite similar (Park, JPediatSurg, 1991; 26:219). It is of interest that unusual bile acids have been demonstrated in the fetus and newborn infant, as compared with adults, and that the number of bile acids in fetuses and newborn infants is close to 40, rather than the 4 of adults (Suchy, SemLivDis, 1987; 7:77). Sophisticated technology now enables us to recognize defective bile acid metabolism in enigmatic and hitherto unexplained liver diseases such as idiopathic neonatal hepatitis (Balistreri, JInherMetDis, 1991; 14:459). Abnormal 27-carbon bile

acids have been shown to accumulate in the bile, serum, and urine of children with paucity of intrahepatic bile ducts (Hanson, JCI, 1975; 56:577). Unusual bile acids, including large amounts of 3β-hydroxy-cholenoic acid, were detected in the sera of children with Alagille's syndrome (Hernanz, CCActa, 1985; 145:289) and fetal type bile acids accumulate in the serum in extrahepatic bile duct atresia (Hata, p.182 in reference 8). Biliary injury resembling that observed in extrahepatic bile duct atresia has been reproduced by administration of certain bile acids (lithocholic acid, chenodeoxycholic acid) to newborn animals or to their mothers in late pregnancy (Jenner, AnnRCSurg, 1978; 60:367).

The concept that damage and involution of the bile ducts may be due to some abnormal intermediate or unusual pathway of bile acid metabolism is worth further consideration.

Reflux of pancreatic juice in the biliary tree

A further possible cause of extrahepatic bile duct atresia is reflux of pancreatic juice into the bile duct system. This could be favoured by abnormal anatomical relationships between the common bile duct and the pancreatic duct in the region of the ampulla of Vater (Suda, ActaPathJpn, 1980; 30:187).

Angiofibromatosis

Histological examination of fibrous remnants of extrahepatic bile ducts and fibrous plaques near the porta hepatis often reveals impressive numbers of blood vessels, giving the impression of an angiofibromatosis (Gautier, ArchPathLabMed, 1981; 105:397). The suggestion has been made that these vascular anomalies might be related causally to extrahepatic bile duct atresia.[4]

Experimental extrahepatic bile duct atresia

Experimental induction of extrahepatic bile duct atresia has been attempted by several means. Induction of ischaemia of the bile ducts in fetal animals has been discussed above. Another hypothesis holds that some cases of biliary atresia and neonatal hepatitis are initiated by an adverse effect of unsaturated monohydroxy bile acids on the fetal and infantile hepatobiliary system. Intravenous injection of lithocholic acid into preterm rabbits produced obstruction within the biliary tract in a minority of newborn rabbits (Jenner, AnnRCSurg, 1978; 60:367).

Intra-abdominal infusion of L-proline in adult mice led to bile duct enlargement; this finding led the authors to suggest that bile duct hypoplasia and atresia may result from a defect in proline metabolism, and that proline administration might possibly be therapeutic during the early phase of extrahepatic bile duct atresia (Vacanti, JPediatSurg, 1979; 14:814). However, injection of proline in pregnant mice did not cause proliferation of bile duct epithelium in newborn mice (Schier, JPediatSurg, 1989; 24:267).

Chemicals used to induce lesions which resemble extrahepatic bile duct atresia include 1,4-phenylene di-isothiocyanate (Ogawa, JPediatSurg, 1983; 18:131), 4,4′-diaminodiphenylmethane (Bourdelat, BullAssAnat, 1983; 67:375), and phorbol meristate acetate (Schmeling, AnnSurg, 1991; 213:350; Schmeling, p.15 in reference 6).

A number of investigators have studied the physiological involution and atresia of the bile ducts in the lamprey during metamorphosis as an animal model of human extrahepatic bile duct atresia (Sidon, JMorphol, 1983; 177:109). The most interesting aspects of this work concern the mechanism of bile duct involution and the adaptation of the liver and the organism to survival without a draining biliary system. An analogous problem of ductless livers is encountered in syndromatic paucity of intrahepatic bile ducts (Alagille's syndrome) and in several long-term survivors of hepatic portoenterostomy.

Clinical features—diagnostic work-up

The goals of diagnostic investigation in infants with protracted hyperbilirubinaemia are to identify specific treatable entities and to define those who may benefit from surgical treatment. Prompt identification of cholestasis is imperative because this condition is never benign, unlike unconjugated hyperbilirubinaemia (Balistreri, JPediat, 1985; 106:171; Mowat, p.14 in reference 2).

Clinical features

Unfortunately, there is no pathognomonic clinical symptom of extrahepatic biliary atresia, since intrahepatic and extrahepatic forms of cholestasis share numerous clinical and biochemical features. Nevertheless, clinical features may aid in the discrimination between extrahepatic bile duct atresia and the numerous other causes of cholestasis in early childhood.

Extrahepatic bile duct atresia occurs more frequently in girls, usually with normal birthweight, whereas 'neonatal hepatitis' appears to be more common in boys (up to 70 per cent). Familial cases are rare in extrahepatic bile duct atresia, whereas a familial incidence is noted in 15 to 20 per cent of patients with neonatal hepatitis. Associated polysplenia syndrome also suggests extrahepatic bile duct atresia (Karrer, JPediatSurg, 1991; 26:524; Davenport, p.11 in reference 8).

In extrahepatic bile duct atresia the stools are consistently acholic, whereas incompletely or intermittently decoloured stools indicate incomplete cholestasis of the intrahepatic type. However, intrahepatic cholestasis may also be severe and complete, causing total absence of bile pigment in stools. In neonatal hepatitis, pathological jaundice follows the physiological hyperbilirubinaemia without interval, and is observed already in the 2nd week of life. In extrahepatic bile duct atresia, neonatal physiological jaundice also persists in 34 per cent of cases; in contrast, in 66 per cent of patients, an intercalated jaundice-free period of about 2 weeks occurs between physiological jaundice and the appearance of pathological icterus.[4] Hepatomegaly is often palpable in the 1st or 2nd week in neonatal hepatitis, whereas liver enlargement usually becomes detectable in extrahepatic bile duct atresia in the 3rd or 4th week of life. In view of the importance of an early diagnosis (Hussein, ArchDisChild, 1991; 66:1177), liver disease should be suspected in any infant jaundiced after 14 days of age (Mieli-Vergani, Lancet, 1989; i: 421; Maller, p.45 in 6). Simple visual stool inspection remains an important diagnostic screening test (Brown, SAMedJ, 1990; 77: 358).

Pathological jaundice (indicating cholestasis) should be considered present in a patient with hyperbilirubinaemia if the conjugated (direct-reacting) fraction comprises more than approximately 20 per cent of the total (Balistreri, JPediat, 1985; 106: 171). In extrahepatic bile duct atresia, direct-reacting bilirubinaemia shows a more progressive rise than in neonatal hepatitis. Serum

enzymes are not very helpful in discrimination. In the first 3 months of life, neonatal hepatitis may cause higher elevations of serum aspartate aminotransferase and alanine aminotransferase, whereas γ-glutamyl transferase is more abnormal in extrahepatic bile duct atresia (Vajaradul, JMedAssThai, 1989; 72:395; Maggiore, JPediatGastrNutr, 1991; 12:21).

Different scoring systems based on clinical and laboratory data have been developed in attempts to achieve better differentiation of extrahepatic bile duct atresia from neonatal hepatitis (Sakurai, p.293 in reference 11). According to Alagille, clinical features and laboratory data allow a differentiation between extrahepatic bile duct atresia and neonatal hepatitis in 83 per cent of cases before the age of 3 months.[18] The following features occur significantly more frequently in infants with neonatal hepatitis than in those with extrahepatic bile duct atresia: male gender (66 compared with 45 per cent); low birth weight (mean 2680 compared with 3230 g); the presence of other congenital anomalies (32 compared with 17 per cent); the onset of jaundice (mean 23 compared with 11 days of age); the onset of acholic stools (mean 30 compared with 16 days); white stools during the first 10 days after admission (26 compared with 79 per cent); and enlarged liver with a firm or hard consistency (53 compared with 87 per cent). Other studies have confirmed the helpful discriminating value of clinical symptoms.[4]

Further investigation of the infant with protracted conjugated hyperbilirubinaemia

Further investigations in the diagnostic work-up for differentiating extrahepatic from intrahepatic cholestasis fall in two general categories: those that measure hepatobiliary secretion, providing information about the patency of the biliary system, and those that attempt to establish a definite diagnosis. A series of additional investigations has been introduced for differentiating extrahepatic from intrahepatic cholestasis, and hence for checking the patency of extrahepatic bile ducts. The discriminating value of such tests was recently evaluated (Maller, p.45 in reference 6; Sunaryo, p.11 in reference 19). There is a consensus that usually a single diagnostic criterion is insufficient to distinguish the various causes of neonatal jaundice (Burton, SouthMedJ, 1990; 83:294; Maller, p.45 in reference 6).

Discriminating tests include: determination of serum α-fetoprotein values; serum values of bile acids; lipoprotein X determination, before and after stimulation of bile flow with cholestyramine; vitamin E and riboflavin absorption tests; duodenal intubation for bilirubin content and bile acid profiles, eventually repeated after injection of cholecystokinin; endoscopic retrograde cholangiopancreatography (**ERCP**); percutaneous transhepatic cholangiography; laparoscopy; determination of excreted radiolabelled (^{131}I) rose bengal; hepatobiliary scintigraphy; ultrasonography; and liver histology (Ikeda, EurJPed, 1989; 148:396; Hsu, JFormosanMedAss, 1991; 90:487; Shirai, AmJGastr, 1993; 88: 536; Sunaryo, p.11 in reference 19).[7]

The most valuable investigations appear to be hepatobiliary scintigraphy when performed under appropriate conditions (Spivak, JPediat, 1987; 110:855) or in combination with the 'string test' (for evidence of radioactive tracer on a swallowed string following radionuclide administration) (Maller, p.45 in reference 6), ultrasonography (since it permits rapid detection of a choledochal cyst

Table 1 Staged evaluation of the infant with suspected cholestasis

1. Clinical evaluation (history, physical examination)
2. Fractionated serum bilirubin or serum bile acid determination
3. Stool colour
4. Index of hepatic synthetic function (prothrombin time)
5. Viral and bacterial cultures (blood, urine, spinal fluid)
6. Viral serology (HBsAg, TORCH) and VDRL titres
7. α_1-Antitrypsin phenotype
8. Thyroxine and thyroid-stimulating hormone
9. Sweat chloride
10. Metabolic screen (urine or serum amino acids, urine-reducing substances)
11. Ultrasonography
12. Hepatobiliary scintigraphy or duodenal incubation for bilirubin content
13. Liver biopsy

Taken from Balistreri WF. SemLivDis, 1987; 7(2), with permission.

and allows identification of associated abnormalities which have an impact on surgical procedures) (Abramson, Radiol, 1987; 163:377), and liver biopsy, because it may provide the most reliable evidence for extrahepatic bile duct atresia (Balistreri, JPediat, 1985; 106: 171; Ridaura Sanz, RevInvestClin, 1992; 44:193; Brough, p.381 in reference 1).[18,20] With further development of instruments specifically designed for paediatric use, ERCP has gained broader applicability (Shirai, AmJGastr, 1993; 88:536).

Diagnostic work-up

The first goal in the management of the newborn infant with jaundice is prompt identification of cholestasis and early differentiation from physiological jaundice induced by breast milk. The next goal is early recognition of specific, treatable, primary causes of cholestasis (Balistreri, JPediat, 1985; 106:171). The need for early surgical correction in patients with extrahepatic bile duct atresia leaves the paediatrician with only a short period for diagnostic evaluation.

The clinical findings usually allow the experienced paediatrician or surgeon to recognize extrahepatic bile duct atresia in a number of patients.[18] A series of additional investigations serve to confirm the diagnosis and/or to identify other causes of neonatal cholestasis (Maller, p.45 in reference 6). Table 1 is an example of a recommended staged evaluation of the infant with suspected cholestasis (Balistreri, SemLivDis, 1987; 7:61). Similar diagnostic protocols have been published by other authors (Altmann, Pediat-Ann, 1985; 14:481; Ferry, ClinPediat, 1985; 24:305). Whichever plan of investigation is chosen, the emphasis must be on early diagnosis, as surgical results are related to the age of the infant at operation (Schweizer, p.88 in reference 2).

Treatment of extrahepatic bile duct atresia

The prognosis of untreated extrahepatic bile duct atresia is very poor. Adelman (JPediatSurg, 1978; 13:389) performed a baseline study for comparison with the results of hepatic portoenterostomy. The rate of apparent cure was 1.1 per cent. The average age at death was 12 months (ranging from 2 months to 4 years); the mean age was 10 months. These findings correlate with other reports,

defining the lifespan of patients with extrahepatic bile duct atresia without corrective surgery as between 1 and 2 years (Schweizer, MonatsschrKinderheilkd, 1992; 140:422).

Hepatic portoenterostomy

Numerous operative techniques have been applied in order to re-establish drainage of bile in 'uncorrectable' types of extrahepatic bile duct atresia.[4] As discussed above, the hepatic portoenterostomy or Kasai procedure revolutionized the treatment of this disease (Kasai, JPediatSurg, 1968; 3:665). The rationale of hepatic porto-enterostomy is the presence of patent ducts at the porta hepatis, at least in the early stages of extrahepatic bile duct atresia. A transection is made in the parenchyma above the fibrous cone of obliterated proximal ducts, and the exposed area of crude liver surface is anastomosed to the intestine (Fig. 2). Healing of the portoenterostomy is complete in about 6 weeks (Takemoto, JPediat-Surg, 1989; 24:271). Kasai's unorthodox approach was initially met with scepticism by surgeons and paediatricians but has nevertheless acquired broad application. It was recognized at an international meeting in 1977[1] as the standard procedure for treatment of extrahepatic bile duct atresia, and was even recommended later for so-called 'correctable' extrahepatic bile duct atresia (Lilly, JPediatSurg, 1987; 22:522).

One of the common and sometimes fatal complications in patients with successful portoenterostomy and adequate drainage of bile is recurrent cholangitis, especially in the first 2 years after operation, with a reported incidence of about 50 to 92 per cent (Howard, BrJSurg, 1983; 70:193; Gottrand, AmJDisChild, 1991; 145:213; Karrer, p.73 in reference 6; Ohi, p.125 in reference 14). The aetiology and pathogenesis of postoperative cholangitis is not entirely clear. It is thought to be due to reflux towards the porta hepatis of intestinal contents from the draining intestinal loop. This has led to several modifications of the original Kasai procedure with construction of external venting conduits. A full discussion of the technical aspects of the various surgical procedures is beyond the scope of this chapter. The most frequently applied techniques (Fig. 2) are the Kasai I, the Kasai II,[9] Suruga I, and Suruga II (Suruga, JPediatSurg, 1981; 16:621) procedures, and the use of a cutaneous double-barrelled enterostomy constructed by the Mikulicz technique (Lilly, WorldJSurg, 1978; 2:581). The usefulness of external diversion of bile for preventing the development of cholangitis after portoenterostomy has been a matter of debate (Burnweit, JPediatSurg, 1986; 21:1143). On the other hand, in the belief that postoperative cholangitis is not of ascending origin, some surgeons recommend lymphatic drainage by omentopexy (Hirsig, JPediatSurg, 1979; 14:142).

Specific modifications of the Kasai operation include the use of microsurgery, extended dissection into the porta hepatis, and use of an intussuscepted ileocolic conduit or special techniques for revision of the portoenterostomy in case of inadequate bile flow.[7] Recently, there has been a return to the original Kasai procedure in order to avoid complicating the technical performance of liver transplantation at a later date in case of failure of the portoenterostomy (Shim, JPediatSurg, 1985; 20:689).

Hepatic portocholecystostomy (Fig. 2) is the method of choice in approximately 25 per cent of patients with obstruction of the common hepatic duct but with patent cystic duct, gallbladder, and

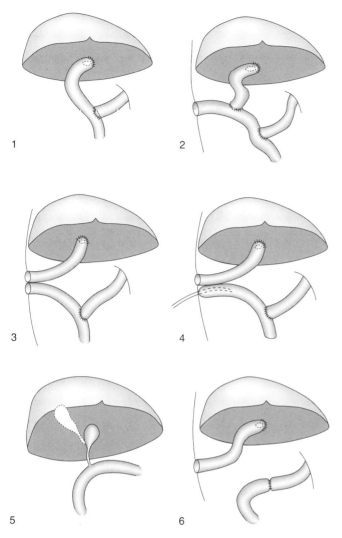

Fig. 2. The most common surgical procedures used for extrahepatic bile duct atresia. 1. Kasai I: the original hepatic portoenterostomy. 2. Kasai II: double Roux-en-Y hepatic portoenterostomy. 3. Suruga I: double-barrelled hepatic portoenterostomy. 4. Suruga II: refinement of Suruga I procedure, to include subcutaneous enterostomy for the distal jejunal limb with the insertion of a jejunal tube. 5. Sawaguchi: hepatic portojejunostomy with external stoma (requires stay in hospital until second operation, substitution of fluid and electrolytes, and reinfusion of bile through gastric intubation). 6. Hepatic portocholecystostomy. (From reference 7 with permission.)

common bile duct. This type of anastomosis, using 'biliary' conduits for re-establishing continuity, has the advantage of preventing the complications of cholangitis (Matory, SGO, 1985; 161:541). The important factors contributing to optimal operative results are: (i) an early operation, preferably within 60 days after birth; (ii) a precise dissection and adequate transection of the porta hepatis; (iii) prevention of postoperative cholangitis; (iv) absence of significant numerical and morphological alterations of the intrahepatic bile ducts; and (v) the experience of the surgeon (Schweizer, p.88 in reference 2). When the operation is carried out before 60 days of age, excretion of bile is obtained in 82 per cent of patients. The ability to achieve good postoperative bile flow decreases with advancing age. Active bile flow is obtained in only 40 per cent of

patients who are older than 90 days at the time of surgery (Kasai, p.79 in reference 19). A large series of reports has been published on the postoperative complications and their treatment, and the overall long-term results (Grosfeld, Surgery, 1989; 106:692; Laurent, Gastro, 1990; 99:1793; Chiba, EurJPaediatSurg, 1992; 2:22; Miyano, WorldJSurg, 1993; 17:332, Caccia, p.246 in reference 8; Miyano, p.87 in reference 8; Callea, p.304 in reference 14).[7]

Over the years, the results of portoenterostomy have gradually improved. It was estimated on the basis of the operative results that about 65 per cent of patients with extrahepatic bile duct atresia can be 'cured' if an adequate corrective operation is carried out before 60 days of age and postoperative cholangitis is prevented (Schweizer, p.88 in reference 2).

Although hepatic portoenterostomy has improved the outcome of patients with extrahepatic bile duct atresia, it has created a population with unique health problems, including recurrent cholangitis, nutritional and growth deficiencies, delayed development, portal hypertension, osteomalacia and osteoporosis, and social and psychiatric difficulties (Barkin, JPediat, 1980; 96:1015). These complications usually respond to aggressive medical therapy and support, which have been detailed in recent reviews (Balistreri, JPediat, 1985; 106:171; Maller, p.45 in reference 6; Balistreri, p.167 in reference 8). The indocyanine green test has been advocated as a reliable indicator of postoperative liver function in extrahepatic bile duct atresia (Kubota, JPediatGastrNutr, 1993; 16:61; Kubota, p.215 in reference 8). However, even successful portoenterostomy is not tantamount to cure (Ryckman, SemLivDis, 1987; 7:134; Grosfeld, Surgery, 1989; 106:692; Alagille, p.233 in reference 3). It appears particularly difficult to determine fully and accurately the ultimate outcome in patients with extrahepatic bile duct atresia because the short- or mid-term cure does not clearly reflect the eventual prognosis of the disease. Perhaps the most disappointing aspect of hepatic portoenterostomy is the failure of resolution of hepatic parenchymal disease in many patients. It is the exceptional patient who shows histological improvement after operation.[4,12] Even in patients with 'correctable' extrahepatic bile duct atresia, that is, with patency of the proximal extrahepatic bile ducts, there is a mortality of 14.6 per cent, although the initial rate of success in establishing drainage of bile is 100 per cent. Thus re-establishment of bile flow does not equate with cure in this disease.

Thirty years have passed since the pioneer period of hepatic portoenterostomy. The following considerations about the usefulness of this type of surgical treatment for extrahepatic bile duct atresia can be made. There is no doubt that some patients with this disease are cured by hepatic portoenterostomy. Kasai's patient with the longest survival is over 37 years of age and is well; four of his patients are married, and two have healthy children (Karrer, p.73 in reference 6). Similar successful results have been published in occasional reports (Raffensperger, JPediatSurg, 1991; 26:176; McMichens, ObsGyn, 1992; 80:492).

Complete clearing of jaundice after surgery is seen in 30 to 60 per cent of children (Karrer, p.73 in reference 6). The 5-year survival ranges from 29 to 66 per cent, with a reported jaundice-free state in 30 to 66 per cent (Karrer, p.73 in reference 6). The 10-year survival in three reported series ranges between 16 and 30 per cent. However, after a 10-year follow-up, only a minority of patients—7.8 per cent (Miyano, WorldJSurg, 1993; 17:332) to 9 per cent (Laurent, Gastro, 1990; 99:1793)—is really cured, free of jaundice and portal hypertension.

Even when bile drainage with the portoenterostomy procedure is achieved, many infants follow a clinical course punctuated by bouts of cholangitis, multiple admissions to hospital for antibiotic therapy or the management of episodic variceal bleeding, progressive cirrhosis, nutritional failure, and delay in development (Knisely, AnnClinLabSci, 1990; 20:113; Hoffman, p.81 in reference 6).

Finally, an important consideration is that the portoenterostomy procedure has entered a static phase with little in the way of technical innovation to be anticipated. It is therefore unlikely to undergo significant improvement (Hoffman, p.81 in reference 6).

Portoenterostomy and liver transplantation

Because of its increasing applicability and success, liver transplantation (Beath, BMJ, 1993; 307:825; Kalayoglu, Surgery, 1993; 114:711) represents a new treatment strategy for the infant with extrahepatic bile duct atresia. In view of the short-term and long-term complications of portoenterostomy, this creates a dilemma about the treatment of choice.

Successful liver transplantation theoretically represents a more complete treatment of extrahepatic bile duct atresia, since it not only assures re-establishment of bilioenteric continuity but also replaces a diseased organ with a healthy one. Until recently, donor organ availability represented a serious logistic problem (Gordon, ClinTranspl, 1991:105). In recent years, the shortage of donor organs has been considerably alleviated by the introduction of reduced-size orthotopic liver engraftment (Bismuth, Surgery, 1984; 95:367; Langnas, Transpl, 1992; 53:387), split-liver engraftment procedures (Bismuth, BrJSurg, 1989; 76:722; Otte, Surgery, 1990; 6:605; Houssin, BrJSurg, 1993; 80:75), and use of living-related partial liver grafts (Broelsch, AnnSurg, 1991; 214:428; Tanaka, p.277 in reference 8). However, it should also be stated that in many respects liver transplantation exchanges one disease (extrahepatic bile duct atresia) for another (the post-transplant immunocompromised state). Multiple hospital stays, particularly in the early period after the initial hospital discharge, are the rule.

There has been a growing consensus that a unified approach to the management of extrahepatic bile duct atresia should be aimed at. It is recognized that both individual treatment strategies comprise imperfect management solutions, and that the complementary and sequential utilization of both methods is necessary (Hoffman, p.81 in reference 6). This attitude has been advocated in several studies (Kasai, JPediatSurg, 1989; 24:851; Wood, JPediatSurg, 1990; 25:153; Martinez-Ibanez, JPediatSurg, 1992; 27:830; Ryckman, JPediatSurg, 1993; 28:382; Hoffman, p.81 in reference 6; Ryckman, p.271 in reference 8; Vacanti, p.229 in reference 8)[21] and is discussed in a particularly thoughtful manner by Pearl (p.62 in reference 6) and Hoffman (p.81 in reference 6) in a recent authoritative monograph on extrahepatic bile duct atresia. In this comprehensive approach, the fundamental precept in the care of the infant with extrahepatic bile duct atresia remains early diagnosis with timely surgical referral and intervention.

Portoenterostomy should be performed before 12 weeks of age. Liver transplantation should be considered for the infant who presents beyond this time limit, particularly in the setting of advanced cirrhosis (Kasai, JPediatSurg, 1989; 24:851).

In view of a possible future liver transplantation, the portoenterostomy procedure should be as simple and tissue-conserving as possible: a simple retrocolic Roux-en-Y portoenterostomy is an appropriate procedure if deemed necessary with an antireflux valve in the Roux limb. Complex variations on the Kasai procedure, the addition of cutaneous venting stomas, and revision portoenterostomies should be avoided, as they amplify the complexity and morbidity of the liver transplant procedure. After portoenterostomy, the child should be followed closely. When signs of failure in bile drainage arise, children should be referred promptly to a liver transplant centre while their hepatic reserve and nutritional status is still adequate. Paediatric liver transplant centres also have an obligation within this sequence: the development of a programme of reduced-size liver engraftment is highly desirable in view of the paucity of suitable whole-organs for transplantation into small recipients. Late referral of the infant for primary portoenterostomy as well as death of the child with failed portoenterostomy on a pretransplant waiting list represent missed opportunities (Hoffman, p.81 in reference 6).

In this comprehensive and sequential approach, the Kasai procedure is viewed as a staging operation, which provides a cure for some and a bridge to liver transplantation for the majority (Pearl, p.62 in reference 6). As such, liver transplantation does not merely represent a therapeutic 'safety net' for rescuing the child with a failed portoenterostomy, but instead is calculated in from the beginning.

Liver alterations after hepatic portoenterostomy

Most reports on long-term follow-up mention some abnormalities in liver enzymes and serum bile salt levels, hepatomegaly, splenomegaly, and often portal hypertension, occasionally with severe bleeding from oesophageal varices (Howard, BrJSurg, 1983; 70:193; Alagille, Hepatol, 1984; 4:7S; Gautier, JPediatSurg, 1984; 19:263; Ohi, JPediatSurg, 1986; 21:271; Ryckman, SemLivDis, 1987; 7:134; Alagille, p.233 in reference 3; Caccia, p.281 in reference 14; Valayer, p.105 in reference 19).[12]

The time-span before appearance of complications such as cirrhosis and portal hypertension varies in different patients. No correlation is found between the development and severity of oesophageal varices and the initial lesions at the time of surgery (Kang, JPediatSurg, 1993; 28:63; Davenport, p.233 in reference 8). In surgical reports, the complication of cirrhosis with portal hypertension is ascribed usually to the occurrence of repetitive episodes of cholangitis. However, there is a growing suspicion that the more serious long-term hepatic complications after portoenterostomy reflect the relentless, slow progression of the intrahepatic component of the basic disease process of extrahepatic bile duct atresia. Hepatic portoenterostomy apparently exerts a beneficial effect on the progression of the intrahepatic lesion, not so much by arresting the basic disease process, as by eliminating the superimposed obstruction caused by the progressive obliteration of the extrahepatic bile ducts. Relief of obstruction saves the patient from rapid deterioration to the stage of secondary biliary cirrhosis, and is responsible for the increased survival of patients whose prognosis is otherwise extremely bad. However, the basic inflammatory process affecting the intrahepatic branches of the biliary system continues to operate in many patients, albeit at variable speeds, comparable with intrahepatic bile duct destruction in adults with primary biliary cirrhosis or primary sclerosing cholangitis. A patient has been reported who had endstage cirrhosis at the age of 33 years after a portoenterostomy was performed in infancy (Bussutil, AmJSurg, 1987; 154:25). The following section summarizes the major findings from histological examination of the liver in follow-up studies after hepatic portoenterostomy, with some suggestions for interpretation.

Description of histological findings

Development of bile duct cysts and bile duct dilatation, mostly after unsuccessful portoenterostomy

In patients with inadequate postoperative flow of bile, or attacks of cholangitis, the development of large bile duct cysts has been demonstrated, possibly as a result of the operative procedure (Werlin, JPediatGastrNutr, 1985; 4:537; Tsuchida, p.147 in reference 8). The pathogenesis of intrahepatic bile duct dilatation and cyst formation remains unclear. The possibility of associated Caroli's disease should be considered (Canty, AmJSurg, 1987; 154:25).

Improvement in liver histology after successful portoenterostomy

In several studies of liver specimens from patients followed after hepatic portoenterostomy (Dessanti, ArchDisChild, 1985; 60: 739), an improvement in hepatic histological alterations was observed in some patients. Such improvement included decrease in parenchymal and ductular cholestasis, ballooning and damage of liver cells, infiltration by inflammatory cells, and periportal fibrosis.

Progressive liver damage observed in long-term follow-up after successful portoenterostomy

Successful portoenterostomy in this context implies adequate postoperative flow of bile, disappearance of jaundice, and a generally good condition of the patient. These patients may suffer from episodes of cholangitis, especially during the first postoperative year, and later develop portal hypertension. A variety of histological abnormalities has been observed in several studies of such patients, followed for up to 5 years and longer (Gautier, JPediatSurg, 1984; 19:263; Callea, p.304 in reference 14; Hadchouel, p.65 in reference 19).

Mild periportal fibrosis

In some patients, only mild periportal fibrosis is observed, with virtual absence of inflammatory infiltration (Plate 5). The lobular parenchyma appears normal. This pattern was observed in 4 of a series of 16 cases (Callea, p.304 in reference 14). In some cases, however, careful analysis often reveals a number of additional abnormalities. Many portal tracts are large and densely 'collagenized'. Histology leaves the impression that a number of smaller 'terminal' portal tracts are missing. An occasional portal tract lacks an identifiable interlobular duct. On PAS–diastase stained sections, the basement membrane of the ducts is more prominent than normal. A few small foci of small ductules are usually found close

to, or even inside, the lobular parenchyma. Almost invariably, some periductular oedema and an occasional neutrophilic polymorph is found, indicating a minimal degree of cholangiolitis.

Rhodanine staining for copper usually yields negative results. On preparations immunostained for an epidermal type of keratin or tissue polypeptide antigen, the foci of ductular proliferation are more clearly revealed. Moreover, the periportal hepatocytes (acinar zone 1) are positive for keratin or tissue polypeptide antigen, indicating an early stage of biliary metaplasia and hence revealing a state of 'latent cholestasis' (Van Eyken, Histopath, 1989; 15:125). Such histological features are observed in patients who are 'cured' clinically. They have normal levels of bilirubin in sera but often have a mild rise in alkaline phosphatase.

When the periportal fibrosis is somewhat more pronounced, the lobular pattern of the liver is accentuated, and the histological appearance at first glance is reminiscent of the normal histology of the pig's liver.

Congenital hepatic fibrosis-like pattern

In clinically 'cured' cases, without jaundice or overt cholestasis, the liver histology may resemble that of 'congenital hepatic fibrosis' (Plate 6). This pattern was observed in 5 of 16 cases (Callea, p.304 in reference 14). The histology is characterized by large portal tracts, with dense collagenized stroma and periportal fibrosis. The portal areas of connective tissue contain an increased number of bile ducts, occasionally showing curved shapes, and even typical circular or near-circular patterns of ductal plates. Closer analysis reveals features of smouldering, low-degree bile duct destruction. Several segments of bile ducts show necrobiosis of their lining cells, with acidophilic condensation of cytoplasm and pyknosis of nuclei. This lesion may affect a few single cells scattered in the section, or the 'melting down' of the bile duct lining may be extensive. Several segments of bile duct are surrounded by thick, hyaline, collagenous sheets. Minute foci of intralobular ductules, often—but not necessarily—at the periphery of the parenchyma, show discrete signs of cholangiolitis. Rhodanine staining for copper is negative or minimally positive. Immunostains for keratin or tissue polypeptide antigen not only emphasize the 'ductal hyperplasia' and show to better advantage the foci of 'ductular reaction', but also reveal the keratin positivity of periportal hepatocytes. A frequently noted feature in such cases is the hypoplastic size of portal vein branches in the portal tracts. Medial smooth muscle cells develop in the wall of the portal vein branches correlating with the degree of portal hypertension (Nio, p.243 in reference 14). A decrease in calibre of the main portal vein was also observed by abdominal sonography in patients with poor hepatobiliary function (Hernandez-Cano, JPediatSurg, 1987; 22:519).

All patients with a congenital hepatic fibrosis-like picture on follow-up biopsy showed ductal plate malformation of the intrahepatic bile ducts at the time of portoenterostomy.

Secondary biliary fibrosis and cirrhosis

In a proportion of clinically 'cured' cases, histological study of late follow-up biopsies reveals extensive fibrosis, with numerous portal–portal connective tissue septa (Plate 7). In some patients, the picture is that of true secondary biliary cirrhosis. The borderline between biliary fibrosis and biliary cirrhosis is unclear, since long-standing cholestasis leads to increasing fibrosis with predominant localization in zone 1. Only in later stages does further development of portal–central septa occur, realizing the complete picture of true biliary cirrhosis.[13] Reports do not always distinguish between advanced biliary fibrosis and secondary biliary cirrhosis (Weinbren, JClinPath, 1985; 38:1013). For this reason, and because of the admitted difficulty in making this distinction clearly on small specimens of tissue, 'advanced biliary fibrosis' and 'biliary cirrhosis' are treated together.

In patients with advanced biliary fibrosis, the basic pattern of connective tissue is similar to that described above in the congenital hepatic fibrosis-like pattern. Connective tissue septa predominate from portal area to portal area. The parenchyma appears as garland-shaped masses between these septa. The portal vein branches in the portal tracts appear hypoplastic. There may be an increased number of dilated lymphatic channels, recognizable by positive staining with *Ulex europeus* lectin and negative results for factor VIII-related antigen of their lining endothelium.[13] Lymphocytic infiltration may be seen, especially in the periphery of the portal tracts, but there is no or only a little piecemeal necrosis. A striking feature is the absence of interlobular bile ducts (Plate 7). This stage corresponds to acholangic biliary fibrosis (and/or cirrhosis). This pattern was observed in 2 of a series of 16 cases.[13] Several small foci of cholangiolitis can be found, in the form of small clusters of ductules near to, or even inside, the parenchyma, associated with some interstitial oedema and a rare neutrophilic polymorph.

In some cases the loss of ducts is not total. An occasional portal tract still contains an interlobular bile duct, showing signs of involution and necrobiosis of its lining cells. Such ducts may have a normal tubular shape or exhibit a ductal plate configuration. Occasionally, the involuting duct is surrounded by lymphocytes ('lymphocytic cholangitis'). This pattern of 'paucity of ducts' was observed in 5 of 16 cases.[13]

The persistence of some remaining ducts or ductal plates creates a pattern intermediate between the picture described above as congenital hepatic fibrosis-like and the pattern classified as acholangic biliary fibrosis (and/or cirrhosis). Even in instances with a total lack of interlobular bile ducts, there is no bilirubinostasis, either in the parenchyma, or in the occasional remaining ducts, or in the ductules.

Rhodanine staining may show some accumulation of copper in peripheral hepatocytes, especially in specimens with complete loss of ducts. Immunostaining for keratin or tissue polypeptide antigen emphasizes the ductopenia, reveals the foci of ductular proliferation much better than routinely stained histological sections, and shows positive staining of peripheral hepatocytes and of cholestatic liver-cell rosettes. The last feature, together with the foci of cholangiolitis, attests to the existence of a mild, smouldering state of cholestasis.

Liver lesions observed near the time of clinical deterioration in patients with long-term clinical cure

Although some patients remain jaundice free for years after successful portoenterostomy, jaundice may reappear after 4 to 7 years. Biopsies taken at this time show active biliary disease, superimposed on one of the patterns described above—seldom periportal fibrosis, more often a congenital hepatic fibrosis-like pattern or biliary fibrosis–cirrhosis pattern. In a series of 21 patients followed over a long period (4 to 7 years), 16 patients were jaundice free.[13] However, 5 further patients showed clinical signs of deterioration

with appearance of jaundice. The follow-up liver specimens of these children showed lesions of acholangic biliary fibrosis and/or cirrhosis displaying the 'active' features described below.[13]

Besides the features already mentioned, these specimens are characterized by an unsharp borderline between the connective tissue and the remaining parenchyma. The irregularity in outline is caused by so-called 'biliary piecemeal necrosis'. The peripheral parenchymal cells are dissociated by interstitial oedema and infiltration with inflammatory cells, including mononuclear and polymorphonuclear leucocytes. The dissociated liver-cell plates may show features of ductular metaplasia and/or cholate stasis. Bilirubinostasis is found in the parenchyma, usually as intercellular plugs of bile and bilirubin staining of hypertrophic Kupffer cells and macrophages. Some parenchymal cells show feathery degeneration. Cholestatic liver-cell rosettes occur to a variable extent. The concurrent presence of these features indicates active (instead of slowly-smouldering) biliary disease, with more severe degrees of progressive cholestatic lesions.

The portal tracts may still contain an involuting bile duct, in tubular or ductal plate configuration, showing atrophy and epithelial involution, and occasionally lymphocytic infiltration ('lymphocytic cholangitis'). Sometimes only lymphoid aggregates are found, possibly indicating the site of a pre-existing duct.

Interpretation of histological findings

In patients with an unsuccessful postoperative course, the liver lesions correspond to those of the underlying liver disease, possibly aggravated by postoperative complications of ischaemia, renewed obstruction, and especially acute cholangitis.

In patients with a successful postoperative course, the spectrum of liver lesions observed allows the formulation of the following hypothesis. The core of the hypothesis is not new and refers to extrahepatic bile duct atresia as a progressive destructive inflammation of intrahepatic and extrahepatic bile ducts (Landing, ProgPediatSurg, 1974; 6:113; Haas, WorldJSurg, 1978; 2:561). It further implies that the underlying basic disease process continues at its own pace and during its own (individually determined) period of time, in spite of successful surgery. Portoenterostomy has relieved the patient from extrahepatic obstruction and its own disastrous effects, but it leaves the patient with his/her intrinsic intrahepatic disease of bile ducts (the 'basic disease process') (Haas, 1978). The basic disease process may heal spontaneously, resulting in a patient clinically and histologically normal. There is not much histological documentation of this course of events. In some, the intrahepatic disease of bile ducts, with its accompanying inflammation and fibrosis, continues for a while, resulting in some periportal fibrotic scarring before it finally heals. This course would apply for those patients who remain clinically well and biochemically normal, but in whom some mild and functionally insignificant periportal fibrosis is found. The only sequel is that the human histological pattern of the liver has moved closer to that of the normal pig's liver.

As discussed above, several cases are characterized by a particular 'fetal' type of 'ductular reaction' in the form of ductal plate formation, and even repetitive ductal plate formation resulting in (often incomplete) concentric rings of bile duct structures ('early severe' extrahepatic bile duct atresia).

When after successful portoenterostomy the basic disease process causing intrahepatic bile duct destruction stops in an early phase, the liver is left in a state characterized by an excess of 'immature' types of bile duct structures. The bile duct destruction stops, but the remodelling of the ductal plate is deranged. This 'bile duct hyperplasia', together with the increased portal and periportal connective tissue which accompanies the later waves of ductal plates, creates the histological appearance described as congenital hepatic fibrosis-like. One may speculate whether 'natural' congenital hepatic fibrosis is brought about by a comparable process of excess stimulation of ductal plate formation with arrest of the normal remodelling process. In this view, congenital hepatic fibrosis would represent a 'fetal type' of biliary fibrosis (Desmet, Histopath, 1992; 20:465). One can further speculate whether the congenital hepatic fibrosis-like pattern in extrahepatic bile duct atresia may not cause the development of portal hypertension in the same way as does 'natural' congenital hepatic fibrosis. Portal hypertension, followed by the complications of oesophageal varices and variceal haemorrhage, is now recognized universally as a late complication of successful hepatic portoenterostomy (Howard, p.167 in reference 3; Okamoto, p.283 in reference 3; Davenport, p.233 in reference 8; Dessanti, p.238 in reference 8; Valayer, p.105 in reference 19), although spontaneous alleviation of portal hypertension has been observed in some patients (Lilly, JPediatSurg, 1984; 19:476).

It appears that the arrest in ductal plate remodelling may be complete or variably incomplete. Complete arrest of remodelling would result in a congenital hepatic fibrosis-like pattern with ductal plate configurations in numerous portal areas. Partial remodelling would result in a congenital hepatic fibrosis-like pattern with ductal plates or ductal plate remnants in some portal tracts, and normally shaped (remodelled) ducts in other portal areas. The variability in degree of ductal plate formations, and the variability in degree of remodelling (or arrest of the latter), might explain the spectrum of lesions in congenital hepatic fibrosis-like patterns and the variation in the time-dependent development of portal hypertension. The mechanisms of development of portal hypertension in congenital hepatic fibrosis are not established, but presumably include the sometimes documented hypoplasia of interlobular branches of the portal vein (Ohuchi, JPediatSurg, 1986; 21:10), and the excess fibrous connective tissue in and around the portal tracts. Whatever the mechanism of development of portal hypertension, the latter may be the only complication in operated patients. The liver parenchyma is normal, and when progressive destruction of the intrahepatic bile ducts has ceased, there is no perpetuation of the state of smouldering cholestasis. Liver function tests are normal. The abnormally shaped intrahepatic bile ducts seem to assure adequate drainage of the bile produced by the liver.

In several patients, however, continued low-grade destruction of intrahepatic bile ducts (in excess numbers and in ductal plate configuration) continues to occur. This is reflected in the histological picture described as a congenital hepatic fibrosis-like pattern, but with superimposed signs of smouldering cholestasis. This low-grade destructive cholangitis may lead—over months and years—to progressive disappearance of intrahepatic bile ducts of whatever shape, mature and immature, resulting in ductless portal tracts expanded by increasing amounts of connective tissue and periportal fibrosis. This gradually leads to the stage of biliary fibrosis and cirrhosis with virtually complete ductopenia. The patient may still be jaundice free. However, the cholestasis will reflect itself in raised serum levels of alkaline phosphatase, γ-glutamyl transferase,

cholesterol, and bile salts. It remains unclear how the liver gets rid of bile pigments. It is possible that drainage occurs through hepatic lymph vessels in the absence of intrahepatic bile ducts.[22] The finding of excess numbers of dilated lymphatic vessels is of interest in this respect (Callea, p.304 in reference 14). This stage may be characterized by portal hypertension due to hypoplasia of intrahepatic portal vein branches, extensive portal and periportal fibrosis, and nodular cirrhotic transformation of the liver architecture.

In some patients, a long-term 'clinical cure' may deteriorate with reappearance of jaundice. This may be due to clinical episodes of cholangitis, as often reported in the surgical literature. However, some authors emphasize the lack of correlation between development of biliary cirrhosis in their patients and presence or absence of repeated episodes of cholangitis (Gautier, JPediatSurg, 1984; 19:263). The cause of this 'deterioration' is not clear. It may be late occlusion of the anastomosis at the porta hepatis or late-stage obliteration of the larger intrahepatic draining ducts due to the basic disease process; it may be a block in lymphatic drainage by slow, progressive fibrosis; or it may be a change in metabolic pathways inside the liver cells. Whatever the mechanism, the clinical deterioration is accompanied by, and—according to two observations—even preceded by, histological changes of 'active' biliary disease as described above. Finally, the non-homogeneous spread of lesions observed in follow-up biopsies of patients after portoenterostomy should be stressed (Hadchouel, p.65 in reference 19). A heterogeneous distribution of the lesions is not surprising in progressive and destructive intrahepatic bile duct disease, in view of the knowledge gained from experience in adults with primary biliary cirrhosis and sclerosing cholangitis.

The lack of homogeneity of lesions throughout the liver, however, causes sampling problems in small percutaneous needle biopsies. This explains why some authors recommend surgical biopsy in order to assure a more representative tissue sample (Gautier, JPediatSurg, 1984; 19:263; Alagille, p.233 in reference 3).

In several studies, the progressive disappearance of interlobular bile ducts in extrahepatic bile duct atresia, even after 'successful' hepatic portoenterostomy, has been documented (Nietgen, Gastro, 1992; 102:2126; Fabbretti, p.70 in reference 8; Nio, p.53 in reference 8; Perez-Atayde, p.60 in reference 8). As discussed in this chapter, we consider this lesion to be a result of the 'basic disease process' in extrahepatic bile duct atresia. Based on the unequal spread of the lesions throughout the liver, other authors have interpreted the progressive ductopenia as resulting from obstruction of some larger ducts at the porta hepatis (Nietgen, 1992; Perez-Atayde, p.60 in reference 8). However, biliary cirrhosis is observed in endstage liver disease following portoenterostomy in spite of patency of larger ducts at the liver hilum, suggesting an important role for the 'basic disease process' of extrahepatic bile duct atresia in the progressive destruction of interlobular ducts (Fabbretti, p.70 in reference 8).

In conclusion, the histological changes observed in liver specimens obtained from patients followed in the long term after hepatic portoenterostomy allow the conclusion that the basic disease process of the intrahepatic bile ducts continues to run its natural course, as has been proposed on several occasions (Haas, WorldJSurg, 1978; 2:561; Howard, BrJSurg, 1983; 70:193; Alagille, p.233 in reference 3; Fabbretti, p.70 in reference 8).[12] The advantage of portoenterostomy is the relief of the extrahepatic bile duct occlusion, which itself is the result of the extrahepatic component of the basic 'sclerosing cholangitis' process. After re-establishment of bilioenteric continuity, the intrahepatic bile duct disease may heal spontaneously or may progress at higher or slower speed.

The pathological mechanisms result in progressive obliteration and disappearance of intrahepatic bile ducts, accompanied by increasing periportal fibrosis, resulting in the endstage of biliary fibrosis and/or cirrhosis. The histological pattern of changes is modulated by the extent to which ductal plate formation and derangement in remodelling of ductal plates has occurred. Presumably this depends largely on an earlier antenatal onset of disease, and persistence of a 'fetal type' of ductular reaction to obstruction during the first 2 months of life.

Atresia of intrahepatic bile ducts
Introduction: terminology and classification

Atresia of the intrahepatic bile ducts is usually not complete, but consists of a reduced ratio of the number of interlobular ducts to the number of portal tracts. This explains the alternative terms: intrahepatic biliary hypoplasia, hypoplasia of interlobular bile ducts, ductular hypoplasia, ductular paucity, and paucity of interlobular (or intrahepatic) bile ducts. The last term has been the most popular in recent years.

A sound morphological diagnosis of paucity of interlobular bile ducts requires a sufficiently large biopsy specimen and morphometric evaluation of bile ducts. Some authors recommend surgical wedge biopsies of the liver (Alagille, JPediat, 1975; 86:63).[10] Others feel that a simple percutaneous needle biopsy may be adequate, on condition that it contains at least six portal tracts (Labrecque, Hepatol, 1982; 2:467).[4] Immunostains for cytokeratins or tissue polypeptide antigen are helpful for better visualization of interlobular ducts (Van Eyken, VirchArchA, 1987; 412: 63). Paucity of interlobular bile ducts is diagnosed if the ratio of interlobular ducts to the number of portal tracts is less than 0.5; in normal children this ratio lies between 0.9 and 1.8 (Alagille, JPediat, 1975; 86:63; Alagille, JPediat, 1987; 110:195; Alagille, p.59 in reference 3). It may be lower in premature infants (Kahn, Hepatol, 1989; 10:21). In the case of premature newborn infants, the fetal age is important for adequate evaluation of the bile duct/portal tract ratio.

The portal areas without bile ducts usually appear hypoplastic as a whole, and the total number of portal tracts per square millimetre of tissue is reduced compared with normal controls (Hadchouel, ArchPathLabMed, 1978; 102:402).

Paucity of interlobular bile ducts may be an isolated defect or associated with other extrahepatic anomalies. This allows patients with this condition to be grouped into two categories: those with syndromic and those with non-syndromic paucity of interlobular bile ducts.

Syndromic paucity of interlobular bile ducts
Definition, clinical features, and evolution

In 1975, Alagille and coworkers described a distinct disorder which can be differentiated from other forms of cholestasis in infancy and childhood (Alagille, JPediat, 1975; 86:63). The entity is now known

Table 2 Syndromic paucity of interlobular bile ducts: major features

Pulmonary artery hypoplasia or stenosis
Chronic cholestasis
Characteristic facial features
Pulmonary artery hypoplasia or stenosis
Butterfly-like vertebral arc defects
Posterior embryotoxon

as Alagille's syndrome, arteriohepatic dysplasia, or syndromic paucity of interlobular bile ducts (Riely, SemLivDis, 1987; 7:119).

Syndromic paucity of interlobular bile ducts is the most common form of familial intrahepatic cholestasis; it occurs worldwide and in various races. Affected children are often of low birthweight. The disorder affects multiple organ systems but can be very variable in expression. Most cases present in infancy, either with jaundice in the neonatal period or for evaluation of congenital heart disease.

Generally, patients with syndromic paucity of interlobular bile ducts have cholestasis which is most severe in infancy and childhood, but which improves, or even resolves clinically, with increasing age. Usually the cholestasis is accompanied by pruritus and jaundice, and often xanthomas. Laboratory tests reveal elevated levels of serum bile acids, alkaline phosphatase, 5'-nucleotidase, γ-glutamyl transferase, and cholesterol. There is attendant fat malabsorption and rickets, vitamin K-deficient coagulopathy, and vitamin E-deficient neuropathy (Riely, SemLivDis, 1987; 7:119).

Further examination reveals a number of extrahepatic abnormalities (Table 2). Most patients have a heart murmur present from birth, due to stenosis of the peripheral pulmonary arteries. The most specific ophthalmological finding is posterior embryotoxon. This is an asymptomatic embryological remnant, corresponding to a thickening of the line formed at the junction of Descemet's membrane with the endothelium of the anterior chamber angle. Examination with a slit lamp or by gonioscopy by an experienced ophthalmologist, in infants under general anaesthesia, is usually required to discover the lesion. The posterior embryotoxon is present from birth, and is found in 90 to 95 per cent of patients with syndromic paucity of interlobular bile ducts. However, it is neither absolutely specific for this syndrome nor constant.

The most common bone defect is an abnormality in the vertebral bodies, with 'butterfly' vertebras or incomplete spina bifida. Other bone anomalies include shortened distal phalanges and a short ulna. Alagille and co-workers (JPediat, 1975; 86:63) reported a typical facial appearance: a flattened nose with bulbous tip, deep-set and widely spaced eyes, a down-turned mouth, and a small mandible with pointed chin. It appears, however, that a similar dysmorphic face is not absolutely pathognomonic for syndromic paucity of interlobular bile ducts.

The five major features of syndromic paucity of interlobular bile ducts vary in their frequency. Thus it is possible to consider a patient to have a complete type if these five major features are present, or a partial type if four or at least three of the features are present (Alagille, p.33 in reference 2). In the complete or partial form, several other less frequently associated abnormalities may be found.

Reported neurological abnormalities include arreflexia, strabismus, poor impulse control, poor school or job performance, and irritability. Renal dysfunction, with diminished creatinine clearance and azotaemia is often part of the syndrome. Other reported renal abnormalities include tubulointerstitial nephropathy and intramembranous and mesangial lipid deposits (Riely, SemLivDis, 1987; 7:119).

Many reports document the familial occurrence of syndromic paucity of interlobular bile ducts. It occurs in sibships and transmission from one generation to the next, even through three or four generations, has been documented (Riely, SemLivDis, 1987; 7:119). The disease appears to be inherited as an autosomal dominant trait.

The pathogenesis remains unknown. No mechanism that is restricted to the liver will successfully explain the pathogenesis of this disorder. The most attractive suggestion to date is a chromosomal anomaly del (20p) (Byrne, AmJMedGen, 1986; 24:673; Legius, AmJMedGen, 1990; 35:532).

The course followed by most patients with syndromic paucity of interlobular bile ducts is clinical improvement, with resolution of the jaundice and the xanthomas, and amelioration of the pruritus as the patients grow up. A still undefined proportion of patients develop liver cirrhosis. However, except for cardiac complications, the syndromic form seems to run a more benign course than non-syndromic types of paucity of intrahepatic bile ducts, in which cirrhogenic evolution is more frequent (Alagille, JPediat, 1987; 110: 195; Alagille, p.33 in reference 2). Detailed clinical discussions of syndromic paucity of interlobular bile ducts or Alagille's syndrome can be found in some excellent reviews (Alagille, 1987; Riely, SemLivDis, 1987; 7:119).

Pathology of syndromic paucity of interlobular bile ducts

The basic lesion in this condition is a diminished number (paucity) of intrahepatic bile ducts; the extrahepatic bile ducts are patent, although often hypoplastic (Hashida, PediatPath, 1988; 8:1). The diminished number of interlobular bile ducts is usually estimated as the bile duct to portal tract ratio, as previously discussed. However, several recent studies have emphasized that syndromic paucity of interlobular bile ducts is a progressive disease with bile duct destruction. Originally, the interlobular bile ducts are present, but are gradually destroyed with advancing age, rendering the morphometric diagnosis of 'paucity' age dependent. Degenerative changes of bile duct epithelial-lining cells and concentric cellular periduct fibrosis accompany the involution of the ducts (Plate 8).

Portal fibrosis is not a feature during infancy, but develops to a variable extent in the following years. It is at present impossible to predict on an early biopsy which patients will eventually develop a greater degree of portal fibrosis. Moderate perisinusoidal fibrosis is frequently observed.

Bilirubinostasis is usually more hepatocellular than canalicular (Hashida, PediatPath, 1988; 8:1). One electron microscopic study suggested a failure in hepatocyte ability to secrete bile into canaliculi (Valencia-Mayoral, Hepatol, 1984; 4:691); another study confirmed the minimal dilatation of bile canaliculi, but also emphasized the marginal difference and the overlap with other cholestatic syndromes (Witzleben, Hepatol, 1987; 7:1262).

There is a statistically significant reduction in the number of portal tracts, indicating a decreased ramification of the portal tracts.

It is of interest that the lesion of the peripheral pulmonary arteries may also be a paucity of their ramification, imparting a 'pruned tree' appearance by angiography (Hashida, PediatPath, 1988; 8:1). Although the aetiology of syndromic paucity of interlobular bile ducts remains unknown, this observation suggests a derangement in vascular ramifications of both portal venous and pulmonary arterial vessels.

The extrahepatic bile ducts in syndromic paucity of interlobular bile ducts are patent, but hypoplastic. Endoscopic retrograde cholangiography has revealed abnormalities in the biliary tree, including focal dilatation such as that seen in primary sclerosing cholangitis. It seems likely therefore that the disease in syndromic paucity of interlobular bile ducts need not be limited to the liver and intrahepatic bile ducts, but can also affect the major extrahepatic ducts (Riely, SemLivDis, 1987; 7:119). This raises intriguing questions about the relationship between extrahepatic bile duct atresia and paucity of intrahepatic bile ducts.[7]

Syndromic paucity of interlobular bile ducts is not an indication for hepatoportoenterostomy. Since operative cholangiography is not infallible, particularly in hypoplasia of extrahepatic bile ducts, several patients with syndromic paucity of interlobular bile ducts with a misdiagnosis of extrahepatic ductal atresia have undergone a Kasai-type operation. In retrospect, it appears that such operative treatment did not adversely affect the pathological course in these patients (Alagille, JPediat, 1987; 110:195; Hashida, PediatPath, 1988; 8:1).

Non-syndromic paucity of interlobular bile ducts

Definition, clinical features, and evolution

Paucity of intrahepatic bile ducts with patent extrahepatic ducts may occur without a set of extrahepatic anomalies. This non-syndromic form is less common than the syndromic variety, and is clearly a heterogeneous disorder. Although the majority of cases are idiopathic, non-syndromatic paucity of interlobular bile ducts may be associated with a variety of diseases such as congenital rubella, α_1-antitrypsin deficiency, familial trihydroxycoprostanic acid excess, Down syndrome, Turner syndrome, trisomy 17/18, and congenital syphilis (Hashida, PediatPath, 1988; 8:1).[23]

Such patients are clinically very similar to those with syndromic paucity of interlobular bile ducts. Often they are of low birthweight, and present with jaundice and pruritus. They have elevated levels of cholesterol, aminotransferases, and alkaline phosphatase. This heterogeneous group as a whole has a worse prognosis than patients with the syndromic condition, since cirrhosis develops in nearly 50 per cent of the patients. The heterogeneity in outcome probably reflects the fact that this category is composed of several disorders of different aetiology (Riely, SemLivDis, 1987; 7:119).

Pathology of non-syndromic paucity of interlobular bile ducts

Again, the degree of 'paucity' can be estimated by calculating the bile duct to portal tract ratio. In the non-syndromic variety of paucity of interlobular bile ducts also, evidence has been found of inflammatory destruction of existing ducts; the picture is further characterized by mild periportal fibrosis (Kahn, Hepatol, 1986; 6:

890). A decrease in number of ducts is already present in the first 3 months of life (Plate 9).

The progressive disappearance of interlobular ducts has not, however, been observed in other series studied (Alagille, p.33 in reference 2), although it should be emphasized that the age of the patients was not mentioned. The aetiology and pathogenesis of the diminished or diminishing number of interlobular bile ducts in non-syndromic paucity of interlobular bile ducts remain unclear. A chronic cholestatic disease in adults has been described as 'idiopathic adulthood ductopenia'. It may represent either an intrahepatic variant of primary sclerosing cholangitis unassociated with ulcerative colitis or, alternatively, a late manifestation of non-syndromic paucity of interlobular bile ducts (Ludwig, JHepatol, 1988; 7:193).

Combined extra- and intrahepatic bile duct atresia

Cases of combined extrahepatic bile duct atresia and paucity of interlobular bile ducts have been described repeatedly (Riely, Sem-LivDis, 1987; 7:119),[7] and more recent studies continue to report patients with extrahepatic bile duct atresia who clearly have Alagille's syndrome or syndromic paucity of interlobular bile ducts. In such patients, the usual finding at laparotomy is the presence of a small, empty gallbladder and cholangiography that documents flow of dye into the duodenum but not back into the intrahepatic radicles.

As discussed above, the extrahepatic bile ducts are often hypoplastic in Alagille's syndrome, and one microscopic study has reported that the histopathological changes of the bile ducts in the porta hepatis were indistinguishable from those seen in fibrous bile duct remnants of extrahepatic bile duct atresia (Kahn, Hepatol, 1983; 3:77).[23] This raises the suspicion that so-called 'hypoplasia' may in fact represent an incomplete or arrested 'atresia' of the extrahepatic bile ducts. A 'sclerosing cholangitis with neonatal onset' has been described which clinically bears striking similarities to extrahepatic bile duct atresia and some forms of non-syndromic paucity of interlobular bile ducts (Amedee-Manesme, JPediat, 1987; 111:225). This new subgroup of patients with sclerosing cholangitis of childhood led the authors to speculate that extrahepatic bile duct atresia, non-syndromic paucity of interlobular bile ducts, and sclerosing cholangitis are different expressions of antenatal or perinatal damage to the bile ducts, and that neonatal sclerosing cholangitis may result from the same type of bile duct injury as in extrahepatic bile duct atresia but without the same extent of damage, thus representing a 'near-miss extrahepatic bile duct atresia' .

It thus appears that further investigations are required in order to establish which factor(s) cause(s) destruction of bile ducts in the antenatal or perinatal period, and which modulating influences determine the predominant involvement of one or other segment of the biliary tree, resulting in recognizable but overlapping clinical syndromes diagnosed today as neonatal sclerosing cholangitis, hypoplasia of extrahepatic bile ducts, or extrahepatic bile duct atresia or paucity of interlobular bile ducts of the syndromic and non-syndromic variety.

References

1. Javitt NB, ed. *Neonatal hepatitis and biliary atresia.* DHEW Publication No (NIH) 79–1296 ed. US Department of Health, Education, and Welfare, 1979.
2. Waldschmidt J, Charissis G, and Schier F, eds. *Cholestasis in neonates.* Munich: W Zuckschwerdt, 1988.
3. Kasai M, ed. *Biliary atresia and its related disorders.* Amsterdam: Excerpta Medica, 1983.
4. Schweizer P and Müller G. *Gallengangsatresie. Cholestase-Syndrome intramuscular Neugeborenen- und Suglingsalter.* Stuttgart: Hippokrates Verlag, 1984.
5. Stein J and Vacanti J. Biliary atresia and other disorders of the extrahepatic biliary tree. In Suchy F, ed. *Liver disease in children.* St Louis: Mosby, 1994: 426–42.
6. Hoffman MA, ed. *Current controversies in biliary atresia.* Austin: RG Landes Company, 1992.
7. Desmet VJ and Callea F. Cholestatic syndromes of infancy and childhood. In Zakim D and Boyer TD, eds. *Hepatology. A textbook of liver disease*, Vol. 2, 3rd edn. Philadelphia: WB Saunders, 1996: 1649–98.
8. Ohi R, ed. *Biliary atresia.* Tokyo: ICOM Associates, 1991.
9. Kasai M. Treatment of biliary atresia with special reference to hepatic porto-enterostomy and its modifications. In Bill AH and Kasai M, eds. *Progress of pediatric surgery*, Vol. 6. Baltimore: University Park Press, 1974: 5–52.
10. Alagille D and Odièvre M. *Liver and biliary tract disease in children.* New York: John Wiley & Sons, 1979.
11. Kasai M and Shiraki K, eds. *Cholestasis in infancy.* Tokyo: University of Tokyo Press, 1980.
12. Ravitch MM, Welch KJ, Benson CD, Aberdeen E, and Randolph JG, eds. *Pediatric surgery*, 3rd edn. Chicago: Year Book Medical Publishers, 1979.
13. Desmet VJ. Cirrhosis: aetiology and pathogenesis: cholestasis. In Boyer JL and Bianchi L, eds. *Liver cirrhosis.* Lancaster: MTP Press, 1987: 101–18.
14. Ohi R, ed. *Biliary atresia.* Tokyo: Professional Postgraduate Services, 1987.
15. Desmet VJ. Vanishing bile duct disorders. In Boyer JL and Ockner RK, eds. *Progress in liver diseases*, Vol. 10. Philadelphia: WB Saunders, 1992.
16. Valayer J. Hepatic porto-enterostomy: surgical problems and results. In Berenberg SR, ed. *Liver disease in infancy and childhood.* The Hague: Martinus Nijhoff Medical Division, 1976: 84–96.
17. Dimmick J and Kalousek D. *Developmental pathology of the embryo and fetus.* Philadelphia: JB Lippincott, 1992: 545–78.
18. Alagille D. Cholestasis in the first three months of life. In Popper H and Schaffner F, eds. *Progress in liver diseases*, Vol. 1. New York: Grune & Stratton, 1979: 471–85.
19. Daum F, ed. *Extrahepatic biliary atresia.* New York: Marcel Dekker, 1983.
20. Mowat AP. Paediatric liver disease: medical aspects. In Wright R, Millward-Sadler GH, Alberti KGMM, and Karran S, eds. *Liver and biliary disease. Pathophysiology, diagnosis, management*, 2nd edn. London: Baillière Tindall, WB Saunders Company, 1985: 1201–18.
21. de Ville DE, Goyet J, and Otte JB. *Place of liver transplantation in biliary atresia.* Dordrecht: Kluwer Academic Publishers, 1992: 265–72.
22. Mallet-Guy D, Michoulier J, and Beau S. Experimental studies on liver lymph flow: conditions affecting bilio–lymphatic transfer. In Taylor W, ed. *The biliary system.* Philadelphia: FA Davis Corporation, 1965: 69–78.
23. Kahn E. Paucity of interlobular bile ducts. Arteriohepatic dysplasia and nonsyndromic duct paucity. In Abramowsky CR, Bernstein J, and Rosenberg HS, eds. *Perspectives in pediatric pathology. Transplantation pathology—hepatic morphogenesis*, Vol. 14. Basel: Karger; 1991: 168–215.

11.2 Non-parasitic cystic diseases of the liver and intrahepatic biliary tree

Jean-Pierre Benhamou and Yves Menu

Non-parasitic cystic diseases of the liver and intrahepatic biliary tree include entities which differ in aetiology, prevalence, manifestations, and severity, but have two common characteristics. First, these diseases result from a congenital malformation, inherited or not inherited, of the intrahepatic bile ducts. Second, the basic lesion consists of cysts, either macroscopic or microscopic. The macroscopic cysts are easily recognized by ultrasonography or computed tomography, which are the main procedures for their diagnosis. The microscopic cysts are not demonstrated by these imaging procedures, but only by histological examination.

Simple cyst of the liver

The simple cysts of the liver are cystic formations, containing a serous fluid, not communicating with the intrahepatic biliary tree. Numerous terms have been used to designate this lesion: non-parasitic cyst of the liver, benign hepatic cyst, congenital hepatic cyst, unilocular cyst of the liver, and solitary cyst of the liver (which is inappropriate because, as mentioned below, the simple cysts are often multiple).

Pathology and pathogenesis

Macroscopically, a simple cyst of the liver has a spherical or ovoid shape with a diameter ranging from a few millimetres to 20 cm or more. The cyst does not communicate with the intrahepatic bile ducts. Small cysts are surrounded by normal hepatic tissue. Large cysts produce atrophy of the adjacent hepatic tissue: a huge cyst may result in complete atrophy of a hepatic lobe with compensatory hypertrophy of the other lobe. Atrophy respects the large bile ducts and blood vessels which therefore appear to be abundant in the atrophic tissue in contact with the cyst. Large bile ducts and blood vessels persisting after atrophy may protrude and form folds over the inner surface of the cyst. There is no septation; the cysts are unilocular. The cystic fluid is clear.

In half the adults having the lesion, there is only one cyst. In the other half, there are two or more cysts (Larsen, ActaPMIScand, 1961; 51:47). In a small number of cases, simple cysts are multiple, resembling the liver cysts of adult polycystic kidney disease.

Microscopically, the cysts appear to be bordered by a single layer of cuboid or columnar epithelial cells, resembling the biliary epithelial cells. The cells are uniform, without any atypia. The stroma is absent in small cysts and reduced to a thin layer of connective tissue in large cysts.

Simple cysts of the liver are regarded as a congenital malformation. An aberrant bile duct would have lost communication with the biliary tree and would dilate progressively. The composition of the fluid, which contains water and mineral electrolytes without bile acids and bilirubin, is close to that of the normal secretion of the epithelium of the bile ducts.

Prevalence and aetiology

Simple cysts have long been considered a rare lesion: up to 1971, only 350 cases had been reported (Flagg, ArchSurg, 1967; 95:964; Moreaux, ArchFrMalAppDig, 1971; 60:203). In fact, symptomatic or complicated simple cysts are uncommon, but asymptomatic simple cysts are found in about 1 per cent of adults at autopsy (Larsen, ActaPMIScand, 1961; 51:47). The prevalence of simple cysts demonstrated by ultrasonography or computed tomography might likewise be about 3 per cent in the adult population (Benhamou, personal observation).

The female-to-male ratio is 1.5:1 in asymptomatic simple cysts demonstrated at autopsy (Larsen, ActaPMIScand, 1961; 51:47) or on ultrasonography or computed tomography (Benhamou, personal observation). However, the female-to-male ratio amounts to 9:1 in symptomatic or complicated simple cysts (Moreaux, ArchFrMalAppDig, 1971; 60:203). Simple cysts are larger in adults over the age of 50 years than in younger individuals (Larsen, 1961). Huge cysts affect almost exclusively women of over 50 years (Larsen, 1961).

In contrast to cysts of the liver that occur in adult polycystic kidney disease, simple cysts of the liver are sporadic, even when multiple. However, in a small number of cases, there is a familial clustering suggesting a genetic transmission. These cases of multiple simple cysts of the liver are genetically different from adult polycystic kidney disease in that the genetic markers, PKD1 and PKD2, of the latter are absent (Pierson, Hepatol, 1996; 23:249).

Manifestations and diagnosis

In the vast majority of cases (all the small cysts, but also most of the large cysts), simple cysts are asymptomatic and fortuitously demonstrated by ultrasonography or computed tomography. Only some of the large cysts produce abdominal pain or discomfort.

Because of the high prevalence of simple cysts in adults, the fortuitous coincidence of this lesion and another hepatic or extrahepatic disease is not uncommon: therefore, the causal relationship between abdominal pain or discomfort and a simple cyst of the liver must be admitted with caution and accepted only if the cyst is large and the other possible causes of the symptoms have been excluded.

At clinical examination, only the large cysts can be palpated as spherical tumours. In most cases, the fluid content of the tumour can be suspected. However, in some cases, the cyst is so tense that it may be taken for a solid tumour. The condition of individuals with simple cysts of the liver is good. Liver function tests are normal.

Ultrasonography is the best procedure for recognizing simple cysts. A simple cyst produces a circular or oval, totally anechoic area, with sharp, smooth borders and strong posterior wall echoes, indicating a well-defined tissue–fluid interface (Spiegel, AJR, 1978; 131:235). There is accentuation of the echoes beyond the cyst compared with echoes at a similar depth transmitted through normal adjacent liver tissue (Spiegel, 1978). This accentuation of echoes, which indicates that the lesion is fluid filled, is observed only when deep tissue transmits ultrasound and is not seen when a total reflector, such as gas or bone, lies behind the cyst. In one-half of the cases, only one cyst can be demonstrated; in the other half, two or more cysts are present. In a few patients, multiple cysts are recognized. Ultrasonography of the kidneys shows no abnormality except for the fortuitous coincidence of one or two simple renal cysts, which is also a common finding in adults.

The other imaging procedures are of less interest for diagnosis than ultrasonography and are generally not required. Computed tomography confirms the presence of one or several, round or oval, water-dense lesions, without septation or intracystic formations; dynamic computed tomography shows that the tumours are avascular. However, in small cysts, recognition of water density may be difficult (the average density of the cyst being masked by the density of the adjacent liver tissue) and an apparent increase in density may be observed after injection of contrast medium. Liver scintiscan shows defects corresponding to the cysts if their diameter is over 3 cm. Angiography shows that the cysts are avascular and, if large, displace the intrahepatic vessels.

If the patient is living or has been living in an area where hydatid disease is endemic, or if there is any doubt about a possible hydatid cyst, serological tests for this parasitic infection must be performed.

Aspiration, after exclusion of a hydatid cyst, has been proposed for confirming the diagnosis by showing a clear fluid, by relieving the symptoms, and by demonstrating the absence of communication with the biliary tree after injection of contrast (Roemer, AJR, 1981; 136:1065). In our experience, this investigation is unnecessary in most cases.

Course and complications

In most cases, simple cysts are asymptomatic and remain silent; repeated ultrasonography usually shows no appreciable changes over years. In some patients, the cysts grow slowly. In a small number of patients, the size of the cysts increases rapidly: such a course, which is associated with severe pain and discomfort, is observed almost exclusively in women over 50 years of age.

The complications are uncommon. The most frequent complication is intracystic bleeding (Moreaux, ArchFrMalAppDig, 1971; 60:203; Frisell, ActaMedScand, 1979; 205:541). The clinical manifestation consists of sudden severe pain and increase in the size of the cyst. In a few cases, pain is mild or even absent. On ultrasonography, echoic material corresponding to clots is present in the cyst; usually this echoic material is mobile, sliding in the inferior part of the cyst. The other complications include rupture, bacterial infection, compression of the inferior vena cava (Frisell, 1979), fistulation into the duodenum (Williamson, BrJSurg, 1978; 65:871), communication with an intrahepatic duct (Perreau, ArchFrMalAppDig, 1965; 54:881), cholestasis due to compression of the bifurcation or the common bile duct (Moreaux, 1971; Santman, Gastro, 1977; 72:325; Cappel, AmJGastr, 1988; 83:93; Kalouch, GastrClinBiol, 1988; 12:80), portal hypertension due to compression of the portal vein (Lebon, ArchFrMalAppDig, 1955; 44:1274), torsion (Soud, PostgradMedJ, 1974; 50:48), and carcinoma (Americks, AnnSurg, 1972; 172:713; Greenwood, JPath, 1972; 107:145; Lynch, AmJGastr, 1988; 83:426).

Differential diagnosis

Simple cysts are easily distinguishable from liver abscesses, necrotic malignant tumours, large haemangiomas, and haematomas. The clinical context of these lesions is different. On ultrasonography and computed tomography, these lesions rarely appear as purely fluid-filled, sharply defined areas. However, a few cases of hepatic metastases of neuroendocrine tumours can be difficult to distinguish from liver cysts because these malignant tumours can be well tolerated and the necrotic areas may be sharply defined.

The distinction between simple cysts and hydatid disease can be difficult. Several characteristics of the simple cyst and hydatid disease, listed in Table 1, usually allow a clear distinction between the two diseases. However, difficulties may be due to the following points: (i) hydatid disease may have been contracted in an area where this parasitic infection is not endemic; (ii) calcifications, septations, and a split wall may be absent in hydatid cysts, which are then indistinguishable from simple cysts; and (iii) septations may be mimicked by contiguous simple cysts.

Multiple simple cysts of the liver must be distinguished from the liver cysts of adult polycystic kidney disease. First, since adult polycystic kidney disease is transmitted as an autosomal dominant trait, it is usual for one parent or sibling to have been recognized as suffering from the disease, whereas in the case of simple cysts of the liver, which are non-inherited malformations, parents and siblings are not affected by the disease. However, because the expression of adult polycystic disease varies, affected individuals may be asymptomatic and therefore unrecognized. Second, multiple renal cysts are constantly associated with liver cysts in adult polycystic kidney disease, whereas renal cysts are absent in multiple simple cysts of the liver. However, as mentioned above, one or a few simple renal cysts may be fortuitously associated with simple cysts of the liver; patients with this fortuitous association must not be regarded as affected with adult polycystic kidney disease.

Treatment

Asymptomatic simple cysts, even when large, need no treatment. Only the large, symptomatic or complicated, cysts have to be

Table 1 Distinctive characteristics of simple cyst and hydatid cyst of the liver

	Simple cyst	Hydatid cyst
Septations	Absent	Common
Calcifications	Absent	Common
Split wall	Absent	Possible
Communication with the biliary tree	Absent	Possible
Serological tests for hydatid disease	Negative	Positive[a]

[a] In most, but not in all, patients with hydatid disease.

treated. Percutaneous aspiration of the fluid content, which can be performed under ultrasonographic guidance, does not provide definitive therapy: after aspiration, the cyst recurs more or less rapidly (Saini, AJR, 1983; 141:559).

Intracystic instillation of alcohol or other sclerosing agent has been employed successfully and may be the treatment of choice in patients with high surgical risk.

Fenestration (partial excision of the external part of the cyst) can be performed by open surgery or, more comfortably for the patient, by coelioscopy. Surgical or coelioscopic fenestration is a very efficient treatment of simple cysts of the liver (Goldstein, AJR, 1976; 127:850; Bean, AJR, 1985; 144:237; Andersson, BrJSurg, 1989; 76: 254; Kairaluoma, AnnSurg, 1989; 210:208). In patients with very numerous cysts, the same procedure as that used in the treatment of liver cysts of adult polycystic kidney disease can be applied: fenestration of most of the liver cysts and resection of the segment invaded by large and numerous cysts (Que, Gastro, 1995; 108:487). Liver transplantation should be reserved for the rare patients with no spared segment of the liver.

Cystadenoma of the liver

Cystadenoma of the liver is a rare tumour which has a strong tendency to recur and has malignant potential. Therefore, differentiation of this tumour from a simple cyst of the liver is important.

Pathology and pathogenesis

Cystadenoma of the liver is a large tumour, measuring from 10 to 20 cm in diameter. It has a globular external surface from which cysts of various sizes bulge outwards. The cut surface shows multiple lobules of various sizes, limited by thin walls. The lobules usually contain a mucinous fluid (Ishak, Cancer, 1977; 39:322).

On microscopic examination, the lobules are limited by a single layer of cuboidal or columnar cells resting on a basement membrane. These cells are uniform, with round or oval nuclei; their cytoplasm is clear or faintly vacuolated; the vacuoles stain positively for mucin. In places, the epithelium forms multiple polypoid or papillary projections. The stroma supporting the epithelium is thick, compact, and cellular, resembling ovarian stroma; it often contains pigmented or foamy macrophages and cholesterol clefts (Ishak, Cancer, 1977; 39:322).

The pathogenesis of cystadenoma is unknown. A congenital origin from an abnormal intrahepatic bile duct or from misplaced germ cells is usually considered. The former hypothesis, although generally accepted, does not account for the mucinous epithelium which borders the lobules. The latter hypothesis would explain the similarity of cystadenoma of the liver to ovarian cysts.

Prevalence and aetiology

Cystadenoma of the liver is a very uncommon tumour. From a review of the literature up to 1955, the prevalence of cystadenoma has been estimated as 20 times less than that of simple cyst of the liver (Geist, ArchSurg, 1955; 71:867). According to our experience, mainly based on the recognition of liver cysts by ultrasonography and computed tomography, the prevalence of cystadenoma of the liver appears to be much lower, probably 1000 times less than that of simple cyst of the liver.

Cystadenoma of the liver mainly affects women of over 40 years (Ishak, Cancer, 1977; 39:322). Only one case has been reported in a child (Alexander, EdinburghMedJ, 1925; 32:61)

Manifestations and diagnosis

The presenting symptoms of cystadenoma are abdominal pain, abdominal discomfort, anorexia, nausea, and abdominal swelling. A large hepatic mass can be palpated. However, in patients with a small cystadenoma, the disease may be asymptomatic and clinical examination may be normal. Liver function tests are usually normal.

Diagnosis of cystadenoma is based mainly on ultrasonography and computed tomography. Ultrasonography shows a large anechoic, fluid-filled, ovoid or globular area with irregular margins; internal echoes are seen, corresponding to septations delimiting multiple lobules of various sizes and to papillary growths originating from the cystic wall or from the septa (Forrest, AJR, 1980; 135:723). Computed tomography demonstrates comparable abnormalities: a low-density area, with internal septations and mural nodules (Frick, AJR, 1982; 139:393).

Other imaging procedures are of less interest for diagnosis. Liver scintiscan shows a defect corresponding to the tumour. Arteriography shows that: the intrahepatic arteries are displaced by the tumour; the tumour itself is avascular; there are multiple clusters of fine vessels in the periphery of the tumour; and accumulation of contrast material in the wall of the cystadenoma, in the septa, and in the papillary growths may be seen in the parenchymal phase (Forrest, AJR, 1980; 135:723; Korobkin, AJR, 1989; 153:507). Endoscopic retrograde cholangiography shows displacement of the

Table 2 Distinctive characteristics of cystadenoma and simple cyst of the liver

	Cystadenoma	Simple cyst
Number of cysts	One	One or several
Septations	Common	Absent
Papillary projections	Common	Absent
Cystic fluid	Mucinous	Serous
Recurrence after partial excision	Common	Very uncommon
Malignant transformation (cystadenocarcinoma)	Possible	Very uncommon

intrahepatic bile ducts by the tumour and no communication between the biliary tree and cystadenoma.

Serological tests for hydatid disease must be performed systematically and are negative. Percutaneous aspiration, after exclusion of hydatid disease, provides a mucinous fluid.

Course and complications

Cystadenoma grows very slowly. Complications, which may be the first manifestations of the tumour, include cholestasis due to compression of the bile duct confluence or the common bile duct (Roekel, JClinGastro, 1982; 4:167), intracystic haemorrhage, bacterial infection, rupture, recurrence after partial excision, and transformation into cystadenocarcinoma.

Cystadenocarcinoma of the liver develops almost exclusively in a pre-existing cystadenoma. Histologically, the malignant epithelium is multilayered, with numerous papillary projections; malignant epithelial cells are dysmorphic and invade the stroma. Malignancies may affect all the epithelium or, more often, only a part of the cystadenoma. Malignant transformation may be suspected by ultrasonography or computed tomography showing abundant and large projections protruding into the lumina of the lobules and septal calcifications (Stanley, GastrRad, 1983; 8:245; Korobkin, AJR, 1989; 153:507). Malignant tissue can be obtained by biopsy under ultrasonographic guidance (Iemoto, Gastro, 1983; 84:399). Cystadenocarcinoma extends progressively in the liver. Extrahepatic metastases can develop.

Differential diagnosis

Cystadenoma of the liver must be distinguished from hydatid cyst and simple cyst of the liver. Cystadenoma resembles hydatid cyst in that septations are present in both diseases; the presence of calcifications and the positive serological tests are good arguments in favour of hydatid disease. The distinctive characteristics of cystadenoma and simple cyst of the liver are listed in Table 2; the distinction between these two diseases is important because their prognosis and treatment are completely different.

Treatment

Cystadenoma of the liver, even when asymptomatic, must be treated by complete excision. Partial excision exposes the patient to the risk of recurrence and to the risk of cystadenocarcinoma (Lewis, ArchSurg, 1988; 123:563).

Congenital hepatic fibrosis

Congenital hepatic fibrosis is an inherited malformation characterized by portal spaces enlarged by fibrosis and multiple bile ductules, the main consequence of which is portal hypertension. The disease was described as fibrocystic disease of the liver by Grumbach (ArchAnatCytolPath, 1954; 30:74). Congenital hepatic fibrosis was the name introduced by Kerr (QJMed, 1961; 30:91).

Pathology and pathogenesis

The lesion of congenital hepatic fibrosis consists of portal spaces markedly increased in size because of abundant connective tissue and numerous bile ductules, more or less ectatic, communicating with the biliary tree. It must be emphasized that congenital hepatic fibrosis is not simply fibrosis and that bile ductular proliferation is an essential component of the lesion. A few portal spaces may remain normal, which explains why congenital hepatic fibrosis may be unrecognized on histological examination of a small specimen taken by liver biopsy. Some clusters of multiple bile ductules surrounded with fibrosis may be present within the lobules, apart from the portal spaces. Some bile ductules are so markedly dilated that they form microcysts, which communicate with the biliary tree. Separation between the fibrotic portal spaces and the rest of the liver parenchyma is sharp. The architecture of the liver remains normal. There is no regenerative nodule.

The primary disorder of congenital hepatic fibrosis is likely to be ductular proliferation, fibrosis being secondarily induced by the multiple bile ductules. The initial lesion may be clusters of multiple bile ductules, namely von Meyenburgh complexes, resembling the initial lesion of the liver cyst associated with adult polycystic kidney disease. However, in congenital hepatic fibrosis, the abnormal bile ductules maintain their communication with the biliary tree and, as a result, only microcysts are formed. In adult polycystic kidney disease, the abnormal bile ductules lose their communication with the biliary tree and, therefore, dilate markedly and form large cysts.

The mechanism for the development of multiple bile ductules in congenital hepatic fibrosis is unknown. It has been suggested that bile ductular proliferation might result from a disproportionate overgrowth of the biliary epithelium (Nakanuma, Liver, 1982; 2: 346). A similar disorder affecting the epithelium of the large bile ducts might account for Caroli's syndrome associated with congenital hepatic fibrosis. A similar mechanism might explain the dilatation of the renal collecting tubules and the dilatation of the pancreatic ducts, two extrahepatic malformations which may be associated with congenital hepatic fibrosis.

Aetiology

Congenital hepatic fibrosis is an inherited malformation, transmitted as an autosomal recessive trait (Kerr, QJMed, 1961; 30:91; Alvarez, JPediat, 1981; 99:370). The parents, presumably heterozygous, are phenotypically normal. Males and females are equally affected and several siblings may have the condition. Consanguinity increases the risk of congenital hepatic fibrosis.

The prevalence of congenital hepatic fibrosis has not been established, but it is certainly very low and might be of the same order of magnitude as that of another autosomal recessive liver disease, Wilson's disease, at an incidence of about 1:100 000.[1] There is no ethnic predominance.

Manifestations and diagnosis

The main consequence of congenital hepatic fibrosis is portal hypertension, which is likely to be present from the patient's birth. The disease is recognized at the first episode of gastrointestinal bleeding due to ruptured oesophageal varices, which occurs usually between the ages of 5 and 20 years, sometimes later. In a few patients, the disease is recognized before any gastrointestinal bleeding, because of blood disorders due to hypersplenism, abdominal discomfort resulting from an enlarged spleen, or the presence of abdominal collateral venous circulation.

On clinical examination, the liver is often, but not constantly, enlarged. Splenomegaly is present in most of the patients. Abdominal collateral venous circulation, Cruveilhier syndrome in some patients, is often visible. Ascites is absent. There is no symptom or sign indicating liver failure, in particular jaundice or spider naevi. The liver function tests are normal, except for moderately increased alkaline phosphatase and γ-glutamyl transferase in a few patients. Endoscopic and/or radiographic examinations demonstrate oesophageal varices. Ultrasonography and/or computed tomography show that the liver is often enlarged, the portal vein is patent (which excludes extrahepatic portal hypertension), the spleen is enlarged, and portacaval collateral circulation is present; the venous phase of coeliac and mesenteric arteriography would provide similar information. Histological examination of a hepatic specimen taken by needle biopsy demonstrates the typical liver lesion in most of the patients; however, especially if the specimen is small, the lesion may be missed because, as mentioned above, some of the portal spaces may be normal.

Course and complications

The course of the disease is dominated by recurrent episodes of gastrointestinal bleeding, the frequency of which varies widely from patient to patient. The episodes of gastrointestinal bleeding are often well tolerated and are usually not followed by hepatic encephalopathy, ascites, or jaundice. The patient's death is due to massive bleeding but not to liver failure. Thus, the course of congenital hepatic fibrosis resembles that of extrahepatic portal hypertension and differs from that of cirrhosis.

In a few patients, in the absence of Caroli's syndrome, congenital hepatic fibrosis is complicated by recurrent episodes of bacterial cholangitis. Uncontrolled, severe bacterial cholangitis may cause the death of such patients.

Associated malformations

Congenital hepatic fibrosis is often associated with Caroli's syndrome, either clinically silent or determining cholangitis (see below).

Congenital hepatic fibrosis is likewise often associated with a renal malformation consisting of ectatic collecting tubules, resembling sponge kidney (Kerr, ClinRadiol, 1962; 12:85); however, dilatation affects both the medullary and cortical portions of the collecting tubules in congenital hepatic fibrosis, whereas dilatation is limited to the medullary portion in sponge kidney (Clermont, CanMedAssJ, 1967; 97:1272).[2] This renal malformation is clinically silent except for haematuria and/or urinary infection in a few patients. Dilatation of the collecting tubules can be demonstrated by intravenous pyelography showing enlarged kidneys and coarse streaking of the medulla (Kerr, ClinRadiol, 1962; 12:85). These radiological abnormalities are present in about two-thirds of the patients (Kerr, ClinRadiol, 1962; 12:85; Alvarez, JPediat, 1981; 99: 370); their presence is good evidence for, but their absence is not an argument against, the diagnosis of congenital hepatic fibrosis. In some patients with a normal intravenous pyelogram, histological examination of the kidneys may show ectatic collecting tubules (Clermont, CanMedAssocJ, 1967; 97:1272).

In most patients, dilatation of collecting tubules remains stable. However, in a few of them, the ectatic segments lose their communications with the urinary tract and transform into large renal cysts; the renal malformation then resembles adult polycystic kidney disease (Dupont, AnnIntMed, 1978; 88:514). This transformation accounts for the large renal cysts detectable by intravenous pyelography or ultrasonography in a certain number of patients with congenital hepatic fibrosis (Alvarez, JPediat, 1981; 99:370). The transformation may be rapid and take place in infancy or, more often, is more progressive, large renal cysts being formed only over 30 or 40 years. In patients with large renal cysts, the renal malformation may cause renal failure and/or arterial hypertension.

Other associated malformations are uncommon and include duplication of the intrahepatic portal vein branches (Odièvre, Radiol, 1977; 122:427), cystic dysplasia of the pancreas (Kerr, QJMed, 1961; 30:91), intestinal lymphangectasia (Chagnon, GastrClinBiol, 1982; 6:326), pulmonary emphysema (Williams, JClinPath, 1964; 17:135), cerebellar haemangioma (Wagenvoort, MayoClinProc, 1962; 37:301), aneurysms of renal and cerebral arteries, and cleft palate (Kerr, QJMed, 1961; 30:91).

Treatment

Active bleeding from ruptured oesophageal varices requires blood transfusions and oesophageal tamponade.

Endoscopic sclerotherapy of oesophageal varices can be recommended for the prevention of recurrent bleedings, although this procedure has not been specifically evaluated in congenital hepatic fibrosis. However, the efficacy of sclerotherapy has been demonstrated for the prevention of variceal bleeding in cirrhosis and can be reasonably expected to be effective in congenital hepatic fibrosis.

In patients in whom sclerotherapy is inefficient, poorly tolerated, or not possible, a surgical portacaval shunt can be considered.

Hepatic encephalopathy and liver failure after a portacaval shunt would be less common in patients with congenital hepatic fibrosis than in those with cirrhosis (Kerr, Gut, 1978; 19:514; Alvarez, JPediat, 1981; 99:370)

Splenectomy, which has been performed in a few patients in whom hypersplenism had not been related to congenital hepatic fibrosis, does not prevent occurrence or recurrence of gastro-intestinal bleeding and may be followed by portal vein thrombosis, preventing a subsequent surgical portacaval shunt (Benhamou, personal observation).

Operations or invasive investigations on the biliary tree, such as cholecystectomy, choledocotomy, T-tube drainage, intraoperative cholangiography, or endoscopic retrograde cholangiography, must be avoided because of the risk of inducing bacterial cholangitis.

Caroli's syndrome

Caroli's syndrome is a congenital malformation characterized by multifocal dilatation of the segmental bile ducts. The main consequence of this malformation is recurrent bacterial cholangitis. The malformation described by Caroli (SemHopPar, 1958; 34:136) is not a single entity and, for this reason, the term Caroli's syndrome is more appropriate than Caroli's disease.

Pathology, classification, and aetiology

The lesion of Caroli's syndrome consists of multifocal dilatation of the segmental bile ducts. The ectatic portions form cysts of various sizes, separated by portions of bile ducts which are normal or regularly dilated. The multifocal dilatation may be diffuse, affecting the whole intrahepatic biliary tree (although it may be more marked in one part of the liver), or may be confined to a part of the liver, often the left lobe or a segment of the left lobe (Caroli, SemHopPar, 1958; 34:488). The number of cysts is large in the diffuse form and limited, usually less than 10, in the localized form.

Multifocal dilatation of the segmental bile ducts is not a single entity. In the majority of cases, it is associated with congenital hepatic fibrosis.[2] In this type of Caroli's syndrome, the distribution of multifocal dilatation is diffuse. The malformation is transmitted as an autosomal recessive trait (as congenital hepatic fibrosis) and may be associated with the same renal malformation as that associated with congenital hepatic fibrosis.

In a small number of cases, multifocal dilatation of the segmental bile ducts is not associated with congenital hepatic fibrosis. In such cases, multifocal dilatation is often confined to one part of the liver. This type of Caroli's syndrome is not inherited and is usually not associated with a renal malformation, but may be associated with other malformations of the biliary tree, in particular choledochal cysts (Loubeau, ArchSurg, 1976; 111:1384).

Manifestations and diagnosis

Caroli's syndrome, which is likely to be present at birth, remains asymptomatic for the first 5 to 20 years of the patient's life, sometimes longer, and in a few cases for the patient's whole life. Asymptomatic Caroli's syndrome is unrecognized, except in patients in whom congenital hepatic fibrosis has been diagnosed and multifocal dilatation of the segmental bile ducts has been suspected and demonstrated by ultrasonography or computed tomography.

In most patients, the first episode of cholangitis occurs in the absence of any apparent cause. In a few, the first episode of cholangitis is the consequence of a surgical operation or an invasive investigation on the biliary tree, such as cholecystectomy, choledochotomy, T-tube drainage, intraoperative cholangiography, or endoscopic retrograde cholangiography (Benhamou, personal observation; Grumbach, ArchAnatCytolPathol, 1954; 30:74; Clermont, CanMedAssJ, 1967; 97:1272; Erlinger, PressMed, 1969; 77:1189).

The main and often the only symptom of cholangitis due to Caroli's syndrome is fever, in contrast to cholangitis complicating common bile duct stones in which fever is usually accompanied by pain and/or jaundice. As a consequence, the first episodes of fever may be not attributed to cholangitis.

On clinical examination, the liver is usually enlarged. There is no sign or symptom indicating liver failure. In patients with Caroli's syndrome associated with congenital hepatic fibrosis, manifestations of portal hypertension are present. Liver function tests are normal except for alkaline phosphatase and γ-glutamyl transferase, which may be moderately increased.

The best procedures for the diagnosis of Caroli's syndrome are ultrasonography and computed tomography, which show cystic formations of various size, diffuse or limited to a part of the liver, and associated or not associated with tubular dilatation of segmental bile ducts. Ultrasonography and computed tomography show tiny dots within dilated intrahepatic bile ducts (the central dot sign); these intraluminal dots correspond to intraluminal portal veins and this finding indicates that the portal radicles are surrounded by dilated intrahepatic bile ducts (Choi, Radiol, 1990; 174:161). Computed tomography after intravenous injection of biliary contrast may show opacification of cysts and dilated segmental bile ducts. Cystic formation may be demonstrated by intraoperative cholangiography, postoperative cholangiography through a T-tube, or endoscopic retrograde cholangiography; these three procedures must not be used in patients with asymptomatic Caroli's syndrome, but can be employed in patients with Caroli's syndrome already complicated by cholangitis.

The other imaging procedures are of less interest for the diagnosis of Caroli's syndrome. Radiocolloid liver scan shows cold areas corresponding to the large cysts. Hepatobiliary scan shows cold areas in the early phase which become hot at a late phase of imaging (Stillman, Gastro, 1981; 80:1295).

Course and complications

The course of Caroli's syndrome is dominated by recurrent episodes of cholangitis, the frequency of which varies widely: some patients experience 10 to 20 episodes a year, whereas others suffer only 1 or 2 episodes a year. In patients with frequent episodes of cholangitis, the prognosis is poor: generally, 5 to 10 years after the onset of recurrent cholangitis such patients die from uncontrolled biliary bacterial infection.

Cholangitis may be complicated by liver abscesses, septicaemia, extrahepatic abscesses, and secondary amyloidosis (Fevery, Gut, 1972; 13:604).

Cholangitis often induces the formation of intracystic stones (Mathias, ActaHepatogastrBelg, 1978; 25:30), which are usually recognized on ultrasonography or endoscopic retrograde cholangiography, but may be missed by computed tomography when not calcified. These stones can migrate from the cysts into the common bile duct and then cause biliary pain, cholestasis, and/or acute pancreatitis (Sahel, NouvPresseMed, 1976; 5:2067). Cholangiocarcinoma develops in some patients with Caroli's syndrome (Dayton, AmJSurg, 1983; 145:41).

Associated malformations

In patients with Caroli's syndrome and congenital hepatic fibrosis, the malformations described in association with congenital hepatic fibrosis alone may obviously be present. In patients affected by Caroli's syndrome with or, more often, without congenital hepatic fibrosis, an associated choledochal cyst is relatively common (Loubeau, ArchSurg, 1976; 111:1384). Exceptionally, Caroli's syndrome is associated with Laurence–Moon–Biedl syndrome (Tsuchiya, ArchSurg, 1977; 112:82).

Treatment

Episodes of bacterial cholangitis are treated by appropriate antibiotics. The prevention of the recurrences of bacterial cholangitis is difficult. Periodic administration of antibiotics seems efficacious in some patients but completely inefficient in others. T-tube drainage is not effective and may be dangerous in patients with associated congenital hepatic fibrosis; large amounts of water and electrolytes, secreted by the multiple bile ductules, may be lost through the T-tube, which may result in severe dehydration (Turnberg, Gastro, 1968; 54:1155). Administration of chenodesoxycholic acid may be useful for the prevention and treatment of intracystic stones. Although this treatment induced the disappearance of intracystic stones in one patient (Kutz, ActaHepatogastrBelg, 1978; 25:398), it was not clearly efficacious in others (Mathias, ActaHepatogastrBelg, 1978; 25:30). Ursodiol seems to be more efficient in the treatment and prevention of intracystic stones and its administration has been recommended to all patients with Caroli's syndrome (Ros, Lancet, 1993; 342:404). Transhepatic intubation and drainage of the biliary tree have been used successfully in a small number of patients (Witlin, Surgery, 1982; 91.205). Surgical biliointestinal anastomoses or endoscopic papillotomy may facilitate the passage of stones into the intestine, but cannot be recommended because these procedures may increase the frequency and severity of the episodes of cholangitis (Watts, ArchSurg, 1974; 108:592). In the localized form of Caroli's syndrome, partial hepatectomy is indicated and excellent results can be expected (Ramond, DigDisSci, 1984; 29:367). In the diffuse form, if the cysts clearly predominate in one part of the liver, partial hepatectomy can also be envisaged. However, in such patients, partial hepatectomy is difficult because of associated congenital hepatic fibrosis and portal hypertension, and the long-term results may be compromised because multifocal dilatation affecting the remaining liver may be the source of recurrent cholangitis (Ramond, 1984). In the diffuse form without predominance of the cysts in any part of the liver, complicated by severe recurrent cholangitis, liver transplantation might be considered.

References

1. Scheimber IH and Sternlieb L. *Wilson's disease*. Philadelphia: Saunders, 1984.
2. Fauvert R and Benhamou JP. Congenital hepatic fibrosis. In Schaffner F, Sherlock S, and Leevy CM. *The liver and its diseases*. New York: Intercontinental Medical Book Corporation, 1974: 283–8.

12

Viral infections of the liver

12.1 Viral hepatitis

12.1.1 Introduction

Mario Rizzetto

Definition of viral hepatitis

Although many viruses can affect liver function and morphology indirectly as a result of systemic infections, only a minority are truly hepatropic, that is, infectious to the liver itself, producing hepatitis as the major clinical manifestation. The term 'viral hepatitis' refers to disease caused by this subgroup. Although, taxonomically it should encompass infections caused by exotic viruses such as yellow fever and disease due to Ebola, Marburg, and Lassa fever viruses, the term 'viral hepatitis' is conventionally used only for a few diseases caused by several viruses, whose discovery and characterization in recent years has constituted one of the most spectacular successes of modern clinical research.

Historical background and nomenclature

Although viral hepatitis is a disease of antiquity and epidemic jaundice is mentioned in the Talmud, the infectious nature of the disease was not recognized until the end of the nineteenth century.

The first description of 'hepatitis B' dates back to 1885 when Lurman, a public health officer in Bremen, Germany, gave a detailed report of an outbreak of jaundice that developed among workers of a local company vaccinated against smallpox with glycerinized human serum (Lurman, KlinWschr, 1885; 22:20).

Transmission studies in human volunteers in the late 1930s and during the Second World War provided the first informations about the infectivity, mode of transmission, and properties of the hepatitis agents; they suggested that two distinct viral agents, lacking cross-immunity, were responsible for military outbreaks, and McCallum (Lancet, 1947; ii:691) introduced the classic terminology of hepatitis A virus (HAV) and hepatitis B virus (HBV).

Faeces were shown to induce hepatitis A (infectious hepatitis) by the oral route; the incubation period was 15 to 30 days. Acute-phase serum was shown to induce hepatitis B (serum hepatitis), after several months, when given by the parenteral route.

Volunteer transmission studies by Krugman and associates in the late 1950s and early 1960s using the newly discovered assays for serum transaminases, contributed significantly to the understanding of the characteristics of the two hepatitis 'viruses' (identified by Krugman as the MS1 strain, causing hepatitis A and the MS2 strain, causing hepatitis B).[1]

When the major breakthrough arrived the ground was already prepared. The discovery of the Australia antigen, now called hepatitis B surface antigen (HBsAg), by Blumberg and his associates in the mid-1960s (Blumberg, JAMA, 1965; 191:541), and the recognition by Prince (PNAS, 1968; 60:814) of its specific relation to hepatitis B, started the contemporary era in the field of hepatitis. Intensive research led quickly to the identification of the mature hepatitis B virion (Dane, Lancet, 1970; i:695), to the recognition of its antigenic complexity (Magnius, JImmunol, 1972; 109:1017) and oncogenic potential (Sherlock, Lancet, 1970; i:1243), to the mapping and cloning of its DNA genome,[2] and later to the development of a safe and effective vaccine.[3]

Research on hepatitis B opened an unexpected new area: in 1977 a discrepancy in immunofluorescence testing for HBV antigens in the liver led Rizzetto and his associates to the discovery of the delta antigen (Rizzetto, Gut, 1977; 18:997), which was subsequently shown to be related to a new RNA virus designated the hepatitis delta virus (HDV).

The lessons learned from work on hepatitis B also helped in the discovery of HAV. Using an immunoelectron-microscopic technique, previously applied to reveal the nucleocapsid of HBV, Feinstone *et al.* (Science, 1973; 182:1026) identified HAV in 1973 in immunocomplexes from faeces to which serum of a patient convalescent from hepatitis A had been added.

When testing for hepatitis A and B was made generally available, it became clear that the two viruses did not explain all causes of viral hepatitis, as many patients lacked markers of either infection. Thus the concept emerged of a new variant of viral hepatitis; it was called 'non-A, non-B hepatitis' to highlight the fact that the diagnosis was based on exclusion criteria, not on specific positive evidence (Feinstone, NEJM, 1975; 292:767). The magnitude of the problem was best seen in relation to blood transfusion: in the wake of the widespread and increasing application of blood transfusion and plasma substitution, hepatitis continued to occur in 5 to 10 per cent of the recipients of blood products, despite almost total control of HBV.

However, efforts to identify the major aetiological agent of endemic non-A non-B hepatitis met with failure or with spurious results until 1989. The breakthrough this time was not fortuitous but resulted from exhaustive research involving the use of sophisticated technological methods. Several thousands clones of genetic material from a serum containing a putative agent of non-A non-B hepatitis were systematically analysed. Houghton and associates (Choo, Science, 1989; 244:359) thus identified a clone that met the criteria for being a new viral genome and provided the key to the characterization of the hepatitis C virus (HCV). Meanwhile a novel agent responsible of outbreaks of epidemic non-A non-B hepatitis in tropical and subtropical areas and named the hepatitis E virus

(HEV) had been identified in the early 1980s by epidemiological analysis and human transmission studies (Khuroo, AmJMed, 1980; 68:818).

The five viruses recognized by the end of the 1980s account for 85 to 90 per cent of viral hepatitides occurring at temperate latitudes. Two new viruses have seen since been proposed to fill the remaining nosological gap. An agent thought to be responsible for sporadic non-A non-E hepatitis transmitted through the orofaecal route was described in 1994 and called the hepatitis F virus (HVF) for its French origin and in accordance with the sequence of hepatitis viruses discovery (Deka, JVirol, 1994; 6:7810). However, the existence of this separate agent has not been further substantiated; an adenovirus-like agent cultivable *in vitro* was present in the basic stool used for the identication of the putative HFV, and the proposed HFV was probably an ubiquitous, non-pathogenic, intestinal resident virus that largely colonizes stools during liver injury.[4] More recently, two different reseach groups have identified a novel hepatotropic flavivirus named GB virus-C by one group (Muerhoff, JVirol, 1995; 69:5621) and hepatitis G virus (HGV) by the other group (Linnen, Science, 1996; 271:505); they appear to be the same virus. Sensitive and specific diagnostic assays based on nucleic acid identification have been developed to detect infected individuals. The role of GBV-C HGV in acute chronic liver disease is under investigation; at present it seems only marginal.

References

1. Krugman S, Giles JP, and Hammond J. Infectious hepatitis; evidence for two distinctive clinical, epidemiological and immunological types of infection. *Journal of the American Medical Association,* 1967; **200**: 365–73.
2. Tiollais P, Charnay P, and Vyas GN. Biology of hepatitis B virus. *Science,* 1981; **213**: 406–11.
3. Szmuness W, *et al.* Hepatitis B vaccine: demonstration of efficacy in a controlled clinical trial in a high risk population. *New England Journal of Medicine,* 1980; **303**: 833–51.
4. Pillot J, Meng J, Maillard P, and Dauguet C. The presumed hepatitis F virus. In Rizzetto M., Purcell RH, Gerin JL, and Verme G, eds. *Viral hepatitis and liver diseases.* Turin, Italy: Minerva Medica, 1997: 399–401.

12.1.2 The viruses of hepatitis

12.1.2.1 Structure, replication, and laboratory diagnosis of hepatitis viruses

Wolfram H. Gerlich and Reiner Thomssen

Introduction
Definition

Five human hepatitis viruses have been identified, the hepatitis A (HAV), B (HBV), C (HCV), D (HDV), and E (HEV) viruses.[1] Recently, a blood-transmissible virus was identified in certain cases of chronic hepatitis and termed GB-virus C (GBV-C; Simons,

NatMed, 1995; 271:505) or hepatitis G virus (HGV; Linnen, Science, 1996; 271:505). Neither its final designation nor its clinical significance as a hepatitis virus have been established, but for the sake of description the term 'HGV' has been provisionally adopted; nevertheless, evidence is accumulating that HGV does not replicate in the liver and does not cause hepatitis.

The hepatitis viruses have a very narrow host range. Although man seems to be their reservoir, the human viruses can be transmitted to chimpanzees, and to a certain extent to other non-human primates. Non-human viruses related to HAV, HBV, and 'HGV' are found in certain other primates. All these hepatitis viruses either do not replicate at all in cell culture (HCV, HEV, HGV) or are difficult to adapt (HAV, HBV, HDV).

Although all hepatitis viruses (except possibly for HGV) are pathogenic *in vivo*, their cytotoxicity for the infected cell appears to be low. Cytotoxic variants may be selected in cell culture (HAV) or evolve spontaneously *in vivo* (HBV, HDV, HGV?). However, it is believed that most of the pathogenicity is contributed by the host's immune system against viral proteins. Cytotoxic T lymphocytes seem to be the major factor both for pathogenicity and/or for the resolution of the infection (HAV, HBV, HCV), but antibodies are also required for virus elimination and may contribute to immune-complex disease if virus replication is not stopped by the T-cell-mediated immune reaction (HBV, HCV).

Taxonomy

In spite of their common organotropism, host range, and disease manifestations, the hepatitis viruses are not phylogenetically related to one another. They have (except for HCV and 'HGV') completely different genomic organizations, mechanisms of replication, and survival strategies in their host population. Table 1 summarizes the taxonomy and some important structural, diagnostic, and biological features of the six viruses. The faecal–oral transmitted HAV and HEV are small, non-enveloped, plus-strand RNA viruses that do not cause persistent infection or chronic hepatitis *in vivo*. The parenterally transmitted HBV/HDV, HCV, and HGV are enveloped, and they may cause persistent viraemia in a large or even predominant proportion of infected individuals. The overall genomic organization and the virion structure of HEV are reminiscent of the family *Caliciviridae* but its non-structural proteins are different; thus it has not been assigned to a known virus family but remains unclassified. 'HGV' or GBV-C is similar to two isolates, GBV-A and -B, from marmoset monkeys (Muerhoff, JVirol, 1995; 69:5621) and these may form their own genus within the family *Flaviviridae*; an official decision has not yet been made on this issue. The following sections describe the structure and replication of the five hepatitis viruses and 'HGV', indications for undertaking diagnostic tests, and finally, a discussion of the significance of the results. Full descriptions of the diseases will be presented in other chapters of this book.

Hepatitis A virus

HAV is the major cause of acute hepatitis world-wide. It is highly prevalent in virtually all areas with suboptimal hygiene of water supply and food production.

Table 1 Classification and biological and clinical properties of human hepatitis viruses

Property	A	B	C	D	E
Virus family Genus[a]	Picornaviridae Hepatovirus	Hepadnaviridae[a] Orthohepadnavirus	Flaviviridae Hepacivirus	Satellites Deltavirus	Not classified
Virion size[b] (nm)	28	42	40–60	36	34
Genome type[c]	RNA^+	ds/ssDNA,c	RNA^+	$RNA,^-c$	RNA^+
Genome size	7.5	3.2	9.3	1.7	7.4
Envelope protein	No	HBsAg, L, M, S	E1, E2	HBsAg, L.M.S	No?
Capsid protein	VP1–VP4	HBcAg	core	HDAg	ORF-2
Transmission	Faecal–oral	Parenteral	Parenteral	Parenteral	Faecal–oral
Maximum titre[d]	10^9/g	10^9/ml	10^6/ml	10^{11}/ml	?
Prevalence	High	High	Moderate	Low regional	Regional
Fulminant course	Uncommon	Uncommon	Uncommon	Common	In pregnancy
Chronic state	No	Often	Very often	Very often	No
Liver cancer	No	Yes	Yes	Yes	No
Therapy	No	Interferon[e] Lamivudin	Interferon[e] Ribavirin	(Interferon)[e]	No
Vaccine	Killed virus	Recombinant HBsAg	No	Recombinant HBsAg	No

[a] All viruses form new genera in their family; *Hepadnaviridae* a new family; [b] all viruses are spherical; [c] + serves also as mRNA; −, mRNA has antigenome sense; ds/ss, double-stranded/single-stranded; c, circular; [d] infectivity per g stool or ml serum, respectively; [e] α-interferon is partially effective in selected patients.

Structure, replication, and course of infection[2,3]

Virus structure and assembly

HAV belongs to the family of *Picornaviridae*, in which it forms its own genus, hepatovirus.[4] Like all picornaviruses, HAV consists of a spherical protein shell (the capsid) with an outer diameter of approximately 27 nm and an inner diameter of approximately 20 nm (Fig. 1). It encapsidates a single-stranded RNA of *c.* 7.5 kb with a small, covalently bound protein (Vpg) at the 5′ end and a poly(A) tail at the 3′ end (Fig. 2). The capsid assembles from a precursor protein, P1, which first forms a 14*s* (Svedberg units) pentamer. Thereafter, the pentamers assemble at the 12 corners of a pentagondodecaeder. During assembly, P1 is cleaved into proteins 1AB, C, and D, which are of similar size. Thus, the capsid is built up of 180 protein subunits that assume the icosahedral, pseudo-T3 symmetry. For maturation and infectivity of the virus, protein 1AB has to cleave itself slowly into the very small 1A and the larger 1B fragments. For historical reasons, the terms VP1 for 1D, VP2 for 1B, VP3 for 1C, and VP4 for 1A are also used for these proteins (see Figs 1 and 2).

The main fraction of the RNA-containing capsids has a buoyant density of 1.32 to 1.34 g/ml in caesium chloride centrifugation and a sedimentation coefficient of 156 to 160*s*. However, particles with higher density and empty particles with lower density also exist.

Stability

It is part of the viral survival strategy to be very resistant to adverse environmental conditions. Virions survive pH 1 for 2 h, which

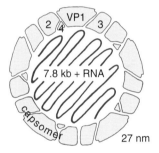

Fig. 1. Schematic presentation of HAV.

favours gastric passage; they are resistant to organic solvents, and to excretion via the bile and the intestine. The particles can withstand dryness and heat (60°C, 10 h), which explains their long survival in the environment. HAV is further stabilized by Mg^{2+} ions and may then survive short heating to even 80°C, in sea water, for example in clam dishes. HAV is, however, sensitive to formaldehyde and to strong oxidants such as chlorine.[2]

Virus attachment and entry

In vivo uptake of the virus occurs orally or, in rare cases, by transfusion of blood or clotting factors. In the latter case the virus can reach the liver directly via the bloodstream. Usually it will have to pass the gastrointestinal tract, but it is not known where it enters the bloodstream or whether primary replication occurs in mucosal cells. Attachment in cell culture is rather inefficient and seems to require calcium (Stapleton, JInfDis, 1991; 164:1098). Recently a novel, mucin-like, membrane glycoprotein was found, which reacts

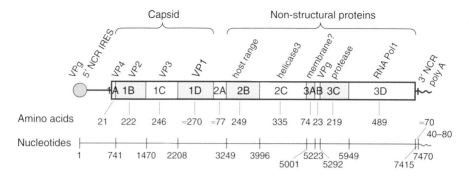

Fig. 2. Genome map of HAV. VPg, genome-linked viral protein; 5′ NCR, 5′ non-coding region; IRES, internal ribosome entry site; VP, viral protein. Sections 1A to 3D represent the cleavage products of the polyprotein precursor.

with monoclonal antibodies that block the susceptibility of cell cultures to infection with HAV (Kaplan, EMBOJ, 1996, 15:4282). It is assumed that the virus is taken up by this and/or other unknown receptors, and that the genome is released from the endosome as is the case with many other viruses. Disassembly and uncoating of the virus seems to be a limiting step for the relatively low replication activity of HAV in cell culture. When released, the genomes enter the replicative cycle.

Genomic organization

All *Picornaviridae* encode one polyprotein by their RNA genome (Fig. 2); the RNA genome can be directly translated by the host cell's machinery for protein synthesis without the involvement of further viral factors. Thus, the RNA is infectious if transferred to the cytoplasm. By definition, such viral genomes are termed plus-strand RNA. In *Picornaviridae* a shorter, subgenomic RNA does not need to be made, in contrast to some other plus-strand RNA viruses such as HEV.

Number and function of genes

The polyprotein precursor of *Picornaviridae* is cleaved by the viral protease(s) into 11 proteins that are derived from three intermediates, P1, P2, and P3. P1 forms the capsid and is subsequently cleaved to form proteins 1A to 1D. P2 is cleaved into proteins 2A, 2B (with unknown function), and 2C, which is probably a GTP-binding protein, and a helicase type III.[4] Protein 2B is important for adaptation in host range and cell culture. In HAV, protein 2A is not a protease as in other picornaviruses and is smaller than originally believed. In fact, the primary cleavage by 3C protease occurs between P2A/B before P1 is cleaved into the structural proteins. Thus, a VPx is generated as a 1D/2A intermediate that is cleaved after encapsidation of the RNA (Bishop, Virology, 1993; 197:616). P3A/B is the precursor of Vpg (3B); 3C is a cystein protease of the chymotrypsin-like protease family, the crystal structure of which has been analysed (Allaire, Nature, 1994; 369:72). Protease 3C cleaves first at P2A/B and later at the other sites except for P1A/D, which is probably cleaved autocatalytically. Protein 3D is the RNA-dependent RNA polymerase present in all supergroup-1, positive-strand viruses. Proteins 3C and 3D may be targets for antiviral therapy, but antiviral substances are not presently available.

Internal ribosomal entry site

The viral RNA genome has to compete with cellular mRNA for the ribosomes. Secondary and tertiary structural elements at the 5′ non-coding region of the RNA bind certain host factors that govern the ribosome to initiate protein synthesis at base 735 or preferably at 741. The structure of the HAV internal ribosomal entry site more closely resembles that of the picornaviral genera cardio- and aphto-viruses than of entero- or rhinoviruses. However, the internal ribosomal entry site of HAV is much less active than that of the cardiovirus, EMCvirus. The internal ribosomal entry site of HAV may contain negative elements because certain mutations enhance its translation activity in cell culture (Schultz, JVirol, 1996; 47:260). Furthermore, defective, interfering RNAs of HAV accumulate and inhibit production of complete HAV (Nüesch, Virology, 1988; 165: 419).

Replication

The 3D polymerase transcribes the genomic plus strand into the RNA minus strand. Since RNA-dependent polymerases require some type of primer, it is assumed that the hydroxyl group of a Tyr in the Vpg serves this function. Alternatively, a 3′ hairpin backfold serves as primer, and is linked after cleavage and transesterification to Vpg.[4] A relatively large number of plus strands is transcribed from the minus strand, resulting in replicative intermediates containing both strands. RNA replication seems to occur at the membrane of the smooth endoplasmic reticulum. The new plus strand may enter another cycle of replication or serve as a template for polyprotein translation. When a critical concentration of P1 has accumulated, procapsids are formed that encapsidate plus-strand RNA.

Virulence

Replication of HAV in cell culture is slow, requiring many days. Cell cultures usually survive and develop persistent infection. The virus remains cell-bound, but does not accumulate to toxic concentrations because its replication is down-regulated, possibly by a host protein that binds to a 3′ terminal stem-loop structure (Kusov, JVirol, 1996; 70:1890). *In vivo* the virus is secreted into bile and blood, resulting in viraemia and virucopria before the onset of liver damage. There seems to be an inverse relation between the ability to grow *in vitro* and virulence *in vivo*. Cell culture-adapted HAV strains from human or non-human primate origin may be used as live, attenuated vaccines because of their low virulence in man (Emerson, JInfDis, 1996, 173:592). In contrast to other picornaviruses, HAV has no 2A or leader protease able to suppress protein synthesis in the host cell.

Variability and genotypes

HAV is one of the genetically most stable viruses known. Its genome has only 28 per cent sequence homology to other picornaviruses, but within various HAV strains the homology is above 85 per cent. A genome region at the junction of the *1D* and *2A* genes is particularly variable; it has been used to define genotypes of HAV with less than 85 per cent nucleotide-sequence identity in this region, and subgenotypes with less than 92.5 per cent identity. Genotype I, with its subtypes A and B, has the highest prevalence world-wide. Genotypes IIIA and B are also rather common; genotypes II and VII are known only from one isolate each. Genotypes IV, V, and VI have only been isolated from various Old World monkeys. Genotype IIIA has also been found in New World monkeys. Intratypic differences are sufficient to follow up infectious chains by reverse transcriptase-PCR (**RT-PCR**) and sequencing (Robertson, JGenVirol, 1992; 73:1369).

Antigenicity

HAV capsids, both complete and empty, are excellent immunogens and antigens. Neutralizing antibodies are induced in high titre by natural infection and often persist at detectable concentrations lifelong. In spite of this heavy immune pressure, antibodies against all isolates, including those from non-human primates, are cross-neutralizing. Escape mutants to neutralizing monoclonal antibodies can be selected in cell culture, although they revert rapidly in infected non-human primates. Most mutations are found around amino acids 65 to 74 of VP3 and 102 to 114 of VP1. Uncleaved P1 and isolated virus proteins do not induce neutralizing antibodies, except for an aminoterminal peptide from VP1. These data suggest that the immunodominant neutralizing epitope(s) are formed by surface-exposed loops from both VP1 and VP3, and are assembled only after proteolytic cleavage of the pentameric precursor (Ping, JVirol, 1992; 66:2208). However, the immunodominant sites can be mimicked by peptide sequences not present in HAV (Mattioli, JVirol, 1995; 69:5294).

Course of infection (see Fig. 3)

About 10 days after uptake, HAV can be found in stools. Titres as high as 10^{-9} infectious virus particles per g stool may be reached during the incubation period. Viraemia parallels virucopria but only reaches infectivity titres of 10^{-4}/ml.[1]

HAV shedding decreases by the time of onset of hepatitis and usually becomes undetectable within a few days. Prolonged viral shedding or viraemia can be observed up to many weeks in about 10 per cent of all cases.

The IgM antibody titre to HAV (**IgM anti-HA**) rises shortly before the onset of symptoms and reaches a peak soon after. It decreases within weeks or months to undetectable concentrations.

The IgG antibody titre to HAV (**IgG anti-HA**) increases during the acute phase and decreases very slowly during convalescence. Even after asymptomatic infection the antibody remains detectable

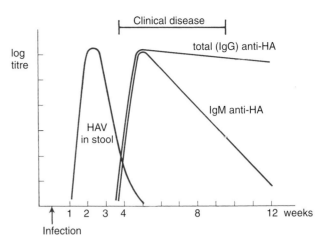

Fig. 3. Schematic course of an HAV infection.

for decades, and only becomes serologically negative in old age. At least a fraction of IgG anti-HA is virus-neutralizing.

Virological diagnosis[2]

Table 2 shows the clinical or epidemiological questions that may be asked about HAV infection and the assays that may provide answers.

Total anti-HA antibody
Diagnostic significance

The universal diagnostic feature is total antibody in serum or plasma (serum IgG, IgA, IgM) against HAV (**anti-HA**). It indicates previous or continuing infection by HAV and resistance to further HAV infection. Healthy individuals with anti-HA are immune. Anti-HA-negative individuals are susceptible to HAV infection. After a recent contact they may experience disease within 4 weeks or develop an asymptomatic infection. Individuals negative for anti-HA can be passively immunized with normal immune globulin if they have just been subjected to an immediate high risk of infection but are still without symptoms.

During acute hepatitis, a negative assay for anti-HA excludes HAV as an aetiological agent. A positive result for anti-HA is virtually always found in acute, symptomatic HAV infection but is not sufficient to diagnose HAV as the aetiological agent of an acute hepatitis. In many areas of the world the majority of the population (especially older individuals) are positive for anti-HA owing to previous infection, which was often asymptomatic. In these areas, acute hepatitis in adults and even in children is often caused by

Table 2 Diagnostic features of HAV infections

Problem	Measure
Any contact with HAV?	Total anti-HAV
Immune or susceptible for HAV?	Total anti-HAV
Active infection with HAV?	
Aetiology of acute hepatitis?	IgM anti-HAV
Asymptomatic HAV infection?	IgM anti-HAV
Incubation period of HAV?	HAV in stool
Infective for HAV?	HAV in stool

other agents. Testing for IgM anti-HA is required for diagnosis in such cases. In regions or age groups with a low prevalence of HAV infection, a positive anti-HA is more likely to indicate that HAV is the actual agent of an acute hepatitis. Even in such cases, the diagnosis should be verified by assay of IgM anti-HA. Some experts advocate assay of IgM anti-HA only for the diagnosis of acute hepatitis A. However, information on immunity or susceptibility to HAV can only be obtained from an assay of total anti-HA, and this is always relevant. Inversely, a positive result for IgM anti-HA should be confirmed by an assay of total anti-HA. Active vaccination with HAV induces transiently low titres of IgM anti-HA.

Passive acquisition

Infants are anti-HA-positive up to 8 months after birth if their mother is anti-HA-positive. Blood transfusion in high-prevalence areas will often transmit detectable quantities of anti-HA, but titres are low and disappear rapidly. Normal immune globulins from unselected plasma pools are required to contain moderate to high concentrations of anti-HA. Special preparations of immune globulin against other agents will usually also contain anti-HA. If anti-HA testing and the administration of immune globulin are scheduled, it is necessary to take a blood sample first.

Enzyme immunoassay of anti-HA

Immune adherence haemagglutination, complement fixation, or immunolectron microscopy are now of historical interest. All commercially available test kits use the same principle: anti-HA in the sample competes with labelled anti-HA (one of the reagents) for binding to HAV, which is fixed to a solid phase (the other reagent). The sample is shown to contain anti-HA if binding of the label to the solid phase is significantly inhibited (Fig. 4(a)).

Plastic beads, wells of microplates, or microbeads are usually used as the solid phase.

Anti-HA IgG is labelled with enzymes; horseradish peroxidase is most commonly used. Quantitative detection of the label is usually done by photometry. Fluorescent or luminescent products of the enzymatic reaction have been recently introduced and allow more sensitive assays than photometry.

The analytical and clinical specificity of the assay is excellent, provided it is done properly, including clean work, good washing procedures, reliable detection of the label, and the use of positive and negative controls. Because of non-specific inhibitory factors in human serum, the sample is usually prediluted.

The analytical sensitivity of the inhibition assay is better than that of complement fixation or immunofluorescence, but poorer than that of direct radio- or enzyme immunoassays for antigens or antibodies (see Fig. 4(b,c)). The assay is sensitive enough to detect anti-HA for decades after symptomatic and even asymptomatic HAV infection. It is not clear whether immunosuppressed individuals always develop anti-HA after infection. The sensitivity of commercially available inhibition assays is not always sufficient to detect protective concentrations of anti-HA after immunization with a killed vaccine (Flehmig, Lancet, 1989; i:1039), but may be optimized (Zuckerman, JVirolMethods, 1996; 56:27).

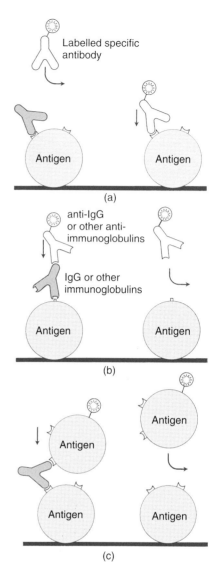

Fig. 4. Schematic explanation of solid-phase assays for viral antibodies. The antibody to be detected is shown in grey. The star stands for the label in the reagent, either a radio-isotope, an enzyme, or a light-emitting substance. The left part of the figures shows a positive case, the right part a case when the analyte is absent. (a) Inhibition assay for total antiviral antibody; an IgG antibody is shown as an example. A solid phase coated with viral antigen (e.g. HAV or HBcAg) is incubated with the serum sample, and subsequently (blocking assay) or simultaneously (competitive assay) reacted with a labelled antibody against the viral antigen. If the sample contains specific antibody, the label is not bound to the solid phase and is washed away. (b) Anti-immunoglobulin assay. The antigen at the solid phase is incubated with the sample and, after washing, with labelled anti-immunoglobulin antibody. IgG and anti-IgG are shown here. In a negative case the label is washed away. The assay is also used to detect antiviral IgM or IgA. (c) Sandwich assay for antiviral antibody. The solid phase is coated with purified virus antigen (e.g. HBsAg). The antigen is incubated with the serum sample and, after washing, with the labelled antigen. In a positive case the label is bound to the solid phase.

Neutralization assays

These measure the blocking of viral growth in cell culture by the preincubation of defined amounts of the test serum with a defined number of infectious doses. The assays are more difficult and test kits are not commercially available. The neutralization assay is important for the development and evaluation of HAV vaccines but unnecessary for diagnosis in the routine laboratory.

Quantitative inhibition assays

These are essential for the quality control of immune globulin preparations, of anti-HA test kits, and for HAV vaccination studies. International standard preparations for anti-HA have been defined. The sensitivity of the assays is between 20 and 200 international units (iu)/l. The concentrations of anti-HA are around 10 000 iu/l after natural infection and a factor of 10 to 100 lower after complete vaccination. The minimal protective concentration of anti-HA is not known, but concentrations above 10 iu/l are probably protective.

Antibodies to non-structural proteins

If it appears necessary to distinguish natural immunity from immunity induced by non-infectious HAV capsids, antibodies against non-structural proteins derived from P2 or P3 may be assayed. Immune precipitation of these proteins labelled during *in vitro* translation showed that antibodies occur in wild-type HAV-infected individuals but not after vaccination (Robertson, JMedVirol, 1993; 40:76). The assay is, however, not very sensitive and is not a routine method.

IgM anti-HA

Significance

Antibodies of the immunoglobulin M (M = macro) class are the first to be formed after the encounter between specific B lymphocytes and an antigen. Thereafter, a switch from IgM to IgG (G = γ) antibodies occurs; the half-life of IgM is only 5 days. Thus, antibodies of the IgM class are considered acute-phase antibodies. They help to distinguish current from previous infections. It has to be kept in mind that continuous or repeat contact with the antigen may also induce IgM antibodies, although at lower concentrations.

Techniques for detection

The classical way of distinguishing between IgM and IgG antibodies is separation by ultracentrifugation through a sucrose gradient, since normal IgM sediments at 19s while IgG sediments at 7s. A similar separation can also be achieved by gel chromatography using wide-pore gels such as 6 per cent agarose. Both techniques are still reference methods, but are time-consuming, expensive, laborious, and not suitable for large numbers of samples.

The anti-μ capture test (Duermeyer, JMedVirol, 1979; 4:25) has gained priority in many fields of application during the last 15 years. Antibodies against human μ-chains of IgM fixed to a solid phase bind a portion of the IgM in serum samples. If the sample contains IgM anti-HA, the HAV reagent is also bound to the solid phase. In the last step a labelled IgG anti-HA of human origin, or a monoclonal anti-HA, are added (Fig. 5).

HAV is able to agglutinate goose erythrocytes. Thus, instead of labelled anti-HA, goose erythrocytes may be added to the solid

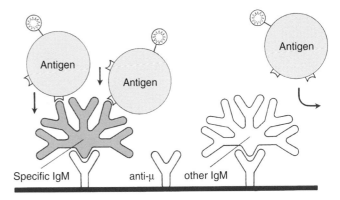

Fig. 5. Anti-μ capture assay for antiviral IgM antibodies. The right part explains the negative reaction, the left the positive. Anti-μ chain-specific antibody is adsorbed to a solid carrier. Dilutions of the serum sample are incubated with the solid phase, and IgM is bound, irrespective of its specificity. If the IgM contains paratopes against a viral antigen (e.g. HAV, HBcAg, HDAg), this antigen will be bound in the next step. The antigen may be labelled either directly (*) or by an additional specific antibody.

phase for detection of bound HAV (Perry, JMedVirol, 1993; 39:23; Summers, JClinMicrobiol, 1993: 31:1299).

The anti-μ capture assay is very sensitive and is not inhibited by IgG anti-HA in the sample. Depending on the origin and nature of the reagents, precautions must be taken to avoid non-specific results produced by rheumatoid factor or by non-specifically adherent IgG anti-HA. Commercial suppliers of test kits usually provide a 'cocktail' in which the serum sample must be diluted. Dilution is also required to reduce the very high sensitivity.

It is unknown whether all inapparent, fresh cases of HAV infection are detected by this test. Samples taken very early or late during the course of the infection may be rated negative, although the signal of the sample may be significantly higher than the negative controls. If IgM anti-HA is negative at the onset of an acute hepatitis, a second test after several days may be advisable (Hirata, AmJGastr, 1995; 90:1168). The reaction of immunosuppressed individuals is not known. If increased sensitivity is desired, the ratio of the signal for the sample to the negative control (S/N) may be requested from the laboratory. Values higher than 2 may indicate recent or beginning HAV infection. Weakly positive, non-specific signals may be obtained in a few individuals suffering from other infectious diseases or from immunological disorders. IgM anti-HA usually appears with the clinical symptoms of acute hepatitis A and disappears within 6 weeks to 6 months. Protracted cases of HAV remain IgM anti-HA-positive longer than 'regular' cases of resolving hepatitis A.

Detection of HAV

Diagnostic significance

The detection of HAV may be useful in contact cases incubating hepatitis A, in the early acute phase, or in protracted cases of hepatitis A. By using very sensitive assays it may be possible to identify HAV directly in contaminated shellfish, drinking water, blood products, or other materials.

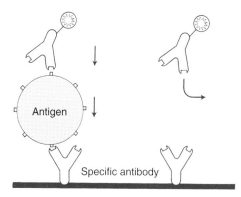

Fig. 6. Detection of viral antigens by a sandwich solid-phase assay. The solid phase is coated with specific (e.g. monoclonal) antibody against the antigen. Since most viral antigens contain many epitopes, a labelled antibody may also bind to the antigen and become linked to the solid phase. In a negative case (right) the labelled antibody is washed away.

Cell culture

Cultivation of the virus in suitable cell cultures is not a diagnostic method, but it may be useful if the agent of an outbreak or of an interesting case is to be studied further in a specialized laboratory. Detection of replicating virus in cells requires specific staining methods, for example immunofluorescence.

HAV antigen

Detection of HAV antigen (**HA-Ag**) is possible in stools at the peak of viral shedding, 10 to 20 days after infection. At the onset of the disease, only 20 to 50 per cent of the stools are positive, but in protracted cases HA-Ag may be detectable even as long as 6 weeks after the onset of the disease. Only the most sensitive detection methods are suitable, i.e. radio- or enzyme immunoassays (Fig. 6); the detection limit of these assays is about 10^7 virus particles/ml suspension. However, stool samples are not obtained as often as blood samples, and HA-Ag testing is thus done less often than indicated.

HAV RNA

Detection of HAV RNA by molecular hybridization (Fig. 7), or preferably by nucleic-acid amplification, is the method of choice for the recognition of HAV in diagnostic samples. HAV RNA is detectable in the patients stools or serum. Detectable HAV RNA in serum correlates with high concentrations of IgM anti-HA, and with a high degree of disease activity (Oren, JMedVirol, 1989; 28: 261). It is not clear whether the assay for HAV RNA in serum is of importance for routine diagnosis.

The PCR after reverse transcription of the RNA genome is the most popular form of nucleic-acid amplification. Because of its sensitivity, contamination with amplified cDNA may be a problem causing false-positive results. However, false-negative results due to inhibitors, wrong RNA extractions, or wrong primers are also possible. Sensitivity and practicability may be improved by prior enrichment of HAV with monoclonal anti-HA (Jansen, PNAS, 1990; 87:2867). In sewage, contaminated drinking water, and other sources with highly diluted HAV, pre-enrichment by precipitation, filtration, or other techniques is required.

The detection of HAV RNA by PCR and sequence identification of the amplificate has been instrumental in the elucidation of sporadic HAV infections caused by contaminated strawberries (Niu, JInfDis, 1992; 166:518) and in blood clotting factor-transmitted HAV (Normann, Lancet, 1992; 340:1232; Purcell, VoxSang, 1994; Suppl. 4:2). The detection of HAV RNA in anti-HA-containing samples does not necessarily mean that infectious HAV is present, because it may be neutralized by anti-HA. However, a small fraction of HAV may escape neutralization by anti-HA due to masking by lipid (Lemon, JGenVirol, 1985; 66:2501). Long-range PCR may be used to amplify the entire HAV genome and to generate infectious HAV RNA directly from the amplicon (Tellier, PNAS, 1996; 93: 4370).

Hepatitis E virus

HEV may cause epidemics of acute, resolving hepatitis in areas where severe faecal contamination of drinking water occurs.

Structure and classification[5]

HEV is a small, spherical, RNA virus without envelope, of approximately 30 nm diameter. It belongs neither to the *Picornaviridae* nor to the *Caliciviridae*. HEV may share some morphological features with the *Caliciviridae*: these have 180 capsomers, which form cup-like indentations characteristic of this virus family (Fig. 8), but

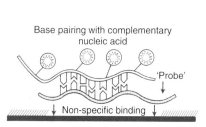

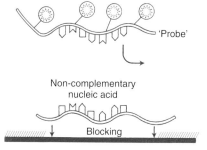

Fig. 7. Filter hybridization assay for detection of nucleic acids (dot-, slot-, Southern, northern blot). The nucleic acid in the sample is, if necessary, first made single-stranded, then adsorbed non- specifically to the filter membrane by blotting from a gel or by filtration through a membrane. Fixation by heat or ultraviolet light may be necessary for certain membranes. Remaining adsorption sites are blocked by the 'prehybridization mix'. A labelled nucleic acid complementary to the sequence to be detected (the 'probe') is then incubated at defined temperature and ionic conditions ('stringency'). After washings, the filter membranes are developed with enzyme-coupled reagents, or by autoradiography if the label was radioactive.

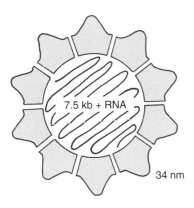

Fig. 8. Schematic presentation of HEV (*Caliciviridae*).

the existence of these indentations has not been proven un-equivocally for HEV. The genomic organization of HEV is also reminiscent of the *Caliciviridae*, showing a non-structural polyp-rotein at the 5′ terminal part and structural protein(s) at the 3′ end that may be encoded by a subgenomic mRNA (Cubitt, ArchVirol, 1995; Suppl. 10:359). However, the order and the type of the genes within the non-structural polyprotein are profoundly different from those of the *Caliciviridae* (Fig. 9), and resemble those of the rubi-like lineage of supergroup 3 of positive-strand RNA viruses to which, for example, rubellavirus belongs (Koonin, PNAS, 1992; 89: 8259).

The 7.5 kb-long, plus-strand RNA of HEV is encapsidated by a capsid protein that is probably the product of the open reading frame 2 of the genome. *In vitro*, a 75-kDa protein has been expressed from this open reading frame (He, JClinMicrobiol, 1995, 33:3308), but in purified virus this protein or its derivatives have not yet been identified, owing to lack of material. The product of open reading frame 2, with 659 or 660 amino acids, contains an aminoterminal, endoplasmic reticulum translocation signal and three potential *N*-glycosylation sites. It can be expressed in transfected cells as an 88-kDa glycoprotein (Jameel, JVirol, 1996; 70:207). However, the structure in HEV-infected cells or in the virus is not known. The function of the open reading frame 3, with 123 or 122 amino acids, is also unknown.

Open reading frame 1 encodes a polyprotein with motifs for a methyltransferase, a papain-like protease, a helicase type I, and a RNA-dependent RNA polymerase of supergroup 3. The presence

of a methyltransferase suggests that the 5′ end of the RNA genome may carry a methylated cap structure, which would facilitate trans-lation. The 5′ non-coding region is very short. The 3′ non-coding region of 65 nucleotides is joined with a poly(A) tail of *c*. 150 to 200 bases.

HEV is supposed to be less stable than HAV, but it seems to survive oral uptake and faecal shedding. Its density in caesium chloride is reported to be 1.35 or 1.39 g/ml, but it may be unstable in this medium. The sedimentation coefficient is 183*s*.

Replication

The virus does not grow well in cell cultures. It has been propagated in primary hepatocyte cultures from HEV-infected macaques (Tam, Virology, 1996; 215:1). Replication in a non-human primate cell line A549 has also been reported (Huang, JMedVirol, 1995; 47:299). Various non-human primate species are susceptible to HEV; cynomolgus macaques have been used most extensively for experimental studies. Intravenous infection is more effective than oral uptake. The receptor for HEV is unknown. Replication takes place in the cytoplasm and seems to involve two coterminal, subgen-omic mRNAs from the 3′ terminal part. Replication occurs via minus-strand RNA synthesis (Panda, JMedVirol, 1994; 42:237), but the details of this process have not yet been studied.

Variability and HEV antigens

HEV may divided into three genotypes, which are found in South-East Asia (Burma), northern and central Asia (China), and North America (Mexico). Variability is moderate, not exceeding 23 per cent in parts of open reading frame 1 and less than 10 per cent in open reading frame 2. The putative capsid antigen of open reading frame 2 seems to be more conserved than the product of open reading frame 3. Cross-challenge experiments in non-human prim-ates suggest that all known HEV isolates induce partial cross-protection and thus belong to one serotype. However, protection by cell-mediated immunity cannot be excluded.

The antigen of HEV open reading frame 2 has been identified indirectly in HEV-infected cynomolgus macaques and seems to be the major antigen recognized by human antisera (Panda, JMedVirol, 1994; 44:212). Antibodies against the antigen of open reading frame 3 have also been found in infected individuals. Antigens of open

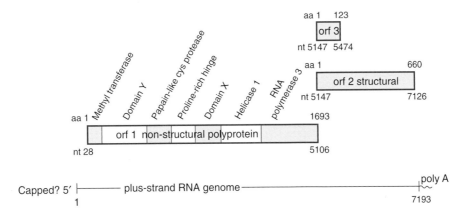

Fig. 9. Genome map of HEV. Orf, open reading frame; aa, amino acid; nt, nucleotide number.

reading frames 2 and 3 have been demonstrated in livers from two patients with fulminant hepatitis (Lau, JHepatol, 1995; 22:605).

Course of infection

The course of HEV infections is similar to that of HAV. Virus shedding from the infected hepatocytes to the bile (and thereafter to faeces) and to blood precedes the symptoms of the disease (Chauhan, Lancet, 1993; 341:149). Viraemia and virucopria begin about 20 days after the inoculation of experimental animals or human volunteers. Symptoms follow about 30 days after infection. IgM and IgG against antigens of open reading frames 2 and 3 appear soon after. Chronic infections are not known.

Diagnosis

HEV particles can be enriched from stool suspensions and visualized by electron microscopy. The identity of such particles can be confirmed by agglutination using antibody in HEV convalescent serum. This method of immunoelectron microscopy has also been used for the detection of anti-HE antibodies. Immunofluorescence quenching exploiting liver sections of infected cynomolgus monkeys as antigen can also be used for the detection of anti-HE; the HEV antigen is stained as fine cytoplasmic dots (Krawczynski, JInfDis, 1989; 159:1042). In contrast to HAV, HEV does not induce high concentrations of easily detectable antibodies. Assays using HEV particles, HEV-containing liver tissues, or recombinant HEV proteins as antigens do not detect IgM and IgG antibodies with complete reliability and for a long period of time. Thus, diagnosis during the acute phase should be complemented by RT-PCR (Clayson, JInfDis, 1995; 172:927; van Cujek-Gandre, AmJTropMedHyg, 1996; 54:134). Enzyme-linked immunosorbent assays for anti-HEV are commercially available in Asia and Europe, but they may be rather insensitive and non-specific. Thus, publications reporting on anti-HEV antibodies in groups without specific risk for HEV should be considered with reservation. Proteins of open reading frames 2 and 3 expressed in insect cells may be better antigens than partial peptides or *Escherichia coli*-derived partial proteins. IgG antibody to open reading frame 3 reportedly disappeared earlier than that for open reading frame 2 (Li, JClinMicrobiol, 1994; 32:2060).

IgG antibody to open reading frame 3 appears to indicate acute hepatitis E, whereas IgM and IgG antibodies to open reading frame 2 appear to be more insensitive and non-specific (Panda, JClinMicrobiol, 1995; 33:2659). The factors that make detection of anti-HEV so unreliable during acute infection and early convalescence are not understood. The classical techniques of immunoelectron microscopy or immunofluorescence using natural HEV in liver or faecal specimens may be too insensitive. Enzyme-linked immunosorbent assays or Western blots using recombinant antigens or peptide should give more sensitive signals, but these antigens may not expose the naturally relevant epitopes. Capsid epitopes would be expected to be conformational, as is the case with HAV or HBV. The presence of a signal peptide suggests chaperone-assisted folding and glycosylation in the endoplasmic reticulum, which would probably not occur in bacteria. Thus, the antibody response may, in fact, be better than is anticipated from the partially unsatisfactory results obtained so far.

Viraemia was detected in most patients using the RT-PCR, in one case up to 112 days after onset (Nanda, Gastro, 1995; 106:225), often in the absence of detectable anti-HEV. Indications to search for HEV RNA in serum and/or stool, and for anti-HEV IgM and IgG antibodies, are non A-D hepatitis, particularly in regions with faecally contaminated water supplies or in returning travellers from such areas. Person-to-person transmission, or transmission by contaminated food, is possible but rare. In cynomolgus macaques, the infectivity titre of faeces was 10^{-6}, similar to the titre in the RT-PCR (Tsarev, JMedVirol, 1994; 43:135).

The presence of HEV RNA or of IgM anti-HEV proves the presence of infection with HEV. Detection of anti-HEV IgG may indicate acute infection or previous exposure and possibly protection against clinical overt hepatitis E. However, at least in monkeys, mild reinfection without disease has been observed in previously infected animals (Pillot, CRAcadSci 3, 1993; 318:1059). Active or passive immunization of cynomolgus monkeys with a partial protein of open reading frame 2 induced protection against the disease but not against reinfection (Tsarev, PNAS, 1994; 91:10198).

It is not clear how long anti-HEV IgG persists. Even in highly endemic regions, for example Pune, India, the prevalence detected with a sensitive enzyme-linked immunosorbent assays did not exceed 40 per cent in age groups over 25 years, whereas the attack rate of acute hepatitis E is low at higher age (Arankalle, JInfDis, 1995; 171:447). Whether older age groups are less exposed or are immune in spite of undetectable anti-HEV is not clear.

Hepatitis B virus
Structure and classification[6-9]

HBV is a spherical, small, DNA virus with an envelope containing the hepatitis B surface antigen (**HBsAg**) and a nucleocapsid containing the core antigen (**HBcAg**) (Fig. 10). Similar viruses are found in woodchucks (marmot-like animals from the eastern United States), ground squirrels, ducks, and grey herons, forming the family of *Hepadnaviridae* (reviewed in ref.[7-9]). This family is subdivided into the genus orthohepadnavirus, which infects mammals, and avihepadnavirus, which infects birds. Both genera cause persistent infections and chronic hepatitis, but also demonstrate some clear differences in structure and biology (Howard, ArchVirol, 1995, Suppl. 10 (Virus taxonomy):179). All hepadnaviruses have a similar genomic organization, as outlined in Fig. 11. Since the *Hepadnaviridae* replicate by reverse transcription, they may be grouped together with *Retroviridae* and the plant-virus families *Caulimoviridae* and *Badnaviridae* into a superfamily of retroid viruses. For certain purposes it may be useful to consider these viruses together with the retrotransposons; in this case the term retroid elements may be used.

Viral proteins

Surface protein
Primary structure

Orthohepadnaviruses have three different but closely related envelope proteins (Heermann, JVirol, 1984; 52:386). The middle-sized (M) and the smallest proteins (S) are identical to

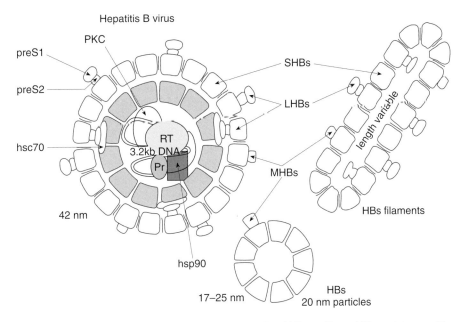

Fig. 10. Schematic models of HBV and HBs particles. SHBs, MHBs, LHBs: small, middle, and large HBs proteins; preS1, preS2: domains of LHBs or MHBs; PKC, protein kinase C; hsp 90, heat-shock protein 90; RT, reverse-transcriptase domain of HBV polymerase; Pr, primase domain.

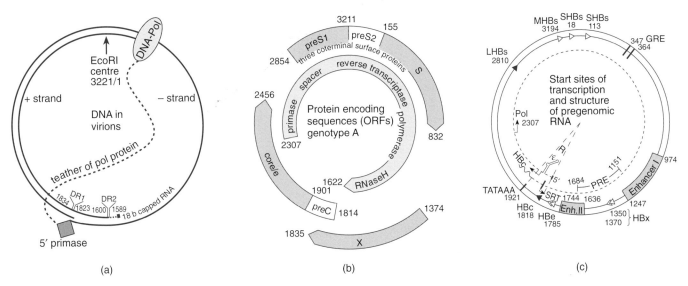

Fig. 11. Organization of the HBV genome. (a) Physical map of the DNA. DRs, direct repeats of 11 bases. DNA-Pol consists of the reverse transcriptase and RNase H. It may fill up the gap *in vitro*. The 5′ end of the minus strand is covalently linked to the primase and starts within DR1, that of the plus strand is linked with a short piece of capped RNA and starts within DR2. Numbering starts at the *Eco*RI cleavage site. (b) Open-reading frames (ORFs) of the HBV genome that are known to be expressed *in vivo*. The core ORF expresses two coterminal proteins, the S ORF three. The largest ORF encodes the polymerase polyprotein with the four indicated domains. (c) Transcription-relevant sites in the HBV genome. Triangles show the start sites of mRNAs for the corresponding proteins. Closed triangles show start sites that depend on liver-specific transcription factors; open triangles correspond to liver-independent start sites. All mRNAs stop behind the TATAAA box (base 1921). As an example, the pregenomic mRNA that encodes HBc and pol protein is shown. SRT, signal for reverse transcription at the 3′ end; ε, stem-loop structure necessary for encapsidation of the pregenome; R, terminal redundancy of the pregenomic RNA; GRE, glucocorticoid-responsive element; PRE, post-transcriptional regulatory element that prevents splicing.

the largest (L), except that segments of amino acids 119 or 176, respectively, are missing at the amino end (Fig. 12). The large protein is not a precursor of the smaller proteins. The three proteins originate from one gene by alternative use of three START codons for protein synthesis. The sequence between the first and the second START codon is termed pre-S1, and between the second and the third, pre-S2; the sequence from the third START codon to the STOP codon is termed S. All three proteins (large, middle, small) are part of the HBsAg. Thus, we suggest the terms **LHBs, MHBs, SHBs**; the terms pre-S1, pre-S2, and S should be reserved for the segments or domains of the whole protein sequence (Fig. 12).

The proteins form doublets in sodium dodecyl sulphate-gel

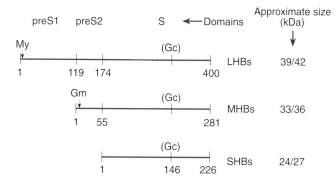

Fig. 12. Map of the three surface proteins of HBV (HBs proteins). LHBs, large HBs protein; MHBs, middle HBs protein; SHBs, small or major HBs protein. Numbers give the codons or amino acids beginning with the first methionine of the S open-reading frame in subtype adw. My, myristic acid at Gly2. Glyc$_h$, hybrid-type glycan at Asn4. Glyc$_c$, complex glycan at Asn146 of domain S. Apparent sizes in sodium dodecyl sulphate-gel electrophoresis are given in kDa. Redrawn after Heermann, JVirol, 1984; 52:396.

electrophoresis because a part of the molecules is glycosylated at Asn146 of the S domain (Gillece-Castro, ArchBiochemBiophys, 1987; 256:194).

Antigenicity of HBs protein

The S domain is highly hydrophobic. After the budding of the particles it crosses the lipid bilayer of the endoplasmic reticulum membrane at least four times (Berting, Intervirology, 1995; 38:8). SHBs and the S domains of MHBs and LHBs are cross-linked by disulphide bonds. The central portion of the S domain (amino acids 100–165) is hydrophilic, and in SHBs it is exposed to the surface. There it forms an antigenic loop that acquires a complicated conformation by several disulphide bonds. Additional S epitopes are formed at the interface of two SHBs molecules. There are very few sequential B-lymphocyte epitopes on SHBs. Most epitopes are lost if natural HBs is treated with reducing reagents. Thus, most antibodies against SHBs (**anti-SHBs**) usually cannot be detected by immunoblot (Heermann, Intervirology, 1987; 28:14). The glycan of the S domain does not contribute essentially to the antigenicity, but it may mask epitopes around Asn146.

Pre-S2 domain

The pre-S2 domain contains only 55 amino acids. It is hydrophilic and is located at the surface of MHBs, but in LHBs it is hidden by the pre-S1 domain. In MHBs it carries a mannose-rich glycan of the hybrid type, linked to Asn4 of the pre-S2 domain (Stibbe, Virology, 1982, 123:436). The B-cell epitopes of pre-S2 are linear, but some of them are glycoside-dependent. Monoclonal antibodies against such epitopes allow for the selective detection of MHBs in the presence of LHBs.

The pre-S2 domain binds a small subfraction of human serum albumin (Krone, Hepatol, 1990; 11:1050). Stronger binding is found if the albumin is polymerized by glutaraldehyde (Machida, Gastro, 1984; 86:910). The biological function of the pre-S2 domain is unknown. *In vitro*, polymerized human serum albumin links HBV to hepatocyte membranes (Pontisso, JVirol, 1989; 63:1981), but it is not known whether this occurs *in vivo*. Bound albumin may cover

pre-S2 epitopes. The pre-S2 sequence (13–19) has been characterized as a major B epitope (Milich, JImmunol, 1986; 137:2703).

Pre-S1 domain

The pre-S1 domain is present on the surface of the virus. It contains sequential and conformational epitopes (Heermann, Intervirology, 1987; 28:14), but together with the pre-S2 domain it is also in a part of the LHBs molecules facing the interior of the particles (Bruss, EMBOJ, 1994; 13:2273). Pre-S1 is linked to myristic acid (a C_{14} fatty acid) as an amide to the Gly2 of pre-S1 (Persing, JVirol, 1987; 61:1388). The pre-S1 sequence (21–47) forms an attachment site of HBV to human hepatocytes (Neurath, Cell, 1986; 46:429; Pontisso, Virology, 1989; 173:522).

Core proteins
Capsid

The capsid of HBV is formed by 240 copies (Crowther, Cell, 1994; 77:943) of one major protein of M_r 22 kDa (Gerlich, JVirol, 1982; 42:761), named **HBc** protein. This protein is able to assemble spontaneously into core particles (34 nm diameter), even in the absence of other viral proteins. The HBc protein has a carboxy-terminal domain of 35 amino acids, very rich in arginines. This domain confers affinity to RNA; core particles enclose RNA during the assembly process (Fig. 13). Although packaging of RNA in HBc-transformed bacteria is non-specific, pregenomic HBV RNA is predominantly packaged *in vivo*. RNA packaging does not occur if the carboxyterminal domain is missing, but assembly is still possible (Gallina, JVirol, 1989; 63:4645).

Antigenicity of core proteins

Core particles of HBV are a potent immunogen. They induce the T-cell-independent production of high anti-HBc titres during natural HBV infection and also in immunized animals (Milich, Science, 1986; 234:1398). The strong antigenicity of the 'core' antigen (HBcAg) depends on the folding and assembly of the HBc protein. Recent studies using cryoelectron microscopy show that the HBcAg loop is formed by dimers at the tip of a four-helix bundle protruding from the core particles (Böttcher, Nature, 1997; 386:88; Conway, Nature, 1997; 386:91). A truncated core protein without a carboxyterminal domain may be exposed and lend further antigenicity, referred to as **HBeAg**. The dissociation of core particles by anionic detergents and proteases destroys much of the HBc antigenicity also, and generates HBe antigen (McKay, JMedVirol, 1981; 8:237).

Foreign B epitopes can be genetically introduced into the *HBc* gene; provided that the insertion does not disturb the symmetry; these epitopes are very efficient inducers of antibody production (Pumpens, Intervirology, 1995; 38:63).

Non-structural proteins
Natural HBe protein

HBeAg is found as soluble protein in the blood of HBV carriers. It correlates with massive viraemia (Zyzik, EurJClinMicrobiol, 1986; 5:330). Natural HBeAg is not a breakdown product of core particles, but a second form of the core protein, which should be termed HBe protein but which is occasionally termed 'precore' protein, even

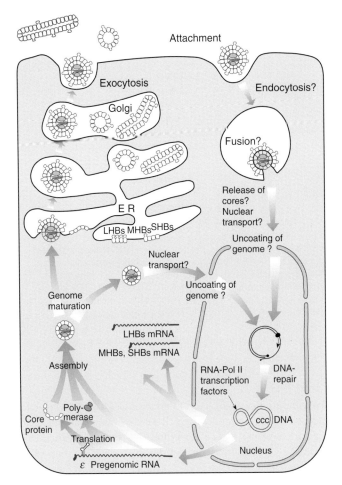

Fig. 13. Schematic view of the lifecycle of HBV (for explanation see text).

though it is not a precursor of core protein. The *HBe* gene is coterminal with the *HBc* gene. In addition, it contains 29 codons in phase upstream of the *HBc* gene. This so-called precore (pre-C) (the designation pre-E would be better) sequence codes for a signal peptide that causes insertion and partial translocation to the lumen of the endoplasmic reticulum (Fig. 14). During the translocation the 19-amino acid signal peptide is removed (Standring, PNAS, 1988; 85:8405). The resulting HBe protein, p23e, can be secreted if the carboxyterminal domain is truncated or completely removed by proteolysis (Bruss, Virology, 1988; 163:268). Part of p23e returns to the cytoplasm and migrates to the nucleus (Ou, JVirol, 1989; 63: 5238). Another part may end in the cellular plasma membrane (Schlicht, JVirol, 1989; 63:5399). HBe protein without signal peptide but with the full carboxyterminal domain forms mixed particles with HBc proteins but suppresses RNA encapsidation (Scaglioni, JVirol, 1997; 71:345). HBe and HBc protein can be expressed by the same cell because a part of the longest viral mRNA starts upstream and another part starts downstream of the initiation codon of the precore sequence (Sells, JVirol, 1988, 62:2836).

The function of the HBe protein is enigmatic, particularly in view of its negative effect on replication. It is predominantly a non-structural viral protein that is unnecessary for HBV infectivity (Schlicht, JVirol, 1987; 61:3701), but, in contrast to the wild type, HBe-negative mutants of woodchuck hepatitis virus do not induce

persistent infection in newborn woodchucks (Chen, JVirol, 1992; 66:5682). Its association with massive viraemia may be secondary to the induction of a partial immune tolerance. HBe/c protein suppresses the induction of interferon-β (Twu, JVirol, 1989; 63: 3065). HBeAg can pass the placenta (at least) in mice and there induce T-cell tolerance to HBcAg (Milich, PNAS, 1990; 87:6599; JImmunol, 1994; 152; 455). It is, however, not known whether such a mechanism is also important in human mother-to-child transmission. HBeAg favours induction of Th2 cells against HBc/e epitopes and may thus suppress the cytotoxicity-inducing Th1 response against HBc/e (Milich, JVirol, 1997; 71:2192).

HBx protein

The product of the X open reading frame is the HBx protein with 154 amino acids. It is difficult to demonstrate HBx protein in infected or transfected cells, but the corresponding X protein from woodchuck hepatitis virus has been found in infected woodchuck liver and carcinoma (Dandir, JVirol, 1996; 70:6246). X protein probably does not exist in avihepadnaviruses. HBx-deficient HBV genomes are replication-competent in transfected cell cultures (Blum, JVirol, 1992; 66:1223) but X-protein-deficient woodchuck hepatitis virus genomes cannot induce infection in transfected woodchucks (Chen, JVirol, 1993; 69:1218; Zoulim, 1994; JVirol, 68: 2026). The biochemical and biological function of HBx is not clear. A possible non-specific, transcription-activating function has been extensively studied, but the data are very variable (Henkler, JViralHepat, 1996; 3:109). An involvement in hepatocarcinogenesis by HBV is likely but not proven (Schaefer, Intervirology, 1995; 38: 143; Caselmann, AdvVirusRes, 1996; 47:253; Hildt, SemVirol, 1996; 7:333).

Replication[7,8]

A survey of the viral lifecycle is presented in Fig. 13.

Viral entry

The first step is attachment to hepatocytes and possibly to other cells. It appears very likely that the pre-S1 sequence (21–47) and possibly elements of pre-S2 are involved in attachment, because anti-pre-S1(21–47) (Neurath, Vaccine, 1989; 7:234) and anti-pre-S2(1–26) (Neurath, Vaccine, 1986; 4:35) are able to neutralize HBV. The S domain can interact with hepatocyte membranes via endonexin II (Hertogs, JVirol, 1994; 68:1516) or indirectly via apolipoprotein H (Mehdi, Virology, 1996; 217:58). Among the numerous cellular proteins that are supposed to interact with the HBV surface, the asialoglycoprotein receptor may mediate uptake of HBV (Treichel, JGenVirol, 1994; 75:3021) because HBV and HBsAg filaments contain terminal galactoses at their glycoproteins. HBV seems to be taken up by human hepatoma cell line HepG2; core particles are released and bound to the nuclear membrane but the cells are not productively infected (Qiao, Virology, 1994; 201: 356). Infectivity for HepG2 cells may be enhanced if the HBV particles are pretreated with Glu-specific protease, possibly due to exposure of a membrane fusion sequence (Lu, JVirol, 1996; 70: 2277). In the duck HBV system, two receptors have been identified (Kuroki, JBiolChem, 1995; 270:15022; Li, JVirol, 1996; 70:6029). They may be involved in an endosomal, but pH-independent, uptake of the duck HBV (Köck, JVirol, 1996; 70:5827). Core

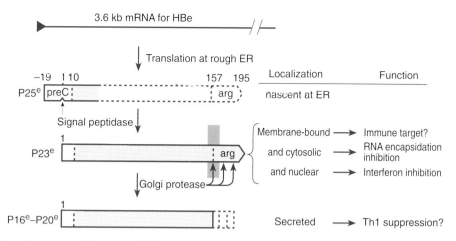

Fig. 14. Biosynthesis of the HBe protein. If the large mRNA of HBV starts upstream of the precore (pre-C) sequence, the HBe precursor p25e is translated, and cleaved at the Ala19. A part of p23e is translocated to the endoplasmic reticulum, clipped at variable carboxyterminal sites, and secreted as p16e or p18e. Another part of p23e goes back to the cytoplasm, where it is modified at the carboxyterminal part, resulting in p24e. This may migrate to the nucleus. Both pathways may possibly contribute to the specific immune tolerance against HBV.

particles derived from entering virus bind to the nucleopore complex and there release the polymerase–DNA complex to the nucleoplasm (Kann, JVirol, 1997; 71:1310).

Genome structure

The genome of HBV is a circular DNA with a peculiar primary structure (Fig. 11(a)). Its size, of about 3200 bases (partly paired, partly single), is very small compared with other viruses. It has, however, a high coding capacity through the multiple use of a given sequence (Fig. 11(b)). Most of the sequence is covered by the gene for the viral DNA polymerase (pol). Within this gene there is, in another phase, the tripartite gene for the HBs proteins (Fig. 12). Upstream of the *pol* gene and partially overlapping is the *hbc/e* gene; downstream of *pol* and also partly overlapping, is the *X* gene. There are two further open reading frames, the function of which is unknown (Miller, Hepatol, 1989; 9:322).

All four functional open reading frames are on the DNA strand that encodes the mRNAs for the corresponding products HBc/e, pol, HBs, and X. Thus, the polarity of this DNA strand is defined as 'minus'. Within the infectious virus the minus DNA strand is complete and even redundant by nine bases at the extreme ends. It carries the viral DNA polymerase covalently linked at its 5′ end.

The plus strand is usually incomplete. It has a fixed 5′ end but a variable 3′ end, leaving a single-stranded gap in the viral DNA. The 5′ end is formed by a short RNA sequence of 18 bases that has a 'cap' structure at its start. Such caps are typical for the 5′ end of mRNAs.

HBV-DNA molecules are brought into a circular configuration because the 5′ terminal parts of 234 bases are complementary in the two DNA strands. At the end of these cohesive regions there are two direct sequence repeats of 11 bp termed DR1 and DR2. The sequence of the DNA minus strand begins within DR1, whereas the RNA piece of the plus strand begins upstream, close to DR2. The peculiar structure of the HBV genome is explained by its mode of replication (Fig. 15).

The complete sequences of numerous HBV isolates are known. Numbering of the bases is unfortunately not standardized. The unique cleavage site of the restriction endonuclease *Eco*RI is often used as zero.

RNA transcription

After entering the nucleus of the infected cell, the DNA is made completely double-stranded by cellular repair enzymes and converted to covalently closed, superhelical circles. Transcription of the various viral mRNAs procedes thereafter with the cooperation of the viral DNA sequence (i.e., *cis*-acting) elements, cellular transcription factors, cellular RNA polymerase II, and viral-transacting products. It appears that the organotropism of HBV partly depends on the organ-specific transcription factors of the cell, which act on sequence elements within the HBV genome (Fig. 11(c)). A part of these sequence elements is clustered in enhancers I and II of the genome (Yuh, JVirol, 1992; 66:4073; Kosavsky, JBiolChem, 1996; 271:21859), but other regions of the DNA sequence also bind positive and negative transcription factors, including steroid receptors (Tur-Kaspa, Virology, 1988; 167:330). DNA sequence elements that govern not only the level but also the start site of RNA synthesis are called promoters.

Expression of the three HBs proteins is regulated at the transcriptional and the translational level. A transcription promoter located upstream of the entire *HBs* gene (SPI) governs synthesis of the mRNA for LHBs. Its sequence contains, as a typical transcription signal, the TATA box. The activity of the SPI promoter depends on the hepatocyte nuclear factors 1 and 3; this explains the liver-specific expression of LHBs (Chang, MolCellBiol, 1989; 9: 5189; Raney, JVirol, 1995; 69:3265). A second promoter without a TATA box is located within the pre-S1 sequence (SPII). It has no obvious organ specificity and governs synthesis of heterogeneous mRNAs initiating slightly upstream or downstream of the START codon of MHBs. Biosynthesis of both MHBs and SHBs is regulated by this promoter (Cattaneo, Nature, 1983; 305:336). The relative predominance of SHBs over MHBs is partially explained by the fact that the initiation of protein synthesis is suboptimal at the START codon of MHBs. Some internal initiation may occur at the START codon of SHBs.

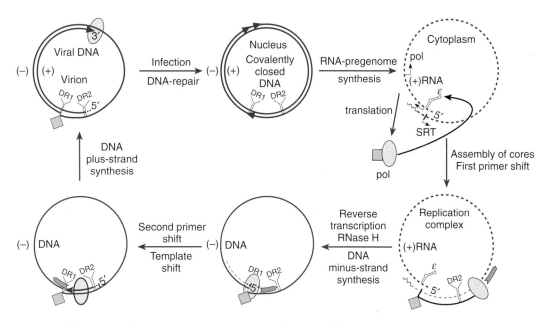

Fig. 15. Replication of the HBV genome. After entry of the virus into the cell, the viral DNA is released into the nucleus, and completed to covalently closed circles. These are transcribed to pregenomic RNA (see also Fig. 11), and translated to HBc and pol proteins. The three components assemble into core particles, and within these particles reverse transcription starts at the primase (■). During elongation of the minus strand, the reverse transcriptase (○) probably remains linked to the primase. The RNase H cleaves the RNA of DNA/RNA hybrids, leaving a complete, single-stranded DNA minus strand. The remaining 18 bases from the 5′ terminal part of the pregenomic RNA are able to shift from DR1 to DR2, where they serve, after a template switch of the reverse transcriptase, as primer for the DNA plus strand. Multiplication of the HBV genome occurs via transcription of the pregenomic mRNA.

Transcription of the HBc mRNA depends on liver-specific factors (Buckwold, JVirol, 1996; 70:5845; Yu, JVirol, 1996; 70:8719). The promoter region for the *hbc/e* genes also contains the liver-specific enhancer II (Chen, JVirol, 1995; 69:3649). Mutations in this promoter decrease the ratio of HBe to HBc protein and enhance virus replication (Baumert, JCI, 1996; 98:2268).

At least five classes of mRNAs for synthesis of the viral proteins are made. Their 5′ end is governed by the various promoters, as shown in Fig. 11c; they all have a common 3′ end.

Pregenome and polymerase

The pregenomic RNA that starts within the precore sequence is essential for genomic replication. The slightly larger HBe mRNA that starts upstream of the precore is not replication-competent. The pregenomic RNA is used for the synthesis of core protein and for the polymerase. The HBV pol polymerase has at least four distinguishable domains (Fig. 11(b)). The aminoterminal domain provides the 5′ terminal protein (primase) of the DNA minus strand, which acts as protein primer for its synthesis (Bartenschlager, EMBOJ, 1988; 7:4185). The next domain, which overlaps with the pre-S1 in the *hbs* open reading-frame domain, is highly variable, and is probably only needed as a spacer. The reverse transcriptase forms the next domain, which overlaps with the S region. It carries sequence elements that are conserved in all known reverse transcriptases. The RNase H domain, which cleaves the RNA in RNA–DNA hybrids soon after reverse transcription, is located at the carboxy end. This domain is necessary for synthesis of the DNA plus strand (Radziwill, JVirol, 1990; 64:613).

Pregenome encapsidation and reverse transcription

In addition to these functions, the polymerase induces specific packaging of itself and of the pregenome (Hirsch, Nature, 1990; 334:552) into core particles. It binds to a secondary structure, element ε (for encapsidation), close to the 5′ end of the pregenomic RNA, which also encodes the core and pol proteins. It initiates, within a bulge of ε, the synthesis of the DNA minus strand for the first three or four bases using Tyr96 as primer (Weber, JVirol, 1994; 68:2994; Zoulim, JVirol, 1994; 68:2026). Thereafter, it is translocated to the signal for reverse transcription (SRT in Figs 11(c) and 15) from where the DNA minus strand is completed. The polymerase has been expressed *in vitro* and can be used as target molecule for antiviral drugs (Wang, Cell, 1992; 71:663; Lanford, JVirol, 1995; 69:6833; Tavis PNAS, 1993; 90:4107). The polymerase requires ε (Tavis, JVirol, 1996; 70:5741) and the cellular heat-shock protein (**hsp**) 90 (Hu, PNAS, 1996; 93:1060) to become an active reverse transcriptase: hsp90 is also encapsided within the core particle (Hu, EMBOJ, 1997; 96:59).

Virus release

A number of the core particles containing mature HBV DNA may migrate to the nucleus and amplify the number of episomal viral genomes (Tuttleman, Cell, 1986; 47:451). Another part is enveloped by the surface proteins and secreted as complete virus. Interaction between the cytosolic, pre-S domain of LHBs protein and the core particles is necessary for viral envelopment in the endoplasmic reticulum (Bruss, JVirol, 1995; 69:6652) and some interactions with S-domain sequences have also been identified (Dyson, PNAS, 1995; 92:2194). During transport the glycans of the HBs proteins must be trimmed. Inhibition of the involved enzyme glucosidase I leads to the retention of HBV and MHBs-containing particles (Block, PNAS, 1994; 91:2285).

Integration of HBV DNA and hepatocellular carcinoma

In contrast to the genuine *Retroviridae*, integration of DNA is not a necessary step in the lifecycle of *Hepadnaviridae*. Correspondingly, the HBV pol protein does not contain a domain with integrase function (Radziwill, JVirol, 1990; 64:613). Nevertheless, the integration of HBV DNA proceeds by non-homologous recombinational events involving cellular enzymes. The integrated DNA is virtually always defective in the sense that vital genes of the virus are deleted, or at least interrupted or rearranged. Thus, reactivation of a silent HBV infection by integrated DNAs is unlikely to occur. However, viral proteins, in particular truncated HBs and HBx proteins, may be expressed by integrated HBV DNA. Because of the integration, truncated virus proteins may be generated and/or fusion with cellular proteins may occur. In one case, such a neoprotein, a retinoic acid receptor (hap), was shown to be involved in hepadnavirus-associated oncogenesis (Dejean, Nature, 1986; 322:70). Integration of HBV DNA was also found within the gene for the cell-cycle control protein, cyclin A; this may lead to uncontrolled growth (Wang, Nature, 1990; 343:555). Truncation of HBV genes may also change the properties of HBV neoprotein. Thus, it was found that a truncated MHBs protein (Kekule, Nature, 1990; 343:457) or a truncated *LHBs* gene from human hepatomas are transcription activators (Caselmann, AdvVirusRes, 1996; 47:253; Hildt, SemVirol, 1996; 7:333). The high oncogenicity of woodchuck hepatitis virus in the host animal is caused by the integration of a fragment of the viral DNA near the host's *Nmyc2* locus, which becomes activated in an uncontrolled manner by the integration (Fourel, EMBOJ, 1994; 13:2526). However, viral factors also seem to be involved because ground squirrels, which also have a cellular *Nmyc2* locus, develop carcinomas much more rarely after infection with their hepatitis virus (Quignon, Oncogene, 1996; 12:2011).

It is possible to transform hepatocytes *in vitro* or transgenic mice by HBV-DNA sequences, in particular with the *X* gene, but the mechanism is not clear (Schaefer, Intervirology, 1995; 38:143). The postulated interaction of HBx with the tumour-suppressor protein p53 is controversial (Henkler, ViralHepatitisRev, 1996; 2:143). Furthermore, it is unclear whether HBV-associated cases of hepatocellular carcinoma are really caused by HBV as an aetiological agent. HCV, cirrhosis, and the fungal toxin aflatoxin B are important cofactors, but there are cases of HBV-associated hepatocellular carcinoma without these.

Destabilization of cellular DNA and chromosomal translocations are frequent in HBV-associated hepatomas. They may be induced by the enhanced activity of cellular topoisomerase I (Wang, JVirol, 1991; 65:2381; Rogler, SemLivDis, 1992; 12:265).

Storage of LHBs may possibly also contribute to the development of hepatomas. Spherical HBs particles are only formed by SHBs and MHBs. If more than a few per cent of HBs proteins are present as LHBs, HBsAg filaments are formed. If the proportion of LHBs is very high, the filaments cannot be secreted. They are stored in the endoplasmic reticulum and generate ground-glass hepatocytes (Dienes, Gastro, 1990; 98:1017). Heavy overexpression of LHBs in transgenic mice induces storage disease and hepatoma (Chisari, Cell, 1990; 59:1145).

HBV genotypes and HBsAg subtypes

The genomes of *Hepadnaviridae* are relatively stable. Owing to the multiple use of the DNA sequence, any point mutation may affect more than one function. Within human HBV isolates, no more than 15 per cent nucleotide-sequence variation is found. The genomes of woodchuck and ground-squirrel HBVs are 60 per cent homologous to human HBV, and certain serological reagents for human HBV cross-react with the woodchuck virus. The human HBV exists in at least six genotypes, A to F, which can be distinguished by typical amino acid combinations within the S domains and other parts of the genome (Magnius, Intervirology, 1995; 38: 24). The known HBsAg subtype determinants *d* or *y*, *w* or *r*, and *w1* to *w4* also correspond to typical alleles within the S domain, but they do not clearly correlate with the genotypes (see Table 3). Notable differences are found in genotype D, which has an 11-amino acid deletion at the amino end of pre-S1, and in genotype A, which has a 2-amino acid insertion in the core protein. The features of a genotype are clearly maintained within an infection chain (Uy, JGenVirol, 1992; 73:3005).

Variants of HBV

Variants of HBV occur in certain patients and are often characterized by functionally changed proteins. One of the best known variants has absent or low-level expression of HBeAg, owing to mutations in the precore region or in the HBe/c promoter/enhancer that may

Table 3 Geographical distribution of HBV genotypes and HBsAg subtypes

Genotype	HBsAg subtype	Areas of high prevalence
A	adw2	North-western Europe
	ayw1	Central Africa
B	adw2	Indonesia, China
	ayw1	Vietnam
C	adw2	East Asia
	adr−	Polynesia
	adrq+	Korea, China, Japan
	ayr	Vietnam
D	ayw2	Mediterranean area
	ayw3	India
E	ayw4	West Africa
F	adw4q−	American natives, Polynesia

also affect the *X* gene (Carman, Intervirology, 1995; 38:95) or the group-specific determinant *a* of the HBsAg (Carmann, Lancet, 1995; 345:1406). Precore and HBs variants have been associated with fulminant hepatitis B (Hasagawa, JVirol, 1994; 68:1651; Bahn, JMedVirol, 1995; 47:336; Kaneko, JMedVirol, 1995; 47:204). Selection of the variants seems to be driven by humoral and cellular immune responses (Bozkaya, JHepatol, 1997; 26:508).

Atypical serology

Not all unusual patterns of serological reaction are due to genetic variants of HBV. HBsAg may be undetectable in serum because of masking by anti-HBs. It could be present in the liver in a form that has not assembled to mature HBsAg (Dienes, Gastro, 1990; 98: 1017). Anti-HBc may be absent in the early incubation phase, or in chronic carriers who are immunodeficient. Low-level replication may be due to host factors, or to concomitant infection with HDV or HCV (Blum, Digestion, 1995; 56:85; and see Chapters 12.1.2.4 and 12.1.2.5).

Diagnosis[8]

Course of HBV infection

For the purpose of this chapter, five clinical courses of HBV infection are briefly considered (Fig. 16).

Subclinical transient infection

After the virus has entered a non-immune host there may be limited replication and rapid development of immunity without clinical disease (Fig. 16, top). This course of infection occurs often in healthy, immunocompetent individuals after mucosal exposure to low doses of the virus, for example after heterosexual contact with a virus carrier.

In these cases, HBsAg may be detectable for a few months after the exposure. Owing to a lack of clinical symptoms, this short period of viraemia is usually missed unless the patient is followed-up closely after exposure. Anti-HBc and anti-HBs appear soon after, with or without moderately elevated transaminases. IgM anti-HBc does not reach high titres (Gerlich, JClinMicrobiol, 1986; 24:288) but remains detectable for a few months (Fig. 16(a)).

Acute hepatitis B

After parenteral exposure to blood containing HBV, clinical manifestations are frequently more severe. The virus replicates massively in liver and possibly in other cells. After a silent interval of from several weeks up to several months depending on the dose of infecting virus, HBsAg, HBeAg, and HBV DNA appear in the blood, and within several weeks increase to very high concentrations without symptoms of disease (Fig. 16(b)). Soon before, or at the onset of, acute hepatitis B, serum HBV DNA, HBeAg, and HBsAg start to decrease. In resolving cases, HBeAg disappears within 6 weeks or less; it may be undetectable at the onset of disease. HBV DNA disappears even more rapidly. HBsAg may persist for up to 6 months, but in resolving cases its concentration decreases by at least a factor of two within the first 4 weeks. In rare cases, HBsAg may be absent in the serum from the beginning of disease.

Total anti-HBc and IgM anti-HBc appear at the onset of clinical symptoms and rapidly reach peak concentrations. The decrease in IgM anti-HBc during convalescence occurs at variable rates. Anti-HBe and subsequently anti-HBs typically appear during late convalescence; they may also remain undetectable (Fig. 17). High titres of HBV DNA, HBeAg, and HBsAg without severe symptoms of acute hepatitis are markers of the late incubation period or of impending chronicity.

Chronic productive HBV infection

This course may develop from an acute hepatitis, more often from a mild or a completely asymptomatic primary infection (Fig. 16(c)). Chronic productive infection sustained by wild-type HBV is characterized by high titres of HBV DNA, HBsAg, and HBeAg; titres of IgM anti-HBc are often moderately high and indicate inflammatory liver disease. Chronic productive infection sustained by precore-minus mutants of HBV is characterized by variable titres of HBsAg, fluctuations of HBV-DNA concentration, and by the finding of anti-HBe instead of the HBeAg.

Similar to acute hepatitis B, the clinical symptoms of chronic hepatitis B are inversely correlated with the titre of infectious HBV and of the viral antigens. Chronic productive infections may last for years or decades.

HBsAg carriership

After a variable duration of productive infection, a selective immune reaction against the HBV and the HBV-expressing hepatocytes develops (Fig. 16(d)). Elimination of these hepatocytes may result in a flare up of transaminases, but control of viral replication may also be effective, without killing. Hepatocytes that carry silent or defective HBV genomes, or that express only HBsAg for various reasons, may obviously be tolerated by the immune system. Thus, the state of the so-called HBsAg carrier develops. Latent HBV genomes, which may reactivate, are apparently controlled by cellular immunity, but under immunosuppression HBV replication may be reactivated.

Hepatocellular carcinoma

Chronic HBV infection is epidemiologically correlated with the development of hepatocellular carcinoma. Tumour cells often contain mono- or oligoclonal inserts of HBV genomic fragments in their chromosomes. Very rarely these fragments express HBsAg or other viral proteins. Non-tumourous surrounding liver tissue usually expresses HBsAg but not complete HBV or HBeAg. Thus, such patients often share the serological picture of lowly symptomatic HBsAg carriers or late-phase chronic hepatitis B, but in some patients HBsAg or even anti-HBc may be missing. Even in the majority of HCV-associated hepatocellular carcinoma, HBV DNA has been detected by Southern blotting.

Selection of diagnostic measures

The diagnostic spectrum for the detection of HBV infections reflects the complex structure and biology of the virus. It is useful to distinguish between screening or 'first-line tests' and follow-up or 'second-line' tests. The various diagnostic or clinical questions to be asked if no previous information on hepatitis infections is available are listed in Table 4. From the different serological courses of HBV infection it is evident that, in most cases, testing for total

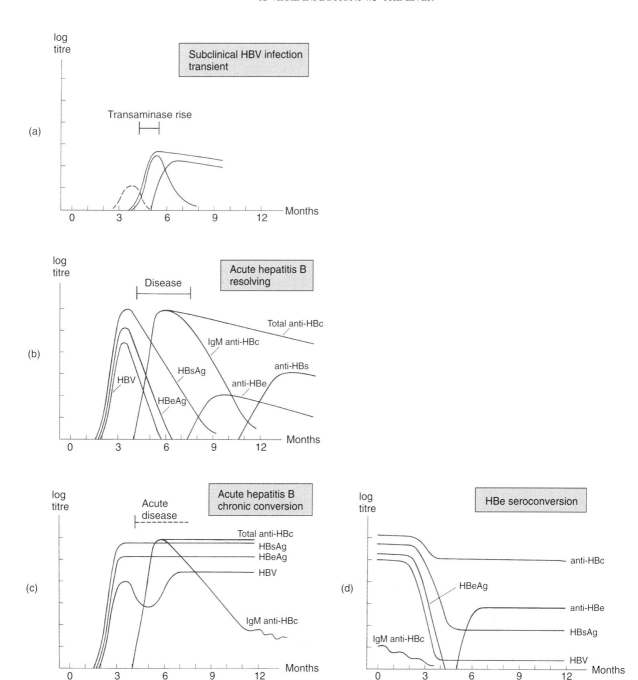

Fig. 16. Schematic serological profiles of HBV infections.

anti-HBc, HBsAg, or both is required. In cases of acute hepatitis, IgM anti-HBc may be tested without waiting for the result of the assay for total anti-HBc. There is no need to monitor HBsAg and anti-HBc to assess the success of hepatitis B vaccination unless exposure to HBV is suspected shortly before or after vaccination.

If a positive result for HBsAg is obtained or is already known from previous testing, additional assays should be performed (Table 5).

1. Although modern immunoassays for HBsAg are highly specific, washing errors and instrument failures may occur, and serum samples may have been mixed up or contaminated. This should be excluded by a second assay of HBsAg and a second serum sample should be requested if an individual has been found to be HBsAg-positive for the first time.

2. Anti-HBc should be assessed if not yet tested. A positive result is good confirmation of the positive HBsAg test.

3. Quantitative assay of IgM anti-HBc will give information on the phase of infection if required.

4. Testing for HBV DNA will help to recognize potential infectivity and viral activity.

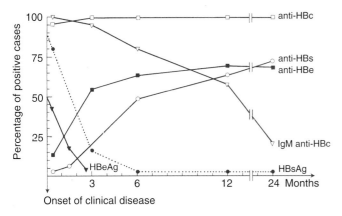

Fig. 17. Serological patterns of viral antigens and antibodies during and after acute hepatitis B. Markers were measured at the times indicated by radio- or enzyme immunoassay. Cases had histologically confirmed acute hepatitis with transient HBsAg or high IgM anti-HBc as markers of HBV infection. Numbers of patients are shown at the top. (Data from a multicentre study on viral hepatitis sponsored by Deutsche Forschungsgemeinschaft.) The assays used for this study had typical sensitivity, except for IgM anti-HBc, which was more sensitive.

5. If an assay for HBV DNA is not available, HBeAg and anti-HBe may give information on infectivity and viral activity; this type of result is, however, less reliable.
6. If HBsAg is repeatedly positive but all the other assays are negative, the specificity of the HBsAg reaction should be checked by neutralization after preincubation with anti-HBs.
7. Optional tests are HBsAg concentration, HBsAg subtype, and the identification of variants.

An anti-HBc-positive result should be joined by the following assays:

(1) HBsAg, if not yet determined;

(2) anti-HBs;
(3) in case of HBsAg-negative hepatitis, IgM anti-HBc;
(4) in case of chronic HBsAg-negative hepatitis, assay of anti-HBe and of HBV DNA by PCR (see below) may give important information.

The assays and the significance of these serological variables are described in more detail below.

Assay of HBsAg

HBsAg has represented the cornerstone in the diagnosis of viral hepatitis since 1968. Virtually all available immunological techniques have been used for its detection. Today, in most countries, sandwich immunoassays (Fig. 6) are used for screening purposes. They are sensitive, rapid, specific, and relatively inexpensive. Automation is available for large numbers of samples. Passive haemagglutination assays may be used as a substitute but they are less sensitive and less specific.

Sandwich immunoassays (Fig. 6) use plastic beads, microplates, test tubes, or suspensions of microbeads as the solid phase. The capturing anti-HBs antibody on the solid phase and the labelled antibody may be affinity-purified or a mixture of monoclonal antibodies. Some assays may produce decreasing signals with increasing HBsAg concentrations if a concentration of about 100 ng/ml is exceeded (prozone or Hook effect). Since most chronic HBsAg carriers and patients with hepatitis B have much higher concentrations of HBsAg, no conclusion as to the amount of HBsAg can be drawn from the signals of sandwich immunoassays unless extensive serial dilutions are tested.

Quantification

Since sandwich assays are not well suited to the quantitation of HBsAg, older and less sensitive assays, including passive haemagglutination, may be used for titration; electroimmunodiffusion

Table 4 Selection of serological markers of HBV for screening tests*	
Problem or question	**Marker**
Any contact with HBV?	Anti-HBc
Immune or susceptible to HBV? (no vaccination)	Anti-HBc
Active infection with HBV?	HBsAg
Aetiology of acute hepatitis	HBsAg and IgM anti-HBc
Aetiology of chronic hepatitis	HBsAg and anti-HBc (optional HBV DNA by PCR)
Asymptomatic infection or non-hepatic manifestation?	HBsAg Anti-HBc optional
Incubation period?	HBsAg
Liver carcinoma	HBsAg and anti-HBc (HBV DNA by PCR)
Potentially infective for HBV?	HBsAg (HBV DNA by PCR)
Immunity after vaccination?	Anti-HBs, quantitative

* In cases of positive anti-HBc or HBsAg, see Table 5. PCR, polymerase chain reaction.

Table 5 Follow-up of positive screening results

(a) *HBsAg-positive*
Repeat HBsAg
Total anti-HBc
IgM anti-HBc

HBV DNA and/or
HBeAg/anti-HBe

Optional:
　HBsAg concentration
　HBsAg subtype

If all other HBV markers absent:
　Specificity control by neutralization

(b) *Anti-HBc-positive*
HBsAg*
Anti-HBs

If HBsAg negative:

Acute hepatitis
IgM anti-HBc

Chronic hepatitis
Anti-HBc titre
Anti-HBe
HBV DNA by polymerase chain reaction

*If positive see above.

using a reference serum is preferable for quantitation (Gerlich, DevelopBiolStandard, 1975; 30:78).

The amount of HBsAg may be given in Paul Ehrlich Institute (**PEI**) units, in international units (iu), defined by the World Heath Organization (**WHO**), or in ng or μg of HBs protein. The PEI unit was defined as 1 ng active HBsAg. Unfortunately, purified HBsAg has lost much of its antigenicity and thus the 'ng' or 'μg' units are undefined overestimates of the true amounts. Reference samples for HBsAg/ayw and HBsAg/adw are available from the PEI. One WHO unit corresponds to 0.5 PEI units of HBsAg/adw.

Specificity and sensitivity

Any, even the slightest, amount of HBsAg is of diagnostic significance; thus the highest sensitivity is required. With current assays the detection limit should be between 0.02 and 1.0 ng/ml. The highest natural serum concentrations observed are in the region of 1 000 000 ng/ml; typical values are between 10 000 and 100 000 ng/ml. The broad range of concentrations creates the problem of cross-contamination between samples during handling. A second problem is that quantitation of HBsAg by simple end-point dilution requires very high dilutions, which are often made inaccurately; in addition, different subtypes may generate different titration curves.

A third problem is that specificity testing by neutralization often requires very large amounts of anti-HBs or several steps of predilution. If other markers of active HBV infection, such as HBeAg, HBV DNA, or IgM anti-HBc, are clearly positive, a specificity control of HBsAg may not be necessary. A preferable way of confirming a positive result for HBsAg is retesting by a less sensitive assay. If electroimmunodiffusion is used for this purpose, a simple and accurate quantitation is simultaneously obtained; approximately 80 to 90 per cent of true positive samples generate a detectable precipitation line in this method. The problem of specificity is not a major one with the sandwich immunoassays in current use, but false-positive findings should be avoided under all

circumstances; thus, the first positive result should be communicated as 'preliminary' and complemented later by the definitive result. Reproducibly false-positive results occur at a frequency of 1: 1000 to 1:10 000 in normal blood donors, depending on the test kit used.

Occasionally, HBsAg and anti-HBs may be present in the same serum. This pattern occurs in approximately 10 to 20 per cent of patients with chronic hepatitis B. It is usually not due to an artefact but to different fine specificities of the HBsAg and anti-HBs. Only the HBsAg is relevant for diagnosis; the anti-HBs in this case does not represent a favourable prognosis.

Subtyping

The determination of HBsAg subtypes is limited to specialized laboratories because monospecific antibodies are not commercially available. Subtypes are usually not of clinical or prognostic importance, but may be useful for the study of infection chains, since the subtype is conserved. Subtypes of HBV may also be determined after the disappearance of HBsAg using the subtype-specific proportion of anti-HBs as marker. The best subtyping of the HBV isolates is done by PCR and subsequent sequencing.

Diagnostic significance of HBsAg

The confirmed and specific finding of HBsAg in the blood or other fluids of an individual usually shows that genes for HBs proteins are present somewhere and expressed in his/her body. Often, but not always, this means that the entire infectious virus genome is also present, replicated, and secreted into the blood. The degree of viraemia may, however, vary from less than one virus per ml to more than 10^9/ml. Thus no conclusion can be drawn from a positive result for HBsAg on the state of health or infectivity of an individual. Such conclusions are possible only if the additional assays mentioned in Table 5 are performed and measures of liver damage are taken into account.

Passive acquisition

HBsAg is passively acquired during vaccination against HBV and is detectable in the serum for several days thereafter. Erroneous transfusion of HBsAg-positive blood may generate detectable concentrations of HBsAg for a few days before it is completely resorbed. The reappearance of HBsAg after several weeks indicates HBV infection. Measurable transfer of HBsAg from a HBV carrier mother to her baby occurs in less than 5 per cent of all cases; in this circumstance, perinatal infection is likely, but a negative HBsAg in the cord blood does not exclude infection of the baby.

Concentration of HBsAg

The concentration of HBsAg may be monitored if a positive result is obtained (Table 5). In acute hepatitis B, a second assay after 3 to 4 weeks allows prognosis: resolving cases show a decrease of more than 50 per cent in HBsAg concentration, but persistent cases show unvaried or increasing concentrations of HBsAg after the peak of transaminases. High HBsAg concentrations of more than 30 000 PEI units/ml are usually associated with massive viraemia and a non-responsiveness to interferon (Burczynska, JHepatol, 1994; 21:1097). The concentration of HBsAg decreases significantly during a response to interferon (Janssen, AntiviralRes, 1994; 23:251).

Incubation phase

During the incubation phase of hepatitis B, HBsAg is the earliest detectable marker amenable to routine testing. After recognized exposure, testing at monthly intervals is advisable.

Negative finding for HBsAg

A negative finding for HBsAg does not exclude the presence of HBV, for the following reasons:

1. The individual may be incubating HBV infection; HBsAg may remain negative for up to 6 months after exposure. HBV DNA may be detected by sensitive tests several weeks before HBsAg.
2. The HBV genomes may be latent and inactive but may potentially reactivate.
3. HBs protein may be expressed but not secreted. This may occur when LHBs is selectively produced. In such cases only a liver biopsy would allow a more reliable diagnosis.
4. HBsAg may be being secreted in quantities too small to be detected by assays in current use.
5. HBsAg is circulating in amounts of more than 1 ng/ml in the blood, but is covered by antibody.

The last two cases occur occasionally and may give rise to discrepancies between immunoassays from different producers. In the early and late phase of an acute infection, and in a few low-level carriers or patients with chronic hepatitis, the HBsAg concentration may be between 0.02 and 2.0 ng/ml; this is the range of detection limits by which current immunoassays may differ. In a few other cases a less sensitive assay is able to recognize an HBsAg sample that is missed by an analytically more sensitive assay. The discrepancy may be explained by partial masking of HBs epitopes by endogenous anti-HBs. Whether the remaining epitopes contribute to the detection of HBsAg depends on the specificity of the anti-HBs reagents. Escape from neutralization may be due to genetic variants with mutation in the HBs proteins.

However, all of these are rare exceptions; as a rule a negative HBsAg finding means that a individual has no active HBV infection and that his/her blood is not infectious for HBV.

Assays for HBV virions

Infectivity

Assays for infectious HBV cannot be performed as widely as they are indicated because the methods are complicated or unsatisfactory. Infectivity assays are costly and of limited use. Besides man, only chimpanzees are susceptible to HBV after intravenous inoculation. Primary hepatocyte cultures can be infected with HBV but the yield of virus is much lower than the original input (Gripon, Virology, 1993; 192:534; Galle, Gastro, 1994; 106:664). Human hepatocyte cultures are difficult to harvest and to maintain; they become refractory to HBV within a very short time. Hepatoma cell lines are not susceptible to HBV infection.

HBV may be visualized by electron microscopy as a double-shelled, round particle of 42 nm (Dane, Lancet, 1970; i:695), but this assay is insensitive, laborious, and has been replaced by assays for HBV DNA.

Endogenous DNA polymerase

This enzyme incorporates labelled deoxynucleotide triphosphates into the HBV genome in vitro by filling up the single-stranded gap in the viral DNA (Fig. 13). The so-called endogenous polymerase reaction was the first proof that the 'Dane' particle contained DNA (Kaplan, JVirol, 1973; 17:885) and provided the key to the isolation and cloning of the HBV genome. The assay has been widely used for monitoring antiviral therapy; it gives quantitative results. The enzyme is heat-labile and sensitive to high salt concentrations or repeated freezing and thawing. For monitoring viral activity in a patient the assay has been replaced by the hybridization assays for HBV DNA; it remains useful for testing antiviral substances that inhibit the HBV DNA polymerase and for identifying drug-resistant variants (Bartholomew, Lancet, 1997; 349:20).

Assay of HBV DNA

Significance

The detection of HBV DNA in serum is not proof of, but is a necessary precondition for, high HBV infectivity. In samples with high titres of HBV DNA the correlation with infectivity is very good (Berninger, JMedVirol, 1982; 9:57). Although a positive test may indicate only defective genomes, degraded or neutralized virus, especially when titres are low, the finding of HBV DNA in serum provides evidence of continuing genomic replication within host cells and of productive infection.

Quantitation

Results may be represented as picograms of HBV DNA per ml, or preferably as HBV genome equivalents/ml. One picogram corresponds to 2.86×10^5 genome equivalents if a mol. wt of 2.1×10^6 is assumed for full-length, double-stranded HBV DNA. Qualitative results of hybridization assays are less useful. A comparison of various test kits for DNA hybridization showed that the tests were not calibrated to the same reference and yielded contradictory results (Janssen, JMedVirol, 1993; 40:307; Zaaijer, JClinMicrobiol,

1994; 32:2088). Two quantitative international reference samples with HBV genotype A and D in plasma have been defined. Using these samples, most assays were found to underestimate the number of HBV-DNA molecules. It has been suggested that HBV carriers with less than 10^6 genome equivalents/ml pose only a low risk of transmission to their contacts (Gerlich, ViralHepatitisRev, 1995; 1: 53).

Filter hybridization (dot- or slot-blot)

In the simplest version of the hybridization assay a serum or plasma sample is lysed by sodium hydroxide and filtered through a porous membrane, where the DNA adsorbs. Thereafter the membrane is incubated with the labelled DNA probe. Specific binding of the probe to the filter occurs if the sample contains homologous HBV DNA (see also Fig. 7). The average sensitivity is between 10^5 and 10^6 genome equivalents/ml (Zyzik, EurJClinMicrobiol, 1986; 5: 330). Semiquantitative assays are possible by visual comparison with a reference dilution series, densitometry, or scintillation counting.

Liquid hybridization

In this technique, HBV DNA, liberated from the virion by lysis, is directly mixed with the labelled HBV DNA probe after adjustment of the buffer to allow for hybridization. ^{125}I has been used as label. Free and hybridized probe are separated by column chromatography. Sensitivity is similar to that of the dot-blot (Kuhns, JMedVirol, 1989; 27:274). A slightly more sensitive, chemoluminescence method has also been described (Urdea, Gene, 1987; 61:253). The assays allow quantitation, are relatively rapid, but are laborious and costly.

Polymerase chain reaction[10]

Purpose

This technique is able to amplify one copy of a given DNA sequence (the amplicon) to a virtually unlimited number of identical copies without needing replication in a living organism. The amplificate is thereafter detected by one of the conventional biochemical assays. The technique is useful in all fields of laboratory medicine. In medical microbiology and virology it has become essential for the discovery and diagnostic determination of infectious agents that cannot be multiplied in non-living growth media or cell culture. Since the PCR is less laborious and dangerous, it has replaced these techniques for many applications, even for those agents that do grow *in vitro*.

Extraction of DNA

This technique for the PCR requires DNA in an accessible form, that is, liberated from cells or viruses. The simplest method of extraction is boiling, but with serum or highly proteinaceous samples this is unsatisfactory. Proteinase K digestion in presence of sodium dodecyl sulphate, extraction with phenol/chloroform, and ethanol precipitation is the best but most laborious way to extract HBV DNA from serum or tissues. Alternatively, the serum sample is diluted with alkali, which disrupts the HBV particles, and is reneutralized. This simple technique, however, allows analysis of only a few microlitres of serum per PCR test.

Primers and extension

Multiplication of the DNA is achieved by annealing a synthetic oligonucleotide (the primer) with 20 to 24 bases to a complementary sequence in a single-stranded DNA to be detected (the template). A DNA polymerase as reagent adds further nucleotides to this primer according to base pairing with the template (extension). The resulting double-stranded DNA is separated by heating to more than 90°C. The separated DNA is thereafter cooled down to the annealing temperature of about 50 to 70°C and a second primer complementary to the newly synthesized strand is annealed; thereafter synthesis starts in the counter direction at 72°C. This will run off at the 5′ end of this new template, which is defined by the first primer. Thereafter, further cycles of strand separation (at more than 95°C), annealing, and extension will result in the duplication of defined DNA molecules in every cycle. The simple realization of this concept has become possible by the use of DNA polymerases from heat-stable bacteria, for example from *Thermus aquaticus* (*Taq* polymerase), which survive heating to 100°C and are active at 72°C, and by the development of inexpensive, programmable thermostats.

Specificity

The specificity of the reaction depends on the length of the primers, the G/C proportion in the primer, which causes stronger binding than A/T, the absence of mismatches, the annealing temperature, and the exact composition of the reaction buffer. The 5′ end of the primers may be linked with biotin, fluorescent groups, or other chemicals in order to facilitate easy detection or further use of the amplificate. It is important to select primers the sequence of which is highly conserved in the genome to be detected. In particular, the 3′ end of the primer must be correct. Minor mismatches within the primer sequence are tolerated if the annealing conditions are not too stringent.

Genotyping

For genotyping purposes a set of primers may be used that is complementary to variable regions and generates amplification products (amplicons) of typical different size. Primers from the variable pre-S region for this so-called multiplex PCR have been used for genotyping HBV isolates (Repp, JClinMicrobiol, 1993; 31: 1095).

Polymerases

Taq polymerase is suitable for the amplification of sequences between 50 to several hundred bases long, but protocols for longrange PCR have been developed using recombinant *Tth* or other polymerases. Full-length HBV genomes have been amplified in a replication-competent form (Günther, JVirol, 1995; 69:5437).

Detection of the amplificate

The amplified DNA may be detected by ethidium bromide staining after agarose gel electrophoresis. The size of the fragment is given by distance of the primer sequences in the original template and thus provides a specificity control. Ethidium bromide staining is relative insensitive and requires 10 to 100 ng of amplificate. In a single reaction with the maximally useful number of 35 cycles, one copy of DNA is not sufficient to generate an amount of amplificate that can be detected by ethidium bromide. Various techniques have been used to improve or simplify the detection of the amplificate. In the so-called nested PCR the amplificate is amplified in a second round with a primer pair located within the sequence of the first amplificate. This technique reliably detects one DNA copy present in the first round if the conditions for the PCR are optimized. Another possibility is to blot the amplificate after gel electrophoresis and to hybridize it to a labelled probe in a Southern blot. Better suited to high through-put applications is the capturing of the amplificate via a biotin group or a specific oligonucleotide to a solid phase. The amplificate can then be made single-stranded by alkali and hybridized with an enzyme-labelled probe. Thus the detection of the amplificate can be handled like an enzyme immunoassay (Erhardt, JClinMicrobiol, 1996; 34:1885). The most modern technique is fluorometric detection during amplification using two sensor oligonucleotides.

Sensitivity

While in theory one viral genome can be detected in a sample, in reality sensitivity may often be unsatisfactory. Samples may contain inhibitors of the PCR causing false-negative results. Extraction of the DNA may be incomplete or the DNA is degraded. The sequence of the primers may not match the target sequence. A standard PCR with subsequent ethidium bromide staining may not detect fewer than 1000 copies. Samples volumes are usually small. Finally, performance and reagents may be suboptimal or insufficient. In a quality-control trial the great majority of the participants failed to detect reliably 20 000 HBV particles/ml plasma (Quint, JClinMicrobiol, 1995; 33:225). When well performed the detection limit approaches one copy per sample, but then the statistics of particle distribution limit sensitivity (Erhardt, JClinMicrobiol, 1996; 34: 1885). With standard techniques (using, for example, 4-μl aliquots of serum or plasma) the presence of fewer than 1000 HBV particles cannot be reliably detected.

Specificity

The specificity of most PCR assays would be close to perfect if there were no problems with contamination. Early studies using the PCR were heavily plagued by uncontrolled transfer of amplificate to negative samples. One expensive way to control the problem is the use of four separate rooms for reagent preparation, sample preparation, the actual PCR, and detection of the amplificate. Of course, cloned target DNA or high-titre virus samples must also not enter these rooms. It is possible to incorporate dUTP instead of dTTP as the precursor nucleotide and to destroy any carry-over of amplificate by pretreatment with uracil N-glycanase. Another way is to use completely closed systems for every sample. Test kits for the PCR are usually safe against carry-over of amplificate, whereas in-house techniques have often lacked the proper precautions.

Distinction between different molecular forms of HBV DNA

In liver samples it is useful to distinguish integrated from free HBV DNA. This can be achieved by Southern blotting. This technique combines size determination of nucleic acids by gel electrophoresis and hybridization with an HBV-specific probe. Integrated HBV DNA is not demonstrable by this technique without prior cleavage

of chromosomal human DNA by restriction enzymes. If a restriction enzyme is used that probably does not cut the HBV genome (e.g. HindIII), the appearance of defined DNA bands shows that the cell sample consists of clonal cells and the number of bands suggests the number of HBV-DNA insertions (Shafritz, NEJM, 1981; 305:1067). Both hepatocellular carcinomas and premalignant cirrhotic nodules consist of mono- or oligoclonal cells and very often contain integrated HBV DNA. Integrated HBV DNA has been observed in liver samples from patients who did not have HBV markers in the serum (Brechot, NEJM, 1985; 312:270). Usually, the integrated HBV genomes are defective, for example genes are missing or rearranged. Sites of frequent viral integration are the direct repeats; no preferred site of cellular integration is known. A functional core gene is usually absent. The X gene is often present, but it is truncated at the 3′ end and is frequently connected with cellular sequences (Nagaya, GenesDevelop, 1987; 1:773). Free episomal HBV DNA and replicative intermediates can be detected by Southern blotting without prior cleavage by restriction enzymes.

Episomal DNA

Episomal DNA may occur in covalently closed circles, open circular double-stranded DNA, circular DNA with a variable gap, and growing single-stranded DNA minus strands. The first two DNA species may occur in the nucleus without active HBV replication (Raimondo, Virology, 1988; 166:103). The last two species occur in the cytoplasm and are a sign of active replication. The growing minus strands form an intense smear of 0.8 to 1.5 kb in the autoradiographs of Southern blots (Scotto, JInfDis, 1985; 151:610). There are rare cases of chronic HBV infections where intrahepatic HBV replication is not accompanied by detectable HBV DNA or HBeAg in the serum (Brechot, NEJM, 1985; 312:270).

Covalently closed circles of HBV DNA may also be detected by a plus strand-specific probe spanning the gap region (Lin, JMedVirol, 1989; 29:284) The Southern blot is not very sensitive, and in practice may be replaced by the PCR; however, reliable distinction between integrated and free HBV DNA still requires this technique. Covalently closed HBV DNA as a precondition of productive infection may be more satisfactorily detected by a modified PCR that bridges the gap/nick region of the genome only if this is covalently closed (Köck, Hepatol, 1996; 23; 405; Lu, JVirol, 1996; 70:2277).

Assay of pre-S1 antigen

The pre-S1 antigen is present on HBV particles in a proportion 10-fold higher than on 20-nm HBs particles (Heermann, JVirol, 1984, 52:396). In acute resolving hepatitis B it disappears more rapidly from blood than HBsAg (Gerken, Gastro, 1987; 92:1864; Delfini, JMedVirol, 1989; 28:169). Pre-S1 was detected by enzyme-linked immunosorbent assay in the serum of 96 per cent of chronic HBsAg carriers irrespective of health status and viraemia, provided a sensitive assay was used (Deepen, MedMicrobiolImmunol, 1990; 179:49). The antigen has two major linear epitope regions from amino acid 12 to 48 and from amino acid 90 to 117 (Neurath, AdvVirusRes, 1988; 34:65).

The assay of pre-S1 antigen in serum does not give much additional information to that provided by assays for HBeAg or HBV DNA. However, in the liver, LHBs may be selectively stored and may generate ground-glass cells, as is often the case in asymptomatic anti-HBe positive carriers of HBsAg. LHBs in liver biopsies can be also detected by immunoblotting (Gerken, JMedVirol, 1989; 29:261) or by immunohistology using monoclonal antibodies against pre-S1 (Dienes, Gastro 1990; 98:1017).

Assay of pre-S2 antigen

Pre-S2 occurs in similar proportions on HBs spheres, filaments, and HBV particles (Heermann, JVirol, 1984; 52:396); 20-nm HBs particles from low-viraemic carriers contain a smaller proportion of MHBs than those from highly viraemic carriers (Stibbe, Virology, 1982; 123:436). Normal human serum, but not animal sera (except from chimpanzees), contain one or more factor(s) that bind to pre-S2, blocking the epitopes on its aminoterminal half. The titre of the inhibiting factor is relatively low. Most HBeAg-positive carriers and anti-HBe-positive carriers with more than 5 μg HBsAg/ml serum have free pre-S2 epitopes (Deepen, MedMicrobiolImmunol, 1990; 170:49). Pre-S2 has a binding site for human serum albumin (Krone, Hepatol, 1990; 11:1050). Albumin polymerized by glutaraldehyde binds much better (Machida, Gastro, 1984; 85:268); this can be used as a capture reagent to the solid phase in an enzyme-linked immunosorbent assay. The assay for pre-S2 antigen does not provide essential information over and above that obtained by conventional HBsAg, HBeAg, and HBV DNA.

HBeAg and anti-HBe
Diagnostic significance

Assaying for these two factors helps to distinguish between asymptomatic HBsAg carriers with high and low viraemia. HBeAg is not suitable as a screening test; sera negative for HBsAg but positive for HBeAg are very rare and most (but not all) are due to false-positive HBeAg reactions. Assaying for HBeAg is thus indicated only in HBsAg-positive sera.

Anti-HBe may occur with or without HBsAg or anti-HBs but never without anti-HBc. Testing for anti-HBe is thus indicated only when anti-HBc is positive. Anti-HBe may give additional information to that provided by anti-HBc in cases of chronic hepatitis and in HBsAg carriers; its appearance during acute hepatitis B points to a good prognosis.

Most HBeAg-positive HBsAg carriers have more than 10^5 HBV genomes/ml serum. The majority have genome numbers around 10^9/ml, and are thus potentially infectious; about 10 to 15 per cent of the HBeAg carriers and most anti-HBe carriers have fewer than 10^5 HBV genomes/ml serum and their infectivity is probably negligible. About 30 per cent of patients with chronic hepatitis B with anti-HBe have more than 10^5 genomes/ml (Zyzik, EurJClinMicrobiol, 1986; 5:330). These patients often have an HBe-minus variant of HBV and very severe liver disease (Carman, Intervirology, 1995; 38:95). Although the existence of infective HBe-minus genomes of HBV emphasizes that the HBeAg/anti-HBe system is not the best indicator of viraemia, these markers are important in the clinical follow-up of chronic HBV infections as they describe the immune status against the HBc/e protein and the prognosis.

HBeAg-positive patients with liver cirrhosis have a worse prognosis than those with anti-HBe (de Jongh, Gastro, 1992; 103:1630; Realdi, JHepatol, 1994; 21:656), in particular if they do not

seroconvert after interferon therapy (Niederau, NEJM, 1996; 334:1422).

Antiviral therapy of chronic hepatitis B can be expected to induce a permanent clinical improvement only when, besides HBV DNA, HBeAg has also cleared from serum (Heijtink, JMedVirol, 1995; 47:245). If assays for measuring the concentration of HBsAg and HBV DNA are not available, testing for HBeAg is helpful in monitoring the outcome of acute hepatitis B. In resolving cases the test should become negative within 6 weeks from the onset of disease. A negative HBeAg test at the onset of an acute hepatitis B suggests in itself a good prognosis, unless the case runs a fulminant course.

Assays for HBeAg/anti-HBe

Sandwich immunoassays are currently the standard techniques. HBeAg is assayed directly, anti-HBe by inhibition of HBeAg. Tests are performed with monoclonal anti-HBe raised against a degraded or truncated HBc/e protein with HBe antigenicity from E. coli (Ferns, JGenVirol, 1984; 65:899). Two non-overlapping HBe epitopes a and b are known; they cover contiguous sequences around amino acids 80 and 120 (Salfeld, JVirol, 1989; 63:798).

The sensitivity of sandwich assays is high; strongly positive sera reach titres of several thousands. Only a few HBsAg-positive sera remain negative in both assays, usually those with a low concentration of HBsAg (less than 1000 ng/ml). Lack of specificity is not a problem, yet it would be difficult to recognize false-positive results; weak results for HBeAg may be confirmed by neutralization with anti-HBe.

Anti-HBc
Diagnostic significance

The presence of this antibody is determined when studying the prevalence of HBV infections, as it is found both in active and resolved HBV infections. A positive result for anti-HBc should therefore be complemented by assays for HBsAg and anti-HBs (see Table 5). As a marker of previous HBV infection, anti-HBc is superior to anti-HBs for the following reasons.

1. Anti-HBs may be induced by vaccination.
2. Anti-HBc is present in the so-called window phase when HBsAg has disappeared and anti-HBs has not yet appeared.
3. About 15 per cent of convalescents from hepatitis B do not develop anti-HBs.
4. After 6 years, about 20 per cent of convalescents have lost anti-HBs but still have anti-HBc.
5. In endemic regions about 20 per cent of HBsAg-negative, anti-HBc-positive individuals do not have anti-HBs; only a few have anti-HBs without anti-HBc.

In single cases, blood reactive only in the anti-HBc test has transmitted hepatitis B to the recipient (Hoofnagle, NEJM, 1978; 298:1379; Niermeijer, NEJM, 1978; 299:958); however, a clear risk of post-transfusion hepatitis from the administration of anti-HBc-positive, HBsAg-negative blood has not been substantiated in prospective studies.

Truly positive anti-HBc reactions are relatively rare in individuals living in regions of low endemicity for hepatitis B; they may indicate that these individuals belong to a group at high risk for blood- or sexually transmitted diseases.

A positive anti-HBc test in cases of clinically apparent acute hepatitis should be followed by an assay for IgM anti-HBc. If IgM anti-HBc is negative or low the hepatitis is probably unrelated to HBV. However, in immunodeficient individuals and children, IgM anti-HBc may remain negative or low in the face of a recent HBV infection with massive viral replication.

The finding of anti-HBc without HBsAg in chronic hepatitis is difficult to interpret as the absence of HBsAg does not invariably exclude an aetiological role for HBV (see above); high titres of anti-HBc support this assumption. Testing for anti-HBe is advisable in such cases. As anti-HBe does not persist for long after the resolution of hepatitis B, the simultaneous presence of high or moderate titres of anti-HBc and anti-HBe suggests that HBc/e protein is being continuously expressed in the liver. This finding can be substantiated by sensitive PCR assays for HBV DNA in serum.

Assays for anti-HBc

Inhibition of HBcAg detection in sandwich immunoassays is widely used (Fig. 4, top): the principle of the test is the same as that used to measure anti-HA, but IgG-binding assays are also available. HBcAg became available on a large scale by cloning and expression of the *hbc* gene in *E. coli* (Stahl, PNAS, 1982; 79:1606). Labelled anti-HBc may be produced from high-titre human IgG or from monoclonal anti-HBc. As all B-cell epitopes of the HBc protein are closely overlapping, the choice of the labelled anti-HBc is not critical (Salfeld, JVirol, 1989; 63:798). Horseradish peroxidase is often used as the enzyme label.

Sensitivity

The analytical sensitivity of the immune blocking assay is moderate. It depends on the amount of HBcAg that must be inhibited, and on the extent of inhibition that is considered significant. Acute HBV infections are virtually never missed. Antibody titres reach 10^4 and more during the acute phase, but may decrease to undetectable concentrations within several years in some (<10 per cent) patients. In chronic HBV infection, titres are usually high unless the individual is immunodeficient, but the generation of HBc/e-negative HBV variants may lead to a decrease or even to the disappearance of anti-HBc.

Specificity

This is the Achilles heel of immunoassays for anti-HBc. Human serum contains variable amounts of a factor that non-specifically inhibits the binding of labelled anti-HBc to recombinant HBcAg. This factor is probably not an immunoglobulin but cross-reactive IgM and IgA specificities have been reported (Sällberg, JClin-Microbiol, 1989; 27:849). Depending on the addition of negative human serum to the antigen and adjustment of the cut-off value, the sensitivity may be reduced and the specificity increased. Non-specific results are often weakly positive, occasionally are borderline negative after repetition, and often cannot be reproduced by another test kit; the sera are usually negative for all other HBV markers.

Non-specific results may be controlled by a direct binding assay (see Fig. 3; Nelles, JVirol, Methods, 1988; 20:219; Yang, VoxSang, 1989; 57:49). Although this assay may also be non-specific, it can be inhibited specifically by anti-HBc of animal origin. The application of this assay has confirmed the suspicion that most borderline results obtained with inhibition assays are non-specific.

IgM anti-HBc

Diagnostic significance

As IgM anti-HBc is always found in clinically overt acute hepatitis B, its presence is a requisite to diagnose this condition. Although cases of acute hepatitis B can usually be recognized from the clinical and biochemical symptoms, and from the presence of HBsAg, IgM anti-HBc is of central importance in some infrequent but significant circumstances, as follows.

1. A chronic HBV carrier who is HBsAg- and anti-HBc-positive may experience a non-B hepatitis infection, for example by HDV or HCV. Low or missing IgM anti-HBc will show that the episode of acute hepatitis is caused by an agent other than HBV. This circumstance occurs more often in high-risk groups and highly endemic areas. In one study about 10 per cent of cases of HBsAg-positive acute hepatitis were not due to HBV (Gerlich, JClinMicrobiol, 1986; 24:288); in highly endemic areas the proportion may be higher (Tassopoulos, Gastro, 1987; 92:1844).
2. Acute hepatitis B may occur without detectable HBsAg. Either the serum was taken too late or the immune elimination was very vigorous, as in cases of fulminant disease. A high IgM anti-HBc titre identifies HBV as the agent of the acute hepatitis in spite of the missing HBsAg. If sensitive HBsAg assays are applied, and blood is taken during the early acute phase, this serological pattern is rare (about 2 per cent). The proportion of IgM anti-HBc-positive, HBsAg-negative cases increases when only mild or subclinical cases of HBV infection are considered, and when serum is taken in the late phase of disease.

As IgM anti-HBc may persist for a long time after the acute phase, and chronic cases of hepatitis B may show fluctuations of the IgM anti-HBc titre, the distinction between chronic and acute HBV infection can be problematic if only qualitative results are obtained. Recently, it has been shown that cases of chronic HBV contain an anti-HBc specificity that cross-reacts with woodchuck hepatitis core (**WHc**) antigen, whereas sera from acute HBV cases do not react with this antigen. Thus unclear results obtained with IgM antiHBc may be complemented by an assay of anti-WHc (Maruyama, Gastro 1994; 106:1006; Milich, SemImmunopathol, 1995; 17:149).

In chronic HBV carriers, low or moderate IgM anti-HBc indicates the continuing production of HBcAg and therefore represents an indirect marker of disease activity. An increased rate of IgM anti-HBc was found in patients with hepatocellular carcinoma from Taiwan (Roggendorf, JHepatol, 1987; 5:268). Healthy carriers are rarely positive, even by the most sensitive assays, but about 50 per cent of patients with chronic hepatitis B are positive. A summary of the significance of various IgM antiHBc titres is given in Table 6.

Assays for IgM anti-HBc

The only test widely used is the anti-μ capture test described in the section on IgM anti-HA (see also Fig. 4). Assays from different producers may vary in specificity and sensitivity. Whether the cut-off value is indeed adjusted to detect only acute hepatitis B cases

Table 6 Significance of IgM anti-HBc titres

IgM anti-HBc (units)	Total anti-HBc	HBsAg	Suggested diagnosis
>600	+	+	Acute hepatitis B
30–600	+	+	(a) Chronic hepatitis B (b) Early acute phase (c) Late acute phase (d) Immune deficiency
<30	+	+	(a) Healthy HBsAg carrier (b) Chronic hepatitis B (c) Immune deficiency
>1200	+	ϕ or −	Acute hepatitis B
150–1200	+	ϕ or −	(a) Mild transient infection (b) Early convalescence
<150	+	ϕ or −	(a) Previous infection (b) Silent seroconversion

needs to be verified. For quantitation it is advisable to select a highly positive serum as an internal reference. A reference serum and a unit for IgM anti-HBc have been defined by the Paul Ehrlich Institute (Langen, Germany).

Anti-HBs

Diagnostic significance

Anti-HBs is not a screening measure like anti-HBc for naturally acquired immunity against HBV or for prevalence of HBV infections. This assay is recommended (i) to monitor the success of hepatitis B vaccination, and (ii) to determine the state of immunity in anti-HBc-positive individuals including convalescents from hepatitis B or patients with chronic liver disease. In HBsAg-negative, anti-HBs-positive convalescents from acute hepatitis B with a strong T-cell immunity, HBV DNA can be detected at low concentrations (Rehermann, NatMed, 1996; 2:1104). Thus the absence of HBsAg and the presence of anti-HBs do not mean a complete absence of intrahepatic HBV replication. This serological constellation indicates, however, that the level of replication (if present) is being controlled successfully at a low level by the immune system. Furthermore, the circulating virus is probably being neutralized by anti-HBs.

HBsAg carriers and patients with chronic hepatitis B usually produce anti-HBs or antipre-S but the excess of circulating HBsAg saturates this antibody, resulting in immune complexes (Madalinski, ClinExpImmunol, 1991; 84:493).

The meaning of the term anti-HBs in the literature is not completely clear. Natural HBsAg contains the three antigenic domains, S, pre-S2, and pre-S1, and theoretically anti-HBs should include all three antibody specificities. In fact, most workers consider as HBsAg only the small HBs protein (i.e., the S domain) and most of the available sandwich assays for anti-HBs do not recognize antipre-S.

Assays for anti-HBs

Owing to the relatively low concentrations of anti-HBs in immune individuals, only sensitive assays are suitable. Sandwich immunoassays are used almost exclusively at present. They employ purified HBsAg linked to a solid phase as the capture antigen and labelled HBsAg as the tracer. Quantitation can be easily achieved, provided that each test run includes a dilution series of a reference serum. For economic reasons, producers suggest the use of only one positive control serum and the assumption of a predefined calibration curve. It is usually unnecessary to titre out the sample in naturally immune individuals. For the evaluation of hepatitis B vaccines it may be desirable to assay a suitable dilution that produces a signal in the zone of proportionality of the test. The WHO has defined an international unit (iu) of anti-HBs measured by quantitative sandwich immunoassays. Originally, international units were meant to be used to control the potency of hepatitis B immune globulins. Preparations of hepatitis B immune globulin for intramuscular injection should contain more than 200 iu/ml. Due to its lower protein content, hepatitis B immune globulin for intravenous application contains less anti-HBs, i.e., 50 iu/ml. One international unit is able physically to bind 0.9 µg HBs particles (Stamm, JBiolStandard, 1980; 8:59). Many investigators prefer to communicate miu/ml instead of iu/ml or iu/l. Conventional immunoassays have a detection limit between 2 and 10 iu/l. Most enzyme and radioimmunoassays reach saturation between 100 and 1000 iu/l.

Specificity

Assays for anti-HBs are not very specific. Anti-HBs is found in approximately 1 per cent of normal individuals who have no other HBV markers (such as anti-HBc) and were not overtly exposed to HBV or HBsAg (i.e., vaccine). This non-specific antibody often belongs to the IgM class and has a very narrow subtype specificity. Animal sera may contain such non-specific IgM antibodies, which appear to be 'natural' antibodies (Berthelot, JMedPrimatol, 1984; 13:119). The artefact may be recognized by the failure to inhibit anti-HBs on addition of an HBsAg-positive serum. This inhibition assay is advisable but it does not always mean that the anti-HBs-like activity is caused by contact with HBsAg. Because of the specificity problem, anti-HBs should not be the sole marker of naturally acquired immunity. A reliable assessment of immunity requires combined testing for anti-HBs and anti-HBc, as the occasionally non-specific anti-HBc activity is apparently independent of the anti-HBs non-specificity. Strongly positive results for anti-HBs are rarely found in non-vaccinated individuals without anti-HBc.

Sensitivity

Even with the most sensitive assays a proportion of convalescents from hepatitis B (approximately 20 per cent) do not develop detectable anti-HBs, and the antibody disappears in another proportion (approximately 20 per cent) within a few years (Fig. 17); therefore its absence during convalescence does not necessarily indicate persistence of the virus or protracted disease. Nevertheless, the majority of convalescents from hepatitis B retain well-detectable concentrations of anti-HBs and anti-HBc. In highly endemic regions or high-risk groups only 10 to 20 per cent of individuals positive for anti-HBc have neither HBsAg nor anti-HBs.

Protective concentrations

In passively immunized individuals, 10 iu/l is considered to be the minimal plasma concentration that protects against HBV infection. Data on protective concentrations in postexposure prophylaxis are contradictory (Iwarsson, Lancet 1989; i:146). The qualitative composition of hepatitis B immune globulin, the type of exposure, and the delay between exposure and the administration of the immune globulin are probably more important than the exact amount of anti-HBs.

In recipients of hepatitis B vaccine, 10 iu/l of anti-HBs is also considered by convention as the minimal concentration for an adequate response. This refers to the antibody concentration 4 weeks after the completion of the vaccination. Non- or low responders who do not reach this concentration or remain antibody-negative are probably not protected and may acquire hepatitis B. In immunocompromised individuals, even concentrations higher than 10 iu/l may not be protective (Stevens, NEJM, 1984; 311:496); however, when HBV infection occurs in this setting it is usually subclinical. The same is true in normal individuals who originally had a titre higher than 10 iu/l but have since lost anti-HBs. Many European countries recommend revaccination if the anti-HBs titre is below 10 iu/l. This results in a sharp increase of anti-HBs (Jilg, JInfDis, 1988; 157:1267).

Subtyping of anti-HBs

This may complement the subtyping of HBsAg in epidemiological investigations. Mixing of the sample containing anti-HBs with serum containing subtypes of HBsAg and the subsequent assaying of residual anti-HBs allows simple subtyping. The homologous subtype of HBsAg inhibits the corresponding anti-HBs completely.

The proportion of subtype-specific anti-HBs over type-specific anti-HBs is important in the evaluation of hepatitis B vaccines. The early anti-HBs response is often subtype-specific and may not protect against other subtypes. After complete vaccination, type-specific anti-HBs/a is always present (Legler, DevelopBiol-Standard, 1983; 54:179). Fortunately, anti-HBs/a protects against all known subtypes of HBV. However, escape mutants from antibodies against the *a* determinant around Gly145 of SHBs were found in neonatally infected vaccine recipients.[12] This

observation suggests that vaccines and reagents that contain all HBs epitopes and possibly several subtypes should be used.

Antipre-S antibodies
Diagnostic significance

Antipre-S1 antibodies are detected very early in resolving acute hepatitis B and are a good prognostic marker (Takai, JImmunolMethods, 1986; 95:23). Antipre-S2 appears soon after antipre-S1, and both usually occur before conventional anti-HBs (Budkowska, in ref. 3, p. 287). Some convalescents who do not develop anti-HBs have detectable antipre-S1. However, many other convalescents with anti-HBs do not have detectable antipre-S (Deepen, MedMicrobiolImmunol, 1990; 179:49). It has been suggested that antipre-S disappears more rapidly than anti-HBs, but it is possible that this is a problem of the sensitivity of the different types of assay. Natural, plasma-derived HBsAg vaccine contains small amounts of pre-S1 and pre-S2 antigen, and a recombinant pre-S2-containing HBsAg vaccine has been introduced to the market (Tron, JInfDis, 1989; 160:199). Pre-S1-containing recombinant vaccines are currently under study. Antipre-S1(12–47) and antipre-S2(1–32) are virus-neutralizing, protective, and possibly more important in protection than anti-SHBs (Neurath, AdvVirusRes, 1988; 34:65). Unfortunately, the convincing detection of antipre-S antibodies after vaccination with such vaccines has not yet been achieved in humans.

Assays for antipre-S

Conventional sandwich assays for anti-HBs do not usually recognize antibodies against the pre-S domains and no generally available assays specific for antipre-S have yet been introduced. The following methods have been described.

1. Direct, IgG-binding, enzyme immunoassays using partial pre-S peptides fixed on a solid phase: sequences of pre-S1(1–50) and pre-S2(1–25) have mostly been used (Coursaget, Vaccine, 1988; 6:357; Kuijpers, in ref. 3, p. 280).
2. Recombinant fusion proteins containing pre-S1, pre-S2, or whole pre-S may be used as antigen for immunoblots or direct, IgG-binding, enzyme immunoassays.
3. Inhibition by the test sample of the binding between natural or recombinant HBsAg containing pre-S and monoclonal mouse antibodies against the pre-S domains (Budkowska, Hepatol, 1986; 6:360). Certain pre-S2 monoclonal antibodiess, such as Q19/10, are, however, also inhibited by normal human serum (Krone, Hepatol, 1990; 11:1050).
4. Most epitopes in the pre-S domains are denaturation-resistant and may be detected by immunoblot using a natural mixture of LHBs, MHBs, and SHBs as antigen. Coexisting anti-SHBs in the sample usually does not react with SHBs in immunoblots because its epitopes are conformation-dependent. Differentiation of antipre-S1 from antipre-S2 is possible if the reaction with LHBs is stronger than with MHBs (Heermann, Intervirology, 1987; 28:149; Shouval, Vaccine, 1994; 12:1453).

Other markers
Anti-HBx

The significance of antibodies against the X protein is not clearly established. Anti-HBx is not a marker for HBV-associated hepatocellular carcinoma, as it is often found during acute and chronic hepatitis B (Abraham, MedMicrobiolImmunol, 1989; 178: 187). However, it may reach very high titres in some cases of hepatocellular carcinoma (Levrero, Virology, 1990; 174:299). No commercial assays are available. Immunoblot or radioimmune precipitation (Pfaff, Virology, 1987; 158:456) of recombinant X protein are used for the detection of anti-HBx.

X protein

The X protein itself is difficult to determine because most of the available anti-HBx reagents, including monoclonal antibodies, are of questionable specificity. Reports on the occurrence and localization of the X protein are controversial. At present this is not a reliable diagnostic or prognostic marker.

Polymerase

The diagnostic value of the HBV DNA polymerase activity was discussed earlier. Direct detection of the pol protein or its components is of theoretical interest only.

Antibodies against the HBV polymerase (**anti-HBp**) may be detected by immunoblot using bacterial fusion proteins with the polymerase (Stemler, JGenVirol, 1988; 69:689; Chang, Hepatol, 1989; 10:332). Anti-HBp can be detected in acute and chronic hepatitis B. It appears that highly viraemic carriers often develop anti-HBp (Kann, JMedVirol, 1993; 40:285).

Hepatitis D virus
History and nomenclature

The 'D' in the virus designation is derived from the original term δ (Greek delta); δ antigen was first described in the livers of certain patients suffering from chronic hepatitis B (see Chapter 12.1.2.4). Soon after it was realized that the expression of δ antigen was dependent on infection with a novel, virus-like agent (δ agent) that was later named HDV (Rizzetto, JInfDis, 1980; 121:590). The corresponding antigen and antibody are **HDAg** and **anti-HD**. HDV is a defective virus that needs HBV as helper in order to acquire an envelope and infectivity. HDV was found to consist of an HBsAg envelope, a HDAg core, and a small, 1.7-kb RNA (Rizzetto, PNAS, 1980; 77:6124). After cloning and sequencing of the HDV RNA, a similarity between HDV and viroids and virusoids (plant pathogens) was recognized (Wang, Nature, 1986; 323:508). Formally, HDV is now classified as genus deltavirus within the family of single-strand RNA satellites (Howard, ArchVirol, 1995; Suppl. 10:493). It does not, however, have much in common with the other satellites except being dependent on a helper virus. Its structure and replication have recently been reviewed.[11,12]

Structure of the virus particle (Fig. 18)

Approximately 70 HD protein subunits form, together with the small RNA genome, a nucleocapsid-like structure (Ryu, JVirol, 1993; 67:3281), but a symmetry of this complex has not been identified and may in fact be absent. The HD protein exists in two forms: a small HD protein (**SHD**) with 195 amino acids and a colinear, large form (**LHD**) with a carboxyterminal extension of 19 amino acids resulting in a length of 214 amino acids. The two

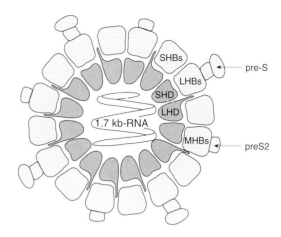

Fig. 18. Schematic model of hepatitis delta virus. The circular RNA genome is highly self-complementary and forms double-stranded rods. SHBs, MHBs, LHBs: small, middle, large hepatitis B surface protein; SHD, LHD: small and large hepatitis delta protein. Pre-S, pre-S2, domains of HBs proteins.

proteins migrate in sodium dodecyl sulphate–gel electrophoresis with M_r 24 and 27 kDa. The envelope consists of SHBs, MHBs, and LHBs. As with HBV, SHBs is the major component and MHBs a minor component. In contrast to HBV, LHBs is also a minor component as in 20-nm HBsAg particles. Assembled HDV has a size of 36 to 43 nm and a density in caesium chloride of 1.24 to 1.25 g/ml. HDAg can be released from HDV by treatment with non-ionic detergents. Since the envelope is required for infectivity, the stability of HDV is probably similar to that of HDV.

Genome structure (Fig. 19)

HDV has a genomic structure unique among the animal viruses. Its RNA forms a covalently closed, single-stranded circle with 1670 to 1685 nucleotides, depending on the isolate. Because of 70 per cent self-complementarity within the RNA sequence, the circle folds to a double-stranded rod with covalently closed ends at base 795 and 1638. By electron microscopy the HDV genome appears as short rod of about 280-nm length that opens under denaturing conditions to circles (Kos, Nature, 1986; 323:558).

The genome and its complementary copy, the antigenome, contain several open reading frames, but only one in the antigenome encodes the HD proteins and is conserved in all HDV isolates. Thus, the genome has minus-strand polarity. It must be transcribed to the antigenome sequence before the HD proteins can be translated.

RNA editing

In order to encode the two forms to HD proteins, HDV has evolved a unique strategy. The replication-competent form of the HDV genome encodes the SHD protein because SHD is required for HDV genomic replication. This S genome carries, at position 1015, a U, and in the antigenome an A, as part of an UAG ('amber') STOP codon for the 195-amino acid, SHD protein. For envelopment and secretion of the HDV, LHD protein is required. In order to encode LHD, the S antigenome is mutated ('edited') by the cellular enzyme, double-stranded RNA adenosine deaminase, at position 1015 from adenosine to inosine. This unusual base is transcribed during RNA

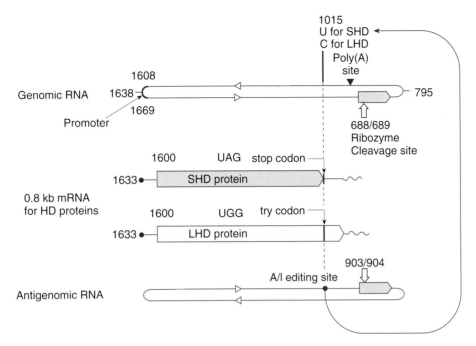

Fig. 19. Genome structure, RNA editing, and expression products of HDV. U, uridine; C, cytidine; A, adenine; I, inosine.

replication to C in the genome strand and to G in the newly produced antigenome sequence. Thus codon 196 of HD protein is no longer a STOP codon, but encodes Trp, and allows for an extension of 19 amino acids until the next STOP codon occurs (Casey, Nature, 1996; 380:454). Since SHD protein is required for genomic replication, an HDV infection can only be established by the S genome, but spread of HDV and the establishment of HD viraemia require partial conversion of S to L genomes.

Ribozyme

The genome and the antigenome contain, similar to viroids, a ribozyme structure that is able to self-cleave and self-ligate its own sequence (i.e., in *cis*). The delta-type ribozymes have a 'pseudoknot', tertiary structure of 84 bases with four short, double-helical structures (Perrotta, Nature, 1991; 350:434). The cleavage occurs at the 5′ end of this minimal structure and may cleave off any sequence upstream. This property of the delta ribozyme has been used as a molecular tool to generate RNAs with exactly defined 3′ ends, which are necessary for the generation of replication-competent, minus-strand RNA viruses (i.e., measles or influenza viruses). Helix I, where the cleavage occurs, allows some sequence flexibility as long as the double-strandedness is maintained, and furthermore the counterstrand connected with helix II in the natural delta ribozyme may originate from another RNA. Thus cleavage can also occur in *trans*. This property could theoretically be used to design ribozymes that could cleave and thus destroy almost any target RNA. However, the ribozyme activity in *trans* has so far been shown only *in vitro*, while the activity in *cis* is an essential part of the viral lifecycle.

Properties of HD proteins (Fig. 20)

A schematic presentation of the various identified functions of HD proteins is shown in Fig. 20. A region between amino acids 31 to 52 forms coils that can interact with each other and mediate oligomerization of the HD proteins. The HD proteins contain a HD proteins inwbipartite, nuclear localization signal. Thus HD proteins are predominantly found in the nucleus. Two Arg-rich motifs support binding of RNA. They are specific for rod-like RNA-structures with closed ends as in the HDV genome. All these features of SHD contribute to the replication of the HDV genome. LHD has, in addition, 19 amino acids, the sequence of which may be rather variable. A Cys-Arg-Pro-Glu motif is conserved at the carboxy end, which is target for a linkage between the Cys and a 15-C farnesyl isoprenoid. This modification is required for the secretion of HD protein within the HBs envelope. LHD has a transdominant-negative effect on the functions of SHD protein, mediated by the coil–coil interaction. Possibly LHD is partially retained by the isoprenylate at the endoplasmic reticulum whereas SHD functions only in the nucleus. Mature virions always contain a mixture of S- and LHD. Both HD proteins are phosphorylated by casein kinase II, SHD also by protein kinase C (Yeh, JVirol, 1996; 70:6190). Protein kinase C activates SHD functions, but LHD is six times more phosphorylated and inhibits SHD functions.

HD proteins are moderately immunogenic. Antibodies react with the nuclear localization signal and the C-terminal sequences of S- and LHDAg (Bichko, JVirol, 1996; 70:5807). Patients' antibodies react well with the HD nucleoprotein complex and with denatured HD proteins in Western blots.

HDV is closely related to the viroids and virusoids of plants but these agents do not encode their own protein. It has been proposed that, in the past, RNA polymerase II has switched on one rare occasion from transcription of a viroid to the mRNA of a cellular HD-protein precursor, thus linking a complementary copy of this mRNA to a viroid. A HD-binding protein with some presumed sequence homology has been found in cells (Brazas, Science, 1996; 274, 90) and is believed to be such a precursor.

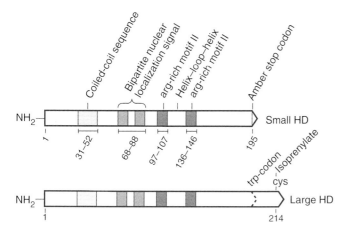

Fig. 20. Functions and motifs of the two HD proteins.

Replication

Host and organ tropism

HDV can infect humans and non-human primates if HBV is also present. Infection of woodchuck hepatitis virus-carrying wood-chucks with HDV of human origin is also possible. In this case the envelope is acquired during replication from woodchuck hepatitis virus. If brought into cells by transfection (e.g., of cDNA), HDV RNA can replicate in various mammalian cells, provided HD protein is present to initiate the replication cycle. Spread from cell to cell and to secretions is only possible in the presence of SHBs and LHBs. In transgenic mice the HDV genome is best expressed in muscle cells (Polo, JVirol, 1996; 69:4880). Thus the natural organ specificity is most likely due to the attachment and penetration mediated by the HBs envelope proteins.

Genome expression (Fig. 19)

After penetration the HDV genome reaches the nucleoplasm, possibly guided by the nuclear localization signal of the HD ribonucleoprotein complex. As with viroids, the cellular RNA polymerase II (against all rules of normal gene expression) is able to accept the HDV RNA genome as a template. The RNA-encoded promoter is formed by sequence 1608 to 1669, which forms a stem-loop region with two bulges. This secondary structure is required for HDV genomic expression and replication (Beard, JVirol, 1996; 70:4986).

Proximal to the 3′ end of the *hd* gene the genome contains a leaky signal for STOP of transcription and polyadenylation. Thus, a 0.8-kb mRNA encoding either SHD or LHD, depending on base 1015, is generated, but only SHD-encoding genomes will be replicated.

Genome replication (Fig. 21)

In the presence of increasing amounts of SHD protein the poly(A) site is suppressed and the entire circular genome is transcribed to a linear, more-than-genome length, antigenomic intermediate. The nascent antigenomic RNA strand has the ability to fold, first, into the ribozyme structure and then to clip the continuously growing

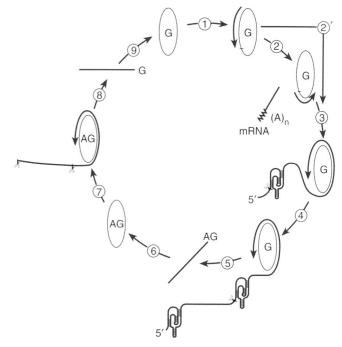

Fig. 21. HDV-RNA replication cycle. The genomic (G) strand is transcribed (1) by RNA polymerase II to a short mRNA (2) and a long, continuously growing strand (3), which cleaves itself first by its ribozyme at the 5′ end (4) and thereafter a second time, resulting in a genome-long linear RNA (5). This antigenome (AG) is able to recircularize (6) and now to repeat the cycle with the genomic transcript (7–9). (From ref. 12 with permission.)

intermediate into genome-long units. This molecule folds back to the rod-like structure and undergoes self-ligation. Host factor(s) prevent, first, folding of the rod structure and then stabilize the ribozyme. After the generation of the circular structure the ribozyme is inactivated by RNA sequences in *cis*, which prevent further self-cleavage of the genome (Lazinski, JVirol, 1996; 69:1190). The clipping and self-ligation is (*in vitro*) reversible and independent of any protein, and thus a true ribozyme reaction. The energy of the phosphodiester bond is conserved in the cleaved state by transesterification of the phosphate from the 5′ group to a 2′, 3′ cyclic monophosphate terminus. The same process now starts with the antigenome, thus generating progeny genomes. Interaction with SHD stabilizes the RNA and facilitates further cycles of replication. The base-paired region around base 1015 of the antigenome is subject to RNA editing: a certain proportion of the genome will finally encode LHD and no longer contribute to replication but to envelopment and secretion.

Assembly

SHD has an affinity for the RNA rods of HDV and it can also form mixed complexes with LHD. LHD interacts in the endoplasmic reticulum with SHBs. Isoprenylation is required for the envelopment of LHD, but the oligomerization is dispensable for this function (Sheu, Virology, 1996; 218:275). In contrast to HBV, LHBs is not required for the envelopment of HDV nucleoprotein. However, mixed assembly of SHBs with LHBs is required for the infectivity of HDV, whereas MHBs is dispensable (as is the case with HBV). The structure and function of the HBs envelope in HDV are different from those of the HBV envelope because the host specificity of HDV is obviously not so narrow and primary cell cultures can be infected more easily.

Genotypes and variability

All selected populations of HDV must contain a mixture of SHD- and LHD-encoding genomes. Editing is not completely restricted to base 1015 but also affects neighbouring bases of the antigenome. The major part of the *hd* gene is rather variable with the exception of essential motifs. Three genotypes, I to III, have been identified, which differ by as much as to 40 per cent in their nucleotide sequences. Genotype I is most frequent and has variable pathogenicity. Genotype II has been found in Japan, causing relatively mild disease, whereas genotype III is associated with HBV genotype F and fulminant hepatitis in South America (Casey, JInfDis, 1996; 174:920).

Cytotoxicity and virulence

A high ratio of LHD- to SHD-encoding genomes at the onset may favour resolution of the disease (Yang, JGenVirol, 1995; 76:3071) because it attenuates HDV replication. Immunopathogenicity seems to play a part in HDV. Furthermore, HDV induces autoantibodies in some patients. Observations in reinfected HBV/HDV carriers after liver transplantation suggest that HDV develops its full pathogenicity only together with overt HBV infection.

Although highly self-complementary, the HDV genome does not possess double-stranded RNA segments of longer than 15 bp and thus should not activate double-stranded RNA-dependent enzymes or factors such as the interferon-induced protein kinase R that inhibits protein synthesis in interferon-responsive cells. However, the HDV genome does paradoxically activate the kinase activity of protein kinase R but it does not inhibit protein translation (Robertson, JVirol, 1996; 70:5611). This observation may explain why interferon is rather inefficient in HDV infection.

Course of the disease

Two states must be distinguished, as follows.

1. Coinfection, where the infectious material contains both HBV and HDV. HDV suppresses, by unknown mechanisms, the replication of HBV; the course of infection is usually self-limiting but the acute phase is of variable severity including many fulminant cases. The infectivity titre of the inoculum is determined by either HBV or HDV, whichever is lower.
2. In superinfection HDV infects an HBV carrier. Owing to the established colonization by HBV, HDV can replicate much more vigorously. Superinfection of HBV carriers usually leads to chronic HDV infection, and may often cause fulminant hepatitis. The infectivity titre of the inoculum is determined only by HDV.

In both circumstances the HD protein first appears in the liver after an incubation period of weeks or months. HDV is secreted into the blood before the onset of clinical disease and starts to decrease during acute hepatitis. Infectivity titres of HDV may reach 10^{11}/ml serum during the early acute phase (Ponzetto, JInfDis,

1987; 155:72) but are, as a rule, lower in persistent infection. Anti-HD antibodies appear during the acute phase and may disappear within a few months after recovery. In persistent infection titres remain high, as is also true for IgM anti-HD.

Diagnosis of HDV infection

HDV infection occurs together with HBV infection. Thus the detection of HDV and anti-HD antibodies is normally indicated only for individuals with markers of active HBV infection. HDV-infected patients who have received a liver transplant are the exceptions to this. In such cases the new liver can be infected in spite of seemingly absent HBV. As a general recommendation an assay of anti-HD should be done as a screening test in all HBsAg-positive individuals and in cases of HBsAg-negative acute hepatitis where no other agent can be identified. Owing to the suppression of HBV by HDV, HBsAg may indeed be absent in some patients during acute HDV infection (Caredda, JInfDis, 1989; 159:997); these patients usually have IgM anti-HBc. In drug abusers and recipients of blood products, testing for anti-HD may be also informative, even when HBsAg is absent.

During early acute hepatitis D as well as during the incubation period, anti-HD may still be negative; in this phase, HDAg may be detectable in detergent-treated serum samples. When anti-HD appears, direct testing for HDAg by immunoassay is no longer useful unless HDV proteins are separated from anti-HD.

Disease activity and infectivity cannot be deduced from the presence of anti-HD but only from the determination of HD protein in serum and liver, or preferably from an assay of HDV RNA.

Determination of anti-HD and HDAg

HDAg and anti-HD were first assayed by immunofluorescence using liver biopsies from chronic HDV carriers as antigen and serum from the carriers as antibody (Rizzetto, Gut, 1977; 18:997). Currently, HDAg in serum is detected by sandwich immunoassays using high-titre IgG anti-HD as the capturing antibody and labelled anti-HD as the tracer. The inhibition of tracer binding to HDAg fixed on a solid phase indicates the presence of anti-HD in the serum sample (Fig. 4). Several test kits for anti-HD and HDAg are available on the market. The HDAg for these anti-HD kits may be derived from various sources such as woodchuck or chimpanzee liver, or serum from acutely ill individuals. Recombinant HDAg may replace natural HDAg (Gowans, JVirolMethods, 1990; 27: 69), and monoclonal antibody may replace the patient's polyclonal immunoglobulin.

As with all inhibition assays the analytical sensitivity is not high, but is sufficient to detect the great majority of productive HDV infections. Naturally extracted HDAg may also contain HBcAg and serum of patients with IgG anti-HD may contain anti-HBc. However, the HBc system does not interfere with the specificity of the anti-HD assay.

IgM anti-HD

The standard anti-μ capture assay is used to detect this antibody. The assay may be applied to the diagnosis of acute infection, but patients with both acute and chronic disease have high titres of IgM anti-HD. IgM anti-HD may be considered an indirect marker of active HDV infection and HDV-associated disease (Farci, JAMA, 1986; 225:1443).

HDV proteins by immunoblot

Detection of HDAg is more informative if anti-HD is removed by denaturation in ionic detergent (sodium dodecyl sulphate) and subsequent separation by gel electrophoresis. The separated proteins are transferred to membranes and detected by the reaction with labelled anti-HD. The sensitivity of the immunoblot assay can be improved if HDV particles are pelleted from serum by ultracentrifugation before sodium dodecyl sulphate-gel electrophoresis. The majority of patients with HDAg in liver biopsies also have HDAg in serum by immunoblot (Smedile, JMedVirol, 1990; 30:20). However, the method is laborious and no test kits are available.

HDV RNA

Various probes for HDV RNA are available from specialized laboratories but not as yet commercially. Dot- or slot-blot hybridization yields sufficiently sensitive results if radiolabelled riboprobes are used (Smedile, JMedVirol, 1990; 30:20). More sensitive is the application of the PCR. The assay is indicated for monitoring chronic patients, especially when antiviral therapies are undertaken. The detection of intrahepatic HDAg is as sensitive; it requires, however, an invasive liver biopsy.

Hepatitis C virus
History and classification

The agent of parenterally transmitted non-A, non-B hepatitis long remained elusive. Its existence was recognized by the transmission of hepatitis to recipients of blood that had been tested for HBsAg (Prince, Lancet, 1974; ii:2418; Feinstone, NEJM, 1975; 292:767) and thereafter by the experimental infection of chimpanzees (Alter, Lancet, 1978; i:459; Tabor, Lancet, 1978; i:463). Filtration experiments showed that the size of the agent was between 50 and 80 nm. Its low density and sensitivity to organic solvents suggested that it was enveloped (Bradley, Gastro, 1985; 88:773).

The typical changes of the endoplasmic reticulum in infected chimpanzee liver (Shimizu, Science, 1979; 205:197; Pfeifer, Virch-Arch, 1980; 33:233) are reminiscent of flavivirus infections. In immunosuppressed chimpanzees rather high titres of the infectious agent (10^6/ml plasma) could be generated. Shotgun-expression cloning of cDNA fragments derived from such plasma by M. Houghton and his coworkers at Chiron Corp. led to a clone termed (5–5–1) expressing a small protein fragment that bound IgG from patients convalescent from non-A, non-B hepatitis. This cDNA clone has eventually allowed the cloning, sequencing, and characterization of the whole HCV genome. It is a single-stranded RNA of 9.5-kb length and of plus polarity, with one open reading frame of 3010 to 3033 amino acids. The genomic organization puts HCV into the virus family *Flaviviridae* (Choo, Science, 1989; 244:359), where it forms its own genus together with the genera flavivirus and pestivirus (Wengler, ArchVirol. 1995; Suppl. 10:415). The prototype virus of this family is the yellow fever virus; other important members are, for example, the viruses of tick-borne

encephalitis, West Nile fever, dengue fever, and Japanese encephalitis, which all belong to the genus flavivirus. The pestiviruses, which cause classical swine fever and bovine viral diarrhoea, are, however, more closely related to HCV. Their genomic organization is more similar, they do not need an insect vector, and they can also cause persistent infection. Houghton has reviewed the virology of HCV,[13] and Rice that of the virus family *Flaviviridae*.[14]

Structure of the virus particles

Infection experiments in chimpanzees characterized the virus as an enveloped particle of moderate size, most probably with an RNA genome. In one experiment the density of the infectious virus was determined at 1.105 g/ml but lower densities could not be excluded (Bradley, JMedVirol, 1991; 34:206). After the identification of HCV sequences, further efforts to characterize the virus used the RT-PCR for the detection of HCV RNA in order to determine the density, size, and abundance of the virus particles. Since HCV cannot be grown efficiently in cell cultures, plasma samples from HCV-infected individuals were analysed. These studies revealed a surprising heterogenicity and variability of the HCV RNA-associated particles. The buoyant density of the particles is between less than 1.02 and 1.25 g/ml in sucrose-gradient centrifugation and varies from patient to patient (Thomssen, MedMicrobiolImmunol, 1992; 181:293; 1993; 192:329). The sedimentation behaviour is difficult to analyse because of this heterogeneous density. Reliable sedimentation of HCV by ultracentrifugation of serum cannot be assumed.

Association with host proteins and lipids

The variable density of the HCV-containing structure is mainly caused by the association of the virus with very low-density, low-density, and high-density lipoproteins. The binding of low-density lipoprotein to HCV occurs at low temperature with most sera but is abrogated if the sera are preincubated at 37°C for 1 h, even if fresh low-density lipoprotein is added. Thus, most sera that have been stored immediately in the cold contain complexes of HCV particles with a very low density (R.Thomssen, unpublished data). Other fractions of HCV RNA-containing particles are associated with IgG and/or IgM.

Size of HCV particles

Even if sera are analysed in which no host proteins are bound to the HCV RNA-containing particles (for example, some individual specimens, or by collecting and centrifuging serum at 37°C), the sedimentation and density profile reveals three classes of particles with diameters of 26 to 32 nm, 39 to 43 nm, and 55 to 60 nm. The small particles can be immunoprecipitated with antibodies against the HCV core protein but have a density of only 1.10 to 1.13 g/ml. This indicates that they must contain, in addition to HCV core protein and RNA, lipid (R.Thomssen, unpublished), because classical virus cores would have a density of more than 1.32 g/ml. Clinical observations suggest that during early phases of infection, particles with low density and without bound antibody prevail whereas in the chronic phase, particles with high density and bound antibody occur (Kanto, Hepatol, 1994; 19:296). Size-exclusion chromatography showed that HCV RNA was associated mainly with particles larger than 150 nm of very low density, and with

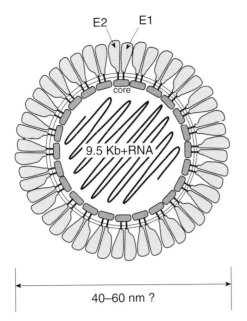

Fig. 22. Schematic model of the HCV particle. Published data suggest that the virus has a diameter of c. 60 nm. The model assumes that the envelope proteins E1 and E2 form a heterodimer and are present in equimolar amounts with the core protein

intermediate particles of 78 nm with intermediate density that may represent free virus (C. Jursch and W.H. Gerlich, unpublished). Membrane filtration of plasmas showed that the infectivity was associated with particles of more than 50 nm and less than 80 nm, but the complete size distribution and the density of the infectious particles could not be analysed. Membrane-filtration experiments found, however, HCV RNA-containing particles smaller than 38.8 nm (Yuasa, JGenVirol, 1991; 72:2021). Figure 22 shows a hypothetical model of HCV assuming a similarity with other *Flaviviridae*.

Electron microscopy

The comparatively low number of HCV particles in serum has made their direct visualization difficult. In order to confirm the specificity of the virus-like structures seen by electron microscopy, these were incubated with antibodies against the HCV envelope protein 2 (**E2**). Particles of 60 to 70 nm were found either directly (Kaito, JGenVirol, 1994; 75:1755) or after the removal of lipoprotein by detergents. Furthermore, 40-nm structures were found in the detergent-treated preparations that were supposed to represent defective viruses (Prince, JViralHepat, 1996; 3:11). HCV RNA-containing particles of 40 nm diameter and intermediate density have been found in cultures of insect cells transfected with the genes for the structural proteins of HCV (T.F. Baumert, unpublished). Cultures of differentiated human hepatocytes transfected with presumably complete HCV cDNA expressed virus-like particles with diameters of between 40 and 60 nm within intracellular vacuoles (M. Kaito, unpublished). At the time of writing the morphology of the virion has not been definitively revealed. Accumulated evidence suggests that the virus may be heterogeneous and have a diameter between. 60 and 80 nm. Larger forms may contain host protein, in particular lipoproteins.

Stability

As an enveloped virus, HCV is sensitive to organic solvents and detergents. Plasmas or blood products treated with various modifications of pasteurization (standard is 10 h, 60°C) are not reliably free of HCV infectivity, although the virus is heat-sensitive. Systematic studies of its sensitivity to disinfectants or inactivating agents are not available because its infectivity cannot easily be determined. The virus of bovine viral diarrhoea has been used as the closest related substitute, but the justification for this model system has not been established. The infectivity of HCV is destroyed by chloroform. This suggests that HCV is sensitive to detergent-like disinfectants.

Reports on the stability of HCV RNA have been highly divergent. This may in part be due to the fact that HCV is itself highly heterogeneous. Thus, some serum samples may contain a large number of defective or temperature-sensitive variants that may rapidly degrade; others may be more stable. For diagnostic purposes it is advisable to store samples frozen at least at $-20°C$. Storage at room temperature or 4°C does not seriously diminish detectability by RT-PCR within 60 h, but at 37°C the titre is reduced by a factor of 100 (R. Thomssen, unpublished).

Genome structure and gene products (Fig. 23)

Much more knowledge than that on virion structure and morphology has been gathered on the sequence of HCV RNA and the products and functions it encodes. The first, almost complete sequence has been published by Chiron (Choo, PNAS, 1991; 88: 2451). The RNA has a total length of c. 9300, depending on the isolate. It has a highly conserved, 5′ non-coding or untranslated region of at least 341 bases, a long open reading frame of 9030 to 9099 bases encoding a polyprotein of 3010 to 3033 amino acids, and a 3′ terminal non-coding region of 200 to 230 bases, which was only recently identified completely (Kolykhalov, JVirol, 1996; 70:3363; Tanaka, JVirol, 1996; 70:3307). Both non-coding regions have a conserved secondary structure similar to that of pestiviruses.

Internal ribosomal entry site

The 5′ non-coding region has the ability (as with the pestiviruses and in contrast to the flaviviruses) to bind ribosomes independently from a 5′ cap structure, that is, an internal ribosomal entry site. The internal ribosomal entry site of HCV forms a complex array of eight hairpin loops (A–H) that bind host factors. The joining sequences encoding the HCV core protein are obviously a part of the internal ribosomal entry site or enhance its efficiency considerably (Lu, PNAS, 1996; 93:1412). The significance of several conserved, very short open reading frames within the internal ribosomal entry site is unclear. The exact function of the internal ribosomal entry site depends on the host cell type (Rijnbrand, Virology, 1996; 226:47).

3′ non-coding region

This genomic segment contains a type-specific sequence of 28 to 40 bases, a variable poly(U) and C/U repeat stretch, and a highly conserved core element (3′ X) of 98 to100 bases with three potential hairpin loops, I–III. The 3′ non-coding region is very probably involved in the binding of the HCV-encoded, RNA-dependent

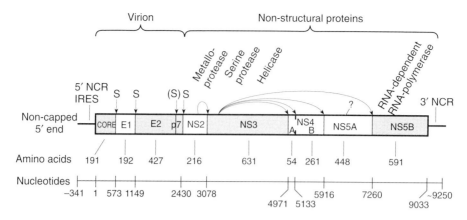

Fig. 23. Genome map of HCV. NCR, non-coding region, IRES, internal ribosomal entry site; E1, E2, envelope proteins 1 and 2; S, cleavage sites by the cellular signal peptidase; NS2–NS5B, non-structural proteins generated by autoproteolytic cleavage (see arrows) from the polyprotein precursor. (Data on polyprotein from Hijikata, PNAS, 1991; 88:5547 completed according to the text.)

RNA polymerase and in initiating synthesis of the HCV minus-strand (Jamada, Virology, 1996; 223:255).

Gene order within the open reading frame

Similar to the replication strategy of *Picornaviridae*, the various gene products of *Flaviviridae* are generated by co- and post-translational cleavage from one polyprotein precursor. The similarity extends to the 5′ terminal position of the structural proteins and the 3′ terminal position of the non-structural proteins. Furthermore, *Picornaviridae* and *Flaviviridae* have the RNA-dependent RNA polymerase at the most 3′ terminal position. The array of the other genes differs, however, between the two virus families and even between the genera of the *Flaviviridae*. Formally, the structure of the HCV gene products is not well established in the natural infection but deduced from studies with transfected cell cultures. The gene order shown in Fig. 23 is likely also to be relevant in human HCV infection: core, envelope protein 1 (**E1**), and E2 each have a hydrophobic signal peptide that inserts into the endoplasmic reticulum membrane. The cellular signal peptidase cleaves at the N-terminus of the signal peptide and generates the three putative HCV structural proteins. Core protein faces the cytosol, whereas E1 and 2 face the lumen of the endoplasmic reticulum. It appears likely that the three proteins interact with the HCV genome and bud into an intracellular vesicle as particles, which are shown schematically in Fig. 22. The non-structural (**NS**) proteins, NS2, NS3, NS4A, NS4B, NS5A, and NS5B, are generated by proteases encoded by the virus. NS2 is a metalloprotease that cleaves, in *cis*, its junction with NS3. NS3 is a serine proteinase that cleaves its junction with NS4A in *cis*, the other junctions in *trans*. The numbering of the NS proteins is derived historically from studies on viruses belonging to the genus flavivirus. HCV and the pestiviruses do not possess an NS1.

Core protein

The protein can be expressed in many bacterial and eukaryotic host-cell systems, and is generated in the presence of vesicles of the endoplasmic reticulum as a membrane-bound, 21-kDa protein from the polyprotein. It forms the ribonucleoprotein of HCV and has been extracted from HCV particles (Takahashi, Virology, 1992; 191:431). However, core-like particles in serum have a lower density

(see above). Multimeres of core protein interact with viral RNA and with E1 (Lo, JVirol, 1996; 70:5177). Since artificially expressed structural proteins encapsidate their own mRNA in the absence of non-structural sequences, it is likely that an encapsidation sequence exists within the structure encoding part of the genome (T. F. Baumert, unpublished work).

Besides its structural function, several biological functions have been attributed to the core protein, as follows.

1. It binds through sequences 36 to 91 to the cytoplasmic domain of the lymphotoxin-B receptor (a member of the cell death-inducing tumour necrosis-factor receptor family) and activates apoptosis (Matsumoto, JVirol, 1997; 71:1301)). Sensitization to *fas*-mediated apoptosis was observed (Ruggieri, Virology, 1997; 229:68). However, inhibition of c-*myc*-induced apoptosis has been also reported (Ray, Virology, 1996; 226:176).
2. It binds to apolipoprotein AII and induces steatosis in naturally infected chimpanzees (Barba, PNAS, 1997; 94:1200).
3. It inhibits HBV replication by interfering with the phosphorylation of viral proteins (Shih, JVirol, 1993; 67:5823).
4. It has been reported to cooperate with the H-*ras* oncogene during the transformation of rat embryo fibroblasts (Ray, JVirol, 1996; 170:4438).

All these properties may contribute to the pathogenicity of HCV *in vivo*, but definite links between these *in vitro* observations and clinical phenomena have not yet been established.

Envelope proteins 1 and 2

E1 forms a glycoprotein (**gp**)31, E2 a gp70, if expressed in animal cells or *in vitro* in the presence of vesicles of the endoplasmic reticulum (Deleersnyder, JVirol, 1997; 71:697). E1 and E2 have binding sites for low-density lipoprotein and E1 additionally for high-density lipoprotein (R.Thomssen, unpublished). E2 has two hypervariable regions (**HRV**) that extend from amino acids 384 to 414 (HRV1; Hijkata, BBResComm, 1991; 175:220) and from amino acids 474 to 480 (HRV2; Kato,VirRes, 1992; 22:107). E1 and E2 are cotranslationally separated from each other before they assume their complex conformation as heterodimers in the endoplasmic reticulum (Dubuisson, JVirol, 1996; 70:778). E1 and E2 or their heterodimers are not secreted and must be extracted from transfected animal cells (Ralston, JVirol, 1993; 67:6753). By fusion of the E2 gene with the gene of a secreted glycoprotein, an E2 protein can be obtained in the supernatant of transfected mammalian cells (Nisihara, Gene, 1993; 129:207), but it is not clear whether this has the same conformation as in the natural E1/E2 complex. Possibly a p7 is also part of the virion (Lin, JVirol, 1994; 68:8147). It cannot be excluded that mature HCV particles have a different structure than that deduced from the data on *in vitro* expression and from analogies with other genera of the *Flaviviridae*; initially it appeared possible that E2 would correspond to the NS1 of the flaviviruses.

NS2

NS2 is a Zn-dependent metalloprotease of 23 kDa with Cys and His residues in the active centre (Hijikata, JVirol, 1993; 67:4665). It is supposedly membrane-associated and seems to interact with the other non-structual proteins. It is involved in the phosphorylation of NS5A (Tanji, JVirol, 1995; 69:3980).

NS3

NS3 is a 70-kDa protein with two domains, an N-terminal protease and a C-terminal α-helicase type II. The protease domain with 181 amino acids has been expressed separately in *E.coli*, crystallized, and the spatial structure elucidated (Kim, Cell, 1996; 87:343; Love, Cell, 1996; 87:331). The protease is chymotrypsin-like, with the classical triad Ser139, His157, and Asp81 in the active centre. The substrate specificity with Cys or Ser in the N-terminus of the cleavage site and an acid residue (Asp or Glu) six amino acids upstream is mediated by the side-chains in the substrate pocket. NS3 has a binding site for NS4A (amino acids 22–33), which is an essential cofactor for the NS3 protease activity. Distal from the active centre is a Zn^{2+}-binding site formed by Cys97, 99, 145, and His149 that contributes to the folding of the enzyme. The accurate knowledge of the spatial structure supports a rational design for protease inhibitors as potential drugs against HCV. Various assays for NS3 protease activity have been developed and allow *in vitro* testing of potential inhibitors (Lin, PNAS, 1995; 92:7622).

A further potential target of drugs against HCV may be the NS3 helicase domain. *In vitro* assays for the nucleotide triphosphatase and nucleic acid strand-separating activity have been developed (Tai, JVirol, 1996; 70:8477). Given the fact that HCV is often associated with liver tumours, the *in vitro* capacity of NS3 to transform NIH 3T3 mouse fibroblasts to malignant growth is remarkable (Sakamuro, JVirol, 1995; 69:3893).

NS4A/B

NS4A is an amphipathic, small protein of 54 amino acids with a hydrophobic N-terminus and a hydrophilic C-terminus. It interacts with membranes, NS3, and possibly other non-structural proteins. The function of the 27-kDa, large NS4B protein is unknown.

NS5A

NS5A occurs in mammalian cells as a variably phosphorylated protein of M_r 56 or 58 kDa. It is associated with a cellular serine/threonine protein kinase (Tanji, JVirol, 1995; 69:3980). NS5A encodes an interferon sensitivity-determining region (Enomoto, NEJM, 1996; 334:77) present in wild-type HCV isolates of genotypes 1b (amino acids 2209–2248) or 2 (2193–2228). In interferon-responsive patients this 1b region usually has several mutations. The probability of response increases with the number of mutations and is very high (84 per cent) with more than three. NS5A seems to interact with the interferon-induced protein kinase R and may thus indeed be an interferon-resistance factor (M. G. Katze, personal communication).

NS5B

NS5B (68 kDa) is the RNA-dependent RNA polymerase. It contains the typical sequence motifs of this enzyme (e.g. GDD). It has been expressed in insect cells, purified, and shown to incorporate nucleoside triphosphatases into a growing RNA strand using a backfold of the 3′ end as primer/template (Behrens, EMBOJ, 1996; 15:12). The authentic RNA replication probably requires further viral and cellular factors. *In vitro* it interacts with NS5A and HCV RNA. The RNA polymerase is another important target for potential drugs against HCV.

Replication

Chimpanzee infection

Infection of chimpanzees was initially the only possibility for determining the infectivity titre and the physical properties of HCV, and to gain material for the cloning of the viral genome, but considerable divergence was observed between the high titres of genome in the RT-PCR and the low titres of infectivity.

Cell cultures

Cell cultures cannot be used for the production or titration of HCV because the yield of progeny virus is extremely low. New infection at very low concentrations is detectable in certain T-lymphocyte cultures (Molt 4Ma, Daudi cells, MT-2, MT-2C) (Shimizu, JVirol, 1994; 68:1494; Mizutani, JVirol, 1996; 70:7219) and in certain primary hepatocyte cultures that were fused with permanent hepatocyte lines (IMY, PH5CH, PH5CH1) or with primary hepatocyte cultures. As proof of infection the synthesis of RNA minus strands is measured. However, precautions have to be taken that the procedure for the RT-PCR is indeed minus strand-specific (Lanford, JVirol, 1996; 69:8079). Adsorption and possibly uptake of HCV occur with many cell lines of human or non-human primate origin, for example fibroblasts (Zibert, Virology, 1995; 208:653), whereas bovine fibroblasts do not adsorb. The H9 lymphocyte line is also an efficiently binding line (Rosa, PNAS, 1996; 93:1759). Both adsorption and/or replication of certain isolates can be neutralized by antibodies against the hypervariable region 1 of E2 protein but the neutralizing specificity is very narrow (Shimizu, Virology, 1996; 223:409). The adsorption of HCV on to human fibroblasts can be inhibited by low-density lipoprotein. Using a human fibroblast cell line devoid of the low-density lipoprotein receptor, no binding of HCV could be found. Transfection of such cells with an low-density lipoprotein expression vector confers the ability to adsorb HCV (Monazahian and Thomssen, unpublished work). This suggests that HCV binds either directly or indirectly via adsorbed low-density lipoprotein to the low-density lipoprotein receptor. However, this binding cannot explain the organotropism of the virus.

In order systematically to study the replication an infectious cDNA clone would be very helpful. Recently, such a clone has been generated, successfully transfected to a chimpanzee, and a full HCV infection obtained (Kolykhalov, Science, 1997; 277:570).

Replication in vivo

In vivo, replication seems to occur mainly in the liver. Leucocytes do take up the virus but probably contribute very little to HCV production. The level of HCV replication may, in fact, be much higher than anticipated from the relatively low number of HCV particles in the blood. HCV probably has a very short half-life (a few hours) in plasma whereas maturation and secretion require several days (Zeuzem, Hepatol, 1996; 23:366).

Molecular events

The molecular events of replication can be derived from general knowledge of *Flaviviridae*. They involve adsorption, penetration, release of genome into the cytosol, and translation of the polyprotein at the rough endoplasmic reticulum with the aid of the internal ribosomal entry site. The NS5B replicase will generate a copy of minus-strand RNA and thereafter progeny plus-strand genomes. These may serve as template for the synthesis of new polyproteins, or may be encapsidated by the structural proteins in an unknown cellular compartment probably between the endoplasmic reticulum and the Golgi network. The liver-specific factors in this process are unknown. Most likely there is no nuclear phase of the replication cycle, but single viral proteins, for example HCV core, could theoretically reach the nucleus (Shih, JVirol, 1993; 67:5823) and have some function there, although this has not been observed *in vivo* (Barba, PNAS, 1997; 94:1200). Synthesis and assembly of the viral components most probably occurs at intracellular membranes (Mizutani, JVirol, 1996; 70:7219). The glycoproteins are not expressed at the cell surface.

Genotypes and variability

More than a thousand HCV RNA isolates have been partially sequenced and several dozens of HCV genomes have been more or less completely sequenced. The overall result indicates extreme genome variability, which parallels that of the human immunodeficiency virus (**HIV**). In contrast to many other highly variable viruses, recombination between various HCV strains seems to occur very rarely or not at all, although coinfection with several genotypes occurs often. Thus genotyping by one genome region allows extrapolation to the entire genome, if these data are informative at all. The different regions of the HCV genome have different variability: the 5′ non-coding region, 3′ non-coding region, core, and NS5 are relatively conserved; E1, E2, NS2, NS3, and NS4 are more variable. There are two hypervariable regions (HVR1 and 2) in E2 (review by Simmonds, Hepatol, 1995; 21:570).

Genotypes and genosubtypes

Pairwise comparison of the percentage sequence homologies of different isolates shows a discontinuous distribution with three peaks: 88 to 100 per cent homologous isolates are considered to belong to the same genotype and genosubtype; 79 to 86 per cent homology indicates a different subtype but identical genotype; less than 70 per cent homology identifies a different genotype. The original proposed genotypic grouping of the HCV isolates using roman numerals (Okamoto, JGenVirol, 1992; 73:673) has been substituted by the nomenclature introduced by Simmonds. Currently, six genotypes of HCV are known, designated by arabic numerals, and a variable number of subtypes distinguished by lower-case letters: genosubtype 1a is the prototype HCV that was originally cloned by the coworkers of Chiron Corp.

Evolution and geographical distribution of genotypes

Studies on the divergence of HCV after the infection of numerous individuals from a common source, such as by HCV-contaminated immunoglobulin, show a nucleotide exchange rate of 10^{-3} to 10^{-2} per nucleotide and year. This high mutation rate suggests that HCV has colonized mankind only in historical times. Genosubtype 1b is estimated to have separated from an ancestral genotype 1 only 65 to 70 years ago, whereas separation of the genotypes was deduced to have occurred 500 years ago (Smith, JGenVirol, 1997; 78:321). Japan and Central Europe have predominantly genosubtype 1b, whereas north-west Europe and the United States have predominantly 1a. Genotype 2 is prevalent all over Europe and may have existed there before. Genotypes 3 and 6 are prevalent in southern and eastern Asia, 4 and 5 in Africa. Genotypes 3, 4, and 6 have many subtypes, which suggests a longer time-span for their evolution than for genotype 1 or 2. Notable is the absence of an indigenous HCV subtype in the Amerind population (in contrast to HBV genotype F or HDV genotype III). This would suggest that HCV entered mankind not earlier that 7000 to 12 000 years ago. Recent intravenous drug abuse has caused a rapid spreading of genotype 3a from southern Asia to Europe. Newly defined genotypes 7 to 11 are probably subtypes of genotype 3 and 6 (Simmonds, JGenVirol, 1996; 77:3013).

Genotyping is important for the identification of infection chains; differences in the pathogenicity of the various genotypes seem to exist. Genosubtype 1b is supposedly more virulent, pathogenic, and interferon-resistant that other geno(sub)types. However, some recent evaluations did not confirm a different pathogenicity or virulence of the various genotypes (Einstein, Hepatol, 1996; 24: 1312; Zeuzem, Hepatol, 1996; 24:1003; Zhou, Hepatol, 1996; 24: 1041).

Individual variability

Besides the overall variability of the HCV genome, hypervariability exists in the 27-amino acid-long HVR1 at the N-terminus of E2, with as many as 1.5×10^{-2} exchanges/year in HRV1 and only 0.9 to 5.2×10^{-3} in E1 (Höhne, ArchVirol, 1994; 137:25). It appears that the variability of this region is due to selection by neutralizing antibodies, similarly to the hypervariable region V3 of HIV gp120 (Weiner, PNAS, 1992; 89:3468). In a patient with agammaglobulinaemia, HCV infection was very severe and no variability in HVR1 was observed (Kumar, Gastro, 1994; 106:1072). During the acute phase after primary HCV infection only a few exchanges are found in comparison to the infecting virus, for example six exchanges in 10 patients (R. Thomssen, unpublished). In an experimental study, two of five chimpanzees cleared the infection rapidly and did not produce variants with altered HVR1. In two of the animals the HVR1 sequence changed gradually during chronic infection in the presence of antibodies against the original HVR1; in the third, chronically infected animal no anti-HVR1 antibodies developed for 6 years, but when anti-HVR1 finally appeared, a new variant with an altered HVR1 was selected (van Doorn, JVirol, 1995; 69:773). Variations in HVR1 probably contribute to the persistence of HCV but cannot be the only mechanism of immune escape.

Most patients harbour a mixture of variants. At any given time and in any individual patient, viruses in general, and highly variable viruses such as HCV and HIV in particular, are not homogeneous but form a quasispecies with most of the replicated genomes being more or less defective.

Antigenicity and immunogenicity of HCV proteins

The antigenicity and immunogenicity of HCV proteins have mostly been studied with overlapping synthetic peptides and partial or complete proteins expressed in various host cells. Recently, the HCV core gene has been directly expressed in mice by injection of a cDNA fragment encoding the HCV core protein. A strong, cytotoxic T-cell response and a weak antibody response were the result (Tokushige, Hepatol, 1996, 24:14).

B-cell epitopes

Historically, a fragment of NS4 was the first HCV antigen immunogenic in HCV-infected individuals. Later, more important epitopes were located in the aminoterminal part of the core protein and in NS3. On using these two antigens, an antibody response can be detected in almost all HCV-infected individuals after a variable period of weeks to months. Only very few develop antibodies against NS4 and NS5 but no antibodies against core or NS3. These antibodies have no protective or neutralizing power.

Antibodies against E1 and E2 are also not clearly correlated with the resolution of infection. The only antibodies that contribute to resolution *in vivo* or the neutralization of HCV binding (**NOB** assay) to cells are directed to defined sequences within the HVR1 (Rosa, PNAS, 1996; 93:1759). Infectivity in cell culture can also be neutralized by animal antibodies that recognize the exact HVR1-sequence (Shimizu, Virology, 1996; 223:409). Naturally infected chimpanzees often remain susceptible to reinfection with the same inoculum. This may be due to outgrowth of different HVR1 variants during the first and second infection. Such animals are protected against reinfection if they contain high titres of NOB antibodies. The same was true for chimpanzees in which protection was induced by immunization with E2 protein. Spontaneously resolving chronic hepatitis C but not acute resolving hepatitis C were also associated with NOB antibodies (Rosa, PNAS, 1996; 93:1759).

Most antibodies from HCV-infected individuals react with conformational epitopes from core or NS3 protein. Conformational epitopes of E1 and E2 are only obtained by expression in animal cells, preferably mammalian cells, but the HVR1 epitopes can be well presented as short synthetic peptides, for example decamers. Core and NS3 proteins contain mostly conserved epitopes, but some partial peptides of the core and protein react with genotype- or even subtype-specificity and may allow serological HCV typing (Machida, Hepatol, 1992; 16:886; Bhattacherjee, JGenVirol, 1995; 76:1737).

T-cell immunity

As with HAV and HBV, CD4+ and CD8+ lymphocytes contribute both to the control and the pathogenesis of HCV infections. In contrast to HAV and HBV, HCV-specific T cells are found in the circulation, though often in low numbers. The recognition of epitopes and the induction of HCV-reactive T cells depends on the processing and presentation of HCV proteins, and on the presence and activity of cytokines and their receptors. Though no clear rule can be made, some findings appear interesting. A major T-helper-cell epitope was found in NS3 (amino acids 1248–1261) that could be presented by at least six different *HLA-DR* alleles (Diepolder, JVirol, 1997; 71:6011). T-helper-cell reactivity to the NS3 peptides was associated with the resolution of acute HCV infection.[1] Similarly, strong T-helper-cell reactions to five different epitopes in the core protein (amino acids 20–44, 39–63, 79–103, 118–156, 148–172) and in three regions of E1 (amino acids 198–252, 308–372, 368–392) were found in healthy blood donors with weak anti-HCV without detectable viraemia. Patients with chronic hepatitis C with viraemia had high anti-HCV titres and a low T-helper-cell reactivity (Botarelli, Gastro, 1993; 104:580; Lechmann, Hepatol, 1996; 24: 790). T-cell reactions against epitopes of NS4 and NS5B were also associated with resolution of the infection (Ferrari, Hepatol, 1994; 19:286). The core-peptide amino acids 132 to 140 are a highly conserved epitope for intrahepatic, cytotoxic T lymphocytes with *HLA-A2* (Ohno, personal communication). Chronically HCV-infected patients less often have major histocompatibility complex class-II alleles *DQB1*0302* and *DQA1*03* than healthy control groups with similar exposure (Congia, Hepatol 1996; 24:1338; Tibbs, Hepatol, 1996; 24:1342). *DRB1*13101-*β_3 and *DRB1*1302* alleles are also more frequent in low-viraemic HCV infections (Thursz and Kutzushita, personal communication) whereas *DRB1*0701* is as associated with high viraemia. However, many T-cell epitopes show very little HLA restriction.

Course of the infection and disease

The source of the infectious material is usually blood, plasma, or serum from infected individuals. The infectivity titre for chimpanzees may reach 10^7 infectious units/ml serum but is usually much lower. However, in another case, a low infectivity, such as 10^2 infectious units/ml, was correlated with a high number of HCV genome equivalents/ml (10^7) (Hijikata, JVirol, 1993; 67:1953). Usually the numbers of HCV particles and the infectivity in serum are high during the incubation phase. Later, the number of particles is highly variable but infectivity is usually lower. HCV is usually both free in the serum and bound to leucocytes, but in some rare cases, leucocytes may contain HCV RNA whereas the serum reacts negatively.

Depending on the dose of the infectious agent and, possibly, the viability of the variants composing the viral quasispecies, HCV will rapidly (within a few weeks or even days) induce a viraemia, detectable by a sensitive RNA-amplification technique, without recognizable symptoms. In contrast to HAV and HBV, serum alanine transaminase rises significantly before HCV antibodies are detectable, usually 5 to 12 weeks after infection (extreme values at 2–26 weeks). Acute disease may result, with resolution within several months. In up to 85 per cent of cases, viraemia persists in the presence of anti-HCV. About 45 per cent of patients with acute

Table 7 Diagnostic questions concerning HCV

Question	Tests		
Active HCV infection:			
Early, or immunocompromised patient	1. HCV RNA	2. Anti-HCV	
Time-point unknown, or chronic hepatitis	1. Anti-HCV	2. HCV RNA	
Indication for interferon therapy	HCV RNA (quantitative), genotype		
	NS5A ISDR sequence, optional		
Monitoring of interferon therapy	HCV RNA		
Monitoring of HCV-positive organ recipients	1. HCV RNA	2. Anti-HCV	
Resolution and 'immunity'	1. Anti-HCV	2. HCV RNA	
Infectivity	HCV RNA (quantitative)		
Infection chain	1. HCV RNA	2. Genotype	3. Sequence
Safety of plasma proteins	HCV RNA		
Prevalence in risk groups	Anti-HCV (ELISA)		
Incidence in risk groups	Seroconversion of anti-HCV		

ELISA, enzyme-linked immunosorbent assay; ISDR, interferon sensitivity-determining region.

hepatitis develop histologically confirmed chronic hepatitis. Chronic hepatitis may proceed with variable activity; it usually takes decades until cirrhosis or hepatic failure become apparent.

Virological diagnosis

The range of diagnostic questions concerning HCV is listed in Table 7; the tools to answer these questions are listed in Table 8. The following text will critically discuss first the problems associated with the diagnostic tasks and then the diagnostic methods.

Diagnostic problems
Active hepatitis C

If clinical symptoms are present or there is a serious suspicion of HCV infection, an anti-HCV test should be done first, using an enzyme-linked immunosorbent assay and a mixture of HCV antigens. If the assay is positive, it should be confirmed by a supplementary assay with separated HCV antigens. If this assay is positive or indeterminate, testing for HCV RNA is advisable. A positive anti-HCV assay together with a positive HCV RNA assay

Table 8 Methods for detection of HCV components and anti-HCV antibodies

Measure	Methods	Remarks
Anti-HCV, screening	EIA	Sensitive, specific, but delayed positivity in recent HCV infection; commercially available
Anti-HCV, supplementary test	RIBA, Dot Matrix, etc. separate antigens on membranes	Potentially less sensitive than EIA; non-quantitative
HCV core antigen	EIA	Moderate or low sensitivity; no routine method
HCV RNA (qualitative)	RT/PCR Amplicor	Commercially available test kit, usually reliable
	Other techniques	Not commercially available; patent problems
	In-house techniques	Quality variable, depending on the laboratory
HCV (quantitative)	Quantiplex (bDNA)	Accurate, moderately sensitive
	RT/PCR with competitor RNA (Amplicor™)	Sensitive, less accurate
	RT/PCR limiting dilution	
HCV genotype	RT/PCR sequencing	Laborious
	Multiplex PCR	Sensitive, somewhat ambiguous
	RT/PCR, hybridization	Commercially available, reliable
	Serotyping by peptide EIA	Technically easiest method, in c. 90% correct results

EIA, enzyme immunoassay; ge, genome equivalents; RT/PCR, reverse transcriptase–polymerase chain reaction.

confirm that HCV is present and replicating, and that the clinical symptoms of acute or chronic hepatitis are being caused by HCV.

If the history of the patient suggests that the HCV infection has recently occurred, or the hepatitis appears to be acute and not chronic, or if a known exposure (for example, an outbreak in a haemodialysis unit) should happen to be followed-up early on, an anti-HCV assay alone is not informative. In these circumstances a sensitive HCV-RNA assay is necessary to exclude an active HCV infection. Suspected infection of newborns at birth or of immunocompromised patients also requires HCV-RNA testing. If the HCV-RNA assay is positive and anti-HCV is negative, an early phase of infection or immunodeficiency must be postulated.

Prognosis and monitoring

The distinction between acute and chronic infection is prognostically relevant because an acute infection has some potential to resolve within a year. If the first sample from a patient is already anti-HCV positive it may be rather difficult to distinguish between an acute and a chronic infection. The determination of IgM anti-HCV is not reliable in this case, because the assays are not well standardized and the clinical differences between acute and chronic phases are not helpful. Antibodies against NS4 antigen are more prevalent in chronic infection. The appearance of anti-HCV in a previously negative individual indicates recent infection.

The appearance of HCV RNA in a previously negative individual (also anti-HCV negative) indicates recent infection and a possible hepatitis to come. The persistence of HCV RNA for more than 6 months suggests chronicity. During convalescence from acute hepatitis C, HCV RNA may disappear and reappear. Thus, testing should be repeated at appropriate intervals (for example 3 months).

Genotyping is not really useful for prognosis. The fine specificity of the immune response may possibly give hints on the prognosis, but the tests are not suitable for routine diagnosis. High genomic diversity appears to be a bad omen.

Perinatal and intrafamilial infection

HCV may be transmitted from an infected mother to her child either through the placenta or perinatally. The frequency of transmission seems to depend on the concentration of HCV RNA and is low (less than 10 per cent) unless HIV or another source of immunodeficiency are also present. Anti-HCV in the child is not informative because initially it is passively transferred from the mother. Furthermore, the immune system of the new-born does not produce its own antibodies. Thus follow-up and testing for at least 1 year by qualitative methods for HCV RNA are necessary. Detectable HCV RNA in the cord blood does not necessarily mean that the child will become infected.

Resolution and immunity

Resolution of the disease with normalization of the alanine aminotransferase and normal liver histology is associated with permanent disappearance of HCV RNA from serum (at a detection limit of 10^3 genome equivalents/ml or less). Titres of anti-HCV seem to decrease thereafter but it is not known whether anti-HCV disapppears completely, nor is it known whether HCV also disappears from the liver. The experience with naturally infected or E2-immunized

chimpanzees suggests that spontaneous or interferon-induced resolution does not mean immunity against another variant of HCV, even in the same inoculum. Nevertheless, one may consider a low (specificity-confirmed) anti-HCV concentration together with a negative HCV-RNA test to be a marker of resolved HCV infection and a marker of immunity against at least the autologous HCV quasispecies.

Infectivity of HCV-positive individuals

This infectivity can only be determined by titration experiments in the chimpanzee. The concentration of HCV RNA is a surrogate measure that gives (if accurately determined) the theoretical upper limit of how many infectious particles there might be in a sample. Concentrations of 10^8 genome equivalents/ml and infectivity titres of 10^6 infective doses/ml have been reported, but very often the infectivity is much lower despite a high genome equivalent/ml. Members of medical staff are more often infected by HCV carriers than by HIV carriers, but less often than by HBV carriers. Infections of patients by surgeons have been reported, but these are rare exceptions.

Reports on the sexual transmission of HCV are controversial. Those studies that find the prevalence of HCV to be associated with a high prevalence of sexual diseases cannot exclude other modes of transmission. In a large study on married couples (where the wife was infected by contaminated intravenous gammaglobulin), no transmissions were observed (Meisel, Lancet, 1995; 345:1209).

Infection chains

In order to stop infectious chains it is important to identify the source of infection in a newly identified or recently infected individual. If a potential source (contact, blood donor, plasma-protein product, physician) has been identified, it is necessary to verify the identity or non-identitiy of the two isolates. Convincing analysis is possible if both the 'donor' and 'acceptor' are HCV RNA-positive. In this case the genotype or serotype should be determined (see below) and, if identical, the HVR1 sequences should be amplified, sequenced, and compared. Identity or high similarity show either transmission from the donor to the acceptor, or, in certain circumstances, that both individuals were both exposed to another common source. Clear non-identity excludes transmission from the suspected source if it exceeds more than 10 per cent within the 91 bases of HVR1 (1151–1243).

Blood-donor screening

Since the introduction of second-generation anti-HCV tests, post-transfusion hepatitis has become very rare. Although the current enzyme-linked immunosorbent assays for the detection of anti-HCV are highly specific (more than 99.7 per cent), the low prevalence and incidence of specific anti-HCV antibodies in many blood-donor populations creates a state in which the majority of reactive results from enzyme-linked immunosorbent assays in blood donors may either be non-reproducible or (if reproducible) turn out to be non-specific when controlled by a supplementary test with separated HCV antigens. Every donor confirmed as positive should be examined for potential liver disease, even if the alanine aminotransferase is normal. In first-time donors in developed countries the prevalence of specific anti-HCV is between 0.1 and 1 per cent.

Two potential gaps in the safety of the procedure remain. First, during the incubation phase of the HCV infection, virus may be present for up to 6 months before anti-HCV becomes detectable. In order to protect recipients, fresh-frozen plasma is stored (quarantined) for 6 months and then the donor is retested. Only if the second anti-HCV assay is available and negative may the plasma be used. The quarantine is not applicable to erythrocytes or thrombocytes because it is not feasible to store them for such a long time. In order to prevent HCV infections from recently infected donors, numerous criteria are applied to identify individuals at risk and to keep them away from donation. Incidence, that is, new HCV infection in repeating donors, is very low in non-paid ('voluntary') donors from rural areas of Europe (less than 1 in 10 000 per year, in many regions less than 1 in 100 000), but has been rather high in paid plasma donors from urban areas in North American in the early 1990s.

A potential second gap may be donors with undetectable anti-HCV, but positive HCV RNA, who never seroconverted or have become negative for anti-HCV. These donors are probably low-level HCV carriers. The magnitude and significance of this group are not known, but presumably they are low.

Testing every donor for HCV RNA is expensive and may, possibly, not be adequate in view of the low remaining risks.

Diagnostic methods

Detection of infectious virus

Chimpanzee hepatocytes can be infected in culture (Lanford, Virology, 1994; 202:606), but replication of HCV is minimal and can only be detected by a RT-PCR for minus-strand RNA. The same is true for all other cell-culture systems.

Detection of HCV RNA

This is the method of choice for the diagnosis of active HCV infection or contamination of materials by HCV. Attention must be paid to the treatment of the blood sample. Plasma is preferable. Centrifugation of EDTA or citrate blood should be done within 6 h at 4°C or room temperature. Serum is also acceptable if it is not stored for longer than 6 h at room temperature before separation from the cells (Miskovski, JClinMicrobiol, 1996; 34:1975). The RNA may be detected qualitatively or quantitatively by various amplification and/or hybridization procedures.

An essential first step is RNA extraction. The liberated RNA is very sensitive to RNases. Thus rapid denaturation or inactivation of these enzymes is essential. Usually the serum or plasma are mixed with chaotropic substances such as guanidinium thiocyanate, phenol/chloroform with or without proteinase K, or the sample is subjected to an RNA extraction/purification kit, for example RNAzol, or RNA clean®. The RNA may be purified further using minicolumns from Quiagen®. The frequently used Amplicor test kit from Hoffmann LaRoche extracts RNA with guanidinium thiocyanate and purifies it by precipitation with isopropanol.

The amplification is done by various techniques. The most established is the RT-PCR. The RNA is first reversibly transcribed to cDNA using a primer complementary to a short sequence in the viral RNA. This cDNA is then amplified in a normal PCR, as described in detail for HBV DNA. The Amplicor test kit uses a heat-stable DNA polymerase (rTth from T. thermophilus) that also has reverse-transcriptase activity. Primers from conserved elements in the 5′ non-coding region are used.

Some techniques combine extraction, purification, and binding to specific primers. By using fluid-phase hybridization the RNA can be directly reacted with a biotinylated primer; thereafter the complex is bound to streptavidin-coated magnetic beads, washed, and used for the PCR (Heermann, JVirolMethods, 1994; 50:43; 1996; 59:33). The ligation-dependent PCR uses first fluid-phase hybridization and thereafter anneals the HCV RNA with two 'hemiprimers' in such a way that only a nick is left between the two primers. This nick is closed with ligase, generating a continuous strand. The hemiprimers contain terminal parts that are HCV-independent. Using primers against these regions the ligated DNA molecule is conventionally amplified by PCR (Hsuih, JClinMicrobiol, 1996; 34:501). The advantage of the method is the well-standardized technique for the PCR.

Strand-displacement amplification generates a normal cDNA but uses special primers with overhanging ends and a unique restriction site in those ends. The amplification is done with a normal DNA polymerase at low temperature, but with thio-dTTP. Cleavage with the restriction enzyme occurs only in the parental strand without thio groups, thus generating a new primer site. The DNA polymerase can then start in the counter direction and replace the parental strand. The procedure allows a cyclic chain reaction without changing temperatures (Walker, PNAS, 1992; 89:392).

Another amplification technique without temperature cycles is the nucleic acid sequence-based amplification. It uses a combination of reverse transcriptase with RNaseH and T7 RNA polymerase. The reverse transcriptase synthesizes a cDNA and the RNA is degraded within the hybrid. The T7 polymerase synthesizes many copies of RNA from the cDNA because the primer contains a T7 promoter in addition to the HCV sequences. Thereafter the reverse transcriptase is again active. The process amplifies by a factor of 10^6 to 10^7 within 2.5 h at 41°C (van Gennem, JVirolMethods, 1993; 43: 177). The transcription-mediated amplification is similar but uses thereafter a fluorescent probe for hybridization.

The detection of the amplicon is often achieved by ethidium bromide staining after gel electrophoresis if in-house tests are used. Commercially available test kits usually employ hybridization of one amplicon strand with an enzyme-labelled probe, and separation of free and bound probe by a solid-phase reagent. The Amplicor system uses one biotin-labelled primer and a capture probe on a microwell plate for the same strand. An avidin–peroxidase reagent then binds to the biotin label and generates a coloured product. Alternatively, digoxigenin-labelled dUTP may be incorporated during the PCR; the labelled amplicon strand is captured via the biotin residue at the primer to the solid phase (Boehringer Mannheim).

One of the most modern ways to detect the amplicon is the TaqMan™ system, in which the amplification is directly coupled to generation of a fluorescent signal that can be measured in a special fluorometer. The amplicon hybridizes in situ with a DNA probe that contains covalently a fluorescent group and a quencher group. The system uses a Taq polymerase with 5′–3′ exonuclease activity that digests the probe into single nucleotides. This happens, however, only if the probe is bound to the specific amplicon strand. The fluorescent group and the quencher are separated by the enzymatic release and fluorescence is generated (information from Perkin Elmer/Applied Biosystems). A combination of one probe with a quencher and one with a fluorescent group is used in the Amplisensor system, but here the signal is generated by strand displacement during amplification. The molecular-beacon technique uses a probe with a fluorescent group at one end and a quencher at the other. In the absence of the amplicon the probe forms a stem-loop structure in which the two groups are in close proximity. After hybridization of the probe to the amplicon the two groups are separated and fluorescence increases (Tyagi, NatureBiotechnol, 1996; 12:303). The fluorescence detection systems have the advantage of easy quantitation over a wide range of concentrations, but they need special equipment and reagents that are not (yet) available in the average polymerase chain-reaction laboratory.

The branched-DNA signal-amplification system (bDNA assay; Quantiplex, Chiron Corp.) functions completely without nucleic-acid amplifications. It is essentially a hybridization assay but its sensitivity is enhanced by the use of branched ('b') DNA probes that are coupled to an enzyme. Sensitivity is further improved by using a chemoluminescence reaction for detection of the enzyme.

Specificity and sensitivity

Several quality-control trials have been performed on assays for HCV RNA. In-house methods have provided excellent results in some laboratories but more often they are plagued by false-positive and -negative results (Damen, JVirolMethods, 1996; 58:175). Initially, commercial systems were also not completely reliable but sufficient sensitivity has now been reached. Besides the technical points mentioned in the section on HBV, the lability of HCV RNA creates some additional problems. The nested PCR without an amplicon-destroying pretreatment is the most endangered by contamination.

Quantitation

Quantitative assays for HCV RNA have been calibrated by using *in vitro*-transcribed HCV RNA as the reference substance. Furthermore, the amplification reactions include a known amount of competitor RNA that uses the same primer but has a different internal sequence that hybridizes with a different probe. Thus the somewhat variable efficiency of amplification can be normalized to the amount of amplicon of the competitor RNA. Nevertheless, the three commercially available assay systems, Amplicor, Quantiplex and NASBA, generated grossly different quantitative results when applied to the EUROHEP panel of samples, thus leaving the 'true' number of HCV genomes in reference samples uncertain by a factor of 100. In the lower concentration range the Amplicor Monitor assay agreed well with a calibrated in-house assay, but at high concentration, above 500 000 genome equivalents/ml, it was unreliable (Roth, JClinMicrobiol, 1996; 34:261). At present the Quantiplex assay seems to be the most adequately calibrated. Furthermore, the Amplicor system seems to be less sensitive for genotype 3 than genotype 1 (Damen, JVirolMethods, 1996; 58:175). A working reagent with several thousand genome equivalents/ml for the control of sensitivity is available (Saldanha, VoxSang, 1996; 70:148). For accurate calibration of quantitative assays, reference panels are recommended (for example, Pelicheck from CLB, Amsterdam based on the results reported by Damen (JVirolMethods, 1996; 58:175).

Antigen detection

Improved detection systems have recently allowed detection of the HCV core antigen in serum with a clinical sensitivity similar to that of the bDNA assay. This improved assay could be useful for monitoring antiviral therapy (Orito, Gut, 1996; 39:876). For the detection of HCV antigens in liver, many monoclonal antibodies of mouse or human origin are available.

Antibody assays

The standard enzyme immunoassay employs recombinant HCV antigens bound to a solid phase, to which bind the anti-HCV IgG antibodies from the sample. Binding is revealed by enzyme-labelled anti-IgG antibodies [the principle is explained in Fig. 4(b)]. The first-generation enzyme immunoassay used the C100 antigen covering the NS4 region. This assay was rather insensitive and nonspecific. It missed *c*. 30 per cent of the true-positive samples and generated false-positive results with problematic sera containing rheumatoid factor or immunoglobulin aggregates The second-generation enzyme immunoassay used recombinant core proteins C22, NS3 (C33), and C100 as an antigen mix. Sensitivity was improved and the assay was very specific (more than 99.8 per cent in normal populations). The variable and occasionally 6 month-long lag phase between the time of HCV infection and the appearance of anti-HCV remained a drawback. Third-generation enzyme immunoassays contain in addition (depending on the supplier) NS5 and/or modified core antigens, but the sensitivity and specificity, or the time of appearance of positive results after infection, have improved only marginally if at all (Vrielink, VoxSang, 1996; 69:14).

Supplementary assays

In blood-bank settings and professional surveillance programmes the number of false-positive results often exceeds the number of true-positive results; in some patients with immune disorders, false-positive results may also occur. Thus, when there is a positive result for anti-HCV in an enzyme immunoassay it should be repeated, preferably in duplicate. Only reproducibly positive results should be considered positive; results with two negative repetitions should be considered negative, unless the findings are all close to borderline. In the latter case, a serum sample taken 1 to 2 weeks later will help to clarify the results. Impending seroconversion will then show up, with a stronger positive result.

Reproducibly positive results in an enzyme immunoassay should be confirmed with assays employing separate HCV antigens. By convention, at least two antigens should bind IgG detectably for a serum to be considered positive. Reaction with one antigen is considered an indeterminate result. One of the most common supplementary tests is the RIBA 3.0®. In blood donors this test may generate a number of false-positive results due to reaction with NS3 or NS5 (Damen, Transfusion, 1995; 35:745) On the other hand, indeterminate results are often (31/59) matched by a positive test for HCV RNA in high-risk groups (Pawlotsky, JClinMicrobiol, 1996; 34:80). Although negative supplementary assays may suggest that the results of the enzyme immunoassay are non-specific, true-positive borderline results in an enzyme immunoassay may be undetectable with assays using separate antigens. Confirmation by the sensitive assay for HCV RNA is, therefore, in any case advisable.

The likelihood of a positive confirmation is much higher in individuals with elevated alanine aminotransferase concentrations or in risk groups. Of note, a negative HCV RNA does not mean that an anti-HCV result is a false-positive. In general, 60 per cent of all anti-HCV-positive blood donors or healthy individuals are HCV RNA-positive, whereas patients with chronic hepatitis are almost always positive.

Antibody patterns and clinical monitoring

It appears that the antibody titres are correlated with disease activity, particularly the titre against core protein; the IgM antibody seems to be most relevant (Löhr, JHepatol, 1996; 25:292). Furthermore, IgM anticore seems to be associated with liver disease and viraemia; however, this assay cannot replace HCV RNA assays because it is less sensitive. The assay for IgM anti-HCV is not suitable for distinction of acute or chronic hepatitis C.

Genotyping

HCV genotypes are important for epidemiological studies, the elucidation of infection chains, and, possibly, for prognosis and indications for therapy. The most accurate procedure is sequencing of the 5′ non-coding region after a RT-PCR (Bukh, SemLiverDis, 1995; 15:41; Toniutto, JClinMicrobiol, 1996; 34:2382). If the identified region is very divergent from known genotypes, a second region, preferably NS5, should be sequenced. Only if this region is also divergent should a new geno(sub)type be postulated and included in the known phylogenetic trees. More than 14 per cent divergence in NS5 suggests a new subtype, more than 28 per cent a new genotype. The program package PHYLIP is very useful for sequences evaluations (Felsenstein J. *PHYLIP inference package*, version 3.5. Seattle: Department of Genetics, University of Washington, 1993).

Less laborious procedures for genotyping are the multiplex PCR with a mixture of geno(sub)type-specific primers (Okamoto, JVirolMethods, 1996; 57:31) or hybridization of the amplicon with genotype-specific probes (Simmonds, JGenVirol, 1996; 77:3013). The line-probe assay for genotyping uses biotinylated amplicons hybridized to solid phase-bound, geno(sub)type-specific probes (i.e., lines), and the bound biotin is detected by a streptavidin–alkaline phosphatase conjugate (Stuyver, JClin Microbiol, 1996; 34:2259). The commercially available version of the line-probe assay (INNO-LIPA HCVII®, Innogenetics) allows distinctions of geno(sub)types 1a, 1b, 1c, 2a, 2b, 2d, 3a, 3b, 3c, 3d, 3e, 3f, 4a, 4b, 4c, 4d, 4e, 4f, 4g, 4h, 4i, 4j, 5a, and 6a.

Serotyping uses typical sequence differences in major HCV-antigen epitopes, preferably in NS4. Genotypes can usually be clearly distinguished; subtypes are not distinguished reliably. The procedure has been used successfully in a large study and is available as the Murex HC02 serotyping assay (Simmonds, JHepatol, 1996; 24:517).

GB-C virus or so-called hepatitis G virus

History of discovery

The successful discovery and great importance of HCV encouraged several pharmaceutical firms to search for further viruses that might be a cause of parenterally transmitted hepatitis. Abbott Laboratories reactivated research that had been started in the early 1960s by F. Deinhardt in Chicago at a time when neither HAV nor HBV had been discovered. In those early attempts a serum from a patient suffering from acute hepatitis (initials G.B.) was inoculated into tamarin monkeys. Their serum was passaged to further animals and there caused hepatitis. Unfortunately, the virus could not be identified and the connection between the hepatitis in the animals and the human disease remained unclear (Parks, JInfDis, 1969; 120: 539). It has, however, been shown that the virus was not identical to the later-identified human hepatitis virus type A–E. Using advanced techniques for amplification and cloning of unknown nucleic acid molecules, Abbott Laboratories succeeded in isolating and sequencing two *Flaviviridae*-like genomes from the monkeys; the viruses were named GB virus (**GBV**) A or B (Simons, PNAS, 1995; 92:3401). On using the most sensitive polymerase chain-reaction techniques, these viruses could not be identified in human cases of presumed non-A-E hepatitis. Individual genotypes of GBV-A RNA were, however, found in several New World non-human primate species: in 13/37 *Sanguinus mystax*, in 7/19 *S. nigricollis*, in 3/12 *S. labiatus*, in 2/4 *S. oedipus*, in 2/2 *Callithrix jacchus*, and in 6/12 *Aotus trivirgatus* (Muerhoff, JVirol, 1995; 69:5621). These viruses cause a non-pathogenic, persistent infection. Inoculation of these primate species with GBV-B, however, caused hepatitis. While GBV-A and -B RNAs could not be found in humans, some human sera reacted in enzyme immunoassays with recombinant GBV-A or -B proteins; this suggested that a related virus existed in man. By using degenerate primers derived from GBV-A and -B, an RNA genome was isolated from human hepatitis patients and termed GBV-C (Simons, NatureMed, 1995; 1:564; Leary, JMedVirol, 1996; 48:60). A second group from Genelabs Technologies, supported by Boehringer Mannheim, took a more direct approach and isolated from a patient with post-transfusion hepatitis of unknown aetiology a very closely related RNA genome, which was called 'hepatitis G virus' or 'HGV' (Linnen, Science, 1996; 271:505).

Structure and classification

The virus particles of GBV-C/HGV (the neutral acronym **G/GBV-C** combining the designations applied in the original descriptions is used here) have not been characterized. The overall genomic structure and organization is that of the *Flaviviridae* (Fig. 24), with more significant differences from the genera flavivirus and pestivirus and some closer relation to HCV. The sequence homology between GBV-A, GBV-B, and G/GBV-C is low, and not much higher than with HCV (Fig. 25). The 5′ non-coding region has between 282 and 552 nucleotides. It contains an internal ribosomal entry site as with the genera hepaci- and pestivirus (Simons, JVirol, 1996; 70: 6126). The open reading frame begins at variable sites depending on the isolate, only 14 to 105 amino acids upstream of the signal peptide for E1, and has correspondingly a variable length of 2842 to 2933 amino acids. A core protein analogous to that of the other *Flaviviridae* including HCV has not yet been found in G/GBV-C isolates (Okamoto, JGenVirol, 1997; 78:737). G/GBV-C shares this strange property with GBV-A, but the hepatotropic GBV-B has a core protein like HCV.

E1 and E2, and NS2 to 5, can be identified by the corresponding sequence motifs. Remarkable is the existence of a metalloprotease

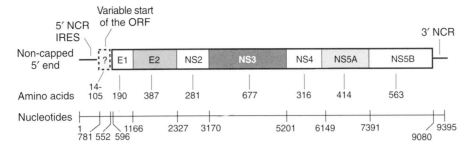

Fig. 24. Genome map of GV; abbreviations are the same as in Fig. 23 (data from Okamoto, JGenVirol, 1997; 78:737).

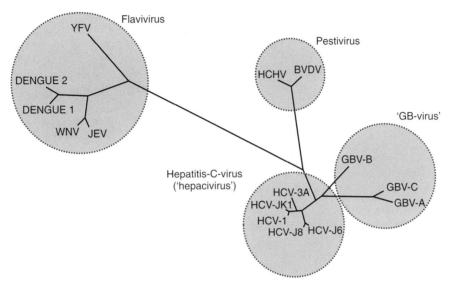

Fig. 25. Phylogenetic tree of selected members of the *Flaviviridae*. YFV, yellow fever virus; WNV, West Nile virus; JEV, Japanese encephalitis virus; HCHV, hog cholera virus (or classical swine fever virus); BVDV, bovine viral diarrhoea virus. The length of the lines between branching points gives an estimate of evolutionary distance.

motif in NS2, which is also found in the other GB viruses, and in HCV, but not in pesti- or flaviviruses. The genome of G/GBV-C has some variability but much less than HCV. There is probably only one genotype but several subtypes with typical geographical distributions. GBV-C and HGV are two different subtypes of the same virus.

Course of infection

G/GBV-C cannot be propagated in cell culture as is the case for HCV and GBV-A or B. It has been experimentally transmitted to chimpanzees. Viraemia appeared after 11 to 12 weeks, persisted, and reached 10^7 RNA molecules/ml; there were no signs of liver damage. G/GBV-C is not pathogenic for tamarins.

After a variable time, G/GBV-C RNA may disappear from the serum and antibodies against the E2 protein appear. This suggests that, in contrast to HCV (and similarly to HBV), the antibodies against the envelope protein are indicative of control of the infection and not of continuing infection. Preliminary evidence suggests that G/GBV-C causes a stronger viraemia than HCV but the titres of G/GBV-C RNA in the liver of double-infected individuals were lower than the corresponding titres of HCV RNA. This observation, if confirmed, suggests that G/GBV-C may not be hepatotropic.

Diagnosis

G/GBV-C is detected by RT-PCR. Detection of the amplificate may be achieved by the nested PCR and ethidium bromide staining, or by a single-round PCR and hybridization with enzyme-labelled probes using the Boehringer system. Primers from the NS3, the NS5, and the 5′ non-coding regions have been used; the last is more sensitive. However, none of the primer sets detected all PCR-positive samples. Quantitation is possible with the bDNA hybridization assay from Chiron.

For prevalence studies the RT-PCR should be complemented by the anti-G/GBV-C-E2 assay (Pilot-Matias, Virology, 1996; 225: 282; Tacke, Lancet, 1997; 349:318). Antigenic regions of GBV-A and B and G/GBV-C were identified in partial-protein sequences expressed in *E. coli* using non-human primate or human antisera; in this system, NS3, NS4, and NS5 have expressed epitopes. GBV-B had also a core antigen (Pilot-Matias, JMedVirol, 1996; 48:329). Inactivated blood products are not known to transmit G/GBV-C; even most recipients of non-inactivated products do not have G/GBV-C infections (Jarvis, Lancet, 1996; 348:1352).

According to current knowledge there is no immediate necessity to test blood donors or patients with hepatitis for G/GBV-C RNA or anti-G/GBV-C-E2 antibodies.

References

1. Zuckermann AR and Thomas HC, eds. *Viral hepatitis.* 1st edn. London: Churchill Livingstone, 1993. (2nd edn in press)
2. Hollinger FB and Ticehurst IR. Hepatitis A virus. In Fields BN, *et al.*, eds. *Virology.* 3rd edn. Philadelphia: Lippincott Raven, 1996: 735–82.
3. Rueckert RR. *Picornaviridae*: the viruses and their replication. In Fields BN, *et al.*, eds. *Virology.* 3rd edn. Philadelphia: Lippincott Raven, 1996: 609–54.
4. Purcell RH. Hepatitis E virus. In Fields BN, *et al.* eds., *Virology.* 3rd edn. Philadelphia: Lippincott Raven, 1996: 2831–44.
5. McLachlan A, ed. *Molecular biology of hepatitis B viruses.* Boca Raton FL: CRC Press, 1991.
6. Ganem D. Hepadnaviridae: the viruses and their replication In Fields BN, *et al.*, eds. *Virology.* 3rd edn. Philadelphia: Lippincott Raven, 1996: 2703–37.
7. Hollinger FB. Hepatitis B virus. In Fields BN, *et al.*, eds. *Virology.* 3rd edn. Philadelphia: Lippincott Raven, 1996: 2738–808.
8. Kann M and Gerlich WH. Hepatitis B. In Collier L, *et al.*, eds. *Topley and Wilson's microbiology and microbial infections.* 9th edn. London: Arnold, 1997.
9. Clewley JP. *The polymerase chain reaction (PCR) for human viral diagnosis.* Boca Raton FL: CRC Press, 1995.
10. Purcell RH and Gerin JL. Hepatitis delta viruses. In Fields BN, *et al.*, eds. *Virology.* 3rd edn. Philadelphia: Lippincott Raven, 1996: 2819–30.
11. Lai MMC. The molecular biology of hepatitis delta virus. *Annual Review of Biochemistry,* 1995; **64**: 259–86.
12. Houghton M. Hepatitis C viruses. In Fields BN, *et al.*, eds. *Virology.* 3rd edn. Philadelphia: Lippincott Raven, 1996: 1035–58.
13. Rice CM. *Flaviridae*: the viruses and their replication. In Fields BN, *et al.*, eds. *Virology.* 3rd edn. Philadelphia: Lippincott Raven, 1996: 931–60.

12.1.2.2 Hepatitis A*

Jules L. Dienstag

Definition and virology

Hepatitis A is an acute, usually self-limited, necroinflammatory disease of the liver resulting from infection with the enterically transmitted hepatitis A virus (**HAV**). Hepatitis A virus is a positive-stranded, non-enveloped, icosahedral, 27-nm RNA virus,[1] now classified as a hepatovirus within the picornavirus family.[2] Unusually resistant to heat, ether, and acid, HAV has an RNA genome of approximately 7500 nucleotides, the protein product of which is post-translationally cleaved to yield three protein precursors of four capsid viral polypeptides, VP1 to VP4. Non-structural proteins include a viral polymerase and proteases. Although genomic heterogeneity of up to 25 per cent exists among virus strains, and although at least seven genotypes have been identified, all isolates appear to be immunologically indistinguishable, that is, only a single serotype exists (Robertson, JGenVirol, 1992; 73:1365). Unique among the human hepatitis viruses, HAV is the only one that can be cultivated in cell culture;[3] however, most strains replicate slowly, and unlike many picornaviruses, HAV is not cytopathic in culture.[4] The entire genome has been cloned and characterized.[5,6] A detailed review of the basic virology of HAV appears in Chapter 12.1.2.1.

Although the virus can be detected in stools within 10 days to 2 weeks after infection, the clinical incubation period, measured to

* This chapter is a revised, updated version of the original chapter written by Ian Gust and Steven Feinstone for the first edition of this text.

the onset of symptoms, is approximately 4 weeks (range 2 to 6). During the late incubation period (10 to 14 days before the onset of clinically apparent illness), the virus is excreted in the stool, but faecal excretion wanes rapidly and rarely lasts beyond the first few days of clinical or subclinical illness;[7] viraemia is very limited, detectable for a few days towards the end of the incubation period. Although some investigators have reported detection of HAV in intestinal cells of experimentally infected animals, the consensus is that HAV replication is limited to the liver; from the liver, the virus is excreted through the bile into the intestine and shed in the stool. Although HAV can be detected in the liver for weeks, and although circulating HAV antigen can be detected in serum by sensitive immunoassays for longer than a week after the onset of clinical illness, infectivity does not extend beyond the first few days of illness (except when it recurs in 'relapsing' cases, see below). A potential exception to such brief faecal shedding of HAV has been reported in a neonatal intensive care unit, in which neonates with hepatitis A were infectious, presumably shedding faecal virus, for 6 months (Rosenblum, JInfDis, 1991; 164:476). Faecal shedding of HAV persisting for months has been documented as well in patients undergoing liver transplantation for fulminant hepatitis A (Fagan, JMedVirol, 1990; 30:131). Protracted hepatitis A and faecal shedding have not been documented in immunocompetent persons.

The primary antibody response to HAV, which is of the IgM class (IgM anti-HAV), lasts only a few months and is replaced ultimately by anti HAV of the IgG class (IgG anti-HAV). After infection with HAV, IgG antibody remains detectable indefinitely and correlates with lasting immunity.

History

The illness we know today as hepatitis A was probably recognized during antiquity, but its link to viral infection was not established until the 1940s.[8] Before the virus was identified and characterized, the illness associated with HAV infection was recognized to occur in epidemics, very common as an affliction of armies during military campaigns, but was mistakenly blamed on overindulgence, excessive use of alcohol, and blockage of bile ducts by mucous secretions ('catarrhal jaundice'). Epidemiological and volunteer studies during and after the Second World War differentiated between 'infectious hepatitis' and 'serum hepatitis' (MacCallum, BrMedBull, 1972; 28: 105) and established that infectious hepatitis was caused by a filterable agent, presumably a virus, that had a short incubation period and was spread predominantly by the faecal–oral route. These volunteer studies were continued in the 1950s and 1960s (Krugman, AmJMed, 1962; 32:717; Krugman, JAMA, 1967; 200: 365) and were supplemented by studies suggesting successful transmission of a viral agent in marmoset monkeys (tamarins) (Deinhardt, JExpMed, 1967; 125:673; Holmes, Science, 1969; 165:816). Ultimately, clinical specimens generated in volunteer and experimental-animal studies provided the reagents that were used to identify HAV.

In 1973 workers at the National Institutes of Health, using immune electron microscopy, found 27-nm virus-like particles that were aggregated by convalescent but not by preinfection serum in the stools of volunteers infected with HAV.[1] This discovery was

Table 1 Epidemiology of hepatitis A virus
Transmission in nature almost exclusively by the faecal–oral route
Percutaneous transmission very rare
Perinatal transmission unlikely
Endemic in developing countries (where infection is predominant in childhood)
Declining in developed countries
Mean age of exposure increasing
Frequency of clinically apparent disease increasing

followed rapidly by the development of serological tests, confirmation of the marmoset model and establishment of the chimpanzee as an experimental model, the cultivation in 1979 of HAV *in vitro*,[3] and the cloning (Ticehurst, PNAS, 1983; 80:5885) and sequencing (Baroudy, PNAS, 1985; 82:2143; Najarian, PNAS, 1985; 82:2627) of the viral genome.[9]

Epidemiology (Table 1)
Mode of transmission

Hepatitis A virus is transmitted in nature almost exclusively by the faecal–oral route. Although viraemia occurs, it is transient and does not contribute to transmission of HAV infection except in very unusual circumstances. As an enteric agent, hepatitis A is spread from person to person or is acquired when a susceptible person ingests water, milk, or food such as bivalve shellfish that has been contaminated with faecal material from an infected person, occasionally in the context of a food-borne outbreak traced to a food handler. Indeed, a massive shellfish-associated outbreak, involving more than 310 000 persons, occurred in Shanghai as recently as 1988 (Halliday, JInfDis, 1991; 164:852). Poor personal and environmental hygiene foster the spread of enteric agents like HAV, both sporadic cases and outbreaks are common, and efficient intrafamilial spread accounts for secondary cases within the household of an infected person. Infectivity peaks during the late incubation period; therefore, the risk of transmission is highest for those in contact with a patient just before clinically apparent illness, rather than for those exposed to the patient during or after the onset of clinical illness. Because HAV does not cause chronic infection and is not associated with a carrier state, perpetuation of infection within populations relies upon person-to-person transmission or environmental contamination; certainly, HAV has been shown to remain stable in the environment for many months (Lednar, AmJEpid, 1985; 122:226). In temperate climates, hepatitis A tended to occur in seasonal waves, concentrated in the late autumn and early winter, and in epidemic waves cycling every 5 to 20 years, relying on the emergence of new susceptible populations; however, in developed countries, the frequency of hepatitis A has been declining regularly during the second half of the twentieth century, and these seasonal and generational cycles are not as apparent.

Groups recognized traditionally as being at high risk for HAV infection include travellers from non-endemic to endemic areas, whose risk has been estimated to be 3 cases per 1000 travellers per month;[10] military personnel stationed in endemic areas; persons working with non-human primates; children, employees, and parents of children in day-care centres; and clients and employees of institutions for the developmentally disabled (Szmuness, JAMA, 1977; 237:1702).[11] In day-care centres, hepatitis A in the children is so mild that clinical recognition is rare; outbreaks become apparent when adults exposed to the children (employees of the centre and parents) become clinically ill (Hadler, JInfDis, 1982; 145:255). Although the role of sexual transmission is not known, homosexual men have an increased risk of HAV infection (Corey, NEJM, 1980; 302:435), probably through faecal exposure. Similarly, intravenous drug users have been found to have an increased risk of HAV infection, not as a result of percutaneous exposure to contaminated needles but rather related to poor hygiene. Recent attention has been focused on outbreaks among staff of neonatal intensive care units, presumably infected by exposure to faecal material from infected neonates (Rosenblum, JInfDis, 1991; 164:476), and among recipients of clotting factors (Mannucci, AnnIntMed, 1994; 120:1). An outbreak of hepatitis A in patients with tumours treated with interleukin 2 and lymphokine-activated killer cells was attributed to contaminated plasma used to dilute the killer cells (Weisfuse, JInfDis, 1990; 161:647). Such rare cases in recipients of blood products notwithstanding, hepatitis A is rarely transmitted by transfusion. Hepatitis A is rarely, if ever, transmitted perinatally from mother to offspring, in spite of one case report (Watson, JInfDis, 1993; 167:567), and health workers do not have a higher prevalence of infection than that of the general population (Gibas, AmJEpid, 1992; 136:603).

Distribution within populations

In the United States and other developed countries, HAV accounts for approximately one-quarter of all reported cases of acute viral hepatitis. Approximately 25 000 cases of acute hepatitis A are reported to the Centers for Disease Control and Prevention in the United States, and unreported cases have been estimated to bring the number of new cases per year to in excess of 130 000,[11] for an annual incidence of approximately 0.05 per cent. Exposure is inversely proportional to socioeconomic status, and seroprevalence surveys show an increase in anti-HAV frequencies with advancing age. The most compelling trend in the prevalence of HAV infection (reflected by anti-HAV frequencies) has been the regular decline in the frequency of infection in developed countries. When populations in the United States, western Europe, and Australia are evaluated at intervals a decade apart, overall prevalences and age-specific prevalences have been documented to fall. In the United States, the most recent survey (Third National Health and Nutrition Examination Survey, NHANES-III, conducted between 1988 and 1991) revealed an anti-HAV prevalence of 33 per cent,[11] which is 5 per cent lower than the prevalence detected during the 1976 to 1980 NHANES-II survey (Shapiro, Vaccine, 1992; 10(Suppl. 1): S59) and 12 per cent lower than the prevalence reported in a survey of New York blood donors in 1976 (Szmuness, NEJM, 1976; 295: 755). In Europe, a north–south gradient exists in relative endemicity of hepatitis A, from negligible in northern, Scandinavian countries, to more common in southern, Mediterranean countries. In the United States, the frequency of acute hepatitis A is higher in western states as well as in certain populations, including Alaskan natives and native Americans (American Indians).[11]

As with other enteric viral infections, hepatitis A is primarily an infection of childhood, but the mean age of exposure increases with

Table 2 Clinical features of HAV infection

- An acute, self-limited illness, with modest morbidity and negligible mortality
- Incubation period 2 to 6 weeks, with a mean of 4 weeks
- Occasional variants include cholestatic and relapsing hepatitis
- Clinical severity and the likelihood of jaundice increase with age
- Fatality rate (fulminant hepatitis) less than 1/1000
- No long-term sequelae, no chronic hepatitis A, no chronic carrier state

improvement in the levels of hygiene and sanitation. Thus, in developing countries, where HAV is endemic, such as Africa, Central and South America, Central Asia, South-East Asia, and the Mediterranean, childhood exposure to HAV is almost universal, and almost all infections, and consequently immunity, are acquired by the age of 10 years. In highly developed countries, the overall prevalence of anti-HAV in the general population may be lower than 20 per cent and the age of acquisition higher. In many countries, as improvements are made in environmental hygiene, the epidemiology of hepatitis A continues to change. As infections in childhood decline, the prevalence of anti-HAV declines. As a result, a population of adults emerges that, having escaped HAV infection in childhood, remains susceptible into adulthood. As this susceptible population matures into adulthood and becomes sufficiently affluent to travel, imported cases of acute hepatitis A begin to emerge in non-endemic areas. Moreover, as infection with HAV becomes less frequent in a population, and as cases are shifted from younger to older segments of the population, a shift occurs as well in clinical presentation. Because infections in young children tend to be subclinical, while infections in adults tend to be clinically apparent and even severe, paradoxically, as the frequency of hepatitis A infections decreases in a population, the occurrence of clinically apparent and severe cases increases.[12,13] Therefore, in developed countries, cases of acute hepatitis A sufficiently severe to require admission to hospital, even fulminant cases, are more common today than they were several decades ago.

Clinical and laboratory features
Clinical features (Table 2)

Infection with HAV may be asymptomatic or may result in acute hepatitis of variable severity, including fulminant hepatitis. Although the severity and duration of acute hepatitis A may vary, HAV does not cause chronic hepatitis, and there is no hepatitis A carrier state.

The symptoms and signs of acute hepatitis A are similar to those for the other types of viral hepatitis. After a clinical incubation period of approximately 4 weeks (range 2 to 6), patients may experience prodromal, non-specific, systemic symptoms, such as fatigue, malaise, headache, low-grade fever, myalgias, arthralgias, nausea and vomiting, loss of appetite, alteration in gustatory and olfactory senses, and weight loss. More hepatitis-specific symptoms, such as pain in the right upper quadrant, dark urine, jaundice, and acholic stools, occur later, as the clinical illness peaks. When jaundice is severe, pruritus may occur. Physical examination usually reveals mildly tender hepatomegaly and, in icteric cases, scleral

icterus and jaundice. Signs of chronic liver disease, such as spider angiomas and splenomegaly, are rare but can be seen transiently. Except in fulminant cases, which are very rare (in the order of 1 in 1000 cases), symptoms and signs subside within several weeks, after which recovery is complete and without sequelae. Clinical and laboratory recovery occurs in approximately one-half of otherwise healthy young adults within 3 weeks, and the remainder recover thereafter; rarely, laboratory abnormalities may persist for months to a year. In a small proportion of cases, fatigue may be prolonged and outlast all other symptoms, signs, and laboratory abnormalities.

Laboratory features

The biochemical hallmark of acute hepatitis is an elevation in the level of serum aminotransferase activities; levels of alanine aminotransferase tend to exceed those of aspartate aminotransferase. Values of several hundred units are common, but, occasionally aminotransferase levels exceed 1000 or 2000 units. Elevations in aminotransferase activity tend to precede elevations of bilirubin, which may continue to climb even as aminotransferase levels decline. Elevations in prothrombin time and reductions in serum albumin are rare, and alkaline phosphatase levels are normal or minimally elevated. Transient neutropenia and atypical lymphocytosis can occur, and an elevation of serum IgM that is not virus specific is recognized commonly, in addition to a mild increase in total gammaglobulin levels.

Diagnosis

Technically, a diagnosis of acute HAV infection can be made by demonstrating virus in stools or serum during the late incubation period; however, faecal shedding and viraemia have usually subsided by the time a patient presents clinically. In the same vein, diagnosis by cultivation of HAV *in vitro* is impractical because of the long latency of the virus in culture. Therefore, a diagnosis is made by relying on serological detection of antibodies to HAV (anti-HAV) (Fig. 1). Antibodies to HAV appear early during acute illness, even while faecal shedding of virus is still occurring and while serum aminotransferase levels are elevated. The early antibody response is of the IgM class, and the presence of IgM anti-HAV establishes the diagnosis with 100 per cent sensitivity and a specificity nearly as good, marred only by rare, confounding, non-specific immunoassay binding in the presence of rheumatoid factor. As tests for IgM anti-HAV are configured, this primary humoral immune response remains detectable for approximately 3 months in most patients, rarely lasting longer. Thereafter, beginning during convalescence and persisting indefinitely, IgG anti-HAV predominates and is associated with life-long immunity to reinfection. In patients presenting with acute hepatitis whose serum contains IgG anti-HAV rather than IgM anti-HAV, the current acute hepatitis is not related to hepatitis A. Because IgM anti-HAV persists for several months after acute infection, IgM anti-HAV testing can be used to make a retrospective diagnosis, for example, in a person suspected as the source of a food-borne outbreak or in a traveller returning after recovery from acute illness. More detailed information on diagnostic tests for HAV infection appears in Chapter 12.1.2.1.

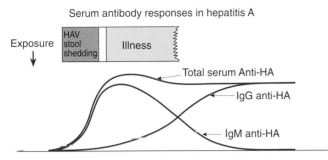

Serum antibody responses in hepatitis A

Fig. 1. Diagrammatic representation of the clinical, serological, and virological events that occur in HAV infection

Pathology

Liver biopsies are almost never indicated in patients with acute hepatitis A, a self-limited disease. The histological hallmarks of acute hepatitis A have been described, however, and share the typical features of all forms of acute viral hepatitis: ballooning of hepatocytes, coagulative necrosis, focal necrosis, portal expansion by a mononuclear infiltrate, periportal inflammation, and Kupffer cell hyperplasia. Cholestasis may be present and, in more severe cases, piecemeal necrosis (erosion of the limiting plate of periportal hepatocytes) and/or bridging necrosis (cell drop-out that spans lobules) may be observed. Although periportal fibrosis may be seen in protracted cases, progression to cirrhosis has not been documented. When liver tissue is available, HAV can be localized by immunohistochemical staining to the hepatocyte cytoplasm (Shimizu, JImmunol, 1978; 121:1671).

Pathogenesis

Hepatitis A virus replicates predominantly in the liver. Although the virus has been detected by some investigators in extrahepatic sites such as the gut (Mathieson, InfectImmun, 1977; 18:524; Kariyannis, JMedVirol, 1986; 18:261), and although virus replication in the intestine has been identified in orally infected monkeys (Asher, JMedVirol, 1995;47:260), the relative magnitude of intestinal HAV replication and its importance in the lifecycle of the virus is not known. Whether hepatocyte receptors are responsible for the hepatotropism of HAV remains unknown. Like other hepatitis viruses, HAV is not a cytopathic agent, and the virus is not cytolytic in cell culture, having no effect on the rate of RNA synthesis of host protein (Locarnini, JVirol,1981; 37:216). As is the case for all the hepatitis viruses, in hepatitis A, liver injury is almost certainly mediated by cellular immune responses to virus-infected hepatocytes. Although the vast majority of published literature on the immunopathogenesis of viral hepatitis relates to hepatitis B, and to a lesser extent hepatitis C, demonstration of cytolytic T-cell responses in acute hepatitis A has been documented (Vallbracht, Hepatol, 1986; 6:1308; Vallbracht, JInfDis, 1989; 160:209; Fleischer, Immunol, 1990; 69:14). In addition, cytolytic T-cell epitopes, potential targets for cytolytic T cells, have been identified on HAV structural proteins.[14] A reasonable hypothesis is that CD8 + cytolytic T cells that recognize HAV antigens complexed with host histocompatibility antigens on the hepatocyte cell surface participate in the immunopathogenesis of hepatitis A by attacking and injuring HAV-infected hepatocytes.

Determinants of severity in acute hepatitis A are not well characterized. Although the size of the virus inoculum varies inversely with the length of the incubation period, inoculum size does not affect the severity of acute hepatitis A. As noted above, age of infection is an important factor in clinical expression of illness; the frequency of clinically apparent hepatitis increases with age. While young children with hepatitis A only rarely have hepatitis-specific symptoms such as jaundice (less than 30 per cent), the majority of adults with hepatitis A become jaundiced (more than 70 per cent), and the morbidity of infection is more profound (Lednar, AmJEpid, 1985; 122:226). Studies of candidate HAV vaccine strains after serial passage in cell culture have shown that the pathogenicity of the virus can be attenuated, and such attenuation has been linked to changes at the genome level (Cohen, JVirol, 1989; 63:5364; Emerson, JVirol, 1992; 66:650; Zhang, Virol, 1995; 212:686); potentially, genetic variation among natural strains of HAV could account for differences in severity as well. To date, however, such interstrain differences in clinical disease severity have not been identified.

Extrahepatic manifestations of acute hepatitis mediated by vascular deposition of immune complexes, such as rash (cutaneous vasculitis) and arthralgias/arthritis, are common in patients with hepatitis B but have been reported only rarely in patients with acute hepatitis A (Inman, AnnIntMed, 1986; 105:700; Scully, AmJGastr, 1993; 88:277). Such manifestations have also been reported in patients with relapsing hepatitis A (see below) (Inman, AnnIntMed, 1986; 105:700; Glickson, Medicine, 1992; 71:14).

Complications

With rare exceptions, all patients with acute hepatitis A recover completely without any lasting sequelae. Neither chronic hepatitis A nor a chronic hepatitis A carrier state has been demonstrated to exist. In addition, recovery from acute hepatitis A is followed by life-long immunity to reinfection. Fulminant hepatitis A, which occurs rarely (approximately 1 in 1000 cases of acute hepatitis A), can lead to death; based on an estimated (not the reported) number of deaths per year in the United States, the Centers for Disease Control estimate a case–fatality rate of 0.3 per cent.[11] In patients older than 50 years the case–fatality rate is higher, 1.8 per cent according to the Centers for Disease Control estimate, and, in patients with underlying chronic liver disease, the risk of fulminant hepatitis A is increased (Akriviadis, AnnIntMed, 1989; 110:838).

Two variants of acute hepatitis A merit special attention—cholestatic hepatitis and relapsing hepatitis. Cholestatic hepatitis A, characterized by persistent jaundice and pruritus, with marked elevation of bilirubin levels, occurs rarely and can be misconstrued for extrahepatic biliary obstruction or chronic cholestatic liver disease. Although symptoms and biochemical abnormalities may persist for many months and even up to a year, cholestatic hepatitis A resolves invariably and is followed by complete recovery. When this syndrome occurs in the setting of acute hepatitis A that is serologically well-documented, the clinician can reassure the patient. Generally, liver biopsy is not required in this setting but, when obtained, liver tissue demonstrates profound centrilobular cholestasis as well as more typical portal inflammation (Gordon, AnnIntMed, 1984; 101:635).

Relapsing hepatitis A can occur in as many as 5 to 10 per cent of patients with acute hepatitis A, usually reflected by an asymptomatic elevation of aminotransferase activity within weeks to months after apparent biochemical recovery (Gruer, Lancet, 1982; ii:163; Bamber, Gut, 1983; 24:561; Jacobson, JMedVirol, 1985; 16:163; Chiriaco, JInfDis, 1986; 153:378; Raimondo, JInfDis, 1986; 153:172; Glickson, Medicine, 1992; 71:14). In a proportion of cases, symptoms and jaundice recur during relapse, and resumption of faecal HAV excretion has been documented during relapse (Sjögren, AnnIntMed, 1987; 106:221). Even when hepatitis A relapses, the disease does not become chronic; this variant, too, resolves invariably without any chronic sequelae.

Other complications during acute hepatitis A are rare, although a host of miscellaneous case reports link hepatitis A in rare instances to Guillain–Barré syndrome (Tabor, JMedVirol, 1987; 21:207), pancreatitis (Davis, AmJGastr, 1992; 87:1648), cholecystitis (Mourani, AnnIntMed, 1994; 120:398), aplastic anaemia, renal failure (Geltner, JClinGastro, 1992; 14:160), and encephalitis (Thomas, AmJGastr, 1993; 88:279), among others.

Although acute hepatitis A does not progress to chronic hepatitis or cirrhosis, isolated cases have been described in which autoimmune hepatitis (with autoantibodies and substantial hyperglobulinaemia) followed acute hepatitis A (Vento, Lancet, 1991; 337:1183; Rahaman, AmJGastr, 1994; 89:106; Huppertz, JHepatol, 1995; 23:204). In such cases, observed as well in patients following acute hepatitis B and C, the hypothesis is that, in the setting of genetically acquired, increased susceptibility to autoimmunity, virus-induced liver injury may provide the environmental trigger that precipitates autoimmune injury.

Management

No specific therapy is required for acute hepatitis A or for its variants, cholestatic hepatitis or relapsing hepatitis A. Because the disease is self-limited, specific antiviral therapy is not required, nor have any antiviral agents been shown to be effective clinically in hepatitis A. Management remains supportive, and admission to hospital is rarely required, except for patients with other concurrent, serious medical problems, those who cannot maintain oral intake, or those with incipient liver failure (for example coagulopathy, mental status changes). Neither bed rest, restrictions of physical activity, nor dietary restrictions are of any benefit (Chalmers, JCI, 1955; 34:1163), but abstaining from alcohol is a reasonable, common-sense approach, albeit one that has not been proven in clinical trials. Corticosteroids are not helpful and should be avoided. For the systemic symptoms of acute hepatitis A, patients may be instructed to take acetaminophen or non-steroidal anti-inflammatory drugs in moderation; rarely, cholestyramine is required to manage severe pruritus. In patients with fulminant hepatitis A, meticulous, intensive supportive care is the only available intervention, short of liver transplantation. In a case report involving four patients with fulminant hepatitis A, interferon-β was administered and followed by recovery (Yoshiba, Lancet, 1994; 343:288), but up to 80 per cent of patients with fulminant hepatitis A managed with supportive care have been reported to survive. Both management of fulminant hepatitis and liver transplantation are addressed in other chapters in this volume.

Prevention

In areas of the world where hepatitis A is endemic and in which most infections are asymptomatic and acquired in childhood, control of hepatitis A requires societal improvements in environmental hygiene, including a clean, safe water supply, adequate disposal of waste, and improvements in living conditions. In developed countries, most people reach adulthood without exposure to hepatitis A, yielding a large, susceptible population. Although hepatitis A vaccines are now available, simple, common-sense hygienic measures (such as hand washing, special training for food handlers) play a role in limiting the spread of hepatitis A. Because HAV is spread by close person-to-person contact, no special precautions are required for classmates and coworkers of patients with acute hepatitis A. Similarly, universal precautions currently practised in hospitals, clinics, and doctors surgeries are sufficient to prevent nosocomial hepatitis A; therefore, additional, cumbersome isolation in a private room as well as the use of gowns and gloves are not required. Travellers to endemic areas should avoid tap water and uncooked food and drinks potentially contaminated with water (salads, ice in drinks).

Currently, both passive immunization with immunoglobulin and active immunization with a killed vaccine are available for prophylaxis against HAV infection

Passive immunization

Until very recently, before hepatitis A vaccines were developed, prophylaxis against hepatitis A relied upon passive immunization with immune globulin prepared from large plasma pools, inactivated by cold ethanol fractionation, and invariably containing anti-HAV. Cold alcohol fractionation has been shown to yield a safe product, free of infectious agents, including HIV. Although the frequency of anti-HAV has been falling in the general population, and although the minimum protective concentration of anti-HAV in immune globulin is not known, all contemporary lots of immune globulin contain sufficient anti-HAV (at least 100 IU/ml) to be protective. The efficacy of immune globulin was first demonstrated in an outbreak at a summer camp in 1944 (Neefe, JAMA, 1945; 128:1063) and confirmed in large-scale studies among American soldiers serving in Europe during the Second World War (Gellis, JAMA, 1945; 128:1062) as well as in persons residing in institutions for mentally handicapped persons (Krugman, JInfDis, 1976; 134:70).

Immune globulin is most effective if given before exposure; for example, in Swedish troops serving in Gaza in 1957, the incidence of hepatitis A was 1 per 1000 among those who received immune globulin and 90 per 1000 among those who did not (Kluge, ActaMedScand, 1963; 174:469). When given pre-exposure, immune globulin is administered intramuscularly at a dose of 0.02 ml/kg for brief expected exposures (1 to 2 months, such as for recreational travel) or 0.06 ml/kg for longer exposures (3 to 5 months, such as for military tours, Peace Corps volunteers). For prolonged exposure, repeat injections of immune globulin at 5- to 6-month intervals was recommended. Now that hepatitis A vaccine is likely to replace immune globulin for pre-exposure prophylaxis, the role of immune globulin may be confined to postexposure prophylaxis. When administered within 2 weeks of exposure, immune globulin has been shown to be at least 85 per cent effective in preventing acute

Table 3 Postexposure prophylaxis against HAV infection with immune globulin

Indications:	Close personal contacts
	Household contacts
	Sexual contacts
	Day-care centres with recognized cases of hepatitis A
	Staff
	Children attending the centre
	Household members of children attending the centre
	Common-source exposure
	Other food handlers besides index case
	Patrons—prophylaxis unlikely to be of benefit unless administered within 2 weeks after exposure
	Schools, factories, offices, hospitals—not recommended routinely
Regimen:	0.02 ml/kg, intramuscularly, as soon after exposure as possible, not beyond 2 weeks of exposure

hepatitis A.[11] Although levels of measurable anti-HAV are low or undetectable after passive immunization, protection lasts for several months (Fujiyama, Hepatol, 1992; 15:983).

The earlier after exposure that immune globulin can be given, the more effective it is likely to be. When administered sufficiently early after exposure, immune globulin prevents HAV infection entirely; however, if administration is delayed into the late incubation period, immune globulin may not abort infection entirely but, instead, attenuate it and render the infection clinically inapparent. Consequently, long-lasting immunity resulting from subclinical infection occurs, rather than transient protection resulting from passive immunization, that is, 'passive–active' immunity. Such postexposure prophylaxis should be given as soon after the exposure as possible (without prior screening for anti-HAV, which would delay immunization unnecessarily and which would add substantial expense) to household, sexual, and institutional contacts of patients with acute hepatitis A; however, prophylaxis is not necessary for casual contacts (such as classmates, office and factory coworkers, hospital employees). Immune globulin has been given routinely to persons exposed to HAV in common-source (such as food-borne) outbreaks; however, by the time such outbreaks are recognized, a full incubation period has elapsed, and prophylaxis may be too late to prevent infection. On the other hand, prophylaxis this late may attenuate clinical illness in some recipients and/or, potentially, limit the number of secondary cases (Table 3).

In some settings (such as in a traveller who does not have sufficient time before embarking to complete a course of hepatitis A vaccine and who expects to travel for an extended period or to travel frequently in the future), a combination of passive immunization with immune globulin plus active immunization with hepatitis A vaccine, at different sites of administration, may be appropriate. Although levels of anti-HAV following a combination of passive and active immunization may be lower than those achieved after vaccination alone (Wagner, Vaccine, 1993; 11:1027), for all practical purposes, the two types of immunization do not interfere with the efficacy of the other. Immune globulin does not interfere with any known killed vaccine but can interfere with immune responses to live, attenuated vaccines; therefore, administration of such live,

attenuated vaccines should be delayed for 5 months or longer after immune globulin administration.[11]

Active immunization

Approaches to the development of live, attenuated hepatitis A vaccines have met with very limited success, while killed vaccines have been shown to be safe, immunogenic, and highly protective (Werzberger, NEJM, 1992; 327:453; Innis, JAMA, 1994; 271:1328). Two commercial, killed hepatitis A vaccines, with alum as an adjuvant, have been approved for use, and analyses based on projections of the kinetics of antibody decay over time suggest that protection after two (in adults) to three (in children) vaccine injections can last for 20 years or longer (Wiens, JMedVirol, 1996; 49:235). Details of the development of hepatitis A vaccines, their immunogenicity and efficacy, and suggested risk groups targeted for vaccination are covered in detail in Chapter 12.1.3.1.

References

1. Feinstone SM, Kapikian AZ, and Purcell RH. Hepatitis A: detection by immune electron microscopy of a virus-like antigen associated with acute illness. *Science*, 1973; **182**: 1026–8.
2. Melnick JL. Properties and classification of hepatitis A virus. *Vaccine*, 1992; **10** (Suppl. 1): S24–6.
3. Provost PJ and Hilleman MR. Propagation of human hepatitis A virus in cell culture *in vitro*. *Proceedings of the Society for Experimental Biology and Medicine*, 1979; **160**: 213–21.
4. Lemon SM. Type A viral hepatitis: new developments in an old disease. *New England Journal of Medicine*, 1985; **313**: 1059–67.
5. Ticehurst JR. Hepatitis A virus: clones, cultures, and vaccines. *Seminars in Liver Disease*, 1986; **6**: 46–55.
6. Cohen JI. Hepatitis A virus: insights from molecular biology. *Hepatology*, 1989; **9**: 889–95.
7. Dienstag JL, Feinstone SM, Kapikian AZ, and Purcell RH. Fecal shedding of hepatitis A antigen. *Lancet*, 1975; i: 763–5.
8. Feinstone SM and Gust ID. Hepatitis A virus. In Richman DD, Whitley RJ, and Hayden FG, eds. *Clinical virology*. New York: Churchill Livingstone, 1997: 1049–72.
9. Hollinger FB and Ticehurst JR. Hepatitis A virus. In Fields BN *et al.*, eds. *Fields virology*. Philadelphia: Lippincott-Raven, 1996: 735–82.
10. Steffen R, Kane MA, Shapiro CN, Billo N, Schoellhorn KJ, and van Damme P. Epidemiology and prevention of hepatitis A in travelers. *Journal of the American Medical Association*, 1994; **272**: 885–9.
11. Centers for Disease Control and Prevention. Prevention of hepatitis A through active or passive immunization: recommendations of the Advisory Committee on Immunization Practices (ACIP). *Morbidity and Mortality Weekly Report*, 1996; **45**(No. RR-15): 1–30.
12. Purcell RH. Hepatitis viruses: changing patterns of human disease. *Proceedings of the National Academy of Sciences* (*USA*), 1994; **91**: 2401–6.
13. Shapiro CN and Margolis HS. Worldwide epidemiology of hepatitis A virus infection. *Journal of Hepatology*, 1993; **18** (Suppl. 2): S11–14.
14. Wunschmann S, Vallbracht A, Flehmig B, Winokur P, Klinzman D, and Stapleton JT. Cytolytic T lymphocyte epitopes are present on hepatitis A virus structural proteins. In Rizzetto M, Purcell RH, Gerin JL, and Verme G, eds. *Viral hepatitis and liver disease*. Turin: Edizioni Minerva Medica, 1997: 51–4.

12.1.2.3 Hepatitis B

Geoffrey Dusheiko

Definition

Hepatitis B virus infection remains an important world-wide disease. Type B hepatitis is caused by the hepatitis B virus (**HBV**), a small, enveloped DNA virus that infects the liver causing hepatocellular necrosis and inflammation.[1] HBV infection can be either acute or chronic, and can range in severity from being asymptomatic and completely resolving to severe and symptomatic with progressive and even fatal illness.

Acute hepatitis B is defined as a self-limiting disease marked by acute inflammation and hepatocellular necrosis in association with a transient HBV infection The diagnosis generally rests upon the finding of hepatitis B surface (s) antigen (**HBsAg**) and IgM antibody to hepatitis B core (c) antigen (anti-**HBc**) in the serum of a patient with clinical and serum biochemical evidence of acute hepatitis.[2] The disease generally lasts 1 to 6 weeks, but may be prolonged and can be fulminant. Not all patients with acute HBV infection develop clinically apparent acute hepatitis B; indeed, the majority (50–70 per cent) never develop symptoms or abnormal liver biochemical tests, but rather have a silent, self-limiting infection and ultimately clear the virus and produce protective antibody (anti-HBs and anti-HBc) (Fig. 1).

Chronic hepatitis B is defined as persistent HBV infection accompanied by evidence of hepatocellular injury and inflammation. The diagnosis is based upon the finding of abnormal concentrations of serum aminotransferases and HBsAg in serum for 6 months or more. Symptoms in chronic hepatitis B, if they are present at all, are typically mild, with intermittent fatigue, muscle aches, and nausea. Laboratory tests show persistent or fluctuating elevations of serum aminotransferases. Serum bilirubin and tests of hepatic function are usually normal unless the disease is severe or cirrhosis has developed. Chronic hepatitis B generally lasts for years, but is not necessarily lifelong. Not all patients with chronic HBV infection develop chronic hepatitis B, and some patients with chronic hepatitis B ultimately enter a phase of remission with an improvement in serum aminotransferases despite the persistence of HBsAg (Fig. 1). These persons are usually referred to as 'healthy' chronic HBsAg carriers (Hoofnagle, Hepatol, 1987; 7:758). However, this term is somewhat misleading, as these patients are at risk of reactivation of active hepatitis, and, if cirrhosis has developed, may ultimately develop hepatocellular carcinoma. Other patients not only show improvement on serum biochemical tests but also ultimately clear HBsAg and develop anti-HBs. Unfortunately, some patients do not resolve their chronic hepatitis B and ultimately develop cirrhosis, portal hypertension, and hepatocellular failure. A proportion also develop hepatocellular carcinoma due to chronic HBV infection.[3]

Introduction

The key breakthrough in understanding hepatitis B came in 1965 with the description of the Australia antigen (Blumberg, JAMA, 1965; 191:541). This antigen was shown to actually represent the

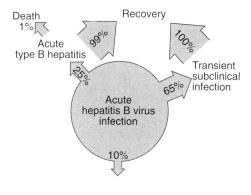

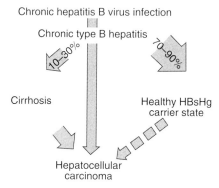

Fig. 1. Outcomes of HBV infection.

envelope or surface antigen of HBV and was accordingly named the hepatitis B surface antigen.

HBsAg provided a sensitive and specific marker for HBV infection, and allowed rapid advances in knowledge about this virus and its disease. After the identification of HBsAg, hepatitis B was clearly linked to the development of cirrhosis and hepatocellular carcinoma (Popper, Hepatol, 1987; 6:764). Subtypes of HBsAg were described (Le Bouvier, JInfDis, 1971; 123:671), the virus and subviral particles were identified in serum,[4] a nucleocapsid core protein (HBcAg) and an associated DNA polymerase activity were described,[5] and the genome of the virus was isolated, characterized as a small, circular molecule of DNA (Summers, PNAS, 1975; 72: 4597; Robinson, JVirol, 1984; 14:384). Although HBV could not be grown in cell culture, the availability of sensitive and specific serological markers of hepatitis B led to a complete characterization of the natural history and course of acute and chronic hepatitis B, and identified its epidemiological features and mode of spread (Szmuness, AmJPath, 1975; 81:629). Importantly, the identification of HBV led to an understanding of the immunology of hepatitis B and the development of vaccines using HBsAg isolated from serum of chronic carriers (Szumness, NEJM, 1980; 303:833).

The development of molecular biological techniques accelerated the already rapid pace of advances in hepatitis B research. By 1978 the genome of the HBV had been cloned and four open reading frames delineating the four gene products of HBV were identified (Galibert, Nature, 1979; 281:646). Furthermore, identification of animal viruses resembling human HBV (Summers, PNAS, 1978; 75:4533; Mason, JVirol, 1980; 36:829) led to the characterization of the replication cycle of this family of viruses, the so-called hepadnaviruses.[6]

The virus exists as a 42-nm, double-shelled particle found in serum (see Chapter 12.1.2.1). HBV has an outer envelope component of HBsAg and an inner nucleocapsid component of HBcAg. In addition to actual virions, incomplete viral particles, 20-nm spheres and tubules, which consist entirely of HBsAg without HBcAg or nucleic acid, are present in serum and actually outnumber virions by a factor of $1:10^3$. The large number of these subviral particles in serum accounts for the finding of large amounts of HBsAg in the blood during acute and chronic hepatitis B. HBsAg can also be detected in the liver, generally in a membranous pattern on the surface of the majority of hepatocytes. In chronic hepatitis B, HBsAg is also found in a homogeneous cytoplasmic location.

The nucleocapsid HBcAg is not found free in serum, but rather inside HBV virions. Inside the core particle is an endogenous DNA polymerase activity with a single molecule of partially double-stranded, circular DNA. DNA polymerase activity and HBV DNA can be detected in serum and used to monitor viral replication. HBcAg can be detected in liver, usually in the nuclei but also in the cytoplasm of hepatocytes. The third HBV antigen is the hepatitis B e antigen (**HBeAg**), which, unlike HBsAg and HBcAg, is not particulate, but rather is detectable as a soluble, 17-kDa protein in serum. The presence and titre of HBeAg correlate rather well with the presence and concentration of virus in serum and HBcAg in liver, making HBcAg a useful marker also for HBV replication.

The genomic structure of HBV DNA is unique and compact.[7–10] It has four open reading frames, all of which appear to represent functional genes. The *S* gene encodes HBsAg, the *C* region encodes HBcAg, the *P* gene encodes the viral polymerase, and the *X* gene encodes a small protein of unclear function (**HBxAg**).

The *S* gene region is complex, in that it is preceded by three functional start codons so that three differently sized polypeptides (having different N-termini) can be produced: large, medium, and major HBsAg (Neurath, Nature, 1985; 315:154).

The *C* region of the HBV genome has two potential start codons yielding a precore and core region. Interestingly, the N-terminus of the precore protein encodes a signal sequence that directs the protein to the endoplasmic reticulum where the signal peptide is removed and, after further modification, the end-product of the precore and core region is secreted as HBeAg. In contrast, the polypeptide synthesized from the core region alone (without precore) is directed to the nucleus and, after post-translational modification, accounts for the HBcAg detected in liver (Ou, PNAS, 1986; 83:1578) and self-assembles into core particles that are incorporated into mature virions.

The HBV replicates largely in the liver (see Chapter 12.1.3.1). Replication has necessarily been studied in the absence of a cell-culture system; these studies still depend upon *in vitro* transfections, duck hepatitis B cell-culture systems, and transgenic mouse models.[9,10] How the virus enters the hepatocyte is unclear, but it probably involves a specific receptor on them for HBV. A number of candidate receptors have been identified, including the transferrin receptor, the asialoglycoprotein receptor molecule, and human liver endonexin.[11,12]

HBV DNA is also present in non-hepatic tissues including pancreas, kidneys, skin, bone marrow, and peripheral blood mononuclear cells. The HBV DNA is integrated into the host genome in these cells, but the method of replication in them is not known.

Epidemiology

The relative ease with which HBV antigens and antibodies can be assayed has greatly expedited study of the transmission and epidemiology of this disease. Infection with HBV is a common problem world-wide (see ref. 2, p. 297). In developed countries, acute hepatitis B is a frequent cause of jaundice in adults and accounts for about 50 per cent of cases of acute viral hepatitis. (Alter, JAMA, 1990; 263:1218). Chronic hepatitis B is relatively uncommon, affecting 1 per cent or less of persons in industrial nations. In contrast, in undeveloped nations, HBV infection is an almost universal infection of childhood and the HBsAg carrier state affects 5 to 15 per cent of adults.[13] World-wide, approximately 5 per cent of the population has chronic HBV infection, an estimated 300 million individuals. The ratio of males to females is usually between 1.5 and 2:1.

Transmission

Transmission of HBV is largely from the parenteral or 'inapparent parenteral' route. For transmission of hepatitis B to occur there must be (i) a source (such as HBsAg-positive blood), (ii) a mode of spread (such as a needlestick), and (iii) a susceptible host. The source of most HBV infection is probably exposure to blood secretions from chronic carriers (Alter, Lancet, 1975; ii:838). Hepatitis B is not highly contagious (as, for instance, is hepatitis A) but the presence of large amounts of virus in the blood and secretions of infected persons over a long time means that even an isolated, single, and minute exposure can transmit this infection. Spread is facilitated by the fact that many chronic HBsAg carriers are asymptomatic and unaware of their infection and potential infectivity.

Highest amounts of HBV are present in blood. Titres of infectivity have been estimated from chimpanzee transmission studies (Barker, JInfDis, 1973; 127:648) and from assays for HBV genome in serum using dot hybridization and the polymerase chain reaction (Bonino, RicClinLab, 1988; 18:121; Kaneko, PNAS, 1989; 86:312). These studies indicate that HBsAg carriers vary immensely in their infectivity from less than 10 to greater than 10^8 virions/ml of plasma. Patients with HBeAg in addition to HBsAg generally have 10^6 virions/ml, which explains why transmission of hepatitis B usually occurs from exposure to an HBeAg-positive person (Perillo, Gastro, 1979; 76:139; Hoofnagle, SemLivDis, 1986; 6:1). It has been suggested that anti-HBe-positive, HBsAg-positive individuals may not be infectious at all. However, anti-HBe-positive persons do have virus, but usually in low titre, so that a larger-volume exposure is necessary. Thus a needlestick exposure to HBsAg-positive, anti-HBe-positive blood often does not result in transmission of hepatitis B, but this is probably because a needlestick may only represent exposure to less than 0.001 ml of plasma, too little if HBV is below 10^3/ml. Thus all HBsAg-positive individuals must be considered infectious, but only those patients with HBeAg or with HBV DNA as detected by routine methods (thus more than 10^5 virions/ml) will spread the disease by minute parenteral exposure. With large-volume exposure such as blood transfusions, however, anti-HBe-positive blood is infectious.

HBV has been transmitted by transfusion with HBsAg-negative, anti-HBc-positive blood, which probably represents low levels of infection such that virus is present but there is too little HBsAg to be detected. Supporting this occurrence has been the finding of HBV DNA by polymerase chain reaction for a time in occasional patients who have cleared HBsAg after the resolution of acute or chronic hepatitis B (Kaneko, PNAS, 1989; 86:312). HBsAg can also be detected in other bodily secretions, even without blood contamination. However, the amount of virus is always 100- to 1000-fold less in these secretions than in blood. Infectivity of saliva and semen has been documented in transmission studies on chimpanzees (Heathcote, Lancet, 1974; i:71; Villarejos, NEJM, 1974; 291:1375). While HBsAg can occasionally be found in urine, breast milk, vaginal secretions, cerebrospinal fluid, sweat, tears, bile, and faeces, the amounts are rather low and these secretions are not provenly infectious. Furthermore, the role of minute blood contamination of any of these secretions cannot be easily assessed.

HBV, unlike many viruses, is a hardy agent. The infectivity of HBsAg-positive plasma is stable after storage at –20°C for many years and the virus resists heating to 60°C for up to 4 h. Heating blood products to 60°C for 10 h will inactivate low concentrations of HBV as occur in albumin products but is inadequate to inactivate all virus in highly infectious serum (Gellis, JCI, 1948; 27:239). HBV also resists drying and storage for a time at room temperature. Because there is no simple tissue-culture or animal model for HBV transmission (the chimpanzee, an endangered species, is the only reliable model for assessing infectivity), the precise inactivation kinetics for HBV is not known. Autoclaving is the only proven means of inactivating all HBV infectious materials. However, thorough cleansing followed by hypochlorite, formalin, or glutaraldehyde appears to be reliable. For instruments that cannot survive such vigorous treatment (such as endoscopes), thorough cleaning and mild glutaraldehyde or steam sterilization appear adequate.

The usual mode of transmission of hepatitis B is parenteral or percutaneous exposure such as with blood transfusions, the use of unpasteurized plasma products, needlestick accidents, and injections with unsterilized instruments such as in tattooing, acupuncture, ear piercing, or dentistry. Outbreaks of nosocomial HBV infection have been ascribed to gynaecological surgery or dentistry (Rimland, NEJM, 1977; 296:153) when the surgeon has been HBsAg- and HBeAg-positive. Recently, transmission from HBeAg-negative, HBV DNA-positive surgeons has also been reported.[14] Hepatitis B from transfusion has become rare since the introduction of routine screening of blood donors for HBsAg (Lettau, JAMA, 1986; 255:934). Isolated cases of post-transfusion hepatitis do still occur, which may be due to the rare blood donor who is a low-level carrier of hepatitis B (without detectable HBsAg) or who is in the incubation or immediate convalescent period of acute hepatitis B. Routine testing of blood for anti-HBc (which was introduced as an indirect means of eliminating non-A, non-B hepatitis) may further decrease post-transfusion hepatitis B, but many countries have chosen not to include anti-HBc screening. Immune serum globulin, if properly manufactured by the cold ethanol fractionation of Cohn and using plasma that has been screened for HBsAg, is not believed to transmit hepatitis B.

Hepatitis B can also be spread by blood products such as factor VIII, factor IX concentrates, cryoprecipitates, fibrinogen, and human thrombin. As a result, patients with haemophilia have a higher incidence of exposure. The introduction of HBsAg screening of plasma donors decreased but did not eliminate HBV from these products. Recently improved techniques of 'dry' or 'wet' heating,

as well as the affinity purification of proteins and the use of donors with a safe pedigree, have further decreased the risk of hepatitis B from these products. The risk still exists, however: these products should only be used in patients who have received HBV vaccine. Hepatitis B is a major complication of accidental needlesticks and therefore a major risk for health-care workers. Not all physicians or nurses with hepatitis B remember an actual percutaneous exposure. HBV contamination of other surfaces can also be a source of infection (such as on paper or glass used to test blood samples). Intravenous drug abuse is an increasing cause of hepatitis B in many areas of the world. Drug paraphernalia is often shared and thus contaminated with HBV.

Careful investigation of cases of acute or chronic hepatitis B does not always uncover a potential parenteral source of transmission. With the development of serological tests for hepatitis B it became clear that this disease could be spread by sexual contact (Szmuness, AnnIntMed, 1975; 83:489). Indeed, in most developed countries of the world the major mode of spread is probably sexual. This accounts for the very high rate of hepatitis B among male homosexuals and in promiscuous heterosexuals (Dietzman, JAMA, 1977; 238:2625). How HBV is spread during sexual activity is not clear. HBV is detectable in semen but spread would seem also to require a break in the skin or mucous membranes of the susceptible host. In this regard, it is significant that the sexual activity most frequently incriminated in HBV transmission has been anal intercourse, especially transmission to the receptive partner. The marked decrease in promiscuity and in rectal intercourse with the onset of the pandemic of acquired immune deficiency disease (AIDS) in the 1980s has resulted in a decrease in hepatitis B among homosexual men.

Sexual spread of hepatitis B among heterosexuals also appears to occur, both female to male and male to female. HBV in semen or vaginal secretions combined with minute penile or vaginal lacerations may account for heterosexual spread of HBV. Actually, HBV appears to be more readily spread by sexual contact than the human immunodeficiency virus (HIV) or hepatitis C virus (HCV), as shown by the higher rates of antibodies to hepatitis B than anti-HIV or anti-HCV among sexual contacts of haemophiliacs and drug addicts (who may have all three chronic infections). It must be pointed out, however, that HBV may be spread by other means among intimate contacts. Use of condoms is an often recommended but unproven means of preventing the spread of hepatitis B.

Hepatitis B is also spread by intimate contact that is not apparently sexual or parenteral. Thus non-sexual intrafamilial spread, while not common, does occur (Szmuness, NEJM, 1973; 289:1162). This type of spread is particularly common if the infected proband is an infant or child, which has been most clearly seen among adoptive parents of chronic HBsAg carrier children. The reasons for this are probably multiple. HBV-infected children typically have very large amounts of virus; children are less careful with secretions and are likely to be touched and fondled. Interestingly, teenage children, probably because of better hygiene and less physical contact, rarely spread hepatitis B to other family members.

Non-sexual intrafamilial spread is best described as inapparent parenteral spread, the vehicle perhaps being saliva, blood-tinged fluid, and fluid from open sores, skin lesions, or scratches. Thus, the non-sexual spread of hepatitis B in families, and particularly amongst small children, as appears to occur in underdeveloped areas of the world, is partially unexplained. Saliva, while potentially infectious, will not spread hepatitis B without parenteral or percutaneous exposure (Ben Aryeh, ArchOralBiol, 1985; 30:97), which may be enhanced by small lesions in the oral mucosa. Thus, in chimpanzee studies, HBsAg-positive blood, saliva, and semen did not transmit hepatitis B when placed on the skin or given orally, nasally, or vaginally. Transmission only occurred when these secretions were injected percutaneously or roughly applied to the vagina in imitation of sexual intercourse. The possible role of biting insects cannot be dismissed, despite the lack of firm evidence (Brotman, Lancet, 1973; i: 1305; Prince, Lancet, 1982; ii:247). In undeveloped areas of the world, poor hygiene, shared utensils, frequent skin diseases, and child-care practices have been cited as means of spread of hepatitis B among children. Other cultural practices, such as tribal and witch-doctor scarification and acupuncture (Stryker, JFamPractice, 1986; 22:155), may spread hepatitis B. A splash of blood in the eye may also transmit the infection (Kew, InfectImmun, 1973; 7:823).

An important mode of transmission of hepatitis B is perinatal spread (Okada, NEJM, 1976; 294:746). New-borns of mothers who are HBeAg-positive are likely to develop HBV infection (Beasley, AmJEpid, 1977; 105:94). Most babies are not HBsAg-positive at birth; the onset of infection is usually 3 months after birth. The acute phase of infection is typically mild, not associated with apparent illness, and accompanied by minimal abnormalities of aminotransferases. However, infection during the neonatal period almost always leads to chronic infection. Maternal–infant spread is an important means by which this virus infection is sustained in populations. It is typically silent, neither the mother nor the infant being ill with the infection at the time. Mothers with HBeAg in addition to HBsAg are the most infectious, and spread the chronic infection to their new-born in over 90 per cent of cases. It is believed that infection is acquired by inoculation of the infant by infected maternal blood and liquor during passage through the vagina at birth, rather than through intrauterine transmission. Although the breast milk of HBsAg-positive mothers is frequently positive, the role of breast feeding in transmitting hepatitis B is unsettled. In a small proportion of cases, particularly in pregnancies accompanied by threatened abortions, intrauterine transmission may also occur. Mothers with anti-HBe are less infectious but do spread the infection in a proportion of cases and indeed occasionally transmit an acute icteric or even fulminant hepatitisB to their new-born. Mothers with acute hepatitis B can transmit the infection to their neonates, but usually only if their hepatitis appears during the third trimester. In any case, new-borns of HBsAg-positive mothers should receive prophylaxis in the form of both hepatitis B immunoglobulin and vaccine. Because of the silent nature of chronic HBV infection, routine screening of pregnant women for HBsAg is now recommended, although it is not always practised. Hepatitis B does not appear to be spread by casual contact. Faeces of chronic HBsAg carriers do not appear to harbour virus and faecal–oral spread has not been documented. Hepatitis B is not spread in the work place (unless blood or secretions are handled in there), or by casual contact such as touching, hugging, kissing or sharing towels, eating utensils, or food.

Epidemiological patterns

Low- (less than 2 per cent), intermediate- (2–8 per cent), and high-prevalence (more than 8 per cent) areas of hepatitis B infection are recognized. The disease is endemic in several regions: these include the Far East and more than 40 countries in the Pacific region, also large parts of Asia and subSaharan Africa. The disease is also prevalent in South America and in a number of foci in other regions, for example eastern Europe and the Arctic. There is a wide distribution within countries and regions, and within some countries with ethnically diverse communities, for example South Africa and New Zealand, where there are differences between the Caucasian and the aboriginal populations. Within endogenous populations, differences are found between rural and urban areas.

These variations probably reflect differences in modes of transmission due to variations in socioeconomic conditions and social practices. In general, the developed, industrialized nations of the world, such as the United States, Canada, United Kingdom, western Europe, South Africa, and Australia (Caucasians), are areas of low endemicity. In these areas, hepatitis B is largely a disease of adults, occurring typically in particular high-risk groups. In these Caucasian populations, the HBsAg carrier rate is low (<1 per cent), cirrhosis from hepatitis B and hepatocellular carcinoma are rare, and maternal–infant transmission is infrequent.

In contrast, in the underdeveloped or less developed nations of the world, such as China, South-East Asia, countries of the Pacific rim, and the indigenous populations of subSaharan Africa, hepatitis B is hyperendemic, the disease is common in children, most adults have serological evidence of continuing or past infection, and the HBsAg carrier state is high (>10 per cent). These areas have a high rate of maternal–infant spread. Furthermore, the complications of chronic HBV infection, cirrhosis and hepatocellular carcinoma, are common.

Some areas have an intermediate endemicity and appear to be in a state of transition from high to low. In some countries, such as Japan, Italy, Spain, Greece, Portugal, countries of eastern Europe, and in South America, the carrier rate amongst adults is 1 to 5 per cent and infections occur in both adults and children. In Southern Europe the incidence of HBV infections has consistently declined in the last decade.

The two extremes of endemicity can probably be accounted for by two separate major patterns of HBV transmission. In highly endemic areas, HBV is spread, in a first wave, by maternal–infant transmission, which creates a cohort of children with chronic hepatitis B who are highly infectious. Variation in HBeAg status determines the rates of mother–infant transmission. In turn, this pattern of childhood infection determines a high rate of chronic infection. Because infection occurs in childhood, the carrier rate is high and the pool of infected individuals is sustained to the next generation (Schweitzer, AmJMed, 1973; 55:762). Because disease complications occur only after decades of chronic infection, the infectious carriers are healthy enough to have offspring and the cycle of infection is continued.

Mother–infant transmission, although relatively common, does not account for at least 50 per cent of infections in children, and horizontal transmission, that is, child–child, is equally important. A second wave of transmission occurs in early childhood when the disease is spread to infants whose mothers were not carriers. In endemic areas in Africa, the prevalence in children is quite low at 1 year of age but increases rapidly thereafter, and in many countries in this region the prevalence reaches a peak in children of 7 to 14 years of age.

Infection of neonates at birth from their infected mothers is common in the Far East and China, whereas horizontal transmission from child to child is more common in Africa (Botha, Lancet, 1984; i:1210; Dusheiko, JInfDis, 1985; 152:566). The patterns of transmission are related to the higher prevalence of HBeAg and hence higher infectivity in Chinese (40 per cent) as compared to African mothers (15 per cent). A changing epidemiological pattern of the disease has been observed in endemic areas, and in urban areas of South Africa infection in the Black population is declining (DiBisceglie, BMJ, 1986; 292:140).

In areas of low endemicity the cycle of maternal–child followed by child–child transmission has been broken or was never established. HBV infection is rare in childhood in these countries but rather is a disease of adults, typically those who are in high-risk occupations or have high-risk habits such as drug abuse or sexual promiscuity. Hepatitis B in adults more frequently leads to acute, icteric hepatitis and rarely causes the carrier state. Thus, in the general population the carrier state is very rare and it exists in high-risk individuals at rates below those in endemic areas. The high-risk groups for hepatitis B can be guessed from the description of the modes of transmission of this disease and include male homosexuals, drug abusers, health-care workers, prostitutes (Goh, IntJEpid, 1986; 15:112), patients who received blood transfusions, renal dialysis patients, haemophiliacs, staff and residents of institutions for the mentally handicapped (Perrillo, AmJEpid, 1986; 123:690), prisoners, and immigrants from areas of the world where hepatitis B is common. These rates will begin to change now that HBV vaccine is available and recommended for these groups. After 1977, all blood transfusions in the United States were limited to voluntary donations, and recruitment of paid donors ceased. This led to a remarkable reduction in hepatitis B infections following transfusion. There is still a background incidence of transmission of HBV by blood transfusion because donors may have concentrations of HBsAg below the level of detection of sensitive radioimmunoassays. In the United Kingdom, annual reports show a declining incidence of acute hepatitis B. Behavioural changes because of concerns about AIDS have been influential. Drug abusers form almost one-quarter of the patients reported, and the remainder is comprised of male homosexuals, those with sexual exposure, medical- and dental-service staff, and those with a history of travel abroad or military assignment to an epidemic geographical region (Gardner, AmJEpid, 1986; 123:464). In general, hepatitis B is not common in the population of developed nations. In the United States there are an estimated 30 000 cases of acute hepatitis B yearly, for an overall incidence of 10/100 000 (Hoff, Gastro, 1973; 64:1194). Investigation of unselected acute viral hepatitis in five different areas in the United States showed that hepatitis B accounted for approximately 50 per cent of cases. Epidemiological characterization of cases suggests that most are attributable to drug abuse, heterosexual contact, transfusion, and occupational exposure. Fully 33 per cent of cases had no history of exposure or high-risk practices. These percentages have been changing over time, probably due to initiation of vaccination programmes, the growth of drug abuse as a social problem, and changes in high-risk sexual practices by

homosexual men. These proportions are, of course, also highly dependent upon the population of cases investigated; different findings would apply to urban rather than suburban or rural populations.

Population-based serological surveys were carried out in the United States before the availability of HBV vaccine. In these studies, antibody to hepatitis B was detected in 20 per cent of Americans. The prevalence of antibody rose with age (6 per cent of those younger than 20 years and 31 per cent of those older than 20 years were positive), and was higher in men than women, in the Hispanic and black rather than the white populations (Cherubin, Lancet, 1972; ii:149; Lander, JAMA, 1972; 220:1079). These findings also indicate that the typical patterns of transmission of hepatitis B do not apply for all locales of the developed world. Thus pockets of high endemic rates of hepatitis B occur in developed countries. A striking example of this is amongst first-and second-generation South-East Asian immigrants, in whom maternal–infant and childhood spread of hepatitis B still occurs.

Several epidemiological studies indicate that the reported rates of hepatitis B infection have declined in western and northern Europe, and the United States; the decline is the result of a number of factors, including safer sexual practices, behavioural changes, safe needle practices, vaccination (but not as a result of widespread adoption of immunization),[15] blood-screening refinements, and the use of viral-inactivated blood components. Treatment may have reduced the infectivity of a proportion of carriers. Universal rather than selective vaccination has been more advantageous.[16] These findings all point to a need for expanding the use of HBV vaccine.

Pathogenesis

Hepatitis B is marked by necrosis of hepatocytes and an accompanying lymphocytic infiltrate. In acute hepatitis the injury is diffuse, necrosis of individual cells is prominent, there is general cellular unrest, and inflammatory cells are found in the parenchyma and portal areas. Although serious or even fatal hepatitis may occur as a result of acute hepatitis B, the optimal outcome is eradication of infected hepatocytes, curtailment of viral replication, and rapid hepatic regeneration. This process may occur in the absence of jaundice and symptoms. However, a proportion of patients exposed to HBV do not clear HBsAg but progress to chronic hepatitis. In chronic hepatitis the cell injury and unrest are less severe, tend to be periportal, and focal and inflammatory cells are predominantly portal.

While acute and chronic infection are undoubtedly due to the viral infection, the nature and pattern of infection suggest that immunological factors are important. Indeed there is little correlation between the severity of illness and the amount or level of viral replication or viral antigen production. Peak HBV replication occurs well before peak cellular injury in acute hepatitis, suggesting that the disease represents immune lysis of infected hepatocytes. Varying levels of HBV replication may be found during chronic infection, but there is a spectrum of disease in patients, ranging from minimal hepatitis to rapidly progressive liver injury and cirrhosis. Patients with the highest concentrations of virus in liver and serum may have the mildest disease. Large amounts of HBsAg and HBcAg can also be found in liver biopsies with minimal or even no evidence of cellular necrosis (Gudat, LabInvest, 1975; 32:1).

These findings suggest that HBV is not cytopathic and that failure of clearance (establishment of chronic infection) is due to a failure of an adequate immune response. The immune response is also responsible for disease pathogenesis during chronic infection. The subsequent expression of the disease involves a poorly understood interplay between viral and host factors.

If cellular injury in hepatitis is immunologically mediated, it remains unclear what specific immune reaction is responsible for cell lysis, or what failure of the immune response leads to viral persistence. Furthermore, it is probably an oversimplification to say that host factors alone determine the outcome of HBV infection, or that the virus is totally non-cytopathic. While definitive evidence is lacking, it appears that the major determinants of cellular injury and clearance of virus are cytotoxic T-cell responses to nucleocapsid (HBcAg) viral products (Mondelli, JImmunol, 1982; 129:2773). Yet the diversity and complexity of the human immune responses make it probable that multiple host factors modulate expression of this disease while viral factors also play a part in its expression. Super-infection by other viruses, and other environmental factors, may also alter the outcome.

Acute hepatitis

In acute hepatitis B, intense lysis of hepatocytes occurs. The observed increase in serum alanine aminotransferase is the discernible manifestation of this phenomenon. Serum bilirubin increases in proportion to the severity of the hepatic damage. There is evidence that HBV replication is maximal before cell lysis occurs, and, as the clinical illness peaks, there is evidence of cessation of HBV replication. Immune lysis is believed to eradicate HBV. Antibodies to pre-S components appear early in the disease, and correlate with the disappearance of serological markers of HBV replication, suggesting a role in immunological clearance of HBV (Milich, Science, 1985; 288:1195; Cupps, JInfDis, 1990; 161:412). Both anti-pre-S1, pre-S2, and anti-HBs have neutralizing activity (Neurath, Cell, 1986; 46:429). Immune complexes may be responsible for some of the manifestations of the acute disease. A mild decrease in serum C3 and C4 occurs in acute hepatitis B, and may reflect the formation of antigen–antibody complexes. The composition and specificity of these complexes are unresolved, but they may contain HBsAg and anti-HBs, or other antigens of HBV complexed with antibody. Autoantibodies, including abnormalities in rheumatoid factor, and antinuclear and antismooth-muscle antibodies, are also detectable in acute hepatitis. In fulminant hepatitis, extremely rapid clearance of HBeAg and HBsAg may occur.

HLA-restricted immune response

The elimination of virus-infected hepatocytes is dependent on the recognition of viral determinants in association with HLA proteins on the infected cells by cytotoxic T cells. Several *in vitro* systems and models have been developed that allow analysis of HBV-specific, cytotoxic T-lymphocyte responses in patients suffering from acute and chronic HBV infections.[17] Findings in most of these systems/ models suggest that, in acute disease, a polyclonal and vigorous cytolytic T-cell response can occur. It is known that HLA class I molecules bind peptide fragments derived from intracellular cytosolic processing of viruses to present to CD8 + T cells, which act to eliminate intracellular virus. HLA class II molecules, in contrast,

generally bind viral peptides derived from extracellular antigens that are processed within antigen-presenting cells. These specialized cells present exogenous viral peptides to HLA class II-restricted, CD4 + T cells that secrete cytokines.

HLA-restricted epitopes from the core, envelope, and polymerase have been identified in acute hepatitis B; in particular, several HLA-A2-restricted, cytotoxic T-cell epitopes have been defined.[18,19] The weight of available evidence suggests that a strong, multispecific T-cell response to several or all the viral proteins accounts for the cellular injury and viral clearance in acute hepatitis B. This response can be detected in the peripheral blood of patients with chronic hepatitis B. The HBcAg epitope located between core amino acids 50 to 69 is most commonly recognized by class II-restricted lymphocytes in patients with acute hepatitis B.[20] Patients with acute, self-limiting hepatitis B also develop a polyclonal, HLA class I-restricted, cytotoxic T-cell response against numerous epitopes in the HBV envelope, nucleocapsid, and polymerase proteins.[21,22] Most of these epitopes thus far identified are HLA-A2-restricted and embody the predicted HLA-A2-binding motif with Leu in position 2 and Val at the C-terminus, for example core 18–27 (FLPSDFFPSV). Additionally, an HBV nucleocapsid epitope (141–151) has been defined from patients with acute viral hepatitis B that is restricted by both HLA-Aw68 and HLA-A31 (STLPETTVVRR). It is of interest that the nuclear localization and genome encapsidation signals of HBcAg are sited in this region.

HLA-protein display is in turn modulated by interferon proteins; interferons may also regulate the lytic processes of cytotoxic T and natural killer cells. However, most investigators have not found detectable levels of α-interferon in the serum of patients with acute hepatitis, and HBV is not an efficient inducer of interferon.

Mechanisms of chronicity: immunological function/persistence

The failure to eradicate HBV reflects an inadequate immune response to the virus, but the precise impairment of humoral and cellular immunity that determines the development and outcome of hepatitis B has not been categorized. Chronic disease is unusual in those patients with acute icteric hepatitis B, and the majority of cases of chronic hepatitis will not have been preceded by an episode of clinically apparent, icteric hepatitis, suggesting that the clearance of HBV requires a hepatitic illness. This in turn demands an appropriate limb of the cellular immune response, the action of neutralizing antibodies, and an interplay between the immune and interferon systems.

The propensity to cause chronic infection is a property of hepadnaviral infections, particularly in those mammalian or avian hosts affected early in life. There is an inverse relation between age at infection and the probability of chronic disease.

The mechanisms that lead to viral persistence are not well understood. In neonates, specific suppression of the cell-mediated immune response may favour infection, perhaps because of exposure to HBeAg inducing tolerance to epitopes that are usually the target of the cytotoxic T-cell response at a time when the immune system is ontogenically 'immature'. Clonal deletion of HBV-specific T cells may occur as as a consequence of transplacental infection of the developing fetus or transplacental passage of viral antigens. While this remains to be proven, in murine transgenic experiments, non-transgenic progeny of HBeAg-positive transgenic mothers are known to be tolerant to both HBeAg and HBcAg at the T-cell level, perhaps due to the thymic deletion of major histocompatibility complex (**MHC**) class II-restricted, HBV nucleocapsid-specific, helper T cells as a result of transplacental exposure to HBeAg.[23]

Alternatively, maternal anti-HBc, which is transported across the placenta, may modulate the lysis of infected hepatocytes by T cells (Thomas, SemLivDis, 1988; 8:342). These theories, while of interest, do not explain the mechanism of chronic infection in children who acquire the disease by horizontal transmission.

In contrast to the vigorous, polyclonal, class I- and class II-restricted T-cell response that can be identified in patients with acute icteric hepatitis B, in chronic disease the HLA class II-restricted response in peripheral blood is relatively weak and focused (oligoclonal), and insufficient to clear replicating virus. This may be the result of an incapacity of the host to mount an antiviral immune response that is sufficiently rapid and efficient to limit the spread of infection. The specific epitopes recognized by B as well as T cells are currently being mapped.

Mutations abrogating recognition of wild-type hepatitis B in patients infected by variants have been recognized. Natural variants of the HBcAg 18–27 core epitope that interfere with recognition of the wild-type epitope and act as T-cell-receptor antagonists have recently been identified in two patients with chronic hepatitis.[24] This antagonism could in theory lead to an active inhibition of epitope recognition at T-cell-receptor contact sites.

The mechanism of the immunological defect in otherwise healthy adult carriers is imprecisely understood. A B-lymphocyte defect may explain impaired synthesis of anti-HBs after induction by non-specific mitogens; *in vitro* synthesis of anti-HBc and immunoglobulin remain normal in chronic carriers (Dusheiko, JCI, 1983; 71:1104). The high concentrations of HBsAg in the serum may lead to a state of tolerance.

Antibody to HBcAg (anti-HBc) may blunt the expression of nucleocapsid antigens on the surface of hepatocytes (Mondelli, JImmunol, 1982; 129:2773). Alternatively, selective killing of antigen-specific B cells delivering HBsAg envelope proteins to class I-restricted, cytotoxic T cells may suppress the antibody response. The immune response may also be blunted by HBV infection in lymphocytes or macrophages (Pontisso, BMJ, 1984; 288:1563).

Interferon production

In chronic HBV infection there is some evidence of a failure of interferon production and activation in the infected liver cells so that synthesis of viral protein is not decreased and there is poor enhancement of HLA-protein display. The production of α-interferon by peripheral blood leucocytes is generally suboptimal in chronic carriers, although there is considerable variation in individual carriers. Production of γ-interferon remains normal. The degree of interferon deficiency does not correlate with the severity of the illness, however (Zachoval, JHepatol, 1989; 6:364).

HBV may have the capacity to down-regulate immunoregulatory molecules (Twu, PNAS, 1988; 85:252). Experimental HBV transfection and integration appear to affect the ability of the cell to respond to interferon. Recent studies suggest that HBcAg can suppress transcription of the β-interferon gene,[25] and that the

HBV polymerase protein can inhibit the cellular response to interferons α and γ.[26] Such a mechanism might result in failure of presentation of HLA antigens on the cell surface, and hence poor presentation of viral peptides to the immune system, reducing recognition of viral antigens.

The mechanism of resistance may reflect nucleotide homology between HBV DNA and sequences regulating the interferon-induced antiviral system, or involve transcription or translation products of HBV (Onji, Hepatol, 1989; 9:92). Arguing against a defect in interferon synthesis or production is the fact that the expression of β_2-microglobulin on hepatocyte membranes, reflecting the display of HLA antigen, has indeed been observed in patients with acute hepatitis, chronic active hepatitis, and cirrhosis, and in those treated with interferon (Nagafuchi, Hepatol, 1986; 6:20). Moreover, there is only partial support for the hypothesis that there is an inherent deficiency in the interferon system in acute or chronic hepatitis B: serial concentrations of 2′,5′-oligoadenylate synthetase did not identify in those patients who progressed from acute to chronic hepatitis, and patients with chronic hepatitis B infection, regardless of the histological appearances of their liver, had normal basal concentrations of lymphocyte 2′,5′-oligoadenylate synthetase (Heathcote, Hepatol, 1989; 9:102). Also, recombinant γ-interferon given to patients with chronic hepatitis B causes an increase in β_2-microglobulin and 2′,5′-oligoadenylate synthetase (Quiroga, JInterferonRes, 1988; 8:755). The immunological role of HBV DNA in bone marrow cells and peripheral blood lymphocytes and leucocytes is unknown (Shen, JMedVirol, 1986; 18:201).

Chronic infection is also more common in immunosuppressed individuals, particularly patients on renal dialysis, kidney transplant patients, children with Down's syndrome, leprosy or leukaemia, and homosexuals with HIV infection. A heterogeneous group of immunoregulatory defects may exist in these groups.

Immunopathogenesis

HBV does not seem to be ordinarily cytopathic to hepatocytes. It would seem that the immune response to HBV-encoded antigens is responsible both for viral clearance and disease pathogenesis when viral eradication fails to occur during chronic infection. This has been difficult to study, however, as 'classical' experimental systems are not available because HBV is not infectious for human cells *in vitro*.

While the frequency of occurrence of HBV-specific, cytotoxic T-lymphocyte precursors is greatly diminished in the peripheral blood of chronically infected patients, such cells are none the less present at very low concentrations in the periphery and in the infected liver.[27] This could explain both the continuing, indolent liver injury and exacerbations of the disease.

Recent experiments indicate that, although many patients will not ordinarily have a discernible cytotoxic T-cell response, a proportion do mount a 'secondary' immune response, associated with seroconversion to anti-HBe and at least a temporary remission in disease. A proliferative T-cell response, measured by analysis of [³H]thymidine uptake in response to a panel of recombinant HBV antigens, is evident in active disease. In addition, an HLA-restricted, cytotoxic T-cell response can be detected around the time of anti-HBe seroconversion during spontaneous or interferon-induced HBeAg clearance, or when there has been an exacerbation of the disease associated with an increase in HBV DNA.[19,28–31] This associated immune response may have implications for the timing of treatment with α-interferon. An understanding of the nature of the immune response in active disease that leads to loss of active HBV replication may produce more specific immunotherapy, for example using the core peptide 18–27 in HLA-A2-positive individuals.

Cytokines are also released in acute and chronic hepatitis.[32] Necrosis of hepatocytes may also be amplified by antigen-non-specific release of cytokines rather than by a direct cytotoxic T-cell response.[33] In transgenic mice, non-cytolytic mechanisms, including the suppression of viral gene expression and replication by a post-transcriptional mechanism mediated by γ-interferon, tumour necrosis factor-α, and interleukin 2, have been observed.[34–38] In these experiments the direct cytopathic effect of cytotoxic T cells is limited to an attack on relatively few hepatocytes; the findings in these transgenic mice suggest that most destruction of hepatocytes is in fact caused by inflammatory cells recruited or activated by the cytotoxic T cells.

T-cell subsets

Regulatory T-helper (**Th**) cells have been categorized into two different major functional subsets, Th1 and Th2, which produce distinct lymphokines. In general, Th1 cells mediate cellular immune responses and Th2 cells mediate humoral immunity. Circulating HBeAg may down-regulate antiviral clearance mechanisms by virtue of eliciting the production of anti-inflammatory, Th-2-like cytokines.[39] Experiments in mice have suggested that a predominance of HBeAg-specific, Th2-type cells may contribute to chronicity in HBV infection.

Because HBeAg may act as a tolerogen during the vertical transmission of chronic HBV infection, a predominance of HBeAg-specific Th2 cells expressing a limited repertoire may influence the initiation or maintenance of the HBV chronic carrier state.[40] The two structural forms of the viral nucleoprotein, the particulate HBcAg and the non-particulate HBeAg, may preferentially elicit different Th-cell subsets. HBcAg-primed Th cells efficiently produce interleukin 2 and γ-interferon, and low concentrations of interleukin 4. Conversely, efficient production of interleukin 4 and lesser amounts of γ-interferon are elicited by HBeAg immunization.

Molecular status of hepatitis B

The natural history of chronic hepatitis is related to varying degrees of immune responsiveness and is inherently variable. A change in the molecular status of the HBV also occurs during the disease, which in part probably reflects a process of both immune selection and molecular variation. Typically, many patients with chronic hepatitis show a gradual or rapid transition from predominantly 'replicative' to predominantly 'non-replicative' infection. In general, predominantly episomal HBV DNA is detectable in hepatocytes in carriers with high levels of viral replication, who are HBeAg-positive, whereas integrated HBV DNA genomes are detectable in those with less active viral replication and long-standing disease, who are anti-HBe-positive. Integrated sequences have been detected in acute HBV infection, but detectable integration may increase

with the duration of infection (Shafritz, NEJM, 1981; 305:1067). Continued production of HBsAg in the absence of high levels of replication may be related to integration of the cohesive end-region of the viral genome, which disrupts the transcription and packaging of nucleocapsid proteins but allows continued transcription of envelope proteins (Brechot, Lancet, 1981; ii: 765).

The immune injury may be modified according to whether the HBV DNA is episomal and active replication within the cells is occurring, the complete virion is packaged, and nucleocapsid antigens presented at the cell membrane, or whether envelope proteins alone are transcribed. In most patients there is a requirement for active viral replication in the pathogenesis of liver injury, and histological improvement follows interferon-induced or spontaneous reductions in viral replication and seroconversion to anti-HBe. Cells that do not express nucleocapsid antigens may be protected from the host immune response.

Most evidence suggests that the nucleocapsid antigens (HBcAg and HBeAg) expressed on the cell membrane are the important target of the immune response and cytolytic T cells. These antigens are products of a single gene region on the virion genome (Stahl, PNAS, 1982; 79:1606). The *C* gene has two initiation codons and therefore two gene regions (precore and core) and two potential molecular forms (HBcAg and HBeAg) can be produced. HBcAg is a 27-nm, particulate, nucleocapsid protein. HBcAg is not detected free in serum, but is an intracellular virion-associated nucleocapsid antigen that is the product of the *C* gene alone. HBeAg has substantial amino-acid homology with HBcAg, and the proteins are cross-reactive at the T-cell level.

The antigenic epitopes of HBcAg and HBeAg have been mapped in inbred mice (Milich, JImmunol, 1987; 139:1223). Studies using recombinant HBcAg and HBeAg have shown that HBcAg is significantly more immunogenic than the particulate or non-particulate forms of HBeAg. This disparity may be explained by the fact that HBcAg can function as a T-cell-independent antigen, whereas HBeAg is a T-cell-dependent antigen (Milich, JImmunol, 1988; 141:3617). HBcAg is able to induce an antibody response in athymic mice, which lack mature T lymphocytes.

HBeAg and HBcAg appear cross-reactive at the T-cell but not at the B-cell level, different peptides leading to anti-HBc and anti-HBe responses. T but not B cells are made tolerant by HBeAg in neonatal mice, and T-cell tolerance elicited by HBeAg also extends to HBcAg-specific T cells (Milich, JImmunol, 1989; 143:3148). The combination of T-cell tolerance to the nucleocapsid antigens in the presence of a B-cell response to HBcAg (anti-HBc) may mimic the outcome in new-borns of chronic carrier mothers. It has been suggested that a peptide fragment of HBeAg or intact HBeAg cross the placenta and induce T-cell tolerance to HBeAg and HBcAg in the new-born (Milich, PNAS, 1990; 87:6599). The tolerance may be overcome in later life, explaining the clearance of HBeAg in some patients.

HBcAg can be demonstrated in both the nucleus and the membrane of the hepatocyte. Membranous or cytoplasmic rather than nuclear expression of HBcAg may correlate with disease activity. Membrane-bound HBeAg has now been detected, and the relative presentation of HBeAg as opposed to HBcAg may modulate immune injury. However, anti-HBc binding can also be detected in patients with minimal or no histological damage. Since circulating anti-HBc is usually universal in acute and chronic HBV infection, the modulation of hepatocytic cytolysis by anti-HBc and anti-HBe may depend upon the relative presentation of HBeAg and HBcAg.

Natural killer cells may be involved, but differences in natural killer function cannot account for the difference in pathology between various categories of chronic HBV infection. The cytotoxicity of peripheral blood lymphocytes is confined primarily to purified, T-cell-enriched fractions.

Investigators seem to agree that CD8+ T lymphocytes predominate in portal and lobular inflammatory infiltrates in the liver in patients with acute and chronic hepatitis B. CD4+ cells predominate in areas of single-cell necrosis and focal inflammation in the hepatic parenchyma (Thomas, Liver, 1982; 2:266). Irrespective of histological classification, HBeAg-positive patients contain predominantly CD8+ cells, whereas in anti-HBe-positive patients, CD4+ helper T cells and B cells are more common in the portal areas. This pattern of mononuclear cell infiltrates in the liver in patients with chronic HBV infection suggests that T-cell-mediated cytotoxicity to HBV-infected hepatocytes is diminished in accordance with the decrease of active HBV replication shown by seroconversion from HBeAg to anti-HBe (Yamada, GastrJap, 1985; 70:441).

Genetic restriction

Viral-antigen (peptide) presentation, physically associated with MHC class I antigens, is a requisite for cytotoxicity by effector T cells. In patients with a high level of HBV replication, nuclear HBcAg has been detected with relatively faint HLA expression. In contrast, in patients with limited virus replication (anti-HBe-positive), nuclear HBcAg is absent and membrane expression of HLA-A, -B, and -C is intense. The finding of increased expression of HLA class I and II in association with cytoplasmic HBcAg and active chronic hepatitis B adds credence to the possibility that nucleocapsid antigens of HBV may be the focus of immunologically mediated injury (Pignatelli, Hepatol, 1986; 6:349).

In males there is an increased likelihood of remaining chronically infected. Renal transplant recipients who are anti-HBs-positive are more likely than anti-HBs-negative recipients to reject a kidney from a male than a female donor. This suggests that the immune response to HBV antigens is influenced by male and female genes. Non-responders to hepatitis vaccine have an increased frequency of HLA-D7 and lack HLA-D1, or possibly a higher frequency of an HLA-linked, immune-suppression gene for HBsAg, in linkage disequilibrium with *HLA-Bw54-DR4-Drw53* haplotype (Wanatababe, HumImmunol, 1988; 22:9).

In vivo antibody production to HBsAg in the mouse is regulated by at least two immune-response genes mapping to different loci. The HBsAg-specific, T-cell proliferative response of congenic mouse strains parallels the *in vivo* production of anti-HBs and may also be genetically restricted (Milich, JImmunol, 1985; 134:4194). The pre-S2 region is significantly more immunogenic than the S region at the T-cell level, and pre-S2 region-specific T-cell activation is regulated by immune-response genes and correlates with genetic restriction of antibody production *in vivo* to the pre-S2 region (Milich, PNAS, 1985; 82:8168). S-region unresponsiveness may be circumvented by immunization with pre-S1- or pre-S2-containing HBsAg particles.

An association of MHC class II alleles (DRB *1302) with lack of persistent HBV infection has been reported from the Gambia.[41] These observed differences may relate to allele-specific peptide binding.

Recently, the correlation between patterns of liver reaction and molecules mediating binding between cells and adhesion molecules involved in the recruitment of lymphocytes has been studied. Intracellular adhesion molecule 1 and lymphocyte-function associated antigen 1, which are not normally found in liver cells, can be up-regulated in acute hepatitis, and in some patients with chronic active hepatitis (Volpes, Hepatol, 1990; 12:59). These molecules may facilitate the accumulation of lymphocytes into inflammatory regions. The reactions, which are enhanced by α-interferon, may be an important facet of a coordinated immune and inflammatory response.

Superinfection

When there is delta virus superinfection in a carrier of chronic HBV, there is an acceleration of the rate of progression of the liver disease (Rizzetto, Hepatol, 1983; 3:729). Superinfection by hepatitis A virus, HIV, and possibly HCV may also affect HBV replication.

Drug treatment and pathogenesis

Hepatic failure may develop after stopping cytotoxic therapy, and drugs that modify the immune response, such as levamisole or corticosteroids, may in fact affect HBV expression. During high-dose prednisolone therapy there is a decrease in immunoglobulin synthesis by peripheral blood mononuclear cells and in lymphocyte proliferation to all mitogens. Following the withdrawal of prednisolone in chronic HBV carriers, lymphocyte function rapidly returns to baseline, and in some carriers is associated with a subsequent rebound increase in serum aminotransferases. This is accompanied by a striking increase in suppressor T-lymphocyte activity without significant changes in either helper T-cell or B-cell function. The close correlation between changes in helper and suppressor T-lymphocyte function and serum aminotransferase activities during and after immunosuppressive therapy suggests that immunoregulatory T lymphocytes may be important in the pathogenesis of chronic type B hepatitis (Hanson, Hepatol, 1986; 6:173).

Experimental systems and conclusion

Overproduction of the HBV large envelope polypeptide in transgenic mice results in chronic liver-cell injury, regenerative hyperplasia, and a secondary inflammatory response. Hepatocellular carcinoma may develop in these mice, and it is suggested that injury-induced regenerations may induce random mutations and result in cellular transformation (Chisari, Cell, 1989; 59:1145).

In conclusion, the complexity of the immune response and cytopathogenicity of hepatitis B infection has defied an easy explanation for the disease spectrum. A large repertoire of factors acting in concert is clearly operative. Improvements in the techniques of molecular mapping, cell culture, and immunopathology should enhance our understanding of this complex disease.

HBV variants

In chronic hepatitis B, defective viral particles are produced in excess, and recent data have suggested that spontaneous mutations in the genome are not uncommon, and might explain the variation in disease expression in some patients. Envelope, precore, and core variants, and more recently a polymerase variant, have been described.

Envelope variants

The finding of HBV DNA in persons negative for all serological markers of HBV has suggested that there are genetic variants of HBV accounting for some cases of non-A, non-B hepatitis. A particularly high prevalence of HBV DNA is found in HBsAg-negative alcoholic patients with hepatocellular carcinoma (Brechot, NEJM, 1982; 306:1384; 1985; 312:270). In addition, HBsAg determinants have been identified in HBsAg-negative sera with monoclonal anti-HBs. Amplification with the polymerase chain reaction will identify HBV DNA in some patients negative for all HBV serological markers. Inoculation of HBsAg-negative but infectious human sera into chimpanzees has been shown to induce acute hepatitis; the subsequent cloning of the chimpanzee isolates after amplification by polymerase chain reaction, and comparison of the nucleotide sequences with that of known HBV subtypes, revealed point mutations in the 3' end of the S gene (Thiers, Lancet, 1988; ii:1273). It is possible that spontaneous mutations of the virus to a form that does not produce immunologically dominant antigens is another mechanism of its persistence.

Unusual serological patterns have been found in Senegalese children, whose serum showed transient reactivity for HBsAg but lacked anti-HBc, anti-HBe, and anti-HBs on follow-up (Coursaget, Lancet, 1987; ii:1354). Pre-S2 reactivity was sometimes found, and virus particles similar to HBV were detected. It was suggested that this was a new HBV-related virus, HBV-2; however, it is possible that these individuals have an aberrant immune response and do not produce anti-HBc.

Envelope antigenic variants may be selected if advantaged over wild type under pressure of immune selection: these have been observed after hepatitis B immunoglobulin and hepatitis B vaccination, and after use of hepatitis B monoclonal and polyclonal immunoglobulin for prophylaxis in liver transplant recipients.[42–44]

Precore region

A number of naturally occurring precore mutations preventing HBeAg synthesis have been identified in HBeAg-negative carriers. These genetic mutants of HBV are found in serum of anti-HBe- and HBV DNA-positive patients who have HBcAg in hepatocytes and histological evidence of chronic active hepatitis but who lack HBeAg in serum (Hadziyannis, Hepatol, 1983; 3:729).

As discussed above, the C gene has two initiation codons and therefore two regions (precore and core); two potential molecular forms (HBcAg and HBeAg) can be produced. Initiation of translation at the first site (nucleotide 1814) produces a 312 amino-acid polypeptide (p25), which has a signal peptide directing it to the endoplasmic reticulum where the signal piece is removed by signal peptidase to cleave the N-terminal 19 aa residues as well as the C-terminal 34 residues. The resultant polypeptide of 150 amino acids is secreted as HBeAg (p15–18), a soluble protein that is the product of 10 residues coded by the precore region and 149 residues coded by the C gene (Ou, PNAS, 1986; 83:1578). Translation from the second initiation codon (nucleotide 1901) results in unprocessed polypeptides (p23, 183 amino acids), which are assembled into core particles within the liver (p21). Amplification by polymerase chain reaction and subsequent sequencing of DNA from virions in serum of patients lacking HBeAg has revealed one or more nucleotide substitutions in the precore region of the HBV genome.

An HBV variant with a G–A mutation at nucleotide 83 in the precore region (mutant HBV) accounts for most cases of HBeAg-defective hepatitis B. A point mutation from G to A creating an in-frame TAG stop codon with or without additional point mutations in succeeding codons (Carman, Lancet, 1989; ii:588; Brunetto, JHepatol, 1990; 10:258) has been described. This mutation induces a Trp at codon 28, and explains the serological absence of HBeAg. It is still not clear how this mutant is associated with HBeAg seroconversion. During disease, HBeAg-defective virus may be selected for by immune pressure. This substitution prevents the production and secretion of HBeAg. It is not clear whether these represent *de novo* infections with a mutant-type virus, or, perhaps more likely, whether these mutations have arisen during infection as a result of pressure of immune selection. Hepatocytes not expressing HBeAg might escape immune elimination: it has been suggested that hepatocytes infected with wild-type HBV produce HBeAg molecules that would be exposed on their surfaces and become the target of the host immune attack, whereas hepatocytes infected with precore defective mutants would not be able to produce HBeAg. Immune selection may thus assist pre-C-defective mutants with an HBeAg-negative phenotype to exceed HBeAg-positive phenotypes. The mechanism of active hepatitis in these patients is not clear: these variants may be cytotoxic, or the immunopathogenicity of the host response may be affected. It has been proposed that cytotoxic T cells primed with anti-HBc/anti-HBe might selectively attack hepatocytes harbouring defective mutants because of the lack of blocking HBeAg. Pre-C-region defects are also found in patients with fulminant hepatitis; these variants may have altered virulence.[45] However, both wild-type and precore mutant strains can be found in patients with fulminant hepatitis B, and other mutations affecting the level of viral replication or antigen expression, or indeed host factors, may be critical.[46–48]

There is an influence of HBV genotype on the prevalence of precore mutations. For example, two precore variants of HBV occur in chronic carriers in Hong Kong Chinese. One variant has a Ser at amino acid 15 while the other has a stop codon at amino acid 28, which inhibits the production of HBeAg. The Ser15 strain produces antigenically normal amounts of HBeAg. These variants are mutually exclusive, probably due to sequence requirements for encapsidation;[49] this exclusivity is probably due to the special role of the 3' part of the bulge as a template for the first nucleotide of the minus-strand DNA in HBV reverse transcription.[50] Thus this mutation is relatively uncommon in HBsAg carriers of North American and west European origin who are infected with genotype A of HBV and who carry a cytosine at position 1858 [rather than a thymine (uracil) at position 1858]. Uracil at position 1858 may form a base pair with either G or A in nucleotide 1896 but cytosine strains do not tolerate a G–A mutation in nucleotide 1896 as this reduces the efficiency of encapsidation and replication.

Mutations in core regions

The core region of hepatitis B can accumulate escape mutations.[51] These tend to be most prevalent in active disease: multiple analyses have shown that the frequency of core gene mutations is significantly associated with mutations of precore stop codons, HBeAg negativity, and active liver disease, but not with patients' age.[52]

Mutations that affect the level of replication of HBV, such as those in the core promoter, perhaps associated with precore mutations, could account for some cases of fulminant hepatitis B.[53] In other cases, mutations have not been observed, or these have been insufficient to explain fulminant disease.[54]

Polymerase-region mutations

Recently, mutations in the polymerase region of the HBV have been observed. These have occurred in immunosuppressed but also in non-immunosuppressed patients treated with the nucleoside analogue, lamivudine. In some cases, patients have been studied before and after liver transplantation. The polymerase domain of the polymerase open reading frame has been sequenced and a Met–Val substitution in the YMDD motif as well as other mutations in the polymerase have been observed. Met–Ile mutations have also been found in the YMDD motif.[55]

Acute hepatitis B
Typical clinical course

Acute hepatitis B resembles other forms of acute hepatitis clinically and cannot be distinguished by history, physical examination, or routine serum biochemical tests [Norkrans, ScaJInfectDis, 1978; 17 (Suppl.):1]. The course is divided into the incubation period, preicteric, icteric, and convalescence phases. From the incubation period to the onset of symptoms or jaundice averages 75 days (range 40–140 days).

The onset of hepatitis B is typically insidious, with non-specific symptoms of malaise, poor appetite, nausea, and pain in the right upper quadrant. This preicteric phase usually lasts 3 to 7 days. A serum sickness-like syndrome appearing during the preicteric phase is more common in hepatitis B than in other forms of viral hepatitis, being particularly common in women. This syndrome consists of fever, arthralgias (or frank arthritis), and skin rash (typically urticaria or a fleeting, erythematous, maculopapular rash) (Alpert, NEJM, 1981; 285:185). These symptoms usually resolve quickly with the onset of icterus or dark urine.

With onset of the icteric phase, symptoms of fatigue and anorexia typically worsen. Jaundice can last from a few days to several months, the average being 2 to 3 weeks. Itching and pale stools may occur. Weight loss of 2 to 10 kg is typical.

The convalescent phase of hepatitis B begins with the resolution of jaundice. A return of good appetite is frequently the first sign of convalescence. Fatigue is generally the last symptom to abate and may persist for many months into convalescence.

The physical signs of typical acute hepatitis B are not prominent. Patients usually look well nourished and otherwise healthy. Fever occurs in the preicteric phase, but is usually intermittent and low grade; it rarely lasts into the icteric period. Variable degrees of jaundice are present. The only other common physical finding in

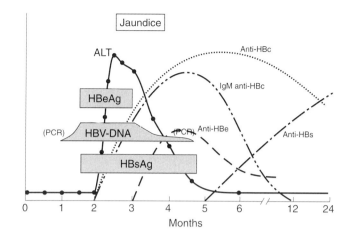

Fig. 2. Serological course of acute hepatitis B. ALT, alanine aminotransferase; PCR, polymerase chain reaction.

acute hepatitis B is a mild and slightly tender hepatomegaly. Mild enlargement of spleen or lymph nodes occurs uncommonly. Wasting, ascites, oedema, palmar erythema, and prominent spider angiomas should suggest the presence of chronic liver disease.

While symptoms and physical signs of acute hepatitis are non-specific and are rarely helpful in diagnosis, the results of routine blood tests are rather accurate in indicating a diagnosis. As in other forms of acute hepatitis, the serum alanine and aspartate aminotransferases are usually markedly elevated and to the same extent (10- to 50-fold). The serum alkaline phosphatase and lactic dehydrogenase are usually only mildly elevated (less than threefold). The bilirubin is variably increased, in both the direct and indirect fractions. Serum albumin rarely falls except with protracted severe disease. The prothrombin time can increase and is the most reliable marker of severity of injury. Blood counts usually do not change unless the disease is prolonged or fulminant. The sedimentation rate is usually normal, and serum immunoglobulins show only a mild increase in the IgG fraction. Various autoantibodies can appear during the course of acute hepatitis B, most typically to smooth muscle.

The results of serological testing provide the means for diagnosis of hepatitis B. The course of a 'typical' case of acute hepatitis B is shown in Fig. 2. The first serological marker to be detectable in the serum is HBsAg, which appears during the incubation period and rapidly rises in titre. By the onset of symptoms, concentrations of HBsAg generally range between 1 and 50 μg/ml (Froesner, EurJClinMicrob, 1982; 1:52). With progression of the illness the titres of HBsAg begin to fall, but in most patients HBsAg persists in the serum throughout the icteric phase and into convalescence. This makes HBsAg a convenient marker for the diagnosis of acute hepatitis B. However, there are several problems with this approach. First, in about 10 per cent of patients, HBsAg is cleared early and may no longer be detectable when the patient is first seen by the physician (see ref. 2, pp. 219–43). Second, patients with chronic hepatitis B also have HBsAg in serum and an acute exacerbation of disease or a superimposed acute hepatitis (such as hepatitis A, C, or D) in an HBsAg carrier can be mistakenly interpreted as acute hepatitis B. For these reasons, other serological markers such as IgM anti-HBc are often used to document acute hepatitis B (Lindsay, Hepatol, 1986; 6:1325).

Concurrent with, or shortly after, the appearance of HBsAg in serum, HBeAg and HBV DNA are detectable and rapidly increase in concentration (Aikawa, NEJM, 1978; 298:439; Krogsgaard, Hepatol, 1985; 5:10). HBV DNA usually reaches 10^5 to 10^8 genome equivalents/ml by the onset of symptoms, after which the concentrations of virus decrease, becoming undetectable within a few days to a few weeks after the onset of symptoms. Indeed, disappearance of these serological markers indicates resolution of viral replication and thus predicts the ultimate resolution of the hepatitis. In patients who develop chronic hepatitis B, in contrast, HBV DNA and HBeAg remain high during the acute phases of illness and/or infection, suggesting that it is the early attainment of high levels of viral replication that leads to chronicity of infection.

HBcAg is not found in the serum but is detectable in the liver in some patients with acute hepatitis B (Mathiesen, Gastro, 1979; 77:623). This marker of viral replication, like serum HBV DNA and HBeAg, is usually cleared early in the infection. These features of the serological course of acute hepatitis B suggest that HBV replication occurs early and that the onset of disease represents the onset of immune clearance of the virus. At the peak of disease severity the direct markers of viral replication, such as HBcAg in liver and HBeAg and HBV DNA in serum, are often no longer detectable. Furthermore, even though still present in the serum, HBsAg is not detectable in hepatocytes (by immunostaining) late in the course of the disease. These features suggest that the persistence of HBsAg in serum into convalescence is not due to continued production but rather to a delay in the clearance of this antigen from the circulation. The first antibody to arise during the course of typical acute hepatitis B is to HBcAg (anti-HBc). This antibody appears in all patients with acute or chronic hepatitis B, arising shortly before, or concurrent with, the onset of symptoms. Initially, most of the anti-HBc is IgM. The IgM anti-HBc generally persists for only a few months after acute disease, making detection of IgM anti-HBc a valuable marker for the diagnosis of acute hepatitis B. IgG anti-HBc generally persists for life; highest titres occur in patients with persistent infection.

Antibody to HBsAg (anti-HBs) usually appears during convalescence, after clearance of HBsAg. It is not clear whether anti-HBs is not produced until convalescence or whether the anti-HBs that is produced earlier is absorbed or complexed out by the large amounts of HBsAg in serum, making it undetectable. In general, anti-HBs is considered a marker of recovery and immunity to hepatitis B. Patients who receive HBV vaccine will have anti-HBs and are protected against infection. Antibody to HBeAg commonly appears with clearance of HBeAg from the serum (Aikawa, NEJM, 1978; 298:439). However, titres of this antibody are generally low in acute hepatitis B and this is not a particularly long-lived antibody.

Other serological markers that have been applied to the study of hepatitis B include DNA polymerase activity[56] and antibody to DNA polymerase, hepatitis B X antigen (**HBxAg**) and antibody (Feitelson, Gastro, 1990; 98:1071), pre-S1 and pre-S2 antigen, and antipre-S1 and antipre-S2 (Kurai, Hepatol, 1989; 9:175). DNA polymerase activity is detected in some sera that have HBV DNA, its measurement being less sensitive and less quantitative of virus in serum than that of HBV DNA. HBxAg is not reliably detected in serum; small amounts are found in some specimens of liver tissue, particularly in chronic HBV infection (Feitelson, Gastro, 1990; 98:1071). Anti-HBx also is not a very reliable serological marker for HBV infection, being present in the minority of patients with acute and chronic disease. Furthermore, the clinical significance of the detection of anti-HBx remains unclear.

The presence and pattern of pre-S antigens and antibodies during acute and chronic hepatitis B have been studied extensively (Kurai, Hepatol, 1989; 9:175), but unfortunately the results have been conflicting. In general, the pre-S antigens can be detected in any serum or liver that has HBsAg; indeed, the genomic structure of HBV indicates that pre-S antigens cannot be present without concurrently detectable HBsAg (there are no stop codons between the pre-S and S regions). However, the highest titres of pre-S antigens are generally detected in patients with HBeAg and high levels of viral replication (HBV DNA in serum), suggesting that these antigens also reflect active viral replication. Some investigators have pointed out that high titres of HBsAg are also found in these same states. Antipre-S has been detected in variable proportions of patients with acute and chronic hepatitis B. Reports that the appearance of anti-pre-S during the course of acute hepatitis B was a favourable prognostic sign have not been confirmed. Detection of pre-S antigens and antibodies adds little clinical information and these remain research-based serological markers of uncertain significance.

Tests for HBV DNA in serum are the most direct markers for assessing viral replication. The usual method for measuring viral genome uses ^{32}P-labelled, cloned HBV DNA for hybridization with immobilized DNA extracted from serum, referred to as dot (or slot) blot hybridization (Krogsgaard, Hepatol, 1985; 5:10). Liquid hybridization techniques using ^{125}I-labelled HBV DNA for the detection of viral DNA in serum and liver have also been developed and are now commercially available. Signal-amplification methods are also available. All these hybridization techniques are capable of detecting as little as 0.1 pg per sample (approximately 1–10 pg/ml or 10^6 genome equivalents/ml). Thus, while very sensitive, hybridization techniques detect HBV DNA only when it is present in rather high concentrations.

The polymerase chain technique for the detection of DNA has been adapted to the detection of HBV DNA in serum and liver (Kaneko, Gastro, 1990; 99:799). This technique is capable of detecting as few as 100 viral genomes per sample and is thus at least 10 000-fold more sensitive than direct hybridization. During acute hepatitis B, less than 50 per cent of patients will have HBV DNA detectable by hybridization by the onset of clinical illness. However, when the polymerase chain reaction is applied to serum samples, HBV DNA is detected in the majority of patients and often persists for as long as HBsAg is present in serum. Thus, the highest concentrations of HBV are present during the preicteric and early icteric phases of infection, but the kinetics of clearance of the virus is such that low concentrations of HBV DNA at least persist for as long as HBsAg is present.

In a number of patients with acute hepatitis B the serological course may be atypical; these patients clear HBsAg rapidly and are negative for this viral marker when first seen by the physician. The diagnosis of acute hepatitis B can be made in these circumstances by detection of IgM anti-HBc, which is present in high titres (Lindsay, Hepatol, 1986; 6:1325).

Complicated clinical course
Subacute hepatic necrosis

In a small proportion of patients with acute hepatitis B the disease may worsen over 1 to 3 months, with increasing jaundice, deteriorating coagulation, ascites, bleeding, and encephalopathy. The serum aminotransaminases may paradoxically improve as the disease worsens. Submassive hepatic necrosis, as the disease is also known, is more common in patients older than 40 years. Histopathological examination may reveal bridging or massive hepatic necrosis. The prognosis is poor.

Cholestatic hepatitis

This is more frequent in type A than type B hepatitis. Clinical cholestasis occurring late in the icteric phase may be seen. The disease is characterized by a prolonged course, pruritus, prolongation of the prothrombin time, and a markedly elevated serum alkaline phosphatase. The outcome is good, although the illness may be protracted and associated with weight loss.

Relapses

Clinical relapses occur in 1 to 3 per cent of patients. These are often attributed to a return to full activity or to alcohol, but the evidence for this is lacking. Acute hepatitis B and D infection may be associated with relapse, sometimes leading to fulminant hepatitis (Govindarajan, Gut, 1986; 27:19).

Posthepatitis syndrome

A percentage of patients who recover from acute hepatitis B are left with chronic symptoms of fatigue, anorexia, nausea, and pain in the right upper quadrant. Liver tests reveal little evidence of liver injury or inflammation. Symptoms can be relieved by reassurance.

Hepatitis during pregnancy

The excessive mortality of viral hepatitis in pregnant women is probably largely related to hepatitis E in developing countries. Hepatitis B in the third trimester of pregnancy may be associated with transmission of hepatitis to the infant, and precautions to immunize the new-born infant should be taken.

Fulminant hepatitis

Fulminant hepatitis B is also an atypical course for this infection, occurring in less than 1 per cent of icteric cases (see Section 19). Fulminant hepatitis refers to a clinical condition with rapid onset and development of acute hepatic failure, with encephalopathy, coma, and death in more than 70 per cent of cases. Data collected by the Acute Hepatic Failure Study Group in the United States showed that of 188 patients with fulminant hepatitis presenting between 1972 and 1979, hepatitis B alone accounted for 56 per cent of cases. The survival rate in those with hepatitis B was greater than for non-A, non-B hepatitis. Hepatitis D coinfection may predispose to fulminant hepatitis. The prevalence is approximately 2/1000 icteric cases. The mortality varies with the age of the patient. The onset of symptoms may also be insidious (Bernuau, SemLivDis, 1986; 6:97). Morphologically the liver shows massive multilobular or bridging necrosis. The development of hepatic encephalopathy is the clinical criterion used for diagnosis of fulminant hepatitis. Encephalopathy may be first manifested by a subtle change in personality, abusive or violent behaviour, confusion, or extreme lassitude. With progressive disease, stuporousness and then coma develop. Physical findings include confusion, asterixis, and stuporousness. Jaundice deepens progressively. With protracted disease, ascites may appear. Serum aminotransferases, while high at the onset of disease, may fall as the patient deteriorates. Serum bilirubin rises and albumin falls progressively. Most ominous, however, is a progressive rise in the prothrombin time reflecting decreases in coagulation factors synthesized by the liver, particularly factors V and VII. Typically, in fulminant disease, HBV DNA and HBeAg become undetectable as hepatic failure supervenes. HBsAg titres also begin to decrease and patients can become HBsAg-negative despite fatal outcome. However, in analyses of large numbers of cases of fulminant hepatitis B, the early clearance of HBsAg has been shown to be a favourable prognostic feature. The pattern of serological markers during the course of fulminant hepatitis B suggests that this outcome is due to a sudden and extreme immunological response to HBV infection (Bernuau, SemLivDis, 1986; 6:97). The features that lead to a fulminant course are not known but may relate to host factors (age, sex, immunological status) as well as viral factors (dose and strain).

Chronic hepatitis

Some patients with acute hepatitis B do not recover normally and may progress to chronic hepatitis. The persistence of abnormal alanine aminotransferase activity for more than 6 months after the onset of acute hepatitis B is indicative of disease progression, and is usually accompanied by serological evidence of continued infection.

Extrahepatic complications

Neuromuscular

Apathy, irritability, difficulty in concentrating, headache, photophobia, and neck rigidity can occur in acute hepatitis. Guillain–Barré syndrome has been observed (Walle, Hepatogast, 1981; 28: 305; Perseghin, ItalJNeurolSci, 1985; 6:447). The clinical course is typical of the classic syndrome. In patients with type B hepatitis, HBsAg may be detectable in cerebrospinal fluid. The prognosis appears to be good. Peripheral neuropathy and cranial nerve involvement have been described in patients with acute viral hepatitis, as has myokymia (Mandal, Lancet, 1972; ii:132; Cargnel, JMedVirol, 1988; 25:245). Minor degrees of peripheral neuropathy may be common with acute hepatitis. A slow, coarse tremor of the extremities has been described in the convalescent phase of type B hepatitis. Neuropsychiatric dysfunction, including behavioural abnormalities, irritability, insomnia, and changes in personality, may occur with fulminant hepatitis, and may be the presenting manifestation of this disease. Posthepatitis syndrome can be often accompanied by persistent depression and alterations in mood. The basis for this is unknown.

Haematological

Mild lymphocytosis may occur in some patients during the course of the illness, as may a minor decrease in the haematocrit. Acute viral hepatitis has been associated with red-cell aplasia, thrombocytopenia, agranulocytosis, and aplastic anaemia (Hagler, Medicine, 1975; 54:139). The majority of patients have been young (mean age

19 years, range 2–74), and two-thirds are male. Pancytopenia usually appears in convalescence. The interval between the onset of jaundice and the appearance of pancytopenia is 2 to 12 weeks. Onset of aplastic anaemia is heralded by the appearance of weakness, fever, fatigue, or bleeding. Several forms of therapy have been used without much evidence of benefit. There are only rare cases of aplastic anaemia with type B hepatitis (McSweeney, AmJMed, 1988; 85:255); the majority have been associated in the past with non-A, non-B hepatitis. A dose-dependent suppression of erythroid colony formation and suppression of haemopoietic progenitor cells by HBV have been observed, which may explain the inhibition of erythrogenesis in vivo by HBV (Zeldis, Hepatol, 1988; 8:755).

Cardiac

Mild degrees of brachycardia and hypertension may occur in patients with acute icteric hepatitis. A variety of electro-cardiographic abnormalities have been described, including atrial fibrillation and ventricular ectopic beats. Significant cardiac complications are rare, but myocarditis has been reported, as has pericarditis (Bell, JAMA, 1971; 218:387; Adler, Pediat, 1978; 61: 716). It is unknown whether these cardiac complications are due to complications of fulminant hepatic failure or to the effects of HBV in these tissues.

Respiratory

Symptoms typical of an upper respiratory-tract infection may be common during the preicteric phase of acute hepatitis. Pleural effusions have developed in patients (Gross, Gastro, 1971; 60:898). The fluid is usually colourless and may contain both HBsAg and HBeAg (Tabor, Gastro, 1977; 73:1157). These effusions decline with improvement in the underlying hepatitis. The cause is obscure.

Gastrointestinal tract

Anorexia, nausea, and vomiting may occur, as can either constipation or diarrhoea. A superficial gastritis is reportedly common in patients with icteric hepatitis. Other uncommon gastrointestinal complications include villous atrophy and possibly haemorrhagic gastritis (Gudmand-Hoyer, ScaJGastr, 1973; 8:377). Severe diarrhoea is more typical of hepatitis A virus infection.

Pancreatic

Acute pancreatitis is a frequent complication of fulminant hepatitis (Wands, JohnsHopkMedJ, 1973; 133:156). Elevations in serum amylase activity are found in between 20 and 30 per cent of patients, and morphological evidence of pancreatitis is present in up to 50 per cent. A few patients with non-fatal hepatitis may also have clinical, biochemical, or radiological evidence of acute pancreatitis, which is usually mild and asymptomatic. The pathogenesis is obscure (Geokas, CalifMed, 1972; 117:1). HBV may replicate in the pancreas, as HBsAg is detectable in pancreatobiliary secretions. HBsAg and HBcAg have also been detected in pancreatic acinar cells in some chronic HBsAg carriers (Halpern, Virology, 1986; 150:276).

Renal

Patients with icteric viral hepatitis may have mild proteinuria and abnormalities of the urinary sediment. The albuminuria typically occurs during the preicteric and early icteric phases. The urinary sediment may contain red cells, hyaline casts, and red blood-cell casts. These abnormalities generally resolve.

Renal failure is common in fulminant hepatitis (Wilkinson, BMJ, 1978; 2:338). Azotaemia develops during the first or second week, and is characterized by increases in blood urea and serum creatinine. Most patients are oliguric. Functional renal failure or acute tubular necrosis can occur; the latter usually resolves with recovery. Dialysis may be necessary.

Dermatological

Urticaria is a characteristic manifestation of the preicteric phase of acute viral hepatitis and a component of the serum sickness-like syndrome (Lockshin, ArchDermatol, 1972; 105:570). Skin biopsy shows a perivascular infiltrate of lymphocytes and histiocytes in the dermis around small to medium-sized vessels. The complication may be caused by deposition of circulating immune complexes of viral antigen and antibody. Other erythematous maculopapular rashes or erythematous patches may appear during the prodromal phase of acute hepatitis. Acne and seborrhoeic dermatitis have been reported. A transient worsening of acne is common during the early convalescent phase of the illness. Pruritus is common with cholestatic hepatitis.

In children with acute type B hepatitis, papular acrodermatitis (Gianotti) syndrome, characterized by erythematous papules on the arms, legs, and face but usually sparing the trunk, has been described (Gianotti, ArchDisChild, 1973; 48:794; Ishimaru, Lancet, 1976; i: 707). The papules do not itch; they persist for 6 to 8 weeks before resolving. The syndrome is most commonly seen in young children aged 1 to 6 years, in Japan [where it is related to a subtype of HBsAg that is unusual in the Orient (ayw)] and in Italy.

Rheumatological

Acute hepatitis B may be accompanied by a serum sickness-like syndrome in 5 to 15 per cent of patients, manifested by low-grade fever, rash, and arthralgias. The rash is usually urticarial but can be maculopapular. The arthralgias typically affect the wrist, elbows, knees, and ankles, and can be quite severe. The syndrome is probably due to immune-complex formation, and is associated with severe depression of total serum haemolytic complement (Alpert, NEJM, 1971; 285:185). Morning stiffness is common. Occasionally there may be a marked tenosynovitis. Muscle pains and even myositis with elevations in serum creatinine phosphokinase may occur. The joint fluid may have elevated protein and lymphocytes, as well as a depression of complement. Rheumatoid factor can develop during the course of viral hepatitis. The arthritis of acute hepatitis usually begins to improve with the onset of jaundice and eventually resolves completely. Permanent deformity and chronic arthritis are not produced. There are rare examples of rheumatoid arthritis, Reiter's syndrome, and polymyalgia rheumatica related to acute hepatitis B, but this may be coincidental. Raynaud's phenomenon, chronic seronegative polyarthritis, and polyarteritis nodosa have been associated with chronic HBV infection (Liang, Lancet, 1976; i:43).

Vasculitis and cryoglobulinaemia

Digital vasospasm and infarction with Raynaud's phenomenon have been reported. An association has been described between polyarteritis nodosa and circulating HBsAg. The liver disease is usually chronic but insignificant. Vasculitis may follow acute HBV infection. The patient presents with fever, polyarthralgia, and rashes. Peripheral neuropathy, hypotension, and azotaemia may develop. There are circulating immune complexes of HBsAg and anti-HBs. HBsAg can be demonstrated in the vessels. Some patients may show hypersensitivity angiitis. Cryoproteins have been demonstrated in small blood vessels. An analysis of polyarteritis in 13 Yupik Eskimos (in whom the annual incidence of HBV-associated polyarteritis nodosa is 7.7 cases per 100 000 population) found all 13 to be HBeAg-positive in diagnosis. A better outcome was found in patients treated with prednisolone and cyclophosphamide than in those treated with prednisolone alone (McMahon, Hepatol, 1989; 9:97).

Chronic hepatitis B: clinical course

Prospective studies conducted by the Copenhagen Hepatitis Study Group have observed that 5 to 10 per cent of adults exposed to the HBV may develop chronic type B viral liver disease (Shah, ArchIntMed, 1985; 145:881). The proportion of symptomatic patients who develop chronic liver disease after acute hepatitis B may be lower than this (Leen, JInfect, 1989; 18:257). In contrast, 90 per cent of neonates infected perinatally will develop chronic hepatitis B (Stevens, NEJM, 1975; 292:771). The incidence in children is inversely related to the age of onset. Males are more likely to become chronic carriers than females. Chronic hepatitis B is rather variable in its clinical course, presentation, progression, and outcome.[57] Only a small percentage of patients with chronic infection give a history of acute hepatitis or jaundice. In most patients with chronic hepatitis B the onset of infection is asymptomatic and mild. As a corollary to this, the majority of patients with acute, icteric hepatitis B resolve the infection and do not develop chronic hepatitis. Thus, for the majority of patients with chronic hepatitis B, the time of onset is unknown, a circumstance that is typical of perinatal and childhood infection in endemic areas.

Most patients with uncomplicated chronic hepatitis B have no symptoms of liver disease. If symptoms are present, they are usually non-specific and mild. The most common symptom is fatigue, which is described variously as lack of energy, poor stamina, lassitude, easy fatiguability, malaise, increased need for sleep, or the feeling that one is ageing. The fatigue of chronic hepatitis tends to be intermittent and worsens with exertion or exercise. It is rarely disabling, tending to affect social life more than work. Myalgias, arthralgias, and transient skin rashes are common extrahepatic manifestations of chronic hepatitis B, which may be due to immune-complex deposition and which occur more frequently in women than men. Other symptoms of chronic hepatitis include nausea, poor appetite, weight loss, abdominal discomfort, weakness, feverishness, dark urine, and jaundice. These symptoms occur largely in patients with severe disease or with an acute exacerbation. With the development of cirrhosis, weight loss, weakness, wasting, abdominal swelling, oedema, dark urine, and jaundice may become progressive problems. Many carriers may be detected through routine screening for HBsAg or through the presence of hepatomegaly and abnormal liver function tests. Older patients may present with complications of chronic active hepatitis and cirrhosis, or even with hepatocellular carcinoma, as occurs typically in Africa. A proportion of patients

may present with an extrahepatic manifestation of HBV infection, for example glomerulonephritis, vasculitis, or polyarteritis (Combes, Lancet, 1971; i:234). HBV is an important cause of glomerulonephritis in tropical areas. Typically, nephritis or nephrotic syndrome associated with HBV infection occurs in those with higher levels of viral replication, and most children with HBsAg-positive membranous nephropathy are HBeAg-positive (Milner, Nephron, 1988; 3:184). Immunoelectron microscopy has been used to localize 'membrane attack complexes' and HBeAg to subepithelial deposits (Akano, VirchArchA, 1989; 414:325).

Physical findings in chronic hepatitis B are also mild and variable. In most patients with uncomplicated disease there are no physical abnormalities. With more severe disease there may be spider angiomas and tender hepatomegaly. Wasting, ascites, peripheral oedema, palmar erythema, pale nails, and bruising suggest advanced disease with cirrhosis. In patients with extrahepatic manifestations there may be oedema from glomerulonephritis and hypoproteinaemia, fleeting urticarial or maculopapular rashes from mucocutaneous vasculitis, or mild tenderness, redness, and synovial thickening from hepatitis B-related arthritis. The features of portal hypertension, such as ascites and bleeding oesophageal varices, are late features of a chronic active hepatitis accompanying cirrhosis.

Laboratory test results in typical, uncomplicated chronic hepatitis B are characteristic, demonstrating increases in alanine and aspartate aminotransferases with little or no increase in alkaline phosphatase, γ-glutamyltranspeptidase, or lactic dehydrogenase. The aminotransferases fluctuate over time, generally ranging from just above normal to between five- and eightfold elevated. Aspartate aminotransferase is usually lower than alanine aminotransferase, the ratio being between 0.5 and 0.8. Serum bilirubin and albumin, the prothrombin time, and the sedimentation rate are normal unless the disease is particularly severe. Serum immunoglobulins may demonstrate mild increases in IgG. Autoantibodies should be nonreactive, even in the face of immune-complex deposition.

The terms used to describe the pathology of chronic hepatitis are being reappraised. The previous definitions of chronic hepatitis, chronic active hepatitis, chronic persistent hepatitis, and chronic lobular hepatitis are no longer widely used. More emphasis is now placed on staging the degree of inflammation and grading the extent of fibrosis. Numerical assessments of liver biopsy findings have been developed as a tool for studying the course of chronic hepatitis B and for judging the efficacy of drugs in clinical therapeutic trials. There is consensus that scoring of the microinflammatory lesions should be separated from scoring of the architectural changes in the liver.

With progressive disease and the development of cirrhosis from chronic hepatitis B, the laboratory test results will change, becoming progressively more abnormal. By and large, the severity of the current injury and hepatitic disease activity is best reflected in the aminotransferase abnormalities, particularly aspartate. As cirrhosis develops, the ratio aspartate aminotransferase:alanine aminotransferase will gradually increase (Williams, Gastro, 1988; 95: 734); the finding of aspartate greater than alanine aminotransferase therefore suggests the presence of cirrhosis. In addition, alkaline phosphatase and γ-glutamyltranspeptidase will increase, serum albumin will fall, and the prothrombin time will become prolonged with the onset of cirrhosis and worsening hepatocellular function. Autoantibodies, particularly smooth-muscle autoantibodies and

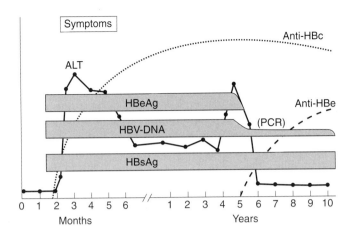

Fig. 3. Serological course of chronic hepatitis B. ALT, alanine aminotransferase; PCR, polymerase chain reaction.

rheumatoid factor, may become detectable, and the immunoglobulins increase in concentration, a raised IgA being particularly suggestive of cirrhosis. Many of these abnormalities occur late in the progression of disease: a fixed hyperbilirubinaemia with depressed albumin and prolonged prothrombin time are poor prognostic findings in chronic hepatitis B.

Serological markers in chronic hepatitis B are helpful in defining the stage of infection and predicting outcome. The course of a 'typical' case of chronic hepatitis B is shown in Fig. 3. The onset of infection is similar to that of acute hepatitis B: HBsAg, HBeAg, and HBV DNA appear in the serum during the incubation period (see ref. 2, pp. 219–42 and Krugman, NEJM, 1979; 300:101). With the onset of serum aminotransferase abnormalities, anti-HBc (both IgG and IgM) arises. At this point, however, a critical event does not occur; viral replication persists, and HBV DNA and HBeAg rise to sustained high titres. The disease accompanying the onset of chronic HBV infection tends to be mild, anicteric, and minimally if at all symptomatic. Serum aminotransferases remain elevated but usually do not reach the heights seen in typical, self-limiting acute hepatitis B. With time the aminotransferases settle to between two- and eightfold elevations.

The subsequent course of chronic hepatitis B is variable. The majority of patients with chronic infection have a relatively benign outcome. Probably only 15 to 20 per cent of patients who acquire this infection in adulthood ultimately develop cirrhosis and any chronic disability. Furthermore, the development of cirrhosis is usually slow, occurring over 5 to 20 years. Infection in childhood may have a different prognosis, with a higher percentage of persons ultimately developing cirrhosis and hepatocellular carcinoma (Beasley, Cancer, 1988; 61:1942). Typically, the infection is mild in childhood and associated with few symptoms and minimal elevations of the aminotransferases. However, the disease may change once adulthood is reached, with marked fluctuations in its activity and the development of cirrhosis in up to 40 per cent of patients. Observations on large numbers of patients with chronic hepatitis B indicate that its course and outcome correlate with serological markers of viral replication (Liaw, Gastro, 1983; 84:216; Pontisso, JMedVirol, 1985; 17:145).[58,59]

The pattern of viral infection changes with time, and this change influences the clinical and pathological progression of the disease. Recent retrospective studies have focused on survival in compensated cirrhosis due to hepatitis B. Notable among these is a European, multicentre, longitudinal study to assess the survival of HBsAg-positive patients with compensated cirrhosis. Three hundred and sixty-six Caucasian HBsAg-positive patients with cirrhosis who had never had clinical manifestations of hepatic decompensation were enrolled and followed for a mean period of 72 months. Death occurred in 23 per cent, mainly from liver failure or hepatocellular carcinoma. The probability of survival was 84 per cent and 68 per cent at 5 and 10 years, respectively. The worst survival was in HBeAg- and HBV DNA-positive individuals (at diagnosis).[60] Thus, progressive disease is associated with persistence of viral replication and remission is associated with loss of active viral replication. As shown in Fig. 3, after years or even decades of persistent infection a spontaneous remission can occur. This remission is marked first by the disappearance of HBV DNA (and DNA polymerase activity) from the serum, followed by the loss of HBeAg and then improvements in the serum aminotransferase activities.[58] In approximately 70 per cent of patients undergoing this type of remission there is a transient worsening of disease activity immediately before the loss of HBeAg (Liaw, Gastro, 1983; 84:216). It is important to recognize this feature, for a sudden worsening of serum aminotransferases and symptoms may be a good rather than a bad prognostic sign in this disease. Once HBeAg is cleared and remission has occurred, serum aminotransferases generally remain normal and symptoms (if present) resolve. In follow-up, a small proportion of patients (10–15 per cent in Western series) experience a reactivation of infection, with a return of HBeAg and HBV DNA in serum associated with marked increases in serum aminotransferases.[61]

The exacerbations associated with the decline in viral replication, or the reactivation of viral replication causing a recurrence of disease, can be severe and life-threatening. Indeed, the pattern of recurrent reactivation with multiple remissions and recurrences is a particularly severe form of this chronic infection, frequently leading to cirrhosis and ultimately hepatic failure.

For many patients who enter either a spontaneous remission or who, after treatment with α-interferon, clear HBeAg and HBV DNA, the remission is sustained, serum aminotransferase activities remain normal, and indeed some ultimately become HBsAg-negative and develop anti-HBs (Lindsay, Hepatol, 1981; 1:586).[62] The loss of HBsAg generally occurs years after that of HBeAg and may be preceded by mild increases in serum aminotransferase activities. The loss of HBsAg in chronic hepatitis B is probably more common in patients with adult-onset disease than in those with childhood-onset infections (more common in Asian and African countries) (Lok, Gastro, 1987; 92:1839). Circulating HBsAg may be lost after acute hepatitis D in a small percentage of carriers (Chin, DigDisSci, 1988; 33:851).

Sensitive assays for HBV DNA in patients with chronic hepatitis B demonstrate that the loss of HBeAg is associated with a decrease rather than complete clearance of HBV DNA in the serum. With loss of HBeAg, HBVDNA usually can no longer be detected by hybridization but is often detectable by polymerase chain reaction (Kaneko, Gastro, 1990; 99:799). Thus, patients with HBeAg in serum usually have HBV DNA of at least 10 pg/ml or 10^5 genome equivalents/ml. After the loss of HBeAg only low concentrations of HBV DNA are detected. These low concentrations probably reflect low levels of HBV replication, but do not appear to be associated with active liver disease in most patients. The continued low level of replication probably explains the persistence of HBsAg in the serum after the loss of HBeAg and other conventional serological markers of active replication. The persistence of low levels of replication may also explain the phenomenon of reactivation as well as the occasional patient without HBeAg in serum who has active liver disease. Finally, in patients who ultimately become HBsAg-negative, HBV DNA is generally no longer detectable, even by polymerase chain reaction.

Occasionally, patients lose HBeAg or are found to be negative for it, yet continue to have active liver disease and HBV DNA detectable in serum by direct hybridization (Pontisso, JMedVirol, 1985; 17:145). Frequently, these patients have been shown to harbour an HBV mutant with a nucleotide substitution in the precore region of the genome, as described above. However, viral replication appears to occur with this mutant despite the lack of HBeAg. These HBeAg-minus mutants are common in Mediterranean countries, particularly Italy and Greece, but are rare in the United States and the United Kingdom. The disease activity associated with the HBeAg-minus mutant can be severe. This form of disease tends to run a relapsing course and is associated with other unusual serological features, such as prominence of HBcAg in the cytoplasm of hepatocytes and relatively low, fluctuating HBV DNA in serum. Mutation rates are highest around the time of active disease.[52] The absence of HBeAg is not always explained by the dominance of HBeAg-minus variants.[63] Not all patients with chronic hepatitis B ultimately seroconvert and lose HBeAg and high concentrations of HBV DNA. In addition, some patients seroconvert and enter a remission in disease activity only after having developed cirrhosis with significant degrees of portal hypertension and hepatocellular dysfunction.

Several large, prospective studies have shown that the relative risk of HBsAg-positive men dying of liver disease is high (30–100-fold). Those with continuing HBV replication appear to have a worse prognosis. The calculated annual rate of development of cirrhosis in HBV carriers is of the order of 1.5 to 2.5 per cent (Fattovich, Hepatol, 1988; 8:1651; Sakuma, Hepatol, 1988; 8:1642). The likelihood of cirrhosis increases with increasing age, and patients may experience hepatic decompensation, including repeated episodes of acute exacerbation, ascites, oedema, variceal haemorrhages, infection, and encephalopathy (Liaw, Hepatol, 1988; 8:493). The 5-year survival rate of HBsAg-positive cirrhotic patients in Child's groups A, B, and C in Taiwan was 83, 79, and 30 per cent, respectively, with the major causes of death being variceal bleeding, hepatic failure, hepatorenal syndrome, infection, and hepatocellular carcinoma (Tsai, JGastHepatol, 1988; 3:583).

Development of hepatocellular carcinoma

Chronic hepatitis B can lead to hepatocellular carcinoma, which is a common form of cancer in many areas of the world where chronic hepatitis B is also common (Beasley, Lancet, 1981; ii:1129; Cancer, 1988; 95:734; Di Bisceglie, AnnIntMed, 1988; 108:390). Furthermore, a large percentage of patients with hepatocellular carcinoma have chronic HBV infection. Epidemiological and clinical studies suggest that hepatocellular carcinoma is a complication of prolonged HBV infection, most patients having had the disease for several decades before diagnosis of the carcinoma. Indeed, the majority of patients with this cancer also have cirrhosis, although it is often mild and inactive (Okuda, Cancer, 1985; 56:98).

In a large European study, hepatocellular carcinoma developed during a mean follow-up of 6 years in 9 per cent of 317 patients with compensated hepatic cirrhosis. Five years after diagnosis the probability of hepatocellular carcinoma appearing was 6 per cent (and that of decompensation 28 per cent). After the first episode of decompensation, the 5-year probability of survival (35 per cent) was poor.[64]

Hepatocellular carcinoma is more common in men than women and appears to be most common in patients who acquire HBV infection in childhood rather than adulthood. These features may explain why it is such a common complication of HBV infection in Asia and Africa, but a somewhat uncommon complication among patients born in the United States and Western Europe (Di Bisceglie, AnnIntMed, 1988; 108:390). Hepatocellular carcinoma rarely presents clinically until it has grown to fairly large size (>10 cm in diameter). The typical symptoms include poor appetite, weight loss, muscle wasting, weakness, and abdominal pain. Any clinical deterioration should raise the question of hepatocellular carcinoma. In endemic areas of HBV infection, HBV carriers frequently have silent disease until the development of advanced hepatocellular carcinoma. A large liver or a large, firm mass may be felt on physical examination. Laboratory tests can be normal or may show slight increases in serum bilirubin, alkaline phosphatase, and aminotransferases. The most sensitive screening test for the presence of hepatocellular carcinoma is abdominal ultrasonography, which can usually detect lesions of 1 cm in diameter or greater (Sheu, Cancer, 1985; 56:660). Small tumours are often hypoechoic; larger tumours may be hyperechoic or have complex shadows. There are several serum tests that can suggest the presence of hepatocellular carcinoma, the most commonly applied being that for α-fetoprotein. This is a small molecular-weight protein produced in high concentrations by the liver during fetal life. Its serum concentrations fall at birth to an adult level below 9 ng/ml by 6 months of age. Thereafter, elevations, outside of pregnancy, are distinctly abnormal, being found in up to 80 per cent of patients with hepatocellular carcinoma and rarely with other tumours.

Elevations of α-fetoprotein can also occur with liver disease, especially in patients with acute hepatitis (during recovery), or with an exacerbation of chronic hepatitis in a patient with cirrhosis. A progressive increase in α-fetoprotein without concurrent activity of the liver disease is highly suggestive of hepatocellular carcinoma (Heyward, Lancet, 1982; ii:889). For these reasons, ultrasonographic examinations and regular determinations of α-fetoprotein can be used to screen for hepatocellular carcinoma in high-risk populations. Of course, the populations at highest risk are men over the age of 40 years who acquired HBV infection during childhood and who have cirrhosis.

A large body of scientific evidence has confirmed a relation between chronic HBV infection and hepatocellular carcinoma (Austin, CancerRes, 1986; 46:962), but the mechanism of oncogenesis is not known. HBsAg-associated hepatocellular carcinoma is a prevalent tumour throughout subSaharan Africa, Asia, the Middle

East, southern Europe, and South America. Prospective and epidemiological studies have shown that male asymptomatic carriers are at substantial risk of hepatocellular carcinoma (Beasley, Cancer, 1988; 61:2554). In Taiwan, the data suggest that HBV infection is the major cause of hepatocellular carcinoma and that hepatocellular carcinoma in the absence of any HBV marker is rare. Prospective surveillance studies using serum α-fetoprotein and real-time ultrasonography in 432 patients with chronic type B hepatitis in Taiwan identified asymptomatic hepatocellular carcinoma with a calculated annual incidence of 826/100 000 (but 2768/100 000, respectively, in patients over the age of 35 years) (Liaw, Gastro, 1986; 90:263). In a separate study of the natural history of hepatocellular carcinoma in HBsAg-positive cirrhotics, the occurrence rate was 5.7 per cent per year (Tsai, JGastHepatol, 1988; 3:583).

Exogenous factors may speed the process of oncogenesis, but chronic HBV infection must be considered an important independent risk factor. The pathogenesis of HBV-associated hepatocellular carcinoma is unknown, however, and may be related to the phasic necrosis, regeneration, and cirrhosis induced as a result of HBsAg infection. Although the molecular mechanism of HBV-associated carcinogenesis is unknown, HBV may have a direct cytogenetic role. Integration of the HBV genome into the hepatocyte DNA may be an important initiating factor, as the consequent disruption of the *C* (core) gene may confer a selective advantage to affected cells not expressing the viral core antigen (HBcAg). Experimental evidence suggests that HBV may directly induce malignant transformation.

HBV sequences are frequently integrated into hepatocellular DNA. It is postulated that the development of hepatocellular carcinoma could be by insertional mutagenesis, or by the production of novel fusion genes, chromosomal deletions, and translocations associated with HBV integration, or by loss of tumour-suppressor alleles, or, as in woodchucks, by c-*myc* oncogene amplification (Hino, PNAS, 1986; 83:8338; Moroy, Nature, 1986; 324:276). A retinoic acid receptor is expressed at high concentration in human hepatocellular carcinoma, in association with a HBV integration (Benbrook, Nature, 1988; 333:669). Nucleocapsid-polymerase fusion proteins have been detected in hepatocellular carcinoma tissues, suggestive of synthesis of a reverse transcriptase (Will, Science, 1986; 231:594).

Recent evidence has suggested that the translational product of the *X* gene, a 17-kDa protein, is a transactivating factor for viral enhancers, and that in cotransfection experiments the *X* gene encodes a protein with the ability to stimulate transcription (Spandau, JVirol, 1988; 62:427). Such a transactivating protein might stimulate heterologous promoters and modulate cellular gene expression.[65] The *X*-gene product does not directly bind DNA but a number of effects of HBx on cell growth and cell-cycle progression have been reported. Exposure to aflatoxin may be important in some geographical regions. A genetic susceptibility to hepatocellular carcinoma associated with genetic variation in enzymatic detoxification of aflatoxin has been reported.[66]

In some parts of the world, codon 249 mutations in p53 are associated with aflatoxin exposure. The increased formation of carcinogen–DNA adducts may represent one mechanism adding to the association between chronic hepatitis B infection and the development of hepatocellular carcinoma.[67]

Transactivating activity has also been detected in the pre-S region of the genome, a region frequently conserved in HBV integrations. Although enhanced expression of *ras* p21 has been detected in a few tumours studied, there is no clear relation between the expression of *ras* and c-*myc* oncogenes and HBV infection in human hepatocellular carcinoma (Lee, Hepatol, 1988; 8:1116).

Overexpression of transforming growth factor-α has been reported in transitional cells.[68] Any oncogenic role for HBV must, however, be reconciled with the knowledge that hepatocellular carcinoma occurs after a long latent period and does not occur in all HBV carriers (Miller, PNAS, 1986; 83:2531). The shortest latent period, to date, has been deduced from the case of a 4-year-old Japanese boy with hepatocellular carcinoma, and HBV integration, in the absence of cirrhosis.

Therapy
Management

The primary approach to the management of hepatitis B should be conservative, with the education of the patient, the avoidance of further injury, and the protection of contacts. Specific therapies have been developed for chronic hepatitis B but are of no apparent benefit in acute hepatitis B.

Acute hepatitis B

Good management includes supportive measures, relief of symptoms, and avoidance of further injury. Most patients can be managed at home and do not require admission to hospital. Bed rest should be recommended as long as jaundice and symptoms are present. Patients should avoid unnecessary activities, exercise, or travel during the period of jaundice and major symptoms. Once the symptoms abate, patients can be allowed to return to their previous activities, and if they feel well should be encouraged to return to exercise or regular amounts of exertion. A generally nutritious diet should be recommended. Patients may find that fatty foods induce nausea, indigestion, or early satiety. To ensure an adequate intake of calories, a high-carbohydrate diet can be recommended. Alcohol should be avoided during the period of jaundice and symptoms, as should all but the most necessary medications. Vitamins should be taken judiciously: in particular, doses of vitamin A in excess of 5000 units/day should not be used. If analgesics are needed, paracetamol (acetaminophen) is preferable to aspirin. Only the mildest of sedatives should be used.

Attention should be given to the protection of contacts of patients with acute hepatitis B. In most countries, hepatitis B is a reportable disease; health officials should be informed of the case. Recommendations on the protection of contacts are not standardized, largely because it has been difficult to demonstrate the efficacy of any method in preventing spread. Hepatitis B vaccine should be provided to all intimate, sexual and household contacts of a patient with acute hepatitis B. Prescreening of vaccinees is prudent, but not necessary. Vaccine can be given in an accelerated schedule of 0, 1, and 2 months. Hepatitis B immune globulin is of unproven benefit for prophylaxis against household and sexual contact with a patient with acute hepatitis B. If it is used, it should be given only to sexual or parenteral contacts. A single injection at the start of vaccination is all that is necessary.

Chronic hepatitis B

Treatment of chronic hepatitis B must be directed at patients with active disease and viral replication, preferably at a stage before cirrhosis or significant injury have occurred. Thus, patients should be treated before the development of symptoms or signs of severe liver disease.

Specific therapies for chronic hepatitis B are now being developed. Good management includes patient education, the protection of contacts, monitoring for infection and disease activity, screening for complications of disease including hepatocellular carcinoma, and specific therapy with α-interferon in certain circumstances. Management of chronic hepatitis B should begin with educating the patient about the nature of the disease, its infectiousness, and prognosis. Patients should be urged to have family members tested for antibody to HBV and receive HBV vaccination if they are not immune. Patients should have instructions on 'safe sex' and modes of spread of disease. Medical personnel should be instructed carefully on barrier practices.

No particular diet or pattern of activity has been shown to be beneficial in chronic hepatitis B. In general, patients without symptoms and evidence of cirrhosis should not have major restrictions placed upon their lifestyle or activities. A generally nutritious diet should be recommended. Patients should be encouraged to exercise regularly if they feel well. Alcohol should be discouraged; however, it need not be proscribed but should be kept to a minimum. A few medications need to be avoided in this disease; chief among these are corticosteroids (such as might be given for allergies).

Monitoring of patients with chronic hepatitis B should be tailored to the stage and severity of the disease. For patients with typical, well-compensated chronic hepatitis B, the serum aminotransferases, albumin, bilirubin, and HBV markers (usually HBsAg and HBeAg) can be measured every 3 to 6 months, depending upon whether therapy is planned. In patients who are healthy HBsAg carriers without aminotransferase abnormalities or HBeAg or HBV DNA in serum, yearly liver tests and monitoring of HBsAg are probably sufficient.

Screening for hepatocellular carcinoma is appropriate for persons at risk for developing this tumour. High-risk factors include age over 40, Asian or African background, the presence of cirrhosis, and a family history of hepatocellular carcinoma. Besides liver function tests, testing for α-fetoprotein and ultrasonographic examination of the liver at 6-monthly intervals are recommended.

Antiviral therapy of hepatitis B

Specific therapy for hepatitis B has now become practical with the demonstration that α-interferon inhibits HBV replication and that prolonged therapy can lead to a remission in disease.[69,70]

Acute hepatitis B

Most cases of acute, icteric disease eventually resolve with clearance of the virus and complete healing of the hepatic injury. There is no evidence that α-interferon speeds this healing or clearance of the virus or that early treatment prevents the development of chronic disease (Tassopoulos, Hepatol, 1989; 9:576). One must be cautious in using any medication with adverse effects in patients with acute hepatitis in whom the hepatic functional reserve is compromised,

drug pharmacokinetics is abnormal, and drug toxicities are common. At present, neither α-interferon nor any other antiviral agent should be used to treat patients with typical acute hepatitis B.

Medical management of fulminant hepatitis B is challenging and difficult (see Section 19). The dire prognosis of this syndrome often leads physicians to apply therapies of unproven benefit. α-interferon has not been found to be beneficial in fulminant hepatitis, and it certainly has side-effects that can complicate management considerably (such as fever, confusion, bone-marrow suppression). Currently, the optimal therapy for fulminant hepatitis B is liver transplantation, once prognostic factors indicate that survival is unlikely. Antiviral agents should not be used outside of prospective, randomized controlled trials.

Chronic hepatitis B

The immediate goal of therapy is to eradicate viral replication and improve the underlying liver disease. α-interferon is clearly beneficial in improving the course of chronic, HBeAg-positive hepatitis B (Dusheiko, Hepatol, 1985; 5:556; Alexander, Lancet, 1987; i:66; Hoofnagle, Gastro, 1988; 95:1318). Therapy with α-interferon is indicated in patients with typical chronic hepatitis B who have HBsAg in serum together with HBV DNA and/or HBeAg and raised aminotransferases (at least twice the upper limit of normal).

The role of newer antiviral agents or immunomodulatory therapies is discussed elsewhere in this volume.

Prevention

Clinical studies have established that hepatitis B vaccination is an effective means of preventing the disease in both adults and neonates. A full discussion of hepatitis B vaccines can be found in Chapter 12.1.3.1.

References

1. Tiollais P, Pourcel C, and Dejean A. The hepatitis B virus. *Nature*, 1985; **317**: 489–95.
2. Hoofnagle JH, *et al*. Serologic response in hepatitis B. In Vyas GN, Cohn E, and Schmid R, eds. *Viral hepatitis. 1978 International Symposium*. Philadelphia: Franklin Institute Press; 1978: 219–42.
3. Beasley R, Lin C, Hwang L, and Chien C. Hepatocellular carcinoma and hepatitis B virus: a prospective study of 22,707 men in Taiwan. *Lancet*, 1981; **ii**: 1129–33.
4. Dane DS, Cameron CH, and Briggs M. Virus-like particles in serum of patients with Australia-antigen-associated hepatitis. *Lancet*, 1980; **i**: 695–8.
5. Kaplan PM, Greenman RL, Gerin JL, Purcell PH, and Robinson WS. DNA polymerase associated with human hepatitis B antigen. *Journal of Virology*, 1983; **12**: 995–1005.
6. Summers J and Mason WS. Replication of the genome of a hepatitis B-like virus by reverse transcription of an RNA intermediate. *Cell*, 1982; **29**: 403–15.
7. Natoli G, *et al. ras-* and *raf*-dependent activation of c-*jun* transcriptional activity by the hepatitis B virus transactivator pX. *Oncogene*, 1994; **9**: 2837–43.
8. Qadri I, Maguire HF, and Siddiqui A. Hepatitis B virus transactivator protein X interacts with the TATA-binding protein. *Proceedings of the National Academy of Sciences (USA)*, 1995; **92**: 1003–7.
9. Offensperger W-B, Offensperger S, Stoll B, Gerok W, and Häussinger D. Effects of anisotonic exposure on duck hepatitis B virus replication. *Hepatology*, 1994; **20**: 1–7.

10. Guidotti LG, Matzke B, Schaller H, and Chisari FV. High-level hepatitis B virus replication in transgenic mice. *Journal of Virology*, 1995; **69**: 6158–69.

11. De Bruin WCC, Leenders WPJ, Moshage H, and Van Haelst UJGM. Species specificity for HBsAg binding protein endonexin II. *Journal of Hepatology*, 1996; **24**: 265–70.

12. Hertogs K, *et al.* Endonexin II, present on human liver plasma membranes, is a specific binding protein of small hepatitis B virus (HBV) envelope protein. *Virology*, 1993; **197**: 549–57.

13. Szmuness W. Recent advances in the study of the epidemiology of hepatitis B. *American Journal of Pathology*, 1975; **81**: 629–49.

14. Heptonstall J, *et al.* Transmission of hepatitis B to patients from four infected surgeons without hepatitis B e antigen. *New England Journal of Medicine*, 1997; **336**: 178–84.

15. Anderson B, Bodsworth NJ, Rohrsheim RA, and Donovan BJ. Hepatitis B virus infection and vaccination status of high risk people in Sydney: 1982 and 1991. *Medical Journal of Australia*, 1994; **161**: 368–71.

16. Da Villa G, Picciotto L, Elia S, Peluso F, Montanaro F, and Maisto T. Hepatitis B vaccination: universal vaccination of newborn babies and children at 12 years of age versus high risk groups. A comparison in the field. *Vaccine*, 1995; **13**: 1240–3.

17. Van Hecke E, *et al.* Hepatitis B virus-specific cytotoxic T lymphocyte responses in patients with acute and chronic hepatitis B virus infection. *Journal of Hepatology*, 1994; **20**: 514–23.

18. Rehermann B, Pasquinelli C, Mosier SM, and Chisari FV. Hepatitis B virus (HBV) sequence variation in cytotoxic T lymphocyte epitopes is not common in patients with chronic HBV infection. *Journal of Clinical Investigation*, 1995; **96**: 1527–34.

19. Rehermann B, *et al.* The cytotoxic T lymphocyte response to multiple hepatitis B virus polymerase epitopes during and after acute viral hepatitis. *Journal of Experimental Medicine*, 1995; **181**: 1047–58.

20. Ferrari C, *et al.* Cellular immune response to hepatitis B virus-encoded antigens in acute and chronic hepatitis B virus infection. *Journal of Immunology*, 1990; **145**: 3442–9.

21. Penna A, *et al.* Cytotoxic T lymphocytes recognize an HLA-A2-restricted epitope within the hepatitis B virus nucleocapsid antigen. *Journal of Experimental Medicine*, 1991; **174**: 1565–70.

22. Chisari FV and Ferrari C. Hepatitis B virus immunopathogenesis. *Annual Review of Immunology*, 1995; **13**: 29–60.

23. Milich DR, Jones JE, Hughes JL, Price J, Raney AK, and McLachlan A. Is a function of the secreted hepatitis B e antigen to induce immunologic tolerance *in utero*? *Proceedings of the National Academy of Sciences (USA)*, 1990; **87**: 6599–603.

24. Bertoletti A, *et al.* Cytotoxic T lymphocyte response to a wild type hepatitis B virus epitope in patients chronically infected by variant viruses carrying substitutions within the epitope. *Journal of Experimental Medicine*, 1994; **180**: 933–43.

25. Whitten TM, Quets AT, and Schloemer RH. Identification of the hepatitis B virus factor that inhibits expression of the beta interferon gene. *Journal of Virology*, 1991; **65**: 4699–704.

26. Foster GR, Goldin RD, Hay A, McGarvey MJ, Stark GR, and Thomas HC. Expression of the terminal protein of hepatitis B virus is associated with failure to respond to interferon therapy. *Hepatology*, 1993; **17**: 757–62.

27. Barnaba V, Franco A, Alberti A, Balsano C, Benvenuto R, and Balsano F. Recognition of hepatitis B virus envelope proteins by liver-infiltrating T lymphocytes in chronic HBV infection. *Journal of Immunology*, 1989; **143**: 2650–5.

28. Jung M-C, *et al.* Activation of a heterogeneous hepatitis B (HB) core and e antigen-specific CD4$^+$ T-cell population during seroconversion to anti-HBe and anti-HBs in hepatitis B virus infection. *Journal of Virology*, 1995; **69**: 3358–68.

29. Tsai SL, *et al.* Acute exacerbations of chronic type B hepatitis are accompanied by increased T cell responses to hepatitis B core and e antigens. Implications for hepatitis B e antigen seroconversion. *Journal of Clinical Investigation*, 1992; **89**: 87–96.

30. Rehermann B, Lau D, Hoofnagle JH, and Chisari FV. Cytotoxic T lymphocyte responsiveness after resolution of chronic hepatitis C virus infection. *Journal of Clinical Investigation*, 1996; **97**: 1655–65.

31. Waters JA, O'Rourke S, Schlicht HJ, and Thomas HC. Cytotoxic T cell responses in patients with chronic hepatitis B virus infection undergoing HBe antigen antibody seroconversion. *Clinical and Experimental Immunology*, 1995; **102**: 314–9.

32. Fukuda R, *et al.* The expression of IL-2, IL-4 and interferon-gamma (IFN-gamma) mRNA using liver biopsies at different phases of acute exacerbation of chronic hepatitis B. *Clinical and Experimental Immunology*, 1995; **100**: 446–51.

33. Ando K, *et al.* Mechanisms of class I restricted immunopathology. A transgenic mouse model of fulminant hepatitis. *Journal of Experimental Medicine*, 1993; **178**: 1541–54.

34. Tsui LV, Guidotti LG, Ishikawa T, and Chisari FV. Posttranscriptional clearance of hepatitis B virus RNA by cytotoxic T lymphocyte-activated hepatocytes. *Proceedings of the National Academy of Sciences (USA)*, 1995; **92**: 12 398–402.

35. Cavanaugh VJ, Guidotti LG, and Chisari FV. Interleukin-12 inhibits hepatitis B virus replication in transgenic mice. *Journal of Virology*, 1997; **71**: 3236–43.

36. Guidotti LG, Guilhot S, and Chisari FV. Interleukin-2 and alpha/beta interferon down-regulate hepatitis B virus gene expression *in vivo* by tumor necrosis factor-dependent and -independent pathways. *Journal of Virology*, 1994; **68**: 1265–70.

37. Guidotti LG, *et al.* Cytotoxic T lymphocytes inhibit hepatitis B virus gene expression by a noncytolytic mechanism in transgenic mice. *Proceedings of the National Academy of Sciences (USA)*, 1994; **91**: 3764–8.

38. Guilhot S, Guidotti LG, and Chisari FV. Interleukin-2 downregulates hepatitis B virus gene expression in transgenic mice by a posttranscriptional mechanism. *Journal of Virology*, 1993; **67**: 7444–9.

39. Milich DR, Schödel F, Hughes JL, Jones JE, and Peterson DL. The hepatitis B virus core and e antigens elicit different Th cell subsets: antigen structure can affect Th cell phenotype. *Journal of Virology*, 1997; **71**: 2192–201.

40. Milich DR, Schödel F, Peterson DL, Jones JE, and Hughes JL. Characterization of self-reactive T cells that evade tolerance in hepatitis B e antigen transgenic mice. *European Journal of Immunology*, 1995; **25**: 1663–72.

41. Thursz MR, Kwiatkowski D, Allsopp CEM, Greenwood BM, Thomas HC, and Hill AVS. Association between an MHC class II allele and clearance of hepatitis B virus in the Gambia. *New England Journal of Medicine*, 1995; **332**: 1065–9.

42. Carman WF, *et al.* Vaccine-induced escape mutant of hepatitis B virus. *Lancet*, 1990; **336**: 325–9.

43. Carman WF, *et al.* Hepatitis B virus envelope variation after transplantation with and without hepatitis B immune globulin prophylaxis. *Hepatology*, 1996; **24**: 489–93.

44. McMahon G, *et al.* Genetic alterations in the gene encoding the major HBsAg: DNA and immunological analysis of recurrent HBsAg derived from monoclonal antibody-treated liver transplant patients. *Hepatology*, 1992; **15**: 757–66.

45. Carman WF, *et al.* Association of a precore genomic variant of hepatitis B virus with fulminant hepatitis. *Hepatology*, 1991; **14**: 219–22.

46. Nakayama J, *et al.* Fulminant hepatitis caused by a hepatitis B virus core region variant strain. *Journal of Hepatology*, 1995; **23**: 199–203.

47. Liang TJ, *et al.* Hepatitis B virus precore mutation and fulminant hepatitis in the United States. A polymerase chain reaction-based assay for the detection of specific mutation. *Journal of Clinical Investigation*, 1994; **93**: 550–5.

48. Hasegawa K, Huang J, Rogers SA, Blum HE, and Liang TJ. Enhanced replication of a hepatitis B virus mutant associated with an epidemic of fulminant hepatitis. *Journal of Virology*, 1994; **68**: 1651–9.

49. Boner W, Schlicht H-J, Hanrieder K, Holmes EC, and Carman WF. Further characterization of 2 types of precore variant hepatitis B virus isolates from Hong Kong. *Journal of Infectious Diseases*, 1995; **171**: 1461–7.

50. Rieger A and Nassal M. Distinct requirements for primary sequence in the 5′- and 3′-part of a bulge in the hepatitis B virus RNA encapsidation signal revealed by a combined *in vivo* selection *in vitro* amplification system. *Nucleic Acids Research*, 1995; **23**: 3909–15.

51. Hosono S, *et al.* Core antigen mutations of human hepatitis B virus in hepatomas accumulate in MHC class II-restricted T cell epitopes. *Virology*, 1995; **212**: 151–62.

52. Akarca US and Lok ASF. Naturally occurring hepatitis B virus core gene mutations. *Hepatology*, 1995; **22**: 50–60.

53. Sato S, *et al.* Hepatitis B virus strains with mutations in the core promoter in patients with fulminant hepatitis. *Annals of Internal Medicine*, 1995; **122**: 241–8.

54. Hsu H-Y, *et al.* Precore mutant of hepatitis B virus in childhood fulminant hepatitis B: An infrequent association. *Journal of Infectious Diseases*, 1995; **171**: 776–81.

55. Ling R, *et al.* Selection of mutations in the hepatitis B virus polymerase during therapy of transplant recipients with lamivudine. *Hepatology*, 1996; **24**: 711–13.

56. Krugman S, *et al.* Viral hepatitis, type B. Studies on the natural history and prevention re-examined. *New England Journal of Medicine*, 1979; **300**: 101.

57. Hoofnagle JH and Alter HJ. Chronic viral hepatitis. In Hoofnagle JH, Vyas GN and Dienstag JL, eds. *Viral hepatitis and liver disease*. New York: Grune and Stratton, 1984: 97–113.

58. Hoofnagle JH, Dusheiko GM, Seeff LB, Jones EA, Waggoner JG, and Bales ZB. Seroconversion from hepatitis B e antigen to antibody in chronic type B hepatitis. *Annals of Internal Medicine*, 1981; **94**: 744–8.

59. Hadziyannis SJ, Lieberman HM, Karvountzis GG, and Shafritz DA. Analysis of liver disease, nuclear HBcAg, viral replication and hepatitis B virus DNA in liver and serum of HBeAg versus anti-HBe positive carriers of hepatitis B virus. *Hepatology*, 1983; **3**: 656–62.

60. Realdi G, *et al.* for EUROHEP. Survival and prognostic factors in 366 patients with compensated cirrhosis type B: a multicenter study. *Journal of Hepatology*, 1994; **21**: 656–66.

61. Davis GL, Hoofnagle JH, and Waggoner JG. Spontaneous reactivation of chronic hepatitis B virus infection. *Gastroenterology*, 1984; **86**: 230–5.

62. Korenman J, Baker B, Waggoner J, Everhart JE, and Di Bisceglie AM. Long-term remission of chronic hepatitis B after alpha-interferon therapy. *Annals of Internal Medicine*, 1991; **114**: 629–34.

63. Niitsuma H, *et al.* Prevalence of precore-defective mutant of hepatitis B virus in HBV carriers. *Journal of Medical Virology*, 1995; **46**: 397–402.

64. Fattovich G, *et al.* Occurrence of hepatocellular carcinoma and decompensation in Western European patients with cirrhosis type B. *Hepatology*, 1995; **21**: 77–82.

65. Caselmann WH. Transactivation of cellular gene expression by hepatitis B viral proteins: a possible molecular mechanism of hepatocarcinogenesis. *Journal of Hepatology*, 1995; **22** (Suppl. 1): 34–7.

66. Gonzalo A, Fernandez M, Navarro J, and Ortuño J. Searching for hepatitis C virus antibodies in chronic primary glomerular diseases. *Nephron*, 1995; **69**: 96.

67. Izzotti A, Scatolini L, Lewtas J, Walsh D, and De Flora S. Enhanced levels of DNA adducts in the liver of woodchucks infected with hepatitis virus. *Chemico-Biological Interactions*, 1995; **97**: 273–85.

68. Schaff Z, Hsia CC, Sarosi I, and Tabor E. Overexpression of transforming growth factor-α in hepatocellular carcinoma and focal nodular hyperplasia from European patients. *Human Pathology*, 1994; **25**: 644–51.

69. Grellier L, *et al.* Lamivudine prophylaxis against reinfection in liver transplantation for hepatitis B cirrhosis. *Lancet*, 1996; **348**: 1212–15.

70. Dusheiko GM. Treatment and prevention of chronic viral hepatitis. *Pharmacology and Therapeutics*, 1995; **65**: 47–73.

12.1.2.4 Hepatitis D

Mario Rizzetto, Antonina Smedile, and Giorgio Verme

Definition

Hepatitis D, also named hepatitis delta, is a disease caused by the hepatitis delta virus (**HDV**), a hepatotropic pathogen requiring, for *in vivo* infection, obligatory helper functions provided by the hepatitis B virus (**HBV**).[1,2]

Introduction

The virion of HDV is a particle of 36 nm diameter coated by the HB surface antigen (**HBsAg**), inside which are sequestered an RNA genome and the HD antigen (**HDAg**) (see Chapter 12.1.2.1). HDV can establish infection only in patients simultaneously infected by HBV; it may modify the natural history of the underlying HBV infections upon which it thrives, aggravating pre-existent hepatitis B or creating hepatitis D in healthy carriers of HBV.[3]

Natural history

As a corollary to its biological requirements, HDV can establish infection only in individuals with continuing HBV infection. Persons susceptible to HBV or already infected by it are susceptible to HDV, and therefore hepatitis D occurs in two settings: in a normal person simultaneously infected by HDV–HBV (coinfection) or in a carrier of HBsAg superinfected by HDV (superinfection). Persons protected from HBV by the acquisition of antibody to HBsAg (**anti-HBs**) appear to be protected from HDV.

As the need for helper HBV is met differently in coinfection and superinfection, the clinical expression and outcome of HDV infection is different in normal persons and in carriers of HBV (Table 1).

Coinfection

Transmission of HDV can be attained by a single inoculation of serum containing both HBV and HDV.[4] Infection with HDV demands that the helper HBV be first activated, thus providing the functions (mainly the HBsAg) necessary for the activation of HDV. As HDV cannot infect until HBV has infected hepatocytes, the expression of the defective virus depends on (and is limited by) the virulence of the associated HBV. Slow spread of HBV to hepatocytes either fails to support HDV, or supports only an abortive infection; rapid spread provides enough vulnerable hepatocytes for the defective virus to be activated to a clinically significant degree.

Because of the complex interactions between the two viruses, the expression of HDV is variable, ranging from incomplete to very virulent infection. However, since the background HBV infection is usually self-limiting and HDV cannot outlive the elimination of its helper virus, acute HBV–HDV coinfections are rarely progressive and cause chronic liver disease in only about 2 per cent of cases (Caredda, JInfDis, 1985; 151:925)

Superinfection

A pre-existing HBV infection (with production of HBsAg) provides the ideal terrain for the activation of superinfecting HDV, affording a highly susceptible substrate that permits the rapid amplification of the defective pathogen; in this setting it establishes infection independently of the virulence of the HBV present in the original inoculum transmitting the HDV, as the helper function necessary for HDV replication is provided by the HBV colonizing the host.[3] A pre-existing HBsAg state may rescue minimal amounts of HDV, and material containing HDV that is not infectious to the normal person can transmit hepatitis D to the carrier of HBsAg (Ponzetto, Hepatol, 1988; 8:1655).

With superinfection, HDV transcapsidates from the HBsAg coat worn in the original inoculum to the coat made available by the HBV infection of the host, a process that also takes place with interspecies passage of HDV to animals infected with hepadna-viruses different from HBV (Ponzetto, PNAS, 1987; 234:47).

Although superinfection can be self-limiting, it most often results in chronic HDV infection.[2] As continuing production of HBsAg secures the indefinite survival of the agent, providing the biological niche in which it can replicate and from which it can seed continuously, the chronic carrier of HBsAg/HDV represents the reservoir of HDV.

Reinfection in liver transplants

Early studies of HDV reinfection in liver transplants suggested that HDV may return very soon after surgery in these patients, without evidence of HBV reinfection detectable with conventional immuno-logical and hybridization-based assays (Ottobrelli, Gastro, 1991; 101:1649; Samuel, Hepatol, 1995; 21:333). However, HBV DNA has been detected in these patients with sensitive, polymerase chain reaction (**PCR**)-based assays (Smedile, Hepatol, 1994; 20:309A). Thus clinically latent HDV infections of liver grafts are not really autonomous but reflect a relatively constant rate of HDV synthesis (detectable with conventional assays) in the presence of very low levels of HBV synthesis (detectable only with sensitive PCR assays). Interestingly, the subsequent reactivation of HBV to full expression of its antigenic and genomic markers has enhanced massive HDV replication and has transformed latent HDV infections into florid hepatitis of the graft (Ottobrelli, Gastro, 1991; 101:1649); this would indicate that HBV plays a critical part and is an essential cofactor in the induction of HDV-related hepatocellular damage (Davies, AmJClinPath, 1992; 98:554).

Diagnosis

The 'gold standard' for diagnosis remains the detection of the HDAg in the liver by immunofluorescence or immunoenzymatic methods; however, this diagnostic approach is relatively impractical because it requires a liver biopsy. Screening for hepatitis D relies on indirect antibody markers that are the expression of the humoral response of the infected host. The clinical significance of recently developed, very sensitive PCR techniques in serum is not yet apparent; they are not generally available but available only to research laboratories (Table 2).

Viral markers

The finding in serum or liver of HDV RNA or of HDAg establishes the presence of active HDV infection. The intrahepatic antigen can be demonstrated by immunohistological techniques in frozen and in fixed liver specimens (Fig. 1);[1] fixed material must be pre-digested with protease (Stochlin, Hepatol, 1981; 1:238).

The intrahepatic distribution of the small and large HDAg is the same (Cullen, Hepatol, 1995; 22:1090). The intrahepatic expression of HDAg decreases as the disease progresses, thus increasing the probability of a false-negative result caused by sampling variation with needle biopsy (Negro, JHepatol, 1988; 6:8). A direct *in situ* hybridization technique has been developed to detect HDV RNA in fixed liver tissue (Negro, Hepatol, 1989; 10:916); non-radioactive procedures to determine intrahepatic HDV RNA have also been developed (Pacchioni, HumPath, 1992; 23:557).

To measure HD antigenaemia, serum must be pretreated with detergent in order to expose antigen within the HBsAg envelope. Conventional (available commercially) solid-phase immunosorbent tests for the measurement of HDAg in serum can detect antigen only during the early stage of primary infection, before the de-velopment of antibody to HDV (**anti-HD**); at the point at which the antibody appears in blood, HDAg is masked in immune com-plexes that render it unavailable to the assay. Thus HD antigenaemia is not demonstrable by straightforward radioimmunoassays or en-zyme-linked immunosorbent assays in patients with chronic HDV infection, who invariably have high serum titres of anti-HD.

Polyacrylamide gel electrophoresis under denaturing conditions allows the HDAg to separate from the respective antibody and the antigen can thus be detected in patients with chronic infection. The method is as sensitive as conventional molecular hybridization assays (Buti, Hepatol, 1989; 10:907). Alternatively, viraemia can be detected with genetic probes that hybridize with complementary HDV RNA. Strand-specific cRNA probes have lowered the de-tection limit to about 10^5–10^6 genome molecules per assay (Negro, JInfDis, 1988; 158:151). With gel-blot hybridization assays, HDV RNA has been detected in the serum of 64 per cent of patients with acute hepatitis D during the first week of illness and in 70 per cent of patients with chronic hepatitis D and intrahepatic HDAg (Smedile, Hepatol, 1986; 6:1297; Rasshofer, JInfDis, 1988; 157:191). The introduction of reverse transcriptase and PCR-based assays (Madejon, JHepatol, 1990; 11:381; Zignego, MolCellProbes, 1990; 4:43; Cariani, Hepatol, 1992; 15:685) has increased the limit

Table 1 Types of HDV infection		
	Coinfection with HBV in the normal individual	**Superinfection in the carrier of HBV**
Helper effect	Provided by coinfecting HBV	Provided by HBV of the carrier
Clinical course of primary infection	Variable	Usually severe
Chronicity	Rare (about 2%)	Frequent (70–80%)

Table 2 Diagnostic tests in hepatitis D virus infection

	Direct assays	Indirect assays
Liver	HDAg (IFL, HRPO) HDV-RNA (Northern blotting, RT-PCR, *in situ* hybridization)	anti-HD IgG anti-HD IgM anti-rHD IgM
Serum	Slot-blot (cDNA hybridization) Riboprobe (RNA hybridization) RT-PCR HDV-RNA Nested PCR HDV-RNA HDV genotyping: PCR direct sequencing, RFLP/PCRs	

IFL = immunofluorescence, HRPO = immunoperoxidase, r = recombinant, PCR = polymerase chain reaction, RT = reverse transcriptase, RFLP = restriction fragment length polymorphism.

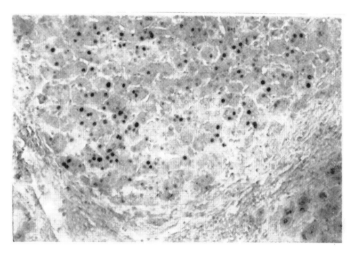

Fig. 1. Hepatitis delta antigen in the liver of a patient with chronic type D hepatitis, demonstrated by immunohistochemistry using a peroxidase-labelled anti-HD human antiserum.

of sensitivity to less than 10 genome molecules per assay [Negro, JHepatol, 1995; 22 (Suppl. 1):S136].

The use of PCR assays has shown that virtually all HBsAg carriers with chronic hepatitis D have continuing HDV replication; there is a strong correlation between the finding of HDAg in liver by immunostaining and of HDV RNA by PCR in blood (Simpson, DigDisSci, 1994; 39:2650).

HDV RNA was detected by PCR in 93 per cent of patients with HBV–HDV coinfection and in 100 per cent of those with HDV superinfection; with conventional dot-blot techniques the viral genome was found only in 60 per cent of the former and 62.5 per cent of the latter (Jardi, Hepatol, 1995; 21:25). The PCR assay is also useful in early diagnosis and in monitoring the effect of therapy with interferon [Madejon, JHepatol, 1993; 17 (Suppl. 3): S157; Tang, JHepatol, 1994; 21: 953]. However, the choice of suitable primers for the amplification of HDV RNA is difficult because of the extensive sequence heterogeneity of the different viral isolates; only a few conserved regions exist in the HDV genome, and secondary and tertiary constraints may further reduce the efficiency of reverse transcription. Amplification of the C-terminal half of the HDAg-coding region assures the highest degree of efficiency [Negro, JHepatol, 1995; 22 (Suppl 1):S136].

Antibody markers

Because of the limits to direct testing, screening for HDV relies primarily on indirect antibody testing. Indirect markers of HDV infection are the IgM anti-HD and total anti-HD.[5,6]

An immunoassay for antibodies against peptides encoded by a newly discovered, small open reading frame of HDV has been developed but its diagnostic significance is unknown (Khudyakov, VirRes, 1993; 27:13). IgM anti-HD is detected transiently in acute hepatitis D with a mean delay of 7 to 15 days from admission; it may be the only serum marker of acute HDV infection (Dimitrakakis, JMedVirol, 1986; 20:305; Aragona, Lancet, 1987; i:478). The IgM antibody persists and increases in titre as hepatitis D progresses to chronicity (Farci, JAMA, 1986; 225:1443).

During primary infections it consists essentially of pentameric 19*S* molecules; in chronic infections, monomeric 7*S* molecules become prevalent (Macagno, Gastro, 1990; 98:1582). The IgM antibody was considered an indicator of HDV-related liver damage (Farci, JAMA, 1986; 225:1443; Buti, Hepatol, 1989; 10:907) but this role has been questioned (Zignego, JHepatol, 1990; 11:102; Lau, JMedVirol, 1991; 33:273).

The IgG antibody is not protective; it is present in all immunocompetent patients with HDV infection and coexists with concurrent replication of HDV. It may also be present as a serological 'scar' in patients whose double HBV–HDV infection has resolved. It usually appears in acute hepatitis D but increases to high titres as HDV infection progresses to chronicity. High titres may help to distinguish chronic hepatitis D from past HDV infection, which is characterized by a low antibody titre.

Pathogenesis

Host immune reactions appear relevant to the pathogenesis of chronic hepatitis D: for example, the degree of cellular infiltration within the portal tracts and of lobular inflammation correlated with the number of HDAg-positive hepatocytes (Negro, JHepatol, 1988; 6:8). CD4 + T-cell clones specific for the repertoire of HDAg peptides have been isolated from patients with chronic hepatitis D, but lymphocyte-mediated cytotoxicity does not seem important in sustaining the infection (Wong, Proc. V Int. Symp. on Hepatitis Delta Virus and Liver Disease. Gold Coast, Australia, 28 August–3 September, 1995: Abstr. D13).

Aberrant humoral immune reactions detectable by immuno-fluorescence occur in many patients with chronic hepatitis D. About 50 per cent have autoantibodies against a 46-kDa antigen (Amengual, ClinExpImmun, 1989; 78:80) present in human thymocytes and in the basal-cell layer of the rodent forestomach (Zauli, Hepatol, 1984; 4:1103; Magnius, JInfDis, 1985; 152:232). A number of patients develop antibodies against nuclear lamin C (Wesierka-Gadek, Hepatol, 1990; 12:1129). About 15 per cent have an auto-antibody reacting with the microsomal membranes of the liver and kidney (Crivelli, ClinExpImmun, 1983; 54:232); this autoantibody has been named LKM3 to distinguish it from the LKM1 auto-antibody characteristic of idiopathic autoimmune hepatitis type 2 and present also in patients with chronic HCV infection (see Chapter 14.3). HDV-associated LKM3 is directed against a 55-kDa microsomal band containing UDP-glucuronyl transferase 1 (Philipp, Lancet, 1994; 344:578; Durazzo, Gastro, 1995; 108:455). The raising of LKM3 does not appear to be pathogenic or to aggravate the underlying chronic hepatitis D.

Direct viral cytotoxicity has been implicated as a major patho-genic mechanism in acute hepatitis D as well as a pathogenic component in cases of chronic disease. Microvesicular steatosis of hepatocytes was observed in epidemics of severe hepatitis D in South America (Popper, Hepatol, 1983; 3:906), in sporadic ful-minant hepatitis in the Western world (Lefkowitch, Gastro, 1987; 82:1262), and in HDV transplants experiencing a recurrence of acute hepatitis D in the graft (David, Gastro, 1993; 104:1122). Cytoplasmic eosinophilia and microvesicular steatosis without an inflammatory infiltrate were also observed in chronic hepatitis D (Verme, Hepatol, 1986; 6:1303). *In vitro* studies suggest that HDAg may be cytotoxic when expressed at high levels within the cell (Cole, Hepatol, 1991; 13:845); in HELA and HepG2 cell lines transfected with HDV-RNA constructs under the inducible control of the metallothionine promoter, the expression of the short form of HDAg caused apoptotic cell death. The cytopathic lesions could also be explained by a derangement in the secretory pathway of the hepatocytes. There are sequence similarities between regions of HDV RNA and regions of the human signal recognition particle (SRP) RNA, a small cytoplasmic protein–RNA complex involved in the correct targeting of secretory and membrane proteins to the membrane of the endoplasmic reticulum; therefore, replicative antigenomic intermediates of HDV RNA could base-pair to the corresponding SRP RNA regions, disturbing cell secretion (Negro, Nature, 1989; 341:111). Massive HDV replication could also in-terfere with the physiological processes directed by cellular RNA polymerases or with DNA replication and cell division. However, a number of observations argue against an intrinsic cytopathic effect of HDV, such as the lack of injury in liver grafts expressing HDAg (Ottobrelli, Gastro, 1991; 101:1649), in hepatocytes of transgenic mice expressing the short or long form of HDAg (Hsiedh, JVirol, 1990; 64:3192), and in hepatocytes of woodchucks expressing HDAg (Cullen, Hepatol, 1995; 22:1090).

Differences in pathogenicity might also depend on genetic factors related to HDV. A comparison of the sequence of a semiconserved region from 14 HDV-RNA isolates[7] has indicated that there are at least three different HDV genotypes, the first characteristic of Europe, North America, the Middle East, South Pacific and Asia, the second identified so far only in Japan, the third isolated from patients with severe hepatitis D in South America. The association of a particular genotype with severe forms of hepatitis D, such as those occurring in the Amazon basin, has led to the suggestion (Casey, JInfDis, 1996; 174:920) that genetic factors related to HDV heterogeneity may be important in determining variations in the clinical characteristics of HDV infections; however, a widely differ-ent spectrum of clinical conditions has been observed in association with HDV genotype 1 in Italy (Niro, Hepatol, 1997; 25:728).

Epidemiology
Transmission

HDV infection is acquired in the same way as HBV infection. Transmission is by the parenteral route, either overtly through blood and its derivatives or inapparently through personal contact. HDV is maintained by transmission through superinfection from carrier to carrier of the HBsAg; secondary extension of the virus to normal, HBsAg-negative individuals occurs in direct proportion to the rate of HBsAg carriers and in reverse proportion to the rate of HBV immunity (presence of anti-HBs) in contacts. Spread to non-carriers has no long-term epidemiological consequences as it results in self-limiting forms of HBV–HDV infection.

Vertical transmission of HDV has been documented rarely (Zanetti, JMedVirol, 1982; 9:139). It is probably a form of super-infection in a baby that has previously acquired HBV. Perinatal HDV transmission is rare because the majority of HDV carrier mothers have inactive, HBV DNA-negative, HBV infections and do not transmit the helper virus necessary for HDV replication.

The relative efficiency of HDV transmission differs from that of HBV. Intravenous drug addicts are the most frequent victims of HDV, as they are of other blood-borne infections. HDV-infected drug addicts are often also infected with the hepatitis C virus (HCV). In this setting the infection is associated with high mor-bidity, and clustered epidemics of fulminant hepatitis D have been reported in drug-abusing communities of the United States and western Europe (Raimondo, Lancet, 1982; i:249; Lettau, NEJM, 1987; 317:1256).

Though clinically obscured by the importance of the im-munodeficiency syndrome, an association has also emerged between HDV and the human immunodeficiency virus (HIV) in drug ad-dicts, haemophiliacs, and homosexuals, among whom both viruses share the same means of transmission (Novick, JInfDis, 1988; 158: 795).

The risk of HDV from blood screened for HBsAg is very low as the control of HBV eliminates virtually all blood containing HDV.[8]

Promiscuous activities, in particular sexual intercourse, that involve exchange of body fluids constitute a risk for HDV transmission; high rates of hepatitis D have been found in heterosexual partners of HDV-infected individuals and among Taiwanese and Greek, HBsAg-posi-tive prostitutes (Liaw, JInfDis, 1990; 162:1170; Tassopoulos, ProgClinBiolRes, 1993; 324:221). The risk of HDV infection in specific settings, such as in medical personnel, haemodialysis units, in-stitutionalized patients, prisoners, and haemophiliacs receiving co-agulation-factor concentrates, has varied depending on the degree of penetration of the virus and on standards of HBV control; with the general improvement of control achieved in recent years in developed countries, HDV infection has declined in these settings also.

Geographical prevalence

HDV infection occurs worldwide, the most important factor influencing its spread being the rate of HBV infection within the population. However, there are large geographical variations independent from the prevalence of HBV. Predictably, the rate of hepatitis D is low in North European and North American countries where the prevalence of HBV is also low. High prevalence rates of HDV infection have been reported in tropical and subtropical areas of Africa and the South American continent where HBV is hyperendemic, yet very low prevalence rates were reported in the Far East and among Alaskan Eskimos despite high local prevalence of HBV.

In the Mediterranean basin the prevalence of HDV infections in the 1970s and 1980s was intermediate between the low of northern Europe and the high of subtropical and tropical areas, with a composite epidemiological pattern resulting form endemic infection in the general population and epidemic outbreaks among drug addicts in urban areas. The infection was peaking around the fourth decade of life (Ponzetto, EurJEpid, 1985; 1:257). Spread occurred within the household (Bonino, JHepatol, 1985; 1:221), facilitated by promiscuity and overcrowding, as well as by cultural practices such as tattooing and acupuncture.[2]

Epidemiological surveys in the 1990s indicate a significant decrease in the prevalence of acute and chronic hepatitis D in many areas of the world and in particular in southern Europe (Hadziyannis, ProgClinBiolRes, 1994; 382:259; Navascuez, AmJGastr, 1995; 90:1981). In this area the increased control of HBV fostered by the impact of public health measures to control the acquired immune deficiency syndrome (**AIDS**) and by the implementation of vaccination has consistently decreased the circulation of HBV infection and, as a consequence, the local prevalence of HDV infection is rapidly decreasing. In Italy, Spain, and Greece the rate of HDV among carriers of the HBsAg with chronic liver disease has diminished to less than 10 per cent from as high as 40 per cent in the 1970s. In a recent survey the incidence rate of acute hepatitis D has dropped in Italy from 3.1/1 00 000 inhabitants in 1987 to 1.2/100 000 in 1992 (Stroffolini, JHepatol, 1994; 21:1123). Aside from the global reduction of HBV infection, a second major determinant of the decrease in HDV infection among the Italian population has been the reduction of family sizes; in Southern Italian families, overcrowding was one of the major risk for the spreading of the HDV in the household (Sagnelli, JHepatol, 1992; 15:211).

Despite the general decline of HDV infection in the Western world, hepatitis D remains a scourge in the developing world, with about 15 000 000 carriers of HBsAg also infected by HDV. In addition, new foci of HDV endemicity have been identified in recent years in Albania (Dalekos, EurJGastroHepatol, 1995; 7:553), in North India (Singh, JViralHepat, 1995; 2:151) in areas of China (Li, Proc. V Int. Symp. on Hepatitis Delta Virus and Liver Disease. Gold Coast, Australia, 28 August–3 September 1995: Abstr. D22), and in Okinawa (Sakugawa, JMedVirol, 1995; 45:312).

Disease
Acute hepatitis D

The clinical manifestations of acute hepatitis D are non-specific and do not differ significantly between coinfections and superinfections.

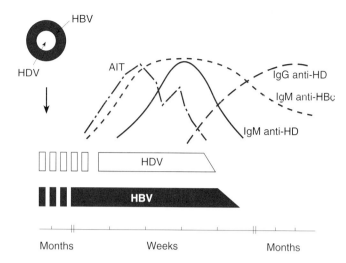

Fig. 2. Course of typical HBV–HDV coinfection; AIT, alanine aminotransferase.

In either condition, severe and fulminant forms of hepatitis occur more frequently than in ordinary acute hepatitis B.[9]

In coinfections the serological picture may show the classic features of acute HBV infection [including IgM antihepatitis B core antigen (**HBc**)] with superimposed markers of HDV (Fig. 2). When HDV expression is minor, the severity of coinfection hepatitis is essentially related to the virulence of the associated HBV infection; HD antigenaemia is not usually detectable and the specific antibody response may be absent. Transient viraemia may be detected by PCR. When HDV expression is conspicuous, the disease may be severe or fulminant; these forms exhibit a full serological response consisting of early HD antigenaemia followed by seroconversion to anti-HD, initially of the IgM and then of the IgG class.

In drug addicts, coinfection frequently tends to run a biphasic course with two peaks of liver necrosis a few weeks apart (Govindarajan, Gut, 1986; 27:19).

The antibody response to HDV is relatively slow; the initial IgM response may be delayed for days to weeks after the onset of hepatitis and the IgG response may first appear during convalescence.[6] Therefore, prolonged monitoring for antibodies to HDV is required to exclude or confirm HDV coinfection in patients presenting with HBsAg-positive hepatitis suspected to have hepatitis D.

The clinical presentation of HDV superinfection in patients chronically infected by HBV depends on whether they were asymptomatic carriers of HBsAg, or whether clinical features of type B hepatitis were present. In the asymptomatic carrier, superinfection appears as an intercurrent hepatitis; in the patient with chronic type B hepatitis it may be mistaken for an exacerbation of the underlying HBV disease (Raimondo, BMJ, 1983; 286:845). In asymptomatic carriers unaware of their HBsAg state, superinfection may mimic classic acute hepatitis B since a positive HBsAg test suggests this diagnosis, if it is first performed after infection with HDV. Clues to the nature of the disease are positive HDV serology and an incomplete or atypical HBV profile (superinfected carriers, unlike patients with acute hepatitis B, may lack the IgM antibody to the HBcAg). Progressive HDV disease developing in superinfected carriers unaware of their state may also mimic progressive hepatitis

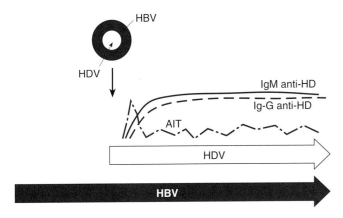

Fig. 3. Course of typical HDV superinfection in HBsAg carriers; AIT, alanine aminotransferase .

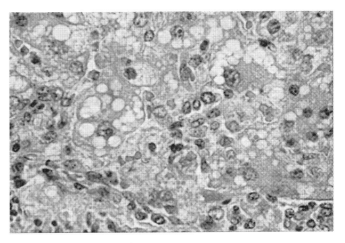

Fig. 4. Small-droplet steatosis in a case of fulminant delta hepatitis in the Amazon basin (by courtesy of Professor L. Da Costa Gayotto, São Paulo, Brazil).

B and is easily confused with this entity (Farci, Gastro, 1983; 85: 669).

In superinfection the antibody response is more uniform and consistent than in coinfection. There is a relatively brisk IgM and IgG anti-HD response; both antibodies increase in a few weeks when superinfection progresses to chronicity, and may persist in high titres as hepatitis D continues (Fig. 3). In patients whose chronic hepatitis D resolves, the IgM antibody disappears rapidly while IgG anti-HD declines slowly. The IgM antibody is absent in carriers of HBsAg who circulate IgG (total) anti-HD, but have no liver disease.

Whether acquired by coinfection with HBV or superinfection in a chronic HBsAg carrier, HDV can precipitate an episode of fulminant hepatitis. The relative role of coinfection and superinfection in the pathogenesis of fulminant hepatitis varies worldwide according to local epidemiological features (Saracco, AnnIntMed, 1988; 108:380). In the tropics, where the rate of HBsAg carriage is very high, most fulminant hepatitides associated with HDV are acquired by superinfection; in industrialized countries they occur predominantly in drug addicts who acquire HDV infection together with HBV. In this setting, HDV RNA may be the only marker of viral infection; it may only be detectable after PCR amplification (Wu, Hepatol, 1994; 19:836). In exotic cases of fulminant hepatitis D the microscopic appearance has resembled microvesicular steatosis (Fig. 4), or a foamy degeneration, similar to that seen in children with Reye's syndrome and in patients with drug-induced injury (Popper, Hepatol, 1983; 3:906); these aspects have been observed only occasionally in fulminant hepatitis D in developed countries (Lefkowitch, Gastro, 1987; 82:1262).

Atypical acute hepatitis D

The course of HDV infection may be confounded by the inhibitory effect exerted by HDV on replication of HBV. In coinfection, early repression of HBV can produce a picture of HBsAg-negative hepatitis resembling a non-B hepatitis (Caredda, JInfDis, 1989; 159: 977). Sequential expression of HBV and HDV may result in a biphasic hepatitis where the first episode is associated with HDV and the second with HBV, or vice versa.[9] The most striking example of HBV suppression is the termination of the HBsAg carrier state by acute superinfection (Moestrup, BMJ, 1983; 286:

87). This event has reported in as many as 10 per cent of superinfected carriers (De Cock, AnnIntMed, 1986; 105:108).

Transient suppression of pre-existing HB viraemia can create diagnostic confusion because, as well as a negative HBsAg test caused by marked inhibition of HBV at the time of superinfection, anti-HBs can temporarily appear in these patients, simulating the resolution of an acute HBV hepatitis (Fig. 5); the HBsAg, however, returns at the termination of the florid HDV infection.[9]

Chronic hepatitis D

Early clinical studies emphasized the link between HDV infection and severe liver disease, leading to the concept that chronic HDV infection is almost invariably pathogenic.[9,10] However, further studies in Greece and in American Samoa, where HDV is endemic, have shown that a large percentage of HBsAg carriers with anti-HD have no clinical or biochemical sign of liver disease.[11] Thus it now appears that HDV infection is associated with a spectrum of clinical conditions ranging from the asymptomatic carriage of the virus to fulminant hepatitis and cirrhosis.

Nevertheless, patients with chronic hepatitis D suffer from a disease that is more serious and progressive than ordinary hepatitis B. Studies conducted in the 1970s and 1980s in Europe and the United States have shown that markers of HDV were more prevalent in HBsAg carriers with chronic hepatitis than in apparently healthy carriers, and in carriers with liver damage the prevalence of

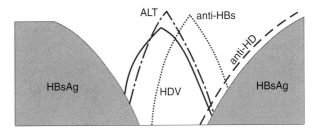

Fig. 5. HDV superinfection inducing repression of HBV to the point where HBsAg becomes temporarily undetectable. A transient anti-HBs reactivity often occurs in this setting. With termination of florid HDV infection the HBsAg returns in serum and anti-HBs disappears.

HDV was higher in those with chronic active hepatitis or cirrhosis than in those with chronic persistent hepatitis;[2] in apparently asymptomatic Italian carriers with anti-HD the liver biopsy often shows occult but significant damage (Arico, Lancet 1985; ii:356).

In about 10 to 15 per cent of patients with hepatitis D the disease rapidly progresses to liver failure (within 6 months to 2 years from exposure to HDV). This rapidly evolving form was described in the 1980s in drug addicts with HDV disease sustained by **HBe** (early)**Ag**-positive (wild-type) HBV infection (Saracco, JHepatol, 1987; 5:274). Many of these cases were probably also infected by HCV; since diagnostic tests for hepatitis C became available in the 1990s, HCV infection has been found in 70 to 80 per cent of HDV-infected drug addicts; thus a proportion of rapidly evolving (subacute) forms of hepatitis D are probably caused by multiple viral infections. In one study, concurrent HCV superinfection tended to suppress detection of HDAg in the liver (Liaw, JMed-Virol, 1992; 37:294). In two other studies, coexistent HBV–HDV infection appeared to have suppressed HCV replication (Coppola, EurJEpid, 1994; 10:79; Simpson, DigDisSci, 1994; 39:2650). The prevalence of HIV infection is high among parenteral drug addicts with chronic hepatitis D. In two series, from New York and Barcelona, 58 and 68 per cent of patients, respectively, had been exposed to HIV (Novick, JInfDis, 1991; 163:1351).

Concomitant HIV infection does not seem to modify the course of hepatitis D when the disease in HIV-positive patients is compared with the natural course of hepatitis D in HIV-negative patients (Castillo, Digestion, 1991; 48:149; Monno, JMedVirol, 1991; 34:199). Immunocompromised patients with AIDS who are also infected with HDV may have blunted IgM HD responses (Monno, JMedVirol, 1991; 34:199). They may exhibit atypical patterns of persistent HD antigenaemia, detectable with straight commercial assays for HDAg, with low or absent anti-HD (Grippon, Lancet, 1987; i:1013; Roingeard, JMedVirol, 1992; 38:191). Serum HDAg or HDV RNA has been found in these patients without detectable HBsAg (Castillo, Digestion, 1991; 48:149).

A survey of 148 Italian patients with chronic hepatitis from 1977 to 1994 has shown two patterns of disease. In about 10 per cent the disease was mild, non-progressive, and characterized at histology by a chronic persistent hepatitis. In the other 90 per cent the disease has been progressive and characterized by chronic active hepatitis or active cirrhosis. Transition to anatomical cirrhosis was usually rapid, with about 30 to 40 per cent of the patients with non-cirrhotic disease at baseline developing cirrhosis within 5 years of follow-up; however, the cirrhotic stage often remained clinically stable for decades, and the course of cirrhosis was asymptomatic over many years (Rosina, Proc. V Symp. on Hepatitis Delta Virus and Liver Disease. Gold Coast, Australia, 28 August–3 September 1995: Abstr. D21; Giustozi, *ibid.*: D19). After the first episode of decompensation the probability of survival at 5 years is no more than 30 per cent.

In children the course of chronic hepatitis D is as progressive as in adults. In two series collected in the early 1980s and the beginning of 1990s (Farci, Gut, 1985; 26:4; Bortolotti, JPediat, 1993; 122:736), the prevalence of HDV infection among children with chronic HBsAg-positive hepatitis with cirrhosis was 34 and 30 per cent, respectively; anti-HD is very rarely seen in childhood carriers of HBsAg without liver disease. In the Mediterranean countries, HDV infection represents one of the most important causes of juvenile cirrhosis.

The clinical features of chronic hepatitis D are not distinctive. Patients with advanced chronic hepatitis D often exhibit a marked enlargement of the spleen. They may develop a variety of auto-antibodies; about 5 per cent have serum autoantibodies against the microsomal membranes of the liver and kidney (Crivelli, ClinExp-Immun, 1983; 54:232). In contrast to the usual lack of past history obtained from ordinary carriers of HBsAg, about 70 per cent of those with chronic HDV disease report an attack of acute hepatitis in the past, probably corresponding to the time of superinfection with HDV.

The pathological aspects of hepatitis D are non-specific; the majority of the patients exhibit necroinflammatory lesions indistinguishable from those induced by ordinary hepatitis B. In 70 per cent of 206 liver biopsies collected in Turin from 1976 to 1984 the histological picture was that of a chronic active hepatitis with a high degree of piecemeal perilobular necrosis, marked lobular involvement, and an eosinophilic granular degeneration of hepatocytes unaccompanied by peripolesis of lymphocytes (Verme, Hepatol, 1986; 6:1303).

In most cases HBV infection is repressed. HBV DNA is often detectable only with sensitive PCR techniques but may be undetectable with these techniques also (Simpson, DigDisSci, 1994; 39:2650; Wu, Gastro, 1995; 108:796). The underlying HBV strain sustaining HDV is usually the 'HBeAg minus' variant and the majority of patients have anti-HBe in serum. Wild-type replicative forms of HBV can also support HDV; although less frequent, this association causes severe liver damage.

In a recent PCR study (Wu, Gastro 1995; 108:796) the virological profile of chronic hepatitis D was shown to consist of three phases: an early phase following superinfection characterized by elevated alanine aminotransferase, active HDV replication, and suppression of HBV: an intermediate phase characterized by moderately elevated alanine aminotransferase, decreasing HDV synthesis, and reactivation of HBV; and a late cirrhotic phase characterized by marked reduction of the synthesis of both HBV and HDV.

The recent changes in the epidemiology of HDV have had a major impact on the medical setting of hepatitis D. In the period 1976 to 1981, 81 per cent of 237 HDV carriers without risk factors for parenteral exposure to hepatitis viruses seen in Turin had a chronic active hepatitis or active cirrhosis; in contrast only 35 per cent of 112 patients collected in the period 1987 to 1992 had an active disease, while the proportion of those with advanced inactive cirrhosis had risen to 40 per cent. The relative increase of the latter subgroup probably represents cohorts of patients who acquired HDV infection in past decades, when HDV was more diffuse; with the recent decline of helper HBV and consequent decline of HDV the early stages characterized by productive HDV infection and inflammation are much less frequently observed. The medical corollary is that the proportion of potentially treatable and reversible chronic hepatitis D is decreasing markedly, while the bulk of the disease is now represented by endstage cirrhosis; throughout the Mediterranean area the number of HDV patients becoming candidates for liver transplantation is disproportionately high compared to the current low epidemiological impact of the infection.

References

1. Rizzetto M, *et al.* Immunofluorescence detection of a new antigen antibody system (delta anti-delta) associated with hepatitis B virus in liver and in serum of HBsAg carriers. *Gut*, 1977; **18**: 997–1003.

2. Rizzetto M, Verme G, Gerin JL, and Purcell RH. Hepatitis delta virus disease. In Popper H and Schaffner E, eds. *Progress in liver disease VIII*. New York: Grune and Stratton, 1986: 417–31.

3. Smedile A, *et al.* Infection with the HBV associated delta agent in HBsAg carriers. *Gastroenterology*, 1981; **81**: 992–7.

4. Rizzetto M, *et al.* Transmission of hepatitis B virus associated delta antigen to chimpanzees. *Journal of Infection Diseases*, 1980; **121**: 590–602.

5. Smedile A, *et al.* Radioimmunoassay detection of IgM antibodies to the HBV-associated delta antigen; clinical significance in delta infection. *Journal of Medical Virology*, 1982; **9**: 131–8.

6. Rizzetto M, *et al.* Incidence and significance of antibodies to delta antigen in hepatitis B virus infection. *Lancet*, 1979; **ii**: 986–90.

7. Casey JL, Brown TL, Colan EJ, Wignall FS, and Gerin JL. A genotype of hepatitis D virus that occurs in northern South America. *Proceedings of the National Academy of Sciences (USA)*, 1993; **90**: 9016–20.

8. Rosina F, Saracco G, and Rizzetto M. Risk of post transfusion infection with the hepatitis delta virus. *New England Journal of Medicine*, 1985; **312**: 1488–91.

9. Rizzetto M, Gerin JL, and Purcell RH. The hepatitis delta virus (HDV) and its infection. *Progress in Clinical and Biological Research*, 1986; **234**: 361–521.

10. Rizzetto M, *et al.* Chronic HBsAg hepatitis with intrahepatic expression of delta antigen. An active and progressive disease unresponsive to immunosuppressive treatment. *Annals of Internal Medicine*, 1983; **98**: 437–41.

11. Smedile A, Rizzetto M, and Gerin JL. Advances in hepatitis D virus biology and disease. In Boyer JL and Ockner RK, eds. *Progress in liver disease XII*. Philadelphia: Saunders, 1994: 157–75.

12.1.2.5 Hepatitis C

Alfredo Alberti and Flavia Bortolotti

Definition

This disease is caused by the hepatitis C virus (**HCV**) (Choo, Science, 1989; 244:359), an RNA virus which shares genomic similarities with the pestiviruses and has been classified within the flaviviridae family (Choo, PNAS, 1191; 88:2451). Significant genomic heterogeneity has been observed among different HCV isolates, leading to the classification of HCV into at least nine distinct genotypes designated by Arabic numerals (i.e. HCV-1, HCV-2, HCV-3, etc.) and into subtypes identified by lower case letters (i.e. HCV-1a, HCV-1b, HCV-1c, etc.) (Simmonds, Hepatol, 1994; 19:1321).

Hepatitis C virus is a bloodborne agent transmitted parenterally. Before the discovery of HCV, blood transfusion was a frequent cause of hepatitis C transmission. With the implementation of anti-HCV screening in blood donors, the risk of post-transfusion hepatitis C has been dramatically reduced, but the infection continues to occur via other modes of apparent and inapparent parenteral transmission.

Hepatitis C has a global distribution. The prevalence of chronic infection is very high in risk groups, such as intravenous drug abusers, patients with haemophilia, and those who have received multiple blood transfusions, and may often exceed 70 to 80 per cent. Infection with HCV often results in chronicity, due to the high propensity of the virus to persist by evading attack by the immune system.

The diagnosis rests upon the detection in serum of a set of antiviral antibodies (anti-HCV) and of viral genomic sequences (HCV RNA). Currently anti-HCV is detected by enzyme-linked immunosorbent assays (anti-HCV **ELISA**) which measure antibodies against a variety of structural and non-structural antigens of HCV. These assays may give non-specific 'false positive' reactions when used for screening 'low-risk' individuals without obvious signs of liver disease; in this context, confirmation of the specificity of the reaction by immunoblotting assays (anti-HCV RIBA) is mandatory.

Serum HCV RNA is detected by the polymerase chain reaction using primers derived from the most conserved 5′ untranslated region (5′UTR) of HCV RNA. This test is not used for screening but is essential for the diagnosis of hepatitis C in a number of clinical settings. Quantification of HCV RNA and characterization of the HCV genotype can be accomplished by a variety of methods, including commercial assays.

HCV causes acute and chronic hepatocellular damage of variable severity and evolution (Fig. 1). Infection may also occur in extrahepatic cells and tissues leading to a spectrum of extrahepatic disorders which include immunological abnormalities, autoimmune phenomena and diseases, cryoglobulinaemia, vasculitis, and possibly other types of immunocomplex disease. Many patients have low titres of autoantibodies in their serum that may be organ or non-organ specific; a small subgroup develops antibodies to liver/kidney microsomal antigens (**anti-LKM**), mimicking the serological profile of type 2 'autoimmune' hepatitis. The relationship of HCV to other disorders such as porphyria cutanea tarda, thyroiditis, sialadenitis, and B-cell non–Hodgkin lymphomas remains unclear.

Acute HCV infection is defined as an infection of less than 6 months duration. Most often, acute infections are asymptomatic and remain clinically unrecognized. Severe and fulminant hepatitis C is extremely rare. Only a few patients with acute hepatitis C recover completely with virus eradication; in most the acute infection progresses to chronicity. Chronic HCV infection is defined as HCV infection lasting more than 6 months with or without clinical manifestations of hepatic or extrahepatic diseases. Carriers of the virus exist with no signs or symptoms of liver disease and with normal levels of serum alanine aminotransferase (**ALT**), but many have underlying chronic liver lesions on liver biopsy. Biochemically active forms of chronic hepatitis C are characterized by variable ALT profiles and by histological changes ranging from mild to severe inflammation and fibrosis. Progression to cirrhosis occurs slowly, and in an unpredictable way in a subgroup of patients who may ultimately die of portal hypertension, hepatic failure, or hepatocellular carcinoma. The downhill course of chronic liver disease is accelerated by a number of aetiological cofactors, including coinfection with hepatitis B virus and alcohol excess. Much remains to be understood about the natural course of chronic hepatitis C and on the causes and markers of disease progression in the individual patient.

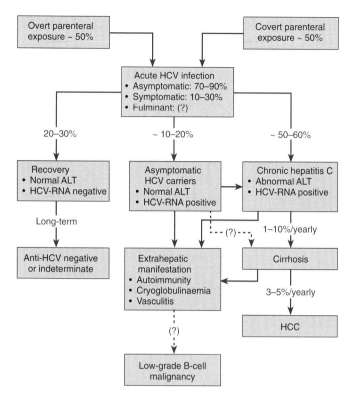

Fig. 1. The spectrum of hepatitis C.

Historical background

Following the development of serological tests for the diagnosis of hepatitis A and B, it became evident in the mid-1970s that there were many cases of 'infectious' hepatitis unrelated to either agent (Alter, Lancet, 1975; ii:838; Feinstone, NEJM, 1975; 292:767; Prince, Lancet, 1975; ii:241; Villarejos, NEJM, 1975; 293:1350).

The name 'non-A, non-B (**NANB**) hepatitis' was coined for a diagnosis based upon exclusion criteria, in the absence of specific assays for the aetiological agent(s). Milestones in the history of hepatitis NANB and of its development into hepatitis C are listed in Table 1. In the late 1970s and early 1980s it became clear that NANB infection was responsible for 15 to 50 per cent of all cases of acute viral hepatitis in adults and that major risk factors for community-acquired NANB hepatitis were blood transfusion, use of parenteral drugs, and occupational (e.g. health personnel) contact with infected patients (Alter, InfectImmunBloodTransf, 1985; 71: 341). It also became obvious that about 40 per cent of all patients in the community with acute NANB hepatitis had no overt parenteral exposure to contaminated materials or other risk factors which could explain the acquisition of the disease (Dienstag, AnnIntMed, 1977; 87:1; Bamber, Gut, 1983; 24:5611; Francis, AmJMed, 1984; 76:69). Successful transmission of NANB hepatitis to experimental animals (Hoofnagle, AnnIntMed, 1977; 87:14; Alter, Lancet, 1978; i:463; Hollinger, IntVirol, 1978; 10:60; Bradley, JMedVirol, 1979; 3:253), together with retrospective analysis of viral hepatitis transmission to human volunteers in the 1950s (Murray, JAMA, 1954; 154:1072; Hoofnagle, AnnIntMed, 1977; 87:14), provided conclusive evidence that NANB hepatitis was caused by transmissible agents. In the attempt to detect NANB agents and markers, many investigators pursued immunological techniques that had proven

successful in the identification of hepatitis A and B viruses and their respective antigen/antibody systems. However, repeated claims of the discovery of specific serological markers and putative virus particles during the decade 1978 to 1988 were not substantiated (Dienstag, Gastro, 1983; 85:743).

With the discovery of the hepatitis C virus in 1989 (Choo, Science, 1989; 244:359) (see Chapter 13.1.3.1) and the development of specific serological tests for the diagnosis of this infection, it became evident that HCV was responsible for most cases of parenterally acquired (Alter, NEJM, 1989; 321:1494; Van Der Poel, Lancet, 1989; ii:297; Mosley, JAMA, 1990; 263:77; Tremolada, AnnIntMed, 1991; 114:277) and community-acquired (Alter, NEJM, 1989; 321:1538; Bortolotti, JHepatol, 1991; 12:176) NANB hepatitis worldwide. These findings were soon confirmed and further completed by data indicating that most patients with chronic NANB (or cryptogenic) liver disease were positive for anti-HCV, including those with cirrhosis and hepatocellular carcinoma (Esteban, Lancet, 1989; ii:294; Jeffers, Hepatol, 1989; 10:644; Parker, Hepatol, 1989; 10:685; Sansonno, Lancet, 1989; ii:798), leading to the conclusion that HCV was the causative agent in the vast majority of non-alcoholic, non-autoimmune, HBsAg-negative cases of chronic liver disease.[1]

Epidemiology

The global prevalence of HCV infection is estimated around 3 per cent in the general population with more than 150 million carriers in the world (WHO, WklyEpidemiolRec, 1997; 72:65). Reported prevalence rates in the community vary depending on the specificity and sensitivity of the method used, but also according to the geographical origin and the characteristics of the population studied. Many prevalence studies have been conducted in blood donors; a few large surveys are available from the general population. Most have not included confirmatory testing and should therefore be interpreted with caution, given the frequent lack of specificity when anti-HCV is screened for in low-risk individuals. High-risk groups with high prevalences of hepatitis C have been identified; the incidence of infection and disease in some of these groups is continually changing as a consequence of changes in the prevailing transmission mode. Hepatitis C is transmitted by apparent and inapparent parenteral routes; the type and size of the inoculum, route of transmision, titre of virus, and immunocompetence of the host may affect the efficiency of transmission.

Geographical distribution of HCV genotypes

The epidemiology of HCV infection was recently studied in relation to the geographical prevalence of the different HCV genotypes (see Chapter 12.1.2.1). These are not uniformly distributed around the world (Tokita, PNAS, 1994; 91:11022; Simmonds, Hepatol, 1995; 21:2; Mellor, JClinMicrobiol, 1996; 34:417). In some areas the range of HCV types is limited but there are many different subtypes (HCV-1 and HCV-2 in West Africa; HCV-3 in India; HCV-4 in Central Africa and Egypt; HCV-6 in South-East Asia). HCV-1, HCV-2, and HCV-3 are common in western Europe, North America, and Australia, while HCV-1 and HCV-2 are predominant in Japan.

Table 1 The history of parenterally acquired NANB (non-A, non-B; type C) hepatitis

Year		References
1974–1975	Recognition that post-transfusion hepatitis is not due to hepatitis A and B	Prince, Lancet, 1975; ii:241; Alter, Lancet, 1975; ii:838; Feinstone, NEJM, 1975; 292:767
1975	First description of NANB hepatitis unrelated to overt parenteral exposure	Villarejos, NEJM, 1975; 293:1350
1977–1978	NANB hepatitis due to transmissible agents	Hoofnagle, AnnIntMed, 1977; 87:14; Tabor, Lancet, 1978; i: 463; Alter, Lancet, 1978; i:459
1980	More that one aetiological agent as a cause of NANB hepatitis	Tsiquaye, JMedVirol, 1980; 5:63; Hollinger, JInfDis, 1980; 142:400
1979–1982	Definition of clinical features and chronic sequelae	Berman, AnnIntMed, 1979; 91:1; Realdi, Gut, 1982; 23:270
1980–1983	Successful chemical inactivation of NANB agents	Tabor, JInfDis, 1980; 142:767; Yoshizawa, Gastro, 1982; 82: 502
1978–1988	A decade of unsuccessful efforts to identify viruses or antigen/antibody systems	Dienstag, Gastro, 1983; 85:743; Alter, TransfusMedRev, 1982; 2:288
1989	Identification of hepatitis C virus, the major agent of parenterally acquired NANB hepatitis	Choo, Science, 1989; 244:359; Kuo, Science, 1989; 244:362

Worldwide prevalence of HCV markers in blood donors and in the general population[2,3]

Table 2 shows prevalence rates of anti-HCV in blood donors and in the general population, using second or third generation assays and supplemental tests to confirm the specificity of the anti-HCV reaction. Low rates are found in North America and western Europe, intermediate rates in Japan, and high rates in some areas of eastern Europe, the Middle East, and South America. The number of infected individuals is very high in Egypt. Reported prevalence rates in blood donors may underestimate the real impact of infection in the general population as blood donors represent a selected group. Few prevalence studies have been performed in the general population. Representative prevalences of anti-HCV positivity around the world are presented in Table 2. In many reports, HCV infection is more common in males; this could reflect a more efficient clearance of HCV by females (Yamakawa, JViralHepat, 1996; 3: 317). There is evidence for an age-related distribution of infection, with prevalences which are minimal in childhood and progressively higher with increasing age (Sirchia, Lancet, 1989; ii:797; Lee, Hepatol, 1991; 13:830; Hepatitis Surveillance Report No 55, CDC, Atlanta, 1994). In the United States, the highest rates of HCV infection were found in adults aged between 30 and 49 years in the third National Health and Nutrition Examination Survey (Alter, AntiviralTher, 1996; 1:9), while community-based surveys conducted in Europe and in the Mediterranean area have detected the highest prevalence rates in the oldest age groups (Guadagnino, JHepatol, 1997; 26(Suppl.1):73; Nalpas, European Survey on Hepatitis C, 1997). In Italy, prevalence of HCV infection in the elderly exceeds 30 per cent in some areas of the south (Guadaquino, Hepatol, 1997; 26:1006).

Prevalence of HCV markers in high-risk groups

Prevalence rates of anti-HCV in risk groups are reported in Table 3. A wide range of prevalence has been reported in different studies, suggesting that geographical origin, race, age, and environment may significantly affect the risk of acquiring HCV by these individuals.

Prevalence of HCV markers in patients with liver disease

The incidence data on symptomatic community-acquired acute hepatitis C in the United States showed an average rate of 8/ 100 000 cases between 1983 and 1989, with a subsequent 63 per cent decline (3/100 000 cases) between 1990 and 1994 (Alter, Hepatol, 1997; 26:62S). In Italy an attack rate around 2/100 000 has been observed in the 1990s (Bortolotti, Infec, 1994; 22:321), and was reduced to 1/100 000 in 1996.

HCV has been proven responsible for 70 to 95 per cent of acute post-transfusion and 5 to 60 per cent of community-acquired acute hepatitis (Alter, JAMA, 1990; 264:2231; Bortolotti, JHepatol, 1991; 12:176; McHutchison, Gastro, 1991; 101:1117; Buti, JHepatol, 1994; 20:589).

The prevalence of chronic HCV infection in patients with chronic hepatitis, cirrhosis, and hepatocellular carcinoma is very high in Europe and Japan (60 to 90 per cent), intermediate in the United States, Australia, and Africa (30 to 60 per cent), and lower in China and in other countries of the Far East (10 to 30 per cent). The highest prevalence of anti-HCV positivity is found in patients who have acquired chronic liver disease from blood transfusion or have a well recognized risk for parenteral contamination in the past history. The prevalence of HCV infection in patients with chronic hepatitis, cirrhosis, and hepatocellular carcinoma varies in the world

Table 2 Prevalence of anti-HCV in blood donors and in the general populations from different geographical areas

	% Anti-HCV positive	References
Studies in blood donors		
Scandinavia	0.01–0.1*	Mathiesen, ScaJGastr, 1993; 28:581; Nordoy, ScaJGastr, 1994; 29:77
United Kingdom	0.01–0.07*	Bow, JMedVirol, 1993; 41:215; Conlon, IrJMedSci, 1993; 162:145
Greece	0.7*	Hadziyannis, JHepatol, 1993; 17:572
France	0.3*	Ranger, Gut, 1993; 34(Suppl. 2):S50
Italy	0.8*	Lai, JMedVirol, 1993; 41:282
Croatia	0.7*	Mihaljevic, VoxSang, 1992; 63:236
Russia	1.4–4.8*	Mikhailov, p. 175 in ref. 4
United States	0.5*	Kleinman, Transfusion, 1992; 32:805
Brazil	2.9*	Patino Sarcinelli, Transfusion, 1994; 34:138
Australia	0.06–0.31*	Archer, MedJAust, 1992; 157:225; National Health and Medical Research Council Report, 1993
New Zealand	0.1*	Jackson, NZMedJ, 1994; 107:10
China, Macau	0.9*	Aach, NEJM, 1991; 325:1325
Japan	1.9*	Yano, Gut, 1993; 34(Suppl. 2):S13
Saudi Arabia	3.2	Abdelaal, Transfusion, 1994; 34:135
Egypt	25	Arthur, Triennal, p. 178 in ref. 4
Ethiopia	1.4	Frommel, AmJTropMedHyg, 1993; 49:435
Studies in the general population		
France	0.68*	Janot, Hepatol, 1995; 21:725
Italy	3.2	Bellentani, Hepatol, 1994; 20:1442
United States	1.4*	Alter, SemLivDis, 1995; 15:5
Peru	0	Hyams, JMedVirol, 1992; 37:127
Africa	0.6–6.5*	Fromel, AmJTropMedHyg, 1993; 49:435; Delaporte, TrRSocTropMedHyg, 1993; 87: 6366; Abdool Karim, SAMedJ, 1993; 83:191
Korea	1	Kim, GastrJap, 1993; 28:17
Yemen	2.6*	Scott, AmJTropMedHyg, 1992; 46:63
Taiwan	5.6	Chien, JGastrHepatol, 1993; 8:574
Japan	5.1	Tajima, Lancet, 1991; 337:1410
China	2.1	Tao, GastrJap, 1991; 26:156

* Data were confirmed by supplemental anti-HCV RIBA and/or HCV-RNA polymerase chain reaction testing.

depending on the hepatitis B virus endemicity. In areas of high HBV endemicity HCV infection is relatively uncommon, whereas in areas of intermediate or low HBV endemicity the prevalence of hepatitis C increases significantly.

In areas of high or moderate HBV endemicity concurrent HBV and HCV infection is seen in patients with chronic liver disease. This association increases in frequency with the severity and stage of liver disease.

Transmission

Early studies in transfusion recipients demonstrated that HCV is efficiently transmitted by blood and blood products. However, in the various studies only 5 to 35 per cent of patients with hepatitis C had been transfused (Alter, JAMA, 1989; 262:201; Zeuzem, JHepatol, 1996; 24:3), a percentage that has much declined after the introduction of anti-HCV screening of blood donors. A major contribution to the pool of acute and chronic HCV infections is provided by intravenous drug abusers, who account for up to 50 per cent of infections in some geographical areas (Table 4). Overall, other identified parenteral routes (haemodialysis, needlestick injuries to health care professionals, and tattooing) accounted for no more than 5 per cent of exposures in the Centers for Disease Control (**CDC**) study of community-acquired, non-A, non-B hepatitis (Alter, JAMA, 1989; 262:1201). Therefore a consistent proportion of patients with hepatitis C have no identifiable percutaneous

exposure. The source of infection and the modes of HCV transmission in this setting remain a matter of debate and concern.[5]

Data from the Centers for Disease Control and Prevention (United States) indicate that between 1991 and 1995 about 30 per cent of patients presenting with acute hepatitis C had no definite risk factors for parenteral exposure during the 6 months preceding onset of the disease, although in many of them detailed evaluation of past history indicated at-risk behaviours (Alter, Hepatol, 1997; 26:62S).

Post-transfusion hepatitis

In the past, recipients of blood or blood products were at significant risk of acquiring HCV infection and HCV was implicated in more than 85 per cent of cases of post-transfusion, non-A, non-B hepatitis. The frequency of transfusion-transmitted disease started to decline in the 1980s, well before anti-HCV testing became available, as a consequence of the exclusion of paid donors, the introduction of anti-HIV screening, and the use of 'surrogate markers' to identify potentially infectious donors. The use of first-generation enzyme immunoassays for HCV screening was associated with an 80 per cent reduction in the risk of infection among transfusion recipients in retrospective and prospective studies (Aach, NEJM, 1991; 325: 1325; Gonzales, Hepatol, 1995; 22:439). Residual post-transfusion cases may be partially explained by the relative insensitivity of first-generation anti-HCV assays used in the early 1990s, and by

Table 3 Prevalence of anti-HCV in risk groups

Risk group	% Anti-HCV positive	References
Thalassaemics	42–83	Ni, PediatRes, 1996; 39:323; Resti, EurJPed, 1992; 151:573
Haemophiliacs	50–95	Kumar, JMedVirol, 1993; 41:205; Jackson, NZMedJ, 1994; 107:10
Haemodialysis patients	10–45	Al Nasser, VoxSang, 1992; 62:94; Nordenfeldt, JMedVirol, 1993; 40:266
Health care professionals	0–10	Germanaud, AmJPublHlth, 1994; 122:84; Klein, Lancet, 1991; 338:1539
Intravenous drug abusers	48–90	Esteban, Lancet, 1989; ii:294; Verbaan, ScaJGastr, 1993; 28:714
Tattooed persons	11	Ko, JMedVirol, 1992; 38:288
Patients with history of blood transfusion or major surgery	21	Kelen, NEJM, 1992; 326:1399
Prisoners	15–46	De Mercato, MinMed, 1995; 86:89; Holsen, EurJClinMicrob, 1993; 12:673
Patients admitted to emergency rooms	18	Kelen, NEJM, 1992; 326:1399
Dentists practising oral surgery	9	Klein, Lancet, 1991; 338:1539
Recipients of transplanted organs from anti-HCV positive donors	62	Pereira, NEJM, 1992; 327:910
Alcoholics	15–25	Verbaan, ScaJGastr, 1993; 28:714; Zarski, JHepatol, 1993; 17:1014
Handicapped or institutionalized individuals	4–7	Pregliasco, EurJEpid, 1994; 10:113; Chang, JMedVirol, 1993; 40:170
Heterosexual partners of HCV carriers	0–18	Everhart, AnnIntMed, 1990; 112:54; Akahane, AnnIntMed, 1994; 120:748
Prostitutes	0.7–6	Hyams, JAIDS, 1993; 6:1353; Lissen, EurJClinMicrobiol, 1993; 12:827
Homosexuals	3–18	Thomas, JInfDis, 1993; 167:66; Quaranta, JMedVirol, 1994; 42:29
Household non-sexual contacts of HCV carriers	0–11	Deny, JHepatol, 1992; 14:409; Ideo, Lancet, 1990; 335:353; Diago, JHepatol, 1996; 25:125
Children of HCV-infected mothers	0–6	Ohto, NEJM, 1994; 330:744; Lam, JInfDis, 1993; 167:572

Table 4 Transmission routes for HCV infection

Proved and highly efficient	Proved or highly suspected but not very efficient	Suspected but not proved
Blood transfusions	Needlestick injury	Haemodialysis facilities
Intravenous drug abuse	Maternofetal or neonatal	Acupuncture
Organ transplantation	Sexual contact	Ear piercing
	Household contact	Intranasal cocaine use
	Tattooing	

transmission from seronegative HCV carriers—acutely infected individuals who are asymptomatic and have not yet seroconverted to anti-HCV. Among donors controlled with the new generation of screening tests, the risk of giving blood during an infectious window period was recently estimated to be 1 in 103 000 (Schreiber, NEJM, 1996; 334:1685). A direct correlation exists between the number of blood products received and the risk of acquiring HCV infection. In the past, before anti-HCV screening of donors, patients with haemophilia who were transfused with untreated or inadequately treated factor concentrates had prevalence rates of anti-HCV exceeding 90 per cent (Brettler, Blood, 1990; 76:254), and up to 65 per cent of patients with thalassaemia receiving multiple transfusions of blood products were anti-HCV positive (Lai, JPediatGastrNutr 1993; 16:458). Modern virus inactivation procedures for pooled plasma products, the production of clotting factors by recombinant DNA technology, and donor screening for anti-HCV have decreased the risk of acquiring HCV infection with blood products. Nevertheless, in 1994 an outbreak of acute hepatitis C caused by intravenous immunoglobulin preparations screened for anti-HCV occurred in Europe. Among patients infected in the United Kingdom (Healey, Gastro, 1996; 110:1120), 82 per cent had HCV RNA in their serum and 79 per cent had abnormal aminotransferase levels within 7 weeks after infection with the contaminated material. Comparison of virus isolates from the infected patients and from the implicated batch showed an identical viral sequence. This incident emphasizes the need to improve further the safety of blood products.

At present, screening of every donor for HCV RNA would be too expensive and difficult to standardize; likewise the HCV RNA results of the final product may be difficult to interpret with regard to infectivity.

Non-transfusional percutaneous transmission

The importance of percutaneous transmission outside the transfusional setting is emphasized by the prominent role of hepatitis C as the cause of acute and chronic liver disease in patients who have never been transfused. Intravenous drug abusers represent a consistent reservoir of HCV infection (Thomas, Medicine, 1995; 74:212). The main route of HCV transmission in this setting is the sharing of contaminated needles. Recently, sharing of straws has been reported as a potential route of transmucosal transmission in nasal cocaine users (Conry-Cantilena, NEJM, 1996; 334:1691). Drug abusers who started to self-infect before the AIDS prevention campaigns and the discovery of HCV have anti-HCV prevalence rates greater than 90 per cent; most have evidence of liver disease. Although in some areas the prevalence of anti-HCV in drug abusers has diminished in the 1990s (Galeazzi, Liver, 1995; 15:209), new infections continue to occur in this setting; with the dramatic reduction of transfusion-associated hepatitis, hepatitis C occurring in drug abusers accounts at present for 40 to 50 per cent of all cases of acute hepatitis C.

HCV is the major cause of acute hepatitis in the population receiving renal dialysis, accounting for over two-thirds of hepatitis cases. The prevalence of anti-HCV in patients on haemodialysis averages 10 to 20 per cent.[6] These patients may have acquired HCV not only through blood transfusions but also by the dialysis procedure. Several studies support this hypothesis (Hardy, Clin-Nephrol, 1992; 38:44; Irie, JHepatol, 1994; 20:557), others found no evidence for transmission related to haemodialysis facilities (Jadoul, Lancet, 1995; 345:189). The application of universal precautions and scrupulous aseptic techniques are recommended to limit the spread of infection in this setting. The issue of the isolation of patients on haemodialysis who are HCV positive is controversial: some authors (Jadoul, 1995) claim that this strategy would be expensive and would fail to prevent HCV transmission by acutely infected patients who have not yet seroconverted, and to avoid superinfection of segregated patients with other HCV genotypes.

Organ transplant recipients are also at risk of HCV infection.[7] About 50 per cent of the recipients of an organ from donors positive for anti-HCV develop hepatitis after transplantation and up to 96 per cent become positive for HCV RNA (Pereira, NephrolDialTranspl,1996; 11:1520). Currently, several organ procurement organizations restrict the use of donors positive for anti-HCV to lifesaving transplants.

Health care professionals in contact with blood or blood products may become exposed to HCV through needlestick injuries or contact with mucous membranes. Seroprevalence rates of anti-HCV in health care providers average 1 per cent in the Western world. Needlestick accidents involving HCV-infected patients lead to virus

transmission in 0.7 to 10 per cent of cases (average 1.8 per cent) (Kiyosawa, AnnIntMed, 1991; 115:367; Mitsui, Hepatol, 1992; 16: 1109; Puro, AmJPublHlth, 1995; 85:1272; Hepatitis Surveillance Report no.56, Atlanta, 1995:3). Certain subsets of workers, such as oral surgeons, dentists, and dental auxiliary personnel, are at greater risk (Klein, Lancet, 1991; 338:1539; Wang, Lancet, 1991; 337:48). Transmission of HCV has been documented from an infected health care professional to patients (Esteban, NEJM, 1996; 334:555).

Transmission from patient to patient, possibly through medical procedures, may be responsible for nosocomial outbreaks of parenterally transmitted hepatitis C on haematology and oncology wards (Allander, Lancet, 1995; 345:603; Widell p.176 in reference 4).

Covert non-percutaneous transmission

A large percentage of patients with acute or chronic hepatitis C have no history of an identifiable parenteral exposure; household, sexual, or maternal–infant transmission is suspected.

A number of studies have raised the possibility of sexual transmission of HCV.[8] A CDC study involving patients with non-A, non-B hepatitis and non-infected controls showed that patients with hepatitis were more likely than the general population to have a history of unprotected sexual contact with a person with hepatitis and multiple sexual partners (Alter, JAMA, 1989; 262:1201). After the discovery of HCV, higher infection rates have been reported among sexually exposed individuals than in the general population. Prevalence rates among heterosexual partners of infected individuals average no more than 5 per cent in Western countries (Bresters, Lancet, 1993; 342:210; Osmond, JAMA, 1993; 269:361).

However, a Japanese study of 154 spouses of patients with index cases of hepatitis C (Akahane, AnnIntMed, 1994; 120:748) reported that 18 per cent were HCV RNA positive; genotype analysis showed that 89 per cent of these spouses had the same genotype as their partners, confirming partner to partner transmission. Sexual transmission of HCV seems enhanced when the partner is coinfected with HIV (Eyster, AnnIntMed, 1991; 115:764); this could be related to the high levels of HCV viraemia induced by HIV-associated immunodeficiency. The prevalence rate of HCV infection in male homosexuals is somewhat higher than in the general population (4 to 8 per cent when corrected for coexistent intravenous drug abuse), but remains well below the prevalence rates for HBV and HIV infections in the same risk group (Osmond, JInfDis, 1993; 167:66; Westh, Infec, 1993; 21:115); no correlation was found between the prevalence of anti-HCV and sexual practices that are thought to enhance viral transmission. The rate of HCV infection is higher among male homosexuals with HIV infection; the same is true for prostitutes, clients of prostitutes, and individuals attending clinics for sexually transmitted diseases.

All these observations indicate that HCV is not spread very efficiently by the sexual route compared with other sexually transmitted viruses. The low virus load associated with HCV infection could partially explain this difference. Data concerning the presence of HCV RNA in semen and saliva of subjects with viraemia are conflicting (Hsu, Hepatol, 1991; 14:763; Fried, Gastro, 1992; 102: 1306; Wang, JMedVirol, 1992; 36:28).

In some studies the prevalence of HCV infection among household non-sexual contacts of HCV-infected individuals was greater than expected in the general population or among family contacts of HCV-negative patients; usually it did not exceed 10 per cent (Ideo, Lancet, 1990; 335:353; Chang, JMedVirol, 1994; 42:91; Diago, JHepatol, 1996; 25:125) and it was lowest in children of patients with index cases (Meisel, Lancet, 1995; 345:1209) and increased with age (Diago, JHepatol, 1996; 25:125). In other studies, household non-sexual contacts did not increase the risk of HCV transmission (Caporaso, JGastro, 1990; 22:281; Coltorti, Infec, 1994; 22:183). Children whose parents are both infected stand an increased risk of infection (Nisiguchi, Lancet 1992; 339:1486); the route of HCV transmission in this setting remains unknown.

The question of perinatal transmission of HCV has been addressed by many investigators.[9] The diagnosis of perinatal infection is made from the persistence of anti-HCV in the serum for more than 12 months after birth (positivity for the first 12 months may be due to passively transmitted maternal antibody) and/or on the detection of HCV RNA in at least two post-delivery samples; however, the antibody-based diagnosis may not be reliable as in a few cases passively transmitted antibodies may persist for longer than 12 months. More compelling evidence for mother to child transmission comes from a high degree of homology of HCV cDNA and HCV RNA sequences in mother–infant pairs, (Inoue, JInfDis, 1992; 166:1425; Ohto, NEJM, 1994; 330:744). Even with stringent diagnostic criteria, however, most epidemiological studies show minimal evidence for mother to infant transmission, the average rate being 5 per cent. Factors that influence vertical transmission appear to be the HCV RNA titre in the mother and maternal coinfection with HCV and HIV. The analysis of HCV RNA titres in mothers positive for anti-HCV indicates that only those with HCV RNA titres higher than 10^6 transmit infection to their babies (Lin, JInfDis, 1994; 169:638; Ohto, NEJM, 1994; 330:744); transmission from highly viraemic mothers occurs in 36 per cent of newborn infants (Ohto, NEJM, 1994; 330:744). Two studies in urban areas of northern Italy (Giovannini, Lancet, 1990; 335:1166; Zanetti, Lancet, 1995; 345:289) have shown a high rate of perinatal transmission (36 to 44 per cent) from drug-abusing mothers coinfected with HCV and HIV, compared with no infection in babies born to mothers circulating HCV alone; however, these data were not confirmed (Lam, JInfDis, 1993; 167:572; Manzini, Hepatol, 1995; 21:328).

All studies were unable to distinguish between intrauterine, perinatal, breast feeding, or other transmission routes; infectivity of breast milk has been suggested but not proved (Ogasawara, Lancet, 1993; 341:561; Gurakan, NEJM, 1994; 331:399; Karauchi, Arch-GynecolObstet, 1993; 253:121) and breast feeding is not considered to increase the risk of HCV infection in infants of mothers with hepatitis C (Dienstag, Hepatol, 1997; 26:665).

As the overall efficiency of sexual, household, or perinatal routes of transmission of HCV seems to be low, the transmission modes of HCV in the community remain controversial. Surreptitious parenteral drug abuse, overlooked transfusions received in infancy, covert routes by which blood may be transported from individual to individual such as acupuncture, tattooing, sharing of toothbrushes and razors, ear piercing, and other means of traumatic contact with objects contaminated with blood have been advocated. Of note, potential exposures such as sexual and household contacts, although of limited transmission efficiency, may occur so frequently as to account cumulatively for large numbers of infected persons.

Pathogenesis

Our knowledge of the biology of HCV including its molecular organization and expression in infected cells[10] and the type and pattern of immune response of the host[11] has significantly advanced in recent years. Nevertheless, the pathogenesis of hepatitis C remains uncertain as to the determinants of virus persistence and to the mechanisms of hepatocellular damage and of extrahepatic involvement. HCV has a strong propensity to establish chronic infection; this justifies the prominent role of this virus in the aetiology of chronic liver diseases worldwide. Circumstantial evidence suggests that chronicity of hepatitis C may depend on (i) non-cytopathic infection of hepatic and non-hepatic cells and/or (ii) evasion of the host's immune response. As is the case for most viral infections, eradication of HCV is likely to involve the interaction of neutralizing antibodies with circulating virions and the activation of cytotoxic T lymphocytes to the killing of infected cells and to the inhibition of intracellular virus through the release of regulatory cytokines. HCV may evade the neutralizing antibody response by rapid mutation of the antigenic composition of its envelope proteins. The hypervariable region near the amino terminus of the NS1/E2 proteins is recognized by circulating antibodies (Spaete, Virology, 1992; 188:819), including neutralizing antibodies (Shimizu, JVirol, 1994; 68:1494). Elevated rates of genetic variation in the envelope proteins are observed among HCV-infected patients and in sequential studies of individual cases, suggesting that HCV has acquired a highly efficient strategy to mutate within this region in order to evade the host immune response and to establish chronicity (Kato, JGenVirol, 1993; 67: 923). This strategy is reflected in the quasispecies nature of HCV, which circulates not as a homogeneous virus population but as a mixture of related but immunologically distinct variants, any of which can become the predominant strain when other coexisting strains are controlled by the immune system. In this scenario, neutralizing antibodies would have limited efficacy; they are nevertheless produced during natural infection, since serum from patients with chronic hepatitis C was shown to neutralize a titrated virus preparation inoculated into chimpanzees (Farci, PNAS, 1994; 91: 7792). Neutralization may have a narrow specificity within the HCV quasispecies, thus making the development of an efficient HCV vaccine problematic.

HCV may also reduce antiviral immune responses by directly infecting the lymphoid cells (Bouffard, JInfDis, 1992; 166:1276; Wang, JInfDis, 1992; 166:1167; Muller, JGenVirol, 1993; 74:669); however, there is no definitive proof that the virus replicates in these cells and controversies still exist about which blood cell subpopulations may harbour the virus.

HCV sequences were detected in CD8+ (Zignego, JHepatol, 1992; 15:382) and CD4+ (Shimizu, PNAS, 1992; 89:5477) T lymphocytes, but also in B lymphocytes (Muller, JGenVirol, 1993; 74:669) and in monocytes (Bouffard, JInfDis, 1992; 166:1276). It is uncertain whether in hepatitis C, like in many viral diseases including several caused by other flaviviruses (Bielefeldt, JGenVirol, 1987; 68:1971), non-cytopathic infection of lymphoid cells is an important determinant of virus presistence. Defective interferon production may also be implicated (Zachoval, JHepatol, 1988; 6: 364).

The mechanisms by which HCV causes hepatocellular damage remain speculative. A direct cytopathic effect of the virus is suggested by the observation that the histological lesions of hepatitis C often consist of prominent degenerative changes with a modest inflammatory infiltrate. Many pathogens of the Flaviviridae family cause cell damage (including liver damage in the case of yellow fever virus) through a direct cytopathic action. However, because of the lack of suitable methods for 'in vitro' culture of the virus, the possibility of direct cytopathic effects has not been properly assessed. Clinical studies have analysed the relation between serum and/or hepatic virus expression and the activity/severity of liver damage in an attempt to clarify whether virus replication and accumulation in the liver may cause disease. The results were controversial, with some reports favouring (Hagiwara, Hepatol, 1993; 17:545) and others opposing (Naito, Hepatol, 1995; 22:407) the hypothesis of a correlation between virus activity and disease severity. Other studies have suggested that some HCV genotypes, namely 1b, may be more cytopathic than others (Dusheiko, Hepatol, 1994; 19:13).

Cell-mediated cytotoxicity also contributes to the pathogenesis of hepatocellular damage in hepatitis C. Cytotoxic T lymphocytes (CD8+) which react in a HLA class I-restricted manner with core and envelope antigens of HCV were identified in the serum and liver of chronically infected individuals with active disease (Koziel, JVirol, 1993; 67:7522; Battegay, JVirol, 1995; 69:2462), often in close contact with infected cells and apoptotic bodies (Ballardini, JCI, 1995; 95:2067); their amount correlates with ALT levels (Hayata, Hepatol, 1991; 13:1022). Helper (CD4+) T lymphocytes recognizing core epitopes of HCV may influence the outcome of HCV infection, as they are detected in patients with a more benign course of disease (Botarelli, Gastro, 1993; 104:580); CD4+ T lymphocytes recognizing non-structural (NS4 and NS5) as well as structural (core protein) epitopes of HCV have been detected in peripheral blood and liver of chronically infected individuals (Ferrari, Hepatol, 1994; 19:286).

The CDF-T cell response to structural and non-structural proteins of HCV is weaker in patients with acute hepatitis C who progress to chronicity compared to recovering cases, suggesting that the vigour of this antiviral response may be an important determinant of disease outcome (Missale, JClinInvest, 1996; 98:706). The pattern of cytokine production is also different in patients who recover after acute hepatitis C and those who develop chronic disease, being mainly of the Th1 type in the former and of the Th2/Th0 type in the latter (Bertoletti, Gastro, 1997; 112:193).

HCV infection has been associated with a number of immunological disorders,[12] for instance cryoglobulinaemia, vasculitis, glomerulonephritis, arthritis, and thyroiditis, as well as with the induction of a number of autoantibodies;[13] the most characteristic finding is the presence of liver/kidney microsomal antibodies (anti-LKM) typical of type 2 'autoimmune' chronic hepatitis. The pathogenesis of HCV-related cryoglobulinaemia and of other types of vasculitis may depend on long-term viral stimulation of the immune system with the induction of oligoclonal/monoclonal antibody reactions and the formation of immune complexes of the IgG/IgM type; alternatively, HCV may infect the lymphoid tissue directly. The chronic stimulation/infection of the immune system may eventually be responsible for the development of B-cell lymphomas

of low-grade malignancy (Ferri, EurJCan, 1994; 30:1591). Anti-LKM antibodies are found in 1 to 10 per cent of cases and evidence has been provided that they are triggered by HCV infection (Mackie, Gastro, 1994; 106:1672). Anti-LKM are directed against conformational and linear autoepitopes on cytochrome P-450 11D6 or other microsomal proteins (Duclos-Vallee, Gastro, 1995; 108.470, Durazzo, Gastro, 1995; 108:455). Antigenic mimicry between autoantigens and HCV antigens may be involved, as shown also for anti-GOR antibodies, another autoimmune reaction frequently observed in HCV-infected individuals. The propensity of HCV to trigger autoimmune reactions remains largely unexplained.

Diagnosis

Infection with HCV can be identified and staged with a variety of diagnostic tools that include tests for antiviral antibodies (anti-HCV) of the IgG and IgM type, direct detection and quantification of the virus genome (HCV RNA) in serum and in infected tissues and cells, and characterization of the genomic sequences of the virus to define the genotype and subtype of the infecting HCV.

Anti-HCV

Tests for serum antibodies against a variety of non-structural and structural HCV antigens are currently used to screen for hepatitis C and to diagnose past and present infection. Commercially available anti-HCV ELISA were initially based on the use of the C100-3 epitope from the non-structural NS4 region of HCV (Kuo, Science, 1989; 244:362). This test had a major impact on the screening of blood donors, leading to a drastic reduction of post-transfusion hepatitis C (Esteban, NEJM, 1990; 323:1107; Donahue, NEJM, 1992; 327:369). However, it had low sensitivity in detecting hepatitis C (Esteban, NEJM, 1990; 323:1107; Alter, Transfusion, 1991; 31:771) and poor specificity in low-risk groups (Weiner, Lancet, 1990; 336:336; Alter, AnnIntMed, 1991; 115:644) and in the presence of hypergammaglobulinaemia (McFarlane, Lancet, 1990; 335:754). Second-generation ELISA were then developed which incorporate multiple viral antigens derived from the NS4 region of HCV (C100-3 epitope) as well as from the NS3 region (C33c epitope) and from the structural core region (C22-3 epitope) (Van der Poel, Lancet, 1991; 337:317; Alter, Hepatol, 1992; 15:350). More recently, a third-generation ELISA has been licensed, with the inclusion of an antigen from the NS5 region and the C22c and C100-3 antigenic components as synthetic peptides (Courouce, Transfusion, 1994; 34:790; VyHendaele, VoxSang, 1994; 34:122). Several ELISA-based tests have been produced by various companies with minimal differences in specificity and sensitivity (Anderson, JViralHepat, 1995; 2:55). New-generation assays have increased sensitivity compared with first-generation ELISA (Klinman, Transfusion, 1991; 32:805; Alter, Hepatol, 1992; 321:350); however, the problems of false negative reactions in infected patients who do not produce significant titres of anti-HCV and of false positive results in low-risk individuals have not been eliminated (Lelie, JMedVirol, 1992; 38:203; Waumans, VoxSang, 1993; 64:145).

The diagnostic reliability of anti-HCV ELISA tests varies greatly in different populations. Hepatitis C may not be identified by anti-HCV ELISA in patients who are in the early phase of infection before seroconversion (Van der Poel, Lancet, 1994; 341:1475), or in immunosuppressed or immunocompromised patients, including those who have received a transplant (Younossi, ViralHepatRev, 1996; 2:161). In these patients, hepatitis C can be diagnosed only with viral assays for serum HCV RNA. A positive anti-HCV ELISA test is diagnostic for hepatitis C in high-risk groups, namely individuals with a well-recognized risk for parenteral contamination, as well as in patients with acute or chronic liver disease and no other aetiological factors; in these cases the use of supplemental anti-HCV tests is not recommended, as it would not be cost-effective. However, up to 50 per cent of anti-HCV ELISA reactivities may be false positive in low-risk individuals, namely those without parenteral exposure or evidence of liver disease (Kleinman, Transfusion, 1992; 32:805; Lelie, JMedVirol, 1992; 38:203). False positive reactions are also seen in patients with hypergammaglobulinaemia, autoimmune reactions and diseases such as primary biliary cirrhosis (Houset, AnnIntMed 1991; 114:251) and systemic lupus erythematosus, alcoholic liver disease (Mendelhall, Hepatol, 1991; 14:581), and metabolic disorders, as well as in pregnant women (Marcellin, DigDisSci, 1993; 38:2151). Improper serum storage increases the risk of false reactions. The introduction of third-generation assays has only partially solved the problems of specificity and in doubtful cases it is essential to use supplemental anti-HCV assays to confirm the diagnosis. The most commonly used assay of this type is the recombinant immunoblotting assay (anti-HCV RIBA, Chiron Corporation, Emeryville, California, USA), but similar assays (Matrix HCV, Abbott Laboratories, Chicago, USA; Innolio, Immunogenetics, Benelux) are also available (Zaaijer, Transfusion, 1994; 34:603). These tests allow visualization of individual antibody reactions against the same non-structural and structural HCV antigens used in the ELISA tests. The antigens are spotted on to nitrocellulose strips and the reaction is recognized as a band in a different position for each antigen. Sera are defined as positive when they react with at least two viral antigens, indeterminate when they react with a single viral antigen, and negative when no band of reaction with HCV antigens is seen.

Up to 30 to 50 per cent of sera positive for anti-HCV ELISA from low-risk individuals screened without a specific diagnostic indication are negative for anti-HCV RIBA and for HCV RNA by PCR (Aach, NEJM, 1991; 325:1325; Waumans, VoxSang, 1993; 64:145; Damen, Transfusion, 1995; 35:745), 20 to 30 per cent are indeterminate, and only 30 to 40 per cent are positive. ELISA-positive, RIBA-negative results should be considered as non-specific reactions in the test system and not indicative of true HCV infection. These cases do not need further assessment or follow-up. RIBA-positive and indeterminate sera should be tested for serum HCV RNA to assess the phase of HCV infection. RIBA-positive individuals often have HCV RNA in their serum and 80 to 90 per cent transmit HCV infection via their blood (Esteban, NEJM, 1990; 323:1107; Alter, AnnIntMed, 1991; 115:644). On the other hand, most RIBA-indeterminate reactions are non-specific and do not indicate ongoing HCV infection (Tobler, Transfusion, 1994; 34:130). However, about 25 per cent of symptomless subjects with a persistent indeterminate RIBA pattern may result positive for serum HCV RNA , particularly when the isolated antibody reactivity is against the core (C22-3) protein of HCV (Zanella, Hepatol, 1995; 21:913).

Methods for detection of IgM antibodies to the different antigens of HCV have been developed recently and tested for their diagnostic and prognostic value in patients with acute and chronic HCV infection.[14] These assays have not proved helpful for the diagnosis of acute infection, due to the inconsistent and unequal appearance of IgM anti-HCV during acute hepatitis C. In chronic infection, IgM HCV has been proposed as a marker to predict response to interferon therapy; a negative anticore IgM test before treatment and disappearance of anti-C100 IgM during therapy were found to be associated with a better chance of response to interferon (Brillanti, Hepatol, 1992; 15:998; Quiroga, Gastro, 1992; 103:1285). However, this conclusion resulted from studies in small and selected groups of patients, and a definitive clinical validation of the significance of the IgM anti-HCV assays remains to be obtained.

Serum HCV RNA

HCV RNA is detected in serum by the polymerase chain reaction (**PCR**), usually with primers derived from the more conserved 5′ untranslated region (5′UTR) of the viral genome.[15] Although theoretically this is the more direct and sensitive way to establish the diagnosis of ongoing HCV infection, the technique is expensive and difficult to standardize, with unsatisfactory specificity and reproducibility in many laboratories (Zaaijer, Lancet, 1993; 341: 722). These problems have been solved only in part following the development of diagnostic kits by the pharmaceutical industry (HCV Amplicor: Roche Molecular Diagnostics Systems; HCV branched DNA assay: Chiron Corporation). These assays still lack optimal specificity, reproducibility, and sensitivity. Serum HCV RNA testing is not superior to anti-HCV testing in establishing a diagnosis of hepatitis C in immunocompetent patients who have evidence of liver disease without other aetiological factors; anti-HCV remains positive over time while viraemia may fluctuate and occasionally falls below the detection limit (false negative). The clinical settings in which testing for serum HCV RNA is recommended for evaluation of hepatitis C are summarized in Table 5. These include:

1. Individuals who are anti-HCV RIBA positive or indeterminate with normal ALT. Serum HCV RNA allows the distinction between current and past infection. Eighty to ninety per cent of RIBA-positive patients are serum positive for HCV RNA. Most of these individuals have histological evidence of chronic hepatitis, despite the normality of liver enzymes. RIBA-positive, HCV RNA-negative subjects are interpreted as cases of past infection if they are confirmed negative for HCV RNA on repeated testing. Patients who are RIBA indeterminate and show isolate reactivity against C33c or C22 may have HCV RNA in their serum as evidence of ongoing infection. In contrast, cases with isolated reactivity against C100-3 or 5-1 epitope are almost invariably HCV RNA negative and the low level ELISA reactivity is most likely non-specific.

2. Patients in the early phase of acute hepatitis C, before anti-HCV seroconversion. All patients with acute hepatitis of unknown origin should be tested for serum HCV RNA to assess whether they have acute infection with HCV.

3. Immunocompromised or immunosuppressed patients in whom hepatitis C may be suspected. These patients may not produce anti-HCV or may develop low antibody titres of doubtful interpretation. This group includes transplant recipients. In patients who have received a liver allograft, the HCV RNA test

Table 5 Recommended diagnostic/clinical use of qualitative (PCR-based) serum HCV RNA tests

Diagnostic/clinical settings	Interpretation
Low-risk individuals with normal ALT and a positive or indeterminate anti-HCV RIBA	HCV RNA positive: ongoing hepatitis C HCV RNA negative: past hepatitis C (?)
Patients negative for anti-HCV with acute hepatitis of unknown aetiology	HCV RNA positive: early acute hepatitis C HCV RNA negative: no hepatitis C
Immunocompromised, immunosuppressed, transplanted patients with hepatitis who are negative for anti-HCV. Anti-HCV negative essential cryoglobulinaemia. Chronic hepatitis of unknown origin	HCV RNA positive: anti-HCV seronegative hepatitis C or HCV infection
Patients positive for anti-HCV with chronic liver disease and present of aetiological cofactors (autoimmunity, alcohol abuse, metabolic disease etc)	HCV RNA positive: HCV is a cofactor of liver damage
Neonates born to anti-HCV mothers	To assess transmission of HCV
Hepatitis C cases treated with interferons/antivirals	To monitor virological responses

is the only reliable method to identify *de novo* infection or recurrence of hepatitis C.

4. Patients negative for anti-HCV with essential mixed cryoglobulinaemia, which is often associated with hepatitis C but may not exhibit anti-HCV in serum (Agnello, NEJM, 1992; 327: 1490).

5. Patients negative for anti-HCV with 'cryptogenic' chronic hepatitis. Some of these patients may have seronegative hepatitis C, identified only by testing serum or liver HCV RNA.

6. Patients positive for anti-HCV with autoimmune disorders, autoimmune reactions, or hypergammaglobulinaemia. The anti-HCV reaction may not be specific or may not be associated with ongoing infection. In patients with autoimmune markers and chronic hepatitis (chronic hepatitis positive for antinuclear or anti-LKM antibodies), testing for serum HCV RNA allows us to define whether liver damage is associated with HCV replication or is mainly due to an autoimmune reaction.

7. Patients positive for anti-HCV with liver disease who have evidence of other aetiological cofactors such as alcohol abuse or metabolic disorders. Testing for serum HCV RNA allows us to define whether HCV contributes to liver damage.

8. Neonates born to mothers who are anti-HCV positive. Anti-HCV is always found as a result of passively transmitted maternal antibodies. Serum HCV RNA testing represents the only way to establish whether transmission of HCV has occurred.

9. Patients with hepatitis C treated with interferons or antivirals. Serum HCV RNA is useful to monitor the response to therapy (see Chapter 12.1.3.2).

Quantification of serum HCV RNA

Serum levels of HCV RNA can be measured by a number of laboratory procedures.[16] Home-made assays include endpoint-detection competitive PCR and coamplification of synthetically mutated target RNA (Brechot, JHepatol, 1993; 17:S35). These approaches are expensive, difficult to standardize, and often lack reproducibility. Commercial assays have also been developed (Urdea, ClinChem, 1993; 39:725). They are very expensive and not fully standardized (Gretch, AnnIntMed, 1995; 123:312); their use in the clinical setting is controversial. They do not appear to give

essential information in the diagnostic and prognostic evaluation of acute and chronic hepatitis C; a correlation between levels of viraemia and the activity or outcome of liver disease has not been established, and viraemia may fluctuate over time in the same individual, with or without a parallel behaviour of serum ALT (Lok, Hepatol, 1997; 26:485). Particularly high levels of HCV RNA are found in the early phase of acute hepatitis C but also in the endstage phase of cirrhosis (Gretch, JInfDis, 1994; 169:1219). Immunosuppressed patients often have high viraemic titres. A 10- to 100-fold increase in HCV RNA is usually observed after liver transplantation in HCV-infected patients, as a consequence of immunosuppression (Charouclleres, Gastro; 1994; 106:994). The response to interferon therapy in chronic hepatitis C is significantly affected by the level of HCV RNA in the pretreatment serum (see Chapter 12.1.3.2).

HCV genotyping

A variety of methods have been developed to define the genotype and subtype of the infecting HCV in the individual patient (Smith, ClinGastroent, 1996; 10:243). These include hybridization with genotype-specific oligonucleotide probes derived from different HCV RNA regions, restriction enzyme analysis, PCR amplification with type-specific primers, and serotyping methods. Although genotyping methods are not used routinely in the clinical assessment of hepatitis C, they may give useful information in specific diagnostic settings.

The prognosis of chronic hepatitis C may depend, at least in past, on the HCV genotype, infection with HCV-1b being associated with a more severe outcome in patients with chronic hepatitis C (Dusheiko, Hepatol, 1994; 19:13) and after liver transplantation (Feray, Gastro, 1995; 108:1088). These data, however, have not been confirmed in other series (Yamada, DigDisSci, 1994; 39:234). HCV-1b was shown to prevail in patients with cirrhosis and with hepatocellular carcinoma; other genotypes, like HCV-2, are more frequently found in asymptomatic carriers of HCV with normal aminotransferases (Silini, Hepatol, 1994; 21:285). While these observations may indicate a different pathogenicity of HCV genotypes, it is also possible that HCV-1b has existed for longer than other genotypes, and has therefore generated a cohort of patients infected with HCV-1b having a longer standing, and therefore more advanced, chronic liver disease (Nousbaum, AnnInt Med, 1995; 122: 161). Further studies are needed to assess the clinical relevance of virus genotyping in hepatitis C.[17] The response to interferon therapy is influenced by the genotype of infecting HCV (Yoshioka, Hepatol, 1992; 16:293; Chemello, Hepatol, 1995; 22:700). Patients with HCV-1, particularly those with HCV-1b, and with HCV-4 have rates of primary and sustained responses significantly lower than those observed in patients with other genotypes.

Clinical use of HCV markers and diagnostic algorithms

Based on the above information the following recommendations can be made for the use of HCV markers by the clinician.

When acute hepatitis C is suspected, the detection of serum HCV RNA by PCR may have diagnostic relevance during the early phase; anti-HCV seroconversion by second- or third-generation anti-HCV ELISA assays should be sought in later phase serum samples. IgM anti-HCV tests give inconsistent results and do not provide additional diagnostic or prognostic information. The outcome after acute hepatitis C can be assessed by sequential HCV RNA testing, and persistence of a positive PCR for more than 6 months after clinical onset is highly suspicious of a chronic evolution; a progressive reduction of anti-HCV titres in patients in whom ALT levels have returned to normal and cleared HCV RNA is indicative of full recovery from the infection.

In patients with a sustained ALT elevation and clinical and/or histological evidence of chronic hepatitis, anti-HCV by ELISA is sufficient to make the diagnosis of hepatitis C; supplemental anti-HCV or HCV RNA testing may not be required.

Quantitative assessment of serum HCV RNA levels and characterization of the type and subtype of HCV may be considered if treatment with interferon is contemplated. In low-risk individuals with normal ALT who are found to be anti-HCV positive by ELISA at occasional testing, or during screening for blood donation, supplemental RIBA testing is necessary to make the diagnosis (Fig. 2). Serum HCV RNA should then be tested by PCR in RIBA-positive and indeterminate cases. Repeated HCV-RNA testing is recommended in those cases initially found negative to exclude intermittent viraemia or false-negative results due to suboptimal testing conditions (Lok, Hepatol, 1997; 26:485). In patients found HCV-RNA positive, ALT should be monitored to identify hepatitis reactivation (Alter, Hepatol, 1997; 26:29S). As for chronic hepatitis C, quantitative assessment of viraemia and HCV genotyping do not have a precise prognostic significance if the patient is not a candidate for interferon therapy.

Natural history and clinical course

The current knowledge of the natural history of acute and chronic HCV infection is largely based on studies of post-transfusion and community-acquired NANB hepatitis, revisited as cases of hepatitis C by retrospective assessment of HCV markers. More recently, these have been complemented by studies on cohorts of HCV-positive patients observed at different stages of the disease. Major obstacles to the full comprehension of the natural history of hepatitis C[18,19] are the silent nature of acute and chronic infections, which

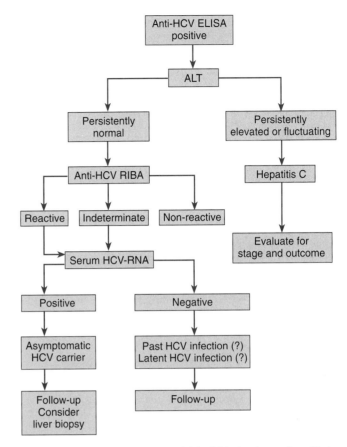

Fig. 2. Diagnostic algorithm in low-risk individuals who are found to be anti-HCV positive at occasional screening.

often impedes detection of the disease in its early stages, and the slow, unpredictable, and often discontinuous progression of the hepatic damage, which appears to take one or two decades to cause serious chronic sequelae.

Acute infection

The average incubation period of acute hepatitis C, as determined in prospective studies of post-transfusion hepatitis, is 7 to 8 weeks (Seeff, Gastro, 1977; 72:111), but the range varies widely (2 to 26 weeks) (Realdi, FrontGastrRes, 1984; 8:158). Shorter incubation periods were frequent in experimental infections and in individuals with haemophilia treated with factor VIII (Hruby, JAMA, 1978; 240:1353; Bamber, Gut, 1981; 22:854); in these patients incubation was described as short as 2 days (Craske, Lancet, 1975; ii:221; Bradley, JMedVirol, 1979; 3:253). In prospectively followed transfusion recipients, viraemia was the first marker to become detectable during acute hepatitis C; it was demonstrated by sensitive PCR as early as 1 week after exposure (Farci, NEJM, 1991; 325:98). Viraemia then persists without an antibody response for a period (window phase) of a few weeks to several months; during this early period, serum HCV RNA titres are higher than those found during the chronic phase.

Using second- or third-generation ELISA assays, anti-HCV seroconversion usually can be detected 4 to 8 weeks after exposure (Aach, NEJM, 1991; 325:1325; Maatbson, ScandJInfecDis, 1992; 24:15), but may be delayed up to several months, with large individual variations. Titres of serum HCV RNA decrease as anti-HCV becomes detectable. The various antiviral antibodies usually do not appear simultaneously, but rather in sequence; most commonly, anticore (C22) is raised first, followed by anti-NS3 (C33c) and anti-NS4 (anti-C100). Other patterns can be seen and not all patients develop the full battery of anti-HCV reactivities (Giuberti, Hepatol, 1994; 20:666; Barrera, Hepatol, 1995; 21:639).

The onset of liver damage, marked by variable ALT elevations, is always delayed with respect to the appearance of viraemia and may either precede or follow seroconversion to anti-HCV.

Patients rarely have prodromic symptoms or fever; some show a mild and brief elevation of ALT. The acute phase of hepatitis C is often mild or inapparent and usually less severe than hepatitis A and B;[20] more than two-thirds of the cases are asymptomatic and anicteric. Only 25 per cent of prospectively followed patients with transfusion-associated hepatitis C were icteric and less than 10 per cent were severely ill, while symptoms and jaundice have been more frequently reported in community-acquired disease (Alter, NEJM, 1992; 327:1899); the difference is probably not real, since in published studies most patients with the latter form were recognized because of clinical symptoms while the former group was identified prospectively during the follow-up of blood recipients. A severe or fulminant course of acute hepatitis C occurs rarely, (Cossart, Lancet, 1982; i:208; Ohori, JMedVirol, 1983; 11:105) except in patients with immunodeficiency, with pre-existing liver disease, or with other cofactors such as hepatitis A or B or drugs (Fagan, Hepatol, 1994; 19:1307). At present the role, if any, of HCV in causing fulminant hepatic failure remains controversial; there may be significant geographical differences, as HCV RNA was detected rarely in fulminant hepatitis cases in Western countries (Feray, Gastro, 1993; 104:549; Liang, Gastro, 1993; 104:556; Fagan, Hepatol, 1994; 19:1307) but frequently in cases in Japan (Yashiba, Hepatol, 1994; 19:829).

The clinical symptoms of acute hepatitis C are those of any type of viral hepatitis and are often indistinguishable from hepatitis A and B. Symptomatic cases present with malaise, dark urine, nausea (with or without vomiting), abdominal discomfort, and/or jaundice. Hepatitis C exhibits several patterns of aminotransferase elevation (Tateda, JInfDis, 1979; 139:511); the most typical is polyphasic, with significant fluctuations of enzyme levels over time. Sometimes, phases of biochemical abnormality are separated by periods of ALT normality. Other patterns of ALT with prognostic implications are: (i) a monophasic pattern with a rapid increase to peak aminotransferase levels, followed by a rapid decline and, eventually, return to normal; and (ii) a plateau pattern, with ALT persistently elevated without significant fluctuations, the acute phase often merging into a chronic outcome. Chronic hepatitis develops frequently in patients with the polyphasic ALT pattern.

Acute hepatitis C displays γ-glutamyl transferase levels somewhat higher than the other forms of viral hepatitis. The IgG fraction of the serum immunoglobulins is often increased without significant changes in the IgM fraction (Tage-Jensen, ScaJGastr, 1980; 15:229; Weiland, ScaJInfectDis, 1981; 13:247); the latter is more affected than IgG in other forms of acute viral hepatitis (Norkrans, Infec, 1980; 8:98; Zhuany, Gastro, 1982; 83:944). The histological features of acute hepatitis C include a few peculiar morphological changes, in addition to the classic features common to viral hepatitis in general (Dienes, Hepatol, 1982; 2:562). Liver biopsies may show eosinophilic clumping of the cytoplasm, macrovescicular steatosis,

marked activation of sinusoidal cells, piling up of bile ductular cells in the lumen, and large numbers of acidophilic bodies (Kryger, ScaJInfecDis, 1980; 12:165; Omata, Liver, 1981; 1:201). These changes coexist with a lymphocytic infiltration that is less prominent than in hepatitis A and B. Despite characteristic findings, a liver biopsy is not recommended for routine diagnosis of acute hepatitis C as none of the histological lesions is specific.[21] A liver biopsy is not essential to identify progression to chronicity; this can be diagnosed by monitoring ALT levels and serum HCV RNA in the months after acute disease. By definition, patients with abnormal ALT values for more than 6 to 12 months have progressed to chronic hepatitis C and may at this point undergo a liver biopsy to establish the histological activity of the disease. Also, patients who remain serum positive for HCV RNA despite ALT levels returning to normal, often have evidence of chronic hepatitis, usually of mild activity, on liver biopsy. A subacute course of hepatitis C with progressive hepatic failure is exceptional and should always stimulate a search for other causes of liver damage.

The most frequent pattern of evolution is that of a progressive reduction of ALT levels after the early acute phase, often with transient prolonged periods of normal levels followed by relapses of enzyme activity. Serum HCV RNA is persistently or intermittently positive. Sequential evaluation of the patient for at least 6 to 12 months is essential to define the outcome of acute hepatitis C correctly.

Three main virological, serological, and biochemical profiles develop during and after acute hepatitis C:

Pattern A

In this type there is full recovery with virus eradication (Fig. 3). This favourable outcome is thought to occur in 10 to 30 per cent of infected individuals. The percentage with self-limited infection has varied in different series, as a consequence of the type of patients included and of the criteria used to define recovery. The persistence of a normal level of ALT after the acute phase is not an acceptable criteria for recovery as chronic infection may develop with normal ALT (Fig. 4). Furthermore, a negative HCV RNA test in a single serum sample may not guarantee virus eradication, because of the possibility of intermittent viraemia during chronic infection (Fig. 4). Some studies have gone to the extreme of denying that full recovery of acute hepatitis C with complete virus eradication is possible; others have described such cases (Table 6). Patients with full recovery become negative for HCV RNA and may loose all anti-HCV reactivities over the long term (Fig. 3). The RIBA pattern may become indeterminate with an isolated reactivity to C22 before anti-HCV becomes negative (Fig. 3). In some studies, recovery was more frequent in patients with community-acquired hepatitis and no overt parenteral exposure compared with post-transfusion hepatitis (Bortolotti, ItalJGastr, 1982; 14:86), but this was not confirmed in other studies (Tassopoulos, Gastro, 1992; 102:969). Resolution of acute hepatitis C may also depend on the viraemic titre and genomic heterogeneity of the quasispecies in the infecting inoculum and on the HCV genotype.

Pattern B

In this type there is persistent viraemia with normal ALT levels. In these patients ALT remains normal after acute hepatitis while serum

Table 6 Outcome of acute hepatitis C

Author	No of cases	Long-term outcome	
		Persistent ALT elevation (%)	Persistent HCV RNA positivity (%)
Barrera, Hepatol, 1995; 21:639	41	77	90
Omata, Lancet, 1991; 338:914	14	78	82
Lampertico, Lancet, 1994; 341:1501	16	63	100
Hwang, Hepatol, 1994; 21:831	17	62	87
Alter, NEJM, 1992; 327:1899	106	62	100
Tassopulos, Gastro, 1992; 102:969	96	62	n.t.
Giuberti, JHepatol, 1994; 20:666	60	77	77

n.t., not tested.

HCV RNA remains continuously or intermittently positive with transition into a chronic HCV carrier state (Barrera, Hepatol, 1995; 21:639) (Fig. 4). About 10 to 20 per cent of patients with acute hepatitis C develop this profile. They usually maintain high anti-HCV titres over the long term. The natural course of chronic infection in these cases is only partially known and will be described under chronic infection.

Pattern C

In this type there is a progression to biochemically active chronic hepatitis (Fig. 4). This is the most frequent pattern, with 40 to 60 per cent of patients with acute hepatitis C progressing to chronic hepatitis C; biochemical activity is shown by the ALT behaviour. The enzyme profile may remain continuously abnormal or exhibit ALT peaks and elevations separated by phases of a normal level that last from months to a few years. Conceivably, the asymptomatic HCV carrier state and biochemically active chronic hepatitis C may represent different phases of the same disease rather than two separate clinical entities. Viraemia may be persistent or intermittent, with large fluctuations in titres often, but not always, mimicking the behaviour of ALT. The long-term outcome in these patients is described under chronic infection.

Chronic infection

Usually chronic HCV infection is not preceded by an overt acute episode. Two different biochemical profiles are recognized: (i) The HCV carrier state with persistent (or intermittent) viraemia and normal ALT, and (ii) chronic hepatitis C with ALT abnomalities.

HCV carrier state

A subgroup of chronic HCV carriers have normal ALT levels despite persistent or intermittent viraemia These individuals were named 'asymptomatic' HCV carriers, but the term is inappropriate, referring to the absence of biochemical (ALT) abnormalities rather than of symptoms. A better definition might be that of 'HCV carriers with normal ALT'. Individuals with HCV RNA in their serum and repeatedly normal (for at least 6 months) ALT values

are often identified at screening for blood donation or at occasional anti-HCV testing. Despite the normality of liver enzymes, most of these HCV carriers have histological signs of liver disease when a liver biopsy is performed; a true healthy carrier state is relatively uncommon (Table 7). Published reports agree that more than two-thirds of the HCV carriers with normal ALT exhibit histological evidence of chronic hepatitis, usually of the mild to moderate type; an occasional patient may have liver cirrhosis (Alberti, Lancet, 1992; 340:697). A completely normal liver biopsy is rarely seen; about 10 to 30 per cent have non-specific histological changes (Hoofnagle, Hepatol, 1997; 26:155). The pathogenesis and natural history of HCV infection in these virus carriers have not been fully defined. Some studies have reported a low prevalence of genotype HCV-1b and a high prevalence of HCV-2 (Silini, Hepatol, 1995; 21:285); likewise, the activity and severity of histological lesions have been associated with the HCV load, patients with milder forms of liver damage displaying lower HCV RNA amounts in serum and liver (Naito, Hepatol, 1994; 19:871).

However, other studies have not confirmed these findings (Shindo, Hepatol, 1995; 22:418). Of note, patients initially identifed as HCV carriers with normal ALT may show reactivation of liver enzymes during the follow-up with transition into a biochemically active chronic hepatitis C; sustained clearance of HCV RNA with resolution of HCV infection is extremely rare, at least at medium-term follow-up. Thus, individuals who are found to be HCV carriers with normal ALT must be monitored carefully with periodic clinical and biochemical evaluation. The indications for a liver biopsy when the ALT level is normal are controversial; most patients will show histological signs of mild chronic hepatitis, but the prognostic value of histological activity scores in this setting has not been defined. Although a liver biopsy may be useful to define the stage of the liver disease, according to the amount and pattern of fibrosis, there is at present no indication to treat with interferon HCV carriers with normal ALT, irrespective of histological activity and stage. Periodic ALT monitoring should be used to identify patients with bio-chemical reactivations and to decide whether to perform a liver biopsy and give treatment.

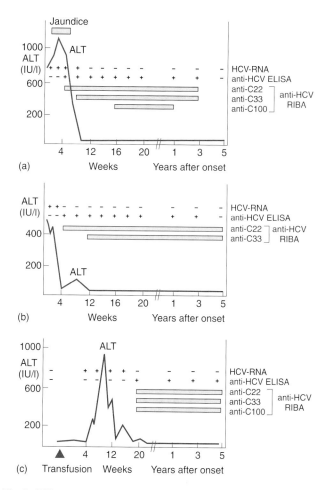

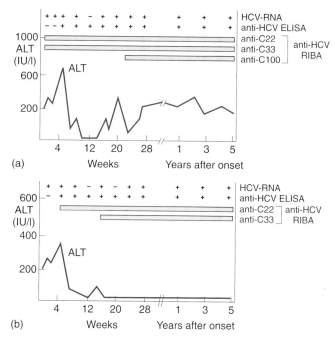

Fig. 4. Chronic evolution of hepatitis C. (a) Evolution into biochemically active chronic hepatitis C. Seroconversion to anti-HCV was delayed with respect to anti-C22 and anti-C33. A transient phase of serum HCV RNA negativity and of normal levels of ALT occurred during the post-acute phase period. (b) Evolution into the chronic HCV asymptomatic carrier state. ALT returned to normal after the acute phase but viraemia persisted.

Fig. 3. Different biochemical and virological profiles in patients with acute hepatitis C showing full biochemical and virological recovery. (a) Symptomatic, community-acquired acute hepatitis C. Early acute phase is positive for serum HCV RNA without anti-HCV. During convalescence the patient developed first anti-C22, followed by anti-C33. Anti-C100 positivity was delayed and short lived. Over the long term all anti-HCV reactivities disappeared. (b) Community-acquired acute hepatitis C without jaundice. Viraemia was limited to the early phase, followed by anti-C22 and anti-C33 seroconversion, without anti-C100. Over the long term the patient developed an indeterminate anti-HCV RIBA pattern with isolated anti-C22 reactivity. (c) Post-transfusion acute hepatitis C. This patient had a prolonged phase of viraemia without anti-HCV throughout the whole period of liver damage. Simultaneous anti-C22, anti-C33, and anti-C100 seroconversion occurred during convalescence and all antibody reactivities remained detectable up to 5 years after onset.

Biochemically active chronic hepatitis C

The course of chronic hepatitis C with ALT elevations is often unpredictable in the individual patient. In a number of patients it progresses slowly to more severe and active liver disease with increasing fibrosis and ultimately with transition to cirrhosis. Cirrhosis may become complicated by severe sequelae, including hepatocellular carcinoma. Progression may take years or decades. Progressive disease is depicted in Fig. 5. In other patients, the liver disease remains stable in a mild or intermediate stage without significant worsening.

Rates of progression from acute hepatitis C to cirrhosis, and from each of the intermediate stages into the next stage (as derived from the limited number of longitudinal studies available to date), are given in Table 8. The speed of advance to endstage liver disease remains controversial. It is obviously affected by the time and disease stage at which the observation is initiated and this starting point is variable in published series.

When the degree of hepatic fibrosis was related to the known duration of HCV infection, chronic HCV carriers could be classified as rapid, intermediate, and slow 'fibrosers' with an estimated time interval between infection and development of cirrhosis of 3 to 10 years, 15 to 30 years, and more than 50 years, respectively, with about one-third of patients falling in each group (Poynard, Lancet, 1997; 349:825). In these studies, rate of fibrosis progression was increased by factors such as male gender, alcohol consumption, and acquisition of HCV after the age of 45 years.

A number of studies have described chronic hepatitis C as a progressive disease, with clinically severe sequelae. In patients presenting with chronic hepatitis C to a tertiary referral centre in the United States, who were followed for a mean period of 4 years, there was a 50 per cent rate of progression to cirrhosis and a 5 per cent progression rate to hepatocellular carcinoma with 15 per cent mortality (Tong, NEJM, 1992; 332:1463). Similar results were obtained in Spain where over a follow-up period of 10 years, 30 per cent of the patients with chronic hepatitis C developed cirrhosis, 2 to 7 per cent hepatocellular carcinoma, and 4.9 per cent died of liver complications (Sanchez-Tapias, unpublished).

In contrast, a study of 568 transfused patients found no overall increase in mortality 18 years after transfusion in patients who had

Table 7 Risk factors and liver histology in asymptomatic HCV carriers with HCV RNA in serum and normal ALT

Author	No. of cases	Risk factors (% cases)				Liver histology (% cases)			
		Blood transfusion	IV drugs	Others	No	Normal or unspecific	CPH	CAH	Cirrhosis
Alberti, Lancet, 1992; 340:697	10	20	—	—	80	—	60	30	10
Van Thiel, JHepatol, 1995; 23:503	21	54	32	—	14	—	10	33	57
Naito, Hepatol, 1994; 19:871	22	60	—	—	40	14	86	—	—
Silini, Hepatol, 1995; 21:285	48		n.r.			35	42	23	—
Prati, Gastro, 1996; 110:178	41	19	6	9	66	31	15	54	—
Prieto, Hepatol, 1995; 22:413	58	23	6	6	65	41	38	21	—
Shindo, Hepatol, 1995; 22:418	21	57	—	—	43	10	90	90	—
Serfaty, Hepatol, 1995; 21:725	85	35	34	—	31	5	35	53	7

n.r., not recorded.
CPH, chronic persistent hepatitis.
CAH, chronic active hepatitis.

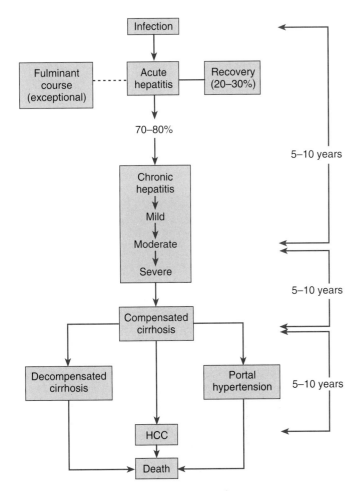

Fig. 5. Natural history of hepatitis C.

individuals who underwent liver biopsy exhibited only a mild form of chronic hepatitis 15 years after the infection (Wiese, JHepatol, 1995; 23:89).

Variables associated with the outcome of chronic hepatitis C are described in Table 9. The ALT levels and profile do not predict the severity of histological lesions (Alberti, Lancet, 1992; 340:697; Alter, NEJM, 1992; 327:1899) although high ALT values (more than 10-fold the upper normal limit) predict a more prominent piecemeal necrosis (Haber, AmJGastr, 1995; 90:1250) and a correlation between the level of serum ALT and liver histological scores has been reported (Hoofnagle, Hepatol, 1997; 28:15S). The age of the patient and the duration of the infection correlate with the stage of liver disease, older patients with longer disease displaying more advanced lesions (Qu, JHepatol, 1994; 21:70; Nousbaum, AnnIntMed 1995; 122:161; Pontisso, JViralHepat, 1995; 2:33). The age and mode of acquisition of HCV infection may also be important; histology and outcome are often more severe in patients infected via blood transfusion than those with community-acquired hepatitis C (Gordon, Hepatol, 1993; 18:1338), possibly as a consequence of a larger virus inoculum and higher levels of HCV replication (Lau, Lancet, 1993; 341:1501). A number of recent studies suggest that the course of chronic hepatitis C may be particularly severe with a more rapid progression to cirrhosis when the infection is acquired at an age of more than 45 or 50 years (Lucidarme, JHepatol, 1997; 26(Suppl.1): 88; Roudot-Thoraval, JHepatol, 1997; 26(Suppl.1):82). Intravenous drug abusers often have mild forms of chronic hepatitis C, if not coinfected by HIV (Booth, Gut, 1995; 36:427), and are more frequently infected by genotype HCV-3 (Pontisso, JViralHepat, 1995; 2:33); a finding that raises the question of whether the HCV type plays a role in determining severity and course of chronic hepatitis C. A number of reports have suggested that in patients with HCV-1b the disease runs a more active and advanced course (Dusheiko, Hepatol, 1994; 19:13; Pozzato, JMedVirol, 1994; 43: 291; Nousbaum, AnnIntMed, 1995; 122:161; Silini, Hepatol, 1995; 21:285). A more rapid evolution was recently documented in patients infected with HCV-1 in a prospective, long-term, follow-up study (Kabayashi, Hepatol, 1996; 23:695), but this is not in

contracted hepatitis C, with a 3.3 per cent mortality rate due to liver disease (Seeff, NEJM, 1992; 327:1905). Likewise, chronic hepatitis C developed in 50 per cent of a homogeneous group of 350 women injected with anti-DIg contaminated with HCV, but all the 345

Table 8 The natural course of hepatitis C

A. Progression rates from acute HCV infection to cirrhosis

	Progression (%)	Mean follow-up (years)
Tong, NEJM, 1995; 332:1463	50	21
Di Bisceglie, Hepatol, 1991; 14:696	24	23
Koretz, AnnIntMed, 1993; 119:110	18	16
Wiese, JHepatol, 1995; 23:89	0	15
Tremolada, JHepatol, 1992; 16:273	32	5
Booth, Gut, 1995; 366:427	30	10

B. Histological progression in patients with chronic hepatitis C

	Yearly rates (%)						
	(1)	(2)	(3)	(4)	(5)	(6)	(7)
CPH → remission	4	—	—	—	—	—	—
CPH → CAH	4	—	—	—	4	—	—
CPH → cirrhosis	0.6	—	—	—	0.9	<1	—
CAH → remission	0	—	—	—	—	—	—
CAH → cirrhosis	23	4	1.2	8	2–10	5	3

C. Liver disease-related mortality in patients with post-transfusion hepatitis C

Author	Follow-up after transfusion (years)	% Death due to liver disease
Tremolada, JHepatol, 1992; 166:273	10	4.8
Tong, NEJM, 1992; 332:1463	~28	15
Seeff, NEJM, 1992; 327:1905	~18	3.3
Di Bisceglie, Hepatol, 1991; 14:696	23	4–9
Sanchez-Tapias (unpublished)	10	3–6

(1) Hopf, JHepatol, 1990; 10:69; (2) Davis, JHepatol, 1990; 11:972; (3) Garcia del Ancos, JHepatol, 1990; 11:S11; (4) Tremolada, JHepatol, 1992; 16:273; (5) Takahashi, AmJGastr, 1993; 88:240; (6) Yano, Hepatol, 1996; 23:1334; (7) Sanchez-Tapias (unpublished).
CPH, chronic persistent hepatitis.
CAH, chronic active hepatitis.

Table 9 Variables influencing the severity and course of chronic hepatitis C

Variable	Type of association	Available evidence
Patient's age	Stage of disease	Consistent
Duration of infection	Stage of disease	Consistent
Mode of transmission	Post-transfusion more severe than others	Controversial
ALT levels and profile	No association with histology	Consistent
Liver histology	Predictive of outcome	Mostly consistent
Viraemia levels	Activity and outcome of liver disease	Mostly controversial
HCV genotype	Activity and outcome of liver disease	Controversial
HCV quasispecies	Activity and outcome of liver disease	Controversial
HBV infection	Activity and outcome of liver disease	Consistent
Alcohol abuse	Activity and outcome of liver disease	Mostly consistent

keeping with other studies (Yamada, DigDisSci, 1994; 39:234; Naito, Hepatol, 1995; 22:407; Takano, Hepatol, 1995; 21:650); possibly the severity of the liver disease often seen in individuals infected with HCV-1b may depend on older age and longer duration of infection rather than on intrinsic virus pathogenicity (Qu, JHepatol, 1994; 21:70; Nousbaum, AnnIntMed, 1995; 122:161). Also controversial is the role of high levels of serum HCV RNA and of the diversity of the HCV quasispecies in influencing the severity and course of chronic hepatitis C.

High levels of viraemia were reported to correlate with more severe histology (Gunji, IntJCanc, 1992; 52:726; Hagiwara, Hepatol, 1993; 17:545; Kato, Hepatol, 1993; 18:16), but this association was negated by others (Magrin, Hepatol, 1994; 19:273; Shindo, Hepatol, 1995; 22:418). The HCV quasispecies was shown both to correlate

Table 10 Clinical features of chronic hepatitis C

Clinical features at presentation	Frequency (%)	
	Post-transfusion hepatitis	Community-acquired hepatitis
Symptoms of disease	39	25
Jaundice	12	0
Hepatomegaly	25	10
Splenomegaly	13	10
Spider naevi	12	0
Portal hypertension	11	0
Biochemical features		
ALT fluctuations	90	75
Raised IgG	35	15
Raised IgM	0	0
Raised γ-glutamyl transferase	90	55
Histological features		
Chronic persistent hepatitis	20	45
Chronic lobular hepatitis	22	25
Chronic active hepatitis	46	30
Active cirrhosis	12	0

(Honda, Hepatol, 1994; 20:1144) and not to correlate (Naito, Hepatol, 1995; 22:407; Shindo, Hepatol, 1995; 22:418) with progression of liver disease. The changes in quasispecies during follow-up were found in one prospective study to correlate with the clinical outcome of acute hepatitis C, with a diminishing number of variants in resolving infection, a stable number of variants in those who progressed to chronic mild disease, and a marked increase in the virus heterogeneity in those with a severe outcome (Farci, Hepatol, 1996; 24:350A). Given the uncertain prognostic value of most biochemical and virological markers, liver histology still represents the most adequate way to assess the stage and prognosis of chronic hepatitis C. In a large cohort of untreated patients, followed for a long period of time, the risk of developing cirrhosis was closely related to the initial degree of portal and periportal fibrosis as well as on the grade of necroinflammatory activity (Yano, Hepatol, 1996; 23:1334). Aetiological cofactors such as coinfection with HBV (Chen, JInfDis, 1990; 162:817; Pontisso, Gastro, 1993; 105:1529; Benvegnù, Cancer, 1994; 74:2442) or with HIV (Eyster, JAIDS, 1993; 6:602), alcohol abuse (Seeff, NEJM, 1992; 327:1906; Yamauchi, AmJGastr, 1993; 88:39; Sato, JViralHepat, 1996; 3:143), and malignancy (Inui, JHepatol, 1994; 21:748) have a definite worsening effect on chronic hepatitis C; in contrast, coinfection with HGV does not seem to affect prognosis (Alter, NEJM, 1997; 336:747). The course of hepatitis C appears to be more severe in patients with hypo/agammaglobulinaemia (Bjoro, NEJM, 1994; 331:1607).

In conclusion, male gender, age and duration of infection, liver histology, presence of aetiological cofactors, particularly HBV and alcohol, and the immunocompetence of the host are important in predicting the course of chronic hepatitis C; the prognostic value of other parameters such as virus load and type needs to be better defined in well conducted and controlled prospective studies.

Clinical features of chronic hepatitis C

The clinical features depend on the stage of the underlying liver disease. Table 10 is a description of some features observed in a large series of patients with chronic post-transfusion or community-acquired hepatitis C. In chronic hepatitis without cirrhosis, about one-third of cases are symptomatic and the symptoms are those of any other chronic liver disease.[20] Mild to intermediate hepatomegaly is found in 30 to 70 per cent of cases and splenomegaly is present in 0 to 15 per cent. The main symptom is fatigue, present in 50 to 100 per cent of patients depending on the stage of disease (Tong, NEJM, 1995; 332:1465). Anorexia, weight loss, and abdominal discomfort are rarely seen initially but become more prominent with the progression of liver disease. Muscle aches, arthralgias, and itching may also be present.

Jaundice is present in no more that 1 per cent of cases (Tong, NEJM, 1995; 332:1465), apart from patients with decompensated, endstage disease. ALT is more sensitive than aspartate aminotransferase in detecting liver damage (Koretz, Gastro, 1985; 88: 1251). It often waxes and wanes with periods of normal or near normal values between reactivations; fluctuations tend to diminish as the disease advances to the cirrhotic stage. The same pattern is seen in patients in whom the biochemical resolution of hepatitis is delayed; vacillation of ALT is typical of the early phase but may not be a feature of long-standing disease. Gammaglobulins are not elevated, or only slightly, in patients without cirrhosis, the increase relating to the IgG fraction (Table 10). γ-Glutamyl transferase activity is usually increased more than in other forms of chronic hepatitis. The histological features of chronic hepatitis C cover a spectrum of lesions ranging from non-specific and mild changes to chronic lobular, chronic persistent, and chronic active hepatitis with, or without, superimposed cirrhosis.[21] Compared with hepatitis B and autoimmune hepatitis, chronic hepatitis C usually displays less portal and periportal inflammatory activity and more lobular and degenerative changes. Bridging necrosis is rare; in analogy with the acute disease, macrovesicular steatosis, sinusoidal cell activation, and eosinophilic granules are frequent. Bile duct lesions, with piling up of ductular epithelial cells in the duct lumen without a break in the basement membrane, have been reported as characteristic

(Poulsen, HumPath, 1972; 3:217), but are inconsistently present (Bamber, JClinPath, 1981; 34:1175; Dienes, Hepatol, 1982; 2:562); in recent studies, they were found in about 25 per cent of patients (Scheuer, Hepatol, 1992; 15:567; Lefkowich, Gastro, 1993; 104: 595). Macrovesicular steatosis is present in 30 to 70 per cent of cases (Bach, Hepatol, 1992; 15:572; Czaja, Gastro, 1993; 105:1824).

Therefore, histological features may be helpful for suspecting and defining chronic hepatitis C, but none are pathognomonic and many cannot be relied upon to establish a morphological diagnosis. Liver biopsy evaluation is nevertheless important for assessing grade, stage, and prognosis of the disease.[22,23]

Semiquantitative methods for scoring liver biopsies of patients with chronic viral hepatitis, including hepatitis C, have been developed (Knodell, Hepatol, 1981; 1:431; Desmet, Hepatol, 1994; 19:1513; French, Hepatol, 1994; 20:15). These methods grade four different features: periportal necrosis, with or without bridging necrosis, parenchymal injury, portal inflammation, and fibrosis. Grading is derived from the summation of the first three parameters while staging is defined by the fibrosis score. High grading scores are associated with more active disease and predict a more rapid future progression. High fibrosis scores indicate more advanced disease. The fibrosis score may allow prediction of when cirrhosis will eventually develop, at least in instances in which the date of onset of hepatitis C is known (Poynard, Lancet, 1997; 349:825). Liver histology is therefore the gold standard for assessing severity and prognosis of hepatitis C.

Clinical course of hepatitis C in special subgroups

The course of acute and chronic hepatitis C is influenced by the immunocompetence of the host and by the effect of aetiological cofactors of liver damage. In the immunocompromised host, hepatitis C may run a more severe course, as is the case in renal transplant recipients in whom the infection is an important cause of liver disease and may significantly reduce survival (Chan, Gastro, 1993; 104:862; Hanafusa, TransplProc, 1995; 27:956). Patients with human immunodeficiency virus (HIV 1) are frequently coinfected with HCV, and HCV replication appears to be enhanced in this setting. Coexisting HIV infection may accelerate the evolution of HCV-related liver disease (Martin, Gastro, 1989; 97:1559); the course becomes particularly aggressive and severe in the presence of low CD4 cell counts (Eyster, JAIDS, 1993; 6:602). However, survival of HIV-positive patients seems not to be significantly affected by coinfection with HCV (Wright, Hepatol, 1994; 20:1152). Patients with malignancy have an increased prevalence of HCV infection; this is particularly frequent in those with haematological tumours because of the frequent use of blood transfusion and blood products. A more severe and progressive course of chronic hepatitis C was reported in Japanese children with severe anaemia compared with cases of benign anaemia (Inui, JHepatol, 1994; 21:748). The presence of pretransplant HCV infection was reported to be a significant risk factor for severe liver disease after bone marrow transplantation (Frickhofen, Blood, 1994; 83:1998), but this was not confirmed (Locasciulli, BoneMTrans, 1997; 19:237). HCV infection did not affect in a significant way the morbidity and mortality of long-term survivors of acute leukaemia, at least in the paediatric

setting (Locasciulli, Blood, 1997; 90:4628). The interaction between hepatitis C and alcohol has been the subject of many studies, most of them concluding that liver disease is more progressive and severe when the two aetiologies coexist (Nalpas, JHepatol, 1991; 12:70; Zignego, Hepatol, 1994; 19:577); this is the basis for recommending avoidance of alcoholic beverages to HCV-infected subjects.

Coinfection with HBV and HCV is not uncommon and is associated with more severe histological liver lesions and more rapid progression towards liver failure (Sanchez Tapias, AnnIntMed, 1990; 112:921; Fong, Hepatol, 1994; 21:509).

HCV and hepatocellular carcinoma

HCV markers are frequently detected in patients with hepatocellular carcinoma, although with significant geographical variations.[24] The highest rates of association are found in Southern Europe (Bruix, Lancet, 1989; ii:1004; Colombo, Lancet, 1989; ii:1006; Ruiz, Hepatol, 1992; 16:637) and Japan (Nishioka, Cancer, 1991; 67:429), intermediate rates in Austria (Baur, ArchVirol, 1992; 2:76), Taiwan (Jeng, JMedVirol, 1991; 34:74), and Saudi Arabia (Al Karawi, JGastHepatol, 1992; 7:237), and low rates in the United States (Di Bisceglie, Hepatol, 1991; 86:335), South Africa (Kew, Lancet, 1990; 335:873), and in some countries of the Far East. Patients positive for anti-HCV with hepatocellular carcinoma almost invariably have an underlying cirrhosis, but there have been occasional reports of patients with hepatocellular carcinoma in a non-cirrhotic liver, and HCV has been implicated in a tumour arising in a normal liver (De Mitri, Lancet, 1994; 345:413). Sequences of HCV RNA are detectable in the tumorous tissue (Gerber, AmJPathol, 1992; 141: 1271; Takeda, Cancer, 1992; 70:2255) and virus replication has also been demonstrated within this tissue (Horrike, JMedVirol, 1993; 41:312). The mechanism by which HCV infection promotes the development of hepatocellular carcinoma is not understood.[25] The effect of the virus may only be indirect, causing cirrhosis which in itself is a risk factor for the development of this tumour; a direct oncogenic effect of HCV and/or virus products cannot be excluded.

The risk for an individual chronically infected with HCV to develop hepatocellular carcinoma was assessed in retrospective and prospective studies.[26] Sequential transition from acute hepatitis C to chronic hepatitis, cirrhosis, and hepatocellular carcinoma in individual patients has been well documented, with a time-lag between infection and the appearance of the tumour of 5 to 30 years (Kiyosawa, AmJGastr, 1984; 79:777; Di Bisceglie, JClinGastro, 1994; 29:222). The annual risk of developing hepatocellular carcinoma is around 0.5 to 1.5 per cent for patients with chronic hepatitis C without cirrhosis and between 3 and 10 per cent for patients with compensated HCV cirrhosis; it is higher in Japanese patients (Oka, Hepatol, 1990; 12:680; Takano, Hepatol, 1995; 21: 650) than in Caucasians (Benvegnù, Cancer, 1994; 74:2994). The continuing biochemical activity of liver disease increases the risk of developing this tumour. Coinfection with HBV and alcohol abuse is associated with an increased risk of hepatocellular carcinoma in those with cirrhosis (Yamauchi, AmJGastr, 1993; 88:39; Benvegnù, 1994).

It has been suggested that patients with HCV-1b may develop hepatocellular carcinoma more frequently than those with other genotypes (Yamauchi, IntHepatolComm, 1994; 2:328); however,

Table 11 Extrahepatic disorders and diseases caused by or associated with hepatitis C

Extrahepatic manifestations	Association with hepatitis C
Essential mixed cryoglobulinaemia Vasculitis Membranoproliferative glomerulonephritis	Strong (HCV most likely has a pathogenetic role)
Porphyria cutanea tarda Low-grade malignant non-Hodgkin's lymphoma	Significant (HCV may act as an aetiological cofactor)
Mooren's corneal ulcers Autoimmune thyroiditis Lichen planus	Possible (further data needed)
Sjögren's syndrome Idiopathic pulmonary fibrosis Aplastic anaemia Polyarteritis nodosa Erythema nodosum	Weak (a pathogenetic role of HCV is unlikely)

definitive evidence that these patients have a significantly increased risk is lacking (Benvegnù, Hepatol, 1997; 25:211).

Extrahepatic manifestations of hepatitis C

Chronic HCV infection has been associated with a variety of extrahepatic manifestations, listed in Table 11. The specificity of the association has been established for essential mixed cryoglobulinaemia, vasculitis, and membranoproliferative glomerulonephritis; it is strong for porphyria cutanea tarda; suspected for some forms of low-grade malignancy B-cell lymphomas, Mooren's corneal ulcers, and autoimmune thyroiditis; and weak and doubtful for Sjögren's syndrome, lichen planus, and idiopathic pulmonary fibrosis.[27] About 50 per cent of patients with chronic hepatitis C have cryoglobulins in their serum at variable concentrations and about 10 to 15 per cent have significant cryocrits (Lunel, Gastro, 1994; 106:1291); cryoglobulinaemia is of type III (polyclonal immunoglobulins) or of type II (mixed monoclonal and polyclonal immunoglobulins). Similarly, the majority of patients presenting with essential mixed cryoglobulinaemia have evidence of liver disease and many are infected by HCV (Misiani, AnnIntMed, 1992; 117:573; Ferri, Blood, 1993; 81:1132); this suggests a major aetiological role of HCV in the development of cryoglobulinaemia. The role of HCV in causing this condition is supported by the presence of HCV RNA in cryoprecipitable immune complexes as well as in the vasculitic lesions (Sansonno, Hepatol, 1995; 21:305). HCV RNA may be found in the serum and cryoprecipitate of patients with type II essential mixed cryoglobulinaemia who are negative for anti-HCV (Agnello, NEJM, 1992; 327:1490). Cryoglobulinaemia is asymptomatic in most patients; 10 to 25 per cent experience the clinical syndrome of essential mixed cryoglobulinaemia, namely a systemic vasculitis characterized by arthralgias, Raynaud's disease, purpura, and weakness, which may become complicated by peripheral neuropathy and glomerulomembranous nephritis. The development of mixed cryoglobulinaemia in chronic hepatitis C does not correlate with virus replication or with the type of infecting HCV but shows a clear relation to the duration of infection and to advanced stages of liver disease.

The observation that cryoglobulins are more frequent in patients with long-standing infection and advanced liver disease suggests that chronic immune stimulation of B cells may be important for the production of immune complexes. As there are geographical differences in the prevalence of cryoglobulinaemia in chronic hepatitis C (higher in southern Europe than in other areas), genetic factors may be involved. Chronic stimulation of the immune system may also explain the progression from mixed type II cryoglobulinaemia towards the low-grade malignancy non-Hodgkin's lymphoma reported in patients with chronic HCV infection (Pozzato, Blood, 1994; 84:3047).

Porphyria cutanea tarda, the most common form of porphyria, is strongly associated with HCV infection; 60 to 80 per cent of affected patients are positive for anti-HCV in serum and up to 100 per cent for HCV RNA in the liver (Fargion, Hepatol, 1992; 16:1322; Navas, Hepatol, 1995; 21:279). Therefore patients with this metabolic defect should always be tested for HCV markers.

A relationship between chronic HCV infection and Sjögren's syndrome was suggested by the detection of anti-HCV in a number of patients with this syndrome, usually in association with cryoglobulinaemia, and by the finding of lymphocytic sialoadenitis in up to 50 per cent of HCV-infected individuals (Haddad, Lancet, 1992; 339:321). This association, however, was not confirmed in other series (King, AmJGastr, 1994; 89:1047). The role, if any, of HCV in other autoimmune and skin diseases[28] in which this virus has been implicated on the basis of an increased prevalence of viral markers in serum remains unproved.

The association between hepatitis C and type II autoimmune hepatitis

Many patients with chronic hepatitis C have low titres of autoantibodies that are organ specific (mainly antithyroid) or non-organ specific (mainly antinuclear and anti-smooth muscle).[29] In the absence of typical features of autoimmune hepatitis or of coexisting autoimmune diseases, these reactions are thought to be epiphenomena without clinical significance. A subgroup (0 to 10 per cent) of patients with chronic HCV infection have serum antibodies against liver/kidney microsomal antigens (anti-LKM-1). In this clinical setting, it is important to distinguish chronic hepatitis C with anti-LKM-1 from autoimmune type 2 hepatitis, but overlapping cases may exist (see Chapter 14.3)

Therapy and prevention

Therapy

This is dealt with in Chapter 12.1.3.2.

Prevention

A vaccine to protect against hepatitis C is not yet available. Effective pre- and postexposure prophylaxis is not currently available and immunoglobulin injection is not recommended. Screening of blood and organ donors prevents the transmission of hepatitis C via transfusion and transplantation, but these types of exposure account for a small minority of infections. The modification of high-risk behaviours among drug abusers is important to reduce the spread of hepatitis C. Carriers of HCV should be told to avoid sharing potentially contaminated objects and counselled on behaviours to minimize the risk of transmitting the disease.[30]

In the health care setting, universal precautions should be adopted to reduce the risk of contamination of medical personnel and patients.

On the basis of available data and according to the general consensus (United States National Institutes of Health, Consensus Development Statement on 'Management of Hepatitis C', March 24 to 26, 1997),[31] condom-protected sexual practices should be encouraged in persons with multiple sexual partners, while this type of precaution is less important in monogamous long-term relationships. Sexual partners of HCV-infected patients should be tested periodically for anti-HCV.

Pregnancy is not contraindicated in HCV-infected women and breast feeding is considered safe.

References

1. Houghton M, *et al.* Molecular biology of the hepatitis C viruses: implications for diagnosis, development and control of viral disease. *Hepatology*, 1991; **14**: 382–8.
2. Alter MJ. Epidemiology of hepatitis C in the West. *Seminars in Liver Disease*, 1995; **15**: 5–14.
3. Mansell CJ and Locarnini SA. Epidemiology of hepatitis C in the East. *Seminars in Liver Disease*, 1995; **15**: 15–32.
4. Rizzetto M, Purcell RH, Gerin JL, and Verme G, eds. *Viral hepatitis and liver disease*. Turin, Italy: Minerva Medica, 1997.
5. Alter HJ. Transmission pattern in hepatitis C virus infection. *Viral Hepatitis and Liver Disease*, 1994; 445–9.
6. Roth D. Hepatitis C virus: the nephrologist's view. *American Journal of Kidney Diseases*, 1995; **25**: 3–16.
7. Terrault NA and Wright TL. Hepatitis C virus in the setting of transplantation. *Seminars in Liver Disease*, 1995; **15**: 92–100.
8. Scott GR. The sexual transmission of hepatitis C virus. *International Journal of STD and AIDS*, 1995; **6**: 1–3.
9. Ruff AJ. Breastmilk, breastfeeding and transmission of viruses to the neonate. *Seminars in Perinatology*, 1994; **18**: 510–16.
10. Matsuura Y and Miyamura T. The molecular biology of hepatitis C virus. *Virology*, 1993; **203**: 297–304.
11. Booth JCL and Thomas HC. Pathogenesis of chronic hepatitis C and associated clinical manifestations. In Alberti A, ed. *Baillière's clinical gastroenterology*, Vol 10. London, 1996: 257–74.
12. Koff RS and Dienstag JL. Extrahepatic manifestations of hepatitis C and the association with alcohol liver disease. *Seminars in Liver Disease*, 1995; **15**: 101–9.
13. Strassburg CP and Manns MP. Autoimmune versus viral hepatitis C. *Liver*, 1995; **15**: 225–32.
14. Alberti A. IgM antibodies to hepatitis C virus. *Journal of Viral Hepatitis*, 1994; **1**: 85–6.
15. Krajden M. Molecular detection of hepatitis C virus: impact of detection methodology on clinical and laboratory correlations. *Critical Reviews in Clinical Laboratory Sciences*, 1995; **32**: 41–66.
16. Lau JYN, *et al.* Significance of serum hepatitis C virus RNA levels in chronic hepatitis C. *Lancet*, 1993; **341**: 1501–4.
17. Simmonds P. Variability of hepatitis C virus. *Hepatology*, 1995; **21**: 570–83.
18. Seeff LB. Natural history of viral hepatitis, type C. *Seminars in Gastrointestinal Disease*, 1995; **6**: 20–7.
19. Sherlock DS. Chronic hepatitis C. *Disease-A-Month*, 1994; **40**: 117–96.
20. Dienstag JL. NANB hepatitis.I. Recognition, epidemiology and clinical features. *Gastroenterology*, 1983; **85**: 439–62.
21. Goodman ZD and Ishak KG. Histopathology of hepatitis C virus infection. *Seminars in Liver Disease*, 1995; **15**: 70–81.
22. Knodell RG, *et al.* Formulation and application of a numerical scoring system for assessing histological activity in asymptomatic chronic active hepatitis. *Hepatology*, 1981; **1**: 431–5.
23. Desmet VJ, *et al.* Classification of chronic hepatitis: diagnosis, grading and staging. *Hepatology*, 1994; **19**: 1513–20.
24. Di Bisceglie AM. Hepatitis C and hepatocellular carcinoma. *Seminars in Liver Disease*, 1995; **15**: 64–9.
25. Brechot C. Hepatitis B and C viruses and primary liver cancer. In Alberti A, ed. *Baillière's clinical gastroenterology*, Vol. 10. London, 1996: 335–73.
26. Benvegnù L and Alberti A. Risk factors and prevention of hepatocellular carcinoma in HCV infection. *Digestive Diseases and Sciences*, 1996; **41**: 33S–39S.
27. Gumber SC and Chapra S. Hepatitis C: a multifaceted disease. *Annals of Internal Medicine*, 1995; **123**: 615–20.
28. Pawlotsky JM, Dhumeaux D, and Bagot M. Hepatitis C virus in dermatology. *Archives of Dermatology*, 1995; **131**: 1185–93.
29. Pawlotsky JM, *et al.* Immunological disorders in C virus chronic active hepatitis: a prospective case–control study. *Hepatology*, 1994; **19**: 841–8.
30. Dusheiko GM, Khakoo S, Soni P, and Grellier L. A rational approach to the management of hepatitis C infection. *British Medical Journal*, 1996; **12**: 357–64.
31. NIH Consensus Development Conference. Management of hepatitis C. *Hepatology*, 1997; **26** (Suppl. 1): 1S–155S.

12.1.2.6 Hepatitis E

K. Krawczynski

Hepatitis E is a form of acute, icteric, self-contained viral hepatitis caused by hepatitis E virus (HEV), a 28 to 34 nm, spherical, non-enveloped, single-stranded, positive-sense RNA virus transmitted by the faecal–oral route. The elimination of virus from the host is associated with the virus-specific immune response manifested by the development of antibody to HEV (anti-HEV). The host–virus interaction results in a syndrome of clinical symptoms associated with pathological changes in the liver. The clinical and epidemiological characteristics of hepatitis E in disease-endemic geographical regions of the Indian subcontinent, Asia, and Africa indicate that hepatitis E is an imporatant cause of morbidity and mortality in humans.

Clinical characteristics, pathology, and pathogenesis

Clinical features

Clinical signs and symptoms of the disease in patients with symptomatic HEV infection are similar to those of acute hepatitis A or B (see Chapters 12.1.2.2 and 12.1.2.3). The acute-phase symptoms include abdominal pain, anorexia, arthralgia, asthenia, clay-coloured stools, dark or tea-coloured urine, diarrhoea, fever, hepatomegaly, jaundice, malaise, nausea, pruritus, rash, splenomegaly, and vomiting.[1] The most commonly reported symptoms have been malaise (95 to 100 per cent), anorexia (66 to 100 per cent), nausea/vomiting (29 to 100 per cent), fever (23 to 97 per cent), and hepatomegaly (10 to 85 per cent).[2–4] Laboratory findings in patients with hepatitis E are also similar to findings in patients with other forms of viral hepatitis and include elevated serum bilirubin, alanine aminotransferase (**ALT**), aspartate aminotransferase, alkaline phosphatase, and γ-glutamyl transferase.

The incubation period in human volunteers after oral exposure was 4 to 5 weeks; incubation periods of 15 to 60 days have been reported during hepatitis E outbreaks (Ticehurst, JMedVirol, 1992; 36:84; Chauhan, Lancet, 1993; 341:149). The acute-phase symptoms are preceded by the prodromal phase, usually characterized by fever and nausea. Most patients with acute hepatitis E have a self-limited course, and resolution of hyperbilirubinaemia and elevated aminotransferase levels generally occurs within 3 weeks (range 1 to 6 weeks) after illness onset. The ratio of clinical to subclinical infections has not been determined; however, lower disease rates for younger age groups, which have been identified in several outbreak investigations, may be the result of anicteric and/or subclinical HEV infections. In most hepatitis E outbreaks, the highest rates of symptomatic disease (jaundice) have been in young to middle-age adults (Arankalle, Lancet, 1988; ii:1199).[5] No evidence of chronic hepatitis has been detected among patients followed up clinically and among those who had liver biopsies after acute hepatitis E (Khuroo, Lancet, 1980; ii:97; Chadha, JAssocPhysInd, 1991; 39:651).[6]

The overall case–fatality ratio for the general population in disease-endemic countries has been from 0.5 to 4 per cent.[7] Case–fatality rates ranging from 5 to 25 per cent have been reported among pregnant women infected during the third trimester.[4,8,9]

Treatment for hepatitis E is supportive. No data are available to evaluate the efficacy of antiviral agents or other specific therapies for treatment of hepatitis E.

Pathology

In most hepatitis E outbreaks, liver tissue specimens have rarely been available for histopathological analysis. Two types of histopathological changes were observed in specimens obtained from an outbreak in Delhi (India) in 1955 to 1956 (Gupta, IndJMedRes, 1957; 45(Suppl.):101). An 'obstructive' or cholestatic type was found in 58 per cent of examined cases, and a 'standard' type was identified in 42 per cent of cases. The cholestatic type was

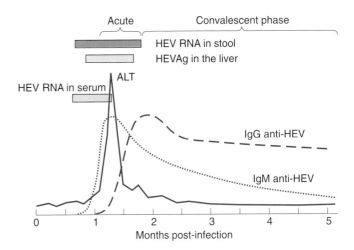

Fig. 1. Clinical course of hepatitis E. The hypothetical summary of HEV infection based on data gathered from outbreaks of hepatitis E among humans and from experimentally infected primates. The separation between the acute and convalescent phases of disease has been arbitrarily established on the basis of the alanine aminotransferase (ALT) curve.

characterized by bile stasis in canaliculi and parenchymal cells, which were arranged in a gland-like fashion. Cholestasis and glandular transformation of liver cell cords were significant in the specimens from an outbreak in West Africa (63 and 93 per cent, respectively) (Morrow, AnnIntMed, 1968; 68:1250). Degenerative changes of liver cells (including acidophilic bodies) and focal necrosis were less frequently seen in the cholestatic type of hepatitis E in the Indian patients. Polymorphonuclear leucocytes were observed both in intralobular infiltrations and in portal tracts in larger amounts than seen in the classic acute viral hepatitis, although in portal tracts monocytes (lymphocytes) remained the predominant cell type. In the 'standard' type of change typically observed in cases of viral hepatitis, ballooned hepatocytes, acidophilic degeneration of hepatocytes, and acidophilic body formation were the most frequently encountered. Similarly, in experimentally induced hepatitis E in primates, the acidophilic type of hepatocytic degeneration was a characteristic morphological feature, especially in cynomolgus macaques. Focal necrosis was observed in both patients and infected primates, with prominent accumulations of mononuclear macrophages and activated Kupffer cells and a much less striking presence of lymphocytes. Lymphocytes prevailed in portal infiltrations both in human and experimentally infected liver specimens.

Elements of pathogenesis

Clinical and pathological features of HEV infection have been characterized using surveys of patients involved in outbreaks of hepatitis E, human volunteers, and experimental models of infection in non-human primates. Data on virus replication in the liver (and perhaps extrahepatically), humoral immune response, and liver pathology related to HEV infection were collected from these studies and used to develop a composite picture of the pathogenetic events of HEV infection (Fig. 1).

In hepatitis E patients, the pathogenic features associated with HEV infection have been characterized in rare volunteer studies (Chauhan, Lancet, 1993; 341:149).[10] Although the mechanism(s) by which HEV initially reaches the liver from the intestinal tract is unknown, genomic sequences of HEV were identified in stools, bile, and sera. In surveys of patients involved in outbreaks of acute hepatitis E, HEV RNA has been detected in faeces of most patients for about 2 weeks (Aggarwal, Lancet, 1992; 340:787),[11] and faecal HEV excretion for as long as 52 days has been reported;[12] however, the correlation of HEV RNA detection with infectivity in stools has not been demonstrated. HEV RNA has regularly been found in serum in virtually all patients within 2 weeks after illness onset.[11] Prolonged periods of HEV RNA positivity in serum ranging from 4 to 16 weeks have also been reported (Schlauder, Lancet, 1993; 341:378).[12]

Both IgM and IgG anti-HEV are generally detectable at the time of illness onset, but the exact time course for the development of an antibody response is not known. It appears that the anti-HEV IgM response begins to develop just before the maximal ALT activity and disappears about 5 months into the convalescent phase of the disease.[13] The IgG response begins to develop shortly after the IgM response and its titre increases throughout the acute phase into the convalescent phase, remaining high from 1 to 4.5 years after the acute phase of the disease (Dawson, JVirolMethods, 1992; 38: 175).[13] Virtually all patients have detectable IgG anti-HEV for at least 20 months after acute infection;[14] however, in one study, less than 50 per cent of persons had detectable antibody approximately 14 years after infection (Khuroo, Lancet, 1993; 341:1355).

The experimental model of HEV infection is reproduced best in cynomolgus macaques, although other non-human primates (chimpanzees, rhesus and owl monkeys, tamarins) were shown to be susceptible to HEV infection (Soe, Liver, 1989; 9:135; Longer, JInfDis, 1993; 168:602).[15-18] In macaques inoculated with HEV intravenously, expression of HEVAg in hepatocytes,[15] indicative of viral replication, is first seen about day 7 postinfection. HEVAg has been detected in 70 to 90 per cent of hepatocytes at the peak of HEV replication and decreases rapidly after the maximum ALT activity (Krawczynski K et al., unpublished data). HEVAg has been detected simultaneously in hepatocyte cytoplasm, bile, and faeces during the second or third week after inoculation, and before and concurrently with the onset of ALT elevation and histopathological changes in the liver (Longer, JInfDis, 1993; 168:602).[17,18] These findings suggest that HEV may be released from hepatocytes into bile and, consequently, in faeces before the peak of morphological changes in the liver.

The humoral immune response in infected animals resembles patterns observed in humans. Both IgM and IgG anti-HEV are detected in serum in assays using immunoreactive epitopes of open reading frame 2 and 3 (**ORF2** and **ORF3**). As in humans, the IgM antibody level decreases rather precipitously, reaching negligible levels in the early convalescent phase. High titres of IgG anti-HEV are detected during convalescence. Anti-HEV has been observed as long as 10 years after inoculation and onset of acute hepatitis E in chimpanzees experimentally infected with serum specimens derived from HEV-infected patients in Tashkent, Pakistan, and Mexico. The profile of anti-ORF3 antibody response in a challenge experiment that followed immunization of cynomolgus macaques with recombinant capsid proteins suggested that the presence of this antibody may be indicative of HEV replication.

The inoculum titration experiments in cynomolgus macaques suggest that the size of the infectious dose may be related to the virological, immunological, and pathological sequelae of the infection.[19] The virus replication, anti-HEV immune response, and acute hepatitis were all observed only when the high-titred inoculum was administered. Clinical and pathological evidence of the liver disease and expression of HEVAg were less conspicuous with the decreasing amounts of inoculated HEV; seroconversion to anti-HEV was also observed with an increasing delay. The infection resulting from the end-point dilution of the infectious inoculum (HEV Mexico strain) was marked only by seroconversion to anti-HEV (Krawczynski K et al., in preparation).

The mechanism responsible for the destruction of hepatocytes during HEV infection remains unknown. However, the onset of ALT elevations and histopathological changes in the liver generally corresponds with the detection of anti-HEV in serum and with decreasing levels of HEVAg in hepatocytes. In addition, infiltrating lymphocytes in the liver of HEV-infected cynomolgus macaques have been found to have a cytotoxic/suppression immunophenotype (Soe, Liver, 1989; 9:135). These findings suggest that liver injury may be largely immune-mediated and result from both a cell-mediated immune mechanism and humoral immunity.

Epidemiology

Epidemiological features of hepatitis E comprise a set of parameters with rather distinguished characteristics (Table 1). HEV is transmitted primarily by the faecal–oral route and faecally contaminated drinking water has been identified as the likely vehicle of transmission in most reported outbreaks. Recurrent hepatitis E epidemics, with a periodicity of 5 to 10 years, have been observed in several parts of the world, including India, north-west China, Indonesia, and the Central Asian Republics of the former Soviet Union (Favorov, VoprVirusol, 1986; 31:65; Zhuang, MonogrVirol, 1992; 19:126; Corwin, TrRSocTropMedHyg, 1995; 89:262). Reasons for this periodicity have not been determined; however, several outbreaks have occurred in a seasonal pattern after heavy rains.[20] Person-to-person transmission of HEV appears to be uncommon, even in settings with poor environmental sanitation, such as refugee camps (Viswanathan, IndJMedRes, 1957; 45(Suppl. 1):1).[3,5,21] Reported secondary attack rates for households with hepatitis E cases have ranged from 0.7 to 2.2 per cent compared with 50 to 75 per cent among susceptible contacts in households with hepatitis A cases (Villarejos, AmJEpid, 1982, 115:577). HEV transmission from mother to infant has not frequently been studied. A small group of children born to women who recovered after infection during the third trimester were found to be infected with HEV during an outbreak in India (Khuroo, Lancet, 1995; 345: 1025).

Areas of the world can be classified as HEV-endemic based on the occurrence of hepatitis E outbreaks, which have been reported throughout Asia, Africa, the Middle East, and Central America. The first extensively studied outbreak of waterborne hepatitis, which involved 29 000 cases of icteric hepatitis, was observed in Delhi (India) between 1955 and 1956 (Viswanathan, IndJMedRes, 1957; 45(Suppl. 1):1) and was serologically documented as non-A, non-B hepatitis several years later (Wong, Lancet, 1980; ii:876). Subsequent outbreaks of epidemic and sporadic hepatitis E in this region occurred in Ahmadabad city (Sreenivasan, IndJMedRes, 1978; 67:197), North India (Tandon, IndJMedRes, 1982; 75:739),

Table 1 Epidemiology of hepatitis E outbreaks

Occurrence in HEV-endemic regions:	Large outbreaks involving thousands of cases
	Sporadic cases*
Mode of transmission:	Faecal–oral
Vehicle of transmission in outbreaks:	Faecally contaminated water
Peak of epidemic:	6 to 7 weeks after primary exposure

Low secondary attack rate among exposed household members
Highest attack rate among individuals between 15 and 40 years of age
High case–fatality ratio among infected pregnant women (20 per cent)

* Sporadic cases are also observed in non-endemic regions, primarily in travellers to HEV-endemic regions.

Kashmir (Khuroo, AmJEpid, 1983; 118:360), and Nepal (Hillis, JNepalMedAss, 1973; 11:145).[22] Many hepatitis E outbreaks have consisted of several thousand cases; the largest reported to date, involving over 100 000 cases, occurred in north-west China between 1986 and 1988 (Zhuang, MonogrVirol, 1992; 19:126). Finally, two small outbreaks of hepatitis E occurred recently on the North American continent in two villages located south of Mexico City (Velázquez, JAMA, 1990; 263:3281).

In many areas where hepatitis E outbreaks have been reported, HEV infection accounts for a substantial proportion of acute sporadic hepatitis in both children and adults (Khuroo, AmJEpid, 1983; 118:360; Hyams, JInfDis, 1992; 165:1001; Khuroo, JMedVirol, 1994; 43:281). In seroprevalence studies conducted in HEV-endemic countries, anti-HEV has been detected in as many as 5 per cent of children less than 10 years of age, and this ratio increases to 10 to 40 per cent among adults more than 25 years of age (Lok, Lancet, 1992; 340:1205; Paul, JInfDis, 1994, 169:801; Arankalle, JInfDis, 1995; 171:447). Hepatitis E may also be endemic in several countries where outbreaks have not been reported, including Hong Kong, Turkey, and Egypt, based on a high incidence of sporadic hepatitis E cases in these countries (Goldsmith, Lancet, 1992; 339: 328; Lok, Lancet, 1992; 340:1205; el-Zimaity, AmJTropMedHyg, 1993; 48:372; Thomas, Lancet, 1993; 341:1561).

In most countries where hepatitis E is not endemic, the disease accounts for fewer than 1 per cent of reported cases of acute viral hepatitis. Most cases of acute hepatitis E reported in these countries have been associated with travel to HEV-endemic regions.[23] However, acute hepatitis E cases have also been reported among persons with no history of travel to disease-endemic countries (Chapman, AustNZJMed, 1993; 23:722; Coursaget, ResVirol, 1994; 145:51; Sallie, JHepatol, 1994; 20:580; Tassopoulus, JMedVirol, 1994; 42:124; Heath, MedJAust, 1995; 162:318). Seroprevalence studies among blood donors in some non-endemic countries have found an anti-HEV prevalence of 1 to 5 per cent (Paul, JInfDis, 1994, 169:801; Moaven, JMedVirol, 1995; 45:326),[14] which is relatively high compared with the low rate of clinically evident disease associated with HEV in these areas. Possible reasons for these findings include subclinical and/or anicteric HEV infection, serological cross-reactivity with other agents, and false positive tests. The geographical distribution of hepatitis E and subclinical HEV infection, which has not yet been fully determined, depends on the availability of specific, sensitive, and practical assays for anti-HEV.

It is possible that an environmental reservoir may exist in disease-endemic geographical regions. Another potential reservoir for HEV in these regions may be serial transmission of the infection among susceptible individuals. Sporadic cases of hepatitis E account for a substantial proportion of acute viral hepatitis in countries where hepatitis E outbreaks have been reported, and these infections may maintain transmission of the virus during interepidemic periods. Finally, HEV has been detected in faeces of wild-caught pigs, anti-HEV has been detected in the serum of pigs, cattle, and sheep in disease-endemic regions, and pigs and lambs were found to be susceptible to experimental HEV infection (Balayan, JMedVirol, 1990; 32:58; Clayson, AmJTropMedHyg, 1995; 53:228).

Prevention

Public health strategies for the prevention of hepatitis E ought to consider the fact that inactivated or live attenuated virus vaccines cannot currently be developed due to the lack of an efficient culture system. The use of immunoglobulin manufactured in the hepatitis E-endemic areas in pre- or postexposure prophylaxis has been evaluated in a few studies only (Joshi, IndJMedRes, 1985; 81: 18; Khuroo, IndJGastro, 1992; 11:113). No statistically significant difference in disease rates was found among persons who received and those who did not receive immunoglobulin preparations. Moreover, the natural history of protective immunity after acute HEV infection has not been fully determined, although the presence of pre-existing IgG anti-HEV was found to prevent hepatitis E in young adults (Khuroo, Lancet, 1993; 341:1355).

Recombinant HEV proteins have recently become available and were used in experiments carried out in cynomolgus macaques for the purpose of evaluating these proteins as potential candidates for a prototype hepatitis E vaccine. In an early study, the *trpE*–C2 fusion protein derived from HEV ORF2 and expressed in *Escherichia coli* was shown to attenuate HEV infection, but has not prevented virus excretion in stools.[24] In two more recent trials, cynomolgus macaques were immunized with recombinant, baculovirus-expressed HEV proteins derived from ORF2 (55 kDa and 62 kDa) and challenged either with the same strain of HEV[25] or with a heterologous HEV strain, divergent from the vaccine source (Krawczynski K *et al.*, in preparation). The immunized animals developed neither hepatitis nor viraemia and HEV RNA was detected only transiently in a single stool specimen. Thus, the HEV vaccine experiments in susceptible primates have demonstrated the practical use of this approach to hepatitis E prevention. However, further modifications of the recombinant immunogen, the use of more efficient adjuvants, and optimization of immunization schedules may all be necessary to induce satisfactory levels of neutralizing antibodies and prevent HEV infection.

Because no products are currently available to prevent hepatitis E, prevention relies primarily on the provision of clean drinking water. No data are available regarding the efficacy of chlorination of water in inactivating HEV, and studies are needed to identify other appropriate environmental control measures. Until such prevention measures are determined, the only prophylactic measures against HEV infection that can be currently recommended and applied are improved sanitation and sanitary handling of food and water. The best prophylaxis in disease-endemic geographical areas is to drink water from safe sources, eat cooked vegetables, and practice adequate personal hygiene.

References

1. Purdy MA and Krawczynski K. Hepatitis E. *Gastroenterological Clinics of North America*, 1994; **23**: 537–46.

2. Khuroo MS. Study of an epidemic of non-A, non-B hepatitis. Possibility of another human hepatitis virus distinct from post-transfusion non-A, non-B type. *American Journal of Medicine*, 1980; **68**: 818–24.

3. Myint H, *et al.* A clinical and epidemiological study of an epidemic of non-A, non-B hepatitis in Rangoon. *American Journal of Tropical Medicine and Hygiene*, 1985; **34**: 1183–9.

4. Song DY, *et al.* Hepatitis E in Hetian City: a report of 562 cases. In Hollinger FB, Lemon SM, and Margolis HS, eds. *Viral hepatitis and liver disease.* Baltimore: Williams & Wilkins, 1991: 528–9.

5. Mast E, *et al.* Hepatitis E among refugees in Kenya: minimal apparent person-to-person transmission, evidence for age-dependent disease expression and new serologic assays. In Nishioka K, Suzuki H, Mishiro S, and Oda T, eds. *Viral hepatitis and liver disease.* Tokyo: Springer-Verlag, 1994: 375–8.

6. Chuttani HK, *et al.* Follow-up study of cases from the Delhi epidemic of infectious hepatitis of 1955–6. *British Medical Journal*, 1966; **2**: 676–9.

7. Mast EE and Alter MJ. Epidemiology of viral hepatitis: an overview. *Seminars in Virology*, 1993; **4**: 273–83.

8. Khuroo MS, *et al.* Incidence and severity of viral hepatitis in pregnancy. *American Journal of Medicine*, 1981; **70**: 252–5.

9. Tsega E, *et al.* Acute sporadic viral hepatitis in Ethiopia: causes, risk factors, and effects on pregnancy. *Clinics in Infectious Diseases*, 1992; **14**: 961–5.

10. Balayan MS, *et al.* Evidence for a virus in non-A, non-B hepatitis transmitted via the fecal–oral route. *Intervirology*, 1983; **20**: 23–31.

11. Clayson ET, *et al.* Viremia, fecal shedding, and IgM and IgG responses in patients with hepatitis E. *Journal of Infectious Diseases*, 1995; **172**: 927–33.

12. Nanda SK, *et al.* Protracted viremia during acute sporadic hepatitis E virus infection. *Gastroenterology*, 1995; **108**: 225–30.

13. Favorov MO, *et al.* Serologic identification of hepatitis E virus infections in epidemic and endemic settings. *Journal of Medical Virology*, 1992; **36**: 246–50.

14. Bryan JP, *et al.* Epidemic hepatitis E in Pakistan: patterns of serologic response and evidence that antibody to hepatitis E virus protects against disease. *Journal of Infectious Diseases*, 1994; **170**: 517–21.

15. Krawczynski K and Bradley DW. Enterically transmitted non-A, non-B hepatitis: identification of virus-associated antigen in experimentally infected cynomolgus macaques. *Journal of Infectious Diseases*, 1989; **159**: 1042–9.

16. Bradley DW, *et al.* Enterically transmitted non-A, non-B hepatitis: serial passage of disease in cynomolgus macaques and tamarins and recovery of disease-associated 27–34 nm viruslike particles. *Proceedings of the National Academy of Sciences (USA)*, 1987; **84**: 6277–81.

17. Ticehurst J, *et al.* Infection of owl monkeys (*Aotus trivirgatus*) and cynomolgus monkeys (*Macaca fascicularis*) with hepatitis E virus from Mexico. *Journal of Infectious Diseases*, 1992; **165**: 835–45.

18. Tsarev SA, *et al.* Variation in course of hepatitis E in experimentally infected cynomolgus monkeys. *Journal of Infectious Diseases*, 1993; **167**: 1302–6.

19. Tsarev SA, *et al.* Infectivity titration of a prototype strain of hepatitis E virus in cynomolgus monkeys. *Journal of Medical Virology*, 1994; **43**: 135–42.

20. Bile K, *et al.* Contrasting roles of rivers and wells as sources of drinking water on attack and fatality rates in a hepatitis E epidemic in Somalia. *American Journal of Tropical Medicine and Hygiene*, 1994; **51**: 466–74.

21. Aggarwal R and Naik SR. Hepatitis E: intrafamilial transmission versus waterborne spread. *Journal of Hepatology*, 1994; **21**: 718–23.

22. Kane MA, *et al.* Epidemic non-A, non-B hepatitis in Nepal: recovery of a possible etiologic agent and transmission studies in marmosets. *Journal of the American Medical Association*, 1984; **252**: 3140–5.

23. Centers for Disease Control and Prevention. Hepatitis E among US travelers, 1989–1992. *Morbidity and Mortality Weekly Report*, 1993; **42**: 1–4.

24. Purdy MA, *et al.* Preliminary evidence that a trpE–HEV fusion protein protects cynomolgus macaques against challenge with wild-type hepatitis E virus (HEV). *Journal of Medical Virology*, 1993; **41**: 90–4.

25. Tsarev SA, *et al.* Successful passive and active immunization of cynomolgus monkeys against hepatitis E. *Proceedings of the National Academy of Sciences (USA)*, 1994; **91**: 10198–202.

12.1.2.7 The new 'hepatitis' virus G or GBV-C

Stephanos J. Hadziyannis

Introduction

Although sensitive and specific tests for the detection of the known hepatitis viruses and their variants are now available, the aetiology of a proportion of post-transfusion and community-acquired or sporadic hepatitis still remains unknown.[1] The same is true for a variable but significant proportion of patients with chronic liver disease of unknown aetiology. Such cases are currently referred to by the terms cryptogenic or non-A–E, the last implicating a viral aetiology beyond the five known hepatitis viruses—A, B, C, D, and E. A new, parenterally transmitted flavivirus provisionally designated hepatitis G virus (**HGV**)[2,3] and a second isolate of the same viral species termed GB virus C (**GBV-C**)[4–6] have been implicated recently as agents of non-A–E liver disease. However, though phylogenetically related to the hepatitis C virus, they do not seem to be highly pathogenic for the liver and appear to account for little if any of non-A–E or cryptogenic liver disease (Alter, NEJM, 1996; 334:1536; Hadziyannis, Hepatol, 1996; 24:2294). The neutral acronymic term **G/GBV-C** combining the designations applied in the original descriptions of the two isolates, omitting the adjective hepatitis, is used.

Several isolates of the G/GBV-C agent have been hitherto identified from various parts of the world.[6,7] They represent single-strand RNA viral genomes of positive polarity about 9400 base pairs long, encoding for a large polyprotein of approximately 3000 amino acids. The new viruses belong to the family flaviviridae (Fig. 1).

Genome organization

The structural organization is reported in Chapter 12.1.2.1.

The structural genes *E1* and *E2* encode for the proteins of the putative envelope of the virus. E2 is cleaved from E1 and from the first non-structural protein NS2 by the host cell signalase.[7] Contrary to HCV, the *E* genes are highly conserved among the various isolates of G/GBV-C and no hypervariable region has been identified.[6] Alignment studies of the E2 proteins of G/GBV-C isolated from four geographically different regions showed sequence identity greater than 90 per cent (Erker, JGenVirol, 1996; 77:2713). The lack of variability in the E2 sequence suggests that G/GBV-C does not possess the ability to escape neutralizing antibodies; in fact, the presence of anti-E2 is almost invariably associated with clearance of G/GBV-C.[8]

The first non-structural protein NS2, like that of HCV, appears to have a zinc-dependent protease.[6,7] The *NS3* gene encodes a protein essential for viral replication that has activities and motifs of helicase. At its N-terminal portion, it contains a chymothrypsin-like serine protease.

The functions of *NS4a* and *b* and *NS5a* are unknown. The *NS5b* gene encodes an RNA-dependent RNA-directed polymerase (RNRP; supergroup II of RNA polymerases). This enzyme is necessary for the replication of all single-stranded, positive-strand RNA viruses, including the Flaviviridae, that have no DNA intermediates and replicate their RNA by synthesizing a negative-strand intermediate.

The G/GBV-C RNA terminates with a translation termination codon, followed by an additional 61 untranslated nucleotides.[7]

Processing of the G/GBV-C polyprotein

The G/GBV-C has a single, large, continuous ORF which is translated into a large polyprotein. The large G/GBV-C polyprotein is cleaved by cellular and viral proteases into the individual viral proteins necessary for the completion of the viral life cycle.[6,7]

Expression of the various G/GBV-C proteins as recombinant peptides and testing by Western blots has led to the identification of at least four epitopes in GBV-C (Pilot-Matias, JMedVirol, 1996; 48:329) which are now applied in diagnostic ELISAs for the detection of the anti-G/GBV-C antibodies.

Diagnostic assays of G/GBV-C infection

Diagnosis of G/GBV-C infection is based on the detection of the RNA of the virus by various RT-PCR techniques using primers from several of its regions. Genelabs Technologies have applied primers from the *NS5* region, Abbott Laboratories from the *NS3* region, but currently most investigators are advocating the use of primers from the 5' UTR.[6,7] The amplicons can be detected in agarose or polyacrylamide gel electrophoresis with ethidium bromide staining; however, confirmation by hybridization to a radio-labelled probe after Southern blotting to nitrocellulose is needed (Schlauder, JMedVirol, 1995; 46:90).[6] Solution hybridization with the use of chemiluminescence in a Perkin-Elmer CD PCR system is an alternative.

Adaptation of the PCR technology to the ligase chain reaction has been successfully incorporated by Abbott Laboratories into a system of semi-automated PCR using a commercially available Lcx instrument. The new technology is easy to perform and can avoid the problem of carry-over by neutralization of the amplicons in a closed system. It is sensitive and the results are identical to those of the most sensitive PCR techniques.

Boehringer Mannheim has developed a PCR method using two primers, one from the *NS5* and the other from the 5' UTR region; by incorporating digoxigenin-labelled triphosphates into the amplicons, the final PCR product can be measured in an immunoanalyser (ES 300) or a microtitre plate system using antibodies to digoxigenin (Schlueter, JClinMicrobiol, 1996; 34:2660). These assays claim a sensitivity level of less than 200 copies/1 ml or 10 copies/50 µl of serum. However, all of the PCR-based methods, except the one in the Lcx analyser, require many manual steps, and contamination of reagents with G/GBV-C amplicons is a constant threat.[6] Moreover, current PCR procedures are still too complex for general introduction into clinical laboratories for screening of a large number of blood units.

A convenient bench-top assay, the branched DNA, which is easier to perform than PCR and much less likely to give false positive results due to contamination (Hendricks, AmJClinPath, 1995; 104:537), has been developed recently.[6] Its detection limit is claimed to be approximately 40 000 copies/1 ml.

An antibody test to the envelope protein E2 of G/GBV-C has recently been developed (Tacke, Lancet, 1997; 349:318). The E2 protein has been expressed in CHO cells and an ELISA assay has been developed to detect anti-E2 in serum using antihuman IgG peroxidase labelled antibodies. As antibodies to E2 are usually undetectable in ongoing G/GBV-C infection, they are likely to represent evidence of recovery or past infection. A commercially available assay for anti-E2 has been produced by Boehringer Mannheim (Germany) and a similar ELISA assay for anti-E2 has been developed by Abbott Laboratories (Chicago, Illinois), but it is not yet clear whether the latter will become commercially available. The sensitivity and specificity of the new serological assays of anti-E2 must be assessed.

So far, three distinct serological patterns can be observed, with the following interpretations:

1. Positive G/GBV-C RNA only, indicating acute-phase or chronic G/GBV-C infection.
2. Positive anti-E2 only, indicating a self-limited episode of G/GBV-C infection followed by development of antibodies. The self-limited episode may have lasted for a short period or for years and the anti-E2 may also be transient or persist for years.

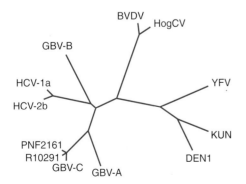

Fig. 1. Phylogenetic tree analysis (unrouted tree) of HGV, GBV-C, GBV-A, GBV-B, HCV, and other pestiviruses (BVDV and HogCV) and flaviviruses (YFN, KUN, DEN1). PNF2161 and R10291 represent the two first isolates of HGV.[2] Data from Kim, *et al.*[3], with permission.

Table 1 World-wide seroprevalence rates of G/GBV-C RNA in high risk groups for parenteral viral exposure (data from 26 studies in 12 countries)

| Risk group | No. of studies | Total no. of individuals | | | G/GBV-C RNA positivity (%)* | | |
		Tested	Positive	(%)	Range	Mean	Median
Haemophiliacs	4	197	35	(17.8)	5.3–32.1	13.3	18.4
Multiphy transfused thalasaemics	5	508	134	(26.4)	17.8–47.0	28.5	27.2
Intravenous drug abusers	13	870	250	(28.7)	15.6–52.0	28.7	32.5
Liver transplant patients	4	176	48	(27.3)	17.4–66.0	37.0	27.8
Haemodialysis patients	6	984	83	(8.4)	3.1–57.4	14.9	7.9
Homosexuals	2	279	63	(22.5)	13.4–33.1	23.3	—
Prostitutes	1	193	27	(14.0)	—	14.0	—

From Hadziyannis S and Hess G[9], with permission.
* Among the reviewed studies.

3. Concomitant positivity of G/GBV-C RNA and of anti-E2, probably signalling the end of a current G/GBV-C infection before clearance of the virus, or G/GBV-C reactivation.

Transmission and epidemiology of G/GBV-C infection

G/GBV-C is a bloodborne virus which is most efficiently transmitted to humans through large or repeated percutaneous exposures to infectious blood and its products (Hadziyannis, JHepatol, 1995; 23(Suppl. 1):784; Masuko, NEJM, 1996; 334:1485). Transmission of G/GBV-C by transfusion of blood from infected donors has been documented by linkage studies between donors and recipients (Alter, NEJM, 1997; 336:747) and by molecular evidence obtained from sequence analysis of the G/GBV-C genome in donor and recipient (Schmidt, Lancet, 1996; 347:909). Infection with G/GBV-C is frequent among patients with thalassaemia who have received multiple transfusions, haemophiliacs, and intravenous drug abusers.[6] Table 1 summarizes the G/GBV-C RNA prevalence rates among various high risk groups. Evidence for G/GBV-C transmission by other routes, collectively referred to as 'inapparent parenteral', comes from the demonstration of vertical transmission from mother to infant (Feucht, Lancet, 1995; 347:615) and from relatively high G/GBV-C prevalence rates among homosexuals, prostitutes, and their steady sexual partners. In vertical transmission, the virus appears to be inoculated during delivery or postpartum and not through the placenta, while the recent finding of the virus in sperm has been associated with sexual G/GBV-C transmission (Persico, JHepatol, 1996; 25(Suppl. 1):77).

Prevalence rates of G/GBV-C RNA among high risk groups significantly underestimate overall exposure rates to the virus. Many individuals infected with G/GBV-C clear the virus over time; transition to chronicity occurs in approximately one-third of the infected individuals (Wang, Blood, 1996; in press). Preliminary studies of anti-E2 have shown seroprevalence rates two to three times higher than the G/GBV-C RNA prevalence in the same group. In multiply transfused individuals the cumulative prevalence of G/GBV-C RNA and of anti-E2 is about 80 per cent, and in intravenous drug abusers almost 100 per cent (Hadziyannis, unpublished work).

The very high frequency of G/GBV-C infection among groups at high risk for parenteral viral transmission (Table 1) implies a relatively large pool of the virus in the general population. Available data, though limited to relatively small numbers of tested individuals, are indeed compatible with high G/GBV-C endemicity rates worldwide (Table 2). G/GBV-C frequencies among volunteer donors and the general population of most developed countries exceed 1 per cent and even 2 per cent. Positivity rates do not seem to be age dependent and no significant difference between males and females has been reported, but data are still very limited. The majority of G/GBV-C infected individuals in the general population or in blood donors have normal levels of alanine aminotransferase and do not admit to any apparent parenteral procedure (Hadziyannis, Hepatol, 1996; 24:229a). In the tropics and subtropics, G/GBV-C seroprevalence rates exceed 5 per cent and even 10 per cent (Table 2). Thus the overall population and burden of cryptogenic, community acquired G/GBV-C infection is for greater than of infection acquired in groups at risk for parenteral transmission (Table 1). The high G/GBV-C frequency in the tropics and subtropics raises the possibility that insects or other vectors are involved in the so-called cryptogenic or sporadic G/GBV-C transmission.

Role of G/GBV-C in the aetiology of acute and chronic liver disease

The role of G/GBV-C as an aetiological factor of acute and chronic hepatitis remains uncertain. Evidence in the original reports on the G and GBV-C isolates[2,3] suggested an aetiological link with acute and chronic, post-transfusion, non-A–E hepatitis and a subsequent study showing high G/GBV-C prevalence in fulminant hepatitis in Japan (Yoshiba, Lancet, 1995; 346:1131) appeared to confirm that the new flavivirus represented the sixth hepatitis virus. However, with further information from various parts of the world, the link with hepatitis became questionable (Alter, NEJM, 1996; 334:1536; Pessoa, Hepatol, 1996; 24:461). In the National Institute of Health's (**NIH**) series of acute non-A, non-B, post-transfusion hepatitis only 3 of 84 cases (3.5 per cent) were associated with G/GBV-C, while 6 additional cases (7 per cent) showed acute G/GBV-C and HCV

Table 2 G/GBV-C RNA prevalence rates in the general population and in blood donors (data from 19 studies in 15 countries)

Author	Country	Population	Tested (n)	G/GBV-C RNA (+) n	%
Moaven LD	Australia	Volunteer donors	120	5	4.2
Tagger A	Cameroon	Bantu and pygmies	34	5	14.7
Eleftheriou A	Cyprus	Blood donors*	275	17	6.2
Corwin AL	Egypt	Paid donors	NS	NS	20.0
Trepo C	France	Anti-HBc(+) donors	31	3	9.7
Heringlake S	Germany	Volunteer donors	106	5	4.7
Kekule AS	Germany	Volunteer donors	NS	NS	1–1.5
Stark K	Germany	Blood donors	90	2	2.2
Papakonstantinou A	Greece	General population	430	7	1.6
Corwin AL	Indonesia	Non-hepatitis controls	21	1	4.8
Fiordalisi G	Italy	Blood donors	145	1	0.6
Masuko K	Japan	Healthy donors	448	4	0.9
Mishiro S	Japan	Blood donors	1772	19	1.1
Nakatsuji Y	Japan	Volunteer donors	114	1	0.9
Saiz JC	Spain	Volunteer donors	200	6	3.0
Lin H	Taiwan	Pregnant women	270	1	0.4
Wang JT	Taiwan	Volunteer donors	400	6	1.5
Dawson GJ	USA	Volunteer donors**	331	9	2.7
Dawson GJ	USA	Plasmapheresis donors	93	12	12.9
Linnen J	USA	Volunteer donors***	1478	24	1.6
Pujol FH	Venezuela	Amerindians	48	3	6.3
Dawson GJ	West Africa	General population	332	49	14.8

From reference 8, with permission.
* Regardless of HBV and HCV status.
** With normal level of alanine aminotransferase (ALT): 0.8%; with increased ALT: 3.9%.
*** No difference between donors with normal and increased ALT levels.

coinfection. Similar data were reported from a series of patients with post-transfusion hepatitis in Taiwan (Wang, Blood, 1996; 88: 181), where the mean peak alanine aminotransferase (**ALT**) in isolated G/GBV-C infections was 31 units compared with 500 in isolated HCV infections. In fact, 80 per cent (20 of 25) of the isolated G/GBV-C infections in the Taiwan series and 79 per cent in the NIH series (by projection) were not associated with ALT or aspartamine aminotransferase abnormalities. Moreover, there were no statistically significant differences in the frequency of G/GBV-C RNA among patients with hepatitis non-A–E (3/13 or 23 per cent) compared with those with minor ALT elevations (12 of 100 or 12 per cent) and those with no biochemical evidence of hepatitis (14/181 or 8 per cent). Chronicity of infection ranged between 35 and 60 per cent. These data taken together with those reported by other investigators clearly confirm that there is a high frequency of transfusion-transmitted G/GBV-C infection, persistence of infection is high, but the association with hepatitis at least in the post-transfusion setting is rather rare. A combined analysis of the results of six studies from various parts of the world revealed that among 103 patients with acute post-transfusion hepatitis that was non-A–E, one-quarter were G/GBV-C RNA positive (Table 3). However, the frequency of infection among transfused controls without hepatitis was unknown.

The failure to establish G/GBV-C causality in non-A–E, transfusion-associated hepatitis is consistent with similar evidence in other clinical and epidemiological forms of acute and chronic liver disease of cryptogenic or non-A–E origin.[9] Data shown in Tables 3 and 4 represent mean, median, and ranges of universal G/GBV-C RNA seroprevalence rates in community-acquired acute non-A–E hepatitis, fulminant hepatitis, and chronic liver disease of non-A–E aetiology deduced from a compilation of the findings of numerous studies reported in the literature (mostly in abstract form). In addition to transfusion-associated non-A–E hepatitis, an overall high G/GBV-C RNA seroprevalence rate (27.3 per cent) has been reported in fulminant hepatitis; however, differences from study to study were striking with positivity ranging from 0 per cent (Kuroki, Lancet, 1996; 347:65; Salice, Lancet, 1996; 347:1552) to 50 and 62.5 per cent (Heringlake, JHepatol, 1996; 25:63).

Patients with fulminant hepatitis, regardless of aetiology, are at high risk for G/GBV-C transmission through transfusions of blood and its products which are given to correct the coagulation abnormalities of hepatitis and/or in transplantation. This was well documented in a study of fulminant hepatitis from Australia; seropositivity to G/GBV-C RNA was 0 per cent in the first blood sample at presentation, but seroconversion to a positive test occurred after transplantation in 67 per cent of patients.[8] However, this was not true in other studies. The possibility has therefore been raised of geographical differences in the aetiology of fulminant hepatitis as well as of genetic variability in G/GBV-C strains associated with the disease. The need for well designed studies with appropriate controls is obvious.

The cumulative data in chronic non-A–E hepatitis, cryptogenic cirrhosis, and hepatocellular carcinoma, presented in Table 4, show rather low frequencies of G/GBV-C infection compared with the

Table 3 Seroprevalence rates of G/GBV-C RNA in acute post-transfusion, community acquired, and fulminant non-A–E hepatitis (data from 24 studies in 13 countries)

Diagnosis	Number of studies	Total no. of patients			G/GBV-C RNA positivity (%)*		
		Tested	Positive	(%)	Range	Mean	Median
Acute post-transfusion hepatitis	6	103	26	(25.2)	12.5–35.3	22.7	21.5
Acute, community acquired**	9	268	22	(7.5)	0.0–34.4	8.7	5.3
Fulminant and subfulminant***	11	139	38	(27.3)	0.0–62.5	25.4	10.0

From Hadziyannis S and Hess G[9], with permission.
  * Among the reviewed studies.
  ** Sporadic or non-defined epidemiologically.
  *** Cryptogenic or sporadic and occasionally post-transfusion.

Table 4 Seroprevalence rates of G/GBV-C RNA in chronic non-A–E hepatitis, cryptogenic cirrhosis, and hepatocellular carcinoma (data from 14 studies in 9 countries)

Diagnosis	Number of studies	Total no. of patients			G/GBV-C RNA positivity (%)*		
		Tested	Positive	(%)	Range	Mean	Median
Chronic non-A–E hepatitis**	11	505	51	(10.0)	0.0–60.0	14.6	14.9
Cryptogenic cirrhosis	4	134	12	(8.9)	5.0–14.3	10.5	11.5
Hepatocellular carcinoma***	5	126	11	(8.7)	3.8–37.5	17.6	7.0

From Hadziyannis S and Hess G[9], with permission.
  * Among the reviewed studies.
  ** Also described as 'cryptogenic' chronic hepatitis.
  *** Mostly on the grounds of cryptogenic cirrhosis.

relatively high frequency of the infection in the general population and in blood donors, thus suggesting that the new flavivirus does not represent an important cause of liver disease. However, the lack of appropriate controls may under- or overestimate the relative risk. Lack of other markers of G/GBV-C infection and of markers diagnostic of host immune reactions to the virus further confound the problem. In view of these conjectures, the role of the new flavivirus in the aetiology of acute, fulminant, and chronic non-A–E hepatitis, cryptogenic cirrhosis, and hepatocellular carcinoma remains uncertain.

G/GBV-C has been detected in low frequencies in patients with various other forms of liver disease of known and unknown aetiology (Hadziyannis, JHepatol, 1995; 23:78), except for those due to HBV, HCV, and HDV.[9] Epidemiological analysis of such patients indicates that dual or triple infections with G/GBV-C and HCV and/or HBV are particularly common among intravenous drug abusers and multiply transfused patients, being related to shared risk factors for parenteral viral exposure. More than 50 per cent of patients with dual or triple infections were found to have a history of blood transfusion or intravenous drug abuse.

In combined infections with G/GBV-C and HCV or HBV, mean G/GBV-C RNA levels did not differ significantly from those in isolated G/GBV-C infections. The same is true for mean HCV RNA levels in dual infections with G/GBV-C and HCV compared with infections with HCV alone (Hadziyannis, Hepatol, 1996; 24: 229A). Moreover, ALT levels do not differ significantly between isolated and dual infections and the same appears to be true regarding the severity of changes in liver histology.

Finally, the response to interferon of HCV infection does not seem to be influenced significantly by the concomitant presence of G/GBV-C.[9]

Taken together, the data suggest that G/GBV-C does not play a major role in the aetiology of acute and chronic liver disease. Whether it may play a minor role or even no role is uncertain. Lack of correlation between the level of G/GBV-C viraemia and indices of hepatocellular damage in the three original cases of post-transfusion non-A–E hepatitis,[2] which were associated with G/GBV-C infection, further suggests that other aetiological factors could be responsible for disease. Therefore, it has been proposed that G/GBV-C represents an innocent bystander in an inflammatory process of other aetiology. While this may be true, the alternative possibility that G/GBV-C is of limited hepatotropism and causes liver damage only under certain conditions has to be carefully evaluated; in this hypothesis, host-related as well as virus factors might be important in determining hepatitis G. The recent identification of G/GBV-C variants associated with fulminant hepatitis (Heringlake, Lancet, 1996; 348:1626) lends some support to this view.

References

1. Alter HJ and Bradley DW. Non-A, non-B hepatitis unrelated to the hepatitis C virus (non-ABC). *Seminars in Liver Disease*, 1995; **15**: 110–20.
2. Linnen J, *et al.* Molecular cloning and disease association of hepatitis G virus: a transfusion transmissible agent. *Science*, 1996; **271**: 505–8.

3. Kim J, *et al.* Molecular cloning and characterization of hepatitis G virus (HGV). In Rizzetto M, Purcell RH, Gerin JL, and Verme G, eds. *Viral hepatitis and liver disease.* Turin: Edizione Minerva Medica, 1997: 341–6.

4. Simons JN, *et al.* Isolation of novel virus-like sequences associated with human hepatitis. *Nature Medicine*, 1995; **1**: 564–9.

5. Muerhoff AS, *et al.* Genomic organization of GB viruses A and B: Two new members of the flaviviridae associated with GB agent hepatitis. *Journal of Virology*, 1995; **69**: 5621–30.

6. Deinhardt F, Holmes AW, Capps PB, and Popper H. Studies on the transmission of disease of human viral hepatitis to marmoset monkeys. Transmission of disease, serial passage and description of liver lesions. *Journal of Experimental Medicine*, 1967; **125**: 673–87.

7. Leary TP, *et al.* Sequence and genomic organisation of GBV-C: a novel member of the Flaviviridae associated with human non-A–E hepatitis. *Journal of Medical Virology*, 1996; **48**: 60–7.

8. Hadziyannis S and Hess G. Epidemiology and natural course of G/GBV-C infection. In Zuckerman A and Thomas H, eds. *Viral hepatitis.* 2nd edn. Livingstone, in press.

9. Karayiannis P, *et al.* Hepatitis G virus infection. Clinical characteristics and response to interferon. *Journal of Viral Hepatitis*, 1997; **4**: 37–44.

12.1.3 Prevention and treatment of viral hepatitis

12.1.3.1(A) Vaccines against hepatitis A

Francis André

Virological and epidemiological considerations

The aetiological agent of hepatitis A is a particularly resistant virus that belongs to the Picornaviridae family and has been classified in the *Hepatovirus* genus.[1] The viral epitope, which elicits neutralizing antibodies that protect against infection, has a three-dimensional conformation obtained by the juxtaposition of binding sites on two capsid polypeptides, VP1 and VP2, which are encoded by the P1 segment of the viral single-stranded open reading frame. Despite the considerable genetic heterogeneity that exist between different strains, there is no significant variation in the conformation of the epitope(s) that determine(s) virus neutralization because polyclonal antibodies cross-neutralize viruses from all genotypes. Therefore, a vaccine containing a strain that induces polyclonal neutralizing antibodies will protect against all strains. As there is no antiviral drug for specific therapy of the infection, treatment is only supportive; prevention is the best medical approach to the considerable disease and economic burden still inflicted by the hepatitis A virus (**HAV**). Avoidance of exposure is theoretically possible, but in practice is usually ineffective except in very hygienic societies (Steffen, Vaccine, 1991; 10(Suppl.1):S69). Passive preexposure or postexposure prophylaxis with immunoglobulin preparations containing HAV antibodies is efficacious, but is logistically impractical and is epidemiologically an ineffective method of control since the protection conferred is short lived and exposure may occur occultly (Stapleton, Vaccine, 1992; 10(Suppl.1):S45). It is evident that the prophylactic use of a vaccine that elicits long-lasting immunity is a preferable modality for disease control.

Development of vaccines

Work on the development of a vaccine started as soon as the causative agent was identified (Hilleman, JHepatol, 1993; 18:S5). At first, HAV could not be propagated in cell culture and viral antigen was prepared from the liver of infected marmosets (Provost, PSEBM, 1978; 159:201). Cultivation of the virus in cells (Provost, PSEBM, 1979; 160:213) was the breakthrough that paved the way to the successful development of several hepatitis A vaccines that have been introduced in recent years. After the introduction, in early 1992, of the first formol-inactivated whole-virion vaccine (André, Vaccine, 1992; 10(Suppl.1):S160)—analogous to the killed (Salk-type) poliomyelitis vaccine—other similar vaccines have been introduced. These vaccines have been shown to be well tolerated and efficacious in extensive clinical studies that have preceded their licensure and commercial introduction. Although few comparative studies have been done with these vaccines, the available evidence suggests that any differences in immunogenicity that may exist between them are likely to be of minor clinical significance as all are highly immunogenic when administered according to the recommended dosages and schedules. The antigen content per vaccine dose is expressed in a variety of units by manufacturers and the recommended vaccination schedules also vary.

A live attenuated vaccine has also been introduced in China.[2] Two controlled field trials have confirmed the high protective efficacy of inactivated vaccines used prophylactically (Werzberger, NEJM, 1992; 327:453; Innis, JAMA, 1994; 271:1328). From mathematical modelling of the decay of vaccine-induced antibodies, the protection conferred is expected to last at least 20 years. Rapid interruption of ongoing hepatitis A outbreaks has also been achieved through vaccination of a significant percentage of susceptibles in whole populations (Prikazsky, JMedVirol, 1994; 44:457; McMahon, ArchPediatrAdolescMed, 1996; 150:733). So far, no safety issue has emerged in the course of routine vaccination of several million persons. The only reactions that can be imputed definitely to the vaccine are mild transient soreness, erythema, and induration at the site of injection in a small percentage of vaccinees, as was shown in clinical studies (André, Vaccine, 1992; 10(Suppl.1):S160). Only very few instances of primary vaccine failure, as evidenced by the absence of vaccine-induced antibodies or the development of hepatitis A, have been documented among persons who have received the vaccine. This extensive experience has shown that the inactivated vaccine appears to be safe. It is well tolerated and highly effective. Although other approaches are possible to develop alternative vaccines against hepatitis A, it is unlikely that these will replace inactivated vaccines in the near future (André, JInfDis, 1995; 171(Suppl.1):S33).

Current use of hepatitis A vaccines

Hepatitis A vaccine is currently available in more than 50 countries; so far, it has predominantly been used to protect travellers from industrialized countries who visit developing regions of the world. It has also been used, in a limited fashion, in some at-risk occupational groups. More recently, particularly in the United States, the vaccine has been used, with success, to interrupt community-wide out-breaks.[3] Such targeted use in at-risk individuals and communities, although beneficial to those who are vaccinated, will not control the disease on a population-wide basis because most cases occur in persons who are not in well-defined risk groups (Shapiro, Vaccine, 1992; 10(Suppl.1):S59). To date, no country has recommended universal vaccination against hepatitis A, no doubt because of the financial implications of such a decision. However, it must be pointed out that because HAV circulates only in humans, disease elimination or even eradication, as for poliomyelitis, can be envisaged (Deinhardt, Vaccine, 1994; 10(Suppl.1):S10).

Future use of vaccine

A safe and efficacious vaccine against hepatitis A has been introduced for routine use in the last few years. So far, it has not shown its effectiveness in controlling the incidence of hepatitis A on a regional or national basis because it has been used sparingly in a selectively targeted fashion; this strategy failed for hepatitis B and led to the re-evaluation of immunization recommendations for this disease (Alter, JAMA 1991; 263:1218). In due course, a similar reappraisal of the use of hepatitis A vaccine will probably take place. The development of combined vaccines with a hepatitis A component, which is already far advanced (a combined hepatitis A and B is already available), should encourage the wider use of hepatitis A immunization in the future. Clearly, just as in the case of hepatitis B, control of the infection in the general population will require a national policy that uses the vaccine in systematic immunization programmes. To reduce disease incidence significantly at a national level, vaccination of whole birth cohorts, either in early chilhood or in adolescence, as well as risk groups, is likely to be necessary. Cost–benefit and cost–effectiveness studies are being undertaken to examine whether the required expenditure can be justified.

References

1. Lemon SM and Robertson BH. Taxonomic classification of hepatitis A virus. In Nishioka K, Suzuki H, Mishiro S, and Oda T, eds. *Viral hepatitis and liver disease*. Tokyo: Springer-Verlag, 1994: 50–3.
2. Mao JS, *et al.* Further studies of attenuated live hepatitis A vaccine (H2 strain) in humans. In Hollinger FB, Lemon SM, and Margolis H, eds. *Viral hepatitis and liver disease*. Baltimore: Williams & Wilkins, 1991: 110–11.
3. Averhoff F *et al.* Use of inactivated vaccine to interrupt a communitywide hepatitis A outbreak. *IX Triennial International Symposium on Viral Hepatitis and Liver Disease, 21–25 April, 1996, Rome*: Abstract subcutaneous 2.

12.1.3.1(B) Hepatitis B vaccines and immunization

Mark A. Kane

Introduction
Hepatitis B virus

Hepatitis B virus (**HBV**) belongs to a closely related group of viruses, pathogenic to a number of species, known as the hepadnaviruses. It is a 42-nm particle with partially double-stranded DNA, composed of an inner 'core' protein, hepatitis B core (c) antigen (**HBcAg**), and an outer surface (s) glycoprotein, **HBsAg**. Excess HBsAg also appears as tubular forms and 22-nm spheres that can be made into hepatitis B vaccine.

Types of vaccine

Hepatitis B vaccines are highly purified preparations of the 22-nm spherical particles of HBsAg, either harvested from the serum of chronic HBV carriers (plasma-derived vaccines) or produced by recombinant DNA techniques in yeast or mammalian cells (recombinant DNA vaccines). Both types of vaccine contain aluminium salts as an adjuvant and are preserved with thymerosal. They are very similar from a chemical and immunological point of view, and have similar characteristics for immunogenicity, efficacy, and safety (Table 1).

Plasma-derived vaccines

In the 1960s it had been shown that boiled serum from patients with 'serum' hepatitis could protect against clinical disease, as could passively transferred serum containing anti-HBs antibody.[1] Traditional methods of making inactivated viral vaccines and live attenuated vaccines were not possible because the virus could not be grown in tissue culture, and because it is oncogenic. Teams in many countries developed vaccines from highly purified preparations of HBsAg from the plasma of HBV carriers using various methods of purification and inactivation.[2–4] These vaccines proved to be safe, highly immunogenic, and effective in preventing disease in various populations, including homosexually active men, [5,6] health-care workers, children in developing countries,[7] infants of HBV carrier mothers,[8] residents of institutions for the retarded,[9] and many other groups.

Plasma-derived vaccines were the first to become commercially available (1982) and are still in common use. Early acceptance of plasma-derived vaccines was harmed by fears that they might contain the (at that time) undiscovered aetiological agent of the acquired immune deficiency syndrome (**AIDS**). However, when the human immunodeficiency virus (**HIV**) was discovered, it was quickly shown that these vaccines could not cause infection with HIV or any other infectious agent (Francis, JAMA, 1986; 256:869), and subsequent experience with over 500 million doses have made experts very confident on this point (McMahon AmJMed, 1992; 92: 254). However, residual fears persist among uninformed individuals and are sometimes exploited by the manufacturers of competing products. Plasma-derived vaccines are now primarily used in Asia, Africa, and the Pacific basin. China can produce up to 70 million doses per year, and large producers in the Republic of Korea sell to other countries. A number of countries have plasma-derived vaccines under development, including Myanmar, Indonesia, Mongolia, and Vietnam. Plasma-derived vaccines sell in public-sector markets in developing countries for between US$ 0.55 and 1.25 per paediatric dose.

DNA recombinant vaccines

A second generation of vaccines, DNA recombinant vaccines, was developed in the 1980s by inserting plasmids containing the HBsAg

Table 1 Types of vaccines

Plasma-derived vaccines

DNA recombinant vaccines

Combination vaccines:
Available
    diphtheria + tetanus + pertussis + hepatitis B (DTP-HB)
    Haemophilus influenzae type B + hepatitis B (Hib-HB)
Under development
    diphtheria + tetanus + acellular pertussis + hepatitis B (DTaP-HB)
    DTaP-HB-Hib
    DTP-Hib-HB-IPV (inactivated polio vaccine)
    hepatitis A-HB

Experimental vaccines
HBsAg expressed in:
    Vaccinia and other viruses
    Salmonella and other bacteria
    Higher plants
HB core particles
Peptide vaccines
Idiotype/anti-idiotype vaccines
DNA vaccine

gene from the virus (with or without the pre-S1 and pre-S2 components) into yeast or mammalian cells. These cells then produce self-assembling, immunogenic HBsAg particles, almost identical to those found in the plasma of HBV carriers.[10–12]

DNA recombinant vaccines are currently produced in Belgium, China, Cuba, France, Japan, the Republic of Korea, Switzerland, and the United States; a number of other countries, including Brazil, the Republic of Korea, Israel, and the United Kingdom, have vaccines under development. Yeast fermentation systems are the most successful economically, and vaccines produced from them have been sold for as little as US$ 1.00 to public-sector programmes of large developing countries, although the cost is much higher in the markets of industrialized countries. Since these vaccines contain only viral coat protein, they cannot transmit HBV or other communicable disease agents.

Combination vaccines

An increasing number of vaccine antigens are becoming available and are being recommended for infant use, and there is concern about how many injections per visit will be acceptable to parents and health workers. Various combination vaccines are being developed to address this issue, and combined diphtheria–tetanus–pertussis–hepatitis B vaccines (**DTP-HB**)[13] and *Haemophilus influenzae* type b-hepatitis B vaccines (**Hib-HB**) are already commercially available. DTP-HB vaccines containing acellular pertussis vaccine, DTaP-HB-Hib, DTP-Hib-HB-IPV (inactivated polio vaccine) (see Table 1), and hepatitis A-hepatitis B vaccines are under development. Aside from fewer injections, combination vaccines have the advantage of fewer vials, fewer syringes, and smaller storage and transport volumes, and may save on staff time and paperwork. One problem is that many developing countries make their own DTP and may not be interested in importing it in the form of DTP-HB vaccine. Some producers in developing countries may develop their own DTP-HB vaccine using either imported or indigenously produced hepatitis B vaccine.

Experimental vaccines

Because the antigen and antibody systems of HBV are well understood, extremely sensitive and specific reagents are commercially available, and the antigen self-assembles into immunogenic particles that induce protective antibody, the HBV has been a favourite system for the development of many types of experimental vaccines. These include HBsAg expressed in vaccinia (Smith, Nature, 1983; 302:490) and other viruses, salmonellae and other bacteria, higher plants, HBV core particles used as vaccines, peptide vaccines, idiotype/anti-idiotype vaccines, and DNA vaccines (Davos, Hum-MolGenet, 1993; 2:1847). Few of these products will become commercially available. Because of the extremely high efficacy and immunogenicity of current plasma-derived and DNA recombinant vaccines, it would be difficult to demonstrate that any of these vaccines were superior to them except in certain conditions such as seroconversion in older adults. Although academic developers claim that some of these approaches could be much cheaper than the current vaccines, the economic realities of vaccine production make it unclear this would actually be the case.

Pre-S1 and pre-S2

Pre-S1 and pre-S2 are antigenically distinct polypeptides found on the surface of the native HBsAg particle and coded for by the pre-S1 and pre-S2 regions of the surface antigen gene. Pre-S1 is involved in viral attachment to the liver cell and pre-S2 attaches to albumin, which may also be involved in viral attachment. By including these segments in the expression vector, it is possible to express them on the surface of the particle in DNA recombinant vaccines, and to induce antipre-S1 and/or antipre-S2 antibodies, which in theory could enhance protection against HBV infection, especially in those who do not respond to vaccines that contain HBsAg alone (Moulia Pelat, Vaccine, 1994; 12:499). Although plasma-derived and DNA recombinant vaccines containing pre-S1 and/or pre-S2 have been around for many years, claims that they add immunogenicity or protective efficacy to the vaccine have not been clearly substantiated.

Vaccine characteristics

Safety

Hepatitis B vaccines have been used since 1982 with an outstanding record of safety.[14] Because these vaccines contain alum, local side-effects such as redness and swelling at the injection site are observed in 10 to 20 per cent of recipients, and fever and malaise lasting less than 24 h are reported in some recipients. However, serious side-effects are rare and, in most cases, cannot be causally linked to the vaccine.[15] In addition, there are no adverse interactions between hepatitis B vaccine and any other vaccine, so they can be administered during the same visit, although at different sites.[16] Hepatitis B and other vaccines should not be combined in the same syringe before injection unless they are part of a licensed combination vaccine.

Immunogenicity

The immunogenicity of hepatitis B vaccine is measured by sero-conversion, which is usually defined as the proportion of susceptible individuals who develop at least 10 million international units (iu)/ml of anti-HBs within 3 months of the third dose of vaccine, and the geometric mean titre of anti-HBs developed in the study population. However, the clinical significance of the geometric mean titre is increasingly being questioned. Expert groups in a few countries have arbitrarily defined other concentrations of anti-HBs (such as 100 million iu/ml) as seroconversion, but these are based on programmatic rather than biological lines of reasoning. Immunogenicity is a complex function of the particular vaccine antigen, the dose and number of doses, the age and immune competence of the recipients, and the schedule, route, and site of administration. By varying these factors it may be possible for any vaccine to give any level of seroconversion and geometric mean titre.[17] The important question for manufacturers, public-health officials, and control authorities is 'how much is enough ?', balancing cost, convenience, and effectiveness. Marketing personnel from each manufacturer try to convince customers of the relative advantage of their product over that of their competitors, and it is important to separate marketing claims from valid issues and concerns.

Immune response to vaccine

Susceptible individuals who receive hepatitis B vaccine will develop anti-HBs but not anti-HBc (or anti-HBe). This distinction permits serological differentiation of the response to immunization from that of natural infection. This is important in serological surveys to determine the prevalence of infection or the impact of immunization in populations, and in pre- and postimmunization testing of persons in certain high-risk groups. Although anti-HBs and anti-HBc antibodies induced by natural infection usually persist for life, vaccine-induced anti-HBs wanes after a certain number of years (usually 5 to 20 years) and the duration of measurable anti-HBs correlates in individuals with the titre of anti-HBs achieved after immunization (Jilg, Hepatol, 1988; 6:201).

Efficacy

In order to understand vaccine efficacy it is necessary to distinguish between protection against infection, as evidenced by the development of an anti-HBc response, and protection against clinical disease and/or the carrier state, which persists longer than detectable anti-HBs. In most cohorts that have been followed for between 10 and 15 years, no cases of clinical hepatitis B, and no or very few chronic carriers, have been reported despite the fact that many or most of the cohort had lost detectable anti-HBs for a number of years (Hadler, NEJM, 1986; 315:276; Wainwright, JInfDis, 1997; 175:674).

Exposure to the virus (or to booster doses of vaccine) provokes a rapid anamnestic response (Hall, BMJ, 1993; 307:276), which is sufficient to protect the individual from significant disease provided that the primary immunization series has induced adequate immunological priming (West, Vaccine, 1996; 14:1019). However, in most studies some individuals develop anti-HBc from a boost of anti-HBs without developing clinical symptoms or the chronic carrier state. Most investigators consider this benign or even positive in that these individuals may have very long-term, even lifelong, protection against disease. A few have raised the possibility that some of these individuals may have silently integrated the viral genome into their liver cells and increased their risk of developing liver cancer, but the minimal rates of liver cancer in anti-HBc- and anti-HBs-positive individuals in studies in Taiwan (Beasley, Lancet, 1981; ii:1129) make this possibility very unlikely.

If long-term protection against clinical disease and the chronic carrier state depends upon properly priming the immune system (circulating memory cells and the anamnestic response) (West, Vaccine, 1996; 14:1019) and not on having high concentrations of circulating anti-HBs, then the necessity for immunization strategies based on inducing and maintaining high anti-HBs may be questioned. These strategies include using high doses of antigen, schedules with four vaccine doses, schedules with gaps of several months between the second and third dose, quantitative postvaccination testing, the use of elevated concentrations of anti-HBs (100 or 200 million iu/ml) to define seroconversion, and the use of booster doses.

Age and vaccine response

Immunogenicity before the age of 40 is excellent (usually 90 to 100 per cent); after 40 years of age the response rates may drop somewhat but are usually greater than 80 per cent. Non-response has been correlated with increasing age, obesity, smoking, male sex, and a variety of conditions related to immunodeficiency, such as HIV infection or renal dialysis (Collier, AnnIntMed, 1988; 109: 101; Shaw, Vaccine, 1989; 7:425). True non-responders remain susceptible to natural HBV infection, and any infection that does occur is equal to the wild-type infection in severity and progression to the carrier state.[6] A small proportion of non-responders have a genetic inability to respond to HBsAg.

Non-responders to three or four doses of vaccine may sero-convert after further doses but their antibody response is usually low and often transient. Many protocols have been proposed to induce seroconversion in health-care workers who have not responded, and some individuals have been subjected to questionable

Table 2 Doses and schedules

Adult doses: ranging from 2.5 to 10 µg
Infants and children doses: ranging from 1.5 to 10 µg

Schedules
0, 1, 2, 12:
1st dose, (1 month)→2nd dose, (1 month)→3rd dose, (10 months)→4th dose
0, 1, 2:
1st dose, (1 month)→2nd dose, (1 month)→3rd dose
0, 1, 6:
1st dose, (1 month)→2nd dose, (5 months)→3rd dose

Childhood immunization:
At birth 1st dose, (1 month)–2nd dose, (several months)→3rd dose with DTP-3 or measles

DTP, diphtheria–tetanus–pertussis.

practices such as receiving more than 12 doses of vaccine, or being removed from work in certain hospital settings.

Dose, route of administration, and storage

Hepatitis B vaccines are not generic products, and the number of micrograms per immunizing dose varies from product to product, by age, and by the immune status of the recipients. Thus 2.5 µg of one product may give the same immune response (seroconversion and geometric mean titre) as 10 µg of another. Recommended doses for infants and children vary from 1.5 to 10 µg per dose.

Appropriate doses are determined in dose titration studies in various age groups. It is the responsibility of the national licensing authority in each country to approve the doses sold by licensed manufacturers.

The vaccine should be administered intramuscularly into the anteriolateral thigh in infants and into the deltoid in older children and adults. Inoculation into the buttock is not acceptable as the immunogenicity of vaccine administered at this site is significantly lower (Shaw, Vaccine, 1989; 7:425), and significant nerve damage from gluteal injections has been reported in children. EPI recommends that the appropriate dose be incorporated in a standard volume of 0.5 ml for childhood immunization.

Hepatitis B vaccines are destroyed by freezing. They should be stored and handled like DTP vaccines, at 4 to 8°C. Hepatitis B vaccines are rather heat-stable, and research into how they may be used beyond the 'cold chain' is in progress.

Schedule

During the development of hepatitis B vaccines, 0, 1, 6 and 0, 1, 2, 12 schedules (Table 2) were studied and adopted by most major producers and approved by national control authorities in most countries. These schedules produce high levels of seroconversion (generally over 90 per cent of children and young adults produce at least 10 million iu/ml of anti-HBs) and good geometric mean titres of antibody. They are used in many countries with good results, but others may be more appropriate or more convenient for situations such as infant immunization schedules that are already well established, or to reach populations that may not be accessible for as

long as 6 or 12 months (e.g. short-term employees, attendees at clinics for sexually transmitted diseases, prisoners, travellers).

A considerable amount of data now suggests that the timing of the three vaccine doses is not critical as long as they are at least 1 month apart (Greenberg, Vaccine, 1996; 14:811). The seroconversion with the 0, 1, 2 schedule is identical to that with the 0, 1, 6 and 0, 1, 2, 12 schedules, but the geometric mean titre reached is somewhat lower for the 0, 1, 2 schedule (Hadler, Vaccine, 1989; 7:106). While the duration of detectable anti-HBs is related to the initial geometric mean titre, current data suggest that this may have little clinical relevance. This flexibility in scheduling makes it easy to combine hepatitis B immunization with other childhood immunizations in any country, so that additional immunization contacts to deliver hepatitis B vaccine are not necessary, which has important cost implications, especially in the developing world.

The first dose of hepatitis B vaccine should be given at birth if possible or, if not, with the first dose of DTP vaccine (DTP-1). The second dose should be given 1 month after the first. The third dose should be given with either DTP-3 or measles vaccine. The timing of the third dose will not change the percentage of children seroconverting, but if the third dose is given several months after the second a higher anti-HBs titre will be achieved.

Higher titres of antibody will persist longer, but it is unclear whether this has any practical significance, since long-term protection lies in memory cells that produce an anamnestic response if challenged with exposure to wild virus or additional doses of vaccine. If significant drop-out occurs between parent visits for DTP-3 and measles vaccination, the vaccine should be administered with DTP-3.

Immunization of previously infected individuals

The hepatitis B vaccine will neither benefit nor harm individuals who have already been infected with HBV, whether they are HBsAg-positive carriers or immune (Dienstag, AnnIntMed, 1982; 96:575). Immune individuals already have anti-HBs and anti-HBc, and lifelong immunity against repeat hepatitis B infection, and do not need vaccination. HBV carriers already have high titres of circulating HBsAg in their plasma, and the addition of a few more micrograms in the form of vaccine has no effect on them. Reports that immunization with a pre-S1- and -S2-containing vaccine can induce carriers to lose HBsAg need confirmation (Pol, Lancet, 1994; 334:442).

Pre- and postvaccination testing for anti-HBs

In certain circumstances, antibody screening to identify immune individuals before vaccination may be cost-effective in avoiding waste of vaccine, depending on the cost of the testing, the cost of the vaccine, and the expected prevalence of 'immunes' in the population. However, such screening has no place in large, national immunization programmes among children.[18]

Postvaccination testing of health-care workers is done in many institutions and has been recommended in some countries for certain risk groups. Health-care workers who have not responded can be offered additional doses of vaccine and appropriately counselled if they do not respond. Although the impact of this strategy on disease and cost-effectiveness can be questioned, it does make infection-control personnel more comfortable and may be useful for medicolegal purposes. However, as in prevaccination screening this strategy has no place in large, national immunization programmes among children.

Pre-exposure prophylaxis

Most children in the world are not born to carrier mothers but to mothers who have either anti-HBs and anti-HBc or no circulating antibody. Infants born to anti-HBs-positive mothers receive passive anti-HBs that lasts for approximately 6 months and anti-HBc that persists somewhat longer (up to 15 months). These infants are protected against infection for much of the first year of life, but this passive protection then wanes, and the children begin to become infected, first by carrier children in their families and later by playmates in the community.

They may also become infected by percutaneous exposures such as injections or other medical or dental procedures using contaminated, unsterilized equipment, transfusion with unscreened blood, or by traditional procedures such as circumcision, tattooing, acupuncture, or scarification.

If they escape infection by these routes, sexual transmission is highly efficient and causes many infections among adolescents and adults.

The prevention of horizontal transmission by using hepatitis B vaccine is highly effective. Most studies show that more than 95 per cent of infants, children, and young adults will seroconvert after three doses of the vaccine, and that virtually all of the seroconverters will be protected against infection. The duration of protection is unknown, since the vaccine has only been in use for a little over 13 years. However, it is clear that, although titres of vaccine-induced anti-HBs wane over a number of years, protection against acute hepatitis B and the development of the carrier state persists well past the loss of detectable anti-HBs in the serum. Because of the long incubation period of the disease, circulating memory cells have time to produce a strong anamnestic antibody response after exposure to the virus, and can abort clinical infection and the development of the carrier state. Some of these individuals do develop anti-HBc, indicating that some cycles of viral replication have occurred in the liver.

Since most carrier states are generated by perinatal and childhood infection before the age of 7 years, and since protection by vaccination lasts at least 10 years, it is likely that, even if infection occurs at a later age, it would follow the adult pattern and rarely develop into the carrier state. Another implication of the effectiveness of the memory cells in aborting infection is that booster doses of vaccine are not indicated at present. Although some recommend booster doses in groups such as health-care workers who have lost antibody, they have no place in large, national, hepatitis B immunization programmes.

Postexposure prophylaxis
Perinatal transmission

An infant infected at birth from an HBeAg-positive-carrier mother (perinatal transmission) has a 70 to 90 per cent chance of becoming a carrier (Stevens, NEJM, 1975; 292:771). Infection is thought to be transplacental in a minority (5–8 per cent) of cases; most infection is thought to occur at the time of birth when the new-born infant is covered with infectious fluids, such as blood, amniotic fluid, and vaginal secretions, that come into contact with the eyes, mucous membranes and skin lesions, and are swallowed (Lee, JInfDis, 1978; 138:668). Since HBeAg-positive carrier mothers have no anti-HBs, there is no passively acquired protective antibody in the child, and infection and the development of the carrier state usually occur (Beasley, AmJEpid, 1977; 105:94).

Transmission and progression to the carrier state can, in most cases, be prevented by passive immunization with hepatitis B immune globulin,[19] administration of hepatitis B vaccine,[8] or a combination of both.[20] Hepatitis B immune globulin is a fractionated blood product prepared from pooled plasma. It is essentially immunoglobulin prepared from donors with high titres of anti-HBs. Intramuscular preparations of hepatitis B immune globulin prepared by the Cohn–Oncly cold ethanol fractionation procedure have not transmitted viral hepatitis of any type, HIV, or any other infectious agent.

Before the advent of hepatitis B vaccine, hepatitis B immune globulin in three doses was shown to have an efficacy of approximately 75 per cent in preventing the carrier state from developing at 1 year of age in the infants of HBeAg-positive carrier mothers.[21]. However, passive protection from this product wanes, and the infants were left unprotected in a household with an HBeAg-positive mother and often one or more HBeAg-positive siblings. In this setting, infection often occurred within a few years.[21] Hepatitis B immune globulin is rather expensive, unavailable in most developing countries, and requires maternal screening during pregnancy to identify carrier mothers in order to treat their new-born infants. Laboratory facilities and a sophisticated prenatal programme to organize this system are also lacking in many developing countries.

When hepatitis B vaccine became available, combinations of hepatitis B immune globulin and the vaccine were investigated in attempts to prevent perinatal transmission and the development of the carrier state. These studies showed excellent (85–95 per cent) efficacy in preventing the carrier state in the infants of HBeAg-positive mothers,[20,22] and combined hepatitis B immune globulin/vaccine protocols are recommended for these infants in most industrialized countries.[23] In developing countries, however, the constraints previously described for hepatitis B immune globulin make this strategy untenable.

It is fortunate that hepatitis B vaccine alone has proved highly effective in preventing the carrier state from developing in the infants of HBeAg-positive mothers, and this is the treatment of choice in most developing countries. The efficacy of vaccine alone is about 75 per cent for the plasma-derived vaccine, but several reports on recombinant DNA vaccines have reported a higher efficacy, approaching that of hepatitis B vaccine plus immune globulin (André, JMedVirol, 1994; 44:144).

In order to prevent the carrier state from developing in the infants of carrier mothers, the first dose of vaccine must be given soon after birth, preferably on the day of delivery. This is feasible when births take place in hospitals or clinics, but may be difficult for home births after which the first contact with the immunization system may not occur for weeks or months. In these settings, investigators have tried several strategies to encourage early immunization, including enhanced birth registration with a visit to the home by a vaccinator, and giving trained birth attendants hepatitis B vaccine to keep at home and administer immediately after the delivery of the baby. Hepatitis B vaccine is rather thermostable and can be kept at ambient temperatures for several weeks without loss of immunogenicity, making such programmes feasible.

The contribution of perinatal transmission to the overall transmission of hepatitis B varies from region to region. This is due to the variation in HBeAg positivity in carrier mothers. In East and South-East Asian countries, approximately 40 per cent of carrier women of child-bearing age are HBeAg-positive, compared with only about 10 to 15 per cent of African and European carrier mothers.[22] The reason for this difference is not well understood. On considering two hypothetical countries with 10 per cent of HBsAg-positive mothers, one in Asia and one in Africa, an infant born in the Asian country has a 4 per cent chance of having an HBeAg-positive carrier mother, while the African child has a 1 per cent chance. If 12 per cent of the population in these countries are carriers, 25 to 30 per cent of carriers in the Asian country and less than 10 per cent of carriers in the African country will be attributable to perinatal transmission.

It is important to understand that other modes of transmission, usually child–child, contribute more than perinatal transmission to the overall prevalence of carriers, even in Asia. Thus, even if perinatal transmission cannot be prevented because early immunization is not feasible, an enormous impact on the carrier prevalence can be achieved by immunization starting at a few months of age.

Booster doses

An additional dose of hepatitis B vaccine given years after the initial series leads to a significant boost in the titre of anti-HBs in almost all recipients who initially responded to the vaccine, whether or not they have lost detectable anti-HBs. Various schemes for delivering booster doses of hepatitis B vaccine have been proposed, including boosting at regular intervals (e.g. every 5 or 10 years), measuring anti-HBs titre after the initial vaccination and boosting a variable number of years later depending on the titre of anti-HBs achieved, testing for anti-HBs at certain intervals and boosting those found to be negative, or not boosting at all (Hadler, AnnIntMed, 1988; 108:457). The vaccine package information in some countries recommends booster doses using one of the above methods. However, the United States Centers for Disease Control[23] and the World Health Organization (WHO) currently feel that booster doses are not necessary; this advice would change if reports on clinical hepatitis B or the development of the carrier state indicate that protection is waning.

Protection against hepatitis D (delta hepatitis)

Hepatitis delta virus (HDV) is a defective, hepatotropic, RNA virus that requires HBsAg as an envelope protein and can only replicate in the presence of active HBV infection. Infection with HDV occurs as a coinfection with HBV or a superinfection of HBV carriers (Rizzetto, Hepatol, 1983; 3:729). When coinfection occurs, HDV infection may be self-limiting, as the virus cannot outlive the transient HBV infection. HDV superinfection in a chronic HBV carrier may lead to fulminant disease, and severe chronic hepatitis with accelerated progression to cirrhosis is more likely to occur. Hepatitis B vaccine, by preventing HBV infection, also protects against delta coinfection. However, the vaccine cannot eliminate the carrier state and thus cannot prevent delta superinfection.

Strategies for use
Routine childhood immunization

The WHO and many other expert groups have recommended that all children receive hepatitis B vaccine as a routine part of childhood immunization, and almost half of all children in the world live in countries that have adopted this policy.[24] The WHO recommends that countries of high and intermediate endemicity (HBV carrier prevalence of 2 per cent or greater) should include hepatitis B vaccine in their infant immunization programmes. This strategy will have the greatest impact on chronic carriers and therefore chronic disease, since most carriers are generated by early childhood infection. In countries of low endemicity (below 2 per cent HBV carriers), adolescent immunization may be added to infant immunization or adolescent immunization done alone. Combined infant and adolescent strategies will lead to the most rapid control of HBV infection in the community, and adolescent immunization can be stopped when cohorts of immunized children reach adolescence.

It is not yet known whether a booster dose will be necessary at adolescence following infant immunization. Most industrial countries now recommend infant and/or adolescent immunization with hepatitis B vaccine, although some in northern Europe are not yet convinced that routine hepatitis B immunization is cost-effective in their populations (Van Damme, BMJ, 1997; 314:1033). Some countries are attempting even more rapid control of HBV infection with 'catch-up' strategies such as immunizing all children under a certain age.

Infants of carrier mothers

Most industrial countries screen all pregnant women for HBsAg so that infants of carrier mothers can be treated at birth with hepatitis B immune globulin and vaccine.[22] Some countries have criteria to screen 'high risk' mothers only, but careful studies have shown that this strategy misses a large proportion of carriers, both because many carrier mothers have no risk factors and because selective screening strategies depend on the knowledge and interest of thousands of individual health-care providers (McQuillan, AmJEpid, 1987; 126:484). Although early studies showed a significant benefit for a combined hepatitis B immune globulin/vaccine strategy, recent studies have shown that the efficacy of vaccine alone approaches that of vaccine plus immune globulin (André, JMedVirol, 1994; 44:144). Developing countries, most of which have severely constrained resources and no extensive laboratory network for testing, are advised to put resources into universal infant immunization, starting at birth if possible, which will prevent much more disease than maternal screening and treatment of newborns of carrier mothers with hepatitis B immune globulin and vaccine.

'High risk' groups

Most countries have recommendations to immunize members of 'high risk' groups defined by lifestyle, occupation, medical conditions, or ethnicity. These include health-care workers, certain public-service workers, sexually active heterosexuals (including attendees at clinics for sexually transmitted diseases and prostitutes), homosexually active men, parenteral drug users, recipients of blood products, haemodialysis patients, residents of institutions for the developmentally disabled, certain travellers and residents of highly endemic areas, and members of certain ethnic groups.

While members of high-risk groups will benefit as individuals from immunization and should receive hepatitis B vaccine, only one of these groups, health-care workers, has received significant amounts of vaccine, and health-care workers represent less than 5 to 10 per cent of reported cases in most countries. Most other high-risk groups are difficult to reach or are not motivated to seek immunization. It is clear that control of HBV infection in the community cannot be achieved by strategies focused on high-risk groups, and this has led most experts to recommend routine immunization of children as the only strategy that will control HBV infection on a community basis.

Impact of immunization

The impact of immunization on groups and populations has exceeded our expectations. No cases of acute hepatitis B or chronic carriage have been reported in adult responders to vaccine (such as health-care workers) even if detectable anti-HBs has been absent for several years. In cohorts of immunized children in developing countries followed for more than 10 years, immunization has reduced the prevalence of carriers to less than 2 per cent (low endemicity), even in populations where the prevaccination prevalence in children exceeded 10 per cent. These results have been reported from all regions of the world, including Africa,[7] China, South-East Asia, the Pacific basin, Alaska, and the Middle East. In addition to almost complete protection of children who receive a complete series of vaccine, decreased rates of HBV infection in non-immunized individuals (herd immunity) are also found (Whittle, Lancet, 1995; 345:1089). Pressure of infection is decreased when there are fewer childhood carriers and because adult carriers naturally lose infectivity as they convert to anti-HBe. In some populations where extensive immunization has taken place, the reported rate of acute HBV infections has fallen to zero and no carriers have been found in cohorts of immunized children (Wainwright, JInfDis, 1997; 175:674).

Economic considerations

Hepatitis B immunization, despite the fact that hepatitis B vaccine is often more expensive than traditional vaccines, has been found to be cost-effective or cost-beneficial in most studies. In one extensive review, 89 per cent of 88 economic studies listed were partially or completely favourable.[25] This was true in countries of low, intermediate, and high endemicity. In one study from The Gambia, the cost per carrier prevented was $35, and the cost per death averted was $150 to $200, putting hepatitis B immunization in the middle of cost-effectiveness of routine childhood immunizations (Hall, TrRSocTropMedHyg, 1993; 87:333), which are themselves recognized to be the most cost-effective interventions in all of medicine. The extremely favourable cost-effectiveness of the addition of hepatitis B vaccine to EPI has also been described by the World Bank.[26] In low-endemicity countries such as western Europe and North America, the cost-effectiveness of the routine use of hepatitis B vaccine has been well established because of the high cost of treating chronic hepatitis B, which may include interferon for carriers and liver transplantation.[27,28]

Mutants

Reports of so-called vaccine-escape mutants have recently generated much interest, but there is no evidence they pose a threat to current vaccination programmes. The mutants of concern to immunization are in the common 'a' determinant of HBsAg, a highly conserved polypeptide loop on the surface of the virus, the 22-nm HBsAg particle, and hepatitis B vaccines. This loop is the antigen that elicits anti-HBs, and mutations in it could theoretically lead to viral 'escape' from vaccine-induced anti-HBs protection, which may be more restricted than the more 'polyclonal' protection induced by wild-type infection that induces anti-HBc, anti-HBe, anti-pre-S etc. There is also concern that these mutants might generate viruses that could not be detected by commercial kits designed to identify HBsAg, which make use of anti-HBs antibody.

Most mutants of this type have been described in infants of HBsAg carrier mothers who have been unsuccessfully treated with hepatitis B immune globulin and vaccine. It has been known for some time that infants of carrier mothers, most of whom get infected before treatment, have a poorer response to hepatitis B vaccine than infants of non-carrier mothers. Virus mutants may partly explain that phenomenon, but there is currently no evidence that these can infect immunized individuals and thus pose a threat to immunization programmes or necessitate a change in the composition of vaccines or reagent kits.

Escape mutants have been found in mothers and other relatives of the infants, as well as carriers in the general population who have never received vaccine. Most are detected by commercial HBsAg kits, although with less sensitivity, and have been found in children who received hepatitis B immune globulin and vaccine, so the 'escape' may have been from the immune globulins and not the vaccine. The mutants are able to infect susceptible (Ogata, JInfDis, 1997; 175:511) but not immunized chimpanzees. It is possible that what has emerged is not new mutants but our ability to identify them. As we apply the new techniques of sequencing to larger populations of carriers, our understanding of the true role of these mutants will be greatly enhanced.

Conclusion

Hepatitis B vaccines have been commercially available since 1982 and have proved themselves to be safe, immunogenic, and effective. More than 90 per cent of recipients develop good immune responses and have been protected against clinical hepatitis B and the carrier state until the present day. Many new concepts are emerging relating to vaccine dose, schedule, duration of protection, the need for booster doses, combination vaccines, and strategies for the most effective use of the vaccine. More than 80 countries now use this vaccine as a routine childhood immunogen, and global control of HBV infection is feasible and has been recommended by the WHO.

References

1. Krugman S, Giles JP, and Hammond J. Viral hepatitis type B (MS-2 strain): studies on active immunization. *Journal of the American Medical Association*, 1971; **217**: 41.
2. Purcell RH and Gerin JL. Hepatitis B subunit vaccine: a preliminary report of safety and efficacy tests in chimpanzees. *American Journal of the Medical Sciences*, 1975; **270**: 395.
3. Hilleman MR *et al*. Purified and inactivated human hepatitis B vaccine. *American Journal of the Medical Sciences*, 1975; **270**: 401.
4. Maupas PAG *et al*. Immunization against hepatitis B in man. *Lancet*, 1976; **i**: 1367–70.
5. Szmuness W, *et al*. Hepatitis B vaccine: demonstration of efficacy in a controlled clinical trial in a high risk population in the United States. *New England Journal of Medicine*, 1980; **303**: 833.
6. Francis DP, *et al*. The prevention of hepatitis B with vaccine; report of the Centers for Disease Control Multi-Center Efficacy Trial among homosexual men. *Annals of Internal Medicine*, 1982; **97**: 362–6.
7. Fortuin M, *et al*. Efficacy of hepatitis B vaccine in the Gambian Expanded Programme on Immunisation. *Lancet*, 1993; **341**: 1129–31.
8. Xu ZY, *et al*. Prevention of perinatal acquisition of hepatitis B virus carriage using vaccine: preliminary report of a randomized, double blind placebo controlled and comparative trial. *Pediatrics*, 1985; **76**: 713–18.
9. Van Damme P, Vranckx R, and Meheus A. Immunogenicity of a recombinant DNA hepatitis B vaccine in institutionalized patients with Down's syndrome. *Vaccine*, 1990; **8**: S53–55.
10. Valenzuela P, *et al*. Synthesis and assembly of hepatitis B surface antigen particles in yeast. *Nature*, 1982; **298**: 347–50.
11. André FE and Safary A. Clinical experience with a yeast derived hepatitis B vaccine. In Zuckerman AI, ed. *Viral hepatitis and liver disease*. New York: Alan R. Liss, 1988.
12. Zajac BA, West DJ, McAleer WJ, and Scolnick EM. Overview of clinical studies with hepatitis B vaccine made by recombinant DNA. *Journal of Infection*, 1986; **13**: 39–45.
13. Papaevangelou G, *et al*. Evaluation of a combined tetravalent diphtheria, tetanus, whole-cell pertussis and hepatitis B candidate vaccine administered to healthy infants according to a three-dose vaccination schedule. *Vaccine*, 1995; **13**: 175–8.
14. Niu MT, Davis DM, and Ellenberg S. Recombinant hepatitis B vaccination of neonates and infants: emerging safety data from the Vaccine Adverse Event Reporting System. *Pediatric Infectious Diseases Journal*, 1996; **15**: 771–6.
15. Institute of Medicine. Hepatitis B vaccines. In Stratton KR, Howe CJ, and Johnston RB, eds. *Adverse events associated with childhood vaccines: evidence bearing on causality*. Washington DC: National Academy Press, 1994: 211–35.
16. Coursaget P, *et al*. Simultaneous injection of hepatitis B vaccine with BCG, diphtheria and tetanus toxoids, pertussis and polio vaccines. In Coursaget P and Tong MJ, eds. *Progress in hepatitis B immunization*. Vol. 194. Colloque INSERM/John Libbey Eurotext, 1990: 319–24.
17. Kane MA. Reduced doses of hepatitis B vaccines: is it a good idea? *Bulletin of the World Health Organization*, 1995; **73**: 529–30.
18. Kane MA, Hadler SC, and Maynard JE. Antibody to hepatitis B surface antigen and screening before hepatitis B vaccination. (Editorial). *Annals of Internal Medicine*, 1985; **103**: 791–3.
19. Beasley R, *et al*. Hepatitis B immune globulin (HBIG) efficacy in the interruption of perinatal transmission of hepatitis B virus carrier state. *Lancet*, 1981; **ii**: 388–93.
20. Beasley RP, *et al*. Prevention of perinatally transmitted hepatitis B virus infection with hepatitis B immune globulin and hepatitis B vaccine. *Lancet*, 1983; **ii**: 1099–102.
21. Beasley RP and Hwang LY. Postnatal infectivity of hepatitis B surface antigen-carrier mothers. *Journal of Infectious Diseases*, 1983; **147**: 185–90.
22. Stevens CE, *et al*. Perinatal hepatitis B transmission in the United States: prevention by passive–active immunization. *Journal of the American Medical Association*, 1985; **253**: 1740–5.
23. Centers for Disease Control. Hepatitis B virus: a comprehensive strategy for eliminating transmission in the United States through universal childhood vaccination: recommendations of the Immunization Practices Advisory Committee (ACIP). *Morbidity and Mortality Weekly Reports*, 1991; **40** (No. RR-13): 1–25.
24. Kane MA. Global status of hepatitis B immunisation. *Lancet*, 1996; **348**: 696.
25. Jefferson T and Demicheli V. Is vaccination against hepatitis B efficient? A review of the world literature. *Health Economics*, 1994; **3**: 25–37.
26. World Bank. *World development report*. Geneva, 1993.
27. Bloom BS, Hillman AL, Fendrick AM, and Schwartz JS. A reappraisal of hepatitis B virus vaccination strategies using cost-effectiveness analysis *Annals of Internal Medicine*, 1993; **118**: 298–306.
28. Margolis HS, *et al*. Prevention of hepatitis B virus transmission by immunization: an economic evaluation of current recommendations. *Journal of the American Medical Association*, 1995; **274**: 1201–8.

12.1.3.2 Therapy of chronic viral hepatitis

Giorgio Saracco and Mario Rizzetto

Introduction

Many drugs and herbs were used to treat viral hepatitis before the era of serology but none has proved efficacious.[1] With the identification of the agents of viral hepatitis in the 1970s and 1980s, the therapeutic approach has become more rational, but of the drugs tested only interferon has gained universal acceptance and has been licensed worldwide for the therapy of chronic viral hepatitis. Table 1 lists drugs that passed preclinical studies but did not prove viable clinically. This chapter deals with interferon therapy of chronic viral hepatitides and with novel forms of therapies that are currently under clinical appraisal.

The interferons

The interferons are a family of cytokines produced by eukaryotic cells under a variety of stimuli.[2] They are biologically multivalent, possessing antiproliferative, antiviral, and immunomodulant properties. Inhibition of viral replication is mediated by the induction of a protein kinase, a $2'$–$5'$-A-endonuclease, a phosphodiesterase, and an oligoadenylate synthetase; the synthetase has been used as a clinical index of interferon activity. The immunomodulant properties of the cytokine are mediated by the induction and maturation of HLA class I and II antigens, an increase of natural killer-cell activity, and the stimulation of T lymphocytes.

There are three types of interferon: α, produced mainly by leucocytes, β, produced mainly by fibroblasts, and γ, produced mainly by T lymphocytes. Interferon-α and -β interact with the same cellular receptor; interferon-γ interacts with a different receptor. Interferon-β and -γ are coded by a single gene; there are at least 15 proteins, coded by 23 genes, that exert the biological functions of interferon-α.

Interferon-γ is ineffective in viral hepatitis (Saez-Royuela, Hepatol, 1991; 13:327). Four types of interferon-α are available commercially, two recombinant (single, pure subtypes of interferon produced by recombinant technology as two variants α2a and α2b) and two natural, lymphoblastoid and leucocyte-derived, produced by the stimulation of lymphoblastoid cells and human leucocytes, respectively.

Interferon-α is administered subcutaneously and intramuscularly. It may by given daily on alternate days, but thrice weekly is generally preferred. The total and single-shot dosage varies according to the virus involved. Single-shot doses usually vary from 3 million units (**MU**) to 10 MU.

Side-effects are proportional to the single-shot dose; they diminish with dose reduction.

Extensive clinical trials have confirmed the efficacy of recombinant interferon-α (both 2a and 2b) and lymphoblastoid interferon in chronic hepatitis B, C, and D.[3] Natural α- (from leucocytes) and β- (from fibroblasts) interferons have been used in Mediterranean countries; their efficacy has been less well documented. Natural interferon-β derived from fibroblasts has been used intravenously (Omata, Lancet, 1991; 338:914; Koff, AmJGastr, 1993; 88:171). Data with a new 'consensus' interferon, expressed from a RNA assembled with therapeutically active genetic fragments from different types of interferons, do not indicate a substantial advantage over conventional interferons in the therapy of hepatitis C (Tong, Hepatol, 1997; 26:747).

Hereafter the term 'interferon' refers to interferon-α.

Contraindications/indications for interferon

Interferon is contraindicated in patients with concomitant severe extrahepatic illnesses, chronic infections, and myelosuppression. Patients with thyroid dysfunction should not be given interferon as it may induce thyroiditis, possibly leading to irreversible functional loss of the gland (Berris, DigDisSci, 1991; 36:1657; Lisker-Melman, Gastro, 1992; 102:2155). Severe psychiatric disorders and underlying autoimmune diseases contraindicate the use of the drug; autoimmune diseases may be exacerbated by the stimulating action of interferon on the antigens of the major histocompatibility complex (Papo, AnnIntMed, 1992; 116:51; Garcia-Buey, Gastro, 1995; 108:1770).

When considering indications for giving interferon to a patient with chronic viral hepatitis, the following points should be kept in mind:

1. Interferon cures disease and eradicates viral infections in only a minority of patients whatever the aetiological factors; most will not respond, or will respond only partially or temporarily. Only patients with a long-lasting response have a clinical benefit; the value of therapy is unclear in transient and partial responders.
2. Therapy needs to be prolonged and often induces side-effects that may occasionally be serious and rarely life-threatening.
3. Our knowledge of the natural history of chronic viral hepatitis is limited and the course of the disease is variable. In many patients with chronic hepatitis C the disease runs an indolent course without symptoms and does not alter their quality of life. Complications affecting survival occur in a subgroup only. Ideally, treatment should be given to those who stand a significant risk of disease progression and a high chance of therapeutic response, but these events are not predictable.

An indication for therapy should emerge from a balance between the presumed risk of morbidity posed by the liver disease, the presumed benefit of therapy, and the risk of important side-effects in the individual clinical setting. For instance, the need to treat is obvious when the risk of clinical expression of the disease is high, as in the young adult with chronic hepatitis C; in such a patient there is a high risk that the indolent and slowly progressive disease will progress to cirrhosis and liver failure over many years. However,

Table 1 Drugs used without success in the therapy of chronic viral hepatitis				
	Type of chronic viral hepatitis			
Drug	**B**	**C**	**D**	**Reasons for failure**
Foscarnet	+		+	Toxic
Fialouridine	+			Toxic
Levamisole	+			Ineffective
Arabinoside monophosphate	+	+	+	Toxic
Phyllantus amarus	+			Ineffective
Steroids	+	+	+	Harmful

because of the therapeutic failures and the inconveniences of therapy, its value seems doubtful in patients in whom chronic hepatitis itself is unlikely to cause a new or an additional medical problem, as in the aged patient or the patient with other advanced chronic illnesses; interferon therapy may be superfluous as they are likely to die of old age or of an unrelated disease rather than of the consequences of hepatitis C (Seeff, NEJM, 1992; 327:1906).

Before treatment is begun a liver biopsy is useful to confirm the nature of the lesion, grade the extent of inflammation, reveal unsuspected, non-viral damage, and stage the degree of fibrosis. The major role of histological investigation is to uncover or confirm an underlying cirrhosis, as this condition diminishes the response to interferon. If cirrhosis is ruled out by appropriate liver function tests, the advantage of a liver biopsy before treatment in patients with well-documented chronic viral hepatitis is relative as therapy is currently recommended for the whole spectrum of non-cirrhotic viral disorders regardless of the degree of enzymatic and inflammatory activity.

The need for a liver biopsy after therapy is questionable; the histological picture is unlikely to have changed in non-responders while it is likely to have improved in responders (response being defined by liver function and virological indices) (Saracco, Drugs, 1997; 53:74). Biopsies should not be performed earlier than 1 year after the completion of interferon therapy because histological improvements are delayed compared to biochemical improvements.

Side-effects

Although deaths due to interferon have been reported (Durand, Lancet, 1991; 338:1268; Marcellin, Lancet, 1991; 338:828; Janssen, BMJ, 1993; 306:107), they are very rare and usually related to decompensation of an unrecognized, advanced cirrhosis. In a recent survey on more than 11 000 patients with chronic viral hepatitis treated with interferon, the incidence of fatalities was 0.04 per cent, of life-threatening adverse reactions 0.07 per cent, and of *de novo* non-hepatic morbidity 1.2 per cent. (Fattovich, JHepatol, 1996; 24: 38).

At the start of therapy, interferon induces mild to moderate side-effects; patients usually complain of headache, myalgia, and asthenia, often accompanied by fever and rigors. Symptoms appear 4 to 6 h after the injection and persist for 6 to 12 h. They gradually diminish and then disappear over 2 to 3 weeks of therapy, are dose-dependent (more troublesome the higher the dosage), and are controlled with paracetamol. During prolonged therapy, patients may complain of fatigue, headache, myalgias, irritability, and loss of appetite, weight, and hair. All these symptoms are reversed with the discontinuation of interferon. Rarely they force withdrawal of therapy; it usually suffices to diminish the dose for a while.

Psychiatric complications are more difficult to evaluate and potentially more dangerous; they include irritability, anxiety, depression, psychosis, and suicidal attempts (Renault, ArchIntMed, 1987; 147:1577; Janssen, JHepatol, 1994; 21:241).

Thyroid dysfunction may occur in 3 to 5 per cent of patients with interferon-treated hepatitis. Rare side-effects include convulsions (Janssen, Lancet, 1990; ii:1580; Obaid Shakil, JHepatol, 1996; 24: 48) acute renal failure, acute myocarditis, and generalized bacterial infections (Renault, SemLivDis, 1989; 9:273).

Monitoring of therapy

Periodic monitoring is required to assess the effect of therapy and to detect unwanted side-effects. Patients should be checked at least once a month during therapy and during the first 6 months after the end of therapy. Responders should then be followed-up once every 3 to 4 months for the next 2 years and yearly thereafter. Monthly testing should include counts of white blood cells and platelets in order to identify dangerous, interferon-induced myelo- and thrombocytopenia. A periodic dosage of thyroid hormones including thyroid-stimulating hormone is advisable in order to detect interferon-induced thyroid disease. There is no need to test systematically for autoantibodies during therapy; they should be looked for if a *de novo* autoimmune disorder is suspected. Virological monitoring is dealt with in each specific chapter.

Interferon therapy of chronic hepatitis B

There are differences in the response to interferon between wild-type dominant (hepatitis B e (**HBeAg**)-positive) and pre-core mutant dominant (HBeAg-negative, anti-HBe-positive) chronic hepatitis B virus (**HBV**) hepatitis, the former responding better than the latter. Response rates have been higher in patients infected with HBV genotype A than in those with genotype D or E (Zhang, JMedVirol, 1996; 48:8). Variations in the core region of HBV may also affect the response to interferon-α (Fattovich, Hepatol, 1995; 22:1355).

Wild-type dominant (HBeAg-positive) chronic hepatitis B

In the average-size adult, optimal therapeutic dosages are 10 MU of interferon given thrice weekly, or 5 MU given daily, for 4 to 6 months; a minimum total of 200 MU of interferon is needed to obtain a response. There is no benefit in prolonging therapy if no response is observed within this period. Some patients may respond after cessation of therapy. Between 15 and 61 per cent of treated patients in different series have reportedly responded (Table 2); the large variations in response are due primarily to the epidemiological and clinical heterogeneity of the patients enrolled in the various trials (Hoofnagle, Gastro, 1988; 95:1318; Brook, BMJ, 1989; 299: 652; Saracco, Hepatol, 1989; 10:336; Perrillo, NEJM, 1990; 323: 295; Lok, Gastro, 1992; 102:2091; Wong, Gastro, 1995; 108:165).

Response is marked by the clearance of serum HBV DNA, and an increase of aminotransferases during the second or third month of therapy, which reflects the immunological response leading to clearance of the virus. The IgM antibody against the HBcAg (IgM anti-HB core) increases after the enzyme flare, and before the normalization of liver enzymes and seroconversion from HBeAg to anti-HBe (Fig. 1); the latter may occur several months after discontinuation of therapy. Clearance of HBsAg and seroconversion to anti-HBs is a late event. One year after completion of therapy, 10 to 15 per cent of responders who seroconverted to anti-HBe have lost HBsAg and seroconverted to anti-HBs (Karayannis, JHepatol, 1990; 10:350); after 4 years this percentage increases to about 70 per cent of those who had initially responded to interferon. Serum HBV DNA is no longer measurable, even with the most sensitive

Table 2 Interferon-α in chronic hepatitis type B (HBeAg +ve)

Author	Interferon	Dosage	Duration (months)	No. of patients	HBeAg clearance Treated	Controls
Hoofnagle	rec	10 MU 3/weekly	4	45	10 (32%)	1 (7%)
Brook	rec	2.5–10 MU 3/weekly	6	44	12 (41%)	0 (0%)
Saracco	lymph	5 MU/m² 3/weekly	6	64	21 (61%)	12 (33%)
Perrillo	rec	5 MU daily	4	84	15 (37%)	3 (7%)
Lok	rec	10 MU 3/weekly	4	75	6 (15%)	3 (8%)
Wong	lymph	5–>10 MU/m² 3/weekly	3	50	6 (24%)	1 (4%)

rec, recombinant; lymph, lymphoblastoid.

polymerase chain reactions (**PCR**), in 80 per cent of these individuals (Korenman, AnnIntMed, 1991; 114:629; Carreno, JHepatol, 1992; 15:102; Kuhns, Gastro, 1992; 103:1649). HBV DNA sequences have been detected in hepatocytes as late as 67 months after seroconversion from HBsAg to anti-HBs; (Marcellin, AnnIntMed, 1990; 112:227); in this context the HBV DNA is probably not transcriptionally active (Kuhns, Hepatol, 1990; 12:904).

Caucasian children tolerate interferon and respond as well as adults to similar doses of the cytokine; when 7.5 MU/m² was given thrice weekly for 6 months, seroconversion from HBeAg to anti-HBe was observed in 30 per cent of children treated (Barbera, Hepatol, 1994; 20:287). Chinese children born to HBeAg-positive mothers do not respond to conventional treatment schedules (Lai, Lancet, 1987; ii:877).

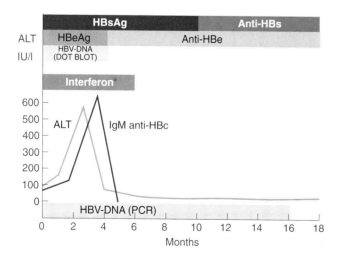

Fig. 1. Typical biochemical, immunological, and virological pattern of a complete response to interferon in chronic HBeAg positive hepatitis B.

Reactivation of HBeAg after interferon-induced seroconversion to anti-HBe is uncommon; it occurs in less than 10 per cent of cases, usually within one year after completion of therapy. HBeAg-negative mutants may be selected by the process of seroconversion to anti-HBe during interferon therapy (Gunther, Virology, 1992; 187:271).

The biochemical improvement is matched by a significant histological improvement and no disease progression is seen in long-term follow-up liver biopsies of sustained responders; the overall histological improvement is better over the long term than that observed within 1 year after withdrawal of therapy (Korenman, AnnIntMed, 1991; 114:629; Perrillo, AnnIntMed, 1991; 115:113). Interferon seems to exert a persistent suppression of serum markers of connective tissue turnover independently of its antiviral and anti-inflammatory effect (Teran, Hepatol, 1994; 19:849).

In a meta-analysis of 10 controlled trials including 496 treated and 255 untreated cases of chronic HBeAg-positive hepatitis B, interferon significantly increased the clearance of HBeAg, with an overall relative rate of 1.76 compared to untreated controls. The effect of therapy was dose-related and the relative rate of HBeAg clearance reached 2.05 in patients treated with at least 200 MU/m² of interferon.[4]

Another meta-analysis of 15 controlled studies has confirmed that elimination of HBeAg is three times greater after interferon therapy than in untreated controls, with a four-fold increase in the loss of HBsAg; the rates of HBeAg clearance and of HBsAg clearance during the first year were, respectively, 38 to 45 per cent and 7 per cent in treated patients, and 9 to 14 per cent and 1.7 per cent in untreated patients. The estimated subsequent annual rates of HBeAg and HBsAg clearance were 7 and 2 per cent, respectively. Progression to cirrhosis was reduced by 13 per cent, decompensation by 9 per cent, and development of hepatocellular carcinoma by 4 per cent.[5]

Studies on survival and the cost–benefit of therapy, based on models predictive of the likely clinical outcome and related medical expenses, have also shown that interferon is able to prolong life in patients with chronic hepatitis B who have HBeAg in their serum, and that benefits exceed costs when an evaluation of life expectancy is included in the analysis (Dusheiko, Hepatol, 1995; 23:1863, Wong, AnnIntMed, 1995; 122:664). More conclusive evidence, based on solid clinical end-points, of the beneficial effect of interferon in this setting has been recently provided. One hundred and three treated patients were followed up for a mean of 50 ± 20 months and compared with 53 untreated controls. The estimated rates of HBeAg and HBsAg clearance at 5 years were 56 and 12.6 per cent in treated patients as compared to 28 and 0 per cent in untreated controls. Survival and quality of life were significantly better in sustained responders who had cleared HBeAg than in non-responders or untreated patients.[6]

Response in selected groups: factors predicting response

Individuals with impaired immune reactivity such as those with chronic renal failure, and transplanted patients, respond less well than immunocompetent patients.[3] Coinfection with human immunodeficiency virus (HIV) and male homosexuality reportedly diminish the response to interferon, but a recent study has shown that interferon is as effective in homosexuals without HIV coinfection as in heterosexuals (Wong, Gastro, 1995; 108:165). Cirrhotic patients respond poorly; if treated at all, those with decompensated cirrhosis should be treated cautiously with low doses (Perrillo, Gastro, 1995; 109:908).

The selection of patients based on immune reactivity, as manifested by higher serum alanine transferase (ALT) and lower serum HBV DNA, improves the response; in most trials, ALT before therapy was significantly higher in responders than in non-responders.[4] High pre-therapy titres of IgM anti-HBc were considered predictive of a response to interferon (Scully, Hepatol, 1990; 12:1111).

There are significant differences between Caucasian and Chinese patients. Chinese patients respond less well, and in one study (Lok, Gastro, 1993; 105:1833) only 21 per cent of those with a sustained response cleared serum HBV DNA as measured with PCR-based assays; very few of those who experienced a sustained loss of HBeAg had delayed clearance of the HBsAg, probably reflecting the integration of the viral genome in the host's genome.

One study (Marinos, Hepatol, 1994; 19:303) found that an index value of IgM anti-HBc higher than 0.3 (IMx core M, Abbott Laboratories, Chicago, Illinois, USA) was superior to ALT in predicting a response. Elevated antibody titres were present in 84 per cent of responders and 25 per cent of non-responders whereas a high ALT was originally present in 53 per cent of responders and 38 per cent of non-responders. However, the predictive role of IgM anti-HBc was not confirmed in a series of child patients (Barbera, Hepatol, 1994; 20:287).

As patients with normal/low ALT and high viraemia (immunotolerant) stand a poor chance of response, it may be convenient to wait for a spontaneous increase of ALT (which is usually accompanied by a concomitant decrease of serum HBV DNA) before treating these patients.

Virological monitoring

Virological monitoring includes testing for HBV DNA, which disappears during successful therapy. However, since serial determinations of the viral genome during therapy may not be practical, monitoring of IgM anti-HBc may be used to determine the expected flare of HBV-related disease activity that heralds seroconversion to anti-HBe.

HBsAg, HBeAg, and HBV DNA should be tested for at the end of therapy and 6 months later.

HBeAg-negative mutant dominant (HBeAg −ve, anti-HBe +ve) chronic hepatitis B

A HBeAg-negative phenotype may be the consequence of a variety of mutations in the precore region. The most common clinically relevant genomic mutation of HBV involves a G–A substitution in the precore region (nt 1896) that results in the transformation of a tryptophan codon at position 28 into a termination codon, with blocking of the synthesis and secretion of HBeAg (Brunetto, ItalJGastr, 1989; 21:151; Carman, Lancet, 1989; ii:588).

This 'HBeAg minus' variant of HBV has become the predominant viral strain in the Mediterranean basin and most therapeutic experience with HBeAg-negative chronic hepatitis B has been gained in this area. The patients usually have a progressive disease characterized by wide fluctuations of aminotransferases and of viraemia. In this setting the primary end-point of therapy is the clearance of HBV DNA; this is often difficult to assess because the natural course of the disease is marked by spontaneous remissions, viral as well as biochemical, which may last several years (Brunetto, PNAS, 1991; 88:4186). Moreover, HBV DNA may be undetectable with commercial assays and testing with PCR assays is expensive and unsuited to monitoring viraemia; semiquantitative dosage of IgM anti-HBc may substitute for the direct measurement of viraemia (Brunetto, JHepatol, 1993; 19:431). As relapses may occur years after the end of therapy, a prolonged follow-up is mandatory.

Dosage has varied from 3 to 10 MU and duration of therapy from 6 to 24 months. The therapeutic results obtained so far are controversial (Table 3). All studies have shown a high initial rate of ALT normalization accompanied by clearance of HBV DNA (67–90 per cent): in three studies this was followed by a high relapse rate among responders (78–85 per cent) (Brunetto, Hepatol, 1989; 10:198; Hadzyiannis, JHepatol, 1990; 11 (Suppl. 1): S133; Pastore, JHepatol, 1992; 14:221), but another study has shown a significant response (37 per cent) also during a 18-month follow-up (Fattovich, Hepatol, 1992; 15:584). Overall, no more than 15 to 20 per cent of patients have maintained a clinical and virological remission 12 to 24 months after cessation of therapy. Discrepancies between the different published reports could be explained by lower dosage of interferon, longer duration of disease, and more severe histological changes in the liver in the patients enrolled into the studies with poor long-term results, when compared to the study with more favourable results.

No consensus has been reached on the optimal protocol for therapy. Although it was suggested (Hadzyiannis, Hepatol, 1994; 19:701) that therapy prolonged for 12 months or more with 3 to 5 MU of interferon is associated with a 40 per cent response rate during long-term follow-up, and with fewer relapses, this was not

Table 3 Interferon-α in chronic hepatitis type B (anti-HBe +ve, HBV-DNA + VC)

Author	Interferon	Dosage (MU)	Duration (weeks)	HBV-DNA clearance (%)	Relapse rate (%)
Brunetto	rec	9 + 3 3/weekly	16 + 8	67	85
Hadziyannis	rec	5 3/weekly	24	80	78
Pastore	rec	10 3/weekly	24	90	85
Fattovich	lymph	10 3/weekly	24	63	27

rec, recombinant; lymph, lymphoblastoid.

confirmed in another long-term trial (Lampertico, Hepatol, 1995; 22:325A). Response is not improved by timing the start of therapy with the onset of relapses.

No clinical measure of response has been identified. An increased proportion of precore as compared to wild-type HBV was proposed to be predictive of response (Brunetto, Gastro, 1993; 105:846) but this has not been confirmed (Fattovich, Hepatol, 1995; 22:1355; Lok, Hepatol, 1995; 21:19).

In patients with chronic HBeAg-negative HBV hepatitis who respond to therapy, the pattern of response is different from that observed in HBeAg-positive patients. There is no sudden peak of ALT during therapy but liver enzymes decrease steadily in a few weeks followed by the disappearance of serum HBV DNA; rarely an ALT flare some months after the end of therapy heralds viral eradication, more often it represents a relapse (Fig. 2). In view of the poor long-term results and the requirement for an aggressive protocol, therapy should be limited to non-cirrhotic patients with relatively early but severe and evolving disease. A short course of interferon may be used to bring under control the periodical hepatitic flares associated with viraemic relapses.

Alternative therapies for chronic hepatitis B

More than 60 per cent of patients with chronic hepatitis B fail to respond to interferon. A second course of interferon is usually ineffective. Combinations of interferon with levamisole (Fattovich, Hepatol, 1996; 16:1115), with zidovudine (Janssen, Hepatol, 1993; 17:383), and with ribavirin (Kakumu, Hepatol, 1993; 18:258), have not given good results and in some cases were harmful to the patient.

To increase viral eradication in immunocompetent patients the combination of a short pulse of steroids followed by the course of interferon has been proposed (Perrillo, NEJM, 1990; 323:295), with the rationale that steroid withdrawal leads to an immunological rebound reflected by an increase in ALT, and that this is followed by a transient decrease of viraemia, both conditions promoting the efficacy of interferon. A meta-analysis[7] has shown that this combination gives no further advantage in patients with high initial ALT but does accelerate the clearance of HBeAg in patients with a low baseline ALT. The therapeutic protocol consists of tapering doses of prednisone (60 down to 20 mg for 4–6 weeks), followed by no therapy for 2 weeks and then by interferon, 5 to 10 MU thrice weekly for 4 to 6 months. The hepatitic flare induced by steroid withdrawal may induce liver decompensation in cirrhotic patients; this combination therapy is therefore contraindicated in patients with a limited hepatic reserve (Perrillo, Hepatol, 1986; 6:1416).

Nucleoside analogues

Nucleoside analogues interact with HBV replication by inhibiting the reverse transcriptase encoded by the *pol* gene of hepadnaviruses. A major limitation in assessing their efficacy is the absence of a cell-culture system; primary cultures of human hepatocytes produce variable results with regard to the extent of HBV replication. As a surrogate, transfection of hepatoma cell lines with HBV DNA has been used to screen antiviral agents against HBV. This *in vitro* technique has shown that the antivirals with the strongest and long-lasting inhibitory effect on HBV DNA are 2′,3′-dideoxy-3′-thiacytidine (3TC, Lamivudine, Epivir), 2′,3′-dideoxy-5-fluoro-3-thiacytidine (FTC), penciclovir-famciclovir and 9–2 (phosphonyl-methoxyethyl) adenine (**PMEA**) (see reference 8, pp. 736–62).[8] Penciclovir and PMEA appear to inhibit all replicative intermediates of HBV, including supercoiled DNA, without any accumulation of viral products occurring (see reference 8, pp.743–8).

Famciclovir and lamivudine are currently the most promising nucleoside analogues under clinical investigation. Both are readily absorbed after oral administration. After absorption, famciclovir is

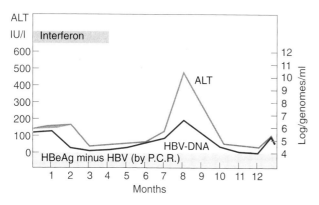

Fig. 2. Late relapse in chronic HBeAg- variant hepatitis B treated with interferon.

transformed into the active molecule penciclovir. Lamivudine acts by inhibiting the synthesis of HBV DNA through chain termination of the nascent proviral DNA. Bioavailability is 80 per cent. Besides activity *in vitro*, it is active in ducklings infected with the duck hepatitis B virus and in chimpanzees infected with the HBV; doses above 5 mg have reproducibly decreased HBV DNA in serum. Serum HBV DNA became negative in 70 per cent of patients given 25 mg and in 100 per cent given 100 or 300 mg of lamivudine for 12 weeks (Dienstag, NEJM, 1995; 333:1657). However, HBV DNA returned in most patients after therapy was completed; 19 per cent of the treated patients had a sustained response and HBeAg disappeared in 12 per cent. Cases of severe reactivation of hepatitis B have been observed after lamivudine therapy (Honkoop, Lancet, 1995; 346:1156). The drug may induce point mutations in the *pol* gene of HBV (Tipples, Hepatol, 1996; 24:714; Bartholomew, Lancet, 1997; 349:20).

While nucleoside analogues can effectively inhibit viral DNA synthesis, the inhibition in humans is only transient and even long-term therapy is unlikely to cure chronic hepatitis B. However, by diminishing HBV viraemia, nucleoside analogues may facilitate the interferon-induced clearance of HBV through the action of the immune response (Averett, ViralHepatitisRev, 1995; 1:129); this is the rationale for the current trials of the combination of lamivudine with interferon.

Adenine arabinoside monophosphate exerts a marked antiviral effect *in vitro* and *in vivo* against HBV, but severe neurotoxic side-effects hinder its clinical use (Jacyna, BrMedBull, 1990; 46:368). To reduce side-effects a conjugate of adenine arabinoside monophosphate and lactosaminated human serum albumin has been developed; the albumin component acts as a hepatotropic drug carrier that is selectively taken up by the hepatocyte (Fiume, Lancet, 1988; ii: 13). Concentration of the conjugate in hepatocytes allows the administration of doses four- to seven-fold smaller than the ordinary dosage of free adenine arabinoside monophosphate (1.5 mg/kg of conjugated drug as compared to 5–10 mg/kg of free drug). The conjugate has been given intravenously for up to 28 days without significant side-effects; it markedly and rapidly diminished the titre of serum HBV DNA in all patients, but in most viraemia increased again when therapy was stopped (Torrani Cerenzia, Hepatol, 1996; 23:357). Recombinant chylomicrons have also been used for the targeting of nucleoside agents to achieve effective intrahepatic concentrations (Rensen, NatureMed, 1995; 1:221).

Immunotherapy

The use of the hepatitis B vaccine has been advocated to overcome the initial inadequate response to the natural infection by widening the immune repertoire against the HBV. In a pilot study, serum HBV DNA disappeared after 6 months in 12 of 46 (26 per cent) patients with chronic hepatitis B given three standard injections of the hepatitis B vaccine; in eight other patients the reduction in viraemia was more than 50 per cent (Pol, Lancet, 1994; 344:342).

Vaccination together with interferon has been advocated in order to potentiate the response to interferon. Serum HBV DNA disappeared in 28 of 46 (60 per cent) patients given vaccine therapy with and without interferon; these results were not, however, different from those obtained in 43 patients given antiviral therapy alone (see reference 8, pp. 775–3).

Subcutaneous injection of thymosin, an immune stimulant that enhances suppressor T-cell activity and *in vitro* B-cell synthesis of IgG, induced the clearance of HBV DNA in a proportion of patients with HBeAg-positive chronic hepatitis B (Mutchnick, Hepatol, 1991; 14:409). Further studies on the efficacy of thymosin in this clinical setting are awaited. Thymosin induced a sustained clearance of viraemia in about 40 per cent of treated patients with anti-HBe-positive chronic hepatitis B (Andreone, Hepatol, 1996; 24:774); it was better tolerated than interferon.

Reconstitution of recipient bone marrow with bone marrow transplants primed to produce anti-HBs resulted in humoral immunity against HBV in the recipient (Shouval, Hepatol, 1993; 17: 995). Bone marrow transplantation from a hepatitis B-immune donor led to the ablation of persistent hepatitis B in another recipient (Ilan, Gastro, 1993; 104:1818). Although a bone marrow transplant from HBV immune donors to HBsAg-positive recipients may facilitate clearance of chronic HBV infection, it can also cause significant liver injury (Hervas, JHepatol, 1995; 23: 79 (Abstr.); Caselitz, JHepatol, 1995; 23: 18 (Abstr.)). Recombinant human granulocyte–macrophage colony-stimulating factor alone or in combination with interferon was used in a pilot study. There was good tolerance and some antiviral effect (Martin, Hepatol, 1993; 18:775); however, this approach has not been pursued.

The finding that patients with acute hepatitis B have a strong, cytotoxic T-cell response against an epitope containing an HLA-A2-binding motif (located between residues 18 and 27 of the HBV core protein) led to attempts to develop a therapeutic vaccine using this peptide as immunogen (Bertoletti, JVirol, 1993; 67:2376). This procedure, and DNA-based immunization using purified plasmid DNA (Whalen, ClinImmunPath, 1995; 75:1), are under appraisal in an animal model. Molecular therapies with ribozymes against pregenomic HBV RNA (Von Weizsacker, BBResComm, 1992; 189: 743) or with antisense oligonucleotides inhibiting the expression of the HBsAg gene (Goodarzi, JGenVirol, 1990; 71:321) are still in experimental stages.

Interferon therapy of chronic hepatitis D

Recombinant and lymphoblastoid interferon induce good biochemical responses (normalization of ALT) in patients with chronic hepatitis D while they are on therapy, but in the great majority of responders there is a relapse after discontinuation (Table 4). There is no consistent effect of therapy on the hepatitis D virus (**HDV**) itself; in most patients the level of viraemia is unaffected.[9]

Liver tests became normal or showed significant improvement after 4 months of therapy in 42 per cent of 31 Italian patients enrolled into an Italian multicentre trial (Rosina, Hepatol, 1991; 13: 1052) who received 5 MU/m^2 interferon thrice weekly for 4 months followed by 3 MU/m^2 for 8 more months. Some patients relapsed while on the lower dosage of interferon; only eight (25 per cent) were in remission when interferon was discontinued and there was a relapse in all but one (3 per cent) during follow-up. More favourable results were obtained with a more aggressive therapeutic protocol (Farci, NEJM, 1994; 330:88). ALT normalized in 10 of 14 (71 per cent) patients receiving 9 MU of interferon for 48 weeks as compared with 4 of 14 (29 per cent) treated with 3 MU and 1 of 13

Table 4 Interferon-α in chronic hepatitis type D

Author	No. of patients	Interferon	Dosage (MU) (3/weekly)	Duration (months)	Primary response (%)	Sustained response (%)
Rosina (1990)	12	rec	5	3	33	8
	12	controls	—	—	17	0
Rosina (1991)	31	rec	5	4		
			3	8	45	25
	30	controls	—	—	27	0
Farci	14	rec	9	12	71	36
	14	rec	3	12	29	0
	13	controls	—	—	8	0
Gaudin	11	rec	5	4		
			3	8	66	9
	11	controls	—	—	36	18

rec, recombinant.

untreated controls (8 per cent). In patients treated with 9 MU the normalization of ALT was associated with marked improvement in histological findings, and no HDV RNA was detected while they were on therapy. In five patients the biochemical response persisted up to 4 years; however, there was no long-term effect of the cytokine on HDV as HDV RNA reappeared in the serum of all responders.

Overall no more than 10 per cent of treated patients exhibit a sustained normalization of ALT and clearance of HDV; only a proportion are permanently cured of the disease. In this minority, IgM anti-HD disappears quickly from serum and HBsAg is cleared within months to years with seroconversion to anti-HBs (Lau, JMedVirol, 1993; 39:292; Rosina, ExpOpinInvestDrugs, 1996; 5: 197). The elimination of HBsAg is the most reliable end-point of successful therapy and the best indicator of when interferon can be stopped (Fig. 3) (Battegay, JMedVirol, 1994; 44:389). Response is no better in children; none of 10 (Craxi, JHepatol, 1990; 11:S175) improved after one year of treatment.

In drug addicts with chronic hepatitis D who were anti-HIV-positive the response to interferon was not different from that expected in immunocompetent patients (Buti, JHepatol, 1989; 9 (Suppl. 1):S131).

The type of underlying HBV infection does not influence the therapeutic response to HDV. Adults and children with chronic hepatitis D associated with HBeAg-positive wild-type HBV infection cleared HBeAg during interferon therapy without significant changes in liver chemistry; this demonstrates that interferon may be efficacious against HBV yet does not affect the associated HDV infection (Craxi, JHepatol, 1990; 11:S175; Rosina, Hepatol, 1991; 13:1052).

High dosages of interferon (between 6 and 9 MU) given thrice weekly for prolonged periods (over 12 months) are currently recommended. Treatment should be maintained for 12 months after normalization of ALT (Rosina, ExpOpinInvestDrugs, 1996; 5:197). With this aggressive protocol, side-effects become important and have often forced the discontinuation of therapy; thyroiditis and depression with suicidal attempts have been reported in HDV patients under high-dose interferon therapy (Gaudin, Liver, 1995; 15:45).

As with other forms of chronic viral hepatitis, a major factor influencing the response to interferon in chronic hepatitis D is the duration of the HDV infection; patients with early disease respond better than those with long-standing fibrosis or cirrhosis (Marzano, ItalJGastr, 1992; 24:119). The improved control of HBV infection brought about in recent years by changes in sexual behaviour as result of HIV prevention, and by vaccination has caused a decrease of satellite HDV infection; thus the current prospects of interferon therapy for HDV disorders appear even less encouraging as there has been an increase of interferon-resistant fibrotic and cirrhotic forms (representing disease of long standing acquired years ago) over interferon-susceptible fresh forms of the disease.

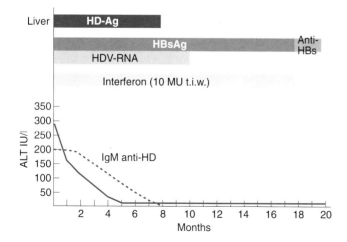

Fig. 3. Temporal behaviour of HDV markers in chronic HBV/HDV hepatitis responding to a prolonged course of interferon.

Interferon therapy of hepatitis C

Following the pioneer work of Hoofnagle *et al.*,[10] many studies have confirmed the value of interferon in the therapy of chronic hepatitis C. The key index defining therapeutic efficacy is the normalization of ALT ('complete response' or simply 'response').

Author	Interferon	Dosage (MU) (3/weekly)	Duration (months)	Primary response (%)	Sustained response (%)	Relapse rate (%)
Davis	rec 2b	1/3	6	45	22	50
Di Bisceglie	rec 2b	2	6	48	10	80
Saracco	rec 2b	1/3	6	46	60	20
Weiland	rec 2b	3	9	58	64	20
Gomez-Rubio	rec 2b	5, 1.5	18	40	33	25
Marcellin	rec 2b	1–3	6	42	44	14
Saez-Royuela	rec 2b	7.5, 5, 2.5	12	50	33	30
Causse	rec 2b	1–3	6	43	70	17
Diodati	rec 2b	6, 3, 1	12	47	40	27
Negro	rec 2a	6 6	9 3+3	46 45	47 60	17 10

Table 5 Interferon-α in chronic hepatitis type C

rec, recombinant.

Early studies also considered it a therapeutic success if there was a fall in the liver enzymes even if they did not return to normal; such a 'partial response' is now considered a therapeutic failure. Response that is maintained until the completion of treatment is defined as end-of-treatment response (ETR). Responses that persist for 6 to 12 months after suspension of interferon are defined as 'sustained responses'; those that persist over the subsequent follow-up are defined as 'permanent responses'.[11,12]

The need for this redundant classification stems from the fact that most studies have taken the sixth or twelfth month after therapy as the end-point to evaluate the efficacy of interferon; however, post-therapy relapses of hepatitis C can occur after several years of biochemical remission.

Ideally, response to therapy should include eradication of hepatitis C virus (HCV) RNA and the disappearance or reduction of the serological reactions associated with HCV infection. In practice the virological response to interferon therapy is complex.

Efficacy of therapy

Most controlled studies have made use of interferon dosages of 3 to 6 MU given on alternate days or thrice weekly for 6 months. Within this therapeutic range the rate of response has varied from 40 to 74 per cent; the spontaneous remission rate is not higher than 10 per cent.

In all studies, suspension of therapy has been accompanied by a significant relapse rate (about 50 per cent of responders) (Table 5). Only 20 to 30 per cent of patients maintain biochemical remission 6 to 12 months after the last dose of interferon (sustained response); however, disease can relapse in 5 to 15 per cent of these sustained

responders over the subsequent 3 years of follow-up and overall no more than 17 to 20 per cent of patients maintain a permanent response (Shindo, Hepatol, 1992; 15:1013; Saracco, Hepatol, 1993; 18:1300). The risk of relapse is higher in the first 6 months after the suspension of therapy; patients with normal ALT 6 months after stopping therapy are likely to have a sustained long-term response (Reichard, Hepatol, 1995; 21:918).

Long-term responses are associated with the sustained loss of HCV RNA in serum (Yokosuka, Gut, 1995; 37:721); in a minority of patients, HCV RNA may remain detectable despite normal ALT (Saracco, Hepatol, 1993; 18:1300; Castillo, Hepatol, 1994; 19:1342). Interferon therapy leads to an improvement in liver function (as measured by the antipyrine clearance test) in responders but not in non-responders; the functional improvement is delayed in onset and is most evident 6 months after stopping therapy (Coverdale, Hepatol, 1995; 22:1065). Little information is yet available on the long-term clinical outcome of therapy. Data from early trials suggest that long-term responders maintain histological improvement, and no further deterioration was reported in patients treated with multiple courses of interferon who responded to therapy but then relapsed (Reichard, ScaJInfectDis, 1994; 26:383). However, long-term evaluation of the efficacy of interferon is difficult because of the lack of knowledge of the natural history of chronic hepatitis C. A critical unanswered question is whether the response to interferon might select patients with milder non-progressive disease, non-responsiveness being a feature of more advanced disease.

It has been suggested that interferon therapy may lower the risk of the development of hepatocellular carcinoma independently from the biochemical or virological response (Nishiguchi, Lancet, 1995;

346:1050; Mazzella, JHepatol, 1996; 24:141). However, in a retrospective study no significant difference in mortality from liver-related causes was found between treated and untreated cirrhotic patients (see reference 8, pp. 787–90). Long-term studies are necessary to resolve this issue.

The efficacy and tolerance of interferon are similar in children (Ruiz-Moreno, Hepatol, 1992; 16:882). In an Italian trial (Bortolotti, Hepatol, 1995; 22:1623), 6 of 14 (43 per cent) children who received 5 MU /m² of interferon thrice weekly for 4 months had a sustained normalization of ALT associated with clearance of HCV RNA, compared with only 1 of 13 (7.5 per cent) untreated controls.

The minimal requirements for therapy remain controversial. In view of the many drawbacks of interferon and its cost, this therapy has been initially recommended only in patients with histologically important but not endstage cirrhotic disease who exhibit ALT at least 1.5 above the upper normal limit (Hoofnagle, JHepatol, 1993; 17:5130); a sizeable elevation of ALT was required in order to follow the effect of treatment, which in most centres could only be monitored by the curve of the liver enzyme. This approach has been challenged on the grounds that there is no relation between liver histology and serum ALT (Esteban, AnnIntMed, 1991; 115: 443), that progression to cirrhosis may occur despite histological findings of mild inflammation (Di Bisceglie, Hepatol, 1991; 14:969), and that testing for HCV RNA can now be used to monitor therapy in most centres; furthermore, decision-modelling techniques suggest that in the setting of mild disease interferon therapy is effective in extending life expectancy at minimal cost (Bennett, Hepatol, 1995; 22:290A).

However, the results of interferon therapy for chronic hepatitis C in patients with normal or near normal ALT have been contradictory. In two studies (Sangiovanni, Hepatol, 1995; 22:290A; Serfaty, Gastro, 1996; 110:291) there was no virological response in HCV carriers with normal ALT treated with 3 MU interferon thrice weekly for 6 months; unwanted ALT flares occurred frequently. In contrast, in a United States study (Van Thiel, JHepatol, 1995; 23: 503), HCV-positive patients with serum ALT less than 1.5 below the upper normal limit who were given daily doses of 5 MU interferon for 6 to 12 months responded well as defined by the clearance of HCV RNA from serum; the overall response rate was 65 per cent in a histologically mixed population including patients with chronic persistent hepatitis, chronic aggressive hepatitis, and active cirrhosis. In a Portuguese study (Areias, Hepatol, 1995; 22: 343A), 33 per cent of the carriers had lost HCV RNA at the end of therapy, and histological features improved in those with underlying disease.

Optimal therapeutic protocol

Doses smaller than 3 MU are usually not sufficient (Causse, Gastro, 1991; 101:497). Several studies have indicated that in the medium-sized adult doses of 3 MU interferon induce rates of responses that are not significantly different from those induced by higher dosages (5–9 MU), provided that interferon is given continuously (on alternate days or thrice weekly) for 6 months or more (Benelux Multicentre Trial Study Group, Gut, 1993; (Suppl.):S119); responses to shorter courses are almost invariably followed by relapses.

A retrospective multivariate analysis of 1831 patients treated with different dosages of interferon for 3, 6, and 12 months showed that the best response rates were obtained with an induction dose of 6 MU given thrice weekly for 3 months followed in responding patients by a maintenance dose of 3 MU thrice weekly for another 3 months (Ryff, JHepatol, 1995; 22 (Suppl. 1):101). However, in recent trials the administration of interferon for 12 to 18 months was followed by a lower relapse rate (less than 10 to 15 per cent) than with 6-month courses (Table 6) (Reichard, Hepatol, 1994; 19: 280; Chemello, Hepatol, 1995; 22:700; Kasahara, Hepatol, 1995; 21: 291; Lin, JHepatol, 1995; 23:487; Poynard, NEJM, 1995; 332:1547). Likewise, the use of an aggressive induction consisting of a dose of 5 MU of interferon given daily for 1 month followed by dose reduction or de-escalation may improve the rate of end-of-treatment responses (Hadziyannis, Hepatol, 1997; 26 (Suppl.2):420A, abstract 1165); in responders, viraemia decreases, quickly disappearing within 14 days of the beginning of therapy (Hadziyannis, Hepatol, 1997; 26 (Suppl.2):420A, abstract 1166; Bekkering, Hepatol, 1997; 26 (Suppl. 2):415A, abstract 1147). A recent meta-analysis evaluating the benefits of higher doses or of longer duration in comparison with a standard interferon regimen[13] found that the best efficacy/risk ratio was in favour of 3 MU thrice weekly for at least 12 months.

Attempts to use different protocols in order to improve the rate of response, contain costs, and diminish side-effects have produced no substantial advantage over the standard protocol. With the administration of interferon in two 3-month cycles separated by a 6-month therapy-free interval the rate of responses was not different from that in controls treated continuously over 9 months (Negro, Gastro, 1994; 107:479). Although intermittent therapy is likely to reduce cost and inconvenience to patients, an unwanted hepatitis peak occurs almost invariably after the conclusion of the first therapeutic cycle. The progressive increase of dosage to 5 to 6 and then 9 to 10 MU in non-responders to 3 MU has not produced a significant increase of responses compared to a fixed 3-MU dosage (Marcellin, Gastro, 1995; 109:156).

Clinical and virological course during therapy

In responders, ALT normalizes within 3 months from the start of therapy and remains normal throughout the course of therapy. The fall of ALT is linear (Fig. 4). Rarely (1–5 per cent of patients) the first doses of interferon may induce an increase of liver enzymes. This paradoxical response may be related to toxicity of interferon and so therapy should be withdrawn. If ALTs have not returned to normal after 3 months of therapy, it is unlikely that they will normalize in subsequent months; the current consensus is to interrupt therapy (Ryff, JHepatol, 1995; 22 (Suppl. 1):101) or to change the protocol.

ALT may increase during therapy after an initial normalization. This event, called 'breakthrough', signals resistance to interferon and is accompanied by the reappearance of HCV RNA in responders who had previously cleared the viral markers. Breakthroughs have been reported in 12 per cent (Roffi Hepatol, 1995; 21:645) to 27 per cent (see reference 8, pp. 800–3) of responders to interferon.

No pretreatment epidemiological, clinical or virological feature appears predictive of breakthrough. Several explanations of breakthrough have been advocated. In some cases it is accompanied by the development, or an increase in titre, of antinuclear or

Table 6 Results of prolonged treatments with interferon-α in chronic hepatitis type C

Author	Interferon	Dosage (MU)	Duration (months)	Primary response (%)	Sustained response (%)	Relapse rate (%)
Chemello	rec	6–3	12	72	36	49
	2a	3	12	55	40	31
		6 (3/weekly)	6	74	62	28
Reichard	rec 2b	3	15	60	37	37
Poynard	rec	3	18	45	22	50
	2b	3–1	18	27	10	63
		3	6	30	8	73
Kasahara	natural	5	6	62	33	46
		5	12	63	53	14
Lin	rec	3	6	61	20	69
	2b	5	6	64	17	73
		3	24	55	59	46

rec, recombinant.

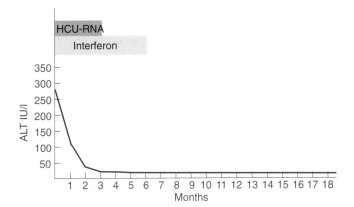

Fig. 4. Biochemical and virological pattern of a sustained response to interferon in chronic hepatitis C.

Table 7 Methods investigated for determining sustained response to treatment and their associated problems

ALT	Discrepancies with viral data
Anti-core IgM	Few data, inconsistent
Loss of HCV RNA in serum	Disease recurrence even if negative
Loss of HCV RNA in liver—RT–PCR	Requires biopsy, false negatives due to inhibitors
Loss of HCV RNA in liver—bDNA	Requires biopsy, few data on responders

From Willber, *Antiviral therapy*, (in press).
ALT, alanine transferase; RT–PCR, reverse transcriptase–polymerase chain reaction.

antiliver–kidney microsomal autoantibodies, which suggests the possibility of an autoimmune reaction induced by interferon. In one study (Roffi, Hepatol, 1995; 21:645), breakthroughs were associated in 50 per cent of cases with the appearance of neutralizing interferon antibodies; similarly in another study (see reference 8, pp. 800–3), interferon antibodies were significantly more frequent in patients who experienced a breakthrough than in responders (46 vs 8 per cent).

Often there is no obvious reason for the escape from the therapeutic effect of interferon; alterations in the patient's immune response or the emergence of HCV strains resistant to interferon are possible explanations; extensive qualitative and quantitative modifications of the quasi-species distribution of HCV were noted under therapy in patients experiencing breakthroughs (Pawlotsky, AnnIntMed, 1995; 122:169).

HCV RNA disappears from serum in over 85 per cent of the patients who respond to interferon (Zeuzem, Hepatol, 1996; 23: 366); this viral marker is usually cleared by the second month of therapy. A biochemical relapse is almost invariable in patients who remain viraemic at the end of therapy despite a persistent

normalization of the liver enzymes throughout the course of treatment. However, the value of the HCV RNA assay in predicting the outcome of therapy is limited (Table 7).

The apparent clearance of HCV RNA during interferon therapy does not prevent subsequent clinical relapse and a return of the virus in the blood (Shindo, AnnIntMed, 1991; 115:700), and HCV RNA may be found in patients with prolonged biochemical remissions (Saracco, Hepatol, 1993; 18:1300; Castillo, Hepatol, 1994; 19:1342). More reliable prognostic information can be obtained by testing HCV RNA in patients who have maintained a normal ALT for 12 months after therapy; in one study, none of 80 non-viraemic patients experienced a relapse in the subsequent 6 to 36 months' follow-up whereas the probability of relapse was 53 per cent in viraemic patients (Chemello, AnnIntMed, 1996; 124:1058). The virus may persist in mononuclear blood cells (Castillo, Hepatol, 1994; 19:1342; Ounadian, JMedVirol, 1995; 45:141) or in the liver (Romeo, AnnIntMed, 1994; 121:276) and escape detection in serum. A complete response without post-therapy relapse appears to be best predicted by the disappearance of genomic HCV RNA both from the liver and from mononuclear cells (Gil, Hepatol, 1993; 18: 1050).

Modifications in the serological profile are slow to occur in successfully treated patients. Total anti-HCV decreases slowly over several years; there is a relatively rapid fall of anti-HCV core protein and of anti-C 100-3 (Saracco, Hepatol, 1993; 18.1300; Yuki, Hepatol, 1993; 17:960); a sustained reduction of anti-HCV core protein appears to reflect virus clearance (Yuki, Hepatol, 1993; 17: 960). IgM anti-HCV diminishes and often disappears rapidly from serum in patients who normalize ALT (Douglas, DigDisSci, 1993; 38:601). It was suggested that the early decline of IgM anti-HCV may help to predict a long-term response (Brillanti, Hepatol, 1992; 15:998); however, in another study (Douglas, DigDisSci, 1993; 38: 601) the disappearance of the IgM antibody did not predict a long-term response, as relapses were also seen in patients who lost IgM anti-HCV during therapy. The prognostic role of IgM anti-HCV is limited; with current assays this antibody is undetectable in about 40 per cent of patients with chronic hepatitis C.

The virological and biochemical normalization induced by therapy is accompanied by histological improvement (David, AmJClin-Path, 1992; 98:397); a significant decrease is observed in the degree of lobular and piecemeal necrosis, and in portal and parenchymal inflammation (Hoofnagle, SemLivDis, 1989; 9:259). The efficacy of interferon in reducing the degree of fibrosis is still controversial (Camps, JHepatol, 1993; 17:390; Manabe, Hepatol, 1993; 18:1344). In non-cirrhotic long-term responders, progression to cirrhosis is probably halted (Saracco, Hepatol, 1993; 18:1300).

In early and presumably still reversible phases of chronic hepatitis, interferon therapy appears capable of interfering biologically with the fibrogenic mechanisms (Guido, JHepatol, 1996; 24:301).

Retreatment

Most of the responders to a first course of interferon who relapse will respond to a second similar course, but only a minority achieve a permanent remission (Saracco, JHepatol, 1990; 11 (Suppl. 1):S43; Weiland, JHepatol, 1990; 11 (Suppl. 1):S57). A change in the type of interferon may offer some benefit to patients exhibiting an ALT breakthrough during the first course (Roffi, Hepatol, 1995; 21:645; Saracco, JHepatol, 1994; 21:278).

The role of more aggressive therapy is controversial. In two studies, higher doses of interferon or more prolonged treatment did not produce any effect in non-responders (Marcellin, JInfDis, 1993; 167:780; Bonkowsky, DigDisSci, 1996; 41:149). However, in another study of 90 patients who did not respond in a sustained fashion to a first therapeutic course, 25 classified as non-responders did not develop a sustained response regardless of whether they received the same schedule or a higher dose or a longer period of therapy; of the other 65 patients classified as relapsers, 20 per cent developed a sustained response upon retreatment; of those who received 3 MU thrice weekly for 6 months and were retreated with 6 MU for 6 months followed by 3 MU for a further 6 months, 41 per cent became sustained responders after retreatment (see reference 8, pp. 727–35).

In patients relapsing after a successful first course, retreatment appears more likely to induce a sustained response in cases with undetectable HCV RNA at the end of the initial cycle (Toyoda, AmJGastr, 1994; 89:1453).

Therapy of acute hepatitis C

In view of the high rate of progression of HCV infections, treatment of acute hepatitis C has been advocated in order to prevent chronicity. Some very good results have been reported (Omata, Lancet, 1991; 338:914). Ten of 11 patients with acute hepatitis C treated with a mean total of 52 MU of interferon-β for 30 days maintained normal ALT after 3 years compared to only 3 of 14 untreated patients; the responders cleared HCV RNA. In a further analysis of the Japanese series (Takano, Gastro, 1994; 107:805), dosage appeared to be important, 6 MU daily of interferon-β providing the best results. Further studies have been less optimistic and also contradictory. In a Spanish study (Viladomiu, Hepatol, 1992; 15: 767), 73 per cent of the patients given 3 MU of interferon thrice weekly for 12 weeks normalized ALT during therapy compared to only 38 per cent of controls, but these differences had disappeared at 6 and 12 months of follow-up. When using the same short-term therapy in Italy (Lampertico, Hepatol, 1994; 19:19), normalization of ALT and clearance of HCV RNA were observed after 18 months of follow-up in 53 and 39 per cent, respectively, of the treated patients, with corresponding figures of 37 and 0 per cent in untreated controls.

Although there is no evidence that treating patients during the primary phase of HCV infection is more beneficial than treating them after the conventional criteria of chronicity have been acquired, there is also no evidence of a diminished or detrimental effect of interferon in patients with acute hepatitis C. Therapy therefore should be instituted as soon as hepatitis C is recognized. The implementation of the test for anti-HCV in the screening of blood donations has made the acquisition of acute hepatitis C by transfusion a very rare event. Consequently, the diagnosis of acute hepatitis C is now made infrequently and such patients are difficult to recruit for clinical trials.

Therapy of HCV-associated cryoglobulinaemia

Efforts to treat cryoglobulinaemia with immunosuppressive drugs such as steroids, cyclophosphamide, 6-mercaptopurine, and methotrexate have not been successful. Plasmapheresis is efficacious, in particular when combined with cyclophosphamide (Ferri, Nephron, 1986; 43:246), but relapses are the rule.

Interferon was first used by Bonomo et al. (AmJMed, 1987; 83:726): therapy led to a reduction of the cryocrit and clinical improvement in seven patients given the drug. In a further study (Casato, Blood, 1991; 78:3142), interferon given every day for 3 months at a dose of 3 MU induced a response as assessed by the reduction of the cryocrit to less than 10 per cent, with amelioration of symptoms in 10 of 21 treated patients. Controlled studies have confirmed the therapeutic role of interferon in HCV-related cryoglobulinaemia. In another study (Misani, NEJM, 1994; 330:751), vasculitis improved and serum HCV RNA disappeared in 15 of 25 treated patients but in none of 26 untreated controls. Other good clinical results during therapy are also reported (Dammacco, Blood, 1994; 84:3336); the best were obtained by combining interferon with prednisone.

Decrease of the cryocrit and amelioration of symptoms caused by cryoglobulinaemia correlate with the normalization of ALT and

Table 8 Predictors of response to interferon in chronic hepatitis C

Factor	Consensus
Low viraemia	+ +
Viral genotype (non-1)	+ +
Non-cirrhotic histology	+
Viral homogeneity	±
Low intrahepatic iron content	+
Short duration of disease	+

+ +, full consensus; +, consensus by most; ±, not fully assessed.

the decline of HCV viraemia; however, relapses are frequent when interferon is interrupted and the loss of HCV RNA during therapy is not predictive of a sustained response.

The response of the underlying liver disease (normal ALT 6 months after stopping therapy) was not different between patients with chronic hepatitis C with and without cryoglobulinaemia (24 vs 27 per cent) (see reference 8, pp. 428–34); severely symptomatic patients with neuropathy, vasculitis or glomerulopathy responded less well than asymptomatic or mildly symptomatic patients (6 vs 35 per cent). The virological factors predictive of response were the same as in non-cryoglobulinaemic patients with hepatitis C; cryoglobulinaemic patients with low serum HCV RNA and with HCV genotype 2 or 3 responded better.

Predictors of response to interferon therapy

Multivariate analysis indicates that several pretreatment variables influence the rate of response to interferon therapy; these so-called predictors of response are listed in Table 8. Predictors of response allow better definition of the chances of response to interferon, but do not provide clear-cut discrimination between responders and non-responders; therefore they are a helpful adjuvant in decision-making in the individual case, but their score should not be considered an absolute measure upon which to base decisions. Response predictors may be useful in tailoring therapy, prompting the use of more aggressive protocols in patients with a poor score.

Histology

Baseline histological features influences the long-term response to interferon (Camps, Gut, 1993; 34:1714; Davis, JHepatol, 1994; 21:1; Pagliaro, Hepatol, 1994; 19:820; Serfaty, JHepatol, 1994; 21:12). Response is better in mild to moderate than in advanced liver disease. The response to therapy becomes very limited in patients with marked fibrosis or cirrhosis (Jouet, Gastro, 1994; 106:686); if they respond, they often relapse.

In cirrhotic patients, interferon may precipitate liver failure and often dangerous complications such as pneumonitis, bacterial peritonitis, and hepatitic relapses. While decompensated cirrhosis is considered a contraindication to interferon therapy, the role of the cytokine in compensated cirrhosis is controversial. Interferon may be used when histologically there is residual inflammatory activity, in order to control inflammation and improve liver function; in this context it is usually used at low dosages.

Duration of disease

Although a long duration of chronic hepatitis is considered an indicator of diminished response, the definition of 'long duration' is often vague; this index may reflect progression of the disease to a fibrotic stage, which itself diminishes the response to therapy. Alternatively, infections of long standing may promote viral heterogeneity, that is, further diversity of the genomic chains that constitute the quasi-species of this virus, which renders the infection resistant to interferon.

Concomitant disease

Concomitant non-viral liver disease (e.g. alcoholic) or a metabolic abnormality affecting the liver (e.g. diabetes) decrease the response. Abnormal quantities of iron in the liver diminish the response to interferon (Van Thiel, JHepatol, 1994; 20:410). In patients with chronic hepatitis C a liver iron concentration higher than 1000 μg/g liver identifies a subgroup of patients who have an 88 per cent probability of not responding (Olyink, Gastro, 1995; 108:1104). Phlebotomy has been proposed to diminish the iron overload and render the patient more susceptible to interferon. The major problem is in polytransfused patients such as those with thalassaemia; control of iron overload by desferrioxamine is relatively poor in this context.

Development of interferon antibodies

In different studies, interferon antibodies appeared in 1 to 20 per cent of patients, depending on the treatment protocol (Lok, Hepatol, 1990; 12:1266), the type of interferon (Antonelli, JInfDis, 1991; 163:882), and on the methods used to determine the antibodies (Itri, Cancer, 1987; 59:668). Recombinant interferons appear to be more prone to induce interferon antibodies than lymphoblastoid and leucocyte-derived interferons (Milella, Liver, 1993; 13:146; Roffi, Hepatol, 1995; 21:645).

The clinical role of interferon antibodies is controversial. It is believed that they may block the therapeutic effect of interferon but that this occurs rarely and only when they are present in high titre; most of interferon antibodies are unable to neutralize the biological activity of the cytokine. The appearance of anti-interferon antibodies should be suspected when there is a breakthrough after an early response to therapy.

Switching from recombinant to natural lymphoblastoid interferon was proposed to restore responsiveness to the cytokine (Roffi, Hepatol, 1995; 21:645).

Virological factors

Viraemia

The level of viraemia can influence the rate of sustained responses to interferon. Several studies (Hagiwara, Gastro, 1993; 104:877; Lau, Lancet, 1993; 341:1501; Camps, JHepatol, 1994; 21:4; Magrin, Hepatol, 1994; 19:273; Mita, DigDisSci, 1994; 39:977; Yamada,

Table 9 HCV genotype and percentage of sustained response to therapy

Genotype	IFN monotherapy (%)	IFN + ribavirin (%)
1a	15–20	?
1b	4–8	20
4	17	17
2	30–40	40
3a	35–50	75

IFN, interferon.

DigDisSci, 1994; 39:441; Booth, Gut, 1995; 36:427; Shindo, Ann-IntMed, 1995; 122:586) have found that long-term responders had a lower baseline HCV RNA; highly viraemic patients responding to the drug tend to relapse more frequently than low-viraemic patients.[11]

Viral genotypes

Many studies have demonstrated that genotypes are important in determining the outcome of interferon therapy (Table 9). Early studies from Japan showed that patients with HCV genotypes 2 and 3 have higher sustained response rates than patients with genotype 1 (Tsubota, JGastHepatol, 1993; 8:535; Matsumoto, DigDisSci, 1994; 39:1273; Tsubota, Hepatol, 1994; 19:1088). These findings have been confirmed (Dusheiko, Hepatol, 1994; 19:13; Qu, JHepatol, 1994; 21:70). Patients infected with genotype 2 were reported to have a lower level of viraemia than those infected with genotype 1b (Yoshioka, Hepatol, 1992; 16:293; Brechot, AmJGastr, 1994; 89:S41; Hino, JMedVirol, 1994; 42:299) but this difference was not confirmed (Mita, JHepatol, 1994; 21:468).

Several studies have also demonstrated the role of HCV heterogeneity in influencing the sustained response to interferon (Okada, Hepatol, 1992; 16:619; Kanazawa, Hepatol, 1994; 20:1121; Koizumi, Hepatol, 1995; 22:30), this being more likely in patients with lesser degrees of HCV diversity. Sequence changes in the hypervariable region of the HCV might be accelerated by the immune attack induced by interferon therapy (Enomoto, JHepatol, 1994; 20:252), and an interferon-resistant quasi-species may be responsible for the breakthrough elevations of ALT during interferon therapy and relapses after therapy is withdrawn. An amino acid sequence associated with sensitivity or resistance to therapy was described (Enomoto, NEJM, 1996; 334:77) in the COOH-terminal half of the NS5A region of the HCV genome.

Therapy of chronic viral hepatitis with associated autoimmune features

Autoantibodies against thyroglobulin and thyroid microsomes are detected in up to 15 per cent of females with chronic hepatitis C (Tran, Hepatol, 1993; 18:253) but only in 2 per cent of those with chronic hepatitis B. Recognition of these autoimmune reactivities is important because interferon treatment can trigger latent auto-immune thyroid disease (Fentiman, Lancet, 1985; i:1166; Schultz, Lancet, 1989; i:1452; Lisker-Melman, Gastro, 1992; 102:2155;

Pateron, JHepatol, 1992; 16:244). Among patients with interferon-induced thyroid dysfunction, hypothyroidism is more frequent than hyperthyroidism; the course is sometimes biphasic with a short phase of hyperthyroidism followed by hypothyroidism. In most cases, thyroid dysfunction is transitory and spontaneously reversible if interferon is stopped promptly (Baudin, ClinEndoc, 1993; 39:657; Marcellin, JHepatol, 1995; 22:364).

De novo autoimmune thyroid dysfunction can occur with interferon therapy in patients in whom antithyroid autoantibodies were not detectable before therapy (Mayet, Hepatol, 1989; 10:24; Saracco, JHepatol, 1990; 11:339; Berris, DigDisSci, 1991; 36:1657; Marcellin, JHepatol, 1995; 22:364). While the presence of antithyroid autoantibodies represents a risk factor for the development of autoimmune thyroid disease, interferon therapy should not be withheld if biochemical tests of thyroid function are normal; the patients must, however, be closely monitored for evidence of thyroid dysfunction and in this event interferon must be withdrawn. Biochemical evidence of thyroid dysfunction accompanied by signs of thyroid autoimmunity is a contraindication to the use of interferon.

Non-organ-specific autoantibodies are detectable in up to one-third of patients with chronic hepatitis C (Abuaf, JHepatol, 1993; 18:359; Clifford, Hepatol, 1995; 21:613), in 10 to 15 per cent of the patients with chronic hepatitis D (Crivelli, ClinExpImmun, 1993; 54:232), and in only a minority of patients with chronic hepatitis B. In most cases they are at low titres and represent laboratory findings without clinical relevance; in some patients, however, they suggest an underlying autoimmune derangement associated with the viral infection.

Autoimmune problems are rarely faced when treating chronic hepatitis B; one patient (Silva, Gastro, 1991; 101:840) developed a severe, delayed ALT flare with an increase of the titre of antinuclear (ANA) and smooth-muscle (SMA) antibodies after interferon-induced resolution of HBV infection and seroconversion to anti-HBe. There are anecdotal reports of hepatitic flares in HDV patients with LKM 3 in serum, but no adverse effect of interferon was noted in ten patients with LKM enrolled in different clinical trials.[9]

The relatively large subset of patients with hepatitis who have positive HCV serology and autoantibodies, that is, patients who may not be classified simply as having liver disease of either autoimmune or viral origin (Schapiro, Hepatol, 1996; 23:647), pose a therapeutic dilemma. Interferon therapy is appropriate if the origin of the disease is viral but may be detrimental if its origin is autoimmune, as the cytokine can trigger the exacerbation of an autoimmune diathesis. Conversely, therapy with steroids is indicated if the basis to the disease is autoimmune but this treatment is bound to increase HCV viraemia (Magrin, Hepatol, 1994; 19:273). There have been anecdotal reports of a hepatitis flare or favourable steroid responses in patients with ANA and SMA treated with interferon (Shindo, Gastro, 1992; 102:1406; Bellary, Ann-IntMed, 1995; 123:33); these patients also had other autoimmune features, such as insulin-dependent diabetes mellitus, rheumatoid arthritis, and increased gammaglobulin.

There is a report (Muratori, JHepatol, 1994; 21:199) of a serious hepatitic flare in three of six patients with chronic hepatitis C and LKM 1 during interferon therapy; ALT fell with subsequent steroid therapy. Steroid therapy was also efficacious initially in seven patients with hepatitis C and ANA/SMA (Zeniya, Liver, 1994; 14:206). However, in more extensive consecutive series, therapy with interferon has been efficacious and largely uneventful in patients with chronic hepatitis C and ANA (Fried, DigDisSci, 1993; 38: 631), in those with LKM 1 (Todros, Hepatol, 1995; 22:1374), and in those with ANA and LKM 1 (Calleja, JHepatol, 1996; 24:308).

Occasionally, ANA or LKM are first found during interferon therapy, and coinciding with the flare up of an autoimmune hepatitis (Saracco, JHepatol, 1990; 11:339; Todros, Hepatol, 1995; 22:1374); this event is relatively rare but in one series it was reported in 5 per cent of interferon-treated patients with chronic hepatitis C (Garcia-Buey, Gastro, 1995; 108:1770).

Based on the experience accumulated so far, the following therapeutic recommendations can be made (see reference 8, pp. 780–2) in patients with chronic hepatitis C and autoimmune features.

1. Borderline ANA or SMA reactivities occur often in all forms of liver disease; their frequency increases with age and with the inflammatory activity of the underlying liver disease. In the absence of other signs of autoimmunity they should be disregarded.
2. In patients with LKM antibodies or significant titres of ANA and SMA (greater than 1:40 in indirect immunofluorescence) the diagnosis of HCV infection should be confirmed by the finding of HCV RNA in serum. If viral markers of HCV are not consistently detected, the disease should first be considered autoimmune and a trial of steroids should be given.
3. In patients with well-documented HCV infections, attention should be given to other autoimmune stigmata such as arthritis, haemolytic anaemia, and a high level of IgG (hypergammaglobulinaemia is unusual in chronic hepatitis C except when the disease has reached the cirrhotic stage). In order to sort out dubious cases one can apply the International Autoimmune Hepatitis Group Scoring System[14] devised to identify autoimmune liver disease. If the aggregate score is non-diagnostic, therapy with interferon (started at low dosage) appears to be safe. If the score points to probable or definite autoimmune hepatitis, steroids appear advisable as the first therapeutic option.

Alternative therapies for chronic hepatitis C

Despite efforts to optimize interferon schedules, interferon therapy alone induces a permanent remission in only a minority of patients with chronic hepatitis C. To improve results, attention has focused on combination therapies. Preliminary studies (Andreone, Hepatol, 1993; 18:659; Gastro, 1994; 106:859) suggest that the concomitant administration of interferon and indomethacin or ketoprofen may induce a sustained response in a significant number of non-responders; larger controlled, randomized trials are needed to confirm these findings. The rationale for the use of this therapeutic association is based upon the observation of the ability of prostaglandin E_2 to reduce lymphokine function (Kunkel, JImmunol, 1986; 136: 186) and to exert a negative feedback mechanism on the cellular immune reactions (Leung, Nature, 1980; 288:597). Thus, non-steroidal anti-inflammatory drugs may act as amplifiers of interferon's antiviral and immune response by inhibiting arachidonic acid metabolites.

As ursodeoxycholic acid may improve liver function in patients with chronic hepatitis C (Takano, Hepatol, 1994; 20:558), the combination of interferon with ursodeoxycholic acid has been tested; ALT remained normal in some patients after stopping

interferon (Boucher, Hepatol, 1995; 21:322), but there was no virological effect or significant histological improvement attributable to the combination.

Two pilot studies using steroids in combination with interferon (Liaw, Liver, 1993; 13:46; Chayama, Hepatol, 1996; 23:953) have shown a marginal benefit over treatment with interferon alone; steroids can, however, markedly increase HCV RNA (Fong, Gastro, 1994; 107:196).

The most promising combination and the one currently undergoing extensive phase II trials is the association of ribavirin with interferon. Ribavirin is a guanosine analogue with a broad spectrum of activity against RNA and DNA viruses. The drug is given orally (1000–1200 mg/day) and is reported to induce few and relatively minor side-effects (mild haemolytic anaemia, hyperuricacidaemia). Patients treated with ribavirin alone exhibited a progressive decrease or ALT, but relapses invariably occurred after withdrawal of therapy (Reichard, Lancet, 1991; 337:1058): in one study (Reichard, JMedVirol, 1993; 41:99) serum HCV RNA was not appreciably altered but in another (Di Bisceglie, Hepatol, 1992; 16:649) viraemia decreased consistently during therapy. The use of ribavirin with interferon combines the presumed antiviral action of the nucleoside with the immunomodulant properties of the cytokine. Pilot studies (Brillanti, Gastro, 1994; 107:812; Schvarcz, JMedVirol, 1995; 46:43) have reported sustained responses in about 40 per cent of patients who relapsed or failed to respond to interferon alone. Further studies have shown that the response to combination therapy is significantly different between patients who have not responded to a previous course of interferon and those who have relapsed after an initially successful course: a sustained response is observed in most interferon relapsers but in only a few interferon non-responders (Brillanti, JHepatol, 1995; 23 (Suppl.2): 13; Schvarcz, JHepatol, 1995; 23 (Suppl. 2):17). Apparently, the success of the combination therapy is not affected by the viral genotype or histological features {Brillanti, JHepatol, 1995; 23 (Suppl. 2):13}.

The efficacy of this combination therapy was recently confirmed by a meta-analysis (Schalm, JHepatol, 1997; 26:961) on 186 patients; they represented 90 per cent of the published reports and included 51 patients treated with ribavirin monotherapy (1000–2000 mg/day) and 78 patients treated with the combination of interferon with ribavirin. Overall the combination was significantly more efficacious than interferon monotherapy regardless of the infecting genotype and of the presence of cirrhosis, with a two- to threefold potentiation of interferon's efficacy. The estimated probabilities of a sustained response after combination therapy were 51 per cent in relapsers after interferon therapy but only 16 per cent in non-responders to this therapy. A small, three-armed, randomized trial conducted in 45 interferon-naive patients (Chemello, JHepatol, 1995; 23 (Suppl. 2):8) has also shown that combination therapy is significantly superior to ribavirin or interferon monotherapy in inducing a sustained response to interferon.

References

1. Koff RS and Galambos JT. Viral hepatitis management. In Schiff L and Schiff ER, eds. *Diseases of the liver*. VIth edn. Philadelphia: Lippincott, 1987: 529–37.
2. Baron S, *et al.* The interferons—mechanisms of action and clinical applications. *Journal of the American Medical Association*, 1991; **266**: 1375.

3. Hoofnagle JH. Therapy of acute and chronic viral hepatitis. *Advances in Internal Medicine*, 1994; **39**: 241–75.

4. Krogsgaard K, *et al.* and the European Concerted Action on Viral Hepatitis (Eurohep). The treatment effect alpha-interferon in chronic hepatitis B is independent of pre-treatment variables. Results based on individual patient data. *Journal of Hepatology*, 1994; **21**: 646–55.

5. Wong DK, *et al.* Effect of alpha-interferon treatment in patients with hepatitis B e antigen-positive chronic hepatitis B. A meta-analysis. *Annals of Internal Medicine*, 1993; **119**: 312–23.

6. Niederau C, *et al.* Long-term follow-up of HBeAg-positive patients treated with interferon alfa in chronic hepatitis B. *New England Journal of Medicine*, 1996; **334**: 1422–7.

7. Cohard M., Poynard T, Mathurin P, and Zarski JP. Prednisone–interferon combination in the treatment of chronic hepatitis B: direct and indirect meta-analysis. *Hepatology*, 1994; **20**: 1390–8.

8. Rizzetto M, Purcell RH, Gerin JL, and Verma G, eds. *Viral hepatitis and liver disease*. Turin: Edizioni Minervc. Medica, 1997.

9. Rosina F and Rizzetto M. Treatment of chronic type D (delta) hepatitis with alpha interferon. *Seminars in Liver Disease*, 1989; **9**: 264–6.

10. Hoofnagle JH, *et al.* Treatment of chronic non-A, non-B hepatitis with recombinant human alpha interferon. A preliminary report. *New England Journal of Medicine*, 1986; **315**: 1575–8.

11. Saracco G and Rizzetto M. The long-term efficacy of interferon alfa in chronic hepatitis C patients: a critical review. *Journal of Gastroenterology and Hepatology*, 1995; **10**: 668–73.

12. Hoofnagle JH, *et al.* Consensus Development Conference Panel Statement: Management of Hepatitis C. *Hepatology*, 1997; **26**(Suppl. 1): 25–105.

13. Poynard T, *et al.* Meta-analysis of interferon randomized trials in the treatment of viral hepatitis C: effects of dose and duration. *Hepatology*, 1996; **24**: 778–9.

14. Johnson PJ and McFarlane IG. Meeting report: International Autoimmune Hepatitis Group. *Hepatology*, 1993; **18**: 998–1005.

12.2 Systemic virosis producing hepatitis

Dieter Neumann-Haefelin, Paul Griffiths, and Mario Rizzetto

A number of viruses are not primarily hepatotropic and are only occasionally associated with hepatitis. These non-classical, 'non-A to E' hepatitis viruses probably cause mild degrees of acute liver dysfunction more often than is attested by the medical literature. They also have a role in clinically overt hepatitis that is significant in neonates and immunocompromised hosts.

Herpesviruses

Herpesviruses are a family of large enveloped DNA viruses persistently infecting all kinds of vertebrates. Eight members commonly infecting humans are known so far.

Infection with herpesviruses occurs worldwide and, for seven of the eight viruses, prevalence rates between 50 per cent and close to 100 per cent are known in all adult populations investigated. Following primary infection these viruses are not cleared by the host but their DNA persists in a latent form and can be reactivated to give rise to infectious virions many months or years later. Another possible type of persistence may be characterized by minimal replication at remote sites in the body. The acquisition of, or resistance to, disease as well as the development and maintenance of latency are determined by the host response to the infection.

α-Herpesvirus subfamily

The viruses in this subfamily infect mucocutaneous epithelia and neuronal cells in the adult immunocompetent host. Only in neonates and immunocompromised hosts can they spread and may also infect hepatocytes and various other cell types, including brain cells.

Herpes simplex virus

Both types of herpes simplex virus (**HSV**-1 and HSV-2) share genomic sequences and antigenic properties.[1] Inclusion bodies (Cowdry, type A) are found in the nuclei where replication of the viruses takes place. The infection may remain latent and reactivate subsequently to reproduce the herpetic lesions; trauma, stress, ultraviolet light, and immunosuppression can induce reactivation.

Primary infection occurs early in life and is subclinical in the great majority of cases. The clinical manifestations of primary and recurrent infection are usually focal, consisting of orofacial, genital, and rectal/perianal vesicular and ulcerative lesions accompanied by regional lymphoadenopathy; constitutional symptoms are present especially in primary infections. Recurrent infection with HSV is a frequent cause of corneal blindness and of sporadic encephalitis.

Generalized infections are usually associated with hepatic lesions. They are most common in the neonate[2] and in immunosuppressed children[3] and may be caused by HSV-1 or HSV-2. Liver involvement consists of hepatocellular necrosis, mild and scattered inflammation, multinucleated hepatocytes, and nuclear inclusion bodies; hepatomegaly, raised serum aminotransferase, and a prolonged prothrombin time are the main clinical manifestations. The condition may deteriorate, mainly due to haemorrhagic complications combined with central nervous system involvement (Hufert, ScaJInfectDis, 1995; 27:627; Kulhanjian, PediatInfectDis, 1992; 11:1069), and is frequently associated with a fatal outcome. Severe liver disease caused by HSV has also been reported in children with kwashiorkor (Becker, SAMedJ, 1963; 37:74).

Most cases of herpes simplex hepatitis in adults have occurred in immunosuppressed patients, particularly in those with liver transplants (Shanley, Transpl, 1995; 59:145) and other solid organ transplants (Elliot, ArchIntMed, 1980; 140:1656; Taylor, Arch-IntMed, 1981; 141:1519; Kusne, JInfDis, 1991; 163:1001) or in abnormal hosts, including patients with severe burns (Foley, NEJM, 1970; 282:652), pemphigus vulgaris (Keane, ArchIntMed, 1976; 136:1312), and postcardiotomy syndrome treated with steroids (Williams, AmHeartJ, 1985; 110:679), Hodgkin's disease (Lee, HumPath, 1972; 3:277), and thymic dysplasia (Sutton, AmJMed, 1974; 56:545). Liver infections with HSV-1 and HSV-2 have also been reported in healthy pregnant women (Stagno, NEJM, 1985; 313:1327; Fink, JClinPath, 1993; 46:968) and in apparently healthy individuals (Goodman, AmJClinPath, 1986; 85:694). The clinical course has been severe, with most patients succumbing to acute liver failure (Manoux, GastrClinBiol, 1983; 7:340; Rubin, JAMA, 1985; 253:1299).

Presentation is characterized by fever, mild or minimal jaundice, and markedly elevated aminotransferase; leucopenia, thrombocytopenia, and coagulopathy are frequent in fulminant cases. Primary mucocutaneous or genital foci of virus were identified in a number but not in all patients. The rapid presumptive diagnosis based on viral culture and polymerase chain reaction (**PCR**) from mucocutaneous lesions is confirmed by liver biopsy; in cases which resolved, histological examination showed well delineated intralobular foci of necrosis surrounded by hepatocytes containing the typical nuclear inclusions (Fewett, Gastro, 1976; 71:500; Nahmias,

NEJM, 1973; 289:667). Characteristic *post mortem* findings in fatal cases are hepatomegaly with multiple areas of coagulation and haemorrhagic necrosis and with scanty inflammatory infiltration of lymphocytes and neutrophils; the liver often shows white nodules.

PCR and immunohistochemical analysis of the liver specimen using monoclonal antibodies to HSV give the specific diagnosis;[1] the nuclear inclusions can be identified and further analysed by electron microscopy. Serological assays are of little use as only a minority of patients exhibit consistently raised antibody levels between acute and convalescent sera. Only retrospectively, assessment of seroconversion may be useful to prove cases due to primary infection.

If infection with HSV is suspected, acyclovir 5 mg/kg three times daily, intravenously, should be given immediately (Alford, AmJMed, 1982; 73:225), which is active against systemic herpes simplex disease, although its effect in herpes simplex hepatitis has not been proven (Tomita, ArchPathLabMed, 1992; 116:173). Since most cases occurred in patients not receiving prophylactic antivirals despite severe immunosuppression, preventive acyclovir should be more generally considered in such patients. In the management of fulminant hepatic failure secondary to HSV hepatitis, liver transplantation was successful in conjunction with high doses of acyclovir (Shanley, Transpl, 1995; 59:145).

Varicella-zoster virus

Varicella (chickenpox), a benign illness of childhood characterized by a vesicular rash, is caused by the primary infection, and zoster by recurrent infections[4] with varicella-zoster virus.

Clinical hepatitis is not observed in children with uncomplicated varicella but liver function tests may be abnormal (Pitel, Pediat, 1980; 65:631; Ey, Pediat, 1981; 67:285). It has been estimated that about a third of normal children experiencing uncomplicated varicella have slightly raised aminotransferase values (Myers, Arch-DisChild, 1982; 57:317). Liver abnormalities are more severe and often have clinical expression in immunocompromised children and adults who develop progressive varicella or disseminated zoster; hepatitis in this setting may be fatal (Morishita, JAMA, 1985; 253: 511; Bensousan, TransplProc, 1995; 27:2512) and requires prevention measures (Kusne, Transpl, 1995; 60:619) such as active and passive immunization as well as acyclovir in case of exposure.

In normal, immunocompetent adults primary varicella is more severe than in children and is not infrequently complicated by pneumonia; hepatitis has been reported in patients with lung involvement (Krugman, NEJM, 1957; 257:843; Sander, Sca-JInfectDis, 1970; 2:231). The histopathology, when reported, invariably showed focal hepatic necrosis. Although varicella often precedes the development of Reye's syndrome (encephalopathy with fatty degeneration of the liver) the pathobiological mechanism linking the viral infection to this syndrome is not understood (Myers, ArchDisChild, 1982; 57:317).

Specific diagnostic tools for the identification of varicella-zoster virus hepatitis are similar to those for HSV—PCR, culture, and immunohistochemistry of liver biopsy or *post mortem* specimens are superior to serological testing, which is of little use especially under conditions of immunological impairment. Therapeutic considerations also resemble those for HSV-related hepatitis, except that high-dose acyclovir (10 mg/kg three times daily, intravenously)

is essential. The more potent compound sorivudine has recently been denied a licence by the United States Federal Drug Administration because a metabolite inhibits the catabolism of 5-fluorouracil and related anticancer drugs, leading to fatal bone marrow aplasia.

The β- and γ-herpesvirus subfamilies

The viruses in these subfamilies lack a distinct tropism, but may spread through the body via peripheral white blood cells at any time following primary infection. Only cytomegalovirus (**CMV**) and Epstein–Barr virus (**EBV**) can cause acute hepatitis as the main clinical picture but more usually they induce few or no symptoms. Both viruses infect well over 50 per cent of the world population so that the majority of patients presenting with hepatitis will have laboratory evidence of past or current infections with CMV, EBV, or both. In most of such cases neither virus is the cause of the hepatitis and particular combinations of laboratory tests specific for each virus are required before either can be implicated aetiologically, as is discussed in more detail below. The most recently identified β-herpesviruses (human herpesviruses 6 and 7) and γ-herpesvirus (human herpesvirus 8) are discussed later.

Cytomegalovirus

Epidemiology and pathogenesis

Primary infection with the β-herpesvirus CMV can be acquired at any age.[5] Between 0.3 and 2.0 per cent of babies are born with congenital infection. The rate of transmission, and even more the rate of prenatally acquired disease, is strongly correlated to the rate of primary CMV infections in the population of pregnant women (Peckham, Lancet, 1983; i:1352; Fowler, NEJM, 1992; 326:663). The virus may be present in infected maternal genital secretions or may be found in breast milk, both of which act as sources of perinatal infection (Stagno, NEJM, 1980; 103:1073). Following perinatal infection, excretion into the urine and saliva continues for many years and transmission between children in play groups, perhaps through the sharing of toys contaminated with saliva, has been described (Pass, NEJM, 1987; 316:1366). Virus acquired in this setting may be transferred to the parents when the children return home and may be a cause for concern if the mother is contemplating pregnancy. It is well recognized that CMV is transmitted within family groups, particularly in those that are socially disadvantaged. In western industrialized countries, approximately 40 per cent of young adults have been infected with CMV and this figure continues to rise by 1 per cent per annum until at least the middle 50s (Griffiths, BrJObsGyn, 1984; 91:307). Virtually all of these primary infections are entirely asymptomatic, although occasional cases of glandular fever syndrome do occur.

Reactivation of CMV from its latent state occurs asymptomatically and is an important means by which the virus can spread horizontally. Such episodes of reactivation are controlled by the body's cell-mediated immune response and it is this response which maintains CMV in its latent state. The major target of cytotoxic T-cells is pp65, the product of the unique long 83 open reading frame (Riddell, Science, 1992; 257:238). CMV infection becomes much more common and lasts longest in patients who are immunocompromised. Thus, CMV can frequently act as an opportunist in allograft patients, in those receiving chemotherapy, and in patients with AIDS (Glenn, RevInfDis, 1981; 3:1151; Pillay, AIDS, 1993; 7:969). Recent studies suggested that in immunocompromised patients CD34$^+$ stem cells can carry CMV as a source of subsequent reactivation (von Laer, Blood, 1995; 86:4086). In all of these individuals, the presence of IgG antibodies acts as a marker for potential reactivation so that those with antibody are at risk of getting the disease. Just as individuals with antibody cannot prevent endogenous virus reactivating, so the presence of antibody does not render a person immune to reinfections from an external source. Reinfections occur particularly where CMV is transmitted by blood products or by a donor organ and can only be identified by typing the DNA of the infecting strains by molecular methods. The distinction between reactivation and reinfection proved that, at least in renal transplant patients, primary infection reinfection produces more CMV disease than does reactivation (Grundy, Lancet, 1988; ii:132).

Virology

Primary infection with CMV can be diagnosed by seroconversion. This provides a possible means of diagnosing CMV mononucleosis in immunocompetent individuals but it cannot be used in neonates due to the passive transfer of IgG antibodies from the mother. The detection of IgM antibodies can support the serological diagnosis of CMV infection but is not reliable in cases of congenital infection and immunosuppression (Griffiths, Pediat, 1982; 69:544). Re-emerging IgM antibodies due to CMV reactivation secondary to various immunomodulating conditions as well as IgM antibody-positive primary infection may lack a clinical correlate. IgM antibodies to CMV are detectable in approximately one-third of renal transplant patients with mild recurrent infections (Kangro, JMcdVirol, 1982; 10:203; Rasmussen, JInfDis, 1982; 145:191). IgM antibodies are not found in some immunocompromised patients, in particular AIDS patients with life-threatening CMV infection. Test results may in this clinical context be false positive. Thus, caution is necessary in the interpretation of CMV IgM antibody results (Galama, JInfect, 1991; 23:175). Therefore, serology should not be used, apart from routine proof of seropositivity or seronegativity, for investigating any of these patients.

The detection of the virus itself or its structural components is the preferred diagnostic strategy. To avoid delays in diagnosing CMV infection due to its slow growth in standard cell cultures, rapid laboratory methods for virus detection have been developed. The widely used rapid culturing technique relies on the detection of fluorescent foci by use of monoclonal antibodies directed against the so-called early and immediate early proteins of CMV (Griffiths, Lancet, 1984; ii:1242; Gleaves, JClinMicrobiol, 1984; 21:217). Reported sensitivities of 70 to 80 per cent make the assays particularly useful. Only overnight incubation is required for this culturing process.

In viraemic patients viral antigens, in particular the matrix phosphoprotein pp65 (Gerna, JClinMicrobiol, 1992; 30:1232), are detectable in polymorphonuclear leucocytes (CMV antigenaemia). The presence of CMV antigenaemia in an individual with normal immunity is strong evidence of disseminated infection and can be used to diagnose CMV hepatitis. To determine that CMV is the cause of disease in children and adults, samples of urine, saliva, and anticoagulated blood should be collected. Urine and saliva are introduced in the rapid culturing process. The blood should be subject to separation of white blood cells by sedimentation through an appropriate medium (van der Bij, JMedVirol, 1988; 25:179) for the subsequently simultaneous assay of antibodies and viral antigens. For detection of congenital infection, urine is the preferred specimen since it contains a high titre of CMV (Stagno, JInfDis, 1975; 132:568).

In immunocompromised patients, surveillance samples of urine, saliva, and anticoagulated blood taken at least weekly should be used routinely to test for the presence of CMV. When this is done, CMV antigenaemia is found so frequently in these patients that the presence of CMV in the blood cannot on its own be used to diagnose CMV hepatitis. The rate of pp65-positive leucocytes (Meyer-Kšnig, ClinDiagVirol, 1995; 3:49) may be used to attempt a quantification of viraemia. Counts in the range of 10 to 100 pp65-carrying cells per 2×10^5 polymorphonuclear leucocytes are regarded as suggestive of clinically relevant disease and correlate well with detectable levels of CMV mRNA in leucocytes (Meyer-Kšnig, JInfectDis, 1995; 171: 705).

PCR is another tool for monitoring CMV infection in immunocompromised patients, especially in those previously seronegative, who have received blood or solid organs from a CMV-seropositive donor. Repeated detection of CMV DNA prior to specific symptoms is judged as a suitable time point for pre-emptive antiviral therapy (Kidd, Transpl, 1993; 56:867; Einsele, Blood, 1995; 86:2815). PCR employing nested primers may be an overly sensitive technique for the detection of clinically relevant CMV disease (Brainard, Transpl, 1994; 57:1753). The high negative predictive value of the PCR technique helps to manage the liver transplant recipient (Wolff, Transpl, 1993; 56:572) and immunocompromised patient with liver dysfunction (Einsele, MedMicrobiolImmunol, 1994; 205:16). One disadvantage of PCR is the difficulty of quantifying viraemia; as in the case of HIV in the course of AIDS, measuring the viral load in patients suspected of CMV-related disease may become important for therapeutic decisions (Fox, JGenVirol, 1995; 76:309; Boivin, JInfectDis, 1996; 173:1304). Methods such as branched DNA signal amplification assay (Cao, AIDSResHumRV, 1995; 11:353) and nucleic acid sequence-based assay, as well as competitive PCR techniques (Lin, JInfectDis, 1994; 170:533), have proven helpful in nucleic acid quantification but evaluation in CMV-related disease is still inadequate.

If possible, a liver biopsy should be performed in cases of suspected CMV hepatitis. *In situ* reactions can be carried out to seek specific proteins or specific nucleic acid sequences of CMV within the liver. Several investigators have attempted to use human immune sera to detect CMV antigens within liver biopsies but because this virus induces Fc receptors for human IgG molecules such methods should no longer be used. Mouse monoclonal antibodies are not affected by the same problem. Only reports using such reagents should be considered (Sacks, Gastro, 1984; 86:346; Paya, Hepatol, 1990; 12:119). Likewise, several false reports of the association between CMV and a variety of medical conditions have appeared in the literature due to the use of DNA probes containing whole genomic molecules. Since CMV contains several regions which are homologous with host cell DNA (Peden, Cell, 1982; 31: 71) only reports using subgenomic fragments for *in situ* hybridization should be considered (Naoumov, Lancet, 1988; i:1361; Espy, DiagMicrobInfDis, 1991; 14:293).

CMV Hepatitis

Clinical features

Danks *et al.*[2] and Watkins *et al.*[6] have reviewed the different types of conditions leading to neonatal jaundice. The cases with CMV infection are found among those with the clinical diagnosis of 'neonatal hepatitis'. Hyperbilirubinaemia is found in both direct and indirect forms and the levels of conjugated bilirubin may be similar to those found in cases of biliary atresia. The unconjugated bilirubin rarely rises to levels requiring exchange transfusion to prevent kernicterus. Haemolytic anaemia may contribute to the jaundice. The levels of serum transaminases are increased only moderately. Clinically, these cases are classified as mild-to-moderate hepatitis and they usually resolve within the first year of life (Berenberg, Pediat, 1970; 46:403).

In adults, primary CMV infection occasionally causes glandular fever syndrome. The patients commonly present with fever, malaise, or tiredness occasionally accompanied by pharyngitis or lymphadenopathy. The hepatitis is mild and self limiting with only mild or moderately raised levels of serum transaminases and alkaline phosphatase (Horwitz, ClinChem, 1980; 26:243). Clinically, it is usually obvious that these cases are glandular fever with liver involvement (Klemola, BMJ, 1965; 2:1099; Carlstom, BMJ, 1968; 2:521; Clarke, AmJMed, 1979; 66:264). In some cases, however, the hepatitis may be so prominent that the diagnosis of acute viral hepatitis is considered (Lamb, Lancet, 1966; ii:1003; Toghill, Lancet, 1967; i:1351; Carter, BMJ, 1968; 3:786). On follow-up the additional features of prolonged fever or mild hepatitis together with the presence of peripheral blood atypical mononuclear cells usually suggests the underlying diagnosis.

In allograft patients, particularly in liver transplant recipients[7] CMV is a common cause of acute hepatitis, being responsible for between 25 and 50 per cent of all episodes (Ware, AnnIntMed, 1979; 91:364; Meyers, JInfDis, 1986; 153:478; Barkholt, ScaJGastr, 1994; 29:553).

Diagnosis

The presence of some characteristic clinical findings may suggest the diagnosis of CMV hepatitis. For example, a spiking fever in a transplant patient associated with arthralgia suggests the diagnosis of CMV infection. Routine haematological tests showing atypical mononuclear cells may also suggest the diagnosis, and marked thrombocytopenia is an alarming sign of severe CMV infection. A full knowledge of the serological status of the donor and recipient should be available in the case of transplant patients; the presence of a seropositive donor suggests that a fever 6 weeks after transplant is most likely due to CMV, especially if the recipient is seronegative. However, in view of the ubiquity of CMV infections in such patients care must be taken in attributing hepatitis to this virus alone. Likewise, congenital CMV infection is so common that some neonates with liver disease due to other causes can also be expected to have concomitant CMV infection.[2]

Histopathology

Congenital CMV hepatitis appears as 'giant cell neonatal hepatitis' with the multinucleated giant cell reaction being an entirely

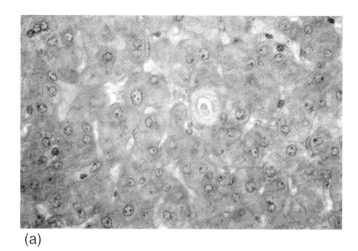

(a)

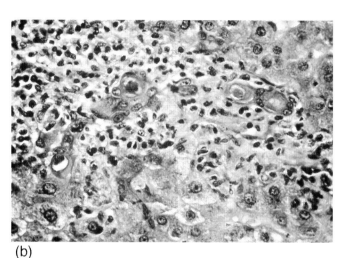

(b)

Fig. 1. CMV liver infection. (a) CMV inclusion in a hepatocyte. (b) CMV inclusions in cholangioles within periportal inflammation. (× 400.)

non-specific response (Stern, BrMedBull, 1972; 28:180). Single, large intranuclear inclusions (Cowdrey type A; so called 'owl's eye') (Fig. 1) may be found in hepatocytes or Kupffer cells but are found with the highest incidence in the biliary tract epithelium (Zupann, JPediatrGastrNutr, 1986; 5:489). The predilection of CMV for bile duct epithelium has led to the suggestion that bile duct atresia could be caused by intrauterine CMV infection (Finegold, HumPath, 1982; 13:662; Openhiemer, AmJPath, 1973; 73:2a). Other investigators have excluded CMV as a cause of congenital biliary atresia[2] or primary sclerosing cholangitis (Mehal, JHepatol, 1992; 15:396). Liver fibrosis secondary to CMV infection, however, has been reported by three independent workers, suggesting that this virus can induce non-cirrhotic portal fibrosis (Drester, JPediat, 1978; 93:887; Riely, JPediat, 1979; 94:1011; Ghishan, Hepatol, 1984; 4:684). It has been suggested (Openhiemer, AmJPath, 1973; 71:2a) that the hepatic fibrosis may be secondary to an inflammatory response but the possibility that the virus releases growth factors for fibroblasts should not be overlooked.

In patients with normal immunity presenting with CMV hepatitis, owl's eye inclusions can be found in some hepatocytes but are more frequent in bile duct epithelium. The formation of non-caseating granuloma has been described (Clarke, AmJMed, 1979; 66:264; Vanstapel, ApplPathol, 1983; 1:41).

There are some differences between the histological appearances seen in immunocompromised patients compared to patients with normal immunity. Inclusion bodies are found more frequently in hepatocytes and are also found in vascular endothelium and bile epithelium (Henson, HumPath, 1974; 5:93; Bombi, ArchPathLabMed, 1987; 111:125; Ten Napel, Liver, 1984; 4:184). The presence of intranuclear inclusions correlates with a poor inflammatory infiltration and with increased liver cell damage suggesting that the virus is directly cytolytic in the liver and that the normal immune response prevents severe damage occurring (Ten Napel, Liver, 1984; 4:184).

Complications

Most investigators agree that CMV is not a cause of chronic hepatitis (Toghill, Lancet, 1967; i:1351) although no definitive study has been performed to exclude this possibility. It is a little worrying to see several reports of hepatic fibrosis following congenital CMV infection, including fatal portal cirrhosis (Drester, JPediat, 1978; 93:887; Riely, JPediat, 1979; 94:1011; Ghishan, Hepatol, 1984; 4:684). A recent report also suggests that the occurrence of CMV infection in liver transplant recipients sharing a well matched HLA haplotype with the donor may predispose to the vanishing bile syndrome (O'Grady, Lancet, 1988; ii:302). While the pathogenesis of this condition is not clear, it is interesting to speculate that the infection together with the sharing of particular HLA antigens may make the donor bile duct epithelium vulnerable to particular types of recipient cell-mediated immune responses.

Treatment

There are no controlled trials of any antiviral agent in proven cases of CMV hepatitis. However, ganciclovir has widely been used for treatment. Anecdotal cases suggest that the drug may be efficacious (Theise, HumPath, 1993; 24:103; Sano, TranspISci, 1994; 4:105); however bone marrow suppression may become a limiting side-effect. CMV frequently becomes resistant to the drug during prolonged administration (Crumpacker, NEJM, 1996; 335:721). Virus resistance due to previous treatment for other CMV-related problems may be an important issue in immunocompromised patients with CMV hepatitis. Ganciclovir resistance is frequently associated with specific amino acid exchanges in the unique long 97 gene coding for a phosphotransferase that is needed for the phosphorylation of the drug (Littler, Nature, 1992; 358:160). Thus, relatively simple restriction enzyme analysis of viral DNA can prove resistance without cumbersome and time-consuming biological testing (Chou, JInfectDis, 1995; 171:576). In such cases, foscarnet is the alternative antiviral in life-threatening CMV infection. Foscarnet seems to be equally effective as estimated mainly from retinitis therapy in AIDS patients (Anonymous, NEJM, 1992; 326:213). However, its use is limited by nephrotoxicity. Until drugs with less toxic side-effects are available, ganciclovir and foscarnet should not be given to patients with underlying normal immunity since it is known that CMV hepatitis in such patients is normally self limiting. Other drugs under development include cidofovir (De Clercq, RevMedVirol, 1993; 3:85), lobucavir, and 1263W94.

Epstein–Barr virus

Epidemiology and pathogenesis

Primary infection with EBV can occur at any age but there is no convincing evidence of intrauterine infection with this virus. Although as a γ-herpes virus[8] EBV is considered lymphotropic, it can be found, at least intermittently, in saliva or in female genital secretions of many adults. The duration of excretion of this virus following primary infection is not known. Most cases in childhood are asymptomatic whereas most cases in adults are accompanied by the typical symptoms of infectious mononucleosis; this difference is attributed to the large dose of virus transmitted between adolescents by deep kissing but could also be due to changes in the immune system. In older adults, abdominal pain may be prominent.

Following acquisition of EBV, the virus replicates in epithelial cells, certainly in the pharynx (Lemon, Nature, 1986; 306:480) and probably on the cervix as well (Sixbey, Lancet, 1986; ii:1122). Peripatetic B-lymphocytes acquire EBV from this site. B-lymphocytes contain complement receptor 2 (C3d) which can be used by the virus as a receptor (Fingeroth, PNAS, 1984; 81:4510). Following infection of B-lymphocytes, the virus genome is expressed and neoantigens appear on the surface of the lymphocytes. Until this moment the patient remains asymptomatic but T-lymphocytes then react against the presence of the neoantigens. The resulting infectious mononucleosis is thus immunopathologically mediated and the peripheral blood atypical mononuclear cells represent reactive T-lymphocytes. In the rare condition of X-linked lymphoproliferative disease (Duncan's syndrome), otherwise healthy male children are unable to mount a cytotoxic T-lymphocyte response and frequently succumb from primary EBV infection (Purtilo, RevMedVirol, 1992; 2:153).

EBV establishes latency and may reactivate in saliva and cervical secretions. At any one time, only a small percentage of seropositive individuals excrete EBV but this figure increases in those who are immunosuppressed (Crawford, Lancet, 1981; i:10). Perhaps surprisingly, this increased excretion is not accompanied by symptoms although patients are at risk of EBV associated B-cell lymphomas (Lipscomb, AIDSRes, 1983; 1:59; Craig, AmJClinPath, 1993; 99:265) and, in the case of AIDS patients, of oral hairy leucoplakia (Greenspan, JInfDis, 1987; 155:475). Latent infection in blood and organ donors represents a potential source of virus. Fortunately, most recipients are immune to EBV and so appear not to develop symptoms (Haque, RevMedVirol, 1996; 6:77).

Serology and virology

Testing by indirect immunofluorescence for the antibody response to viral antigens expressed in EBV-infected cells allows specific proof or exclusion of acute or past EBV infection. The sequential appearance of antibodies against the various EBV-specific antigens present in Burkitt's lymphoma cells is shown in Fig. 2. Most patients with EBV hepatitis are already viral capsid antigen IgG-positive at the time of presentation and so viral capsid antigen IgM antibodies should be sought in addition. In this acute phase, the patient should be anti-Epstein–Barr virus nuclear antigen-1-negative and a follow-up check 2 to 3 months later will confirm the primary infection by showing seroconversion against Epstein–Barr virus nuclear antigen-1. Unfortunately, certain cases do not conform

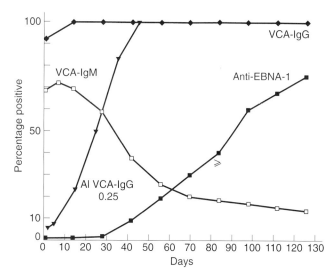

Fig. 2. Temporal appearance of antibodies following primary infection with Epstein–Barr virus (From: Avidities of IgG directed against viral capsid antigen or early antigen: Useful markers for significant Epstein–Barr virus serology. Andersson A, Vetter V, Kreutzer L, and Bauer G, JMedVirol, 1994; 43:238, reprinted by permission of Wiley-Liss). Positivity rates are based on 82 individual case histories. AI = avidity index (anti-viral capsid antigen IgG titre by indirect immunofluorescence read after 3 min washing with 6 M urea divided by titre read after conventional washing). The probability of antibody maturing to AI ≥ 0.25 was calculated from assays in 105 sera available from 52 patients.

to this diagnostic approach. A substantial proportion (up to 25 per cent) of patients experiencing primary EBV infection will not have detectable IgM antibodies at the time they develop symptoms, nor at subsequent controls. Some patients may fail to raise or sustain Epstein–Barr virus nuclear antigen-1 antibodies due to impaired immune response, and nevertheless harbour stable non-primary EBV infections in a well balanced clinical state (Henle, CancerRes, 1981; 41:4222; Vetter, ClinDiagVirol, 1994; 2:29). Thus, a considerable number of fresh infections might be missed and others incorrectly diagnosed.

In most cases, a solution to the dilemma is warranted by measuring the avidity of IgG—that is the stability of antibody binding to specific antigen in the presence of urea (Hedman, JClinImmunol, 1988; 8:214). This method was evaluated for EBV viral capsid antigen IgG in suspected cases of infectious mononucleosis that were antibody negative for viral capsid antigen IgM and Epstein–Barr virus nuclear antigen-1 (Andersson, JMedVirol, 1994; 43:238). Recent infection is invariably characterized by low avidity values of IgG, whereas subsequent controls show the increased avidity of the matured antibody generation that is typical of past infection (Fig. 2).

Though inexpensive and technically simple, these classical immunofluorescence assays are so far available only in specialized laboratories (Henle, HumPath, 1974; 5:551; Bauer, ClinLab, 1995; 41:623); they require a fair effort for standardization. Enzyme immunoassay variants of these procedures have been developed and evaluated (Gorgievski-Hrisoho, JClinMicrobiol, 1990; 28:2305) so that specific serology is now more widely available.

In a patient who is already seropositive, reactivation of EBV should be diagnosed by detecting the virus. Methods such as

immortalization of cord blood cells and hybridization assays with DNA extracted from tissues are expensive and time consuming. (Donhuijsen-Ant, BrJHaemat, 1990; 74:557; Ablashi, IntVirol, 1987; 27:25). Infected B-cells containing EBV can be found in patients with various unrelated diseases and thus the detection of the virus by sensitive PCR in blood or solid tissues is of limited clinical use due to its ubiquitous presence. However, the use of DNA probes for the detection of EBV-encoded small RNA has provided some progress, especially with *in situ* applications (Randhawa, NEJM, 1992; 327:1710; Hubscher, Hepatol, 1994; 20: 899). Recurrent infections are often sought serologically by detection of antibodies against the various early antigens of EBV (Schooley, NEJM, 1983; 308:307; Jones, AnnIntMed, 1985; 102:1). Such diagnoses are unsound in patients in whom polyclonal B-cell activation may occur and where abnormal immune responses should be expected, such as AIDS patients or transplant recipients.

EBV hepatitis

Clinical features

In adolescents and adults, primary EBV infection can present with fever, pharyngitis, malaise, and lymphadenopathy typical of infectious mononucleosis (Hoagland, AmJMedSci, 1960; 240:55; Mason, AmJMedSci, 1958; 236:447). Clinically the hepatitis is mild.[9] In some adults over 40 years of age, atypical presentations have been described with prominent abdominal pain, together with persistent fever, moderate abnormalities of transaminases and alkaline phosphatase, and only minor lymphadenopathy (Horowitz, Medicine, 1983; 62:256; Ansari, AmJGastr, 1984; 79:471; Jacobson, AmJGastr, 1984; 79:628). Haemolysis and cholestasis may contribute to the jaundice (Fuhrman, ArchIntMed, 1987; 147:850; Whitelaw, BrJClinPract, 1995; 49:212). In children, EBV hepatitis may mimic a chronic active hepatitis (Lloyd-Still, PediatPath, 1986; 5:337).

Diagnosis

The diagnosis of infectious mononucleosis with liver involvement is readily made in most cases by detecting heterophile agglutinins using Paul–Bunnell or monospot tests (Hoagland, AmJMedSci, 1960; 240:53; Mason, AmJMedSci, 1958; 236:447). Abdominal pain may be prominent in older patients and biliary tract disease may be mimicked.

Histopathology

The liver biopsy shows no change in liver architecture. There may be portal and sinusoidal mononuclear cell infiltration with little hepatic necrosis (Nelson, AmJMed, 1956; 21:26; Kilpatrick, ArchIntMed, 1966; 117:47). Frozen sections can be stained for the Epstein–Barr virus nuclear antigen with monoclonal antibodies and assayed for EBV-encoded small RNA by *in situ* hybridization (Clemens, MolBiolRep, 1993; 17:81).

Complications

Although most cases of EBV hepatitis resolve in a few weeks, fatigue and abnormal laboratory tests may persist for months (Aceti, Lancet, 1995; 346:1603). Fatal cases of EBV hepatitis have been described (Davies, PostgradMedJ, 1980; 56:794; Papatheodoridis, JHepatol,

1995; 23:348). The hypersplenism associated with infectious mononucleosis may lead to splenic rupture and death. A case of chronic hepatitis associated with EBV has also been reported (Tanaka, JPediatGastrNutr, 1986; 5:467). The haemophagocytic syndrome has been associated with EBV infection (Sullivan, Blood, 1985; 65: 1097). Patients with infectious mononucleosis may develop a rash if given ampicillin.

Special attention should be given to the occurrence of EBV hepatitis and EBV-associated post-transplant lymphoproliferative disease, especially in liver grafts (Langnas, AmJGastr, 1994; 89: 1066). From experience with 585 cases it was concluded that the disease is infrequent (2 per cent), closely related to the use of antilymphocyte preparations (OKT3), and may be treated successfully.

Treatment

There have been no controlled trials of any antiviral agent in proven cases of EBV hepatitis. Acyclovir inhibits EBV *in vitro* and suppresses viral excretion in the oropharynx without affecting latent infection. Anecdotal cases suggest that it can cause the regression of oral hairy leucoplakia in AIDS patients (Resnick, JAMA, 1988; 259:384), whereas a controlled trial in primary EBV infection showed little or no effect on the disease course, with or without steroids (Tynell, JInfDis, 1996; 174:324). Nevertheless, in serious cases of EBV hepatitis, for example post-transplant, it is imperative to give a trial of intravenous acyclovir in high dose albeit an empirical basis; immunosuppression has to be minimized or discontinued in such patients.

Human herpesviruses 6, 7, and 8

Human herpesviruses 6 and 7 (**HHV-6** and **HHV-7**) are two closely related β-herpesviruses isolated from peripheral blood mononuclear cells of patients with lymphoproliferative disorders and healthy adults, respectively. These viruses grow in cultures of stimulated primary T-cells and have been adapted to T-cell lines. Although their T-lymphotropic properties are well established,[10,11] a role in haemato-oncological disease has not been demonstrated. Both viruses are highly prevalent in young children, with rates of >90 per cent for HHV-6 by the age of 3 years. HHV-6 was identified as the causative agent in exanthema subitum, also named roseola (Yamanishi, Lancet, 1988; i:1065). Most children, however, experience subclinical primary infection or febrile illness with varied clinical manifestations.

No case of liver involvement was noted among 34 culture-proven HHV-6 infections in a prospective study on 243 acutely ill children aged 2 years or less (Pruksananonda, NEJM, 1992; 326:1445) or in a large study of febrile children (Hall, NEJM, 1994; 331:432). Anecdotal reports have associated primary HHV-6 infection in newborns and infants with fulminant hepatitis (Mendel, PediatInfectDis, 1995; 14:993; Asano, Lancet, 1990; 335:862) and with exacerbation of pre-existing hepatic disease (Tajiri, Lancet, 1990; 335:863). HHV-6 was also found in a 20-month-old child with relapsing liver dysfunction who had experienced primary HHV-7 infection 3 months previously. Both viruses were detected by PCR in a subsequent liver biopsy (Hashida, Pediat, 1995; 96: 783); an interaction between these closely related herpesviruses resulting in cross reactivation has been suggested.[11]

Although all the cited reports are based on sound diagnostic methods of HHV-6 and HHV-7 infection (viral culture, PCR, viral neutralization, and immunofluorescence), the causative role of these agents in hepatitis remains questionable due to the ubiquity of primary infections at a young age. Also in adults, the detection of HHV-6 infection in coincidence with hepatitis (Sobue, NEJM, 1991; 324:1290; Dubedat, Lancet, 1989; ii:1463) rises the question of viral persistence and reactivation rather than unambiguously revealing the aetiology. In a surveillance study on 58 cardiac transplant patients, HHV-6 reactivation was suggested by serology in 14 cases but could not be related to post-transplant hepatitis (Robert, PressMed, 1994; 23:1209). Probably, OKT-3 therapy acts as a reactivating factor for HHV-6.[10] Even in liver transplant recipients, no specific hepatic complication due to HHV-6 was proven, except coagulopathy (Singh, AnnIntMed, 1996; 124:1065), though reactivation of the virus is common in this setting.

Further diagnostic approaches to the question as to whether hepatitis can be associated with HHV-6 or HHV-7 should not rely on serology, which has been of little use so far. Instead, the established methods of virus detection in peripheral blood mononuclear cells (Collandre, JVirolMethods, 1991; 31:171; Cone, JClinMicrobiol, 1993; 31:1262; Clark, JGenVirol, 1996; 77:2271; Kidd, JInfDis, 1996; 174:396) should be combined with *in situ* analyses in biopsy specimens (Fox, Lancet, 1990; 336:590).

Both, ganciclovir and foscarnet are effective against HHV-6 *in vitro* (Burns, JInfectDis, 1990; 162:634). Although clinical studies have not been carried out, a therapeutic trial should be considered when HHV-6 pathogenesis is implicated in the immunocompromised.

The discovery of Kaposi's sarcoma-associated human herpesvirus 8 (HHV-8) has only recently been followed by virus isolation and propagation in cell culture (Renne, NatureMed, 1996; 2:342). The virus was grown in a B-cell line and was classified in the γ-herpesvirus subgroup, since its DNA sequence is related to EBV and the non-human primate herpesvirus saimiri (Moore, JVirol, 1996; 70:549). The methodology needed for epidemiological studies is currently being developed (Kedes, NatureMed, 1996; 2:918; Gao, NEJM, 1996; 335:233). The potential of HHV-8 to affect liver tissue is not known, except for the occurrence of Kaposi lesions in the visceral type of the disease. As other herpesviruses might be responsible for HHV-8 liver involvement at the time of primary infection, this should be further defined by investigations in the groups at risk of HHV-8 infection (Gao, NatureMed, 1996; 2:925; Lennette, Lancet, 1996; 348:858).

Measles virus

Measles is an acute febrile eruption caused by an RNA virus classified as a paramyxovirus.[12] The patient presents with malaise, irritability, fever, conjunctivitis, photophobia, and nasal discharge. Koplick's spots (small red lesions with a blue-white centre) appear 1 to 8 days before the rash in the oral mucous membrane. The rash appears first on the forehead and spreads downward. Florid disease is accompanied by leucopenia. Serological confirmation can be obtained with complement fixation, enzyme immunoassays, immunofluorescence tests, and haemagglutination inhibition tests. The current standard diagnostic procedure is the demonstration of specific IgM by ELISA simultaneously with occurrence of the rash.

Viraemia may persist beyond this time point, since the virus infects blood monocytes which carry the virus to the liver and other organs (Esolen, JInfectDis, 1993; 168:47).

Abnormalities of liver chemistry, mainly increases in aminotransferases, occur in up to 80 per cent of adult patients admitted to hospital[13] but less frequently in paediatric patients; the incidence of clinical liver dysfunction is much lower, probably of the order of 5 per cent of the total number of unadmitted patients with average illnesses. In a recent review of the literature[14] 27 cases of measles-associated hepatobiliary disease were reported. Changes in liver chemistry are usually self limited and subclinical. Occasionally, however, hepatitis may be a salient clinical manifestation (Siegel, ArchIntMed, 1977; 137:1178; McLellan, JAMA, 1982; 247:2000). In a study of two epidemics of measles in Jerusalem, five out of 60 patients admitted to hospital had clinical jaundice;[13] in this study a correlation was observed between severity of hepatic involvement and occurrence of secondary bacterial infection. In a child who died of severe ileocolitis complicating measles, liver histological changes were lymphocytic infiltration with small foci of hepatocellular necrosis (Monif, AmJDisChild, 1970; 120:245).

Rubella virus

Rubella (German measles) is a febrile exanthema caused by a togavirus transmitted via the nasopharynx.[15] Prodromal symptoms such as malaise, headache, conjunctivitis, and lymphadenopathy may precede the exanthem, which starts in the face and spreads to the trunk and extremities. As a rule the rash is accompanied by regional adenopathy; postauricular and suboccipital nodes are those more overtly involved. The acquired disease is benign; however, when it occurs in the first trimester of pregnancy it may cause infection and congenital malformations in the fetus with fatal outcome in many cases either *in utero* or *post partum*.

In surviving babies congenital rubella is manifested by heart malformations, cataract, deafness, and mental retardation. Hepatomegaly is a temporary finding (Korones, GenPractitioner, 1967; 35:78). Cholestatic jaundice may be observed 1 or 2 days after birth. Alkaline phosphatase and bilirubin levels are increased more than aminotransferase levels but acute hepatitis may also occur; the lesions include focal hepatocellular necrosis and giant cell hepatitis (Esterly, JPediat, 1967; 71:676; Stern, Lancet, 1966; i:293). The virus can be identified in the liver. The course of disease is usually self limited.

Enteroviruses

Coxsackieviruses A and B and echoviruses have been implicated as causes of liver impairment in neonates.[16]

Coxsackieviruses

Group A coxsackieviruses cause herpangina, aseptic meningitis, and respiratory infections; infection has only occasionally been associated with hepatitis (Morris, NEJM, 1962; 267:1230). Although different viral types have been isolated in stools of patients with infectious hepatitis, a direct pathogenic link between these common enteric viruses and liver disease was not established.

Group B coxsackieviruses cause a variety of syndromes, including pleurodynia, myocarditis, and aseptic meningitis. Generalized infections affecting several organs mostly occur in the newborn but hepatitis is a rare clinical feature (Kaplan, RevInfectDis, 1983; 5:1019). Liver involvement ranging from dysfunction to severe coagulapathy and fatal multiorgan failure has been reported in a number of children with coxsackie B1 infections (Chou, ActaPaedSin, 1995; 36:296; Kulhangian, PediatInfectDis, 1992; 11:1069). An anicteric form of hepatitis occurred in an 8-year-old child in association with coxsackie B2 infection (Lansky, JPediat, 1979; 94:64) and a Reye-like syndrome was observed in an 11-month-old infant in whom coxsackie B2 virus was isolated from the cerebrospinal fluid (Kaul, JPediat, 1979; 94:67); histological examination showed foci of centrilobular necrosis and patchy steatosis but cellular infiltrate was scarce and the appearance of the portal areas was unremarkable. Two cases of neonatal, fatal, systemic infection associated with hepatitis have been related to coxsackie B4 virus (Kibrick, Pediat, 1958; 22:857).

Hepatitis has also been reported in adults with generalized infections (Sun, NEJM, 1966; 274:190; Gregor, MtSinaiMedJ, 1975; 42:575). However, in recent years there have been no reports of an association between cocksackievirus B infection and hepatitis; errors due to previously unknown hepatitis viruses cannot be excluded in the older literature.

Echoviruses

Echoviruses are a frequent cause of simple febrile illnesses and aseptic meningitis. Disease in adults is most usually benign and self limited; it may be severe in patients with B-cell deficiency syndromes (Lederman, Medicine, 1985; 64:145; Ross, RevInfDis, 1987; 9:334). Echoviruses have rarely been associated with liver disease in adults (Schleissner, AnnIntMed, 1968; 68:1315). Neonates, however, are uniquely susceptible to infection with echoviruses and often have clinical liver disease. In a review of 61 neonates with infection of echoviruses reported before 1985, severe hepatitis occurred in 68 per cent, associated in 27 per cent of cases with meningitis or meningoencephalitis; 83 per cent of the patients with severe hepatitis died (Modlin, RevInfDis, 1986; 8:918). In neonates with fatal hepatitis, the near totality of the liver parenchyma was necrotic (Hughes, AmJDisChild, 1972; 123:61). Fulminant and fatal cases were more frequent when the disease was associated with echovirus 11 (Gitlia, WestJMed, 1983; 138:260; Modlin, Pediat, 1988; 66:775; Speer, JPediatSurg, 1984; 19:591). It is probable that milder forms of liver disease are very common; anicteric hepatitis has been reported in a young infant infected with echovirus 3 (Leggiadro, AmJDisChild, 1982; 136:744).

Adenoviruses

Adenoviruses are ubiquitous DNA viruses currently classified in 47 human serotypes.[17] They are endemic in the paediatric age group (Chanock, PrevMed, 1974; 3:466). They cause rhinitis, lymphoadenopathy, keratoconjunctivitis, and pharyngoconjunctivitis in man. Canine and avian adenoviruses induce hepatitis in their natural hosts (Wigton, Blood, 1976; 47:278; Grimes, AvianDis, 1977; 21: 26).

In most individuals, infection is subclinical or mild and self limited. It may be severe and even fatal in immunocompromised subjects; in this setting hepatitis is a frequent complication, second only to respiratory tract disease.

Severe hepatitis caused by adenoviruses has been described in patients (mostly children) with inherited immunodeficiency syndromes, such as lymphoid depletion (Benyesh-Melnick, JPediat, 1964; 64:83), thymic alymphoplasia (Wigger, NEJM, 1966; 275: 870), thymic dysplasia (Aterman, VirchArchA, 1973; 360:155), acute lymphoblastic leukaemia (Carmichel, AmJClinPath, 1979; 71:352), Hodgkin's disease (Zahradnick, AmJMed, 1988; 68:725; Bonabdallah, AnnMedIntern, 1990; 141:81), severe combined immunodeficiency (Rodriguez, AmJClinPath, 1984; 82:615; Ohbu, ActaPathJpn, 1987; 37:655), and following paediatric liver transplantation (Koneru, TransplProc, 1990; 22:1547; Michaels, JInfDis, 1992; 165:170). Probably allograft reactions, graft-versus-host as well as host-versus-graft, render the organ susceptible to adenoviral infection and virulence. Monoclonal OKT3 or polyclonal antithymocyte antibody treatment for graft rejection episodes may further enhance the development of severe hepatitis with case fatality rates up to 30 per cent (Cames, JPediat, 1992; 120:33). Reactivation of persisting adenovirus as well as donor-associated transmission may be relevant in these cases. Adenovirus types 1, 2, and 5 were frequently identified, with type 5 being most common.

Less severe forms of liver dysfunction associated with adenoviruses are probably common in immunosuppressed patients; enzyme abnormalities were detected in 43 out of 51 patients who underwent bone-marrow transplantation from whom adenoviruses were isolated (Shields, NEJM, 1985; 312:529) and an acute self-limited hepatitis caused by adenoviruses has been reported in an adolescent with severe burns (Fruttaldo, MinMed, 1989; 80:501).

The pathological picture has been fairly consistent in cases of fatal hepatitis. Electron microscopy shows widespread focal necrosis with hepatocytes containing Feulgen-positive nuclear inclusion and crystalline arrays of virions; adenovirus antigens have been detected in the nuclear inclusion by indirect immunofluorescence (Ohbu, ActaPathJpn, 1987; 37:655). In addition to *in situ* methods, adenovirus isolation in human diploid cells, Hela cells, or, most efficiently, human embryonic kidney cell cultures should be used for diagnosis from stool and liver tissue. Adenovirus serology is of little help and PCR should be used very critically if at all, since persistent infection may give positive results lacking clinical relevance (Allard, JMedVirol, 1992; 37:149). No specific therapy for adenovirus infections is known; immunosuppression has to be reduced or discontinued when associated with diseases of adenoviral origin.

Reoviruses, parvovirus B19, and 'other viruses'

Reoviruses,[18] including the rotavirus genus,[19] induce hepatitis in mice. In immunodeficient children with life-long persisting rotavirus-related diarrhoea, a viral non-structural protein was traced in the kidney and the liver using immunostaining with polyclonal antibodies (Gilger, JPediat, 1992; 120:912). However, specific hepatic lesions were not demonstrated and the conclusion that rotavirus

infection extends beyond the intestinal tract in such cases awaits further confirmation.

The hypothesis of an association of neonatal biliary atresia with reovirus 3 (Richardson, JGastHepatol, 1994; 9:264) or rotavirus (Riepenhoff-Talty, JInfDis, 1996; 174:8) is doubtful. In the infants investigated, these infections may have occurred as a secondary event favoured by the underlying anatomical abnormality rather than being the cause of the morphological changes in the liver.

The role of parvoviruses[20] in inducing hepatitis has been studied in the rat (Kilham, AmJPath, 1966; 47:457), and human parvovirus B19 is found in liver tissue from cases of hydrops fetalis (Anand, NEJM, 1987; 316:183). This is not unexpected, since liver is a major site of prenatal erythropoiesis and erythroblasts are identified as the main targets of the virus.[20] Recent reports on parvovirus B19 infection associated with aplastic anaemia and fulminant hepatitis in children (Langnas, Hepatol, 1995; 22:1661; Yoto, Lancet, 1996; 347:868; Naides, Lancet, 1996; 347:1563) imply that also cells other than haematopoietic cells are targets of the virus. This is supported by the finding that globoside acts as a receptor for parvovirus B19 (Brown, Science, 1993; 262:114). Reports of parvovirus-related liver dysfunction in adults (Naides, ClinRes, 1987; 35:859A; Tsude, AmJGastr, 1993; 88:1463) remain controversial.

Liver involvement may be seen in various other viral infections—some associated with organ dysfunction due to unknown mechanisms and many related to AIDS pathogenesis (as discussed in Chapter 12.3) or acquired in an 'exotic' environment (Chapter 12.4).

References

1. Whitley RJ. Herpes simplex viruses. In Fields BN, *et al.*, eds. *Virology*, 3rd edn. Philadelphia: Lippincott-Raven, 1996: 2297–342.
2. Danks DM, Campbell PE, Jack I, *et al.* Studies of the aetiology of neonatal hepatitis and biliary atresia. *Archives of Diseases of Childhood*, 1977; **52**: 360–7.
3. Kipps A, *et al.* Fatal disseminated primary herpes infection in children: epidemiology based on 93 non-neonatal cases. *South African Medical Journal*, 1967; **41**: 647–51.
4. Arvin AM. Varicella-zoster virus. In Fields BN *et al.*, eds. *Virology*, 3rd edn. Philadelphia: Lippincott-Raven, 1996: 2547–86.
5. Britt WJ and Alford CA. Cytomegalovirus. In Fields BN, *et al.*, eds. *Virology*, 3rd edn. Philadelphia: Lippincott-Raven, 1996: 2493–524.
6. Watkins JB, Katz AJ, and Grand RJ. Neonatal hepatitis: A diagnostic approach. *Advances in Pediatrics*, 1977; **24**: 399–454.
7. Kanj SS, *et al.* Cytomegalovirus infection following liver transplantation: review of the literature. *Clinical Infectious Diseases*, 1996; **22**: 537–49.
8. Rickinson AB and Kieff E. Epstein-Barr virus. In Fields BN, *et al.*, eds. *Virology*, 3rd edn. Philadelphia: Lippincott-Raven, 1996: 2397–446.
9. Markin RS. Manifestations of Epstein-Barr virus-associated disorders in liver. *Liver*, 1994; **14**: 1–13.
10. Pellett PE and Black JB. Human herpesvirus 6. In Fields BN, *et al.*, eds. *Virology*, 3rd edn. Philadelphia: Lippincott-Raven, 1996: 2587–608.
11. Frenkel N and Roffman E. Human herpesvirus 7. In Fields BN, *et al.*, eds. *Virology*, 3rd edn. Philadelphia: Lippincott Raven, 1996: 2609 22.
12. Griffin DE and Bellini WJ. Measles virus. In Fields BN *et al.*, eds. *Virology*, 3rd edn. Philadelphia: Lippincott-Raven, 1996: 1267–312.
13. Gavish D, Kleinman Y, Morag A, and Tova-Chajek S. Hepatitis and jaundice associated with measles in young adults. *Archives of Internal Medicine*, 1983; **143**: 674–7.
14. Khatib R, *et al.* Measles associated hepatobiliary disease: An overview. *Infection*, 1993; **21**: 112–14.

15. Wolinsky JS. Rubella virus. In Fields BN, *et al.*, eds. *Virology*, 3rd edn. Philadelphia: Lippincott-Raven, 1996: 899–930.

16. Abzug MJ. Perinatal enterovirus infections. In Rotbart HA, ed. *Human enterovirus infections.* Washington, DC: ASM Press, 1995: 221–38.

17. Horwitz MS. Adenoviruses. In Fields BN *et al.*, eds. *Virology*, 3rd edn. Philadelphia: Lippincott-Raven, 1996: 2149–72.

18. Tyler KL and Fields BN. Reoviruses. In Fields BN *et al.*, eds. *Virology*, 3rd edn. Philadelphia: Lippincott-Raven, 1996: 1597–624.

19. Kapikian AZ and Chanock RM. Rotaviruses. In Fields BN, *et al.*, eds. *Virology*, 3rd edn. Philadelphia: Lippincott-Raven, 1996: 1657–708.

20. Young NS. Parvoviruses. In Fields BN, *et al.*, eds. *Virology*, 3rd edn. Philadelphia: Lippincott-Raven, 1996: 2199–220.

12.3 Hepatitis and human immunodeficiency virus infection in homosexual men and injecting drug users

Richard Gilson and Ian Weller

Introduction

The major causes of liver disease in homosexual men and injecting drug users are acute and chronic viral infections. Owing to their similar modes of transmission, infection with the human immunodeficiency virus (**HIV**) often coexists, leading to interactions affecting the natural history and response to treatment of chronic viral hepatitis. Other causes of liver disease associated with HIV infection include opportunistic infections, tumours, and reactions to drugs used in treatment and prophylaxis. The first part of this chapter describes the epidemiology and clinical features of hepatitis in relation to homosexual men and injecting drug users.

Hepatitis in drug users and homosexual men

Hepatitis B virus infection

Soon after sensitive tests for hepatitis B virus (**HBV**) infection had been developed, it was suggested that male homosexual behaviour might be associated with increased risk of acquiring HBV infection (Vahrman, Lancet, 1970; ii:774). Studies of attendees at clinics for sexually transmitted diseases in Europe and North America showed that 50 to 75 per cent of male homosexuals had evidence of past or current infection, with an HBV carrier rate of 1.5 to 4 per cent,[1] five to ten times the rate in heterosexuals. HBV infection is an important cause of acute hepatitis in this group, and the most common cause of chronic hepatitis. A fall in the incidence of reported cases of acute hepatitis B in the United Kingdom and United States since the mid-1980s has been associated with changes in sexual behaviour since the emergence of the HIV epidemic. Unprotected anal intercourse is the major risk factor for transmission.[2] Hepatitis B surface antigen (**HBsAg**) and HBV DNA have been demonstrated in semen; HBsAg is detectable in swabs from superficial, asymptomatic, rectal mucosal lesions, as well as from unaffected mucosa, and in faeces (Reiner, AnnIntMed, 1982; 96:170).

The prevalence of HBV infection among drug users is similar to that in homosexual men,[3] although prevalence estimates vary, partly due to over-representation of patients with acute infection in some studies. The major route of transmission is by the sharing of needles and syringes, but other injecting equipment such as filters may also be contaminated. Sexual transmission is also important, particularly to non-drug-using partners, and where drug use is associated with commercial sex.

Hepatitis A virus infection

An excess of cases of hepatitis not caused by HBV in men aged 20 to 40 years was reported in San Francisco in 1979 (Owen, WestJMed, 1979; 130:236). A study of attenders at a clinic for sexually transmitted diseases in Seattle, United States (Corey, NEJM, 1980; 302:435) showed that homosexual men with multiple sexual partners had a higher prevalence (30 per cent) of antibodies (anti-HAV) to hepatitis A virus (**HAV**) than heterosexual controls (12 per cent) enrolled in a study of recurrent genital herpes. During 6 to 9 months of follow-up the annual attack rate in homosexual men was 22 per cent, with no infection in the controls. Further support for sexual transmission was provided by a documented epidemic in Scandinavia (Christenson, AmJEpid, 1982; 116:599). The most likely transmission is by oral–anal contact. However, seroprevalence studies have not found a higher prevalence of past exposure to HAV in homosexual men than in heterosexual controls, suggesting that sexual transmission does not contribute substantially to the risk of infection in this group (Nandwani, GenitourinMed, 1994; 70:325).

Among drug users, epidemics of HAV infection have been reported from Scandinavia[4,5] and the United States,[6] and a seroprevalence four times greater than that in the general population has been recorded (Scheutz, ScaJInfectDis, 1983; 15:139). The most likely mode of transmission is the faecal–oral route, due to poor personal hygiene under adverse social conditions. Blood-borne transmission by contamination of shared needles and equipment is probably rare, because of the short period of viraemia in acute disease and the absence of chronic carriage.

Acute HAV infection may be more severe in homosexual men and injecting drug users than in other adults, but this may be related to the presence of underlying chronic liver disease caused by chronic viral hepatitis or alcohol (Reiner, AnnIntMed, 1982; 96:170; Laskin, AnnIntMed, 1989; 110:845).

Hepatitis D virus infection

Hepatitis D virus (**HDV**; delta virus) infection is an important additional cause of acute and chronic hepatitis in drug users in Europe and North America,[7,8] and now affects other regions where the prevalence of drug use is increasing (Duraisamy, MedJMalaysia, 1994; 49:212). Among HBV-infected drug users in Europe the prevalence of HDV infection is 60 to 80 per cent.[9-13] In a surveillance study in Italy, half the cases of HDV infection were coinfections with HBV, and half were superinfections in HBV carriers (Stroffolini, JHepatol, 1994; 21:1123).

Sexual transmission of HDV occurs, but is less efficient than parenteral transmission.[14,15] In homosexual men with newly diagnosed HBV infection (acute or chronic) in the United States, 1 to 2 per cent had HDV markers (Weisfuse, Hepatol, 1989; 9:872). In Europe the prevalence was also low, 0 to 3 per cent,[9,16-18] although some small studies have suggested higher prevalences of 14 to 40 per cent (Mele, EurJEpid, 1988; 4:488; Pol, Hepatol, 1989; 10:342); it is important to consider undisclosed drug use in such cases.

Hepatitis C virus infection

Hepatitis C virus (**HCV**) infection accounts for at least 80 per cent of the cases of non-A, non-B hepatitis, recognized as the main cause of chronic liver disease in injecting drug users.[19] Although most patients with antibodies to HCV do not have a history of acute hepatitis, HCV is the cause of up to 50 per cent of cases of acute hepatitis in this group. Half of injecting drug users with HCV antibodies, of whom 80 to 90 per cent have detectable HCV viraemia, have raised transaminase activities and more have histological evidence of chronic hepatitis. Most have no symptoms.

Sexual transmission of hepatitis C is well documented. Population-based studies in the United States showed that at least 10 per cent of cases of acute non-A, non-B hepatitis were acquired by sexual or household contact.[20] Studies among homosexual men show a small excess risk over heterosexual controls, with a prevalence of 1 to 3 per cent. A cumulative incidence rate of 4 per cent was reported from a cohort study of homosexual men in Denmark (Melbye, BMJ, 1990; 301:210).

Other hepatitis virus infections

Hepatitis E virus is an important cause of sporadic and epidemic acute hepatitis in parts of Asia. Transmission is by the faecal–oral route, mainly through contamination of water supplies. Sexual transmission is not thought to contribute substantially. Limited epidemiological studies do not suggest that either homosexual men or drug users are at increased risk.

Hepatitis G virus (also identified as GB virus type C) is related to HCV. While it is certainly transmissible by blood and blood products, and is associated with persistent viraemia, it is less clear to what extent it is a cause of acute or chronic hepatitis.

Epidemiological studies are required to determine the contribution of hepatitis G to chronic viral hepatitis in homosexual men and injecting drug users.

Epstein–Barr virus and cytomegalovirus infection

Either may cause abnormality of liver function tests in association with a glandular fever syndrome. Clinical hepatitis due to either virus is rare, despite the high seroprevalence of cytomegalovirus infection among homosexual men (typically 90 to 95 per cent compared to 50 to 60 per cent in age-matched heterosexual controls).

Other causes of liver disease in drug users and homosexual men

The prevalence of abnormal liver function tests and liver histology in drug users is high, typically 50 to 60 per cent.[3] Infection with HBV, HAV, HDV, Epstein–Barr virus or cytomegalovirus contributes, but most is caused by hepatitis C. Alcohol abuse is common and may exacerbate other causes of liver disease (Novick, AlcoholClinExpRes, 1986; 10:500). A variety of drugs and toxins have also been implicated.

Experimental studies in animals and man have not shown a direct hepatotoxic effect of morphine. Studies of cocaine in mice have shown several patterns of liver injury, including periportal and multizonal necrosis, the former being seen after both acute and chronic administration. Acute, fatal hepatotoxicity has been observed in man following cocaine use. The histological appearances include zone-1 necrosis and well-demarcated zone-3 necrosis indistinguishable from paracetamol poisoning (Wanless, Gastro, 1990; 98:497). Acute hepatitis related to the use of the stimulant drug 'ecstasy' (3,4-methylenedioxymethamphetamine, MDMA) has also been reported (Skopp, DeutschMedWoch, 1995; 120:1165).

Intercurrent hepatitis

A common clinical problem is the diagnosis of an episode of intercurrent hepatitis (Table 1). Patients with chronic hepatitis may suffer episodes in which the results of liver function tests show deterioration, with or without associated symptoms of acute hepatitis. The clinical history may indicate whether the patient has been at risk of acquiring a new infection, for example by needle sharing, sexual exposure, or travel to an endemic area. The cause of pre-existing chronic hepatitis is important. An HBeAg-positive hepatitis B carrier may present with an intercurrent hepatitis preceding seroconversion to anti-HBe. HCV infection is more commonly associated with spontaneous relapses and remissions, possibly related to fluctuations in viral replication.

Interactions between HIV and hepatitis virus infections

The routes of transmission of HBV and HCV are shared by HIV (sexual, parenteral, perinatal), although the relative efficiencies of transmission differ. Dual infection with HIV and HBV is common in homosexual men and heterosexuals, especially in sub-Saharan Africa and Asia, and in the new-born of HIV-infected women. Injecting drug users and recipients of blood products are more likely

Table 1 Causes of intercurrent hepatitis

HBV carrier (HBeAg + ve)	HBeAg to anti-HBe seroconversion
HBV carrier (HBeAg − ve)	Reactivation to HBeAg + ve from HBeAg − ve
Chronic hepatitis	Exacerbation or progression of chronic liver disease
New infection	Any cause of acute hepatitis in susceptible individuals
Drugs	e.g. ketoconazole, antituberculous drugs, antidepressants
Toxins	Alcohol
HIV infection	Any cause of HIV-related liver disease (see text)
Other sexually transmitted diseases	e.g. rare complication of syphilis
Other causes of chronic hepatitis	e.g. autoimmune chronic hepatitis

to have coinfection with HIV and HCV. Important interactions may occur (Table 2).

The prevalence of HBV markers in HIV-positive homosexual men and drug users is higher than in HIV-negative controls. A high prevalence of HIV infection has been reported in patients with acute hepatitis B.[21] This is consistent with these infections having common risk factors, such as unprotected sex with multiple homosexual partners, and sharing injecting equipment, which predispose to HBV as well as HIV infection. It is possible that an increased susceptibility to acute HBV infection may exist in HIV-infected patients, but this has not been proved.

HBV and the immune system

HBV infects lymphocytes of both the CD4 + (helper-inducer) and CD8 + (suppressor-cytotoxic) subgroups (Laure, BrJHaemat, 1987; 65:181). A decrease in CD4 counts in peripheral blood accompanied by a reduction in autologous mixed-lymphocyte reactions was demonstrated in HBeAg-positive HBV carriers (Mazzetti, AmJGastr, 1987; 82:130), although HIV coinfection was not excluded in this study. Another study found lowered CD4:CD8 ratios due to increased numbers of CD8 cells (Novick, JHepatol, 1986; 3:363). Whether these changes are specifically related to HBV infection or could be associated with concomitant herpesvirus infection in homosexual men is not certain. If such an effect exists, the course of HIV disease might be affected. However, studies of the determinants of HIV disease progression have not identified hepatitis B as an independent predictor of the rate of progression.

Table 2 Interactions between infection with HIV and HBV

↓ HBV attack rate because of changing behaviour
↑ Rate of chronic carriage following acute infection
↑ Infectivity of HBV carriers
↓ Rate of spontaneous clearance of HBeAg
↓ Hepatic inflammatory activity in HBV carriers
↓ Response rate to hepatitis B vaccine
↑ Loss of natural and vaccine-induced antibodies
↓ Response to antiviral treatment
? Effect on risk of cirrhosis and hepatocellular carcinoma

A cytotoxic T-cell response to HBV core proteins in hepatocytes is important in the hepatic parenchymal inflammatory response to HBV replication. Pre-existing HIV infection would be expected to modify this response. This would explain the effect of HIV infection on the rate of chronicity after infection with HBV. Twenty per cent of HIV-infected adults become chronic carriers compared to 5 per cent or less of HIV-uninfected patients.[22,23]

It is not known whether HIV infection affects the incidence of fulminant hepatitis B. Immunosuppression might be expected to reduce the severity of immune-mediated liver-cell death but higher levels of virus replication might have an opposite effect.

Effect of HIV on the chronic carrier state

In chronic HBV carriers, HIV coinfection is associated with lower transaminase activities and less severe hepatitis histologically.[24–27] Markers of HBV replication, including serum HBV-DNA polymerase activity and HBV DNA, are higher in HBeAg-positive patients with HIV infection. In addition there is increased hepatocyte HBcAg and HBeAg. Therefore despite higher levels of viral replication, the associated liver disease may be less severe.

There are conflicting reports on the effect of HIV infection on the natural history of HBV replication as determined by the rate of spontaneous loss of HBeAg or serum HBV DNA. One study[26] showed a significantly lower rate of clearance of HBV DNA in HIV-infected carriers (4 per cent vs 20 per cent), but only a trend towards a lower rate of loss of HBeAg. Of the more recent larger studies using survival analysis methods, one failed to show an effect of HIV on loss of HBeAg (Loke, Gut, 1988; 29:A1464), while two others have shown a reduction from 12 to 5 per cent per year.[27,28] Concomitant HIV infection, by prolonging the HBeAg-positive state, extends the period of high infectivity. Consistent with this is the observation that HIV-infected HBV carriers have a decreased response rate to antiviral therapy.[29]

The list of variables that may affect the spontaneous decrease in productive viral replication and loss of HBeAg now includes HIV infection, ethnic origin, length of infection, sex, perhaps sexual orientation, degree of hepatitis inflammatory activity, level of pre-existing HBV replication, intercurrent hepatotropic virus infection, and corticosteroid treatment.[30]

The effect of HIV on the longer-term sequelae of HBV infection is not known. The reduction in hepatic inflammatory activity could reduce the risk of endstage liver disease and hepatocellular carcinoma, but HIV infection is associated with an increased risk of several malignancies. Such considerations become more relevant as the survival of patients with HIV infection improves, including some long-term survivors with well-preserved immunological functions (Learmont, Lancet, 1992; 340:863).

HIV and HBV reactivation

HIV-infected homosexual men and drug users are at risk of reactivation of HBV infection. HBV carriers who have anti-HBe may revert to HBeAg-positivity, usually associated with a rise in transaminases and occasionally symptoms of acute hepatitis.[3,21, 26] Spontaneous reactivation is rare in the absence of immunosuppression. Reactivation also occurs in patients who have become immune to hepatitis B by conventional criteria, with the development of anti-HBs. Loss of detectable anti-HBs is accelerated by HIV (Biggar, NEJM, 1987; 316:630). As with reactivation in HBV carriers, the reappearance of active viral replication, HBsAg- and HBeAg-seropositivity may occur without symptoms or be accompanied by a severe, even fatal, hepatitis (Lazizi, JInfDis, 1988; 158:666; Vento, Lancet, 1989; i:332). Some patients never develop a detectable anti-HBs response after recovery from acute infection. Reactivation of HBV infection or reinfection by an HBV strain with a different HBsAg subtype may occur in patients with anti-HBc as their only HBV serological marker.[31]

Interaction between HIV and HCV infection

Patients coinfected with HIV and HCV have higher rates of HCV replication, measured by the amounts of HCV RNA in serum, than patients with HCV alone (Cribier, AIDS, 1995; 9:1131). Their antibody responses are also diminished. More HIV-coinfected patients have indeterminate test results for HCV antibody; rarely there is no detectable antibody response. HCV RNA rises after HIV seroconversion and increases as CD4 counts decline (Eyster, Blood, 1994; 84:1020). There may also be an increased rate of progression of HCV-related liver disease in HIV-infected patients: this has been observed principally in HCV-HIV coinfected haemophiliacs (Eyster, JAIDS, 1993; 6:602), although further controlled studies are required.

HIV infection affects the rate of transmission of HCV infection. Among pregnant women the reported risk of vertical transmission of HCV to their child is in the range of 0 to 20 per cent. HIV-HCV coinfected mothers have a higher rate of transmission in all studies, although the absolute rate is still uncertain due to the small size of the population samples. No transmissions were found among 94 babies of mothers with HCV alone, but 36 per cent (8 of 22) among HIV-coinfected mothers.[32] There is also evidence of a greater risk of sexual transmission of HCV when the source partner is HIV coinfected. In a study of sexual partners, 9.2 per cent of the partners of HIV-coinfected patients were HCV infected compared with 4.1 per cent of the partners of HIV-uninfected patients (Lissen, EurJClinMicrobInfDis, 1993; 12:827). Homosexual contacts are more likely to be infected than heterosexual contacts according to a study in the United States.[33] HCV infection does not affect the

rate of progression of HIV infection (Dorrucci, JInfDis, 1995; 172: 1503).

Treatment of chronic hepatitis B and C in HIV-coinfected patients

HBeAg-positive HBV carriers, including those coinfected with HIV, may be considered for treatment with α-interferon. Most clinical trials of interferon have excluded HIV-coinfected patients, after early indications that they were less likely to respond and to simplify the interpretation of the trial results. There are therefore few data to inform treatment decisions in coinfected patients. A review from one centre of factors associated with response to a variety of agents including interferon (Novick, Hepatol, 1984; 1:29) suggested that homosexual men were less likely to respond. None had AIDS, but the study predated the availability of HIV antibody tests. A study of adenine arabinoside monophosphate found no difference in response between heterosexual and homosexual patients (Marcellin, Hepatol, 1989; 10:328). Several small studies have shown that HBeAg to anti-HBe seroconversion may occur with interferon treatment in HIV-coinfected patients, but larger studies indicate that the response rate is low (di Martino, JViral-Hepat, 1996; 3:253). In a dose-comparison study of interferon in which 38 of 43 subjects were homosexual men, none of the 14 HIV-infected patients lost HBeAg with treatment whereas 33 per cent of the HIV-uninfected control group did (McDonald, Hepatol, 1987; 7:719). In another study of 50 patients, half of whom were HIV infected, seroconversion was seen in 1 of 12 HIV-infected and 5 of 13 HIV-uninfected patients treated, compared to none of 12 and 1 of 12 untreated controls, respectively (Wong, Gastro, 1995; 108: 165). The study groups were small and the difference in response rate between HIV-infected and HIV-uninfected patients was not significant (the response rate in the HIV-infected group was no better than in the untreated control group). Adverse effects of interferon in HIV-infected patients have not differed from those seen in HIV-uninfected patients. However, a combination of interferon with zidovudine for the treatment of HIV disease was poorly tolerated, with anaemia and neutropenia being the most common problems.

Although interferon is currently the only licensed treatment for chronic hepatitis B, patients coinfected with HIV may be given antiretroviral treatments that have activity against HBV infection. Lamivudine (3TC), the (−)-enantiomer of 3′-thiacytidine, a nucleoside analogue in use for the treatment of HIV infection, also suppresses HBV replication (Dienstag, NEJM, 1995; 333:1657). Among HIV-infected patients, few seroconvert (from HBeAg-positive to anti-HBe-positive) after a short course of treatment with lamivudine, but higher seroconversion rates may be obtained with longer treatment (Benhamou, Lancet, 1995; 345:396). Whether lamivudine-containing antiretroviral combinations should be used routinely in HIV-coinfected patients is not known. Other antiretroviral nucleoside analogues currently in use do not have appreciable activity against HBV. Adefovir dipivoxil is an adenine nucleotide analogue that is being given in phase III studies to examine its antiretroviral and antiherpesvirus activity. A phase II study in HBeAg-positive HBV carriers suggests that it is active in both HIV-uninfected and HIV-infected patients (Gilson, Hepatol, 1996; 24:281A). Other agents active against herpesviruses have activity against HBV. Famciclovir is used in the treatment and prophylaxis of herpes simplex infections and has activity against HBV, and ganciclovir, licensed for the treatment of cytomegalovirus disease, also has some anti-HBV activity.

The response rate to interferon in chronic hepatitis C in HIV-coinfected patients is lower than the response seen in HIV-uninfected patients. Again, few HIV-coinfected patients have been treated in trials. Treatment may be considered most appropriate in patients with progressive liver disease and preserved immune function. None of the current range of antiretroviral agents has activity against HCV.

Prevention of viral hepatitis

Hepatitis B vaccine offers the hope of eliminating hepatitis B as an infectious disease among homosexual men and drug users. In the first 5 years of its availability there was no impact on the recorded incidence of HBV infection in the United States.[34] Although the majority of cases in the United States occur in homosexual men, drug users, and heterosexual contacts, it has been estimated that less than 15 per cent of the doses of vaccine reached these groups. The first vaccine was purified HBsAg obtained from the sera of HBV carriers. It was expensive and its supply limited. In most parts of the world it has been replaced by synthetic HBsAg vaccines made by recombinant yeast technology. Even when the cost of vaccine was high, a study in the United Kingdom showed that it would be cost-effective to vaccinate homosexual men because of the reduction in health-care and other costs related to acute hepatitis.[35] This study did not include the costs associated with the late sequelae of infection. A study in the United States also indicated a reduction in health-care costs.[36] Despite this, the coverage with this vaccine has been slow to gain momentum (Loke, BMJ, 1989; 298:234). It is questionable whether a targeted vaccine policy, as is still operated in some countries including the United Kingdom, can achieve sufficient coverage to reduce substantially HBV infection rates. In many countries, particularly those with high prevalence rates for HBV, a policy of universal immunization of infants is being promoted with additional support from the World Health Organization. Adolescent immunization is being given in some countries to provide an earlier impact on adult infection rates. In all regions, immunization of high-risk adult groups such as homosexual men and drug users is recommended.

The incidence rate of HBV infection has fallen in recent years in most developed countries. In homosexual men the fall is probably due to changes in behaviour since the beginning of the HIV epidemic. The effect of HIV in prolonging the period of high infectivity could reverse this trend. In addition, the response to the vaccine is diminished in HIV-positive patients, with both a reduction in the proportion responding and in the mean titre of anti-HBs. The proportion with at least 10 iu (international units)/l of anti-HBs is reduced from 90–95 per cent, as observed in the early studies,[37] to around 50 per cent (Carne, BrMedJClinRes, 1987; 294:866; Collier, AnnIntMed, 1988; 109:101).

Hepatitis A vaccines are available that, in contrast to passive immunization with immunoglobulin, provide long-term protection. The vaccines, which are inactivated, whole-virus preparations, are highly immunogenic and offer high levels of protection. The development of multivalent vaccines combining HBV and HAV immunogens may lead to wider use, but the routine immunization of homosexual men or injecting drug users against HAV infection has not been promoted. There is a stronger case for immunizing chronic carriers of hepatitis B or hepatitis C against HAV infection to prevent an acute hepatitis on a background of chronic liver disease.

There is no hepatitis C vaccine available yet, and no evidence for protection by passive immunization.

An important component of prevention strategies for all types of viral hepatitis is risk reduction by appropriate health education. This is also essential for the prevention of HIV transmission. For injecting drug users, advice on safe injecting practices must include the importance of not sharing filters and other equipment as well as needles and syringes. Needle-exchange schemes can have an important role in helping to reduce the risk of infection, and provide an opportunity for health education and access to other services.

Liver disease in HIV/AIDS

Liver disease occurs commonly in patients with HIV disease but is usually seen when patients already have a diagnosis of AIDS or other serious HIV-related complications. The disease process may be complex with several components, including pre-existing disease such as chronic viral hepatitis, the side-effects of multiple drug therapy, the effects of systemic disease and malnutrition, and parenchymal or biliary, AIDS-related opportunistic infections or neoplasms. In one series of 1800 patients seen in an HIV clinic, 18 per cent had evidence of liver dysfunction; viral hepatitis and alcohol-related liver disease were the most common diagnoses (Fortgang, AmJGastr, 1995; 90:1433).

A better understanding of liver disorders in AIDS may contribute to our knowledge of hepatic disease mechanisms in general, particularly in the area of the balance between the direct pathogenicity of organisms and the host immune response.

Clinical features and investigation

The most common syndrome is one of fever, hepatomegaly, and abnormal liver function tests. Pain in the right upper quadrant in this context tends to occur in those with biliary disease, as discussed below. Splenomegaly is a feature of HIV infection and therefore may not reflect portal hypertension.

Serological tests for hepatitis viruses should be performed on all patients. Ultrasonography may detect enlargement of the liver due to parenchymal disease or infiltration, or the dilatation of the intra- or extrahepatic biliary tree found in sclerosing cholangitis (further investigated by endoscopic retrograde cholangiopancreatography). Filling defects may be due to tumours such as Kaposi sarcoma, or to abscess formation. Enlarged lymph nodes may be part of the persistent, generalized lymphadenopathy of HIV infection, or due to infection, particularly by mycobacteria, or infiltration by Kaposi sarcoma or lymphoma.

Liver biopsy in patients with abnormal liver function tests may result in the diagnosis of a specific infection in up to 60 per cent of cases. The most common finding is mycobacterial disease caused by *Mycobacterium avium-intracellulare* (Cappell, AmJMed, 1990; 88: 123).

Differential diagnosis of liver disease in HIV/AIDS

Granulomatous hepatitis

The most common histological finding in AIDS patients undergoing liver biopsy is a granulomatous hepatitis for which the two principal causes are atypical mycobacteria and drugs.[38]

Mycobacteria

Atypical mycobacteria of the *M. avium-intracellulare* complex are the most common opportunistic organisms to be identified on liver biopsy.[39,40] Their presence is usually associated with fever, night sweats, and weight loss, as well as elevated serum alkaline phosphatase and transaminases, with or without hepatomegaly. Liver biopsy will confirm the diagnosis in almost all cases (Plate 1); however, this is usually a disseminated infection and examination and culture of bone marrow, lymph-node aspirates or blood will often give the diagnosis, avoiding the need for liver biopsy. Granuloma formation is often scanty, so examination of smears and culture of biopsy tissue is essential. Response to treatment, particularly in patients with advanced disease, is often poor, and maintenance therapy is required to prevent relapse.

There is also an increased incidence of *M. tuberculosis* among HIV-infected patients, particularly drug users and patients from developing countries. Extrapulmonary disease is more common than in HIV-uninfected patients. Tuberculosis has been added to the latest surveillance case definition of AIDS.[41] Response to treatment is good but maintenance treatment may be required and the frequency of drug reactions is high compared to HIV-uninfected patients (Soriano, AIDS, 1988; 2:429; Chaisson, JInfDis, 1989; 159: 96).

Drugs

Sulphonamides are some of the most widely used drugs in patients with HIV infection. High-dose intravenous co-trimoxazole is used to treat *Pneumocystis carinii* pneumonia; low-dose oral co-trimoxazole is used in primary and secondary prophylaxis. Sulphadiazine with pyrimethamine are used in the treatment of toxoplasmosis, the most common cause of a space-occupying cerebral lesion. Adverse reactions to sulphonamides usually occur after about 10 days of high-dose treatment, when there is persistence or recrudescence of fever and a generalized erythematous eruption. If the liver is involved there is an increase in aminotransferases, with or without a rise in alkaline phosphatase. Histologically there are granulomas, but in contrast with *M. avium-intracellulare* infection, no organisms are found and there are more eosinophils in the infiltrate.

Antituberculous drugs, particularly isoniazid and rifampicin, may cause abnormal liver function tests, the former being associated with granuloma formation.

Other infections

Infection with *Cryptococcus neoformans*, *Histoplasma capsulatum*, and *Leishmania donovani* may cause a granulomatous hepatitis. Granulomatous hepatitis has been described in association with hepatic infection by the microsporidian protozoa *Encephalitozoon*

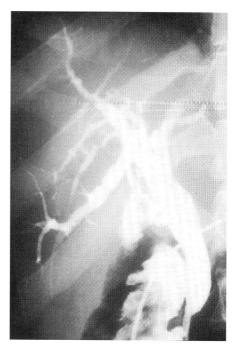

Fig. 1. AIDS sclerosing cholangitis: endoscopic retrograde cholangiopancreatogram showing dilated common bile duct with a stricture at the lower end and irregularities of both extra- and intrahepatic ducts.

cuniculi (Terada, AnnIntMed, 1987; 107:61). Hepatitis associated with disseminated pneumocystosis has been reported occasionally in AIDS patients and may cause a chronic hepatitis with raised alkaline phosphatase (Poblete, AnnIntMed, 1989; 110:737; Merkel, JClinGastro, 1992; 15:55).

Biliary disease

In patients presenting with any combination of pain in the right upper quadrant, fever, and elevated serum alkaline phosphatase, a diagnosis of AIDS sclerosing cholangitis should be considered.[42]

Biliary disease was first described in AIDS in 1984, when cytomegalovirus, cryptosporidia, and campylobacter were identified in the gallbladders of AIDS patients with acalculous cholecystitis (Blumberg, AmJMed, 1984; 76:1118). Reports followed of patients with abdominal pain and raised alkaline phosphatase who had cholangiographic appearances similar to those of primary sclerosing cholangitis (Margulis, AnnIntMed, 1986; 105:634). In contrast to primary sclerosing cholangitis, dilatation of the common bile duct may be a feature, and pain was more, and jaundice less, frequent. AIDS sclerosing cholangitis may present as a painless cholestasis or an acute bacterial cholangitis.

In a series of 26 AIDS patients[43] with clinical and biochemical features of AIDS sclerosing cholangitis, 20 (77 per cent) had cholangiographic abnormalities. There were four patterns of abnormality: sclerosing cholangitis with papillary stenosis (50 per cent), papillary stenosis alone (15 per cent), intrahepatic sclerosing cholangitis alone (20 per cent), and long strictures of the extrahepatic bile duct with or without intrahepatic abnormalities (15 per cent) (Fig. 1).

Endoscopic sphincterotomy has relieved pain in some cases, suggesting that it might be related to duct hypertension and/or dysfunction of the sphincter of Oddi, similar to 'biliary dyskinesia'. Computed tomography and ultrasonography often demonstrate biliary dilatation and thickening of the bile duct and/or gallbladder wall, which may be considerable. Histological studies on material taken *in vivo* or at autopsy show deep, focal, mucosal ulceration with chronic inflammation. Liver biopsy may reveal portal fibrosis with distorted interlobular bile ducts, sparse evidence of a lymphocytic inflammatory infiltrate, and bile-duct abnormalities including paucity in number, intraepithelial lymphocytic deposits, and epithelial nuclear and cytoplasmic abnormalities.

The cause of AIDS sclerosing cholangitis is not known, but it seems likely that an opportunistic infection is involved. Cases of sclerosing cholangitis with associated cryptosporidiosis have been documented in patients with other forms of immunodeficiency (Davis, AmJGastr, 1987; 82:1196). Infection of the biliary and pancreatic ducts by cryptosporidia has also been documented in animals. The organism does not invade the mucosa so, as with small-bowel cryptosporidiosis, the mechanism of any injury is unknown. Cytomegalovirus and/or cryptosporidia have been present in most patients in the reported series of AIDS sclerosing cholangitis: 75 per cent have had evidence of intestinal cryptosporidial infection and 62 per cent cytomegalovirus infection. Cytomegalovirus and cryptosporidia have been found in the gallbladders of some AIDS patients with acute acalculous cholecystitis. Cytomegalovirus is thought to be involved in some cases of posttransplant biliary stricturing (Martineau, Surgery, 1972; 72:604) and it has been detected periductally at autopsy in some cases of AIDS sclerosing cholangitis.

There is conflicting evidence for the role of a double-stranded RNA virus, reovirus type 3, in some cases of neonatal extrahepatic biliary atresia and neonatal hepatitis. It has been suggested that this agent may also be implicated in AIDS sclerosing cholangitis but this has not been confirmed. A syndrome of cholestasis and hepatitis in early infancy associated with perinatally acquired HIV infection has been described; the aetiology is not known.[44]

Other causes of hepatitis in AIDS

Drugs

AIDS patients are often exposed to polypharmacy in order to treat and prevent the numerous manifestations of their disease. The physician should be aware of the altered pharmacokinetics that results from underlying chronic viral hepatitis, the drugs that may cause liver disease, and the potential for drug interactions.[45] Drugs causing granulomatous hepatitis have been discussed already. Co-trimoxazole, as well as causing a granulomatous hepatitis due to the sulphonamide component, may be associated with an intrahepatic cholestasis due to either the sulphonamide or the trimethoprim components. There is a report of fatal fulminant hepatitis as part of the 'sulfone syndrome' (fever, rash, haemolytic anaemia, hepatitis) associated with dapsone therapy in an HIV-infected woman (Chalasani, SouthMedJ, 1994; 87:1145). Ketoconazole is used as systemic treatment for oesophageal and recurrent oral candidiasis. It may cause a hepatitis with elevation of transaminases, and less commonly a pure cholestasis.[46,47] Hepatitis appears to be less common with fluconazole. Abnormalities of liver function tests have also been reported with intravenous pentamidine used to treat *Pneumocystis carinii* pneumonia.

Antiretroviral therapy with nucleoside analogues has been associated with signs of hepatotoxicity. In one report an acute cholestatic hepatitis developed in a patient taking zidovudine and recurred when the patient was rechallenged (Dubin, AnnIntMed, 1989; 110:85). The mechanism is not known but studies on rats have confirmed hepatic toxicity related to the duration of treatment (Corcuera, PatholResPract, 1996; 192:182). Zidovudine is metabolized to the glucuronide, and in patients with chronic liver disease this is reduced, which may lead to increased toxicity (Bareggi, JClinPharm, 1994; 34:782). Similarly, abnormal liver function tests were described in phase I studies of dideoxyinosine (DDI) and subsequently, cases of fulminant hepatitis with lactic acidosis were reported (Bissuel, JIntMed, 1994; 235:367). Hepatic toxicity, characterized by asymptomatic elevation of aminotransferases, has been described in patients taking stavudine.[48]

Unexplained abnormalities of liver function tests, usually without symptoms, are found in HIV-infected patients. A diversity of histological features has been described but no specific, HIV-induced hepatic disorder identified.

Cytomegalovirus

Antibodies to cytomegalovirus are present in almost all AIDS patients. Like other herpesviruses, cytomegalovirus causes latent infection and most episodes of disease in patients with AIDS are caused by reactivation, usually when immunosuppression is advanced (CD4 count $<50–100 \times 10^6/l$). The difficulty is to establish whether cytomegalovirus is the cause of disease. The finding of cytomegalovirus in cultures of urine, throat swabs, and biopsies from the gastrointestinal tract is common in AIDS patients, even without clinical features of cytomegalovirus disease. Cytomegalovirus inclusions on liver histology, together with abnormal liver function tests, and without evidence of another cause of hepatitis, are taken as confirmation of the diagnosis.

Hepatitis viruses

These should always be considered as a cause of acute or chronic hepatitis in patients with HIV disease. However, acute HBV infection is uncommon in patients with AIDS. Most will have already been exposed or no longer at risk. Reactivation can occur, as discussed above.

HDV infection should be considered in exacerbations of chronic hepatitis B, particularly in drug users, but in this group, chronic HCV infection, as discussed above, remains the more common problem.

Liver tumours

Kaposi sarcoma

The majority of cases of Kaposi sarcoma are diagnosed by the appearance of typical skin lesions (Plate 2). Endoscopic and radiographic studies suggest that the gastrointestinal tract is also affected in about 40 per cent of cases at the time of diagnosis. It is not known what proportion have liver involvement at first diagnosis. Analysis of a series of liver biopsies carried out because of fever, hepatomegaly, or elevated liver function tests, or a combination of these, revealed a few cases of hepatic Kaposi sarcoma but cutaneous lesions are usually present (Plate 3). At autopsy, liver involvement is found to be more common but lesions are also present elsewhere. It seems likely that sampling error accounts for a proportion of the negative liver biopsies in patients with extensive cutaneous disease. Liver function tests usually show abnormality of both alkaline phosphatase and transaminases. Systemic chemotherapy with cytotoxic agents or interferon is used in patients with extensive visceral or cutaneous disease, but liver involvement is unlikely to be the deciding factor in either choice of treatment or outcome.

Lymphoma

HIV infection is associated with an excess of cases of non-Hodgkin's lymphoma and to a lesser extent also Hodgkin's disease. The non-Hodgkin's lymphoma characteristic of AIDS is of intermediate or high-grade, B-cell type. Unlike non-Hodgkin's lymphoma in other patients, extranodal disease is very common: 74 per cent in one series, with 31 per cent being extranodal only.[40,49] After the central nervous system and bone marrow, the gut and liver are the most common extranodal sites involved. Non-Hodgkin's lymphoma may be the presenting feature of HIV disease or occur in patients with a preceding diagnosis of AIDS (27 of 84 patients in one series). Lymphoma has been described affecting the liver alone without evidence of disease elsewhere.

Patients usually present with fever, anaemia, and an extranodal mass, or rapidly increasing or asymmetrical lymphadenopathy. Most cases are diagnosed by biopsy of a lymph node, extranodal mass, or bone marrow. The prognosis for non-Hodgkin's lymphoma in AIDS is poor, with a median survival of 3 to 6 months. There is a wide variation, however, with better survival in patients with nodal disease alone and good immune status with high CD4+ counts. The optimal therapy has not been established, but most patients are given chemotherapy, which in about 50 per cent will obtain an initial response.[50,51]

Involvement of the biliary tract is rare in non-Hodgkin's lymphoma. One report described non-Hodgkin's lymphoma mimicking sclerosing cholangitis in a patient without a preceding diagnosis of AIDS, who presented with fever, intermittent jaundice, and pain in the right upper quadrant (Kaplan, AnnIntMed, 1989; 110:161). Histological examination of the common bile duct revealed a small, non-cleaved-cell lymphoma.

References

1. Schreeder MT, *et al*. Hepatitis B in homosexual men: prevalence of infection and factors related to transmission. *Journal of Infectious Diseases*, 1982; **146**: 7–15.
2. Szmuness W, *et al*. On the role of sexual behavior in the spread of hepatitis B infection. *Annals of Internal Medicine*, 1975; **83**: 489–95.
3. Weller IV, *et al*. Clinical, biochemical, serological, histological and ultrastructural features of liver disease in drug abusers. *Gut*, 1984; **25**: 417–23.
4. Widell A, Hansson BG, Moestrup T, Serleus Z, Mathiesen LR, and Johnsson T. Acute hepatitis A, B and non-A, non-B in a Swedish community studied over a ten-year period. *Scandinavian Journal of Infectious Diseases*, 1982; **14**: 253–9.
5. Widell A, Hansson BG, Moestrup T, and Nordenfelt E. Increased occurrence of hepatitis A with cyclic outbreaks among drug addicts in a Swedish community. *Infection*, 1983; **11**: 198–200.
6. Centers for Disease Control. Hepatitis A among drug abusers. *Morbidity and Mortality Weekly Reports*, 1988; **37**: 297–305.
7. Raimondo G, Smedile A, Gallo L, Balbo A, Ponzetto A, and Rizzetto M. Multicentre study of prevalence of HBV-associated delta infection and liver disease in drug-addicts. *Lancet*, 1982; i: 249–51.
8. Centers for Disease Control. Delta hepatitis—Massachusetts. *Morbidity and Mortality Weekly Reports*, 1984; **33**: 493–4.
9. Buti M, *et al*. Epidemiology of delta infection in Spain. *Journal of Medical Virology*, 1988; **26**: 327–32.
10. de Miguel J, Collazos J, Mayo J, Lopez de Goicoechea MJ, Echaniz C, and Mendarte U. Seroprevalence of delta virus and hepatitis C virus in patients with chronic infection with hepatitis B virus. *Revista Clínica Española*, 1994; **194**: 897–900.
11. Navascues CA, *et al*. Epidemiology of hepatitis D virus infection: changes in the last 14 years. *American Journal of Gastroenterology*, 1995; **90**: 1981–4.
12. Coppola RC, Manconi PE, Piro R, Di Martino ML, and Masia G. HCV, HIV, HBV and HDV infections in intravenous drug addicts. *European Journal of Epidemiology*, 1994; **10**: 279–83.
13. Smith HM, Alexander GJ, Webb G, McManus T, McFarlane IG, and Williams R. Hepatitis B and delta virus infection among 'at risk' populations in south east London. *Journal of Epidemiology and Community Health*, 1992; **46**: 144–7.
14. Liaw YF, Chiu KW, Chu CM, Sheen IS, and Huang MJ. Heterosexual transmission of hepatitis delta virus in the general population of an area endemic for hepatitis B virus infection: a prospective study. *Journal of Infectious Diseases*, 1990; **162**: 1170–2.
15. Wu JC, *et al*. Sexual transmission of hepatitis D virus infection in Taiwan. *Hepatology*, 1990; **11**: 1057–61.
16. Weller IV, *et al*. Significance of delta agent infection in chronic hepatitis B virus infection: a study in British carriers. *Gut*, 1983; **24**: 1061–3.
17. Leon P, Lopez JA, Contreras G, and Echevarria JM. Antibodies to hepatitis delta virus in intravenous drug addicts and male homosexuals in Spain. *European Journal of Clinical Microbiology and Infectious Diseases*, 1988; **7**: 533–5.
18. Hess G, Bienzle U, Slusarczyk J, Hansson BG, and Meyer zum Buschenfelde KH. Hepatitis B virus and delta infection in male homosexuals. *Liver*, 1986; **6**: 13–6.
19. Alter MJ. Community acquired viral hepatitis B and C in the United States. *Gut*, 1993; **34**: S17–19.
20. Alter MJ, *et al*. Risk factors for acute non-A, non-B hepatitis in the United States and association with hepatitis C virus infection. *Journal of the American Medical Association*, 1990; **264**: 2231–5.
21. Arendrup M, Lindhardt BO, Krogsgaard K, Gaub J, and Nielsen JO. Antibody to HIV in patients with acute hepatitis B in the period 1975–1984. *Scandinavian Journal of Infectious Diseases*, 1987; **19**: 167–72.
22. Hadler SC, *et al*. Outcome of hepatitis B virus infection in homosexual men and its relation to prior human immunodeficiency virus infection. *Journal of Infectious Diseases*, 1991; **163**: 454–9.
23. Bodsworth NJ, Cooper DA, and Donovan B. The influence of human immunodeficiency virus type 1 infection on the development of the hepatitis B virus carrier state. *Journal of Infectious Diseases*, 1991; **163**: 1138–40.
24. Rustgi VK, *et al*. Hepatitis B virus infection in the acquired immunodeficiency syndrome. *Annals of Internal Medicine*, 1984; **101**: 795–7.
25. Perrillo RP, Regenstein FG, and Roodman ST. Chronic hepatitis B in asymptomatic homosexual men with antibody to the human immunodeficiency virus. *Annals of Internal Medicine*, 1986; **105**: 382–3.
26. Krogsgaard K, *et al*. The influence of HTLV-III infection on the natural history of hepatitis B virus infection in male homosexual HBsAg carriers. *Hepatology*, 1987; **7**: 37–41.
27. Bodsworth N, Donovan B, and Nightingale BN. The effect of concurrent human immunodeficiency virus infection on chronic hepatitis B: a study of 150 homosexual men. *Journal of Infectious Diseases*, 1989; **160**: 577–82.
28. Gilson RJC, *et al*. Interactions between human immunodeficiency virus and hepatitis B virus in homosexual men: effects on the natural history of infection. *AIDS*, 1997; **11**: 597–606.
29. Lane HC. Interferons in HIV and related diseases. *AIDS*, 1994; **8** (Suppl. 3): S19–23.

30. Weller IV, *et al.* Spontaneous loss of HBeAg and the prevalence of HTLV-III/LAV infection in a cohort of homosexual hepatitis B virus carriers and the implications for antiviral therapy. *Journal of Hepatology*, 1986; **3** (Suppl. 2): S9–16.

31. Waite J, *et al.* Hepatitis B virus reactivation or reinfection associated with HIV-1 infection. *AIDS*, 1988; **2**: 443–8.

32. Zanetti AR *et al.* Mother-to-infant transmission of hepatitis C virus. Lombardy Study Group on Vertical HCV Transmission. [See Comments]. *Lancet*, 1995; **345**: 289–91.

33. Thomas DL, *et al.* Sexual transmission of hepatitis C virus among patients attending sexually transmitted diseases clinics in Baltimore—an analysis of 309 sex partnerships. *Journal of Infectious Diseases*, 1995; **171**: 768–75.

34. Centers for Disease Control. Update on hepatitis B prevention. *Morbidity and Mortality Weekly Reports*, 1987; **36**: 353–60; 366.

35. Adler MW, Belsey EM, McCutchan JA, and Mindel A. Should homosexuals be vaccinated against hepatitis B virus? Cost and benefit assessment. *British Medical Journal*, 1983; **286**: 1621–4.

36. Mulley AG, Silverstein MD, and Dienstag JL. Indications for use of hepatitis B vaccine, based on cost-effectiveness analysis. *New England Journal of Medicine*, 1982; **307**: 644–52.

37. Szmuness W, *et al.* Hepatitis B vaccine: demonstration of efficacy in a controlled clinical trial in a high-risk population in the United States. *New England Journal of Medicine*, 1980; **303**: 833–41.

38. Lebovics E, Dworkin BM, Heier SK, and Rosenthal WS. The hepatobiliary manifestations of human immunodeficiency virus infection. *American Journal of Gastroenterology*, 1988; **83**: 1–7.

39. Orenstein MS, *et al.* Granulomatous involvement of the liver in patients with AIDS. *Gut*, 1985; **26**: 1220–5.

40. Kahn SA, Saltzman BR, Klein RS, Mahadevia PS, Friedland GH, and Brandt LJ. Hepatic disorders in the acquired immune deficiency syndrome: a clinical and pathological study. *American Journal of Gastroenterology*, 1986; **81**: 1145–8.

41. Centers for Disease Control. 1993 revised classification system for HIV infection and expanded surveillance case definition for AIDS among adolescents and adults. *Morbidity and Mortality Weekly Reports*, 1992; **41**: 1–19.

42. Dowsett JF, *et al.* Sclerosing cholangitis in acquired immunodeficiency syndrome. Case reports and review of the literature. *Scandinavian Journal of Gastroenterology*, 1988; **23**: 1267–74.

43. Cello JP. Acquired immunodeficiency syndrome cholangiopathy: spectrum of disease. *American Journal of Medicine*, 1989; **86**: 539–46.

44. Persaud D, *et al.* Cholestatic hepatitis in children infected with the human immunodeficiency virus. *Pediatric Infectious Disease Journal*, 1993; **12**: 492–8.

45. Heylen R and Miller R. Adverse effects and drug interactions of medications commonly used in the treatment of adult HIV positive patients. *Genitourinary Medicine*, 1996; **72**: 237–46.

46. Stricker BH, Blok AP, Bronkhorst FB, Van Parys GE, and Desmet VJ. Ketoconazole-associated hepatic injury. A clinicopathological study of 55 cases. *Journal of Hepatology*, 1986; **3**: 399–406.

47. Lake Bakaar G, Scheuer PJ, and Sherlock S. Hepatic reactions associated with ketoconazole in the United Kingdom. *British Medical Journal*, 1987; **294**: 419–22.

48. Skowron G. Biologic effects and safety of stavudine: overview of phase I and II clinical trials. *Journal of Infectious Diseases*, 1995; **171** (Suppl. 2): S113–17.

49. Ziegler JL, *et al.* Non-Hodgkin's lymphoma in 90 homosexual men. Relation to generalized lymphadenopathy and the acquired immunodeficiency syndrome. *New England Journal of Medicine*, 1984; **311**: 565–70.

50. Kaplan LD, *et al.* AIDS-associated non-Hodgkin's lymphoma in San Francisco. *Journal of the American Medical Association*, 1989; **261**: 719–24.

51. Rubio R, *et al.* Non-Hodgkin's lymphomas associated with the acquired immunodeficiency syndrome. A multicenter clinical study of 77 cases. *Medicina Clinica Barcelona*, 1995; **104**: 481–6.

12.4 Exotic virus infections of the liver

Anna Lucchini and Paolo Gioannini

The term exotic means 'originating in a foreign country'; in the context of exotic virus infections of the liver it refers to infections acquired in the tropics. Many infections now defined as 'exotic' were widely distributed in Europe and northern America up to the beginning of the twentieth century. Nowadays they are mainly encountered under tropical and sub-tropical conditions; however, they are not confined to these regions.

The increase in international travel and in the speed of transportation has made it possible for many exotic diseases to be exported to countries where they are not endemic. Physicians and health officials should be aware of this possibility and should learn to recognize signs and symptoms of unusual infections and to face the possible public health consequences of the introduction of these infections in their countries.

The liver is often affected by exotic virus infections: sometimes it is the primary target organ, but often it is only marginally affected. In very few cases, the exotic infection is only hepatotropic.

Yellow fever

Yellow fever was first recognized in the seventeenth century in Central America. It was one of the great epidemic scourges of mankind until the twentieth century.

Yellow fever virus probably originated from West Africa and was transported to the Americas by slave ships carrying the infected mosquitoes. In the past, temperate regions of North America, as far north as Baltimore and Philadelphia, have been affected by epidemics. Epidemics have also been described in Cadiz (Spain) and Lisbon (Portugal), but yellow fever has never been established in Asia, Australia, or Oceania.[1]

In 1900 the combined efforts of Findley, Reed, and Gorgas led to the discovery that yellow fever is caused by a filterable agent transmitted by *Aedes aegypti* mosquitoes. The virus was isolated in 1927 and effective vaccines were developed in the 1930s.

Mass vaccination campaigns carried out in endemic areas of West Africa by colonial health services led to the virtual disappearance of the disease. However, newly independent African states were unable to afford the vaccine; as a consequence, yellow fever has re-emerged across Africa and in South America, with a dramatic increase in official reports of the infection.[2] Since the 1980s epidemics have occurred in all endemic African countries.

Far from being under control, yellow fever seems to be extending its endemic zone to include new areas (Robertson, JAMA, 1996; 276:1157).

Aetiological agent and epidemiology

Yellow fever virus is the prototype Flavivirus, family Flaviviridae. It is an enveloped, spherical virus, 30 to 60 nm in diameter, with a single-stranded, positive-sense RNA. Short spikes protrude from the viral surface. Nucleotide sequence analysis of the genome has led to the identification of several strains. The genome encodes three structural proteins (C, capsid; M, membrane; E, envelope) and at least seven non-structural proteins.[3] The E glycoprotein is exposed on the surface and contains the most important antigenic sites. Monoclonal antibodies to the virus envelope protein distinguish different strains of wild and vaccine virus (Schlesinger, Virology, 1983; 125:8).

Nucleotide sequence variations in the envelope genes of different isolates from Africa and South America identify two major evolutionary yellow fever virus lineages, designated E genotypes I and II. E genotype I contains viruses isolated from East and Central Africa; E genotype II is divided in two sublineages: IIA from West Africa and IIB from America. The close genetic relatedness of genotypes IIA and IIB supports the theory of dissemination of the yellow fever virus from Africa to America (Chang, JVirol, 1995; 69:5773).

Viral replication occurs within the cytoplasm of infected cells. Assembly and morphogenesis take place in intracellular vesicles; subsequent fusion of these vesicles with the cell plasma membrane leads to release of the virions.[3]

Yellow fever is enzootic in the tropical forests of Africa, South and Central America. There are two modes of transmission, the sylvatic cycle and the urban cycle. In the former, transmission occurs primarily among non-human primates by an arthropod vector. In Africa the most important vector of sylvatic yellow fever is *Aedes africanus*, while in South America the forest vectors are mosquitoes of the genera *Haemagogus* and *Sabethes*.[1] Humans are infected when they enter forested areas where they are fed upon by infectious mosquitoes. However, the greatest risk for human epidemics is when viraemic individuals return to urban areas and are fed upon by competent domestic mosquito vectors, especially *Aedes aegypti*, which then transmit the virus to other humans, initiating the urban cycle (WHO, WklyEpidemiolRec, 1996; 71:313). The reinfestation of tropical and subtropical cities by *Aedes aegypti*, mainly due to poor environmental conditions, is increasing the risk of urban epidemics and is a cause for concern (WHO, WklyEpidemiolRec, 1995; 70:65).

Mosquitoes are infected when they bite a viraemic animal or human, and they then become infectious after 4 to 18 days, depending on the local temperature. Mosquitoes remain infectious for life. Replication of virus in invertebrate hosts does not seem to result in any significant pathology. Transovarial transmission has been demonstrated for some species of *Aedes* in natural conditions: this would make them ideal vectors and reservoirs of the infection. Other arthropods may function as vectors but their epidemiological significance is uncertain.[1]

The susceptibility to yellow fever varies in different species of primates: howler monkeys in South America die in large numbers during the recurring epizootics, while African vervet monkeys, colobus, mangabeys, and baboons develop inapparent infections.[1]

Person-to-person transmission does not occur, but human blood is infective in the first 3 to 4 days of illness. Handling infected tissues, monkeys, or mosquitoes can be dangerous.[1]

Pathology and pathogenesis

Yellow fever virus appears to injure infected cells directly. Experimental observations in monkeys suggest that, after inoculation by mosquitoes, the virus replicates in draining lymph nodes. Following this early replication, the virus spreads to internal organs by the haematogenous route (Monath, RevInfDis, 1987; 9:165). The liver is the main target organ, but other tissues become infected, such as spleen, pancreas, bone marrow, heart, and skeletal muscles, where replication occurs and from which the virus is released into the blood, mantaining the viraemia.[4] In the liver, Kupffer cells are initially infected. Hepatocytes are subsequently infected through the haematogenous route or by direct spread from Kupffer cells. Hepatocytes show fatty degeneration throughout the lobule, with necrosis affecting the midzone but sparing cells around the central vein and the portal area (Monath, RevInfDis, 1987; 9:165). Councilman bodies are often observed. The inflammatory response is very mild or completely absent.[1]

Typical lesions may not be found in patients who recover from yellow fever. In fatal cases, amorphous masses (Torres bodies) are seen within the degenerating hepatocyte nuclei. Small, granular, yellow bodies (Villela bodies) can also be seen free in the sinuses or phagocytosed by Kupffer cells. Neither Villela nor Torres bodies are diagnostic. Even in fatal cases, the liver is not shrunken and the morphological injury rarely is as severe as in fulminant viral hepatitis.[4]

In the kidneys, the tubular epithelium shows fatty changes and necrosis.[1] Viral antigen is present in glomeruli of experimentally infected monkeys (Monath, RevInfDis, 1987; 9:165). Myocarditis and fatty changes are seen in the sino-atrial node and in the bundle of His. In the brain, perivascular haemorrhages and cerebral oedema are observed.[1] Haemorrhages occur in severe cases, due to decreased synthesis of clotting factors and to disseminated intravascular coagulation.[4]

Clinical manifestations

Most infections are probably inapparent. Only 1 in 5 to 20 gives clinical manifestations. The incubation period is 3 to 6 days. The onset is sudden with fever, headache, myalgia and back pain, prostration, nausea, and vomiting. A characteristic bradycardia in relation to the temperature is observed (Faget sign);[3] conjunctival injection and dry tongue with red edges are also present. This early phase corresponds to the so-called 'period of infection' during which viraemia is detectable. After 3 days the patient may recover

or transiently improve ('period of remission') but after a few hours (up to 24) the fever remits and systemic symptoms appear. At this time, the so-called 'period of intoxication', the virus is no longer circulating in the blood and specific antibodies appear. Jaundice becomes evident; albuminuria and oliguria occur and may lead to renal failure. Haemorrhages are common, with haematemesis ('black vomit'), melaena, and bleeding from nose, mouth, eyes, bladder, or other organs.[1] Myocardial involvement may give rise to hypokinetic heart failure and alterations of the electrocardiogram.[1] Central nervous system complications may occur with signs and symptoms suggesting encephalitis, such as slurred speech, tremors, intractable hiccup; delirium, stupor and coma are terminal signs.

In fatal cases, death occurs following shock, generally between the seventh and the tenth day of illness. Recovery may be rapid, in 3 to 4 days, or may take more than 2 weeks. Jaundice can last for months.[4]

Suppurative parotitis and bacterial pneumonia may complicate the course of the disease. Late deaths are rare and are generally due to myocardial damage with arrhythmias or heart failure.[4] The overall case fatality rate does not exceed 5 per cent; however, when jaundice is present the prognosis is poor with a mortality approaching 50 per cent.[3]

Laboratory findings

Leucopenia, thrombocytopenia, and prolonged clotting time are common features. Liver enzymes and direct bilirubin are markedly increased in patients with jaundice but may be normal in other cases.[1] Albuminuria and granular casts in the urine are often observed. A rising azotaemia generally predicts a bad outcome.[3]

Diagnosis

Differential diagnosis of yellow fever should include viral hepatitis, falciparum malaria, leptospirosis, relapsing fever, typhoid fever, and other viral haemorrhagic fevers associated with jaundice (Rift Valley fever, Crimean/Congo haemorrhagic fever, and dengue haemorrhagic fever with jaundice).

The yellow fever virus can be isolated from the blood during the first 3 to 4 days of illness, or later from liver tissue.[1] The virus grows on a variety of cell lines, on chick or mouse embryos, or in mosquitoes after intrathoracic inoculation (Ludwig, InVitro, 1993; 29:296).

Direct yellow fever antigen identification may be performed by enzyme-linked immunosorbent assay (**ELISA**) in serum; a polymerase chain reaction (**PCR**)-based test is also available to detect viral sequences in biological samples. Tissue samples may be studied with immunohistochemical methods to detect yellow fever antigen (De Brito, PatholResPract, 1992; 188:177).

The serological diagnosis relies on several tests: the IgM antibody-capture ELISA is rapid and easy to apply under field conditions. IgM antibodies generally disappear after weeks or months, thus being a reliable marker of recent infection. Complement fixation antibodies behave in the same way, while haemagglutination-inhibiting antibodies and neutralizing antibodies persist longer: only paired acute and convalescent serum samples with rising antibody titres provide a confirmatory diagnosis. There is some degree of crossreaction with other flaviviruses (Monath, AmJTropMedHyg, 1984; 33:151).

Treatment

Treatment is only symptomatic. No specific antiviral drug is available. Analgesics are utilized to control headache and severe myalgias. Antiemetics may be used, and antacids, cimetidine, or ranitidine are given to reduce the risk of gastric bleeding. If severe bleeding occurs, blood transfusions and fresh frozen plasma are indicated. Oxygen should be administered and the patient monitored to detect any sign of shock: hypotension, oliguria, or electrolyte imbalance. If renal failure develops, the patient should undergo dyalisis. Heparin may be given to cases with strong evidence of disseminated intravascular coagulation, but its use is controversial (Monath, RevInfDis, 1987; 9:165).

Prevention

Patients with yellow fever do not need to be isolated as interhuman transmission does not occur. They should be nursed in conditions that guarantee isolation from mosquitoes to prevent further spread of the disease.

Yellow fever is a preventable disease. Since the 1930s, two vaccines have been developed. The French neurotropic vaccine was widely used in French-speaking African countries up to 1961 but vaccination was associated with an unacceptably high risk of encephalitis in children.[5]

The 17D vaccine, derived by serial passages of the Asibi strain of yellow fever virus in mouse and chick embryo tissues and replicated in developing chick embryos, was first used in South America in 1938. In 1945 WHO set manufacturing standards.[5] Yellow fever 17D vaccine is a safe, live-attenuated vaccine, that has been used extensively. The most serious side-effect is vaccine-induced encephalitis, which occurs almost exclusively in infants and young children (Tsai, JInfDis, 1993; 49:214). Since 1945, only 18 cases of post-vaccine encephalitis have been described, and only one fatal case, in a previously healthy 39-month-old child. Analysis of the virus isolated from this case indicated that a single epitope mutation on the envelope E protein had occurred, leading to a fully virulent, neurotropic virus. The reason for such a mutation is not clear. Two other similar cases have been reported, but in-depth viral studies were not performed (Jennings, JInfDis, 1994; 169:512).

Currently, yellow fever vaccination is not recommended for children below 6 months of age and for pregnant women. Yellow fever 17D vaccine virus can pass the placenta and infect the fetus (Tsai, JInfDis, 1993; 49:214). However, in a follow-up study of women who had been vaccinated during pregnancy, no adverse event was described in their offspring; in particular there was no congenital abnormality, encephalitic event, or sign of congenital infection. Pregnant women show much lower antibody responses than non-pregnant women of comparable age (Nasidi, TrRSoc-TropMedHyg, 1993; 87:337).

Vaccination is recommended for international travellers to endemic countries of Africa and South America. At the same time, travellers may be vaccinated against other diseases such as viral hepatitis A (Receveur, BullSocPath, 1993; 86:406) and B, typhoid fever (Ambrosch, Vaccine, 1994; 12:625), and polio (Coursaget, Vaccine, 1994; 12:625) without any interference between the immune responses and with no increase in adverse reactions. Although the immunity is certified for 10 years, neutralizing antibodies may persist for 35 to 40 years and vaccine immunity is now presumed to be lifelong.[5]

In endemic African countries, discontinuation of mass immunization in the 1960s led to a dramatic increase in yellow fever outbreaks that now involve a large proportion of children. For this reason the WHO Expanded Programme on Immunization has recommended the inclusion of yellow fever vaccine in the childhood immunization programmes of 33 African countries at risk for the disease (WHO, WklyEpidemiolRec, 1996; 71:313). Routine vaccination would significantly reduce morbidity and mortality and its cost-effectiveness exceeds that of the present policy of epidemic-driven control by mass vaccination campaigns.[5] Measles and yellow fever vaccines are administered together to 9-month-old children with full efficacy of each of the components (CDC, MMWR, 1990; 39:RR6).

New vaccine approaches are under study: a recombinant vaccinia virus expressing portions of the 17D yellow fever virus (prM and E) is able to induce high titres of neutralizing antibodies in mice and is protective against intracranial challenge with neurotropic strains of the virus (Pincus, Virology, 1992; 187:290).

Vector control plays an important role in the prevention of urban yellow fever. Proper environmental management with reduction of breeding sites of the peridomestic vector, Aedes aegypti, is a key factor. During urban epidemics, emergency vector control, aimed at rapid reduction of adult mosquitoes, can be carried out by fogging with insecticides. Larvicides should be used at the same time to inhibit the emergence of new adult mosquitoes. The efficacy of vector control measures in sylvatic yellow fever is controversial: insecticide aerial spraying has been applied to control epidemics involving wild vectors but results were not evaluated.[4]

Other Flaviviridae

Other members of the Flaviviridae can cause liver damage even though the liver is not the primary target organ.

Dengue fever

Dengue fever is the most important arbovirus disease in humans, both in terms of morbidity and mortality. It is caused by one of four serotypes of dengue virus, an enveloped, single-stranded RNA virus, 50 nm in size, transmitted by Aedes mosquitoes.

Dengue viruses have a widespread distribution in the tropics, where they may potentially infect up to 100 million persons annually. Transmission occurs throughout the year, but seasonal variations are generally observed with increased attack rates in the rainy season in relation to vector population densities (Halstead, SE-AsianJTropMedPublHlth, 1990; 21:636).

In its milder form, dengue fever presents as a biphasic febrile illness of sudden onset, frequently accompanied by rash, severe muscle pain, headache, and prostration (break bone fever). In a few cases the liver is enlarged; abnormal levels of transaminases are found in the majority of patients (Kuo, AmJTropMedHyg, 1992; 47:265).

After a first dengue infection, or in newborn babies with maternal IgG dengue antibody, a subsequent sequential infection with a different serotype of the virus may promote the development of dengue haemorrhagic fever. The presence of circulating antibody, crossreacting with the second infecting dengue virus but unable to neutralize it, has been shown to enhance virus replication inside mononuclear cells (Halstead, CurrOpinInfDis, 1990; 3:434). This, along with the effect of several cytokines released by activated T-lymphocytes (Hober, AmJTropMedHyg, 1993; 48:324), contributes to the immunopathogenesis of dengue haemorrhagic fever and of its most severe manifestation, dengue shock syndrome.

Dengue haemorrhagic fever/ dengue shock syndrome (**DHS/ DSS**) has been a recurrent problem in South-East Asia but the syndrome has been observed only recently in Latin America. The presence of DHF/DSS in some, but not all, areas of the global distribution of dengue viruses remains a mystery; it seems, however, that only strains originating from South-East Asia are associated with this severe form of the infection.[2]

Clinically, DHF/DSS is characterized by severe capillary leak-age, leading to hypovolaemic shock and death. Disseminated intra-vascular clotting can occur and is responsible for severe bleeding. In the course of DHF/DSS there is often a tender hepatomegaly; the liver shows focal necrosis of hepatic and Kupffer cells with formation of Councilman bodies. Treatment is supportive; there is no vaccine available even though several candidates (inactivated, attenuated, or recombinant) are currently being evaluated (Putnak, AmJTropMedHyg, 1996; 55:504).

Focal liver necrosis is also seen in two other viral haemorrhagic fevers caused by flaviviruses: Omsk haemorrhagic fever and Ki-asanur forest disease. Both are transmitted by ticks; interhuman transmission has also been reported for Omsk haemorrhagic fever. The blood of patients is potentially infective. These diseases have a limited geographical distribution: Omsk haemorrhagic fever occurs in the Omsk area of Siberia, while Kiasanur forest disease is found only in the central-western region of India.

Lassa fever

Lassa fever was originally described as a highly contagious, severe infection, with a high mortality rate. The first outbreak was recorded in 1969 in a hospital in northern Nigeria; additional hospital out-breaks were then described in Nigeria, Liberia, and Sierra Leone (Monath, JInfDis, 1987; 155:433). Since then, it has become ap-parent that Lassa fever is more prevalent and less frequently fatal than was supposed at first (Clegg, TrRSocTropMedHyg, 1984; 78:307).

Aetiological agent and epidemiology

The causative agent, Lassa fever virus, is a member of the Arena-viridae. It is an enveloped particle, 80 to 150 nm in size, containing a single-stranded RNA and a number of electron-dense granules, approximately 20 nm in diameter, giving a distinct 'sandy' ap-pearance under the electron microscope. This granularity prompted the use of the name arenavirus from '*arena*', the Latin word for sand. The viral envelope, formed from the plasma membrane of the infected cell, contains surface club-shaped projections 5 to 10 nm long. During virus maturation, the particle forms by extrusion of the plasma membrane: surface projections become visible and ribosome granules become arranged regularly below the thickened, extruding membrane (Howard, TrRSocTropMedHyg, 1984; 78:299).

Lassa fever virus grows readily in cell cultures (Vero cells) where it induces the formation of distinct intracytoplasmatic inclusion bodies, preceding gross cytopathological alterations.

Lassa fever is endemic in West Africa, causing an estimated 300 000 infections and 5000 deaths annually (McCormick, JInfDis, 1987; 155:437). It is prevalent in all countries from Nigeria to Senegal. However, the ease of international travel makes it possible for the infection to occur anywhere in the world.

All arenaviruses can cause acute or persistent infections of rodents, usually benign. *Mastomys natalensis*, a common rat around human habitations in Africa, is the host of enzootic Lassa fever virus. The virus is spread to humans primarily through direct contact with infected rats in households or by direct contact with food or water contaminated by rodent urine. Both sexes and all age groups appear to be affected (McCormick, JInfDis, 1987; 155:437). Person-to-person transmission occurs and is responsible for nosocomial outbreaks through contact with contaminated blood or other infectious body fluids (Holmes, NEJM, 1990; 323:1120).

The concentration of virus in the blood of patients varies; the virus is less frequently recovered from throat swabs and only sporadically from urine of patients, but late shedding is recorded (Johnson, JInfDis, 1987; 155:456). No instance of secondary trans-mission to medical staff or contacts has been recorded from patients with Lassa fever imported into developed countries (Johnson, NEJM, 1990; 323:1139). In endemic countries poor medical prac-tices appear to be responsible for most cases acquired in the hospital setting: parenteral inoculation via unsterilized equipment, unprotected contact with infected body fluids, and, in a few in-stances, aerosols are considered potentially dangerous (Fisher-Hoch, BMJ, 1995; 311:857).

Pathology and pathogenesis

Lassa virus is pantropic, causing lesions and probably dysfunction of multiple organ systems. In experimentally infected animals, the highest concentration of virus is found in the liver, but the virus can be recovered in titres significantly higher than those in blood from many visceral tissues: lungs, adrenal glands, pancreas, spleen, kidneys, and lymph nodes. The central nervous system appears, on the contrary, to contain lower concentrations of virus than the blood (Jahrling, JInfDis, 1980; 141:580).

The placenta of infected pregnant women contains extremely high viral titres: the virus can be isolated from fetal blood. Mis-carriage is the rule, but cases of congenital infection have been described (Monson, TrRSocTropMedHyg, 1984; 78:549). Lassa virus is also found in the milk of nursing mothers (Monson, AmJTropMedHyg, 1987; 36:408).

High levels of viraemia are consistently associated with increased probability of a fatal outcome (Johnson, JInfDis, 1987; 155:456).

In the liver, four principal, and sometimes concurrent, alterations are observed: focal cytoplasmic degeneration of hepatocytes; ran-domly distributed multifocal hepatocellular necrosis with Coun-cilman bodies; monocytic reaction to confluent necrotic hepatocytes; and hepatocellular mytoses (McCormick, AmJTropMedHyg, 1986; 35:401).

Infected hepatocytes, containing large quantities of Lassa viral antigens, are randomly distributed throughout the parenchyma. Neither the degree of liver disfunction nor the extent of tissue necrosis are sufficient to incriminate liver failure as a cause of death in Lassa fever. There is also no correlation between the titre of virus in blood or liver tissue and the various histological measures of liver damage (McCormick, AmJTropMedHyg, 1986; 35:401).

The marked elevation of aspartate aminotransferase observed in these patients may not be solely hepatic in origin but may also be of muscular origin: alanine aminotransferase, a more specific marker of hepatic dysfunction, is only slightly elevated and prothrombin time only marginally affected. Jaundice is rarely observed. These observations have led to the conclusion that Lassa fever is not primarily a clinical hepatitis (Fisher-Hoch, JInfDis, 1987; 155:465). Haemorrhages are seen in fewer than 20 per cent of patients and do not explain the profound shock typical of fatal disease. More subtle changes in vascular function are likely to be responsible. Although the endothelium does not appear histologically to be damaged by viral replication, its physiological functions are impaired and platelets fail to aggregate in *in vitro* tests. The picture suggests a capillary leakage syndrome (Fisher-Hoch, JInfDis, 1987; 155:465).

The raising of antibodies does not seem to be associated with either recovery from disease or a reduction in viraemia. Cell-mediated immunity seems to be central to virus clearance and protection and may be, at least transiently, impaired by the virus itself. Effector substances, possibly released from macrophages and neutrophils, may play a role in the functional disturbance of endothelium, platelets, and T cells (Fisher-Hoch, JInfDis, 1987; 155:465).

Clinical manifestations

Lassa fever is a disease with a remarkable spectrum of clinical manifestations as well as severity. Most Lassa virus infections in Africa are mild or asymptomatic, as shown by serosurveys (McCormick, JInfDis, 1987; 155:437). Only 10 to 30 per cent of infections are associated with a clinical illness. In hospitalized patients, the case fatality rate ranges between 15 and 25 per cent, a much lower figure than reported in earlier nosocomial outbreaks. Data from serological surveys suggest that the mortality due to Lassa virus infection may be only 1 to 2 per cent (McCormick, JInfDis, 1987; 155:437).

After an incubation period of 7 to 18 days, Lassa fever begins gradually with fever, weakness, and general malaise. By the third or fourth day of illness, most patients develop a severe retrosternal chest pain and a lower back pain. Two-thirds of patients develop a dry, non-productive cough. Severe headache and a sore throat are common, starting on the fourth or fifth day. At this time vomiting and diarrhoea, often accompanied by abdominal pain, are reported in more than half of the patients. Signs include a low systolic blood pressure, pharyngitis, which may be exudative in half of the patients, and conjunctivitis. In patients with more severe disease, conjunctival haemorrhages, bleeding of gums and nose, and oedema of the face and neck are commonly observed. Pleural and pericardial effusions are not uncommon and may be associated with an interstitial pneumonitis (McCormick, JInfDis, 1987; 155:445).

Recovery generally begins within 8 to 10 days of onset, with lysis of fever and resolution of headache, sore throat, and chest pain. A persistent weakness is often reported.[1]

More severe cases progress rapidly during the second week of disease to respiratory distress, hypovolaemic shock, pulmonary oedema, and, sometimes, massive pleural effusions and ascites. Bleeding is often associated with severe disease but its magnitude is not enough to produce shock. There may be clinical signs of encephalopathy with coma and seizures.

During the second or third week of illness, eighth nerve deafness, which may be unilateral or bilateral, may appear. Its severity ranges from complete to mild loss of high frequencies; in a few patients deafness may improve, but usually it is not reversible (McCormick, JInfDis, 1987; 155:445). Haemorrhages, pleural and pericardial effusions, orchitis, and uretritis may also occur at this time.

The case fatality rate in pregnant women is much higher than in non-pregnant adults. Miscarriage is common and congenital infection may occur (Monson, TrRSocTropMedHyg, 1984; 78: 549). Clinical manifestations in children include a distinctive syndrome characterized by widespread oedema, abdominal distension, and bleeding, which affects children less than 2 years old and carries a poor prognosis. The case fatality rate in hospitalized children is higher than among adults (Monson, AmJTropMedHyg, 1987; 36: 408).

Laboratory findings

Two reliable predictors of the outcome of the infection are the concentration of virus in blood and the aspartate aminotransferase level. Patients with high levels of aspartate aminotransferase (>150 UI/litre) combined with high viraemia have a 78 per cent fatality rate, compared to 17 per cent in patients who do not present with these features (Johnson, JInfDis, 1987; 155:456).

Other laboratory parameters are not distinctive. The haematocrit is often elevated; proteinuria is common; lactic dehydrogenase and creatine phosphokinase are abnormal, with a level of aspartate aminotransferase disproportionately higher than the level of alanine aminotransferase (McCormick, JInfDis, 1987; 155:445).

Diagnosis

The differential diagnosis of Lassa fever in endemic countries should include malaria, typhoid fever, pneumonia, gastroenteritis, pelvic inflammatory disease, influenza, and infections with arboviruses such as dengue or chikungunya (Monson, TrRSocTropMedHyg, 1984; 78:549).

Lassa virus is readily cultivated on Vero cells: viraemia is detected in virtually all fatal cases where it persists until death. Viraemia is detectable in up to 70 per cent of survivors and declines progressively after the sixth day of illness (Johnson, JInfDis, 1987; 155: 456). Lassa virus is less frequently isolated from throat swabs and urine where it may nevertheless persist for several weeks. Viral isolation should be performed only in high-containment laboratories.

Antigen detection by ELISA has proved very useful in the early diagnosis of Lassa fever. It is rapid and can be carried out on β-propiolactone-treated sera, reducing the biohazard of manipulating Lassa virus. Either Lassa antigen or IgM antibodies can be detected in the blood of virtually all acutely ill patients (Jahrling, Lancet, 1985; i:250).

Recently, two PCR-based techniques were developed to detect Lassa virus (Trappier, AmJTropMed Hyg, 1993; 49:214). The best results are obtained with a reverse transcription PCR (**RT–PCR**), showing complete concordance with virus culture. In one study,

80 per cent of patients with confirmed Lassa fever were RT–PCR positive on admission and all became positive by the third day (Demby, JClinMicrobiol, 1994; 32:2898).

Serodiagnosis of Lassa fever is based on the detection of IgM antibodies by immunofluorescent antibody or ELISA tests. However, IgM may be present in only one-third of patients on admission (Jahrling, Lancet, 1985; i:250). A fourfold or greater rise in IgG antibody titres is considered diagnostic, but it requires serum pairs and therefore it is not suitable for early diagnosis (Frame, TrRSocTropMedHyg, 1984; 78:656).

Treatment

Early reports suggested that convalescent plasma may be effective in the treatment of patients with Lassa fever (Frame, TrRSoc-TropMedHyg, 1984; 78:319). However, these results have not been confirmed. Specific antibody is detected early in the disease but this does not affect its course. Selected convalescent plasma, containing higher than usual titres of neutralizing antibody, might be effective as adjunctive therapy in very serious cases (McCormick, NEJM, 1986; 314:20).

The treatment of choice is based on ribavirin, a nucleoside compound with broad antiviral properties. Ribavirin can reduce mortality in patients with Lassa fever, especially when the drug is given intravenously before day 7 of the disease. Both oral and intravenous ribavirin appear to be effective, but the oral drug is less well-tolerated in patients with gastroenteric symptoms and the intravenous preparation may have more therapeutic efficacy. Treatment starts with a 2 g loading dose followed by 1 g every 6 h for 4 days, then reduced to 0.5 g every 8 h for another 6 days. The only adverse effect observed is haemolysis, which is usually reversible and requires no transfusion (McCormick, NEJM, 1986; 314:20).

Fluid and electrolyte balance should be maintained and cautious volume replacement should be started before signs of clinical shock appear.[1]

Prevention

The nursing of Lassa fever patients requires the use of meticulous barrier procedures and universal precautions to prevent contact with contaminated blood or other body fluids. Recommendations suggesting total isolation have been discarded following observation in endemic situations (Johnson, NEJM, 1990; 323:1139). However, as infectious aerosols might transmit the virus, it is advisable to place patients in single rooms and, wherever possible, in rooms with isolated negative pressure airflow. All specimens and refuse should be double-bagged (WHO, WklyEpidemiolRec, 1995; 70:249).

Laboratory-acquired infection is a major concern, thus any work with Lassa virus should be conducted in laboratories having maximum biological containment. Close contacts of patients with Lassa fever should be carefully monitored for any sign of fever. For high-risk contacts or needle-stick injuries, prophylaxis with oral ribavirin is recommended (5 mg/kg three times daily for 2 to 3 weeks).[6]

Inactivated Lassa virus elicits non-protective immune responses in monkeys (McCormick, JMedVirol, 1992; 37:1). Experimental evidence in animal model systems suggests the possibility of a vaccine based on related, apparently non-pathogenic viruses, such

as Mopeia (Clegg, TrRSocTropMedHyg, 1984; 78:307). Vaccinia-vectored Lassa genes, coding for nucleocapsid proteins, have been shown to be protective in experimental animals (Clegg, Vaccine, 1992; 10:89).

Other Arenaviridae

The taxon Arenaviridae contains 16 members, all with a unique morphology and sharing antigenic components (Howard, TrRSoc-TropMedHyg, 1984; 78:299). Only six members have been implicated as causes of naturally acquired human disease: lymphocytic choriomeningitis virus, Lassa fever virus, Flexal, Junin, Machupo, and Guaranito viruses. The last three are endemic in South America, where they cause severe haemorrhagic fever with a mortality rate of 10 to 15 per cent. Recently two cases of another lethal arenavirus infection, Sabia virus, have been described in Brazil (Coimbra, Lancet, 1984; 343:391).

Junin virus is the aetiological agent of Argentinian haemorrhagic fever, endemic in the pampas north of Buenos Aires. The main reservoir rodent is Calomys masculinus, which breeds in maize fields. Transmission occurs through direct contact with rodents during the harvesting season, when most cases are recorded. Indirect transmission from contaminated food is possible, but person-to-person spread is rare (WHO, WklyEpidemiolRec, 1993; 68:233).

Machupo virus is the cause of Bolivian haemorrhagic fever, first recognized in 1959 in the north-eastern region of Bolivia. The reservoir rodent is Calomys callosus, living in grasslands but readily entering houses in the small towns and villages of the region. Transmission occurs by aerosol contact or by food contaminated with rodent urine. Person-to-person transmission is possible but rare (WHO, WklyEpidemiolRec, 1995; 70:16).

Guanarito virus was recognized in 1989 as the causative agent of haemorrhagic fever in Venezuela. Major implicated reservoirs are the cotton rat, Sigmodon alstoni, and the cane mouse, Zygodontomys brevicauda, living in fields, pasture, and peridomestic habitats (Tesh, AmJTropMedHyg, 1993; 49:227).

After an incubation period of 5 to 19 days, all of these viruses can cause a clinical illness with an insidious onset, characterized by fever, malaise, back pain, retro-orbital pain, and conjunctival injection. A petechial rash with enanthem is present in most patients. After 6 to 8 days of illness there may be a sudden deterioration with multiple mucosal haemorrhages, signs of capillary leakage, proteinuria, neurological disturbances, narrowing pulse pressure, and clinical shock.[1]

There is no evidence of a distinctive pathological process playing a role in the clinical illness. No vasculitis is observed; there is no inflammatory response and only small focal haemorrhages can be found on mucosal surfaces. Focal hepatic necrosis, with Councilman bodies, is present but less severe than in Lassa fever.[1] Treatment is supportive. Immune plasma has been shown to be effective in Argentinian haemorrhagic fever when administered within 8 days of onset, with a reduction of the case fatality rate to 1 per cent or less (WHO, WklyEpidemiolRec, 1993; 68:233).

A live-attenuated Junin virus vaccine has been developed, which is safe, well-tolerated, and immunogenic. Efficacy has been clearly established in a small number of human volunteers and a large prospective trial is now under way to document persistence of protection, duration of serum antibody, and the possible occurrence of low-frequency adverse events (WHO, WklyEpidemiolRec, 1993; 68:233).

Marburg and Ebola virus diseases

Marburg and Ebola viruses are members of the family Filoviridae. Their public health importance lies in their high mortality rate rather than in the frequency and total number of human infections recorded since their identification.[7]

Marburg virus was isolated in 1967 when an epidemic of severe haemorrhagic fever occurred among workers handling a shipment of African green monkeys in Marburg, Germany and Belgrade, former Yugoslavia. Twenty-five primary cases and six secondary cases were described, with a case fatality rate of 23 per cent.[7] Since then, only sporadic cases have been reported, mostly acquired in Uganda and Kenya, i.e. the areas from which the monkeys were shipped in 1967 (Smith, Lancet, 1982; i:816). Only in one instance, was circulation of the Marburg virus proven outside these areas: this was in Zimbabwe, where a traveller acquired the disease and then infected two other persons while under medical care in South Africa (Gear, BMJ, 1975; 4:489).

Ebola virus was first recognized in 1976 when two simultaneous, unrelated epidemics occurred in Zaire and in Sudan with a case fatality rate of about 90 per cent and 60 per cent, respectively.[7] Another smaller outbreak occurred in the same area of Sudan in 1979. Only isolated cases were reported up to 1995 when the re-emergence of Ebola in Kikwit, Zaire, caused 315 cases (WHO, WklyEpidemiolRec, 1995; 70:241). Since then, Ebola virus has been associated only with a few isolated cases and with two small outbreaks in Gabon, in 1996 (WHO, WklyEpidemiolRec, 1996; 71: 125).

Great apprehension was caused by the discovery of another Ebola virus subtype in cynomolgous monkeys imported to the United States and Italy from Mindanao, the Philippines, in 1989. Four individuals who had contact with the infected animals sero-converted without a febrile illness; nevertheless the infection proved to be highly pathogenic for monkeys (Jahrling, Lancet, 1990; 335: 502).

Aetiological agents and epidemiology

Filoviruses owe their name to their characteristic thread-like appearance (from 'filo', Latin for filament). They are enveloped, single-stranded RNA viruses, 80 nm in diameter; their length varies, ranging from 790 to 970 nm for the replicative forms of Marburg and Ebola virus, respectively (Ellis, JMedVirol, 1979; 4:213). The helical nucleocapsid is surrounded by a membrane formed as the virus buds from the host cell. Intracytoplasmic inclusions of nucleocapsid aggregates can be visualized by electron microscopy in infected cells; in ordinary sections they appear as red-stained masses.[8]

Sequence analysis of the Ebola virus genome indicates that it is organized in a similar way as Rhabdoviruses and Paramyxoviruses and is virtually the same as Marburg virus. The structural proteins of Ebola and Marburg viruses contain large regions of homology despite the absence of serological crossreactivity (Sanchez, VirRes, 1993; 29:215).

Marburg virus isolates belong to one of several strains, called, for example, Popp, Musoki, and Ravn. While they are indistinguishable by cross-neutralization testing, comparison of nucleotide sequences suggests that Ravn is a different subtype of Marburg virus (Johnson, ArchVirolSuppl, 1996; 11:101).

There are three known subtypes of Ebola virus, which differ significantly from one another: the Sudan, Zaire (Cox, JInfDis, 1983; 147:272), and Reston subtypes. Comparison of genomic sequences shows more than a 40 per cent nucleotide difference between any pair of them. While there is no serological cross-reactivity between Marburg and Ebola viruses, the three Ebola subtypes largely crossreact by immunofluorescence or ELISA.[8]

There is no known animal reservoir of filoviruses. Extensive research and serosurveys of many primates, rodents, bats, birds, and insects in the areas affected by Ebola epidemics failed to identify a reservoir host (WHO, WklyEpidemiolRec, 1995; 70:241). There is now clear evidence that Ebola virus can infect animals in the wild, such as chimpanzees, which were the identified source of infection of several human cases in Ivory Coast (WHO, WklyEpidemiolRec, 1995; 70:137) and in Gabon (WHO, WklyEpidemiolRec, 1996; 71: 125). However, as these animals were seriously ill and died of the disease, it is improbable that they represent the true reservoir of the virus.[7] It is possible that chimpanzees live in close association with the primary maintenance reservoir and occasionally become infected (Johnson, TrRSocTropMedHyg, 1993; 87:536).

Transmission of Marburg virus to humans takes place only through close contact with blood, body fluids, or tissues of infected monkeys. Secondary cases have mainly affected hospital staff following a blood exposure. A single case was apparently transmitted by sexual intercourse.[1] Interhuman transmission of Ebola virus occurs through direct contact with body fluids of infected, symptomatic individuals. During the African epidemics, the disease was spread among medical staff, due to inadequate measures of containment and improper nursing techniques. Transmission to household contacts was associated with nursing of sick patients or preparation of bodies for burial (WHO, WklyEpidemiolRec, 1995; 70:149).

Airborne transmission has been documented between monkeys in quarantine facilities (Reston incident) or under laboratory conditions, but this route seems irrelevant to the natural spread of human infection, even under conditions of close proximity.[7]

Data from serosurveys in Africa suggest that filoviruses may be less pathogenic in their natural settings than commonly thought. Most human filovirus disease has been described in epidemic settings, which may involve atypical modes of exposure. Sero-epidemiological surveys clearly document the occurrence of non-fatal filovirus infection without apparent disease. However, circulation of crossreactive, non-pathogenic members of the filovirus family cannot be excluded (Johnson, TrRSocTropMedHyg, 1993; 87:530). A high antibody prevalence seems to be associated with the hunter–gatherer subsistence strategy, in populations that frequently come into contact with freshly killed animals, especially feral monkeys (Johnson, TrRSocTropMedHyg, 1993; 87:536).

Pathology and pathogenesis

Marburg and Ebola viruses cause a severe haemorrhagic disease in humans and primates. They are pantropic virus infections with invasion of cells and necrotic lesions in all organs.[1] In the liver, irregularly confluent necrosis of single hepatocytes with fatty degeneration are observed. Eosinophilic cytoplasmic inclusions resembling Councilman bodies are common. The basic architecture of the liver remains intact with a minimal inflammatory response. Histological lesions are found also in kidneys, lungs (haemorrhages), heart, bone marrow, and spleen (Baskerville, JPath, 1985; 147:199), but all known histological and pathophysiological parameters of the disease are not sufficient to explain the devastating symptoms. Haemorrhages, activation of coagulation, and shock, all clinical features of the disease, suggest damage to the endothelium with loss of its important regulatory functions. Marburg virus has been shown to replicate in human endothelial cells, supporting the hypothesis that viral replication is the cause of destruction of these cells (Schnittler, JCI, 1993; 91:1301).

Marburg virus also replicates in human monocytes/macrophages, resulting in cytolytic infection and release of infectious virus particles. Monocytes/macrophages are activated by Marburg virus infection to release tumour necrosis factor-α (TNF-α), which plays a critical role in mediating the increased permeability by formation of interendothelial gaps. The endothelial damage contributes significantly to the fatal haemorrhages and fulminating shock syndrome so frequently seen (Feldmann, JVirol, 1996; 70: 2208).

The antibody response does not seem to provide effective protection.[8] Ebola virus expresses an immunosuppressive amino acid sequence associated with its envelope glycoprotein, which may explain the failure to mount an effective immune response (Volchkov, FEBSLett, 1992; 305:181).

Viraemia is present during the acute illness and generally disappears with clinical improvement. However, relapses can occur in Marburg virus infections; in one case the virus was isolated from semen 12 weeks after the onset of illness.[1]

Clinical manifestations

The proportion of symptomatic infections is unknown: inapparent infection can occur, but in most cases the symptoms that do develop are severe. Only 32 human cases of Marburg virus disease have been described, with a case fatality rate of 25 per cent. Ebola virus disease is more common; mortality rates varied from 50 to 60 per cent in the Sudan epidemic to 80 per cent in Zaire.[7,8]

The clinical picture of the two infections is indistinguishable. The incubation period is from 2 to 21 days. The illness has a sudden onset with fever, severe headache, often periorbital or frontal, weakness, muscle pain, and sore throat with herpetic lesions on the mouth and pharynx. A prominent feature is a watery, sometimes bloody, diarrhoea, lasting for several days; its entity is a measure of the severity of the disease. Vomiting, abdominal pain, chest pain, cough, conjunctival injection, and jaundice are common features.[1]

Widespread haemorrhages occur in most cases and generally appear on the fifth day of disease. Bleeding from mucous membranes such as gingivae, nasopharynx, gastrointestinal tract, and vagina is associated with petechiae and ecchymoses on the skin. Five to seven days after onset, a maculo-papular rash develops, more prominent on the trunk and back.[8] The central nervous system is often involved, with delirium, coma, or hemiplegia.

Death occurs from severe blood loss and shock, with multiple organ failure most commonly in the second week of disease. If the patient survives, fever will decrease and the general conditions will improve markedly. The convalescence is generally protracted and may be characterized by local complications such as uveitis, orchitis, and hepatitis.[1,8]

Laboratory findings

Common features are leucopenia, raised aminotransferases levels, especially aspartate aminotransferase, and thrombocytopenia. Hypoproteinaemia and albuminuria are present and virocytes can be observed following the initial leucopenia.[1]

Diagnosis

The differential diagnosis is from yellow fever, Lassa fever, and other haemorrhagic fevers. Filoviruses are readily cultivated on Vero cells or monkey kidney cells, from blood, serum or biopsy specimens of patients. Viraemia persists throughout the entire acute stage of the illness.[8] Viral culture should be carried out only in maximum biological containment laboratories (WHO, Wkly-EpidemiolRec, 1995; 70:149).

An ELISA is available to detect Ebola virus antigens, both in serum and tissue homogenates of patients (Ksiazek, JClinMicrobiol, 1992; 30:947). Viral RNA can also be detected by reverse transcription PCR (WHO, WklyEpidemiolRec, 1995; 70:149). Serological results obtained with the immunofluorescent antibody test allow for differentiation between Ebola and Marburg. However, false positives and unreproducible results may create problems, especially when the test has been used for serosurveys of apparently healthy human populations.[8] The ELISA for IgM and IgG antibody is reliable and reproducible. However, specific antibody appears late in the disease and may be negative on admission.[8]

Treatment

There is no specific treatment available for filovirus infections. The management of patients is mainly supportive. Replacement of blood, coagulation factors, and platelets, together with careful maintenance of hydration, are the mainstay of therapy (WHO, Wkly-EpidemiolRec, 1995; 70:149). Use of convalescent serum is not indicated.

Prevention

No vaccine is available. Strict barrier nursing and avoidance of all at-risk procedures, such as needle sharing, use of unsterilized equipment, and unprotected handling of excreta or of dead bodies, are adequate measures to avoid epidemics in health facilities of endemic countries. Whenever feasible, isolation should be applied (WHO, WklyEpidemiolRec, 1995; 70:249). Strict quarantine procedures for imported animals and application of methods to prevent contamination of vaccines or cell cultures greatly reduce the risk of filovirus spread in non-endemic countries.[8]

Rift Valley fever

Rift Valley fever is a viral disease affecting animals and humans throughout most of Africa. It was first described in Kenya in 1931.[1] Until 1977 epidemics occurred only in subSaharan Africa; in 1977 there was the first massive epidemic in Egypt with an estimated number of 200 000 human cases and nearly 600 deaths (Turell, AmJTropMedHyg, 1996; 54:136); a second smaller outbreak was recorded in 1993 (WHO, WklyEpidemiolRec, 1994; 69: 74).

Aetiological agent and epidemiology

Rift Valley fever is caused by a virus of the genus *Phlebovirus*, family Bunyaviridae. Like other members of the family, it possesses a single-stranded, tripartite RNA genome composed of a large, a medium, and a small segment. It is a spherical, enveloped virus, 90 to 110 nm in diameter, with spikes protruding from the external surface. Replication occurs in the cytoplasm of the infected cells and mature virions bud from the endoplasmic reticulum and also through the outer membrane of hepatocytes (Anderson, Virology, 1987; 161:91). There is generally high conservation of genetic and phenotypic characteristics among wild strains of Rift Valley fever virus isolated in different locations. However, specific amino acid sequence variations have been identified which may be involved in virus neutralization and may contribute to the virulence characteristics of the virus. Certain viral isolates can be differentiated by their pathogenicity for laboratory rodents (Battles, AmJTropMedHyg, 1988; 39:617).

Rift Valley fever is common in most subSaharan African countries; it is not found outside Africa. However, its recent appearance in Egypt suggests that it might spread to other regions such as the Middle East or Central Asia.

Rift Valley fever is mostly a zoonotic disease, with epizootics generally preceding the observation of human cases. Epizootics cause high mortality and abortion rates among domestic animals, especially sheep and cattle (Mariner, AmJTropMedHyg, 1995; 53: 217). It is not known whether any of the many animals susceptible to Rift Valley fever virus infection serves as the maintenance reservoir host. Domestic animals can serve as amplifiers of the infection during epizootics (Battles, AmJTropMedHyg, 1988; 39:617).

Among animal hosts, the virus is transmitted by mosquitoes. Several groups of mosquitoes have been shown to be competent vectors: *Eretmapodites*, *Coquillettidiae*, *Mansonia*, *Aedes*, and *Culex*. *Aedes* and *Culex* mosquitoes are of particular relevance as they may function as bridge vectors from domestic animals to humans under epidemic conditions (Turell, AmJTropMedHyg, 1996; 54:136). Vertical, transovarial transmission has been proposed as a possible mechanism of maintenance of the infection in mosquitoes during inter-epizootic periods, but this has not been confirmed by experimental studies (Turell, JMedEntomol, 1992; 29:792).

Experimentally, Rift Valley fever virus may be transmitted by a wide array of other arthropod vectors, such as ticks (*Hyalomma truncatum*) (Linthicum, AmJTropMedHyg, 1989; 41:491) or sandflies (*Phlebotomus duboscqi*) (Turell, AmJTropMedHyg, 1990; 42: 185), but the relevance of this transmission in natural conditions is unknown.

Veterinarians, shepherds, farmers, and abattoir workers are at special risk of acquiring the disease by the aerosol route or by close contact with the blood or carcasses of infected animals, especially during epizootics. However, during epidemics the most important route of transmission to humans is from mosquito bites.[9] Person-to-person transmission does not occur, but the blood of patients during the acute illness is highly infectious.[1]

Pathology and pathogenesis

The liver is the main target organ. The virus directly invades hepatocytes, causing midzonal hyaline degeneration leading to necrosis and formation of Councilman bodies.[1] The virus also invades endothelial cells and is responsible for a vasculitis leading to damage of all internal organs and to haemorrhages. Antigen–antibody immune complexes may play a role in the pathogenesis of visceral damage.[1]

Clinical manifestations

Most humans infected by Rift Valley fever virus develop a non-specific, self-limiting febrile illness.[9] The incubation period is 2 to 7 days. The onset is sudden with fever, headache, retro-orbital pain, joint and muscle pain. There may be nausea, vomiting, and diarrhoea, but in most cases a complete recovery follows. Sometimes recrudescences are observed and convalescence may take several weeks.[1]

In fewer than 5 per cent of the patients, the disease is much more severe: extensive haemorrhages develop with purpura and gastrointestinal bleeding. Jaundice is often observed. The prognosis is poor and death usually occurs following shock and hepatic failure. Viral invasion of the central nervous system leads to a severe, often fatal, meningoencephalitis which generally develops after the end of the acute febrile illness.[9] A small proportion of patients may present with ocular disease consisting of retinal damage due to several factors: retinitis, retinal haemorrhages, vasculitis, and retinal detachment. Vision may improve with time but the damage may be permanent with residual blindness.[1] During the 1993 outbreak in Egypt, the predominant clinical presentation was visual impairment (WHO, Wkly EpidemiolRec, 1994; 69:74). The overall mortality rate is less than 1 per cent.[1]

Laboratory findings

There is no typical finding. The white cell count may be initially decreased or slightly increased. Liver function tests are abnormal in severe cases. When encephalitic complications develop, the cerebrospinal fluid shows increased protein levels and lymphocytic pleocytosis.

Diagnosis

The differential diagnosis is simple during epidemics and when the three typical clinical forms occur together in the same area (haemorrhagic, encephalitic, and ocular disease).[1]

The virus is easily isolated from the blood of patients during the acute illness. It can be cultured on several cell lines, such as Vero cells or BHK, or may be inoculated intracerebrally in suckling mice.[9] As the virus is highly infectious by aerosol, isolation should be carried out exclusively in high-containment laboratories.[9]

Antigen detection by ELISA is a promising technique.[9] Antibodies to Rift Valley fever virus appear 5 to 10 days after the onset of disease and may be detected by several methods: immunofluorescence, ELISA, haemagglutino-inhibition, plaque-reduction neutralization test, complement fixation. ELISA detection of IgM antibodies is reliable for rapid diagnosis. Neutralizing antibodies are the only specific response, while other antibodies may be crossreactive with different viruses of the genus *Phlebovirus* (Niklasson, JClinMicrobiol, 1984; 19:225).

Treatment

Studies *in vitro* and in experimental animals show that ribavirin may be effective in the treatment of Rift Valley fever. Limited clinical experience seems to confirm the efficacy of the drug (Peters, AntiviralRes, 1986; 6:285).

In experimental models, substances able to induce interferon production have been shown to be effective in the treatment and prophylaxis of the infection (Sidwell, AnnNYAcadSci, 1992; 653: 344; Zvilich, AntiviralRes, 1995; 27:389; Frese, JVirol, 1996; 70: 915). The use of immune convalescent serum has been recommended in severe cases of Rift Valley fever.[1]

Prevention

During epizootics the movement of animals from areas where the infection has been detected should be restricted. Immunization of animals should be carried out to establish a '*cordon sanitaire*' around the infected area (WHO, WklyEpidemiolRec, 1994; 69:258). Two vaccines are available for use in animals, a live-attenuated and an inactivated vaccine. Both are active and have been shown to be effective (WHO, BullWHO, 1983; 61:261).

Veterinarians, abattoir workers, and laboratory personnel may be immunized with an inactivated vaccine that is safe and effective (Niklasson, Vaccine, 1985; 3:123).

During epizootics, attempts should be made to control mosquito populations (WHO, WklyEpidemiolRec, 1994; 69:258).

Patients are not contagious, but in transmission areas should be nursed under conditions of isolation from mosquitoes. Barrier nursing to avoid contact with infectious human blood is recommended.[1]

Crimean/Congo haemorrhagic fever

The first description of human cases of haemorrhagic fever in soldiers and peasants from the Crimean peninsula goes back to the 1940s; however, it is believed that the disease had been circulating in Central Asia for centuries. In 1956, a virus named Congo was isolated from a child in that country and subsequently, in 1969, it was demonstrated that the two viruses were identical: hence the virus was called Crimean/Congo haemorrhagic fever virus (Hoogstraal, JMedEntomol, 1979; 15:307).

Aetiological agent and epidemiology

Crimean/Congo haemorrhagic fever virus belongs to the genus *Nairovirus* of the family Bunyaviridae. As all Bunyaviruses, it is a spherical, enveloped virus, 90 to 100 nm in diameter with a negative sense, single-stranded RNA genome divided into three segments of different size: large, medium, and small (Schwarz, AmJTropMedHyg, 1996; 55:190). Only the small segment encoding the viral nucleoprotein has been sequenced so far (Marriott, Virology, 1992; 189:795). The virus presents numerous surface projections which are arranged hexagonally. The virions mature inside the endoplasmic reticulum into vescicles that are released on disintegration of the host cell.

Crimean/Congo haemorrhagic fever virus is widely distributed throughout the arid regions of south and eastern Europe, Africa, the Middle East, and Asia. The infection is transmitted by ticks of the genus *Hyalomma* and is enzootic in many animal species, such as sheep, cattle, goats, and camels, where it is mostly asymptomatic (Hoogstraal, JMedEntomol, 1979; 15:307). Ticks may also be infected sexually and transovarially and this mechanism may contribute to the maintenance of transmission in nature (Gonzalez, ResVirol, 1992; 143:23).

Close contact with infected animals may be hazardous. Transmission may occur through exposure to infected blood, respiratory secretions, and excreta of patients in the hospital setting (Burney, AmJTropMedHyg, 1980; 29:941). Crushing infected ticks has been reported to be dangerous.[9]

Pathology

Crimean/Congo haemorrhagic fever resembles many other viral haemorrhagic fevers. The liver is often involved, with focal necrosis, often localized in the midzonal areas, and with the presence of Councilman bodies.[1] Necrosis and haemorrhages can be found in the kidneys and spleen.[1]

Clinical manifestations

In epidemic settings, Crimean/Congo haemorrhagic fever is a severe haemorrhagic fever with a mortality rate ranging from 10 to 80 per cent in different outbreaks.[1] Mild or asymptomatic infections may occur, as proved by serosurveys in populations of central Africa (Johnson, TrRSocTropMedHyg, 1993; 87:530). The disease has a milder, self-limiting course when occurring sporadically.[1]

After an incubation period of 3 to 7 days, the onset is abrupt, with fever, headache, nausea, and vomiting. A petechial rash accompanied by gingival bleeding may be observed. In some patients, after 4 or 5 days, severe haemorrhages develop with massive bleeding, leading to hypotensive shock and death. There may be an acute, icteric hepatitis, and in some cases disseminated intravascular coagulation.[1] Leucopenia, thrombocytopenia, and abnormal liver function tests are common laboratory findings.

Diagnosis

The differential diagnosis is mainly with the other viral haemorrhagic fevers.

The diagnosis of acute infection relies on virus isolation in cell cultures utilizing Vero or BHK cells, or by inoculation in the brain of suckling mice (Schwarz, AmJTropMedHyg, 1996; 55:190). Virus isolation requires high-containment laboratories.[9]

An antigen-capture ELISA is available for detection and quantification of Crimean/Congo haemorrhagic fever virus in both humans and ticks (Saluzzo, JClinMicrobiol, 1987; 25:922). Recently, an RT–PCR has been developed, with good results (Schwarz, AmJTropMedHyg, 1996; 55:190). Several methods for demonstrating antibody to Crimean/Congo haemorrhagic fever virus are available. The antibody response usually develops 5 to 14 days after the onset of symptoms and is rarely detected in the patients who die of the disease (Burt, EpidInf, 1994; 113:551). Indirect immunofluorescence and ELISA can be used to detect IgM and

IgG antibodies; as handling the virus to prepare reagents may be hazardous, recombinant antigens have been proposed to detect the antibody response by ELISA (Marriott, JGenVirol, 1994; 75:2157).

Treatment

Studies *in vitro* and in experimental animals suggest that ribavirin may be effective in the treatment of Crimean/Congo haemorrhagic fever. Recently three patients were successfully treated with oral ribavirin, supporting its use in the treatment of this disease (Fisher-Hoch, Lancet, 1995; 346:472).

Prevention

No vaccine is available. Strict barrier nursing and, if feasible, isolation under negative pressure of patients is indicated to prevent in-hospital spread of the disease by aerosol or contact with blood and other body fluids (WHO, WklyEpidemiolRec, 1995; 70:249). Tick control is extremely difficult; personal measures to avoid tick bites (such as tick repellents) are of limited value.[9]

References

1. Simpson DIH. Arbovirus infections. In *Manson's tropical diseases*. London: Saunders, 1996: 615–65.
2. Halstead SB. Dengue, yellow fever and rabies. *Current Opinion in Infectious Disease*, 1994; 7: 559–63.
3. Monath TP. Flaviviruses. In *Principles and practice of infectious diseases*. New York: Churchill Livingstone, 1995: 1465–74.
4. Monath TP. Yellow fever. In *Tropical and geographical medicine*. New York: McGraw Hill, 1990: 661–74.
5. Monath TP and Nasidi A. Should yellow fever vaccine be included in the Expanded Program of Immunization in Africa? A cost-effectiveness analysis for Nigeria. *American Journal of Tropical Medicine and Hygiene*, 1993; **48**: 274–99.
6. Peters CJ and Johnson KM. Lymphocytic choriomeningitis virus, Lassa virus and other Arenaviruses. In *Principles and practice of infectious diseases*. New York: Churchill Livingstone, 1995: 1472–9.
7. Clegg JCS and Lloyd G. Ebola haemorrhagic fever in Zaire, 1995: a perspective. *Current Opinion in Infectious Disease*, 1995; 8: 225–8.
8. Peters CJ. Marburg and Ebola virus hemorrhagic fevers. In *Principles and practice of infectious diseases*. New York: Churchill Livingstone, 1995: 1543–6.
9. Peters CJ and Johnson KM. California encephalitis viruses, Hantaviruses and other Bunyaviridae. In *Principles and practice of infectious diseases*. New York: Churchill Livingstone, 1995: 1567–72.

13

Other infections of the liver

13.1 Bacterial and rickettsial infections

13.1.1 Bacterial infection and the liver

Christopher C. Kibbler and Jose Maria Sánchez Tapias

Introduction

Bacteria may affect liver function either as a result of parenchymal or biliary invasion, or as a systemic manifestation of bacteraemia or toxaemia. There is a wide spectrum of involvement from minimally abnormal results in liver function tests to frank jaundice and hepatocellular failure. Certain organisms, such as *Leptospira interrogans* serovar *icterohaemorrhagiae*, are more consistently associated with liver dysfunction than others. However, because of the large numbers of different bacteria and clinical conditions that may be involved, the presentation of abnormal liver function tests in an apparently septic patient has a large differential diagnosis.

The spectrum of typical results for liver biochemistry seen in the infections discussed in this chapter is shown in Table 1; an appreciation of these can be helpful in reaching a diagnosis.

Liver dysfunction in extrahepatic infection

Definition

Sepsis is the systemic response to infection, which may be confirmed by the detection of bacteraemia and/or the identification of a primary source.[1] Bacteraemia implies the isolation of an organism from one or more sets of blood cultures. The term covers a multitude of clinical syndromes from an asymptomatic condition to septic shock. In most writing on this subject bacteraemia and septicaemia are synonymous. It is important to identify the source of the bacteraemia, if possible, as some sites of sepsis are more frequently associated with abnormal liver function tests (particularly the lung and urinary tract) and, more importantly, identification of the source will affect management in terms of choice of antibiotics and the need for concomitant surgical procedures.

Introduction

Jaundice in patients with pneumococcal pneumonia, with or without bacteraemia, was first described in 1836 (Garvin, SouthMedSurg, 1896; 15:36). Since then, deranged liver function has been noted with a variety of organisms isolated from extrahepatic sites or in blood cultures.

Epidemiology

There have been few published studies in which the incidence of liver dysfunction in extrahepatic infection has been assessed. Most have been of cases selected because of jaundice or biochemical abnormalities, or studies in particular populations in which jaundice might be expected to be more common (for example, Black Africans, in whom haemolysis may occur in those deficient in glucose 6-phosphate dehydrogenase). In addition, definitions of jaundice vary between studies. Taking these factors into account, the incidence of jaundice in community-acquired bacteraemia in patients without underlying liver disease has ranged from 0.6 to 34 per cent (Zimmerman, JLabClinMed, 1950; 35:556; Bernstein, Pediat, 1962; 29:873; Fahrlander, Gastro, 1964; 47:590; Eley, BMJ, 1965; 2:75; Neale, BMJ, 1966; 31:382; Vermillion, ArchIntMed, 1969; 124:611; Theron, JPath, 1972; 106:113; Miller, Gastro, 1976; 71:94; Tugwell, QJMed, 1977; 46:97; Zimmerman, Gastro, 1979; 77:362). In a large prospective study, the incidence of jaundice (conjugated bilirubin >20 μmol/l) was 7.8 per cent in a mixed South African population with community-acquired pneumonia (Rayner, QJMed, 1988; 69:907). Another study (Franson, RevInfDis, 1985; 7:1) prospectively examined the liver function of 100 patients with positive blood cultures and found that 54 per cent had a total bilirubin above 1.0 mg/l; in 34 per cent it was above 2.0 mg/l; there were no significant sex differences in this series. In an earlier study, liver dysfunction was present in all patients with septic shock and multiple organ failure (Cerra, Surgery, 1979; 137:409).

Jaundice occurs commonly with bacteraemia in childhood, particularly in infants, where the source may be umbilical sepsis, pneumonia, urinary-tract infection, spontaneous group B streptococcal bacteraemia, otitis media, or exchange blood transfusion. In the prospective study mentioned above, 42 per cent of bacteraemic children under 12 years of age had a total bilirubin above 2.0 mg/l and 80 per cent of these were under the age of 1 month (Franson, RevInfDis, 1985; 7:1).

Pathogenesis and pathology

The cause of the biochemical abnormalities is not clear. The pattern of jaundice occurring in patients in different series is variable and it appears that it can be caused by more than one factor. Several investigators have proposed that the jaundice is cholestatic in nature, as their patients showed marked hyperbilirubinaemia with marginal changes in liver enzymes. Histological sections of liver have shown intrahepatic cholestasis with occasional focal necrosis, fatty change, and periportal cell infiltrates (Zimmerman, JLabClinMed, 1950; 35:

Table 1 Liver function tests in bacterial infections

Disease	Alkaline phosphatase	AST	Total bilirubin
Sepsis syndrome	+	+	+ +
Pneumococcal pneumonia	+	+	+ +
Liver abscess	±	Normal	Normal
Toxic shock syndrome	+	+ +	+ + +
Gas gangrene	+	+ +	+ + +
Listeriosis	+	+ +	+/+ +
Legionnaires' disease	+	+ +	+
Brucellosis	+	+	+
Melioidosis	+	+	+/+ +
Typhoid fever	Normal	+ +	+
Tularaemia	Normal	+ + +	+
Secondary syphilis	+ + +	+ +	+
Lyme disease (stage 1)	Normal	+	±
Leptospirosis	+	+ + +/+ + + +	+ +/+ + + +
Relapsing fever	±	+ +	+ + +
Q fever	+	+	±
Rocky Mountain spotted fever	+	+	+
Chlamydia infection	±	+ +	±
Mycoplasma pneumoniae infection	±	+ +	±
Cat-scratch disease	±	Normal	Normal
Tuberculosis	±	Normal	Normal

Modified after Cunha BA. Systemic infections affecting the liver. *Postgraduate Medicine*, 1988; 84:148–68.
AST, aspartate aminotransferase.

556; Miller, Gastro, 1976; 71:94). Miller suggested that, because the serum concentrations of most substances normally excreted in the bile were either normal or only marginally elevated, there is an isolated defect of excretion of conjugated bilirubin. On the other hand, in another study, mean serum concentrations of the aminotransferases and alkaline phosphatase were elevated in proportion to the serum bilirubin, suggesting that the jaundice might be hepatocellular in nature (Rayner, QJMed, 1988; 69:907).

Endotoxaemia may play some part in the impairment of liver function in Gram-negative infections. In studies with isolated, perfused rat liver, endotoxin caused a dose-dependent decrease in bile flow (Utili, JLabClinMed, 1977; 89:471), and this was associated with a reduction in the excretion of organic ions (Utili, Gastro, 1976; 70:248); the reduction in bile flow appeared to be due to a selective reduction in the bile salt-independent fraction. Endotoxin dose-dependently inhibited Na^+/K^+-ATPase in rat liver plasma membranes enriched with bile canaliculi, but did not seem to affect the activity of other membrane-associated enzymes such as 5-nucleotidase (Utili, JInfDis, 1977; 136:583). These effects of endotoxin might explain the high incidence of jaundice in neonates with Gram-negative infection as they have a low bile salt-dependent flow (Watkins, Gastro, 1975; 69:706), but jaundice can occur during sepsis in which endotoxaemia is absent (Gimson, IntensCareMed, 1987; 13:162). In addition, patients with multiple organ failure following severe trauma have a pattern of liver impairment similar to that seen with intra-abdominal sepsis, suggesting a common mechanism (Goris, ArchSurg, 1985; 120:1109). In both sepsis and trauma, hepatic blood flow is apparently depressed (Garrison, Surgery, 1982; 92:713; Gottlieb, JTrauma, 1983; 23:836), and a concomitant reduction in hepatic oxygen supply has been demonstrated in the rat with sepsis (Fitch, CirculShock, 1983; 10:51). However, other studies have shown an increase in hepatic blood flow and

oxygen consumption during early sepsis and it may be that circulatory changes only become important in the later stages of infection (Wilmore, AnnSurg, 1980; 192:491; Lang, AmJPhysiol, 1984; 246:R331).

The production of tumour necrosis factor during sepsis activates neutrophils, resulting in the release of neutrophil elastase. This has been shown to have a cytotoxic effect on hepatocytes *in vitro*, causing release of lactate dehydrogenase (Oka, JSurgRes, 1993; 55:1). Tumour necrosis factor-α and interleukin 1 appear to be the main mediators responsible for upregulation of intercellular adhesion molecule-1 mRNA in the liver during endotoxaemia. The upregulation of intercellular adhesion molecule-1 and the CD11b/CD18 neutrophil receptor (Mac-1) is necessary for neutrophil-induced liver injury to occur in endotoxaemic mice (Essani, Hepatol, 1995; 21:163).

Certain organisms (such as *Staphylococcus aureus* and *Clostridium perfringens*) produce other toxins that cause abnormalities of liver function and these will be dealt with in subsequent sections. Liver dysfunction in a septic patient may also be coincidental, as a result of the administration of hepatotoxic drugs, total parenteral nutrition, halothane anaesthesia, cardiopulmonary bypass surgery (Gimson, IntensCareMed, 1987; 13:162), or blood transfusion.

Clinical features

The majority of patients are febrile (temperature >37°C) and some may have rigors, confusion, and sweating. Jaundice usually follows the onset of infection by 2 or 3 days. In patients who are frankly jaundiced pruritus is rare; there is painless hepatomegaly in more than 50 per cent of cases. The most common sources of bacteraemia in these patients are pneumonia, urinary-tract infection, and soft-tissue infection, although organisms may also originate from pelvic infection, peritonitis, meningitis, lung abscess, septic abortion, and

Table 2 Blood-culture isolates associated with abnormal liver function tests

Aerobic Gram-negative bacteria:
   Escherichia coli
   Klebsiella spp.
   Salmonella typhi
   Pseudomonas aeruginosa
   Pseudomonas spp.
   Burkolderia pseudomallei
   Alkaligenes spp.
   Neisseria meningitidis
   N. gonorrhoeae
   Brucella spp.
   Yersinia spp.
   Fransiscella tularensis
Aerobic Gram-positive bacteria:
   Streptococcus pneumoniae
   Staphylococcus aureus
   β-Haemolytic streptococci (Lancefield groups A, B, and C)
   Coagulase-negative staphylococci
Anaerobic bacteria:
   Bacteroides spp.
   Clostridium perfringens

tracheitis. There have been reports of jaundice in association with meningococcal septicaemia and meningitis in which patients had an initial history suggestive of viral hepatitis, with high serum concentrations of the transaminases (Cowan, JTropMedHyg, 1987; 90:95). A list of the blood-culture isolates that have been associated with liver dysfunction is shown in Table 2.

Complications in these patients reflect those seen in non-jaundiced patients with bacteraemia and include acute renal failure, adult respiratory distress syndrome, and disseminated intravascular coagulopathy. The overall mortality is up to 45 per cent.

Investigations

Liver function tests have shown varying patterns in different studies (Zimmerman, JLabClinMed, 1950; 35:556; Fahrlander, Gastro, 1964; 47:590; Eley, BMJ, 1965; 2:75; Neale, BMJ, 1966; 31:382; Vermillion, ArchIntMed, 1969, 124:611; Miller, Gastro, 1976; 71: 94; Tugwell, QJMed, 1977; 46:97; Zimmerman, Gastro, 1979; 77: 362; Franson, RevInfDis, 1985; 7:1; Rayner, QJMed, 1988; 69:907). The overall picture is that of a marked conjugated hyperbilirubinaemia with moderate elevation of alkaline phosphatase and aspartate aminotransferase (**AST**). The serum bilirubin does not correlate with mortality. Blood cultures and samples from probable primary sites of infection should be taken before commencing antibiotic therapy.

Treatment

Resolution of abnormal liver function appears to follow the response of sepsis to appropriate antibiotic therapy. Choice of treatment will obviously depend upon the antibiotic sensitivities of the causative organisms, if isolated. However, the severely ill septic patient requires empirical therapy, which should be governed by the source of sepsis.

Patients admitted with community-acquired pneumonia should be treated initially with an intravenous cephalosporin such as cefotaxime (2 g 8-hourly) and erythromycin (1 g 6-hourly) until the causative organism is established. Advice on the treatment of life-threatening urinary-tract infection should be sought from the microbiology department, as there is considerable variation in local patterns of antibiotic sensitivity. Those patients with uncomplicated urinary-tract infections may be treated with an aminoglycoside or a second- or third generation cephalosporin. Patients with complicated urinary-tract infections, or those who have had recent instrumentation of the urinary tract (including an indwelling urinary catheter), may be infected with organisms resistant to the commonly used antibiotics, including *Pseudomonas aeruginosa*. Hence these infections should be treated with agents such as an aminoglycoside (e.g. gentamicin), a carbapenem (e.g. imipenem/cilastatin, meropenem), a quinolone (e.g. ciprofloxacin, ofloxacin), piperacillin/tazobactam or an antipseudomonal cephalosporin. Patients with jaundice and soft-tissue infection usually require therapy for staphylococci, streptococci, or both. Hence treatment with benzylpenicillin and flucloxacillin is appropriate. However, it should be borne in mind that certain necrotizing soft-tissue infections associated with multiorgan failure are multibacillary in nature, and that severely immunocompromised patients may suffer soft tissue infections with Gram-negative organisms, particularly *Ps. aeruginosa*.

Pyogenic liver abscesses
Definition

Pyogenic liver abscesses result from bacterial infection of the liver parenchyma and subsequent infiltration of the area with neutrophils and other phagocytes to form a collection of pus. In some cases the wall of the abscess may be formed by biliary epithelium, for example in patients with ectatic ducts, or by the lining of an hydatid cyst that has become secondarily infected.

Introduction

The condition was recognized by the ancient Greeks, who classified it separately from other causes of liver cysts. The first large series was reported more than 100 years ago, when 11 cases were found among 257 patients with appendicitis (Fritz, AmJMedSci, 1886; 91: 321).

Epidemiology

There has been a change in the age distribution of liver abscess in recent years. It used to be most common during the third and fourth decades of life, but the peak incidence is now in patients aged 60 to 70 years. Based upon surveys of hospital admissions (Neoptolemos, ActaChirScand, 1982; 148:415) and autopsy series, the condition is found in less than 0.5 per cent of patients.[2-4]

Pathogenesis and pathology

Bacteria cause liver abscesses by three routes: (i) biliary-tract infection, (ii) haematogenous infection, (iii) extension of contiguous infection into the liver.

In adults, biliary-tract infection following obstruction of the common bile duct is associated, in as many as 40 per cent of cases of liver abscesses (Lazarchick, MayoClinProc, 1973; 4:349; Pitt,

Table 3 Organisms isolated from pyogenic liver abscesses

Aerobes:
   Escherichia coli
   Klebsiella pneumoniae and other species
   Enterobacter spp.
   Pseudomonas spp.
   Staphylococcus aureus
   Streptococci:
      Group D
      α-haemolytic
      Microaerophilic (*Strep. milleri*)
   Yersinia enterocolitica
   Listeria monocytogenes
   Salmonella spp.
   Gardnerella vaginalis
   Calymmatobacterium granulomatis (the cause of
     granuloma inguinale)
Anaerobes:
   Bacteroides fragilis
   Bacteroides spp.
   Fusobacterium necrophorum
   F. nucleatum
   Fusobacterium spp.
   Clostridium perfringens
   C. septicum
   Peptostreptococcus spp.
   Actinomyces spp.
Yeasts

References: Kahn, ArchSurg, 1972; 104:209; Chogle, JAssocPhysInd, 1981; 29:73; Jenkins, Gut, 1987; 28:1661; Ezzell, AmJGastr, 1988; 83:1409; other references in text.

SGO, 1975; 140:228; Greenstein, AmJGastr, 1984; 79:217). These are usually multiple and present in both lobes of the liver. Systemic bacteraemia is thought to be the most common cause of liver abscesses in infants and young children (Barnes, Medicine, 1987; 66:472), and is responsible for between 10 and 20 per cent of cases in adults.[2,3] The lesions are typically multiple microabscesses distributed in both lobes of the liver. Bacteraemia may cause infection and abscess formation in tumours, accounting for up to 16 per cent of liver abscesses (Lazarchick, MayoClinProc, 1973).[3] Transcatheter arterial chemoembolization as therapy for hepatic tumours is also associated with subsequent liver abscess formation in approx. 3 per cent of cases (Ishikawa, JpnJCancer-Chemother, 1994; 21:2233).

Portal bacteraemia is responsible for up to 17 per cent of cases, [2,3] although in the era before antibiotics it may have been the most common cause, particularly following acute appendicitis. The abscesses are usually large, occur mainly in the right lobe, and may be single or multiple. The primary sources of such abscesses include peritonitis, diverticulitis, intra-abdominal abscesses, pancreatitis, portal thrombophlebitis, neonatal sepsis of the umbilical vein, and inflammatory bowel disease. Formation of liver abscess may follow direct extension of infection from cholecystitis, pancreatitis, perihepatic abscess, or penetrating gastric or duodenal ulcers. Blunt trauma to the liver may be followed by abscess, presumably as a result of bacteraemia with consequent infection of haematoma or necrotic tissue (Haight, SouthMedJ, 1994; 87:811). There may be no obvious underlying cause in as many as 25 per cent of cases.[4]

The causative organisms (Table 3) vary according to the primary site of infection. Abscesses following cholangitis or intra-abdominal sepsis are frequently polymicrobial and usually involve enteric Gram-negative organisms and anaerobes, which may be cultured in up to 50 per cent of these cases (Greenstein, AmJGastr, 1984; 79: 217; Barnes, Medicine, 1987; 66:472).[4] Systemic bacteraemia usually causes infection with a single organism, chiefly *Staph aureus*, streptococci, or aerobic Gram-negative organisms. *Klebsiella pneumoniae*, one of the most common of the latter organisms causing liver abscesses, has a strong association with diabetes mellitus and with metastatic infection, particularly endophthalmitis (Han, WorldJMed, 1995; 162:220). *Yersinia enterocolitica* characteristically causes liver abscess in patients with diabetes mellitus, haemochromatosis, or cirrhosis (Bouza, AmJClinPath, 1980; 74:404; Viteri, Gastro, 1981; 81:592; Fothergill, PostgradMedJ, 1982; 58:371; Alberti-Flor, Digestion, 1984; 29:250). Although granuloma inguinale is usually confined to the anogenital area, the liver may be affected following bacteraemia; there may be small abscesses, sometimes multiple, and typical Donovan bodies may be seen histologically (Lyford, BullJHopkHosp, 1946; 79:349). Hepatic granulomas have also been described with this infection.[5]

Clinical features

Patients typically present with slow onset of fever and pain in the right upper quadrant, although there may be rapid clinical deterioration with systemic signs of sepsis, jaundice, and shock in cases associated with cholangitis. In addition, there is usually loss of appetite and weight. Symptoms may have been present for several months before the diagnosis is made.[4] Pain in the shoulder tip or pleuritic chest pain are features suggestive of diaphragmatic involvement. Rarely the patient may present acutely with the signs and symptoms of a perforated viscus as a consequence of the perforation of a gas-containing liver abscess (Matsuyama, Surg-Today, 1994; 24:63).

Investigations

Pyogenic liver abscesses do not produce a characteristic pattern of liver function tests, although the alkaline phosphatase may be elevated.[6] The majority of patients have a neutrophil leucocytosis, a mild anaemia, and a raised erythrocyte sedimentation rate. Blood cultures are positive in up to 60 per cent, and as many as 50 per cent of isolates may be anaerobes.[4,6,7] There is elevation of the right hemidiaphragm in up to 50 per cent of patients on chest radiograph, and right-sided pleural effusions or basal infiltrates may be seen in up to 40 per cent (Pitt, SGO, 1975; 140:228; Greenstein, AmJGastr, 1984; 79:217).[4] Imaging of the liver to allow confirmation of the diagnosis and aspiration of abscess contents is now usually done by means of ultrasonography or CT scanning. The latter is the most sensitive of the two (Barreda, CritRevDiagImag, 1992, 33:29),[6] although MRI scanning and radioisotope imaging are increasingly used. Positive cultures from the abscess contents are obtained in between 73 and 88 per cent of patients, of which more than half are of anaerobes (Greenstein, AmJGastr, 1984; 79: 217; Barnes, Medicine, 1987; 66:472).[4,7,8]

Differential diagnosis

The differential diagnosis is that of any cystic lesions of the liver and includes: (i) hydatid disease, (ii) amoebic liver abscesses,

(iii) primary and secondary malignancies, and (iv) fibropolycystic disease.

Treatment

Pyogenic liver abscesses require aspiration or drainage and treatment with appropriate antibiotics, depending on the organisms isolated. Percutaneous aspiration may be adequate, although laparotomy may be necessary for the relief of biliary obstruction or management of the primary site of sepsis.[4,6,7] Laparoscopic drainage has also recently been shown to be effective (Cappuccino, SurgLapEndosc, 1994, 4:234; Yanaga, BrJSurg, 1994, 81:1022). Antibiotics alone, without drainage, have been used successfully in patients infected with a variety of organisms,[4] although others have reported a high mortality following such treatments.[9] It would seem, therefore, that this management should be reserved for those patients in whom surgical and percutaneous drainage procedures are not feasible. Aspiration carries a small risk of bleeding and pneumothorax, and drainage catheters have caused abscess rupture and subsequent peritonitis.[6]

In view of the wide range of possible organisms, every attempt should be made to make a microbiological diagnosis. Empirical antibiotic therapy should include antibiotics active against the aerobic Gram-negative bacteria, the streptococci (and enterococci), and the anaerobes. There have been no randomized studies of antibiotic therapy, but options include a third-generation cephalosporin, such as ceftriaxone or cefotaxime (with or without ampicillin) plus metronidazole, co-amoxiclav, piperacillin/tazobactam, or a carbapenem, such as imipenem/cilastatin or meropenem. Duration of therapy is probably dependent upon the success of drainage/aspiration. Intravenous therapy for at least 2 weeks until fever and leucocytosis respond, followed by oral antibiotics for a further 4 weeks, appears effective.[6] The need for repeat aspiration of the abscess should be evaluated by means of follow-up scans. One study using ultrasound-guided percutaneous needle aspiration plus antibiotics demonstrated a cure rate of 98 per cent (Giorgio, Radiol, 1995, 195:122), although others, treating higher-risk patients with greater numbers of postsurgical abscesses, were less successful (Lambiase, Radiol, 1992, 184:167; Baek, AJR, 1993, 160:799).

Untreated abscesses are uniformly fatal. Even with effective therapy the condition still carries a mortality of more than 10 per cent. The prognosis is worse in elderly people, in those with multiple abscesses, in the presence of malignancy and severe underlying disease, in cases secondary to biliary-tract disease, and following delay in diagnosis.

Complications

Liver abscesses may rupture, or be associated with bacteraemia or septic emboli. Rupture or embolization occurs in fewer than 10 per cent of patients.[9]

Liver dysfunction following infection with specific organisms

Staph. aureus and toxic shock syndrome

In addition to the effects of staphylococcal sepsis on the liver that have already been described, hepatic dysfunction is common in cases of toxic shock syndrome.

Definition

Toxic shock syndrome is a severe, multisystem disorder occurring in patients colonized or infected with a strain of *Staph. aureus* producing specific toxin(s) including toxic shock syndrome toxin 1 (**TSST-1**).

Introduction

Toxic shock syndrome was first described in the United States in 1978 (Todd, Lancet, 1978; ii:1116). In 1981, two independent groups identified a previously undescribed staphylococcal toxin from more than 90 per cent of *Staph. aureus* strains tested in toxic shock syndrome. This is now called TSST-1 and is distinct from the epidermolytic (exfoliatin) toxin, produced by phage-group II staphylococci and associated with the 'scalded skin syndrome'.

Epidemiology

After the first few cases of toxic shock syndrome it became apparent that most occurred in adult females, and that 90 per cent were associated with the onset of menstruation. The vast majority of these were tampon-related. In one study the incidence of toxic shock syndrome was estimated as 6.2 cases per 100 000 menstruating women per year.[10] Strains of *Staph. aureus* isolated from these patients were predominantly of phage-group 1, lysed by phage 29 and resistant to penicillin.

More recently, active surveillance methods employed in the United States have shown a fall in the incidence of the disease, particularly in the incidence of menses-associated infection. This is thought to be due to the withdrawal of the 'Rely' brand of tampon from the market in 1980 and the elimination of polyacrylate from tampon constituents in 1985. Hence, in 1986 only 54 per cent of cases in the United States were menstrually related [Gaventa, RevInfDis, 1989; 11(Suppl. 1):S28]. In the United Kingdom 64 per cent of confirmed or probable cases of toxic shock syndrome in 1992–1993 were associated with menstruation (CDR, 1994, 4:1)

Pathogenesis and pathology

Liver dysfunction might be produced in toxic shock syndrome as a result of hypoperfusion, circulating exotoxins, or circulating endotoxin. With the hypotension of toxic shock syndrome one would expect elevations of serum AST and bilirubin, but they tend to be higher in patients with shock than those with toxic shock syndrome (Gourley, Gastro, 1981; 81:928).

TSST-1 acts as a superantigen, binding to class II molecules of the major histocompatibility complex, at a site distinct from the antigen-binding groove, on the antigen-presenting cell and the Vβ region of the T-cell receptor. This allows large numbers of T cells (having a receptor Vβ region belonging to the same family) to be activated. The consequence of this is the excess production of T-cell-derived cytokines, particularly interferon-γ, interleukin 1, interleukin 6, and tumour necrosis factor, and other monokines and lymphokines (Kotb, ClinMicroRev, 1995; 8:411). It has also been proposed that damage to the intestinal epithelium by staphylococcal exotoxins might allow portal toxaemia or even Gram-negative bacteraemia, thus potentiating the effect of the circulating exotoxin.[11]

Histological examination of tissue from various organs, including liver, from patients with toxic shock syndrome have shown evidence of vasculitis (Abdul-Karim, HumPath, 1981; 12:16) and microvesicular steatosis (McKenna, MayoClinProc, 1980; 55:663). In one series, which included six cases of toxic shock syndrome, all patients were found to have inflammation of the intrahepatic bile ducts and canaliculi. Some showed necrosis and even rupture of the ducts. Infiltration of the portal tracts with neutrophils, eosinophils, monocytes, and lymphocytes was seen as well as microvesicular steatosis. Only 50 per cent of the cases had evidence of centrilobular cholestasis.[11]

Clinical features

The disease is characterized by fever (>38°C), an erythematous rash causing desquamation of the palms and soles 1 to 2 weeks later, hypotension (systolic blood pressure <90 mmHg), and involvement of at least three of the following systems: (i) gastrointestinal tract (diarrhoea and vomiting), (ii) renal tract (elevation of urea/creatinine twice normal), (iii) liver [bilirubin, AST or alanine aminotransferase (**ALT**) twice normal], (iv) central nervous system (disorientation or an alteration in level of consciousness), and (v) blood (platelets $<100 \times 10^9$/l). [For a more detailed description of the clinical features of toxic shock syndrome, see Chesney, RevInfDis, 1989; 11 (Suppl 1): S1.] The syndrome has been reported in many different clinical settings involving colonization or infection with *Staph. aureus*, and as a complication of surgical procedures, trauma, and local infections. Unusual clinical features have also been observed in patients with the acquired immune deficiency syndrome (Strausbaugh, PostgradMed, 1993; 94:107).

An overall mortality of 8 per cent has been reported in the United States, and up to 30 per cent of patients experience more than one episode of toxic shock syndrome.

Hepatic dysfunction is most marked in the first few days in hospital, with serum bilirubin returning towards normal within a week in the majority of cases.

Investigations

The diagnosis of toxic shock syndrome is based on clinical criteria. Liver function tests usually show an elevation of serum transaminases to between two and three times normal in the first few days of the illness. The alkaline phosphatase is often normal initially, rising to between one-and-a half and three times normal by the end of the first week.[10] The total bilirubin may exceed 3.0 mg/100 ml during the first 3 days of the illness, with at least 50 per cent being conjugated (Gourley, Gastro, 1981; 81:928).[11] Serum albumin is typically low and remains so for at least 10 days (Gourley, Gastro, 1981; 81:928).

A moderate leucocytosis is usually found, with thrombocytopenia (see above) in some cases. A high urea and creatinine, and disordered electrolytes, form part of the diagnostic picture.

Staphylococcus aureus is rarely recovered from blood cultures but is often isolated from vaginal swabs and less commonly from other sites. Isolates should be sent to reference laboratories in order to demonstrate toxin production. TSST-1 has been demonstrated in serum by an enzyme-linked immunosorbent assay, but this is not routinely available (Miwa, JClinMicrobiol, 1994; 32:539).

Differential diagnosis

The differential diagnosis is that of a multisystem disease with fever, hypotension, and rash; it includes: scarlet fever, meningococcaemia, erythema multiforme, drug eruption, leptospirosis, Rocky Mountain spotted fever, and Kawasaki disease.

Treatment

The treatment of toxic shock syndrome is primarily supportive and includes the removal of potentially infected foreign bodies and drainage of infected sites, correction of hypoperfusion with fluids and inotropes, the management of adult respiratory distress syndrome, if present, and the management of renal and hepatic failure. Antistaphylococcal antibiotics are given, although their role in recovery from toxic shock syndrome in patients without foci of infection is uncertain. Intravenous immunoglobulin has high concentrations of antibody to TSST-1 and inhibits the activation of T cells by TSST-1 (Takei, JCI, 1993; 91:602). Hence consideration should be given to its early use in severe cases.

Clostridium perfringens

Although *C. perfringens* is most likely to affect the liver in the form of an abscess (see above), patients with infections due to the presence of the organism at other sites may suffer jaundice.

Definition

The organism is a Gram-positive, spore-forming anaerobe. It is found in soil, and in the gut and female genital tract in humans. It is an important cause of food poisoning, is responsible for enteritis necroticans (or 'pig-bel'), and may be involved in a variety of suppurative infections including those of skin and soft tissue.

Epidemiology

With the exception of food poisoning and gas gangrene following war wounds, the majority of infections due to *C. perfringens* are probably endogenous in nature.

Pathogenesis and pathology

Clostridium perfringens produces at least 17 toxins, of which the four major ones (α, β, ϵ, and ι) are lethal in animal models.[12] α-Toxin is a phospholipase C that splits lecithin to form phosphoryl choline and a diglyceride; it is responsible for the Nagler reaction used in the identification of the organisms. α-Toxin is also produced by other clostridial species, and is the most important toxin in the initiation of gas gangrene.

The site of action of α-toxin is the lecithin and sphingomyelin in cell membranes; it is more active on membrane-bound rather than free lipid. The protein is fixed at the site of inoculation,[13] and its effects appear to be exerted almost exclusively locally, except in postabortion septicaemia and in occasional cases of gas gangrene, where there is massive haemolysis and consequent jaundice, haemoglobinaemia, and renal impairment, with hydrolysis of the plasma phospholipids.

Clinical features

Gas gangrene may develop on the same day as the initiating event (trauma or surgery) or be delayed for up to 20 days. There is typically an increase in pain in the wound, which then becomes tense and oedematous, and there is often a watery discharge, which may contain tiny bubbles of gas. Gas in the tissues is difficult to detect on palpation. At the same time the patient develops systemic signs of tachycardia, circulatory collapse, and progression to renal failure, with or without haemolysis and jaundice.

Uterine gas gangrene usually follows septic abortion 2 to 3 days later. The initial symptoms include vaginal bleeding, suprapubic and back pain, and rigors. Jaundice may appear within hours of the onset of illness and is the result of massive haemolysis. Progression to circulatory collapse, adult respiratory distress syndrome, and renal failure is common.

Investigations

The diagnosis of gas gangrene is based on clinical features. The causative organism is commonly isolated from wound swabs or specimens from the genital tract and is only rarely acting as a pathogen at these sites, although a pure heavy culture is strong support for the diagnosis. Patients with uterine gas gangrene may have a *C. perfringens* bacteraemia. Haemolytic anaemia is present and haemoglobinuria is detectable. There is usually a neutrophil leucocytosis. Radiographs of the affected site may show air in the tissues.

The serum bilirubin may be very high and is chiefly unconjugated. The AST is usually markedly elevated while the alkaline phosphatase is little affected (Cunha, PostgradMed, 1988; 84:148).

Treatment

Immediate surgical intervention, in the form of radical debridement of tissues or uterine curettage, is probably the most important part of therapy. Intravenous benzylpenicillin, 2 to 3 MU 4-hourly, should also be given. Patients allergic to penicillin may be treated with metronidazole, clindamycin or chloramphenicol.

The use of antitoxin is controversial but is more logical in these patients with circulating α-toxin than in those without features of haemolysis. Removal of the damaged red cells by exchange transfusion may also have some effect. The benefits of hyperbaric oxygen are open to question and there are conflicting data on its use.

The mortality in these patients is up to 60 per cent.

Listeria monocytogenes
Definition

Infection with *L. monocytogenes* characteristically causes a meningo-encephalitis, although pneumonitis, endocarditis, conjunctivitis, pyoderma, and hepatic infection may also occur. The organism is a Gram-positive, aerobic bacillus.

Introduction

The organism was first isolated from man in 1929 (Nyfeldt, CSoc-Bio, 1929; 101:590). It is widely distributed in nature, being found in water, soil, and plant material, but rarely causes infection in man and then usually only in pregnant women, immunocompromised patients or neonates.

Epidemiology

The incidence of human infection in the United Kingdom increased until the end of the 1980s when it was estimated to be approx. 1 case per 230 000 of the total population per year and 1 case per 9700 births (McLauchlin, Lancet, 1988; i:177). In recent years the importance of food-borne transmission has been recognized, with outbreaks ascribed to pasteurized milk, coleslaw, pâté, and soft cheeses (Anon, Lancet, 1985; ii:364; Gill, JInfect, 1988; 17:1).[14] Following the introduction of guidelines for pregnant women by the Chief Medical Officer the incidence has fallen in the United Kingdom and a similar fall has taken place in the United States after the imposition of food-monitoring policies (Tappero, JAMA, 1995; 273:1118).

Faecal carriage in the general population is approx. 5 per cent but may be as high as 29 per cent in poultry workers. Direct transmission has been described in veterinary surgeons (Owen, NEJM, 1960; 262:1026), abattoir workers, and farmers (Bojsen-Moller, ActaPMIScand, 1972; 229:1).

Pathogenesis and pathology

In order to produce an infection the organism survives and grows within macrophages. The mechanisms by which it avoids intracellular killing are still only poorly understood, but appear to be related to the secretion of extracellular bacterial products. α-Listeriolysin (a cytotoxin antigenically related to streptolysin O) and β-listeriolysin are associated with pathogenicity, possibly by disrupting the phagosome and allowing release of organisms into the cytoplasm of the phagocyte.[14] Lipopolysaccharide produced by listeria also an immunosuppressive effect (Galsworthy, ClinInvestMed, 1984; 7:223).

In most of the reported cases of disseminated listeriosis with apparent liver involvement, the patients had an underlying liver disease that might be considered at least partly responsible for the hepatic dysfunction.[15] In the few cases in which liver histology was reported, microabscesses,[15] granulomas (Henderson, PostgradMedJ, 1967; 43:794; Gros, MedKlin, 1968; 63:241), and cholestatic hepatitis with 'focal subacute liver dystrophy' were found.

Clinical features

Most cases of listeriosis in adults are symptomless (Anon, Lancet, 1985; ii:364). Approximately 70 per cent of adults with symptomatic disease have underlying predisposing causes that include haematological neoplasia, immunosuppressive drugs (usually corticosteroids, and particularly in transplant recipients), and alcoholism; recently, cases have been identified in patients with infection by the human immunodeficiency virus type 1 (Ridgway, JInfect, 1989; 19:167).

Although infection in pregnancy may lead to abortion, stillbirth, or premature delivery and consequent neonatal sepsis, the mother usually only suffers a mild, influenza-like illness. In the non-pregnant adult, meningitis occurs in approximately 50 per cent, while encephalitis and other neurological syndromes, primary bacteraemia, endocarditis, pneumonia, endophthalmitis, oculoglandular, or cutaneous infection affect the remainder (Barza, NEJM, 1985; 312:438; Gill, JInfect, 1988; 17:1).

Hepatitis is more common in neonatal listeriosis.[15] In adults the presentation may mimic that of viral hepatitis; there may be gradual onset of symptoms over several weeks, although the patient will usually have a high fever.[15] In more severe cases the history is much shorter and the patient may rapidly become moribund. The liver may or may not be palpable and tender; splenomegaly is usually absent.

Investigations

Abnormal liver function tests are common in bacteraemia (see above). However, patients with listeriosis presenting with overt hepatitis characteristically have high serum transaminases (Tschumper, SchweizerMedWochen, 1987; 117:2010)), with the AST elevated to more than 10 times normal.[15] The amount of conjugated bilirubin in the serum is variable and may be less than 30 per cent.[15]

The white-cell count is typically elevated, with a neutrophilia, although it may be normal.[15] The cerebrospinal fluid in patients with meningitis most commonly has a neutrophil leucocytosis with elevation of protein and reduction in glucose, although some patients may have a lymphocytosis or monocytosis.

The diagnosis is confirmed by isolation of the organism from blood, cerebrospinal fluid, pus, or tissue cultures.

Differential diagnosis

The differential diagnosis includes: viral hepatitis, bacteraemia with other organisms, legionnaires' disease, and liver disease with encephalopathy

Treatment

Ampicillin in high dosage is considered the drug of choice for the treatment of listeriosis and is probably best combined with an aminoglycoside (usually gentamicin), with which it may be synergistic. Other agents that may be used in patients with penicillin allergy are erythromycin, rifampicin or co-trimoxazole.[14] Cephalosporins are not effective.

Legionella pneumophila
Definition

Legionella pneumophila causes legionnaires' disease, a pneumonia characterized by multisystem involvement, and Pontiac fever, an acute upper respiratory-tract infection associated with fever, chills, myalgia, and headache. The organism is a fastidious, aerobic, Gram-negative rod and has at least 14 serogroups. Serogroup 1 is the most common cause of disease in man.

Introduction

The disease was first characterized following an outbreak of pneumonia amongst delegates of an American Legion convention in Philadelphia in 1976. The causative organism was isolated post mortem from the lung tissue of four patients, and serological responses to this organism were found in 101 of the 182 patients involved in the outbreak (McDade, NEJM, 1977; 297:1197). Since that time there have been many outbreaks as well as sporadic cases.

Epidemiology

The highest incidence of infection is in the 40- to 70-year-old age group. Men are more commonly affected than women and the disease is rare in children. Patients at risk include those who are smokers or alcoholics, those with chronic illnesses including diabetes mellitus, and those receiving immunosuppressive therapy. Most cases are sporadic but outbreaks have been traced to the following sources:[16] (i) cooling-water systems used for air-conditioning; (ii) cooling-water systems used for industrial purposes; (iii) domestic hot-water systems; (iv) domestic spas and whirlpools; (v) industrial coolants used for grinding and lubrication; and (vi) respiratory therapy equipment. The peak incidence of infection in the United Kingdom is during the summer and autumn months.

Pathogenesis and pathology

The organism spreads directly to adjacent respiratory epithelium and there is invasion of lymphatics and blood vessels by phagocytes containing bacteria, and by free organisms. Hence organisms and antigen can be widely disseminated, and indeed, have been detected in kidney, bone marrow, spleen (Weisenberger, ArchPathLabMed, 1981; 105:130), myocardium (White, ArchPathLabMed, 1980; 104:287), brain (Gatell, Lancet, 1981; ii:202), peritoneum (Dournon, Lancet, 1982; i:1363), and liver (Schurmann, ZblBakteriolMikrobiolHyg, 1983; 255:120). The mechanisms that produce tissue damage in legionnaires' disease are largely unknown. Several potential toxins have been identified, including low molecular-weight exotoxins and proteases.[16] It is thought that cell-mediated immunity plays the major part in the prevention of infection with *L. pneumophila*. Hence patients with defects of cellular immunity are at higher risk of the disease. It may be that the organism is able to evade host defences by multiplying within monocytes.

Most of the pathological changes are seen in the lungs and pleura. Consolidation similar to that of pneumococcal pneumonia can be seen macroscopically in lung sections, and abscesses may be found in 25 per cent of cases. Histological examination of lung tissue reveals accumulation of intra-alveolar exudate together with focal intra-alveolar haemorrhage.

Although a variety of different histological appearances have been described in the liver in legionnaires' disease, the most frequent findings are non-specific, consisting of mild portal infiltration (Winn, HumPath, 1981; 12:401), and neutrophil invasion of the sinusoids (Weisenburger, ArchPathLabMed, 1981; 105:130). Kupffer-cell hyperplasia and centrilobular necrosis have also been described (Weisenburger, ArchPathLabMed, 1981; 105:130). There are case reports of macroscopic and microscopic liver abscesses (Cutz, JPediat, 1982; 100:760), and small hepatic granulomas (Gump, ScaJInfectDis, 1982; 14:75). Verneau (GastrClinBiol, 1987; 11:254) described a patient presenting with cholestatic jaundice in whom the liver was histologically normal except for margination of mitochondria in the hepatocytes; it was suggested that this might be a specific feature of legionnaires' disease.

Clinical features

Legionella pneumophila causes two distinct clinical syndromes, Pontiac fever, an acute self-limiting febrile illness, which will not be discussed further, and legionnaires' disease, which has an incubation period of 2 to 10 days and a very variable clinical presentation. More than 90 per cent of patients have a fever, which may reach 40°C in 50 per cent. A non-productive cough occurs in about 75 per cent of patients and may be associated with mild haemoptysis.

Tachypnoea is common, but chest signs may be unimpressive in the initial phase of the illness. Headache is frequent and up to 30 per cent of sufferers may have a degree of confusion (Yu, AmJMed, 1982; 73:357). Peripheral neuropathy and cerebellar ataxia have also been described. Other features of multisystem involvement include diarrhoea, endocarditis, pericarditis, rhabdomyolysis, and rash.

Hepatomegaly is uncommon (Edelstein, Chest, 1984; 85:114) and, although biochemical evidence of liver involvement is often seen, frank jaundice is unusual (Verneau, GastrClinBiol, 1987; 11: 254).

Investigations

Abnormalities of liver function tests are frequent. In one study,[17] roughly half of affected patients had a raised serum AST (up to 15 times normal) and alkaline phosphatase (up to 9 times normal), and 15 per cent had hyperbilirubinaemia (up to 4.5 mg/100ml).

The white-cell count is raised in up to 78 per cent of cases, proteinuria and haematuria are common, and hyponatraemia is found in more than 60 per cent of patients.[17] Chest radiographic findings are abnormal in approx. 90 per cent (Dietrich, Radiol, 1978; 127:577; Kirby, Chest, 1979; 76:562).

The diagnosis is confirmed serologically in most cases. In the United Kingdom the rapid microagglutination test or immunofluorescent antibody test are most commonly used. The organism may be demonstrated by direct immunofluorescence in sputum or tracheal aspirate or bronchoscopy specimens, or it may be isolated from cultures using charcoal–yeast extract medium. Methods for demonstrating serogroup-1 antigen in the urine include radio-immunoassay (Kohler, AnnIntMed, 1981; 94:601), latex agglutination (Sathapatayuvongs, AmRevRespDis, 1983; 127:559), and enzyme-linked immunosorbent assay (Bibb, JClinMicrobiol, 1984; 20:478; Birtles, JClinPath, 1990; 40:685). A DNA probe for detection of the organism in clinical specimens has similar sensitivity to direct immunofluorescence (Edelstein, JClinMicrobiol, 1987; 25: 1022).

Differential diagnosis

The disease needs to be distinguished from other causes of pneumonia in which abnormal liver function tests may be found and hence the differential diagnosis includes: acute bacterial pneumonia, mycoplasma infection, psittacosis, and Q fever.

Treatment

The drug of choice, based on experimental and clinical evidence, remains erythromycin. For mild infection, 500 mg 6-hourly may suffice, but for severely ill patients the drug should be given intravenously, 1 g 6-hourly, together with rifampicin, 300 to 600 mg 12-hourly.[16] Clarithromycin shows promise in the treatment of this infection; other alternatives include ciprofloxacin and doxycycline (Roig, Drugs 1993; 46:63).

Brucella spp.
Definition

Brucellosis is a zoonosis that occasionally affects man and is caused by a small, Gram-negative coccobacillus of the genus *Brucella*.

There are three important species pathogenic for man: *B. melitensis*, *B. abortus*, and *B. suis*.

Introduction

Brucella melitensis was first isolated in 1887 by Sir David Bruce from the spleens of patients who had died of Malta fever. The organism was obtained from the liver of a patient dying with multiple liver abscesses in 1904 (Eyre, Guy'sHospRep, 1904; 59: 207), and granulomas in the liver in patients with brucellosis were first described in 1937 (Von Albertini, FrankZeitschriPathol, 1937; 51:69).

Epidemiology

Brucellosis is widely distributed in the world. *Brucella abortus* mainly causes disease in cattle and is found in the more temperate zones, particularly those of North and South America. *Brucella melitensis* causes infection in goats and cattle, and is found around the shores of the Mediterranean and in South, East, and West Africa and the Middle East. *Brucella suis* infection in man is contracted from pigs and is mainly found in North America.

The disease is an occupational infection affecting farmers, herdsmen, meat packers, veterinary surgeons, and laboratory workers. Infection is also transmitted in unpasteurized milk, particularly goats' milk in the Mediterranean area and the Middle East.

Pathogenesis and pathology

Organisms enter the body through the skin or oropharynx and spread to the regional lymph nodes. Following multiplication there is a bacteraemic phase, during which the organisms are taken up by macrophages and become localized in the reticuloendothelial tissue of the liver, spleen, lymph nodes, and bone marrow.

The subsequent histological changes appear to be related to host cellular immune responses. The typical findings are those of multiple granulomas consisting of epithelioid cells, lymphocytes, and giant cells. Caseation may occur, with the formation of abscesses, and intracellular organisms may remain latent for months or even years before causing signs of infection.

Histological changes have been seen in the liver in patients with and without clinical or biochemical evidence of hepatic involvement. Small granulomas, indistinguishable from those in sarcoidosis, tuberculosis, and histoplasmosis, are the most common finding. They have been found in patients with infections due both to *B. melitensis* (Masana, AnnIntMed, 1980; 92:709)[18-20] and *B. abortus* (Young, AnnIntMed, 1979; 91:414),[18-20] although Young proposed that the two species differed in their pathogenesis and that *B. melitensis* was not associated with granuloma formation. The granulomas appear to occur in active or acute brucellosis and are rarely found beyond 100 days of the disease,[19] while infiltration and fibrosis of the portal tract are found at all stages, particularly in long-standing infection. A case of *B. abortus* hepatitis that progressed to micronodular cirrhosis in the absence of other causes has been described (McCullough, ArchIntMed, 1951; 88:793).

Liver abscesses are extremely uncommon and, although they may result from infection with any of the three species of brucellae under discussion, they occur most frequently with *B. suis*.[18]

Clinical features

There are clinical differences between infections with the three species. *Brucella melitensis* tends to cause the most severe infections with the greatest risk of chronicity, whereas *B. abortus* infections are generally milder. *Brucella suis* more often causes suppurative lesions.

Brucellosis has an incubation period of 1 to 3 weeks, although the appearance of symptoms may be delayed for much longer.

The disease may take several forms.

Acute brucellosis

There is an abrupt onset with a swinging fever, rigors, and sweats. Arthralgia, typically involving the larger joints, and low back pain are common. Headache, insomnia, and occasional depression may occur, and weight loss is common. Moderate hepatomegaly has been described in up to one-third of cases (more than two-thirds of cases with biochemical evidence of liver involvement)[19] and splenomegaly in more than 26 per cent. Frank jaundice is rare.

Subacute brucellosis

The acute phase may be followed within 3 months by recurring episodes of pyrexia, rising and falling over a 2-week period, or there may be no acute illness, the subacute condition having a gradual onset. The episodes are accompanied by fatigue, malaise, and occasional symptoms of organ involvement. The patient is usually well in between these febrile periods and most infections recover spontaneously.

Chronic brucellosis

Less than 20 per cent of patients suffer recurring symptoms that may continue for years. They are usually afebrile but suffer recurring headaches, malaise, anorexia, weight loss, cough, and sweating. There may be lymphadenopathy, and some patients have minimal hepatomegaly or splenomegaly.

Localized brucellosis

The disease may present chiefly with features of localized infection, particularly in bone. Less frequently there may be endocarditis, bronchopneumonia, epididymo-orchitis, renal infection, meningitis, or meningoencephalitis. Stigmata of chronic liver disease have been found in a few cases.[19]

Investigations

Liver function tests are impaired in up to 38 per cent of cases.[18, 19] The AST is typically raised to between two and three times normal, as is the alkaline phosphatase, the concentration of which does not appear to be influenced by the presence or absence of granulomas (Young, AnnIntMed, 1979; 91:414).

The total white-cell count is usually normal, with a relative lymphocytosis, and atypical lymphocytes may be present. There may be a leucopenia in some cases (Spink, 1956; The Nature of Brucellosis, University of Minnesota Press).

Abscess formation may be demonstrated by CT or ultrasound scanning, and transient focal hepatic lesions up to 3 cm across may be seen in acute brucellosis using the same techniques (Cassani, ItalJGastr, 1985; 17:40).

The organism can be isolated from blood in the acute illness. Although special media, particularly using the Castaneda technique, have been recommended in the past, *Brucella* spp. will grow in modern blood-culture broths. Cultures should be maintained for at least 3 weeks. In chronic or subacute disease, blood cultures are usually sterile but the causative organism may be isolated from bone marrow or tissue specimens.

Agglutinating antibodies appear after the second week of the illness. The disease is most commonly diagnosed by demonstrating rising titres to the standard agglutination test. The standard agglutination test will cross-react with *Franciscella tularensis*, *Yersinia enterocolitica* or *Vibrio cholerae* (including after vaccination), and a prozone phenomenon is commonly seen with high titres. IgM may be measured using radioimmuno- or enzyme immunosorbent assays. This usually peaks in the first few weeks but may persist after recovery from infection.

Differential diagnosis

The acute disease must be distinguished from typhoid fever, tuberculosis, and malignant causes of persistent fever. The differential diagnosis in a patient with hepatic granulomas (see Chapter 14.2) includes: tuberculosis, sarcoidosis, syphilis, Q fever, leishmaniasis, Hodgkin's disease, fungal infection, parasitic infection, cytomegalovirus infection, infectious mononucleosis, inflammatory bowel disease, and drug reactions.

Treatment

Tetracyclines remain the drugs of choice for the treatment of brucellosis. The World Health Organization regimen is doxycycline, 200 mg/day, plus rifampicin, 600 to 900 mg/day, for 6 weeks. Defervescence of fever usually occurs in 4 to 5 days. More than 90 per cent of cases respond to this regimen (Bertrand, NouvPresse-Med, 1980; 2:283). Streptomycin has been added to a tetracycline for the treatment of endocarditis.

Co-trimoxazole (960 mg 12-hourly for 4 weeks) is an alternative therapy, but appears to be associated with a higher relapse rate and should be combined with rifampicin.

Neisseria gonorrhoeae

Definition

Neisseria gonorrhoeae usually causes a urethritis or cervicitis in humans. One of the complications of infection is a perihepatitis known as the Curtis–Fitz-Hugh syndrome, which also results from infection with *Chlamydia trachomatis* (see later). The causative organism is a fastidious, aerobic, Gram-negative diplococcus.

Introduction

Gonococcal perihepatitis was first described in 1930 by Curtis (JAMA, 1930; 94:1221) and subsequently by Fitz-Hugh (JAMA, 1934; 102:2094).

Epidemiology

Gonococcal infection continues to be common among young, sexually active people. Pelvic inflammatory disease is estimated to occur in 9 to 15 per cent of patients with cervical gonorrhoea (Cano, AmJGastr, 1984; 79:280), although only a small number of these will develop Curtis–Fitz-Hugh syndrome. Factors contributing to the development of pelvic inflammatory disease include a large number of sexual contacts, the use of intrauterine devices, young age, and a past history of the disease. Almost all patients with Curtis–Fitz-Hugh syndrome are female, although there have been case reports of the condition occurring in male homosexuals (Kimball, NEJM, 1970; 282:1082).

Pathogenesis and pathology

Peritonitis and perihepatitis probably result from direct spread of the organism from the genital tract in the female. Since the condition has been described in men it is possible that the organism reaches the peritoneum via blood or the lymphatics. The condition follows localized (or generalized) peritonitis that causes the formation of adhesions between the parietal and visceral peritoneum overlying the liver. Histologically these adhesions show fibrinous changes that involve the liver capsule, but the liver parenchyma is usually normal (Cano, AmJGastr, 1984; 79:280).

Clinical features

The typical presentation is in a young female, who has severe pain in the right upper quadrant, often following lower abdominal pain with, or without, vaginal discharge. In addition there may be vomiting, fever, sweating, and headache. She is usually febrile and has tenderness in the right upper quadrant, with or without guarding. The findings on pelvic examination may be unremarkable.

Investigations

Liver function tests are usually normal. The white-cell count is often raised, although it may be normal, and the erythrocyte sedimentation rate is usually raised. Laparoscopy reveals the typical 'violin string' adhesions between the anterior surface of the liver and the anterior abdominal wall (Muller-Schoop, BMJ, 1978; 1: 1022). The adhesions may be seen on CT scans (Haight, AmJGastr, 1988; 83:323). The syndrome is best confirmed by isolating *N. gonorrhoeae* from peritoneal samples but this is rarely achieved. Isolation of the organism from endocervical or urethral swabs provides support for the diagnosis.

Differential diagnosis

The differential diagnosis includes: cholecystitis, acute appendicitis, and perihepatitis due to *C. trachomatis.*

Treatment

Division of the adhesions by means of biopsy forceps (Cano, AmJGastr, 1984; 79:280) or cautery (Reichert, JAMA, 1976; 236: 266) may provide immediate relief of abdominal pain. The infection is best treated with a regimen suitable for pelvic inflammatory disease, using agents such as doxycycline and amoxycillin or clindamycin and gentamicin; antibiotic therapy should be for 10 to 14 days. Contact tracing, investigation, and relevant therapy of partners should also be carried out.

Burkholderia pseudomallei

Definition

Burkholderia (Pseudomonas) pseudomallei is the cause of melioidosis. This is an infectious disease of man and animals that resembles glanders. The causative organism is a small, Gram-negative, motile, aerobic bacterium that grows well on standard culture media.

Introduction

The organism was first isolated from cases in Rangoon by Whitmore and Krishnaswarmi (IndMedGaz, 1912; 47:262). Since that time most cases have occurred in South-East Asia.

Epidemiology

The organism is found in the environment, in soil and water, in endemic areas. Infection in man results from contamination of wounds and skin abrasions or through inhalation, and, although the disease occurs in sheep, goats, horses, pigs, and seals, these do not appear to be a source of infection for man.

Although the disease is endemic in south-east Asia, particularly in Vietnam, Cambodia, Laos, Thailand, Malaysia, and Burma, cases have occurred in China, Madagascar, India, Bangladesh, Australia, Central America, and South America.

Patients with diabetes mellitus and renal failure are especially predisposed to infection with *B. pseudomallei* (Chaowagul, JInfDis, 1989; 159:890; Vatcharapreechasakul, ClinInfDis, 1992; 14:412). In endemic areas there is a marked seasonal variation, with most infections occurring in the rainy season.

Pathogenesis and pathology

As already mentioned, the pathogenicity of *B. pseudomallei* depends on the immune status of the host. Seroprevalence studies demonstrate that many fit, healthy people have asymptomatic infections whereas immunocompromised ones may suffer fulminant disease. A heat-labile exotoxin and a protease have been identified and are thought to contribute to the virulence of the organism. In addition, endotoxin is presumably responsible for many of the features of severe disease.

Burkholderia pseudomallei is capable of survival within the phagocytes of the reticuloendothelial system. This may contribute to abscess formation in the liver and spleen in recrudescent forms of the disease.

The histological features depend on the clinical form of the disease. In acute melioidosis, focal lesions are most often seen in lung, liver, spleen, and lymph nodes. The typical findings are those of suppurative inflammation. The liver contains many small abscesses, 2 to 3 mm in diameter. These are filled with neutrophils, organisms, and some macrophages, and are surrounded by a zone of necrosis (Piggott, ArchPath, 1970; 90:101). With progression of the disease, the abscesses coalesce. The lesions of chronic melioidosis are granulomatous. The granulomas consist of epithelioid and giant cells, and have central zones of necrosis that may be caseous, resembling tuberculous lesions, or contain purulent exudate (Piggott, ArchPath, 1970; 90:101). Organisms are rarely seen in these lesions, which most commonly involve lung, lymph nodes, liver, spleen, and skin.

Clinical features

The disease may present in a wide variety of forms, varying from asymptomatic cases to overwhelming septicaemia. The incubation period may be as short as 2 days and infection may remain latent for as long as 26 years (Mays, Chest, 1975; 68:261). The acute form of the disease most commonly presents with pulmonary infection. There may be sudden or gradual onset of fever, rigors, headache, myalgia, and anorexia, together with a cough, which may be associated with haemoptysis. Chest signs are minimal, and in the non-disseminated forms of the disease the liver and spleen are not enlarged. In disseminated cases there is a sudden onset of high fever, headache, pharyngitis, diarrhoea, and the development of skin pustules. The patient may also develop tender, swollen joints, and signs of meningitis (Chaowagul, JInfDis, 1989; 159:890); such patients may also have enlargement of the liver and spleen. Occasionally, cholangitis has been reported.[21]

In chronic disease, patients are often afebrile and symptoms are referable to the affected organ. They most commonly present with clinical features suggestive of pulmonary tuberculosis.

Investigations

Approximately 40 per cent of patients with bacteraemic melioidosis have a serum bilirubin greater than 5 mg/100 ml and 30 per cent have elevated AST. However, in a comparative study these measures were not found to be significantly different from those in patients with bacteraemia caused by other bacteria (Chaowagul, JInfDis, 1989; 159:890). In a study from Thailand of patients with liver abscesses, jaundice and pain in the right upper quadrant were more common in patients with liver abscesses from other bacteria (Vatcharapreechasakul, ClinInfDis, 1992; 14:412).

The white-cell count may be normal or elevated to more than $20 \times 10^9/l$. Chest radiographs may reveal cavitating lesions and abscess cavities may be demonstrated in the liver by ultrasonography.[21] Multiple hypoechoic areas are characteristic of liver abscesses caused by this organism and patients are more likely to have associated splenic abscesses (Vatcharapreechasakul, ClinInfDis, 1992; 14:412).

The diagnosis is best made by culture of *B. pseudomallei* from blood or pus. Rising titres of antibody measured by haemagglutination, complement fixation, or agglutination are helpful in diagnosis. Several immunoassays, both enzyme immunosorbent and latex agglutination, have been shown to be useful for the diagnosis of melioidosis using urine and serum samples (Ismail, JMedMicrobiol, 1987; 23:353; Desakorn, AmJTropMedHyg, 1994; 51:627; Smith, JClinPath, 1995; 48:174).

Differential diagnosis

Melioidosis should be considered in any patient presenting with severe sepsis, pyrexia of unknown origin, or suppurative disease who is from, or who has visited, an endemic area. Hence the differential diagnosis includes: (i) other bacterial causes of severe sepsis; (ii) other causes of liver abscess; and (iii) tuberculosis.

Treatment

Until recently, conventional therapy consisted of chloramphenicol or tetracycline, or combination therapy consisting of chloramphenicol plus doxycycline plus co-trimoxazole. However, the organism is susceptible to ceftazidime *in vitro* and a comparative trial from Thailand showed that ceftazidime was superior to the then recommended combination therapy (White, Lancet, 1989; ii: 697). Ceftazidime, 120 mg/kg per day in divided intravenous doses, reduced mortality to 37 per cent as compared with 74 per cent seen with the standard regimen and should now, therefore, be the treatment of choice for at least the first 7 days; treatment is then changed to an oral regimen in an attempt to prevent relapse. The optimal choice (and duration) for this is still not clear, but co-amoxyclav may provide some benefit (White, Lancet, 1989; ii:697).

Hepatic involvement in infections with bacterial enteric pathogens
Shigella spp.

Shigellae were first isolated from the liver at autopsy in 1910 (Knox, JohnsHopkHospRep, 1910; 14:1). Since that time there have been isolated case reports of hepatic involvement in shigellosis. In a case of cholestatic jaundice that occurred during infection with *S. sonnei*, the liver biopsy showed a cholestatic hepatitis with some focal necrosis and both portal and periportal infiltration with neutrophils and mononuclear cells (Horney, AmJGastr, 1976; 66:146). A more recent report of a patient with fever and diarrhoea, and from whom *S. flexneri* was isolated from stool and splenic abscesses, described hepatitis with jaundice, although no liver biopsy was performed (Squires, JPediat, 1981; 98:429). Liver dysfunction has also been seen in patients with *S. dysenteriae* type 1 infection (Levine, WestJMed, 1974; 121:501).

Liver function tests show raised alkaline phosphatase and AST in most cases, although the latter is not always elevated initially. The liver enzymes and serum bilirubin return to normal with effective treatment of the shigellosis, usually within 2 to 3 weeks.

Treatment

Appropriate therapy in such cases includes ampicillin (500 mg 6-hourly), co-trimoxazole (960 mg 12-hourly), and the fluoroquinolones, such as ciprofloxacin (500 mg 12-hourly), but there is widespread transferable drug resistance among the shigellae and it is important to check the sensitivity of the isolate.

Differential diagnosis

The differential diagnosis includes any diarrhoeal illness in which disturbance of liver function may occur: (i) other causes of bacterial enterocolitis, (ii) bilharzial colitis, (iii) pseudomembranous colitis, (iv) haemolytic–uraemic syndrome, and (v) inflammatory bowel disease with sclerosing cholangitis or portal pyaemia.

Verotoxin-producing Escherichia coli

This organism [also known as enterohaemorrhagic *E. coli* (EHEC)] causes haemorrhagic colitis and haemolytic–uraemic syndrome. The unconjugated hyperbilirubinaemia that characteristically develops after several days of bloody, watery diarrhoea may be confused with liver dysfunction, but is the consequence of haemolysis. Cholestasis has been described in this syndrome but is rare (Jeffrey, Gut, 1985; 26:315).

The diagnosis is made by isolating the causative organism from the stool, using sorbitol–MacConkey agar. The majority of strains have the O157:H7 serotype. The diagnosis can also be confirmed by detecting serum antibodies to the verotoxin.

Treatment

The treatment of haemorrhagic colitis and haemolytic–uraemic syndrome is supportive. Antibiotics have not been shown to be of benefit, but are usually administered in an attempt to eliminate the organism.

Differential diagnosis

The differential diagnosis includes any diarrhoeal illness in which disturbance of liver function may occur: (i) other causes of bacterial enterocolitis, (ii) bilharzial colitis, (iii) pseudomembranous colitis, and (iv) inflammatory bowel disease with sclerosing cholangitis or portal pyaemia.

Campylobacter spp.

A mild degree of liver dysfunction may be relatively common in *Campylobacter* infection. In a series of 63 cases from the Mayo Clinic, 10 per cent of patients had mild elevations of alkaline phosphatase and 24 per cent mildly raised AST (Drake, Mayo-ClinProc, 1981; 56:414). However, there are very few reports of severely deranged liver function or histological changes in *Campylobacter* infection. Cases of hepatitis, with or without hepatomegaly, have been described during infection with *C. coli* (Amperlas, NouvPresseMed, 1982; 11:593), *C. foetus* (Wyatt, JPediat, 1977; 91:441), and *C. jejuni* (Reddy, JClinGastro, 1983; 5:259). The appearances of liver biopsy specimens are those of non-specific hepatitis, with focal necrosis and infiltration with neutrophils and monocytes.

Besides causing hepatitis, *C. foetus* (Verbruggen, BrJSurg, 1986; 73:46) and *C. jejuni* (Mertens, Lancet, 1979; i:1092) have also been isolated from bile during episodes of cholecystitis in association with gallstones.

Treatment

Erythromycin has been the drug of choice for severe *Campylobacter* infections. Cases have responded to 500 mg 6-hourly for 7 days, with improvement in liver function tests taking up to 3 weeks (Reddy, JClinGastro, 1983; 5:259). The fluoroquinolones are also effective.

Differential diagnosis

The differential diagnosis includes any diarrhoeal illness in which disturbance of liver function may occur: (i) other causes of bacterial enterocolitis, (ii) bilharzial colitis, (iii) pseudomembranous colitis, (iv) haemolytic–uraemic syndrome, and (v) inflammatory bowel disease with sclerosing cholangitis or portal pyaemia.

Salmonella spp.

Whilst a variety of *Salmonella* species may cause cholangitis, cholecystitis, and liver abscesses, parenchymal liver dysfunction is the result of infection with those species causing enteric fever. Hepatomegaly in typhoid fever was first reported by Osler in 1899 (Osler, JohnsHopkHospRep, 1899; 8:373) and since that time the incidence of hepatomegaly has ranged from 13 to 65 per cent (Stuart, ArchIntMed, 1946; 78:629; Butler, ArchIntMed, 1978; 138:407; Kabbaj, GastrClinBiol, 1979; 3:651).[22,23] Abnormal liver function tests are seen in up to 60 per cent of cases (Stuart, ArchIntMed 1946; 78:629; Nasrallah, AmJGastr, 1978; 69:63). Hyperbilirubinaemia (serum bilirubin >1.8 mg/100 ml) is present in up to 17 per cent[23] and the most frequent abnormality is a moderate rise in the serum AST. A prolonged prothrombin time has been documented in up to 25 per cent, although this is not usually of clinical significance.[23]

Hepatic dysfunction in enteric fever is most likely to occur in patients with anaemia, malnutrition, and poor health, and is then more likely to be severe. It is also more likely to be severe in those with relapsed infection.[23]

The liver in cases of enteric fever most often shows the histological appearances of non-specific reactive hepatitis.[22] However, some cases may show evidence of 'typhoid nodules' in which there is granuloma formation, consisting of infiltration with mononuclear cells around a central area of necrosis.[22,23] Immunofluorescent studies, using conjugated anti-IgG, -IgM, -IgA, and -C3, have demonstrated the presence of these antibodies and complement components in the epithelial cells of the bile canaliculi, suggesting a role for immune complexes in the pathogenesis of 'hepatitis typhosa'.

Treatment

Ciprofloxacin (500 mg twice a day) has become the treatment of choice for enteric fever and should be given for 10 to 14 days. Chloramphenicol (50 mg/kg per day while febrile, reducing to 500 mg 6-hourly when afebrile) is still widely used and should be given for at least 2 weeks, although relapse occurs in about 15 per cent of cases so treated. Alternative antibiotics include ampicillin, amoxycillin, co-trimoxazole, and trimethoprim.

Differential diagnosis

The condition requires differentiation from: (i) malaria, (ii) viral hepatitis, (iii) other bacteraemic illnesses, and (iv) tuberculosis.

Yersinia spp.

Disseminated yersinial infections have mainly been described in association with iron overload and most are due to *Y. enterocolitica* (Rabson, JInfDis, 1975; 131:447; Editorial, Lancet, 1984; i:84). However, they rarely cause hepatic dysfunction. The most common complication affecting the liver is the formation of abscesses following bacteraemia with *Y. pseudotuberculosis* or *Y. enterocolitica* (Dubois, NouvPresseMed, 1982; 11:1619). A few cases of granulomatous hepatitis or hepatitis with necrosis and cholestasis have also been reported (Dubois, NouvPresseMed, 1982; 11:1619). Such patients do not always have hepatomegaly or splenomegaly and may be anicteric. There is usually a rise in both serum AST and alkaline phosphatase. In the granulomatous form of the disease, histological examination of the liver reveals well-formed granulomas consisting of epithelioid cells with giant-cell formation and occasional eosinophils (Dubois, NouvPresseMed, 1982; 11:1619). Liver biopsy in more severe cases may show a neutrophil inflammatory infiltrate, with areas of focal necrosis and evidence of cholestasis.

There are also reports of patients with symptoms suggestive of recurrent cholecystitis in whom abdominal pain associated with abnormal liver function tests and elevated *Y. enterocolitica* antibody titres have been described. Such patients are thought to have chronic hepatic involvement (Saebo, ActaChirScand, 1977; 143:445).

Treatment

Yersinia spp. are often resistant to penicillins and first-generation cephalosporins because of β-lactamase production.[24] *Yersinia enterocolitica* is usually sensitive to aminoglycosides, tetracyclines, chloramphenicol, and third-generation cephalosporins, and a combination of gentamicin and doxycycline is appropriate therapy for adult bacteraemic cases until the results of sensitivity tests are available (Cover, NEJM, 1989; 321:16). The fluoroquinolones are increasingly being used with good effect.

Differential diagnosis

The condition requires differentiation from: (i) other causes of bacteraemia, (ii) cholecystitis, (iii) viral hepatitis, and (iv) other causes of granulomatous hepatitis.

Hepatic involvement in infections with other pathogens

Franciscella tularensis

Definition

Franciscella tularensis is a small, non-motile, Gram-negative rod. It causes tularaemia, an infectious disease of rodents, which may be transmitted to man by insect bites, directly from infected animals, or from drinking contaminated water.

Introduction

The disease was first described in 1911 when a plague-like illness was reported in ground squirrels in Tulare County, California; the causative organism was subsequently identified by the same workers (McCoy, JInfDis, 1912; 10:61). The first human case with clinical involvement of the liver was reported in 1924 (Verbryke, JAMA, 1924; 82:1577).

Epidemiology

The disease occurs in four main areas of the world: North America, Europe (excluding the United Kingdom), the Russian Federation, and Japan. In North America the main animal reservoirs are jack-rabbits and hares. Infection is usually acquired by hunters and farmers, from infected animals or from tick and deer-fly bites, and is most common in the summer months. In Europe the hare is the main reservoir of the disease, whilst in Sweden the lemming is responsible for many cases (hence the name 'lemming fever') through the contamination of water supplies. The water-rat and musk-rat are responsible for the spread of infection in the Russian Federation.

Pathogenesis and pathology

Following entry to the body via the gastrointestinal tract, the skin, the conjunctiva or the oropharynx, the organism multiplies locally and then spreads to the regional lymph nodes and occasionally via the bloodstream to other organs. In such cases the lungs are affected in approx. 90 per cent, the liver in 75 per cent, and the spleen in about 70 per cent of patients (Gundry, AnnIntMed, 1933; 7:837). Granulomas may be found in the lymph nodes early in the infection and have also been found in the liver. However, the typical pathological findings in the liver are multiple focal areas of coagulative necrosis with a surrounding chronic inflammatory infiltrate, consisting of lymphocytes, monocytes, and occasional neutrophils (Foshay, Medicine, 1940; 19:1); giant and epithelioid cells are uncommon.[25]

Clinical features

The incubation period is between 1 and 10 days, and up to 32 per cent of infections may be subclinical (Dahlstrand, ScaJInfectDis, 1971; 3:7). Five types of tularaemia were defined by Francis: ulceroglandular, oculoglandular, oropharyngeal, glandular, and typhoidal. The infrequent clinical involvement of the liver in recent years is thought to be because of the use of antibiotics preventing dissemination of organisms, and hepatomegaly probably occurs in less than 16 per cent of cases now (Ortego, Gastro, 1986; 91:461). Ascites has been reported in occasional cases (Foshay, Medicine, 1940; 19:1).

Other complications of the infection include pericarditis, peritonitis, osteomyelitis, and rashes (Gourdeau, CanMedAssJ, 1983; 129:1286).

Investigations

Liver function tests have shown a four-fold rise in ALT, AST, and alkaline phosphatase in 10.2 per cent, 7.7 per cent, and 3.8 per cent of patients, respectively (Evans, Medicine, 1985; 64:251). The presence of hepatic abscesses may be demonstrated by ultrasonography (Gourdeau, CanMedAssJ, 1983; 129:1286).

The organism may be isolated from the blood, skin lesions, or other sites of infection. It is difficult to grow and specimens should be cultured on cystine agar. The diagnosis is otherwise made serologically. Agglutinating antibodies appear in the second week but these may cross-react with *B. abortus* or *B. melitensis*.

Differential diagnosis

The condition must be differentiated from plague, enteric fever, and other causes of granulomatous liver disease.

Treatment

The treatment remains streptomycin, 30 to 40 mg/kg per day in two divided doses for 3 days, continuing with half of this dose for another 7 days.[26] Alternative drugs include tetracycline or gentamicin.

Treponema pallidum (syphilis)

Definition

Syphilis is an infectious, multisystem disease capable of latency and chronicity, which, if left untreated, passes through a series of clinical stages. It is caused by the spirochaete *T. pallidum* subsp. *pallidum*, which is a microaerophilic Gram-negative bacterium, 6 to 15 μm in length and 0.1 to 0.2 μm wide. Jaundice as a complication was first described by Paracelsus in 1585 in association with the clinical features of secondary syphilis (Wile, JAMA, 1917; 68:1311).

Epidemiology

Until recently, syphilis in most Western countries had become a disease chiefly affecting homosexual and bisexual men. However, the last decade has seen an increase among the heterosexual population in urban areas of the United States (CDC, MMWR, 1988; 37:486). The possible reasons for these changing epidemiological patterns are discussed elsewhere (CDC, MMWR, 1988; 37:35), but it seems that the disease may be undergoing a resurgence.

The estimated incidence of liver disease in cases of syphilis has varied from less than 1 per cent to 12 per cent (Wile, JAMA, 1917; 68:1311; Feher, Lancet, 1975; ii:896), but abnormal liver function tests may occur in up to 50 per cent of those with secondary syphilis (Petersen, AmJMed, 1983; 75:166). The patients' age ranges from the neonate with congenital infection to the elderly with gummatous disease, whereas syphilitic hepatitis is primarily a disease of young and middle-aged adults. The great majority are male.

Liver involvement is present at various stages of disease and probably results from different mechanisms at these stages (Stokes, *Modern clinical syphilology*. Philadelphia: Saunders, 1926). Although jaundice is occasionally seen in primary syphilis, this appears to be due to coincidental viral hepatitis and is not a feature of the primary disease (Mulder, NedTGeneesk, 1980; 124:973).

Congenital syphilis

Pathogenesis and pathology

The disease may be transmitted to the fetus at any stage of pregnancy but lesions of congenital syphilis are only found after 16 weeks' gestation when the immune system has begun to develop. Hence, although the liver may be teeming with spirochaetes, it seems that the disease may be mediated by immunopathological mechanisms rather than a direct toxic effect of *T. pallidum*. Certainly such mechanisms seem to be responsible for the glomerulopathy of congenital syphilis.

There is evidence that penicillin may potentiate hepatic involvement in congenital syphilis. The incidence of hepatitis appears to have increased since the advent of penicillin therapy. Thus 15 out of 16 fatal cases in infants who had been treated with penicillin had histological abnormalities of the liver (Oppenheimer, JohnsHopkMedJ, 1971; 129:63) In addition, there are reports of infants who have developed liver dysfunction following the administration of penicillin,[27] although these may represent cases of the Jarisch–Herxheimer reaction.

Biopsy of the liver in the early stages reveals a diffuse hepatitis, and spirochaetes may be demonstrated by silver staining (Wright,

BrJVenerDis, 1974; 50:241) or electron microscopy (Brooks, ArchPathLabMed, 1978; 102:502). The treponemes are mostly extracellular, within the space of Disse. Several studies have demonstrated the presence of multinucleate giant cells (Oppenheimer, JohnsHopkMedJ, 1971; 129:63).[27] In the later stages, portal and pericellular fibrosis develops, resulting in a pericellular cirrhosis.

Clinical features

Affected infants are typically premature, of low birth weight, and born to young unmarried women who have not had adequate antenatal care and are from lower socioeconomic groups (Lane, MedJAust, 1988; 148:171). The majority of cases have no liver involvement at birth. Only 25 per cent of those with congenital syphilis are diagnosed during the first year of life. Severe early disease may result in stillbirth or death in the early neonatal period. Besides the characteristic mucocutaneous lesions, osteitis, and osteochondritis seen in those with early manifestations of congenital syphilis, the infant usually has hepatosplenomegaly and mild jaundice,[27] which may be partly the result of haemolysis.

Late manifestations of congenital syphilis occur after the second year of life. They most commonly present between the ages of 7 and 15 years, but the condition may occur as early as the third year of life or be delayed until adulthood. Abnormal liver function is not a feature of this condition, but hepatic gummas may be present.

Investigations

In early disease, the conjugated serum bilirubin usually exceeds 40 per cent of the total serum bilirubin, which may be greater than 20 mg/100 ml.[27] Peak serum aminotransferases may be up to 150 times higher than normal and the AST is typically higher than the ALT.[27]

The diagnosis of congenital syphilis may be confused by the presence of maternal antibodies in young infants. A rising reagin antibody titre, either the rapid plasma reagin (RPR) or Venereal Diseases Reference Laboratory (**VDRL**) test, confirmed by specific antibody tests such as the *T. pallidum* haemagglutination (**TPHA**) and fluorescent treponemal antibody absorption (**FTA-ABS**) tests, detectable reagin antibody in the cerebrospinal fluid, or a dark-field examination positive for treponemes, provides conclusive evidence of congenital syphilis (Ingall. In Remington and Klein, eds. *Infectious diseases of the fetus and newborn infant*. Philadelphia: Saunders, 1976:420). Enzyme-linked immunosorbent assays for detecting IgG antibodies against specific treponemal antigen are beginning to replace the older tests in many laboratories (Silletti, JClinMicrobiol, 1995; 33:1829).

The detection of FTA-IgM antibodies is further support for the diagnosis, but these may be absent for several months following delivery, and false positives may occur.

Differential diagnosis

The conditions that should be considered in the differential diagnosis of an infant with liver dysfunction resulting from early congenital syphilis include the following: (i) physiological jaundice, (ii) acute bacterial sepsis, (iii) total parenteral nutrition, (iv) infection with cytomegalovirus, rubella, coxsackie, herpes simplex, and hepatitis B viruses, (v) hypothyroidism, (vi) biliary atresia, (vii) galactosaemia, (viii) α_1-antitrypsin deficiency, (ix) cystic fibrosis, (x) tyrosinosis, (xi) hereditary fructose intolerance, and (xii) congenital hepatic fibrosis.

Secondary syphilis

Pathogenesis and pathology

The aetiology of jaundice in secondary syphilis has caused much debate. It seems likely that some of the published cases are the result of coincidental viral hepatitis (Veeravahu, ArchIntMed, 1985; 145:132). Several other mechanisms have been proposed to explain the jaundice, including obstruction of portal lymph nodes by syphilitic adenitis, and intestinal and biliary condylomas (Wile, JAMA, 1917; 68:1311). Most cases, however, appear to be the result of a true hepatitis and the mechanisms for this are unclear. Spirochaetes are only infrequently found in the liver, making a direct toxic effect of the organism on hepatocytes difficult to support. The detection of autoantibodies (Mustakallio, IntArchAllApplImmunol, 1967; 31: 417) and evidence of immune-complex disease (Braunstein, AmJMed, 1970; 48:643) in secondary syphilis suggest that immunopathological mechanisms underlie the hepatitis. There appears to be an increased frequency of syphilitic hepatitis in homosexual men with primary anal or rectal lesions, and it has been suggested that these lesions might allow direct invasion of the portal venous system and consequent hepatic involvement (Schlossberg, AmJ Gastr, 1987; 82:552).

The histological appearances of the liver have differed in various series. Some studies have demonstrated necrotic areas extending from portal to central zones (Baker, NEJM, 1971; 284:1422; CDC, MMWR, 1988; 37:35), with a mononuclear and polymorphonuclear infiltrate in the portal tracts. Others have described the presence of granulomas together with areas of inflammation and necrosis (Hahn, AmJSyphGonVenDis, 1943; 27:529; Longstreath, ArchDermatol, 1976; 112:1451; Bansal, ArchDermatol, 1978; 114:1228; Morrison, DigDisSci, 1980; 25:87; Scully, NEJM, 1983; 309:35). Cholestatic changes are also occasionally found (Veeravahu, ArchIntMed, 1985; 145:132).

Clinical features

The patient typically presents with a history of anorexia, weight loss, pale stools, and dark urine. Some may suffer pruritus (Sarkany, ProcRoySocMed, 1973; 66:237). Jaundice is mild to moderate, but may be occasionally absent. The rash of secondary syphilis is usually present, but it may be masked by the presence of jaundice or racial pigmentation. The primary chancre has often healed by the time of presentation but may be present in the anus or rectum. There is usually a degree of tender hepatomegaly, and splenomegaly is occasionally present.

Investigations

The white-cell count is usually within normal limits but the erythrocyte sedimentation rate is typically elevated to between 40 and 90 mm/h.

The reaginic antibody tests for syphilis are positive in high titre and the specificity of these results is confirmed by positive TPHA, IgG enzyme-linked immunosorbent assay, and FTA-ABS tests (Table 4). Liver function tests show considerable variation. The

serum bilirubin may be normal or moderately elevated. Where data are available both conjugated and unconjugated bilirubinaemia are usually recorded (Baker, NEJM, 1971; 284:1422; Lee, NEJM, 1971; 284:1423; Parker, BrJVenerDis, 1972; 48:32; Campisi, ArchIntMed, 1979; 139:365; Sarkany, ProcRoySocMed, 1973; 66:237). AST, ALT, and glutamyl transpeptidase may be variably raised, but the alkaline phosphatase is usually disproportionately elevated (Campisi, ArchIntMed, 1979; 139:365), sometimes by as much as 10 times normal (Lee, NEJM, 1971; 284:1423; Schlossberg, AmJGastr, 1987; 82:552).

Ultrasonography may reveal hypoechoic lesions up to 3 cm in diameter within the liver parenchyma, and these appear as attenuated areas in CT scans that fail to enhance with intravenous contrast medium (Vas, DiagnosImagingClinMed, 1985; 54:1).

Differential diagnosis

The following conditions may either be the cause of hepatitis in patients with secondary syphilis, or may mimic the rash and liver dysfunction of the disease: (i) hepatitis B, (ii) hepatitis C, (iii) hepatitis A, (iv) Epstein–Barr virus infection, (v) cytomegalovirus infection, and (vi) coxsackievirus infection.

Tertiary syphilis

Pathogenesis and pathology

The granulomatous nature of the lesions of tertiary syphilis, and the fact that few, if any, treponemes can be demonstrated within them, suggest that they result from cell-mediated hypersensitivity to treponemal antigen.

Histological examination reveals a non-specific granulomatous infiltration with central necrosis. Epithelioid and giant cells, together with fibroblastic cells, may be seen in the surrounding area, forming a fibrous capsule. The small vessels show evidence of perivasculitis and endarteritis obliterans, the cause of the central necrosis.

Clinical features

Gummas of the liver are usually discovered incidentally at laparotomy or autopsy. Occasionally, however, they may be confused with cirrhosis or more frequently with metastatic malignancy. The liver is often enlarged in the early stages, but, as hepar lobatum ensues (Symmers, ArchPath, 1946; 42:64), the contour of the liver becomes nodular. Although most cases are asymptomatic, there may be weight loss, pain, and tenderness in the right hypochondrium, and even jaundice.

Investigations

Investigations, including liver function tests (which are often normal), are unhelpful and the multiple filling defects seen on axial CT scans may resemble those of metastatic carcinoma (Rodriguez, JInfDis, 1988; 157:606).

The VDRL test may be negative in up to one-third of patients with tertiary syphilis, but the TPHA or FTA-ABS tests are usually positive (Table 4). Examination of liver biopsy tissue is essential to confirm the diagnosis.

Table 4 A summary of serological responses in syphilis

Clinical diagnosis	VDRL/RPR	TPHA	FTA–ABS
No serological evidence of syphilis	Neg	Neg	Neg
Biological false positive	±/+	Neg	Neg
Untreated primary syphilis	Neg	Neg	±
	±	Neg	Neg
	+	Neg	+
Untreated early syphilis	+/++	±/+	+
Treated early syphilis	Neg	+	Neg/+
Untreated late syphilis	+/±/Neg	+	+
Treated late syphilis	±/Neg	+	+

Neg, negative.
Based on Sequira PJL. Syphilis. In Jephcott AE, ed. *Sexually transmitted diseases. A rational approach to their diagnosis.* London: PHLS.

Treatment of the condition with penicillin may produce a reduction in size of the lesions.

Differential diagnosis

The differential diagnosis of gummatous disease involving the liver is that of a space-occupying lesion and includes: (i) primary and secondary carcinoma, (ii) benign cysts, (iii) hydatid disease, and (iv) liver abscess.

The Jarisch–Herxheimer reaction

This is a systemic condition thought to be due to the release of large quantities of endotoxin when spirochaetes are killed by antibiotics. It is seen in approx. 90 per cent of cases of secondary syphilis, but is rare in late disease. It usually begins within 4 to 12 h after the first injection of antibiotic and may last for up to a day. The patient feels unwell, and may experience pyrexia, vasodilatation, and worsening of existing skin lesions. The reaction, although rare, may have fatal consequences in neurosyphilis and cardiovascular syphilis. In secondary disease it is usually of minor importance, but liver dysfunction may be exacerbated as part of the reaction. A rise in serum AST and ALT has been reported, while the bilirubin and alkaline phosphatase remain unchanged (Young, AmJGastr, 1974; 61:476).

Treatment

The treatment of all stages of syphilis is summarized in Table 5. There is, as yet, no evidence that *T. pallidum* has become resistant to penicillin (Guinan, JAMA, 1987; 257:359). It is clear that treatment in patients with human immunodeficiency virus infection is less effective and there is currently no consensus for 'standard' therapy in these patients [Rolfs, ClinInfDis, 1995; 20 (Suppl. 1): S23].

It is preferable that syphilis be treated jointly by genitourinary physicians and others to facilitate follow-up and appropriate tracing of contacts.

Other treponemal diseases

The important treponemal diseases other than syphilis are: yaws, bejel, pinta, dichuchwa, and endemic (non-venereal) syphilis. These are mentioned here because they may give rise to problems with the diagnosis of syphilis. They are all caused by organisms morphologically and serologically indistinguishable from *T. pallidum*. Hence, serological responses in the primary, secondary, and tertiary stages of all these diseases are very similar to those of syphilis (Table 4). Positive serological tests for syphilis can, therefore, only be taken as evidence of treponemal disease. For a full description of these infections, see Robertson DHH, McMillan A, and Young H, eds. *Clinical practice in sexually transmitted diseases.* 2nd edn. London: Churchill Livingstone, 1989.

Borrelia burgdorferi (Lyme disease)
Definition

Lyme disease is a zoonosis, transmitted by ticks, which takes the form of a chronic, multisystem disorder. The causative organism is the microaerophilic spirochaete *B. burgdorferi*. This is a helical, motile, Gram-negative bacterium, 5 to 25 μm in length.

Introduction

Lyme arthritis was first recognized in 1975 in children from the town of Old Lyme in Connecticut (Steere, ArthRheum, 1977; 20: 7). Burgdorfer and his colleagues subsequently identified spirochaetes in the midgut of *Ixodes dammini* ticks (Burgdorfer, Science, 1982; 216:1317), and the same organism was then isolated from blood, skin lesions, and cerebrospinal fluid from patients with Lyme disease in 1983 (Benach, NEJM, 1983; 308:740; Steere, NEJM, 1983; 308:733).

Epidemiology

Since the first cases in Connecticut the disease has been found to have a worldwide distribution. In the United States it is endemic in three areas: the North-East from Massachusetts to Maryland, the mid-West in Wisconsin and Minnesota, and the West in California and Oregon (Steere, AnnIntMed, 1979; 91:730; CDC, MMWR, 1982; 31:367). Elsewhere, cases have been described in Germany, Switzerland, France, the United Kingdom, and Australia. In the United Kingdom, cases of Lyme disease have been reported from Hampshire, Yorkshire, East Anglia, the Lake District, and Scotland (Glover, JInfect, 1987; 14:99; O'Connell, BMJ, 1995; 310:303). The distribution of the disease is dependent on the prevalence and geographical distribution of the ixodid tick vector. In the United

Table 5 Treatment of syphilis

Stage	Antibiotic	Dose	Duration
Congenital:			
Early	Benzylpenicillin	30 mg/kg b.d. i.m.	10–14 days
	or procaine penicillin	30 mg/kg o.d. i.m.	10–14 days
Late	Procaine penicillin	900 mg o.d. i.m.*	14 days
Primary and secondary	Procaine penicillin	900 mg o.d. i.m.	10 days
	or benzathine penicillin	1800 mg single dose	
Latent disease (>1 year)	procaine penicillin	900 mg o.d. i.m.	14 days
	or benzathine penicillin	1800 mg weekly × 3	
Tertiary	Procaine penicillin	900 mg o.d. i.m.	20 days
Patients allergic to penicillin:			
Early syphilis	Tetracycline	500 mg q.d.s. by mouth	14 days
If pregnant	Erythromycin	500 mg q.d.s. by mouth	14 days
Syphilis >1 year	Tetracycline	500 mg q.d.s. by mouth	28 days
If pregnant	Erythromycin	500 mg q.d.s. by mouth	28 days

b.d., twice daily; o.d., once daily; q.d.s., four times a day; i.m., intramuscular.
* Adult dose—dose should be adjusted for age in children.
In patients with late neurosyphilis or cardiovascular syphilis try to minimize possible Herxheimer reactions by starting corticosteroids the day before the first injection.
Based on Center for Disease Control U.S. Public Health Service, STD Treatment Guidelines. *Morbidity and Mortality Weekly Reports*, 1993; 42:27–46; and Robertson DHH, McMillan A, and Young H. *Clinical practice in sexually transmissible diseases.* Edinburgh: Churchill Livingstone, 1989.

States the vectors are *I. dammini* and *I. pacificus*, and in Europe *I. ricinus*.

The organism has been isolated from white-footed mice, white-tailed deer, and racoons, and specific antibody has been detected in grey squirrels, chipmunks, opossums, white-footed mice, racoons, dogs, and deer (Bosler, Science, 1983; 220:321; Magnarelli, JMedEntomol, 1984; 21:52).

Patients' ages range from 2 to 88 years, with little difference in the numbers of males and females affected. There is some evidence of a genetic predisposition in that those who develop neurological or chronic joint disease have an increased frequency of HLA-DR2.

The incidence of the disease shows a seasonal variation, with onset between May and November.

Pathogenesis and pathology

Following inoculation of the skin of the host by the ixodid tick the organism appears to multiply locally before spreading outwards in the skin, causing erythema chronicum migrans, and disseminating to regional lymph nodes and the major organs and joints (Johnston, AmJPathol, 1985; 118:26). Initially almost all patients have circulating immune complexes, but, following the development of arthritis, immune complexes are found in joint fluid but no longer in blood. The mechanism by which the organism produces disease is not clear; immune-complex deposition may well be involved. However, the fact that some patients may be cured by antibiotics implies that viable organisms are important, perhaps in order to maintain the presence of antigen rather than to cause direct toxic effects. In addition, it has been suggested that the recurrent nature of the disease might be the result of antigenic variation of the outer membrane proteins of the spirochaete, similar to the process that occurs in relapsing fever (Steere, AnnIntMed, 1987; 107:725).

Hepatic involvement is more commonly seen in the early stages of the disease and moderate inflammation of the portal tracts has been described (Steere, AnnIntMed, 1983; 99:76). Although the causative organism has been isolated from the livers of infected animals, it has not been found in human liver in the early stages. However, there are reports of recurrent Lyme disease in which hepatitis was a prominent feature and silver staining has revealed spirochaetes within the hepatic sinusoids and parenchyma (Goellner, AnnIntMed, 1988; 108:707). Histologically the liver showed ballooning of hepatocytes, considerable mitotic activity, hyperplasia of Kupffer cells, prominent microvesicular fat, and infiltration of sinuses with mononuclear cells and neutrophils.

Clinical features

The disease follows three clinically distinct stages.

Erythema chronicum migrans is the characteristic presenting feature, which develops 3 to 32 days after the infected tick bite in up to 50 per cent of cases. The lesion is an area of redness that starts as a papule or macule and slowly expands, with central clearing, taking up to 8 weeks to fade. The thigh, axilla, and groin are common sites. In 20 per cent of these patients no further symptoms develop, but the other 80 per cent go on to suffer joint symptoms and involvement of other systems (Steere, AnnIntMed, 1987; 107:725). Other features besides skin involvement include evidence of meningeal irritation, mild encephalopathy, fatigue and lethargy, sore throat, generalized lymphadenopathy, non-productive cough, testicular swelling, migratory musculoskeletal pain, hepatosplenomegaly, and hepatitis (biochemical hepatitis may persist for several weeks).

Stage 2 follows weeks to months later. Approximately 15 per cent of patients develop neurological syndromes, and about 8 per cent develop cardiac involvement (Steere, AnnIntMed, 1980; 93:8). These features may persist for up to 6 weeks and may recur.

In the third stage, approximately 60 per cent of patients develop arthritis, as long as 2 years after the initial infection. About 10 per cent of these patients develop chronic erosive arthritis, which may resemble rheumatoid arthritis.

Investigations

The diagnosis is usually confirmed serologically by enzyme-linked immunosorbent assay and an indirect immunofluorescent antibody test. Unfortunately, only one-third of patients have raised antibody titres in the first few weeks of the infection and the tests may cross-react with other spirochaetal diseases. The use of immunoblotting allows 80 per cent of patients with disease to be diagnosed in the first few weeks (Anon, Lancet, 1989; ii:198). Titres of specific IgM antibody reach a peak between 3 and 6 weeks after the onset of the disease. IgG antibodies appear to be universally detectable in stage-3 disease. Some patients treated during stage-1 disease may fail to develop an antibody response but have clinical evidence of persistent infection in the form of chronic fatigue, headache, arthritis, or neuroborreliosis. In such cases, specific T-cell responses to *B. burgdorferi* (Dattwyler, NEJM, 1988; 319:1441) or the production of specific antibody in cerebrospinal fluid may be demonstrated (Anon, Lancet, 1989; ii:198). The use of the polymerase chain reaction has also proved useful in difficult cases (O'Connell, BMJ, 1995; 310:303).

Moderate elevation of serum AST and ALT is common in early disease (Steere, AnnIntMed, 1977; 86:685; 1983; 99:76). In addition to the cases of frank hepatitis already described, a patient with Lyme disease and hepatitis was noted to have an eosinophilia and porphyrinuria (Prinz, ZblBakteriolMikrobiolHyg, 1986; 263:389). Other abnormal results may include an elevated erythrocyte sedimentation rate, mild anaemia, and a raised white-cell count.

Differential diagnosis

The differential diagnosis of a patient with Lyme disease and liver involvement is limited: (i) viral hepatitis (especially hepatitis B), (ii) systemic lupus erythematosus, (iii) rheumatoid arthritis, and (iv) infectious mononucleosis.

Treatment

In adults with early disease the drug of choice is doxycycline, 100 mg twice daily for 10 to 21 days. In children, phenoxymethylpenicillin, 50 mg/kg per day in divided doses for 10 to 21 days, is appropriate. Erythromycin, 30 mg/kg per day in divided doses for 15 to 20 days, has been used in penicillin-allergic patients, but seems less effective, and azithromycin may be more beneficial (Weber, Lancet, 1995; 343:1017). Roughly 10 per cent of patients experience a Jarisch–Herxheimer reaction.

Patients with neuroborreliosis will usually respond to intravenous benzylpenicillin, 20 MU/day for 14 to 21 days, although those with motor deficits may require up to 8 weeks of therapy. Ceftriaxone (Dattwyler, JInfDis, 1987; 155:1322) and cefotaxime (Pal, Lancet, 1988; i: 50) have also proved successful in the treatment of refractory neuroborreliosis.

Patients with established arthritis have been treated with high-dose benzylpenicillin. More than 50 per cent treated with 20 MU/day for 10 days were prevented from suffering further symptoms over a mean follow-up period of 33 months (Steere, NEJM, 1985; 312:869), although 14 to 21 days' treatment is probably more effective.

Borrelia recurrentis

Definition

Borrelia recurrentis is a motile, microaerophilic spirochaete, 10–30 μm long. It is the cause of louse-borne relapsing fever, a multisystem disorder characterized by recurrent febrile episodes that resolve spontaneously. Other species of *Borrelia* are responsible for tick-borne relapsing fever, which is generally less severe.

Introduction

The disease has occurred in epidemic form in association with war and famine over the centuries.

Epidemiology

There is no animal reservoir of louse-borne relapsing fever. The body louse, *Pediculus humanus*, becomes infected when feeding on the blood of infected humans. The disease is then transmitted in conditions of overcrowding and poor hygiene when the louse feeds on others. Infection is then usually acquired by inoculating infected haemolymph when the individual scratches. There are endemic foci of infection in Ethiopia, the Far East, and South America.

Organisms causing tick-borne relapsing fever are found in rodents, insectivores, and bats, and in the soft ticks that transmit this disease to man. There are reservoirs of infection in Africa, North, Central and South America, and the Middle East.

Pathogenesis and pathology

Following an initial bacteraemia associated with fever and other clinical features, a variety of antibodies is produced, which clear the organisms from the blood. Subsequent relapses arise as the result of the production of new, variable, major protein antigens by remaining spirochaetes, allowing evasion of existing antibodies and further bacteraemia. The cause of the fever is still not entirely clear. Although the sequence of events is suggestive of endotoxin release, endotoxin has not been consistently demonstrated in patients or in sonicates of the organism (Hardy, PSEBM, 1983; 174:47). Instead it is possible the fever is the result of a heat-stable pyrogen produced by the spirochaete (Butler, JInfDis, 1979; 140:665).

The majority of patients suffer a perivascular, histiocytic, interstitial myocarditis. Follicular splenic abscesses are common and these may be associated with splenic rupture. There are widespread petechial haemorrhages and there may be cerebral haemorrhage. The findings in the liver are those of a non-specific hepatitis with areas of focal necrosis and haemorrhage.

Clinical features

There is an incubation period of 4 to 18 days. The patient suffers sudden onset of rigors, headache, anorexia, myalgia, arthralgia, nausea, vomiting, photophobia, and high fever. A macular or petechial rash is common and there may be petechial conjunctival haemorrhages. Symptoms progress to include cough and upper abdominal pain, and hepatosplenomegaly may be found in as many as 80 per cent of cases.[28] Jaundice occurs in up to 80 per cent (Bryceson, QJMed, 1970; 39:129; Horton, ArchIntMed, 1980; 145: 871).

Between 3 and 10 days after the onset of the illness the episode resolves by crisis. The patient becomes flushed and hypotensive and may die at this point from cardiovascular collapse. After a further period of up to 10 afebrile days there is a relapse that resembles the initial episode. In severe cases, patients may suffer cardiac failure, hepatic failure, and haemorrhagic complications as a consequence of thrombocytopenia and disseminated intravascular coagulopathy.

It is important to bear in mind that both typhus and enteric fever may occur at the same time as relapsing fever, particularly in epidemics (Anderson, AmJPathol, 1955; 31:1083).

Investigations

Liver function tests typically show hepatitic changes with raised AST and ALT, and the serum bilirubin may be as high as 16 mg/100 ml.[28] Although the white-cell count is usually normal or slightly raised initially, it falls during crisis. Thrombocytopenia is a very common finding. Electrocardiographic abnormalities are also frequent, as a result of the myocarditis.

The diagnosis is made by demonstrating *Borrelia* in thick and thin blood films during a febrile episode. The organism may be found in the blood of young mice injected with the blood or cerebrospinal fluid of an infected patient, within 14 days of injection, and it can also be cultured in Kelly broth. Serological tests have been employed for epidemiological studies, but they are not generally available for diagnostic purposes.

Differential diagnosis

There is a wide differential diagnosis and, as previously noted, the possibility of dual infection should be borne in mind. The following must be considered: (i) falciparum malaria, (ii) enteric fever, (iii) typhus, (iv) yellow fever, (v) dengue fever, (vi) rat-bite fever, and (vii) leptospirosis.

Treatment

Various penicillin preparations have been used with some success, but they may fail to prevent relapses, particularly with tick-borne disease, which is probably best treated with oral tetracycline, 500 mg 6-hourly for 10 days. Children and pregnant women may be given oral erythromycin (125–250 mg 6-hourly for 10 days and 500 mg 6-hourly for 10 days, respectively).[29]

Louse-borne infection may be effectively treated with a single dose of tetracycline (500 mg by mouth or 250 mg intravenously) or erythromycin (500 mg by mouth or 300 mg intravenously) (Butler, JInfDis, 1978; 137:573).

The Jarisch–Herxheimer reaction occurs during treatment in almost all cases. It appears to be related to the speed with which spirochaetes are cleared from the blood, and may be severe with penicillin and tetracycline. Although corticosteroids do not prevent it in relapsing fever, they do reduce the concurrent fever and hypotension (Butler, JInfDis, 1978; 137:573). Opioid antagonists also reduced the severity of Jarisch–Herxheimer reactions, suggesting a possible role for endorphins (Teklu, Lancet, 1983; i:837).

Coxiella burnetii

Definition

Coxiella burnetii causes Q fever, an acute illness that typically presents with a sudden onset of fever, malaise, headache, and symptoms of pneumonitis. Hepatic involvement is common. The disease may become chronic in some cases, usually causing infective endocarditis. The causative rickettsia is a Gram-negative, obligate intracellular bacterium.

Introduction

Q fever was first described in Australia by Derrick in 1937 (Derrick, MedJAust, 1937; 1:281). The organism was then identified in ticks in Montana in 1938 (Davies, PubHlthRepWash, 1938; 53:2259). Liver involvement was first reported in 1956 (Gerstl, Gastro, 1956; 30:813).

Epidemiology

The first cases were described in farmers and abattoir workers, and it became apparent that the source of infection is infected sheep, goats, or cattle. Infection may result from contact with livestock, ingestion of contaminated unpasteurized milk, or inhalation of the organism in dust-laden air. The disease has a worldwide distribution and chiefly affects adult males. Outbreaks involving more than 100 people have been documented (Smith, Lancet, 1989; ii:557).

Pathogenesis and pathology

The organism has been found in hepatic lesions or in heart-valve vegetations, but the mechanisms by which it produces disease are not clear. It seems that variation in the phase-I lipopolysaccharide antigens affects pathogenicity. Thus strains of *C. burnetii* isolated from patients with endocarditis possessed different lipopolysaccharides from those of strains isolated from patients with acute Q fever (Hackstadt, InfectImmun, 1986; 52:337).

Liver biopsy usually reveals granulomatous hepatitis. The lesions, which have been described as 'doughnut lesions', [30] are composed of neutrophils, monocytes, eosinophils, and occasional multinucleate giant cells surrounding a central lipid-filled space (Okun, AmJClinPath, 1979; 71:117; Pellegrin, HumPath, 1980; 11:51).[31] These granulomas disappeared over a period of 3 months following antibiotic therapy.[31]

Clinical features

There is an incubation period of 14 to 26 days. This is followed by onset of headache, chills, fever, malaise, myalgia, and anorexia. A dry cough with or without chest pain is a common feature, but physical signs are few. In one study, 65 per cent of patients with acute Q fever had hepatomegaly and the liver was tender in 11 per cent, whilst 4 per cent were jaundiced (Powell, AustAnnMed, 1961; 10:52). Q fever may present as acute hepatitis with no involvement of the respiratory tract.[30]

The disease may be prolonged in approx. 20 per cent of patients, and of these it has been estimated that roughly one-third develop hepatitis with overt jaundice.[32] Endocarditis also develops in a small number of patients, 1 to 20 years after the acute infection.

Death from acute Q fever is rare, but death from hepatic failure has been described (Berkovitch, HelvPaedActa, 1985; 40:87).

Investigations

Liver dysfunction is common in Q fever. In one study, abnormal liver function tests were found in 85 per cent of 72 consecutive patients with the disease.[31] Serum AST may be elevated by up to three times normal and is the most common abnormality, whilst concentrations of alkaline phosphatase are seldom more than twice normal.[30] The total white-cell count is often normal. The erythrocyte sedimentation rate is typically raised and may be greater than 100 mm/h in patients with hepatitis.[30]

The diagnosis is confirmed by detection of antibody to *C. burnetii* phase-I or phase-II antigens by means of complement fixation or immunofluorescent antibody tests. Phase-II antibodies are raised in acute self-limiting disease whereas phase-I antibody titres exceed phase-II antibodies only in patients with chronic Q fever.[30]

Differential diagnosis

The acute hepatitic illness needs to be distinguished from acute viral hepatitis, whereas the differential diagnosis of histologically confirmed granulomatous hepatitis (see Chapter 14.2) includes: (i) tuberculosis, (ii) sarcoidosis, (iii) syphilis, (iv) brucellosis, (v) Hodgkin's disease, (vi) fungal infection, (vii) parasitic infection, (viii) cytomegalovirus infection, (ix) infectious mononucleosis, (x) inflammatory bowel disease, and (xi) drug reactions.

Treatment

Tetracyclines are currently the treatment of choice for the condition, but cannot be recommended for acute Q fever in children or pregnant women. In adults and children aged 12 years or more, tetracycline, 25 mg/kg per day in divided doses for 2 weeks (or doxycycline 100 mg 12-hourly in adults), is suitable. Erythromycin is an appropriate alternative in children, but is less effective than doxycycline (Sobradillo, Thorax, 1992; 47:276).

Recently developed vaccines have been shown to be efficacious in at-risk individuals (Reimer, ClinMicroRev, 1993; 6:193).

Rocky Mountain spotted fever

Definition

Rocky Mountain spotted fever is a tick-borne, multisystem disease caused by *Rickettsia rickettsii*. The organism is an obligate, pleomorphic, intracellular bacterium, most closely resembling a Gram-negative bacterium in biochemical and structural characteristics.

Introduction

The first clinical description of Rocky Mountain spotted fever was in 1899 by Maxey (MedSentinel, 1899, 7:433), although the first cases attributable to the disease probably occurred in 1873 among settlers in the Bitterroot Valley in Montana.

The causative organism, *R. rickettsii*, was first seen under the light microscope by Wolbach in 1916; he noted its presence in ticks and infected vascular endothelial cells (Wolbach, JMedRes, 1916; 34:121). Transmission by ticks was demonstrated in 1908 (McCalla, MedSentinel, 1908; 16:87), using human volunteers, although Ricketts had earlier suggested this mode of transmission.

Epidemiology

The disease is distributed according to the habitat of the various tick species that are the natural hosts of *R. rickettsii*. In the Rocky Mountains the organism is found in the wood tick, *Dermacentor andersoni*. Elsewhere in the United States it is found in the American dog tick, *D. variabilis*.

The disease has its highest incidence among children as they play out of doors and with dogs.

Pathogenesis and pathology

Only the adult tick feeds on humans. Following the blood meal the rickettsiae undergo activation to a virulent state, which takes up to 48 h. The organism spreads via the bloodstream and the lymphatics to involve all the major organs. Invasion of, and proliferation within, endothelial cells is the cause of the clinical disease. The organism is able to kill invaded cells directly *in vitro* (Walker, InfectImmun, 1982; 37:301). It may be that immunopathological mechanisms, such as lysis of infected cells by γ-interferon and cytotoxic T cells observed *in vitro* (Wisseman, JExpMed, 1983; 158:1780), are also important *in vivo*.

Cell-membrane damage appears to be a function of phospholipase A activity in *R. prowazekii* (Winkler, InfectImmunol, 1989; 57:36), and *R. rickettsii*-mediated cell lysis is decreased by agents that inhibit phospholipase activity or block the attachment of *R. prowazekii* to red cells (Walker, InfectImmunol, 1983; 40:840). Effects on the endothelial cell membrane result in adherence of platelets and activation of the clotting cascades (Clements. In Gorbach, Bartlett, Blacklow, eds. *Infectious diseases*. Philadelphia: Saunders, 1992:1304). It appears that this is responsible for the generation of thrombi, haemorrhagic skin lesions, and increased vascular permeability seen in the disease.

The predominant hepatic lesion is an infiltration of the portal tracts with mononuclear cells and neutrophils. Although hepatocellular necrosis may be found, it does not have a characteristic distribution. These features reflect the presence of rickettsiae in the portal tracts, which can be demonstrated by immunofluorescence.[33]

Clinical features

It is uncertain whether asymptomatic infection exists. Most patients suffer moderate or severe illness. The incubation period ranges from 2 to 14 days. Only 60 per cent of patients give a history of tick bite. Initial symptoms include fever, malaise, headache, muscle aches, anorexia, nausea, vomiting, and abdominal pain, followed by a rash on day 3 of the illness. This blanches in the early stages of the disease, but the spots later become haemorrhagic. The rash characteristically appears first on the limbs and involves the palms and soles. However, it is absent in up to 12 per cent of cases, does not have a haemorrhagic component in 50 per cent, and does not always involve the palms and soles when it is present.[34]

Signs and symptoms of encephalitis occur in up to 28 per cent of patients and pneumonitis in 17 per cent.[34]

In a retrospective survey of patients who had died of Rocky Mountain spotted fever, only 33 per cent were clinically jaundiced. All patients were found to have hepatomegaly at autopsy.[33] The incidence of jaundice in other autopsy studies has varied between 16 and 80 per cent (Ramphal, ArchIntMed, 1978; 138:260), but there are few reports detailing the incidence of jaundice in patients who survive. The disease may produce symptoms of cholecystitis as a result of vascular involvement with the organism in the gall-bladder wall (Walker, ArchIntMed, 1985; 145:2194).

Before the availability of antirickettsial drugs, Rocky Mountain spotted fever carried a mortality of more than 20 per cent. In recent years this has fallen to 3 per cent.[34]

Investigations

In the retrospective, autopsy study of Adams and Walker all patients had elevated concentrations of total and conjugated serum bilirubin. Where enzyme concentrations were measured the most consistent abnormality was a moderate rise in the AST.[33]

The organism can be isolated from blood and tissues in a variety of antibiotic-free cell lines including Vero and primary chicken embryo fibroblasts.[34] In the majority of patients the diagnosis is made serologically. In recent years the Weil–Felix test using the agglutination of strains of *Proteus vulgaris* has been superseded by tests using specific antigens of *R. rickettsii*. Indirect immunofluorescent antibody assay and latex agglutination methods are widely available and are extremely sensitive (positive in up to 100 per cent of cases). Unfortunately, neither gives positive results during the acute phase of the disease, the latex test becoming positive 7 to 9 days after the onset of illness and falling to non-diagnostic titres within 2 months.

Differential diagnosis

In the initial stages of the illness the differential diagnosis is large and includes: (i) viral infection (especially measles and entero-viral infection), (ii) meningococcaemia, (iii) gastroenteritis, (iv) appendicitis, (v) acute cholecystitis, (vi) pneumonia, and (vii) meningoencephalitis.

Treatment

Early, empirical therapy is important in reducing the severity and mortality. By the time liver dysfunction has developed, antibiotics may be too late to prevent death. Appropriate agents include doxycycline (100 mg 12-hourly), tetracycline (50 mg/kg per day in four divided doses) or chloramphenicol (50 mg/kg per day in four divided doses). Chloramphenicol should be used for children and pregnant women.

Other rickettsial infections

These include epidemic or louse-borne typhus (caused by *R. pro-mazekii*), endemic or murine typhus (*R. typhi*), scrub typhus (*R. tsutsugamushi*), rickettsialpox (*R. akari*), and tick typhus or bou-tonneuse fever (*R. conorii*). Hepatic involvement has been documented in the last infection.

Rickettsia conorii has a wide distribution and is found in the Mediterranean basin, Kenya, South Africa, and elsewhere along the coasts of Africa and India. It is transmitted to man by the dog tick, *Rhipicephalus sanguineus*.

Tick typhus presents as a febrile illness with arthralgia and myalgia, followed by the eruption of a button-like rash (hence the name boutonneuse fever) on the trunk and limbs. An eschar is found in 80 per cent of cases. The condition usually has a benign course, although central nervous involvement, pneumonitis, or skin necrosis may occur. Investigations may show an elevation of the AST to as much as 10 times normal while the alkaline phosphatase may be up to twice normal.[35] The serum bilirubin is only modestly raised (<2 mg/100 ml).[35]

In one series of patients with tick typhus, five had had liver biopsies, which showed granulomas in three.[35] The granulomas were poorly organized, with no giant cells. In addition, there were small foci of parenchymal collapse with infiltration by macrophages, neutrophils, and lymphocytes. Portal involvement was only slight.

Tetracyclines are the treatment of choice for the condition but cannot be recommended for children. In adults and children aged 12 years or more, tetracycline, 25 mg/kg per day in divided doses for 1 week (or doxycycline 100 mg 12-hourly in adults), is appropriate. Chloramphenicol is also effective.

Ehrlichiosis

Definition

Human ehrlichiosis is a tick-borne infection caused by a Gram-negative, pleomorphic organism in the family Rickettsiaceae.

Introduction

Infection with *Erhlichia* spp. was initially recognized in dogs. The first human case of ehrlichiosis was reported from Japan in 1954 (Tachibana, In Leive, ed. *Microbiology*. Washington, DC: ASM, 1986; 205). The first case of human ehrlichiosis reported in the United States occurred in 1986 (Maeda, NEJM, 1987; 316:853) and it subsequently became clear that hepatitis was a feature of the condition.

Epidemiology

The form of the infection first described, caused by *E. sennetsu*, is thought to be confined to western Japan and Malaysia. In the United States, infection due to a closely related species, *E. chaffeensis*, is found in the south-central and south Atlantic states. Recently the disease has been reported from Europe. The vector of transmission in the United States is thought to be *Amblyomma americanum*.

Pathogenesis and pathology

Infection due to *E. chaffeensis* is primarily of the haemopoietic and lymphoreticular systems. Following injection by a tick the organisms spread via the lymphatics and blood vessels and invade macrophages, monocytes, and lymphocytes. Infected cells have been found in peripheral blood, bone marrow, liver, spleen, kidney, and cerebrospinal fluid (Dumler, NEJM, 1991; 325:1109).

The organism causes cytopathic effects in cell culture, but some of the features of the infection may be the consequence of host response.

Affected tissues notably show perivascular infiltrates of lymphocytes, macrophages, and plasma cells. Focal hepatocellular necrosis is seen on histological examination of the liver, and other organs may have necrotic areas (Dumler, NEJM, 1991; 325:1109).

Clinical features

The incubation period is approx. 7 days, and patients present with fever, headache, myalgia, and malaise. Up to 50 per cent will develop a maculopapular rash. Those with severe disease may develop respiratory failure, acute renal failure, gastrointestinal haemorrhage, and neurological complications. Fatal cases have been described (Walker, Proc. and Abstr., 89th meeting of the American Society for Microbiology, 1989; 95).

Investigations

Patients typically have leucopenia and thrombocytopenia. Elevated transaminases are seen in up to 80 per cent of cases, although far fewer are jaundiced. The condition is usually diagnosed by indirect immunofluorescence assay using cells infected with *E. chaffeensis*.

Differential diagnosis

The differential diagnosis is very broad and depends upon the presenting features. It includes: (i) viral infection (including hepatitis, measles and enteroviral infection), (ii) meningococcaemia, (iii) Rocky Mountain spotted fever, (iv) relapsing fever, (v) tularaemia, (vi) Lyme disease, (vii) tick typhus, (viii) Q fever, (ix) leptospirosis, (x) gastroenteritis, (xi) pneumonia, and (xii) meningoencephalitis.

Treatment

Tetracycline, 25 mg/kg per day in four divided doses, or doxycycline, 100 mg 12-hourly, have been used successfully, and rifampicin is active *in vitro*.

Chlamydial infections
Definition

Chlamydiae are non-motile, Gram-negative, obligate intracellular bacteria. In man they most commonly infect the eye, the genital tract, and the respiratory tract.

Introduction

Human chlamydial disease has, until recently, been thought to be due to two species, *Chlamydia trachomatis* and *C. psittaci*. Man is an atypical host of *C. psittaci* and a new species has recently been described that causes an epidemic form of acute respiratory disease in man (Kleemola, JInfDis, 1988; 157:230). This was initially designated **TWAR** (from the first isolates TW 183 and AR 39) (Grayston, NEJM, 1986; 315:161) and has subsequently been named *C. pneumoniae*.

Hepatic involvement was first described in two cases of psittacosis in 1959 (Yow, AmJMed, 1959; 27:739). The association between perihepatitis and infection with *C. trachomatis* was first reported in 1978 (Muller-Schoop, BMJ, 1978; 1:1022).

Infections with *C. trachomatis*
Epidemiology

The organism is distributed worldwide and is transmitted either by sexual contact (serotypes D–K and L1, L2, and L3) or by flies, fomites, or hand–eye contact (serotypes A, B, Ba, and C). Hepatic involvement, in the form of the Curtis–Fitz-Hugh syndrome, may follow sexually transmitted disease.

Pathogenesis and pathology

Chlamydiae are able to inhibit phagolysosomal fusion within phagocytes and ultimately cause cell damage, but the means by which this is achieved are uncertain. Immediate cytotoxicity can be demonstrated when macrophages ingest viable or ultraviolet-inactivated elementary bodies. This effect is heat-labile and can be blocked by type-specific antibody. In some conditions, cell death requires growth of the organism and might be the result of competition for ATP. Phagocyte death and immunopathological mechanisms are thought to be responsible for the inflammation and scarring that occur in these infections.

It appears that peritonitis and perihepatitis result from direct spread of the organism from the genital tract in the female. Cases have been described in which there is no evidence of salpingitis (Muller-Schoop, BMJ, 1978; 1:1022), although it is assumed that the organism reached the peritoneum via the fallopian tubes. Certainly *C. trachomatis* has been isolated from ascitic fluid in such patients (Marbet, BMJ, 1986; 293:5). Since the condition has also been described in men (Dan, Gut, 1987; 28:1514), it is possible that the organism can also reach the peritoneum via blood or the lymphatics. The disease is the result of localized (or generalized) peritonitis, which causes the formation of adhesions between the parietal and visceral peritoneum overlying the liver. Histological examination of these adhesions reveals fibrinous changes that involve the liver capsule, but the liver parenchyma is usually normal (Wolner-Hanssen, Lancet, 1980; i:901). A case has been described of a 16-year-old male with prolonged fever in whom a liver biopsy revealed mild inflammatory changes in the portal tracts and an isolated granuloma; *C. trachomatis* was isolated from the liver tissue (Dan, Gut, 1987; 28:1514).

Clinical features

The condition typically presents in a young female with severe pain in the right upper quadrant, often following lower abdominal pain with or without vaginal discharge. The pain is exacerbated by coughing, deep inspiration, or truncal movement and may radiate to the right shoulder (Poynard, GastrClinBiol, 1982; 6:321).

The patient is usually febrile and has tenderness in the right upper quadrant, with or without guarding. Pelvic examination may be unremarkable.

Although symptoms usually respond rapidly to therapy, patients may improve without appropriate antibiotic treatment (Muller-Schoop, BMJ, 1978; 1:1022).

Investigations

Liver function tests are usually normal. The white-cell count is often moderately elevated, although it may be normal, and the erythrocyte sedimentation rate is usually raised. Laparoscopy reveals the typical 'violin string' adhesions between the anterior surface of the liver and the anterior abdominal wall (Muller-Schoop, BMJ, 1978; 1:1022). The adhesions may be seen on CT scans of the liver (Haight, AmJGastr, 1988; 83:323).

The syndrome is best confirmed by isolating the organism from peritoneal samples, but this is rarely achieved. Isolation of *C. trachomatis*, or detection of antigen by enzyme-linked immunosorbent assay or immunofluorescence from endocervical or urethral swabs, provides support for the diagnosis, but such swabs may be negative. The diagnosis has been confirmed in many cases by serological means. High IgG titres are usually found by micro-immunofluorescence, with or without raised IgM titres (Muller-Schoop, BMJ, 1978; 1:1022; Poynard, GastrClinBiol, 1982; 6:321), and a rise or fall in titres may be demonstrable (Muller-Schoop, BMJ, 1978; 1:1022).

Differential diagnosis

The disease requires differentiation from: (i) cholecystitis, (ii) acute appendicitis, and (iii) perihepatitis due to *N. gonorrhoeae*.

Treatment

The majority of patients have been treated with tetracyclines. Tetracycline, 500 mg 6-hourly (or doxycycline, 100 mg 12-hourly) is appropriate, and treatment should probably be continued for at least 2 weeks.

Infections with *C. psittaci* and *C. pneumoniae*

Epidemiology

Psittacosis was first described by Ritter in Switzerland in 1879.[36] Although the first cases were contracted from tropical birds, out-breaks have been reported following exposure to non-psittacine species, and the condition has become an occupational disease of veterinarians, pet-shop workers, poultry workers, and pigeon fanciers. The infection is transmitted by the respiratory route following inhalation of dried excreta from infected birds. Person-to-person spread has also been reported.

Following an outbreak of mild pneumonia in teenagers and young adults in Finland due to TWAR (Saikku, JInfDis, 1985; 151: 832), other epidemics, also unrelated to bird exposure, have been described and found to be due to this agent. Initially, TWAR was thought to be a strain of *C. psittaci*, but subsequent studies of the biology of this organism have led to the designation of a new species, *C. pneumoniae*.[37]

Pathogenesis and pathology

Chlamydia psittaci and *C. pneumoniae* invade the respiratory mucosa and interstitial macrophages, and are transported to the Kupffer cells and macrophages of the liver and spleen. Replication then occurs, followed by haematogenous dissemination to the lungs and other tissues.

Whilst histological examination of the lung often reveals areas of necrosis with haemorrhage, the most common hepatic lesion in infection with *C. psittaci* is a mild, non-zonal, focal necrosis, with or without Kupffer-cell hyperplasia (Lillie, NIHBull, 1933; 161:1). Other cases have been described with mild central atrophy and collapse, together with portal lymphocytic infiltration (Yow, AmJMed, 1959; 27:739), or with granulomas (Ragnaud, GastrClinBiol, 1986; 10:234).

Clinical features

The incubation period is between 7 and 15 days (up to 3 weeks in infections due to *C. pneumoniae*). The patient often becomes ill suddenly, with high fever, but the disease can have a more gradual onset over several days. Headache, malaise, anorexia, myalgia, and arthralgia are common, and there may be a pale macular rash

(Horder's spots). There is usually a dry cough, although there may be a mild degree of haemoptysis. Pleuritic chest pain is uncommon. Towards the end of the first week of the illness confusion may develop, usually associated with hypoxia.

On examination there are relatively few chest signs. Fine crepitations may be heard over the lower chest and pleural or pleuro-pericardial rubs may be present. Up to 20 per cent of patients with infection by *C. psittaci* may have non-tender hepatomegaly (Schaffner, AmJPathol, 1962; 40:653; Ragnaud, GastrClinBiol, 1986; 10:234), although frank jaundice usually occurs only in patients who are severely ill. Splenomegaly may be present in up to 70 per cent of cases with this infection.

Infection with *C. pneumoniae* presents as an acute respiratory infection or as pharyngitis in most cases. Some patients have suffered myocarditis during their infections but liver involvement does not appear to be a typical feature.[37] Cases of severe systemic infection have been reported in which there was hepatomegaly (Grayston, PediatInfectDis, 1994; 13:675).

Investigations

Abnormal liver function tests are found in up to 40 per cent of patients with psittacosis; the AST and ALT may be raised to more than seven times normal, whilst the alkaline phosphatase is often unaffected or only slightly raised (Ragnaud, GastrClinBiol, 1986; 10:234). Serum bilirubin is often within normal limits, although cases with severe psittacosis in which the bilirubin was more than 7.0 mg/100 ml have been reported (Yow, AmJMed, 1959; 27:739; Ragnaud, GastrClinBiol, 1986; 10:234).

The white-cell count and the erythrocyte sedimentation rate are often normal. Chest radiographs typically show bilateral, soft, patchy opacities radiating from the hilar regions and in the lower lung fields. The diagnosis is confirmed either by isolation of *C. psittaci* (and less frequently of *C. pneumoniae*) or more usually by demonstration of a serological response. A four-fold or greater rise in complement-fixing antibody titres is diagnostic. The complement fixation test cross-reacts with antibodies to *C. trachomatis* and *C. pneumoniae*, but the two diseases can be differentiated on the basis of specific microimmunofluorescence antibody tests.[37]

Differential diagnosis

The differential diagnosis is that of atypical pneumonia or a pyrexia of unknown origin and includes: (i) mycoplasma infection, (ii) Q fever, (iii) legionnaires' disease, (iv) viral pneumonia, (v) typhoid fever, (vi) tuberculosis, (vii) fungal infections including *Pneumocystis carinii* (in immunocompromised patients), and (viii) bacterial pneumonia.

Treatment

Tetracyclines are considered the most effective agents for therapy of infection with either organism. Tetracycline, 500 mg 6-hourly, should be given for at least 10 days after the patient becomes afebrile, in order to prevent relapse. Erythromycin is a suitable alternative and the newer macrolides may prove to be effective.

Mycoplasma pneumoniae

Definition

Pneumonia caused by *M. pneumoniae* usually involves both lungs and chest radiographic signs are typically more extensive than the physical signs. The condition has also been known as primary atypical pneumonia, virus pneumonia, and Eaton's agent pneumonia. The causative organism is highly pleomorphic because it lacks a rigid cell wall. It is a host-specific intracellular parasite but can be grown on cell-free medium.

Introduction

The name 'primary atypical pneumonia' was first given by Reimann in 1938 to a group of respiratory diseases that differed from typical bacterial pneumonia (Reimann, JAMA, 1938; 111:2377). Eaton produced disease in cotton rats in 1944 using filtered secretions from infected patients, and the causative organism was finally identified in 1962 (Chanock, PNAS, 1962; 48:41).

Epidemiology

The organism has a worldwide distribution and is probably spread by the respiratory route. The disease is most common amongst younger people, particularly schoolchildren and military recruits, and it is rare in the over-40 age group. The majority of patients are males. It appears that the disease spreads initially among schoolchildren and is then introduced into families, where it spreads among non-immune family members.

Pathogenesis and pathology

Following transmission, the organism becomes attached to respiratory epithelial cells at specific receptors. These are glycoproteins containing neuraminic acid (Hu, Science, 1982; 38:598). In the lung, *M. pneumoniae* remains extracellular. Local cytopathic effects have been ascribed to the production of peroxide. Spread of the organism outside the respiratory tract is rare and it therefore seems that extrapulmonary disease may have an immunopathological basis, perhaps as the result of the production of autoantibodies (Biberfeld, ClinExpImmun, 1971; 8:319), or circulating immune complexes (Biberfeld, JImmunol, 1974; 112:413). Liver histology is studied infrequently in cases of atypical pneumonia. Biopsies taken in the acute phase of the disease have usually revealed a non-specific reactive hepatitis (Suzuyama, YaleJBiolMed, 1983; 56:487). Chronic liver disease has been reported in the case of a bone-marrow transplant recipient from whom the organism was isolated in marrow cultures, in association with rising antibody titres against the strain. The liver biopsy revealed massive hepatocellular necrosis with an inflammatory infiltrate, as well as piecemeal necrosis (Jansson, Lancet, 1972; i:1395).

Clinical features

The disease has an incubation period of 9 to 21 days. The onset of the illness is usually with symptoms of an upper respiratory-tract infection. It has been estimated that only 5 per cent of all cases develop pneumonia (Murray, AmFamilyPhysician, 1988; 37:127). The other common presentations include tracheobronchitis, pharyngitis, and myringitis.

Pallor and jaundice are often seen in the second and third week of the illness in patients with significant titres of cold agglutinin (Jacobson, AmJMed, 1973; 54:514). The hyperbilirubinaemia is chiefly unconjugated, and the AST and alkaline phosphatase are typically normal or near normal.

The incidence of true hepatitis is estimated to be approx. 2 per cent in adults (Ali, QJMed, 1986; 58:241), but may be as high as 6 per cent in children (Ruiz-Contreras, AnEspPediat, 1986; 24:15). Liver involvement is usually of little clinical consequence, being detectable biochemically in most cases.

Investigations

Liver function tests in those patients with liver involvement usually show an elevation of AST, to more than five times normal in some cases; alkaline phosphatase is only modestly raised and the total bilirubin is usually less than 1.0 mg/100 ml (Murray, AmJMed, 1975; 54:229).

In the majority of cases the white-cell count is normal and the erythrocyte sedimentation rate is variable. The chest radiograph typically shows soft, patchy, bilateral shadowing, radiating from the hilar regions. Cold agglutinins may be detected in up to 50 per cent of cases by the end of the first week. The disease is usually confirmed by the demonstration of a rise in complement-fixing antibodies, which normally occurs in 2 to 4 weeks.

Differential diagnosis

The disease requires differentiation from other causes of atypical pneumonia. Hence the differential diagnosis includes: (i) psittacosis, (ii) Q fever, (iii) legionnaires' disease, (iv) viral pneumonia, (v) tuberculosis, (vi) fungal infections including *Pn. carinii* (in immunocompromised patients), and (vii) bacterial pneumonia.

Treatment

Treatment is with tetracycline, 500 mg 6-hourly, or erythromycin, 500 mg 6-hourly. The newer macrolides also appear effective. Therapy should be continued for at least 10 days. Relapse may occur but is usually amenable to retreatment.

Cat scratch disease

Introduction

Cat scratch disease was first described in 1950 (Debré, BullMemSocMedHopParis, 1950; 66:76), and since then over 2000 cases have been recorded (Carithers, AmJDisChild, 1985; 139:1124; Margileth, JInfDis, 1987, 155:390). Hepatic dysfunction and hepatomegaly appear to be relatively uncommon. An association with granulomatous hepatitis has been described (Lenoir, Lancet, 1988; i: 1132).

Definition

The disease takes the form of a regional lymphadenitis following an inoculation injury, usually inflicted by a cat. The clinical diagnosis requires fulfilment of three of the four following criteria (Lenoir, Lancet, 1988; i:1132):

(1) a history of contact with an animal (cat or dog) and a skin or eye lesion;

(2) a positive cat-scratch disease skin test;

(3) exclusion of other causes of lymphadenopathy;

(4) characteristic lymph-node histology.

Additional supportive evidence includes the presence of silver-staining bacteria in affected tissue. A positive culture of *Bartonella henselae* from affected tissue, or significant antibody titres to *Bartonella* spp. (this test is not generally available), are suitable substitutes for the skin test.

Epidemiology

Over 90 per cent of cases are associated with exposure to, or scratches by, cats (Margileth, Pediat, 1968; 42:803), although in one series 95 per cent of children had been exposed to dogs and only 90 per cent to cats (Carithers, JAmMedWomAssoc, 1959; 14:19). The majority of cases occur in the autumn and winter. Hepatic involvement has chiefly been described in children and teenagers.

Pathogenesis and pathology

The presence of bacteria in the lymph nodes of patients with cat scratch disease was first demonstrated using the Warthin–Starry silver stain (Wear, Science, 1983; 221:1403). The organisms show branching and are characteristically found around blood vessels. Such organisms have also been found in skin and conjunctival inoculation lesions and in liver biopsy specimens from patients with cat scratch disease (Lenoir, Lancet, 1988; i:1132). Cultures of affected tissue or pus have yielded *B. henselae* (previously designated *Rochalimaea henselae*) in most cases, although *Afipia felis* has also been proposed as the putative cause of cat scratch disease. However, serological evidence supports *B. henselae*.

Histological examination of these sites demonstrates granulomas with caseating or even suppurative centres. Liver biopsies have shown a dense fibrous reaction surrounding bile ducts and containing discrete granulomas.

Clinical features

The onset of the disease is usually 1 to 2 weeks after skin puncture. A single papule develops at the site of inoculation in 50 to 95 per cent of cases.[38] At the same time, tender enlargement of regional lymph nodes occurs, but this may be delayed for up to 7 to 10 weeks.[38] In up to 40 per cent of cases, suppurative lymphadenopathy develops. The nodes usually remain enlarged for 4 to 6 weeks, but resolution may occasionally take more than 2 years (Daniels, JAMA, 1954; 154:1247). A low-grade fever occurs in up to 30 per cent of cases and general malaise in approx. 40 per cent (Rocco, Gastro, 1985; 89:1400). Other common symptoms include headache, anorexia, and fatigue.

Clinically apparent hepatic involvement is uncommon. Hepatomegaly or anicteric hepatitis has been described in less than 1 per cent of cases.

Investigations

In the few cases of hepatic involvement in cat scratch disease, liver function tests have either been completely normal (Lenoir, Lancet, 1988; i:1132) or only mildly deranged (Rocco, Gastro, 1985; 89:1400). The peripheral white-cell count may be raised, as may the erythrocyte sedimentation rate (Lenoir, Lancet, 1988; i:1132). CT

scanning has revealed focal defects of variable size within the liver (Rocco, Gastro, 1985; 89:1400; Lenoir, Lancet, 1988; i:1132).

Differential diagnosis

The differential diagnosis is that of the causes of regional lymphadenopathy and granulomatous hepatitis and therefore includes: (i) mycobacterial infection, (ii) lymphoma, (iii) toxoplasmosis, (v) infectious mononucleosis, (v) brucellosis, (vi) sarcoidosis, (vii) tularaemia, (viii) yersiniosis, and (ix) secondary syphilis.

Treatment

The disease is typically self-limiting, resolving spontaneously over 2 to 4 months, and usually requires no specific therapy, although fatal cases have been reported.[38] In patients with severe disease, antibiotic therapy is warranted; the most effective agents appear to be rifampicin and ciprofloxacin (Margileth, PediatInfDisJ, 1992; 11:474).

Whipple's disease

This is another disease that has been thought of as infective in nature but for which, until recently, no causative pathogen had been identified. Electron microscopy has demonstrated the presence of bacilli in affected tissues, and sequencing of ribosomal RNA has shown it to be a Gram-positive actinomycete, provisionally named *Tropheryma whippelii* (Relman, NEJM, 1992; 327:293). However, the organism has yet to be cultured.

Whipple's disease is important as a rare bacterial infection of the liver causing granulomatous lesions. The condition is most common in middle-aged men, who typically present with a history of intermittent arthralgia followed by the development of steatorrhoea and weight loss. However, the disease is usually considered when biopsies reveal the characteristic histological appearances of infiltrates of macrophages that stain strongly with periodic acid–Schiff reagent. The small bowel is usually involved, but occasional cases occur where other organs, such as the brain, are affected in the absence of intestinal involvement. The diagnosis is confirmed by electron microscopy, which reveals the intracellular bacilli.

The treatment of choice is co-trimoxazole, 960 mg 12-hourly, and this is effective in infection of the central nervous system (Ryser, Gastro, 1984, 86:745; Keinath, Gastro, 1985, 88:1867). Therapy should be given for a year to prevent relapse. Patients unable to tolerate co-trimoxazole can be given phenoxymethyl penicillin, although this may not be as effective for central nervous disease. Other alternatives include ceftriaxone, chloramphenicol, and tetracyclines, particularly for relapses.

Mycobacterial infections

Involvement of the liver is common in patients with mycobacterial infections. The frequency of hepatic tuberculosis varies widely, depending on the geographical area and the type of patient studied, being highest in those with miliary dissemination and less common with chronic tuberculosis. In a few cases, extensive clinical investigation may fail to demonstrate involvement of other organs and the liver appears to be the only organ affected (García Díaz, RevClinEsp, 1988; 182:261). Until recently the incidence of tuberculosis had been declining in developed countries but the emergence

Table 6 Pathology of the liver in mycobacterial infections

Hepatic granuloma
Hepatic tuberculoma
Tuberculous cholangitis
Drug-induced hepatitis
Non-specific changes (fatty infiltration, reactive hepatitis)
Granulomatosis from BCG immunization

of the acquired immune deficiency syndrome (**AIDS**) has led to renewed interest in liver disease related to mycobacterial infection. In this setting, in addition to *M. tuberculosis*, other species, for example *M. avium-intracellulare* or, more rarely, *M. genavense*, may be involved (Gordon, JHepatol, 1986; 2:475; Schneiderman, Hepatol, 1987; 7:925; Mascheck, AmJClinPathol, 1994; 101:95). *Mycobacterium avium-intracellulare* typically affects HIV-infected patients with advanced immunosuppression and causes symptoms related to disseminated infection, whereas hepatic tuberculosis often occurs in those with less severe immunocompromise.[39] Mycobacterial infection of the liver occasionally occurs in immunosuppressed patients after solid organ transplantation (Meyers, Transpl, 1994; 58:301).

The clinical spectrum of liver disease due to *Mycobacterium* spp. ranges from the absence of liver symptoms to severe hepatitis with jaundice and liver failure. Granuloma formation within the hepatic parenchyma is the most common lesion, but granulomas may also affect the intrahepatic and extrahepatic biliary tree or may involve lymph nodes at the porta hepatis and cause biliary obstruction. Granulomas may coalesce and form tuberculomas. Beside these specific lesions, patients with tuberculosis often show non-specific changes in the liver, such as steatosis, reactive hepatitis or, rarely, amyloidosis. They may also present with drug-induced hepatic lesions caused by antituberculous drugs. In patients with AIDS, many agents, including hepatotropic and other viruses, fungi, parasites, alcohol abuse, neoplasms, hepatotoxic drugs, iron deposition, and others, can cause liver damage, which should be distinguished from that related to mycobacterial infection (Lefkowitch, DigDis, 1994; 12:321). Table 6 summarizes the diverse hepatic lesions that may occur in these infections.

Granulomatous hepatitis may develop after immunization with bacille Calmette–Guérin (**BCG**), particularly when used as immunostimulant therapy in patients with melanoma (Hunt, Lancet, 1973; ii:820) or after vaccination in children infected by HIV (Besnard, PediatInfectDisJ, 1993; 12:993). A few cases of granulomatous hepatitis have also been reported after therapeutic intravesical instillation of BCG in patients with carcinoma of the bladder (Proctor, AmJGastr, 1993; 88:1112).

Hepatic granulomatosis

Tuberculosis is a frequent cause of granuloma formation in the liver.[40,41] The number of granulomas varies greatly, being highest in miliary tuberculosis. Localization is also variable, but granulomas are more common in lobular than in portal or periportal areas. Tuberculous granulomas do not have specific morphological features and cannot easily be differentiated from other granulomas morphologically. In most cases the granulomas are small, less than 2 mm in diameter, and consist of an aggregate of epithelioid cells

that is surrounded by mononuclear inflammatory cells and contains a few multinucleated giant cells. Caseation is seen in less than half of the cases and is not specific. Demonstration of acid-fast bacilli is diagnostic, although Ziehl–Nielsen staining is successful in less than 15 per cent of cases.[42] *Mycobacterium tuberculosis* may be isolated from the biopsies in about one-third of cases.

In patients with immunodeficiency infected with atypical mycobacteria, granulomas are poorly formed and consist of inconspicuous aggregates of lymphocytes and pale, foamy macrophages filled with abundant acid-fast bacilli that can be identified with Ziehl–Nielsen staining.

Clinical features

Hepatic involvement usually produces no symptoms in patients with chronic tuberculosis and the clinical manifestations are those of extrahepatic disease. Hepatomegaly and minor abnormalities of liver function tests, particularly elevation of alkaline phosphatase and γ-glutamyl transpeptidase, are frequent incidental findings. Liver function is well preserved. Occasionally, patients may present with loss of weight, general malaise, or fever. Jaundice is rare, and may be due to involvement of the biliary tree (Alvarez, DigDisSci, 1983; 28:193). Ascites may appear, but is usually associated with peritoneal tuberculosis. Portal hypertension and bleeding from oesophageal varices may occur in rare cases (Bruguera, RevIntHep, 1968; 18:895).

The liver is involved in most patients with miliary tuberculosis and in some cases is massively invaded. Occasionally there is no evidence of tuberculosis elsewhere, a condition that was erroneously termed primary tuberculosis of the liver. Symptoms are usually obscured by those of generalized tuberculosis; nevertheless, abdominal pain, jaundice, or ascites may appear. Several cases of acute liver failure, mimicking fulminant hepatitis, have been reported, suggesting that this form of hepatic tuberculosis is not as exceptional as once believed (Sharma, AmJGastr, 1981; 76:153; Asada, HumPath, 1991; 22:92; Godwin, Chest, 1991; 99:752; Hussain, Gut, 1995; 36:792). Disseminated mycobacterial infection of the liver is a frequent finding in HIV-infected patients with abnormal liver function tests and fever of otherwise unexplained origin (Cavichi, ClinInfectDis, 1995; 20:606).

Suspicion of liver involvement must be based on clinical data or on abnormal biochemical findings. Ultrasonographic findings are often non-specific (Wetton, ClinRadiol, 1993; 47:36). Confirmation of the diagnosis requires histological examination and demonstration of mycobacteria by appropriate acid-fast staining, or by culture of liver tissue. Recently, amplification of mycobacterial DNA sequences by the polymerase chain reaction has gained increasing diagnostic relevance. Further refinement of molecular biological techniques allows identification to species level (Kulski, JClinMicrobiol, 1995; 33:668). Alternatively, diagnosis can be made when liver abnormalities coexist with proven infection of other organs or in patients who respond satisfactorily to specific therapy. Noninvasive techniques, such as ultrasound, CT, MRI, usually do not provide specific data but may help to rule out other lesions. Plain radiographic examination may show multiple calcifications in the hepatic area in patients with chronic tuberculosis. Peritoneoscopy is rarely indicated, but it may be useful if granulomas reach the surface of the liver surface and also to exclude peritoneal involvement.

Tuberculoma

The terms tuberculous hepatic abscess or pseudotumoral hepatic tuberculosis are also used to describe this condition. Coalescent granulomas may form large abscesses that are surrounded by fibrous tissue and contain caseum. They may be single or multiple and usually develop in patients with other tuberculous foci, either pulmonary or abdominal.[43] Tuberculous abscesses are being described with increasing frequency in patients with AIDS (Moreno, AnnIntMed, 1988; 109:437; Roig, RevClinEsp, 1995, 195: 89).

Clinical manifestations include prolonged fever, loss of weight, general wasting, and upper abdominal pain (Lupatakin, ClinInfDis, 1992; 14:1040). However, symptoms may not be very apparent and a tuberculous abscess can be discovered following an incidental finding of elevated alkaline phosphatase (Achem, JClinGastro, 1992; 14:72). Lesions have been demonstrated by scintigraphy, or, more recently, by ultrasonography, CT or MRI. The picture may mimic other processes such as liver-cell or metastatic carcinoma, lymphoma or actinomycosis. Percutaneous biopsy with ultrasound or CT guidance offers a good diagnostic alternative to laparotomy or peritoneoscopy. Histological examination reveals granulomas; *M. tuberculosis* can be identified by acid-fast staining and culture.

Tuberculosis of the biliary tract

This condition is very rare. Tuberculous cholangitis, which possibly results from rupture of a caseating granuloma or tuberculoma into the lumen of the bile ducts, may affect the intrahepatic or the extrahepatic branches of the biliary tree (Abascal, AmJGastr, 1988; 83:1183). Clinically, apart from the general symptoms of tuberculosis, there may be obstructive jaundice. Obstruction of bile flow may be caused by compression of bile ducts by tuberculous adenitis at the hilum of the liver (Wee, ActaCytol, 1995; 39:559). Tuberculous cholecystitis, which is usually associated with gallstones, is exceedingly rare (Leader, AnnInt, 1952; 37:594).

Immunization against bacterial infections in liver disease

It is important to review the role of immunization in patients with chronic disease for several reasons.

1. The patient may suffer adverse reactions to certain vaccines that are not experienced by the normal patient.
2. The patient may produce a poor humoral or cell-mediated response to particular bacterial vaccines.
3. The patient may be more prone to infection with particular organisms than the normal patient and hence require additional immunization.

Vaccines are currently available in the United Kingdom for immunization against the following bacterial infections: (i) diphtheria, (ii) tetanus, (iii) pertussis, (iv) tuberculosis, (v) typhoid, (vi) cholera, (vii) meningococcal infection, (viii) pneumococcal infection, (ix) *H. influenzae* type b (**Hib**) infection, and (x) anthrax. Whilst specific contraindications for some of these vaccines have been identified in patients with certain underlying conditions (such as HIV infection), no adverse effects peculiar to patients with acute or chronic liver disease appear to occur. The present recommendations of the Joint Committee on Vaccination and Immunization (Joint Committee. *Immunisation against infectious disease*. London: HMSO, 1996) do not include liver disease among the contraindications for the use of any of these vaccines.

Immunoglobulin synthesis does not seem to be impaired in liver disease. Indeed, concentrations of the different classes are usually higher than in the normal population and this is the result of increased production (Havens, JImmunol, 1954; 73:256). There have been relatively few studies on the immunological effects of bacterial vaccines in patients with liver disease. No significant difference was found between cirrhotic patients and non-cirrhotic individuals in their responses to primary immunization with tetanus toxoid; likewise, a second dose of toxoid given within 2 years of the first produced a similar response in the two groups (Cherrick, NEJM, 1959; 261:340). An earlier study on alcoholic cirrhotics had demonstrated an exaggerated response to secondary stimulation with tetanus toxoid (Havens, NEJM, 1957; 257:637). The same workers also found antibody concentrations that were three times higher in patients with chronic liver disease than in healthy individuals following a dose of diphtheria toxoid (Havens, JImmunol, 1951; 67:347). A more recent study using a single subcutaneous dose of 14-valent pneumococcal polysaccharide vaccine showed that there were no significant differences in antibody production between patients with alcoholic cirrhosis and a group of healthy controls (Pirovino, Hepatol, 1984; 14:946). In addition, the decline in antibody concentrations following immunization was similar in both groups.

Patients with cirrhosis and alcoholic liver disease are at increased risk of death from pneumococcal infection (Austrian, AnnIntMed, 1964; 60:759; Mufson, ArchIntMed, 1974; 134:505). Immunization with the currently available pneumococcal vaccine is, therefore, recommended for this at-risk group (Swartz, AnnIntMed, 1982; 96: 208). Patients undergoing splenectomy for any reason should also receive pneumococcal vaccine, as well as Hib vaccine, and meningococcal vaccination should be considered for patients travelling to high-risk areas.

Whilst tuberculosis is more common in the alcoholic population, the disease that occurs is usually recrudescence of latent infection and the use of BCG in these patients is probably of little benefit.

References

1. Members of the American College of Chest Physicians/Society of Critical Care Medicine Consensus Conference Committee. American College of Chest Physicians/Society of Critical Care Medicine Consensus Conference: definitions for sepsis and organ failure and guidelines for the use of innovative therapies in sepsis. *Critical Care Medicine*, 1992; **20**: 864–74.
2. Rubin RH, Swartz MH, and Malt R. Hepatic abscess: changes in clinical, bacteriologic and therapeutic aspects. *American Journal of Medicine*, 1974; **57**: 601–10.
3. Miedema BW and Dineen P. The diagnosis and treatment of pyogenic liver abscesses. *Annals of Surgery*, 1984; **200**: 328–35.
4. Perera MR, Kirk A, and Noone P. Presentation, diagnosis and management of liver abscess. *Lancet*, 1980; **ii**: 629–32.
5. Simson IW and Gear JHS. Other viral and infectious diseases. In McSween RN, Anthony PP, and Scheuer PJ, eds. *Pathology of the liver*. 2nd edn. Edinburgh: Churchill Livingstone, 1987.
6. Stain SC, Yellin AE, Donovan AJ, and Brien HW. Pyogenic liver abscess. Modern treatment. *Archives of Surgery*, 1991; **126**: 991–6.

7. McDonald MI, Corey GR, Gallis HA, and Durack DT. Single and multiple pyogenic liver abscesses. Natural history, diagnosis and treatment, with emphasis on percutaneous drainage. *Medicine*, 1984; **63**: 291–302.

8. Sabbaj J, Sutter VL, and Finegold SM. Anaerobic pyogenic liver abscess. *Annals of Internal Medicine*, 1972; **77**: 629–38.

9. Bjornson HS. Biliary tract and hepatic infections. In Finegold SM and George WL, eds. *Anaerobic infections in humans*. London: Academic Press, 1989.

10. Davis JP, Chesney PJ, Wand PJ, and La Venture M. Toxic-shock syndrome: epidemiologic features, recurrence, risk factors and prevention. *New England Journal of Medicine*, 1980; **303**: 1429–35.

11. Ishak KG and Rogers WA. Cryptogenic acute cholangitis–association with toxic shock syndrome. *American Journal of Clinical Pathology*, 1981; **76**: 619–26.

12. Smith LDS. Virulence factors of *Clostridium perfringens*. *Reviews of Infectious Diseases*, 1979; **1**: 254–60.

13. Smith LDS. *The pathogenic anaerobic bacteria*. Illinois: Thomas, 1975.

14. Lamont RJ, Postlethwaite R, and MacGowan AP. *Listeria monocytogenes* and its role in human infection. *Journal of Infection*, 1988; **17**: 7–28.

15. Yu VL, Miller WP, Wing EJ, Romano JM, Ruiz CA, and Bruns FJ. Disseminated listeriosis presenting as acute hepatitis. *American Journal of Medicine*, 1982; **73**: 773–7.

16. Bartlett CLR, Macrae AD, and Macfarlane JT. *Legionella infections*. London: Arnold, 1986: 90–119.

17. Kirby BD, Snyder KM, Meyer RD, and Finegold SM. Legionnaires disease: report of sixty-five nosocomially acquired cases and review of the literature. *Medicine*, 1980; **59**: 188–205.

18. Williams RK and Crossley K. Acute and chronic hepatic involvement of brucellosis. *Gastroenterology*, 1982; **83**: 455–8.

19. Cervantes F, Bruguera M, Carbonell J, Force L, and Webb S. Liver disease in brucellosis. A clinical and pathological study of 40 cases. *Postgraduate Medical Journal*, 1982; **58**: 346–50.

20. Spink WW, Hoffbauer FW, Walker WW, and Green RA. Histopathology of the liver in human brucellosis. *Journal of Laboratory and Clinical Medicine*, 1949; **34**: 40–58.

21. Leelarasamee A and Bovornkitti S. Melioidosis: review and update. *Reviews of Infectious Diseases*, 1989; **11**: 413–25.

22. Ramachandran S, Godfrey JJ, and Perera MVF. Typhoid hepatitis. *Journal of the American Medical Association*, 1974; **230**: 236–40.

23. Khosla SN, Singh R, Singh GP, and Trehan VK. The spectrum of hepatic injury in enteric fever. *American Journal of Gastroenterology*, 1988; **83**: 413–16.

24. Butler T. *Yersinia* species (including plague). In Mandell GL, Douglas RG, and Bennett JE, eds. *Principles and practice of infectious diseases*. 4th edn. New York: Wiley, 1995: 2070–8.

25. Fauci AS and Hoffman GS. Granulomatous hepatitis. In Mandell GL, Douglas RG, and Bennett JE, eds. *Principles and practice of infectious diseases*. 4th edn. New York: Wiley, 1995: 1159–64.

26. Isaacson M. Tularaemia. In Geddes AM, Gilles HM, and Wood MJ, eds. *Medicine international*. Oxford: Medicine Education (International), 1984.

27. Long WA, Ulshen MH, and Lawson EE. Clinical manifestations of congenital syphilitic hepatitis: implications for pathogenesis. *Journal of Pediatric Gastroenterology and Nutrition*, 1984; **3**: 551–5.

28. Plorde JJ. Relapsing fever. In Petersdorf RG, Adams RD, Braunwald E, Isselbacher KJ, Martin JB, and Wilson JD, eds. *Harrison's principles of internal medicine*. 10th edn. London: McGraw-Hill, 1983.

29. Warrell DA. Borrelia infections. In Weatherall DJ, Ledingham JGG, and Warrell DA, eds. *Oxford Textbook of Medicine*. Oxford University Press, 1987.

30. Sawyer LA, Fishbein DB, and McDade JE. Q fever: current concepts. *Reviews of Infectious Diseases*, 1987; **9**: 935–46.

31. Hofmann CE and Heaton JW. Q fever hepatitis. Clinical manifestations and pathological findings. *Gastroenterology*, 1982; **83**: 474–9.

32. Woodward TE. The rickettsioses. In Petersdorf RG, Adams RD, Braunwald E, Isselbacher KJ, Martin JB, and Wilson JD, eds. *Harrison's principles of internal medicine*. 10th edn. London: McGraw-Hill, 1983.

33. Adams JS and Walker DH. The liver in Rocky Mountain spotted fever. *American Journal of Clinical Pathology*, 1981; **75**: 156–61.

34. Walker DH. Rocky mountain spotted fever: a disease in need of microbiological concern. *Clinical Microbiology Reviews*, 1989; **2**: 227–40.

35. Guardia J, *et al.* The liver in boutonneuse fever. *Gut*, 1974; **15**: 549–51.

36. Schacter J and Dawson CR. *Human chlamydial infections*. Massachusetts: Wright-PSG, Littleton, 1978.

37. Grayston JT, Wang SP, Kuo CC, and Campbell LA. Current knowledge on *Chlamydia pneumoniae*, strain TWAR, an important cause of pneumonia and other acute respiratory diseases. *European Journal of Clinical Microbiology and Infectious Disease*, 1989; **8**: 191–202.

38. Warwick WJ. Cat scratch disease. In Braude AI, ed. *Medical microbiology and infectious diseases*. Philadelphia: Saunders, 1981: 1852–6.

39. Cappell MS. Hepatobiliary manifestations of the acquired immune deficiency syndrome. *American Journal of Gastroenterology*, 1991; **86**: 1–15.

40. Guckian J and Perry J. Granulomatous hepatitis. An analysis of 63 cases and review of the literature. *Annals of Internal Medicine*, 1966; **65**: 1081–100.

41. Sartin JS and Walker RC. Granulomatous hepatitis: a retrospective review of 88 cases at the Mayo Clinic. *Mayo Clinic Proceedings*, 1991; **66**: 914–18.

42. Lee RG. Other inflammatory patterns and infectious disorders. In *Diagnostic liver pathology*. St. Louis: Mosby, 1994: 195–236.

43. Essop AR, Posen JA, Hodkinson JH, and Segal I. Tuberculous hepatitis: a clinical review of 96 cases. *Quarterly Journal of Medicine*, 1984; **77**: 465–77.

13.1.2 Leptospirosis

L. Carlos Da Costa Gayotto, Luiz Caetano da Silva, and V. A. Ferreira Alves

Definition

Leptospirosis designates the whole spectrum of disease caused by *Leptospira interrogans*, regardless of its serovar (formerly serotype) or the clinical picture. Previously, various syndromes were described and linked to a specific serovar, such as Weil's disease for icteric leptospirosis caused by the serovar *Icterohaemorrhagiae*. The overlap of clinical syndromes and serovars led to designations such as canicola fever, mud fever, autumn fever, Fort Bragg fever, field fever, seven-day fever, Andaman fever, canine typhus, swineherds' disease, and even Weil's disease.

Leptospirosis is a zoonosis that attacks domestic and wild animals as well as humans and, in this respect, its epidemiology is closely related to environmental and occupational factors. Leptospirosis is endemic all over the world and can become epidemic, for example during floods.

Introduction

Icterohaemorrhagic leptospirosis was first described in 1886 in Heidelberg by Weil, who published the cases of four young males with fever, headache, muscular pain, vomiting, bloody diarrhoea, renal involvement, hepatosplenomegaly, and jaundice. In 1887, Goldschmidt called it Weil's disease.[1] In 1916, Inada *et al.* (JExpMed, 1916; 23:377) identified a spirochaete in the liver of guinea pigs injected with the blood of a miner who had a clinical picture of infectious jaundice. This was considered the aetiological agent of the infection and was called *Spirochaeta icterohaemorrhagiae*. In 1918, Noguchi showed that the micro-organism had more spirals, a different motility in agar, and a higher resistance in 1 per cent saponin solution, and therefore classified it in a new genus, *Leptospira* (from the Greek *lepto* meaning thin and *spira*, spire). The same author observed morphological similarities with *Spirochaeta biflexa*, a saprophyte described in 1914 by Wolbach and Binger (Noguchi, JExpMed, 1918; 27:575). In 1907, Stimson described in the kidney of a patient, presumably who had died of yellow fever, a spirochaete with hooked ends resembling question marks, and for that reason he called it *Spirochaeta interrogans*. It was only in 1940 that Sellards recognized from photographs that this micro-organism was really a leptospire (TrRSocTropMedHyg, 1940; 33:545).

The family Leptospiraceae belongs to the order Spirochaetales and has a single genus, *Leptospira*. Although there are two main species, *L. interrogans* (pathogenic) and *L. biflexa* (saprophytic), others have been described: *L. inadai* (Schmid, JClinMicrobiol, 1986; 24:484), *L. parva*, and *L. illini*;[2] the last corresponds to a new genus *Leptonema*, proposed by Houvind-Hougen (IntJSystBacteriol, 1979; 29:245).

On an immunological basis, *L. interrogans* has been divided into 19 serogroups, and these serogroups into 170 serovars. For *L. biflexa*, 65 serovars distributed in 38 serogroups have been described, whereas there is currently only one serovar for *L. inadai*, one for *L. parva*, and two for *L. illini*.[2] Although the serovar is currently used instead of the species in the designation of leptospires, this should be avoided. Thus, the correct designation should be *L. interrogans* serovar *canicola* and not *L. canicola*. The severity of the clinical picture varies with the serovar of *L. interrogans*, the most common ones are *icterohaemorrhagiae*, *canicola*, *autumnalis*, *hebdomadis*, *australis*, and *pomona*.

The most recent classifications are based on the sequences of the bacterial DNA; a species, according to this classification, is a group of strains whose DNA has 70 per cent or more homology at an ideal temperature of association, or 55 per cent at a temperature of dissociation, with 6 per cent or less non-matched bases. On these grounds, *L. parva* and *L. illini* have been confirmed as species, whereas it has been proposed that *L. interrogans* should be split into five new species and *L. biflexa* into two.[2]

Epidemiology

L. interrogans and its various serovars occur world-wide, in urban as well as rural areas. There is a higher rate of infection in underdeveloped and developing countries and none in the polar areas.[3] In Asia, cases have been reported only in Israel, Sri Lanka, Japan, and South-East Asia. In São Paulo State, Brazil, 239 cases of leptospirosis were reported in 1986, while in the whole of the United States the annual number of cases varied from 40 to 110 between 1974 and 1984 (CDC Annual Summary 1984, MMWR, 1986;33).

High-risk groups are made up chiefly of workers exposed to contaminated water, such as miners, sewer workers, soldiers, and farmers, mainly in rice and sugar-cane plantations. Twelve per cent of sewer workers in Quebec, Canada (De Serres, OccupEnvironMed 1995; 52:505) and 10.4 per cent of Brazilian workers in environmental health (Almeida, RevSaúdePúbl, 1994; 28:76) are seropositive for antileptospira antibodies. Workers who handle animal tissues or fluids are also at risk, for example veterinarians, butchers,

Table 1 Serovars of 159 cases of leptospirosis reported in São Paulo, Brazil, 1986

Serovar	No. of cases (%)
Icterohaemorrhagiae	101 (63.5)
Copenhageni	17 (10.7)
Canicola	15 (9.4)
Andamana	13 (8.2)
Cynopteri	9 (5.7)
Brasiliensis	5 (3.1)
Grippotyphosa	4 (2.5)
Autumnalis	4 (2.5)
Shermani	3 (1.9)
Bataviae	2 (1.3)
Pyrogenes	1 (0.6)
Various	4 (2.5)

fishermen, slaughterhouse workers, and laboratory personnel; exposure to leptospires can also occur during recreational activities.

The serovar *icterohaemorrhagiae* is by far the most common; Correa identified this type in 1935 of 2237 (86.5 per cent) positive cases between 1947 and 1972 (RevInstAdolfoLutz, 1973; 33:55). In 190 of the cases of leptospirosis reported in 1986 in the State of São Paulo, Brazil, 31 had negative serology; in 159 cases the serovars shown in Table 1 were found. In 19 cases the reaction was positive for two serovars.

Prevention and control[3]

The following precautions should be taken.

1. Identification and drainage of contaminated water and soil.
2. Protection of high-risk workers with boots and gloves. Lighting of bonfires before sugar-cane harvesting.
3. Elimination of rodents from houses, especially in rural areas.
4. Isolation of infected domestic animals.
5. Education programmes on the transmission of leptospirosis.
6. Immunization with vaccines prepared against the most common serovars in the country. The immunization of farm and domestic animals prevents disease but not infection and subsequent contamination of urine.
7. During outbreaks, the source of contamination must be sought; proven cases should be notified to health authorities. There is no need for isolation of the patients, concurrent disinfection, quarantine, or immunization of contacts.

Pathogenesis
Lifecycle

There are many hosts of leptospires that can pass on the infection via urine. Mammals (wild or domestic) are the most common hosts and act as reservoirs, can excrete the bacteria, and are a lifetime source of infection. The most important hosts are rodents, although the animal reservoir depends upon geographical distribution and serogroups involved. In some countries, such as the United States, domestic animals are important reservoirs, especially dogs, swine, and cattle.[4] Wild animals, such as skunks, raccoons, mongooses, muskrats, opossums, and nutrias can also harbour the infection.

Besides domestic and wild mammals, birds, especially migratory species, and tortoises may occasionally become carriers capable of transmitting leptospirosis.[5] In Brazil, Hyakutake *et al.* (RevInstMedTropSP, 1976; 18:10) demonstrated that harmless and venomous snakes, the latter of genera *Bothrops* and *Crotallus*, were often reactive in microscopic seroagglutination for the serovar *andamana*. Fish have been infected experimentally; ticks and other arthropods do not seem to be involved in the transmission of leptospirosis.[5]

Infection in animals can be demonstrated by serological means and by identification of the spirochaetes using dark-field examination of urine and kidney emulsions. Culture and inoculation in guinea pigs and hamsters are also effective means. In many species, such as opossum, skunk, raccoon, and fox, infectivity ratios range from 10 to 50 per cent.[1] Seventy-eight per cent of rats captured in Curitiba, in the southern region of Brazil, were shown to be infected with leptospires.[5]

When contaminated urine is discharged, some environmental conditions favour the survival of leptospires, the most important being stagnant water. Other factors include humid soil, neutral or slightly alkaline pH, and temperatures around 30°C. Humans are infected when there is contact of contaminated soil and/or water with abraded skin or mucosal surfaces, mainly of the digestive tract; it is unlikely that leptospires can penetrate intact skin.[1] Under special conditions, infection can be transmitted through the bite of domestic or wild animals, especially dogs and rats. The teeth of these animals are contaminated by biting other infected animals or, if they are already infected, by licking their own genitals.

Susceptibility is the same for both sexes. In Brazil, 90 per cent of patients are males, obviously due to occupational risk. Ninety per cent were between 10 and 50 years of age.

There is a marked variation in the incubation period: the usual range is 7 to 13 days, with an average of 10 days. However, after immersion, or accidental laboratory exposure, extremes of 2 to 26 days have been reported.[1] In the lifecycle of leptospires, man is an occasional host and very seldom acts as a source of infection.

Pathology

Leptospirosis has an early septicaemic phase in which spirochaetes can be found by silver impregnation or immunohistochemistry in the central nervous system, muscles, spleen, kidney, and liver, without any apparent cellular reaction. During the localization phase, kidney and liver are the most affected organs, but there is widespread vascular damage involving the skin, vascular lesions contributing with an erythematous hue to the jaundice. In the lungs, increased vascular permeability leads to alveolar and bronchiolar haemorrhage; excess fluid is rapidly reabsorbed, as shown by radiological monitoring of the patient.

In the digestive tract, increased vascular permeability leads to formation of petechiae and diffuse haemorrhage, especially of the mucous membranes of the stomach and small bowel; this may cause hypovolaemia, shock, impaired renal function, and eventually death. Hypovolaemia also aggravates the renal lesions; the disease produces the most severe damage in the kidneys. In the majority of autopsies of leptospirosis, there is focal myocarditis with oedema and mononuclear aggregates composed of prominent histiocytes. These aggregates occur mainly around the thinnest branches of the coronary arteries (De Brito, AnnTropMed, 1987; 81:207). Similar alterations are found in the leptomeninges and striated muscle, in which large mononuclear cells form aggregates. In muscle, they surround foci of hyaline necrosis, involving single fibres, where leptospiral antigens can be demonstrated by immunohistochemistry.

Kidney lesions

The pattern of renal injury is non-specific and is proportional to the severity of the disease. There are generally scattered areas of involvement, and within severely damaged areas, preserved nephrons can be seen. In the swollen interstitium, there are foci of an inflammatory infiltrate composed mainly of mononuclear leucocytes, especially histiocytes. There is a preferential periglomerular and perivenular distribution of the lesions. Haemorrhage is also focal and vascular damage is due mainly to swollen endothelial cells.

Glomeruli, however, are usually well preserved, although some slight focal alterations have been described, including mesangial hyperplasia and swelling of endothelial cells. Electron microscopy shows fusion of the foot processes.[6] The main targets of leptospirosis in the kidney are the convoluted tubules and Henle's loop. Several degrees of cellular damage are seen, from cloudy swelling to overt tubular necrosis. There is tubular dilatation, flattening of the epithelium, and disruption of the tubular architecture. Within the lumen of dilated tubules, there are casts of coagulated protein, bile, and haemoglobin or myoglobin. Histochemical studies show a considerable decrease in enzymatic activity of succinic dehydrogenase and of phosphatases (acid and alkaline). Under electron microscopy, mitochondria show alterations in size, crista, and matrix, reduction of the ribonucleoprotein granules, irregular dilatation of the cisternas of both the smooth endoplasmic reticulum and Golgi complex, and alteration of the brush border with reduction and distortion of the microvilli.[6] The collecting tubules are seldom affected and the degree of the inflammatory infiltrate is proportional to tubular damage.

Leptospires can be seen in the renal tissue by the silver impregnation technique of Whartin and Starry or, more specifically, through immunohistochemistry, either at autopsy or in renal biopsies.[7] Leptospiral antigens are found throughout the renal parenchyma, from the interstitium to the luminal border of endothelial and tubular epithelial cells, and in the cytoplasm of a few macrophages; however, they are not detected in the glomeruli. In the most severe forms a 'total antigen' as well as a glycolipoprotein fraction are found adhered to cell membranes (Alves, ExpPath, 1991; 42: 81).

Microperfusion studies in the guinea pig have shown tubular changes leading to potassium secretion probably due to a decrease in proximal tubule reabsorption; the inability to concentrate urine could result, at least partially, from the resistance of the inner medullary collecting duct to vasopressin (Magaldi, Nephron, 1992; 62:332).

Younes *et al.* (CRAcadSci, 1995; 318:619) have identified the glycoprotein fraction of an endotoxin capable of inhibiting Na^+, K^+-ATPase activity in tubular epithelium of rabbit kidney. Although claimed as one of the possible mechanisms of acute renal failure, rhabdomyolysis was not correlated with the severity of disease in the Brazilian patients studied by Martinelli *et al.* (RevInstMedTropSP, 1994; 36:111).

Liver lesions

In leptospirosis the liver is enlarged, with congestion and a mottled green appearance due to cholestasis. Light microscopic alterations are less striking than in the kidney, and often disproportionate to the severity of the clinical picture. The lobular architecture and the limiting plate are always preserved; the main cellular alterations are found in zone III of the Rappaport acinus. Liver cells are either swollen or shrunken and Councilman acidophilic bodies are seen. An outstanding feature of leptospirosis in the liver is the mitotic activity of hepatocytes, a rare finding in normal liver and in other liver diseases.[8] Regeneration, however, is moderate, as evidenced by twin liver-cell plates. Cholestasis is prominent in human specimens, and bile pigment is found as granules in the cytoplasm of swollen liver-cells, as plugs in slightly dilated canaliculi, and in Kupffer cells. These are usually hypertrophied and hyperplastic throughout the lobule and may show erythrophagocytosis and scanty haemosiderin. In portal tracts, oedema is mild or moderate; the inflammatory infiltrate is composed mainly of lymphocytes and histiocytes but a few polymorphonuclear eosinophils are also seen. In autopsy studies, a common finding is disarray of liver-cell plates with loss of cohesion between hepatocytes. This feature is seldom seen in biopsy specimens, and has been explained as a consequence of severe damage, of a terminal change, or even as an artefact due to autolysis (Popper, ArchPathol, 1948; 46:132). More recent evidence, however, suggests that these phenomena are genuine and due to the presence of leptospires or products of their lysis in liver tissue (Fig. 1).[7]

From the histochemical point of view, no significant alterations were found when the activity of some enzymes such as succinodehydrogenase and cytochrome-oxidase was measured, while alkaline phosphatase activity was increased in liver cells, and acid phosphatase in Kupffer cells.[8] Under electron microscopy, liver cell changes are irregularly distributed, and more intense in severe cases. They are not specific and are similar to those found in viral hepatitis. Granules and filaments were described within swollen mitochondria and De Brito et al.[8] reported alterations and sometimes disappearance of the microvilli of the sinusoidal wall. In the canaliculi, the alterations of the microvilli do not differ from those usually found in extra- and intrahepatic cholestasis.

In 1917, Kaneko and Okuda, using the Levaditi method, could identify leptospires in liver tissue of 23 out of 43 autopsy cases (JExpMed, 1917; 26:325). With the Whartin and Starry method, which also utilizes silver impregnation (for embedded material), leptospires are seen less frequently in human leptospirosis.

An immunohistochemical technique developed by Alves et al. has identified leptospire antigens in all samples of liver tissue obtained from nine autopsies and six biopsies.[7] Leptospires could be demonstrated in the extracellular space of periportal areas, within the sinusoids and portal venous branches, as well as in Kupffer cells and portal histiocytes. The presence of the antigen in Kupffer cells was associated with the resolution of the clinical picture.

Alves et al. (ExpToxPath, 1992; 44:425) have elucidated the pattern of distribution of leptospires and their antigens along the course of the experimental infection of guinea pigs. Intact leptospires are initially found in the portal tracts; in the most severe lesions, granules that probably result from inefficient phagocytosis, together with granular glycolipoprotein antigens, are seen in centrilobular areas. These granular factors could exert a cytotoxic effect

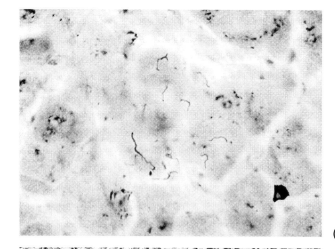

(a)

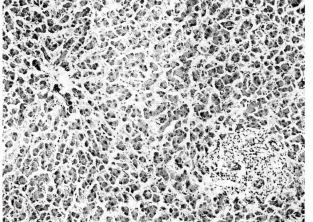

(b)

Fig. 1. Autopsy case of human leptospirosis. (a) The leptospiral antigen is attached to the cytoplasmic membranes of liver cells. In portal tracts it is seen in the interstitium and in histiocytes (immunoperoxidase); (b) lobular structure conserved, hepatocyte plates interrupted, mild cellular infiltration of the portal tracts, and numerous binucleated cells (haematoxylin and eosin × 100).

on endothelial and liver-cell membranes, further leading to the final disarray of liver-cell plates.

Experimental models

Experimental models have contributed to a deeper knowledge of the pathology and pathogenesis of leptospirosis. Studies in humans *in vivo* are limited, since liver biopsies are obtained only when there is diagnostic doubt, and provided that the haemorrhagic phase has subsided. Therefore, most information available comes from autopsy material.

The choice of an animal model may influence the pathological alterations, as these depend on the serovar of *L. interrogans* and the nature of the host species. The severity of the disease appears to increase with the position of the animal in the phylogenetic scale. The pattern of the infections varies with different animal groups. Rodents, especially mice and rats, the most important reservoirs of leptospires, constitute a group of animals without overt disease. Animals with subclinical disease form a second group, including swine and felines. A third group is formed by canines and cattle, in which there is an acute septic form very similar to that found in humans. Finally, in horses the infection can become chronic.[9]

In animals such as the rabbit, inoculation causes a rapid production of protecting antibodies which prevent the clinical picture. This allows production of antibodies for immunological studies. The guinea pig is undoubtedly the best experimental model for the study of leptospirosis, especially if weanling animals are used. Several inoculation routes are effective, such as intraperitoneal, intradermic and subcutaneous, intracardiac, and intraocular. The digestive route is much less effective and intracerebral inoculation is completely ineffective (Stavitsky, JInfDis, 1945; 76:179).

The virulence of *L. interrogans* serovar *icterohaemorrhagiae* can be increased by repeated passages in guinea pigs, and eventually the clinical and pathological picture presented by the animal can mimic very closely the human pattern, with fever, jaundice, haemorrhage, and renal failure. The animals die from the fifth to the seventh day after inoculation.

Clinical aspects and complications

Most natural infections appear 7 to 13 days after exposure. The clinical picture is protean, and the severity of illness varies widely. At one extreme, leptospirosis is asymptomatic; at the other, it is a severe illness characterized by jaundice, renal failure, and haemorrhage, known as Weil's disease. Many anicteric infections go undetected, although there is increasing recognition of mild forms of the disease.[4]

Anicteric leptospirosis

This benign form is the most common presentation; it is usually characterized by a biphasic course accompanied by a biphasic temperature curve. During the first phase, leptospires are present in the blood or cerebrospinal fluid. This phase lasts from 4 to 7 days and is characterized by fever, headache, muscular pain or tenderness, meningism, conjunctival suffusion, nausea, vomiting, anorexia, and severe prostration. Fever is constant, usually above 38°C, sometimes up to 40°C, and is frequently accompanied by rigors or a chilly sensation. Symptoms, particularly fever, have an abrupt onset so that the patient often can identify precisely when the illness started. Headache is severe and generalized, and signs of meningeal involvement may be observed. In the presence of headache, high fever, and neck stiffness, suggesting meningitis, an acellular spinal fluid in the first 5 to 7 days points towards a diagnosis of leptospirosis. Nevertheless, leptospires can be cultured from the cerebrospinal fluid, in which a scanty mixed cellular infiltrate may sometimes be detected.

Muscle pain, a hallmark of leptospirosis, is localized mainly in the calves. The severity of myalgia may even prevent the patient from standing. Muscular lesions are responsible for a striking increase of serum creatine phosphokinase, a valuable biochemical clue to the disease (Johnson, JAMA, 1975; 233:981). Conjunctival suffusion, a characteristic physical sign, usually appears on the third or fourth day of illness. In about 70 per cent of patients with mild disease, abnormalities of the urinary sediment, characterized by proteinuria, pyuria, or haematuria, are observed (Berman, AnnIntMed, 1973; 79:167).

Table 2 Clinical features of Weil's disease and viral hepatitis

	Weil's disease	Viral hepatitis
Onset	Sudden	Variable
Fever	Constant	Variable
Headache	Constant	Occasional
Muscle pain	Severe	Mild
Conjunctival injection	Present	Absent
Concomitant jaundice and renal failure	Frequent	Rare
Prostration	Severe	Mild
Early haemorrhagic diathesis	Common	Rare
Serum aminotransferase elevation	Slight or moderate	Intense
Serum creatine phosphokinase	Elevated	Usually normal
Leucocyte count	Normal or elevated neutrophilia	Lymphocytosis

Based on Sherlock S. *Diseases of the liver and biliary system.* 8th edn. Oxford: Blackwell, 1989, with permission.

The second phase generally appears after a relatively asymptomatic interval of 1 to 3 days. This phase is called the 'immune phase' or period of localization because of the appearance of serum antibodies. Leptospires disappear from the blood but can then be cultured in urine. This phase is characterized by marked variability of the clinical picture, in contrast with the more uniform pattern of the first stage. It lasts from 2 to 4 days in most patients and is characterized by lower fever, less severe myalgia, and milder gastrointestinal symptoms. However, meningitis and iridocyclitis are more common in this phase. Meningitis seems to be the expression of an antigen–antibody reaction rather than of direct injury to the meninges by leptospires.[10]

Sometimes fever and pains recur after the end of the immune phase, between the second and fourth weeks. The pathogenesis of this phase, called the convalescent phase by some clinicians, is not understood.

Icteric leptospirosis

Severe leptospirosis, or Weil's disease, is characterized by jaundice, usually associated with renal damage, changes in haemostasis, anaemia, and neurological disturbances. The onset of this disease is identical to that of milder forms of anicteric leptospirosis. The distinctive features of this form are jaundice and renal failure, which make their appearance on the second or third day of the illness, but generally do not reach a peak until the second week.[11] Serum bilirubin levels may exceed 1000 mmol/l (60 mg/dl), but in two-thirds of patients the levels are less than 330 mmol/l (20 mg/dl) with predominance of the conjugated fraction;[4] high levels of bilirubin are usually seen when there is concomitant renal failure. The duration of jaundice varies from a few days to several weeks. During the immune phase, a deepening jaundice with increasing renal and myocardial damage is observed.

In some patients, differentiation from viral hepatitis may be difficult. Table 2 compares the main features in both diseases.

Signs of renal involvement can appear simultaneously with jaundice, are important for an early diagnosis, and point toward a poor prognosis. In some patients, the renal insufficiency is due to prerenal factors and responds well to fluid administration. Others, however, have features of acute tubular necrosis; death can result from acute renal failure but rarely, if ever, from acute liver failure.

Myocardial involvement begins usually in the septicaemic phase of the disease and is not uncommon. The clinical expression may vary from isolated electrocardiographic changes to heart failure and severe arrhythmias. Acute coronary arteritis is a frequent lesion, and its presence correlates significantly with myocarditis and inflammation of the conductive system, thus being a significant part of the leptospiral cardiomyopathy (De Brito, AnnTropMed, 1987; 81:207). Heart involvement may be severe enough to cause death in some patients with leptospirosis. Pulmonary manifestations, usually cough or chest pain are relatively common but not very prominent. Radiology of the thorax may show pulmonary infiltrates or a picture of interstitial pneumonia.

The demarcation between stages in Weil's disease is rarely as clear-cut as in the anicteric form of leptospirosis.[10] Thus, jaundice may appear from the second to the ninth day and leptospires can be isolated from the blood of patients who had been icteric for 24 to 48 h (Hall, AnnIntMed, 1951; 35:981). These data show that jaundice is not a reliable index in determining the phase of the illness. The early appearance of some features of Weil's disease, particularly jaundice and renal damage, would suggest that they are related to leptospiraemia rather than to immunity.

The main bleeding manifestations of this syndrome are gastro-intestinal haemorrhage, epistaxis, and petechiae or ecchymosis. Haemorrhage correlates with the severity of the disease and seems to be due mainly to a diffuse vasculitis. Thrombocytopenia is often observed in the course of severe leptospirosis, but is not related to the presence of platelet-associated antibodies or to disseminated intravascular coagulation. The role played by thrombocytopenia in haemorrhagic phenomena in Weil's disease is not well established. Interestingly, thrombocytopenia tends to be more frequent in patients with high serum urea levels and in such cases the incidence of haemorrhage is significantly higher.

The frequency of Weil's disease has been reported to vary widely; some authors report 1 to 10 per cent,[1,10] others up to 90 per cent of cases of leptospirosis (Hinrichsen, Thesis, Univ. Fed. Pernambuco, 1987). These discrepancies can be attributed to factors such as serovar, cause of admission to hospital, time, and accuracy of the diagnosis. Serovar *icterohaemorrhagiae* accounts for 40 to 90 per cent of cases of this disease. Infection by the serovars *icterohaemorrhagiae* and *canicola* is often associated with more severe forms.[4] However, other serovars can also be responsible for Weil's disease.

Laboratory findings

Leucocyte counts are either normal or may be slightly elevated (up to 15 000/mm^3), usually due to neutrophilia. Striking leucocytosis (more than 15 000/mm^3) may be present in patients with liver involvement. Leucopenia is rarely found. In prolonged leptospirosis, anaemia is common, due mainly to blood loss secondary to disturbed coagulation or angiopathy. The erythrocyte sedimentation rate is elevated.

Early in the illness, 80 per cent of patients have abnormal urine findings, such as microscopic haematuria, pyuria, proteinuria, and sometimes casts. In anicteric infections these abnormalities disappear after the first week, but in the icteric cases they are more pronounced and azotaemia may be observed. Blood urea and creatinine are elevated in about 90 per cent of cases; serum potassium is usually normal or even decreased.

Coagulation studies may show a prolonged prothrombin time, but this test is frequently normal. Thrombocytopenia is often seen in the course of severe leptospirosis, which is most probably one of the factors leading to respiratory distress in a few patients.[14]

The serum enzyme pattern is characterized by a slight to moderate increase of aminotransferases (5 to 10 times the upper reference limit). A sharp increase of creatine phosphokinase is observed in about 50 per cent of patients; as this is not seen in viral hepatitis, it is useful for the differential diagnosis. γ-Glutamyl transferase is increased up to 10 times and alkaline phosphatase up to 3 times the upper reference limits.

Diagnosis

Early diagnosis of leptospirosis is important because appropriate intensive care is lifesaving in severe cases; specific antimicrobial therapy is probably effective only if started within 2 to 4 days from the onset of illness. The diagnosis should be suspected on the basis of the clinical features discussed above.

In view of the recognition of renal and lung involvement in infections due to Hantavirus,[12] this viral infection must be considered in the differential diagnosis of either renal or lung syndromes presumably due to leptospiral infections. Hantavirus infection presents similar epidemiological conditions as leptospirosis, and outbreaks of this infection have been reported from the United States[12] as well as from Brazil (Iversson, RevAssMedBras, 1994; 40:85). Groen (EpidInf, 1995; 114:373) found Hantavirus-specific antibodies in 1 per cent of Dutch patients suspected of having acute leptospirosis and in 10 per cent of patients with 'acute nephropathy'.

Leptospires can be isolated during the first phase from the cerebrospinal fluid and blood, and in the second phase from urine. Dark-field examination of urine or plasma has been employed for direct identification of leptospirosis, although the method demands a skilled professional; even so, filaments of fibrin and other artefacts can lead to a high rate of false-positive cases (Smith, AmJClinPath, 1979; 72:459).

For blood culture, a liquid (Stuart's) or semisolid (Fletcher's) medium can be used. Culture of leptospires has proven useful in French Polynesia (Jeandel, BullSocPath, 1982; 75:367); however, in Brazil the positivity rate is low.

Animal inoculation is also effective when leptospirosis is suspected. A guinea pig should be inoculated intraperitoneally with 3 ml of oxalated blood. When the rectal temperature reaches 39°C, or on the 15th day, the animal should be sacrificed and fragments of liver and kidney taken for: (i) direct examination of leptospires in dark field, (ii) culture in Fletcher's medium, (iii) imbedding in paraffin for identification of leptospires by the Whartin–Starry method, and (d) reinoculation in young guinea pigs.

In the second phase, serological methods are valuable. Agglutination tests are divided into microscopic and macroscopic. The former are more complex, can give information about the serovar, and are more effective when frequent determinations show a rise in the agglutinin titres. This test can be applied to cerebrospinal fluid, and pleural and synovial exudates.

Macroscopical agglutination or slide test is a more practical test for screening but can give false-negative results and is not serogroup specific. For both agglutination tests it is worth comparing early with convalescent serum samples.

Other serological tests include passive haemagglutination, indirect immunofluorescence, and more recently, an enzyme-linked immunosorbent assay (**ELISA**). Passive haemagglutination, employing sheep red blood cells sensitized with a polysaccharide antigen of serovar *patoc*, was shown to be very useful for the early diagnosis of acute human leptospirosis (Ribeiro, RevInst-AdolfoLutz, 1981; 41:135).

Silva *et al.*[13] developed specific ELISA tests for IgM, IgG, and IgA antibodies in human leptospirosis. IgM antibodies were detected starting on day 2 of symptoms. IgA antibodies were found in some patients on day 5 and in all patients on day 15, persisting up to the 9th month. The authors claim that an anti-IgA ELISA is of value in seroprevalence studies.

Early diagnosis of leptospirosis can also benefit from the recent development of polymerase chain reaction assays, either on urine (Bal, JClinMicrobiol, 1994; 32:1894) or on blood samples (Merien, JInfDis, 1995; 172:281)

Treatment and prognosis

Data concerning the efficacy of antibiotics in human beings are conflicting. Antibiotics such as penicillin and chloramphenicol do not seem to influence the outcome. A favourable response from antibiotics is obtained only if they are used at the very beginning of the disease, during the leptospiraemic phase. Penicillin treatment may result in a Jarish–Hersheimer reaction with a sharp rise in temperature, myalgia, headache, and malaise a few hours after onset of therapy (Winearls, QJMed, 1984; 53:487).

In a randomized, double-blind, controlled trial, doxycycline, in an oral dose of 100 mg twice a day for 7 days, was shown to be effective when begun early in anicteric leptospirosis. Doxycycline reduced the duration of illness by 2 days and favourably affected fever, malaise, headache, and myalgias. Treatment prevented leptospiruria and had no adverse effects (McClain, AnnIntMed, 1984; 100:696). However, the effectiveness of doxycycline or other antibiotics in modifying the illness in patients with Weil's disease is unknown.

Doxycycline is also an efficient chemoprophylatic agent against leptospirosis. This antibiotic, when administered orally on a weekly basis, decreased the attack rate of the infection significantly among American soldiers in Panama (Takafuji, NEJM, 1984; 310:497).

Prognosis is closely related to the presence of jaundice, advanced age, and the coexistence of unrelated disease, such as hepatic cirrhosis, cardiovascular disease, and diabetes mellitus. In the experience of Heath *et al.* no death occurred in the absence of jaundice,

whereas the mortality among patients with jaundice was 17 per cent.[4]

The usual pattern of renal failure in leptospirosis is similar to that of acute tubular necrosis, namely acute oliguric or non-oliguric renal failure followed by gradual return of renal function over 2 to 3 weeks, with a polyuric phase heralding recovery. As a result of improved management of acute renal failure (the principal cause of death), mortality has been lowered. Thus, in 1978 the mortality from Weil's disease was only 5 per cent compared with 15 to 40 per cent in the previous decade.[11]

Patients with the severe forms of leptospirosis who survive have an excellent prognosis with complete recovery and without sequelae. Some patients can continue to harbour the spirochaetes and eliminate them in the urine, thus acting as a reservoir of leptospires.

References

1. Sanford JP. Leptospirosis. In Schiff L and Schiff ER, eds. *Diseases of the liver*. Philadelphia: JB Lippincott Co., 1987: 1197–202.
2. Yasuda PH, Steigerwalt AG, Sulzer KR, Kaufmann AF, Rogers F, and Brenner DJ. Deoxyribonucleic acid relatedness between serogroups and serovars in the family Leptospiraceae, with proposals for seven new Leptospira species. *International Journal of Systematic Bacteriology*, 1987; **37**: 407–15.
3. Benenson AS, ed. *El control de las enfermedades transmisibles en el hombre*. Washington: PAHO and WHO, 1983: 258–61.
4. Heath CW Jr, Alexander AD, and Galton MM. Leptospirosis in the United States. Analysis of 483 cases in man, 1949–1961. *New England Journal of Medicine*, 1965; **273**: 915–22.
5. Corrêa MOA, Veronesi R, De Brito T, Hyakutake S, Santa Rosa CA, and Edelweiss EL. Leptospirose. In Veronesi R, ed. *Doenças infecciosas e parasitárias*. Rio de Janeiro: Editora Guanabara Koogan SA, 1982: 573–92.
6. De Brito T, Penna DO, Pereira VG, and Hoshino S. Kidney biopsies in human leptospirosis: a biochemical and electron microscopy study. *Virchows Archiv für Pathologische Anatomie und für Klinisches Medizin*, 1967; **343**: 124–35.
7. Alves VAF, Vianna MR, Yasuda PH, and De Brito T. Detection of leptospiral antigen in the human liver and kidney using an immunoperoxidase staining procedure. *Journal of Pathology*, 1987; **151**: 125–31.
8. De Brito T, Machado MM, Montans SD, Hoshino S, and Freymuller E. Liver biopsy in human leptospirosis: a light and electron microscopy study. *Virchows Archiv für Pathologische Anatomie und für Klinisches Medizin*, 1967; **342**: 61–9.
9. Gsell O. Epidemiology of the leptospiroses. In *Symposium on Leptospiroses*. Medical Science Publication No. 1, Washington: US Government Printing Office, 1953: 34–56.
10. Edwards GA and Domm BM. Human leptospirosis. *Medicine*, 1960; **39**: 117–56.
11. Jacobs R. Leptospirosis—Medical Staff Conference. University of California, San Francisco. *Western Journal of Medicine*, 1980; **132**: 440–50.
12. Zaki SR *et al.* Hantavirus pulmonary syndrome—pathogenesis of an emerging infectious disease. *American Journal of Pathology*, 1995; **146**: 552–79.
13. Silva MV *et al.* Behaviour of specific IgM, IgG and IgA class antibodies in human leptospirosis during acute phase of the disease and during convalescence. *Journal of Tropical Medicine and Hygiene*, 1995; **98**: 268–72.
14. Nicodemo AC, Duarte MIS, Alves VAF, Takakura CFH, Santos RTM, and Nicodemo EL. *American Journal of Tropical Medicine and Hygiene*, 1997; **56**: 181–7.

13.2 Fungal infections affecting the liver

R. J. Hay

The human fungal infections include a number of common diseases, such as ringworm or dermatophyte infections, superficial candidosis, and pityriasis versicolor, that are confined to epithelial surfaces, as well as deep or systemic infections that may involve internal organs including the liver. Pathogenic fungi are relatively large micro-organisms that range in size from 2 to 250 µm in diameter. There are two morphologically distinct pathogenic forms, known as yeasts and moulds. The yeast fungi, which include organisms such as *Cryptococcus*, multiply by budding and are usually intracellular parasites. Mould fungi such as *Aspergillus* spp. form long chains of cells, hyphae, which are not easily engulfed by a single macrophage. Some fungi, such as *Histoplasma capsulatum*, are dimorphic, existing in either yeast or hyphal form at different phases of their lifecycle.

The liver becomes a target for infection in certain systemic fungal infections for several reasons. First, fungi of the appropriate size, such as *H. capsulatum*, are taken up by reticuloendothelial cells. Secondly, because of the volume of blood flow through the liver, fungi disseminated through the bloodstream commonly involve this organ. Thirdly, certain fungi, notably *Candida albicans* and *C. tropicalis*, are thought to penetrate the gastrointestinal mucosa in severely ill, neutropenic patients and spread directly to the liver via the portal vein before invading other organs. Despite this, the liver is not commonly reported as a site of fungal infection. In many cases this may be a simple oversight due to lack of confirmatory autopsy and pathological support. It also probably reflects the fact that symptoms due to invasion of other sites such as the central nervous system or lung may dominate the clinical picture. The mycoses most frequently associated with invasion of the liver are shown in Table 1. They include the systemic fungal infections histoplasmosis, coccidioidomycosis and paracoccidioidomycosis, and less frequently blastomycosis. One recently described infection seen mainly in patients with the acquired immune deficiency syndrome (**AIDS**) in South-East Asia, penicillinosis due to *Penicillium marneffei*, may also affect the liver. Of the opportunistic fungal pathogens, both *Aspergillus* and *Cryptococcus* may spread to this site, but liver infection is more often seen in disseminated candidosis as well as rarer diseases such as trichosporonosis.

The other important way in which fungi may cause damage to hepatocytes is via mycotoxicosis produced by ingestion of fungal toxins. Many of the aflatoxins produced by a range of environmental fungi such as *Aspergillus* spp. may cause hepatic necrosis or cirrhosis.

Other mycotoxins, such as patulin and ochratoxin A, affect the liver in laboratory animals, although the contribution made by these substances to human disease is largely unproven. There is no evidence that fungi which cause invasive disease produce mycotoxins *in vivo*.

Candidosis

Definition

Infections caused by fungi of the genus *Candida*, known as candidosis or candidiasis, may be either superficial or systemic.[1] Liver involvement follows dissemination via the circulation, either after direct introduction of the organisms through a contaminated intravenous line or intravenous injection in a drug abuser, or after invasion via the gastrointestinal tract. While hepatic infection may pass virtually unrecognized amongst the other manifestations of fulminant systemic candidosis, in certain patients *Candida* infection of the liver and spleen produces a characteristic syndrome called hepatosplenic candidosis (chronic disseminated candidosis).

Introduction

Although superficial infection by *Candida* has been recognized for centuries, the more serious systemic forms of the disease have only been diagnosed since the latter part of the nineteenth century. It is only in the last 30 years that systemic *Candida* infections have become a relatively frequent occurrence in certain groups such as neutropenic cancer or postoperative patients. Infection of the liver

---

Table 1 Liver involvement has been reported in the following deep fungal infections

Opportunistic mycoses
Candidosis—includes hepatosplenic candidosis
Cryptococcosis
Less common: aspergillosis, mucormycosis, trichosporonosis

Pathogenic mycoses
Histoplasmosis—disseminated (classical) histoplasmosis
Paracoccidioidomycosis
Less common: coccidioidomycosis, African histoplasmosis, blastomycosis, penicillinosis

Table 2 Factors predisposing to candidosis

Infancy, pregnancy, old age
Immunological defects
Neutropenia (primary or secondary to therapy or disease)
T-lymphocyte defects (primary or secondary to disease such
   as AIDS, lymphoma)
Endocrine disease, e.g. diabetes mellitus
Therapy, e.g. contraceptive pill, antibiotics
Nutritional, e.g. zinc, iron deficiency
Abnormal surfaces: epithelial, foreign surfaces
Miscellaneous, e.g. intravenous drug abuse

has been a consistent finding in many autopsy surveys of systemic candidosis.

Epidemiology

Candidosis has a world-wide distribution.[1] The most common species that causes human infection is *Candida albicans*, although others such as *C. tropicalis*, *C. parapsilosis*, and *C. (Torulopsis) glabrata* may also be implicated. There do not appear to be great differences in the epidemiology and manifestations of disease caused by each of these species, although *C. tropicalis* is a more common cause of infection in neutropenic patients in the United States than in Europe. *Candida krusei is* usually resistant to the antifungal drug fluconazole.

Candida spp. are common commensal organisms, being carried by a significant proportion of the healthy population in the mouth (25 per cent), gastrointestinal tract (16 per cent), and vagina (22 per cent). The organisms become pathogenic under appropriate conditions, a change often associated with the development of hyphae. These conditions range from abnormalities of epithelial surfaces to physiological changes, endocrine or metabolic disease, and primary or secondary immunodeficiency states. These are shown in Table 2.

Pathogenesis and pathology

Candida causes disease by invasion of tissue. There are various potential routes of systemic invasion. The organisms may be directly introduced into the bloodstream by injection, a form of disease seen in intravenous drug addicts, in whom fungi cause infection of the eyes, hair follicles, and bones. *Candida* may also gain entry via an intravenous drip site by contamination of intravenous fluids or the skin. A major route of entry in neutropenic patients is via the gastrointestinal (probably jejunal) mucosa. This may follow invasion of the mucosa, or a process known as persorption where particles such as *Candida* cells rapidly cross an intact mucosal wall. This is based on evidence in man that non-pathogenic yeasts can appear rapidly in the bloodstream after oral administration, and in neonatal mice transfer of yeasts from the bowel lumen to the circulation appears to occur in the jejunum.

In tissue *C. albicans* is normally found in both yeast and hyphal forms in small abscesses and there are usually many organisms present. However, in patients with hepatosplenic candidosis, where the infection may persist for weeks despite a return of white-cell counts to the normal range, few organisms are seen in the later stages of infection and the tissue response may be granulomatous or mixed, with granulomas surrounding neutrophil abscesses. Hyphae are seldom produced in tissues by *Candida* spp. other than *C. albicans*.

Clinical features and complications

Systemic candidosis usually has few clinical features that can be used to separate it from other septicaemic illnesses in severely ill patients. Patients present with pyrexia, usually after abdominal surgery or during neutropenia. Occasionally there are helpful signs that may give a clue to the diagnosis, such as the appearance of multiple skin nodules, muscle pains, or retinal deposits. However, generally none of these is specific and the aetiological background has to be confirmed. The liver may be enlarged in such cases but this is very variable. Hepatic lesions are usually found incidentally at autopsy. A number of risk factors have been associated with fungal liver infection in bone-marrow transplant recipients. These include deep fungal infection after transplantation, colonization or superficial fungal infection after transplantation, and severe liver dysfunction through veno-occlusive disease or graft-versus-host disease (Rossetti, ClinInfDis, 1995; 20:801).

Hepatosplenic candidosis

In recent years, increasing numbers of patients have been described with a syndrome whose principal feature is *Candida* infection of the liver and spleen (Bodey, Cancer, 1969; 24:417). The main characteristics of these patients were reviewed by Odds (Table 3).[1] Most have leukaemia and have had a prolonged episode of neutropenia. The infection is most often caused by *C. albicans*. Unlike other forms of candidosis the signs may appear after the patient appears to be in remission from the primary disease. The main clinical features are high, swinging pyrexia and chills, with right upper abdominal pain. Appetite is poor and patients show a variable degree of malaise. Progress is variable, but in untreated patients the infection persists over weeks. It is also notoriously resistant to therapy (Baztley, PediatInfectDis, 1982; Miller, Radiol, 1982; 142: 373; Tashjian, RevInfDis, 1984; 6:689; Linker, MedPediatOncol, 1989; 12:380; 1:317). The names hepatosplenic or chronic disseminated candidiasis have been used for this syndrome.

Diagnosis and differential diagnosis

Systemic candidosis may be difficult to diagnose, particularly in the immunocompromised patient. Blood cultures should be set up and repeated if necessary; cultures of intravenous-line tips may also be helpful. Blood cultures are positive in a high proportion of patients after surgery but in less than 20 per cent of those with neutropenia. Other methods of diagnosis include serology, which is often only available in specialized centres. There are a few commercial kits available for the detection of *Candida* antibodies or antigen. Both investigations may be contributory but should not be regarded as diagnostic, particularly in the absence of any other evidence of *Candida* infection. The most reliable method of diagnosis is by biopsy and histopathological examination of appropriate lesions such as skin nodules. Percutaneous liver biopsy has not been widely used, except in hepatosplenic candidosis, where it is the definitive method of diagnosis (Miller, Radiol, 1982; 142:373).

Table 3 Clinical and pathological features of hepatosplenic candidosis

Feature	Details	Percentage with feature
Sex distribution	Male:female	45.2:54.8
Age distribution (years)	<1	0
	1–9	25.0
	10–29	25.0
	30–49	34.1
	50–69	13.6
	>70	2.3
Underlying diseases	Acute leukaemia	86.3
	Aplastic anaemia	5.9
	Other	7.8
Diagnostic features	Fever	100.0
	Upper quadrant abdominal pain	96.3
	Raised alkaline phosphatase	100.0
	Blood leucocytosis	81.0
	CT scan abnormalities	93.8
	Ultrasound abnormalities	66.7
Sites affected	Liver alone	23.5
	Spleen alone	13.7
	Both liver and spleen	62.7
Causative organism	*Candida albicans*	88.2
	C. tropicalis	5.9
Outcome	Patient died	43.2

(Data taken from Table 22.3 in Odds FC, *Candida and candidosis*. London: Baillière Tindall, 1988; 196–205, with permission.)

Hepatosplenic candidosis

In this syndrome a number of approaches to diagnosis in addition to biopsy may also be contributory. The most consistent results are seen with CT scans, which will show liver or spleen granulomas and abscesses (Bartley, PediatInfectDis, 1982; 1:317; Linker, Med-PediatOncol, 1984; 12:380). Ultrasonography has been less helpful but is an alternative. Radionucleotide scanning with technetium-99 or gallium-67 has produced variable results. To prove the identity of the infection it may be necessary to attempt liver biopsy with echo guidance or open biopsy at laparotomy. It is important to submit biopsy samples for both histopathological examination and culture as there may be few organisms in the lesions and these may not grow on culture. Serological tests may be positive in some of these patients and in many such cases antibody rather than antigen titres may be considerably elevated. Liver enzymes are usually elevated, although the most consistent abnormality has been in alkaline phosphatase.

Investigation and other diagnostic considerations

There are few totally satisfactory methods of confirming the diagnosis of systemic candidosis and the early institution of treatment often depends on clinical suspicion. In neutropenic patients it is better to initiate antifungal treatment on incomplete diagnostic evidence rather than to withhold or delay treatment. In hepatosplenic candidosis the presence of a high, swinging pyrexia should alert the attending physician. Some workers consider that the demonstration of circumscribed hepatic or splenic abscesses on CT scans of febrile, seriously immunocompromised patients is an important clue to this diagnosis (Bartley, PediatInfectDis, 1982; 1: 317).

Treatment and prognosis

The mainstay of treatment for systemic *Candida* infections is intravenous amphotericin B (0.5–1.0 mg/kg body wt). Other choices include amphotericin B combined with flucytosine, itraconazole (oral), and fluconazole (oral or intravenous). There is a high mortality in proven infections affecting neutropenic patients; therapy should be continued where possible until there is recovery of white-cell numbers and, at any rate, for a minimum of 2 to 3 weeks. Treatment of hepatosplenic infections is also difficult and many patients fail to respond to long courses of amphotericin B and flucytosine or fluconazole (Tashjian, RevInfDis, 1989; 6:689). Some successes have been achieved with a new approach using liposome-encapsulated amphotericin B (Lopez-Berestein, ClinOncol, 1987; 5:310). By using this formulation it is possible to increase the daily dose of amphotericin B to at least 3.0 mg/kg or even higher. Newer lipid-associated forms of amphotericin B are liposome-based (AmBisome), a colloidal dispersion (ABCD or Amphocil) or a lipid complex (ABLC or Abelcet). Once again there are a few case reports on these new compounds in hepatosplenic candidosis (Sharland, ArchDisChild, 1994; 70:546). Hepatosplenic candidosis is not necessarily a contraindication to bone marrow transplantation, provided that recipients are treated with amphotericin B both before and after engraftment until the graft is established (Bjerke, Blood, 1994; 84:2811).

Other opportunistic fungal infections

On occasions other opportunistic fungi may invade the liver in the course of disseminated infection. Invasive aspergillosis may be associated with solitary or multiple liver abscesses in 13 to 41 per cent of cases.[2] The usual pattern of infection is the invasion of tissue, with scattered fungal hyphae penetrating necrotic liver parenchyma. Occasionally the fungus may form into a fungus ball, or aspergilloma, in this site (Baker, AmJClinPath, 1962; 37:358). Likewise, liver abscesses have been recorded with systemic infections caused by other fungi such as *Trichosporon beigelii* (Haupt, JInfDis, 1983; 147:199). Mucormycosis, invasive zygomycosis, has only occasionally been recorded as causing liver disease, largely because it is often rapidly fatal even with localized infection of a distal site. All these infections are treated in much the same way as systemic candidosis, usually with amphotericin B and/or flucytosine.

Cryptococcosis

Cryptococcosis is caused by *Cryptococcus neoformans,* a yeast that is found in the environment in association with pigeon excreta.[3] There are two varieties of the organism: *C. neoformans neoformans,* which causes disease in Europe and parts of the United States in otherwise healthy people and immunocompromised patients including those with AIDS, and *C. neoformans gattii,* which is seen mainly in non-AIDS patients in Africa and the Far East. An important feature of *Cryptococcus is* the presence of a large mucoid capsule composed of xylomannan. Infection usually follows inhalation. Previously healthy individuals may be infected, particularly in the tropics, but in many parts of the world cryptococcosis is seen mainly in patients with defective T-lymphocyte function, including those with Hodgkin's disease, AIDS, systemic lupus erythematosus, and patients on steroid therapy as well as those receiving immuno-suppression after organ transplants.

The primary focus of infection is the lung but the most common clinical manifestation of the disease is meningitis. Skin or bone lesions may also occur. About 10 to 15 per cent of patients have some evidence of pulmonary involvement, indicating that the prim-ary focus often heals, despite dissemination. Liver infiltration during disseminated cryptococcosis is not common, but has been reported, particularly in patients with AIDS, where enlargement of the liver is not infrequent (Zuger, AnnIntMed, 1986; 104:234; Dismukes, JInfDis, 1988; 157:624). Confirmation of the diagnosis by liver biopsy is seldom obtained in such cases and in the absence of confirmatory biopsy or autopsy evidence, liver involvement must be assumed. In non-AIDS patients, other patterns of liver in-filtration have been recorded rarely. These include focal granu-lomatous hepatitis, which may mimic viral hepatitis, and on occasion widespread infiltrates resulting in hepatic failure (Sabesin, ArchIntMed, 1963; 11:661). Another rare method of presentation is with obstructive jaundice secondary to sclerosing cholangitis,

where the yeasts can be identified in the common bile duct (Bucuvalas, Gastro, 1985; 88:1055). In at least one such case there has been histological evidence of pre-existing cirrhosis.

The best method of laboratory diagnosis is direct microscopic examination of smears, sputum, or cerebrospinal fluid. The samples can be stained with the India ink or nigrosin, both of which emphasize the capsule. Cultures can also be taken and are usually positive in infected cases. There is a rapid antigen detection test using the agglutination of latex particles coated with antibody that can be performed on serum or cerebrospinal fluid.

In most patients the most appropriate therapy is amphotericin B with or without flucytosine given in doses of 0.3 to 0.6 mg/kg daily and 150 mg/kg daily, respectively. Therapy in patients with AIDS is associated with a high relapse rate (over 70 per cent), and it is usually necessary to give long-term treatment at weekly intervals after induction of remission. Some results with the new drugs fluconazole and itraconazole are encouraging. Fluconazole produced significant remissions in a dose of 400 mg daily in comparison with amphotericin B, but there was a somewhat higher frequency of early suppressive deaths in the fluconazole group. It is not clear whether higher doses of fluconazole would produce equal efficacy even in the group with poor prognosis. However, fluconazole is effective as a long-term treatment after initial remission. It has the advantage of being an oral compound. Likewise, itraconazole has been used as an oral suppressive agent for patients in post-primary remission. The most appropriate dosage is still under investigation and higher dosages than those usually prescribed (100–200 mg daily) should probably be used. Combinations of fluconazole or itraconazole with flucytosine are under evaluation.

Histoplasmosis
Definition

Histoplasmosis is a systemic infection caused by *Histoplasma cap-sulatum,* a dimorphic organism that can be found in the environment in soil or material contaminated with bird or bat excreta.[4] Infection follows inhalation, and, in most people, is overcome without the appearance of disease, the only evidence of past exposure being the appearance of delayed-type cutaneous sensitization to histoplasmin. Occasionally the infection may disseminate from the lungs to involve other organs, notably those rich in macrophages. The liver is affected in disseminated infections. This type of infection is known as classical or small-form histoplasmosis and is caused by a specific variant of the fungus, *H. capsulatum capsulatum.* The small-form disease is characterized by the presence of tiny yeasts (2–4 μm diameter) in tissue macrophages; it has a worldwide distribution.

A second type of histoplasmosis, African or large-form histo-plasmosis, caused by another variant of *H. capsulatum,* named *H. capsulatum* var. *duboisii,* is seen in central regions of Africa. The clinical appearances of this infection differ from the classical variety, with skin and bone sites being most frequently involved. Liver infection is not commonly recorded in this form of disease. The tissue yeast forms in African histoplasmosis are large (10–12 μm diameter) and are found in foreign-body giant cells; but small- and large-form *H. capsulatum* are culturally indistinguishable. African histoplasmosis will be discussed separately.

Asymptomatic (sensitization):	Positive delayed-type hypersensitivity to fungal antigen
Acute pulmonary:	Acute pulmonary infection after high-dose exposure
Chronic pulmonary (a) Inactive:	Asymptomatic pulmonary nodule(s)
(b) Active:	Chronic consolidation or cavitary lung disease
Disseminated* (a) Acute:	Widespread extrapulmonary dissemination
(b) Chronic:	Focal slowly progressive dissemination
Primary cutaneous:	Skin lesion and lymphadenopathy following inoculation

* The progress and extent of dissemination in deep mycoses varies depending on the infection and the underlying condition of the patient.

Prevalence and epidemiology

Histoplasmosis (classical) has a well-defined endemic area, being found in the east and central regions of the United States as well as Central and South America, Africa, the Indian subcontinent, and the Far East. Exposure, as assessed by conversion rates on the histoplasmin skin test, is highest in the United States and northern South America. In parts of the United States over 90 per cent of the healthy populace are skin-test positive. A lower prevalence of positive skin test (under 20 per cent) is seen in Africa and the Far East. These findings suggest that the infection is usually asymptomatic and self-healing, and that symptomatic disease is not common. Infection follows inhalation of the organism, which can be isolated from the natural environment. It is particularly associated with large accumulations of bird droppings in roosting sites and old buildings. In the tropics, important sites of potential exposure are bat-infested caves or buildings housing bat colonies.

Pathogenesis

Most of the systemic mycoses follow a common pattern of infection shown in Table 4. Subclinical infection is common but the primary infection may be symptomatic where it is associated with massive exposure to a natural source of the fungus, for instance in a cave (cave fever). Chronic infection of the lungs may develop in those with pre-existing pulmonary disease, such as emphysema.

Some studies indicate that the infection is a frequent, self-healing event, even in subclinical cases, as in endemic areas splenic or hepatic calcification of the site of healed metastatic lesions, some of which contain *H. capsulatum*, is common. In addition to this, dissemination may be progressive, particularly in patients with defective resistance. In rapidly disseminated forms of histoplasmosis, liver involvement may be more common, but it is also a feature of the indolent, chronic form of disseminated histoplasmosis where the main clinical abnormalities are oral ulceration, hepatic

enlargement, or adrenal insufficiency (Sarosi, AnnIntMed, 1971; 75:511).

Clinical features

The clinical features of histoplasmosis are largely determined by the site of infection. Acute and chronic pulmonary histoplasmosis are dominated by respiratory symptoms such as cough, weight loss, chest pain, and fever. Disseminated disease is also associated with weight loss and fever, but in the chronic forms of infection oral or laryngeal ulcers or adrenal insufficiency may appear. These are described in detail elsewhere.[4]

Symptomatic hepatic involvement may be seen in the rapid-onset, disseminated form of *Histoplasma* infection. Studies indicate that as many as 66 per cent of patients have hepatomegaly.[5,6] The enlarged liver may be tender and the spleen is frequently enlarged also. Lesions are usually diffusely distributed through the liver, with multiple granulomas or parenchymal infiltration with many macrophages being stuffed with organisms (Sarosi, AnnIntMed, 197; 75:511). Abnormalities of liver function may also occur. In patients with AIDS, liver enlargement has also been a common feature in those presenting with histoplasmosis (Symmers, AnnSoc-BelgeMedTrop, 1972; 52:435; Mandell, AmJMed, 1986; 81:974; Huang, ArchIntMed, 1987; 147:1181).

The liver may also be involved in chronic disseminated forms of the infection. Here there may be only slight hepatic enlargement. Interestingly, the most common pathological pattern is diffuse granuloma formation and in many of these lesions organisms cannot be found (Wheat, AmJMed, 1985; 78:20).

Investigations

Histoplasma capsulatum is very small and difficult to demonstrate in pathological material without experience. Giemsa- or methenamine silver-stained sections or biopsies may show the organisms. *Histoplasma* can be cultured from such cases. In disseminated forms the bone marrow, lymph nodes or even blood cultures may be positive, but occasionally fungi may be cultured from liver biopsies. Liver biopsies may also be a source of histopathological material (Christian, AmJMed, 1952; 13:689). Serological tests (immunodiffusion and complement fixation) are useful procedures for diagnosis and monitoring therapy. Two very specific precipitin bands, H and M, are found in histoplasmosis, the former being a more reliable indicator of active disease. In AIDS patients an antigen detection assay is helpful. The histoplasmin skin test has no diagnostic value as it simply indicates sensitization, and in many patients with disseminated disease it may be negative as they show anergy associated with severe infection.

Therapy

The treatment of the patient with histoplasmosis affecting the liver is the same as that used for disseminated infections. Amphotericin B is the main treatment and is given in doses of 0.8 to 1.0 mg/kg daily. The duration of treatment varies but may need to be continued until a total dose of 2.0 g is achieved. Itraconazole is effective in some forms of histoplasmosis and is probably the treatment of choice in chronically disseminated forms of the disease; it is also effective in patients with AIDS both for initial therapy at 200 to

400 mg daily and for long-term suppressive therapy (cf. cryptococcosis) at 100 to 200 mg daily.

African histoplasmosis

African histoplasmosis is an uncommon disease. Patients mainly present with disseminated lesions affecting the skin, bones and lymph nodes. Pulmonary involvement is rare. There are few reports of liver involvement in the course of African histoplasmosis.[7]

Paracoccidioidomycosis

Definition

Paracoccidioidomycosis is a systemic fungal infection caused by the dimorphic fungus *Paracoccidioides brasiliensis*.[8] The infection is seen only in parts of South and Central America, and Mexico. The organism causes either a widely disseminated infection or one localized to one or two sites, particularly the oral mucosa or lungs. Involvement of the liver is infrequently recognized, although it is probably common in widespread infections.

Introduction

Paracoccidioides brasiliensis is a dimorphic agent that occurs in human tissue in yeast phase. The yeast forms are very characteristic as the organism forms multiple buds that develop around the periphery of the parent cell. At room temperature, for instance on primary isolation, it is a mould fungus.

Epidemiology and pathogenesis

Paracoccidioidomycosis is a New World infection, although imported cases have been described outside this area in Japan and Europe. While it is believed that *P. brasiliensis* is found in nature, it has only been identified in the natural environment on a few occasions and therefore its true ecological niche is unknown.

Cases of the infection are not common, even in endemic areas, and are mainly seen in adult males. This is thought to be due to an unusual effect of human androgens on the conversion of the organism to the yeast phase. There have been several surveys which suggest that exposure to the organism is fairly widespread in the population of endemic areas, although only occasionally have more than 20 to 25 per cent of the community been found to be skin-test positive to intradermal antigens of *P. brasiliensis*. Infection probably follows inhalation, although some workers believe that direct inoculation of the organism into the mucosa may be responsible for some cases of the infection.

Clinical features

Paracoccidioidomycosis is a multisystem disease involving the lungs and the lymphatic system. It is often classified, as with the other systemic mycoses, into pulmonary and disseminated forms, or by location into pulmonary, lymphatic, mucocutaneous, and mixed depending on the predominant site(s) of clinical involvement. Like histoplasmosis a proportion of those exposed to this organism appear to develop asymptomatic infection, and the process resolves with the only evidence of infection being a positive skin test. It is not clear whether there is a self-resolving type of acute pulmonary infection and generally all pulmonary forms of this disease are treated. They may also coexist with extrapulmonary infection, particularly ulcerative lesions of the oral or genital mucosa as well as adjacent skin. Lymph-node involvement is also common.

Evidence for hepatic involvement is largely based on autopsy surveys, in which between 24 and 56 per cent of those who die with paracoccidioidomycosis are found to have liver involvement (Pinto, Mycopathologia, 1961; 15:90; Teixera, Histopath, 1978; 2:23). In some series over 40 per cent of those with disseminated forms of infection have had hepatomegaly. The liver in these cases is said to be enlarged diffusely with unchanged consistency. Jaundice is rare and is found in less than 6 per cent of cases (Raphael, RevAssMedBras, 1964; 10:151). Biopsy shows lesions ranging from small granulomas to diffuse infiltration of yeast forms and fibrosis. The bile ducts are commonly involved. The earliest signs are changes in aminotransferase concentrations; changes in alkaline phosphatase or bilirubin tend to occur in late disease. Hepatic involvement is usually dominated by the other manifestations of the condition, even though it may be common.

Investigations

The diagnosis is confirmed by the demonstration of the organism in tissue and its isolation in culture. *Paracoccidioides brasiliensis* characteristically produces multipolar buds around the circumference of a yeast cell and these can be seen in direct examination of smears. The organisms grow well in primary culture in Sabouraud's agar but should be converted to yeast form on enriched media such as brain–heart infusion agar. Serodiagnosis may be very helpful, and immunodiffusion and complement fixation tests are available for this disease.

Therapy

The most appropriate therapy available at present is itraconazole, which is given in doses of 100 to 200 mg daily for 3 to 6 months or longer if necessary. The older azole antifungal, ketoconazole, is also very active. Other methods include intravenous amphotericin B and sulphonamides. Relapse after using the latter is very common.

Coccidioidomycosis

Coccidioidomycosis is an infection caused by *Coccidioides immitis*, a soil organism found in the arid western parts of the United States in California, Arizona, Texas, and New Mexico as well as certain areas in South and Central America (northern Argentina, Colombia, Uruguay).[9] Infection follows inhalation of the fungus and, like histoplasmosis, many of those exposed simply become sensitized without infection. Like histoplasmosis, acute or chronic pulmonary infections may result or the disease may spread from the primary lung focus to involve other sites including the liver.

The main features of infection are therefore respiratory, and patients present with acute or chronic cough, malaise, and fever. In some cases of primary infection, patients may develop erythema multiforme or nodosum along with fever and cough. Dissemination often occurs in immunocompromised patients and is also more frequently seen in certain ethnic groups such as Indians or Negroes. The principal sites for dissemination are the meninges, joints, and skin. In severe and widely disseminated infections, involvement of the liver is common and one autopsy survey suggested that hepatic foci could be found in at least half of those with this type of disease.[10] The pattern of liver involvement ranges from focal granuloma formation to diffuse inflammatory infiltration.[10,11] Liver enlargement can occur together with changes in liver enzymes. Liver involvement has also been reported in patients with AIDS who develop coccidioidomycosis.[12]

This infection is diagnosed by culture or by finding the characteristic *Coccidioides* spherules in smears or histologically. The organism grows well in laboratory culture but is a potential laboratory hazard through inhalation. Laboratory staff should be warned about a possible diagnosis of coccidioidomycosis if they are attempting cultures. Serology (immunodiffusion, enzyme immunoassay, or counter-immunoelectrophoresis) is very helpful both for establishing the diagnosis and monitoring the course of disease. Liver biopsy has been reported as a diagnostic procedure in coccidioidomycosis.[11]

Although the management of some forms of coccidioidomycosis may be relatively simple, disseminated infections are difficult to treat. Amphotericin B is the mainstay of therapy, although some patients with soft-tissue disease may respond to ketoconazole, itraconazole, or fluconazole.

Other systemic mycoses

Blastomycosis due to the dimorphic fungus, *Blastomyces dermatitidis*, is occasionally associated with liver infiltration in disseminated forms.[13] The geographical range of this disease is fairly wide, cases being found in north and central United States and Canada, Africa, the Middle East, and occasionally elsewhere. As with histoplasmosis the main route of infection is respiratory, and liver involvement occurs after dissemination from the lungs. It is uncommon and has only occasionally been reported in disseminated infections in immunocompromised patients (Recht, AmRevRespDis, 1982; 125:359). In one study in such groups, two of six patients with chronic myeloid and chronic lymphocytic leukaemia, respectively, had diffuse infiltrations of leukaemic cells and *B. dermatitidis* in the liver at autopsy.

Penicillinosis due to *Penicillium marneffei* is a disease recently reported from South-East Asia and in individuals who have visited that area. The organism naturally causes infection in bamboo rats. Its mode of transmission, and pathogenesis, are unknown, but widespread disseminated forms of the disease have been seen, with foci of infection in bone marrow, spleen, lung, and liver (Supparatpinyo, Lancet, 1994; 344:110). The organism can be recognized histologically and isolated in culture. In tissue, *P. marneffei* may resemble *Histoplasma* small forms, but it does not form buds and individual cells divide by transverse fission. In the liver the fungi are found within macrophages and there is usually a granulomatous response. This infection can be treated with itraconazole or amphotericin B.

Actinomycete infections

The actinomycetes are filamentous bacteria that may cause a variety of different diseases. By convention two of these, actinomycosis and nocardiosis, are usually considered with the fungal infections. One of the features of both these organisms is their ability to form into large aggregates in infections. These aggregates or grains (granules) are composed of a mesh of filaments.

In forming these structures the organisms may undergo certain changes. *Nocardia* spp., for instance, may lose cell walls to form l-forms. In the case of the *Actinomyces* spp. the outer layer of the aggregate is coated with refractile eosinophilic material that is composed of both host and bacterial components including immunoglobulin. In liver infections, *Actinomyces* may form into granules whereas this is unusual for *Nocardia*, which is normally present in this site in individual filaments.

Actinomycosis

Actinomycosis is an infection caused by actinomycetes of the genus *Actinomyces*, notably *A. israelii*, *A. bovis*, and *A. naeslundii*. More rarely other actinomycete species are involved. Infections often occur in specific sites such as the mouth (cervicofacial), abdomen, thorax, or uterus (pelvic). In the pelvic site of infection there has been an association with certain intrauterine contraceptive devices. Actinomycosis is now uncommon in many parts of the world, largely because early treatment of dental sepsis has prevented the development of the cervicofacial form, the most common clinical variety. However, sporadic cases still occur.

Infection is thought to follow local proliferation of organisms. In many cases it appears that aggregates of *Actinomyces* are associated with other bacteria such as coliforms. The part played by these bacteria in the pathogenesis of the infection is unknown. Actinomycosis is mainly seen in otherwise healthy patients. The hallmark of the infection is the formation of inflammatory masses containing granules. Such masses encroach on other structures, and where there is communication with the skin or a cavity, multiple draining sinuses are formed. These may involve the jaw, the chest, or the pelvis and can be confused with a range of other conditions such as mycetoma or tumours. Infection of the liver is unusual but has been recorded.

In about 15 per cent of cases of abdominal actinomycosis, itself a rare condition, the liver is affected.[14] The route of infection to this site is unknown, but it has been suggested that spread follows passage through the portal vein after appendicitis or surgery.[15] Most commonly it presents as a solitary liver abscess and may spread to affect adjacent sites such as the bowel and the diaphragm. The liver may appear enlarged, but jaundice is rare. The course of this infection may be very slow (over 2 years).

There are no characteristic clinical features of actinomycosis of the liver. The diagnosis is made on the basis of cultures after aspiration or biopsy. CT scans show single or multiple, poorly defined areas of increased density.[15] The material should be cultured. In a few centres it is possible to measure the antibody. The main treatment is penicillin given parenterally ($2–12 \times 10^6$ units daily in adults), the dose depending on the site. Alternatives include erythromycin or tetracycline.

Nocardiosis

Nocardia asteroides, *N. brasiliensis*, and *N. caviae* are aerobic actinomycetes that may cause human disease.[16] There are two main clinical varieties: mycetoma, a subcutaneous infection due to implantation, and systemic nocardiosis, an invasive disease seen in both immunocompromised and healthy patients. In the former disease, *Nocardia* spp. form granules in tissue, whereas in the latter the organisms are in filamentous phase. Liver invasion is occasionally seen in disseminated nocardiosis. The primary portal of infection is thought to be the lung, and patients may present with primary lung disease and pulmonary infiltrates or with clinical lesions due to extrapulmonary dissemination, for instance to the brain or skin. The liver is a rare target in disseminated nocardiosis. In one survey of 230 cases of disseminated nocardiosis only 3 per cent of patients had proven hepatic lesions, either solitary or multiple abscesses. In one instance the diagnosis was established by CT-guided needle aspiration of a subcapsular abscess (Cockerill, AmJMed, 1984; 77:558). Most patients with disseminated *Nocardia* infections have some form of underlying disease affecting T-lymphocyte function, such as lymphoma or AIDS, or are receiving immunosuppressive regimens including corticosteroids.

The diagnosis is confirmed by culture, although the presence of partially acid-fast filaments in smears or histopathological sections is helpful. Nocardiosis often responds to treatment with co-trimoxazole. Alternative drugs include minocycline, ampicillin, amikacin, and impipenem.

References

1. Odds FC. *Candida and candidosis*. London: Baillière Tindall, 1988: 196–206.
2. Barbosa Lemos L and Jensen AB. Pathology of aspergillosis. In Al-Doory Y and Wagner GE, eds. *Aspergillosis*. Springfield: Thomas, 1985: 156–95.
3. Hay RJ. Cryptococcosis in the immunocompromised patient. In Warnock D and Richardson MA, eds. *Fungal infection in the immunocompromised patient*. Chichester: Wiley, 1982: 93–118.
4. Schwarz J. *Histoplasmosis*. New York: Praeger, 1981.
5. Ruben H, Furcolow ML, Yates JL, and Brasher CA. The course and prognosis of histoplasmosis. *American Journal of Medicine*, 1959; **27**: 278–88.
6. Redding PA, Gorelick DF, Brasher CA, and Larsh H. Progressive disseminated histoplasmosis seen in adults. *American Journal of Medicine*, 1970; **48**: 629–36.
7. Williams AO, Lawson EA, and Lucas AO. African histoplasmosis due to *Histoplasma duboisii*. *Archives of Pathology*, 1971; **92**: 306–18.
8. Del Negro G, Lacaz C da S, and Fiorillo AM. *Paracoccidioidomicose*. Sao Paulo, Brazil: Sarvier-EDUSP, 1982.
9. Stevens DA, ed. *Coccidioidomycosis*. New York: Plenum, 1981.
10. Huntington RW, Waldman WJ, Sargent JA, O'Conell H, Wybel R, and Croll D. Pathologic and clinical observations of fatal coccidioidomycosis with necropsy. In Ajello L, ed. *Coccidioidomycosis*. Tucson: University of Arizona Press, 1967: 143–63.
11. Ward JR and Hunter RC, Disseminated coccidioidomycosis demonstrated by needle biopsy of the liver. *Annals of Internal Medicine*, 1958; **48**: 157–63.
12. Graybill JR. Coccidioidomycosis. In Hay RJ, ed. *Baillières tropical medicine: Tropical fungal infections*. London: Baillière Tindall, 1989: 125–52.
13. Sarosi GA and Davies SF. Blastomycosis. *American Reviews of Respiratory Disease*, 1979; **120**: 911–38.
14. Putnam HC, Dockerty MB, and Waugh JM. Abdominal actinomycosis. *Surgery*, 1950; **28**: 781–800.
15. Mongiardo N, de Rienzo B, Zonchetta G, Lami G, Pellegrino F, and Squadrini F. Primary hepatic actinomycosis. *Journal of Infection*, 1986; **8**: 65–9.
16. Palmer DL, Harvey RL, and Wheeler RL. Diagnostic and therapeutic considerations in *Nocardia asteroides* infection. *Medicine*, 1974; **53**: 391–401.

13.3 Protozoal infections

13.3.1 Amoebiasis, giardiasis, and cryptosporidiosis

Adolfo Martínez-Palomo

Amoebiasis

Definition

Amoebiasis is an infection of the human gastrointestinal tract by the protozoan parasite *Entamoeba histolytica*. The motile form of the parasite, the trophozoite, lives in the lumen of the large intestine, where it multiplies and differentiates into the cyst, the resistance form, responsible for the transmission of the infection. *Entamoeba histolytica* is the cause of invasive amoebiasis, which is prevalent in certain developing countries. Trophozoites may invade the colonic mucosa and produce dysentery, and through bloodborne spread give rise to extraintestinal lesions, mainly liver abscesses. The course of dysentery is usually self-limiting, but amoebic liver abscess is potentially fatal, unless it is diagnosed promptly and treated appropriately.[1,2] Many asymptomatic intestinal infections formerly attributed to 'non-pathogenic' strains of *E. histolytica*, particularly in countries where invasive amoebiasis is uncommon, are now considered to be caused by a morphologically similar, but non-invasive, species of amoeba, designated as *E. dispar* (Diamond, JEukaryotMicrobiol, 1993; 40:340).

Introduction

The works of Hippocrates frequently allude to dysentery, the most common disorder associated with amoebiasis, but it was not until the second half of the nineteenth century that Lesh, in St Petersburg, recorded a fatal case of dysentery in which amoebas of an unknown species were detected. In 1890, William Osler reported the case of a young physician who contracted dysentery and developed a hepatic abscess that led to his death. One year later, Councilman and Lafleur conducted a detailed study at Johns Hopkins Hospital of patients with dysentery and hepatic abscesses, most of whom were born in Poland and worked as longshoremen in Baltimore. They confirmed the pathogenic role of amoebas and created the term 'amoebic dysentery', as well as the one, not entirely correct, of 'amoebic liver abscess' (Stilwell, Gastro, 1955; 28:606).[3] The lifecycle of the parasite and of other amoebas that may infect the human intestine was carefully analysed by Dobell in London. His excellent monograph (Dobell, *The amoebae living in man*. London: John Bale and Danielsson, 1919) is still a valuable source of information. Thus,

the basic early research on this typical 'tropical' disease was carried out in settings rather remote from the tropics.

The undeniable causal role of *E. histolytica* in many symptomatic cases and its apparently innocuous role in others generated an unsolved dispute that has lasted for more than a century. Although universal agreement has not yet been achieved, during the last 20 years evidence has grown that many asymptomatic intestinal infections formerly attributed to 'non-pathogenic' strains of *E. histolytica* are in fact due to a different species of amoebae, *E. dispar*, as suggested by Brumpt in 1925.[4]

Epidemiology

Invasive amoebiasis is still a major health and social problem in certain areas of Africa, Asia, and Latin America. A high incidence of symptomatic intestinal amoebiasis may be frequent in all age groups, while liver abscesses are mostly seen in adult males. Conditions may have actually deteriorated during recent years as rural populations have tended to migrate to urban areas. Unless prompt diagnosis is followed by adequate treatment, invasive amoebiasis, particularly liver abscess, may be fatal. In most industrialized countries, however, the number of severe cases of amoebiasis is much lower. Nevertheless, knowledge of the disease in these regions is also important since the failure to identify an amoebic infection may result in a lethal outcome, for example intestinal amoebiasis may be treated as chronic ulcerative colitis. In addition, high infection rates can exist among certain immigrant groups, and epidemic outbreaks can occur in institutions such as schools or mental hospitals.

The increase in intestinal amoebic infections in male homosexuals in several large cities of the United States, Canada, and England has reached hyperendemic levels with point-prevalence rates varying from 20 to 31 per cent. In these homosexual populations, most reported cases are asymptomatic, probably because they are caused by *E. dispar* (Allason Jones, NEJM, 1986; 315:353). In countries such as Japan, however, cases of invasive amoebiasis due to *E. histolytica* are not uncommon in male homosexuals (Takeuchi, TrRSocTropMedHyg, 1990; 84:250).

In areas of high prevalence, invasive amoebiasis characteristically occurs in endemic form, probably due to constant reinfection with *E. histolytica*. Epidemic outbreaks are uncommon, and when present are due to a heavily contaminated water supply.[5] In 1984 it was estimated that 40 million people developed disabling colitis or liver abscesses. At least 40 000 deaths that year were attributable to amoebiasis, mostly as a consequence of liver abscesses.[6] Therefore, on a global scale, amoebiasis comes third among all parasitic causes of death, behind malaria and schistosomiasis.

The most common modes of transmission are by food contaminated with cysts of *E. histolytica* or from person to person. The greatest risk is associated with cyst passers, especially if they are engaged in preparation and handling of food. In endemic areas a variety of conditions, including ignorance, poverty, overcrowding, inadequate and contaminated water supplies, and poor sanitation, favour direct faecal–oral transmission from one person to another. Several studies have demonstrated family clustering of amoebic infections, and have implicated intrafamilial spread as a factor of transmission (Martínez-Palomo, ClinTropMedCommDis, 1986; 1: 587).[7]

The main reservoir of *E. histolytica* is man, although morphologically similar amoebas may be found in non-human primates, dogs, and cats. Experimental infections were produced in man with inocula of 2000 to 4000 cysts. The median incubation period was reported to be 21.4 days, but the infection in man has a prepatent period ranging from 2 days to 4 months. The communicability period of untreated intestinal infections is variable, and cysts have been demonstrated in faeces for as long as 2 years (Beaver, AmJTropMedHyg, 1956; 5:1000).[8] The cysts may remain viable and infective for a few days in faeces. Since they are killed by desiccation, cyst-laden dust is not infective. They are also killed by temperatures higher than 68°C, so that boiled water is safe. The amount of chlorine needed to purify ordinary water is insufficient to kill cysts; high concentrations of chlorine are effective, but the water must be subsequently dechlorinated before use.

Prevention and control

Invasive amoebiasis could be controlled by the improvement of living standards and the establishment of adequate sanitary conditions in countries where the disease is prevalent. Since these actions require radical social and economic changes in overpopulated societies where the susceptible population is bound by poverty and ignorance, very little interest has been shown in the implementation of specific control programmes. Strategies should aim at: (i) the community, through the improvement of environmental sanitation including water supply, food safety, and health education to prevent faecal–oral transmission; (ii) the individual, through early detection and treatment in cases of infection and/or disease. Cases of invasive amoebiasis require prompt chemotherapy and asymptomatic carriers should be treated if infected with *E. histolytica*. Mass chemotherapy of high-risk populations has been attempted, with only partial success. Individual or collective chemoprophylaxis is not indicated.[5,9] The introduction of protective immunity has given promising results, but so far only in experimental animal models.

Pathogenesis and pathology

The lytic and invasive characteristics of pathogenic strains of *E. histolytica* are related to the striking motility and phagocytic capacity of the trophozoites, and to the possible release of a membrane pore-forming protein and proteases that produce contact-dependent lysis of target cells, including inflammatory and epithelial cells. Upon contact with extracellular components, amoebas liberate potent enzymes that degrade the extracellular matrix (Martínez-Palomo, ParasitolToday, 1987; 3:111).

Invasion of the colonic and caecal mucosa by *E. histolytica* begins in the interglandular epithelium. Inflammatory cells around invading amoebas are rapidly lysed, leading to tissue necrosis; thus,

acute changes are seldom found in biopsy samples or in scrapings of rectal mucosal lesions. Ulcerations may deepen and progress under the mucosa to form typical 'flask ulcers' that extend into the submucosa producing abundant microhaemorrhages. This explains the finding of haematophagous amoebas in stool specimens or in rectal scrapings, still the best indication of the amoebic nature of a case of dysentery or bloody diarrhoea. Macroscopically, the ulcers are superficial initially, with hyperaemic borders, a necrotic base, and normal mucosa between the sites of invasion. Further progression of the lesions may produce a loss of the mucosa and submucosa covering the muscle layers, and eventually lead to the rupturing of the serosa.[10,11]

Complications of intestinal amoebiasis include perforation, direct extension to the skin, and dissemination, mainly to the liver. Amoebas probably spread from the intestine to the liver through the portal circulation. The presence and extent of liver involvement bears no relation to the degree of intestinal amoebiasis, and these conditions do not necessarily coincide. The early stages of hepatic amoebic invasion have not been studied in humans. In experimental animals, inoculation of *E. histolytica* trophozoites into the portal vein produces multiple foci of neutrophil accumulation around parasites, followed by focal necrosis and granulomatous infiltration. As the lesions extend in size, the granulomas are gradually substituted by necrosis, until the lesions coalesce and necrotic tissue occupies progressively larger portions of the liver. Hepatocytes close to the early lesions show degenerative changes that lead to necrosis, but direct contact of liver cells with amoebas is very rarely observed. The lesion can eventually develop into large areas of liquefied necrotic material surrounded by a thin capsule of fibrous appearance. These experimental results suggest that *E. histolytica* trophozoites do not produce liver abscesses through direct lysis of hepatocytes. Rather, tissue destruction is the result of the accumulation and subsequent lysis of neutrophils and macrophages surrounding the amoebas (Tsutsumi, AmJPathol, 1984; 117:81; Tsutsumi, AmJPathol, 1988; 121:112). Human liver abscesses consist of areas in which the parenchyma has been completely substituted by material, usually of a semisolid or liquid consistency, composed of necrotic debris and a few cells. Neutrophils are generally absent, and amoebas tend to be located at the periphery of the abscess (Fig. 1). Liver abscesses may heal, rupture, or disseminate.

Invasive amoebic lesions in humans, whether localized in the large intestine, liver or skin, almost invariably heal without the formation of scar tissue if properly treated. The absence of fibrotic tissue following necrosis is particularly striking in the liver.[11]

Lifecycle

Trophozoites, the motile forms of *E. histolytica*, dwell in the colon where they multiply and encyst, producing typical four-nucleated cysts, which are found in the formed stools of carriers as round or slightly oval hyaline bodies, 8 to 20 μm in diameter, with a refractive wall. Cysts never develop within tissues. Trophozoites are short-lived outside the body and do not survive in the upper gastrointestinal tract; thus, they are not important in the transmission of the disease. In contrast, cysts remain viable and infective for several days in faeces and water.

Until recently, biological and epidemiological data were taken to indicate that there are two forms of *E. histolytica*, 'pathogenic' and

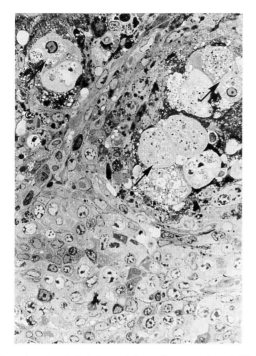

Fig. 1. Amoebas located at the periphery of an experimental liver abscess.

'non-pathogenic'.[12] The first reported biochemical difference between isolates obtained from cases of invasive amoebiasis and amoebas cultured from the stools of asymptomatic carriers was the striking agglutinability of the former with the lectin concanavalin A (Martínez-Palomo, NatureNB, 1973; 245:186). Subsequently, the isoenzyme technique using starch or polyacrylamide gel electrophoresis has shown that amoebas cultured from samples of well-characterized cases of invasive amoebiasis are clustered into distinct enzymatic banding patterns, or zymodemes, which are different from those of amoebas isolated from carriers (Sargeaunt, Lancet, 1982; i:1386). Although the technique is too cumbersome and time-consuming to be used in clinical practice for the identification of amoebas, it has been valuable in demonstrating that most amoebas found in carriers, particularly in countries where invasive amoebiasis is not endemic, have 'non-pathogenic' zymodemes. Antigenic differences between 'pathogenic' and 'non-pathogenic' strains reported with the use of monoclonal antibodies, as well as genetic differences found with DNA and RNA probes, suggest that *E. histolytica* consists of two morphologically identical, but genetically distinct, species (Strachan, Lancet, 1988; i:561; Tannich, PNAS, 1989; 86:5118; Edman, JExpMed, 1990; 172:879; Tachibana, InfectImmun, 1990; 58:955; Clark, MolBiochemParasitol, 1991; 47:297). The 'pathogenic' amoebas retain the name *E. histolytica* Schaudinn 1903, while the 'non-pathogenic' amoebas are now widely considered as the species *E. dispar* Brumpt 1925 (Diamond, JEukaryotMicrobiol, 1993; 40:340).

Clinical features and diagnosis

Intestinal amoebiasis

The clinical spectrum of intestinal *E. histolytica* infection ranges from an asymptomatic carrier state to acute or fulminant colitis with perforation, depending on the nutritional status, the susceptibility of the host, including age, and, probably, on differences in the degree of virulence of amoebic strains. Invasive intestinal amoebiasis usually presents as acute rectocolitis. Most patients present a non-toxic dysenteric syndrome and constitutional symptoms are not as prominent as in shigella dysentery. The onset of acute rectocolitis is gradual, and 85 per cent of patients complain of intense abdominal pain. Initially there are loose, watery stools that rapidly become blood-stained with mucus. Tenesmus occurs in half of the patients and is always associated with rectosigmoidal involvement. Watery diarrhoea or loose stools without blood may be present for few days, particularly when distal regions of the colon are involved. Rectosigmoidoscopy and colonoscopy of benign cases show small ulcerations with linear or oval contours, 3 to 5 mm in diameter, covered by a yellowish exudate containing many trophozoites.[2,13]

Rectosigmoidoscopy and immediate microscopic examination of rectal smears for the presence of motile, haematophagous trophozoites of *E. histolytica* are the most important diagnostic procedures, but the microscopic examination of amoebas has several drawbacks, including the requirement for a skilled technician. Reliable and sensitive assays such as immunoassay or hybridization using gene probes are still in the research phase (Aguirre, TrRSoc-TropMedHyg, 1995; 89:187). Cyst detection usually requires concentration methods including flotation or sedimentation. In cases of colonic invasive amoebiasis the serological detection of antiamoebic antibodies is positive in approx. 75 per cent of cases.[13,14]

Amoebic liver abscess

This is the most common extraintestinal form of invasive amoebiasis. Amoebic abscesses may be found in all age groups, but are 10 times more frequent in adults than children, and show a higher frequency in males than females. They are more common in the poorest sectors of urban populations. Even though liver abscesses develop after infection of the intestine, the patients rarely have associated amoebic rectocolitis; however, colonization of the large intestine with *E. histolytica* may be found in more than 70 per cent of cases of amoebic liver abscess. Lesions are usually single, and most are found in the right lobe of the liver in the posterior, external, and superior portions (Sukov, AmJRadiol, 1980; 134:911).[2,14,15]

In most patients, mainly young individuals less than 30 years old and children, the clinical presentation and course of the disease are typical (Table 1). The onset is abrupt, with pain in the upper abdomen and high fever. The pain is intense and constant, radiating to the scapular region and right shoulder; it increases with coughing, deep breathing, or when the patient rests on the right side. When the abscess is located in the left lobe, the pain tends to be felt in the epigastrium and may radiate to the left shoulder. Fever is present in most cases; it varies between 38 and 40°C, frequently in spikes but sometimes constant over several days, with rigors and profuse sweating. There is anorexia and rapid weight loss; approximately one-third of the patients have non-productive cough. Nausea and vomiting may occur, and in some cases diarrhoea or dysentery may be present. Physical examination reveals a pale, wasted patient with an enlarged, tender liver. Digital pressure in the right lower intercostal spaces will produce intense pain and there is often marked tenderness on percussion over the right lower ribs in the posterior region. Movement of the right side of the chest and

Table 1 Clinical and laboratory finding in amoebic liver abscess

	Percentage (range)
Duration of symptoms (weeks):	
<2	37–66
2–4	20–40
4–12	16–42
>12	5–11
Fever	71–98
Abdominal pain	62–98
Diarrhoea	14–66
Cough	10–32
Weight loss	33–53
Tender liver	80–95
Hepatomegaly	43–93
Epigastric tenderness	22
Rales, ronchi	8–47
Jaundice	10–25
White blood-cell count $>10 \times 10^9/l$	63–94
Haemoglobin <2 g/dl	25–90
Elevated transaminases	26–50
Elevated alkaline phosphatase	38–84
Elevated bilirubin	10–25
Increased erythrocyte sedimentation rate	81

Source of data, reference 2.

diaphragm is greatly restricted, as well as the intensity of respiratory sounds. Older individuals may present a chronic and milder non-specific febrile illness, with hepatomegaly, anaemia, and abnormal liver function tests (Dehesa, RevInvestClin(Mex), 1975; 27:129; Katzenstein, Medicine, 1982; 61:237).[2,15]

Investigations and other diagnostic considerations

The diagnosis of amoebic liver abscess should be particularly suspected in endemic areas, or when there is a history of travel to these countries, in patients who present with spiking fever, weight loss, and abdominal pain in the upper right quadrant or epigastrium with tenderness in the liver area. Other signs include leucocytosis, elevated alkaline phosphatase, and an elevated right diaphragm in chest films. In this situation, liver imaging techniques are indicated; sonography or CT scanning are preferred. Hepatic MRI gives information comparable that from less-expensive imaging procedures (Elizondo, Radiol, 1987; 165:795; Ralls, Radiol, 1987; 165:805). Liver imaging will demonstrate a space-occupying lesion in 75 to 95 per cent of the cases, according to the procedure and the course of the illness. Once the presumptive diagnosis of a space-occupying lesion in the liver is made, the next step is serological investigation to detect antiamoebic antibodies. This test is accurate in more than 90 per cent of cases; techniques currently used are indirect haemagglutination, counterimmunoelectrophoresis, and enzyme immunoassays. Serology is very useful in amoebic liver abscess since antibodies are present at high titres in most patients. The antibody response is directly related to the duration of the illness. It may be negative during the first week after onset; titres reach a peak by the second or third month, decreasing to lower, still detectable levels by 9 months.[2,14]

Differential diagnosis

When a space-occupying mass is found in the liver, the differential diagnosis of an amoebic liver abscess should include a pyogenic abscess and a neoplasm. The pyogenic abscess is more frequent in older patients with a previous history of hepatobiliary diseases, abdominal sepsis, appendicitis, diverticulitis, or abdominal surgery. These patients are more likely to present with jaundice, pruritus, and septic shock; hepatomegaly and an elevated diaphragm in the chest radiographs are uncommon, and amoebic serology is negative. In the presence of a space-occupying lesion with negative serology, aspiration is indicated for microscopy and culture (Conter, SGO, 1986; 162:114; Barnes, Medicine, 1987; 66:472).[2,14]

A liver neoplasm enters in the differential diagnosis when the patient is febrile and wasted, with vague abdominal discomfort. Neoplasms exhibit distinct images, particularly in the CT scan; tumour markers such as α-fetoproteins or carcinoembryonic antigen may be positive. Stool microscopy for the identification of trophozoites or cysts of *E. histolytica* is of value for the diagnosis of amoebic liver abscess, since many patients have associated asymptomatic intestinal amoebiasis.

Complications

Amoebic liver abscesses commonly produce thoracic complications, particularly pleurisy with a non-purulent pleural effusion, manifested by a non-productive cough, thoracic pain, and dyspnoea related to the extent of the effusion. The rupture of a liver abscess into the bronchial tree can be accompanied by the sudden development of a cough and the discharge of an abundant, anchovy sauce-like exudate in the sputum. Less commonly, the liver abscess may rupture into the pleural cavity, accompanied by sudden sharp pain and severe dyspnoea, with impending shock. The least frequent thoracic complication is amoebic pericarditis, which may be present when the abscess is in the left lobe of the liver and is characterized by intense precordial pain, anxiety, dyspnoea, tachycardia, dilatation of the jugular veins, and softened cardiac sounds; a paradoxical pulse and shock may also occur.

Rupture into the abdomen occurs in approximately 8 per cent of patients with amoebic liver abscess. The onset is abrupt, with signs of generalized peritonitis. Only rarely do abscesses rupture into the gallbladder, stomach, duodenum, colon, or inferior vena cava. Occasionally an abscess may erode the abdominal wall and reach the skin. Secondary infection of amoebic liver abscesses is an uncommon complication that is suspected when a severe toxi-infectious state is present, together with lack of response to anti-amoebic chemotherapy.[2,14]

Therapy

Nitroimidazole amoebicides have contributed greatly to decreasing the morbidity and mortality of amoebiasis; in addition to the advantage of having an oral route of administration, they are the most effective therapeutically. They are reasonably well tolerated. In spite of their reported carcinogenic effect in rodents and their mutagenic potential in bacteria, no such effects have been reported in humans. For these reasons, metronidazole and related compounds are the drugs of choice in the treatment of invasive amoebiasis.[2,16] Emetine hydrochloride and dehydroemetine, which act in the liver, intestinal wall, and other tissues, and chloroquine, which acts only in the liver, are seldom used at present.

Amoebic liver abscess should be treated with chemotherapy; surgery is rarely indicated. The treatment of choice is with nitro-imidazoles, orally or, when not tolerated, intravenously. The recommended oral dosage for metronidazole and related compounds is 1 g twice daily for 5 to 10 days for an adult, and 30 to 50 mg/day in three divided doses for 10 days for children. The intravenous route is highly effective in patients with complicated hepatic abscesses; the recommended dosage in those cases is 500 mg every 6 h for 5 to 10 days. In many cases of amoebic hepatic abscess, a favourable response is obtained after the third day of treatment; however, in order to secure an 85 per cent cure rate, treatment should be continued for a minimum of 5 days and administration of the drug for 10 days raises the rate of cure to nearly 95 per cent.[15, 16] Other nitroimidazole derivatives may be effective in 1 to 3 days, but in view of the clinical severity of amoebic liver abscesses there is little reason to shorten therapy. In one study, failure in the treatment of amoebic liver abscess with metronidazole was reported in up to 10 per cent of cases (Thomson, RevInfDis, 1985; 7:171). It is questionable, however, whether a true metronidazole resistance exists in some cases of invasive amoebiasis; treatment was considered a failure when there was a lack of response at 72 h on the assumption that response should be dramatic and immediate. It is therefore unknown whether prolonged treatment of these cases could have resulted in cure. *In vitro* studies and experiments with animal models of liver abscesses have not demonstrated the existence of metronidazole-resistant strains of amoeba. In 85 per cent of cases, liver imaging reveals resolution of amoebic abscesses within 6 months of treatment; the remaining 15 per cent still show imaging defects 3 years after treatment.

Only rarely are the side-effects of metronidazole sufficiently severe to merit suspension of the drug. However, oral administration is occasionally accompanied by symptoms of gastrointestinal upset such as epigastralgia, nausea, and vomiting; additionally, patients often report a metallic taste and a brownish discoloration of the urine. Undesirable reactions are observed when alcoholic beverages are ingested during the course of metronidazole therapy. These effects appear due to the inhibition of alcohol dehydrogenase by the amoebicide. Metronidazole and its derivatives should not be given during the first trimester of pregnancy and should only be prescribed under strict supervision during the second and third trimesters, owing to their ability to cross the placental barrier and enter the fetal circulation. The effect of these drugs on fetal development is unknown. Similarly, because of their elimination in breast milk, they are not recommended for nursing mothers; breast feeding should be suspended if treatment with metronidazole is prescribed. Despite the various side-effects and precautions, metronidazole and related compounds are reasonably safe and effective amoebicidal agents.[16] Although it was generally believed that combined therapy with dehydroemetine is more effective than the nitroimidazole alone, particularly in severe cases, there are no well-controlled comparative studies that demonstrate this point. To prevent recurrences and transmission, patients with amoebic liver abscess treated with metronidazole should also be treated with a luminal amoebicide, because up to two-thirds may have asymptomatic intestinal colonization with *E. histolytica* (Irusen, ClinInfDis, 1992;

14:889). The most frequently used amoebicides with luminal action are diloxanide furoate, diiodohydroxyquin, and paromomycin.

Over the years, the treatment of lesions produced in the liver by amoebic disease has been substantially modified. The former abuse of surgery, including aspiration, arose from the erroneous supposition that the treatment of hepatic abscesses should be approached like that of any other suppurating lesion, and 'pus' should be withdrawn immediately by surgical means (Harries, JRSM, 1982; 75:190). However, amoebic abscesses are basically formed of necrotic material produced by the process of liquefaction, and only exceptionally are they contaminated with bacteria. The introduction of metronidazole in 1970 substantially reduced the frequency of surgical interventions and produced a sizeable reduction in mortality. In the nineteenth century, mortality of amoebic liver abscess was probably well over 90 per cent; the introduction of aspiration reduced this figure to 80 per cent. The subsequent joint approach of aspiration and emetine chemotherapy further decreased the mortality rate to 25 per cent after 1922. A decline in the number of surgical interventions lowered the mortality rate to approximately 12 per cent, with a further reduction after the introduction of metronidazole to less than 2 per cent.[2,14,15]

At present, indications for percutaneous drainage are the imminent rupture of a large abscess, as a complementary therapy to shorten the course of the disease when response to chemotherapy has been slow, or the suspicion of a pyogenic or mixed infection. Drainage should be done under ultrasound or CT guidance; catheters should not be left for drainage and should be rapidly removed to avoid contamination of the track and skin. Indications for surgical drainage include imminent rupture of inaccessible liver abscesses, especially of the left lobe, risk of peritoneal leakage of necrotic fluid after aspiration, or rupture of a liver abscess.[16]

Monitoring of condition of the patient

A prompt diagnosis and an adequate chemotherapy will control most cases of liver abscesses produced by *E. histolytica*. In general, full clinical recovery and the disappearance of liver lesions as confirmed by CT scanning can be obtained in uncomplicated cases. Prognosis is favourable in the absence of the following features: severe malnutrition or alcoholism; age over 50; ultrasonographic or CT scans showing multiple lesions; signs of peritonitis; evidence of toxaemia, or history of surgery for amoebiasis. A poor prognosis is associated with the development of ascites and/or coma, especially if these conditions are present in a patient that is over 50 years old, or has severe jaundice, signs of peritonitis, or toxaemia.[14]

Giardiasis

Giardiasis is a common infection of the human small intestine by the protozoan parasite *Giardia lamblia*. Most individuals are asymptomatic, but an unspecified percentage of those infected may develop acute or chronic symptoms. The acute symptoms include the sudden onset of explosive, watery, foul diarrhoea with flatulence, cramps and abdominal distension, and virtual absence of blood, mucus, or cellular exudate in stools. Subacute or chronic infections may be accompanied by flatulence, mushy foul stools, cramps, and abdominal distension, among other symptoms. Spontaneous resolution of the infection seems to be common. Diagnosis is made by the finding of trophozoites or cysts in the microscopic examination of stools. Treatment is usually effective with metronidazole, quinacrine, or furazolidone. Metronidazole is the drug of choice.[17,18]

Extraintestinal complications of giardiasis are rare and may include chronic cholecystitis with pain in the right upper quadrant of the abdomen, perhaps as a consequence of the presence of trophozoites in the gallbladder (Soto, AmJGastr, 1977; 67:265; Goldstein, AmJDigDis, 1978; 23:559). In addition, granulomatous hepatitis and cholangitis have been reported in association with chronic diarrhoea, weight loss, fever, hypoalbuminaemia and anaemia, and attributed to giardiasis (Roberts-Thomson, Gastro, 1982; 83:480). In all these reports, eradication of the parasite with specific chemotherapy produced rapid improvement of symptoms and resolution of histological changes when liver biopsy was performed.

Cryptosporidiosis

Cryptosporidium, an intestinal protozoan parasite of domestic and wild animals, has been recently found to be an uncommon cause of debilitating diarrhoea in humans. In immunocompetent patients the infection is usually self-limiting and symptoms include diarrhoea, abdominal pain, nausea, vomiting, and anorexia. In contrast, in immunocompromised patients, particularly in acquired immune deficiency disease (**AIDS**), symptoms may last for several months and produce profound weight loss. The diagnosis is based on the microscopic finding of *Cryptosporidium* in stool samples using acidfast stains to differentiate the parasite from yeasts. An effective treatment for cryptosporidiosis in humans is not available at present, although paromomycin has given promising results (Navin, RevInfDis, 1984; 6:313; Jokipii, NEJM, 1986; 315:1643; Sterling, ParasiticProtozoa, 1993; 6:159; Clinton White, JInfDis, 1994; 170: 419).

Cryptosporidium infection of the gallbladder and biliary tract has been found in 10 to 26 per cent of AIDS patients, resulting in acalculous cholecystitis, stenosis of the extrahepatic bile duct, and sclerosing cholangitis. Sonographic or CT imaging show an enlarged gallbladder with a thickened wall, dilated or irregular intra- and extrahepatic biliary ducts, and a normal or stenotic, distal common bile duct. Diagnosis is made histologically after cholecystectomy or ampullary biopsy, or by examination of the bile for oocysts. When patients infected with the human immunodeficiency virus are exposed to *Cryptosporidium*, those with CD4 + cell counts of less than 50/mm^3 are at increased risk for biliary symptoms and for death within 1 year after the infection. Paromomycin treatment decreases stool frequency and oocyst excretion, but biliary disease progresses despite long-term therapy. Surgical treatment includes cholecystectomy and sphincterotomy, with variable therapeutic success (Teixidor, Radiol, 1991; 180:51; Vakh, NEJM, 1996; 334:19).

References

1. Martínez-Palomo A. *The biology of* Entamoeba histolytica. Chichester: University Research Press/Wiley, 1982.
2. Martínez-Palomo A and Ruíz-Palacios G. Amebiasis. In Mahmoud AAF and Warren KE, eds. *Tropical and geographical medicine*. 2nd edn. New York: McGraw-Hill, 1989.
3. Martínez-Báez M. Historical introduction. In Martínez-Palomo A, ed. *Amebiasis*. Amsterdam: Elsevier Biomedical, 1986: 1–9.
4. Brumpt E. Étude sommaire de l''Entamoeba dispar' n. sp. Amibe à quistes quadrinucléés, parasite de l'homme. *Bulletin de l'Académie de Médecine (Paris)*, 1925; **94**: 943–52.
5. Martínez-Palomo A and Martínez-Báez M. Selective primary health care: strategies for control of disease in the developing world. X. Amebiasis. *Reviews of Infectious Diseases*, 1983; **5**: 1093–102.
6. Walsh JA. Prevalence of *Entamoeba histolytica* infection. In Ravdin JI, ed. *Amebiasis. Human infection by* Entamoeba histolytica. New York: Wiley, 1988: 93–105.
7. Walsh JA and Martínez-Palomo A. Control of amebiasis. In Martínez-Palomo A, ed. *Amebiasis*. Amsterdam: Elsevier Biomedical, 1986; 241–60.
8. Feachem RG, Bradley DJ, Garelick H, and Mara DD. *Sanitation and disease. Health aspects of excreta and water management*. Chichester: Wiley/World Bank, 1983: 3337–47.
9. World Health Organization. *Prevention and control of intestinal parasitic infections*. Technical Report Series 749, 1987.
10. Prathap K and Gilman R. The histopathology of acute intestinal amebiasis. A rectal biopsy study. *American Journal of Pathology*, 1970; **60**: 229–45.
11. Pérez-Tamayo R. Pathology of amebiasis. In Martínez-Palomo A, ed. *Amebiasis*. Amsterdam: Elsevier Biomedical, 1986: 45–94.
12. Martínez-Palomo A. The Biology of *Entamoeba histolytica*. In Martínez-Palomo A, ed. *Amebiasis*. Amsterdam: Elsevier Biomedical, 1986: 11–43.
13. Adams EB and MacLeod IN. Invasive amebiasis. I. Amebic dysentery and its complications. *Medicine*, 1977; **56**: 315–23.
14. Sepúlveda B and Treviño-García M. Clinical manifestations and diagnosis of amebiasis. In Martínez-Palomo A, ed. *Amebiasis*. Amsterdam: Elsevier Biomedical, 1986: 170–88.
15. Adams EB and MacLeod IN. Invasive amebiasis. II. Amebic liver abscess and its complications. *Medicine*, 1977; **56**: 325–34.
16. Guarner V. Treatment of amebiasis. In Martínez-Palomo A. ed. *Amebiasis*. Amsterdam: Elsevier Biomedical, 1986: 189–212.
17. Farthing MJG. *Giardia lamblia*. In Blaser MJ, Smith PD, Ravdin JI, Greenberg HB, and Guerrant RL, eds. *Infections of the Gastrointestinal Tract*. New York: Raven, 1995: 1081–105.
18. Hill DR. *Giardia lamblia*. In Mandell GL, Bennet JE, and Dolin R. *Principles and practice of infectious diseases*. New York: Churchill Livingstone, 1995: 2487–92.

13.3.2 Malaria

David A. Warrell and Nick Francis

Definition

In humans, malaria is an infection by one or more of four species of *Plasmodium* (*P. falciparum*, *P. vivax*, *P. ovale*, and *P. malariae*) and very rarely by monkey malarias (*P. knowlesi*, *P. simium*, or *P. cynomolgi*). The hepatocyte is the only site of initial invasion and multiplication of sporozoites injected into the bloodstream by the bite of female *Anopheles* mosquitoes. Subsequent infection of erythrocytes results in rheological, metabolic, and immunological changes and release of mediators, any of which may affect the structure and function of the liver.

Introduction[1,2]

Fever and splenomegaly in marshy areas have been recognized since the time of the Ebers Papyrus (1570 BC). Ancient Greek writers described fevers which may have been malaria, but they did not connect them with mosquito bites. Hippocrates' tertian and quartan fevers and the marsh agues of seventeenth- and eighteenth-century Britain, Holland, and southern Europe were probably malaria. A cure for these illnesses, cinchona or fever tree bark, was discovered in Peru in the seventeenth century and brought to Europe. Laveran discovered the malaria parasite in erythrocytes in unstained blood smears from patients in Constantine in 1880. Marchiafava, Bignami, and their colleagues made extensive clinical and pathological descriptions of malaria ('aestivo-autumnal fevers') in patients infected in the Pontine marshes near Rome.[3] Ross described the sexual mosquito cycle of *Plasmodium* in 1898, while the hepatic exoerythrocytic cycle was first observed by Garnham in *Hepatocystis kochi* in monkeys in 1947.

The generic name, *Plasmodium*, was adopted from the name of the vegetative state of a slime fungus, while *falciparum* is a contraction of the Latin '*falcipariendum* '('sickle producing'), referring to the sickle-shaped gametocytes of this species.

Epidemiology

The endemic area extends through tropical areas of Latin America, Haiti and the Dominican Republic, Africa, the Middle East, Asia, Indonesia, and the islands of the western Pacific. *Plasmodium vivax* is replaced by *P. ovale* in West Africa, *P. falciparum* is absent from the eastern Mediterranean, while *P. vivax* is the dominant species in most parts of the Indian subcontinent. In parts of Africa, Papua New Guinea, and elsewhere, *Anopheles* species are such efficient vectors that children are frequently infected and gradually acquire immunity. In this situation, severe disease is found only in infants and young children. Immunity will lapse in people who live outside the endemic area for several years, such as Indians who emigrate to Britain and are therefore vulnerable to infection when they return home on holiday. Epidemics of malaria have occurred in countries from which malaria had been eradicated for several years, when mosquito control lapsed, and when non-immune populations (for example 'highlanders') were moved into endemic areas. Transmission is often seasonal, usually during or immediately after the rainy season. Except in highly immune populations, malaria is unusually severe in pregnancy, and is a major cause of maternal mortality. In all populations placental malaria is deleterious to the fetus. Genetic factors conferring resistance include absence of Duffy blood group antigen for *P. vivax* and sickle-cell trait, α-thalassaemia, glucose 6-phosphate dehydrogenase deficiency, and South-East Asian ovalocytosis for *P. falciparum*. Attempts are being made to develop vaccines against the different stages of the lifecycle of *P. falciparum* and the gametocytes of *P. vivax*. Only in the case of the exoerythrocytic stage in the liver is there the possibility of inducing a cytotoxic lymphocyte response. The induction of protective immunity against malaria is made difficult by antigenic variation and diversity.

The annual global incidence of malaria is though to be about 250 000 000 clinical cases, with an estimated annual mortality between 1 and 2.5 million. About 2000 cases of imported malaria are reported in Britain each year, with 2 to 12 deaths. In France and the United States similar numbers are reported.

Prevention and control

Attempts to eradicate malaria have been replaced by national control programmes aimed at reducing the number of mosquitoes, protecting individuals by encouraging the use of insecticide-impregnated mosquito nets and domestic insecticides, and by the limited use of chemoprophylaxis in high-risk populations, such as women attending antenatal clinics in the endemic area.

Advice to those travelling to malarious areas

Travellers are advised to protect themselves against mosquitoes by using permethrin-impregnated mosquito nets, protective clothing during the transmission period from dusk to dawn, insect repellents, and insecticides in the home. Malaria must be excluded if they develop a feverish illness, especially during the first 4 to 6 weeks after their last exposure. Specific advice about chemoprophylaxis must be based on assessment of the intensity and duration of potential exposure and the side-effects of antimalarial drugs. No chemoprophylactic agent can be relied on entirely. The combination of 200 mg of proguanil daily and 300 mg of chloroquine base weekly for adults is still safe and reasonably effective in some parts of the world. Chloroquine-resistant strains of *P. falciparum* are now prevalent in all parts of the endemic area except Central America, Haiti and the Dominican Republic, and some areas of West Africa and the Middle East. In some countries the use of potentially more toxic agents such as mefloquine (Lariam®), doxycycline (Vibramycin®), and pyrimethamine–dapsone (Maloprim®) is justified. Travellers may carry a therapeutic course of an antimalarial drug such as quinine, pyrimethamine sulphadoxine (Fansidar®), or mefloquine to be taken if malarial symptoms develop when they are far from medical care.

Pathogenesis, pathology, and pathophysiology

Lifecycle

Sporozoites of all four species are injected into the bloodstream by female *Anopheles* mosquitoes (Fig. 1). They disappear rapidly into hepatocytes, perhaps via Kupffer cells (Meis, Parasitol, 1983; 86: 231). Schizonts develop and the liver cell nucleus may be displaced but there is no associated inflammation. After 6 to 16 days (the 'prepatent' period, during which the parasites are not susceptible to many antimalarial drugs) merozoites are released into the blood and invade erythrocytes. The development of some sporozoites of *P. vivax* and *P. ovale* becomes arrested and they remain dormant as hypnozoites, 5 to 6 μm in diameter, capable of causing relapses months or years later. These have been found in human liver biopsies (Short, BMJ, 1948; 1:547) and in hepatocytes cultured *in vitro*.[4] *Plasmodium falciparum* and *P. malariae* have no persisting hepatic phase but may survive in the blood to give rise to recrudescent infections. Inside erythrocytes, the parasites develop from 'ring' forms through trophozoites to multinucleated schizonts which rupture, releasing merozoites which can infect new erythrocytes but cannot reinvade the liver. Some become gametocytes which, when taken up by mosquitoes, complete a sexual cycle, producing sporozoites to infect a new human host. The prepatent

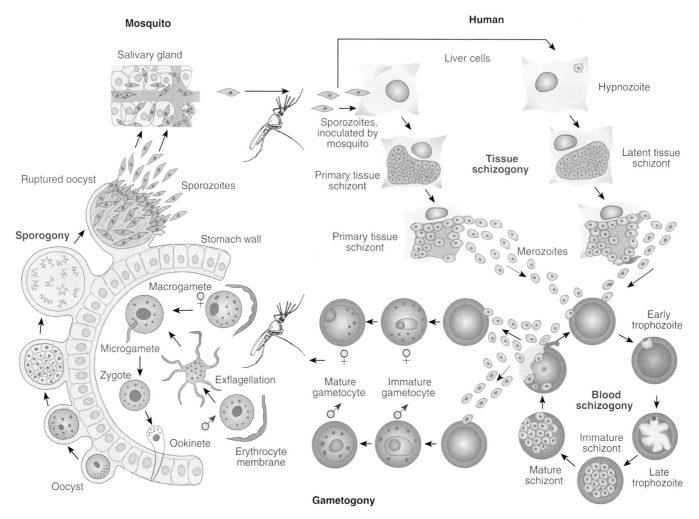

Fig. 1. Development cycle of *Plasmodium* (redrawn by permission of F. Hoffman-la-Roche Ltd, Basel).

period (interval between the infecting mosquito bite and the appearance of parasitaemia) is usually 9 to 10 days for *P. falciparum*, 8 to 13 days for *P. vivax*, 9 to 14 days for *P. ovale*, and 15 to 16 days for *P. malariae*. Incubation periods (intervals between bite and first symptom) are a few days longer.

Pathophysiology[5]

Malaria parasites are confined to hepatocytes (exoerythrocytic stages) and erythrocytes (erythrocytic stages) and are phagocytosed by cells of the reticuloendothelial system, particularly in the liver and spleen. Pathological changes result from microcirculatory disturbances caused by the sticking (cytoadherence), rosetting, and sequestration of erythrocytes containing mature forms of *P. falciparum* in some deep vascular beds, notably in the brain, retina, kidney, liver, intestine, bone marrow, skin, and placenta. Cytoadherence is caused by a specific interaction between malarial antigens expressed on the erythrocyte surface as knob-like protuberances, probably the variable proteins PfEMP-1, and endothelial receptors, such as intercellular adhesion molecule-1 (**ICAM-1**), CD36, thrombospondin, E-selectin, and vascular cell adhesion molecule-1 (**VCAM-1**) (Berendt, Parasitol, 1994; 108:S19). The

secondary effects of sequestration include hypoxia and local production of lactate by sequestered parasites. Schizont rupture produces fever by releasing a malarial pyrogen which activates macrophages to release cytokines such as tumour necrosis factor-α and interleukin-1.

Pathophysiology of hepatic abnormalities in malaria

In uncomplicated falciparum malaria, hepatic blood flow is increased as in other infective fevers, but in severe falciparum malaria blood flow is reduced to below 50 per cent of the convalescent value and there are abnormalities of intestinal absorption of sugars consistent with reduced splanchnic blood flow (Molyneux, AmJTropMedHyg, 1989; 40:470; Pukrittayakamee, ClinSci, 1992; 82:63). In rhesus monkeys infected with *P. knowlesi*, there is evidence of vasoconstriction of hepatic veins mediated by the sympathetic nervous system (Ray, IndJMedRes, 1958; 46:367; Skirrow, AnnTropMed, 1964; 58:502). Evidence of hepatic dysfunction in malaria includes conjugated hyperbilirubinaemia, hypoalbuminaemia, impaired gluconeogenesis resulting in hypoglycaemia and lactic acidosis, and reduction in hepatic synthesis of clotting factors, reflected by prolonged clotting times and elevated INR. Caffeine clearance is reduced in acute severe falciparum malaria, indicating impaired hepatic microsomal metabolism (Wilairatana, AnnTropMedParasit, 1994; 88:13). Venous lactate concentrations are inversely related to liver blood flow in acute severe falciparum malaria, suggesting that reduced blood flow may contribute to abnormal hepatic lactate clearance (Pukrittayakamee, ClinSci, 1992; 82:63). Hepatic metabolism of antimalarial drugs may also be impaired in malaria. In humans, parasitized erythrocytes are found blocking sinusoidal vessels and small vessels in the submucosa of the gastrointestinal tract. Ischaemia of the bowel may be responsible for mucosal changes (even ulceration) and the passive absorption from the lumen of endotoxin. Endotoxaemia is detectable in some cases, especially in those with high parasitaemias, and may contribute to release of cytokines and inhibition of hepatic gluconeogenesis. Antimalarial drugs may damage the liver. Quinine may cause granulomatous hepatitis, and Fansidar® and amodiaquine have caused hepatitis. Amodiaquine hepatotoxicity is attributable to a quinoneimine metabolite together with an antiamodiaquine antibody.

Tropical splenomegaly syndrome is an abnormal immune response to recurrent malaria infections, with excessive IgM production, formation of macromolecular IgM aggregates, and hypertrophy of the splenic reticuloendothelial system which phagocytoses these immune complexes. There are some differences between the condition in Africa and in Papua New Guinea and Indonesia. In Africa, peripheral lymphocytosis results from increased circulating B lymphocytes, whereas T-cell numbers are normal. In Indonesia, T8 were reduced and there was no increase in B-cell numbers. In Ghana, some patients developed a malignant lymphoproliferative disorder with circulating villous lymphocytes (Bates, Lancet, 1991; 337:505).

Pathology

The persistent exoerythrocytic (hepatic) cycle of vivax and ovale malarias is not thought to produce pathological changes in the hepatocyte, except for the presence of hypnozoites. However, severe generalized fatty metamorphosis has been described in an asymptomatic child who moved to the United States after spending the first 30 months of his life in Papua New Guinea. Electron microscopy revealed large and small cytoplasmic vacuoles with normal organelles (Ghishan, AmJGastr, 1980; 74:532). The liver is enlarged by oedema and is soft, congested, and coloured pink, tan, brown, grey, or even black, the slaty-grey colour resulting from the hyperplasia of Kupffer cells containing malarial pigment. In acute infection the liver may be friable, becoming firmer with chronicity. Lobular accentuation is caused by pigment in the portal tracts.

The findings are similar in all forms of malaria but tend to be more severe in *P. falciparum* infection. The major changes are in sinusoids and lining cells, with relatively little damage to hepatocytes. Since there is no direct infection of hepatocytes during the symptomatic phase of malaria we consider the term 'hepatitis' inappropriate.

In early infection there is sinusoidal dilatation and congestion, with Kupffer cell hyperplasia (initially in the periportal zone), parasitized red cells, and fine pigment in red cells and Kupffer cells. There is phagocytosis of both parasitized and non-parasitized red cells by Kupffer cells, endothelial cells, and sinusoidal macrophages,

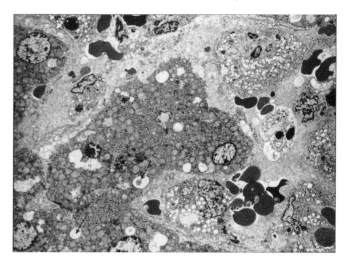

Fig. 2. Liver sinusoids containing numerous parasitized erythrocytes, with swollen endothelial cells and fat droplet formation within hepatocytes (arrow) (electron micrograph, × 1080).

which are increased in number and probably recruited from the spleen. Parasitized red cells fill the sinusoids (Fig. 2). Small areas of central liver cell necrosis are difficult to separate from effects of coexistent shock or disseminated intravascular coagulation, and may not be directly attributable to the parasites. However, individual hepatocyte necrosis, in association with fatty change, has been described. There is often reduced hepatocyte glycogen, on periodic acid–Schiff (**PAS**) staining and ultrastructurally, which may partly explain some cases of hypoglycaemia. In general, the histological severity does not correlate well with abnormalities of liver function.[6]

Later in the disease pigment becomes clumped, macrophages are increased in the sinusoids, and there is a chronic inflammatory infiltrate and pigment deposition in the portal tracts.

Ultrastructurally, most of the parasitized red cells contain trophozoites and may be knobbed or knobless. Parasitized red cells are seen in Kupffer cells and endothelial cells. Characteristic rectangular crystalline malarial pigment granules (see below) are seen in these cells and in parasitized red cells. The crystals are soluble in alkaline lead citrate and therefore appear as electron-lucent areas.[7] Partially degenerate parasitized and non-parasitized red cells are also seen. Sites of 'attachment' between knobbed parasitized red cells and phagocytic cells can be demonstrated (Fig. 3). The hepatocytes, apart from containing lipofuscin and sometimes haemosiderin (see below), show some fat droplet formation (Fig. 2), swollen mitochondria with eventual depletion, narrowing of the space of Disse with loss of microvilli, and loss of microvilli of the bile canaliculi. These last two features have been suggested as the basis of hepatic dysfunction and cholestasis.[8,9]

In cases with disseminated intravascular coagulation, fibrin may be seen in sinusoids; and when there is associated anaemia, haemopoietic elements may be seen, predominantly in the periportal area.

Tropical splenomegaly syndrome (hyper-reactive malarial splenomegaly)

In this syndrome more than 80 per cent of cases show a characteristically dense lymphocyte infiltration of the sinusoids,

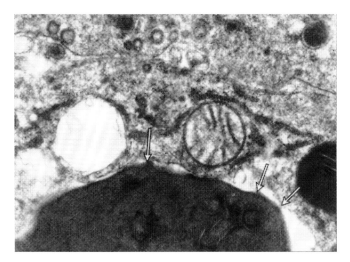

Fig. 3. Sites of attachments between parasitized 'knobby' red-cell and endothelial-cell cytoplasm (arrow) (electron micrograph, × 21 335).

suggesting leukaemia, as well as Kupffer cell hyperplasia with occasional pigment and variable portal tract chronic inflammation. Parasitized red cells are not usually seen. This hepatic sinusoidal lymphocytosis is not essential for a diagnosis of tropical splenomegaly syndrome (see below) and is not diagnostic. Most of the cells are T lymphocytes and there is evidence of sensitization to hepatic antigens.[10]

Pigments

Malarial pigment is an acid haematin related to formalin pigment. These are indistinguishable by light microscopy in formalin-fixed tissue. Fixation in buffered formalin will allow distinction as artefactual formalin pigment is not produced but malarial pigment is preserved. Iron in its ferric form, as in haemosiderin pigment, appears as golden-brown granules, which may be distinguished from formalin or malarial pigment by their positive reaction with Perls' prussian blue. Other forms of complexed iron can only be demonstrated by pretreatment with hydrogen peroxide. Lipofuscins are probably derived from breakdown products of oxidation of lipids and lipoproteins and exist in several forms. They may be widespread in human tissues where they appear as small, brownish granules and may be demonstrated by the PAS, Schmorl's, or Sudan Black B methods of staining.

Clinical features and complications

Gastrointestinal symptoms are quite common in malaria. They include nausea, vomiting, abdominal pain, which may be colicky, and watery diarrhoea without blood or pus cells (Hills, AmJMedSci, 1946; 212:45).

Tender enlargement of the liver and spleen is a common finding in all human malarias, especially in young children or non-immune adults. In children less than 3 years old infected with *P. vivax* in India, 83 per cent had splenomegaly and 68 per cent hepatomegaly (Patwari, ArchDisChild, 1979; 54:139). Forty-one per cent of Korean war veterans in America with relapsing vivax malaria had hepatomegaly and 52 per cent splenomegaly. Jaundice generally indicates severe disease and is more common in adults than in

children. Nineteen per cent of patients with falciparum malaria in eastern Thailand were jaundiced, but in those with parasitaemias of more than 100 000/ml, 45 per cent were jaundiced (Hall, AnnProgrRepSEATOMedResLab, 1974–5; 234). In vivax malaria jaundice is much less common. Hepatic failure has not been attributed convincingly to malaria. Published reports of hepatic encephalopathy (Joshi, Liver, 1986; 6:357) and hepatic necrosis (Gupta, JAssocPhysInd, 1984; 32:921) are more suggestive of cerebral malaria, acute fatty change of late pregnancy, or associated viral hepatitis. Other complications of severe falciparum malaria include anaemia, hyperpyrexia, renal failure, pulmonary oedema, massive intravascular haemolysis ('blackwater fever'), and lactic acidosis. Vivax malaria may be complicated by anaemia and splenomegaly (predisposing to splenic rupture). *Plasmodium malariae* infection may lead to quartan malarial nephrosis. The effect of chronic hepatic dysfunction on the outcome of severe malaria has not been investigated.

Tropical splenomegaly syndrome (hyper-reactive malarial splenomegaly), also known as 'big spleen disease', is defined by the presence of splenomegaly, elevation of serum IgM, and clinical and immunological response to antimalarial prophylaxis. Evidence of immunity to malaria and hepatic sinusoidal lymphocytosis (see above) are additional criteria. Some individuals in the malaria-endemic region, especially in tropical Africa and PapuaNew Guinea, show a progressive, sometimes massive, enlargement of the spleen, instead of the usual reduction in splenic size after childhood. Symptoms include a vague dragging sensation and occasional episodes of severe sharp pain with peritonism, suggesting perisplenitis or splenic infarction. Anaemia may become severe enough to cause the features of high output cardiac failure, and acute haemolytic episodes are described especially in pregnancy. The spleen may be enormous, filling the left iliac fossa, extending across the midline and anteriorly, producing a visible mass with an obvious notch. In 80 per cent of patients there is non-tender hepatomegaly, especially of the left lobe. The untreated mortality is high and usually attributable to overwhelming infection arising in the skin or respiratory system.

Investigations

Malaria is diagnosed by finding parasites in thick or thin films stained with Giemsa, Field's stain, or one of the other Romanowsky stains. Preparation of thick blood films, a simple concentration method, is essential for the diagnosis or exclusion of malaria. Anaemia is common and thrombocytopenia is found in falciparum and vivax infections. The white count may be low in mild infections but in severe malaria neutrophil leucocytosis is associated with a poor prognosis. Bilirubinaemia is predominantly of the unconjugated (van den Bergh indirect) type, indicating haemolysis (Wilairatana, TropMedParas, 1994; 45:298), but in severe falciparum malaria there is an increase in conjugated (direct) bilirubin, indicating hepatocellular damage. Some patients with blackwater fever show evidence of cholestasis. In severe falciparum malaria, other evidence of hepatic dysfunction includes moderate (five- to tenfold) elevation in levels of serum aminotransferases and 5'-nucleotidase, prolonged prothrombin time, decreased serum albumin concentration, lactic acidosis, hypoglycaemia and changes in triglycerides, phospholipids, free fatty acids, cholesterol, and esterified cholesterol and non-esterified fatty acids. Bromsulphthalein, indocyanine green, and caffeine clearances are reduced in acute severe malaria.

In tropical splenomegaly syndrome the blood picture is that of 'hypersplenism'; that is, normochromic, normocytic anaemia, reticulocytosis, thrombocytopenia, leucopenia but, especially in West Africa, peripheral lymphocytosis (which may cause confusion with chronic lymphatic leukaemia) and lymphocytic infiltration of the bone marrow. The raised serum IgM is polyclonal. Immune complexes, cryoglobulins, rheumatoid factor-like antiglobulins, and other autoantibodies have been detected. Levels of both IgM and IgG antimalarial antibodies are raised.

Diagnosis and differential diagnosis[11]

Malaria should be considered in the differential diagnosis of any patient with fever who may have visited a malarious area, or has received a blood transfusion, organ transplant, or contaminated intravenous injection. The combination of acute fever, jaundice, and tender hepatosplenomegaly, with or without a bleeding tendency, may also suggest viral hepatitis, yellow fever, viral haemorrhagic fevers, leptospirosis, and relapsing fevers (borreliosis). 'Viral hepatitis' is a common and potentially dangerous misdiagnosis in travellers with severe falciparum malaria returning to Western countries. The diagnosis of malaria can only be confirmed by finding parasites in thick or thin blood films, but parasites may not be found despite repeated examinations in some patients with severe disease. If there is reasonable suspicion of severe malaria, a therapeutic trial of quinine should be started without delay.

Tropical splenomegaly syndrome must be distinguished from other causes of chronic painless massive splenomegaly, including leukaemias, lymphomas, myelofibrosis, thalassaemias, haemoglobinopathies, visceral leishmaniasis (examine bone marrow, liver biopsy, or splenic aspirate), and schistosomiasis (examine stool, liver biopsy, or rectal snip). Normal or low IgM and impaired cellular immune responses distinguish chronic lymphatic leukaemia. Hepatic sinusoidal lymphocytosis is also seen in non-tropical idiopathic splenomegaly (in which the serum IgM is normal) and Felty's syndrome.

Treatment and prognosis[11]

The choice of antimalarial drug and the route of administration depends on the species of malaria, the geographical origin of *P. falciparum* infections and the severity of the infection (see Tables 1, 2,3). Supportive treatment includes anticonvulsant treatment and correct nursing for cerebral malaria, blood transfusion for severe anaemia, correction of hypovolaemia while avoiding fluid overload, the risk of pulmonary oedema, and the treatment and prevention of metabolic acidosis, pulmonary oedema, renal failure, shock, and secondary bacterial infections, and monitoring for and treatment of hypoglycaemia and acute renal failure. In patients with *P. falciparum* hyperparasitaemia (>10 per cent) or deterioration despite optimal chemotherapy, exchange blood transfusion should be considered. Two possible consequences of hepatic dysfunction may require treatment: hypoglycaemia not associated with quinine-induced

Table 1 Chemotherapy of malaria

Species	
P. falciparum (or unknown)	Quinine/quinidine ± tetracycline (Sulphonamide–pyrimethamine) (Mefloquine)
P. vivax[a] *P. ovale*[a] *P. malariae*	Chloroquine

[a] A course of primaquine is required to eliminate hepatic hypnozoites.

Table 2 Chemotherapy of uncomplicated malaria: patients who can swallow tablets (adult doses)

Chloroquine	Day 1, 300 mg BASE × 3 Days 2 and 3, 300 mg × 1
Quinine	600 mg SALT thrice daily (±250 mg tetracycline four times daily)[a] for 7 days
Sulphonamide–pyrimethamine	Fansidar® (sulfadoxine 500 mg + pyrimethamine 25 mg) × 3
Mefloquine	250 mg BASE × 2, after 6–8 h 250 mg × 2
Primaquine	15 mg/day, days 4–17 (after chloroquine) OR 45 mg/week for 8 weeks

[a] Not in pregnant women and children younger than 8 years.

Table 3 Chemotherapy of severe malaria: parenteral regimens

Quinine dihydrochloride
IV infusion 20 mg SALT/kg over 4 h (loading)
THEN 10 mg SALT/kg over 4 h every 8–12 h for 7 days[a]
OR IM (anterior thigh) same dose
Quinidine gluconate
IV infusion 10 mg SALT/kg over 1–2 h
THEN 0.02 mg SALT/kg/min by infusion pump for 72 h[a]
Artemether[b]
IM injection 3.2 mg/kg
THEN 1.6 mg/kg/day for 6 days
Artesunate[b]
IV injection 2 mg/kg (loading) followed by 1 mg/kg after 12 h
THEN 1 mg/kg/day for 6 days

[a] Or until patient can complete a 7-day course with oral quinine followed by tetracycline (see Table 2).
[b] Not licensed in some countries.
IM, Intramuscular(ly); IV, intravenous.

hyperinsulinaemia, and lactic acidosis. The mortality of severe falciparum malaria is still between 10 and 50 per cent, but deaths from other malarial species are rare, except in small children or severely debilitated patients. However, chronic quartan malarial nephrosis carries a bad prognosis.

Most patients with tropical splenomegaly syndrome respond within 12 months of starting antimalarial chemoprophylaxis. The spleen eventually shrinks to normal size and there is a fall in serum

IgM. Prophylaxis should be continued as long as the patient remains in the malarial endemic area. Splenectomy, splenic irradiation, and antimitotic agents are dangerous and unnecessary. Folic acid supplements may be required.

References

1. Garnham PCC. History of discoveries of malaria parasites and of their life cycles. *History and Philosophy of the Life Sciences*, 1988; **10**: 93–108.
2. Bruce-Chwatt LJ. History of malaria from prehistory to eradication. In Wernsdorfer WH and McGregor I, eds. *Malaria principles and practice of malariology*. Edinburgh: Churchill Livingstone, 1988: 1–59.
3. Marchiafava E, Bignami A. *On summer–autumn malarial fevers.* Translated from the 1st Italian edn. by JH Thompson. London: The New Sydenham Society, 1894: 112–17.
4. Hollindale MR. Malaria and the liver. *Hepatology*, 1985; **5**: 327–35.
5. Warrell DA. Pathophysiology of severe falciparum malaria in man. *Parasitology*, 1987; **94**: S53–S76.
6. McMahon AE, Kelsey JE, and Derauf DE. Hepatitis of malarial origin. *Archives of Internal Medicine*, 1954; **93**: 379–86.
7. Rosen S, Roycroft DW, Hano JE, and Barry KG. The liver in malaria: electronmicroscopic observations on a hepatic biopsy obtained 15 minutes post mortem. *Archives of Pathology*, 1967; **83**: 271–7.
8. de Brito T, Barone AA, and Faria RM. Human liver biopsy in *Plasmodium falciparum* and *Plasmodium vivax*. *Virchows Archives*, 1969; **348**: 220–9.
9. Bhamarapravati N, Boonpucknavig S, Boonpucknavig V, and Ya-emboonruang C. Glomerular changes in acute *Plasmodium falciparum* infection. *Archives of Pathology*, 1973; **96**: 289–93.
10. Gilles HM and Warrell DA. *Bruce–Chwatt's essential malariology*, 3rd edn. London: Edward Arnold, 1993.
11. Bradley DJ, Newbold CI, and Warrell DA. Malaria. In Weatherall DJ, Ledingham JGG, and Warrell DA, eds. *Oxford textbook of medicine*. Oxford: Oxford University Press, 1996; **1**: 835–63.

13.3.3 Visceral leishmaniasis

A. D. M. Bryceson and Robert N. Davidson

Definition

Visceral leishmaniasis (kala-azar) is a systemic infection with the protozoan *Leishmania donovani*, or the closely related *L. infantum* (called *L. chagasi* in the Americas). Occasionally, *L. tropica* can cause typical or atypical visceral leishmaniasis.[1] Visceral leishmaniasis is distinct from cutaneous leishmaniasis, and from mucocutaneous leishmaniasis, which are caused by other species of *Leishmania*. *Leishmania infantum* may, less commonly, cause simple, self-healing sores and *L. donovani* causes post-kala-azar dermal leishmaniasis.

Introduction

Epidemics of kala-azar (black sickness), Burdwan fever, Dumdum fever etc. were well recognized in Assam, Bihar, and Bengal long before the discovery of the parasite, at autopsy, by Leishman (Leishman, BMJ, 1903; 1:1252) and its illustration by Donovan, who found it in the spleens of patients in Madras (Donovan, BMJ, 1903; 2:1401). Christophers demonstrated the cycle in the sandfly in 1925. Treatment with trivalent antimonials was introduced

by Vianna in 1912, and with pentavalent antimonials by Brahmachari in the 1920s. Definition of the geographical limits, and clinical effects, of the 15 or so species of *Leishmania* that infect humans has been achieved by detailed epidemiological investigation supported more recently by isoenzyme and DNA technology and the use of monoclonal antibodies and polymerase chain reaction (**PCR**). All aspects of the leishmaniases have been reviewed extensively.[2]

Epidemiology

Leishmania are parasites of a wide range of vertebrate hosts, and are transmitted by several species of sandfly (Table 1). The epidemiological pattern of human disease reflects the nature of contact with infected sandflies, which may in turn reflect an underlying zoonosis. Sandflies require a precise microclimate, that may only be provided in precise locations of each endemic focus at certain seasons of the year. Sandfly numbers fluctuate widely, depending on climate and competing species. Populations of animal reservoirs and immunity of human populations also change. Thus visceral leishmaniasis is commonly sporadic or epidemic rather than steadily endemic. In general, males are affected four times more often than females.

Visceral leishmaniasis is found in four main geographical zones (Fig. 1). A country-by-country review has been published recently by WHO.[3]

In the belt that embraces the Mediterranean littoral and stretches across the Middle East and Central Asia into northern and eastern China, *L. infantum* causes a zoonosis among dogs, foxes, and jackals. Typically, canine cases outnumber human cases by more than 1000 to 1. Human disease is endemic in many places, and children under 5 years of age are especially affected. Non-immune adults such as tourists, hunters, and soldiers are susceptible. The total number of cases in Europe among immunocompetent patients is probably less than 1000 per annum; an increasing number of visceral leishmaniasis patients are, in addition, found to be co-infected by human immunodeficiency virus (**HIV**), see below.

The Ganges and Brahmaputra valleys of India and Bangladesh are the homes of epidemic visceral leishmaniasis or kala-azar, caused by *L. donovani*. The disease appeared every 15 to 20 years until 1947, when DDT spraying during the national Malaria Eradication Programme reduced vector densities. Visceral leishmaniasis often spreads from India into Bangladesh (>10 000 cases in 1990) and other parts of the continent. *Phlebotomus argentipes* rests in cattle sheds in the villages and bites humans in the houses at night. In the interepidemic period the parasite survives in the skin of patients with post-kala-azar dermal leishmaniasis. Most cases are more than 15 years old. Incidence rates may be as high as 6 per cent, focally. In the state of Bihar alone over 100 000 cases were reported in 1977, and 54 000 in 1990—this is perhaps a fivefold underestimate. Mortality varies from 1 to 80 per cent, depending upon the stage of the epidemic and the availability of treatment.[4]

In Africa, visceral leishmaniasis is highly endemic in Sudan; a major epidemic in the western Upper Nile since 1988 has affected perhaps 100 000 cases. In Kenya, visceral leishmaniasis has increased since 1980, with six endemic foci, and outbreaks occur especially in older children. Skin test surveys suggest that up to 30 per cent of the population become infected, usually subclinically.

Table 1 Features of visceral leishmaniasis

Clinical features of visceral leishmaniasis in the Sudan

Age	22% <9 years, 44% <15 years
Fever	81–100%
Family history of visceral leishmaniasis	63–76%
Duration of symptoms	2–4 months (shorter in children)
Wasting	70–100%
Loss of appetite	62–74%
Spleen uncomfortable	81–88%
Cough	72–83%
Epistaxis	44–55%
Diarrhoea	25–55%
Vomiting	2–37%
Splenomegaly	93–98%
Hepatomegaly	55–65%
Lymphadenopathy	55–86% (uncommon outside of Africa)
Jaundice	2–7%
Oedema	2–7%

Laboratory findings in Sudanese and Indian patients with visceral leishmaniasis

Anaemia	61–92%
Leucopenia	84%
Thrombocytopenia	73%
Albumin <30 g/l	88%
Globulin >30 g/l	98%
Elevated bilirubin	17%
Elevated AST or ALT	22%
Elevated alkaline phosphatase	40%

Diagnostic tests

Positive DAT or IFAT	95%
Parasitologically proven	96%

Outcome with antimonial treatment

Deaths during treatment	3%
Response to treatment	90%
Self-reported relapse after treatment	4–7%
PKDL after treatment	5–55%

Sources: Perea *et al*. (1991), 100 patients [13]; Zijlstra *et al.* (1992), 43 children, 45 adults [14]; Zijlstra *et al.* (1991), 693 patients [15]; Zijlstra *et al.* (1992), 91 patients [10]; Aggarwal *et al.* (1990), 60 patients [16].
DAT, Direct agglutination test; IFAT, indirect immunofluorescence test; PKDL, post-kala-azar dermal leishmaniasis.

In South America the disease is most common in north-eastern Brazil, where the infection is becoming urbanized.[5] As in Europe, canines are the reservoirs: the usual rate of infection in domestic dogs is 3 to 13 per cent. In one endemic area, 7.5 per cent of children under the age of 15 years were seropositive: 60 per cent of these remained subclinical. Undernutrition is associated with progression to clinical disease.[6]

Rare modes of transmission

Visceral leishmaniasis may be transmitted by blood transfusion from subclinical cases. It may be found unexpectedly in immuno-suppressed individuals, for example after renal transplantation, immunosuppressive therapy, or AIDS,[7] many years after exposure to infection. The frequent finding of visceral leishmaniasis among AIDS patients in southern Europe, many of whom were injecting drug users, suggests that contaminated needles and syringes could be a route of transmission. Congenital visceral leishmaniasis has occasionally been reported.[8]

Prevention and control

Where humans are the only reservoir (as in Africa and India), case-finding and treatment of patients with visceral leishmaniasis and post-kala-azar dermal leishmaniasis are important. Early case-finding has been helped by the use of an enzyme-linked immunosorbent assay (**ELISA**)[9] and direct agglutination[10] tests which are suit-able for field use. Domestic biting sandflies may be controlled by residual insecticide spraying. Where dogs are the reservoir, destruction of all unlicensed dogs may be helpful. Elsewhere, measures to avoid bites from sandflies may be the only preventive measure. Long sleeves and trousers, insect repellents, and the impregnation of mosquito nets and clothing (Soto, ClinInfect Dis, 1995; 21:599) with permethrin are helpful. There is no vaccine.

Pathogenesis and pathology
Lifecycle

Leishmania multiply in the gut of the female sandfly in their promastigote form (elongated, motile, and with an anterior

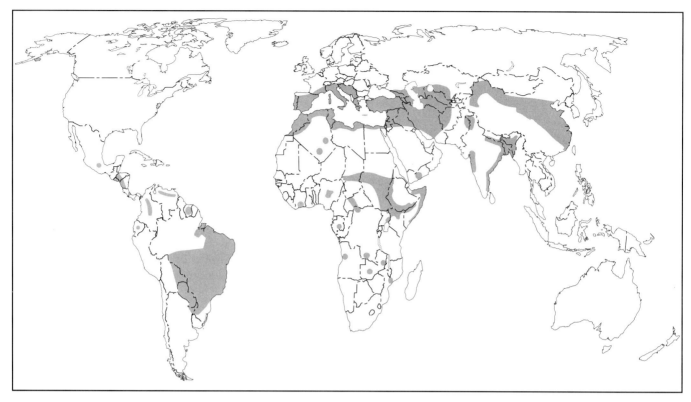

Fig. 1. Map showing geographical distribution of visceral leishmaniasis, showing the four main zones and sporadic human cases.

flagellum). Promastigotes migrate into the pharynx and proboscis after about 10 days of maturation. Promastigotes are inoculated intradermally while the fly is taking a blood meal. They enter macrophages and dendritic cells, in which they multiply in their amastigote or non-flagellate form as round or oval bodies 2 to 3 mm in diameter. The nucleus and kinetoplast stain deeply with Giemsa and give the organism its characteristic appearance (Fig. 2).

Early and subclinical infection

The majority of infections (perhaps 60–95 per cent) are subclinical. Parasites are eliminated either in the skin or liver. In others, a transient mild febrile illness develops, seroconversion confirms the infection, and parasites may be seen briefly in hepatic granulomata.[11] An unknown proportion of infections with *L. infantum* produce localized nodules in the skin, which crust, ulcerate, and heal after some months, without causing visceral disease. All these forms of infection seem to confer lifelong immunity against re-infection, but the parasite is not eliminated and may reappear if immunity is suppressed. Healing is accompanied by evidence of cell-mediated immunity: the leishmanin test becomes positive and lymphocytes transform *in vitro* to leishmanial antigens. Histology of skin and liver lesions shows tuberculoid granulomas. Antibody titres are low and transient.

Established disease

Established visceral leishmaniasis is characterized by failure of specific cellular immunity. The leishmanin test is negative and lymphocytes do not respond to leishmanial antigens. The parasite multiplies freely in macrophages and reticuloendothelial cells in spleen, bone marrow, lymphoid tissues, and jejunal mucosa. In the liver Kupffer cells are parasitized.[12] There is an interstitial pneumonitis of mononuclear cells, some of which are parasitized (Duarte, TrRSocTropMedHyg, 1989; 83:73). In the spleen especially, there is massive reticuloendothelial hyperplasia and infiltration with plasma cells and Russell bodies. Small splenic infarcts may develop. Globulins are overproduced, particularly IgG, some of which is specific antileishmanial antibody and some autoantibody, especially rheumatoid factor. Complement is activated and immune complexes, commonly containing IgM, circulate in high titre. Surprisingly, these events seldom cause much physiological disorder. Immune-complex-mediated nephritis is rare. At autopsy, kidneys show tubular cloudy swelling and sometimes thickening of the glomerular mesangium or amyloid deposition.

Biochemical tests of hepatic function are usually virtually normal. The low plasma albumin may reflect an intestinal lesion, or the switch of hepatocyte protein synthesis to acute phase proteins (Wasunna, TrRSocTropMedHyg, 1995; 89:678). About half the patients have mild malabsorption of xylose and vitamin A, but seldom diarrhoea. The cause of occasional jaundice in visceral leishmaniasis is obscure: it is more usually due to intercurrent viral hepatitis than visceral leishmaniasis itself or drugs. Spontaneous bleeding is unusual, and is associated with hypoprothrombinaemia. Cardiopulmonary function, though never measured, seems unimpaired unless anaemia is very severe.

Visceral leishmaniasis is characterized by anaemia, leucopenia, and thrombocytopenia. These cells are destroyed in the spleen and their circulating half-life is reduced. Complement activation is thought to damage erythrocytes, and in a few cases in which severe haemolysis develops rapidly early in the disease, anti-red cell

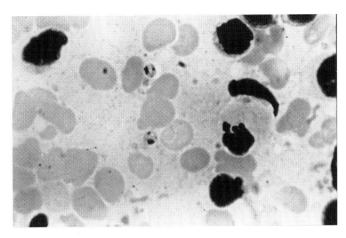

(a)

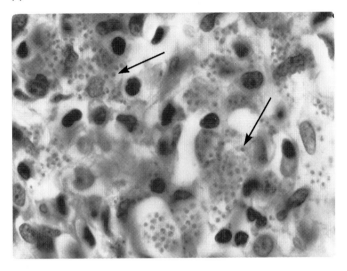

(b)

Fig. 2. (a) Two amastigotes of *L. donovani* in the splenic aspirate of a patient with visceral leishmaniasis. Parasites are usually extracellular in smears, because the macrophages that contain them rupture when the smear is made: they are intracellular in tissue sections. (b) *L. donovani* in Kupffer cells in the liver (× 1000).

antibodies have been demonstrated. The bone marrow is usually hyperplastic, but may show features of maturation arrest and deficiencies of iron or folate if these are locally endemic.

There is also a general suppression of cell-mediated immune responses, characterized by cutaneous anergy to intradermal antigens. *In vitro*, lymphocytes fail to respond to these antigens and their response to phytohaemagglutinin is reduced. It is presumed that this suppression, the leucopenia, and the hypoalbuminaemic malnutrition underlie the susceptibility to secondary infection that so often kills the patient with visceral leishmaniasis.

Clinical features and diagnosis

The incubation period is usually between 2 and 8 months. In endemic areas the onset is usually ill-defined, and several months elapse before the patient seeks help because of fever, discomfort from an enlarged spleen, abdominal swelling, weight loss, cough, or diarrhoea. Classically, the fever spikes twice daily, usually without

rigors, but daily, irregular, or undulant fevers are common. Europeans and Americans, who have acquired the disease while visiting an endemic area, more commonly experience an abrupt onset with high fever and rapid progression of illness with toxaemia, weakness, dyspnoea, and acute anaemia. Physical signs (Table 1) depend to some extent on the duration of the disease, the pre-existing nutritional state of the patient, and the presence of complications. Early cases, detected during field surveys, have only symptomless splenomegaly. Late cases are thin, with wasted muscles. One-third of cases show hair changes and pedal oedema typical of hypoalbuminaemia, but ascites is rare. Hyperpigmentation of face, hands, feet, and abdomen is characteristic of visceral leishmaniasis in India (kala-azar means black sickness). Occasionally in Africa leishmanial nodules may be found in the palate or nares. The spleen is massively enlarged, often reaching the left or even right iliac fossa. It is smooth and non-tender unless there has been a recent infarct. The liver is moderately enlarged in one-third of cases. Generalized lymphadenopathy is present in many African patients, but is less common in India or Europe. Jaundice, mucosal and retinal haemorrhage, and episcleritis are found occasionally. Visceral leishmaniasis should be considered in any person with fever of more than 4 weeks' duration and splenomegaly, who has lived in or travelled through an endemic area.

VL/HIV co-infections

Most patients co-infected with HIV and visceral leishmaniasis have advanced immunosuppression, with fewer than 200 CD4+ T lymphocytes per mm^3. Clinical features are often atypical: symptoms may be vague, laboratory abnormalities may be less severe, and hepatosplenomegaly may be absent or unimpressive. Amastigotes may be found unexpectedly in bone marrow aspirates of oligosymptomatic HIV-positive patients, or in unusual cells, such as circulating neutrophils or gut mucosa. *Leishmania* serology is negative in a third of immunosuppressed patients. Such patients may respond well to antileishmanial treatment, only to relapse 2 to 12 months later; alternatively, response to treatment may be incomplete, or the patient may be totally non-responsive, or suffer exaggerated drug toxicity.[7]

Viscerotropic Leishmania tropica infections

A few US soldiers who served in the Persian Gulf area in 1990–1991 were found to have systemic infection caused by viscerotropic *L. tropica*, normally the cause of urban cutaneous leishmaniasis in the Middle East.[1] The manifestations among these soldiers included an acute to subacute febrile illness with fatigue, arthralgia, and diarrhoea. Some soldiers recovered spontaneously, whereas others progressed to a more chronic condition, associated with adenopathy or splenomegaly. Most responded to treatment with pentavalent antimonials.

Investigations
Parasitological diagnosis

Leishmania may be isolated from material taken from reticuloendothelial tissue. Some of the sample is smeared on to glass slides, stained with Geisma, Wright's, or Leishman's stain, and

Table 2 Differential diagnosis of visceral leishmaniasis

Stage of disease	Diagnosis	Test
Acute	Malaria	Blood smears
	Typhoid	Blood cultures
Chronic	Malaria	Blood smears
	Schistosomiasis	Liver ultrasound, faeces, serology
	Tuberculosis	Liver biopsy and culture
	Brucellosis	Blood cultures
	Lymphoma	Lymph node and marrow biopsy

Table 3 Complications of visceral leishmaniasis

Anaemia, leucopenia, thrombocytopenia
Malnutrition
Immune suppression: specific and non-specific
Secondary infection
Epistaxis and other bleeding
Post-kala-azar dermal leishmaniasis
Relapse
Death

examined for amastigotes. Care, patience, and experience are needed to identify the parasite, and to distinguish it from platelets and debris. The rest of the sample is inoculated on to NNN (Novy–MacNeal–Nicolle's), supplemented Schneider's, or other suitable media, and cultured at 26 to 28 °C for up to 2 weeks. Bone marrow aspiration is most commonly used, but the technique is painful, requires special needles, and is insensitive in early cases.

Splenic aspiration is simple, painless, and safe if prothrombin time is normal and platelet count is above $40 \times 10^9/l$. Palpate the spleen and mark its outline.[17] Using a $1\frac{1}{2}$ inch $\times$ 21 gauge $(0.8 \times 40 \text{ mm})$ needle attached to a 5 ml syringe, penetrate the skin over the spleen, withdraw the plunger 1 ml and plunge the needle into the spleen upwards at an angle of 45° and withdraw immediately, maintaining suction. The liver may be aspirated in the same way. The tiny amount of material obtained is sufficient for culture and smear. Positive yields from smears of aspirates are of the following order:[10] spleen, greater than 95 per cent; bone marrow or liver, 70 to 85 per cent; lymph node (Africa), 58 to 65 per cent; and from a buffy coat preparation of blood, up to 70 per cent. Cultures yield about another 10 per cent in good hands.

Biopsies and histology

Histological examination is an inefficient way to establish the diagnosis. Parasites may be scanty and difficult to identify; in two series, 16/18 and 10/18 liver biopsies were positive.[16,18] Without them the pattern is not diagnostic. Typically, in the liver Kupffer cells are hypertrophied, hyperplastic, and heavily parasitized; a careful search may reveal occasional parasitized hepatocytes as well. Portal tracts are infiltrated with histiocytes, lymphocytes, and plasma cells. Hepatocytes may show some fatty or ballooning degenerative change. In other cases focal collections of histiocytes, lymphocytes, and plasma cells may be seen in lobules and portal tracts, with few, if any, parasites. In cases with few parasites, intralobular proliferation of reticulin and collagen fibres may be

seen. In repeat biopsies a week after the end of treatment, parasites are absent but the mononuclear inflammatory infiltrate persists. Recent studies found focal fibrosis, but no cirrhosis. Occasionally the diagnosis is made by chance from lymph node, jejunal, or skin biopsy.

Immunological diagnosis

Antileishmanial antibodies are present in high titre. Indirect immunofluorescence is suitable for individual cases, using amastigotes or promastigotes as antigen. There is some cross-reactivity, but at low titre, with antinuclear antibodies. Complement fixation was popular in the past, but sera are often anticomplementary. ELISA or direct agglutination tests are suitable for field diagnosis; they are over 95 per cent specific and sensitive[10] (Table 1). The leishmanin test is negative.

Other findings (Table 1)

The haemoglobin is below 7 g/dl (1.12 µmol/l) in half the patients, with a normochromic, normocytic picture without reticulocytosis. Leucopenia and thrombocytopenia are characteristic. Serum albumin is typically about 20 g/l, and globulin about 70 g/l. IgG and IgM are approximately three times and twice the normal population values, respectively. Complement levels (C4 and C3) are normal but Clq and immune complexes are raised. Hepatic enzymes are usually normal or slightly raised, and prothrombin and partial thromboplastin times are usually normal until late in the disease.

Differential diagnosis

The common differential diagnoses are given in Table 2, although the list of causes of febrile splenomegaly is much longer, and visceral leishmaniasis may coexist with other endemic infections.

Complications (Table 3)

Over several months the patient becomes emaciated and exhausted, with a huge protuberant spleen. Intercurrent infections are common, especially pneumococcal otitis, pneumonia and septicaemia, tuberculosis and measles, and other locally important infections such as brucellosis and dysentery. Untreated, 80 to 90 per cent of patients die. Although early studies reported cirrhosis as a complication, especially in India, recent series find intralobular fibrosis rather than true cirrhosis,[16,18,19] and it is likely that earlier studies included patients with chronic hepatitis B or C.

Table 4 Monitoring of Sb^v treatment in visceral leishmaniasis

Assessment as inpatient weekly for 4–6 weeks, then as out-patient after 6 weeks and 6 months

Fever should resolve within 10 days of therapy

Serum albumin and haemoglobin start to rise in the second week, normal by 6 weeks

ESR starts to fall in second week, normal by 3 months

Splenic size (measured in centimetres from costal margin at anterior axillary line to tip) starts to reduce in 3–4 weeks, impalpable or barely palpable by 6–12 months

Leishmanin skin test becomes positive by 6 months in 75–90% of patients

Post-kala-azar dermal leishmaniasis

Twenty per cent of Indian patients and 5 to 55 per cent of African patients develop a rash after spontaneous or natural recovery, on the face and extensor surfaces of the arms and legs. In India the rash begins after an interval of 1 to 2 years and progresses over many years: pale macules become erythematous plaques of nodules resembling lepromatous leprosy, and almost all the body surface may be involved. Histology shows macrophages with a variable degree of parasitization, and a structureless infiltrate of lymphocytes and plasma cells. In Africa the rash appears while the patient is recovering, often before leaving hospital, as discrete nodules which show a tuberculoid histology. It may heal spontaneously within 6 months but, if disfiguring or involving the mucosa of the mouth (more common in infants), it requires treatment. Post-kala-azar dermal leishmaniasis very rarely visceralizes, yet the parasite is enzymatically indistinguishable from its viscerotropic parent.

Treatment

Chemotherapy

Pentavalent antimonials

Pentavalent antimonials (Sb^v) are the traditional first-line drugs. Sodium stibogluconate (Pentostam®, Glaxo-Wellcome, UK; sodium antimony gluconate, Albert David Ltd, Calcutta) containing 100 mg Sb^v per ml, or meglumine antimoniate (Glucantime®, Rhone, Spain and Specia, France; Glucantim®, Farmitalia Carlo Erba, Milan) containing 85 mg Sb^v per ml are the two preparations available.[20, 21] They are given in a single daily dose of 20 mg Sb^v/kg body weight, for a minimum of 20 days. Intravenous injections are less painful than intramuscular. The drug is administered slowly through a fine needle to reduce the risk of superficial venous thrombosis. In this dosage toxic effects are uncommon and not serious, comprising anorexia and muscle aching. Primary resistance to Sb^v is seen in about 1 per cent of cases in Africa and over 10 per cent in Bihar. Relapse rates should be less than 5 per cent but secondary resistance is likely to develop in relapsed patients unless they are treated very thoroughly. In relapsed or immunosuppressed patients a full 20 mg Sb^v/kg or 20 mg Sb^v/kg twice daily should be given, for 4 weeks longer than it takes to eliminate parasites from splenic aspirates. Recently, hyperamylasaemia and frank pancreatitis have been recognized as complications of Sb^v (Gasser, ClinInfDis, 1994; 18:83). The ECG shows unimportant T-wave changes, and occasionally prolongation of QT interval which might predict the onset of a serious arrhythmia. In one study, systolic and diastolic blood pressure fell, and the heart rate increased, but there were no echocardiographic changes and no arrhythmias (Hepburn, QJMed, 1994; 87:465). If toxicity develops, interrupt Sb^v treatment for 1 or 2 days, and reduce the dosage by 2 mg/kg.

Amphotericin B

In India, amphotericin B is being increasingly regarded as a first-line drug for visceral leishmaniasis, partly because of an increase in Sb^v-resistant cases, and partly because of an appreciation that the toxicity of amphotericin B is lower than reputed. The dose of amphotericin B which will reliably cure Indian kala-azar is variously given as 14 doses of 0.5 mg/kg[22] and 20 doses of 1 mg/kg.[23, 24] Liposomal amphotericin B (AmBisome®) has been highly successful and non-toxic in treatment of visceral leishmaniasis in Europe (Davidson, QJMed, 1994; 87:75; Davidson, ClinInfDis, 1996) and of value in Sudan.[25] The recommended regimen is a total dose of 21 to 30 mg/kg AmBisome® given in seven or more daily doses of 2 to 4 mg/kg over a period of 10 days. Individual doses should be in multiples of 50 mg to avoid wastage of this expensive drug. Amphotericin B cholesterol dispersion (Amphocil®) has been used in Brazilian visceral leishmaniasis (Dietze, ClinInfDis, 1993; 17:981; Dietze, TrRSocTropMedHyg, 1995; 89: 309). A regimen of 2 mg/kg per day for 7 or 10 days appears suitable. Adverse events, including fever, chills, and respiratory distress, were common in children less than 3 years old, and were partly preventable by pretreatment with non-steroidal anti-inflammatory drugs.

Supportive treatment

Intercurrent infections must be sought and treated. Haemorrhage is usually associated with hypoprothrombinaemia, and may be corrected with vitamin K. Blood transfusion is rarely needed, but a protein-rich diet and supplements to replace specific nutritional deficiencies should be provided.

Monitoring

After starting treatment, patients usually feel better and fever stops in a few days. Other useful indices of recovery are given in Table 4. Patients who become leishmanin positive are probably immune for life. The significance of persisting anergy, in terms of relapse or reinfection, is not known. It is not usually necessary to obtain parasitological proof of cure, provided the clinical and laboratory features improve steadily. In relapsed or immunosuppressed patients, who will respond more slowly to treatment, and in whom the parasite might prove resistant to Sb^v, splenic aspiration should be performed weekly and parasites enumerated on a logarithmic scale.[17]

References

1. Magill AJ, Grogl M, Gasser RA, Sun W, and Oster CN. Visceral infection caused by *Leishmania tropica* in veterans of Operation Desert Storm. *New England Journal of Medicine*, 1993; **328**: 1383–7.

2. Peters W and Killick-Kendrick R, eds. *The leishmaniases in biology and medicine*. London: Academic Press, 1987.

3. WHO. *Information on the epidemiology and control of the leishmaniases by country or territory*. P. Desjeux, WHO/LEISH/91.30. Geneva: World Health Organization, 1991.

4. Thakur CP. Epidemiological, clinical and therapeutic features of Bihar kala-azar (including post kala-azar dermal leishmaniasis). *Transactions of the Royal Society of Tropical Medicine and Hygiene*, 1984; **78**: 391–8.

5. Cunha S, *et al.* Visceral leishmaniasis in a new ecological niche near a major metropolitan area of Brazil. *Transactions of the Royal Society of Tropical Medicine and Hygiene*, 1995; **89**: 155–8.

6. Cerf BJ, Jones TC, Badaro R, Sampaio D, Teixeira R, and Johnson WD Jr. Malnutrition as a risk factor for severe visceral leishmaniasis. *Journal of Infectious Diseases*, 1987; **156**: 1030–3.

7. Report on the Consultative Meeting on *Leishmania*/HIV coinfection, Rome, 6–7 September 1994. WHO/LEISH 95/35. Geneva: World Health Organization.

8. El-Toum IA, *et al.* Congenital kala-azar and leishmaniasis in the placenta. *American Journal of Tropical Medicine and Hygiene*, 1992; **46**: 57–62.

9. Ho M, Leeuwenburg J, and Mbugua G. An enzyme-linked immunosorbent assay (ELISA) for the field diagnosis of visceral leishmaniasis. *American Journal of Tropical Medicine and Hygiene*, 1983; **32**: 943–6.

10. Zijlstra EE, *et al.* Kala-azar: a comparative study of parasitological methods and the direct agglutination test in diagnosis. *Transactions of the Royal Society of Tropical Medicine and Hygiene*, 1992; **86**: 505–7.

11. Pampiglione S, Manson-Bahr PE, La Placa M, Borgatti MA, and Musumeci S. Studies in Mediterranean leishmaniasis. 3. The leishmanin skin test in kala-azar. *Transactions of the Royal Society of Tropical Medicine and Hygiene*, 1975; **69**: 60–8.

12. Duarte MIS and Corbet CEP. Histopathological patterns of the liver involvement in visceral leishmaniasis. *Revista do Instituto de Medicina Tropical de São Paolo*, 1987; **29**: 131–6.

13. Perea WA, Ancelle T, Moren A, Nagelkerke M, and Sondorp E. Visceral leishmaniasis in southern Sudan. *Transactions of the Royal Society of Tropical Medicine and Hygiene*, 1991; **85**: 48–53.

14. Zijlstra EE, *et al.* Clinical aspects of kala-azar in children from the Sudan: a comparison with the disease in adults. *Journal of Tropical Pediatrics*, 1992; **38**: 17–20.

15. Zijlstra EE, *et al.* Kala-azar in displaced people from southern Sudan: epidemiological, clinical and therapeutic findings. *Transactions of the Royal Society of Tropical Medicine and Hygiene*, 1991; **85**: 365–9.

16. Aggarwal P, Wali JP, and Chopra P. Liver in kala-azar. *Indian Journal of Gastroenterology*, 1990; **9**: 135–6.

17. Chulay JD and Bryceson ADM. Quantitation of amastigotes of *Leishmania donovani* in smears of splenic aspirates from patients with visceral leishmaniasis. *American Journal of Tropical Medicine and Hygiene*, 1983; **32**: 475–9.

18. El Hag IA, Hashim FA, El Toum IA, Homeida M, El Kalifa M, and El Hassan AM. Liver morphology and function in visceral leishmaniasis (kala-azar). *Journal of Clinical Pathology*, 1994; **47** (6): 547–51.

19. Corbett CE, Duarte MI, and Bustamante SE. Regression of diffuse intralobular liver fibrosis associated with visceral leishmaniasis. *American Journal of Tropical Medicine and Hygiene*, 1993; **49**: 616–24.

20. Bryceson ADM. Therapy in man. In Peters W and Killick-Kendrick R, eds. *The leishmaniases in biology and medicine*. London: Academic Press, 1987: 848–907.

21. WHO. *The leishmaniases*. Report of a WHO Expert Committee. Technical Report Series 701. Geneva: World Health Organization, 1984.

22. Mishra M, Biswas UK, Jha DN, and Khan AB. Amphotericin B versus pentamidine in antimony-unresponsive kala-azar. *Lancet*, 1992; **340**: 1256–7.

23. Thakur CP, Sinha GP, Pandey AK, Barat D, and Singh RK. Daily versus alternate-day regimen of amphotericin B in the treatment of kala-azar: a randomized comparison. *Bulletin of the World Health Organization*, 1994; **72**: 931–6.

24. Mishra M, Biswas UK, Jha AM, and Khan AB. Amphotericin versus sodium stibogluconate in first-line treatment of Indian kala-azar. *Lancet*, 1994; **44**: 1599–600.

25. Seaman J, *et al.* Liposomal amphotericin B (AmBisome) in the treatment of complicated kala-azar under field conditions. *Clinics in Infectious Diseases*, 1995; **21**: 188–93.

13.3.4 Toxoplasmosis

José M. Miró and José M. Gatell

Definition

Toxoplasma gondii infection is a zoonosis that occurs worldwide. The term toxoplasmosis describes the clinical or pathological disease caused by *Toxoplasma gondii* and is distinct from toxoplasma infection, which is asymptomatic in the vast majority of immunocompetent patients.[1] A chronic or latent infection (persistence of cyst forms) develops in all infected people after an acute infection (with or without clinical manifestations that may include mild and transient abnormalities of liver function tests).[1] An acute maternal infection during pregnancy may result in disseminated infection and liver involvement in the neonate.[2] Toxoplasmosis occurs almost exclusively in severely immunosuppressed patients (those with AIDS or malignancies, or transplant recipients, including liver transplant recipients) as result of a reactivation of the chronic infection and less often due to rapid progression of a newly acquired infection (when a seronegative transplant recipient receives an organ from a seropositive donor).[3] The central nervous system (encephalitis), the lung (pneumonitis), and the eye (retinochoroiditis) are the organs most frequently affected.[1,3] Disseminated forms with liver involvement have also been reported. Without adequate therapy, mortality approaches 100 per cent.[1,3]

History

T. gondii was discovered in the liver of a North African rodent by Nicolle and Manceaux in 1908 (Nicole, CRAcadSci,1908; 146:207). The first infection in humans was described in 1923.[4] In the 1940s the organism was recognized as a significant cause of acquired and congenital disease. In 1948, Sabin and Feldman described the dye test (Sabin, Science, 1948; 108:660), which is still used as the laboratory reference test for detecting toxoplasma antibodies. Reynolds *et al.* (Reynolds, ArchIntMed, 1966; 118:401) described the first case of toxoplasmosis in a solid organ transplant recipient and Vietzke *et al.* (Vietzke, Cancer, 1968; 21:816) reported the first cases of toxoplasmic encephalitis in patients with malignancies. It was not until the 1980s, as a result of the outbreak of AIDS,[5] that the disease was widely recognized; thousands of cases were reported, and a better knowledge of its pathogenesis, clinical manifestations, prophylaxis, and treatment was achieved.

Aetiology and epidemiology

T. gondii is an ubiquitous intracellular parasite of humans and animals.[1,6] There is only one species although strain-dependent differences in virulence have been reported. Cats are the definitive hosts, maintaining the enteroepithelial sexual cycle and producing oocysts which are excreted to the environment.[1,6] Other animals and humans are incidental hosts; the parasite has an extraintestinal asexual cycle which produces tachyzoites and tissue cysts. There are thus three lifeforms of *T. gondi*.[1,6]

1. Oocysts (10–12 μm) that are excreted in cats' faeces and contain sporozoites. Appropriate environmental conditions of temperature and humidity are required for their maturation (sporulation) and infectivity. Sporulation occurs only between 4 and 37°C. Oocysts remain viable for up to 18 months in moist soil.
2. Tachyzoites (3–7 μm) are the asexual invasive forms of the parasite and can invade almost all mammalian cells, multiplying in the cytoplasm within a parasitophorous vacuole by division every 4 to 6 h. They can lyse the host cell and invade adjacent cells; if the host has an adequate immunological response, a tissue cyst will form. Tachyzoites can be identified in tissue sections with haematoxylin and eosin, Wright–Giemsa, or immunoperoxidase stains.
3. Tissue cysts (10–200 μm) contain thousands of bradyzoites that can persist for life, and are responsible for chronic or latent infection. Bradyzoites can be identified with periodic acid–Schiff, Wright–Giemsa, Gomori, or immunoperoxidase stains. The cyst walls stain with Gomori or immunoperoxidase.

Cysts can develop in any organ, but the brain, heart, and skeletal muscles are the most common locations. They are relatively resistant to digestive juices, but are killed by radiation and by high or low (freezing) temperatures. The most common source of primary infection in humans is the oral route through ingestion of undercooked or raw meat (especially pork and lamb) which contains tissue cysts, or by ingestion of water and food contaminated with oocysts from cat faeces.[1,6] Other routes of infection in humans are congenital, transplanted organs from seropositive donors to previously uninfected recipients, and whole blood or leucocyte transfusions from donors with acute or disseminated infection.[1,6]

Seropositive prevalence among the general population is higher in warm countries and lower in cold countries. In western European countries (France, Spain, Switzerland), prevalence ranges between 50 and 90 per cent.[1,5] Seroprevalence above 50 per cent is also observed in Africa and South and Central America.[1,5] In the United States and Australia, seroprevalence is 3 to 30 per cent and 20 to 40 per cent respectively (Carr, JAIDS, 1993; 6:56).[1,5]

Pathogenesis

After an acute infection, which is asymptomatic in the majority of immunocompetent hosts, a chronic or latent infection develops in all patients and *T. gondii* persists in the cyst form.[1,5] Cellular immunity, macrophage activity, and some cytokines such as γ-interferon play an important role against *T. gondii* infection.[1,2] All patients with an impairment of these functions are at risk of developing toxoplasmosis.

Toxoplasmosis in HIV-infected patients almost always represents reactivation of a chronic (latent) infection and is considered an AIDS-defining disease.[5] Almost all cases of central nervous system toxoplasmosis appear in severely immunodepressed HIV-infected patients, usually with a CD4+ lymphocyte count of less than 100 cells/μl.[5] Up to 50 per cent of HIV-infected, toxoplasma seropositive patients will develop central nervous system toxoplasmosis when their CD4 cell counts drop below 100 cells/μl.[5,7] The incidence of toxoplasmosis among AIDS patients correlates with the prevalence of chronic *T. gondii* infection in a given population (see above), ranging from 5 to 10 per cent in AIDS patients from the United States and 15 to 50 per cent in southern European countries.[5]

Toxoplasmosis in non-AIDS immunodeficient patients appears in individuals with lymphoproliferative or myelopoietic malignancies, [3,8] or in bone marrow or solid organ (including liver) transplant recipients (Salt, JClinPath, 1990; 43:63; De la Loma, EnfermInfectMicroClin, 1990; 8:252).[3,9–14] The disease is usually a reactivation of a chronic infection in patients with malignancies or in bone marrow transplant recipients,[3,8,9] while in heart–lung, liver, or kidney transplant recipients it is a rapidly progressive, newly acquired infection.[10–13] Toxoplasmosis appears in seronegative recipients who receive an organ from a seropositive donor.[3,10–13] The risk depends on the type of solid organ transplant,[13] and is greater in heart or heart–lung transplant recipients (57 per cent) than in liver transplant recipients (5–20 per cent), and much lower in kidney recipients (<1 per cent) (Salt, JClinPath, 1990; 43:63; De la Loma, EnfermInfectMicroClin, 1990; 8:252).[12–14] The risk also is very low (<1 per cent) in bone-marrow transplant recipients,[9] although in some endemic areas such as France, the incidence may be higher (up to 5 per cent).[9] In our institution, three cases of central nervous system toxoplasmosis were diagnosed among 552 bone marrow transplant recipients (0.5 per cent), two cases in 352 liver transplant recipients (0.5 per cent), two cases in 1500 kidney transplant recipients (<0.1 per cent), and none in 100 pancreas transplant recipients (unpublished data). In bone-marrow and solid organ transplant recipients toxoplasmosis usually appears within the first 6 months after transplantation (mainly between 30 and 90 days).[3]

Pathology

Lymph nodes and eyes are most commonly involved in immunocompetent patients.[1] The histopathological changes of toxoplasmic lymphadenitis (Piringer–Kuchinka's lymphadenitis) are usually diagnostic of this infection.[1,15] The presence of a reactive follicular hyperplasia, irregular clusters of epithelioid histiocytes encroaching on and blurring the margins of the germinal centres, and focal distension of sinuses with monocytoid cells are very characteristic.[1,15] Eye infection produces acute chorioretinitis characterized by severe inflammation and necrosis and is considered a late manifestation of a congenital infection.[1] Although in immunocompetent patients hepatic involvement is unusual in acute acquired toxoplasmosis, several cases of acute granulomatous hepatitis have been reported (Vischer, Lancet, 1967; 2:919; Weitberg, NEJM, 1979;

300:1093; Ortego, AmJGastr, 1990; 85:1418; Martinez-Vazquez, SemHôpParis, 1975; 51:963).

The central nervous system (especially the brain and the retina), the lungs, and the heart are most commonly involved in immunodeficient patients.[1,3,5,8,16] Skeletal muscle, gastrointestinal tract, liver, pancreas, prostate, adrenals, kidneys, and bone marrow can also be involved. Brain abscesses are the typical lesions in central nervous system toxoplasmosis.[1,3,5,8] There is usually more than one lesion in basal ganglia, although cerebellar and brainstem lesions can also occur.[1,5] Diffuse toxoplasmosis has also been described.[1,5] Chorioretinitis is characterized by segmental panophthalmitis and areas of necrosis.[1] Pulmonary toxoplasmosis can appear as interstitial pneumonitis and less often as necrotizing pneumonitis or consolidation.[1,5] Myocarditis is a frequent finding at autopsy but is clinically inapparent. Focal necrosis with oedema and an inflammatory infiltrate is typical; also characteristic is the presence of myocytes packed with tachyzoites without an inflammatory response.[1] Liver involvement is characterized by focal hepatocellular necrosis (Brion, ClinInfectDis, 1992; 15:183).[16] Tachyzoites and pseudocysts can be detected in liver cells and to a lesser degree in bile duct epithelia, Kupffer cells, or mesenchymal cells of the portal tracts. Pancreatic involvement is characterized by necrotizing pancreatitis with a moderate lymphohistiocytic inflammatory infiltration.[1,5,16] Tachyzoites and pseudocysts can be detected in the necrosis, in macrophages, in epithelia of the exocrine, and occasionally in the endocrine pancreas and in the mesenchymal stroma cells. The entire gastrointestinal tract from oesophagus to colon may be involved.[1,5,16] The cellular reaction to the presence of tachyzoites may vary remarkably in different parts of the gastrointestinal tract. Haemorrhagic gastritis and colitis with virtually no inflammatory reaction in the infected oesophagus and small intestine have been described. The presence of tachyzoites is required for the diagnosis of an acute infection while the presence of cysts only represents a chronic infection.[1,3,5]

Clinical manifestations

The clinical manifestations of toxoplasmosis differ greatly with the immunological status of the host or if infection is transmitted from mother to fetus.[1–3,5,8]

Toxoplasmosis in immunocompetent patients

Acute acquired toxoplasmosis in immunocompetent patients is asymptomatic in 80 to 90 per cent.[1] An asymptomatic lymphadenopathic syndrome may be the only finding at physical examination.[1] There are usually enlarged lymph nodes in the cervical region. If patients have symptoms, the clinical course is benign and self limited in most cases and mimics a mononucleosis-like syndrome.[1] It is characterized by the presence of fever, malaise, night sweats, myalgias, sore throat, maculopapular rash, and hepatosplenomegaly. Transient abnormalities in liver function tests and/or a small number of atypical lymphocytes (<10 per cent) may be present. However, some patients can have an acute hepatitis (Vischer, Lancet, 1967; ii:919; Weitberg, NEJM, 1979; 300:1093; Ortego, AmJGastr, 1990; 85:1418; Martinez-Vazquez, SemHôpParis,1975; 51:963; Roca, MedicinaClin, 1992; 99:595; Lesur, GastrClinBiol,

1994; 18:798). When the eye is affected in adult patients, *T. gondii* chorioretinitis is usually a reactivation of a congenital infection.[1]

Toxoplasmosis in immunodeficient patients

Toxoplasmosis in AIDS patients usually involves the central nervous system (brain), followed by the eye (chorioretinitis), and the lung (pneumonitis).[1,5,17] Some AIDS patients have multiorgan involvement with acute respiratory failure, shock, and a high mortality rate (Albrect, ScaJInfectDis, 1995; 27:71). Toxoplasmosis is by far the most frequent cause of focal central nervous system lesions.[1,5] The clinical picture is usually subacute with focal neurological signs (hemiparesis, sensory or speech abnormalities, cerebellar signs) although some patients can have an acute presentation with seizures. Headache and fever are not always present. Meningeal signs are uncommon. Cerebrospinal fluid is normal. Computed tomography (**CT**) and magnetic resonance imaging (**MRI**) are the standard tools for clinical diagnosis. CT scan shows multiple bilateral cerebral lesions in 70 to 80 per cent of cases. Lesions are located at the corticomedullary junction, frequently involving the basal ganglia. They are characteristically hypodense with ring-enhancement after intravenous contrast administration. Up to 5 per cent of AIDS patients with central nervous system toxoplasmosis have a normal CT scan, the lesions being apparent only on MRI (Knobel, AmJMed, 1995; 99:220). MRI has a higher sensitivity than CT. Lesions on MRI appear as a low-signal abnormalities on T_1-weighted imaging and as high-signal abnormalities on T_2-weighted imaging, after gadolinium uptake. Differential diagnosis in AIDS patients includes lymphoma and, less often, tuberculoma, cryptococoma, or fungal infections.[1,5] Brain positron emission tomography (**PET**) or single photon emission computed tomography (**SPECT**) can be very useful for rapid differential diagnosis between cerebral toxoplasmosis and lymphoma (Pierce, AnnIntMed, 1995; 123:594; Lorberboym, JNuclMed, 1996; 37:1150). There may be extraneurological involvement simultaneously or independently in about 20 to 30 per cent of cases.[17] Toxoplasma chorioretinitis is second in frequency to brain involvement.[1,5] Fundoscopic examination usually demonstrates necrotizing lesions that may be multifocal or bilateral. Overlying vitreal inflammation is often present and may be extensive. These findings are very different from those in cytomegalovirus retinitis, the most common eye infection in AIDS patients. Toxoplasma chorioretinitis is associated with concurrent toxoplasmic encephalitis in up to 50 per cent of cases. Pulmonary disease due to *T. gondii* is increasingly recognized in patients with AIDS (Pomeroy, ClinInfectDis, 1992; 14:863).[1,5,17] The clinical picture is very similar to that in *Pneumocystis carinii* pneumonia. Extrapulmonary disease may be present in about 50 per cent of cases and mortality may be as high as 35 per cent. The differential diagnosis includes *Pneumocystis carinii* pneumonia and *Mycobacterium tuberculosis* pulmonary infection. Gastrointestinal tract (abdominal pain, ascites, diarrhoea), liver (acute hepatic failure), and pancreatic (pancreatitis) involvement have been described but are uncommon (<5 per cent).[1,3,5,16,17]

Toxoplasmosis in immunocompromised patients without AIDS occurs in those with malignancies, in transplant-recipient (including liver) patients, and, less frequently, in patients with systemic lupus erythematosus or other collagen–vascular diseases, or in patients receiving corticosteroids.[1,3,8] Most patients with malignancies have

Hodgkin's lymphoma.[3,8] Other predisposing malignancies are non-Hodgkin's lymphoma, and acute or chronic lymphocytic or myelogenous leukaemia; toxoplasmosis has also been reported anecdotally in a wide variety of non-haematological malignancies.[3,8] In transplant-recipient patients, toxoplasmosis has been reported (by decreasing order of frequency) in recipients of heart or heart–lung, bone marrow, liver, and renal transplants.[3,9–13] The central nervous system is most frequently involved, followed by the heart and the lung.[1,3] Liver and pancreatic involvement is diagnosed in 5 to 15 per cent and 5 per cent of cases respectively.[3] The gastrointestinal tract or peritoneum is rarely affected. Eye involvement has also been reported (Singer, Retina, 1993; 13:40; Derouin, PressMed, 1992; 21:1853). The clinical picture is very similar to that described in AIDS patients. Toxoplasmosis may simulate organ rejection in organ-transplant recipients.[3,10]

Congenital toxoplasmosis

Diagnosis

Clinical diagnosis of toxoplasmosis can be difficult and requires a high index of suspicion. Laboratory methods can assist the diagnosis of *T. gondii* infection by demonstrating the presence of specific antibodies against the parasite and can also be used to identify tachyzoites or isolate *T. gondii* from clinical specimens.

Diagnosis of T. gondii infection

Serological tests for the demonstration of specific antibodies against *T. gondii* is the method of choice. After infection by *T. gondii* IgM, IgA, and IgG antibodies can be detected within 1 to 2 weeks of infection (peak at 1 to 2 months) and fall at variable rates.[1] IgM and IgA antibodies can persist up to 2 years. IgA will decrease before IgM antibodies. IgG antibodies usually persist for life although at low titres. The most frequently used tests for the detection of IgG antibodies are the Sabin–Feldman dye test, the indirect fluorescent antibody (**IFA**) test, enzyme-linked immunosorbent assay (**ELISA**), immunosorbent agglutination assay (**ISAGA**), or the direct agglutination test.[1] IgM antibodies can be detected using ELISA, the IFA test, or the agglutination test.[1] IgA antibodies can be detected using ELISA or ISAGA.[1] It is important to remember that all serological tests may show false-positive or false-negative results.

As toxoplasmosis in immunodeficient patients is usually due to reactivation of a chronic infection, early detection of IgG antibodies is essential for management.[1,3,5] Serological tests are also very important in the assessment of transplant-recipient patients.[1,3] Seronegative recipients should be identified before transplantation to avoid receiving an organ (particularly a heart) from a seropositive patient, because of the high risk of developing toxoplasmosis. If identification is impossible, the patient should receive prophylactic treatment to avoid infection. In general serological tests are not useful for diagnosis of toxoplasmosis in immunodeficient patients, especially in individuals with AIDS.[5] IgG titre is usually low and tests for IgM and IgA may be negative.[5]

The diagnosis of acute acquired *T. gondii* infection in pregnant immunocompetent mothers is made by the same serological methods used for immunocompetent patients.[1,2] Identification of an acute infection in pregnancy requires examination of the fetus in order to detect congenital toxoplasmosis.

Diagnosis of toxoplasmosis

Toxoplasmosis, as a consequence of acute infection or reactivation of chronic infection in an immunodeficient host, can be diagnosed by isolation of *T. gondii* from blood, body fluids, or tissue samples, demonstration of tachyzoites in histological sections or in cytological preparations, or the demonstration of tissue cysts in the placenta, fetus, or neonate.[1] There are two clinical situations in which the diagnosis of toxoplasmosis can be accepted without these criteria:

1. The characteristic histology of toxoplasmic lymphadenitis is demonstrated.[1,15]
2. AIDS patients with positive IgG antibodies against *T. gondii* and single or multiple cerebral lesions (Fig. 1(a)) which disappear after specific antitoxoplasma therapy can be diagnosed as having central nervous system toxoplasmosis.[5]

Demonstration of tachyzoites in tissue sections (brain, lung, heart, or liver biopsies) (Fig. 1(b)) or in cytological preparations of body fluids (cerebrospinal, bronchoalveolar lavage, pleural, peritoneal, or amniotic fluids) establishes the diagnosis.[1] However, it is often difficult to identify tachyzoites in stained tissue sections. They can be seen with haematoxylin and eosin or Wright–Giemsa stains, but it is probably better to use fluorescent antibodies or peroxidase–antiperoxidase methods.[1] The identification of tissue cysts by themselves do not permit diagnosis of acute toxoplasmosis because their presence suggests chronic or latent infection. The cyst wall can be stained with Gomori or immunoperoxidase stains.

Isolation of *T. gondii* from blood, body fluids (cerebrospinal fluid, bronchoalveolar lavage, pleural, peritoneal, or amniotic fluids), or tissue samples establishes the diagnosis of acute infection.[1] *T. gondii* can be isolated by inoculation of specimens into the peritoneal cavity of mice or, more usually, by cellular culture (Derouin, PressMed, 1992; 21:1853; Kusne, Transpl, 1987; 44:457).[1] Polymerase chain reaction (**PCR**) is a very promising diagnostic tool (Lamoril, JClinPath, 1996; 49:89; Guy, JInfectDis, 1995; 172:319). PCR can detect *T. gondii* DNA in blood, body fluids (cerebrospinal fluid, bronchoalveolar lavage, or amniotic fluids), or tissue samples allowing diagnosis of congenital, ocular, or disseminated toxoplasmosis.[1]

Treatment

Treatment of toxoplasmosis differs greatly between immunocompetent and immunocompromised patients. Immunocompromised patients may be candidates for primary or secondary prophylaxis to prevent reactivation of chronic *T. gondii* infection because available drugs are very active against tachyzoites but not against cyst forms.

Acute acquired T. gondii infection in the immunocompetent patient

Immunocompetent adults with mononucleosis-like syndrome or toxoplasmic lymphadenitis do not usually require treatment unless they have severe disease.[1] Such patients require treatment with sulphadiazine plus pyrimethamine plus folinic acid (see Table 1) for

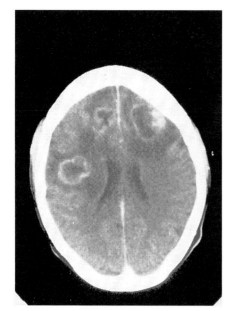

(a)

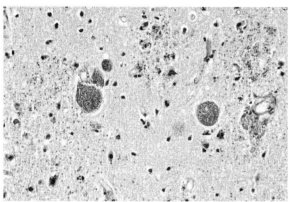

(b)

Fig. 1. (a) Initial CT scan of a 62-year-old woman who underwent liver transplantation 3 months earlier and who was admitted because of seizures and decreased level of consciousness. Several large frontal and parietal ring-enhancing lesions with oedema are visible. (b) Brain biopsy from the same patient showing several *Toxoplasma gondii* pseudocysts and many extracellular tachyzoites (haematoxylin and eosin, × 250; by courtesey of T. Ribalta).

3 to 4 weeks. Clinical and laboratory follow-up is necessary to confirm resolution of the symptoms and to avoid drug toxicity.

Pregnant women with acute acquired *T. gondii* infection should be treated with spiramycin (3 g/day) throughout pregnancy.[1,2] This regimen reduces the risk of fetal transmission by 60 per cent and is currently recommended for this purpose.[1,2] If fetal infection is identified, sulphadiazine (50–100 mg/kg per day), plus pyrimethamine (0.5–1.0 mg/kg per day), plus folinic acid should be substituted for spiramycin which does not cross the placenta.[1,2] Therapeutic abortion should be offered to pregnant women only when fetal infection has been confirmed by prenatal testing.[2]

Acute toxoplasmosis in AIDS patients
Treatment in acute cases

Patients with acute central nervous system toxoplasmosis (see Table 1) are usually treated with a combination of sulphadiazine (4–6 g/day), plus pyrimethamine (50–75 mg/day), plus folinic acid (15 mg/day) over 4 to 8 weeks (Dannemann, AnnIntMed, 1992; 116: 33; Katlama, ClinInfectDis, 1996; 22:268).[1,5] Sulphadiazine is replaced by clindamycin 2.4 g/day if patients develop sulphadiazine intolerance (Dannemann, AnnIntMed, 1992; 116:33; Katlama, ClinInfectDis, 1996; 22:268).[1,5] Corticosteroids can be given if patients have cerebral oedema.[1,5] Evidence of clinical and radiographical improvement with both regimens is usually seen within 10 to 14 days in most patients who respond (Luft, NEJM, 1993; 329:995).[1,5] Other regimens evaluated as effective in small numbers of patients are trimethoprim-sulphamethoxazole, dapsone-pyrimethamine, atovaquone alone, azithromycin or clarithromycin or doxycycline plus pyrimethamine, and clarithromycin plus minocycline.[1,5,18] Median survival after an episode of central nervous system toxoplasmosis is about 1 year and has not improved in recent years.[1,5,18] Although there is less experience with the disseminated or extraneurological forms of toxoplasmosis, the recommended acute and maintenance therapy for them is the same as that for central nervous system toxoplasmosis.[17]

Secondary prophylaxis after an acute episode of central nervous system toxoplasmosis

Because antitoxoplasma drugs are not active against *T. gondii* cysts, 50 to 80 per cent of patients will relapse shortly after successful treatment of an acute episode of central nervous system toxoplasmosis unless secondary prophylaxis is administered (Walckenaer, AnnMedIntern, 1994; 145:181; Podzamczer, AnnIntMed, 1995; 123:175).[1, 5] To avoid relapse a suppressive antitoxoplasma regimen (secondary prophylaxis) is continued for the rest of the patient's life.[1,5,18] It is usual practice to administer lower doses of the drugs used for acute therapy. The regimen of choice for secondary prophylaxis of central nervous system toxoplasmosis in AIDS patients is daily administration of 25 mg of pyrimethamine, plus 2 g of sulphadiazine, plus 15 mg of folinic acid orally (see Table 1) (Katlama, ClinInfectDis, 1996; 22:268; Podzamczer, AnnIntMed, 1995; 123:175).[1,5] With this regimen the relapse rate is less than 10 per cent at 1 year. The combination is also effective in preventing *Pneumocystis carinii* pneumonia (Podzamczer, AnnIntMed, 1995; 123:175).[18] Alternative regimens for sulphonamide-intolerant patients are daily administration of pyrimethamine alone or combined with clindamycin, new macrolides (azithromycin, clarithromycin), dapsone or doxycycline, clarithromycin plus minocycline, or atovaquone (De Gans, JAIDS, 1992; 5:137).[1,5,18]

Acute toxoplasmosis in non-AIDS immunodeficient patients

Therapeutic regimens used for AIDS patients are recommended for acute central nervous system or multiorgan toxoplasmosis in transplant-recipient patients, including liver transplant recipients or in patients with malignancies.[1,3] It is not clear whether a suppressive antitoxoplasma regimen (secondary prophylaxis) is required in these patients after the treatment of the acute episode. Whenever possible, concomitant immunosuppressive regimens should be minimized but it is probable that secondary prophylaxis should be given to transplant-recipient patients using the same drugs at half doses during the 6 to 12 months after transplantation, or longer in cases of

Table 1 Recommendations for treatment of acute toxoplasmosis and secondary prophylaxis

Acute episode of toxoplasmosis

First choice regimen
Pyrimethamine 100–200 mg single dose, followed by 50–75 mg/day
Sulphadiazine 4–6 g/day
Folinic acid 15 mg/day

In case of sulphnamide allergy[a]
Clindamycin 2.4 g/day

Duration of therapy
Immunocompetent patients: 2–4 weeks[b]
Immunodeficient patients: 4–8 weeks[c]

Secondary prophylaxis after an acute episode
(only in immunosuppressed patients)

First choice regimen
Pyrimethamine 25 mg/day
Sulphadiazine 2 g/day
Folinic acid 15 mg/day

In case of sulphonamide allergy[a,d]
Clindamycin 1.8–2.4 g/day[e]

In case of sulphonamide and clindamycin allergy
Pyrimethamine 50–75 mg/day[e]

Duration of therapy
AIDS patients: for life.
Transplant patients: not well defined. It is recommended during the first year after transplantation or longer in cases in which the severe immunosuppression persists.

[a] To substitute clindamycin for sulphadiazine.
[b] Only in severe cases or in patients with eye involvement.
[c] In cases of central nervous system toxoplasmosis may be necessary to use corticosteroids.
[d] To try sulphonamide desensitization.
[e] Add 300 mg of aerosolized pentamidine monthly for preventing *Pneumocystis carinii* pneumonia.

Table 2 Recommendations for primary prophylaxis of toxoplasmosis

HIV-infected patients (<200 CD4 cell/µl and positive serology)

First choice regimen
Trimethoprim-sulphamethoxazole 1 double strength tablet per day or three times per week

Alternative regimens
Pyrimethamine + dapsone
Pyrimethamine 50 mg once a week plus dapsone 50 mg per day, or pyrimethamine 25–50 mg plus dapsone 100 mg two times per week
Fansidar 1 tablet (sulphadoxine 500 mg/pyrimethamine 25 mg) 2 times per week

If sulphonamide allergy is present
Pyrimethamine 50 mg three times per week[a]

Duration of primary prophylaxis: life-long prophylaxis

Transplant-recipients[b] recipient seronegative; donor seropositive
Pyrimethamine 25 mg/day[c]

Duration of primary prophylaxis: 6 weeks

Add in all cases folinic acid for preventing bone marrow suppression.
[a] In AIDS patients add 300 mg of aerosolized pentamidine monthly for preventing *Pneumocystis carinii* pneumonia.
[b] Prophylaxis recommended in heart or heart–lung transplant recipients. As the incidence of toxoplasmosis in seropositive bone marrow transplant recipients and in seronegative non-heart/lung transplant recipients from seropositive donors is much lower, trimethoprim-sulphamethoxazole prophylaxis given for preventing *Pneumocystis carinii* pneumonia (see text) probably is also effective for preventing toxoplasmosis. However seronegative liver/kidney transplant recipients should be followed closely to detect seroconversion to *T. gondii* and it seems reasonable to treat those patients who seroconverted (see Table 1).
[c] In addition to receiving prophylaxis with pyrimethamine, seronegative recipients should be closely monitored for seroconversion (with or without symptoms) and chemotherapy with pyrimethamine plus sulphadiazine plus folinic acid at full doses (see Table 1) should be given for 4–6 weeks if seroconversion takes place.

chronic rejection and continued immunosuppression.[1,3] Maintenance therapy with sulphadiazine (2 g/day), plus pyrimethamine (25 mg/day), plus folinic acid is also useful for preventing *Pneumocystis carinii* pneumonia.

Prevention

Prevention of T. gondii *infection in seronegative patients*

All pregnant women, HIV-infected patients and other immunodeficient patients, and transplant recipients and donors must be screened serologically for *T. gondii* antibodies.[1–3] The following preventative measures must be taken to avoid acquisition·of primary infection.[1]

1. Wash food and surfaces which may be contaminated by cat faeces carefully, to eliminate oocysts and then wash the hands (use gloves if necessary).
2. Cook meat above 66°C or freeze it to below –20°C to destroy cysts.

Primary prophylaxis in immunodeficient patients

HIV-infected patients

All HIV-infected patients with positive antitoxoplasma serology must be considered at risk of developing active toxoplasmosis when their CD4 cell count falls below 200/μl.[1,5,19] Patients with a CD4 cell count of 100/μl or less[7] or an IgG antitoxoplasma titre of 150 IU/ml or higher have a greater risk of developing central nervous system toxoplasmosis (Derouin, AIDS, 1996; 10:1521). A count of 200 CD4 cells/μl should be regarded as the threshold for the start of primary prophylaxis against *Pneumocystis carinii* pneumonia.[19,20] Table 2 summarizes drug recommendations and dosage schedules for primary prophylaxis of toxoplasmosis and *Pneumocystis carinii* pneumonia in HIV-infected patients with a count of less than 200 CD4 cells/μl.[1,5,19]

Trimethoprim-sulphamethoxazole is the drug of choice for the prevention of *Pneumocystis carinii* pneumonia and toxoplasmosis.[1, 5,19,20] A double-strength tablet (trimethoprim 160 mg, sulphamethoxazole 800 mg) administered daily or even 3 days/week is effective.[1,5,19,20] In general, tolerance is good and most side-effects (gastrointestinal symptoms and hypersensitivity reactions) appear during the first month of prophylaxis.[1,5,19] For intolerant patients, dapsone plus pyrimethamine is an alternative.[19,20] The combination of pyrimethamine and sulphadoxine (Fansidar) is also effective against both infections.[1,5,19] For those not able to tolerate sulphonamides, pyrimethamine (plus aerosolized pentamidine) is the only acceptable alternative.[7] The efficacy of atovaquone has not yet been assessed. Macrolides and clindamycin are ineffective.[1,5,19]

Non-HIV-infected patients

Trimethoprim-sulphamethoxazole is also widely used to prevent *Pneumocystis carinii* pneumonia in bone-marrow and solid organ transplant recipients (Momin, AnnIntMed, 1995; 123:205; Petri,

ClinInfectDis, 1994; 18:141).[21,22] As in HIV-infected patients, the combination is also useful for preventing toxoplasmosis in seropositive bone-marrow transplant recipients and in seronegative solid organ transplant recipients from seropositive donors, at least in low-risk populations (non-heart transplants). Low dose trimethoprim-sulphamethoxazole (480 mg/day or 980 mg two/three times per week) is highly effective in preventing *Pneumocystis carinii* pneumonia and is almost free of toxic side-effects (Momin, AnnIntMed, 1995; 123:205; Petri, ClinInfectDis, 1994; 18:141).[21,22] It is not clear how long prophylaxis should continue, but almost all cases of *Pneumocystis carinii* pneumonia and toxoplasmosis occur in the first 6 months after transplantation; most authors prescribe prophylaxis for 6 to 12 months and it should be reinstituted whenever the patient's level of immunosuppression is about to be increased for more than a few days.[21,22] None of the 98 liver transplant recipients who received trimethoprim-sulphamethoxazole (960 mg/day, orally) during the first year of transplantation in our institution between 1991 and 1994 developed *Pneumocystis carinii* pneumonia or toxoplasmosis.[23] [T]he combination of pyrimethamine and sulphadoxine (Fansidar) plus folinic acid, one tablet on a weekly basis during the first 6 months after grafting or longer if immunosuppression persisted, was also useful against *Pneumocystis carinii* pneumonia and toxoplasmosis in 69 French bone-marrow transplant recipients with positive *T. gondii* serology (Foot, BoneMTrans, 1994; 14:241). In sulphonamide-allergic or intolerant patients, dapsone, pyrimethamine, or atovaquone may be used against *Pneumocystis carinii* pneumonia and toxoplamosis although there is little published experience with these drugs.

Seronegative recipients of heart or heart–lung transplant from seropositive donors have special requirements (Petri, ClinInfectDis, 1994; 18:141).[21,22] These patients have the highest risk for developing toxoplasmosis and all should receive primary prophylaxis.[1, 3,13,17] Pyrimethamine (25 mg/day, orally for 6 weeks) has been effective in preventing the development of acute toxoplasmosis in seronegative heart transplant recipients from seropositive donors (Wreghitt, TransplInt, 1992; 5:197). In addition to prophylaxis with pyrimethamine, seronegative recipients should be closely monitored for seroconversion (with or without symptoms) and pyrimethamine plus sulphadiazine plus folinic acid at full doses (see Table 1) should be given for 4 to 6 weeks if seroconversion takes place.[21,22] As the incidence of toxoplasmosis in seronegative non-heart transplant recipients from seropositive donors is much lower, trimethoprim-sulphamethoxazole prophylaxis against *Pneumocystis carinii* pneumonia is probably effective in preventing toxoplasmosis.[13,21] However, these seronegative solid organ transplant recipients should be followed closely for detection of seroconversion to *T. gondii* and it seems reasonable to treat those who seroconvert (see Table 1).

References

1. Beaman MH, McCabe RE, Wong SY, and Remington JS. *Toxoplasma gondii.* In Mandell GL, Douglas RG, and Bennett JE, eds. *Principles and practice of infectious diseases.* New York: Churchill Livingstone, 1994: 2455–75.
2. Wong SY and Remington JS. Toxoplasmosis in pregnancy. *Clinical Infectious Diseases*, 1994; **18**: 853–62.
3. Israelski DM and Remington JS. Toxoplasmosis in the non-AIDS immunocompromised host. *Current Clinical Topics in Infectious Diseases*, 1993; **13**: 322–56.

4. Janku J. Pathogenesis and pathologic anatomy of congenital coloboma of the macula lutea in an eye of normal size, with microscopic detection of parasites in the retina. In Kean BH, Mott KEE, and Russell AJ, eds. *Tropical medicine and parasitology: classical investigations*. New York: Cornell University Press, 1978: 274–82.

5. Wong SY and Remington JS. Toxoplasmosis in the setting of AIDS. In Broder S, Merigan TC Jr, and Bolognesi D, eds. *Textbook of AIDS medicine*. Baltimore: Williams and Wilkins, 1993: 223–57.

6. Wong SY and Remington JS. Biology of *Toxoplasma gondii. AIDS*, 1993; **7**: 299–316.

7. Leport C, Chêne G, Morlat P, *et al*. Pyrimethamine for primary prophylaxis of toxoplasmic encephalitis in patients with human immunodeficiency virus infection: A double-blind, randomized trial. *Journal of Infectious Diseases*, 1996; **173**: 91–7.

8. Israelski DM and Remington JS. Toxoplasmosis in patients with cancer. *Clinical Infectious Diseases*, 1993; **17** (Suppl. 2): S423–35.

9. Derouin F, Devergie A, Auber P, Gluckman E, Beauvais B, Garin YJF, and Lariviere M. Toxoplasmosis in bone marrow-transplant recipients: report of seven cases and review. *Clinical Infectious Diseases*, 1992; **15**: 267–70.

10. Michaels MG, Wald ER, Fricker FJ, del Nido PJ, and Armitage J. Toxoplasmosis in pediatric recipients of heart transplants. *Clinical Infectious Diseases*, 1992; **14**: 847–51.

11. Mayes JT, O'Connor BJ, Avery R, Castellani W, and Carey W. Transmission of *Toxoplasma gondii* infection by liver transplantation. *Clinical Infectious Diseases*, 1995; **21**: 511–5.

12. Luft BJ, Naot Y, Araujo FG, Stinson EB, and Remington JS. Primary and reactivated toxoplasma infection in patients with cardiac transplants. *Annals of Internal Medicine*, 1983; **99**: 27–31.

13. Speirs GE, Hakim M, Calne RY, and Wreghitt TG. Relative risk of donor-transmitted *Toxoplasma gondii* infection in heart, liver and kidney transplant recipients. *Clinical Transplantation*, 1988; **2**: 257–60.

14. Wreghitt TG, Hughes M, and Calne R. A retrospective study of viral and *Toxoplasma gondii* infections in 54 liver transplant recipients in Cambridge. *Serodiagnosis and Immunotherapy*, 1987; **1**: 219–39.

15. Cabe RE, Brooks RG, Dorfman, and Remington JS. Clinical spectrum in 107 case of toxoplasmic lymphadenopathy. *Clinical Infectious Diseases*, 1987; **9**: 754–74.

16. Jautzke G, Sell M, Thalmann U, Janitschke K, Gottschalk J, Schürmann D, and Ruf B. Extracerebral toxoplasmosis in AIDS. Histological and immunohistological findings based on 80 autopsy cases. *Pathological Research Practice*, 1993; **189**: 428–36.

17. Rabaud C, May T, Amiel C, Katlama C, Leport C, Ambroise-Thomas P, and Canton P. Extracerebral toxoplasmosis in patients infected with HIV. *Medicine* (Baltimore), 1994; **73**: 306–14.

18. Miró JM and Gatell JM. Secondary prophylaxis of toxoplasmosis in HIV-infected patients. *HIV and AIDS Current Trends*, 1995; **1**: 8–10.

19. Miró JM and Gatell JM. Primary prophylaxis of toxoplasmosis in HIV-infected patients. *HIV and AIDS Current Trends*, 1995; **1**: 1–4.

20. Podzamczer D, Salazar A, Jiménez J, Consiglio E, Santín M, Casanova A, *et al*. Intermittent cotrimoxazole versus dapsone-pyrimethamine for the simultaneous primary prophylaxis of *Pneumocystis carinii* pneumonia and toxoplasmosis in HIV-infected patients. *Annals of Internal Medicine*, 1995; **122**: 755–61.

21. Rubin RH and Tolkoff-Rubin NE. Antimicrobial strategies in the care of organ transplant recipients. *Antimicrobial Agents and Chemotherapy*, 1993; **37**: 619–24.

22. Rubin RH. Infection in the organ transplant recipient. In Rubin RH and Young LS, eds. *Clinical approach to infection in the compromised host*. New York: Plenum Medical, 1994: 629–706.

23. Moreno A, Rimola A, Claramont X, *et al*. Trimethoprim-sulfamethoxazole in the prevention of *Pneumocystis carinii* pneumonia (PCP) in liver transplant recipients. *36th Interscience Conference on Antimicrobial Agents and Chemotherapy (ICAAC), 1996, New Orleans*. Washington DC: American Society for Microbiology, abstract no. J124.

13.4 Helminthiasis

13.4.1 Blood flukes (schistosomes) and liver flukes

K. S. Warren

Blood flukes

Definition

It is with regret that we must record the death of Dr K. S. Warren during the preparation of this edition.

Blood flukes or schistosomes are trematodes or flatworms, which inhabit the venous circulation of their definitive hosts. The principal species infecting man are *Schistosoma mansoni*, *S. japonicum*, and *S. haematobium*. The habitat of the former two species is the intestinal venules from which they may affect the liver, and that of the latter is the vesical venules where they damage the urinary bladder and the ureters. Two other species, which are rather localized in their geographical distribution, are *S. intercalatum* from West Africa and *S. mekongi* from South-East Asia; both may cause liver disease. Schistosome infection is not synonymous with disease, as the worms do not multiply in their definitive hosts and illness usually occurs only in those with heavy infections. The *S. mansoni* and *S. japonicum* blood flukes are the major cause of parasite-induced liver disease.[1] The liver flukes which inhabit the bile ducts will be discussed below.

Introduction

The schistosomes were discovered by Theodore Bilharz, a German pathologist, in the portal vein of a young Egyptian in Cairo in 1852. He originally called them *Distoma*, but since it was observed that these organisms had one mouth and one sucker they were soon renamed both *Schistosoma* (cleft body) and *Bilharzia*, the former taking precedence.

It was not until 60 years later that the complex means of transmission of these digenetic trematode parasites was worked out. An important step in the process was the discovery of the lifecycle of the liver fluke, *Fasciola hepatica* (the first trematode to be described, in 1379), by both an Englishman and a German in 1881, which revealed digenetic transmission involving asexual reproduction in a freshwater snail intermediate host and sexual reproduction in the definitive host—sheep, and on occasion, man.

In 1913 the digenetic lifecycle of *S. japonicum* was discovered in Japan by Miyairi and Suzuki. Based on their research, Leiper worked out the transmission of both *S. mansoni* and *S. haematobium* several years later.

An early contribution was the development of the first effective antischistosomal drug, tartar emetic, in the Anglo-Egyptian Sudan in 1916. This highly toxic, intravenous drug was essentially not superseded until the 1970s, when a single-dose, non-toxic, oral drug, praziquantel, also effective against liver flukes, was introduced. The pathogenesis of schistosomiasis was not established until the 1960s and 1970s when the schistosome eggs trapped in the liver of the mammalian host were shown definitively to be the parasitic aetiological agent, and the immunological response of the host to the egg was found to be an essential factor. It was not until this era also that disease was shown to occur largely in those with heavy infections, and simple quantitative faecal egg counts enabled the determination of worm burdens. This, in combination with single-dose, non-toxic drugs, has led to a cost-effective strategy of targeted mass treatment to control disease.

Epidemiology

Globally, 200 million people are infected with schistosomes. Of these about two-thirds carry the flukes which reside in the portal and mesenteric venous systems of the gut, *S. mansoni* and *S. japonicum*. Egypt and Nigeria, two of the most populous countries in Africa, and Brazil, the largest country in Latin America, consider schistosomiasis mansoni to be one of their principal health problems, as does China for schistosomiasis japonica. *S. mansoni* is endemic in most countries of Africa south of the Sahara. In the New World the infection is of significance in the Caribbean islands of Puerto Rico, Dominican Republic, Guadeloupe, Martinique, and St Lucia; in South America it is endemic in Venezula, Surinam, and Brazil. *S. japonicum* is prevalent in China, the Philippines, and Sulawesi in Indonesia; it has virtually died out in Japan. *S. intercalatum* occurs in parts of West Africa and *S. mekongi* (a japonicum-like organism) is found sporadically in parts of South-East Asia.

Schistosomiasis mansoni occurs almost exclusively in man, while schistosomiasis japonica is a zoonosis which involves many domestic and wild animals, the principal reservoirs being cattle and rats. The freshwater snail intermediate hosts of *S. mansoni* (*Biomphalaria* spp.) are aquatic while those of *S. japonicum* (*Oncomelania* spp.) are amphibious. Transmission is often seasonal and varies with the ecology; thus on the mountainous island of St Lucia the snails are flushed into the sea in the rainy season, and are concentrated in pools in the dry periods. In Egypt, before the damming of the Nile, transmission decreased when the canals dried out, but now that they always contain water it remains unchanged throughout the year.

Infection takes place principally at certain times of the day, the infective form of *S. mansoni* (cercariae) being shed in large numbers by snails between noon and 2 p.m.; in contrast, *S. japonicum* cercariae are shed in very small numbers in the evening; both survive under natural conditions for only a few hours.

Since schistosomes do not replicate in the definitive host, have a mean lifespan of approximately 5 years, and repeated infection occurs on exposure to water, prevalence which begins in childhood may reach almost 100 per cent in areas of heavy transmission and often remains high throughout the human lifespan. Areas of low prevalence tend to low intensity, while those of high prevalence show heavier infections. Females tend to have a somewhat lower prevalence of infection. With respect to intensity of infection (the number of worms carried by the host), a peak is reached in the teens from which it falls drastically thereafter. This change appears to be related largely to a decrease in exposure to infected water, but also may be associated with some degree of immunity occurring after prolonged infection. The distribution of schistosomes within their definitive hosts is overdispersed with only a small percentage (often less than 10 per cent) of infected individuals carrying heavy worm burdens. Disease, as manifested by hepatomegaly and splenomegaly, is largely seen in those with heavy infections.

Prevention and control

Until recently, the major method of control of schistosomiasis has been the use of molluscicides to destroy the snail intermediate host. While the treatment of the definitive host with antischistosome drugs was tried as a method of control, the agents available required multiple doses and were highly toxic. Another approach has been to provide water supplies and latrines as a means of reducing transmission. China's success in delimiting infection is related largely to the massive application of all of these approaches. The comparative efficacy of these three methods was determined in a 16-year study on the island of St Lucia. Use of the newer drugs, which became available while the study was in progress, was clearly the most cost-effective means of controlling infection. It was also highly effective in controlling disease by sharply reducing the intensity of infection.[2]

It is now possible to target treatment to the most heavily infected sectors of the population and, thereby, prevent the occurrence of hepatosplenic disease at relatively low cost.

Pathogenesis and pathology
Lifecycle

The schistosomes are called digenetic trematodes because their lifecycle includes an asexual phase in freshwater snail 'intermediate hosts' and a sexual phase in mammalian 'definitive hosts', including humans (Fig. 1).

Parasite eggs passed in the faeces of the definitive host hatch in freshwater into ciliated miracidia which penetrate into specific species of snails. Within the snail they undergo several developmental stages multiplying asexually into thousands of tailed, free-swimming cercariae which escape from the snail into water. Schistosome cercariae penetrate the skin of the definitive host directly, those of *S. mansoni* doing so in 5 to 10 min and those of *S. japonicum* as rapidly as 1 min.

Within the definitive host the schistosomes migrate from the skin to the lungs and subsequently to the portal venules where they develop into adult male and female worms, 10 to 30 mm in length. The paired worms then migrate to the mesenteric venules: *S. mansoni* produce about 300 and *S. japonicum* 3000 eggs daily. Approximately half of these eggs pass through the intestinal mucosa and are excreted in the faeces.

Inflammation and fibrosis

Blood fluke disease is due to inflammation and fibrosis elicited by the parasites and their products, and is clearly related to intensity of infection as shown in both experimental models and at autopsy. In the case of the schistosomes the lesions occur primarily in the presinusoidal venules of the liver.

In schistosomiasis the adult worms reside in the intestinal venules and produce large numbers of eggs. The *S. mansoni* eggs are produced at a rate of 300 per worm pair per day and the *S. japonicum* eggs at 3000 per day. Within a tanned protein eggshell with ultramicroscopic fenestrations lies a living embryo contained within a semipermeable membrane. The embryo uses host metabolites in its growth and development, which occurs over a period of 6 days. The mature embryo (the miracidium stage infective to snails) secretes a variety of antigenic molecules including enzymes.

While approximately 30 per cent of the eggs pass through the mucosa into the lumen of the intestines, the remainder stay within the mammalian host, many breaking free in the mesenteric venules where they pass into the liver via the portal venous system and become trapped in the presinusoidal venules. They survive in this milieu for approximately 3 weeks. During this period the host tissues react to the substances secreted by the eggs by the formation of a circumscribed granulomatous reaction of the kind seen in tuberculosis. This lesion has been shown to be essentially a cell-mediated immunological response of the delayed hypersensitivity type on the basis of the occurrence of an anamnestic reaction which is specific to antigens contained within the egg and can be transferred by cells but not by serum. Furthermore, the granulomas can be suppressed by a variety of inhibitors of cell-mediated immunological reactivity, and do not occur in nude, athymic mice.[3]

These granulomatous lesions are dynamic in that the response does not begin until the eggs are embryonated and ceases when they die and the miracidium is resorbed. Furthermore, they depend on the immunological reactivity of the unsensitized, sensitized, or desensitized host. With respect to the latter, the granulomatous response around living eggs declines in chronic infections due to specific modulation of the cell-mediated response. In the last few years there has been a spate of papers on the role of cytokines in granulomatous reactivity. The results have been confusing because they have not been associated with the lesions but have been related to recently discovered subsets of T-helper cells, T_{H1} and T_{H2}. The former has simplistically been correlated with cell-mediated and the latter with antibody-mediated responses. However, a recent review has concluded that both subsets, which apparently overlap, are required in the waxing and waning of this cell-mediated immunological response[4] involving not only mononuclear cells but large numbers of eosinophils.

Investigations of granuloma formation around eggs both *in vivo* and *in vitro* have demonstrated a high rate of collagen synthesis. This is later balanced by collagen degradation, fibrosis being the net result of both a high intensity of infection and an imbalance

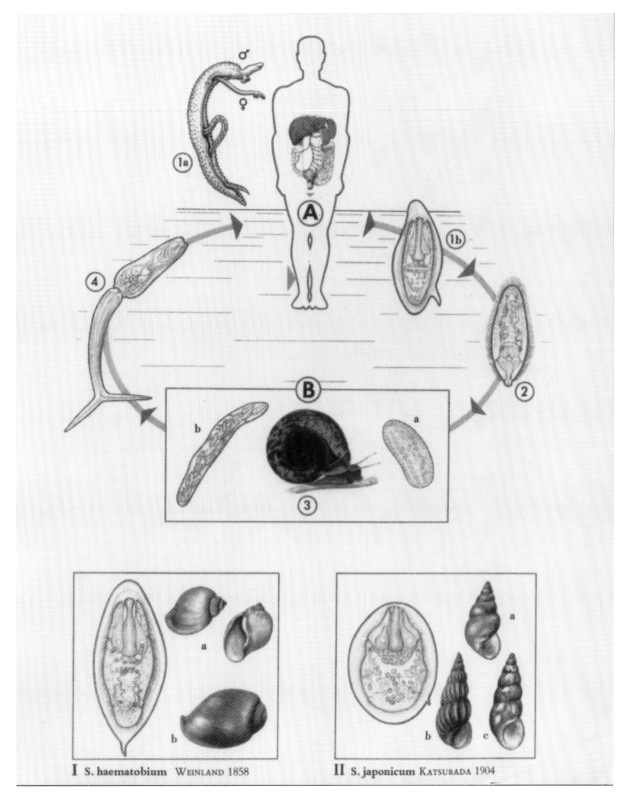

I **S. haematobium** WEINLAND 1858   II **S. japonicum** KATSURADA 1904

Fig. 1. Lifecycle of the schistosome.

toward collagen synthesis. Following treatment, collagen tends to be resorbed, but at a higher rate in early than in late infections. The role of growth factors, cytokines, and parasite egg factors in the pathogenesis of fibrosis in schistosomiasis is under intensive study.

Investigations of the microcirculation in the liver of experimental animals have revealed that the eggs alone do not cause significant obstruction, but that the granulomas and subsequent fibrosis block portal venous circulation. This leads to portal hypertension,

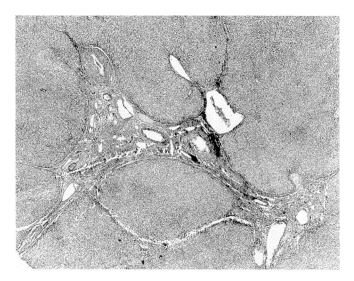

Fig. 2. Surgical liver biopsy showing periportal fibrosis in a patient with hepatosplenic schistosomiasis (haematoxylin and eosin × 20).

splenomegaly, and the development of oesophageal varices. In spite of severe portal venous obstruction, total liver blood flow remains within normal limits due to compensatory neovascular formation of arterial vessels in the areas of inflammation and fibrosis. The following is an excellent description of the human liver in advanced hepatosplenic schistosomiasis (see also Fig. 2).[5]

'Pipestem fibrosis is the only human liver disease directly attributable to schistosome infection. Its precursor stages, observed incidentally at autopsy and in experimental infections of chimpanzees, begin with diffuse inflammatory infiltration around portal radicles proximal to presinusoidal vessels containing egg granulomas. Next, the affected triads become fibrotic and enlarged. First, smaller, then larger portal vein branches become blocked by granulomas and disrupted by inflammation and fibrosis, or by organizing thrombi. Eggs and egg granulomas accumulate around these blockage sites, further contributing to portal enlargement. Simultaneously, the hepatic arteries enlarge and send out neovascular branches. Some portal vessels become dilated to angiomatoid proportions. Kupffer cells become prominent and pigment-laden but the liver parenchyma preserves its lobular and trabecular architecture showing only scattered and mild hepatocytic damage. In full-blown schistosomal liver fibrosis the enlarged, whitish, fibrous triads surrounding portal vein lumina resemble the cross-sections of clay pipestems. The parenchyma between portal fields lacks the nodularity seen in Laennec's cirrhosis.'

The spleen may become grossly enlarged and is firm in consistency, fibrotic, and congested. It may be associated with hypersplenism with its attendant anaemia and pancytopenia.

Clinical features and complications

Clinical manifestations of schistosomiasis may occur in the acute stages of infection and are useful for later diagnostic purposes. These include swimmer's itch, a maculopapular, pruritic rash following penetration of the skin by cercariae. It appears to be a sensitization phenomenon and occurs most frequently following infection by avian schistosomes. When there is a heavy primary infection, acute schistosomiasis, or Katayama fever, may be seen several weeks

following exposure. This appears to be a serum sickness-like reaction with fever, hepatosplenomegaly, lymphadenopathy, and eosinophilia.

Chronic schistosomiasis mansoni and japonica have been associated with a variety of systemic symptoms including weakness, abdominal pain, and diarrhoea. Extensive field studies have revealed that these manifestations are seen only in the small proportion of individuals with heavy infections. These findings have been corroborated away from endemic areas in investigations of many patients seen over a period of years at a hospital for tropical diseases in the United Kingdom.

Hepatomegaly, and particularly splenomegaly, is also seen largely in those with heavy infection. Both organs are firm to hard in texture and non-tender. Many cases are picked up incidentally on physical examination, or following an episode of haematemesis. Since the liver parenchyma is not involved in the pathogenic process, jaundice and the stigmas of chronic liver disease are not seen. Liver function tests are usually within or close to normal limits. Schistosomiasis occurs in many parts of the world where hepatitis is rife. Thus, patients with this parasitic infection and evidence of liver parenchymal dysfunction (so-called decompensated hepatosplenic schistosomiasis) are often seen, but a synergistic interaction between the infections has only been demonstrated in experimentally infected mice. There has been a recent flurry of interest in hepatitis C infection and schistosomiasis in Egypt.[6]

Patients with splenomegaly may show anaemia, leucopenia, and thrombocytopenia. Eosinophilia is often observed in schistosome infections as in other helminth infections. Oesophageal varices are frequently found in those with splenomegaly. Haematemesis may occur erratically or fairly frequently. In those with pure hepatosplenic schistosomiasis, portal-systemic encephalopathy is not observed during bleeding episodes.

Complications of hepatosplenic schistosomiasis include chronic salmonellosis, pulmonary schistosomiasis and cor pulmonale, glomerular involvement and nephrosis, and central nervous system disease. Susceptibility to *Salmonella* appears to occur in infection with all species of human schistosome. Clinical pulmonary disease is seen only after hepatosplenic schistosomiasis results in collateral circulation carrying schistosome eggs to the pulmonary arterioles. This results in granuloma formation and fibrosis which block blood flow and lead to cor pulmonale. Central nervous system involvement is rare. In the case of schistosomiasis mansoni the lower spinal cord is the site of granulomatous lesions leading to the development of paraplegia. In schistosomiasis japonica the cerebrum is the site of the lesions, resulting in focal seizures or generalized encephalopathy. There is evidence that adult egg-laying worms have been found *in situ* leading to granulomatous inflammation and fibrosis.

Diagnosis and differential diagnosis

Diagnosis of schistosomiasis must be considered in terms of both the infection and the disease. Most cases of the infection do not manifest overt disease because of the overdispersed distribution of the parasite in the host, with the great majority of individuals having low intensity infections. Conversely, it is possible to have the disease without the infection. This is because hepatosplenic disease usually takes one or two decades to develop while the mean lifespan of the worms is less than 5 years.

In endemic areas the prevalence of schistosome infection varies from low to high percentages of the population. Intensity usually varies with the degree of prevalence. In non-endemic areas a key factor is the physician's suspicion based on travel to or immigration from an endemic area. Other grounds for suspicion are eosinophilia suggesting a helminth infection, hepatomegaly, splenomegaly, or in the most extreme case, haematemesis. A geographical history is of great importance, not only in terms of which country but where in the country. Exposure to freshwater is essential; schistosomiasis is not transmitted in salt water or in chlorinated swimming pools. If both a geographical history and significant water contact are present, a definitive diagnosis can be made by the demonstration of eggs in the patient's faeces. For this purpose a simple stool smear can be done, with a search at low power for the characteristic eggs of *S. mansoni* and *S. japonicum*, the former oval (60×160 mm) with a pronounced lateral spine, the latter rounder (60×85 mm) with a small knob. To diagnose light infections more elaborate concentration techniques can be used, or in some cases rectal biopsy has been recommended. Since the pathogenesis of schistosomiasis is clearly related to intensity of infection over a prolonged period of time, and most of those with hepatosplenic disease have moderate to heavy infections, determining intensity by egg counts is of great importance.

The best technique for egg counting is the Kato thick smear which is itself a form of faecal concentration. A 50-mg sample of faeces that has been pressed through 105-mesh, stainless steel bolting cloth is placed on a glass slide and covered with a cellophane coverslip impregnated with 50 per cent glycerine. The slide is inverted and pressed on to a bed of filter paper, turned face up, and left for a period of 24 h during which time the faecal matter clears. For more rapid diagnosis it should be noted that a 20-mg faecal sample will clear in 15 min. Although the embryo within the egg clears, the characteristic shape of the eggshell can easily be seen, and the eggs in the sample can be counted. Multiplication of the 50-mg sample by 20 gives the number of eggs per gram of faeces. Patients with less than 100 eggs/g are considered to have light infections, those with counts between 100 and 400, moderate infections, and those with counts greater than 400, heavy infections.

A wide variety of immunological tests, both serological and intradermal, have been used. While many of them are highly sensitive, they are not quantitative and suffer from frequent false-positive reactions. If eggs cannot be detected in the faeces, the intensity of infection is so low that it is unlikely to contribute to disease, the one exception being schistosomiasis of the central nervous system.

With respect to disease, liver enlargement may be observed in acute schistosomiasis 3 to 6 weeks after primary exposure, along with fever, lymphadenopathy, and splenomegaly. This is essentially a transient syndrome, although occasionally it is fatal. Eggs may not be found in the faeces until 2 or 3 weeks after onset of symptoms. In chronic schistosomal disease the liver is enlarged, smooth, firm, and non-tender. As the disease progresses the spleen enlarges, in some cases extending well below the umbilicus and is very firm in texture. It may be associated with a dragging sensation. Jaundice, emaciation, and stigmas of liver parenchymal damage are not present. Liver function tests including bilirubin, enzymes, serum proteins, and even sensitive procedures such as bromosulphthalein retention tend to be within normal limits.

Needle biopsies of the liver are rarely diagnostic because of the focal nature of the lesions. Recently, it has been found that ultrasonography provides a very sensitive and virtually specific means of early diagnosis of hepatic fibrosis by revealing thickened fibrosed portal tracts and narrowed portal blood vessels. This method can also determine the patency of the portal, splenic, and superior mesenteric vessels. Another means of studying these vessels is by splenoportography. The presence of oesophageal varices can be determined by barium swallow and oesophagoscopy. Following anthelmintic treatment, ultrasonography reveals regression of hepatic lesions.[4]

Differential diagnosis of hepatosplenic schistosomiasis includes portal vein thrombosis and rare granulomatous diseases of the liver such as sarcoidosis. A syndrome known as decompensated hepatosplenic schistosomiasis has been seen in endemic areas. These patients, infected with schistosomes, demonstrate a picture similar to cirrhosis of the liver with jaundice, stigmas of liver parenchymal damage, and deranged liver function tests. Many of them are suffering primarily from other forms of liver disease, such as hepatitis, with concurrent schistosomiasis.

Treatment and prognosis

Treatment has been greatly simplified by the development of an excellent non-toxic drug, praziquantel.[7] The recommended single dose for *S. mansoni* and *S. japonicum* infection is 40 mg/kg. Cure rates are 60 to 90 per cent for schistosomiasis mansoni and 60 to 80 per cent for schistosomiasis japonica. In those in whom a cure is not achieved, intensity of infection, as measured by reduction in egg count, is reduced by 95 per cent after 1 year. There is a significant reversal of parasite-induced morbidity after treatment, and enlarged livers and spleens tend to regress in size. Praziquantel therapy is well tolerated, the incidence of side-effects usually ranging from 10 to 15 per cent. They include abdominal pain or discomfort, nausea, vomiting, anorexia, and diarrhoea. There may also be headache, vertigo, dizziness, fever, urticarial rash, and lassitude. On the basis of praziquantel's effectiveness and lack of significant toxicity it is recommended that all patients with schistosomiasis, even those with light infections, be treated.

It may occasionally be necessary to resort to splenectomy to control hypersplenism, but this should not be done until after drug treatment to determine if there is amelioration of this syndrome. Bleeding oesophageal varices should be treated by standard means. It is important to realize that portal-systemic encephalopathy does not occur in patients with pure hepatosplenic schistosomiasis. Repeated bleeding episodes may require oesophagoscopal or surgical means of treating the varices. Portacaval shunting is associated with a high incidence of encephalopathy; splenorenal shunts are preferable.

It is worthy of note that the development of schistosomal disease in endemic areas can be prevented by periodic chemotherapy aimed at keeping the intensity of infection low. In one area of high prevalence and intensity of infection there is evidence that, following a single treatment with praziquantel, hepatosplenic disease does not occur. Furthermore, there is enormous activity going on in laboratories all over the world to develop vaccines for schistosomiasis. The genes for many different protective antigens, not only those on the surface of the parasites but also structural proteins and a wide variety of enzymes, have been isolated and cloned.

Liver flukes

Definition

The liver flukes, whose habitat is the bile ducts, are also a significant cause of hepatic disease. The principal species involved are *Opisthorchis viverrini*, *O. felineus*, *Clonorchis sinensis*, and *Fasciola hepatica*. *Dicrocoelium dendriticum* infections have also been observed in humans.

Introduction

As noted above, *Fasciola hepatica*, a trematode or fluke which causes disease in cattle and sheep and, incidentally, in humans, was first described in 1379. The discovery in 1881 of its unusual lifecycle, oscillating between asexual reproduction in freshwater snail intermediate hosts and sexual reproduction in humans, opened up the study of fluke biology and transmission. The prinicipal liver flukes of humans, *Clonorchis* and *Opisthorchi*, are most prevalent in Asia.

Epidemiology

The liver flukes fall into two groups: those transmitted by eating raw freshwater fish (*Clonorchis* and *Opisthorchis*), which are confined largely to Asia, eastern Europe, and Siberia; and *Fasciola hepatica*, largely a disease of sheep and cattle, which infects humans in most parts of the world. *Clonorchis* and *Opisthorchis* have an overdispersed distribution in their definitive hosts, similar to schistosomes, with only a small proportion of parasitized individuals bearing the heavy infections associated with disease.[8] *Fasciola*, on the other hand, may cause severe symptoms in relatively mildly infected individuals during the acute, migratory phase of the larvae in the host liver. Chronic biliary tract disease, however, is related to intensity of infection.

Prevention and control

Fish-transmitted liver flukes could be easily controlled by changing eating habits to cooked rather than raw or smoked fish. The use of latrines would also prevent transmission of these parasites to their intermediate hosts. Unfortunately, these means of control are not effective in poor rural areas. The availability of an excellent, single-dose, oral antitrematode drug, praziquantel, and the overdispersed distribution of this infection enables the targeting of heavily infected individuals, thereby controlling disease. *Fasciola hepatica* is relatively resistant to treatment and is best controlled by limiting ingestion of watercress from areas where cattle and sheep are maintained.

Pathogenesis and pathology

Lifecycle

Parasite eggs pass out of the bile ducts and are voided in the faeces of the definitive human and animal hosts. They hatch in freshwater into ciliated miracidia which enter into specific species of snails. An exception is *Opisthorchis*, where the eggs are ingested by the snail. Multiplying asexually, they pass through several developmental stages within the snail and pass out into the water as thousands of free-swimming cercariae. The liver flukes *Clonorchis* and *Opisthorchis* penetrate into the flesh of freshwater fish which are infective to mammals when eaten raw. *F. hepatica* cercariae encyst on plants, particularly watercress, and are infective upon ingestion (Fig. 3) .

The adult liver flukes, which are hermaphroditic, range in length from the relatively small *Clonorchis* and *Opisthorchis* (11 to 20 mm) to *F. hepatica*, which is 20 to 30 mm. Upon ingestion of infective larvae the former two genera pass from the gut directly into the bile ducts through the ampulla of Vater. However, *Fasciola* penetrates the gut wall, passes into the peritoneum, and then enters the liver where it migrates through the tissues for a period of several weeks before it penetrates into the bile ducts. The worms produce large numbers of eggs, which pass out of the bile ducts into the intestinal lumen and are excreted in the faeces.

Dicrocelium dendriticum, another fluke of the bile ducts, is a cosmopolitan parasite of sheep, but very few human infections have been reported. It is one of the rare trematodes that use a terrestrial snail as an intermediate host. Cercariae leave the snail in slime balls which are ingested by ants and in turn are infective to man on either accidental or deliberate ingestion.

Inflammation and fibrosis

For liver flukes as for the blood flukes, disease is due to inflammation and fibrosis elicited by the parasites and their products, and is clearly related to intensity of infection as shown in both experimental models and at autopsy. *Clonorchis* and *Opisthorchis* directly enter the bile ducts and cause lesions confined largely to the biliary system. While it is generally believed that the pathogenesis is due to mechanical irritation caused by the flukes and by their toxic secretions, studies in Thailand have recently revealed predominant and highly immunogenic antigens in the eggs of *Opisthorchis*.[8] It has also been demonstrated that animals depleted of T cells show amelioration of the periductular inflammatory response to the parasites. Studies in man have revealed hyperplasia of the epithelial cells lining the biliary tract, periductal fibrosis, thickening of the duct wall, dilatation, and obstruction. Secondary infection occurs due to biliary stasis which results in chronic recurrent suppurative infections. Cholangiocarcinoma has been linked with infection with both of these parasites.

Fasciola hepatica infection may be associated with an acute clinical syndrome which is characterized by prolonged fever, hypochondrial pain, and eosinophilia. This occurs during the period of migration of the fluke larvae in the liver parenchyma, with localized destruction of liver parenchymal cells and resultant inflammation. Heavy infection of the bile ducts in humans is very rare; its pathology is similar to that of the other liver flukes.

Clinical features and complications

The majority of cases of opisthorchiasis and clonorchiasis are symptomless, and are diagnosed on routine stool examination. Although controlled studies have not been done, it is believed that mild cases of disease are associated with dyspepsia, flatulence, diarrhoea or constipation, and dull pain in the right hypochondrium. In more advanced cases lassitude, anorexia, and weight loss may be found. Liver enlargement tends to be found in patients over the age of 40 years. The organ is firm and non-tender. Severe manifestations, which occur only in a minority, include symptoms and signs of relapsing cholangitis and cholecystitis. Cholangiocarcinoma, gallstones, and obstructive jaundice are usual associations.

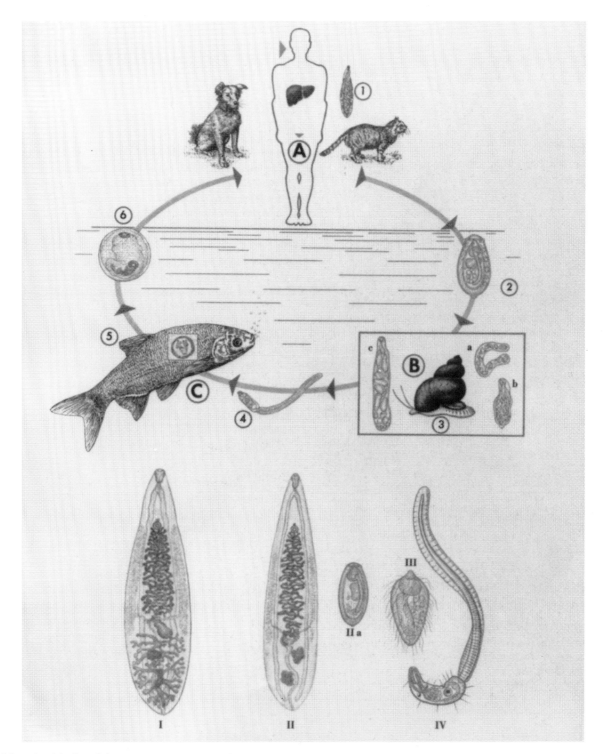

Fig. 3. Lifecycle of the liver fluke.

Fascioliasis has two different clinical stages, larval migration in the liver parenchyma followed by the chronic phase of the flukes in the bile ducts. During the acute stage there may be dyspepsia, anorexia, nausea, vomiting, abdominal pain in the epigastrium and right upper quadrant, fever, headache, hepatomegaly and tenderness, urticaria, and pronounced eosinophilia. After the flukes lodge in the biliary passages there are few symptoms. Reports of

biliary obstructive disease are scant, the worms usually being found incidentally at autopsy.

Diagnosis and differential diagnosis

The diagnosis of *Fasciola* and *Opisthorchis* infections may be done by the quantitative Kato thick-smear technique, as described for schistosomiasis. Differential diagnosis includes other causes of cholangitis and obstructive jaundice. A history of eating raw freshwater fish or using uncooked fish sauce should be elicited. For acute fascioliasis, intense eosinophilia is a frequent occurrence. A careful history should elicit consumption of wild watercress. Cases often occur in clusters.

Treatment and prognosis

For treatment of *Clonorchis* infection the dose of praziquantel is 25 mg/kg three times daily for 2 days. For opisthorchiasis the treatment is 25 mg/kg three times in 1 day. The cure rates have ranged between 73 and 100 per cent. Intensities of infection have been greatly reduced in those not cured. In those with obstructive jaundice a modified Longmire bypass operation may be used for palliation. Praziquantel has not so far proved successful for the treatment of fascioliasis. The current drug of choice remains bithional given orally in a dose of 1 g three times daily for 15 days. Side-effects may be nausea, vomiting and diarrhoea. Triclabendazole, a promising new single dose veterinary drug for fascioliasis, is undergoing clinical trials.[7] For liver fluke infections, as in schistosomiasis, periodic anthelmintic treatment in endemic areas should also prevent disease. Unfortunately, little effort is being devoted to vaccine development.

References

1. Mahmoud AAF and Abdel Wahab MF. Schistosomiasis. In Warren KS and Mahmoud AAF, eds. *Tropical and geographical medicine*. 2nd edn. New York: McGraw-Hill, 1990: 458–72.
2. Warren KS. The control of helminths: non-replicating infectious agents of man. *Annual Review of Public Health*, 1981; **2**: 101–16.
3. Warren KS. The secret of the immunopathogenesis of schistosomiasis: *in vivo* models. *Immunological Reviews*, 1982; **61**: 189–213.
4. McKerrow JH and Sun E. Hepatic schistosomiasis. *Progress in Liver Disease*, 1994; **12**: 121–35.
5. Von Lichtenberg F. Consequences of infections with schistosomes. In Rollinson D and Simpson AJG, eds. *The biology of schistosomes: from genes to latrines*. London: Academic Press, 1987: 185.
6. Koshy A, al-Nabib B, al-Mufti S, Madda JP, and Hira PR. Anti-HCV-positive cirrhosis associated with schistosomiasis. *American Journal of Gastroenterology*, 1993; **88**: 1428–31.
7. World Health Organization. *WHO model prescribing information: drugs used in parasitic infections*. 2nd edn. Geneva: World Health Organization, 1995: 146.
8. Upatham ES, *et al.* Morbidity in relation to intensity of infection in opisthorchiasis viverrini: study of a community of Khon Kaen, Thailand. *American Journal of Tropical Medicine and Hygiene*, 1982; **31**: 1156–63.

13.4.2 Echinococcosis of the liver

Solange Bresson-Hadni, J. P. Miguet, and Dominique A. Vuitton

The two main larval cestode diseases observed in man are hydatid cyst echinococcosis and alveolar echinococcosis. Despite the similarity of the two causative taenias the two diseases are completely different and therefore need to be described separately, except for immunodiagnosis and chemotherapy which share many points.

Hydatid cysts of the liver
Epidemiology
Lifecycle

The adult cestode or 'tapeworm' develops in the small intestine of the definitive host which is a carnivore. This cestode, not exceeding 1 cm in length, has three or four segments (proglottids). The last segment contains eggs which are released into the intestine and dispersed on the grass with the stools of the host. Eggs, with a diameter ranging from 30 to 40 mm, consist of a hexacanth embryo (oncospheres) surrounded by many envelopes. When eggs are eaten by the intermediate host (usually a mammal) the hexacanth embryo with its three pairs of cephalic hooks is released into the duodenum; it passes through the intestinal wall into the portal and lymphatic systems, and then most usually to the liver. Domestic dogs are the most common definitive hosts. Sheep, cattle, swine, or (accidentally) humans serve as intermediate hosts. Dogs are infected by eating raw infective offal containing hydatid larvae. Man becomes infected by eating eggs shed in the stools of infected dogs, either by touching dogs with contaminated hair or by ingesting infected vegetables or water. Besides this domestic cycle, there is a much less common cycle which involves a wild carnivore such as the wolf, jackal, or coyote as definitive host and a wild herbivore such as the elk, caribou, or reindeer as intermediate host.

Prevalence

Echinococcus granulosus occurs worldwide. However, the prevalence of hydatid cyst in humans appears directly related to a low level of sanitation. The disease is prominent in rural areas where humans, dogs, and cattle coexist closely, with poor housing conditions. The incidence of surgical cases in man per 100 000 population per year ranges from 1.4 in Italy to 27.1 in Dalmatia.[1] Recent survey data indicate that infection in man is most common in the regions of the world where the raising of livestock is a major industry.[1] These countries include the entire Mediterranean littoral, New Zealand, southeast Australia including Tasmania, southern and central former USSR, north and northwestern China, and parts of South America, particularly Uruguay, Argentina, and Chile.[1,2]

Prevention and control

Control of *Echinococcus granulosus* in its dog–sheep transmission is a realistic objective. In New Zealand and Tasmania, human incidence of hydatid cyst decreased after control strategies were undertaken.[3] In Tasmania, the annual incidence decreased from 15 cases per 100 000 before 1965 to 1.4 per 100 000 in 1978. In New Zealand the prevalence in dogs has diminished from 12.7 to 0.22 per cent and the prevalence in aged sheep from over 50 to 3.4 per cent (McConnel, AustVetJ, 1979; 55:140). Iceland had the world's highest prevalence of hydatidosis during the nineteenth century, with up to a third of all autopsies disclosing hydatid cyst; the country is currently hydatid free.[3]

Preventive measures include treatment of dogs with praziquantel or destruction of stray dogs. The most efficient measures involve

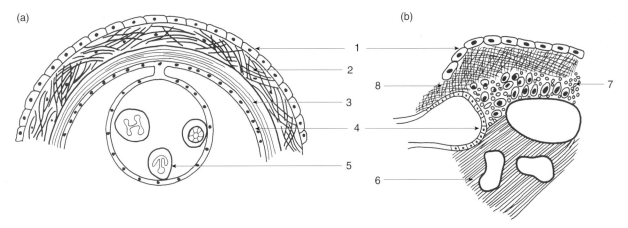

Fig. 1. (a) Diagrammatic structure of an *Echinococcus granulosus* cyst. The following details can be identified: 1 host organ parenchyma; 2 connective tissue layer; 3 laminated membrane; 4 germinative membrane; 5 protoscolices inside a brood capsule. (b) Diagrammatic structure of alveolar echinococcosis of the liver. The following details can be identified: 1 host organ parenchyma; 6 fibrosis; 7 granuloma; 8 necrosis.

education campaigns, active steps to prevent access by dogs to infective offals, and the development of safe livestock slaughtering facilities.[4]

Pathogenesis

Man ingests infective eggs accidentally. In the duodenum, the hexacanth embryos are released and using their hooklets pass through the mucosa and reach the blood vessels. They reach the liver or the lungs via the portal vein and then other organs or tissues via a venous or a lymphatic pathway (Heath, IntJParasitol, 1971; 145:1). The embryos of *Echinococcus granulosus* develop into a parent cyst which is formed by two membranes or layers. The inner, fertile layer is called the germinative membrane. Many brood capsules containing numerous protoscolices (the future head of the adult cestode) develop by budding of the epithelium of the germinative membrane. The outer hyaline membrane is derived from host tissue and is called the laminated membrane. This outer layer is surrounded by a fibrous wall which is sometimes calcified, and limits the extension of the cyst. Outside this wall the liver appears normal (Fig. 1(a)).

The cyst grows at a rate of about 0.3 cm/year and does not usually give clinical symptoms until it has reached 10 cm in diameter; a mass is rarely palpable before the diameter attains 20 cm. Cysts may remain static or spontaneously disappear, as occurs in 7 per cent of cases (Romig, Lancet, 1986; i:861). The cysts are filled with fluid under pressure and contain protoscolices (called hydatid sand), granula (which gave the parasite the name granulosus), and occasionally daughter cysts.

The cysts may be located in any area of the liver, it may be of any size, and solitary or multiple. The right lobe is involved in 75 per cent of cases, and one-third of cysts are solitary.[2] Amongst 1802 patients in an Australian hydatid register, 63 per cent of lesions were located in the liver, 25 per cent in the lungs, 25 per cent in muscle, 3 per cent in bone, 2 per cent in kidney, 1 per cent each in spleen and brain;[2] involvement of multiple organs was observed in 20 per cent of patients.[2] Bone, chest, and brain localizations have been extensively studied (Porat, IsrJMedSci, 1978; 14:223; Xanthakis, Thorax, 1972; 27:517; Abbassioun, JNeurosurg, 1978;

49:408). Exceptionally, cysts have occurred in the heart, biliary tract, thyroid and parotid gland, tongue, tooth, broad ligament, prostate, bladder, tonsil, pulmonary artery, and inferior vena cava.[3]

Clinical features and complications

The hydatid cyst may remain clinically silent for a long time. Very often it is discovered incidentally during routine abdominal ultrasound examination. Occasionally the patient complains of vague right upper quadrant pain, urticaria, and episodes of itching. Exceptionally he may notice the appearance of a right upper quadrant tumoural mass. More often the diagnosis is made when a complication occurs—mainly jaundice. In endemic areas, mass population screening programmes with ultrasound and/or serology are becoming a new way to discover hydatid cyst of the liver (Saint-Martin, JClinUltrasound, 1988; 16:233).

Physical examination of the liver may be normal or may disclose an enlarged and regular liver when the cyst is located in superior, central, or posterior parts. If the cyst is located in the anterior area of the liver, a round, painless tumour can be recognized during physical examination. Exceptionally, a hydatid thrill may be elicited.[2] Sometimes the disease is disclosed when a complication occurs. Compression of the common bile duct, portal or hepatic veins, or inferior vena cava is uncommon, whereas rupture of the cyst (usually into the bile ducts) is much more common. At the time of diagnosis, 36 to 40 per cent of hepatic cysts have ruptured or become secondarily infected.[3] Cysts located near the diaphragm can erode and perforate into the pleural and pericardial cavities, the lung, or the bronchi. Cysts close to the peritoneal cavity may perforate into the peritoneum or into the duodenum, the stomach, the colon, or the right renal pelvis. These ruptures may lead to the development of extrahepatic hydatic cysts, and also may cause allergic symptoms such as a sudden increase of blood eosinophils, itching urticaria, and anaphylactic shock. More commonly, the rupture of hydatid cyst occurs into bile ducts, and is revealed by cholestatic jaundice, cholangitis, or biliary pain. Some ruptures into bile ducts may be clinically silent, and are thus only disclosed during an operation.

Diagnosis

The two key procedures for diagnosis are ultrasonography and serology.

Plain films of the abdomen may sometimes show arc-shaped calcifications which are highly suggestive of the diagnosis. Chest radiography can disclose characteristic deformation of the diaphragm and sometimes images evoking hydatid cyst of the lungs or mediastinum.

Ultrasonography has the best diagnostic efficiency because it can be used to recognize cysts as small as 1 cm in diameter. It can show one or several round masses with a well-defined contour, which may be empty or filled with echogenic structures corresponding to daughter cysts. Ultrasonography can be used to recognize the rupture of the germinative membrane by showing a folded, detached endocyst. When cysts become infected, they are diffusely hyperechogenic and no longer exhibit characteristic ultrasonography features (Lewal, Radiol, 1985; 155:773). In 1981, an ultrasonographic classification was proposed by Gharbi et al. (Gharbi, Radiol, 1981; 139:459) based on a correlation between five ultrasonographic types and pathological findings of the cyst:

Type 1 consists of a rounded fluid collection with well-defined contours.
Type 2 is a type 1 cyst with a mobile inner membrane.
Type 3 is a multiseptated cyst.
Type 4 is heterogeneous with a pseudotumoural appearance.
Type 5 is a calcified cyst.

On computed tomography (**CT**), the unilocular cyst with its spherical or oval structure of near-water density is easily recognized. Conversely, multilocular cysts may have several CT patterns depending on the space occupied by daughter cysts inside the mother cyst; however, the CT densities of viable daughter cysts are always lower than those of mother hydatid cyst and this difference in density appears to be a useful diagnostic sign (Kalovidouris, ComputAssistTomogr, 1986; 10:428). None of the CT findings are pathognomonic, and abscesses or necrotic tumours may mimic some aspects of hydatid cyst. In such circumstances, particularly with negative serological results, only aspiration cytology can establish the diagnosis of hydatid cyst.[5,6] Although hydatid cyst puncture is contraindicated because of a risk of anaphylaxis and peritoneal dissemination, in two large series of hydatid cyst aspiration with a fine needle under ultrasound guidance anaphylaxictic complications were not provoked.[5,6] Diagnostic punctions were systematically followed by the intracystic injection of a scolicid solution.

Surgical treatment

Except for small and multiple hydatid cyst of the liver, cysts should be treated by surgery because of the risks of rupture or secondary infection. The objective is to remove all parasitic cysts and fluid completely. The two surgical alternatives are cystectomy and hepatic resection.

Cystectomy and pericystectomy

These procedures permit the complete removal of the parasite without the risks of liver resection and should be undertaken in most patients.[6]

In a series of 69 patients who underwent surgery for hydatid disease of the liver there were no deaths, and postoperative morbidity was low and equally distributed whether surgery was radical or conservative (Morel, Surgery, 1988; 104:859). In order to avoid intra-abdominal hydatidosis by spillage of the contents of the hepatic cyst, the peritoneal cavity must be carefully protected during cyst evacuation, either by suturing a plastic drape to the cyst wall before opening it[6] or by using a cryogenic cone which seals the cyst wall (Saidi, NEJM, 1971; 284:1346).

The contents of the cyst are first sterilized by injection of scolicidal agents and then evacuated. Formalin and hypertonic saline should no longer be used because of the risk of caustic sclerosing cholangitis (Belghiti, ArchSurg, 1986; 121:1162; Prat, GastrClinBiol, 1988; 12:867). Chlorhexidine, H_2O_2, 80 per cent alcohol, or 0.5 per cent cetrimide are safer alternatives to sterilize the cyst.[6] Intracystic injection of scolicide should not be used if preliminary aspiration gives bile-stained fluid or if there is any radiological or clinical evidence to suspect a biliary communication (Dawson, BrJSurg, 1988; 75:946). Pretreatment of patients with benzidimidazole compounds may make scolicidal agents obsolete.[7] After the liver overlying the cyst has been incised, attempts should be made to excise the laminated membrane intact; generally the membrane is removed piecemeal.

Hepatic resection

Resection is recommended for central cysts of a left lateral segment. The rate of recurrence after hepatic surgery is variable, ranging from 8 to 22 per cent (French, EAMedJ, 1984; 61:113).[7],[8] It appears higher in regions with high endemic rates (Morris, BrJSurg, 1987; 74:805). The rate of recurrence decreases in patients treated with mebendazole and surgery (French, EAMedJ, 1984; 61:113). Orthotopic liver transplantation is indicated for patients with acute parasitic Budd–Chiari syndrome, complicated biliary cirrhosis, or secondary cholangitis (Moreno-Gonzalez, Transpl, 1994; 58:797).

Instrumental treatment: punction–aspiration–injection–reaspiration (PAIR)

Recently, percutaneous treatment of hydatid cyst has been proposed as an alternative to surgery. After percutaneous puncture under ultrasonographic guidance, a complete aspiration is performed; the residual cavity is then completely filled with hypertonic saline, which is reaspired 10 min later.

No anaphylactic shock or secondary dissemination have been reported. This technique can only be proposed for type 1, 2, and 3 cysts. There is no particular contraindication except for a communication of the cyst with the biliary tree. Some authors recommend pre- and postbenzimidazoles therapy to avoid parasitic spillage. In experienced hands, it represents the first choice of treatment, especially for inoperable patients and in cases with a high surgical risk (Khuroo, Gastro, 1993; 104:1452);[9] some authors associate drainage with PAIR (Filice, Radiol, 1992; 184:579). In some endemic areas, especially in developing countries, PAIR, which is less costly, is under evaluation as an alternative to surgery. So far only one centre has published long-term results of percutaneous treatment;[10] in this series of 31 patients with 57 liver hydatid cysts, the mean follow-up period after PAIR was 32.5 months (range 17–48) and the recurrence rate was 2 per cent. This promising new approach should not be used widely unless more experience and longer follow-ups have been achieved.

Treatment of complications

Cholangitis is usually treated by biliary surgical drainage after removal of the cyst. In some instances, papillotomy during endoscopy may be proposed (Dumas, GastrClinBiol, 1989; 13:A247).

The rupture of an hepatic cyst into the peritoneal cavity remains difficult to cure. Despite the surgical removal of cyst contents from the peritoneal cavity, remaining protoscolices form daughter cysts lead to almost inevitable recurrence. Mebendazole or albendazole are strongly indicated in such situations.

Alveolar echinococcosis of the liver

Alveolar echinococcosis of the liver is an uncommon parasitic disease which is due to the intrahepatic growth of the larva of *Echinococcus multilocularis*. The disease is also called alveolar hydatid disease. Alveolar echinococcosis behaves as a liver cancer and is always fatal unless completely removed by surgery.

Epidemiology

Lifecycle

A cycle in wild animals allows the parasite to subsist in nature. The adult worm develops in the small intestine of the definitive host—a fox. This cestode, which does not exceed 3 mm in length, has four or five segments. The last segment contains eggs which are released into the intestine; these disperse on the ground with the stools of the host where they contaminate the grass and, in particular, wild fruits. Eggs, with a diameter ranging from 30 to 40 mm, have three pairs of cephalic hooks. Eggs are surrounded by an envelope which allows them to resist very low temperatures (to −40°C) but they die at +60°C. When eggs are eaten by the intermediate host, usually a wild rodent, the hexacanth embryo is released into the duodenum. It enters the intestinal wall, travels to the liver, and thence can reach lungs, brain, and bones. In the liver alveolar echinococcosis develops; in rodents it consists of a mass of small vesicles each lined by the germinal membrane from which enormous numbers of protoscolices develop.[8] The lesion produced by a single hexacanth embryo attains a diameter of 1 cm, but the lesions produced by several embryos may coalesce and can thus occupy a considerable part of the liver.[11] The lifecycle is completed when the intermediate host, containing infected larvae, is eaten by a suitable host, usually red foxes. In eastern France, 25 per cent of foxes have been found to be contaminated and the prevalence of the disease in rodents has been evaluated at 0.05 per cent.[12] Less commonly, coyotes, domestic dogs, or domestic cats can also serve as definitive hosts and may become potential sources of infection for man (Eckert, TropMedParas, 1974; 25:334).

Prevalence

Humans, accidental intermediate hosts, become infected either by eating contaminated wild fruit or by touching foxes. This explains why 30 per cent of patients from a large series were hunters;[13] most patients were farmers although all kinds of occupations were included. Hence, besides the classical risk factors such as eating unwashed wild fruits and hunting, eating raw vegetables harvested in a kitchen garden near a forest might also represent an important risk factor for the disease.[12] The fact that familial cases are exceptional, despite shared risk factors, could imply the existence of individual and/or immunological factors conditioning the susceptibility to contamination.[12]

The majority of patients are between 30 and 50 years of age. A mean delay of 20 years is usual between contamination and symptoms revealing the disease,[13] although disease has been disclosed in a 5-year-old girl suggesting that its progression might sometimes be faster than is usually thought.[13]

The male:female ratio is 1:1. The main endemic regions for alveolar echinococcosis in humans are central Europe (southern Germany, western Austria, eastern France), the greater part of the former Soviet Union, Turkey, Japan, the Kurile Islands, China, and North America (Alaska, northern Canada). Reports of adult or larval cestodes in north central America (Iowa, Minnesota, Montana, North and South Dakota, southern Canada) suggest that in the United States the parasite is still moving south and east.[11] In north and northwestern China, the prevalence of alveolar echinococcosis can be as high as 16 per cent in some villages (Graig, Lancet, 1992; 340:826).[2]

Prevention and control

Preventive measures are limited to educational programmes aimed at warning the population in endemic areas of the hazards of touching foxes and eating wild fruits. It might be advisable to enclose a kitchen garden located near a forest. Extermination of foxes is not a realistic objective, and could be deleterious. Past experience in rabies control has shown that fox-culling results in an incursion of foxes from neighbouring territories and exacerbates the spatial spread of a disease.[4] Vole trapping might be feasible[4] but an assessment of its effect on the reciprocal host population is required. A third option could be mass dosing of foxes with praziquantel, possibly by the aerial distribution of treated baits.[4] A pilot study on a possible control of the parasite by such a mean was performed in southern Germany (Schelling, MittOstGest-TropMedParas, 1990; 27:70). Six treatments, performed during 14 months, led to a drastic reduction in the prevalence of *E. multilocularis* in foxes in the control area. This suggests that control measures are able to reduce the prevalence of *E. multilocularis* in foxes but control can only be expected if the drug regimen is repeated or distributed over a large surface and for prolonged periods of time.

Praziquantel provides a 100 per cent elimination of the parasite from dogs when given in doses of 5 mg/kg of body weight; it should therefore be given regularly to domestic dogs.

Pathogenesis

In man, the hepatic lesions generally consist of a unique mass of fibrous tissue which displays a multitude of cavities, ranging from a few millimetres to a few centimetres in size (Fig. 2). *Echinococcus multilocularis* also produces hepatic necrosis allowing the parasite to invade the liver step by step in a similar way to a liver carcinoma. The lesions are never limited by a fibrous shell. The parasitic tissue

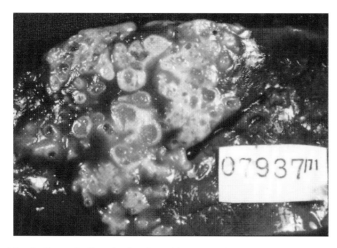

Fig. 2. Gross findings in alveolar echinococcosis: numerous cavities of variable sizes within fibrous tissue. There is no clear demarcation with healthy liver parenchyma.

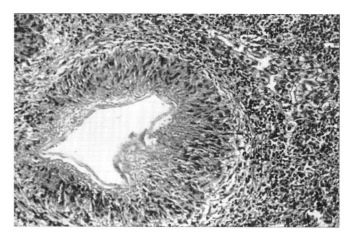

Fig. 3. Characteristic histological findings in alveolar echinococcosis. Thin cuticle with germinative membrane demarcating a small cavity; beyond the cuticle, from inside to outside, cellular reaction with a necrotic zone, a zone of epithelioid cells, and a zone of lymphocytes.

electively involves and destroys the bifurcation of intrahepatic bile ducts. It may also invade major hepatic vessels and inferior vena cava.[13] Usually the lesions are prominent in the right lobe of the liver.

Necrosis and fibrosis (Fig. 1(b)) are the most characteristic damages caused by *Echinococcus multilocularis* in the human liver. The abundance of immunological cells close to the parasite suggests that the lesions are due to a conflict between the parasite and lymphocytes of the host.[12]

Microscopically, the lesions consist of an unique cuticle, usually devoid of a germinative membrane. Scolices are observed in 15 per cent of cases. Apart from the cuticle there is always an intense immune-cell proliferation composed of lymphocytes and histiocytes arranged in a fence pattern. Thus, the histological picture is characteristic of a granuloma (Fig. 3). Despite the absence of a germinative membrane and scolices, it is usually easy to infect rodents with parasitic material obtained from human lesions.[16] We succeeded in infecting each of 20 rodents using parasitic material obtained from patients who underwent surgery (Liance, IntJ-Parasitol, 1990; 20:83). This parasitic granuloma (absent in hydatid cyst disease) leads to a scarring fibrosis which compresses and completely destroys the hepatic vessels and the bile ducts. A necrotic process ensues and leads to the formation of huge cavities containing parasitic and hepatic debris, blood, bile, and sometimes pus.

Clinical features and complications

Very few large series of the disease have been reported.[12,15,16] Our own series of 80 cases illustrates the major features of the disease.[9] Of the 80 patients observed from 1973 to 1988, the 30 cases collected from 1983 are reported separately because the conditions of diagnosis have changed in the meanwhile.

Classical data

Eighty per cent of the patients suffer vague upper abdominal pains for many years before diagnosis. The two major revealing symptoms are cholestatic jaundice in half of the cases and an enlarged and irregular liver without jaundice in the others. Cholestatic jaundice

is usually very similar to that observed in intrahepatic bile duct carcinoma.

Pruritus is commonly observed. In patients with cholestatic jaundice, operative, transhepatic percutaneous, or endoscopic cholangiography shows a more or less complete stenosis of the intrahepatic biliary convergence with a dilatation of the biliary tree upstream. The absence of dilatation of the biliary tree in a few patients with intense jaundice is usually the consequence of a secondary biliary cirrhosis—the fibrotic liver does not allow the biliary tree to expand. Less often, jaundice is associated with colicky abdominal pains, chills, and fever. Such cholangitic forms are related either to intrahepatic stones or, more commonly, to an abscess of the liver. In this case, necrosis causes a large cavity from which debris migrates through the common bile duct and behaves as gallstones. An enlarged liver without jaundice is the presenting symptom in half of the cases. There is a contrast between a huge hepatomegaly mimicking a hepatic carcinoma and the maintenance of good clinical status. Such lesions can sometimes be taken for a malignant tumour, including intraoperatively. Thus, a biopsy is mandatory before diagnosing a carcinoma of the liver in regions where alveolar echinococcosis is endemic. Anaphylactic reactions have never been reported after needle biopsy in alveolar echinococcosis, perhaps because there is usually a lack of protoscolices and germinative membranes. Spontaneous anaphylactic reactions are exceptional; we reported a case of allergy secondary to pulmonary embolism with parasitic thrombi.[17]

Current data

A notable, recent change is the apparent increase in the diagnosis of less severe and asymptomatic case. Sixty per cent of the 30 cases observed between 1983 and 1988 were disclosed by ultrasonography performed for slight pain in the upper abdomen. Only 30 per cent of cases are currently revealed by jaundice; this trend continued in the 55 new cases observed since 1988.

It has been shown that mass screening programmes using immunodiagnostic tests can lead to diagnosis of the disease in its early stages and can thus increase the number of surgically curable cases.[16] In a survey in our endemic region in eastern France, with an enzyme-linked immunosorbent assay (**ELISA**) using a specific antigen of *Echinococcus multilocularis*, eight cases of patients with active parasitic lesions and five of abortive calcified lesions of the liver were found out of 7884 screened sera.[18] Using an ELISA test with a purified *Echinococcus multilocularis* antigen, 35 subjects were found positive in Alaska out of a population of 1103 screened (Gottstein, Lancet, 1985; ii:1097); there was also a significant prevalence of abortive lesions in this series.

Laboratory findings

Total and conjugated bilirubin are increased in proportion to the degree of jaundice. γ-Glutamyl transferase and alkaline phosphatase are markedly increased in jaundiced patients as well as in patients without jaundice. In most of our patients, γ-glutamyl transferase and alkaline phosphatase were greater than 20 and six times the upper limits, respectively. Conversely, serum transaminases are usually normal except for a few patients with a necrotic process in the liver, in whom a two- to four-fold increase is usual. Eosinophilia of greater than 7 per cent is found in about 10 per cent of patients.

A high level of C-reactive protein is highly suggestive of a latent biliary infection.[12] Prothrombin time and factor V are usually normal. In 80 per cent of patients, serum gammaglobulin levels are higher than 30 g/l; electrophoresis shows a polyclonal, and only exceptionally a monoclonal, gammopathy. All three classes of immunoglobulins (G, A, M) are increased.

Complications

Complications rarely reveal the disease but they invariably occur during follow-up. The most frequent complication is biliary infection with septicaemia and septic shock in some instances. Infections occur either when intrahepatic stones are present or when the biliary drainage becomes inefficient. Another frequent complication is bleeding from oesophagogastric varices related to portal hypertension of various origins. This is becoming rarer with the introduction of prophylaxis of variceal bleeding with β-blockers. The commonest cause of portal hypertension is a secondary biliary cirrhosis, and more rarely a chronic Budd–Chiari syndrome or a parasitic portal thrombosis. In two patients from our series, bleeding came from the rupture of jejunal varices which developed on the hepaticojejunostomy. Metastases occur in 10 per cent of the patients; pulmonary metastases being more common than brain or bone metastases.[17] Unusual metastases have been reported in kidneys causing haematuria (Levrat, AnnGastroHep, 1973; 9:37), in the eye with decreased visual acuity (Williams, ArchOphthalmol, 1987; 105: 1107), in the lacrymal gland (Levrat, AnnGastroHep, 1973; 9: 37), in the peritoneum (Levrat, AnnGastroHep, 1973; 9:37), and abdominal lymph nodes. Skin localization via adjacent progression of the larvae has been recently reported (Bresson-Hadni, JAmAcadDermatol, 1996; 34:873). Amyloid and immune complex deposits in renal and hepatic parenchyma have been found in patients with alveolar echinococcosis of the liver (Ali-Khan, AnnTropMed, 1987; 81:381). Amyloidosis is probably secondary to chronic infection. Two patients of our series had a cardiac localization (Etievent, JCardiovascSurg, 1986; 27:671);[17] two others suffered a biliary fistula with the bronchi. Causes of death are cachexia, septic shock, bleeding, hepatic insufficiency, respiratory distress, or strokes.

Morphological findings

In 50 per cent of cases, abdominal radiography shows punctiform, flame-like calcifications which never form a circle, as is usually the case in hydatid cyst. The most useful method for diagnosis and for determining the extension of lesions is ultrasonography (Fig. 4).[15] The ultrasound features are usually characteristic, showing a liver mass with irregular and ill-defined contours. Because of the small size of the cavities, ultrasonography does not disclose cysts but shows a characteristic association of echogenic areas due to fibrosis and transonic zones due to necrosis inside the parasitic mass.[19] In 50 per cent of cases, there are calcifications, shown by an increased echogenicity with accompanying acoustic shadows. Less often, a transonic pseudocystic necrotic zone with debris is disclosed.[19] Ultrasonography may also show hilar involvement and biliary dilatation, with the classical 'shotgun' images, or stenosis of the portal vein or the inferior vena cava with parasitic lesions.

The CT scan shows a typical geographical map pattern with irregular contours.[19] Inside the mass, hypodense areas due to necrosis are associated with hyperdense zones due to calcifications (Fig. 5).[19] No significant enhancement is observed within the lesions after bolus administration of intravenous contrast medium.[19] Magnetic resonance imaging (**MRI**) is used to define the relation of the parasitic mass to large vessels, diaphragm, and heart (Claudon, JComputAssistTomogr, 1990; 14:608). Twenty-five of our patients with liver alveolar echinococcosis lesions underwent MRI examination; the results were compared with a CT scan. MRI imaging characterized well the different components of the parasitic lesions and precisely delineated the necrosis area. It showed the parasitic vesicles in high signal on T2-weighted sequence. It was able to identify a multilocular aspect with multiple parasitic cysts less than 1 cm in high signal on T2 weighted sequence—this honeycomb-like pattern can be considered pathognomonic of alveolar echinococcosis. MRI was more sensitive than CT for disclosing an early case as a homogenous nodule. It was also superior to CT for demonstrating invasion of vena cava, hepatic veins, and diaphragm (Bartholomot, unpublished data).

Percutaneous transhepatic cholangiography and hepatic angiography are generally useful only before surgery.

Treatment

The sole efficient treatment is partial hepatectomy when the lesions are sufficiently localized.[13,15,20] Because the intrahepatic common bile duct is usually involved, it is often necessary to remove the bifurcation and to reconstruct the biliary tract.[12,21] To this purpose, a trisegmentectomy is followed by an anastomosis between the left hepatic duct and a Roux-en-Y loop. In our series from 1983 onwards, such a major hepatectomy has been performed in 30 per cent of the patients as compared to 10 per cent before 1983. Because the right part of the liver is most commonly involved, a left hepatectomy was undertaken in only one of ten cases.

Multiple bilobar lesions may be resectable.[15] 'Atypical' resection, although not curative, was shown to be beneficial in a large series of 119 resections (Al'Perovich, Khirurgia, 1975; 10:47). A review of 66 cases has shown that 42 per cent of the patients were surviving 5 years after surgical excision compared to a 5-year survival rate of 20 to 26 per cent after palliative procedures (Akovbiantz, SchMedWoch, 1978; 108:1104).

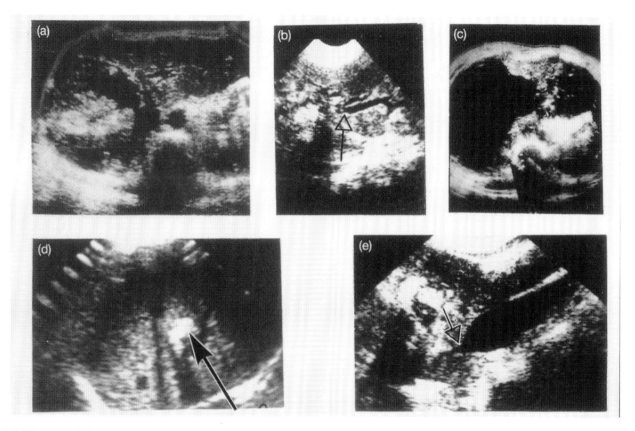

Fig. 4. (a) Transversal ultrasound section showing typical lesions combining hyperechogenic and hypoechogenic zones within a mass with uneven 'map-like' contours; (b) dilatation of intrahepatic ducts (shotgun sign, arrow); (c) large cavity due to retreat of the parasite; (d) hepatic calcifications (arrow) with a cone-shaped acoustic shadow; (e) sagittal section showing narrowing of the inferior vena cava by the parasitic lesion (arrow).

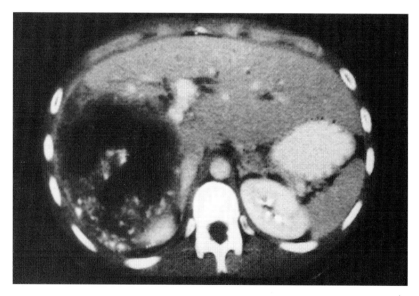

Fig. 5. CT scan section showing lesions with uneven contours and a mosaic of densities extending from the density of water to that of bone.

For unresectable patients, only palliative procedures associated with medical treatment or orthotopic liver transplantation are available. Palliative procedures consist of left or right hepaticojejunostomy, portosystemic shunts, and internal or external drainage of liver abscess.[12] Less invasive procedures, such as sclerotherapy of oesophageal varices and endoprotheses introduced into bile ducts by a percutaneous transhepatic technique,[17] should be used to limit the number of laparotomies before orthotopic liver transplantation; we chose this intervention policy in young patients for whom a liver transplantation may become indicated in the future.

Among the 210 patients with liver transplant from our centre, 21 were transplanted due to alveolar echinococcosis; a report on 17 of these patients has been published.[23] In these patients, nearly all the main relative contraindications for orthotopic liver transplantation were present: multiple palliative surgical procedures had been carried out in ten; six had external biliary and purulent fistulas; the diaphragm and pericardium were invaded in eight and three respectively; the inferior vena cava was involved in eight; untreatable bacterial cholangitis was life-threatening in nine; all but two had portal hypertension—due to secondary biliary cirrhosis in eight, to Budd–Chiari syndrome in five, and to portal thrombosis in four. However, the results have shown that, despite all these contraindications, orthotopic liver transplantation can be performed successfully in patients with terminal alveolar echinococcosis.

It is of note that in 50 per cent of the patients transplantation was only a palliative procedure because of residual areas of parasitic tissue or lung metastases. We have observed the progression of residual alveolar echinococcosis under immunosuppressive therapy. Three patients had a graft-recurrence of alveolar echinococcosis (between the second and the fourth year postorthotopic liver transplantation) originating from residual parasite in the foci diaphragmatic, one of which was symptomatic. In one patient a splenic localization was disclosed 2 years postorthotopic liver transplantation and in one case cerebral metastases disclosed four years postorthotopic liver transplantation led to the death of the patient 1 year later. The serological follow up of IgG against a crude *Echinococcus granulosus* antigenic extract appeared useful in distinguishing between 'palliative' and 'curative' orthotopic liver transplantation; anti-Em2 IgG follow up was not useful in this context (Bresson-Hadni, Hepatol, 1993; 16:279). In our series, the 5-year survival rate after orthotopic liver transplantation for incurable alveolar echinococcosis is currently 46 per cent.

Immunodiagnosis of echinococcosis

Numerous immunodiagnostic tests are currently available for hydatid cyst and alveolar echinococcosis. A cross reactivity is observed between the two cestodes, and immunological tests for hydatid disease can be used for the diagnosis of alveolar echinococcosis.

Serological tests

These are based on the detection of specific antibodies in serum by using an antigen obtained from *Echinococcus granulosus* (hydatid fluid or hydatid sand) or *Echinococcus multilocularis* (protoscolices or parasitic extracts). The complement fixation test is no longer used because of its poor sensitivity and specificity. It has been advantageously replaced by the indirect haemagglutination test and the latex test, using hydatid fluid or crude extracts of *Echinococcus multilocularis*. In hepatic hydatid cyst and alveolar echinococcosis these tests have up to 80 per cent and 85 per cent sensitivity, respectively[24,25] and both have good specificity. Among humoral tests, the latex test is widely used as a screening test because of its simplicity and low cost. Conversely, immunoelectrophoresis is mainly used as a confirmation test because of its high specificity,

particularly when it discloses the precipitation arc.[5,24] A positive latex test needs to be confirmed by immunoelectrophoresis or an indirect immunofluorescence test using hydatid sand as source of antigen.[24] However, an ELISA test, using either fraction 5 of *Echinococcus granulosus* or the Em2 fraction of *Echinococcus multilocularis*, appears currently to be the most sensitive and specific serological test, with up to 90 per cent positivity in both diseases (Gottstein, Experientia, 1982; 38:1372); it can also be used as a screening test.

Besides their diagnostic value, serological tests are also useful in establishing cure. Usually the period just after surgery is characterized by a temporary increase of antibody levels; afterwards a progressive decrease continues for 1 to 2 years before negative results are achieved. The persistence of raised levels or a further increase is suggestive of residual disease or a recurrence (Cesbron, GastrClinBiol, 1986; 10:415).

Several other tests have been proposed to improve sensitivity or specificity; these are the detection of circulating antigens (Graig, AnnTropMed, 1984; 78:219), monoclonal antibodies for antigen 5 (Di-Felice, ParasitolToday, 1987; 3:25), and Western blot (Auer, ZblBaktHyg, 1988; A268:416). A hydatid antigen dot immunobinding assay also seems interesting—in view of its simplicity it will probably be suitable for large-scale field screening (Mistrello, ImmunolLet, 1995; 47:79). In alveolar echinococcosis, a new test called 'Em2 +' ELISA will also probably be of great interest for large-scale, seroepidemiological surveys (Gottstein, J Clin Microbiol, 1993; 31:373).

The analysis of the immunoglobulin G subclass-specific responses in hydatid cyst and alveolar echinococcosis revealed that the predominant antibody response consists mainly of the IgG1 and IgG4 subclasses (Wen, AmJTropMedHyg, 1994; 51:741). Monitoring these responses may increase the specificity of immunodiagnosis and permit improved prognosis following therapy.

Detection of specific IgE antibodies

A radio–allergo–sorbent test detected echinococcosis-specific IgE antibodies in sera from three out of four patients with hydatid cyst and in 50 per cent of patients with alveolar echinococcosis.[26] It has been claimed that specific IgE antibodies are useful in the follow-up of patients treated by chemotherapy (Wilson, AnnRevRespDis, 1978; 118:747) but this has not been confirmed in large series.[26]

The human basophil degranulation test detects the presence of fixed, specific IgE on basophil cells in the presence of hydatid antigen. The test correlates with the viability of the parasite, and has a sensitivity of 91 per cent in hydatid cyst of the liver[27] and close to 100 per cent in alveolar echinococcosis.[26] The human basophil degranulation test is up to 95 per cent specific.[27] *In-vivo* degranulation of mast cells in the presence of parasitic antigens is also the basis of the historical intradermal test developed by Casoni in 1911.

Cellular tests

The specific lymphocyte proliferation of peripheral blood mononuclear cells with hydatid antigen was shown to be positive in seronegative patients both in hydatid cyst (Siracusano, ClinExpImmun, 1988; 72:400) and alveolar echinococcosis.[28] These tests are not applicable for routine diagnosis but should be used in cases where the diagnosis is difficult. In alveolar echinococcosis a reduced responsiveness was observed in patients with chronic disease whereas patients harbouring abortive alveolar echinococcosis lesions exhibited a high *in vitro* lymphoproliferative response to *E. multilocularis* antigen (Gottstein, AmJTropMedHyg, 1991; 45:734).

Medical treatment of echinococcosis of the liver
Mebendazole

Mebendazole, a member of the benzimidazole family effective for many nematode infections, is also active on cestode larval infections such as *E. granulosus* and *E. multilocularis*.

Pharmacokinetics

Mebendazole has low bioavailability due to a poor intestinal absorption related to its low solubility (Bekhti, BrJPharm, 1987; 24:390). Massive oral dosages (up to 4 g/day) and concomitant intake with a fatty meal are necessary.[29] Elimination half-lives range from 2.8 to 9.0 h and mean plasma concentrations from 17.5 to 500 ng/ml; mebendazole is highly bound to plasma proteins (Braithwaite, EurJClinPharm, 1982; 22:161), metabolized by the liver, and largely excreted by the biliary route (Witassek, EurJClinPharm, 1983; 25:85). Caution should be observed in administering mebendazole in patients with liver disease and/or impairment of biliary excretion (Witassek, EurJClinPharm, 1983; 25:81); it is recommended that the plasma concentration is monitored during therapy. It is necessary to attain a plasma level above 100 mmol/l. Mebendazole behaves as an enzyme inducer of the hepatic microsomal oxidizing system in humans (Bekhti, BrJClinPharm, 1986; 21:223; Bekhti, BrJPharm, 1987; 24:390). No reduction in dose is necessary in patients with renal failure.[29] As mebendazole has been shown to be embryotoxic and teratogenic in rats, its use is contraindicated during pregnancy and contraceptive methods should be used during therapy.

Results of treatment with mebendazole in hydatid cyst of the liver

After an initial enthusiastic paper reporting the disappearance of hepatic hydatid cyst in four patients,[30] numerous series of patients receiving mebendazole for hydatid disease have been less conclusive.[31] In 37 patients with an unresectable cyst who received 1.0 to 10.0 g/day of mebendazole for a period ranging from 3 to 6 months, success or partial success (assessed by the disappearance or significant decrease in the size of the cyst) was obtained in only 14 per cent.[33] In another series, predictive factors of efficiency of mebendazole appeared to be the young age of the patient, the young age of the cyst, small size and small numbers of cysts, and, particularly, the extrahepatic localizations (for example in the lungs) (Gil-Grande, AmJGastr, 1983; 78:584). The continued serological monitoring was not reliable in the assessment of the efficiency of mebendazole. Surgery remains the main treatment for hydatid cyst of the liver. Mebendazole is of value as a palliative procedure (Bryceson, TrRSocTropMedHyg, 1982; 76:510) and exceptionally as a curative treatment in inoperable patients. It can also be given

to avoid recurrence of the disease after surgery, and has been proposed as a preoperative treatment to sterilize cysts and prevent parasitic spillage during surgery (Ronconi, IntSurg, 1982; 67:405).

Results of treatment with mebendazole in alveolar echinococcosis of the liver

In 54 patients with alveolar echinococcosis receiving 1.5 to 10 g/day of mebendazole orally for a period ranging from 1 to 12 years, the dose was adapted to obtain a plasma concentration 4 h after the morning dose above 250 mmol/l.[32] After observation for longer than 3 years, stabilization of the lesions was observed in 77 per cent of patients.[32] In another series of patients who had recurring hepatic lesions after surgery, a high oral dosage of mebendazole given for a median duration of 4.5 years was shown to slow down the parasitic growth (Luder, JHepatol, 1985; 1:369). A 10-year clinical trial of continuous treatment with mebendazole showed that life expectancy increased as compared to untreated historical controls.[14] All symptomatic patients had subjective improvement and half of the patients had a reduction of 50 per cent or more in the diameter of hepatic lesions.[14] More recently, the effect of chemotherapy on the parasitic mass and the long-term course of alveolar echinococcosis was evaluated in a series of 37 patients treated for a period ranging from 1.5 to 10.7 years (34 with mebendazole, 3 with albendazole). Marked regression of larval tissue occurred in 18 patients, lesions were stationary in 13 patients, and progression was found in six patients. Severe, late complications were observed in patients with hilar involvement, in most cases this was probably related to post-therapy fibrosis of hilar structures (Amman, Hepatol, 1994; 19:735).

As in hydatid cyst, continued serological assessment did not appear to be a reliable tool in assessing the efficiency of mebendazole (Müller, Hepatogast, 1982; 29:236). Most studies conclude that mebendazole is relatively efficient (Müller, Hepatogast, 1982; 29:236)[14,32,33] as it behaves as a parasitostatic drug; lifetime, or at least long-term, treatment is recommended.

Side-effects of mebendazole

The main side-effects consist of mild anaemia, and mild leucopenia, alopecia, gastrointestinal discomfort, and often a frequent increase of serum transaminases.[32] In three alveolar echinococcosis cases with portal hypertension, we observed alopecia associated to severe anaemia or granulocytopenia.

Clinical hepatitis with jaundice is exceptional. The lack of hypersensitivity manifestations associated with hepatitis, and the close dose–effect relationship between serum concentration of mebendazole and increase of serum transaminase, are interpreted as consequences of a direct hepatotoxic effect of the drug rather than an immunoallergic reaction (Beckhti, GastrClinBiol, 1987; 11:701).

Albendazole
This also acts on cestode infection in man.
Parmacokinetics

Albendazole is characterized by a low bioavailability related to an important effect of hepatic first-pass and a fast liver metabolism. Its metabolite, albendazole sulphoxide, is detectable in serum (Rossignol, GastrClinBiol, 1984; 8:569); the half-life of the sulphoxide averages 8.3 h, and in patients with hydatid disease, high concentrations of albendazole sulphoxide were found in the liver tissue as well as in the hydatid hepatic cyst fluid 12 h after the last dose.[30] High concentrations have also been found in the bile.[34] The level of albendazole sulphoxide in serum varies between patients, and blood concentrations should be carefully monitored during therapy by using an HPLC method.[34] It was recently found that albendazole can behave as an inducer of cytochromes P-450 in rat liver (Amri, JPharmExpTher, 1988; 246:758) but, conversely, the *in vivo* assessment of microsomal hepatic metabolism in humans suggest that it can behave as an inhibitor of the hepatic microsomal drug-oxidizing system (Steiger, GastrClinBiol, 1989; 13:A214).

Results of treatment with albendazole in hydatid cyst of the liver

Since the introduction of albendazole is more recent than mebendazole, there are fewer available studies. Although a preliminary study with albendazole given in 30-day courses separated by 2-week intervals at a dosage of 10 mg/kg per day showed that the drug could cure patients with hydatid cyst of the liver,[34] subsequent larger series were less conclusive, in particular regarding the hepatic localizations of hydatid disease.[32] In a series of 30 patients, 47 per cent of whom had hydatid cyst located only in the liver, a decrease in the size of the cyst was observed in 30 per cent.[32] In another series, albendazole appeared more effective in pleural and peritoneal localization than in hepatic hydatid cyst.[35]

Treatment with a dosage of 10 mg/kg per day for 1 month or more before operation in patients with hepatic hydatid cyst permitted the sterilization of cysts; most of the scolices were found to be dead (Morris, BrJSurg, 1987; 74:805). Medical treatment of hydatid cyst with albendazole appears more efficient than treatment with mebendazole[32] but because of the low efficiency of the former, it is necessary to use mebendazole in inoperable cases, before surgery, or perhaps in the future before treatment by puncture. Needle evacuation of lung hydatid cyst has become a treatment procedure in regions of high prevalence (Megherbi, JChir, 1988; 125:358).

Results of treatment with albendazole in alveolar echinococcosis of the liver

Series of patients treated with albendazole are uncommon, and are often very limited. However, in our experience, albendazole was as effective as mebendazole (unpublished data). From a series of seven patients receiving short-term therapy with albendazole, it was not possible to demonstrate the viability of the parasite by inoculation into red-backed voles with vesicles of larval *E. multilocularis* obtained from surgical tissues of two patients in whom the parasite could be reasonably thought be alive before treatment.[15] These results may be attributable to a therapeutic, and possibly parasitocidal, effect of albendazole in alveolar echinococcosis.[15] However, such effects were never observed in our series (Liance, IntJParasitol, 1990; 20:83).

Side-effects of albendazole

In our series albendazole was well tolerated with few side-effects, except for patients with portal hypertension and/or cholestasis in whom leucopenia and alopecia were not uncommon. Besides these complications, the main side-effect is an increase of serum transaminase which was observed with a prevalence ranging from 3 to 16 per cent.[35] Clinical hepatitis with jaundice was exceptional.[35] The hepatotoxic reaction did not appear to be dose related, nor was it likely to have been due to a hypersensitivity reaction. If AST or ALT levels rise to between 200 and 300 IU/l, discontinuation of therapy should be a major consideration.

Future prospects in medical treatment of echinococcosis of the liver

Two approaches are under current investigations to increase the oral bioavailability of benzimidazoles: combined therapy with cimetidine as an inhibitor of mebendazole metabolism and liposomal albendazole therapy. Preliminary animal studies are encouraging (Wen, BrJClinPharm, 1993; 35:565).

References

1. Schantz PM and Schwabe C. Worldwide status of hydatid disease control. *Journal of the American Veterinary Association*, 1969; **155**: 2104–21.
2. Wen H, New RRC, and Graig PS. Diagnosis and treatment of human hydatidosis. *British Journal of Clinical Pharmacology*, 1993; **35**: 565–74.
3. Radford AJ. Hydatid disease. In Weatherall DJ, Ledingham JGG, and Warrell DA, eds. *Oxford textbook of medicine*. Oxford: University Press, 1987: 5.561–5.
4. Gemmel MA, Lawson JR, and Roberts MG. Towards global control of cystic and alveolar hydatid diseases. *Parasitology Today*, 1987; **3**: 144–51.
5. Hira PR, Lindberg LG, Francis I, *et al*. Diagnosis of cystic hydatid disease: role of aspiration cytology. *Lancet*, 1988; **ii**: 655–7.
6. Bret PM, Fond A, Bretagnolle M, *et al*. Percutaneous aspiration and drainage of hydatid cysts in the liver. *Radiology*, 1988; **168**: 617–20.
7. Langer JC, Rose DB, Keystone JS, Taylor BR, and Langer B. Diagnosis and management of hydatid disease of the liver. A 15-year North American Experience. *Annals of Surgery*, 1984; **199**: 412–17.
8. Little JM, Hollands MJ, and Ekberg H. Recurrence of hydatid disease. *World Journal of Surgery*, 1988; **12**: 700–4.
9. Felice C, Pirola F, Brunetti E, Dughetti S, Strosselli M, and Foglieni CS. A new therapeutic approach for hydatid liver cysts. *Gastroenterology*, 1990; **98**: 1366–8.
10. Akhan O, Ozmen MN, Dinçer A, Sayek I, and Goçmen A. Liver hydatid disease: long term results of percutaneous treatment. *Radiology*, 1996; **198**: 259–64.
11. Lydden Polley L. Visceral larva migrans and alveolar hydatid disease. Dangers real or imagined. *Veterinary Clinics of North America*, 1978; **8**: 353–78.
12. Bresson-Hadni S, Miguet JP, Vuitton D, *et al*. L'echinococcose alveolaire hepatique humaine. Revue generale propos de 80 cas. *Semaine des Hôpitaux*, 1988; **64**: 2691–701.
13. Miguet JP and Bresson-Hadni S. Alveolar echinococcosis of the liver. *Journal of Hepatology*, 1989; **8**: 373–9.
14. Rausch RL, Wilson JF, McMahon BJ, and O'Gorman MA. Consequences of continuous mebendazole therapy in alveolar hydatid disease with a summary of a ten-year clinical trial. *Annals of Tropical Medicine and Parasitology*, 1986; **80**: 403–19.

15. Wilson JF and Rausch RL. Alveolar hydatid disease: a review of clinical features of 33 indigenous cases of *Echinococcus multilocularis* infection in Alaskan eskimos. *American Journal of Tropical Medicine and Hygiene*, 1980; **29**: 1340–55.

16. Kasai Y, Koshino I, Kawanishi N, Sakamoto H, Sasaki E, and Kumagai M. Alveolar echinococcosis of the liver. Studies on 60 operated cases. *Annals of Surgery*, 1980; **191**: 145–52.

17. Bresson-Hadni S, Vuitton D, Didier D, *et al.* Metastases pulmonaires de l'echinococcose alveolaire. Frequence et mecanismes de survenue. *Presse Medicale*, 1989; **18**: 83.

18. Bresson-Hadni S, Laplante JJ, Lenys D, *et al.* Seroepidemiologic screening of *Echinococcus multilocularis* in a European area endemic for alveolar echinococcosis. *American Journal of Tropical Medicine and Hygiene*, 1994; **5**: 837–46.

19. Didier D, Weiler S, Rohmer P, *et al.* Hepatic alveolar echinococcosis: correlative US and CT study. *Radiology*, 1985; **154**: 179–86.

20. Wilson JF, Rausch RL, and Wilson FR. Alveolar hydatid disase. Review of the surgical experience in 42 cases of active disease among Alaskan Eskimos. *Annals of Surgery*, 1995; **221**: 315–23.

21. Mosimann F. Is alveolar hydatid disease of the liver incurable? *Annals of Surgery*, 1980; **192**: 118–23.

22. Bret PM, Paliard P, Partensky C, Bretagnolle M, and Blanchut P. Le traitement de la cholestase par stenose des voies biliaires intrahepatiques au cours de l'echinococcose alveolaire. Essai de drainage biliaire par voie percutanée transhepatique. *Gastroenterologie Clinique et Biologique*, 1984; **8**: 308–13.

23. Bresson-Hadni S, Franza A, Miguet JP, *et al.* Orthotopic liver transplantation for incurable alveolar echinococcosis of the liver: report of 17 cases. *Hepatology*, 1991; **13**: 1061–74.

24. Wattre P, Capron M, Bekhti A, and Capron A. Diagnostic immunologique de l'hydatidose. 139 observations. *Nouvelle Presse Medicale*, 1980; **9**: 305–9.

25. Vuitton D, Lassegue A, Miguet JP, *et al.* Humoral and cellular immunity in patients with hepatic alveolar echinococcosis. A 2-year follow- up with and without flubendazole treatment. *Parasite Immunology*, 1984; **6**: 329–34.

26. Vuitton DA, Bresson-Hadni S, Lenys D, *et al.* IgE-dependent humoral immune response in *Echinococcus multilocularis* infection: circulating and basophil-bound specific IgE against echinococcus antigens in patients with alveolar echinococcosis. *Clinical Experimental Immunology*, 1988; **71**: 247–52.

27. Huguier M, Leynadier F, Houry S, Lacaine F, and Dry J. Human basophil degranulation test in liver hydatidosis. *Digestive Diseases and Sciences*, 1987; **32**: 1354–7.

28. Bresson-Hadni S, Vuitton DA, Lenys D, Liance M, Racadot E, and Miguet JP. Cellular immune response in Echinococcus multilocularis infection in humans: (1) lymphocyte reactivity to Echinococcus antigens in patients with alveolar echinococcosis. *Clinical Experimental Immunology*, 1989; **78**: 61–6.

29. Edwards G and Breckenridge AM. Clinical pharmacokinetics of anthelmintic drugs. *Clinical Pharmacokinetics*, 1988; **15**: 67–93.

30. Bekhti A, Schaaps JP, Capron M, Dessaint JP, Santoro F, and Capron A. Treatment of hydatid disease with mebendazole: preliminary results in four cases. *British Medical Journal*, 1977; **2**: 1047–51.

31. Schantz PM, Van den, Bossche H, and Eckert J. Chemotherapy for larval echinococcosis in animals and humans: report of a workshop. *Zeitschrift für Parasitenkunde*, 1982; **67**: 5–26.

32. Davis A, Pawlowski ZS, and Dixon H. Multicentre clinical trials of benzimidazolecarbamates in human echinococcosis. *Bulletin of the World Health Organization*, 1986; **64**: 383–8.

33. Ping-Li Y. Liver alveolar hydatidosis in Xinjiang autonomous region. *World Journal of Surgery*, 1983; **7**: 511–18.

34. Saimot AG, Cremieux AC, Hay JM, *et al.* Albendazole as a potential treatment for human hydatidosis. *Lancet*, 1983; **ii**: 652–6.

35. Morris DL, Dykes PW, Marriner S, *et al.* Albendazole-objective evidence of response in human hydatid disease. *Journal of the American Medical Association*, 1985; **253**: 2053–7.

13.4.3 Ascariasis, visceral larva migrans, capillariasis, strongyloidiasis, and pentastomiasis

L. Carlos Da Costa Gayotto, Luiz Caetano da Silva, and P. P. Chieffi

Ascariasis

Definition

Ascariasis is a helminthic infection of the small bowel caused by a roundworm, *Ascaris lumbricoides*, that usually produces only vague and mild symptoms. Respiratory manifestations may occur due to the migration of the larvae through the lungs. Serious complications are protean and include intestinal obstruction, appendicitis, peritonitis, and penetration of the biliary and pancreatic trees. Liver involvement may be due to the migration of larvae towards the lungs, or to the obstruction of the biliary tree by adult worms; this can lead to cholangitis, liver abscesses, and formation of calculi around remnants of the parasite.

Introduction

The genus *Ascaris* (from the Greek *askaris*—worm) was first described by Linnaeus in 1758 and its counterpart in the pig, *Ascaris suum*, by Goeze in 1781. This roundworm was known by ancient peoples as a parasite of man. The Greeks called it *Imins stronggyle* and the Romans *lumbricusteres* (lumbricus—worm, teres—round).[1]

It has long been recognized that 'the diagnosis of gallbladder or of biliary duct disorders due to migration of *Ascaris lumbricoides* is not easy', and that 'in the case of an individual who is seized with hepatic colic-pain, accompanied with vomiting of *Ascaris lumbricoides*, migration of the parasite into the biliary ducts or the gallbladder should be considered' (Aviles, SGO, 1918; 27:459).

Epidemiology

The distribution of ascariasis is worldwide, with the highest prevalence in tropical countries, where humidity and temperature favour the maturation of the eggs. It is estimated that one of every four inhabitants of our planet is infected. The percentage varies from country to country and in different areas of the same country; the age group between 8 and 11 years is most heavily affected. Urban areas are less affected than rural ones. The infection depends on poor conditions of personal and general hygiene which result in a heavily contaminated soil.[2]

In highly endemic areas, quantitative stool examinations usually identify a high number of individuals with a low faecal egg output and a few with a high worm burden. The latter group is epidemiologically important and is usually named 'wormy people'; they represent the main source of soil contamination by the eggs (Anderson, AdvParasit, 1985; 24:1).

The penetration of the worm into the biliary tree usually occurs in areas of high prevalence of the infection. The worm was demonstrated in 36.7 per cent of 109 patients with biliary colic prospectively studied in India.[3]

In 14 of 15 patients with intrahepatic stones described in South Africa, the cause of the calculi was probably *A. lumbricoides* (Schulman, Radiol, 1987; 162:425), and in Hong Kong the presence of ova of *Ascaris* and/or remnants of degenerated worms was reported in the stones of 16 of 42 patients with recurrent pyogenic cholangitis (Teoh, JPatholBacteriol, 1963; 86:123).

Children repeatedly infected by *A. lumbricoides*, as well as by other enteric helminths, may exhibit altered reactivities to a number of allergens as a consequence of a marked polyclonal activation leading to high IgE levels (Hagel, ParasiteImmunol, 1993; 15:311). Treatment with anthelmintics restores the normal response to the allergens (Lynch, JAllClinImmunol, 1993; 92:404).

Prevention and control

Contamination of soil can be avoided by adequate disposal of stools. In rural areas, latrines should be used and children should be instructed on basic hygienic habits such as hand washing before eating. It is advisable that contacts are monitored for the infestation, particularly within the household.[2]

Mass treatment in high endemicity areas has been recommended as a means to decrease the morbidity of the disease as well as to prevent soil contamination by eggs of *A. lumbricoides*. (Stephenson, AmJTropMedHyg, 1989; 41:78)

Pathogenesis and pathology

Lifecycle

The adult worm measures from 15 to 35 cm and occasionally reaches 48 cm. On average, females are longer than males and can lay 200 000 eggs per day. The eggs are highly resistant to environmental factors; within 10 to 12 days the first-stage larvae are formed.[4] When the third-stage larvae are formed, the eggs become infectious (Araujo, RevInstMedTropSP, 1972; 14:83). After ingestion, eggshells are broken in the duodenum and the larvae migrate to the caecum; they penetrate the bowel wall and are carried by the bloodstream or the lymphatic system to the liver or heart. The larvae reach the lungs 4 to 5 days after infection through the pulmonary artery; in the alveoli they are transformed into fourth-stage larvae. These larvae are expelled through the bronchial tree and most are swallowed, returning to the intestines as fifth-stage larvae or as young adults 20 to 30 days after the infection. Sex organs develop, females are fertilized, and oviposition starts again, 2 to 3 months after the beginning of the lifecycle.[4]

Adult worms may be found in unusual sites such as the peritoneal cavity after traversing operative suture lines of the gastrointestinal tract, gangrenous patches of the small bowel filled with worm boluses, or sometimes through no apparent pathway. *Ascaris* can migrate to the stomach, oesophagus, and pharynx, penetrate the eustachian tube, enter the nasolacrimal duct, and emerge at the inner cantus of the eye (Daya, SAMedJ, 1982; 62:820). The worm can also emerge at the anus, mouth, nose, or even at the external ear through a perforated tympanus. *A. lumbricoides* has been found

in the urinary bladder,[5] the fallopian tubes (Sterling, JAMA, 1936; 107:2046), Meckel's diverticulum (Fernando, JTropPed, 1958; 4:61), and the right cavities of the heart from where it obstructed both pulmonary arteries (Daya, SAMedJ, 1982; 62:820).

In the liver, third-stage larvae are either destroyed or progress to the heart; clinical manifestations are minor. Hepatobiliary symptoms are caused by the migration of the adult worm through the papilla to the biliary tree (Fig. 1); this may also occur after cholecystectomy or choledochostomy (Aquino, OHospital, 1967; 71:191). The living worms can cause an obstruction of the common duct. Motile worms can migrate back to the intestines as demonstrated by serial ultrasonography;[6] others die, become fragmented, and act as a nidus for stone formation.

Although the majority of the parasites found in the biliary tract on operation are single and alive, cases with numerous worms (up to 48) have been described;[7] dead worms are found in 40 per cent of cases.[8]

The lesions

In experimental animals previously unexposed to the worm, the migrating larvae produce no inflammatory reaction in liver sinusoids; in animals previously exposed to the infection, there may be an inflammatory infiltrate composed of polymorphonuclear neutrophils and eosinophils. If the larvae die, their fragments can elicit a granulomatous response.[9]

In biliary ascariasis, the operative findings include enlargement of the liver and scars on its surface, attesting to previous episodes of inflammation. The common duct is thickened and often dilated to the diameter of a thumb. The branches of the biliary tree are irregularly dilated, with amputation of many at cholangiography (Fig. 2); this is due to mechanical obstruction and severe inflammation of the bile ducts.

Hepatobiliary symptoms are due to the migration of the worms through the papilla. Obstruction is produced when they reach the common duct where they are more often found.[8] They can move further, to thinner branches of the biliary tree, pervade the liver parenchyma, perforate the Glisson's capsule, and exit into the subdiaphragmatic space.

When the roundworm is trapped in the intrahepatic bile ducts, the disintegration of its body and release of a large amount of eggs can produce suppurative cholangitis with compromise of the vein radicles and erosion of the surrounding parenchyma. Pylephlebitis is one of the most dreaded complications of biliary ascariasis. Hepatic abscesses can thus be produced. In the necrotic centres there is pus, remnants of the bodies of the worms, and/or their ova. In the walls there is a dense inflammatory infiltrate composed of mono- and polymorphonuclear leucocytes including many eosinophils. From pus aspirated from liver abscesses, *Escherichia coli* can often be grown.

Fragments of dead worms or eggs, deposited in the thinnest branches of the biliary tree, can elicit a granulomatous response and be phagocytosed by very large giant cells (Fig. 3). It is interesting that segmented ova can be seen within the granulomas, although it is widely accepted that their maturation occurs only after they leave the body and meet adequate conditions of humidity and temperature.

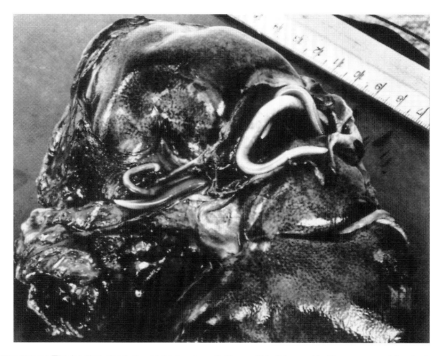

Fig. 1. Biliary ascariasis at autopsy. The bodies of adult worms are seen in the gallbladder and in the common bile duct.

Destruction of periportal parenchyma and lesion of the limiting plate leads to fibroplasia, formation of fibrous septa linking neighbouring portal tracts, and sometimes secondary biliary cirrhosis.

The bile ducts in heavily infected cases show ectasia, periductal fibrosis and oedema, degenerative changes of the biliary epithelium, and areas of ulceration, especially in sites where remnants of the worms adhere to the ductal wall. There is also irregular epithelial hyperplasia, with several mitotic figures and occasional formation of intraductal papillomas (Fig. 4). The epithelial cells show a considerable variation of morphological patterns; mucus secretion increases producing both neutral and acid mucopolysaccharides (Gayotto, RevInstMedTropSP, 1990; 32:91).

Several properties of *A. lumbricoides* favour stone formation: inorganic components of the shells of fertilized eggs are very similar to those found in bile, especially in the presence of inflammation. The same composition is also found, with slight variations, in pigment stones (Asakura, TohokuJExpMed, 1956; 64:117). The albuminoid membrane that covers the eggs of *A. lumbricoides* may also initiate precipitation of calcium compounds.

Clinical features and complications

During the pulmonary migration of the larvae there is cough and a clinical picture of pneumonitis or asthmatic bronchitis; symptoms are more pronounced during reinfection. In children, infection is often massive and the clinical features may be severe; shock and acute abdominal pain, leading to surgical intervention, can develop. In a Brazilian series of 71 cases of biliary ascariasis, Damerau showed that 70 per cent of the patients were less than 30 years old and 60 per cent were females.[8]

Penetration of the biliary tree can be asymptomatic; symptoms vary, depending on the number of migrating parasites. The chief complaint is constrictive epigastralgia; in some cases the pain is so intense that the patient becomes unconscious. The intensity and location of the pain varies from patient to patient; it is either referred to the upper right quadrant and periumbilical area or shows no precise location. The pain may be referred, in decreasing order, to the back, right shoulder, forechest, and left shoulder.[7] Nausea and vomiting are present in one-third of patients and in one-quarter there is elimination of the worm either orally or anally.[8]

Fever is present in 20 to 30 per cent of patients; unexpectedly (in a context of large duct biliary obstruction), jaundice only appears in less than 20 per cent of cases.[7] The low frequency of jaundice could be due to the intermittent nature of the obstruction, as the parasites enter and leave the common duct. In Damerau's series,[8] physical examination showed tenderness to palpation of the epigastric area and/or right upper quadrant in 60.5 per cent of patients and contracture of the abdominal wall in 8.5 per cent; hepatomegaly was present in 12.7 per cent.

Leucocytosis above 10 000/mm³ is present in patients with jaundice. Blood eosinophilia is present in the majority of cases, but the relative count shows striking variations from 8 to 42 per cent. Blood eosinophilia is marked during larval migration; after the development of mature worms it becomes relatively insignificant, [9] unless repeated reinfections by *Ascaris* or simultaneous infections by other worms occur.

Parasitological examination of stools can be negative in cases of biliary ascariasis; the finding of the parasite has a low value in terms of diagnostic specificity.

The penetration of the biliary system by *A. lumbricoides* may represent the starting event that triggers recurrent pyogenic cholangitis (Khuroo, GastrEnd, 1993; 39:674). In 500 patients with hepatobiliary or pancreatic damage from *A. lumbricoides*, Khuroo *et*

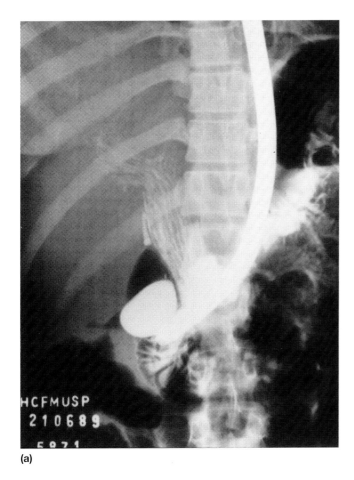

(a)

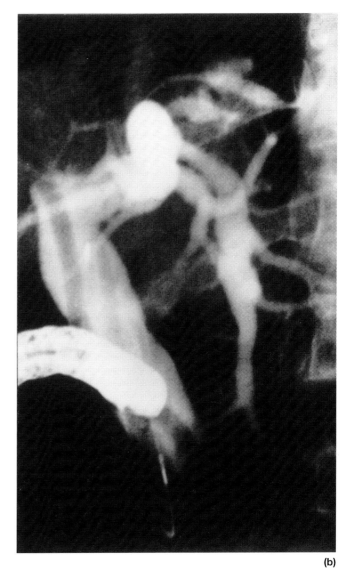

(b)

Fig. 2. Endoscopic retrograde cholangiopancreatography in a case of biliary ascariasis showing filling defects that identify adult worms in a dilated common bile duct. There is amputation of several branches of the biliary tree. (By courtesy of Dr Ernesto Damerau.) (a) Endoscopic retrograde cholangangiopancreatography in a case of biliary ascariasis. (b) In a markedly dilated common bile duct filling defects show many bodies of adult worms. In this case 76 worms were removed from the biliary tree. (By courtesy of Dr Marcel Machado.)

al.[10] observed five clinical forms: acute cholecystitis in 64, acute cholangitis in 121, biliary colic in 280, acute pancreatitis in 31, and hepatic abscess in 4.

Cholangitis occurs in about 25 per cent of patients; it can lead, after repeated bouts, to secondary biliary cirrhosis. Other complications include acute cholecystitis, pancreatitis, and hepatic abscesses. Empyema subsequent to hepatic abscess is accompanied by a high mortality rate (Gomez, JPediat, 1954; 45:478)

Diagnosis

In 85.7 per cent of patients with a clinical diagnosis of biliary ascariasis, ultrasonography can detect worms in the biliary tree.[6] In anicteric cases, oral cholecystography is often unrewarding, but ultrasonography can show living worms in the gallbladder (Cerri, Radiol, 1983; 146:753). Real-time ultrasonography equipment

should be used as the movement of the worms helps to make the diagnosis (Kamath, Gastro, 1986; 91:730). Sonographic features of the worms are long, linear, occasionally curved, echogenic structures, which are single or multiple, with or without acoustic shadowing. Inside the body of the worm a longitudinal anechoic tube, probably representing its digestive tract, can be seen. This structure with a central sonolucent line may exhibit slow movements (Aslam, JUSMed, 1993; 12:573). Liver abscesses, either single or multiple, and oedematous pancreatitis associated with biliary ascariasis can also be detected.[6]

Endoscopic retrograde cholangiopancreatography (**ERCP**) and computed tomography (**CT**) are also useful methods for diagnosis; in the former the roundworms appear as smooth, long, linear defects with tapering ends.[3]

In rare instances, the diagnosis of biliary ascariasis can be made by a liver biopsy showing granulomas within which are typical eggs.

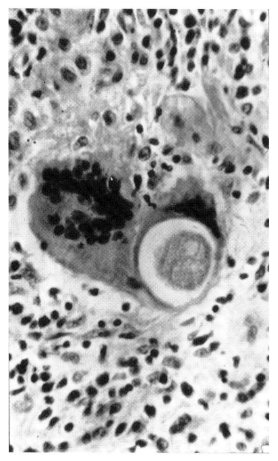

Fig. 3. An egg of *A. lumbricoides* is phagocytosed by a foreign-body giant cell around which there is an eosinophilic infiltrate (haematoxylin and eosin).

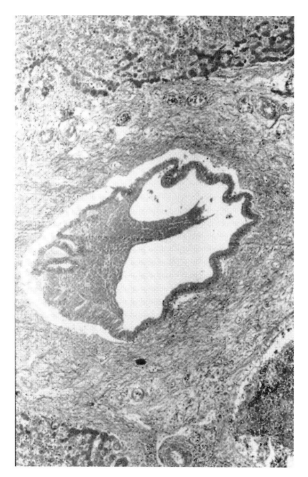

Fig. 4. Remnants of a dead worm mixed with cellular debris are tightly adhered to the hyperplastic epithelial lining of a bile duct. The portal tract shows fibrosis, inflammation, and erosion of the limiting plate (Masson's trichrome).

Treatment and prognosis

Supportive therapy includes intravenous fluids, antibiotics to treat cholangitis, and antispasmodics to relieve pain. The specific treatment of intestinal ascariasis consists of the administration of levamisole or tetramisole, in a single oral dose of 150 mg for adults and 80 mg for children; the cure rate is above 90 per cent. In the case of an association with other intestinal parasites, either mebendazole in oral doses of 100 mg twice daily for 3 days or albendazole in a single dose of 400 mg should be given, as levamisole is active only against *A. lumbricoides*. Pyrantel pamoate is a good substitute for mebendazole. In cases of intestinal obstruction, piperazine is the drug of choice; acting at the myoneural junction of the worm, it produces paralysis and facilitates the elimination of the bolus.

Although in cases of biliary ascariasis the instillation of ascaricides such as piperazine into the biliary tract has been recommended, the administration of an anthelmintic agent can cause paralysis or death of a worm that otherwise would spontaneously move out from the biliary tract into the duodenum. Furthermore, a trapped dead worm can become fragmented and act as a nidus for stone formation. It is preferable, therefore, that biliary ascariasis be treated by conservative means and the anthelmintic agents be administered orally. Worms that migrate out of the biliary tree become susceptible to anthelmintic therapy and are thereafter expelled by the peristaltic activity of the intestines (Zargar, Gastro, 1987; 93:668).

Successful endoscopic extraction can be achieved with or without sphincterotomy (Leung, GastrEnd, 1988; 34:318). ERCP can incidentally relieve bile stasis. Cholecystectomy is indicated when there is concomitant acute cholecystitis or cholelithiasis.[8] Exploration of the biliary tract is needed when trapped worms induce the formation of intrahepatic stones.[3]

When there is multiple invasion of smaller branches of the biliary tree, a suction cannula connected to an aspirator has been recommended as a useful means for removing the worms (Consoni, RevAssMedBras, 1958; 4:54). Complications occur in 15 per cent of patients undergoing operation, the most frequent being biliary fistulas.[8]

Symptoms disappear after successful treatment, biochemical tests return to normal, and control ultrasonography and ERCP show no worms left within the biliary tract.[3]

Visceral larva migrans
Definition

Visceral larva migrans in humans is caused basically by the larvae of the dog ascarid, *Toxocara canis*. In non-natural (paratenic) hosts, such as the man, the development of the parasite is blocked in the larval stage. The larvae may cause lesions in different organs, including the liver.

Introduction

In 1952 Beaver *et al.* (Pediat, 1952; 9:7) identified larvae of *T. canis* in a liver biopsy and proposed the term visceral larva migrans for this condition. Though both *T. canis* and *T. cati* are considered capable of producing human infection, nearly all reported human cases of toxocariasis have been associated with the former.[11-13]

Some authors consider only *T. canis* in the aetiology of visceral larva migrans, because of the peculiar pattern of tissue migration and the capacity to survive for a long period in non-natural hosts.[4, 12] Furthermore, it is unlikely that *T. cati* would behave as a real larva migrans as its whole lifecycle takes place in the intestinal lumen without visceral migrations.[4]

From studies on the larvae of *T. canis* in experimental animals, and observations on their behaviour, distribution, persistence, and pathogenicity in man, it is evident that the kind of infection produced by this species differs markedly from that of most other nematodes.[14] Although some helminths such as *Ascaris suum* and *Capillaria hepatica* can cause an illness clinically indistinguishable from *T. canis* infection, they should not be considered in the aetiology of visceral larva migrans because their development in man resembles that which occurs in the natural host rather than in a paratenic one. Other helminth species such as *Gnathostoma spinigerum* may rarely cause a similar clinical picture in humans, who act as paratenic host.

Epidemiology

T. canis infects canids in tropical and temperate regions of the world and may occasionally infect non-canid carnivores, such as the cat, tiger, and lynx.[14] The incidence of human toxocariasis is unknown because it is not a reportable disease and the infection can be oligo- or asymptomatic. As *T. canis* larvae are retained in visceral tissues and destroyed locally, neither worms nor eggs are passed in human faeces and results of biopsy are often uninformative despite widespread invasion.

Up to 1979, 1920 cases had been reported from 48 countries throughout the world and only 17.7 per cent of cases were in adults.[15] The prevalence of the infection has been determined by serology, based mainly on the enzyme-linked immunosorbent assay (**ELISA**) technique.[16] Data on seroprevalence in different countries are given in Table 1; antibodies to *T. canis* were found in 1 to 5 per cent of the general population. More consistent figures were described in high-risk groups, such as children (Maizels, JImmunol, 1987; 139:207) and in persons in contact with dogs.[11] However, these frequencies may reflect exposure rather than current infection.

As females of *T. canis* can produce 200 000 eggs per day and intestinal parasites may be numerous, infected animals contaminate the environment with millions of eggs per day.[11] The density of the dog population represents a risk factor. In France there are 250 dogs per 1000 rural inhabitants and 40 per 1000 urban inhabitants, and proportions are similar in the United States and United Kingdom.[14] In São Paulo, Brazil, the estimated proportion is 100 animals per 1000 inhabitants.[17]

Control and prevention[2]

Control measures should include:

(1) prevention of contamination of the ground by faeces from dogs and cats in areas where children play and around houses;
(2) adequate disposal of faeces;
(3) treatment of puppies at 3 weeks of age and periodically thereafter;
(4) sanitary education.

The lack of an efficient treatment of pregnant bitches represents an obstacle to the control of the disease.

Pathogenesis and pathology
Lifecycle

Eggs eliminated by dogs in the faeces are not embryonated and are not infective. Under ideal conditions of temperature and humidity, the embryo develops within 2 to 5 weeks and the eggs become infective.[11] Transmission to humans occurs by ingestion of materials contaminated with eggs. The consumption of raw or poorly cooked meat of animals that may act as paratenic hosts of *T. canis* (such as rabbits and poultry) has been incriminated as another possible mechanism of human contamination (Sturchler, JInfDis, 1990; 162:571). The lifecycle of the parasite is not completed in the human host. Upon hatching from ingested fertile eggs, the larvae penetrate the intestinal mucosa, enter the portal circulation, and eventually become trapped in various organs, including the liver; they are therefore prevented from returning to the intestinal lumen to mature into adult worms, and neither eggs nor larvae are passed into the faeces.

The lesions

The pathological changes result from the presence of larvae of *Toxocara* tunnelling through the tissues. Macroscopically, the liver is enlarged and at laparoscopy its surface shows typical diffuse sinuous lesions, 2 to 5 cm long. Sometimes the lesions are circular, slightly prominent, and can appear as numerous nodules on the surface of the liver (Llanio, SemHopPar, 1972; 48:1223) (Fig. 5). Microscopically, an extensive inflammatory process is produced, with areas of necrosis, surrounded by a dense inflammatory infiltrate composed predominantly of eosinophils, among which, crystals of Charcot–Leyden may be found. Sometimes eosinophilic abscesses are produced.

An important aspect of the histopathology of visceral larva migrans is that the inflammatory reaction around the larvae is much larger than the organism itself. Consequently, many histological sections may be required to demonstrate the parasite or its remnants. A reactive process may be found in the neighbourhood of the nodules, with Kupffer cell hyperplasia and portal inflammatory infiltration. Granulomas composed of histiocytes, giant cells, lymphocytes, plasma cells, and eosinophils eventually progress to fibrous nodules with a soft core. Such lesions are found at operation or at autopsy, after the process is burnt out.

In one of our cases in which the suspicion of a neoplastic process had been raised by ultrasonography, granulomas and an eosinophilic abscess with remnants of the worm were demonstrated in a liver biopsy taken during laparoscopy (Fig. 6).

Table 1 Seroprevalence of *Toxocara* infection in some regions of the world			
Location	No. tested	Seroprevalence (%)	Reference
Brazil	2025	3.6	17
France			
Urban	166	4.8	18
Rural	89	14.5	18
United Kingdom	922	2.6	Woodruff, BMJ, 1978; ii:1747
United States	8457	2.8	11
Venezuela	281	1.8	13
Slum dwellers and rural farmers	146	20–25.6	13

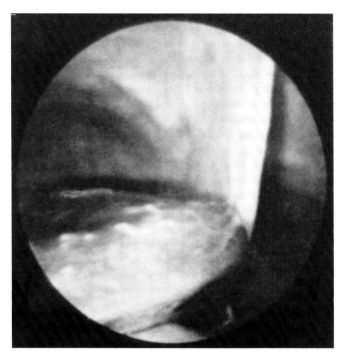

Fig. 5. Laparoscopic view of the liver surface in a case of visceral larva migrans. Typical serpiginous lesions are seen. (By courtesy of Dr Raimundo Llanio.)

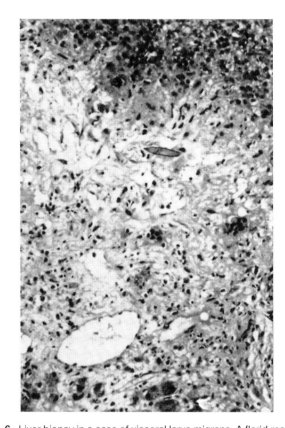

Fig. 6. Liver biopsy in a case of visceral larva migrans. A florid reaction is made up of extensive necrosis of the liver parenchyma, an eosinophilic infiltrate, and many fragments of larval bodies, some phagocytosed by foreign-body giant cells (haematoxylin and eosin).

Clinical aspects and complications

The clinical picture of visceral larva migrans varies widely with the parasitic load, the duration of infection, the presence of larvae in critical locations, and other factors as yet poorly understood.[14] Mild infections may be asymptomatic and probably occur in all age groups. This would explain the discrepancy between the relatively low number of cases reported in the literature and the great number of individuals with positive serological reactions (Table 1).

The symptomatology is protean, but a hypereosinophilic syndrome with fever and hepatomegaly is the usual presentation. In adults, non-specific clinical symptoms such as weakness, pruritus, rash, or urticaria are frequently found.[18] Patients may have digestive symptoms such as abdominal pain, nausea, vomiting, and diarrhoea.

The most severe form of the disease is observed in children. Symptoms include high fever, anorexia, weight loss, urticarial rashes, coughing with wheezing, and even convulsions.[9] Among children, pica is found in 90 per cent of the patients (Huntley, Pediat, 1965; 36:523). Splenomegaly is reported in up to 45 per cent of patients in different series (Abe-Jacob, Pediatria, 1987; 9:9).

An uncommon clinical form of toxocariasis affects mainly females and resembles chronic fatigue syndrome (Magnaval, PressMed, 1987; 16:151). Occasionally, human toxocariasis may be confused with more severe diseases, such as lymphomas, raising problems of differential diagnosis (Wolach, IsrJMedSci, 1995; 31:689)

Laboratory changes include leucocytosis with eosinophilia, hypergammaglobulinaemia, and slight elevations of serum enzymes such as alkaline phosphatase and γ-glutamyl transferase. High anti-A and anti-B isohaemagglutinin titres are frequently detected because *Toxocara* larvae contain surface antigens that stimulate isohaemagglutinin production.

Diagnosis

The diagnosis of visceral larva migrans should be especially suspected in children who have a history of geophagia or close contact with puppies. A high eosinophilic count, often exceeding 5000/mm³, is always found and is particularly elevated in children.[15] Ultrasound examination shows necrotic areas or areas corresponding to the tunnelling of the larvae through the liver parenchyma. CT scans likewise show hypodense areas or areas reflecting necrotic foci. Blind liver biopsy, although a specific method for diagnosis, has a very low sensitivity; sampling errors are a major problem in most cases. Echoguided liver biopsy has a much higher sensitivity.

De Brito and colleagues have demonstrated immunohistochemically the presence of *T. canis* antigens in hepatic lesions, even in the absence of worm remnants.[19]

Serodiagnosis is of particular importance, and an ELISA technique based upon the use of excretory–secretory antigen from *Toxocara* larvae has proved of great value.[13] The specificity of the reaction can be improved by preventing cross-reactivity through absorption of non-specific antibodies with soluble non-homologous parasite extracts (Lynch, ParasiteImmunol, 1988; 10:323). Detection of larva-specific IgE could represent an alternative approach to the clinical diagnosis (Brunello, TrRSocTropMedHyg, 1983; 77:279).

Other serological tests (indirect haemagglutination, bentonite flocculation, and double diffusion in agar) have a much lower sensitivity. Increased titres of isohaemagglutinins, although not specific, are useful. In areas where fascioliasis is endemic, serological tests for this parasite, the manifestations of which closely resemble those of visceral larva migrans, should be performed to exclude this parasitosis.

A Western blotting technique has been reported to increase the specificity of the serological diagnosis. This technique can be used to confirm ELISA-positive cases. (Magnaval, ParasitolRes, 1991; 77:697).

Treatment and prognosis

In spite of the severity of clinical symptoms in some patients, the disease is usually benign. Thiabendazole has been used in the treatment of *T. canis* infections in humans, yielding prompt clinical improvement in some patients. Although thiabendazole has a negligible larvicidal effect, it produces marked inhibition of the migration of the larvae in tissues of infected mice (Abdel-Hameed, JParasitol, 1984; 70:226). The inhibitory effect of the drug on the migrating larvae helps to explain its therapeutic effects in human infections, in which larval migration plays a major role. Ivermectin, albendazole, fenbendazole, and particularly levamisole kill or paralyse the larvae in the liver as shown by experimental infection in mice (Abo-Shehada, ResVetSci, 1984; 36:87). The recommended oral dose of thiabendazole in humans is 25 mg/kg twice a day for at least 5 to 10 days. Diethylcarbamazine is also considered an effective drug. The recommended dose is 2 to 6 mg/kg per day for 1 to 3 weeks.[15]

Despite the usual benign character of the disease, on occasions it may show a severe course, probably due to hypersensitivity. In these cases corticosteroids are useful[14] and produce a drop in the eosinophil count (Huntley, Pediat, 1965; 36:523). Corticosteroids

are also beneficial in the treatment of severe pulmonary involvement.[12]

Symptoms disappear within a few weeks if reinfection is prevented, but the eosinophilia and high antibody titres may persist for some years. Ultrasonographic and CT scan abnormalities of the liver may persist for several months and even for 1 or 2 years. Visceral larva migrans is rarely fatal. Death results from extensive involvement of the heart or central nervous system or from an exaggerated immunological response.[11] Larvae entering the eye may cause blindness due to posterior endophthalmitis.

The hepatic lesions tend to heal and small fibrous cysts or scars can be found on the surface of the liver during laparotomy or in the course of autopsy.

Capillariasis

This uncommon human infection is caused by *Capillaria hepatica*, a worm frequently found in the liver of rats and squirrels. This nematode belongs to the superfamily Trichuroidea. It may also be found in mice, hares, beavers, dogs, muskrats, and some species of monkey.[9] Man is the natural host of another species, *C. philippinensis*, which lives in the intestinal mucosa and may cause diarrhoea.[1]

The non-embryonated eggs of *C. hepatica* are usually released from the carcasses of infected animals. Ova can also be discharged intact in the faeces of animals and humans who ingest contaminated material. After exposure to the air and to moisture in the soil, embryos are formed and the eggs become infective 2 to 6 weeks later.

Ingestion of embryonated eggs occurs particularly in children who live in poor hygienic conditions and practise geophagia. The eggs hatch in the caecum and the free larvae migrate to the liver via the portal system. Maturation to the adult stage occurs in about 3 weeks; after a few weeks the female worm dies and large numbers of eggs are released in the liver.[20]

Pathology

The liver is enlarged and its surface shows many yellowish or grey nodules measuring between 0.1 and 0.2 cm in diameter surrounded by an area of grey induration up to 3 cm in diameter. Bodies of adult worms can be found in liver tissue surrounded by a granulomatous reaction, which can also be elicited by ova of the parasite. These can also be demonstrated in scrapings of fresh liver tissue.[21] The granulomas are composed of epithelioid histiocytes and giant cells; polymorphonuclear eosinophils are conspicuous. The eggs are barrel shaped and bioperculated with double-layer striated shells. The shell is birefringent under polarized light.

Epidemiology

In view of the high prevalence of the infection among domestic rodents and the poor housing and hygienic conditions prevailing in many populations of the developing world, *C. hepatica* may cause human infection at higher rates than is usually assumed.[22]

Clinical picture

The most common manifestations are fever, hepatomegaly, splenomegaly, and eosinophilia, which occur in up to 85 per cent of cases.[21] Some authors emphasize that the clinical picture is similar to that seen in visceral larva migrans. The occurrence of asymptomatic cases is probable.

Laboratory tests show marked leucocytosis with eosinophilia, an increased erythrocyte sedimentation rate, and a slight elevation of serum bilirubin, alkaline phosphatase, and aminotransferase levels.

Diagnosis

Eggs of the parasite are rarely found in human faeces (Coimbra, MemInstOswaldoCruz, 1981; 76:299). The diagnosis is therefore based on morphological data from liver biopsies, where the eggs and bodies of the worm are seen surrounded by granulomas. The operculated and striated ova of *Capillaria* are diagnostic. The worms and ova are more likely to be demonstrated in liver biopsies than those causing toxocariasis.[20]

Treatment

There is no established therapy for this infection. A good response was reported in an acutely ill adult treated with a combination of prednisone, pyrantel tartrate, and disophenol.[21]

Strongyloidiasis

Strongyloides stercoralis lives in the gastrointestinal tract of a substantial proportion of the world's population. In most people the infection is associated with few, if any, symptoms.[2]

The lifecycle of *S. stercoralis* in humans has different patterns; for infection, however, it is essential that filariform (infective) larvae penetrate the skin or mucosa. The worms develop through a pulmonary cycle and adults are found at all levels of the intestines, especially in the duodenum and upper part of the jejunum. From the eggs laid by parthenogenetic or fertilized females, rhabditoid larvae develop; in the intestines, occasionally they can be transformed into filariform larvae.[1] Liver involvement depends upon autoinfection, a process by which filariform larvae invade the walls of the lower portions of the ileum or the colon, entering the portal system and then the lungs. Filariform larvae passed in freshly evacuated stools can also cause autoinfection upon contact with the perianal and perineal skin.

This process is considerably enhanced in immunocompromised patients, resulting in hyperinfection; under these circumstances rhabditoid larvae can also cross the bowel wall and become infective. Sometimes the alveolocapillary wall is not ruptured and the larvae are driven through the pulmonary veins and the general circulation to atypical locations such as the brain, genitourinary tract, or choroid plexus.[1] The disseminated form of strongyloidiasis with liver involvement has been described in patients with severe malnutrition, under corticoid therapy, and with the acquired immunodeficiency syndrome.[23]

The tissue damage is caused directly by the invading worms or by secondary infection with the intestinal micro-organisms. In the liver the larvae are found in portal tracts, occasionally within the veins, or in periportal areas. They are surrounded by an eosinophilic infiltrate or by a granulomatous reaction in which eosinophils are also present. Miliary granulomas can be seen in liver tissue, often without larvae of *S. stercoralis* (Fig. 7). Liver cell damage is usually slight; fatty degeneration and mild cholestasis can be seen. Diagnosis

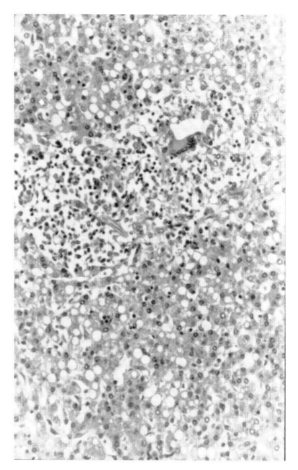

Fig. 7. Miliary granulomas in the liver of a patient with the disseminated form of strongyloidiasis: a giant cell, a few epithelioid cells, a dense eosinophilic infiltrate, and fragments of the larva compose a loose arrangement. There is fatty change in the surrounding parenchyma (haematoxylin and eosin). (By courtesy of Dr Maria de Fatima Araujo.)

of strongyloidiasis in the liver can be made when typical larvae, showing double lateral alas that extend from about the nerve ring to the tail, are found (Poltera, JPath, 1974; 113:241).

Patients with the hyperinfection syndrome present with gastrointestinal and respiratory complaints, such as nausea, vomiting, meteorism, diarrhoea, anorexia, dyspnoea, wheezing, and cough. Fever, malaise, and weakness are also common. Symptoms may be attenuated in those receiving corticosteroids (Wong, AmJMed, 1984; 76:479). Biliary manifestations of strongyloidiasis are rare. Biliary obstruction due to papillary stenosis, resolving with treatment with thiabendazole, has been described (Astagneau, Gut, 1994; 35:705).

Evidence of liver involvement, including hepatomegaly and more rarely jaundice, may be found in the disseminated form of the disease; direct-reacting bilirubin and alkaline phosphatase activity are elevated. Repeated examination of the faeces by the Baermann technique is the simplest diagnostic procedure; the positivity increases if the contents of the duodenum are also examined. Better results have been achieved with agar plate coprocultures (Sato, AmJTropMedHyg, 1995; 53:248). Various serological tests for the diagnosis of human strongyloidiasis have been recommended, such as indirect immunofluorescence (Grove, AmJTropMedHyg, 1981; 30:344), ELISA (Neva, JInfDis, 1981; 144:427), and agglutination with gelatin particles (Sato, TrRSocTropMedHyg, 1991; 85:515). However, they are indicated only for seroepidemiological surveys because of the low specificity of the tests. Conway and colleagues improved specificity through the previous absorption of sera with filariae and *Necator americanus* antigen (Conway, TrRSoc-TropMedHyg, 1993; 87:173).

Treatment is based on the oral administration of thiabendazole at 25 mg/kg twice a day for 3 to 5 days. Ivermectin may be an alternative treatment, in particular for the disseminated form. The optimal duration of treatment of *S. stercoralis* infection in patients with AIDS or in other immunodeficient patients has not yet been defined.

Pentastomiasis (porocephalosis)

Pentastomiasis is an infection produced by Pentastomida, worm-like blood-sucking endoparasites which belong to the phyllum Arthropoda. Two families are of medical interest: Linguatulidae and Porocephalidae.[24]

Epidemiology

The adult parasites live in the respiratory passages of carnivorous animals (*Linguatula serrata*) and snakes (*Armillifer* or *Porocephalus armillatus*). *L. serrata* with a serrated cuticle and a flattened body is present only in the Western hemisphere.[25] In its larval stage it has been found occasionally in humans in Panama, Switzerland, Germany, and Brazil.[4] Cysts with *A. armillatus* larvae have been found in the Unites States and Canada (Guardia, ArchPathLabMed, 1991; 115:515).

Human pentastomiasis has been reported mainly from West Africa and the Congo basin (Zaire); snakes are implicated as vectors.[26] Autopsy records from Ibadan, Nigeria, show an *Armillifer* infestation rate of 2.2 per cent, with porocephalosis as the third most common cause of hepatic granulomas.[25]

Lifecycle

Eggs excreted in the nasal secretions of snakes and carnivorous animals, such as the dog and the fox, may be ingested by an intermediate host, including man. The eggs hatch in the intestines and the primary larvae can reach the liver where they undergo nine moults in a period of about 6 months[24] to form the third-stage larvae or infective nymphs, which are encysted. During these moults the volume of the encysted larvae can increase up to 1000-fold and sometimes, therefore, produces a space-occupying syndrome. In humans the process comes to a dead end at this point and it is accepted that the larvae die within 2 years, eliciting a prominent inflammatory reaction and eventually undergoing calcification. However, in rare instances the infective larvae can emerge from their cysts and invade the peritoneal cavity.[27]

Pathology

Various types of lesions are seen in the liver. Sometimes the encysted nymph is surrounded by dense fibrous tissue and multiple, characteristic, annular thickenings are observed.[27,28] The calcified nymphs may be detected through abdominal radiological examination. Other liver lesions consist of the cuticular remnant surrounded by granulomas or dense fibrous tissue. Necrotic granulomas are the most common lesion seen in porocephalosis: they are due to the disintegration of the parasite in amorphous debris, which eventually undergoes calcification.[24]

It is generally accepted that pentastomid parasites do little harm, being found incidentally at radiological investigations, surgery, and autopsy. Under some circumstances the nymphs may cause disease because of their location, the large numbers involved, or by tissue migrations.[25]

Clinical picture

The clinical picture varies widely from a subclinical disease to a serious illness.[26] This may include pneumonitis, peritonitis, meningitis, and obstructive jaundice and has been ascribed to heavy pentastomid infection. Eosinophilia is not a salient feature.[25] The diagnosis is morphological.

References

1. Faust EC, Russell PF, and Jung RC, eds. *Craig and Faust's clinical parasitology*. Philadelphia: Lea & Febiger, 1970.
2. Benenson AS, ed. *El control de las enfermedades transmisibles en el hombre*. Washington: PAHO and WHO, 1983.
3. Khuroo MS and Zargar SA. Biliary ascariasis. A common cause of biliary and pancreatic disease in an endemic area. *Gastroenterology*, 1985; **88**: 418–23.
4. Pessoa SB and Martins AV. *Pessoa parasitologia médica*, 11th edn. Rio de Janeiro: Guanabara Koogan, 1982.
5. Beaver PC, ed. *Clinical parasitology*, Philadelphia, Lea & Febiger, 1984.
6. Khuroo MS, Zargar SA, Mahajan R, Bhat RL, and Javid G. Sonographic appearances in biliary ascariasis. *Gastroenterology*, 1987; **93**: 267–72.
7. Hsu FH. Clinical observation on 110 cases of *Ascaris* invasion into the biliary tract. *Nagoya Journal of Medical Science*, 1962; **24**: 215–33.
8. Damerau E. PhD Thesis, Universidade Federal de Santa Catarina, Brasil, 1974.
9. Marcial MA and Marcial-Rojas RA. Parasitic diseases of the liver. In Schiff L and Schiff ER, eds. *Diseases of the liver*. Philadelphia: JB Lippincott Co., 1987: 1171–96.
10. Khuroo MS, Zargar SA, and Mahajan, R. Hepatobiliary and pancreatic ascariasis in India. *Lancet*, 1990; **335**: 1503–6.
11. Glickman LT and Schantz PM. Epidemiology and pathogenesis of zoonotic toxocariasis. *Epidemiologic Reviews*, 1981; **3**: 230–50.
12. Zinkham WH. Visceral larva migrans. A review and reassessment indicating two forms of clinical expression: visceral and ocular. *American Journal of Diseases of Childhood*, 1978; **132**: 627–33.
13. Lynch NR, Eddy K, Hodgen AN, Lopez RI, and Turner KJ. Seroprevalence of *Toxocara canis* infection in tropical Venezuela. *Transactions of the Royal Society of Tropical Medicine and Hygiene*, 1988; **82**: 275–81.
14. Beaver PC. The nature of visceral larva migrans. *Journal of Parasitology*, 1969; **55**: 3–12.
15. Ehrhard T and Kernbaum S. *Toxocara canis* et toxocarose humaine. *Bulletin de l'Institut Pasteur*, 1979; **77**: 225–87.
16. Glickman L, Schantz P, Dombroske R, and Cypess R. Evaluation of serodiagnostic tests for visceral larva migrans. *American Journal of Tropical Medicine and Hygiene*, 1978; **27**: 492–8.
17. Chieffi PP, *et al.* Visceral larva migrans: a seroepidemiological survey in five municipalities of São Paulo State, Brazil. *Revista do Instituto de Medicina Tropical de São Paulo*, 1990; **32**: 204–10.
18. Glickman LT, *et al.* Visceral larva migrans in French adults: a new disease syndrome? *American Journal of Epidemiology*, 1987; **125**: 1019–34.

19. De Brito, *et al.* Immunohistochemical detection of toxocaral antigens in human biopsies. *International Journal of Surgery and Pathology*, 1994; **2**: 117–24.

20. Ong GB. Helminthic diseases of the liver and biliary tract. In Wright R, Millward-Sadler GH, Alberti KGMM, and Karran S, eds. *Liver and biliary disease. Pathophysiology, diagnosis, management*. London: WB Saunders Co., 1985: 1523–56.

21. Pereira VG and França LCM. Successful treatment of *Capillaria hepatica* infection in an acutely ill adult. *American Journal of Tropical Medicine and Hygiene*, 1983; **32**: 1272–4.

sc<BIB ID = "hep078-r22">22. Galvão VA. Estudos sobre *Capillaria hepática*: Uma avaliação do seu papel patogênico para o homem. *Memórias do Instituto Oswaldo Cruz*, 1981; **76**: 415–33.

23. Haque AK, Schnadig V, Rubin SA, and Smith JH. Pathogenesis of human strongyloidiasis: autopsy and quantitative parasitological analysis. *Modern Pathology*, 1994; **7**: 276–88.

24. Prathap K, Lau KS, and Bolton JM. Pentastomiasis: a common finding at autopsy among Malaysian aborigines. *American Journal of Tropical Medicine and Hygiene*, 1969; **18**: 20–7.

25. Smith JA, Oladiran B, Lagundoye SB, Lawson EAL, and Francis TI. Pentastomiasis and malignancy. *Annals of Tropical Medicine and Parasitology*, 1975; **69**: 503–12.

26. Self JT, Hopps HC, and Olufemi Williams A. Pentastomiasis in Africans. *Tropical and Geographical Medicine*, 1975; **27**: 1–13.

27. Hopps HC, Keegan HL, Price DL, and Self JT. Pentastomiasis. In Marcial-Rojas RA, ed. *Pathology of protozoal and helminthic diseases with clinical correlation*. Baltimore: Williams & Wilkins, 1971: 970–89.

28. Simson IN and Gear JHS. Other viral and infectious diseases. In MacSween RNM, Anthony PD, and Scheuer PJ, eds. *Pathology of the liver*. Edinburgh: Churchill Livingstone, 1987: 224–64.

Abbreviated journal titles as used in the text

AbdImag .... *Abdominal Imaging*
ActaAnaesthScand .... *Acta Anaesthesologica Scandinavica*
ActaAnat .... *Acta Anatomica (Basel)*
ActaBiolMedGerm .... *Acta Biologica et Medica Germanica*
ActaChemScand .... *Acta Chemica Scandinavica*
ActaChirBelg .... *Acta Chirirurgica Belgica*
ActaChirScand .... *Acta Chirurgica Scandinavica*
ActaChirScandSuppl .... *Acta Chirurgica Scandinavica
　　　　　　　　　　　　　 Supplementum*
ActaClinBelg .... *Acta Clinica Belgica*
ActaCytol .... *Acta Cytologica*
ActaDermVen .... *Acta Dermato-Venereologica*
ActaDiabetol .... *Acta Diabetologica*
ActaEnd .... *Acta Endocrinologica*
ActaEndoscop .... *Acta Endoscopica*
ActaGastroBelg .... *Acta Gastroenterologica Belgica*
ActaGyn .... *Acta Gynecologica*
ActaHaem .... *Acta Haematologica (Basel)*
ActaHepatogastrBelg .... *Acta Hepatogastroenterolgica Belgica*
ActaHepatoGastroenterol .... *Acta Hepato-Gastroenterologica*
ActaHepatolJpn .... *Acta Hepatologica Japonica*
ActaHepatoSplenol .... *Acta Hepato-Splenologica*
ActaHistochem .... *Acta Histochemica*
ActaMedAustr .... *Acta Medica Austriaca*
ActaMedCroatica .... *Acta Medica Croatica*
ActaMedOkayama .... *Acta Medica Okayama*
ActaMedScand .... *Acta Medica Scandinavica*
ActaMedScandSuppl .... *Acta Medica Scandinavica
　　　　　　　　　　　　　 Supplementum*
ActaMedSocUpsal .... *Acta Societatis Medicorum
　　　　　　　　　　　　　 Upsaliensis*
ActaMorphHung .... *Acta Morphologica Academiae
　　　　　　　　　　　　　 Scientiarum Hungaricae*
ActaNeurolBelg .... *Acta Neurologica Belgica*
ActaNeurolScand .... *Acta Neurologica Scandinavica*
ActaNeuropath .... *Acta Neuropathologica*
ActaObGyn .... *Acta Obstetrica et Gynaecologica
　　　　　　　　　　　　　 Scandinavica*
ActaOncol .... *Acta Oncologica*
ActaOphthalm .... *Acta Ophthalmologica*
ActaOrthScand .... *Acta Orthopaedica Scandinavica*
ActaOtolaryngol .... *Acta Otolaryngologica*
ActaPaedScand .... *Acta Paediatrica Scandinavica*
ActaPaedScandSuppl .... *Acta Paediatrica Scandinavica
　　　　　　　　　　　　　 Supplementum*
ActaPaedSin .... *Acta Paediatrica Sinica*
ActaPathJpn .... *Acta Pathologica Japonica*
ActaPharmTox .... *Acta Pharmacologica et Toxicologica*

ActaPhysiolHung .... *Acta Physiologica Academiae
　　　　　　　　　　　　　 Scientiarum Hungaricae*
ActaPhysiolScand .... *Acta Physiologica Scandinavica*
ActaPMIScand .... *Acta Pathologica, Microbiologica, et
　　　　　　　　　　　　　 Immunologica Scandinavica*
ActaPMScandA .... *Acta Pathologica et Microbiologica
　　　　　　　　　　　　　 Scandinavica, Section A:
　　　　　　　　　　　　　 Pathology*
ActaPsychNeurol .... *Acta Psychiatrica et Neurologica*
ActaPsychScand .... *Acta Psychiatrica Scandinavica*
ActaRadiol .... *Acta Radiologica*
ActaSocMedUps .... *Acta Societatis Medicorum
　　　　　　　　　　　　　 Upsaliensis*
ActaUnioIntContra .... *Acta Unio Internationalis Contra
　Cancrum　　　　　　　　　 Cancrum*
AcuteCare .... *Acute Care*
AddicBiol .... *Addiction Biology*
Addiction .... *Addiction*
AdvAlcSubstAb .... *Advances in Alcohol and Substance
　　　　　　　　　　　　　 Abuse*
AdvBiochem .... *Advances in Biochemistry and
　Psychopharmacol　　　　　 Psychopharmacology*
AdvCarbChemBiochem .... *Advances in Carbohydrate Chemistry
　　　　　　　　　　　　　 and Biochemistry*
AdvClinChem .... *Advances in Clinical Chemistry*
AdvClinEnzym .... *Advances in Clinical Enzymology*
AdvEnz .... *Advances in Enzymology*
AdvEnzymReg .... *Advances in Enzyme Regulation*
AdvExpMedBiol .... *Advances in Experimental Medicine
　　　　　　　　　　　　　 and Biology*
AdvImmunol .... *Advances in Immunology*
AdvIntMed .... *Advances in Internal Medicine*
AdvLipRes .... *Advances in Lipid Research*
AdvMyocardiol .... *Advances in Myocardiology*
AdvNephrol .... *Advances in Nephrology*
AdvParasit .... *Advances in Parasitology*
AdvPediat .... *Advances in Pediatrics*
AdvPharmacol .... *Advances in Pharmacology*
AdvProteinChem .... *Advances in Protein Chemistry*
AdvSurg .... *Advances in Surgery*
AdvVirusRes .... *Advances in Virus Research*
AerospaceMed .... *Aerospace Medicine*
Age .... *Age*
AgeAgeing .... *Age and Ageing*
AgentsActions .... *Agents and Actions*
Agressol .... *Agressologie*
AIDS .... *AIDS*
AIDSRes .... *AIDS Research*

AIDSResHumRV .... *AIDS Research and Human Retroviruses*
AJR .... *American Journal of Roentgenology*
AlcAlc .... *Alcohol and Alcoholism*
AlcHealthResW .... *Alcohol Health and Research World*
Alcohol .... *Alcohol*
AlcoholClinExpRes .... *Alcoholism: Clinical and Experimental Research*
Alcoholism .... *Alcoholism*
AlcoholTreatQ .... *Alcoholism Treatment Quarterly*
Alcologia .... *Alcologia*
AlimPharmTher .... *Alimentary Pharmacology and Therapeutics*
Alkfrag .... *Alkoholfraagen*
AMAArchPath .... *AMA Archives of Pathology*
AmFamilyPhysician .... *American Family Physician*
AmHeartJ .... *American Heart Journal*
AmIndHygAssJ .... *American Industrial Hygiene Association Journal*
AmJAnat .... *American Journal of Anatomy*
AmJCard .... *American Journal of Cardiology*
AmJClinNutr .... *American Journal of Clinical Nutrition*
AmJClinOnc .... *American Journal of Clinical Oncology*
AmJClinOncCanClin .... *American Journal of Clinical Oncology and Cancer Clinical Trials*
    Trials
AmJClinPath .... *American Journal of Clinical Pathology*
AmJCritCareMed .... *American Journal of Critical Care Medicine*
AmJDisChild .... *American Journal of Diseases of Childhood*
AmJDrugAlcAb .... *American Journal of Drug and Alcohol Abuse*
AmJEmergMed .... *American Journal of Emergency Medicine*
AmJEpid .... *American Journal of Epidemiology*
AmJGastr .... *American Journal of Gastroenterology*
AmJHemat .... *American Journal of Hematology*
AmJHospPharm .... *American Journal of Hospital Pharmacy*
AmJHumGen .... *American Journal of Human Genetics*
AmJHumMet .... *American Journal of Human Metabolism*
AmJHypertension .... *American Journal of Hypertension*
AmJIndMed .... *American Journal of Industrial Medicine*
AmJInfecControl .... *American Journal of Infection Control*
AmJKidneyDis .... *American Journal of Kidney Diseases*
AmJMed .... *American Journal of Medicine*
AmJMedGen .... *American Journal of Medical Genetics*

AmJMedSci .... *American Journal of the Medical Sciences*
AmJNephrol .... *American Journal of Nephrology*
AmJObsGyn .... *American Journal of Obstetrics and Gynecology*
AmJPathol .... *American Journal of Pathology*
AmJPedHemOnc .... *American Journal of Pediatric Hematology and Oncology*
AmJPerinat .... *American Journal of Perinatology*
AmJPhysAnthropol .... *American Journal of Physical Anthropology*
AmJPhysiol .... *American Journal of Physiology*
AmJPrevMed .... *American Journal of Preventive Medicine*
AmJPsychiat .... *American Journal of Psychiatry*
AmJPublHlth .... *American Journal of Public Health*
AmJReprodImmunol .... *American Journal of Reproductive Immunology*
AmJRespirCellMolBiol .... *American Journal of Respiratory Cell and Molecular Biology*
AmJRoent .... *American Journal of Roentgenology*
AmJRoentRadTher .... *American Journal of Roentgenology, Radiation Therapy and Nuclear Medicine*
    NuclMed
AmJSportsMed .... *American Journal of Sports Medicine*
AmJSurg .... *American Journal of Surgery*
AmJSurgPath .... *American Journal of Surgical Pathology*
AmJSyphGonVenDis .... *American Journal of Syphilis, Gonorrhea, and Venereal Disease*
AmJTropMedHyg .... *American Journal of Tropical Medicine and Hygiene*
AmLabClinSci .... *American Laboratory and Clinical Science*
AmRevRespDis .... *American Review of Respiratory Disease*
AmSci .... *American Scientist*
AmSurg .... *American Surgeon*
AmyloidIntJExp .... *Amyloid: The International Journal of Experimental and Clinical Investigation*
    ClinInvest
Anaesth .... *Anaesthesia*
AnalBioch .... *Analytical Biochemistry*
AnalChem .... *Analytical Chemistry*
AnalQuantCytolHistol .... *Analytical and Quantitative Cytology and Histology*
AnalSci .... *Analytical Sciences*
AnatEmbryol .... *Anatomy and Embryology*
AnatRec .... *Anatomical Record*
Andrologia .... *Andrologia*
AnEspPediatr .... *Anales Espanoles de Pediatrica*
AnesthAnalg .... *Anesthesia and Analgesia*
AnesthClinNAm .... *Anesthesia Clinics of North America*
Anesthesiol .... *Anesthesiology*
AnaesthIntCare .... *Anaesthesia and Intensive Care*
AngewChemIntEdEngl .... *Angewandte Chemie International Edition in English*
Angiol .... *Angiology*

AnnAllergy .... *Annals of Allergy*
AnnBiolClin........................ *Annales de Biologie Clinique (Paris)*
AnnChir............................. *Annales de Chirurgie (Paris)*
AnnChirGyn........................ *Annales de Chirurgie Gynecologique*
AnnChirThoracCardiovasc.. *Annales de Chirurgie Thoracique et Cardio-Vasculaire*
AnnClinBioch .... *Annals of Clinical Biochemistry*
AnnClinLabSci .... *Annals of Clinical and Laboratory Science*
AnnClinRes .... *Annals of Clinical Research*
AnnDermatolVenereol......... *Annales de Dermatologie et de Venereologie*
AnnEmergMed .... *Annals of Emergency Medicine*
AnnEndocr .... *Annales d'Endocrinologie (Paris)*
AnnGastroHep.................... *Annales de Gastroenterologie et d'Hepatologie (Paris)*
AnnHemat .... *Annals of Hematology*
AnnHumGenet .... *Annals of Human Genetics*
AnnInstPasteurMicrobiol .... *Annales de l'Institut Pasteur Microbiologie*
AnnIntMed........................ *Annals of Internal Medicine*
AnnItalMedInt................... *Annali Italiani di Medicina Interna*
AnnMed .... *Annals of Medicine*
AnnMedIntern.................... *Annales de Médecine Interne (Paris)*
AnnMedInterna(Fenn)........ *Annales Medicinae Internae Fenniae*
AnnMedSectPolAcadSci ..... *Annals of the Medical Section of the Polish Academy of Sciences*
AnnNeurol......................... *Annals of Neurology*
AnnNuclMed...................... *Annals of Nuclear Medicine*
AnnNutrAliment................. *Annals of Nutrition and Alimentation*
AnnNutrMetab .... *Annals of Nutrition and Metabolism*
AnnNYAcadMed .... *Annals of the New York Academy of Medicine*
AnnNYAcadSci................... *Annals of the New York Academy of Sciences*
AnnOccupHyg.................... *Annals of Occupational Hygiene*
AnnOncol .... *Annals of Oncology*
AnnPath............................. *Annales de Pathologie*
AnnPediat .... *Annales de Pediatrie*
AnnPharmacother .... *Annals of Pharmacotherapy*
AnnProgrRepSEATO.......... *Annual Progress Report of the*
   MedResLab   *SEATO Medical Research Laboratory*
AnnRadiol.......................... *Annales de Radiologie*
AnnRCSurg .... *Annals of the Royal College of Surgeons*
AnnRepMedChem .... *Annals of Reproductive Medicine and Chemistry*
AnnRevBiochem .... *Annual Review of Biochemistry*
AnnRevCellBiol .... *Annual Review of Cell Biology*
AnnRevGenet .... *Annual Review of Genetics*
AnnRevImmunol................. *Annual Review of Immunology*
AnnRevMed .... *Annual Review of Medicine*
AnnRevMicro .... *Annual Review of Microbiology*
AnnRevNutr .... *Annual Review of Nutrition*
AnnRevPharmTox .... *Annual Review of Pharmacology and Toxicology*

AnnRevPhysiol .... *Annual Review of Physiology*
AnnRevRespDis................. *Annual Review of Respiratory Disease*
AnnRheumDis .... *Annals of the Rheumatic Diseases*
AnnSaudiMed..................... *Annals of Saudi Medicine*
AnnSocBelgeMedTrop .... *Annales de la Societé Belge de Médecine Tropicale*
AnnSurg .... *Annals of Surgery*
AnnThorSurg .... *Annals of Thoracic Surgery*
AnnTropMed...................... *Annals of Tropical Medicine and Parasitology*
AnnTropMedHyg............... *Annals of Tropical Medicine and Hygience*
AnnTropPaediat................. *Annals of Tropical Paediatrics*
AntibiotChemo .... *Antibiotics and Chemotherapy*
AntiCancDrugs................... *Anti-Cancer Drugs*
AntiCancerRes .... *Anticancer Research*
AntimicrobAgents .... *Antimicrobial Agents and*
   Chemother   *Chemotherapy*
AntiviralNews .... *Antiviral News*
AntiviralRes .... *Antiviral Research*
AntiviralChemother .... *Antiviral Chemotherapy*
AnzSchaed .... *Anzeiger für Schaedlingskunde*
ApheresisBull..................... *Apheresis Bulletin*
Appetite .... *Appetite*
ApplBiochemBiotechnol...... *Applied Biochemistry and Biotechnology*
ApplEnvironMicrobiol .... *Applied Environmental Microbiology*
ApplPathol......................... *Applied Pathology*
ArbmedSozmedArbhyg .... *Arbeitsmedizin, Sozialmedizin, Arbeitshygiene*
ArchAnatCytolPath............. *Archives d'Anatomie et de Cytologie Pathologiques*
ArchBiochemBiophys.......... *Archives of Biochemistry and Biophysics*
ArchDermatol .... *Archives of Dermatology*
ArchDermRes .... *Archives of Dermatological Research*
ArchDisChild..................... *Archives of Diseases of Childhood*
ArchEnvironHlth .... *Archives of Environmental Health*
ArchExpPatholPharmakol ... *Archiv für Experimentelle Pathologie und Pharmakologie*
ArchFamMed .... *Archives of Family Medicine*
ArchFrancPediat .... *Archives Françaises de Pediatrie*
ArchFrMalAppDigNutr...... *Archives Françaises des Maladies de l'Appareil Digestif*
ArchGenPsychiatr............... *Archives of General Psychiatry*
ArchGerontolGeriat .... *Archives of Gerontology and Geriatrics*
ArchGewerbepath .... *Archiv für Gewerbepathologie und*
   Gewerbehyg   *Gewerbehygiene*
ArchHistCyt .... *Archives of Histology and Cytology*
ArchIndHlth .... *Archives of Industrial Health*
ArchIndHyg....................... *Archives of Industrial Hygiene*
ArchInternatPharmTher ..... *Archives Internationales de Pharmacodynamie et de Thérapie*
ArchIntMed....................... *Archives of Internal Medicine*
ArchIntPhysiolBioch........... *Archives Internationales de Physiologie et de Biochemie*

ArchJpnChir .... Archiv für Japanische Chirurgie
ArchMalAppDigNutr .... Archives des Maladies de l'Appareil Digestif et des Maladies de la Nutrition
ArchMalCoeur ....,.... Archives des Maladies du Coeur et des Vaisseaux
ArchMalProf...................... Archives de Maladies Professionelles, Hygiene et Toxicologie Industrielles
ArchNeurol........................ Archives of Neurology
ArchGynaecolObstet .... Archives of Gynaecology and Obstetrics
ArchOphthalmol .... Archives of Ophthalmology
ArchOralBiol...................... Archives of Oral Biology
ArchPathLabMed .... Archives of Pathology and Laboratory Medicine
ArchPathol........................ Archives of Pathology
ArchPediat .... Archives de Pédiatrie
ArchPediatrAdolescMed ..... Archives of Pediatrics and Adolescent Medicine
ArchPharmacol .... Archives of Pharmacology
ArchPharm .... Archiv der Pharmazie
ArchSexBehav.................... Archives of Sexual Behaviour
ArchSurg .... Archives of Surgery
ArchToxicol .... Archives of Toxicology
ArchVirol.......................... Archives of Virology
ArchVirolSuppl.................. Archives of Virology. Supplementum
ArkivKemi .... Arkiv foer Kemi
ArqGastroSaoPaulo........... Arquivos de Gastroenterologia
ArthRheum........................ Arthritis and Rheumatism
ArtifOrg............................ Artificial Organs
Artscler .... Arteriosclerosis
ArzForsch .... Arzneimittel-Forschung
Atheroscl........................... Atherosclerosis
ASAIOTrans...................... ASAIO Transactions
ATLA .... ATLA - Alternatives to Laboratory Animals
AustAnnMed .... Australasian Annals of Medicine
AustClinRev .... Australian Clinical Review
AustDrugAlcRev................ Australian Drug and Alcohol Review
AustJDermatol .... Australian Journal of Dermatology
AustJExpBiolMedSci .... Australian Journal of Experimental Biology and Medical Sciences
AustNZJMed..................... Australian and New Zealand Journal of Medicine
AustNZJObsGyn .... Australian and New Zealand Journal of Obstetrics and Gynaecology
AustNZJSurg..................... Australian and New Zealand Journal of Surgery
AustPaedJ .... Australian Paediatric Journal
AustRadiol .... Australian Radiology
AustVetJ........................... Australian Veterinary Journal
AutoImmun .... Autoimmunity
AvianDis .... Avian Diseases

BacteriolRev...................... Bacteriological Reviews
BailClinGastr .... Bailliere's Clinical Gastroenterology
BasicLifeSci .... Basic Life Sciences
BBActa .... Biochimica et Biophysica Acta

BBResComm .... Biochemical and Biophysical Research Communications
BDOAS .... Birth Defects, Original Article Series
BehavBrainRes................... Behavioural Brain Research
BehavGen .... Behavior Genetics
BehavResTher.................... Behavior Research and Therapy
BeitrPath.......................... Beitrage zur Pathologie
BeitrPatholAnat .... Beitrage zur Pathologischen Anatomie und Allgemeinen Pathologie
BiblCardiol........................ Bibliotheca Cardiologica
BiblioNutrDiet................... Bibliotheca 'Nutritio et Dieta'
Biochem........................... Biochemistry
BiochemCellBiol .... Biochemistry and Cell Biology
BiochemGen .... Biochemical Genetics
BiochemGen .... Biochemical Genetics
BiochemInt .... Biochemistry International
BiochemJ.......................... Biochemical Journal
BiochemMed...................... Biochemical Medicine
BiochemMolBiolInt .... Biochemistry and Molecular Biology International
BiochemMolMed .... Biochemical and Molecular Medicine
BiochemPharm................... Biochemical Pharmacology
BiochemSocSymp .... Biochemical Society Transactions
BiochemZ .... Biochemische Zeitschrift
Biochim .... Biochimie
BioconjugChem.................. Bioconjugate Chemistry
BioEssays .... Biological Essays
BiolCell............................ Biology of the Cell
BiolChemHS .... Biological Chemistry Hoppe-Seyler
BiolNeon........................... Biology of the Neonate
BiolPharmBull .... Biological and Pharmaceutical Bulletin
BiolRepro......................... Biology of Reproduction
BiolTraceElemRes.............. Biological Trace Element Research
Biomark .... Biomarkers
BiomedChromatogr .... Biomedical Applications of Gas Chromatography
Biomedicine .... Biomedicine
BiomedPharmacoth .... Biomedicine and Pharmacotherapy
BioMedRes .... Biomedical Research
Biometrika .... Biometrika
BiopharmDrugDispos .... Biopharmaceutics and Drug Disposition
BiophysJ .... Biophysical Journal
BiosciRep .... Bioscience Reports
Blood .... Blood
BloodCells........................ Blood Cells
BloodCellsMolDis.............. Blood Cells, Molecules and Diseases
BloodCoagFibrinol............. Blood Coagulation and Fibrinolysis
BloodRev .... Blood Reviews
Blut.................................. Blut
BMJ................................. British Medical Journal
Bone .... Bone
BoneMTrans...................... Bone Marrow Transplantation
BoneMineral .... Bone and Mineral
Brain................................ Brain
BrainDev .... Brain and Development

BrainRes .... *Brain Research*
BratislLekListy .... *Bratislavske Lekarske Listy*
BrazJMedBiolRes.............. *Brazilian Journal of Medical and Biological Research*
BrHeartJ .... *British Heart Journal*
BrJAddic............................ *British Journal of Addiction*
BrJAlcAlc........................... *British Journal of Alcohol and Alcoholism*
BrJAnaesth........................ *British Journal of Anaesthesiology*
BrJCanc .... *British Journal of Cancer*
BrJClinPharm .... *British Journal of Clinical Pharmacology*
BrJClinPract .... *British Journal of Clinical Practice*
BrJDermatol .... *British Journal of Dermatology*
BrJDisChest...................... *British Journal of Disease of the Chest*
BrJExpPath....................... *British Journal of Experimental Pathology*
BrJHaemat .... *British Journal of Haematology*
BrJHospMed...................... *British Journal of Hospital Medicine*
BrJIndMed .... *British Journal of Industrial Medicine*
BrJIntensCare .... *British Journal of Intensive Care*
BrJNutr .... *British Journal of Nutrition*
BrJObsGyn .... *British Journal of Obstetrics and Gynaecology*
BrJPharmacool .... *British Journal of Pharmacology*
BrJPsychiat .... *British Journal of Psychiatry*
BrJPsychol .... *British Journal of Psychology*
BrJRadiol .... *British Journal of Radiology*
BrJRheum .... *British Journal of Rheumatology*
BrJSportsMed.................... *British Journal of Sports Medicine*
BrJSurg............................. *British Journal of Surgery*
BrJUrol............................. *British Journal of Urology*
BrJVenerDis...................... *British Journal of Venereal Diseases*
BrMedBull......................... *British Medical Bulletin*
BrMedJClinRes.................. *British Medical Journal of Clinical Research*
BrVetJ .... *British Veterinary Journal*
BullAcadNatMed .... *Bulletin de l'Academie Nationale de Medicine (Paris)*
BullAssAnat .... *Bulletin de l'Association des Anatomistes*
BullCanc .... *Bulletin du Cancer (Paris)*
BullExpBiolMed .... *Bulletin of Experimental Biology and Medicine*
BullJHopkHosp................. *Bulletin of the Johns Hopkins Hospital*
BullMemSocChirParis .... *Bulletin et Mémoires de la Societé des Chirurgiens de Paris*
BullMemSocMedHôp......... *Bulletins et Mémoires de la Societé*
  Paris *Medicale des Hôpitaux de Paris*
BullNYAcadMed................ *Bulletin of the New York Academy of Medicine*
BullSocIntChir.................. *Bulletin de la Societé International de Chirurgie*
BullSocMedChir................ *Bulletin de la Societé Médicale des*
  Indochine *Chirurgiens de Indochine*

BullSocPath .... *Bulletin de la Societé de Pathologie Exotique*
BullWHO .... *Bulletin of the World Health Organization*
CalcifTissInt .... *Calcified Tissue International*
CalcifTissRes .... *Calcified Tissue Research*
CalifMed........................... *Californian Medicine*
CanAnaesthSocJ................ *Canadian Anaesthetists Society Journal*
CancChemoPharm .... *Cancer Chemotherapy and Pharmacology*
CancChemoRep .... *Cancer Chemotherapy Reports*
Cancer .... *Cancer*
CancerBiochBiophys .... *Cancer Biochemistry Biophysics*
CancerCauseContr .... *Cancer Causes and Control*
CancerDetectPrev .... *Cancer Detection and Prevention*
CancerDrugDeliv............... *CancerDrugDelivery*
CancerGenetCytogen .... *Cancer Genetics and Cytogenetics*
CancerImmunTher .... *Cancer Immunology and Immunotherapy*
CancerInvest .... *Cancer Investigation*
CancerLett......................... *Cancer Letters*
CancerMetRev .... *Cancer Metastasis Reviews*
CancerRes.......................... *Cancer Research*
CancerSurv .... *Cancer Survey*
CancerTreatRep................. *Cancer Treatment Reports*
CanJBiochCellBiol .... *Canadian Journal of Biochemistry and Cell Biology*
CanJBiochem .... *Canadian Journal of Biochemistry*
CanJCard .... *Canadian Journal of Cardiology*
CanJGastr .... *Canadian Journal of Gastroenterology*
CanJMicrobiol.................... *Canadian Journal of Microbiology*
CanJNeurSci...................... *Canadian Journal of Neurological Sciebces*
CanJPhysPharm .... *Canadian Journal of Physiology and Pharmacology*
CanJPsychiat..................... *Canadian Journal of Psychiatry*
CanJSurg .... *Canadian Journal of Surgery*
CanMedAssJ .... *Canadian Medical Association Journal*
CarbohydrRes .... *Carbohydrate Research*
Carcinogenesis .... *Carcinogenesis*
Cardiol.............................. *Cardiology*
CardiolClin .... *Cardiology Clinics*
Cardiologia........................ *Cardiologia*
CardiovascDrugRes............. *Cardiovascular Drug Research*
CardiovascDrugTher .... *Cardiovascular Drugs and Therapy*
CardvascIntRadiol.............. *Cardiovascular and Interventional Radiology*
CasLekCesk .... *Casopis Lekaru Ceskych*
CCActa .... *Clinica Chimica Acta*
CDCSurvSumm .... *CDC Survey and Summary*
CDR .... *Communicable Disease Reports*
Cell .... *Cell*
CellBiolIntRep .... *Cell Biology International Reports*
CellBiolRep....................... *Cell Biology Reports*

CellCalcium .... *Cell Calcium*
CellDeathDiffer .... *Cell Death and Differentiation*
CellGrowthDiff.................. *Cell Growth and Differentiation*
CellHepSin .... *Cells of the Hepatic Sinusoid*
CellImmunol...................... *Cellular Immunology*
CellMolecBiol .... *Cellular and Molecular Biology*
CellStructFunc .... *Cell Structure and Function*
CellTissKinet.................... *Cell Tissue Kinetics*
CellTissRes....................... *Cell Tissue Research*
CentrAfrMedJ.................... *Central African Medical Journal*
ChemBiolInteract............... *Chemico-Biological Interactions*
Chemosphere .... *Chemosphere*
Chemother .... *Chemotherapy*
ChemPharmBull .... *Chemical and Pharmaceutical*
                                Bulletin
ChemPhysLip .... *Chemistry and Physics of Lipids*
ChemResTox .... *Chemical Research in Toxicology*
Chest .... *Chest*
ChinJGastro...................... *Chinese Journal of Gastroenterology*
ChinJIntMed .... *Chinese Journal of Internal Medicine*
ChinJPhysiol .... *Chinese Journal of Physiology*
ChinMedJ .... *Chinese Medical Journal*
Chirurgie .... *Chirurgie*
ChungHuaFuChan.............. *Chung-Hua Fu Ch'an K'o Tsa Chih*
CibaSymp .... *Ciba Foundation Symposium*
CircRes .... *Circulation Research*
Circul............................... *Circulation*
CircShock .... *Circulation and Shock*
CleveClinJMed .... *Cleveland Clinic Journal of*
                                Medicine
CleveClinQ........................ *Cleveland Clinic Quarterly*
ClinAutonomRes................ *Clinical Autonomic Research*
ClinBioch.......................... *Clinical Biochemistry*
ClinCard .... *Clinical Cardiology*
ClinChem .... *Clinical Chemistry*
ClinDiagVirol.................... *Clinical and Diagnostic Virology*
ClinEndMetab .... *Clinics in Endocrinology and*
                                Metabolism
ClinEndoc......................... *Clinical Endocrinology*
ClinExpDerm .... *Clinical and Experimental*
                                Dermatology
ClinExpImmun .... *Clinical and Experimental*
                                Immunology
ClinExpMet .... *Clinical and Experimental*
                                Metastasis
ClinExpPharmPhys............. *Clinical and Experimental*
                                Pharmacology and Physiology
ClinExpRheumatol............. *Clinical and Experimental*
                                Rheumatology
ClinGastroent .... *Clinics in Gastroenterology*
ClinGenet .... *Clinical Genetics*
ClinHaem .... *Clinics in Haematology*
ClinicsAnesthesiol .... *Clinics in Anesthesiology*
ClinImmunAllergy .... *Clinics in Immunology and Allergy*
ClinImmunPath .... *Clinical Immunology and*
                                Immunopathology
ClinInfDis......................... *Clinical Infectious Diseases*
ClinInvest .... *Clinical Investigator*

ClinInvestMed .... *Clinical and Investigative Medicine*
ClinLabHaemat.................. *Clinical and Laboratory*
                                Haematology
ClinMicroRev .... *Clinical Microbiology Reviews*
ClinNephrol....................... *Clinical Nephrology*
ClinNeurolNeurosurg .... *Clinical Neurology and Neurosurgery*
ClinNeuropathol .... *Clinical Neuropathology*
ClinNeuropharmacol .... *Clinical Neuropharmacology*
ClinNuclMed...................... *Clinical Nuclear Medicine*
ClinNutr .... *Clinical Nutrition*
ClinObstetGynecol............. *Clinical Obstetrics and Gynecol*
ClinOncol.......................... *Clinical Oncology*
ClinOrthopRelRes.............. *Clinical Orthopedics and Related*
                                Research
ClinPediat .... *Clinical Pediatrics*
ClinPharmacokin................ *Clinical Pharmacokinetics*
ClinPharmTher................... *Clinical Pharmacology and*
                                Therapeutics
ClinPhysiol .... *Clinical Physiology*
ClinPhysPhysiolMeas .... *Clinical Physics and Physiological*
                                Measurement
ClinRadiol......................... *Clinical Radiology*
ClinRes .... *Clinical Research*
ClinRheum .... *Clinical Rheumatology*
ClinSci.............................. *Clinical Science*
ClinSciMolMed .... *Clinical Science and Molecular*
                                Medicine
ClinTher............................ *Clinical Therapeutics*
ClinToxicol .... *Clinical Toxicology*
ClinTranspl........................ *Clinical Transplantation*
ClinTropMedCommDis....... *Clinics in Tropical Medicine and*
                                Communicable Diseases
Coagulation .... *Coagulation*
CollRelRes .... *Collagen and Related Research*
CompBiochPhys.................. *Comparative Biochemistry and*
                                Physiology
Complement .... *Complement*
ConnMed........................... *Connecticut Medicine*
ConnTissRes...................... *Connective Tissue Research*
ContactDerm .... *Contact Dermatitis*
ContempSurg..................... *Contemporary Surgery*
ContribNephrol .... *Contributions to Nephrology*
ControlledClinTrials .... *Controlled Clinical Trials*
CRAcadSci........................ *Comptes Rendus de l'Academie des*
                                Sciences (Paris)
CritCareMed...................... *Critical Care Medicine*
CritRevBiochem................. *Critical Reviews in Biochemistry and*
                                Molecular Biology
CritRevClinLabSci.............. *Critical Reviews in Clinical*
                                Laboratory Sciences
CritRevDiagImag .... *Critical Reviews in Diagnostic*
                                Imaging
CritRevImmunol................. *Critical Reviews in Immunology*
CritRevOnc/Hemat .... *Critical Reviews in Oncology/*
                                Hematology
CritRevTherDrugCarrSys... *Critical Reviews in Therapeutic Drug*
                                Carrier Systems
CritRevTox .... *Critical Reviews in Toxicology*

CRSocBio .... *Comptes Rendus des Séances de la Société de Biologie et des Filiales (Paris)*
Cryobiology .... *Cryobiology*
CryoLett .... *Cryo Letters*
CSHarbSymQBiol .... *Cold Spring Harbor Symposia on Quantitative Biology*
CurrAlc .... *Currents in Alcoholism*
CurrBiol .... *Current Biology*
CurrMedResOpin .... *Current Medical Research and Opinion*
CurrModBiol .... *Currents in Modern Biology*
CurrOpinCellBiol .... *Current Opinion in Cell Biology*
CurrOpinGenetDevelop ...... *Current Opinion in Genetics and Development*
CurrOpinGastro .... *Current Opinion in Gastroenterology*
CurrOpinLipidol .... *Current Opinion in Lipidology*
CurrOpinImmunol .... *Current Opinion in Immunology*
CurrOpinInfDis .... *Current Opinion in Infectious Disease*
CurrOpinNephrolHypert .... *Current Opinion in Nephrology and Hypertension*
CurrOpinRheum .... *Current Opinion in Rheumatology*
CurrProbCardiol .... *Current Problem in Cardiology*
CurrProbPediat .... *Current Problem in Pediatrics*
CurrProbSurg .... *Current Problems in Surgery*
CurrTherRes .... *Current Therapeutic Research: Clinical and Experimental*
CurrTopHaemat .... *Current Topics in Haematology*
Cutis .... *Cutis*
Cytobios .... *Cytobios*
Cytochem .... *Cytochemistry*
CytogenetCellGenet .... *Cytogenetics and Cell Genetics*
Cytokine .... *Cytokine*
Cytopath .... *Cytopathology*

DanMedBull .... *Danish Medical Bulletin*
Dermatologica .... *Dermatologica*
Dermatology .... *Dermatology*
DeutschApothekZeit .... *Deutsch Apotheka Zeitung*
DeutschArchKlinMed .... *Deutsches Archiv für Klinische Medizin*
DeutscheZVerdauStoff .... *Deutsche Zeitschrift für Verdaungs und Stoffwechselkrankheiten*
DeutschMedWoch .... *Deutsche Medizinische Wochenschrift*
DeutschZNervenh .... *Deutsche Zeitschrift für Nervenheilkunde*
DevBiol .... *Developmental Biology*
Development .... *Development*
DevDyn .... *Developmental Dynamics*
DevelopBiolStandard .... *Developments in Biological Standardization*
DevPharmacolTher .... *Developmental Pharmacology and Therapeutics*
DiabetAnn .... *Diabetes Annual*
DiabetCare .... *Diabetes Care*
Diabetolog .... *Diabetologia*
DiabeteMetab .... *Diabetes Metabolism*

Diabetes .... *Diabetes*
DiabetMed .... *Diabetes Medicine*
DiabetMetabRev .... *Diabetes-Metabolism Reviews*
DiabetNutrMetab .... *Diabetes Nutrition and Metabolism*
DiabetRes .... *Diabetes Research*
DiabetResClinPract .... *Diabetes Research and Clinical Practice*
DiabetStoffw .... *Diabetes und Stoffwechsel*
DiagCytopathol .... *Diagnostic Cytopathology*
DiagIntervRadiol .... *Diagnostic and Interventional Radiology*
DiagMicrobInfDis .... *Diagnostic Microbiology and Infectious Disease*
DiagTherEndosc .... *Diagnostic and Therapeutic Endoscopy*
DiagnosHistopath .... *Diagnostic Histopathology*
DiagnosImagingClinMed .... *Diagnostic Imaging in Clinical Medicine*
Differentiation .... *Differentiation*
DigDis .... *Digestive Diseases*
DigDisSci .... *Digestive Diseases and Sciences*
Digestion .... *Digestion*
DigSurg .... *Digestive Surgery*
DisChest .... *Diseases of the Chest*
DisColRec .... *Diseases of the Colon and Rectum*
DisHeartCircul .... *Diseases of the Heart and Circulation*
DisMon .... *Disease-a-Month*
DMedWoch .... *Deutsche Medizinische Wochenschrift*
DNA .... *DNA*
DrugAlcDep .... *Drug and Alchohol Dependence*
DrugDel .... *Drug Delivery*
DrugDevRes .... *Drug Development Research*
DrugInvest .... *Drug Investigations*
DrugMetDisp .... *Drug Metabolism and Disposition*
DrugRes .... *Drug Research*
Drugs .... *Drugs*
DrugSafety .... *Drug Safety*
DrugsExpClinRes .... *Drugs under Clinical and Experimental Research*
DrugsMetabolRev .... *Drug Metabolism Reviews*
DtschGesInnMed .... *Deutsche Gesellschaft fur Innere Medizin*
DtshGesundhwesen .... *Deutsche Gesundheitswesen*
DtschZVerdau Stoffwechselkr .... *Deutsche Zeitschrift fur Verdaungs- und Stoffwechselkrankheiten*
EcotoxEnvirSafety .... *Ecotoxicology and Environmental Safety*
EdinburghMedJ .... *Edinburgh Medical Journal*
EJPTox .... *European Journal of Pharmacology, Environmental Toxicology and Pharmacology Section*
ElectroencephalogrClin Neurophys .... *Electroencephalography and Clinical Neurophysiology*
Electroencephalogr Neurophysiol .... *Electroencephalography and Neurophysiology*
Electrophoresis .... *Electrophoresis*
EMBOJ .... *EMBO Journal*

EndMetClinMedNAm .... *Endocrinology and Metabolism Clinics of North America*
Endocrinol .... *Endocrinology*
EndocrinolJpn .... *Endocrinologia Japonica*
EndocrRev .... *Endocrine Reviews*
Endoscopy .... *Endoscopy*
Endothelium .... *Endothelium*
EnfermInfecMicroClin .... *Enfermedades Infecciosas y Microbiologia Clinica*
EnvironHlthPerspect .... *Environmental Health Perspectives*
EnvirRes .... *Environmental Research*
Enzyme .... *Enzyme*
EnzymolBiolClin .... *Enzymologia Biologica et Clinica*
EpidInf .... *Epidemiology and Infection*
EpidRev .... *Epidemiologic Reviews*
EurArchPsychNeurSci .... *European Archives of Psychiatry and Neurological Sciences*
EurCytokineNet .... *European Cytokine Network*
EurHeartJ .... *European Heart Journal*
EurJAnaesth .... *European Journal of Anaesthiology*
EurJBioch .... *European Journal of Biochemistry*
EurJCan .... *European Journal of Cancer*
EurJCanClinOnc .... *European Journal of Cancer and Clinical Oncology*
EurJCellBiol .... *European Journal of Cell Biology*
EurJClinChemClinBioch ..... *European Journal of Clinical Chemistry and Clinical Biochemistry*
EurJClinInv .... *European Journal of Clinical Investigation*
EurJClinMicrobInfDis .... *European Journal of Clinical Microbiology and Infectious Disease*
EurJClinNutr .... *European Journal of Clinical Nutrition*
EurJClinPharm .... *European Journal of Clinical Pharmacology*
EurJDMPharm .... *European Journal of Drug Metabolism and Pharmacokinetics*
EurJEndocr .... *European Journal of Endocrinology*
EurJEpid .... *European Journal of Epidemiology*
EurJGastroHepatol .... *European Journal of Gastroenterology and Hepatology*
EurJHumGenet .... *European Journal of Human Genetics*
EurJImmunogenet .... *European Journal of Immunogenetics*
EurJImmun .... *European Journal of Immunology*
EurJNucMed .... *European Journal of Nuclear Medicine*
EurJObsGynReprodBiol ...... *European Journal of Obstetrics, Gynaecology, and Reproductive Biology*
EurJPed .... *European Journal of Pediatrics*
EurJPaediatSurg .... *European Journal of Paediatric Surgery*
EurJPharm .... *European Journal of Pharmacology*
EurJRadiol .... *European Journal of Radiology*
EurJRespDis .... *European Journal of Respiratory Diseases*

EurJRheumInflamm .... *European Journal of Rheumatic Inflammation*
EurJSurg............................ *European Journal of Surgery*
EurJSurgOnc .... *European Journal of Surgical Oncology*
EurNeurol.......................... *European Neurology*
EurRespJ .... *European Respiratory Journal*
EurSurgRes........................ *European Surgical Research*
ExpAgeRes......................... *Experimental Ageing Research*
ExpCellRes .... *Experimental Cell Research*
Experientia........................ *Experientia*
ExpBiol .... *Experimental Biology*
ExpGerontol .... *Experimental Gerontology*
ExpMolPath....................... *Experimental Molecular Pathology*
ExpParasit .... *Experimental Parasitology*
ExpPath .... *Experimental Pathology*
EXS................................... *EXS*
ExpToxPath .... *Experimental and Toxicologic Pathology*

FASEBJ .... *Federation of American Societies for Experimental Biology (FASEB) Journal*
FEBSLett .... *FEBS Letters*
FedProc .... *Federation Proceedings of American Societies for Experimental Biology*
FertSter .... *Fertilization and Sterilization*
FetDiagTher....................... *Fetal Diagnosis and Therapy*
Fibrinolysis .... *Fibrinolysis*
FOBrMedBull..................... *Foreign Office British Medical Bulletin*
FolHistochemCytol .... *Folia Histochemica et Cytochemica*
FolMed.............................. *Folia Medica*
FolPsychNeurolJapon .... *Folia Psychiatrica et Neurologica Japonica*
FoodChemTox.................... *Food and Chemical Toxicology*
FoodCosmTox .... *Food and Cosmetics Toxicology*
FoodNut .... *Food and Nutrition*
FortschrMed....................... *Fortschritte der Medizin*
FortschrNeurolPsychiatr ..... *Fortschritte der Neurologie-Psychiatrie*
FortschrRoentg .... *Fortschritte der Roentgenologie*
FrankZeitschriPathol .... *Frankfurter Zeitschrift fur Pathologie*
FreeRadicBiolMed .... *Free Radical Biology and Medicine*
FreeRadRes........................ *Free Radical Research*
FreeRadicResComm............ *Free Radical Research Communications*
FrontGastrRes .... *Frontiers in Gastroenterological Research*
FundApplTox .... *Fundamental and Applied Toxicology*

Gann................................. *Gann*
GastrClinBiol..................... *Gastroenterologie Clinique et Biologique*
GastrClinNAm .... *Gastroenterological Clinics of North America*
GastrEnd .... *Gastrointestinal Endoscopy*
GastrInternat .... *Gastroenterology International*

GastrJap.............................. *Gastroenterologia Japonica*
Gastro................................. *Gastroenterology*
Gastroenterologia .... *Gastroenterologia*
GastroHepato...................... *Gastroenterologia y Hepatologia*
GastrRad............................ *Gastrointestinal Radiology*
GazIntMedChir .... *Gazzetta Internazionale di Medicina e Chirurgia*
GClinMed .... *Giornale di Clinica Medica (Bologna)*
GegenbaursMorphJahrb...... *Gegensbaurs Morphologisches Jahrbuch*
Gene................................... *Gene*
GenesDevelop...................... *Genes Developments*
GenetEpid .... *Genetic Epidemiology*
Genetics.............................. *Genetics*
GenetRes .... *Genetical Research*
GenitourinMed .... *Genitourinary Medicine*
Genomics............................ *Genomics*
GenPharmacol .... *General Pharmacology*
GenPractitioner.................. *General Practitioner*
GeogMed............................ *Geographia Medica*
Geriat .... *Geriatrics*
Geront .... *Gerontology*
GItalDermVener .... *Giornale Italiano di Dermatologia e Venereologia*
GItalMedLav .... *Giornale Italiano di Medicina del Lavoro*
GlycoconjugJ .... *Glycoconjugate Journal*
Gut..................................... *Gut*
Guy'sHospRep.................... *Guy's Hospital Reports*
GynecolObsInvest............... *Gynecologic and Obstetric Investigation*
GynOncol .... *Gynecologic Oncology*

Haematol(Pavia) .... *Haematologica (Pavia)*
Haemostasis .... *Haemostasis*
Hautarzt............................. *Hautarzt*
HealthEducJ .... *Health Education Journal*
Heart .... *Heart*
HelvChirActa..................... *Helvetica Chirurgica Acta*
HelvMedActa...................... *Helvetica Medica Acta*
HelvPaedActa .... *Helvetica Paediatrica Acta*
HelvPharmActa.................. *Helvetica Pharmacologica Acta*
Hemat/OncolClinNAm ...... *Hematology/Oncology Clinics of North America*
HemOnc .... *Hematological Oncology*
Hepatogast .... *Hepato-Gastroenterology*
Hepatol .... *Hepatology*
HiroshimaJMedSci.............. *Hiroshima Journal of Medical Sciences*
Histochem.......................... *Histochemistry*
HistochemCytochem........... *Histochemisty and Cytochemistry*
HistochemJ .... *Histochemical Journal*
HistocompTest.................... *Histocompatibility Testing*
Histopath .... *Histopathology*
HoppeSeylerZBiolChem ..... *Hoppe-Seylers Zeitschrift für Biologische Chemie*

HoppeSeyler .... *Hoppe-Seylers Zeitschrift für Physiologische Chemie*
ZPhysiolChem
HormCellReg...................... *Hormones Cell Regulation*
HormMetRes .... *Hormone and Metabolic Research*
HormRes .... *Hormone Research*
HospPract .... *Hospital Practice*
HPBSurgery .... *Hepato Pancreatico Biliary Surgery*
HumExpToxicol .... *Human and Experimental Toxicology*
HumGenet.......................... *Human Genetics*
HumGeneTher .... *Human Gene Therapy*
HumHere............................ *Human Heredity*
HumImmunol...................... *Human Immunology*
HumMolGenet .... *Human Molecular Genetics*
HumNutrAN .... *Human Nutrition. Clinical Nutrition*
HumPath .... *Human Pathology*
HumRepro.......................... *Human Reproduction*
Hypertension .... *Hypertension*
Hypotheses .... *Hypotheses*

IARCEvalCarcinogRisk .... *IARC Evaluation of Carcinogenic Risk of Chemicals for Humans Monographs*
ChemHumMonogr
IARCSciPubl .... *IARC Scientific Publications*
Iatriki................................ *Iatriki*
IEEETrBiomedEng............. *IEEE Transactions on Biomedical Engineering*
Immunity............................ *Immunity*
Immunobiology................... *Immunobiology*
Immunogenet...................... *Immunogenetics*
Immunol .... *Immunology*
ImmunolAllergPract........... *Immunology and Allergy Practice*
ImmunolCommun.............. *Immunological Communications*
ImmunoLett .... *Immunology Letters*
ImmunolRev....................... *Immunological Reviews*
ImmunolToday.................... *Immunology Today*
IndJGastro .... *Indian Journal of Gastroenterology*
IndJMedRes........................ *Indian Journal of Medical Research*
IndJMedSci .... *Indian Journal of Medical Sciences*
IndJPhysiolPharmacol .... *Indian Journal of Physiology and Pharmacology*
IndMedGaz .... *Indian Medical Gazette*
IndMedSurg .... *Indian Medical Survey*
IndPaediat......................... *Indian Paediatrics*
Infec .... *Infection*
InfectImmun...................... *Infection and Immunity*
InnMed.............................. *Innere Medizin*
IntAbstrSurg...................... *International Abstracts of Surgery*
IntArchAllApplImmunol..... *International Archives of Allergy and Applied Immunology*
IntArchOccupEnvirHlth ..... *International Archives of Occupational and Environmental Health*
IntensCareMed .... *Intensive Care Medicine*
IntensCareWorld............... *Intensive Care World*
Internist .... *Internist*
Intervirology .... *Intervirology*

IntHepatolComm .... *International Hepatology Communications*

IntJAddict .... *International Journal of Addiction*

IntJArtifOrg .... *International Journal of Artificial Organs*

IntJAndrol .... *International Journal of Andrology*

IntJBiochem .... *International Journal of Biochemistry*

IntJBiochemCellBiol .... *International Journal of Biochemistry and Cell Biology*

IntJCanc .... *International Journal of Cancer*

IntJCardiol .... *International Journal of Cardiology*

IntJClinLabRes .... *International Journal of Clinical and Laboratory Research*

IntJClinPharmacol.............. *International Journal of Clinical Pharmacology*

IntJClinPharmRes .... *International Journal of Clinical Pharmacological Research*

IntJDermatol...................... *International Journal of Dermatology*

IntJEatingDis..................... *International Journal of Eating Disorders*

IntJEpid............................ *International Journal of Epidemiology*

IntJExpPathol .... *International Journal of Experimental Pathology*

IntJFert............................ *International Journal of Fertility*

IntJGynObs .... *International Journal of Gynecology and Obstetrics*

IntJHlthServ .... *International Journal of Health Services*

IntJObes............................ *International Journal of Obesity*

IntJParasitol .... *International Journal of Parasitology*

IntJPediatriNephrol .... *International Journal of Pediatric Nephrology*

IntJPeptProteinRes .... *International Journal of Peptide and Protein Research*

IntJPharmaceut .... *International Journal of Pharmaceutics*

IntJRadiatBiol .... *International Journal of Radiation Biology*

IntJRadiatOncolBiolPhys..... *International Journal of Radiation, Oncology, Biology, Physics*

IntJSportsMed .... *International Journal of Sports Medicine*

IntJSystBacteriol .... *International Journal of Systematic Bacteriology*

IntJVitNutrRes................... *International Journal for Vitamin and Nutrition Research*

IntMed .... *Internal Medicine*

IntRevCytol .... *International Reviews of Cytology*

IntRevExpPath................... *International Reviews of Experimental Pathology*

IntSurg .... *International Surgery*

IntUrolNephrol.................. *International Urology and Nephrology*

IntVirol .... *International Virology*

InvasMetast....................... *Invasion and Metastasis*

InvestRadiol .... *Investigative Radiology*

InvestUrol.......................... *Investigative Urology*

Invitro................................ *In Vitro Cell Development Biology*

InvOphthalmolVisSci .... *Investigative Ophthalmology and Visual Science*

IRCSJMedSci .... *IRCS Journal of Medical Science*

IrJMedSci .... *Irish Journal of Medical Science*

IrMedJ.............................. *Irish Medical Journal*

ISIAtlasSci:Pharmacol .... *ISI Atlas of Science: Pharmacology*

IsrJMedSci......................... *Israeli Journal of Medical Sciences*

ItalJGastr .... *Italian Journal of Gastroenterology*

ItalJNeurolSci .... *Italian Journal of Neurological Sciences*

ItalJPediat .... *Italian Journal of Pediatrics*

ItalJSurgSci........................ *Italian Journal of Surgical Sciences*

JAIDS................................ *Journal of Acquired Immune Deficiency Syndromes and Human Retrovirology*

JAllClinImmunol .... *Journal of Allergy and Clinical Immunology*

JAMA .... *Journal of the American Medical Association*

JAmAcadDermatol.............. *Journal of the American Academy of Dermatology*

JAmCollCard .... *Journal of the American College of Cardiology*

JAmCollNutr .... *Journal of the American College of Nutrition*

JAmCollSurg .... *Journal of the American College of Surgeons*

JAmDietAssoc.................... *Journal of the American Dietetics Association*

JAmGeriatSoc.................... *Journal of the American Geriatrics Society*

JAmMedWomAssoc .... *Journal of the American Medical Women's Association*

JAmSocNephrol.................. *Journal of the American Society of Nephrology*

JAnat .... *Journal of Anatomy*

JAntimicChemo .... *Journal of Antimicrobial Chemotherapy*

JApplPhysiol .... *Journal of Applied Physiology*

JApplTox .... *Journal of Applied Toxicology*

JAssocPhysInd .... *Journal of the Association of Physicians of India*

JAutonNervSyst................. *Journal of the Autonomic Nervous System*

JAutonPharmacol .... *Journal of Autonomic Pharmacology*

JBacteriol .... *Journal of Bacteriology*

JBC................................... *Journal of Biological Chemistry*

JBehavTherExpPsych .... *Journal of Behavior Therapy and Experimental Psychiatry*

JBioch .... *Journal of Biochemistry*

JBiochem(Tokyo) .... *Journal of Biochemistry (Tokyo)*

JBioenergBiomembr .... *Journal of Bioenergetics and Biomembranes*

JBiolStandard..................... *Journal of Biological Standardization*

JBoneJtSurg .... *Journal of Bone and Joint Surgery*

JBoneMinRes...................... *Journal of Bone and Mineral Research*

JCanAssocRadiol .... *Journal of the Canadian Association of Radiologists*

JCanMedAssoc................... *Journal of the Canadian Medical Association*

JCancResClinOnc............... *Journal of Cancer Research and Clinical Oncology*

JCardiolPharmacol .... *Journal of Cardiology and Pharmacology*

JCardiovascSurg.................. *Journal of Cardiovascular Surgery*

JCellBiochem .... *Journal of Cellular Biochemistry*

JCellBiol .... *Journal of Cell Biology*

JCellPhysiol .... *Journal of Cellular Physiology*

JCellSci.............................. *Journal of Cell Science*

JCerebBloodFlowMetab ...... *Journal of Cerebral Blood Flow and Metabolism*

JChildNeurol .... *Journal of Child Neurology*

JChir................................. *Journale de Chirurgie*

JChromatogr .... *Journal of Chromatography*

JChromatogrB.................... *Journal of Chromatography, B. Biomedical Applications*

JChronDis.......................... *Journal of Chronic Diseases*

JCI..................................... *Journal of Clinical Investigation*

JClinChemClinBioch.......... *Journal of Clinical Chemistry and Clinical Biochemistry*

JClinDysmorph .... *Journal of Clinical Dysmorphism*

JClinElectronMicrosc.......... *Journal of Clinical Electron Microscopy*

JClinEndoc .... *Journal of Clinical Endocrinology and Metabolism*

JClinEndocrinol .... *Journal of Clinical Endocrinology*

JClinGastro....................... *Journal of Clinical Gastroenterology*

JClinEpidemiol .... *Journal of Clinical Epidemiology*

JClinImmunol .... *Journal of Clinical Immunology*

JClinInvest........................ *Journal of Clinical Investigation*

JCiinLabAnal .... *Journal of Clinical Laboratory Analysis*

JClinLabImmunol.............. *Journal of Clinical and Laboratory Immunology*

JClinMicrobiol .... *Journal of Clinical Microbiology*

JClinNeurophys .... *Journal of Clinical Neurophysiology*

JClinNutrGastro .... *Journal of Clinical Nutrition and Gastroenterology*

JClinOncol........................ *Journal of Clinical Oncology*

JClinPath .... *Journal of Clinical Pathology*

JClinPharm .... *Journal of Clinical Pharmacology*

JClinPsych .... *Journal of Clinical Psychology*

JClinPsychpharm .... *Journal of Clinical Psychopharmacology*

JClinSurg........................... *Journal of Clinical Surgery*

JClinUltrasound................. *Journal of Clinical Ultrasound*

JCommDis......................... *Journal of Communicable Diseases*

JComputAssistTomogr .... *Journal of Computer Assisted Tomography*

JCutPath .... *Journal of Cutaneous Pathology*

JDermatol .... *Journal of Dermatology*

JDrugDevel........................ *Journal of Drug Development*

JDrugTarget....................... *Journal of Drug Targeting*

JEgyptSocParasitol............. *Journal of the Egyptian Society of Parasitology*

JElectronMicrosc .... *Journal of Electron Microscopy*

JEMTech .... *Journal of Electron Microscopy Techniques*

JEmbrExpMorph .... *Journal of Embryology and Experimental Morphology*

JEndocr............................. *Journal of Endocrinology*

JEndocrMetab.................... *Journal of Endocrinology and Metabolism*

JEndocrInv .... *Journal of Endocrinological Investigation*

JEpidCommHlth................. *Journal of Epidemiology and Community Health*

JEukaryotMicrobiol............ *Journal of Eukaryotic Microbiology*

JEurTox .... *Journal Européen de Toxicologie*

JExpBiol .... *Journal of Experimental Biology*

JExpImmunol .... *Journal of Experimental Immunology*

JExpMed .... *Journal of Experimental Medicine*

JExpPath........................... *Journal of Experimental Pathology*

JFamPractice..................... *Journal of Family Practice*

JForensicSci....................... *Journal of Forensic Science*

JFormosanMedAss............. *Journal of the Formosan Medical Association*

JGastHepatol .... *Journal of Gastroenterology and Hepatology*

JGastro .... *Journal of Gastroenterology*

JGenPhysiol .... *Journal of GeneralPhysiol*

JGenVirol.......................... *Journal of General Virology*

JGeront............................. *Journal of Gerontology*

JGynObsBiolReprod .... *Journal de Gynecologie Obstetrique et Biologie de la Reproduction*

JHeartLungTranspl............ *Journal of Heart and Lung Transplantation*

JHepatobilPancrSurg.......... *Journal of Hepatobiliary and Pancreatic Surgery*

JHepatol............................ *Journal of Hepatology*

JHered .... *Journal of Heredity*

JHistochemCytochem .... *Journal of Histochemistry and Cytochemistry*

JHospInf............................ *Journal of Hospital Infection*

JHumNutrDiet .... *Journal of Human Nutrition and Dietetics*

JHyg .... *Journal of Hygiene*

JHypert.............................. *Journal of Hypertension*

JikeikaiMedJ .... *Jikeikai Medical Journal*

JImmunol........................... *Journal of Immunology*

JImmunolMethods............. *Journal of Immunological Methods*

JImmunother .... *Journal of Immunotherapy with Emphasis on Tumor Immunology*

JIndHygTox....................... *Journal of Industrial Hygiene and Toxicology*

JInfDis.............................. *Journal of Infectious Diseases*

JInfect............................... *Journal of Infection*

JInherMetDis..................... *Journal of Inherited Metabolic Diseases*

JIntChir .... *Journal International de Chirurgie*
JInterferonRes.................... *Journal of Interferon Research*
JIntMed............................ *Journal of Internal Medicine*
JIntMedRes........................ *Journal of International Medical Research*
JInvDermatol .... *Journal of Investigative Dermatology*
JIrishMedAss .... *Journal of the Irish Medical Association*
JJapSurgSoc...................... *Journal of the Japanese Surgical Society*
JKurumeMedAssoc............. *Journal of the Kurume Medical Association*
JKuwaitMedAssoc.............. *Journal of the Kuwait Medical Association*
JLabClinMed .... *Journal of Laboratory and Clinical Medicine*
JLeukBiol........................... *Journal of Leukocyte Biology*
JLipRes............................. *Journal of Lipid Research*
JMed................................ *Journal of Medicine*
JMedAssThai..................... *Journal of the Medical Association of Thailand*
JMedChem .... *Journal of Medicinal Chemistry*
JMedEntomol .... *Journal of Medical Entomology*
JMedGenet .... *Journal of Medical Genetics*
JMedMicrobiol .... *Journal of Medical Microbiology*
JMedPrimatol .... *Journal of Medical Primatology*
JMedVirol .... *Journal of Medical Virology*
JMembrBiol .... *Journal of Membrane Biology*
JMentalDeficRes .... *Journal of Mental Deficiency Research*
JMicrosc .... *Journal of Microscopy*
JMolBiol .... *Journal of Molecular Biology*
JMolEndocr .... *Journal of Molecular Endocrinology*
JMolMed .... *Journal of Molecular Medicine*
JMorph .... *Journal of Morphology*
JMRI .... *Journal of Magnetic Resonance Imaging*
JNatProd.......................... *Journal of Natural Products*
JNCI................................ *Journal of the National Cancer Institute*
JNepalMedAss .... *Journal of the Nepalese Medical Association*
JNervMentDis .... *Journal of Nervous and Mental Disease*
JNeuroch .... *Journal of Neurochemistry*
JNeurol .... *Journal of Neurology*
JNeurolNeurosurgPsych...... *Journal of Neurology, Neurosurgery, and Psychiatry*
JNeurolSci .... *Journal of the Neurological Sciences*
JNeuropathExpNeurol .... *Journal of Neuropathology and Experimental Neurology*
JNeurosci .... *Journal of Neuroscience*
JNeurosurg .... *Journal of Neurosurgery*
JNuclMed .... *Journal of Nuclear Medicine*
JNutr .... *Journal of Nutrition*
JNutrSciVitaminol .... *Journal of Nutritional Science and Vitaminology*

JObsGynBrCommonw .... *Journal of Obstetrics and Gynaecology of the British Commonwealth*
JObstetGynaecolBrEmp ..... *Journal of Obstetrics and Gynaecology of the British*
JOccMed........................... *Journal of Occupational Medicine*
JOklStatMedAssoc .... *Journal of the Oklahoma State Medical Association*
JohnsHopkHospBull .... *Johns Hopkins Hospital Bulletin*
JohnsHopkHospRep........... *Johns Hopkins Hospital Reports*
JohnsHopkMedJ .... *Johns Hopkins Medical Journal*
JObsGyn .... *Journal of Obstetrics and Gynaecology*
JOralPathol .... *Journal of Oral Pathology*
JParasitol .... *Journal of Parasitology*
JParentSciTech .... *Journal of Parenteral Science and Technology*
JPath............................... *Journal of Pathology*
JPatholBacteriol .... *Journal of Pathology and Bacteriology*
JPediat .... *Journal of Pediatrics*
JPediatChildHlth .... *Journal of Pediatrics and Child Health*
JPediatGastrNutr .... *Journal of Pediatric Gastroenterology and Nutrition*
JPediatSurg .... *Journal of Pediatric Surgery*
JPEN .... *Journal of Parenteral and Enteral Nutrition*
JPerinatMed...................... *Journal of Perinatal Medicine*
JPharmacbioDyn .... *Journal of Pharmacobiodynamics*
JPharmaceutSci.................. *Journal of Pharmaceutical Sciences*
JPharmacokinBiopharm....... *Journal of Pharmacokinetics and Biopharmaceutics*
JPharmExpTher.................. *Journal of Pharmacology and Experimental Therapeutics*
JPharmPharmacol............... *Journal of Pharmacy and Pharmacology*
JPhysiol............................ *Journal of Physiology*
JPhysiolPharmacol .... *Journal of Physiology and Pharmacology*
JpnJAllergy .... *Japanese Journal of Allergology*
JpnJAnesth........................ *Japanese Journal of Anesthesiology*
JpnJCancerChemother .... *Japanese Journal of Cancer and Chemotherapy*
JpnJCancerRes .... *Japanese Journal of Cancer Research*
JpnJClinMed...................... *Japanese Journal of Clinical Medicine*
JpnJClinOncol.................... *Japanese Journal of Clinical Oncology*
JpnJClinPath...................... *Japanese Journal of Clinical Pathology*
JpnJClinRadiol................... *Japanese Journal of Clinical Radiology*
JpnJExpMed .... *Japanese Journal of Experimental Medicine*
JpnJGastro .... *Japanese Journal of Gastroenterology*
JpnJMed .... *Japanese Journal of Medicine*

JpnJNuclMed	*Japanese Journal of Nuclear Medicine*
JpnJPhysiol	*Japanese Journal of Physiology*
JpnJStudAlc	*Japanese Journal of Studies in Alcoholism*
JpnJSurg	*Japanese Journal of Surgery*
JPostgradMed	*Journal of Postgraduate Medicine*
JPsychiatRes	*Jouranl of Psychiatric Research*
JRadioanalChem	*Journal of Radioanalytical Chemistry*
JRadiol	*Journal de Radiologie*
JRArmyMedCorp	*Journal of the Royal Army Medical Corps (London)*
JRCollSurgEdinb	*Journal of the Royal College of Surgeons Edinburgh*
JReprodMed	*Journal of Reproductive Medicine*
JRheum	*Journal of Rheumatology*
JRoyCollPhys	*Journal of the Royal College of Physicians*
JRSM	*Journal of the Royal Society of Medicine*
JSocMed	*Journal of Social Medicine*
JSterBioch	*Journal of Steroid Biochemistry*
JStructBiol	*Journal of Structural Biology*
JStudAlc	*Journal of Studies on Alcohol*
JSubsAbus	*Journal of Substance Abuse*
JSubsAbuseTreat	*Journal of Substance Abuse Treatment*
JSupramolStruct	*Journal of Supramolecular Structure*
JSurgOncol	*Journal of Surgical Oncology*
JSurgRes	*Journal of Surgical Research*
JTheorBiol	*Journal of Theoretical Biology*
JThoracCardiovascSurg	*Journal of Thoracic and Cardiovascular Surgery*
JTraceElemMedBiol	*Journal of Trace Elements in Medicine and Biology*
JTrauma	*Journal of Trauma*
JTropMedHyg	*Journal of Tropical Medicine and Hygiene*
JTropPed	*Journal of Tropical Pediatrics*
JUltrastructRes	*Journal of Ultrastructural Research*
JUrol	*Journal of Urology*
JUrologie	*Journal d'Urologie*
JUSMed	*Journal of Ultrasound in Medicine*
JVascSurg	*Journal of Vascular Surgery*
JVirol	*Journal of Virology*
JViralHepat	*Journal of Viral Hepatitis*
JVirolMethods	*Journal of Virological Methods*
JVit	*Journal of Vitaminology*
KeioJMed	*Keio Journal of Medicine*
Khirurgia	*Khirurgia*
KidneyInt	*Kidney International*
KlinMonatsblAugenheilkd	*Klinische Monatsblatter für Augenheilkunde*
KlinPadiatr	*Klinische Pädiatrie*
KlinWschr	*Klinische Wochenschrift*
LabInvest	*Laboratory Investigation*
Lancet	*Lancet*
Lakartid	*Läkartidningen*
LangArchChir	*Langbecks Archiv für Chirurgie*
LavUmano	*Lavoro Umano*
LebMagDarm	*Leber, Magen, Darm*
LifeChem Rep	*Life Chemistry Reports*
LifeSci	*Life Sciences*
LilleMed	*Lille Medical*
Lipids	*Lipids*
Liver	*Liver*
LiverTransplSurg	*Liver Transplantation and Surgery*
LondMedGaz	*London Medical Gazette*
Lupus	*Lupus*
LymphokineRes	*Lymphokine Research*
Lymphology	*Lymphology*
LyonChirurg	*Lyon Chirurgical*
Maandschr Kindergeneeskd	*Maandschrift voor Kindergeneeskunde*
MagnesBull	*Magnesium Bulletin*
Magnesium	*Magnesium*
MagResImag	*Magnetic Resonance Imaging*
MammGenome	*Mammalian Genome*
MatMedPol	*Materia Medica Polona*
Matrix	*Matrix*
MatrixBiol	*Matrix Biology*
MayoClinMonogr	*Mayo Clinic Monographs*
MayoClinProc	*Mayo Clinic Proceedings*
MedAnnualDC	*Medical Annual DC*
MedBiol	*Medical Biology*
MedChirDig	*Médecine et Chirurgie Digestives*
MedClinNAm	*Medical Clinics of North America*
MedHypothes	*Medical Hypotheses*
MedicinaClin	*Medicina Clinica*
Medicine	*Medicine*
MedicinskiArhiv	*Medicinski Arhiv*
MedJAust	*Medical Journal of Australia*
MedJMalaysia	*Medical Journal of Malaysia*
MedJOsakaUniv	*Medical Journal of Osaka University*
MedKlin	*Medizinische Klinik*
MedLav	*Medicina del Lavero*
MedMicrobiolImmunol	*Medical Microbiology and Immunology*
MedMonatschr	*Medizinische Monatsschrift*
MedOncTumPharm	*Medical Oncology and Tumour Pharmacology*
MedPediatOncol	*Medical and Paediatric Oncology*
MedSentinel	*Medical Sentinel*
MedSciSportsExer	*Medicine and Science in Sports and Exercise*
MedTher	*Médecine Thérapeutique*
MedToxicol	*Medical Toxicology*
MedWelt	*Die Medizinische Welt*
MemInstOswaldoCruz	*Memorias do Instituto Oswaldo Cruz*
MetabolBrainDis	*Metabolic Brain Disease*
Metabolism	*Metabolism: Clinical and Experimental*
MethodsEnz	*Methods in Enzymology*

Microbiology	*Microbiology*
MicrobiolRev	*Microbiological Reviews*
MicrovascRes	*Microvascular Research*
MilitMed	*Military Medicine*
MinDietGastro	*Minerva Dietologica e Gastroenterologica*
MinElecMetab	*Mineral and Electrolyte Metabolism*
MinMed	*Minerva Medica*
MittGrenzgebMedChir	*Mitteilungen aus den Grenzgebieten der Medizin und Chirurgie*
MittOstGestTrop MedParas	*Mitteilungen der Österreichischen Gesellschaft für Tropenmedizin und Parasitologie*
MMWR	*Morbidity and Mortality Weekly Report*
ModPathol	*Modern Pathology*
MolAspMed	*Molecular Aspects of Medicine*
MolBiochemParasitol	*Molecular and Biochemical Parasitology*
MolBiolEvol	*Molecular Biology and Evolution*
MolBiolMed	*Molecular Biology and Medicine*
MolBiolRep	*Molecular Biology Reports*
MolCarcinog	*Molecular Carcinogenesis*
MolCellBiochem	*Molecular and Cellular Biochemistry*
MolCellBiol	*Molecular and Cellular Biology*
MolCellEndocrinol	*Molecular and Cellular Endocrinology*
MolCellProbes	*Molecular and Cellular Probes*
MolEndocrin	*Molecular Endocrinology*
MolImmunol	*Molecular Immunology*
MolMed	*Molecular Medicine*
MolMembBiol	*Molcular and Membrane Biology*
MolPharm	*Molecular Pharmacology*
MonatsschrKinderheilkd	*Monatsschrift fur Kinderheilkunde*
MonogrCancerRes	*Monographs in Cancer Research*
MonogrVirol	*Monographs in Virology*
MonthlyJMedSci	*Monthly Journal of Medical Science*
MorpholIgazOrvSz	*Morphologiai es Igazsagugyi Orvosi Szemle*
MovementDisorders	*Movement Disorders*
MtSinaiMedJ	*Mount Sinai Medical Journal*
MunchMedWoch	*Munchener Medizinische Wochenschrift*
Mutagenesis	*Mutagenesis*
Mycopathologia	*Mycopathologia*
NatlCancerInstMonogr	*National Cancer Institute, Monograph*
Nature	*Nature*
NatureGen	*Nature Genetics*
NatureMed	*Nature Medicine*
NatureNewBiol	*NatureNewBiol*
Naunyn-Schmiedb ArchPharm	*Naunyn-Schmiedberg's Archives of Pharmacology*
NedTGeneesk	*Nederlands Tijdschrift voor Geneeskunde*
NEJM	*New England Journal of Medicine*
Neoplasma	*Neoplasma*
Nephrol	*Nephrology*
NephrolDialTranspl	*Nephrology Dialysis Transplantation*
Nephron	*Nephron*
Nervenarzt	*Nervenarzt*
NethJMed	*Netherlands Journal of Medicine*
NeurochemRes	*Neurochemistry Research*
Neurology	*Neurology*
Neuropediatrics	*Neuropediatrics*
Neuropharmacol	*Neuropharmacology*
Neuroradiol	*Neuroradiology*
NeurosciLett	*Neuroscience Letters*
NewCompBiochem	*New Compounds in Biochemistry*
NIHBull	*National Institutes of Health Bulletin*
NipponGekaGakkaiZass	*Nippon Geka Gakkai Zasshi*
NipponKyobuShikkai GakkaiZasshi	*Nippon Kyobu Shikkai Gakkai Zasshi*
NipponShokGakkaiZass	*Nippon Shokakibyo Gakkai Zasshi*
NorthwestMed	*Northwest Medicine*
NoShinkeiGeka	*No Shinkei Geka*
NouvPresseMed	*Nouvelle Presse Medicale*
NouvRevFrHemat	*Nouvelle Revue Française d'Hématologie*
NucAcidRes	*Nucleic Acids Research*
Nucleonics	*Nucleonics*
NuclMedComm	*Nuclear Medicine Communications*
NutrBioch	*Nutrition and Biochemistry*
Nutrition	*Nutrition*
NutrCanc	*Nutrition and Cancer*
NutrMetab	*Nutrition and Metabolism*
NutrRepInt	*Nutrition Reports International*
NutrRes	*Nutrition Research*
NutrResRev	*Nutrition Research Reviews*
NutrRev	*Nutrition Reviews*
NutrRevInt	*Nutrition Reviews International*
NYStateJMed	*New York State Journal of Medicine*
NZMedJ	*New Zealand Medical Journal*
ObsGyn	*Obstetrics and Gynaecology*
ObsGynSurv	*Obstetrics and Gynaecology Survey*
OccupEnvironMed	*Occupational and Environmental Medicine*
OkajimasFAnatJap	*Okajimas Folia Anatomica Japonica*
Oncogene	*Oncogene*
OncogeneRes	*Oncogene Research*
Oncol	*Oncology*
Ophthalmologica	*Ophthalmologica*
OralSurg	*Oral Surgery*
OsteoporosisInt	*Osteoporosis International*
Pancreas	*Pancreas*
PapuaNGuineaMedJ	*Papua and New Guinea Medical Journal*
ParasiteImmunol	*Parasite Immunology*
ParasiticProtozoa	*Parasitic Protozoa*
Parasitol	*Parasitology*
ParasitolRes	*Parasitology Research*
ParasitolToday	*Parasitology Today*

Pathobio	*Pathobiology*
Pathology	*Pathology*
PatholAnn	*Pathology Annual*
PathInt	*Pathology International*
PatholResPract	*Pathological Research Practice*
Pediat	*Pediatrics*
PediatAnn	*Pediatric Annals*
PediatClinNAm	*Pediatric Clinics of North America*
PediatInfectDis	*Pediatric Infectious Disease*
PediatPath	*Pediatric Pathology*
PediatrDermatol	*Pediatric Dermatology*
PediatRes	*Pediatric Research*
Pediatria	*Pediatria*
PediatrNeurol	*Pediatric Neurology*
PediatrPulmonol	*Pediatric Pulmonology*
PediatrRadiol	*Pediatric Radiology*
Peptides	*Peptides*
PerspectPedPathol	*Perspectives of Pediatric Pathology*
PfleugersArchPhysiol	*Pfleugers Archiv für die Gesamte Physiologie des Menschen und der Tiere*
PharmaceuWeekbl	*Pharmaceutisch Weekblad*
Pharmacogenet	*Pharmacogenetics*
Pharmacol	*Pharmacology*
PharmacolToxicol	*Pharmacology and Toxicology*
PharmBiochBehav	*Pharmacology, Biochemistry, and Behavior*
PharmRes	*Pharmaceutical Research*
PharmResComm	*Pharmacological Research Communications*
PharmRev	*Pharmacology Reviews*
PharmTher	*Pharmacology and Therapeutics*
PhTrRoySoc	*Philosophical Transactions of the Royal Society*
Physiologist	*Physiologist*
PhysiolRev	*Physiological Reviews*
PhysMedBiol	*Physics in Medicine and Biology*
PhysSportsMed	*Physician and Sports Medicine*
Placenta	*Placenta*
Plasma	*Plasma*
PNAS	*Proceedings of the National Academy of Sciences*
PolTygLek	*Polski Tygodnik Lekarski*
PoliclinicoSezMed	*Policlinico- Rome-Sezione Medica*
PopTrends	*Population Trends*
PostgradMed	*Postgraduate Medicine*
PostgradMedJ	*Postgraduate Medical Journal*
PoumonCoeur	*Poumon et le Coeur*
PracovLek	*Pracovni Lekarstvi*
Praxis	*Praxis*
PrenatalDiagn	*Prenatal Diagnosis*
PrescribersJ	*Prescribers' Journal*
PressMed	*Presse Medicale*
PrevMed	*Preventive Medicine*
ProbRéan	*Problèmes de Réanimation*
ProcAmAssocCancerRes	*Proceeding of the American Association for Cancer Research*
ProcAmSocClinOncol	*Proceedings of the American Society of Clinical Oncology*
ProcAmSocTransplSurg	*Proceedings of the American Society of Transplant Surgery*
ProcAmWoodPreservAss	*Proceedings of the American Wood Preservative Association*
ProcAnnMeetAmAssoc CancerRes	*Proceedings of the Annual Meeting of the American Association for Cancer Research*
ProcAssResNervMentDis	*Proceedings of the Association for Research into Nervous and Mental Disorders*
ProcBostonSocNatHist	*Proceedings of the Boston Society of Natural History*
ProcEDTA	*Proceedings of the European Dialysis and Transplant Association*
ProcMayoClinic	*Proceedings of the Mayo Clinic*
ProcNatlSciCounc RepubChina	*Proceedings of the National Science Council of the Republic of China*
ProcNutrSoc	*Proceedings of the Nutrition Society*
ProcRoySocB	*Proceedings of the Royal Society. Series B: Biological Sciences*
ProcRoySocMed	*Proceedings of the Royal Society of Medicine*
ProgBiochemPharm	*Progress in Biochemical Pharmacology*
ProgChemFibrinThromb	*Progress in Chemical Fibrinolysis and Thrombolysis*
ProgClinBiolRes	*Progress in Clinical and Biological Research*
ProgCollPolymerSci	*Progress in Colloid and Polymer Science*
ProgGrowthFactorRes	*Progress in Growth Factor Research*
ProgLivDis	*Progress in Liver Diseases*
ProgMedVirol	*Progress in Medical Virology*
ProgNeurobiol	*Progress in Neurobiology*
ProgNucAcidResMolBiol	*Progress in Nucleic Acid Research and Molecular Biology*
ProgPediatSurg	*Progress in Pediatric Surgery*
ProgrCardiovascDis	*Progress in Cardiovascular Disease*
ProgrDerm	*Progress in Dermatology*
ProgrHepatol	*Progress in Hepatology*
ProsLeukMed	*Prostaglandins, Leukotrienes and Medicine*
Prostagl	*Prostaglandins*
ProteinSci	*Protein Science*
PSEBM	*Proceedings of the Society for Experimental Biology and Medicine*
Psychodynamics	*Psychodynamics*
Psychopharm	*Psychopharmacology*
PublHlthRec	*Public Health Record*
PublHlthRep	*Public Health Reports*
PublHlthRepWash	*Public Health Report Washington*
QJExpPhysiol	*Quarterly Journal of Experimental Physiology*
QJMed	*Quarterly Journal of Medicine*

QJStudAlc	*Quarterly Journal of Studies on Alcohol*
Radiol	*Radiology*
RadiolClinNA	*Radiological Clinics of North America*
RadiothOnc	*Radiotherapy and Oncology*
RCollSurg(Edin)	*Royal College of Surgeons of Edinburgh*
ReanimUrg	*Reanimation Urgences*
ReaSoinsIntensMedUrg	*Réanimation, Soins Intensifs et Médecine d'Urgence*
RecDevAlc	*Recent Developments in Alcoholism*
Receptor	*Receptor*
RecProgHormRes	*Recent Progress in Hormone Research*
RecProgMed	*Recenti Progressi in Medicina (Roma)*
RecResCancRes	*Recent Results in Cancer Research*
RegulPeptides	*Regulatory Peptides*
RenFail	*Renal Failure*
ReprodMed	*Reproductive Medicine*
ResAging	*Research on Aging*
ResCommChemPath Pharm	*Research Communications in Chemical Pathology and Pharmacology*
ResCommMolPathPharm	*Research Communications in Molecular Pathology and Pharmacology*
ResExpMed	*Research in Experimental Medicine*
ResImmunol	*Research in Immunology*
RespEnfApDig	*Revista Espanola de las Enfermadades del Aparato Digestivo*
RespirCircul	*Respiration and Circulation*
RespirPhysiol	*Respiratory Physiology*
ResPublResNervMentDis	*Research Publications - Association for Research in Nervous and Mental Disease*
ResVetSci	*Research in Veterinary Science*
ResVirol	*Research in Virology*
Retina	*Retina*
RevAssMedBras	*Revista da Associacao Medica Brasileira*
RevBiochTox	*Reviews in Biochemical Toxicology*
RevClinEsp	*Revista Clinica Espanola*
RevEspEnfermAparDig	*Revista de las Enfermedades del Aparato Digestivo*
RevEspFisiol	*Revista Espanola de Fisiologia*
RevFrGynObs	*Revue Francaise de Gynecologie et d'Obstetrique*
RevFrMalResp	*Revue Francaise des Maladies Respiratoires*
RevGastrMex	*Revista de Gastroenterologia de Mexico*
RevInfDis	*Reviews of Infectious Diseases*
RevInstAdolfoLutz	*Revista do Istituto Adolfo Lutz*
RevInstMedTropSP	*Revista do Instituto de Medicina Tropical de Sao Paulo*
RevIntHep	*Revue Internationale d'Hepatologie*
RevInvestClin(Mex)	*Revista de Investigacion Clinica (Mexico City)*
RevLyonMed	*Revue Lyonaise de Médecine*
RevMaladEnfance	*Revue des Maladies de l'Enfance*
RevMedChile	*Revista Medica de Chile*
RevMedChirMalFoie	*Revue Medico-Chirurgical des Maladies du Foie*
RevMedInt	*Revue de Médecine Interne*
RevMedMicrobiol	*Reviews in Medical Microbiology*
RevMedVirol	*Reviews in Medical Virology*
RevNeurol	*Revue Neurologique*
RevPhysiolBiochem Pharmacol	*Reviews of Physiology, Biochemistry, and Pharmacology*
RevSaúdePúbl	*Revista de Saúde Pública*
RheumDisClinNAm	*Rheumatic Disease Clinics of North America*
RheumInt	*Rheumatology International*
Rhumatologie	*Rhumatologie*
RicClinLab	*Ricerca in Clinica e in Laboratorio*
RinshoByori	*Rinsho Byori*
RinshoShin	*Rinsho Shinkeigaku*
ROFO	*Fortschritte auf dem Gebiete der Rontgenstrahlen und der Nuklearmedizin*
RPARNMD	*Research Publications – Association for Research in Nervous and Mental Disease*
SAJSurg	*South African Journal of Surgery*
SAMedJ	*South African Medical Journal*
Sante	*Sante*
Sarcoid	*Sarcoidosis*
SbornikVedPraciLek HradKra	*Sbornik Vedeckych Praci, Lekarske Fakulty Karlovy University v Hradci Kralove*
ScaJCLI	*Scandinavian Journal of Clinical and Laboratory Investigation*
ScaJGastr	*Scandinavian Journal of Gastroenterology*
ScaJHaematol	*Scandinavian Journal of Haematology*
ScaJImmunol	*Scandinavian Journal of Immunology*
ScaJInfectDis	*Scandinavian Journal of Infectious Diseases*
ScaJRheum	*Scandinavian Journal of Rheumatology*
ScaJStatist	*Scandinavian Journal of Statistics*
ScaJThorCardiovascSurg	*Scandinavian Journal of Thoracic and Cardiovascular Surgery*
ScaJUrolNephrol	*Scandinavian Journal of Urology and Nephrology*
ScaJWorkEnvirHlth	*Scandinavian Journal of Work Environment and Health*
ScandStudCriminol	*Scandinavian Studies in Criminology*
ScanMicrosc	*Scanning Microscopy*
SchMedWoch	*Schweizerische Medizinische Wochenschrift*

SchRundMed	*Schweizerische Rundschau für Medizin*
SchrVerWaBoLufthyg	*Schriftenreihe des Vereins für Wasser-, Boden-, und Lufthygiene*
SciAm	*Scientific American*
Science	*Science*
SciTotalEnv	*Science of the Total Environment*
ScotMedJ	*Scottish Medical Journal*
SEAsianJTropMed PubHlth	*South East Asian Journal of Tropical Medicine and Public Health*
SemaineMed	*Semaine Medicale*
SemArthrRheum	*Seminars in Arthritis and Rheumatism*
SemCellBiol	*Seminars in Cell Biology*
SemDiagPath	*Seminars in Diagnostic Pathology*
SemGastroDis	*Seminars in Gastrointestinal Disease*
SemHemat	*Seminars in Hematology*
SemHepatol	*Seminars in Hepatology*
SemHopPar	*Semaine des Hôpitaux Paris*
SemImmunopathol	*Seminars in Immunopathology*
SemIntRadiol	*Seminars in Interventional Radiology*
SemLivDis	*Seminars in Liver Disease*
SemNuclMed	*Seminars in Nuclear Medicine*
SemOnc	*Seminars in Oncology*
SemPediatSurg	*Seminars in Pediatric Surgery*
SemRoent	*Seminars in Roentgenology*
SemSurgOncol	*Seminars in Surgery and Oncology*
SemThrombHaemost	*Seminars in Thrombosis and Haemostasis*
SeronoSymposiaRev	*Serono Symposia Review*
SGO	*Surgery, Gynecology and Obstetrics*
SkeletalRadiol	*Skeletal Radiology*
SocNeurosciAbstr	*Abstracts - Society for Neuroscience*
SomCellMolGen	*Somatic Cell and Molecular Genetics*
SouthMedJ	*Southern Medical Journal*
SouthMedSurg	*Southern Medicine and Surgery*
SovHlthcareKirgiz	*Soviet Healthcare Kirgizii*
SportsMed	*Sports Medicine*
SpringerSem Immunopathol	*Springer Seminars in Immunopathology*
SSIEM	*Society for the Study of Inborn Errors of Metabolism*
StatMed	*Statistics in Medicine*
Steroids	*Steroids*
Stroke	*Stroke*
SubcellBioch	*Sub-cellular Biochemistry*
SubsAlcActMis	*Substance and Alcohol Actions/ Misuse*
SurgAnnu	*Surgery Annual*
SurgClinNAm	*Surgical Clinics of North America*
SurgEndosc	*Surgical Endoscopy*
Surgery	*Surgery*
SurgForum	*Surgical Forum*
SurgGastr	*Surgical Gastroenterology*
SurgLapEndosc	*Surgical Laparoscopy and Endoscopy*
SurgToday	*Surgery Today*
SympSocExpBiol	*Symposia of the Society for Experimental Biology*
SyndIdent	*Syndrome Identification*
TexasMed	*Texas Medicine*
Therapie	*Therapie*
Therapiewoche	*Therapiewoche*
TherDrugMonit	*Therapeutic Drug Monitoring*
Thorax	*Thorax*
ThrombDiathHaemorrh	*Thrombosis et Diathesis Haemorrhagica*
ThrombHaem	*Thrombosis and Haemostasis*
ThrombRes	*Thrombosis Research*
Thymus	*Thymus*
TIBS	*Trends in Biological Sciences*
TissAnt	*Tissue Antigens*
TohokuJExpMed	*Tohoku Journal of Experimental Medicine*
TopClinNutr	*Topics in Clinical Nutrition*
ToxApplPharmacol	*Toxicology and Applied Pharmacology*
Toxicol*InVitro*	*Toxicology* in Vitro
Toxicology	*Toxicology*
ToxicolLett	*Toxicology Letters*
ToxicolPath	*Toxicologic Pathology*
ToxRev	*Toxicity Review*
TrAAP	*Transactions of the Association of American Physicians*
TraceElemElectrol	*Trace Elements and Electrolytes*
TraceElemMed	*Trace Element Medicine*
TraceSubEnvirHlth	*Trace Substances Environment and Health*
TrAmNeurolAss	*Transactions of the American Neurological Association*
TrAmSocArtOrg	*Transactions – American Society for Artificial Internal Organs*
TransConfChemother Tuberc	*Transactions – Conference on Chemotherapy of Tuberculosis*
TransfusMed	*Transfusion Medicine*
Transfusion	*Transfusion*
TransfusMedRev	*Transfusion Medicine Reviews*
TransJpnPathSoc	*Transactions of the Japanese Pathological Society*
Transpl	*Transplantation*
TransplBull	*Transplantation Bulletin*
TransplImmunol	*Transplantation Immunology*
TransplInt	*Transplantation International*
TransplMediz	*Transplantationsmedizin*
TransplSci	*Transplantation Science*
TransplProc	*Transplantation Proceedings*
TransplRev	*Transplantation Review*
TreatConnTissDis	*Treatment of Connective Tissue Diseases*
TrendsBiochemSci	*Trends in Biochemical Sciences*
TrendsCellBiol	*Trends in Cell Biology*
TrendsEndocrinMetab	*Trends in Endocrinology and Metabolism*
TrendsNeurosci	*Trends in Neurosciences*

TrendsPharmacolSci	*Trends in Pharmacological Sciences*
TrNYAcadSci	*Transactions of the New York Academy of Sciences*
TropGastr	*Tropical Gastroenterology*
TropGeogMed	*Tropical and Geographical Medicine*
TropMedParas	*Tropical Medicine and Parasitology*
TrRSocTropMedHyg	*Transactions of the Royal Society of Tropical Medicine and Hygiene*
Tubercle	*Tubercle*
TumBiol	*Tumour Biology*
TumTarg	*Tumor Targeting*
UltrastructPathol	*Ultrastructural Pathology*
UnionMedCan	*Union Médicale du Canada*
UpdateIntensCare EmergMed	*Update in Intensive Care and Emergency Medicine*
Urol	*Urology*
UrolClinNAm	*Urology Clinics of North America*
UrolRes	*Urological Research*
USImag	*Ultrasonic Imaging*
USMedBiol	*Ultrasound in Medicine and Biology*
Vaccine	*Vaccine*
VerDschGesInnMed	*Verhandlungen der Deutschen Gesellschaft für Innere Medizin*
VerDschGesPath	*Verhandlungen de Deutschen Gesellschaft für Pathologie*
VetHumTox	*Veterinary and Human Toxicology*
VetPathol	*Veterinary Pathology*
VetRec	*Veterinary Record*
ViralHepatRev	*Viral Hepatitis Reviews*
VirchArchA	*Virchows Archiv. A Pathological Anatomy and Histopathology*
VirchArchCP	*Virchows Archiv. B Cell Pathology*
VirolMon	*Virology Monographs*
Virology	*Virology*
VirRes	*Virus Research*
VitHorm	*Vitamins and Hormones*
VoprVirusol	*Voprosy Virusologii*
VoxSang	*Vox Sanguinis*
WestJMed	*West Indian Journal of Medicine*
WHOChron	*World Health Organization Chronicle*

WienKlinWoch	*Wiener Klinische Wochenschrift*
WienMedWoch	*Wiener Medizinische Wochenschrift*
WIMedJ	*West Indian Medical Journal*
WisMedJ	*Wisconsin Medical Journal*
WklyEpidemiolRec	*Weekly Epidemiological Record*
WorldMedJ	*World Medical Journal*
WorldJSurg	*World Journal of Surgery*
WRevNutrDiet	*World Review of Nutrition and Dietetics*
Xenobiot	*Xenobiotica*
YaleJBiolMed	*Yale Journal of Biology and Medicine*
Zacchia	*Zacchia*
ZblAllgPath	*Zentralblatt für Allgemeine Pathologie und Pathologische Anatomie*
ZblArbMed	*Zentralblatt für Arbeitsmedizin und Arbeitsschutz und Prophylaxe*
ZblBakteriol MikrobiolHyg	*Zentralblatt für Bakteriologie, Microbiologie, und Hygiene (Stuttgart)*
ZblBaktHyg	*Zentralblatt für Bakteriologie und Hygiene*
ZblChir	*Zentralblatt für Chirurgie*
ZGastr	*Zeitschrift für Gastroenterologie Verhandlungsband*
ZGesamExpMed	*Zeitschrift für die Gesamte Experimentalle Medizin*
ZGesHyg	*Zeitschrift für Gesundheitstechnik und Staedtehygiene*
ZImmunitat	*Zeitschrift für Immunitatsforschung*
ZKardiol	*Zeitschrift für Kardiologie*
ZKinderchir	*Zeitschrift für Kinderchirurgie*
ZKinderheilk	*Zeitschrift für Kinderheilkunde*
ZKlinChemKlinBiochem	*Zeitschrift für Klinische Chemie und Klinische Biochemie*
ZKlinMed	*Zeitschrift für Klinische Medizin*
ZKrebsf	*Zeitschrift für Krebsforschung*
ZMikroskAnatForsch	*Zeitschrift für Mikroskopisch-Anatomische Forschung*
ZPhysiolChem	*Zeitschrift für Physiologische Chemie*
ZRheumatol	*Zeitschrift für Rheumatologie*

Index

Page numbers in **bold** refer to major sections of the text.

Page numbers in *italics* refer to pages on which tables may be found.

Indexing style / conventions used

Alphabetical order. This index is in letter-by-letter order, whereby hyphens, en-rules and spaces within index headings are ignored in the alphabetization. Terms in brackets are excluded from initial alphabetization.

Cross-references. Cross-reference terms in *italics* are either general cross-references, or refer to subentry terms within the same main entry (the main entry term is not repeated, in order to save space) i.e. they are not main entry terms.

Abbreviations used without explanation

DNA	deoxyribonucleic acid
EGF	epidermal growth factor
HBV	hepatitis B virus
HCV	hepatitis c virus

HDV	hepatitis D virus
NADP	nicotine–adenine diphosphate
RNA	ribonucleic acid

A

Aagenae's syndrome
hepatic abnormalities 2101
infant 1613
abdomen
ascites 712
cholecystectomy, and gallstones 1621
cirrhosis 492
computed tomography in metastases 1554
discomfort and pain 481–2
epigastrium 492
examination of 489–96
abdominal wall veins 490
adhesions 490
ascites 489–90
Budd–Chiari syndrome 490
inferior vena caval obstruction 490
oedema 490
palpation 490–4
portal hypertension 490
gallbladder 491–2
gallstones 492
hypochondrium 491–2
liver 491–2
palpation of 490–4
porphyria, pain in 1419
pulsatile liver 492
radiotherapy for liver injury 1335
recti 492
rigidity 491
surgery in unsuspected liver disease 2014–15
jaundice 2015
morbidity 2014–15
swelling 482–3
ultrasound examination 492
aberrant artery
ultrasonography 549
abetalipoproteinaemia 1449
apolipoprotein B 1449
microsomal triglyceride transfer protein 1449

abetalipoproteinaemia *(continued)*
very low density lipoprotein 1449
vitamin K deficiency 1449
abscess
in the elderly 1897
pyogenic liver 991–3
antibiotic 1654
aspiration 993
cholangitis 1650–1, 1654
clinical features 992
organisms isolated from *992*
pathogenesis 991–2
treatment 993
acaeruloplasminaemia 1386
Wilson's disease 1377
acalculous cholecystitis, acute 1659
acalculous, burns 1336
acamprosate, alcoholic liver disease 1227
acanthocytes
acanthocytosis 1786
echinocytes 1785–6
spur-cell anaemia 1785–6
access bowel loop, hepatobiliary trauma 2038
acebutol, causing acute hepatitis 1278
acetaldehyde
acetaldehyde–acetaldehyde adducts, covalent binding of 1170–1
adducts, antibodies against 1171
alcohol dehydrogenase 1163
aldehyde dehydrogenase 1165
inhibitors 1166
blood acetaldehyde concentrations 1165–6
elevated 1166
Orientals 1166
ethanol, perivenular hepatotoxicity of 1172
protein–acetaldehyde adducts 1170
Schiff's base 1170
hepatotoxicity associated with microsomal ethanol oxidizing system 1171

acetaldehyde *(continued)*
lipid peroxidation
free radicals 1171–2
glutathione 1171
malondialdehyde 1171
metabolism of 1165–6
changes in 1167–8
dehydrogenase, decrease in activity 1167–8
ethanol oxidation increase 1167–8
mitochondria 1167
reduction in oxidized acetaldehyde 1167–8
pathway to acetate 1165
toxicity of 1170–1
see also alcohol; ethanol
acetaminophen *see* paracetamol
acetate
acetaldehyde 1165
metabolism of 1166
ethanol oxidation 1166
acetone and liver injury 2084
acetyl-CoA carboxylase, cytokines 171
***N*-acetylcysteine**
acute hepatitis 1358, 1364
cholestasis and neonatal jaundice 1414
paracetamol overdose 1325, 1357
***N*-acetylglucosaminidation**, bile acids 250
***N*-acetyltransferase**
drug metabolism 157–9
isoniazid 158
xenobiotic mediation *158*
acid–base balance
acidosis 2013
fructose 285
fulminant hepatic failure 1347
hyperlactaemia 2013
hypochloraemic acidosis 2013
hypokalaemia 2013
lactate metabolism 2013
pH regulation 332
problems in anaesthesia 2020

acid–base balance *(continued)*
protein secretion 348
urea and electrolytes 517–518
acidosis 517–518,
alkalosis 517–518
acid β-glucosidase, measurement of activity in Gaucher's disease 1446
α$_1$-acid glycoprotein 364
control of malaria virulence 364
cytokines 170
drug binding 364
immunomodulation 364
inhibition of platelet aggregation 364
acidophil
condensation 463
necrosis 464
acidosis
anaesthesia 2013
urea and electrolytes 517–518
acinar
organization and bile formation 80
heterogeneity in intracellular binding 119
taurodeoxycholate 119
transport of anions and cations
glycocholate 124
taurolithocholate 124
uptake of organic ions and cations 117
acinus zonal heterogeneity, drugs 94–5
acitretin causing acute hepatitis 1278
acromegaly 1723
octreotide 1723
trans-splenoidal hypophysectomy 1723
acrylonitrile and liver injury 2084
actin cytoskeleton, endothelial cells 36
actin microfilament and bile formation 1592
actinomycosis, affect on liver 1031
activated partial thromboplastin time (APTT)
liver biopsy 541
liver disease 1809